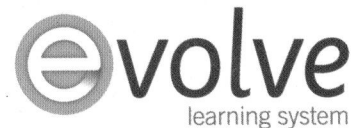
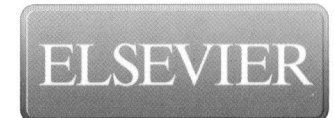
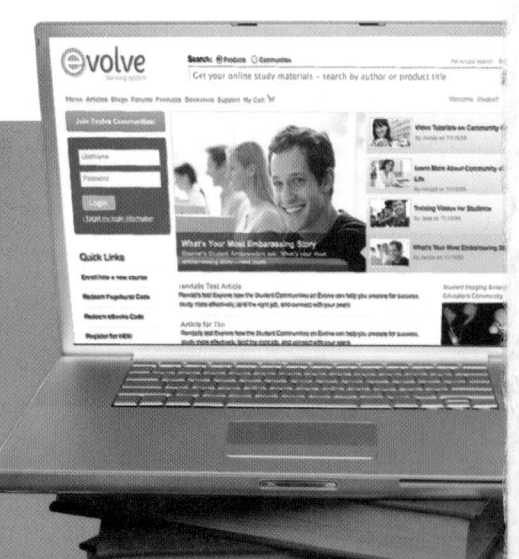

BASIC NURSING

SEVENTH EDITION

Patricia A. Potter, RN, MSN, PhD, FAAN
Research Scientist
Siteman Cancer Center at Barnes-Jewish Hospital
and Washington University School of Medicine
St. Louis, Missouri

Anne Griffin Perry, RN, EdD, FAAN
Professor and Associate Dean
School of Nursing
Southern Illinois University Edwardsville
Edwardsville, Illinois

Patricia A. Stockert, RN, BSN, MS, PhD
Professor, Dean Undergraduate Program
Saint Francis Medical Center College of Nursing
Peoria, Illinois

Amy Hall, RN, BSN, MS, PhD
Professor and Chair
Dunigan Family Department of Nursing and Health Sciences
University of Evansville
Evansville, Indiana

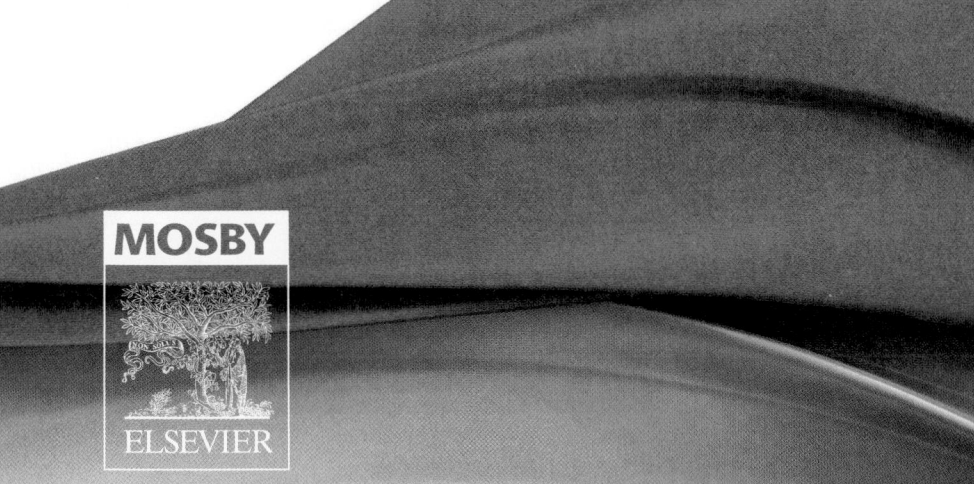

MOSBY

ELSEVIER

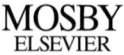

MOSBY
ELSEVIER

3251 Riverport Lane
St. Louis, Missouri 63043

Notice

Knowledge and best practice in this field are constantly changing. As new research and experience broaden
our knowledge, changes in practice, treatment, and drug therapy may become necessary or appropriate.
Readers are advised to check the most current information provided (i) on procedures featured or (ii) by
the manufacturer of each product to be administered, to verify the recommended dose or formula, the
method and duration of administration, and contraindications. It is the responsibility of the practitioner,
relying on personal experience and knowledge of the patient, to make diagnoses, to determine dosages and
the best treatment for each individual patient, and to take all appropriate safety precautions. To the fullest
extent of the law, neither the Publisher nor the Authors assume any liability for any injury and/or damage to
persons or property arising out of or related to any use of the material contained in this book.

The Publisher

Library of Congress Cataloging-in-Publication Data
Basic nursing / Patricia A. Potter . . . [et al.].—7th ed.
        p. ; cm.
   Includes bibliographical references and index.
   ISBN 978-0-323-05891-9 (hardback : alk. paper) 1. Nursing 2.
Nursing—Study and teaching. I. Potter, Patricia Ann.
   [DNLM: 1. Nursing. 2. Nursing Care. 3. Nursing Process. WY 100
B3113 2011]
   RT41.P84 2011
   610.73076—dc22   2010000233

Editor: Tamara Myers
Associate Developmental Editor: Tina Kaemmerer
Publishing Services Manager: Anne Altepeter
Senior Project Manager: Beth Hayes
Design Direction: Kim Denando

Printed in the United States of America

Working together to grow
libraries in developing countries

www.elsevier.com | www.bookaid.org | www.sabre.org

ELSEVIER   BOOK AID International   Sabre Foundation

Last digit is the print number: 9 8 7 6 5 4 3 2

Contributors

Marjorie Baier, RN, PhD
Associate Professor
School of Nursing
Southern Illinois University Edwardsville
Edwardsville, Illinois

Lois Bentler-Lampe, MS, RN
Director of Professional Development
OSF Saint Francis Medical Center
Peoria, Illinois

Jeri Burger, PhD, RN
Assistant Professor
University of Southern Indiana
Evansville, Indiana

Janice C. Colwell, MS, RN, CWOCN, FAAN
Clinical Nurse Specialist
University of Chicago Medical Center
Chicago, Illinois

Eileen Costantinou, RN, MSN, BC
Practice Specialist, Senior Coordinator
Barnes-Jewish Hospital
St. Louis, Missouri

Ruth M. Curchoe, RN, MSN, CIC
Director, Infection Prevention
Unity Health System
Rochester, New York

Christine Durbin, PhD, JD, RN
Assistant Professor
School of Nursing
Southern Illinois University Edwardsville
Edwardsville, Illinois

Margaret Ecker, MS, RN
Director, Nursing Quality
Kaiser Permanente Los Angeles Medical
   Center
Los Angeles, California

Susan J. Fetzer, RN, BA, BSN, MSN,
   MBA, PhD
Associate Professor
College of Health and Human Services
University of New Hampshire
Durham, New Hampshire

Victoria N. Folse, APN, PMHCNS-BC,
   LCPC
Director and Associate Professor
Illinois Wesleyan University
Bloomington, Illinois

Lori Klingman, MSN, RN
Faculty
Ohio Valley Hospital School of Nursing
McKees Rocks, Pennsylvania

Jerrilee LaMar, RN, PhD
Assistant Professor of Nursing
Dunigan Family Department of Nursing
   and Health Sciences
University of Evansville
Evansville, Indiana

Deborah L. Marshall, RN, MSN
Assistant Professor of Nursing
Dunigan Family Department of Nursing and
   Health Sciences
University of Evansville
Evansville, Indiana

Wendy R. Ostendorf, MS, EdD
Associate Professor
Neumann University
Aston, Pennsylvania

Elizabeth S. Pratt, MSN, RN, ACNS-BC
Clinical Nurse Specialist
Barnes-Jewish Hospital
St. Louis, Missouri

Marilyn Schallom, MSN, CCRN, CCNS
Surgical Critical Care CNS
Barnes-Jewish Hospital
St. Louis, Missouri

Ann Tritak, RN, EdD
Dean of Nursing
Saint Peters College School of Nursing
Jersey City, New Jersey

Janis Waite, RN, MSN, EdD
Professor
Saint Francis Medical Center College
   of Nursing
Peoria, Illinois

Ellen Wathen, PhD, RN, BC
Staff Development Specialist
Deaconess Hospital, Inc.
Evansville, Indiana

Jill Weberski, MSN, CNS
Saint Francis Medical Center College
   of Nursing
Peoria, Illinois

Terry L. Wood, PhD, RN, CNE
Clinical Assistant Professor
Southern Illinois University Edwardsville
Edwardsville, Illinois

Rita Wunderlich, RN, MSN, PhD
Director, Baccalaureate Nursing Program
Saint Louis University School of Nursing
St. Louis, Missouri

Valerie Yancey, PhD, RN, CHPN, HNC
Associate Professor
Southern Illinois University Edwardsville
Edwardsville, Illinois

Reviewers

Pamela Adamschick, PhD, RN, MSN,
   PMHCNS, BC
Assistant Professor of Nursing
Moravian College
Bethlehem, Pennsylvania

Liz Allibone, PGCTLCP, BSc, RN
Nurse Teacher
Royal Brompton and Harefield NHS Trust
London, United Kingdom

Suzanne L. Bailey, MSN, CNS
Associate Professor of Nursing
University of Evansville
Evansville, Indiana

Doris Bartlett, BSN, MS
Adjunct Professor
Bethel College
Mishawaka, Indiana

Janet Bitzan, BSN, MS, PhD
Clinical Associate Professor
UWM College of Nursing
Milwaukee, Wisconsin

Linda M. Cason, MSN, RN, CCRN,
   CNRN, BC
Adjunct Faculty
University of Evansville
Evansville, Indiana

Brigitte Casteel, RN, MSN
Professor of Nursing
Director, Practical Nursing Program
Mountain Empire Community College
Big Stone Gap, Virginia

Mariah Charles, BSN, CNRN, MSN-FNP
Clinical Nurse Coordinator in Neurology
Barnes-Jewish Hospital
St. Louis, Missouri

Kim Clevenger, MSN, RN, BC
Assistant Professor of Nursing
Morehead State University
Morehead, Kentucky

Patricia B. Conley, BSN, MSN
Cardio-Pulmonary Telemetry Staff Nurse
Research Medical Center
Kansas City, Missouri

Suzanne M. Costello, RN, BSN, MSN
Professional Nurse Educator
Educational Specialist – Allied Health
    Education
Jameson Hospital School of Nursing
New Castle, Pennsylvania

**Laura M. Criddle, PhD, ACNS-BC, CEN,
    CCRN, CCNS, CFRN, CNRN, RN, BC**
Clinical Nurse Specialist
Laurelwood Consulting
Scappoose, Oregon

**Neva Crogan Pomilla, PhD, GCNS-BC,
    GNP-BC, FNGNA**
Associate Professor
University of Arizona College of Nursing
Tucson, Arizona

Judy Ann Dahl, MSN, RN
Associate Professor of Nursing
Dunigan Family Department of Nursing
    and Health Sciences
University of Evansville
Evansville, Indiana

Lynn M. Derickson, BS, MS, APRN, P/MH
Assistant Professor
WorWic Community College
Salisbury, Maryland

Barbara Derwinski, MSN, RNC, WH, BC
Associate Professor
Bozeman College of Nursing
Montana State University
Billings, Montana

Sylvia A. Duraski, MSN
Nurse Practitioner
Rehabilitation Institute of Chicago
Chicago, Illinois

Kay L. Elmore, MSN, CMSRN
Clinical Nurse Educator
St. Anthony's Medical Center
St. Louis, Missouri

Jessica Estes, BS, MSN, ANCC
Associate Dean of Nursing
Psychiatric and Mental Health Nurse
    Practitioner
Owensboro Community and Technical
    College
OMHS Outpatient Counseling
Owensboro, Kentucky

Linda Fluharty, MSN, RNC, ACLS
Associate Professor
Ivy Tech State College of Indiana
Indianapolis, Indiana

Cira Fraser, PhD, MSN, BSN, RN
Associate Professor and Graduate Faculty
Monmouth University
West Long Branch, New Jersey

Marcia Gardner, PhD, RN, CPNP, CPN
Clinical Associate Professor and Assistant
    Dean
University College of Nursing and Health
    Professions
Philadelphia, Pennsylvania

Margaret Gingrich, RN, MSN
Professor
Harrisburg Area Community College
Harrisburg, Pennsylvania

Yvette Glenn, MSN, FNP-C, CWS
Wound Care Manager – Nurse Practitioner
VA Illiana Health Care System
Danville, Illinois

Stephanie C. Greer, RN, BSN, MSN
Associate Degree Nursing Instructor
Southwest Mississippi Community College
Summit, Mississippi

Cherona Hajewski, MSN, RN, NEA-BC
Vice President Patient Care Services
    and CNO
Deaconess Hospital, Inc.
Evansville, Indiana

Kathy L. Ham, EdD, RN
Associate Professor
Southeast Missouri State University
Cape Girardeau, Missouri

Elisabeth D. Harvey, RN, MSN, CWOCN
Memorial Medical Center
Modesto, California

Patricia Jane Hutchison, MSN, RN, CDE
Education Coordinator
Grove City Medical Center
Grove City, Pennsylvania

Jane H. Kelley, PhD, RN
Adjunct Professor
School of Nursing
University of Mississippi Medical Center
Jackson, Mississippi

Laura Kelly, PhD, MS, ANCC
Assistant Professor
Monmouth University
West Long Branch, New Jersey

T. Camille Killough, RN, BSN
Department of Nursing
Pearl River Community College
Hattiesburg, Mississippi

Pamela D. Korte, RN, MS
Professor of Nursing
Monroe Community College
Rochester, New York

Mary Kotsokalis, EdD, MSN, BSN, AND
Nursing Faculty
Central Piedmont Community College
Charlotte, North Carolina

Kathryn A. Lever, BSN, MSN, WHNP-BC
Associate Professor of Nursing
Dunigan Family Department of Nursing
    and Health Sciences
University of Evansville
Evansville, Indiana

Laura Logan, CNS, RN
Faculty
Stephen F. Austin State University
Nacogdoches, Texas

Rosemary Macy, PhD, RN
Associate Professor
Boise State University
Boise, Idaho

Diana R. Mager, MSN, DNP RN-C
Director of Robin Kaharek Learning
    Resource Center
Fairfield University
Fairfield, Connecticut

B. Gail Marshall, RN, MSN, MEd
Professor
Luzerne County Community College
Nonticoke, Pennsylvania

Barbara Maxwell, MSN, MS, BSN, RN, LNC
Associate Professor of Nursing
State University of New York Ulster
  Community College
Stone Ridge, New York

Lesia D. McBride, BSN, RN
Clinical Research Coordinator and Clinical
  Educator
Community Hospital – Anderson
Anderson, Indiana

Cindy Mulder, RNC, MS, MSN, CNP
Associate Professor
University of South Dakota
Sioux Falls, South Dakota

Bernadette O'Halloran, RN, MSN
Clinical Instructor
Naugatuck Valley Community College
Waterbury, Connecticut

Rebecca Otten, RN, MSN, EdD
Assistant Professor
California State University – Fullerton
Fullerton, California

Rita Peters, RN, BSN, MSN
Nursing Instructor
Hesston College
Hesston, Kansas

Susan Porterfield, PhD, FNP-C
NP Coordinator and Assistant Professor
Florida State University
Tallahassee, Florida

Cherie Rebar, MSN, MBA, RN, FNP
Chair, AS Nursing Program
Kettering College of Medical Arts
Dayton, Ohio

Anita K. Reed, MSN, RN
Clinical Instructor
Community Coordinator
St. Elizabeth School of Nursing
Saint Joseph's College
Lafayette, Indiana

Jill Reed, APRN, MSN
Instructor
College of Nursing
University of Nebraska Medical Center
Kearney, Nebraska

Doreen Rogers, MSN, RN, CCRN, CNE
Instructor
St. Elizabeth College of Nursing
Utica, New York

Mary Jane Ruhland, BSN, MSN, BC
Performance Improvement Engineer
Progress West Healthcare Center
St. Peters, Missouri

Julie Ryhal, RN, BSN, MEd, LCCE
Education Coordinator
Grove City Medical Center
Grove City, Pennsylvania

Maura C. Schlairet, RN, MSN, EdD
Assistant Professor
College of Nursing
Valdosta State University
Valdosta, Georgia

Susan Parnell Scholtz, RN, BSN, MN, DNSc
Associate Professor of Nursing
Moravian College
Bethlehem, Pennsylvania

Ruth E. Schumacher, BSN, MSN, RN
Pediatric Nursing Instructor
College of Nursing
University of Illinois – Chicago
Chicago, Illinois

Debra Servello, RNP, MSN
Assistant Professor of Nursing
Rhode Island College School of Nursing
Providence, Rhode Island

Gale Sewell, RN, MSN, CNE
Assistant Professor
Indiana Wesleyan University
Marion, Indiana

Cynthia Sheppard, RN, MSN, NP, CNS
Associate Professor of Nursing
Schoolcraft College
Livonia, Michigan

Tamara Shields, RN, MS, FNP-BC
St. Elizabeth School of Nursing
Lafayette, Indiana

Patti Simmons, RN, MN, CHPN
Assistant Professor of Nursing
North Georgia College and State University
Dahlonega, Georgia

**Janet Somlyay, MSN, CNS, CPNP-AC/PC,
  CNE, PMHNP-BC**
Assistant Lecturer
University of Wyoming
Laramie, Wyoming

Ann D. Sprengel, EdD, MSN, RN
Professor
Southeast Missouri State University
Cape Girardeau, Missouri

Kathleen A. Stevens, PhD, RN, CRRN
Director of Nursing Education
Rehabilitation Institute of Chicago
Chicago, Illinois

**Marianne Swihart, BSN, MEd, MSN, CRNI,
  CWON, PCCN**
Assistant Professor of Nursing
Pasco-Hernando Community College
New Port Richey, Florida

Mary Tedesco-Schneck, BS, MSN, CPNP
Assistant Professor
Husson University
Bangor, Maine

Scott C. Thigpen, RN, MSN, CCRN, CEN
Associate Professor of Nursing
South Georgia College
Douglas, Georgia

**Donna L. Thompson, MSN, CRNP, FNP-BC,
  CCCN**
Assistant Professor
Neumann University
Aston, Pennsylvania

Linda Toelke, RN, BSN, MSN, CRRN, CARN
Staff Nurse and Nurse Educator
Rehabilitation Institute of Chicago
  Center for Pain Management
Chicago, Illinois

Mary Grace Umlauf, RN, PhD, FAAN
Professor of Nursing
Capstone College of Nursing
University of Alabama
Tuscaloosa, Alabama

Cindy Woods Vardeman, MSN, CWOCN
South Georgia Medical Center
Valdosta, Georgia

Anne Vaughan, MSN, BSN, RN
Post-Masters Nurse Practitioner Student
Spalding University
Louisville, Kentucky

Patricia S. Waldemer, MSN, CMSRN
Clinical Educator
SSM St. Mary's Health Center
St. Louis, Missouri

Janet Willis, RN, MS
Professor
Harrisburg Area Community College
Harrisburg, Pennsylvania

Margaret Wilson, RN, MSN, EdD
Professor of Nursing, Entry Level Masters
  Program
California State University – Fullerton
Fullerton, California

Paige Wimberley, MSN, CNS, CNE
Assistant Professor of Nursing
Arkansas State University
Jonesboro, Arkansas

Gail L. Withers, RN, MSN, ARNP-CNS, CNE
Dean of Nursing and Allied Health
Pratt Community College
Pratt, Kansas

Cynthia A. Worley, BSN, CWOCN
University of Texas MD Anderson Cancer
  Center
Houston, Texas

Toni C. Wortham, RN, BSN, MSN
Professor
Madisonville Community College
Madisonville, Kentucky

Jean Yockey, MSN, FNP-BC, CNE
Associate Professor
University of South Dakota
Vermillion, South Dakota

Contributors to Previous Editions

Jeanette Spain Adams, RN, PhD, CRNI, APRN
Faculty
University of Miami School of Nursing
  and Health Sciences
Coral Gables, Florida

Elizabeth A. Ayello, RN, BSN, MS, PhD, CS, CETN
Clinical Assistant Professor of Nursing
New York University School of Education,
  Nursing
Clinical Associate, Enterostomal Therapy
  Service
New York University Medical Center
New York, New York

Sylvia Baird, RN, BSN, MM
Manager, Patient Safety
Spectrum Health
Grand Rapids, Michigan

Julia Balzer Riley, RN, MN, AHN-C, CET
Adjunct Faculty
University of Tampa
Tampa, Florida
President, Constant Source Seminars
Ellenton, Florida

Peggy Breckenridge, MSN, FNP
Associate Professor of Nursing
College of Health Sciences
Roanoke, Virginia

Judith C. Brostron, RN, BA, JD, LLM
Attorney
Lashly & Baer, P.C.
St. Louis, Missouri

Victoria M. Brown, RN, BSN, MSN, PhD, HNC
Professor of Nursing
Georgia College and State University
Milledgeville, Georgia

Gale Carli, MSN, MSHed, BSN, RN
Assistant Professor
Ohlone College
Fremont, California

Kelly Jo Cone, RN, BSN, MS, PhD
Associate Professor
Graduate Program
Saint Francis Medical Center College
  of Nursing
Peoria, Illinois

Roslyn Corcoran, RN, BSN
Registered Nurse
Barnes-Jewish Hospital
St. Louis, Missouri

Rick Daniels, RN, BSN, MSN, PhD
Professor of Nursing
Oregon Health Science University
  at Southern Oregon University
Ashland, Oregon

Carolyn Ruppel D'Avis, RN, BSN, MSN
Director, Baccalaureate Program, Adjunct
  Assistant Professor
The Catholic University of America, School
  of Nursing
Washington, DC

Sharon J. Edwards, RN, BSN, MSN, PhD
Assistant Professor
University of South Florida
Tampa, Florida

Martha Keene Elkin, RN, MSN, IBCLC
Lactation Counselor
Stephens Memorial Hospital
Norway, Maine

Linda Fasciani, RN, BSN, MSN
Assistant Professor of Nursing
County College of Morris
Randolph, New Jersey

Leah Frederick, MS, RN, CIC
Consultant
Infection Control Consultants
Scottsdale, Arizona

Cynthia S. Goodwin, RN, BSN, MSN
Instructor, School of Nursing at Health
  Professions
University of Southern Indiana
Evansville, Indiana

Lois C. Hamel, BS, MS
Assistant Professor of Nursing
Westbrook College – University
  of New England
Portland, Maine

Maureen Huhmann, MS, RD
Clinical Nutrition Instructor
University of Medicine and Dentistry
  of New Jersey
Newark, New Jersey

Judith Ann Kilpatrick, RN, MSN, DNSc
Assistant Professor
Widener University
Chester, Pennsylvania

Carl A. Kirton, RN-C, BSN, MA, ACRN, ANP
Clinical Assistant Professor, Adult Nurse
  Practitioner
New York University
New York, New York

Mary Kay Knight Macheca, RN, BSN, MSN(R), CS, CDE
Certified Adult Nurse Practitioner
The Health Care Group of St. Louis/Unity
  Medical Group
St. Louis, Missouri

Kristine L'Ecuyer, RN, MSN, CCNS
Assistant Professor
Saint Louis University
St. Louis, Missouri

Ruth Ludwick, RN, BSN, MSN, PhD, RN-C
Associate Professor
School of Nursing
Kent State University
Kent, Ohio

Rita G. Mertig, RNC, MS, CNS
Professor of Nursing
John Tyler Community College
Chester, Virginia

Mary Dee Miller, RN, BSN, MS, CIC
Regional Director, Epidemiology Services
Mercy Regional Health System
Cincinnati, Ohio

Elaine Neel, BSN, MSN
Nursing Instructor
School of Nursing
Graham Hospital
Canton, Illinois

Geralyn A. Ochs, RN, AND, BSN, MSN
Instructor of Nursing
School of Nursing
Saint Louis University
St. Louis, Missouri

Marsha Evans Orr, RN, MS, CS, CNSN
Zone Clinical Manager
Apria Healthcare
Phoenix, Arizona

Dula F. Pacquiao, EdD, RN, CTN
Professor and Director
Transcultural Nursing Institute and MSN
    Program
Kean University
Union, New Jersey

Nancy Panthofer, RN, BSN, MSN
Lecturer
Kent State University
Kent, Ohio

Janice J. Rumfelt, BSN, MSN, EdD, RNC
Assistant Professor of Nursing
Southern Illinois University Edwardsville
Edwardsville, Illinois

Sharon Souter, RN, BSN, MSN
Nursing Program Director
New Mexico State University – Carlsbad
Carlsbad, New Mexico

Elizabeth Speakman, RN, EdD
Associate Professor of Nursing
Community College of Philadelphia
Philadelphia, Pennsylvania

Rachel E. Spector, BS, MS, PhD, CTN, FAAN
Associate Professor
Boston College, School of Nursing
Chestnut Hill, Massachusetts

Susan Speraw, RN, PHD, CNP
Associate Professor of Pediatrics
University of Tennessee, College of Medicine
    Chattanooga Unit
Chattanooga, Tennessee

Riva Touger-Decker, PhD, RD, FADA
Associate Professor and Program Director
Graduate Programs in Clinical Nutrition,
Department of Primary Care, SHRP
Division of Nutrition, Department
    of Diagnostic Sciences
New Jersey Dental School
Newark, New Jersey

**Pamela Becker Weilitz, RN, MSN(r), BC,
ANP, M-SCNS**
Private Practice
Adult Nurse Practitioner
St. Louis, Missouri

Joan Domigan Wentz, MSN, RN
Assistant Professor
Barnes-Jewish College
St. Louis, Missouri

Barbara Yoost, RN, BSN, MSN, CNS
Lecturer, Fundamentals Course Coordinator
College of Nursing
Kent State University
Kent, Ohio

My professional career has been blessed with having been associated with many learned, creative, and dedicated professional nurses. Each in their own way has influenced the ideas and ultimate presentation that makes Basic Nursing *a credible and informative textbook. I thank each of them.*
Patricia A. Potter

To the nursing faculty at Southern Illinois University and Saint Louis University. Your commitment to nursing and nursing education inspires us all to be the guardians of the discipline.

To my granddaughters, Cora Elizabeth Bryan and Amalie Mary Bryan.
Anne Griffin Perry

To my parents, James and Evelyn Clark, who provided my basic nursing education and the foundation for my professional life.

To my husband, Drake, and daughters, Sara and Kelsey—thank you for all your support and understanding while I am reading, writing, and editing. I could not have done it without you. I am blessed to have you all in my life.
Patricia A. Stockert

To my parents, Kay and Larry, whose never-ending support and guidance taught me the importance of thinking critically, teaching enthusiastically, living life fully, and loving others unconditionally. And to the nursing faculty, staff, and students at the University of Evansville, your commitment to excellence in nursing education inspires me every day and fuels my continued passion for the profession of nursing.
Amy Hall

Student Preface

Basic Nursing was developed to provide you with all of the fundamental nursing concepts and skills in a visually appealing, easy-to-use format. We know how busy you are and how precious your time is. As you begin your nursing education, it is very important that you have a resource that includes all the information you need to prepare for lectures, classroom activities, clinical rotations, and examinations—and nothing more. We have designed this text to meet all of those needs. This book has been designed to help you succeed in this course and prepare you for more advanced study. In addition to the readable writing style and abundance of color photographs and drawings, we have incorporated numerous features to help you study and learn. We have made it easy for you to pull out important content. **Check out the following special learning aids:**

Media Resources sections detail the electronic resources available for every chapter.

Learning Objectives begin each chapter to help you focus on the key information that follows.

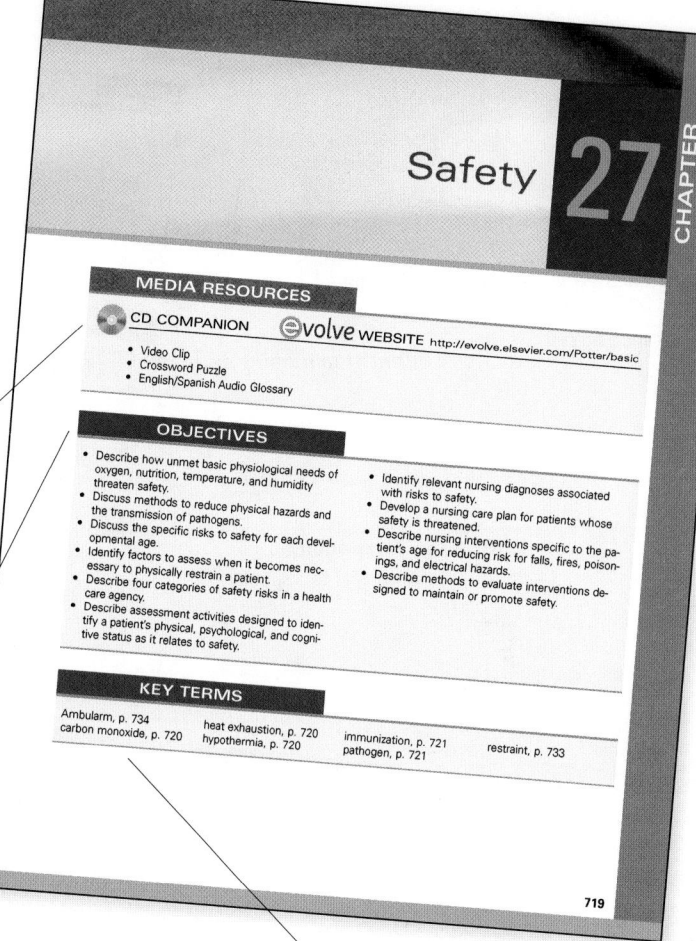

Chapters provide a list of **Key Terms** and the page number where each term is introduced.

Progressive Case Studies introduce you to patients, families, and nurses. These engaging scenarios illustrate the nursing process in action and help you develop critical thinking skills.

Best Practices boxes summarize the results of research studies and indicate how current evidence can be applied to nursing practice.

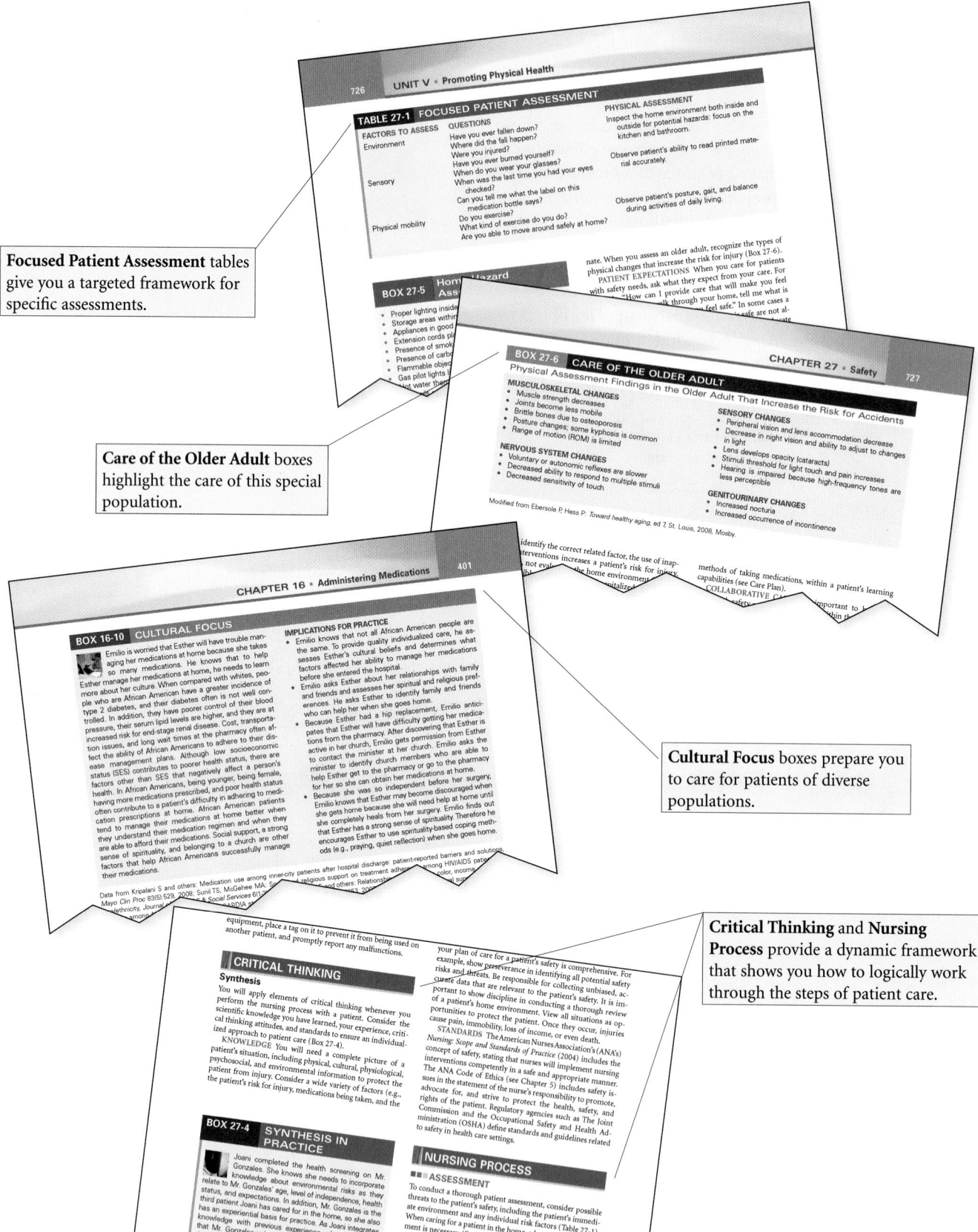

Focused Patient Assessment tables give you a targeted framework for specific assessments.

Care of the Older Adult boxes highlight the care of this special population.

Cultural Focus boxes prepare you to care for patients of diverse populations.

Critical Thinking and **Nursing Process** provide a dynamic framework that shows you how to logically work through the steps of patient care.

Nursing Care Plans incorporate the nursing process and highlight defining characteristics, goals, NIC interventions, NOC expected outcomes, and evaluations.

Nursing Interventions Classification and **Nursing Outcomes Classification** terminologies are used in the care plans to build your knowledge of nursing concepts.

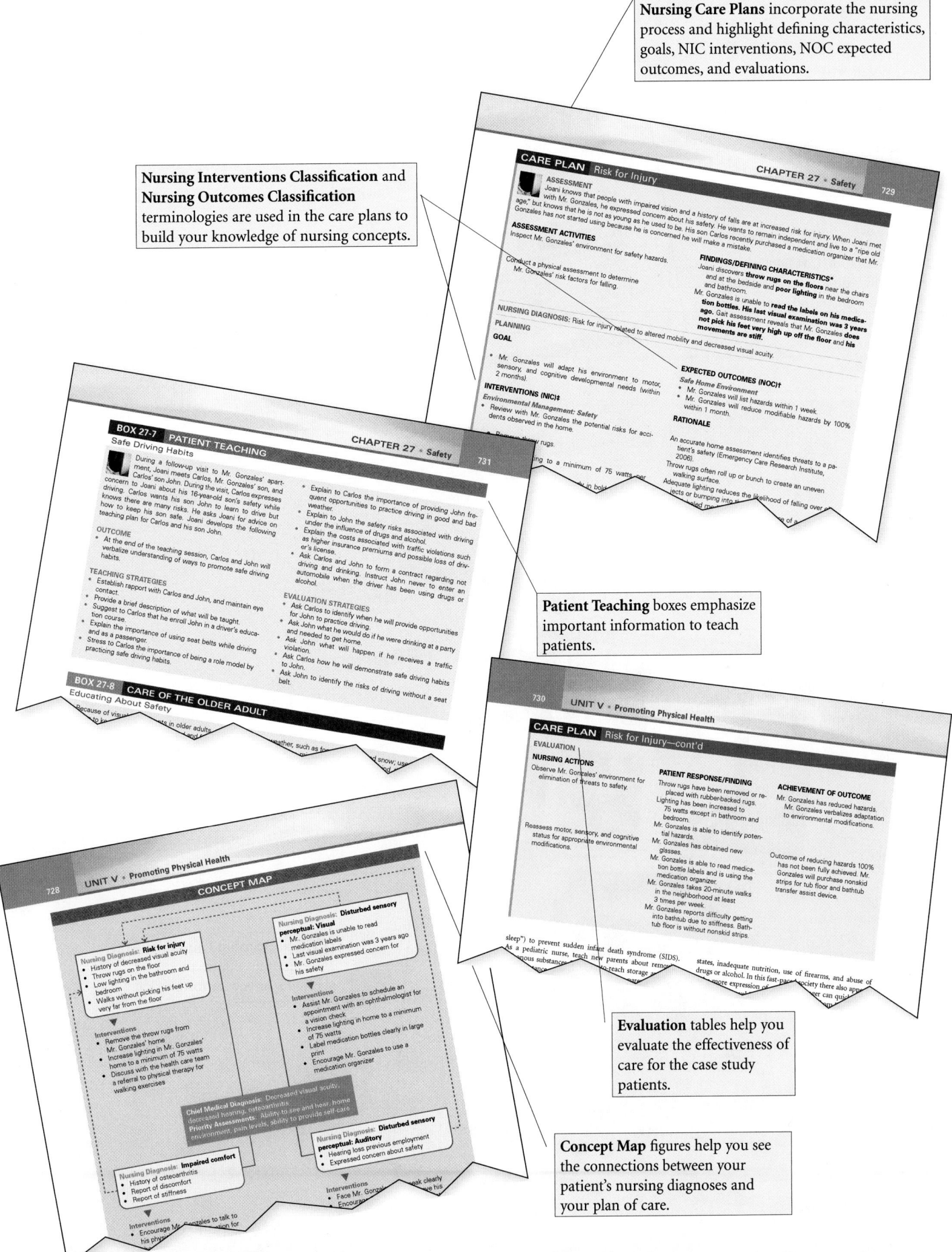

CARE PLAN Risk for Injury   CHAPTER 27 • Safety   729

ASSESSMENT
Joani knows that people with impaired vision and a history of falls are at increased risk for injury. When Joani met with Mr. Gonzales, he expressed concern about his safety. He wants to remain independent and live to a "ripe old age," but knows that he is not as young as he used to be. His son Carlos recently purchased a medication organizer that Mr. Gonzales has not started using because he is used to.

ASSESSMENT ACTIVITIES
Inspect Mr. Gonzales' environment for safety hazards.

Conduct a physical assessment to determine Mr. Gonzales' risk factors for falling.

NURSING DIAGNOSIS: Risk for injury related to altered mobility and decreased visual acuity.

PLANNING
GOAL
• Mr. Gonzales will adapt his environment to motor, sensory, and cognitive developmental needs (within 2 months)

INTERVENTIONS (NIC)‡
Environmental Management: Safety
• Review with Mr. Gonzales the potential risks for accidents observed in the home.

FINDINGS/DEFINING CHARACTERISTICS*
Joani discovers **throw rugs on the floors** near the chairs and at the bedside and **poor lighting** in the bedroom and bathroom.
Mr. Gonzales is unable to **read the labels on his medication bottles. His last visual examination was 3 years ago.** Gait assessment reveals that Mr. Gonzales does **not pick his feet very high up off the floor** and his **movements are stiff.**

EXPECTED OUTCOMES (NOC)†
Safe Home Environment
• Mr. Gonzales will list hazards within 1 week
• Mr. Gonzales will reduce modifiable hazards by 100% within 1 month.

RATIONALE
An accurate home assessment identifies threats to a patient's safety (Emergency Care Research Institute, 2006).
Throw rugs often roll up or bunch to create an uneven walking surface.
Adequate lighting reduces the likelihood of falling over objects or bumping into ...

BOX 27-7 PATIENT TEACHING   CHAPTER 27 • Safety   731
Safe Driving Habits
During a follow-up visit to Mr. Gonzales' apartment, Joani meets Carlos, Mr. Gonzales' son, and Carlos' son John. During the visit, Carlos expresses concern to Joani about his 16-year-old son's safety while driving. Carlos wants his son John to learn to drive but knows there are many risks. He asks Joani for advice on how to keep his son safe. Joani develops the following teaching plan for Carlos and his son John.

OUTCOME
• At the end of the teaching session, Carlos and John will verbalize understanding of ways to promote safe driving habits.

TEACHING STRATEGIES
• Establish rapport with Carlos and John, and maintain eye contact.
• Provide a brief description of what will be taught.
• Suggest to Carlos that he enroll John in a driver's education course.
• Explain the importance of using seat belts while driving and as a passenger.
• Stress to Carlos the importance of being a role model by practicing safe driving habits.

• Explain to Carlos the importance of providing John frequent opportunities to practice driving in good and bad weather.
• Explain to John the safety risks associated with driving under the influence of drugs and alcohol.
• Explain the costs associated with traffic violations such as higher insurance premiums and possible loss of driver's license.
• Ask Carlos and John to form a contract regarding not driving and drinking. Instruct John never to enter an automobile when the driver has been using drugs or alcohol.

EVALUATION STRATEGIES
• Ask Carlos to identify when he will provide opportunities for John to practice driving.
• Ask John what he would do if he were drinking at a party and needed to get home.
• Ask John what will happen if he receives a traffic violation.
• Ask Carlos how he will demonstrate safe driving habits to John.
• Ask John to identify the risks of driving without a seat belt.

BOX 27-8 CARE OF THE OLDER ADULT
Educating About Safety

Patient Teaching boxes emphasize important information to teach patients.

---

730   UNIT V • Promoting Physical Health

CARE PLAN Risk for Injury—cont'd

EVALUATION

NURSING ACTIONS
Observe Mr. Gonzales' environment for elimination of threats to safety.

Reassess motor, sensory, and cognitive status for appropriate environmental modifications.

PATIENT RESPONSE/FINDING
Throw rugs have been removed or replaced with rubber-backed rugs.
Lighting has been increased to 75 watts except in bathroom and bedroom.
Mr. Gonzales is able to identify potential hazards.
Mr. Gonzales has obtained new glasses.
Mr. Gonzales is able to read medication bottle labels and is using the medication organizer.
Mr. Gonzales takes 20-minute walks in the neighborhood at least 3 times per week.
Mr. Gonzales reports difficulty getting into bathtub due to stiffness. Bathtub floor is without nonskid strips.

ACHIEVEMENT OF OUTCOME
Mr. Gonzales has reduced hazards.
Mr. Gonzales verbalizes adaptation to environmental modifications.

Outcome of reducing hazards 100% has not been fully achieved. Mr. Gonzales will purchase nonskid strips for tub floor and bathtub transfer assist device.

sleep") to prevent sudden infant death syndrome (SIDS). As a pediatric nurse, teach new parents about remov... ... states, inadequate nutrition, use of firearms, and abuse of drugs or alcohol. In this fast-pac... society there also app...

Evaluation tables help you evaluate the effectiveness of care for the case study patients.

---

728   UNIT V • Promoting Physical Health

CONCEPT MAP

Nursing Diagnosis: **Risk for injury**
• History of decreased visual acuity
• Throw rugs on the floor
• Low lighting in the bathroom and bedroom
• Walks without picking his feet up very far from the floor

Interventions
• Remove the throw rugs from Mr. Gonzales' home
• Increase lighting in Mr. Gonzales' home to a minimum of 75 watts
• Discuss with the health care team a referral to physical therapy for walking exercises

Nursing Diagnosis: **Disturbed sensory perceptual: Visual**
• Mr. Gonzales is unable to read medication labels
• Last visual examination was 3 years ago
• Mr. Gonzales expressed concern for his safety

Interventions
• Assist Mr. Gonzales to schedule an appointment with an ophthalmologist for a vision check
• Increase lighting in home to a minimum of 75 watts
• Label medication bottles clearly in large print
• Encourage Mr. Gonzales to use a medication organizer

Chief Medical Diagnosis: Decreased visual acuity, decreased hearing, osteoarthritis.
Priority Assessments: Ability to see and hear, home environment, pain levels, ability to provide self-care

Nursing Diagnosis: **Impaired comfort**
• History of osteoarthritis
• Report of discomfort
• Report of stiffness

Interventions
• Encourage Mr. Gonzales to talk to his phys...

Nursing Diagnosis: **Disturbed sensory perceptual: Auditory**
• Hearing loss previous employment
• Expressed concern about safety

Interventions
• Face Mr. Gonza... ...k clearly
• Encour...

Concept Map figures help you see the connections between your patient's nursing diagnoses and your plan of care.

Nursing Skills are presented in a clear, two-column format with steps and rationales so you learn why as well as how. The skills in each chapter begin with a **Safety Guidelines** section that will help you focus on safe and effective skill performance.

Delegation Considerations guide you in delegating tasks to nursing assistive personnel.

Video Icons indicate video clips associated with specific skills that are available on the free Companion CD and Evolve Student Resources website.

Equipment lists show specific items needed for each skill.

Clear, close-up **photographs** help you learn to perform important techniques.

Critical Decision Points alert you to important information to consider as you perform a skill.

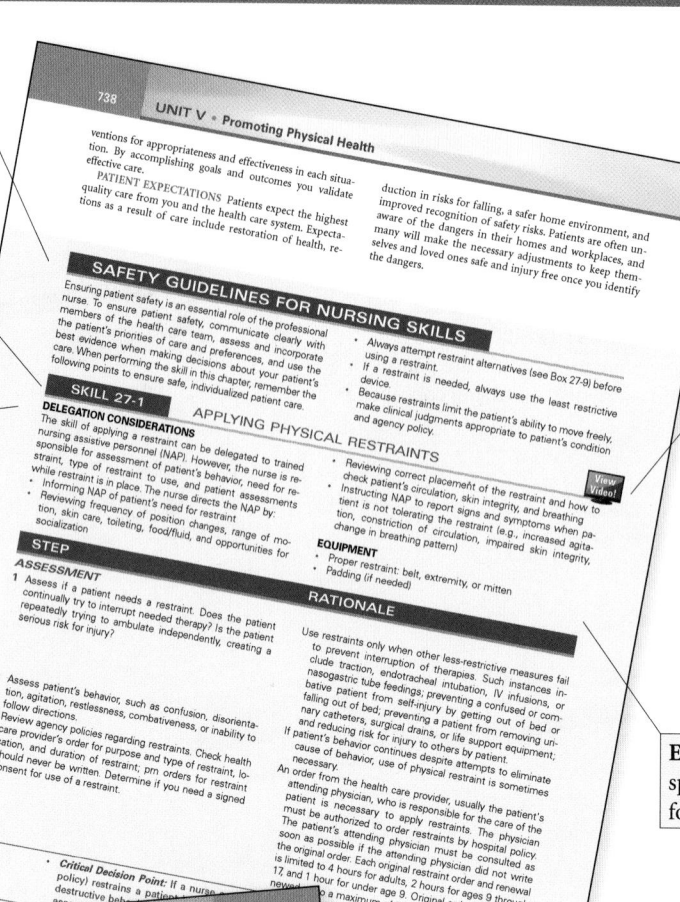

sion of restraint, depending on hospital's Medicare status (see agency policy).

3 After 24 hours, before writing a new order, a physician or health care provider who is responsible for the patient's care must see and assess the patient.

Ensures restraint application continues to be medically appropriate.

4 Observe IV catheters, urinary catheters, and drainage tubes to determine that you positioned them correctly.

5 Provide appropriate sensory stimulation, and reorient patient as needed.

Reinsertion is uncomfortable and increases risk for infection or interruption of therapy.
Use of restraints further increases disorientation.

RECORDING AND REPORTING

- Record patient behaviors before you applied restraints.
- Record restraint alternatives you attempted and the patient's response.
- Record patient and/or family's understanding of and consent to restraint application.
- Record type and location of the restraint and time applied.
- Record times that you performed assessments and releases while patient in restraints.

- Record findings from your assessments related to orientation, oxygenation, skin integrity, circulation, and positioning.
- Record patient's behavior and expected or unexpected outcomes after you applied the restraint.
- Record patient's response when you removed restraints (e.g., calm, cooperative).
- Also see behavioral restraint flow sheet (Figure 27-4).

UNEXPECTED OUTCOMES AND RELATED INTERVENTIONS

- Skin integrity becomes impaired.
  - Reassess need for continued use of restraint and if alternatives can be used.
  - If restraint is necessary, make sure you apply restraint correctly and provide adequate padding.
  - Assess skin, provide appropriate therapy, or remove restraints more frequently.
  - Change wet or soiled restraints.
- Patient becomes more confused and agitated after you apply restraints.
  - Determine the cause of the behavior, and eliminate the cause, if possible.
  - Determine the need for more or less sensory stimulation.
  - Reorient as needed, and/or attempt other restraint alternatives.

- Neurovascular status of an extremity is altered, manifested by cyanosis, pallor, edema, or coldness of skin, or patient complains of tingling, pain, numbness, or loss of ROM.
  - Remove the restraint immediately, stay with the patient, and notify the physician.
  - Protect extremity from further injury.
- Patient releases the restraint and suffers a fall or other injury.
  - Attend to patient's immediate physical needs.
  - Notify the physician, and reassess type of restraint and correct application.

Recording and Reporting provides guidelines for what to chart and report.

Unexpected Outcomes and Related Interventions identify possible undesired results and provide appropriate nursing actions.

BOX 27-10 PROCEDURAL GUIDELINES

Intervening in Accidental Poisoning

1 Assess for signs or symptoms of ingestion of harmful substances, such as nausea, vomiting, foaming at the mouth, drooling, difficulty breathing, sweating, and lethargy.

2 Terminate the exposure by emptying the mouth of pills, plant parts, or other material.

3 If poisoning is due to skin contact or eye contact, irrigate the skin or eye with copious amounts of tap water for 15 to 20 minutes. In the case of an inhalation exposure, safely remove the victim from the potentially dangerous environment.

4 Identify the type and amount of substance ingested to help determine the correct type and amount of antidote needed.

5 If the victim is conscious and alert, call the local poison control center or the national toll-free poison control center number (1-800-222-1222) before attempting any intervention. Poison control centers have information needed

to treat poisoned patients or to offer referral to treatment centers. The administration of ipecac syrup is no longer recommended for routine home treatment of poisoning (American Academy of Pediatrics, 2003).

6 If the victim has collapsed or stopped breathing, call 911 for emergency transportation to the hospital. Initiate CPR, if indicated, until emergency personnel arrive. Ambulance personnel will be able to provide emergency measures if needed. In addition, parent or guardian is sometimes too upset to drive safely.

7 Position victim with head turned to side to reduce risk for aspiration.

8 Never induce vomiting if the victim has ingested the following poisonous substances: lye, household cleaners, hair care products, grease or petroleum products, and furniture polish, paint thinner, or kerosene.

9 Never induce vomiting in an unconscious or convulsing victim because vomiting increases risk for aspiration.

CPR, Cardiopulmonary resuscitation.
Modified from Hockenberry MJ: *Wong's essentials of pediatric nursing*, ed 8, St. Louis, 2009, Mosby; American Academy of Pediatrics, Committee on Injury, Violence and Poison Prevention: Poison treatment in the home, *Pediatrics* 112(5):1182, 2003.

Procedural Guidelines provide streamlined, step-by-step instructions for performing the most basic skills.

KEY POINTS

- A safe environment in a health care agency is comfortable; maintains the patient's privacy; and reduces the risks for injury, infection, and negative effects of treatment or medications.
- In the community a safe environment means basic needs are achievable, physical hazards are reduced, transmission of pathogens and parasites is reduced, pollution is controlled, and sanitation is maintained.
- The transmission of pathogens and parasites is reduced through medical and surgical asepsis, food sanitation, insect and rodent control, and disposal of human wastes.
- Every developmental stage involves assessment of specific safety risks.
- The school-age child is at risk for injury at home, at school, and traveling to and from school.

- Adolescents are at risk for injury from motor vehicle accidents and the effects of drug and alcohol abuse.
- Threats to an adult's safety are frequently associated with lifestyle habits.
- Risks of injury for older adults are directly related to the physiological changes of the aging process.
- Risks to patient safety within a health care agency include falls and patient-inherent, procedure-related, and equipment-related accidents.
- Individualize nursing interventions for promoting safety for developmental stage, lifestyle, and the environment.
- Continually evaluate the nursing care plan to promote safety in order to identify new or continued risks to the patient.
- Use physical restraints only as a last resort, when patients' behavior places them or others at risk for injury.

Key Points and **Critical Thinking Exercises** sections help you review and apply essential content from the chapter.

CRITICAL THINKING EXERCISES

Mr. Gonzales is visiting his widowed sister, Mrs. Pruitt, a 73-year-old who recently had a colectomy to remove a mass in her colon. Mrs. Pruitt did very well after her surgery. Although morphine has been effective in relieving her pain, during your assessment she appears agitated and restless and is picking at her tubes. Mr. Gonzales tells you that he is worried because this is unusual behavior for his sister. You are also concerned that Mrs. Pruitt is at risk for removing her nasogastric tube and IV catheter.

1. What are possible sources for Mrs. Pruitt's unusual behavior?

2. How will you prioritize your interventions when addressing these potential sources?

3. What factors about restraints and their safety implications affect your decision to use a restraint on Mrs. Pruitt?

4. If a restraint is necessary to avoid disruption of therapy, what interventions are necessary to ensure Mrs. Pruitt's safety while in restraints?

5. After application of upper extremity restraints, nursing assistive personnel report that Mrs. Pruitt repeatedly tries to remove the restraints. What actions do you take after hearing this report? Select all that apply. Explain your answers.
   a. Notify the physician or health care provider.
   b. Instruct the nursing assistive personnel to continue hourly checks.
   c. Immediately assess Mrs. Pruitt's behavior.
   d. Instruct the nursing assistive personnel to remove the restraints.

REVIEW QUESTIONS

1. The nurse discovers an electrical fire in a patient's room. Which action should the nurse take first?
   1. Turn off the oxygen to the unit.
   2. Evacuate any patients/visitors in immediate danger.
   3. Close all doors and windows.
   4. Use the nearest fire extinguisher.

2. A parent calls the pediatrician's office frantic about the bottle of cleaner that her 2-year-old child drank. Which of the following is the most important instruction the nurse gives to this parent?
   1. Contact the local poison control center.
   2. Take the child to the nearest emergency department.
   3. Give the child milk.
   4. Give the child syrup of ipecac.

3. During the nursing assessment of a 52-year-old man, he reports increased alcohol consumption secondary to stress at work. One of the expected outcomes for this patient is to:
   1. Contact the local health department for stress management classes
   2. Decrease his alcohol intake during stress
   3. Decrease stress in his life
   4. Adopt sleep hygiene measures to promote sleep

4. The nurse has just completed a gait assessment on a 78-year-old woman. The assessment reveals shuffling gait, decreased balance, and instability. Based on these data, which one of the following nursing diagnoses indicates an understanding of the assessment findings?
   1. Activity intolerance
   2. Impaired bed mobility
   3. Disturbed sensory perception
   4. Risk for falls

5. The nurse has just found a 68-year-old woman wandering in the hallway and exhibiting confused behavior. The patient says she is looking for the bathroom. Which interventions are appropriate to ensure the safety of the patient? Select all that apply.
   1. Ask the physician or health care provider to order a vest restraint.
   2. Insert a urinary catheter.
   3. Provide scheduled toileting rounds every 2 to 3 hours.
   4. Assign a nurse to stay with the patient.
   5. Keep the bed in low position with the upper side rails up.
   6. Keep the pathway from the bed to the bathroom clear.

Multiple-choice questions in the **Review Questions** at the end of each chapter help you evaluate learning and prepare for your course examination.

Preface to the Instructor

"Traditional nursing" is a thing of the past. Today's nurses must be prepared to adapt to the continual changes occurring in health care. They play a vital role in the delivery of multidisciplinary health care services. The practice arena continues to change—moving increasingly more to the community setting. The focus of care is changing as well—more emphasis is being placed on health promotion and restorative care. Even the patients are changing—more cultural diversity exists and the percentage of older adult patients continues to increase. Patients are far more involved in and informed about health care.

Despite these changes—or perhaps because of these changes—it is essential that the basics of nursing must remain the foundation of practice. Nurses must be knowledgeable and professional. They must be both technically proficient and personally caring. And they must be able to synthesize a broad array of knowledge and experiences when providing care for their patients.

We continue to cover all of the fundamental nursing concepts, skills, and techniques that students must master before moving on to other areas of study. We address changes in practice that affect how and where nurses use the skills and knowledge they acquire.

FEATURES

We have designed this text to welcome the new student to nursing, communicate our own love for the profession, and promote learning and understanding. We know that today's students are busy and, too often, overwhelmed by all that they must learn and do. They want their texts to focus on the most current, factual, and essential content and skills. We want to ensure that these students are ready to continue with their education and will, ultimately, be prepared for all of the challenges of practice. To this end, we have included the following key features:

- Students will appreciate the **clear, engaging writing style.** The narrative actually addresses the reader, making this textbook more of an active instructional tool than a passive reference. Students will find that even complex technical and theoretical concepts are presented in a language that is easy to understand.
- The **attractive, functional design** will appeal to today's visual learner. The clear, readable type and bold headings make the content easy to read and follow. Each special element is consistently color-keyed so students can readily identify important information.
- Hundreds of **large, clear, full-color photographs and drawings** reinforce and clarify key concepts and techniques.
- The **five-step nursing process** serves as the organizing framework for all clinical chapters. This logical, consis-

tent framework for narrative discussions is further enhanced by special boxes that highlight assessment, care plans, and evaluation of outcome achievement.

- **Critical thinking** is presented in its own chapter, but is also incorporated as a consistent partner to the nursing process in each clinical chapter. This application of critical thinking provides a practical, clinical decision-making guide that is easy for even the beginning student to understand.
- **Ongoing case studies** in each chapter introduce "real-world" patients, families, and nurses. The chapter follows the case study through the steps of the nursing process, helping students see how to apply the process, along with critical thinking, to the care of patients. Cases take place in both acute and community settings, and include patients and nurses from a variety of cultural backgrounds.
- **Expected outcomes** are addressed in care plans, special boxes, and narrative to help students understand and apply these key clinical measures.
- Implementation narrative consistently addresses health promotion, acute care, and restorative and continuing care to reflect the current focus on **community-based nursing** and **health promotion.**
- **More than 40 nursing skills** are presented in a clear, two-column format with steps and rationales. Skills include delegation guidelines and critical decision points that alert students to steps requiring special assessment or specific technique for safe and effective administration.
- **Procedural guidelines** provide streamlined step-by-step instructions for performing very basic skills.
- Care of the **older adult** and **patient teaching** are stressed throughout chapter narratives, as well as highlighted in special boxes.
- **Learning aids** to help students identify, review, and apply important content in each chapter include Objectives, Key Terms, Key Points, Critical Thinking Exercises, and Review Questions.

New to This Edition

- **New chapter on Evidence-Based Practice** addresses a growing market demand and highlights how research contributes to nursing knowledge and provides implications for continued nursing practice.
- **New section on Informatics** addresses an emerging trend in nursing. The section focuses on data, knowledge, and information being integrated to support specific patient needs.
- A **Safety Guidelines** paragraph precedes each skill section. This helps students focus on safe and effective skill performance.
- **Concept maps** included in each clinical chapter help the student to think critically about nursing diagnoses and interventions in real-life situations.

- **Best Practices** boxes summarize the results of research studies and indicate how evidence can be applied to nursing practice.
- **Skills sections** were moved to the end of the chapter for easier use, better text flow, and readability.
- **Briefer coverage of higher-level concepts** provides just the right amount of detail on research, theory, professional roles, and management to maintain a strong "essentials" focus.

TEACHING AND LEARNING PACKAGE

In recognition of the incredible challenges faced by both students and educators, we have developed an unsurpassed array of teaching and learning materials.

- Each text is packaged with a free **Companion CD** that contains Butterfield's Fluids and Electrolytes tutorial, an audio glossary, video clips, and crossword puzzles.
- The **Evolve Resources for Instructors** includes a TEACH manual, which links all parts of the educational package by providing the instructor with customizable lesson plans and lecture outlines based on learning objectives, a comprehensive Test Bank, an impressive collection of PowerPoint lecture slides and an image collection to enhance classroom lectures, i-Clicker questions and answers to improve student participation, nursing skills online reading assignments, and answers to the Study Guide questions.
- The **Evolve Resources for Students** provides review questions and answers from the book, competency checklists, audio summaries, an audio glossary, crossword puzzles to improve nursing vocabulary, Butterfield's Fluids and Electrolytes tutorial, video clips to highlight common skills, answers to the critical thinking questions in the book, and content updates that inform students of critical changes in practice.

- **Mosby's Nursing Skills Video Series** provides engaging, action-packed demonstrations of how to perform key nursing procedures in real-life clinical situations. Actual nurses perform each skill as they work through contemporary concepts such as delegation, critical thinking, patient rights, and communication techniques.
- **Study Guide** by Patricia A. Castaldi provides students with a wide variety of exercises and activities to enhance learning and comprehension. This study guide features case studies with related questions; chapter review sections with matching, fill-in-the-blank, and multiple-choice questions; study group questions; instructions for creating and using study charts; and skills performance checklists.
- **Virtual Clinical Excursions** is an exciting workbook and CD-ROM experience that brings learning to life in a virtual hospital setting. The workbook guides students as they care for clients, providing ongoing challenges and learning opportunities. Each lesson in *Virtual Clinical Excursions* complements the textbook content and provides an environment for students to practice what they are learning. This CD/workbook is available separately or packaged at a special price with the textbook.
- **Simulation Learning System** is an online toolkit that helps instructors and facilitators effectively incorporate medium- to high-fidelity simulation into their nursing curriculum. Detailed patient scenarios promote and enhance the clinical decision-making skills of students at all levels. The system provides detailed instructions for preparation and implementation of the simulation experience, debriefing questions that encourage critical thinking, and learning resources to reinforce student comprehension. Each scenario in *Simulation Learning System* complements the textbook content and helps bridge the gap between lectures and clinicals. This system provides the perfect environment for students to practice what they are learning in the text for a true-to-life, hands-on learning experience.

Acknowledgments

The seventh edition of *Basic Nursing* is the result of a new collaboration. Creating a textbook of the caliber of *Basic Nursing* is a challenge. Having professional colleagues to work with and trust is a gift. Dr. Amy Hall and Dr. Patricia Stockert are new members of the author team. Their insight, professionalism, attention to detail, and commitment to a quality product are unmatched. Having a sense of humor and being willing to respond to issues at a minute's notice are assets as well. They have made the writing of this textbook a true pleasure.

In addition, this textbook would not have been realized without the support, guidance, and creative direction from our editorial team, designer, and production staff. Likewise, no book is successful without the hard work and dedication of its marketing team. We are also very fortunate regarding the manner in which staff from the electronic media division of Elsevier has produced products that complement the text and ensure its success.

Each of these divisions and the individuals within these groups contributed their time, talent, and energy to create a textbook that remains cutting edge with respect to the science and art of professional nursing. We wish to make special mention of some important individuals.

Tamara Myers, Editor, Nursing Division, is the new editor on the Fundamentals of Nursing team. She is a dedicated professional who challenges the author team to create a state-of-the-art revision and creates an environment for the editorial and production teams to develop a textbook that is creative and reflects contemporary nursing practice.

Tina Kaemmerer is our Associate Developmental Editor. Her professionalism and organization skills ensure that this project remains on target. She effectively tracks the manuscript through the publication process and is an invaluable resource for authors, contributors, and the production team.

Kim Denando, our Book Designer, contributed to a clear, logical, and visually distinctive textbook design. She helped us achieve the goal of creating a text that is visually appealing yet easy for our readers to use. Kim is also credited for her creativity and vision for the design of the cover art and her direction in implementing the overall design of the text.

Many thanks and gratitude go to members of the Production Team.

- Beth Hayes, Senior Project Manager, is a tireless and dedicated professional. As an accomplished production editor, she keeps us on deadline while ensuring consistency in formatting, presentation, and style. Her sense of humor and ability to always remain calm under pressure are invaluable attributes.
- Anne Altepeter, Publishing Services Manager, has contributed support throughout the editing and final pages.

To Dennis Scanio for his photographic excellence and to Progress West Healthcare Center, O'Fallon, Missouri, for the generous use of their facility for our photo shoot.

A tip of the hat must always go to the sales and marketing team, headed by Pat Crowe and Jamie Kitsis, who provided us direction early on in the planning stage of *Basic Nursing*. Their knowledge of market trends and needs helps us to make revisions of high quality.

To Tricia Kinman, readability specialist, whose editing expertise and knowledge of literacy concepts help us to create a text that is informative, clear, and concise for all of our students.

To our contributors, clinicians, and educators who share their experiences and knowledge about nursing practice in helping to create informative, accurate, and current information. Their knowledge of their own clinical specialties ensures we have a state-of-the-art textbook. We are fortunate to be associated with excellent nurse authors who are able to convey standards of nursing excellence through the printed word.

To our many reviewers, for their expertise, candor, knowledge of the literature, and astute comments that assist us in developing a text with high standards that reflect professional nursing practice today.

After more than 25 years of collaboration, we find ourselves very fortunate and humble. *Basic Nursing* and the other textbooks we have been able to develop have made important contributions to nursing practice. It remains a work of love.

Patricia A. Potter
Anne Griffin Perry

Contents

CHAPTER 1

Health and Wellness

MEDIA RESOURCES

 CD COMPANION 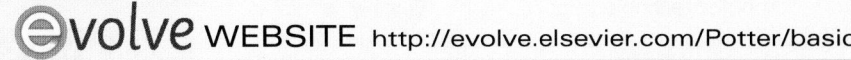 WEBSITE http://evolve.elsevier.com/Potter/basic

- Crossword Puzzle
- English/Spanish Audio Glossary

OBJECTIVES

- Discuss the health belief, health promotion, basic human needs, and holistic health models of health and illness to understand the relationship between patients' attitudes toward health and health practices.
- Describe the variables influencing health beliefs and health practices.
- Describe health promotion and illness prevention activities.

- Explain the three levels of prevention.
- Discuss four types of risk factors and the process of risk factor modification.
- Describe the variables influencing illness behavior.
- Explain the impact of illness on the patient and family.
- Discuss the nurse's role in health and illness.

KEY TERMS

active strategies of
   health promotion,
   p. 7
acute illness, p. 11
chronic illness, p. 11
health, p. 2
health belief model,
   p. 2

health beliefs, p. 2
health promotion, p. 7
health promotion model,
   p. 3
holistic health, p. 5
illness, p. 11
illness behavior, p. 12
illness prevention, p. 7

Maslow's hierarchy of
   needs, p. 4
passive strategies of
   health promotion,
   p. 6
primary prevention,
   p. 7

risk factor, p. 8
secondary prevention,
   p. 7
tertiary prevention,
   p. 8
wellness education,
   p. 7

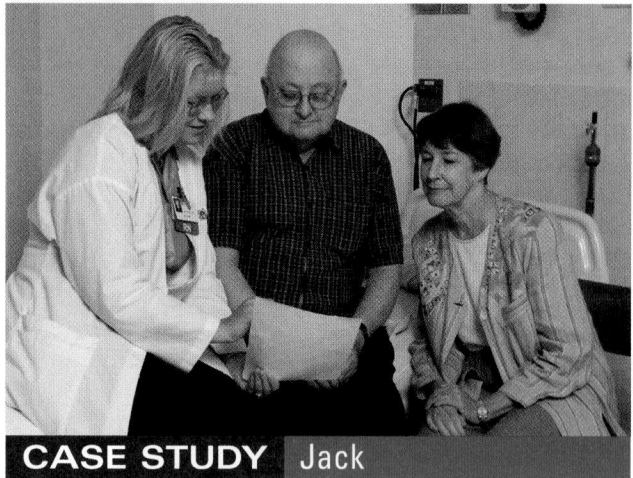

CASE STUDY Jack

Jack is a 59-year-old man with a history of type 2 diabetes, hypertension, and obesity. He is married and works in a computer technology position. He typically works 50 to 60 hours per week. His wife works the same number of hours, although she tends to travel more with her job and sometimes works the night shift. Therefore both Jack and his wife have a hard time fitting exercise into their daily routine, and they often eat at restaurants.

Jack comes into the clinic today for a routine follow-up visit for his diabetes. Sally, the diabetes nurse educator, is working with Jack for the second time. Jack's laboratory data reveal that his blood glucose level is consistently running high. His blood pressure is on the high side of normal. Sally knows she wants to find a way to get Jack's blood glucose levels down to avoid the long-term complications of diabetes. She plans to talk with Jack to determine his understanding of diabetes and to evaluate his readiness for the lifestyle behavior changes needed to manage his health.

In the past most individuals and societies viewed good health or wellness as the opposite or absence of disease. We now understand that some conditions of health lie between disease and good health. Therefore we view health from a broader perspective. As a nurse, you will use concepts of health, health promotion, wellness, and illness to assist your patients in achieving and maintaining an optimal level of health. You will use models of health and illness to understand and explain these concepts. In addition, you will assist patients in making changes to their current health state to bring about improved health and wellness.

DEFINITION OF HEALTH

Defining health is difficult because each person has his or her own personal concept of health. The World Health Organization (WHO) defines health as a "state of complete physical, mental and social well-being, not merely the absence of disease or infirmity" (WHO, 1947). Individual views of health vary among different age-groups, genders, races, and cultures (Pender, 1996; Pender, Murdaugh, and Parsons, 2006). Pender (1996) explains that "all people free of disease are not equally healthy." **Health** is a state of being that people define in relation to their own values, personality, and lifestyle. Pender and others (2006) suggest that for many people, conditions of life rather than pathological states are what define health. Nurses consider the total person, as well as the person's environment, to individualize nursing care and help patients identify and reach their health goals. Therefore health is a complex concept and means more than the absence of disease. People's thoughts about their health and how they take care of themselves influence individuals' definitions of health. For example, many healthy older Americans view health as primarily "a state of mind." Their outlook on life, social health, and physical health all affect their "state of mind" (van Maanen, 2006).

MODELS OF HEALTH AND ILLNESS

A model is a theoretical way of understanding a concept or an idea. Models represent various ways of approaching complex issues. Because health and illness are complex concepts, you need to use models to understand the relationships between health and illness and your patients' attitudes toward health and health practices. Health beliefs influence health practices. **Health beliefs** are a person's ideas, convictions, and attitudes about health and illness. They may be based on facts or misinformation, common sense or myths, or reality or false expectations. Because health beliefs influence health behavior, they can positively or negatively affect a patient's level of health. Nurses develop and use a variety of health models to understand patients' beliefs, attitudes, and values about health and illness to provide effective health care. These models allow you to understand and predict patients' health behavior, including how they use health services, participate in recommended therapy, and care for themselves.

Health Belief Model

Rosenstoch's (1974) and Becker and Maiman's (1975) **health belief model** (Figure 1-1) addresses the relationship between a person's beliefs and behaviors. It provides a way of understanding and predicting how patients will behave in relation to their health and how successful they will be in following health care therapies or regimens. Positive health behaviors are activities related to maintaining, attaining, or regaining good health and preventing illness. Common positive health behaviors include getting immunizations, maintaining proper sleep patterns, getting adequate exercise, and eating healthy foods. Implementation of positive health behaviors is dependent on an individual's awareness of how to live a healthy life and the person's ability and willingness to carry out such behaviors in a healthy lifestyle. Negative health behaviors include activities that are harmful to health, such as smoking, abusing drugs or alcohol, following a poor diet, and refusing to take necessary medications.

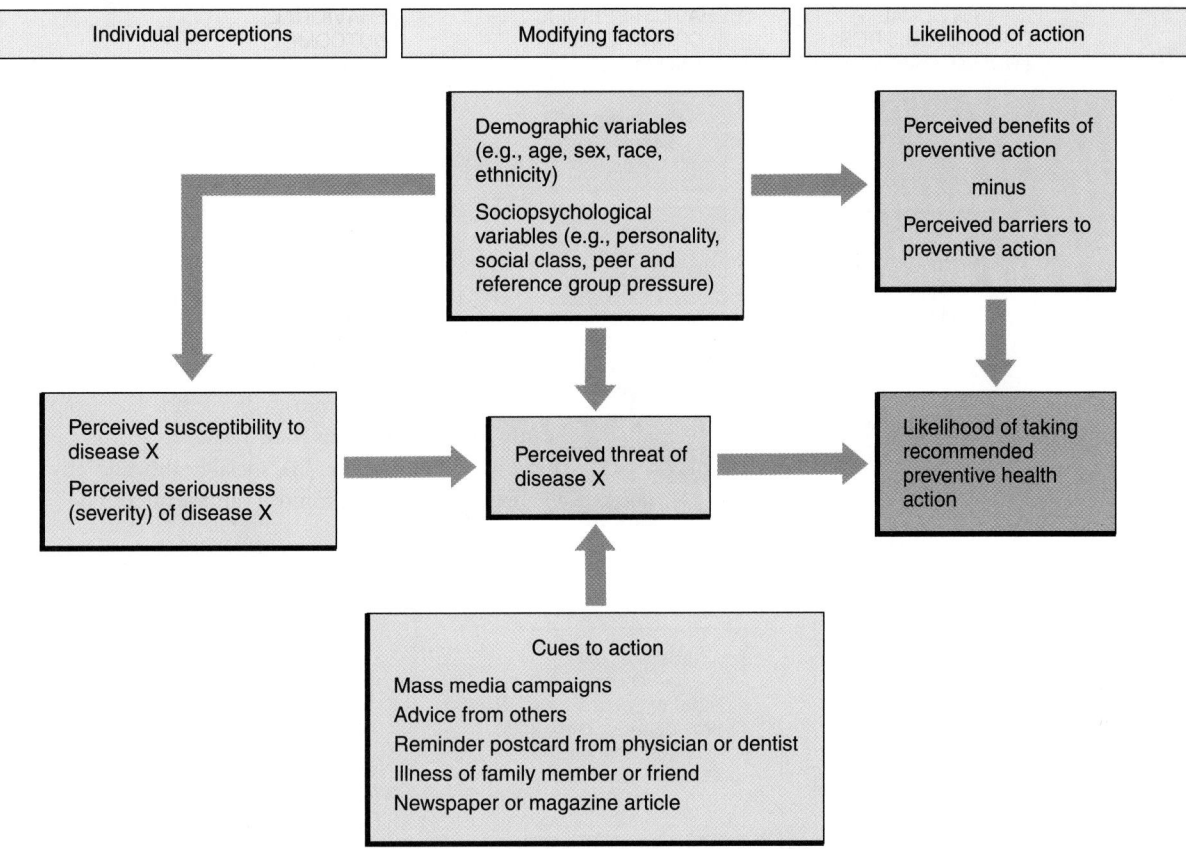

Figure 1-1 ■ Health belief model. (Data from Becker MH, Maiman LA: Sociobehavioral determinants of compliance with health and medical care recommendations, *Med Care* 13[1]:10, 1975.)

The first component of the health belief model involves the individual's perception of susceptibility to an illness. For example, a patient needs to recognize the familial link for coronary artery disease. After recognizing this link, the patient will perceive a personal risk for heart disease. The second component is the patient's perception of the seriousness of the illness. Demographic and sociopsychological variables, perceived threats of the illness, and cues to action (e.g., mass media campaigns and advice from family, friends, and medical professionals) all influence and modify this perception. The third component, the likelihood that the patient will take preventive action, such as following a low-fat diet, results from the patient's perception of the benefits of and barriers to taking action. Preventive actions include lifestyle changes, increased participation in recommended medical therapies, and a search for medical advice or treatment.

The health belief model helps you understand factors influencing patients' perceptions, beliefs, and behavior and to plan care that will most effectively assist patients in maintaining or restoring health and preventing illness. Understand that each patient's views of health and wellness and individual belief systems influence the ability to make lasting changes in health status. Do not make judgments when you encounter views and beliefs that differ from your own individual philosophies of health and wellness.

Health Promotion Model

The health promotion model proposed by Pender (1982, 1996; Pender, Murdaugh, and Parsons, 2002, 2006) (Figure 1-2) defines health as a positive, dynamic state, not merely the absence of disease. The model was proposed as a framework for integrating the perspectives of nursing and behavioral science and the factors that influence health behaviors (Pender and others, 2002). Health promotion is behavior motivated by the desire to increase well-being and actualize human health potential, whereas health protection is behavior that is motivated by a desire to avoid illness, detect it early, or maintain function within the constraints of an illness (Pender and others, 2002). The **health promotion model** describes the multidimensional nature of people as they interact within their environment to pursue health (Pender and others, 2006). This model focuses on three areas:

1. Individual characteristics and experiences
2. Behavior-specific cognitions and affect
3. Behavioral outcomes

The model also organizes cues into a pattern to explain the likelihood of a patient developing health promotion behaviors (Pender, 1993, 1996). The purpose of this model is to explain the reasons that individuals engage in health activities

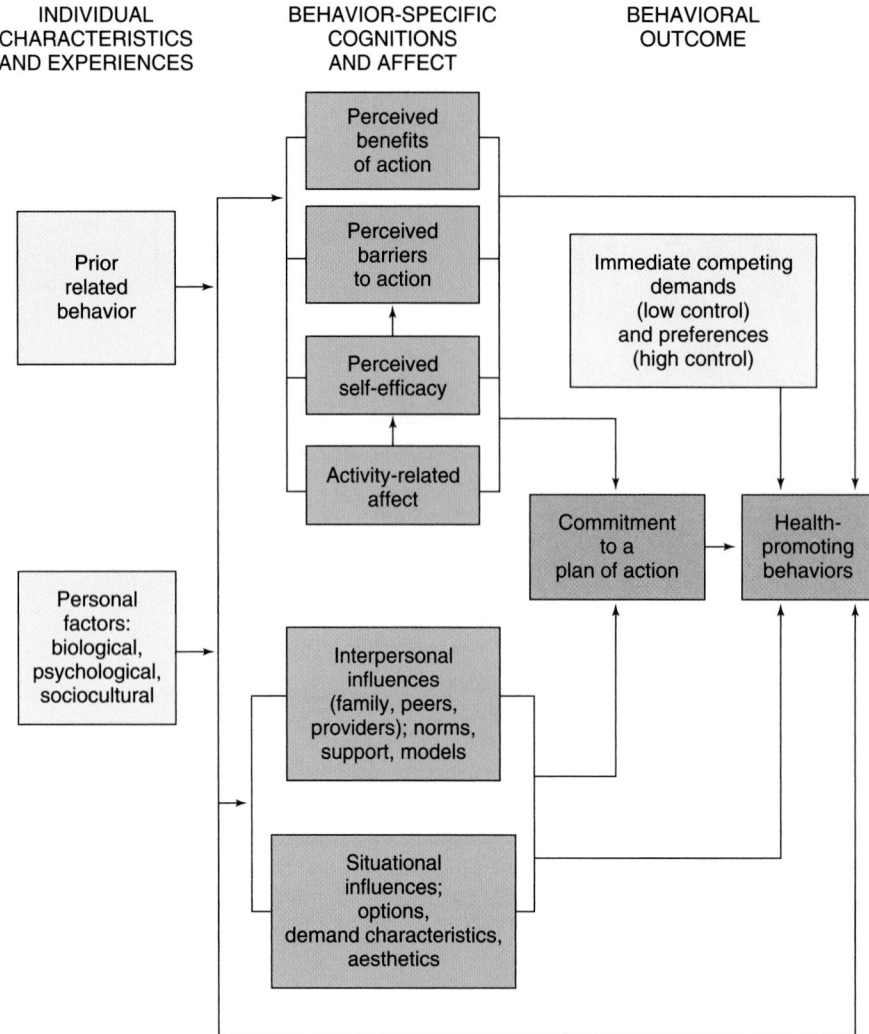

INDIVIDUAL CHARACTERISTICS AND EXPERIENCES   BEHAVIOR-SPECIFIC COGNITIONS AND AFFECT   BEHAVIORAL OUTCOME

Figure 1-2 ■ Health promotion model. (From Pender NJ, Murdaugh CL, Parsons MA: *Health promotion in nursing practice,* ed 5, Upper Saddle River, NJ, 2006, Prentice Hall.)

and is not for use with families or communities. You will use this model to help your patients carry out healthy behaviors in their daily lives.

Basic Human Needs Model

One way to understand an individual's motivation to achieve optimal health is to review Abraham Maslow's hierarchy of needs (1954). This model helps you understand the needs of patients and families, their behaviors, and their readiness to take part in health promotion activities. Maslow's model describes human needs using a pyramid divided into five levels. As people meet the needs of one level, they move up to the next level. According to **Maslow's hierarchy of needs** (Figure 1-3), individuals have to meet lower-level needs before they are able to satisfy higher-level needs. Unsatisfied needs motivate human behavior.

The lowest level of needs on the hierarchy consists of very *basic physiological needs,* such as water, food, sleep, and sex. When these needs are not met, the affected person feels sick or irritated or complains of pain or discomfort. Those feelings motivate the individual to satisfy the need (Maslow,

1970, 1987). The second level on the hierarchy of needs consists of *safety needs,* which include establishing stability and consistency. These psychological needs include the security of a home and a family. For example, a woman living in an abusive home is unable to move to the next level of love and belongingness because she is constantly concerned for her safety. The third level on the hierarchy is *love and belongingness,* which is a desire to belong to groups. It consists of the need to feel love by others and to be accepted. The fourth level deals with the need for *self-esteem.* Self-esteem results from mastery of a task and also includes the recognition gained from others. The highest level of needs on the hierarchy is *self-actualization,* which is the desire to become everything that one is capable of becoming. Individuals at this level are concerned with maximizing their potential.

An understanding of Maslow's hierarchy of needs provides you with a framework to meet patient needs and prioritize care for your patients. Realize that unless a patient's basic needs have been met, higher levels in the pyramid are not relevant and that patients of different generations approach life differently (Wieck, 2007). When using this model,

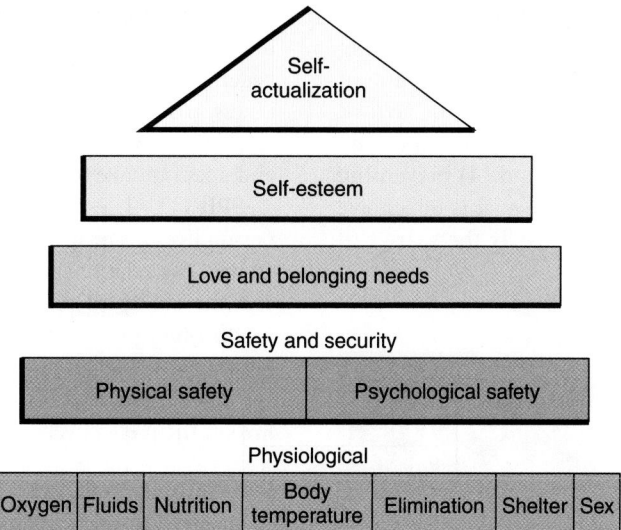

Figure 1-3 ▓ Maslow's hierarchy of needs. (From Maslow AH: *Motivation and personality*, ed 3, Upper Saddle River, NJ, 1987, Prentice Hall.)

you first ensure that basic needs of individuals are met. For example, Jack has a good relationship with his wife, but he is having trouble identifying ways to adjust his eating habits to fit a diabetic diet. Sally works with Jack and his wife to develop a realistic meal plan. The requirements to satisfy the needs of each level on the hierarch vary from person to person. Needs are greater or lesser for different persons. Therefore a thorough and individualized assessment of needs is an important aspect of patient care. For example, in caring for patients with psychological issues, such as depression or risk for suicide, safety and security needs are a priority. As a nurse, you want to provide the patient with physical and psychological safety.

In addition, wellness activities involving health promotion and illness prevention strategies help patients achieve and maintain an optimal level of health. Nurses identify actual and potential risk factors that predispose a person or a group to illness. People have different attitudes and reactions to illness. Medical sociologists call the reaction to illness *illness behavior*. When you understand how patients react to illness, you are able to minimize the effects of illness and assist patients and their families in maintaining or returning to the highest level of functioning.

Holistic Health Model

Health care is taking a more holistic view of health by considering emotional and spiritual well-being, as well as other dimensions of an individual, as important aspects of physical wellness. **Holistic health** is generally a comprehensive view of the person as a biopsychosocial and spiritual being (Edelman and Mandle, 2006). The intent of the holistic health model is to empower patients to engage in their own recovery, thereby assuming some responsibility for health maintenance (Edelman and Mandle, 2006).

The holistic health model incorporates a variety of techniques based on recognition that personal health choices have a powerful impact on an individual's health. Some of the most widely used holistic interventions include aromatherapy, biofeedback, breathing exercises, massage therapy, meditation, music therapy, relaxation therapy, therapeutic touch, and guided imagery (see Chapter 31). Most holistic therapies are easy to learn and apply to almost any nursing setting and to all stages of health and illness. For example, you use reminiscence to help relieve anxiety for an older patient dealing with memory loss or meditation with a patient dealing with the difficult side effects of chemotherapy. Surgical nurses use music therapy in the operating room to create a soothing environment. Relaxation therapy is useful in any setting to distract a patient during a painful procedure, such as a dressing change. You will help patients recognize the many options available and assist them in making choices to enhance health.

HEALTHY PEOPLE DOCUMENTS

Since the 1970s there has been a nationally focused initiative toward better health for the American people. *Healthy People* provides evidenced-based objectives to (1) achieve increased quality and years of healthy life and (2) eliminate health disparities. These objectives are updated every 10 years to meet a wide range of health needs, encourage collaboration in communities, help individuals make informed health decisions, and measure the impact of prevention activities. There are currently three influential documents that outline specific national goals for improving the physical health of Americans: *Healthy People: The Surgeon General's Report on Health Promotion and Disease Prevention* (U.S. Department of Health and Human Services [USDHHS], 1979); *Healthy People 2000: National Health Promotion and Disease Prevention Objectives* (USDHHS, 1990); and *Healthy People 2010: Understanding and Improving Health* (USDHHS, 2000). In January 2010, it is anticipated that the Healthy People 2020 objectives will be released along with guidance for achieving the new 10-year targets (USDHHS, 2008).

Healthy People 2010 includes 467 objectives written in 28 focus areas to provide direction for health care efforts on an individual, community, and national level. The document comprises four areas: (1) promoting healthy behaviors, (2) promoting healthy and safe communities, (3) improving systems for personal and public health, and (4) preventing and reducing diseases and disorders. The goal is to achieve or make improvements for each objective by the year 2010 (USDHHS, 2000).

VARIABLES INFLUENCING HEALTH BELIEFS AND HEALTH PRACTICES

Peoples' beliefs about their own health, as well as their health practices and the manner in which they care for themselves, will ultimately influence their health status. Health beliefs are a person's ideas and attitudes about health. These beliefs often directly influence health practices whether there is evidence to support them or not. Health practices are those activities that individuals perform to care for themselves. Health practices include activities of daily living such as bathing and brushing teeth and formal activities such as taking medications and visiting the health care provider for routine checkups. Today, health care focuses on the role of patients and their responsibility for self-care. The ability to care for oneself is as important for healthy living as managing a complex medical regimen for a chronic illness. Many variables influence patients' health beliefs, health practices, and self-care. Internal and external variables influence how a person thinks and acts and how a person will deal with an illness. Consider the impact of these variables, and be able to incorporate appropriate interventions based on the person's unique characteristics. Internal variables include a person's developmental stage, intellectual background, and emotional and spiritual factors. External variables include family practices, socioeconomic factors, and cultural background.

Internal Variables

DEVELOPMENTAL STAGE A person's concept of illness depends on the person's developmental stage (see Chapter 21). Knowledge of the stages of growth and development will help you predict your patient's response to an actual illness or the threat of future illness. Your educational interventions need to be age appropriate to be effective. For example, use different techniques to teach healthy diet choices to a child and to an adult.

INTELLECTUAL BACKGROUND A person's beliefs about health are shaped in part by knowledge (or misinformation) about body functions and illnesses, educational background, and past experiences. Cognitive abilities shape the *way* a person thinks, including the ability to understand factors involved in illness and to apply knowledge of health and illness to personal health practices.

EMOTIONAL FACTORS A person's degree of anxiety or stress influences health beliefs and practices. The manner in which a person handles stress throughout each phase of life influences the way the person reacts to illness. A person who generally is very calm often has little emotional response during illness, whereas a person normally unable to cope with stress either overreacts to illness or denies the presence of symptoms and does not take therapeutic action (see Chapter 24).

SPIRITUAL FACTORS Spirituality is reflected in how a person lives his or her life, including the values and beliefs exercised, the relationships established with family and friends, and the ability to find hope and meaning in life. Spiritual health often provides motivation during times of change in health status. Religious practices are one way people exercise spirituality. You need to understand patients' spiritual beliefs to involve them effectively in nursing care (see Chapter 20).

External Variables

FAMILY PRACTICES The way that families use health care services generally influences their health practices. Perceptions of the seriousness of diseases and history of preventive care behaviors (or lack of them) influence how patients think about health. For example, a person raised in a family that believed in the importance of preventive care, such as dental checkups twice a year, is more likely to continue those health practices as an adult.

SOCIOECONOMIC FACTORS Social and economic factors increase the risk for illness and influence the way in which a person defines and reacts to illness. Socioeconomic variables in part also determine how and where patients access medical care and receive treatment as well as how they pay for their health care and the potential reimbursement to the health care agency or patient. Economic variables affect a patient's level of health by increasing the risk for disease and influencing how or at what point the patient enters the health care system. In addition, economic status also affects a person's participation in treatment to maintain or improve health. A person who has high utility bills, a large family, and a low income tends to give a higher priority to food and shelter than to costly drugs or treatment or expensive foods for special diets.

CULTURAL BACKGROUND Cultural background influences a person's beliefs, values, and customs. It influences the approach to the health care system, personal health practices, and the nurse-patient relationship. You need to recognize and understand cultural patterns of behavior and beliefs to effectively interact with the patient (see Chapter 19).

HEALTH PROMOTION, WELLNESS, AND ILLNESS PREVENTION

Health promotion activities are either passive or active. With **passive strategies of health promotion,** individuals gain from the activities of others without acting themselves. For example, the city puts fluoride in the municipal drinking water or milk manufacturers fortify homogenized milk with vitamin D. These are passive health promotion strategies.

With **active strategies of health promotion,** individuals adopt specific health programs. Weight reduction and smoking cessation programs require patients to be actively involved in measures to improve their present and future levels of wellness while decreasing the risk for disease.

You need to emphasize health promotion, wellness strategies, and illness prevention activities as important forms of health care because they help patients maintain and improve health. **Health promotion** activities, such as routine exercise and good nutrition, help patients maintain or enhance their present levels of health and reduce their risks for developing certain diseases. **Wellness education** teaches people how to care for themselves in a healthy way and includes topics such as physical awareness, stress management, and self-responsibility (Box 1-1). **Illness prevention** activities, such as immunization programs, protect patients from actual or potential threats to health. The concepts of health promotion, wellness, and illness prevention are closely related and in practice overlap to some extent. All are focused on the future; the differences between them involve motivations and goals. Health promotion activities motivate people to act positively to reach more stable levels of health. Wellness strategies help patients achieve new understanding and control of their lives. Illness prevention activities motivate people to avoid declines in health or functional levels.

Illnesses, particularly chronic illnesses, often increase the cost of health care. Therefore health care has become increasingly focused on health promotion, wellness, and illness prevention. The rapid rise of health care costs has motivated people to seek ways of decreasing the incidence and minimizing the results of illness or disability. Improving self-management, preventive services, and curative services reduces health care needs and costs. You have an important role in educating patients about improving their ability to manage their health. You do this by helping them recognize their responsibility in the health-related choices they make and by helping them understand the effect their choices have on disease prevention. In the case study of Jack and the diabetes educator Sally, there is an obvious need for greater education for Jack. Sally teaches him the importance of diet and exercise to manage his diabetes and prevent long-term complications. Health promotion, wellness activities, and illness prevention are all strategies aimed at decreasing the incidence of illness and minimizing the negative results of that illness or disability.

The Three Levels of Prevention

Nursing care directed at health promotion, wellness, and illness prevention can be understood in terms of health activities on primary, secondary, and tertiary levels (Table 1-1).

Primary prevention is true prevention. It precedes disease or dysfunction and applies to patients considered physically and emotionally healthy. The purpose of primary prevention is to decrease the vulnerability of the individual or population to an illness or dysfunction (Edelman and Mandle, 2006). Primary prevention includes passive and active strategies of health promotion. You provide it to an individual or to a general population, or you focus on individuals at risk for developing specific diseases. Primary prevention aimed at health promotion includes health education programs, immunizations, and physical and nutritional fitness activites. In the case study of Jack, primary prevention means simply wearing shoes at all times because Jack has diabetes and is at risk for infection and alterations in perception of pain in his extremities. These problems increase Jack's risks for experiencing skin breakdown in his feet and altered wound healing. Therefore Jack needs to make additional efforts to prevent injury to his feet.

Secondary prevention focuses on people who are experiencing health problems or illnesses and who are at risk for developing complications or worsening conditions. You direct activities at diagnosis and prompt intervention, thereby reducing severity and enabling the patient to return to a normal level of health as early as possible (Edelman and Mandle,

---

BOX 1-1 PATIENT TEACHING

Encouraging Exercise

 Because Jack occasionally exercises, Sally decides to focus her teaching on the importance of routine exercise to improve Jack's health and help with the management of his diabetes. Sally finds out that 6 months ago Jack was using his treadmill for 20 minutes on most mornings. Since then, he has gotten out of the habit because he now tries to arrive at work 30 minutes earlier.

OUTCOME
- By the end of the visit, Jack will verbalize two reasons it is helpful for him to stay physically active and one new strategy for exercise he is willing to try.

TEACHING STRATEGIES
- Practice active listening and determine what Jack understands regarding health risks related to poor lifestyle (Vanderhoff, 2005).
- Ask Jack what barriers and benefits he perceives with the planned lifestyle change of consistently exercising (Vanderhoff, 2005).
- Help Jack set achievable goals for change.
- Work with Jack to establish realistic time lines for modification of exercise lifestyle habits.
- Reinforce the process of change with Jack.
- Use written resources at an appropriate reading level (Vanderhoff, 2005).
- Include Jack's wife to support the lifestyle change.
- Identify community resources available to Jack (e.g., walking track, fitness facilities, etc.).

EVALUATION STRATEGIES
- Have Jack maintain an exercise log to track adherence and provide positive reinforcement, and evaluate log at the next visit.
- Ask Jack to discuss his success with lifestyle changes, such as minutes spent in activity.
- Have Jack identify community resources used in making change.

TABLE 1-1   The Three Levels of Prevention

PRIMARY PREVENTION		SECONDARY PREVENTION		TERTIARY PREVENTION
HEALTH PROMOTION	**SPECIFIC PROTECTION**	**EARLY DIAGNOSIS AND PROMPT TREATMENT**	**DISABILITY LIMITATIONS**	**RESTORATION AND REHABILITATION**
• Health education • Good standard of nutrition adjusted to developmental phases of life • Attention to personality development • Provision of adequate housing and recreation and agreeable working conditions • Marriage counseling and sex education • Genetic screening • Periodic selective examinations	• Use of specific immunizations • Attention to personal hygiene • Use of environmental sanitation • Protection against occupational hazards • Protection from accidents • Use of specific nutrients • Protection from carcinogens • Avoidance of allergens	• Case-finding measures: individual and mass screening surveys • Selective examinations • Cure and prevention of disease process to prevent spread of communicable disease, prevent complications, and shorten period of disability	• Adequate treatment to arrest disease process and prevent further complications • Provision of facilities to limit disability and prevent death	• Provision of hospital and community facilities for training and education to maximize use of remaining capacities • Education of the public and industries to use rehabilitated persons to the fullest possible extent • Selective placement • Work therapy in hospitals

Modified from Leavell HR, Clark AE: *Preventive medicine for doctors in the community,* ed 3, New York, 1965, McGraw-Hill.

2006). A large portion of secondary level nursing care is in homes, hospitals, or skilled nursing facilities. It includes screening techniques and treating early stages of disease to limit disability by delaying the consequences of advanced disease. Screening activities also become a key opportunity for health teaching as a primary prevention intervention (Edelman and Mandle, 2006).

Tertiary prevention occurs when a defect or disability is permanent, irreversible, and stabilized. It involves minimizing the effects of long-term disease or disability by interventions directed at preventing complications and deterioration (Edelman and Mandle, 2006). Activities are for rehabilitation rather than diagnosis and treatment. Care at this level helps patients achieve as high a level of functioning as possible, despite the limitations caused by illness or impairment. This level of care is called *preventive care* because it involves preventing further disability or reduced functioning. Tertiary prevention for Jack includes continual monitoring and management of blood glucose levels and control of his diabetes. Tight control of blood glucose levels prevents further complications of his diabetes, such as coronary artery disease.

RISK FACTORS

A **risk factor** is any situation, habit, environmental condition, physiological condition, or other variable that increases the vulnerability of an individual or a group to an illness or accident. The presence of risk factors does not mean that a

disease will develop, but risk factors increase the chances that the individual will experience a particular disease. Risk factors play a major role in how you identify a patient's health status. Risk factors also influence health beliefs and practices if a person is aware of their presence. Risk factors are in the following interrelated categories: genetic and physiological factors, age, physical environment, and lifestyle.

Genetic and Physiological Factors

Physiological risk factors involve the physical functioning of the body. For example, physical conditions such as pregnancy or obesity place increased stress on physiological systems (e.g., the circulatory system), increasing susceptibility to illness.. Heredity or genetic predisposition to specific illness is a major physical risk factor. In the case study, Jack has a family history of diabetes mellitus and therefore was at risk for developing the disease. Other examples of genetic risk factors include family histories of cancer, heart disease, and kidney disease.

Age

Age increases susceptibility to certain illnesses. The risks for birth defects and complications of pregnancy increase in women bearing children after age 35. Many kinds of cancer pose a greater risk for persons over age 45 than for younger persons. The risk for heart disease increases with age for both genders. Box 1-2 discusses the importance of health promotion in older adults. Age risk factors are often closely associated with other risk factors, such as family history and personal

BOX 1-2 CARE OF THE OLDER ADULT
Importance of Health Promotion

- Because individuals are living longer, health promotion activities are important to help maintain function and independence and improve quality of life.
- Focusing on self-care abilities and practices that foster health while aging are important nursing interventions (Pender and others, 2006).
- Emphasize the social value of encouraging older adults to participate in group activities (Runciman and others, 2006).
- Monitor older patients, especially those 75 years of age and older, for high blood pressure, obesity, and diabetes (Mokdad and others, 2004b).

- Physical activity extends years of active independent life, reduces disability, and improves the quality of life for older persons (Chodzko-Zajko, 2006).
- Promote self-care activities that maintain and improve functional status, including safe mobility and prevention of falls (Pender and others, 2006).
- Health care interventions often do not correspond with the patient's readiness to change. Use the stages of behavior change model (see Table 1-3, p. 11) to identify older adults who are open to participating in health promotion activities. The easiest way to determine the patient's readiness to change is to ask the patient which stage of change best describes him or her (Reicherter and Greene, 2005).

habits. You need to educate patients about the importance of regularly scheduled checkups for their age-group. The Agency for Healthcare Research and Quality, through the U.S. Preventive Services Task Force, has developed guidelines for screening, counseling, and immunizations by age and gender. You can access scientific evidence, recommendations on clinical prevention services, and information on how to implement recommended preventative services into practice at http://www.ahrq.gov/clinic/prevenix.htm.

Physical Environment

The physical environment in which a person works or lives increases the likelihood that certain illnesses will occur. A person's home environment often includes conditions that pose risks, such as unclean, poorly heated or cooled, or overcrowded dwellings. These conditions often increase the likelihood that a person will contract and spread infections and other diseases. Also, some kinds of cancer and other diseases are more likely to develop when industrial workers are exposed to certain chemicals or when people live near toxic waste disposal sites. Screening for these environmentally based risk factors is directed at the short-term effects of the exposure and the potential for long-term effects (Edelman and Mandle, 2006).

Lifestyle

Lifestyle practices and behaviors have positive or negative effects on health. Practices with potential negative effects are risk factors. Examples of risk factors include overeating or poor nutrition, insufficient rest and sleep, and poor personal hygiene. Other habits that put a person at risk for illness include tobacco use, alcohol or drug abuse, and activities involving a threat of injury such as skydiving or mountain climbing. Some habits are risk factors for specific diseases. For example, excessive sunbathing increases the risk for skin cancer, and being overweight increases the risk for cardiovascular disease. Mokdad and others (2004a) identified modifiable behavioral risk factors that are leading causes of mortality in the United States (Table 1-2). Their analysis showed that although smoking remains the leading cause of mortal-

TABLE 1-2	Actual Causes of Death in the United States in 1990 and 2000	
ACTUAL CAUSE	NO. (%) IN 1990*	NO. (%) IN 2000†
Tobacco	400,000 (19)	435,000 (18.1)
Poor diet and physical inactivity	300,000 (14)	400,000 (16.6)
Alcohol consumption	100,000 (5)	85,000 (3.6)
Microbial agents	90,000 (4)	75,000 (3.1)
Toxic agents	60,000 (3)	55,000 (2.3)
Motor vehicle	25,000 (1)	43,000 (1.8)
Firearms	35,000 (2)	29,000 (1.2)
Sexual behavior	30,000 (1)	20,000 (0.8)
Illicit drug use	20,000 (<1)	17,000 (0.7)
Total	**1,060,000 (50)**	**1,159,000 (48.2)**

*Data from McGinnis JM, Foege WH: Actual causes of death in the United States, *JAMA* 270:2207, 1993.
The percentages are for all deaths.
†From Mokdad AH and others: Actual causes of death in the United States, 2000, *JAMA* 291(10):1238, 2004.

ity, poor diet and physical inactivity will soon be the leading cause of death. These data reflect the importance of a need for emphasis on preventive care and show the economic effect lifestyle choices have on our health care system.

The effect of lifestyle behavior on the risk for developing disease has implications across the life span of a person. Understand that patients of all ages are vulnerable to the influences of unhealthy lifestyle patterns. You are able to influence the choices your patients make by preventing unhealthy behaviors and promoting healthy lifestyle patterns. Parents, caretakers, school nurses, and teachers all influence the lifestyle practices of young children. Many adolescents encounter issues of seat belt use, gun possession, alcohol and drug use, and sexual promiscuity. Therefore you need to understand the relation-

BOX 1-3   BEST PRACTICES

Nursing Interventions for Smoking Cessation

SUMMARY OF EVIDENCE

People who smoke greatly increase their risk for many health problems, but smoking cessation is difficult. Because nurses spend a great amount of time with patients, nurses are in an ideal position to advise their patients to improve their health by stopping smoking. A systematic review of the research regarding nursing interventions for smoking cessation suggests that smoking cessation interventions by nurses are effective, especially if they are not too brief. The interventions are most effective when provided by a nurse whose main role is health promotion or smoking cessation. An opportunity also exists for helping patients in the hospital develop a plan to stop smoking. The efficacy of smoking cessation interventions for hospitalized patients are most effective when patients receive support for at least 1 month after discharge.

APPLICATION TO NURSING PRACTICE

- Determine if your patients smoke during your initial assessment.
- Identify specific ways that smoking negatively affects your patients' health (disease, financial, cosmetic, etc.).
- Collaborate with your patients on a plan to begin to quit smoking.
- Use a health promotion theory such as the stages of behavior change whenever possible.
- Provide ongoing support to your patients for success with smoking cessation through follow-up phone calls, office visits, support groups, and mailed information.
- Monitor success/failure rates to continually improve your approach to smoking cessation.

REFERENCE

Rice VH, Stead LF: Nursing interventions for smoking cessation, *Cochrane Database Syst Rev* 2008(1):CD001188, DOI: 10.1002/14651858. CD001188.pub3.

ship between growth and development and lifestyle behaviors and your patients' health status. Use evidence-based interventions when teaching your patients and the public about wellness-promoting lifestyle behaviors (Box 1-3).

Risk Factor Identification

The goal of risk factor identification is to help patients understand those areas in their lives that they need to modify or even eliminate to promote wellness and prevent illness. You will perform comprehensive health risk appraisals, using a variety of available health risk appraisal forms, to estimate a person's specific health threats based on the presence of various risk factors (Edelman and Mandle, 2006). You need to link findings from a health risk appraisal with educational programs and other community resources available to patients to provide a way for them to make necessary lifestyle changes and risk reduction. You will often find risk factors documented in the patient's medical record. Risk factors are often linked to the patient's age. For example, when caring for adolescents, evaluate parenting practices, schools, neighborhoods, and the community in general to identify at-risk youth (Riesch, Anderson, and Krueger, 2006).

RISK FACTOR MODIFICATION AND CHANGING HEALTH BEHAVIORS

Identifying risk factors is the first step in health promotion, wellness education, and illness prevention activities. Once you identify risk factors, implement health education programs that help a person to change a risky health behavior. This is called *risk factor modification*. Risk factor modifica-

tion, health promotion, or any program that attempts to change unhealthy lifestyle behaviors is a wellness strategy because it teaches patients to care for themselves in healthier ways. You need to emphasize wellness strategies because they have the ability to decrease the potential high costs of unmanaged health problems.

Aim your attempts to change a patient's behavior at stopping a health-damaging behavior (e.g., tobacco use or alcohol misuse) or adopting a healthy behavior (e.g., healthy diet or exercise) (Pender and others, 2006). Changing health behavior is difficult, especially those behaviors that have become habits in people's lifestyle. Many times, adopting healthy behaviors and reducing risk factors require your patients to change. As a nurse, you will be challenged to motivate and facilitate health behavior change in working with individuals, families, and communities (Edleman and Mandle, 2006).

An understanding of the process of change helps you support difficult health behavior change in your patients. Current research shows that change involves movement through a series of five stages of behavior change (Table 1-3), ranging from precontemplation, when a person has no intention to change, to the maintenance stage, when a person maintains a changed behavior (Norcross and Prochaska, 2002). Most people acting on their own do not successfully get through all the stages on their first attempt (Norcross and Prochaska, 2002). As an individual attempts to change behavior, relapse and recycling through the stages occurs frequently. When relapse occurs, the person will return to the contemplation or precontemplation stage before attempting change again. Relapse often feels like a failure, but the person needs to view it as a learning process. What the person learns from relapse can be applied to the next attempt to change. You need to be able to identify your patient's stage of change to implement appropriate care (Box 1-4). Health promotion

TABLE 1-3 Stages of Behavior Change

STAGE	DEFINITION
Precontemplation	Does not intend to make changes within the next 6 months. Patient is unaware of the problem or underestimates it. "There is nothing that I really need to change."
Contemplation	Considering a change within the next 6 months. Patient says he or she is seriously considering a change. "I have a problem, and I really think I need to work on it."
Preparation	Has tried to make changes, but without success. Intends to take action in the next month. "I started to exercise regularly, but it didn't last long. I will probably try again in a few weeks."
Action	Actively engaged in strategies to change behavior. This stage sometimes lasts up to 6 months. This stage requires commitment of time and energy. "I am really working hard to stop smoking."
Maintenance	Sustained change over time. This stage begins 6 months after action has started and continues indefinitely. Important to avoid relapse. "I need to avoid people who smoke so I am not tempted to start smoking again."

BOX 1-4 Application of the Stages of Behavior Change Model

 Sally wants to apply the stages of behavior change with Jack. By using this model, Sally will work with Jack regarding what he is ready to do rather than simply telling Jack to be more active. To do this, she first asks Jack how he feels about exercise and what his plans are. When asked this, Jack states, "I know that exercise would be good for me and I should probably work on it." This tells Sally that Jack is in the contemplation stage. She targets her teaching to helping Jack see the benefits of exercise, how it could fit into his schedule, and what kinds of things he likes to do. She asks Jack to bring a list of benefits of exercise for him and three or four options for exercise to their next appointment. With this process, she hopes to move Jack into the preparation stage of behavior change for exercise at their next visit.

interventions have a greater effect if you time them appropriately to match the patient's specific stage of change. For example, you will not be effective if you teach your patient who is in the contemplation stage and does not routinely eat fruits and vegetables to eat five fruits and vegetables a day. It is better to get your patient thinking about the benefits of fruits and vegetables to encourage moving into the preparation stage.

The health care industry needs to do further work to design interventions and wellness strategies for people in all stages of behavior change. For example, patients are sometimes motivated to adopt needed health behaviors when health care professionals advise that a change in diet and an increase in exercise will prevent further problems. A patient can maintain changes over time only if you integrate the health behavior changes into the patient's overall lifestyle. In addition, understand that true change comes from the pa-

tient's desire to change. Maintenance of healthy lifestyles prevents hospitalizations and potentially lowers the cost of health care. Your advice and support may help patients adapt to a changed and healthier lifestyle.

ILLNESS

Illness is a state in which a person's physical, emotional, intellectual, social, developmental, or spiritual functioning is diminished or impaired compared with previous experience. Cancer is a disease process, but some patients with leukemia who are responding to treatment continue to function as usual. Some patients with breast cancer feel well physically but experience spiritual distress. Of interest, many patients find health within illness. An experience with illness sometimes motivates an individual to adopt more positive health behaviors.

Illness therefore is not synonymous with disease. Although you need to be familiar with different kinds of diseases and their treatments, be concerned more with illness, which includes not only the disease but also the effects on functioning and well-being in all dimensions.

Acute and Chronic Illness

Acute and chronic illness are two general classifications of illness used in this chapter. Both types of illness affect functioning in many dimensions. An **acute illness** is usually short term and severe. The symptoms appear abruptly, are intense, and often subside after a relatively short period. A **chronic illness** usually lasts longer than 6 months. Patients fluctuate between maximal functioning and serious health relapses that are sometimes life threatening.

Because of successes in public health, medicine, and biomedical technology, acute and infectious diseases are no longer major causes of death, disease, and disability in the United States. Many health care analysts believe that the heaviest burden of illness today is due to chronic diseases that are largely preventable. Beyond the prevention of these diseases, a major role for you as a nurse is to provide patient education that helps patients manage their illnesses or disabilities to reduce the occurrence of symptoms and improve the tolerance of symptoms (tertiary prevention). This education enhances wellness and improves quality of life for patients living with chronic illnesses or disabilities. Use a holistic approach when helping patients who have chronic illnesses better manage their care (Kralik, Koch, and Price, 2004). Self-management involves learning about responses to illnesses through daily life experiences and also as a result of trial and error. Taking responsibility for living well with illness strengthens patients. Therefore encourage patients to question the direction of their health care and to make choices about their health care. The process of learning self-management skills is crucial to the transition of learning to live with a chronic illness. The management of chronic illnesses promotes health within illness and also addresses human comfort and quality of life. You as a nurse are able to reduce the impact of chronic illness on the individual, as well as on society, by providing quality, comprehensive, patient-centered care to patients living with chronic illness (Cumbie, Conley, and Burman, 2004).

ILLNESS BEHAVIOR

People who are ill generally adopt **illness behaviors.** These behaviors affect how people monitor their bodies, define and interpret their symptoms, take remedial actions, and use the health care system (Mechanic, 1982). Personal history, social situations, social norms, and the opportunities and limits of community institutions all affect illness behaviors (Mechanic, 1995). Although there is a large variability in the way people react to an illness, patients often use illness behavior displayed in sickness to manage life's difficulties (Mechanic, 1995). If people perceive themselves to be ill, illness behaviors act as coping mechanisms. Illness behavior often results in patients being released from roles, social expectations, or responsibilities. For example, a young mother who is receiving chemotherapy for treatment of breast cancer is very tired and not expected to cook for her family every day. Instead, the members of her church bring her family cooked meals, giving the mother more time to rest, heal, and be with her family.

Variables Influencing Illness Behavior

Just as internal and external variables affect health behavior, they affect illness behavior as well. The influences of these variables affect the likelihood of seeking health care and the participation in therapy, which ultimately affect health outcomes. Based on an understanding of these variables and behaviors, you individualize care to assist patients in coping with their illnesses at various stages. The goal of nursing is to promote optimal functioning in all dimensions throughout an illness.

INTERNAL VARIABLES Internal variables influence the way patients behave when they are ill. These are the patient's

perceptions of symptoms and the nature of the illness. If patients believe that the symptoms of their illnesses disrupt their normal routine, they are more likely to seek health care assistance than if they do not perceive the symptoms as disruptive. If patients believe that the symptoms are serious or perhaps life threatening, they are also more likely to seek assistance. Persons awakened by crushing chest pains in the middle of the night generally view this symptom as potentially serious and life threatening and will probably be motivated to seek assistance. However, sometimes such a perception also has the opposite effect. Some patients fear serious illness and react by denying it and not seeking medical assistance.

The nature of the illness, either acute or chronic, also affects a patient's illness behavior. Patients with acute illnesses are likely to seek health care and adhere readily with therapy. On the other hand, a patient with a chronic illness, in which the symptoms are not curable but only partially relieved, is sometimes not motivated to adhere with the therapy plan. Patients with chronic illnesses sometimes become less actively involved in their care, experience greater frustration, and adhere less readily with care. You will generally spend more time than other health care professionals with patients who have chronic illnesses. You are in the unique position of being able to assist these patients in overcoming problems related to illness behavior.

EXTERNAL VARIABLES External variables influencing a patient's illness behavior include the visibility of symptoms, social group, cultural background, economic variables, accessibility of the health care system, and social support. The visibility of the symptoms of an illness affects body image and illness behavior. A patient with a visible symptom is more likely to seek assistance than a patient who does not have visible symptoms.

Patients' social groups assist them in recognizing the threat of illness or support the denial of potential illness. Families, friends, and co-workers all influence patients' illness behavior. Patients often react positively to social support while practicing positive health behaviors. Cultural and ethnic background teaches a person how to be healthy, how to recognize illness, and how to be ill. The effects of disease and its interpretation vary according to cultural circumstances.

Economic variables influence the way a patient reacts to illness. Because of economic constraints, a patient will delay treatment and in many cases continue to carry out daily activities. Patients' access to the health care system is closely related to economic factors. The health care system is a socioeconomic system that patients enter, interact within, and exit. For many patients, entry into the system is complex or confusing, and some patients seek nonemergency medical care in an emergency department because they do not know how to obtain health services otherwise. The physical proximity of patients to a health care agency often influences how soon they enter the system after deciding to seek care.

IMPACT OF ILLNESS ON PATIENT AND FAMILY

An illness of a family member affects the function of the entire family unit. The patient and family commonly experience behavioral and emotional changes and changes in body image, self-concept, family roles, and family dynamics.

Behavioral and Emotional Changes

Individual behavioral and emotional reactions depend on the nature of the illness, the patient's attitude toward it, the reaction of others to it, and the variables of illness behavior. Short-term, non–life-threatening illnesses evoke few behavioral changes in the functioning of the patient or family. A husband and father who has a cold, for example, lacks the energy and patience to spend time in family activities and is irritable and prefers not to interact with his family. This is a behavioral change, but the change is subtle and does not last long. Some even consider such a change a normal response to illness.

Severe illness, particularly one that is life threatening, leads to more extensive emotional and behavioral changes, such as anxiety, shock, denial, anger, and withdrawal. These are common responses to the stress of illness. You develop interventions to assist the patient and the family in coping with and adapting to this stress, because the stressor itself cannot usually be changed.

Impact on Body Image

Body image is the subjective concept of physical appearance. Our perception of body image changes as we grow and develop (see Chapter 22). Some illnesses result in changes in physical appearance, and patients and families react differently to these changes. These reactions of patients and families to changes in body image depend on the type of changes (e.g., the loss of a limb or an organ), the adaptive capacity of the family, the rate at which changes take place, and the support services available.

When a change in body image occurs, such as results from a leg amputation, the patient generally adjusts by experiencing phases of the grief process (see Chapter 25). Initially the change or impending change shocks the patient. As the patient and family recognize the reality of the change, they become anxious and sometimes withdraw. As the patient and family acknowledge the change, they gradually move toward accepting their loss. At the end of the acknowledgment phase, they accept the loss. During rehabilitation the patient is ready to learn how to adapt to the change in body image.

Impact on Self-Concept

Self-concept is your mental self-image of all aspects of your personality. Self-concept depends in part on body image and roles but also includes other aspects of psychology and spirituality. Self-concept is important in relationships with other family members. A patient whose self-concept changes because of illness is sometimes no longer able to meet family expectations, leading to tension or conflict. As a result, family members change their interactions with the patient. In the course of providing care, you are able to observe changes in the patient's self-concept (or in the self-concepts of family members) and develop a care plan to help the patient adjust to the changes resulting from the illness (see Chapter 22).

Impact on Family Roles and Family Dynamics

People have many roles in life, such as wage earner, decision maker, professional, and parent. When an illness occurs, the roles of the patient and family change (see Chapter 23). Such a change is either subtle and short term or drastic and long term. Patients and their families generally adjust more easily to subtle, short-term changes. Long-term changes, however, require an adjustment process similar to the grief process (see Chapter 25). The patient and family often require specific counseling and guidance to assist them in coping with the role changes.

Family dynamics is the process by which the family functions, makes decisions, gives support to individual members, and copes with everyday changes and challenges. Because of the effects of illness, family dynamics often change. Role functions stop or are delayed. Another family member sometimes needs to assume the patient's usual roles and responsibilities. This often creates tension or anxiety in the family. Role reversal is also common. If a parent of an adult becomes ill and is unable to carry out usual activities, the adult child often assumes many of the parent's responsibilities. Such a reversal leads to conflicting responsibilities for the adult child or direct conflict over decision making. You will view the whole family and plan care to help the family regain the maximal level of functioning and well-being (see Chapter 23).

KEY POINTS

- Health and wellness are not merely the absence of disease and illness. Many variables determine the health status of an individual or community. A person's state of health, wellness, or illness depends on individual values, personality, and lifestyle.
- Unsatisfied needs motivate human beings. Basic human needs must be met before an individual is able to focus on higher-level needs.

- The health promotion model focuses on behaviors motivated by the desire to increase well-being and actualize human potential.
- Holistic health models of nursing promote optimal health by incorporating active participation of the patient in improving the health state. Holistic nursing interventions complement standard medical therapy.

- Internal and external variables influence health beliefs and practices, and you consider these when planning care.
- Health promotion activities maintain or enhance health. Wellness education teaches patients how to care for themselves. Illness prevention activities protect against health threats and thus maintain an optimal level of health.
- Nursing incorporates health promotion, wellness, and illness prevention activities rather than simply treating illness.
- The three levels of prevention are primary, secondary, and tertiary.

- Risk factors threaten health, influence health practices, and are important considerations in illness prevention activities. Risk factors involve genetic or physiological variables, age, physical environment, and lifestyle.
- Improvement in health often requires a change in health behaviors.
- Illness behavior influences how patients use the health care system.
- Illness has many effects on the patient and family, including changes in behavior and emotions, family roles and dynamics, body image, and self-concept.

CRITICAL THINKING EXERCISES

Jack and his wife have another appointment with Sally. In preparation for the visit, Sally reviews Jack's medical record.

1. **a.** Based on what you know about Jack throughout this chapter, identify risk factors that increase Jack's susceptibility to problems with his diabetes and other diseases. What questions would you ask Jack to determine all of his risk factors?
   b. Using the health belief model, identify two individual health perceptions that may be influencing Jack.
2. What is the impact of Jack's disease on his wife?

3. As Sally begins the appointment, Jack says, "I saw there was a sale on walking shoes. If I'm going to start walking, do you think I need to get new shoes? Next week I am taking a week of vacation, just doing things around the house, and I thought this would be a good time to start."
   a. Using the stages of behavior change model, which stage best describes Jack's desire to change?
   b. What goals could Sally help Jack set during this visit?

ⓔvolve *Answers to Critical Thinking Questions can be found on the Evolve website.*

REVIEW QUESTIONS

1. You are caring for a patient on an inpatient psychiatric unit. He was admitted after a severe anxiety attack. He tells you he feels very out of control and does not know how to deal with these feelings. According to Maslow's hierarchy of needs, with which level of needs are you most concerned?
   1. Physiological
   2. Safety and security
   3. Love and belonging
   4. Self-actualization
2. The nurse is working with a 16-year-old in the management of type 1 diabetes. While going through the educational process, the nurse keeps in mind that this adolescent is beginning to assert his independence and allows him to make decisions when possible. Which internal variable is the nurse recognizing?
   1. Developmental stage
   2. Intellectual background
   3. Emotional factors
   4. Spiritual factors
3. Your patient tries to walk for 30 minutes on most days of the week and includes fruits and vegetables with her meals. This is an example of:
   1. Illness prevention activities
   2. Wellness education
   3. Health promotion activities
   4. Illness behavior

4. A patient has decided to eat five fruits and vegetables a day and is exercising at least 3 days a week. What level of prevention is this patient practicing?
   1. Primary prevention
   2. Secondary prevention
   3. Tertiary prevention
   4. Rehabilitation prevention
5. A hospital has an influenza immunization program in which all employees are encouraged to get a yearly influenza shot. This is an example of:
   1. Primary prevention
   2. Secondary prevention
   3. Tertiary prevention
   4. Rehabilitation
6. Your patient realizes he is at risk for type 2 diabetes because his mother and brother have diabetes. Which type of risk factor is this?
   1. Genetic
   2. Age
   3. Physical environment
   4. Lifestyle
7. A 28-year-old male patient travels frequently with his job. He often eats meals high in fat, gets very little exercise, and smokes 1 pack of cigarettes a day. What type of risk factors for heart disease is he experiencing?
   1. Genetic
   2. Age
   3. Physical environment
   4. Lifestyle

8. Your patient smokes 1 to 2 packs of cigarettes per day. He says to you, "I know smoking isn't good for me. I think I am ready to think about quitting." According to the stages of behavior change model, which stage of change is your patient in?
   1. Precontemplation
   2. Contemplation
   3. Preparation
   4. Action

9. You have been working with a patient on a smoking cessation plan for the past 3 months. At your next visit, the patient states, "Even though I've tried and haven't been able to quit smoking in the past, I want to try again. My thirtieth birthday is in 2 weeks, and that is when I'm going to quit." According to the stages of behavior change model, which stage of change is your patient in now?
   1. Precontemplation
   2. Contemplation
   3. Preparation
   4. Action

10. A female patient says to her nurse, "Why should I exercise? We're all going to die of something anyway. I'm too busy for exercise." According to the stages of behavior change model, the nurse's best response is:
    1. "I want you to start walking 30 minutes a day every day of the week."
    2. "It is hard to find time. What things are important to you now? What do you want to make sure you can do 5 years from now? Are there any activities you enjoy doing?"
    3. "That's too bad you are so busy. Maybe you'll have more time in the future."
    4. "That's fine. Exercise isn't that important anyway."

Answers to Review Questions can be found on pages 1197-1198.

REFERENCES

Agency for Healthcare Research and Quality: *Preventive services*, http://www.ahrq.gov/clinic/prevenix.htm, accessed December 29, 2008.

Becker MH, Maiman LA: Sociobehavioral determinants of compliance with health and medical care recommendations, *Med Care* 13(1):10, 1975.

Chodzko-Zajko W: *National blueprint: increasing physical activity among aged 50 and older*, American College of Sports Medicine-Active Aging Partnership, http://www.agingblueprint.org/overview.cfm, accessed July 28, 2006.

Cumbie SA, Conley VM, Burman ME: Advanced practice nursing models for comprehensive care with chronic illness: model for promoting process engagement, *Adv Nurs Sci* 27(1):70, 2004.

Edelman CL, Mandle CL: *Health promotion throughout the life span*, ed 6, St. Louis, 2006, Mosby.

Kralik D, Koch T, Price K: Chronic illness self-management: taking care to create order, *J Clin Nurs* 13(2):259, 2004.

Leavell HR, Clark AE: *Preventive medicine for doctors in the community*, ed 3, New York, 1965, McGraw-Hill.

Maslow AH: *Motivation and personality*, New York, 1954, Harper & Row.

Maslow AH: *Motivation and personality*, ed 2, New York, 1970, Harper & Row.

Maslow AH: *Motivation and personality*, ed 3, Upper Saddle River, NJ, 1987, Prentice Hall.

Mechanic D: The epidemiology of illness behavior and its relationship to physical and psychological distress. In Mechanic D: *Symptoms, illness behavior, and help seeking*, New York, 1982, Prodist.

Mechanic D: Sociological dimensions of illness behavior, *Soc Sci Med* 41(9):1207, 1995.

Mokdad AH and others: Actual causes of death in the United States, 2000, *JAMA* 291(10):1238, 2004a.

Mokdad AH and others: Changes in health behaviors among older Americans, 1990-2000, *Public Health Rep* 119:356, 2004b.

Norcross JC, Prochaska JO: Using the stages of change, *Harv Ment Health Lett* 18(11):5, 2002.

Pender NJ: *Health promotion and nursing practice*, Norwalk, Conn, 1982, Appleton-Century-Crofts.

Pender NJ: Health promotion and illness prevention. In Werley HH, Fitzpatrick JJ, editors: *Annual review of nursing research*, New York, 1993, Springer.

Pender NJ: *Health promotion in nursing practice*, ed 3, Stamford, Conn, 1996, Appleton & Lange.

Pender NJ, Murdaugh CL, Parsons MA: *Health promotion in nursing practice*, ed 4, Upper Saddle River, NJ, 2002, Prentice Hall.

Pender NJ, Murdaugh CL, Parsons MA: *Health promotion in nursing practice*, ed 5, Upper Saddle River, NJ, 2006, Prentice Hall.

Reicherter E, Greene R: Wellness and health promotion: educational applications for older adults in the community, *Top Geriatr Rehabil* 21(4):295, 2005.

Rice VH, Stead LF: Nursing interventions for smoking cessation, *Cochrane Database Syst Rev* 2008(1):CD001188, DOI: 10.1002/14651858.CD001188.pub3.

Riesch SK, Anderson LS, Krueger HA: Parent–child communication processes: preventing children's health-risk behavior, *J Spec Pediatr Nurs* 11(1):41, 2006.

Rosenstoch I: Historical origin of the health belief model, *Health Educ Monogr* 2:334, 1974.

Runciman P and others: Community nurses' health promotion work with older people, *J Adv Nurs* 55(1):46, 2006.

U.S. Department of Health and Human Services: *Developing healthy people 2020*, 2008, http://www.healthypeople.gov/hp2020/, accessed July 25, 2008.

U.S. Department of Health and Human Services, Public Health Service: *Healthy people: the Surgeon General's report on health promotion and disease prevention*, Washington, DC, 1979, U.S. Government Printing Office.

U.S. Department of Health and Human Services, Public Health Service: *Healthy people 2000: national health promotion and disease prevention objectives*, Washington, DC, 1990, U.S. Government Printing Office.

U.S. Department of Health and Human Services, Public Health Service: *Healthy people 2010: understanding and improving health*, Washington, DC, 2000, U.S. Government Printing Office.

van Maanen HMTh: Being old does not always mean being sick: perspectives on conditions of health as perceived by British and American elderly, *J Adv Nurs* 53(1):54, 2006.

Vanderhoff M.: Patient education and health literacy, *PT—Magazine of Physical Therapy* 13(9):42, 2005.

Wieck KL: Motivating an intergenerational workforce: scenarios for success, *Orthop Nurs* 26(60):366, 2007.

World Health Organization Interim Commission: *Chronicle of WHO*, Geneva, 1947, The Organization.

2 The Health Care Delivery System

MEDIA RESOURCES

 CD COMPANION 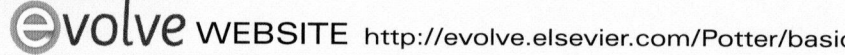 evolve WEBSITE http://evolve.elsevier.com/Potter/basic

- Crossword Puzzle
- English/Spanish Audio Glossary

OBJECTIVES

- Describe the six levels of health care.
- Explain the relationship between levels of health care and levels of prevention.
- Discuss the types of settings in which professionals provide various levels of health care.
- Discuss the role of nurses in different health care delivery settings.
- Differentiate primary care from primary health care.

- Explain the advantages and disadvantages of managed health care.
- Compare the various methods for financing health care.
- Discuss the implications that issues challenging the health care system have for nursing.
- Discuss opportunities for nursing within the changing health care delivery system.

KEY TERMS

acute care, p. 20
adult day care centers, p. 27
assisted living, p. 26
capitation, p. 18
case management, p. 22
critical pathway, p. 22
diagnosis-related groups (DRGs), p. 18
discharge planning, p. 22

evidence-based practice, p. 28
extended care facility, p. 25
globalization, p. 32
home care, p. 24
hospice, p. 27
independent practice association (IPA), p. 19
integrated delivery networks (IDNs), p. 20
managed care, p. 18

Medicaid, p. 24
Medicare, p. 24
Minimum Data Set (MDS), p. 26
nursing-sensitive outcomes, p. 29
patient-centered care, p. 29
primary care, p. 21
professional standards review organizations (PSROs), p. 17

prospective payment system (PPS), p. 18
rehabilitation, p. 25
respite care, p. 26
restorative care, p. 20
skilled nursing facility, p. 25
utilization review (UR) committees, p. 18
vulnerable populations, p. 32

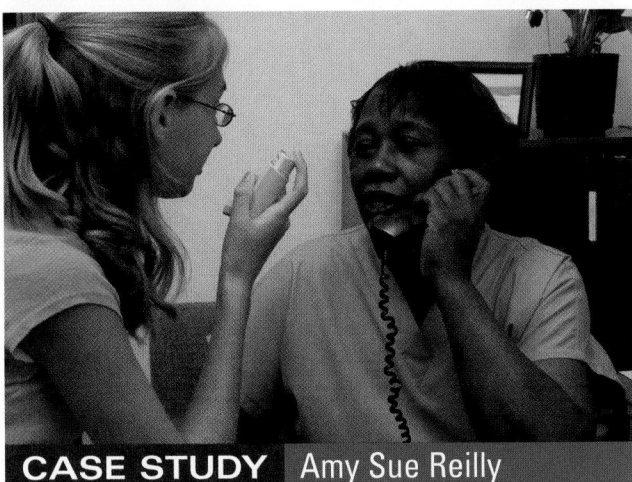

CASE STUDY   Amy Sue Reilly

Amy Sue Reilly is a 15-year-old white female of Irish descent. She is a freshman at a Catholic high school. Her parents are divorced. Her mother, Anne, is a cashier at a local grocery store, and her father, Joseph, is a lawyer. She has two brothers and lives at home with her mother. Although her parents are divorced, Amy Sue reports that her family is very close and that her parents work together to meet all their children's needs.

Amy Sue has had asthma since she was 5 years old. She has been able to control her asthma by taking oral medications and by using her inhalers when needed. However, she recently has had some difficulty breathing, especially during gym class.

Corrine is a 45-year-old African American nurse, who recently accepted a job as a school nurse for the four Catholic schools in the area. Three of the schools are grade schools, and there is one high school. Before she took this job, Corrine worked at a pediatrician's office. Amy Sue's difficulty managing her asthma is significant for Corrine because Corrine's oldest daughter has asthma. In addition, because of her job in the pediatrician's office, Corrine has had experience with caring for children with asthma and with helping patients access the health care delivery system.

A s you begin your career in nursing, you will quickly realize that the U.S. health care system is very complex and is constantly changing. Although health professionals offer a broad variety of services to the public, gaining access to services is difficult for those with limited health care insurance. Uninsured patients present a challenge to health care and nursing because they are more likely to skip or delay treatment for acute and chronic illnesses and die prematurely (Thompson and Lee, 2007). The continuing emergence of new technologies and medications contributes to ever-increasing costs of health care. Pressures to reduce costs come from declining reimbursement by third-party payers and from health care institutions being managed more as businesses than as service organizations. The challenges faced in reducing the costs of health care make it difficult for health care providers to maintain high-quality care for their patients. Many patients who would have

been hospitalized for their condition 20 years ago are now treated in outpatient facilities, in part to reduce the costs resulting from lengthy hospitalization. As a result, hospitalized patients are sicker, and their treatment involves a higher level of technological care. Patients are discharged from hospitals sooner, often leaving families with the burden of providing care in the home setting. Nurses also face significant challenges of keeping individuals healthy and well within their own homes and communities.

Nursing is a caring discipline. The values of our profession are rooted in helping persons to regain, maintain, or improve their health; prevent illness; and find comfort and dignity. The health care system of the new millennium has become less service oriented and much more business oriented because of cost-saving initiatives. The Institute of Medicine (2001) calls for a health care delivery system that is safe, effective, patient centered, timely, efficient, and equitable. The National Priorities Partnership is a group of 28 organizations from a variety of health care disciplines that have joined together to work toward transforming health care (National Priorities Partnership, 2008). The group has set the following National Priorities for health care transformation:

- Patient and Family Engagement—providing patient-centered, effective care
- A Healthy Population—bringing increased focus on wellness and prevention
- Safety—focusing on eliminating errors whenever and wherever possible
- Care Coordination—providing patient-centered, high-value care
- Palliative Care—providing appropriate and compassionate care for patients experiencing advanced illnesses
- Overuse—focusing on waste reduction to achieve effective, affordable care

As a result of the transformations occurring in the health care system, the practice of nursing is changing. Nursing needs to lead the way in change and retain its values for patient care while meeting the challenges of new roles and new responsibilities.

HEALTH CARE REGULATION AND COMPETITION

Through most of the twentieth century, there were few incentives for controlling health care costs. If a patient needed to be in the hospital a few extra days for a wound to heal or for the family to prepare to take care of him or her at home, there were few obstacles. Whatever a physician or health care provider chose to order for a patient's care and treatment, insurers (third-party payers) paid for. However, as health care costs continued to rise out of control, regulatory and competitive approaches attempted to control health care spending. For example, **professional standards review** organizations (PSROs) review the quality, quantity, and cost of health care services provided through Medicare and Medicaid (Sultz and Young, 2006). Medicare-qualified hospitals are required to have physician-supervised **utilization review (UR) committees** to review admissions, diagnostic testing, and treatments provided by physicians or health care providers to patients. The purpose is to identify and eliminate overuse of diagnostic and treatment services. Many hospitals have added nursing case managers to help meet the guidelines established by Medicare, Medicaid, and other payers.

One of the most significant factors that influenced health care payments, costs, and competition was the **prospective payment system (PPS).** Established by Congress in 1983, the PPS eliminated cost-based reimbursement. Hospitals serving Medicare patients were no longer paid for all costs incurred to deliver care to a patient. Instead, inpatient hospital services for Medicare patients were combined into 468 **diagnosis-related groups (DRGs).** Each group has a fixed reimbursement amount with adjustments for case severity, rural/urban/regional costs, and teaching costs. Hospitals receive a set dollar amount for each patient based on the assigned DRG, regardless of the patient's length of stay or use of services in the hospital. Box 2-1 provides a hypothetical scenario, showing how the DRG PPS determines reimbursement for a patient's care. Most health care providers (e.g., health care networks or managed care organizations) now receive capitated payments. **Capitation** is the payment mechanism in which providers receive a fixed amount per patient or enrollee of a health care plan (Gosden and others, 2005). The purpose of capitation is to build a payment plan for select diagnoses or surgical procedures that includes the best standards of care, including essential diagnostic and treatment procedures, at the lowest cost.

Capitation and prospective payment influence the way health care professionals deliver care in all types of settings. The health care industry makes an effort to manage costs through efficiency and effectiveness so that the organizations will remain profitable. For example, when patients are hospitalized for lengthy periods, hospitals absorb the portion of costs not reimbursed. This simply adds more pressure to ensure that patients are managed effectively and discharged as soon as reasonably possible. Soon after implementing prospective payment, hospitals began to increase discharge planning activities, and hospital lengths of stay began to shorten. Because patients are discharged home as soon as possible, home care agencies now provide complex technological care, including intravenous (IV) therapy, mechanical ventilation, and long-term parenteral nutrition.

The term **managed care** describes health care systems in which there is administrative control over primary health care services for a defined patient population. The provider or health care system receives a predetermined capitated payment for each patient enrolled in the program. In this case, the managed care organization bears financial risk in addition to providing patient care. The organization's focus of care shifts from individual illness care to concern for the

---

BOX 2-1   Clinical Scenario of a DRG Example

Mr. Truman, a 70-year-old man, went to his cardiologist because he was experiencing chest pain and shortness of breath. He had cardiac surgery 10 years earlier but was beginning to have recurrent chest pain, even at rest. He has a history of hypertension and emphysema. Mr. Truman has smoked 1 pack of cigarettes a day for 54 years and does not follow a low-fat diet. He has been counseled to quit smoking, but he has been unwilling to stop. He was hospitalized late in the afternoon on November 1 after having a chest x-ray examination and laboratory work done at an outpatient testing center. He had an echocardiogram on November 2. Early in the morning on November 3, Mr. Truman had a cardiac catheterization, and the cardiologist determined he did not need surgery. He was discharged on the evening of November 3. During his hospital stay, Mr. Truman received usual and customary care and experienced no complications.

Principal diagnosis: Chest pain, not otherwise specified (NOS)

Secondary diagnosis: Hypertension NOS, hyperlipidemia, tobacco use disorder, other lung disease, history of past noncompliance

Principal procedure: Left heart cardiac catheterization

DRG assigned: DRG 125: Circulatory disorders except acute myocardial infarction with cardiac catheterization without complex diagnosis

Average length of stay: 2.8 days

Actual length of stay: 2 days

Expected payment from Medicare (based on 2.8 days): Estimated national average hospital base rate × relative weight for DRG = $4430 × 1.146 = $5077

Actual hospital charges for Mr. Truman: $11,700

Actual reimbursement from Medicare: $5300

Loss for hospital: $6400

Data from Ingenix and others: *DRG expert,* ed 21, Clifton Park, NY, 2005, Thomson Delmar Learning.

DRG, Diagnosis-related group.

---

health of its covered population. If people stay healthy, the cost of medical care declines. Systems of managed care focus on containing or reducing costs, increasing patient satisfaction, and improving the health or functional status of the individual (Sultz and Young, 2006).

In theory, if people stay healthy, the cost of medical care declines. The purpose of managed care is to increase access to care while decreasing costs. However, health care spending continues to rise. Increases in health care spending are related to rising health care wages, increased costs of prescription drugs, higher insurance premiums, improved technology, and consumer demands.

You do not have to be a health care financing expert in your role as a nurse. However, it is important for you to understand the basics of health care financing to recognize the effects on employers and patients. Table 2-1 summarizes the most common types of health care plans.

TABLE 2-1 Health Care Plans

TYPE	DEFINITION	CHARACTERISTICS
Managed care organization (MCO)	Provides comprehensive, preventive, and treatment services to a specific group of voluntarily enrolled persons. Structures include a variety of models: *Staff model:* Physicians are salaried employees of the MCO. *Group model:* MCO contracts with single group practice. *Network model:* MCO contracts with multiple group practices and/or integrated organizations. **Independent practice association (IPA):** MCO contracts with physicians who usually are not members of groups and whose practices include fee-for-service and capitated patients.	Focus on health maintenance, primary care. All care provided by a primary care physician. Referral needed for access to specialist and hospitalization.
Medicare MCO	Program same as MCO but designed to cover health care costs of senior citizens.	Premium generally less than with supplemental plans.
Preferred provider organization (PPO)	One that limits an enrollee's choice to a list of "preferred" hospitals, physicians, and providers. An enrollee pays more out-of-pocket expenses for using a provider not on the list.	Contractual agreement exists between a set of providers and one or more purchasers (self-insured employers or insurance plans). Comprehensive health services at a discount to companies under contract.
Exclusive provider organization (EPO)	One that limits an enrollee's choice to providers belonging to one organization. Sometimes able to use outside providers at additional expense.	Focus on health maintenance. Limited contractual agreement. Less access to select specialists.
Medicare	A federally administered program by the Commonwealth Fund or the Centers for Medicare and Medicaid Services (CMS); a financially funded national health insurance program in the United States for people 65 years and older. Part A provides basic provision for medical, surgical, and psychiatric care costs based on diagnosis-related groups (DRGs). Part B is a voluntary medical insurance; covers physician and certain outpatient services. Part C is a managed care provision that provides a choice of three insurance plans. Part D is a Prescription Drug Improvement (Berkowitz, 2005-2006).	Payment for plan deducted from monthly individual Social Security check. Covers services of nurse practitioners. Does not pay full cost of certain services. Supplemental insurance is encouraged.
Medicaid	Federally funded, state-operated program that provides (1) health insurance to low-income families; (2) health assistance to low-income people with long-term care (LTC) disabilities; and (3) supplemental coverage and LTC assistance to older adults and Medicare beneficiaries in nursing homes. Individual states determine eligibility and benefits.	Finances a large portion of maternal and child care for the poor. Reimburses for nurse midwifery and other advanced practice nurses (varies by state). Reimburses nursing home funding.
Private insurance	Traditional fee-for-service plan. Payment computed after services are provided on basis of number of services used.	Policies typically expensive. Most policies have deductibles that patients pay before insurance pays.
Long-term care insurance	Supplemental insurance for coverage of long-term care services. Policies provide a set amount of dollars for an unlimited time or for as little as 2 years.	Very expensive. Good policy has a minimum waiting period for eligibility, payment for skilled nursing, intermediate or custodial care, and home care.

LEVELS OF HEALTH CARE

The health care industry is moving toward health care practices that emphasize managing health rather than managing illness. The premise is that in the long term, health promotion reduces health care costs. A wellness perspective focuses on the health of populations and the communities in which they live rather than just on finding a cure for an individual's disease. Larger health care systems have attempted to develop **integrated delivery networks (IDNs)** that include a set of providers and services organized to deliver a coordinated continuum of care to the population of patients served at a capitated cost (Oodyke, 2004). An integrated system reduces duplication of services, coordinates care across settings, and ensures that patients receive care in the most appropriate setting.

The health services pyramid (Figure 2-1) is a model of improving health care. The pyramid shows that the population-based health care services provide the basis for preventive services. Achievements in the lower tiers of the pyramid contribute to the improvement of health care delivered at the higher levels of the pyramid. An emphasis on wellness and health of populations and the environment has enhanced quality of life (Merzel and D'Afflitti, 2003).

The health care system has six levels of care: preventive, primary, secondary, tertiary, restorative, and continuing care. Levels of care describe the scope of services and settings in which health care is offered to patients in all stages of health and illness. For example, the secondary level of care is the traditional **acute care** setting in which patients who have signs and symptoms of disease are diagnosed and treated. **Restorative care** includes those settings and services in which patients who are recovering from illness or disability receive rehabilitation and supportive care. Levels of care are not the same as levels of prevention (see Chapter 1). Levels of prevention describe the focus of health-related activities: avoiding disease (health promotion and disease prevention), curing disease (secondary prevention), and diminishing complications (tertiary prevention). At any level of care, nurses and other health care providers offer a variety of levels of prevention. For example, the nurse working in an acute care, tertiary setting, monitors the recovery of a patient who has had open heart surgery while also providing health promotion information to the family concerning diet and exercise.

It is important for you to understand how the health care industry organizes and delivers different levels of care. Each level creates different requirements and opportunities for your role as a nurse. Box 2-2 highlights the types of services available to patients and families at each level of care. Changes unique to each level of care developed as a result of health care reform. For example, the health care industry now places

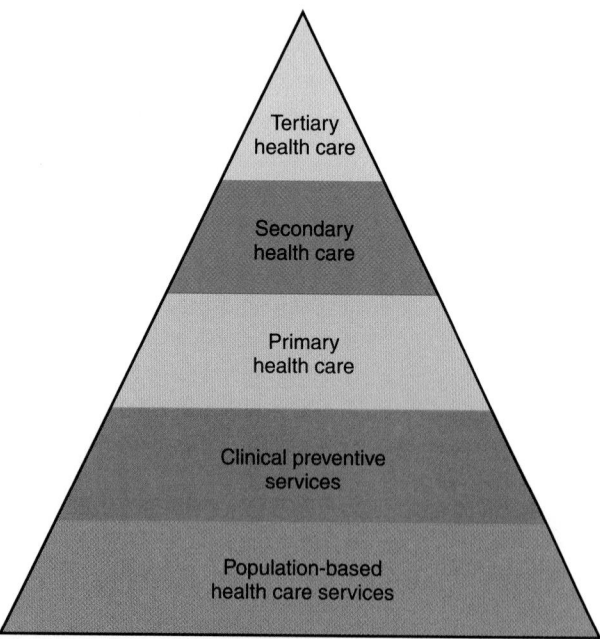

Figure 2-1 ■ Health services pyramid. (U.S. Public Health Service: *The core functions project*, Washington, DC, 1994/update 2000, Office of Disease Prevention and Health Promotion. From Stanhope M, Lancaster J: *Public health nursing*, ed 7, St. Louis, 2008, Mosby.)

BOX 2-2   Examples of Health Care Services

PREVENTIVE CARE
- Blood pressure and cancer screening
- Immunizations
- Poison control information
- Mental health counseling and crisis prevention
- Community legislation (seat belts, air bags, bike helmets)

PRIMARY CARE (HEALTH PROMOTION)
- Prenatal care
- Well-baby care
- Nutrition counseling
- Family planning
- Exercise classes

SECONDARY ACUTE CARE
- Emergency care
- Acute medical-surgical care
- Radiological procedures

TERTIARY CARE
- Intensive care
- Psychiatric facilities

RESTORATIVE CARE
- Cardiovascular and pulmonary rehabilitation
- Sports medicine
- Spinal cord injury programs
- Home care

CONTINUING CARE
- Assisted living
- Psychiatric and older adult day care

greater emphasis on wellness; thus the health care industry directs more resources toward primary and preventive care. Nursing has the chance to provide leadership to communities and health care systems that are coordinating resources to better serve their populations. The ability to find strategies to better address patient needs at all levels of care is critical to the success of improving the health care delivery system.

Preventive and Primary Health Care Services

In the settings that deliver preventive and **primary care**, such as schools, physicians' or health care providers' offices, occupational health clinics, and nursing centers, health promotion is a major theme (Table 2-2). Health promotion is a key to good-quality health care. Successful programs help patients acquire healthier lifestyles. The focus of health promotion is to keep people healthy through personal hygiene, good nutrition, clean living environments, regular exercise, rest, and the adoption of positive health attitudes. Health promotion programs lower the overall costs of health care by reducing the incidence of disease and minimizing complications, thus reducing the need to use more expensive health care resources. In contrast, preventive care is more disease oriented and focused on reducing and controlling risk factors for disease through activities such as immunization and occupational health programs.

Health care providers at the primary level of health care build interventions that lead to improved health outcomes for an entire population. The primary level of health care includes medical and health care services as well as health education, nutritional counseling, maternal/child health care, family planning, and control of diseases. Successful community-based primary health care programs take societal and environmental factors into consideration when addressing the health needs of communities (Merzel and D'Afflitti, 2003). Chapter 3 provides a more comprehensive discussion of primary health care in the community.

Secondary and Tertiary Care

The diagnosis and treatment of illness are traditionally the reason for the most commonly used services of the health care delivery system. With managed care, these services are now often delivered at the primary level of care. For example, more physicians are performing simple surgeries in office surgical suites. However, if a patient develops a problem that the physician or health care provider is not able to care for, the patient will need a medical specialist. Care from a special-

TABLE 2-2   Preventive and Primary Care Services

TYPE OF SERVICE	PURPOSE	AVAILABLE PROGRAMS/SERVICES
School health	Comprehensive programs integrate health promotion principles throughout a school's curriculum. Services stress program management, interdisciplinary collaboration, and community health principles.	Positive life skills Nutritional planning Health screening Counseling Communicable disease prevention Crisis intervention
Occupational health	A comprehensive program geared to health promotion and accident or illness prevention. Goal is to increase worker productivity, decrease absenteeism, and reduce use of expensive medical care.	Environmental surveillance Physical assessment Health screening Health education Communicable disease control Counseling
Physicians' offices	Provide primary health care (diagnosis and treatment). Beginning to focus more on health promotion practices. Advanced nurse practitioners often partner with a physician in managing patient population.	Routine physical examination Health screening Diagnostics Treatment of acute and chronic ailments
Nursing centers	Nurse-managed clinics provide nursing services with a focus on health promotion and health education, chronic disease assessment management, and support for self-care and caregivers.	Day care Health risk appraisal Wellness counseling Employment readiness Acute and chronic care management
Block and parish nursing	Nurses living within a neighborhood provide services to older patients or those unable to leave their home. Provides services that are not available in traditional health care system.	Running errands Transportation Respite care Homemaker aides Spiritual health
Community centers	Outpatient clinics that provide primary care to a specific patient population (e.g., well-baby, mental health, diabetes) that lives in a specific community. Sometimes affiliated with a hospital, medical school, church, or other community organization.	Physical assessment Health screening Disease management Health education Counseling

ist sometimes requires hospitalization of the patient. Typically secondary care and tertiary care (also called *acute care*) are quite costly, particularly if patients wait to seek health care until after symptoms have developed.

HOSPITALS Hospital emergency departments, urgent care centers, critical care units, and inpatient medical-surgical units are sites that provide secondary and tertiary levels of care. When you work in these settings, you will be challenged to work closely with all members of the health care team. Your ability to think critically and to identify patients' changing problems quickly and accurately will be essential. Planning and coordination of care are necessary to deliver services in a competent and timely manner. You will need to apply nursing research findings when selecting nursing interventions to improve patient outcomes. You will constantly evaluate whether care is effective and how to improve it.

Quality, safe care is the focus of most acute care organizations. Patient satisfaction becomes a priority in a busy, stressful location such as an inpatient nursing unit. Patients expect you to treat them courteously and respectfully and to involve them in daily care decisions. As a nurse, you play a key role in bringing respect and dignity to the patient (Vlasses and Smeltzer, 2007). It is necessary for acute care nurses to be aware of patient needs and expectations early to form effective partnerships that ultimately enhance the level of nursing care given.

Managed care organizations expect patients who are hospitalized with a medical diagnosis or who enter the hospital to have surgery to be cared for and discharged within a projected time period. Therefore, if you work in a hospital, you will need to use resources efficiently to help your patients successfully recover and return home. To contain costs, it is important that the hospital be used appropriately as the source for health care (Gold, 2007). Many hospitals have redesigned nursing units to make more services available on nursing units, thus minimizing the need to transfer and transport patients across multiple diagnostic and treatment areas.

Hospitalized patients are acutely ill and need comprehensive and specialized tertiary health care. The services provided by hospitals vary considerably. Some small rural hospitals offer only limited emergency and diagnostic services, as well as general inpatient services. In comparison, large urban medical centers offer comprehensive, state-of-the-art diagnostic services, trauma and emergency care, surgical intervention, intensive care units, inpatient services, and rehabilitation facilities. Larger hospitals hire professional staff from a variety of specialties such as social service, respiratory therapy, physical and occupational therapy, and speech therapy. The focus in hospitals is to provide the highest quality of care possible so that patients are discharged early but safely to the home or another health care facility that will adequately manage any remaining health care needs.

Because of the need to contain costs, many hospitals use a **case management** model of care. In this model a case manager, who is usually a nurse or a social worker, coordinates the efforts of all disciplines to achieve the most efficient and appropriate plan of care for the patient (see Chapter 12). The case manager follows patients across settings. One focus of case management is discharge planning.

DISCHARGE PLANNING **Discharge planning** is a centralized, coordinated, multidisciplinary process that ensures that the patient has a plan for continuing care after leaving a health care agency. *Discharge planning begins the moment a patient is admitted to a health care facility.* You will play a large role in discharge planning if you choose to work in a hospital. Discharge planning provides continuity of care within an acute care hospital. To achieve continuity of care, you use critical thinking skills and apply the nursing process (see Chapters 7 and 8). You anticipate and identify the patient's needs and work with all members of the multidisciplinary health care team to develop a plan of care that moves the patient from the hospital to another environment, such as the patient's home or a nursing home.

One tool available in some acute care settings for coordinating patients' care is a critical pathway. A **critical pathway** is a multidisciplinary treatment plan that shows what treatments or interventions patients need to have for a specific condition while they are in the hospital. For example, some hospitals have critical pathways for patients who have pneumonia or congestive heart failure. The critical pathway includes interventions from different members of the health care team. A pathway promotes collaboration, which enables the patient to be discharged in an appropriate time frame.

Because patients leave hospitals as soon as their physical condition allows, they often have continuing health care needs when they go home or to another facility. For example, a patient still requires wound care after surgery, or a patient who has had a stroke still requires ambulation training. Patients and families worry about how they will care for the patient's needs and manage illness over the long term. As a nurse, you will help by anticipating and identifying patients' continuing needs before the actual time of discharge and by coordinating health team members in achieving an appropriate discharge plan.

Some patients are more in need of discharge planning because of the risks they present. For example, some patients have limited financial resources or limited family support, whereas others may have long-term disabilities or chronic illness. Early discharge teaching is especially important as a way to decrease readmission to the hospital for older adults (Hickman and others, 2007). However, any patient who is discharged from a health care facility with remaining functional limitations or who must follow certain restrictions or therapies for recovery needs discharge planning. All caregivers who care for a patient with a specific health problem participate in discharge planning. The process is truly multidisciplinary. For example, a patient with diabetes visiting a diabetes management center requires the collaboration of a nurse educator, dietitian, and physician or health care provider to ensure that the patient returns home with the right information to manage the condition. A patient who had a stroke will not be discharged from a hospital until caregivers have established plans with physical and occupational therapists to begin a program of rehabilitation.

Effective discharge planning often requires referring patients to various health care disciplines. In many agencies, patients need a physician's or health care provider's order for a referral, especially when specific therapies are planned (e.g., physical therapy). It is best to have patients and families participate in referral processes so that they are involved early in any necessary decision making. Some tips on making the referral process successful include the following:

- Involve the patient and family in the referral process, including selecting the necessary referral. Explain the service to be provided, the reason for the referral, and what to expect from the referral's services.
- Make a referral as soon as possible.
- Inform the care provider receiving the referral of as much information about the patient as possible. This avoids duplication of effort and exclusion of important information.
- Determine what the referral discipline (e.g., physical therapy, social work, diet and nutrition, radiology) recommends for the patient's care, and incorporate this into the treatment plan as soon as possible.

Successful discharge planning involves the patient from the beginning, uses the strengths of the patient in planning, provides resources to meet the patient's limitations, and focuses on improving the patient's long-term outcomes. Discharge planning depends on comprehensive patient and family education (see Chapter 11). Patients need to know what to do when they get home, how to do it, and what to watch for when problems develop. The Joint Commission (2008) requires the following when patients are discharged from health care facilities or transferred to other levels of care:

- A process that addresses the need for continuing care, treatment, and services after discharge or transfer.
- The transfer or discharge of a patient to another level of care, treatment, and services, different professionals, or different settings is based on the patient's assessed needs and the hospital's capabilities.
- When patients are transferred or discharged, appropriate information related to the care, treatment, and services provided is exchanged with other service providers.

INTENSIVE CARE An intensive care unit (ICU) or critical care unit is a hospital unit in which critically ill, unstable patients receive close monitoring and intensive medical care. ICUs have advanced technologies, such as computerized cardiac monitors and mechanical ventilators. Although many of these devices are on regular nursing units, the patients hospitalized within ICUs are monitored and maintained on multiple devices. Nursing and medical staff within an ICU are educated on critical care principles and techniques. An ICU is the most expensive delivery site for medical care because each nurse is usually assigned to care for only one or two patients at a time and because of all the treatments and procedures the patients in the ICU require.

PSYCHIATRIC FACILITIES Patients who have emotional and behavioral problems such as depression, violent behavior, and eating disorders often require special counseling and treatment in psychiatric facilities. Located in hospitals, independent outpatient clinics, or private mental health hospitals, psychiatric facilities offer inpatient and outpatient services, depending on the seriousness of the problem. Patients enter these facilities voluntarily or involuntarily. Hospitalization involves relatively short stays with the purpose of stabilizing patients before transfer to outpatient treatment centers. Patients with psychiatric problems receive a comprehensive multidisciplinary treatment plan that involves them and their families. Medicine, nursing, social work, and activity therapy collaborate to develop a plan of care that enables patients to return to functional states within the community. At the time of discharge from inpatient facilities, patients usually receive referrals for follow-up care at clinics or with counselors.

RURAL HOSPITALS Access to health care in rural areas has been a serious problem. Most rural hospitals have experienced a severe shortage of primary care providers. Many have been forced to close because of economic failure. In 1989 the Omnibus Budget Reconciliation Act (OBRA) directed the U.S. Department of Health and Human Services (USDHHS) to create a new health care entity, the rural primary care hospital (RPCH). An RPCH provides 24-hour emergency care, with no more than six inpatient beds for providing temporary care for 72 hours or less to patients needing stabilization before transfer to a larger hospital. Physicians, nurse practitioners, or physician assistants staff the RPCH. The RPCH provides inpatient care to acutely ill or injured persons before transferring them to better-equipped facilities. Basic radiological and laboratory services are also available.

With health care reform, more big-city health care systems are branching out and establishing affiliations or mergers with rural hospitals. The rural hospitals provide a referral base to the larger tertiary care medical centers. Nurses who work in rural hospitals or clinics often function independently in the absence of a physician. Competence in physical assessment, clinical decision making, and emergency care is essential. Advanced practice nurses (e.g., nurse practitioners or clinical nurse specialists) use medical protocols and establish collaborative agreements with staff physicians.

Restorative Care

Patients recovering from acute illnesses or who have chronic illnesses or disabilities usually require services designed to restore the patient's level of health. Care is necessary until patients return to their previous level of function or reach a new level of function limited by their illness or disability. The goal of restorative care is to assist an individual with regaining maximal functional status, thereby enhancing the individual's quality of life. The goal is to promote patient independence and self-care. With the emphasis on early discharge from hospitals, most patients require some level of restorative care. For example, some surgical patients require ongoing wound care and activity and exercise management until they

BOX 2-3   Home Care Services

WOUND CARE

Sterile dressing changes, debridement and irrigations, packing, and instructing patients and families in wound care techniques

RESPIRATORY CARE

Oxygen therapy, mechanical ventilation, suctioning, and care of tracheostomies

VITAL SIGNS

Monitoring blood pressure and cardiopulmonary status; instructing patients and families in vital sign measurement

ELIMINATION

Ostomy care, appliance application, skin care, and irrigation; insertion of indwelling and intermittent urinary catheters, irrigation, and instructing families in catheter management; home dialysis

NUTRITION

Administration of enteral feedings; assessment of nutrition and hydration status; instructing patients and families in tube feedings

REHABILITATION

Ambulation and gait training, use of assistive devices, range-of-motion exercises, and instructing patients and families in transfer techniques

MEDICATIONS

Monitoring compliance; administering injections; and instructing patients and families in drug information, medication preparation, and steps to take in the event of side effects

INTRAVENOUS THERAPY

Administration of blood products, analgesic and chemotherapeutic agents, and long-term hydration and instructing patients and families in use of intravenous devices, steps to take in the event of disconnection or accidental fluid infusion, and side effects

LABORATORY STUDIES

Blood glucose monitoring (including patient and family instruction) and drawing blood for specific diagnostic purposes

---

have recovered to a point at which they are able to resume normal activities of daily living independently.

The intensity of care has increased in restorative care settings, because patients leave hospitals earlier. It is common to have patients in a home or rehabilitation setting still receiving intravenous fluids (see Chapter 17), enteral nutrition (see Chapter 32), and pain control (see Chapter 31). The restorative health care team is an interdisciplinary group of health care professionals that includes the patient and family or significant others. In restorative settings, nurses recognize that success is dependent on effective and early partnering with patients and their families. Patients and families require a clear understanding of goals for physical recovery, the rationale for any physical limitations, and the purpose and potential risks associated with therapies. The more patients and families are involved in restorative care, the more likely that they will be motivated to follow treatment plans and that patients will be able to achieve optimal functioning.

HOME CARE **Home care** is the provision of medically related professional and paraprofessional services and equipment to patients and families in their homes. Services provided include health maintenance, education, illness prevention, diagnosis and treatment of disease, palliation, and rehabilitation. Patients in home care use nursing services more than any other service. However, home care also includes medical and social services; physical, occupational, speech, and respiratory therapy; and nutritional therapy. A home care service also coordinates the access to and delivery of home health equipment, or durable medical equipment (DME), which is any medically related product adapted for home use.

Home care agencies provide almost every type of health care service in the patient's home. Health promotion and education are traditionally the primary objectives of home care, yet at present, most patients receive professional services on the basis of some medically related need. The focus is on patient and family independence. Home care addresses recovery from and stabilization of illness in the home, where problems related to lifestyle, safety, environment, family dynamics, and health care practices are identified.

Home care agencies provide skilled and intermittent professional services and home care aide services. These services usually are delivered once or twice a day, up to 7 days a week. Box 2-3 summarizes some of the services offered by home care agencies. Approved home care agencies usually receive reimbursement for services from the government (such as **Medicare** and **Medicaid** in the United States), private insurance, and private payers. The government has strict regulations that govern reimbursement for home care services. An agency cannot simply charge whatever it wants for a service and expect to receive full reimbursement. Government programs set the cost for reimbursement of most professional services.

If you choose to work as a home care nurse, you will provide individualized care and have one-on-one contact with patients and families. You will have your own caseload and help patients adapt to many permanent or temporary physical limitations so that they are able to assume a more normal daily home routine. Home care requires a strong knowledge base in many areas, such as family dynamics (see Chapter 23), cultural practices (see Chapter 19), spiritual values (see Chapter 20), and communication principles (see Chapter 10).

REHABILITATION **Rehabilitation** is the use of multiple therapies, such as physical, psychological, occupational, speech and social services, to help restore a person to the fullest physical, mental, social, vocational, and economic usefulness possible (Stanhope and Lancaster, 2004). Patients require rehabilitation after a physical or mental illness, injury, or chemical addiction. Rehabilitation was once available primarily for patients with illnesses or injury to the nervous or musculoskeletal system, but the health care delivery system has expanded its scope of such services. Today, specialized rehabilitation services, such as cardiovascular and pulmonary rehabilitation programs, help patients and families adjust to necessary changes in lifestyle and learn to function with the limitations of their disease. Drug rehabilitation centers help patients become free from drug dependence and return to the community.

Ideally rehabilitation begins the moment a patient enters a health care setting for treatment. For example, some orthopedic programs now have patients undergo physical therapy exercises before major joint repair to enhance their recovery postoperatively. Initially rehabilitation focuses on the prevention of complications related to the illness or injury. As the condition stabilizes, rehabilitation maximizes the patient's functioning and level of independence.

Rehabilitation occurs in many health care settings, including specific rehabilitation institutions, outpatient settings, and the home. Frequently patients needing long-term rehabilitation (e.g., patients who have had strokes and spinal cord injuries) have severe disabilities affecting their ability to carry out the activities of daily living. For rehabilitation services delivered in outpatient settings, patients get treatment at specified times during the week but remain at home the rest of the time. Specific rehabilitation strategies are applied to the home environment to help the patient achieve maximal levels of function and independence. Nurses and other members of the health care team visit homes and help patients and families learn to adapt to illness or injury.

EXTENDED CARE FACILITIES An **extended care facility** provides intermediate medical, nursing, or custodial care for patients recovering from acute illness or patients with chronic illnesses or disabilities. Extended care facilities include intermediate care and skilled nursing facilities. Some include long-term care and assisted living facilities (see later discussion of continuing care). At one point, extended care facilities primarily cared for older adults. However, because hospitals discharge their patients sooner, there is a greater need for intermediate care settings for patients of all ages. For example, a young patient who has experienced a traumatic brain injury resulting from a car accident typically transfers to an extended care facility for rehabilitative or supportive care until discharge to the home becomes a safe option. The growth of extended care facilities will increase as the number of older adults grows.

An intermediate care or **skilled nursing facility** offers skilled care from a licensed nursing staff. This often includes administration of IV fluids, wound care, long-term ventilator management, and physical rehabilitation. Patients receive extensive supportive care until they are able to move back into the community or into residential care.

Extended care facilities provide around-the-clock nursing coverage. If you choose to work in this setting, you will need nursing expertise that is similar to that of nurses working in acute care inpatient settings along with a background in gerontological nursing principles (see Chapter 21).

Continuing Care

Continuing care describes a variety of health, personal, and social services provided over a prolonged period to persons who are disabled, who never were functionally independent, or who suffer a terminal disease. The need for continuing health care services is growing in the United States. People are living longer, and many of those with continuing health care needs have no immediate family members to care for them. A decline in the number of children families choose to have, the aging of care providers, and the increasing rates of divorce and remarriage complicate this problem. Continuing care is available within institutional settings (e.g., nursing centers or nursing homes, group homes, and retirement communities), communities (e.g., adult day care and senior centers), or the home (e.g., home care, home-delivered meals, and hospice) (Meiner and Lueckenotte, 2006). Elder care services that offer companionship, assistance with activities of daily living, and food preparation are another alternative for patients who do not need nursing care but need some assistance to stay independent.

NURSING CENTERS OR FACILITIES The language of long-term care is confusing and constantly changing. The nursing home has been the dominant setting for long-term care (Meiner and Lueckenotte, 2006). With the Omnibus Budget Reconciliation Act of 1987, the term *nursing facility* became the term for nursing homes and other facilities that provide long-term care. Now, *nursing center* is the most appropriate term. A nursing center typically provides 24-hour intermediate and custodial care for residents of any age with chronic or debilitating illnesses. Care provided usually includes nursing, rehabilitation, dietary, recreational, social, and religious services. In some cases, patients stay in nursing centers for room, food, and laundry services only. The majority of persons living in nursing centers are older adults. A nursing center is a resident's temporary or permanent home with surroundings made as homelike as possible (Sorrentino, 2007). Residents receive a planned, systematic, and interdisciplinary approach to care to help them reach and maintain their highest level of function.

The nursing center industry has become one of the most highly regulated industries in the United States. The Omnibus Budget Reconciliation Act of 1987, also known as the Nursing Home Reform Act, raised the standard of services provided by nursing centers. To receive payment from Medicare and Medicaid, nursing centers have to comply with the Act of 1987 and its minimal requirements for nursing homes. There currently are 18 requirements included in this law. Examples of the requirements include having sufficient nursing staff, developing a comprehensive plan of care for each

BOX 2-4 Minimum Data Set and Examples of Resident Assessment Protocols

MINIMUM DATA SET
- Resident's background
- Cognitive, communication/hearing, and vision patterns
- Physical functioning and structural problems
- Mood, behavior, and activity pursuit patterns
- Psychosocial well-being
- Bowel and bladder continence
- Health conditions
- Disease diagnoses
- Oral/nutritional and dental status
- Skin condition
- Medication use
- Special treatments and procedures

RESIDENT ASSESSMENT PROTOCOLS (EXAMPLES)
- Delirium
- Falls
- Pressure ulcers
- Psychotropic drug use

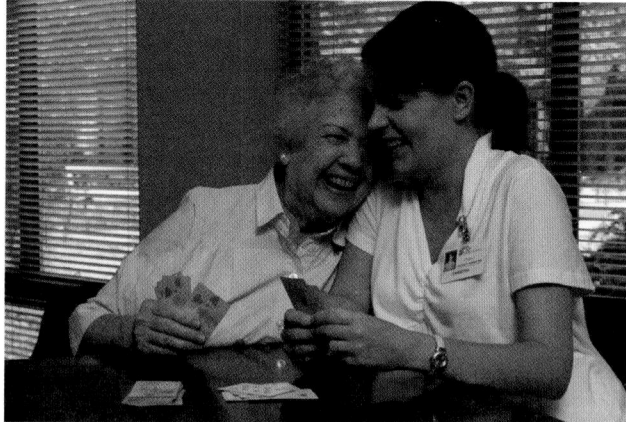

Figure 2-2 ■ Providing nursing services in assisted living facilities promotes physical and psychosocial health.

resident, maintaining dignity and respect for each resident, and providing services needed to maintain personal safety, nutrition, grooming, and personal hygiene (Health Care Financing Administration [HCFA], 2004; Nursing Home Abuse and Neglect Resource Center, 2008).

Interdisciplinary functional assessment of residents is the cornerstone of clinical practice within nursing centers (Meiner and Lueckenotte, 2006). Government regulations require that staff in nursing centers assess each resident comprehensively, with care planning decisions made within a prescribed period. A resident's functional ability (e.g., ability to perform activities of daily living and instrumental activities of daily living) and long-term physical and psychosocial well-being are the focus. The facility needs to complete the Resident Assessment Instrument (RAI) on all residents. The RAI consists of the **Minimum Data Set (MDS)** (Box 2-4), Resident Assessment Protocols (RAPs), and utilization guidelines of each state. The RAI ultimately provides a national database for nursing facilities so that policy makers will better understand the health care needs of the long-term care population. In addition, the MDS is a rich resource for nurses in determining the best type of interventions to support the health care needs of this growing population.

ASSISTED LIVING **Assisted living** is one of the fastest-growing industries within the United States. There are approximately 38,000 assisted living facilities that house about 975,000 people in the United States (National Center for Assisted Living [NCAL], 2008). Assisted living offers an attractive long-term care setting with a homier environment and greater resident autonomy. Patients require some assistance with activities of daily living but remain relatively indepen-

dent within a partially protective setting. A group of residents live together, but each resident has his or her own room and shares dining and social activity areas. Usually people keep all of their personal possessions in their residences. Facilities range from hotel-like buildings with hundreds of units to modest group homes that house a handful of seniors. Assisted living provides independence, security, and privacy all at the same time (Ebersole and others, 2008). These facilities promote independence and physical and psychosocial health (Figure 2-2). Services in an assisted living facility include medication management, exercise and educational activities, social activities, laundry, assistance with meals and personal care, 24-hour oversight, and housekeeping (NCAL, 2008). Some facilities provide assistance with medication administration. Assisted living facilities do not directly provide nursing care services, although a home care nurse is able to visit a patient in an assisted living facility.

Unfortunately, most residents of assisted living facilities pay privately. The average monthly fee is $2627 (NCAL, 2008). With no government fee caps and little regulation, assisted living is not always an option for individuals with limited financial resources.

RESPITE CARE The need to care for family members within the home creates great physical and emotional burdens for adult caregivers, especially when the family member is limited either physically or cognitively. The caregiver is usually an adult who not only has the responsibility for providing care to a loved one (e.g., spouse, parent, or sibling) but often maintains a full-time job, raises a family, and manages the routines of daily living as well. **Respite care** is a service that provides short-term relief or time off for persons providing home care to an ill, disabled, or frail older adult (Meiner and Lueckenotte, 2006). Adult day care is one form of respite care. Trained volunteers in the home also provide respite care. The family caregiver is able to leave the home for errands or some social time while a responsible person stays in the home to care for the loved one. Alternatively, some patients stay temporarily in a nursing center to provide the family relief.

ADULT DAY CARE CENTERS **Adult day care centers** provide a variety of health and social services to specific patient populations who live alone or with family in the community. Services offered during the day allow family members to maintain their lifestyles and employment and still provide home care for their relatives (Meiner and Lueckenotte, 2006). Day care centers are associated with a hospital or nursing home or exist as independent centers. Frequently the patients of such centers do not require hospitalization but need continuous health care services while their families or support persons work. These patients include older adults needing daily physical rehabilitation, individuals with emotional illnesses needing daily counseling, and individuals with chemical dependence problems who are involved in rehabilitation programs. The centers usually operate 5 days per week during typical business hours and usually charge on a per diem basis. Adult day care centers allow patients to retain more independence by living at home, thus potentially reducing the costs of health care by avoiding or delaying an older adult's admission to a nursing center.

Additional services offered in day care settings include transportation to and from the facility, assistance with personal care, nursing and therapeutic services (e.g., counseling and rehabilitation), meals, and recreational activities (Meiner and Lueckenotte, 2006). Nurses working in day care centers provide continuity between care delivered in the home and in the center. For example, nurses ensure that patients continue to take prescribed medication and treatments such as dressing changes. Knowledge of community needs and resources is essential in providing adequate support of patients, who often spend only a few hours a week in the day care setting (Ebersole and others, 2008).

HOSPICE A **hospice** is a system of family-centered care that allows patients to live and remain at home with comfort, independence, and dignity while alleviating the strains caused by terminal illness. The focus of hospice care is palliative care, not curative treatment (see Chapter 25). A hospice benefits patients in the terminal phase of any disease, such as cardiomyopathy, multiple sclerosis, acquired immunodeficiency syndrome (AIDS), or cancer.

A patient entering a hospice is at the terminal phase of illness, and the patient, family, and physician agree that no further treatment will reverse the disease process. Staff members collaborate to provide care that ensures death with dignity in the patient's home. Hospice care is available 24 hours a day, 7 days a week, and services continue without interruption if the patient's care setting changes. Occasionally a patient is admitted to a hospice unit within a hospital. The patient and family need to accept the fact that the hospice will not use emergency measures such as cardiopulmonary resuscitation to prolong life. The focus is on symptom management and ensuring the patient's comfort. The hospice's multidisciplinary team works together continuously with the patient's physician to develop and maintain a patient-directed individualized plan of care.

If you decide to be a hospice nurse, you will work in institutional and community settings. Hospice nurses are committed to the philosophy and objectives of the facilities for which they work. They provide care and support for the patient and family during the terminal phase and at the time of death and continue to offer bereavement counseling and follow-up to the family after the patient's death. Many hospice programs provide respite care, which is important in maintaining the health of the primary caregiver and family.

ISSUES IN HEALTH CARE DELIVERY

The climate in health care today influences health care professionals as well as consumers. As a nurse in the midst of an evolving health care system, be prepared to participate fully and effectively within the managed care environment. Those who provide patient care are the most qualified to make changes in the health care delivery system. As you face issues of how to maintain health care quality while reducing costs, you will need to acquire the knowledge, skills, and values necessary to practice competently and effectively. It will also become more important than ever before to collaborate with your colleagues in health care in designing new approaches for patient care delivery.

Competency

The Pew Health Professions Commission (1998) is a national and interdisciplinary group of health care leaders that recommended 21 competencies for health care professionals in the twenty-first century. These competencies emphasized the importance of public service, caring for the health of communities, and developing ethically responsible behaviors. In addressing the continued challenges facing the health care system, the Institute of Medicine (2001) identified five interrelated competencies that are essential for all health care workers in the twenty-first century (Box 2-5). The Institute of Medicine also identified 10 important rules of performance for a health care system to follow in order to better meet patient needs (Box 2-6) (IOM, 2003).

The health care practitioner competencies are an excellent tool for measuring how well you practice nursing. They also provide guidance as you grow within the nursing profession. A consumer of health care expects that the standards of nursing care and practice in any health care setting are appropriate, safe, and effective. Ongoing competency is your responsibility. Health care organizations ensure good-quality care by establishing policies, procedures, and protocols that are scientifically valid and follow national accrediting standards. Your responsibility is to follow policies and procedures and to know the most current practice standards. As you progress in your career, it becomes your responsibility to obtain necessary continued education and to earn certifications when you choose to practice in specialty areas.

BOX 2-5 Institute of Medicine Competencies for the Twenty-First Century

PROVIDE PATIENT-CENTERED CARE
- Recognize and respect differences in patients' values, preferences, and needs
- Relieve pain and suffering
- Coordinate continuous care
- Effectively communicate with and educate patients
- Share decision making and management
- Advocate for disease prevention and health promotion

WORK IN INTERDISCIPLINARY TEAMS
- Cooperate, collaborate, and communicate
- Integrate care to ensure that care is continuous and reliable

EMPLOY EVIDENCE-BASED PRACTICE
- Integrate best research with clinical practice and patient values
- Participate in research activities as possible

APPLY QUALITY IMPROVEMENT
- Identify errors and hazards in care
- Practice using basic safety design principles
- Measure quality in relation to structure, process, and outcomes
- Design and test interventions to change processes

UTILIZE INFORMATICS
- Use information technology to communicate, manage knowledge, reduce error, and support decision making

Modified from the Institute of Medicine: *Crossing the quality chasm: a new health system for the 21st century,* Washington, DC, 2001, National Academies Press; Institute of Medicine: *Health professions education: a bridge to quality,* Washington, DC, 2003, National Academies Press.

BOX 2-6 Ten Rules of Performance in a Redesigned Health Care System

1 Care is based on continuous healing relationships.
2 Care is individualized based on patient needs and values.
3 The patient is the source of control participating in shared decision making.
4 Knowledge is shared, and information flows freely.
5 Decision making is evidence based with care based on the best available scientific knowledge.
6 Safety is a system property and focused on reducing errors.
7 Transparency is necessary through sharing information with patients and families.
8 Patient needs are anticipated through planning.
9 Waste is continuously decreased.
10 Cooperation and communication among clinicians is a priority.

Modified from the Institute of Medicine: *Crossing the quality chasm: a new health system for the 21st century,* Washington, DC, 2001, National Academies Press; Institute of Medicine: *Health professions education: a bridge to quality,* Washington, DC, 2003, National Academies Press.

Evidence-Based Practice

As you enter the nursing profession, it will be a challenge to stay familiar with new information in order to provide the highest quality of patient care. Nursing practice is dynamic and always changing because of new information coming from research studies, practice trends, technological development, and social issues affecting patients. **Evidence-based practice** is a problem-solving approach to clinical practice that integrates the conscientious use of best evidence in combination with a clinician's expertise and patient preferences and values in making decisions about patient care (Melnyk and Fineout-Overholt, 2005; Sackett and others, 2000). The goal of evidence-based practice is to apply evidence-based data when providing patient care in order to improve patient outcomes. Evidence-based practice will help you resolve problems that arise in the clinical setting. It will also help you provide innovative health care that exceeds quality standards. Using evidence-based practice will also help you provide

consistent patient care using effective and efficient decision-making processes (Spector, 2005) (see Chapter 6).

Quality Health Care

Quality health care is the "degree to which health services for individuals and populations increase the likelihood of desired health outcomes and are consistent with current professional knowledge" (IOM, 2001). Safety is a critical part of quality health care (Tzeng and Yin, 2007). For example, use of infection control standards and fall precautions reduces the incidence of infection and patient injury. Health care providers define the quality of their services by measuring health care outcomes that show how a patient's health status has changed. Examples of outcomes that are monitored are readmission rates for patients who have had surgery, functional health status of patients after discharge (e.g., ability and time frame for returning to work), and the rate of infection after surgery. As a nurse, you will play an important role in gathering and analyzing quality outcome data.

More and more health care institutions are focused on improving processes as a way to improve. Many use strategies such as Six Sigma or value stream analysis. Six Sigma is a data-driven approach to process improvement that reduces variations in processes. It is a measure of quality (isixsigma, 2008). For example, the nursing unit sets up a project to collect data on the process of administering the first dose of an ordered chemotherapy. The audit reveals delays from getting the drug from the pharmacy to the nursing unit. Using Six Sigma, the collected data are analyzed and unnecessary steps in the process are identified. Based on this analysis, the process is streamlined to decrease time from ordering to administration. Value stream analysis is another method that focuses on improvement of processes through studying each step of a process to determine if the step does not add value and costs the health care organization time and resources (Burger, 2008). The aim is to eliminate unnecessary, costly steps.

Health plans throughout the United States rely on the Health Plan Employer Data and Information Set (HEDIS) as a quality measure. The National Committee for Quality Assurance (NCQA) created HEDIS as a tool to collect various data to measure the quality of care and services provided by different health plans. HEDIS compares how well health plans perform on 71 measures across 8 domains of care related to quality of care, access to care, and patient satisfaction (NCQA, 2008). The Joint Commission (2008) requires health care organizations to determine how well an organization meets patient needs and expectations. Organizations are using outcomes such as patient satisfaction as a basis to redesign how to manage and deliver care to improve quality.

PATIENT SATISFACTION Almost every major health care organization measures certain aspects of patient satisfaction. The Hospital Consumer Assessment of Healthcare Providers and Systems (HCAHPS) is a standardized survey developed to measure patient perceptions of their hospital experience (HCAHPS, 2008). HCAHPS was developed by the Center for Medicare and Medicaid Services and the Agency for Healthcare Research and Quality (AHRQ) as a way for hospitals to collect and report data publicly for comparison purposes. The survey has 27 questions that ask patients to respond about communication with nurses and physicians, responsiveness of hospital staff, pain management, communication about medications, discharge planning, cleanliness and quietness of the environment, overall satisfaction, and willingness to recommend the hospital (HCAHPS, 2008).

The Picker Institute (2008) has identified eight dimensions of **patient-centered care** (Box 2-7) that most affect patients' experiences with health care. The eight dimensions cover much of the scope of nursing practice. This is no surprise because nurses are involved in almost every aspect of a patient's care in a hospital. When you look closely, you see that most of the dimensions reflected in patient satisfaction apply to almost any health care setting.

The Picker Institute surveys patient satisfaction in all eight dimensions. The survey looks globally at patient perceptions of care in an attempt to understand how all hospital departments influence patient satisfaction. Like other companies that distribute patient satisfaction surveys, the Picker Institute mails surveys to patients. Staff involved in patient care receive the satisfaction scores as feedback regarding their success in meeting patient expectations. It is the responsibility of staff to identify the unique issues that influence patient satisfaction for their area. For example, nurses working on an oncology unit will have different patient satisfaction issues around physical comfort than nurses caring for new mothers. Patient satisfaction findings become the basis for many quality improvement studies.

It is important for you to recognize the need to identify patient expectations. The eight dimensions of care provide a useful guide. By learning early what a patient expects with regard to information, comfort, and availability of family and friends, you will plan better patient care. When do you ask about a patient's expectations? It will become a routine question when the patient first enters a health care setting, while care continues, and when a patient is ultimately discharged from your care. Patient expectations are an important measure of the evaluation of nursing care.

MAGNET RECOGNITION PROGRAM The American Nurses Credentialing Center (ANCC) established the Magnet Recognition Program to recognize health care organizations that achieve excellence in nursing practice (ANCC, 2008b). In the United States approximately 5% of health care organizations have achieved Magnet status (ANCC, 2008b). Health care organizations that decide to apply for Magnet status must demonstrate quality patient care, nursing excellence, and innovations in professional practice. The professional work environment must allow nurses to practice with a sense of empowerment and autonomy to deliver quality nursing care (Box 2-8). The newly developed Magnet model has five components that are affected by global issues that are challenging nursing today (ANCC, 2008a). The five components are Transformational Leadership; Structural Empowerment; Exemplary Professional Practice; New Knowledge, Innovation, and Improvements; and Empirical Quality Outcomes. Institutions achieve Magnet status through an appraisal process that requires them to present evidence showing achievement of the 14 "Forces of Magnetism" (Box 2-9). Magnet status requires nurses to collect data on specific nursing-sensitive quality indicators or outcomes and to compare their outcomes against a national, state, or regional database to demonstrate quality of care.

NURSING-SENSITIVE OUTCOMES **Nursing-sensitive outcomes** are changes in patients' symptom experiences, functional status, safety, psychological distress, and costs as a result of nursing interventions. Nurses assume accountability and responsibility for the consequences of these outcomes. Examples include pressure ulcers, restraint prevalence, and falls. The National Database of Nursing Quality Indicators (NDNQI) (Box 2-10, p. 32) was developed by the American Nurses Association to measure and evaluate nursing-sensitive outcomes with the purpose of improving patient safety and quality care (NDNQI, 2008). The NDNQI reports quarterly results on nursing outcomes at the nursing unit level. This provides a database for individual hospitals to compare their performance against nursing performance nationally (Kurtzman and Jennings, 2008). Chapter 6 describes approaches for measuring outcomes.

Nurses assume responsibility for a variety of outcomes that include individuals, family caregivers, the family, and the community. A research-based outcomes classification system, the Nursing Outcomes Classification (NOC), helps nurses better define and measure the impact of their interventions (Moorhead and others, 2008). NOC emphasizes patient out-

BOX 2-7   Principles of Patient-Centered Care

RESPECT FOR PATIENT'S VALUES, PREFERENCES, AND EXPRESSED NEEDS

- Patients expect you to treat them with dignity and respect.
- Patients want you to inform and involve them in decisions about their care.
- Patients' perceptions of needs should not be completely different from those identified by a care provider.
- A setting that respects the patient focuses on quality of life.

COORDINATION AND INTEGRATION OF CARE

- A competent and caring staff reduces patients' feelings of powerlessness.
- Patients look for someone to be in charge of care and to communicate clearly with other health team members.
- Patients look to have services and procedures well coordinated.
- Patients need to know at all times whom to call for help.

INFORMATION COMMUNICATION AND EDUCATION

- Patients expect to receive accurate and timely information about their clinical status, progress, or prognosis.
- Patients and families need to be informed of major changes in therapies or status.
- Patients need tests and procedures explained clearly in language they understand.
- Patients and family members want to know how to manage their own care.

PHYSICAL COMFORT

- Physical care that comforts patients is one of the most elemental services caregivers provide.
- Nurses need to respond in a timely and effective way to any request for pain medication, to explain the extent of pain for patients to expect, and to offer alternatives for pain management.
- Patients expect privacy and to have their cultural values respected.
- Patients often need help to complete activities of daily living.
- The health care setting environment needs to be clean and comfortable.

EMOTIONAL SUPPORT AND ALLEVIATION OF FEAR AND ANXIETY

- Patients look to care providers to help reduce anxiety and concerns about health status, medical treatment, and prognosis of illness.
- Patients need to understand the impact illness will have on their ability to care for themselves and their family.
- Patients worry about their ability to pay for their medical care. Are there staff members who will help with those concerns?

INVOLVEMENT OF FAMILY AND FRIENDS

- Care providers need to recognize, respect, and meet the needs of the patients' family and friends.
- Patients have the right to determine if they want family members involved in decisions about their care.
- Patients expect you to properly inform family or friends who will provide physical support and care after discharge.

CONTINUITY AND TRANSITION

- Patients want information about medications to take, dietary or treatment plans to follow, and danger signals to look for after hospitalization or treatment.
- Patients expect to have their continuing health care needs met after discharge with well-coordinated services.
- Patients and family members expect access to any necessary health care resources (e.g., social, physical, financial) after discharge.

ACCESS TO CARE

- Patients want to get to hospitals, clinics, and physicians' offices easily and without hassle.
- Patients need to be able to find transportation when going to different health care settings.
- Patients want to schedule appointments at convenient times without difficulty.
- Patients want to be able to go see a specialist when a referral is made.
- Patients expect to receive clear instructions on how to get referrals to other health care providers.

Data from Picker Institute: *Principles of patient-centered care,* 2008, http://www.pickerinstitute.org/about/about/html.

comes that nursing interventions affect most. However, all health care disciplines are able to use this system.

Because of the importance of nursing-sensitive outcomes, the AHRQ has funded several nursing research studies that looked at the relationship of nurse staffing levels to adverse patient outcomes. These studies found that higher levels of staffing by registered nurses (RNs) in hospitals were associated with fewer adverse patient outcomes. These studies also found that increased levels of nurse staffing positively affected nurse satisfaction. Future studies will evaluate the effect of nurse workload on patient safety and the relationship between nurses' working conditions and patient outcomes.

Other studies are investigating how nurses' working conditions affect medication safety. Measuring and monitoring nursing-sensitive outcomes will help you improve your patients' outcomes. Nurses and health care facilities use nursing-sensitive outcomes to improve nurses' workloads, enhance patient safety, and develop sensible policies related to nursing practice and health care.

Technology in Health Care

Technological advances are influencing health care organizations and changing where and how nurses provide care to patients (Vlasses and Smeltzer, 2007). Sophisticated equipment

BOX 2-8 BEST PRACTICES

Nurses' Work Environment

SUMMARY OF EVIDENCE

Excellence in the professional nursing practice environment is important to the achievement of Magnet Recognition status. The practice environments need to provide nurses autonomy and empowerment that allows them to provide quality patient care. It is also important to have a positive work environment because characteristics of the work environment have been shown to contribute to nursing job and life satisfaction, nursing turnover, and retention. Factors that contributed to the nurses' perception of a positive work environment are Magnet status of the hospital, increased level of education, experience, and type of unit. Positive work environments were perceived more often in Magnet hospitals, by nurses who had increased education, who had increased years of experience, and who worked in critical care areas where collaboration among health care workers was high. Other factors that were associated with a positive work environment included high levels of involvement of the nurses on the unit, high levels

of peer cohesion, high levels of collaboration, skilled communication, meaningful recognition programs for nurses, involvement of nurses in decision making at all levels, commitment of nurses to their job, and good support for the staff from the nursing manager through authentic leadership. Findings also showed that nurses who cared for themselves through adopting healthy behaviors had higher levels of satisfaction, which led to decreased job dissatisfaction and increased retention.

APPLICATION TO NURSING PRACTICE

- Attend seminars, workshops, and educational programs to increase your nursing knowledge base.
- Participate in your unit level committees and professional nursing shared governance programs.
- Develop a relationship with an experienced nurse to serve as your mentor as you begin your nursing career.
- Take care of yourself through good health promotion activities.

REFERENCES

American Association of Critical-Care Nurses: AACN standards for establishing and sustaining health work environments: a journey to excellence, *Am J Crit Care* 14(3):187, 2005.

Kotzer AM, Arellana K: Defining an evidence-based work environment for nursing in the USA, *J Clin Nurs* 17:1652, 2008.

Krebs JP, Madigan EA, Tullaie-McGuinness S: The rural nurse work environment and structural empowerment, *Policy Polit Nurs Pract* 9(1):28, 2008.

Nemcek MA, James GD: Relationships among the nurse work environment, self-nurturance and life satisfaction, *J Adv Nurs* 59(3):240, 2007.

Schmalenberg C, Kramer J: Types of intensive care units with the healthiest most productive work environments, *Am J Crit Care* 16(5):458, 2007.

Schmalenberg C, Kramer J: Essentials of a productive nurse work environment, *Nurs Res* 57(1):2, 2008.

BOX 2-9 Magnet Model and Forces of Magnetism

MAGNET MODEL COMPONENTS	FORCES OF MAGNETISM
Transformational Leadership—a vision for the future and the systems and resources to achieve the vision are created by nursing leaders	• Quality of Nursing Leadership • Management Style
Structural Empowerment—structures and processes provide an innovative environment where staff are developed and empowered and professional practice flourishes	• Organizational Structure • Personnel Policies and Programs • Community and the Health Organization • Image of Nursing • Professional Development
Exemplary Professional Practice—establishment of strong professional practice and demonstration of accomplishments of the practice	• Professional Models of Care • Consultation and Resources • Autonomy • Nurses as Teachers • Interdisciplinary Relationships
New Knowledge, Innovations and Improvements—contributions to the profession in the form of new models of care, use of existing knowledge, generation of new knowledge, and contributions to the science of nursing	• Quality Improvement
Empirical Quality Outcomes—focus on structure and processes and demonstration of positive clinical, workforce, patient, and organizational outcomes	• Quality of Care

Modified from American Nurses Credentialing Center: *A new model for ANCC's Magnet Recognition Program*, 2008a, http://www.nursecredentialing.org/Magnet/NewMagnetModel.

such as electronic IV infusion devices, cardiac telemetry equipment (a device that monitors a patient's heart rate wherever the patient is on a nursing unit), and electronic medical records are just a few examples changing the way providers deliver health care. In many ways, technological systems make your work easier, but they do not replace your judgment. For example, it is your responsibility when managing an IV infusion pump to monitor the device to be sure it infuses on time and without complications. An electronic infusion device provides a constant rate of infusion, but you must be sure you calculate the rate correctly. The device will set off an alarm if the infusion slows, making it important for you to respond to the alarm and to troubleshoot the problem. Technology does not replace a nurse's astute, critical eye and clinical judgment.

Computerized clinical information systems have replaced the traditional printed medical record. A comprehensive electronic record of a patient's medical problems, treatment, diagnostic procedures, and nursing care offers a rich source of information to clinicians who provide patient care. The health information system is decreasing health care costs by collecting and organizing data that provide valuable information for research and quality improvement activities (Vlasses and Smeltzer, 2007). For example, a nurse manager who wishes to track a nursing staff's progress in timely assessment of patients' pain is able to examine a database to review actual patient assessments and the time they occurred.

Documentation on a clinical information system minimizes free text entries and allows you to enter information quickly on specially designed flow sheets, pop-up screens, and nursing care plans. The computer displays important data in a way that allows you to follow your patient's progress and course easily. An electronic system does not make you less responsible for

---

BOX 2-10   NDNQI Nursing Quality Indicators

- Patient falls
- Patient falls with injury
- Pressure ulcers—community acquired, hospital acquired, unit acquired
- Staff mix
- Nursing hours per patient day
- RN surveys on job satisfaction and practice environment scale
- RN education and certification
- Pediatric pain assessment cycle
- Pediatric IV infiltration rate
- Psychiatric patient assault rate
- Restraint prevalence
- Nurse turnover
- Hospital-acquired infections of ventilator-associated pneumonia, central line–associated bloodstream infection, catheter-associated urinary tract infection

Data from National Database of Nursing Quality Indicators: *NDNQI: transforming data into quality care*, 2008, http://www.nursingquality.org.

IV, Intravenous; *RN*, registered nurse.

---

ensuring that you document clinical information about a patient accurately and completely in a timely manner. All members of the health care team usually are able to gain access to the electronic record; thus you have to make information accessible as soon as possible (see Chapter 9).

Globalization of Health Care

Globalization, the increasing interconnection of the world's economy, culture, and technology, is reshaping the health care delivery system (Oulton, 2007). Advances in communication, primarily through the Internet, allow nurses, patients, and other health care providers to talk with others worldwide about health care issues. Improved communication, easier air travel, and easing of trade restrictions are making it easier for people to engage in "health tourism." Health tourism is the travel to other nations to seek health care.

Many problems affect the health status of people around the world. For example, poverty is still deadlier than any disease and is the most frequently cited reason for death in the world today. Poverty increases the disparities in health care services among **vulnerable populations** (Crigger, 2008). Nations and communities that experience poverty have limited access to vaccines, clean water, and standard medical care. The growth of urbanization also is currently affecting the world's health. As cities become more densely populated, problems with pollution, noise, crowding, inadequate water, improper waste disposal, and other environmental hazards become more apparent. Children, women, and older adults are vulnerable populations most threatened by poverty and urbanization. As a nurse, you work toward improving the health of all populations (Crigger, 2008). Although globalization of trade, travel, and culture improves the availability of health care services, the spread of communicable diseases such as tuberculosis and severe acute respiratory syndrome (SARS) has become more common. Finally, the results of global environmental changes and disasters affect health. Changes in climate and natural disasters threaten food supplies and often allow infectious diseases to spread more rapidly (Simpson, 2004).

As a nurse, you need to understand how worldwide communication and globalization of health care affect your practice. Health care consumers demand quality and service and have become more knowledgeable. They often search the Internet about their health concerns and medical conditions. They also use the Internet to select their health care providers. As a result of globalization, it is necessary for physicians and health care providers to make their services more accessible. Because of advances in communication, nurses and other health care providers practice across state and national boundaries. Furthermore, there is currently a nursing shortage in health care institutions across the United States. In an effort to provide high-quality care, health care institutions are recruiting nurses from around the world to work in the United States. The hiring of nurses from other nations has forced U.S. hospitals to better understand and work with nurses from different cultures who have different needs (Nash and Gremillion, 2004).

Nursing's unique focus on caring helps nurses begin to address the issues presented by globalization. You and your fellow nurses will help overcome these issues by working together to improve nursing education throughout the world, by retaining nurses and recruiting people to be nurses, and by being advocates for changes that will improve the delivery of health care (Simpson, 2004). Be prepared for your future in health care. As a leader, you will need to take control of this situation and be proactive in developing solutions before someone outside of nursing takes control (Nash and Gremillion, 2004).

THE FUTURE OF HEALTH CARE

This discussion on the health care delivery system began with the issue of change. Change threatens many of us, but it also opens up opportunities for improvement. The ultimate issue in designing and delivering health care is the health and welfare of our population. Health care in the United States and around the world is not perfect. Many patients do not receive continuity of care when they see multiple health care providers. Many patients are uninsured or underinsured and are unable to gain access to necessary services. However, health care organizations are striving to become better prepared to deal with the challenges in health care. Many health care organizations are changing how they provide their services, reducing unnecessary costs, improving access to care, and trying to provide high-quality patient care. Professional nursing is an important player in the future of health care delivery. Finding the solutions necessary to improve the quality of health care depends on the active participation of nursing and the nursing community.

KEY POINTS

- Increasing costs and decreasing reimbursement are driving changes in health care, forcing health care institutions to deliver care more efficiently without sacrificing quality.
- In a managed care system, the provider of care receives a predetermined capitated payment regardless of services used by a patient.
- Levels of health care describe the scope of services and settings in which health care is offered to patients in all stages of health and illness.
- Occupational health nursing includes reducing exposure to environmental hazards, health education, and helping workers return to work safely.
- Successful community-based health programs involve building relationships with the community and incorporating cultural and environmental factors.
- Hospitalized patients are more acutely ill than in the past, requiring better coordination of services before discharge.
- Rehabilitation allows an individual to return to a level of normal or near-normal function after a physical or mental illness, injury, or chemical dependency.

- Nurse-managed clinics offer primary care delivered by advanced practice nurses with a focus on helping patients assume more responsibility for their health.
- Home care agencies provide almost every type of health care service with an emphasis on patient and family independence.
- Discharge planning begins at admission to a health care facility and helps in the transition of a patient's care from one environment to another.
- Health care organizations are evaluated on the basis of outcomes such as prevention of complications, patients' functional outcomes, and patient satisfaction.
- Consumers of health care should be guaranteed that services are provided by competent health care professionals.
- Nurses need to remain knowledgeable and proactive about issues in the health care delivery system to provide quality patient care and positively affect health.

CRITICAL THINKING EXERCISES

One day during gym class, Amy Sue starts to have more breathing problems than usual. Corrine decides that Amy Sue needs to see her physician today. Corrine calls and notifies Anne, Amy Sue's mother, of the change in Amy Sue's health and the need for medical treatment.

1. On the phone Anne states, "Our insurance company just switched from an exclusive provider organization (EPO) to a preferred provider organization (PPO)." How should Corrine explain the difference in the two plans to Amy Sue's mother?

2. Amy Sue's mother tells Corrine that the hospital they now have to use is a Magnet hospital. She tells Corrine she is not sure what that means. How should Corrine explain a Magnet hospital to Amy Sue and her mother?

Mary Reilly, Amy Sue's 65-year-old widowed grandmother, lives at home. She came to the emergency department and was hospitalized this morning because she experienced a stroke. Currently she has lost movement on her left side but was able to speak clearly. Mrs. Reilly is stabilized, and she was transferred to the general neurology unit. She is participating in occupational and physical therapy, but her left side continues to be weaker than the right, and she is having difficulty walking independently. The advanced practice nurse is hopeful that Mrs. Reilly will overcome her impaired physical mobility. However, Mrs. Reilly must be discharged from the hospital.

3. What type of discharge planning should be started at this time for Mrs. Reilly?

4. After several months, Mrs. Reilly returns home. A home care nurse visits her every other week to monitor her safety and continued progress at home. Which of the following will help Mrs. Reilly avoid future hospitalizations? Select all that apply.
   a. Medication education
   b. Explaining symptoms that indicate Mrs. Reilly should call her physician or health care provider immediately
   c. A pass to ride the city bus so Mrs. Reilly can get to her daughter's house
   d. Verification of Mrs. Reilly's current medication list and reconciliation of any discrepancies
   e. Food stamps

ⓔvolve   *Answers to Critical Thinking Questions can be found on the Evolve website.*

REVIEW QUESTIONS

1. Which health care activity is an example of primary care?
   1. A patient visits the emergency department following a fall at home.
   2. The home care nurse visits the patient twice a week for wound care.
   3. An older couple visits their physician for their annual influenza vaccine.
   4. A patient makes an appointment for routine screening mammography.

2. You are evaluating the work environment on a nursing unit. Which behavior is most indicative of a positive work environment?
   1. The nurse manager tells the nurses that the hospital has decided to have all nurses work 12-hour shifts.
   2. The unit nursing council meets regularly and presents changes in practice based on evidence to the unit.
   3. Each nurse is allowed to attend one education program a year.
   4. The nurse manager decided that the mentoring program was not working and discontinued the program.

3. You are caring for a hospitalized patient who requires transfer to a skilled nursing facility. Which of the following interventions **best** facilitates a referral to the skilled nursing facility?
   1. Provide instructions to the patient that will support the patient's independence and facilitate return to function.
   2. Provide options to the patient and family for possible skilled nursing facilities, and allow them to select the skilled nursing facility.
   3. Match the services provided at the skilled nursing facility with the patient's needs.
   4. Provide accurate information about the patient to the skilled nursing facility so the nurses at the facility will better understand the patient's needs.

4. Which of the following are examples of secondary acute care health services? Select all that apply.
   1. Setting an appointment with the nurse practitioner after having pregnancy confirmed
   2. Outpatient surgery for repair of inguinal hernia
   3. Repair of laceration of arm in the emergency department
   4. Attending the blood pressure screening fair at the mall
   5. Wound care done weekly by the home care nurse

5. As a nurse, you recognize which of the following patients to be a member of a vulnerable patient population?
   1. A single mother who is raising two adolescents
   2. An older adult who is unable to pay for monthly drug prescription costs
   3. A patient who has suffered a traumatic spinal cord injury and is unable to walk
   4. A cancer patient who has decided to undergo experimental treatment for his tumor

6. Which of the following persons is most likely to benefit from participation in respite care?
   1. Mr. Wilson, who was discharged last week with a new colostomy
   2. Mrs. Allen, who is the sole caregiver for her husband with Alzheimer's disease
   3. Mrs. Bradley, who is the mother of a 6-year-old child with asthma
   4. Mr. Hilliard, who has diabetes mellitus and a foot ulcer

7. Which of the following are examples of nursing-sensitive quality indicators or outcomes? Select all that apply.
   1. RN job satisfaction
   2. Catheter-associated urinary tract infections
   3. Pressure ulcers
   4. Influenza cases
   5. Patient falls
   6. Postoperative wound infections
8. A patient is receiving health care by a health care provider who is a salaried employee. Which type of managed care organization does the patient belong to?
   1. Group model
   2. Network model
   3. Independent practice association
   4. Staff model
9. A patient asks you about Medicare drug benefits. To help explain this benefit, you provide the patient with an information handout on which Medicare part?
   1. Part A
   2. Part B
   3. Part C
   4. Part D
10. A nurse working in primary care would work in which of the following settings?
   1. Hospice unit
   2. Intensive care unit
   3. Occupational health clinic
   4. Cardiac rehabilitation center

Answers to Review Questions can be found on pages 1197-1198.

REFERENCES

American Association of Critical-Care Nurses: AACN standards for establishing and sustaining healthy work environments: a journey to excellence, *Am J Crit Care* 14(3):187, 2005.

American Nurses Credentialing Center: *A new model for ANCC's Magnet Recognition Program*, 2008a, http://www.nursecredentialing.org/Magnet/NewMagnetModel.

American Nurses Credentialing Center: *Magnet program overview*, 2008b, http://www.nursecredentialing.org/ magnet/programOverview.html.

Berkowitz E: Medicare and Medicaid: the past as prologue, *Health Care Finance Rev* 27(2):11, 2005-2006.

Burger G: *The 5 whys: a simple tool in value stream analysis*, 2008, http://www.isixsigma.com/library/content/c070910a.asp.

Crigger NJ: Towards a viable and just global nursing ethics, *Nurs Ethics* 15(1):17, 2008.

Ebersole P and others: *Toward healthy aging: human needs and nursing response*, ed 7, St. Louis, 2008, Mosby.

Gold KS: Crossing the quality chasm: creating the ideal patient care experience, *Nurs Econ* 25(5):293, 2007.

Gosden T and others: Capitation, salary, fee-for-service and mixed systems of payment: effects on the behavior of primary care physicians, *Cochrane Database Syst Rev* 2005(3).

HCAHPS: *HCAHPS fact sheet (CAHPS Hospital Survey)*, 2008, http://www.hcahpsonline.org/facts.aspx.

Health Care Financing Administration, Department of Health and Human Services: Requirements for states and long term care facilities, 42 CFR 483 Subpart B (483.1-75), 2004, http://a257. g.akamaitech.net/7/257/2422/12feb20041500/edocket.access.gpo.gov/cfr_2004/octqtr/42cfr483.1.htm.

Hickman L and others: Best practice intervention to improve the management of older people in acute care settings: a literature review, *J Adv Nurs* 60(2):113, 2007.

Ingenix and others: *DRG expert*, ed 21, Clifton Park, NY, 2005, Thomson Delmar Learning.

Institute of Medicine: *Crossing the quality chasm: a new health system for the 21st century*, Washington, DC, 2001, National Academies Press.

Institute of Medicine: *Health professions education: a bridge to quality*, Washington, DC, 2003, National Academies Press.

Isixsigma: *What is Six Sigma?* 2008, http://www.isixsigma.com/sixsigma/six_sigma.asp.

Kotzer AM, Arellana K: Defining an evidence-based work environment for nursing in the USA, *J Clin Nurs* 17:1652, 2008.

Krebs JP, Madigan EA, Tullaie-McGuinness S: The rural nurse work environment and structural empowerment, *Policy Polit Nurs Pract* 9(1):28, 2008.

Kurtzman ET, Jennings BM: Trends in transparency: nursing performance measurement and reporting, *J Nurs Adm* 38(7/8):349, 2008.

Meiner SE, Lueckenotte A: *Gerontologic nursing*, ed 3, St. Louis, 2006, Mosby.

Melnyk BM, Fineout-Overholt E: *Evidence-based practice in nursing and healthcare: a guide to best practice*, Philadelphia, 2005, Lippincott Williams & Wilkins.

Merzel C, D'Afflitti J: Reconsidering community-based health promotion: promise, performance and potential, *Am J Public Health* 93(4):557, 2003.

Moorhead S and others: *Nursing outcomes classification (NOC)*, ed 4, St. Louis, 2008, Mosby.

Nash MG, Gremillion C: Globalization impacts the healthcare organization of the 21st century: demanding new ways to market product lines successfully, *Nurs Adm Q* 28(2):86, 2004.

National Center for Assisted Living: *Assisted living facility profile*, 2008, http://www.ncal.org/about/facility.cfm.

National Committee for Quality Assurance: *What is HEDIS?* 2008, http://www.ncqa.org/tabid/187/Default.aspx.

National Database of Nursing Quality Indicators: *NDNQI: transforming data into quality care*, 2008, http://www.nursingquality.org.

National Priorities Partnership: *National priorities and goals: aligning our efforts to transform America's healthcare*, Washington, DC, 2008, National Quality Forum.

Nemcek MA, James GD: Relationships among the nurse work environment, self-nurturance and life satisfaction, *J Adv Nurs* 59(3):240, 2007.

Nursing Home Abuse and Neglect Resource Center: *Federal regulations and nursing homes*, 2008, http://www.nursinghomealert.com/stoppingabuse/federalregulations.html.

Oodyke RJ: *Why is the integrated delivery network one of your keys to success in healthcare?* 2004, http://www.hcfi.net/040504.pdf.

Oulton J: Nursing in the international community: a broader view of nursing issues. In Mason DJ and others: *Policy and politics in nursing and health care*, St. Louis, 2007, Saunders.

Pew Health Professions Commission, The Fourth Report of the Pew Health Professions Commission: *Recreating health professional practice for a new century*, 1998, The Commission.

Picker Institute: *Principles of patient-centered care*, 2008, http://pickerinstitute.org/about/about/html.

Sackett DL and others: *Evidence-based medicine: how to practice and teach EBM*, London, 2000, Churchill Livingstone.

Schmalenberg C, Kramer J: Types of intensive care units with the healthiest most productive work environments, *Am J Crit Care* 16(5):458, 2007.

Schmalenberg C, Kramer J: Essentials of a productive nurse work environment, *Nurs Res* 57(1):2, 2008.

Simpson RL: No-borders nursing: how technology heals global ills, *Nurs Adm Q* 28(1):55, 2004.

Sorrentino S: *Mosby's textbook for nursing assistants*, ed 7, St. Louis, 2007, Mosby.

Spector N: *Evidence-based health care in nursing regulation*, 2005, http://www.ncsbn.org/pdfs/Evidencebased_NSpector.pdf.

Stanhope M, Lancaster J: *Community and public health nursing*, ed 6, St. Louis, 2004, Mosby.

Sultz HA, Young KM: *Health care USA: understanding its organization and delivery*, ed 5, Sudbury, Mass, 2006, Jones & Bartlett.

The Joint Commission: *Comprehensive accreditation manual for hospitals: the official handbook*, Oakbrook Terrace, Ill, 2008, The Commission.

Thompson JA, Lee V: The effect of health insurance disparities on the health care system, *AORN J* 86(5):745, 2007.

Tzeng H, Yin C: No safety, no quality: synthesis of research on hospital and patient safety (1996-2007), *J Nurs Care Qual* 22(4):229, 2007.

Vlasses FR, Smeltzer CH: Toward a new future for healthcare and nursing practice, *J Nurs Adm* 37(9):375, 2007.

3 Community-Based Nursing Practice

MEDIA RESOURCES

 CD COMPANION 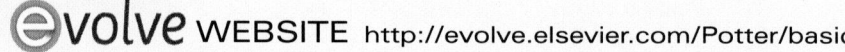 WEBSITE http://evolve.elsevier.com/Potter/basic

- Crossword Puzzle
- English/Spanish Audio Glossary

OBJECTIVES

- Explain the relationship between public health and community health nursing.
- Differentiate community health nursing from community-based nursing.
- Describe the role of the community health nurse.
- Discuss the role of the nurse in community-based practice.

- Explain the characteristics of patients from selected vulnerable populations that influence a nurse's approach to care.
- Describe selected competencies important for success in community-based nursing practice.
- Describe elements of a community assessment.

KEY TERMS

community-based nursing, p. 40
community health nursing, p. 39

incidence rates, p. 37
population, p. 39

public health nursing, p. 39

vulnerable populations, p. 41

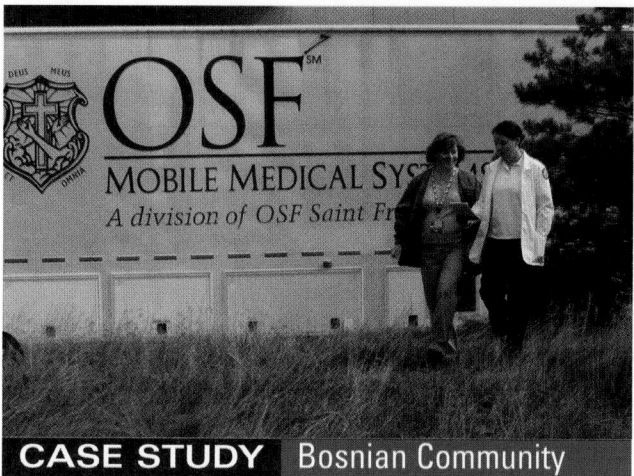

CASE STUDY Bosnian Community

Kim Callahan is a student in a community health nursing course. She is working in a community nursing service within a large city. The majority of patients in this agency are Bosnian immigrants. A major care initiative in this agency is to provide well-child examinations and immunizations to get the children ready to enter the public school system.

In addition, Kim and her classmates conducted an assessment of the community's health care needs and health care practices. This is a close community facing many challenges. Although there is an absence of chronic disease, there is a lack of general preventive health care practices. This includes routine immunizations, well-baby examinations, well-women examinations, and basic screenings for diabetes, hypertension, and cholesterol.

Community-based care focuses on health promotion, disease prevention, and restorative care. Because patients do not usually stay in acute care settings for a long time, there is a growing need to organize health care delivery services where people live, work, socialize, and learn. One way to achieve this goal is through a community-based health care model. Community-based health care is a collaborative, evidence-based model designed to meet the health care needs of the community (Downie, Ogilvie, and Wichmann, 2004). A healthy community includes elements that maintain a high quality of life and productivity. For example, safety and access to health care services are elements that enable people to function productively in their community (U.S. Department of Health and Human Services [USDHHS], 2001a). As community health care partnerships develop, nursing is in a strategic position to play an important role in health care delivery and to improve the health of the community.

The focus of health promotion and disease prevention is essential to the holistic practice of professional nursing. Throughout nursing's history, many nurses have established and met the public health goals of their patients and their families. Within community health settings, nurses are leaders in assessing, implementing, and evaluating the types of public and community health services their communities need. Community health nursing and community-based nursing are components or parts of health care delivery necessary to improve the health of the general public.

COMMUNITY-BASED HEALTH CARE

Community-based health care is a model of care that reaches everyone in the community, including the poor and underinsured. It focuses on primary rather than acute care and provides knowledge about health and health promotion. It occurs outside traditional health care institutions, such as hospitals and nursing homes. Community-based health care provides services for acute and chronic conditions to individuals and families within the community (Stanhope and Lancaster, 2006).

Today there are many challenges in community-based health. Social lifestyles, political policy, and economic ambitions have all influenced some of the major public health problems, including the following: an increase in sexually transmitted infections, environmental pollution, underimmunization of infants and children, and the appearance of pandemics or life-threatening diseases (e.g., swine flu, human immunodeficiency virus [HIV], and other emerging infections). More than ever before, the health care system needs a commitment to reform and bring attention to the health care needs of all communities.

Achieving Healthy Populations and Communities

The U.S. Department of Health and Human Services Public Health Service designed a program to improve the overall health status of people living in this country (see Chapter 1). The *Healthy People Initiative* was first created to establish ongoing health care goals (Figure 3-1). The overall goals of *Healthy People 2010* are to increase the life expectancy and quality of life and to eliminate health disparities through an improved delivery of health care services (USDHHS, 2001b).

Improved delivery of health care occurs through the assessment of the health care needs of individuals, families, or members of the community; development and implementation of public health policies; and improved access to care. Assessment includes systematic data collection about the population, monitoring the population's health status, and accessing information about the community (Stanhope and Lancaster, 2008). A systematic community assessment leads to community health programs, such as teen smoking cessation, exercise programs for school-aged children to reduce the risks for childhood obesity, and nutrition education for expectant mothers. In addition, the assessment helps to gather information on **incidence rates,** such as the identifying and reporting of new infections, determining adolescent pregnancy rates, and reporting the number of motor vehicle collisions by teenage drivers.

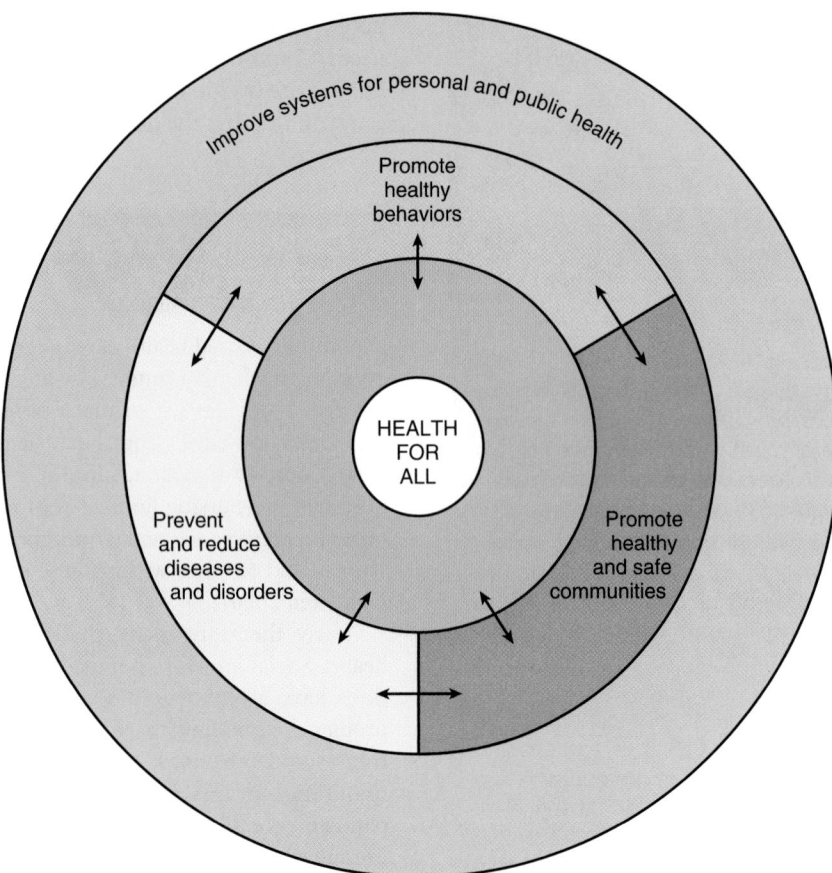

Figure 3-1 ■ *Healthy People 2010:* Healthy People in Healthy Communities. (From Stanhope M, Lancaster J: *Foundations of nursing in the community: community-oriented practice*, ed 2, St. Louis, 2006, Mosby.)

Community health professionals are involved in public policy development and implementation designed to improve the health of the community. Research-based findings help in designing and implementing policies. For example, data identify an increased incidence in motor vehicle collision fatalities when the driver is between 16 and 18 years old and driving after midnight. Community health professionals work with the legislature to develop driving restrictions for new teenage drivers to reduce motor vehicle fatalities.

Improved access to care ensures that essential community-wide health services are available and accessible to the total community (Stanhope and Lancaster, 2006). Examples include prenatal care and well-baby immunization programs for the uninsured. Population-based public health programs focus on disease prevention, health protection, and health promotion. This focus provides the foundation for health care services at all levels (see Chapter 2).

The five-level health services pyramid is an example of how to provide community-based services within the existing health care services in a community (see Figure 2-1, Chapter 2, p. 20). For example, a rural community has a hospital to meet the acute care needs of its patients. However, during a community assessment you notice that there are few services to meet the needs of expectant mothers, to reduce teenage smoking, or to provide nutritional support for older adults. Community-based programs that provide these services improve the health of the specific populations, as well as the population of the community. When the lower-level services are accessible and effective, there is a greater likelihood that the higher tiers will contribute to the total health of the community (U.S. Public Health Service, 1995/2000). For example, when mosquito control is inadequate, it becomes more difficult to enforce health promotion efforts and to prevent mosquito-borne diseases. On the other hand, when a community has the resources for providing childhood immunizations, primary preventive care services are able to focus on higher-tier services, such as child developmental problems and child safety.

The principles of public health practice focus on achieving a healthy environment for all individuals to live in. These principles apply to individuals, families, and the communities in which they live. Nursing plays a role in all levels of the health services pyramid. By using public health principles, you will be able to better understand the types of environments in which patients live and the types of interventions necessary to help keep patients healthy.

BOX 3-1 SYNTHESIS IN PRACTICE

 Many members of the Bosnian community are suspicious of the low cost and/or free care of the community agency and doubt that the examinations and results are confidential. One of the priorities of the community agency is to reach out to the community leaders to create an environment of trust and safety, which will hopefully lead to an increase use of the services. Kim is participating in these community meetings with her community nurse preceptor. These meetings will help explain the role of the community nurses in the delivery of care to the community and reinforce the privacy and confidentiality of the services provided.

Kim and her preceptor meet with community leaders to assess the beliefs and concerns of the community. Together they identify a lack of understanding in the community regarding health care practices in this country. In addition, the community has some misunderstandings and fear of health care services that the community agency and van provide.

Kim recognizes that members of this community came from a war-ravaged county where resources for health promotion were nonexistent. As a result, she understands the concerns and lack of understanding about community care and how this affects the use of services. She operates under the ethical principle of beneficence and wants to do the most good for the most people in this case. She respects the community's beliefs and their current level of health care knowledge. Kim wants to assist the community agency with meeting the health care needs of the Bosnian community.

If she views the community as a patient, Kim will focus her care on the total community. She continually assesses the community's knowledge and acceptance of the health care services provided. In addition, Kim identifies community leaders to serve as key persons or contacts in educational programs designed to meet the health care needs of the community. These programs will also help to change the community's misconceptions and fear of the services provided.

COMMUNITY HEALTH NURSING

Frequently you hear the terms *community health nursing* and *public health nursing* used interchangeably (SmithBattle, Diekemper, and Leander, 2004a, 2004b). There are some similarities. A **public health nursing** focus requires understanding the needs of a **population,** or a collection of individuals who have in common one or more personal or environmental characteristics (Stanhope and Lancaster, 2006). Examples of populations include high-risk infants, older adults, and a cultural group such as Native Americans.

Public health nurses understand factors that influence health promotion and health maintenance of groups. They also understand the trends and patterns influencing the incidence of disease within populations, environmental factors contributing to health and illness, and the political processes used to affect public policy. A public health nurse requires preparation at the basic entry level, and sometimes a public health nurse requires a baccalaureate degree in nursing that includes educational preparation and clinical practice in public health nursing. A specialist in public health is prepared at the graduate level with a focus in public health sciences (American Nurses Association [ANA], 2007).

Community health nursing is nursing care provided in the community, with the primary focus on the health care of individuals, families, and groups in the community. The goal is to preserve, protect, promote, or maintain health (Stanhope and Lancaster, 2006). The emphasis is on improving the quality of health and life within that community. In addition, the community health nurse provides direct care services to subpopulations within that community. These subpopulations are often a clinical focus in which the nurse has gained expertise. For example, a case manager follows older adults recovering from stroke and sees the need for community rehabilitation services, or a nurse practitioner gives immunizations to patients with the objective of managing communicable disease within the community. By focusing on subpopulations, the community health nurse cares for the community as a whole and considers the individual or family to be only one member of a group at risk.

Competence as a community health nurse requires the ability to use interventions that include the broad social and political context of the community (Stanhope and Lancaster, 2006). The educational requirements for entry-level nurses practicing in community health nursing roles are not as clear-cut as those for public health nurses. Not all hiring agencies require an advanced degree. However, nurses with a graduate degree in nursing who practice in community settings are community health nurse specialists, regardless of their public health experience (Stanhope and Lancaster, 2006).

Nursing Practice in Community Health

Community-focused nursing practice requires a unique set of skills and knowledge (Box 3-1). The expert community health nurse comes to understand the needs of a population or community through experiences with individual families and working through their social and health care issues. Critical thinking becomes important for the nurse, who applies knowledge of public health principles, community health nursing, family theory, and communication to find the best approaches in partnering with families (Eide and others, 2006). In a classic study, Diekemper, SmithBattle, and Drake (1999) interviewed community health nurses to hear their stories and to understand what population-focused practice involves. Often community health nurses see their practice evolve "naturally" as they serve families and communities. The best situation for this is when the working environment allows the nurse to work closely with members of the community.

Successful community health nursing practice involves building relationships with the community and responding to changes within the community (Diekemper and others, 1999; Ervin, 2007). For example, when there is an increase in the number of grandparents assuming child care responsibilities, establishing an educational program in cooperation with local schools assists and supports grandparents in this caregiving role.

The community health nurse becomes an active part of a community. This means knowing the community's members, needs, and resources and then working to establish effective health promotion and disease prevention programs. Community health nurses often work with highly resistant systems (e.g., welfare system) and encourage them to be more responsive to the needs of a population. Skills of patient advocacy, communicating people's concerns, and designing new systems in cooperation with existing systems help to make community nursing practice effective.

COMMUNITY-BASED NURSING

Community-based nursing care takes place in community settings such as the home or a clinic; however, the focus is nursing care of the individual or family (Feenstra, 2000). It involves acute and chronic care of individuals and families and enhances their ability for self-care and independent decision making (Stanhope and Lancaster, 2006). Use critical thinking and decision making for the individual patient and family—assessing health status, selecting nursing interventions, and evaluating outcomes of care. Because you will provide direct care services where patients live, work, and play, it is important that you know the diverse needs of the individual and family and appreciate the values of a multicultural community (Neuman, 2005). Through such knowledge,

community nursing practice provides a means to improve, protect, and enhance the quality of health of all who reside in a specific community (Sakamoto and Avilla, 2004).

Community-based nursing centers are the first level of contact between members of a community and the health care delivery system. Ideally, you will provide care close to the patient's residence. This approach helps to reduce the cost of care and improve access to health care services (Pastor, 2005).

Community-based nursing recognizes the interaction of the patient family unit within the community, both of which operate within the sociopolitical system (Figure 3-2). The patient exists within the larger systems of family, community, and society. The social interaction units seen in the figure depict three circles: the inner circle of the patient and family, the second circle of the local community and its values and policies, and the outer circle of larger social political systems, such as government, schools, and churches (Stanhope and Lancaster, 2008).

As a nurse in a community-based practice setting, you need to understand the interaction of all of the units while caring for your patients and their families. Usually you provide care for your patient in the area of the first two circles. For example, in your community practice clinical experience you are working with a home care nurse who has a patient newly diagnosed with diabetes. You work closely with the patient and family to create a comprehensive plan for the patient's health. As the nurse-patient relationship evolves, you begin to understand your patient's habits or lifestyle patterns. You learn how these change when the patient is with friends and co-workers. Knowing the community and available resources (e.g., medical supply shops for glucose monitoring supplies and local diabetes association support groups) helps you to provide comprehensive support for the patient's needs.

With the individual and family as patients, the context of community-based nursing is family-centered care within the community. This focus requires you to be knowledgeable

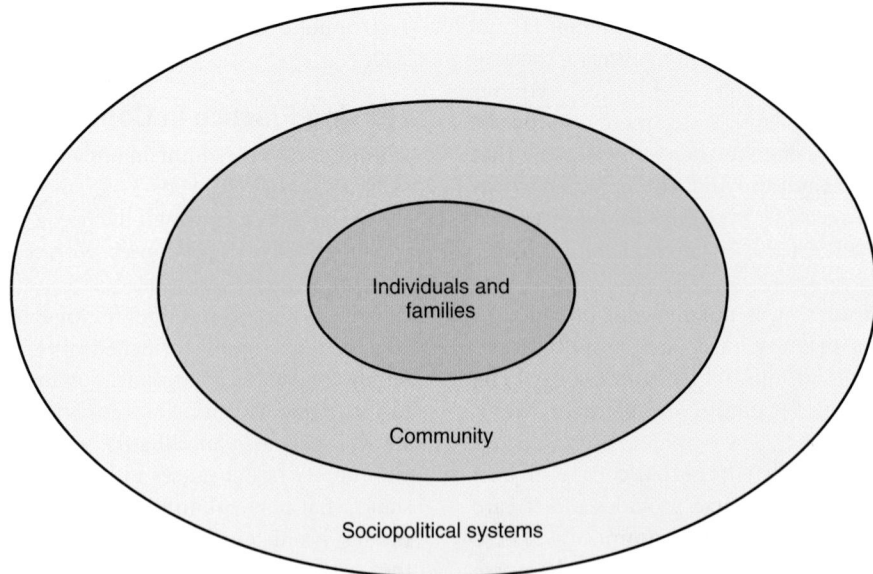

Figure 3-2 ■ Multilevel intervention. (From Stanhope M, Lancaster J: *Public health nursing,* ed 7, St. Louis, 2008, Mosby.)

about family theory (see Chapter 23); principles of communication (see Chapter 10), group dynamics, and cultural diversity (see Chapter 19). This knowledge helps you to partner with patients and families and to understand their health care needs. Ultimately you help your patients and their families assume responsibility for their health care decisions. The families become involved in planning, decision making, implementation, and evaluation of health care approaches.

Vulnerable Populations

In the community you will care for patients from diverse cultures and backgrounds and with various health conditions. However, changes in the health care delivery system have made high-risk groups the community health nurse's principal patients. For example, it is unlikely that you will visit low-risk mothers and babies. Instead, you are more likely to make home visits to adolescent mothers or mothers with substance abuse problems.

Vulnerable populations are groups of patients who are more likely to develop health problems as a result of excess risks. They are also likely to have limits in access to health care services and are usually dependent on others for care. Individuals living in poverty, older adults, homeless persons, individuals in abusive relationships, people who abuse chemical substances, people with mental illnesses, and new immi-

grants are examples of vulnerable populations (Shi and Stevens, 2007). Vulnerable individuals and their families often belong to more than one of these groups, and health care vulnerability affects all age-groups (Sebastian, 2006).

Frequently, vulnerable patients come from varied cultures, have different beliefs and values, face language barriers, and have few sources of social support (see Chapter 19). Their special needs create challenges for nurses in caring for increasingly complex acute and chronic health conditions. You need to determine their specific needs and community-appropriate interventions that will be successful in improving their level of health. Your communication skills and caring practices are critical in identifying and understanding your patients' perceptions of their problems and planning successful health care strategies.

Vulnerable populations typically experience poorer outcomes than those patients with ready access to resources and health care services (Haldenby, Berman, and Forchuk, 2007; Schanzer and others, 2007). It is important to learn your patients' strengths and resources for coping with stressors. Box 3-2 summarizes guidelines to follow when assessing members of vulnerable population groups. Although it is not the intent of this chapter to present all types of vulnerable populations and their health care needs, this section does present the vulnerabilities of selected populations: the im-

---

BOX 3-2 Guidelines for Assessing Members of Vulnerable Population Groups

SETTING THE STAGE
- Create a comfortable, nonthreatening environment.
- Obtain information about the culture so you have an understanding of their practices, beliefs, and values that affect their health care.
- Understand the meaning of the patient's language and nonverbal behavior to complete a culturally competent assessment (Chapter 19).
- Be sensitive to the fact that your patients often have priorities other than their health care. This includes financial, legal, or social issues. Help them with these concerns before you begin a health assessment.
- Work together with other health care and social need providers. If your patient needs financial assistance, consult a social worker. If there are legal issues, provide your patient with a resource. Do not attempt to provide financial or legal advice yourself.

NURSING HISTORY OF AN INDIVIDUAL OR FAMILY
- Because you often have only one opportunity to conduct a nursing history, obtain an organized history of all of the essential information you need to help the individual or family during that visit.
- Collect data on a comprehensive form that focuses on the specific needs of the vulnerable population with whom you work. However, remember to be flexible so that you do not overlook important health information. For example, if you are working with an adolescent

mother, obtain a nutritional history on both the mother and baby. Be aware of the developmental needs of the adolescent mom and listen to her social needs as well.
- Identify the patient's developmental needs, as well as health care needs. Remember, your goal is to collect enough information to provide family-centered care.
- Identify any risks to the patient's immune system. This is especially important for vulnerable patients who are homeless and sleep in shelters.

PHYSICAL EXAMINATION AND HOME ASSESSMENT
- It is important that you complete as thorough a physical and/or home assessment as possible. However, only collect data that you will use and is important to providing care to your patient and family.
- Be alert for signs of physical abuse or substance abuse (e.g., inadequately clothed to hide bruising, underweight, runny nose).
- Sharpen your observation skills when assessing your patient's home. Is there adequate water and plumbing? What is the status of the utilities? Are foods and perishables stored properly? Are there signs of insects or vermin? Look at the walls. Is the paint peeling? Are the windows and doors adequate? Are there water stains on the ceiling, evidence of a leaky roof? What is the temperature? Is it comfortable? What does the outside environment look like: Are there vacant houses/lots nearby? Is there a busy intersection? What is the crime level?

Modified from Stanhope M, Lancaster J: *Community and public health nursing,* ed 6, St. Louis, 2008, Mosby.

BOX 3-3   BEST PRACTICES

Health Care Needs and Practices of the Poor and Homeless

SUMMARY OF EVIDENCE

The populations of the poor and homeless are increasing, leading to an increase in their health care needs. The health care needs of the poor and homeless include chronic illnesses, emerging infections, human immunodeficiency virus (HIV), cancer risks, physical abuse, substance abuse, and mental health disorders. The newly homeless are at greatest risk for changes in health status. This is due to the struggle between residential instability and changes in their physical and/or mental status.

The homeless adolescent is usually without a nuclear family and has greater health care risks because of immaturity and risky behaviors. The adolescent alone has trouble coping with homelessness. However, newly homeless adolescents frequently maintain their prehomeless relationships. The continuation of these relationships is an important resource to maintain health and healthy practices, especially sexual practices, in this age-group. Females are at greater risk for threats to their physical safety. Males have more risky sexual behaviors and are less likely to use community health care resources.

Community health centers provide a health safety net for the poor and homeless population. Many of these centers provide primary and urgent care services. Within these community health centers, there are resources to determine the health care needs of the community, identify health education needs, and provide child care and parenting classes. These centers are successful when they assess for and respect the needs of the target community; provide safe, effective primary and urgent care services; and assist their patients to safe shelters or into transitional housing arrangements.

APPLICATION TO NURSING PRACTICE

- Prompt identification and assessment of the newly homeless assist in timely health and social interventions and enhances the chance for improved health status
- Obtain an ongoing, comprehensive listing of homeless shelters and transitional housing that is age and gender appropriate and know which resources to use to help a newly homeless person obtain placement in an appropriate residence.
- Provide access to "safe sex" behaviors (e.g. condom use, safe sex education, sexually transmitted infection, and HIV prevention).
- Identify existing prehomeless social relationships, and assist the individual in maintaining them.
- Work with the patient to identify his or her personal and social resources.

REFERENCES

Decker S and others: From the streets to assisted living: perceptions of a vulnerable population, *J Psychosoc Nurs Ment Health Serv* 44(6):18, 2006.

Haldenby AM, Berman H, Forchuk C: Homelessness and health in adolescents, *Qual Health Res* 17:1232, 2007.

Rew L and others: Interaction of duration of homelessness and gender in adolescent sexual health indicators, *J Nurs Scholarsh* 40:109, 2008.

Schanzer B and others: Homelessness, health status, and health care use, *Am J Public Health* 97:464, 2007.

Shi L, Stevens GD: The role of community health centers in delivering primary care to the underserved, *J Ambul Care Manage* 30(2):159, 2007.

migrant population, the poor and homeless, patients with mental illnesses, and older adults.

IMMIGRANT POPULATIONS The immigrant population is expected to continue to grow each year through 2050 (U.S. Census Bureau, 2008). This growth creates multiple health issues that lead to many health care needs and pose significant legal and health policy issues. For some immigrants access to health care is limited because of language barriers and lack of benefits, resources, and transportation. In addition, some immigrant populations have specific health care risks such as for hepatitis B, tuberculosis, and dental problems (Stanhope and Lancaster, 2006). Frequently the immigrant population practices nontraditional healing practices. It is important that you understand how these practices interfere with or complement traditional therapies.

Because some immigrant populations left their homes as a result of political oppression, war, or natural disaster, it is important to be sensitive to the physical, psychological, and safety needs of the population. Help the community identify and use appropriate resources when providing culturally sensitive health care to an immigrant population.

POOR AND HOMELESS PERSONS People who live in poverty are more likely to live in hazardous or dangerous environments, work at high-risk jobs, eat less-nutritious diets, and have multiple stressors in their lives (Box 3-3). Patients with low income levels not only lack financial resources, but also sometimes live in poor environments and face practical problems such as poor or unavailable transportation.

Homeless patients have even fewer resources than the poor. They are usually jobless, do not have the advantage of shelter, and must cope with finding a place to sleep at night and finding food. Chronic health problems worsen because they do not get nutritious meals and have no place to store medications, if they can afford them. In addition, they lack a healthy balance of rest and activity because of walking throughout the day to meet basic needs (Schanzer and others, 2007). In the community setting it is important that you help these patients identify available resources, eligibility for assistance, and interventions to improve their health status.

PERSONS WITH MENTAL ILLNESS You need to explore health and socioecomic problems when caring for patients with mental illnesses such as depression, bipolar disorder, and personality disorders (e.g., schizophrenia, obsessive-compulsive, antisocial). When a patient suffers from a pervasive mental illness, the illness affects many aspects of the patient's life and requires medication therapy, counseling,

TABLE 3-1	Major Health Problems in Older Adults and Community Health Nursing Roles and Interventions
PROBLEM	**COMMUNITY HEALTH NURSING ROLES AND INTERVENTIONS**
Hypertension	Monitor blood pressure and weight; educate about nutrition and antihypertensive drugs; teach stress management techniques; promote a good balance between rest and activity; establish blood pressure screening programs; assess patient's current lifestyle and promote lifestyle changes; promote dietary modifications by using techniques such as a diet diary.
Cancer	Obtain health history; promote monthly breast self-examinations and yearly Pap smears and mammograms for older women; promote regular physical examinations; encourage smokers to stop smoking; correct misconceptions about processes of aging; provide emotional support and quality of care during diagnostic and treatment procedures.
Arthritis	Educate adult about management of activities, correct body mechanics, availability of mechanical appliances, and adequate rest; promote stress management; counsel and assist the family to improve communication, role negotiation, and use of community resources; help adult avoid the false hope and expense of arthritis fraud.
Visual impairment (e.g., loss of visual acuity, eyelid disorders, opacity of the lens)	Provide support in a well-lighted, glare-free environment; use printed aids with large, well-spaced letters; assist adult with cleaning eyeglasses; help make arrangements for vision examinations and obtain necessary prostheses; teach adult to be cautious of false advertisements.
Hearing impairment (e.g., presbycusis)	Speak with clarity at a moderate volume and pace, and face audience when performing health teaching; help make arrangements for hearing examination and obtain necessary prostheses; teach adult to be cautious of false advertisements.
Cognitive impairment	Provide complete assessment; correct underlying causes of disease (if possible); provide for a protective environment; promote activities that reinforce reality; assist with personal hygiene, nutrition, and hydration; provide emotional support to the family; recommend applicable community resources such as adult day care, home care aides, and homemaker services.
Alzheimer's disease	Maintain high-level functioning, protection, and safety; encourage human dignity; demonstrate to the primary family caregiver techniques to dress, feed, and toilet adult; provide frequent encouragement and emotional support to caregiver; act as an advocate for patient when dealing with respite care and support groups; protect the patient's rights; provide support to maintain family members' physical and mental health; maintain family stability; recommend financial services if needed.
Dental problems	Perform oral assessment and refer to dentist as necessary; emphasize regular brushing and flossing, proper nutrition, and dental examinations; encourage patients with dentures to wear and take care of them; calm fears about dentist; help provide access to financial services (if necessary) and to dental care facilities.
Drug use and abuse	Get drug use history; educate adult about safe storage, risks for drug, drug-drug, and drug-food interactions; give general information about drug (e.g., drug name, purpose, side effects, dosage); instruct adult about presorting techniques (using small containers with one dose of drug that are labeled with specific times to take drug).
Substance abuse	Arrange and monitor detoxification if appropriate; counsel adults about substance abuse; promote stress management to avoid need for drugs or alcohol; encourage adult to use self-help groups such as Alcoholics Anonymous and Al-Anon; educate public about dangers of substance abuse.

Data from Stanhope M, Lancaster J: *Community and public health nursing*, ed 7, St. Louis, 2008, Mosby; Baas LD and others: The challenge of managing the care of older heart transplant recipients, *AACN Clin Issues* 13(1):114, 2002; Hwang SW: Mortality among men using homeless shelters in Toronto, Ontario, *JAMA* 283(16):2152, 2000; Hwang SW, Bugeja AL: Barriers to appropriate diabetes management among homeless people in Toronto, *Can Med Assoc J* 163(2):161, 2000.

housing, and vocational assistance. Many patients with pervasive mental illnesses are homeless or have poor housing. Others lack the ability to maintain employment or to even care for themselves on a daily basis (Cunningham, McKenzie, and Taylor, 2006). In addition, these patients are at greater risk for abuse and assault (Eckert, Sugar, and Fine, 2002).

Patients who are mentally ill are no longer routinely hospitalized in long-term psychiatric institutions. Instead, the goal is to offer resources within their community. Although comprehensive service networks are in every community, many patients with mental illnesses still go untreated or they are left with fewer and more fragmented services, with little skill in surviving and functioning within the community. Collaboration with multiple community resources is a key to helping people with pervasive mental illnesses receive adequate health care.

OLDER ADULTS Because people are living longer, there is an increase in the older adult population. This means more patients suffer from chronic diseases and there is a greater demand for health care services provided in a community setting (Table 3-1). Successful disease management and symptom control of chronic conditions helps patients to maintain or increase their quality of life. For the older adult population it is important to view health promotion and disease management within a broad context. This begins with your understanding of what health means to older adults and the steps they can take to maintain their own health.

COMPETENCY IN COMMUNITY-BASED NURSING

A nurse in community-based practice needs a variety of skills and talents to be successful. In addition to assisting patients with their health care needs and developing relationships within the community, the community health nurse needs skills in health promotion, disease prevention, and caring for the community's health. Use the nursing process and a critical thinking approach (see Chapters 7 and 8) to ensure individualized nursing care for specific patients and their families. As a student, your clinical practice in a community-based care setting will probably be in partnership with a community nurse. This section will provide you information about selected competencies, such as caregiver, case manager, and educator, used in the community-based setting. You will have an opportunity to observe some of these competencies.

Caregiver

Most important is the caregiving role. In the community setting you manage and care for the community. Using the nursing process and critical thinking skills, develop appropriate, individualized nursing care for specific patients and their families. In addition, you individualize care within the context of the patient's community to achieve long-term successful health outcomes. Work with the patient and family to develop a caring partnership to recognize actual and potential health care needs and identify needed community resources. As a caregiver, you also help build a healthy community that is safe and helps the population achieve and maintain an improved quality of life and optimal health status.

Case Manager

In community-based practice, case management is an important competency. Case management means making an appropriate plan of care based on assessment of patients and families and coordinating needed resources and services for the patient's well-being across a continuum of care (see Chapter 2). Generally, a community-based case manager assumes responsibility for the case management of multiple patients. This usually involves patients who need coordination of different health care services (e.g., patients with neurological disease, patients who have experienced trauma, patients with mental illnesses, and patients with complex medical conditions). The greatest challenge is coordinating the activities of many different providers and payers, in different settings, throughout a patient's continuum of care. An effective case manager eventually anticipates obstacles and opportunities that exist within the community that will influence the ability to find solutions for the patient's and family's needs. Case management with individual patients and families reveals the overall picture of health services and the health status of a community.

Educator

Community-based nurses teach their patients individually or in groups. With the goal of helping patients assume responsibility for their own health care, the role of educator is important in a community-based setting. Patients and families need to acquire certain knowledge and skills to care for themselves (see Chapter 11). The community-based nurse assesses a patient's learning needs and readiness to learn, adapts teaching skills to instruct within the home setting, and makes the learning process meaningful. You assess learning by reviewing skills, following up with phone calls, and referring the patient to community support and self-help groups. Evaluation of patient learning occurs over time, requiring patience and commitment.

COMMUNITY ASSESSMENT

When practicing in a community setting, it is important for you to learn how to assess the community at large. Community assessment requires you to systematically collect data about a population to allow you to monitor the population's health status and make information available about the health of the community (Stanhope and Lancaster, 2006). This is the environment in which your patients live and work. Without an adequate understanding of that environment, any effort to promote the patient's health and to institute necessary change is unlikely to be successful. The community has three components or parts: structure or locale, the people, and the social systems. A complete assessment involves a careful look at each component to begin to identify needs for health policy, health program development, and service provision (Box 3-4).

When assessing the structure or locale, travel around the neighborhood or community and observe its design, the location of services, and the locations where residents meet. A public library or the local health department is a great source for accessing statistics to assess the demographics of the community. To get information about existing social systems, such as schools or health care facilities, visit various sites and learn about their services.

Once you have a good understanding of the community, perform individual patient assessments against that background (Box 3-5). For example, you are assessing a patient's home for safety. Does the patient have secure locks on doors? Are windows secure and intact? Is lighting along walkways and entryways working? As you conduct the assessment, be aware of the level of community violence and the resources that are available to the patient when help is necessary. No individual patient assessment should occur in isolation from the environment and conditions of the patient's community.

BOX 3-4   Community Assessment

STRUCTURE
- Name of community or neighborhood
- Geographical boundaries
- Emergency services
- Water and sanitation
- Housing
- Economic status (e.g., average household income, number of residents on public assistance)
- Availability of public transportation system

POPULATION
- Age distribution
- Gender distribution
- Growth trends
- Density
- Educational level
- Predominant ethnic groups
- Predominant religious groups

SOCIAL SYSTEM
- Educational system
- Government
- Communication system
- Welfare system
- Volunteer programs
- Health system

BOX 3-5   EVALUATION

Kim spent the last 12 weeks working with the community agency and leaders in the Bosnian community. The goal was to provide educational programs to explain how the clinic provides services and the confidentiality of the services. The program also explained the fact that the services were low cost and/or free to patients without adequate insurance or financial resources. Kim presented a series of three programs in the homes of four Bosnian leaders. Kim worked with the leaders on the design of the educational programs and continued to evaluate the community's response to the programs and health care needs. Throughout this period there was a gradual increase in the use of the services within the agency. In addition, young women within the community asked for prenatal classes.

Kim perceived a greater acceptance within the community. After the first 3 weeks following Kim's class, there were fewer "missed" appointments, and the members of the community shared more relevant health care concerns with her. Finally, Kim felt a sense of confidence and competence in developing community health care programs. She learned the importance of including the community and the community leaders in all aspects of program building from the assessment of needs through program development and evaluation.

CHANGING PATIENTS' HEALTH

In community-based practice you will care for patients from diverse backgrounds and in diverse settings. It is relatively easy over time to become familiar with the resources that are available within a particular community practice setting. With practice you learn how to identify the unique needs of individual patients. However, the challenge is how to promote and protect a patient's health within the context of the community. Can a patient with lung disease, for example, have the quality of life necessary when the patient's community has a serious environmental pollution problem? Likewise, it is important to bring together the resources necessary to improve the continuity of care that patients receive. Be a leader in reducing the duplication of health care services and locating the best services for a patient's needs.

Perhaps the most important theme for an effective community-based nurse is to understand patients' lives. This begins when you are able to establish strong, caring relationships with patients and their families (see Chapter 18). This is a challenge when you have little time available to spend with patients. However, as your expertise grows, you are able to advise, counsel, and teach effectively. As you gain an understanding of the needs of the community, you also gain an awareness of what truly makes your patients unique. The day-to-day activities of family life are the variables that influence how you adapt your nursing interventions. Here are a few examples of factors you will consider in community-based practice: the time of day a patient goes to work, the availability of the spouse and patient's parents to provide child care, and the family values that shape views about health. Once you acquire a picture of a patient's life, you introduce interventions to promote health and prevent disease so that the picture becomes enhanced.

KEY POINTS

- The principles of public health nursing practice focus on helping individuals acquire a healthy environment in which to live.
- Essential public health functions include assessment, policy development, and access to resources.
- When population-based health care services are effective, there is a greater likelihood of the higher tiers of services contributing efficiently to health improvement of the population.
- The community health nurse considers the individual or family to be only one member of a group while providing care to the community as a whole.

- A successful community health nursing practice involves building relationships with the community and being responsive to changes within the community.
- The special needs of vulnerable populations form the backdrop for the challenges nurses face in caring for patients' increasingly complex acute and chronic health conditions.
- Chronic health problems are common and worsen among the homeless because they have few resources.
- Essential competencies for a community-based nurse include caregiving, case management, and patient education.
- Assessment of a community includes three elements: structure or locale, the people, and the social systems.

CRITICAL THINKING EXERCISES

Within the Bosnian community there are many single-parent families, usually widows with school-age children. One of the families that Kim met is composed of Katrina Dudek, a 30-year-old widow, and her two children, a 6-month-old and a 3-year-old. Mrs. Dudek arrived in the community 5 months ago. Her husband was killed in a raid in their home in her native country. She is very fearful when anyone other than her close neighbors and friends enter her home. Kim and the community health nurse work with Mrs. Dudek to determine the health care needs of her children and herself. To date the community health agency has not been successful in providing well-child care or immunizations to a large part of the community or any care to Mrs. Dudek

and her children. Kim and Mrs. Dudek talk about the need to have her children immunized and set that as a goal.

1. What information does Kim need about this Bosnian community?
2. What key element would be helpful for initiating care for this family?
3. Mrs. Dudek is fearful about providing an immunization history about her children. What should be Kim's action?
4. What factors within her community increase Mrs. Dudek's vulnerability to health care problems?

evolve   *Answers to Critical Thinking Questions can be found on the Evolve website.*

REVIEW QUESTIONS

1. When health care is provided in a community-based practice setting, the overall goal of *Healthy People 2010* is to:
   1. Assess the health care needs of individuals, families, and communities
   2. Develop and implement public health policies and improve access to care
   3. Gather information on incidence rates of certain diseases and social problems
   4. Increase life expectancy and quality of life and to eliminate health disparities
2. Community health nursing is a nursing approach that merges knowledge from professional nursing theories and which of the following? Select all that apply.
   1. Population sciences
   2. Public health sciences
   3. Environmental sciences
   4. Mental health sciences

3. You are caring for an immigrant community. During a community assessment you identify that the children are undervaccinated. In addition, you note that there is a health clinic within a 5-mile radius. You meet with the community leaders and explain the need for immunizations, the location of the clinic, and the process for accessing health care resources. Together you and the community leaders develop a plan for improving the rate of vaccinations. Which of the following practices are you providing? Select all that apply.
   1. Educating about community resources
   2. Teaching the community about illnesses
   3. Promoting autonomy and decision making
   4. Improving the health care of the community's children
4. A patient has a history of asthma with six hospitalizations over the past 2 years. She tries to control her illness and appropriately uses her inhalers and other prescribed medications. What level of prevention corresponds to her disease management?
   1. Primary prevention
   2. Secondary prevention
   3. Tertiary prevention
   4. Health promotion

5. Vulnerable populations are those who are more likely to develop health problems as a result of:
   1. Chronic diseases, homelessness, and poverty
   2. Poor nutrition and being dependent on others for transportation
   3. Excess risks and increased rates of smoking cigarettes
   4. Limited access to health care and lack of transportation

6. Major health care problems in older adults in community settings include:
   1. Polypharmacy, sensory loss, and chronic illness
   2. Acute illness and abandonment
   3. Poverty and inadequate support systems
   4. Acute illness, inadequate support systems, and poverty

7. Which of the following information categories is not part of a community system?
   1. The structure of the community
   2. The population of the community
   3. The social system of the community
   4. Building codes of the community

8. A high school in the community has an increase in the number of adolescent parents. You work with the school district to design and teach classes about infant care, child safety, and time management. This an example of which community nursing competency?
   1. Caregiver
   2. Case manager
   3. Consultant
   4. Educator

9. What three elements do you need to include in a community assessment?
   1. Individuals and families, community, and sociopolitical system
   2. People, neighborhoods, and social systems
   3. Geographical boundary, neighborhoods, and social systems
   4. Geographical boundary, health care systems, and political systems

10. Following a community assessment, you identify an area of increased respiratory illnesses. It is near an industrial park. The community asks you to come and speak about industrial risks associated with respiratory disease and how the community can reduce these risks. This is an example of which competencies? Select all that apply.
    1. Caregiver
    2. Case manager
    3. Consultant
    4. Educator

Answers to Review Questions can be found on pages 1197-1198.

REFERENCES

American Nurses Association: *Public health nursing scope and standards of practice*, Washington, DC, 2007, The Association.

Baas LD and others: The challenge of managing the care of older heart transplant recipients, *AACN Clin Issues* 13(1):114, 2002.

Cunningham P, McKenzie K, Taylor EF: The struggle to provide community-based care to low-income people with mental illnesses, *Health Affairs* 25(3):694, 2006.

Decker S and others: From the streets to assisting living: perceptions of vulnerable population, *J Psychosoc Nurs Ment Health Serv* 44(6):18, 2006.

Diekemper M, SmithBattle L, Drake MA: Bringing the population into focus: a natural development in community health nursing practice, part I, *Public Health Nurs* 16:3, 1999.

Downie J, Ogilvie S, Wichmann H: A collaborative model of community health nursing, *Contemp Nurse* 20:180, 2004.

Eckert LO, Sugar N, Fine D: Characteristics of sexual assault in women with a major psychiatric diagnosis, *Am J Obstet Gynecol* 186(6):1284, 2002.

Eide PJ and others: The population focused analysis project for teaching community health, *Nurs Educ Perspect* 27(1):22, 2006.

Ervin NE: Clinical specialist in community health nursing: advanced practice fit or misfit? *Public Health Nurs* 24(5):458, 2007.

Feenstra C: Community based and community focused: nursing education in community health, *Public Health Nurs* 17(3):165, 2000.

Haldenby AM, Berman H, Forchuk, C: Homelessness and health in adolescents, *Qual Health Res* 17:1232, 2007.

Hwang SW: Mortality among men using homeless shelters in Toronto, Ontario, *JAMA* 283(16):2152, 2000.

Hwang SW, Bugeja AL: Barriers to appropriate diabetes management among homeless people in Toronto, *Can Med Assoc J* 163(2):161, 2000.

Neuman DM: A community nursing center for the health promotion of senior citizens based on the Neuman Systems Model, *Nurs Educ Perspect* 26:221, 2005.

Pastor DK: An action plan for community hospice nurse leaders, *J Hosp Pall Nurs* 7:107, 2005.

Rew L and others: Interaction of duration of homelessness and gender in adolescent sexual health indicators, *J Nurs Scholarsh* 40:109, 2008.

Sakamoto SD, Avilla A: The public health nursing practice manual: a tool for public health nurses, *Public Health Nurs* 21(2):179, 2004.

Schanzer B and others: Homelessness, health status, and health care use, *Am J Public Health* 97:464, 2007.

Sebastian JG: Vulnerability and vulnerable populations: an overview. In Stanhope M, Lancaster J: *Foundations of nursing in the community: community oriented practice*, ed 2, St. Louis, 2006, Mosby.

Shi L, Stevens GD: The role of community health centers in delivering primary care to the underserved, *J Ambul Care Manage* 30(2):159, 2007.

SmithBattle L, Diekemper M, Leander S: Getting your feet wet: becoming a public health nurse, part I, *Public Health Nurs* 21(1):3, 2004a.

SmithBattle L, Diekemper M, Leander S: Moving upstream: becoming a public health nurse, part II, *Public Health Nurs* 21(2):95, 2004b.

Stanhope M. Lancaster J: *Public health nursing*, ed 7, St. Louis, 2008, Mosby.

Stanhope M, Lancaster J: *Foundations of nursing in the community: community-oriented practice*, ed 2, St. Louis, 2006, Mosby, http://www.us.elsevierhealth.com/product.jsp?isbn59780323066556

U.S. Census Bureau: *Immigration*, updated April 2008, http://www.census.gov/popest/estimates.php, accessed June 2008.

U.S. Department of Health and Human Services, Public Health Service: *Healthy people in healthy communities: a community planning guide using Healthy People 2010*, Office of Disease Prevention and Health Promotion, Office of Public Health and Science, Department of Health and Human Services, 2001a, http://www.healthypeople.gov/Publications/HealthyCommunities2001/default.htm, accessed June 18, 2008.

U.S. Department of Health and Human Services, Public Health Service: *Healthy People 2010: a systematic approach to health improvement*, Washington, DC, 2001b, U.S. Government Printing Office, http://www.healthypeople.gov/implementation, accessed June 18, 2008.

U.S. Public Health Service: *The Core Functions Project*, Washington, DC, 1995/2000, Office of Disease Prevention and Health Promotion.

4 Legal Principles in Nursing

MEDIA RESOURCES

 CD COMPANION 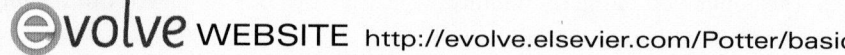 WEBSITE http://evolve.elsevier.com/Potter/basic

- Crossword Puzzle
- English/Spanish Audio Glossary

OBJECTIVES

- Describe the legal obligations and role of nurses regarding federal and state laws that affect health care.
- Explain the legal concepts of standard of care and informed consent.
- List sources for standards of care for nurses.
- Explain the concept of negligence and identify the elements of professional negligence.

- Define the legal relationships of nurse-patient, nurse–health care provider, nurse-nurse, and nurse-employer.
- Identify nursing interventions to improve patient safety.

KEY TERMS

assault, p. 50
battery, p. 50
common law, p. 49
criminal law, p. 49
defendant, p. 50
felony, p. 50
Good Samaritan laws, p. 52

informed consent, p. 53
intentional torts, p. 50
living wills, p. 55
malpractice, p. 50
misdemeanor, p. 50
negligence, p. 50

never events, p. 52
Nurse Practice Acts, p. 49
occurrence report/ incident report, p. 52
plaintiff, p. 50
power of attorney for health care, p. 55

regulatory agencies, p. 49
risk management, p. 52
standard of care, p. 50
statutory law, p. 49
tort, p. 50

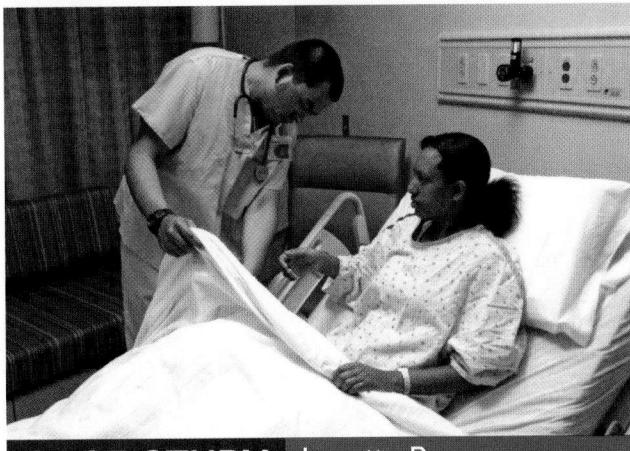

CASE STUDY Lynette Donovan

Lynette Donovan, a 15-year-old female African American, was a passenger in a motor vehicle collision and is now admitted to the hospital with a fractured right femur. The emergency department health care provider applied a cast to the affected leg with insufficient padding. Lynnette told the nurses that her right leg felt numb, was swollen, and looked discolored. The nurses recognized that these symptoms indicated impaired circulation in the extremity with the cast. The nurses were unable to reach Lynette's health care provider despite several calls. The nurses have not notified the nursing supervisor of the patient's situation.

David Ortiz is a 23-year-old nursing student newly assigned to the nursing division and to Miss Donovan. His initial assessment notes that the patient's right leg is swollen, slightly blue, and slightly malodorous. Lynette seems very anxious and upset.

Darling v. Charleston Community Memorial Hospital, 33 Ill.2d 326, 331, 211 N.E.2d 253 (1965).

Safe and competent nursing care includes critical thinking skills and an understanding of the legal boundaries within which you will practice. Frequently nurses practice under several sources and jurisdictions of health care law simultaneously. In addition to understanding the federal laws that apply to health care, it is also important to know the law in your own state and the rules and regulations of your state's **regulatory agencies.** Nurses' familiarity with the law enhances their ability to be patient advocates. If you have specific questions, consult with your own attorney or with your employing institution's attorney.

LEGAL LIMITS OF NURSING

An understanding of the law coupled with sound judgment helps to ensure safe and appropriate nursing care. You need to understand the legal limits or standards that affect nursing practice to know your responsibilities as a nurse and to protect patients from harm.

Sources of Law

Laws that apply to nursing practice today originally derived from two sources: common law and statutory laws. **Common laws** are based on judicial decisions or case law precedent, whereas **statutory laws** are rules codified by legislative bodies of government (Garner, 2006; Martin, 2006; Wacks, 2008). An example of a judicial decision that guides health care practice is *Roe v. Wade* (410 U.S. 113, 1973), in which the U.S. Supreme Court identified time periods in which elective termination of a pregnancy is legal. Statutory laws are frequently made following judicial decisions at the federal or state level. An example of a federal statute that affects health care practice is the Americans with Disabilities Act (ADA), which protects the rights of handicapped individuals (ADA, 1995). **Nurse Practice Acts** are examples of statutes enacted by state legislatures to regulate the practice of nursing. The Nurse Practice Acts of each state define the scope of nursing practice and expanded nursing roles, set educational requirements for nurses, and distinguish between nursing practice and medical practice. Nurse Practice Acts establish a regulatory agency (Martin, 2006), such as the State Board of Nursing, which uses the principles of administrative law (Garner, 2006) to guide the regulation of nursing practice. Nurse Practice Acts permit the State Board of Nursing to set rules, regulations, and guidelines that specifically define the standard of care in nursing practice. An example is the guidelines a nurse uses to avoid patient abandonment (Missouri State Board of Nursing Position Statement, 2006). To practice nursing, you must be licensed by the State Board of Nursing of the state in which you wish to practice. To be licensed in your state, you must have a passing score on the National Council Licensure Examination (NCLEX®) to obtain your initial license and meet the educational requirements set by the state. Many states require obtaining continuing education units for relicensure.

The State Board of Nursing has the power to suspend or revoke a nurse's license if the nurse's conduct violates provisions of the licensing statute. Criminal law violations, even if unrelated to nursing, may jeopardize your license status. Because the nursing license is a common law property right under the law, the State Board must fulfill the constitutional duty of due process in any suspension or revocation situation. Due process (Garner, 2006) requires the State Board to notify the nurse of the listed charges or violations and to conduct a hearing at which the nurse may hear the evidence of the charges and the nurse may offer a defense with or without the assistance of legal counsel. In license hearings, a panel of members of the State Board of Nursing conducts the hearing instead of a judge. Depending on your state's administrative law rules, you may file an appeal of the State Board of Nursing judgment in a court of law. In any licensing proceeding, nurses should exercise the right to legal counsel to ensure full protection of their rights (Karno, 2005).

Criminal Law

Criminal laws are federal or state statutory laws that define as a crime certain actions that inflict or threaten substantial harm to individuals or the public interest without justification (Wacks, 2008). Criminal laws are separated into misdemeanors or felonies. A **misdemeanor** is a crime that while injurious, does not inflict serious harm (Garner, 2006). A misdemeanor usually has a penalty of a monetary fine, forfeiture, or brief imprisonment. A **felony** is a serious offense that results in significant harm to another person or to society in general. Felony crimes may carry penalties of monetary restitution, imprisonment for greater than 1 year, or death (Garner, 2006). Examples of Nurse Practice Act violations that may carry criminal penalties include practicing nursing without a license and misuse of controlled substances.

Torts

Nursing practice is also regulated by the common law or judicial case law of torts. **Torts** are civil wrongful acts or omissions against a person or a person's property that are compensated by awarding monetary damages to the individual whose rights had been violated (Martin, 2006). Torts are characterized as either intentional or unintentional.

Intentional torts are deliberate acts that violate another person's rights (Garner, 2006). An example of an intentional tort in health care is assault and battery. Even though assault and battery can be criminal statutory violations, they may also be tort injuries in health care. The definitions of assault and battery are the same in both criminal and tort law. **Assault** is an intentional threat toward another person that gives that person a reasonable fear of harmful contact (Garner, 2006). No actual contact is required for an assault to occur. An example of an assault in nursing practice is to threaten to restrain a patient for an x-ray procedure when the patient has refused consent. **Battery** is any intentional touching without consent or lawful justification (Garner, 2006). The touching may be harmful to the patient by causing an injury, or it may be merely offensive to the patient's dignity. Battery generally always includes an assault. This is why the law routinely combines the terms *assault* and *battery*. An example of a battery in health care is when the patient has consented to a right knee surgery and the surgeon performs surgery on the patient's left knee. An example of an assault and battery is to threaten to restrain a competent patient for an unconsented x-ray procedure and then to actually restrain the patient.

Negligence is an unintentional tort. **Negligence** is conduct that falls below the generally accepted standard of care of a reasonably prudent person (Garner, 2006). The definition of negligence has evolved over time through common law and case law to be the failure to use the degree of care that a reasonable person would use under the same or similar circumstances. An example of negligence is a driver's failure to stop at a clearly identified stop sign. Malpractice is an example of negligence, sometimes referred to as professional negligence. The law defines nursing **malpractice** as the failure to use that degree of care that a reasonable nurse would use under the same or similar circumstances. To establish the elements of malpractice, the patient or **plaintiff** must prove the following: (1) the nurse **defendant** owed a duty to the patient, (2) the nurse breached that duty, (3) the patient was injured because of the nurse's breach of duty, and (4) the patient has

BOX 4-1	Common Sources of Negligence

Be aware of the common negligent acts that have resulted in lawsuits against hospitals and nurses:
1 Medication errors that result in injury to patients
2 Intravenous therapy errors resulting in infiltration or phlebitis
3 Burns to patients caused by equipment, bathing, or spills of hot liquids and foods
4 Falls resulting in injury to patients
5 Failure to use aseptic technique when required
6 Errors in sponge, instrument, or needle counts in surgical cases
7 Failure to give a report, or giving an incomplete report, to oncoming shift personnel
8 Failure to adequately monitor a patient's condition
9 Failure to notify a health care provider of a significant change in a patient's status

accrued damages as a result of the injury. Negligent acts may result in lawsuits against hospitals and nurses (Box 4-1). The negligent act may be as simple as failing to check a patient's armband and then administering medication to the wrong patient. Failure to monitor the patient's condition appropriately and communicate changes in the patient's condition to the health care provider that result in injury to the patient are examples of negligent acts that may result in malpractice. The best way to avoid being liable for malpractice is to give nursing care that meets the generally accepted standard of care. In a malpractice lawsuit the law uses nursing standards of care to measure nursing conduct and to determine whether the nurse acted as any reasonably prudent nurse would act under the same or similar circumstances. Box 4-2 describes the steps of a typical malpractice lawsuit.

STANDARDS OF CARE

Standards of care are legal guidelines for minimally safe and adequate nursing practice (Garner, 2006). Standards of care are defined by the following: (1) State Nurse Practice Acts, (2) state and federal hospital licensing laws and accreditation rules (The Joint Commission [TJC], 2008b), (3) professional and specialty organizations (ANA, 2001), and (4) written policies and procedures of the nurse's health care facility. Written policies and procedures of the nurse's health care facility are specific guidelines and directions for nursing care and are usually found on every nursing unit in a policy and procedure manual.

It is important that you know the policies and procedures of your employing health care facility because these will be the standards of care to which your actions will be compared in a malpractice trial. If you are a specialized nurse such as a nurse anesthetist, intensive care nurse, certified nurse midwife, or operating room nurse, you will be held to the standard of care and skill exercised by professionals in the specialty area. Nurs-

BOX 4-2   Anatomy of a Lawsuit

Petition—elements of the claim: The plaintiff outlines what the defendant nurse did wrong and how as a result of that alleged negligence the plaintiff was injured. In the case study, the petition would state that the nurses failed to provide adequate care to the patient by failing to appropriately treat the changing condition.

Answer: The nurse admits or denies each allegation in the petition. Anything that is not admitted must be proved. The nurses will admit or deny that they were able to provide further appropriate care to the patient to meet the standard of care during her change in condition.

Discovery: The process of uncovering all the facts of the case. Involves using interrogatories, full access to the medical records in question, and depositions. The patient and all health care staff will be asked questions by counsel for the plaintiff and the defense. They will answer under oath, and their testimony will be recorded and kept for reference in the trial.

Interrogatories: Written questions requiring answers under oath. Usual questions concern witnesses, insurance experts, and which health care providers the plaintiff saw before and after the event.

Medical records: The defendant obtains all of the plaintiff's relevant medical records for treatment before and after the incident. Everything written by the nurses and the health care provider in the medical record is open to examination by both the plaintiff and the defendants.

Witnesses' depositions: Questions are posed to the witnesses under oath to obtain all relevant, nonprivileged information about the case.

Parties' depositions: The plaintiff and defendants (health care provider, nurse, and hospital personnel) are almost always deposed.

Other witnesses: Factual witnesses, both neutral and biased, are deposed to obtain information and their version of the case. This may include family members on the plaintiff's side and other medical personnel (e.g., nurses) on the defendant's side.

Treating health care providers' depositions: Before subsequent treating, health care providers' depositions may be taken to establish issues such as those concerning preexisting conditions, causation, the nature and extent of injuries, and permanency.

Experts: The plaintiff selects experts to establish the essential legal elements of the case against the defendant. The defendant selects experts to establish the appropriateness of the nursing care. Nursing experts will be asked to testify to the reasonableness or inappropriate actions of the health care staff once the patient's condition began to change. The expert will be asked to compare the actions of the nursing staff to the standard of care, which is what the reasonably prudent nurse in the same situation would have done.

Trial: The trial usually occurs at least 1 to 3 years after the filing of the petition. Approximately 5% of cases are actually tried before a judge. Most are dismissed or settled. Settlement means that compensation has been paid for the case to be dismissed.

PROOF OF NEGLIGENCE
- The nurse owed a duty to the patient.
- The nurse did not carry out the duty or breached the duty (failed to use that degree of skill and learning ordinarily used under the same or similar circumstances by members of the profession).
- The patient was injured.
- The patient's injury was caused by the nurse's failure to carry out that duty.
- The patient's injury resulted in compensable damages that can be quantified, such as medical bills, lost wages, pain, and suffering.

---

ing experts are used to testify to the appropriate standard of care as indicated by the policy and procedure manual, your professional organization, or the State Nurse Practice Act, and then compare your conduct to these standards. A few states have developed "apology statutes" that encourage the health care provider to disclose errors or unexpected outcomes to the patient/family without admitting liability. These statutes are designed to decrease litigation (Atwood, 2008). It is always important to be up to date regarding state and federal laws, current legal issues, and any new rules, regulation, or case law that will affect your nursing practice.

Malpractice Insurance

Two percent of all medical malpractice claims in 2005 were made against nurses. Malpractice payments made for non–advanced practice nurses have doubled in the last decade (Chervenak, 2008). Malpractice insurance provides you with an attorney, the payment of attorney's fees, and the payment of any judgment or settlement if a patient sues you for malpractice. If you work for a health care facility, that facility's insurance will cover you during your employment. If you plan on practicing nursing outside of your employing facility, you will need to purchase additional malpractice insurance. For example, if a family friend asks you to provide nursing care in his or her home, the hospital malpractice insurance does not cover you if the family friend files suit against you. Malpractice insurance carriers are required by federal law to report all malpractice insurance verdicts and settlements made to the National Practitioner Data Bank. Unlike in licensing disputes, nurses have no due process rights in the reporting of their name to the Data Bank (Bolin, 2005).

Documentation

It is necessary to document patient assessments, interventions, and evaluations and to develop a caring rapport with the patient to avoid liability. Frequently the nurses' notes are the first thing an attorney reviews when a lawsuit is filed. As a nurse, you chart facts, not assumptions, about patient behavior. In addition, you document as fully as possible the health care provider notifications made regarding the patient. Simply charting "physician notified" is insufficient information when presenting a chart in court. Your assessments and the reporting of significant changes in the assessments are very important factors in defending a lawsuit. Your documentation of your nursing care is your only record of what actually was done for a patient and will serve as proof that you acted reasonably and safely. Trials over health care disputes that involve using the medical record as a source of factual information generally take 2 to 3 years to occur. Most individuals have flawed recall of events over a period of time. Therefore your nursing notes, written at the time of the event, are seen as better evidence of the facts of the event as opposed to any one person's memory. Nurses' notes written carelessly and without regard to detail or hospital standards of documentation do not reflect well on the health care provider's credibility or appearance of accountability to a judge or jury (Monarch, 2007). Make sure your documentation is thorough, accurate, and done in a timely manner.

When there is a deviation from the standard of care, such as when a patient or visitor falls or an error is made, you make specific documentation of the event or incident in the form of an **occurrence report/incident report.** You should complete an occurrence report when anything unusual happens that could potentially cause harm to a patient, visitor, or employee. Most health care facilities provide specific forms for this purpose (Chapter 9). Objectively record the details of the event and any statements the patient makes. An example is as follows: "Patient found lying on floor on right side. Abrasion on right forehead. Patient stated, 'I fell and hit my head.'" At the time of the event, always assess the patient thoroughly, then contact the health care provider to examine the patient. After examining the patient, you and the health care provider document assessment findings in the progress notes. The health care provider orders follow-up care or treatment when necessary. Document any problematic effects caused by the event. Do not include subjective assumptions and statements assigning blame or fault in the nurses' notes or the occurrence report. Occurrence reports are not kept in the patient's medical record, although they may be evidence in lawsuits in some jurisdictions (*In re Intracare Hospital*, 2007). Do not document in the nurses' notes that an occurrence report was completed. Follow your agency's policy to determine what to do with the occurrence report after it is completed. Also be sure to report the occcurrence to the appropriate person (e.g., the charge nurse, your manager).

Risk Management and Quality Assurance

The underlying rationale for quality improvement and risk management programs is the development of an organizational system of ensuring appropriate, quality health care. **Risk management** involves several components, including identifying possible risks, analyzing them, acting to reduce the risks, and evaluating the measures taken to reduce the risks. The Joint Commission (2008b) requires the use of quality improvement and risk management procedures. Both quality improvement and risk management require good documentation.

One tool used in risk management is the occurrence report or incident report. By reviewing occurrence reports, administrators determine areas of patient risk. For example, if a certain kind of problem has occurred repeatedly, such as patients falling when being transferred to stretchers, you use educational methods to help prevent the problem in the future.

Patient safety and improved care are the ultimate goals of risk management and quality assurance. Patient safety issues are the focus of attention by accrediting agencies such as The Joint Commission (2008c) and public interest groups such as the Institute of Medicine. The Institute of Medicine report *To Err Is Human* (Kohn and others, 2000) focused attention on health care providers and agencies and promoted more disclosure of potentially harmful errors or "never events." **Never events** are preventable errors, which may include falls, urinary tract infections from improper use of catheters, and pressure ulcers (Carpenter, 2007). Recently the federal government and health care insurance companies developed policies to withhold reimbursement for preventable medical errors (Brown and others, 2008). Becoming involved in developing and monitoring the policies and procedures of the facility in which you work helps to develop a system and a culture of patient safety.

GOOD SAMARITAN LAWS

Good Samaritan laws exist in almost every state to encourage nurses and other health care providers to assist in emergency situations. These laws limit liability and offer legal immunity if a nurse helps at the scene of an accident. For example, if you stop at the scene of an automobile accident and give appropriate emergency care such as applying pressure to stop hemorrhage, you are acting within accepted standards, even though proper equipment was not available. If the patient subsequently develops complications as a result of your actions, you are immune from liability as long as you acted without gross negligence (Good Samaritan Law, 1998). The statutes also provide that a nurse is able to assist a minor in an emergency at the scene of an accident or a competitive sports event before obtaining the parent's consent. However, although Good Samaritan laws provide immunity to the nurse who does what is reasonable to save a person's life, if you perform a procedure for which you have no training, you will be liable for any injury resulting from that act. Therefore provide only care that is consistent with your level of expertise (Dachs and Elias, 2008). In addition, once you have committed to providing emergency care to a patient, you are responsible for following through, that is, to safely transfer the care of the patient to someone who can provide needed care, such as emergency medical technicians (EMTs) or emergency department staff. Otherwise, you will be liable for abandonment of the patient and responsible for any injury suffered after you left the patient (Dachs and Elias, 2008). Three states (Louisiana, Minnesota, and Vermont) have enacted "failure-to-act" laws that make it a crime not to provide Good Samaritan care (Dachs and Elias, 2008).

CONSENT

A signed consent form from your patient is necessary for all routine treatment, hazardous procedures such as surgery, some treatment programs such as chemotherapy, and participation in research studies (Cady, 2005). A patient will sign a general consent form for treatment when the patient is admitted to the hospital or other health care facility. A patient or the patient's representative has to sign separate special consent forms before anyone performs specialized procedures. Box 4-3 outlines the general guidelines for legal consent to medical treatments. Take special consideration and care regarding the patient who is deaf, illiterate, or speaks a foreign language. In each instance, take steps to ensure that the patient understands the document being signed (Cady, 2005; Johnstone and Kanitsaki, 2006). It is

---

BOX 4-3 Statutory Guidelines for Legal Consent for Medical Treatment

Those who may consent to medical treatment are governed by state law but generally include the following:

I Adults

A Any competent individual 18 years of age or older for himself or herself

B Any parent for his or her unemancipated minor

C Any guardian for his or her ward

D Any adult for the treatment of his or her minor brother or sister (if an emergency and parents are not present)

E Any grandparent for a minor grandchild (if an emergency and parents are not present)

II Minors (younger than 18 years of age)

A Ordinarily minors may not consent for medical treatment without a parent. Emancipated minors, however, may consent to medical treatment without a parent. Emancipated minors include the following:

1 Minors who are designated emancipated by a court order

2 Minors who are married, divorced, or widowed

3 Minors who are in active military service

B Unemancipated minors may consent to medical treatment if they have specific medical conditions:

1 Pregnancy and pregnancy-related conditions (Various states differ in characterizing a pregnant minor as either emancipated or unemancipated. Know your state's rules in this matter.)

2 A minor parent for his or her custodial child

3 Sexually transmitted infection (STI) information and treatment

4 Substance abuse treatment

5 Outpatient and/or temporary sheltered mental health treatment

C The issue of emancipated or unemancipated minor does not relieve the health care provider's duty to attempt to obtain meaningful informed consent (Vukadinovich, 2004).

---

also important to be sensitive to the cultural issues of consent and to understand the way in which patients and their families communicate to make important decisions. The cultural beliefs and values of your patients are sometimes very different from your own or the culture in which you are comfortable. Show respect by not imposing your own cultural values on your patients or their families. For example, traditional Islamic and Jewish cultures have strict guidelines in consent for postmortem examinations and handling of the dead. In general, decision making by a member of a traditional Asian or Hispanic culture is done by the family together and not by the individual seeking treatment. In a situation in which your patient refuses a treatment, it is necessary to make the patient aware of the consequences of his or her refusal (Clifford, 2008).

When a competent patient refuses care or treatment, it is important to recognize that this act is legitimately his or her right. The nurse should inform the health care provider of the patient's refusal to receive care and document the situation in the medical record.

Informed Consent

Informed consent is a patient's agreement to allow something to happen, such as surgery, based on a full disclosure of the risks, benefits, alternatives, and consequences of refusal (Garner, 2006). Informed consent requires that you ensure the patient has all relevant information required to make a decision, that the patient is capable of understanding the relevant information, and that the patient actually gives consent. If you or a health care provider performs a procedure on a patient without informed consent, the person who performed the procedure will possibly be liable for battery. You do not need to have written informed consent when performing most nursing care. However, it is important that you explain to the patient what you are going to do and ensure that the patient accepts the care you are going to provide. Written informed consent is needed when a patient is going to have an invasive medical procedure, such as surgery. Documentation of written informed consent includes the following:

- The patient's signature
- The witnesses' signatures
- The date and time of signing
- Verification that the patient voluntarily signed the consent, that the patient discussed the risks, benefits, alternatives, and the right to refuse the procedure with the health care provider
- Verification that the patient understands the procedure and has had all questions answered satisfactorily (Cady, 2005)

Because nurses do not perform surgery or direct medical procedures, providing information about the procedure and obtaining a patient's informed consent for the procedure does not fall within a nurse's responsibility. Even though a nurse assumes the responsibility for witnessing the patient's signature on the consent form, the nurse does not legally assume the duty of obtaining informed consent. The health care provider performing the procedure assumes that responsibility (Clifford, 2008). When you provide consent forms for patients to sign, ask them if they understand the procedures for which they are giving consent. If patients deny any understanding, or if you suspect that they do not understand, notify the health care provider and your nursing supervisor. A patient refusing surgery or other medical treatment must be informed about any harmful consequences of refusal. If the patient persists in refusing the treatment, make sure the rejection is written, signed, and witnessed (Cady, 2005).

Parents are normally the legal guardians of pediatric patients, and therefore they are the persons who will sign consent forms for treatment. If the parents are divorced, the parent with legal custody gives consent. When a parent refuses medically necessary treatment for a child, health care providers sometimes petition the court to intervene on the child's behalf. Using the standard known as "the best interests of the child," courts may overrule parental decisions (Kon, 2006). Children, most often adolescents under the age of 16, may be characterized as emancipated or unemancipated minors. This characterization refers to their legal standing as a competent adult. An emancipated minor, even though he or she has not achieved the legal age of consent, may give consent for procedures and treatment. Emancipation is certified by a legal document. Some states may characterize some adolescents as emancipated when certain conditions such as pregnancy exist. In this case, the adolescent mother is considered competent to consent to treatment for herself and her child. When there is a question about an adolescent's capacity to consent to a procedure, contact the nursing supervisor for guidance.

If the patient is unconscious, you need to obtain consent from a person legally authorized to give consent on the patient's behalf. In an emergency situation, health care providers may provide care to a patient without consent as long as no evidence exists to indicate that the patient or legal representative would refuse treatment (Cady, 2005). A patient who is legally incompetent in a judicial proceeding needs to have the consent of the legal guardian. If a mentally ill person refuses treatment, involuntary admission is limited to situations in which the patient is determined to be dangerous to himself or others (Cady, 2005). A patient's consent for voluntary psychiatric unit admission is also required. These patients retain the right to refuse treatment until a court has determined that they are incompetent to decide for themselves (Cady, 2005).

Restraints

You need to know when and how to use restraints correctly. The Resident's Rights section of the Omnibus Budget Reconciliation Act (1988) regulates the use of physical or chemical restraints in nursing facilities. In addition, The Joint Commission (2008a, 2008b) has set guidelines for the use of restraints. These regulations set the standard that all patients have the right to be free from seclusion and physical or chemical restraints except to ensure the patient's safety in emergency situations. They further describe the procedures to follow in order to restrain any patient, including who orders restraints, when to write the order, and how often to renew the written order. The standards specifically prohibit

restraining patients for staff convenience, punishment, or retaliation (Ludwick and others, 2008). The regulations also describe documentation of restraint use and follow-up assessments. In particular, the documentation needs to describe all of the less-restrictive interventions attempted before employing a physical or chemical restraint (Evans and Cotter, 2008) (see Chapter 27). Liability for improper or unlawful restraint, as well as liability for patient injury from unprotected falls, lies with the nurse and the health care facility.

Death and Dying

You also need to know your legal responsibilities concerning the process of death and dying. Carefully document all events that occur when you are caring for the dying patient. There are two standards for the determination of death: cardiopulmonary or whole brain (Uniform Determination of Death Act, 1980) (Box 4-4). The cardiopulmonary standard requires failure of a patient's circulatory and respiratory functions. The whole brain standard requires irreversible failure of all functions of the entire brain, including the brain stem. The reason for the development of the two definitions is to set the legal standard for determining death in all situations. The definitions are helpful when there is a question of whether to

---

BOX 4-4 Federal Statutes in Nursing Practice

Americans With Disabilities Act (ADA) (1995)—A civil rights law protecting the disabled regarding access to public services, health care, and employment. Extended to include individuals with HIV infection.

Emergency Medical Treatment and Active Labor Act (EMTALA) (1986)—"Antidumping" law that requires screening of patients in an emergency department and appropriate stabilization before transfer of the patient to another facility.

Health Insurance Portability and Accountability Act (HIPAA) (1996)—Protects a patient from losing health insurance because of preexisting illnesses when changing jobs. Also sets rules regarding release of a patient's protected health information and carries both civil and criminal penalties for violations.

Patient Self-Determination Act (PSDA) (1991)—Requires health care facilities to provide information to all patients regarding advance directives and to document advance directives in the medical record.

Federal Nursing Home Reform Act (1987)—Gives nursing home residents the right to be free of unnecessary and inappropriate restraints.

National Organ Transplant Act (1984)—Prohibits purchase or sale of organs. The act provides immunity from civil and criminal actions against the hospital and health care providers, as well as immunity from liability for the donor's estate.

Mental Health Parity Act (1996)—Prohibits health plans from placing lifetime or annual limits on mental health benefits.

HIV, Human immunodeficiency virus.

continue life support or when the discussion of organ donation is appropriate.

You are legally obligated to treat your deceased patient's remains with dignity and care. Wrongful handling causes emotional harm to survivors. In one litigated case, survivors sued when a mislabeling of bodies led to an Orthodox Jewish person being prepared for a Roman Catholic funeral and a Roman Catholic person being prepared for an Orthodox Jewish burial (*In re Schiller*, 1977).

ADVANCE DIRECTIVES You will encounter legal issues associated with caring for patients who are terminally ill, severely debilitated, or in a persistent vegetative state (permanently comatose). One of these legal issues involves the right to refuse medical treatment and the withholding of food and nutrition. The doctrine of informed consent ensures that the patient has the right to refuse treatment. The Supreme Court has held that a competent person has the right to refuse medical treatment, including lifesaving food and nutrition (*Cruzan v. Director Missouri Department of Health*, 1990).

Many times the decision regarding lifesaving treatment is in writing in the patient's living will or advance directive. **Living wills** are documents instructing the health care provider to withhold or withdraw life-sustaining procedures in patients who are terminally ill. If the patient has executed a durable **power of attorney for health care,** the document will designate an individual who is able to give consent for health care treatment when the patient is no longer able. State law may designate a surrogate decision maker, such as a spouse, who acts as a substitute when no documented preference exists. Each state providing for living wills or advance directives has its own requirements for executing them. In general, you need two witnesses who are not a relative or the health care provider when the patient signs the document. Only a competent patient is able to revoke living wills, advance directives, and durable power of attorney for health care statements. Health care providers who ignore valid living wills, advance directives, or the directions of a health care power of attorney may be subject to civil liability. The Patient Self-Determination Act (1991) requires health care institutions to inquire whether a patient has created an advance directive, to give patients information on advance directives, and to document whether the patient states he or she has an advance directive.

If a health care provider has documented in the progress notes that the patient is deteriorating and the health care provider and the patient have made the decision not to administer cardiopulmonary resuscitation, the health care provider should write a "do not resuscitate" (DNR) order. A DNR order is written, not given verbally. Health care providers need to regularly review DNR orders in case the patient's condition warrants a change. Be familiar with your institution's policies and procedures concerning DNR orders.

ORGAN AND TISSUE DONATION A signed consent is necessary before donating a patient's body, tissues, or organs for medical use. In some states a patient signs the back of his or her driver's license in the presence of witnesses, indicating consent to having his or her body donated. Consent is valid unless the driver's license is revoked, canceled, or suspended,

and the person has to give consent each time the license is renewed. Generally a hospital is not liable for honoring a patient's consent for organ donation despite the family's objection. However, in practice, health care institutions will honor the family's wishes even if they conflict with the patient's organ donation consent. State laws provide whether a nurse is able to witness the consent of an individual donating his or her body, organs, or tissues for medical use. Be aware of the policies and procedures of your employing institution and your state's laws when someone asks you to serve as a witness for a person who is giving consent for organ donation.

In most states there is a law requiring that at the time of death a qualified health care provider ask the patient's family members to consider organ or tissue donation (National Organ Transplant Act, 1984). You approach individuals in the following order: (1) the spouse, (2) adult son or daughter, (3) parent, (4) adult brother or sister, (5) grandparent, and (6) guardian. The person in the highest class makes the donation unless he or she knows of a refusal or contrary indication by the decedent (Uniform Anatomical Gift Act, 1987). In addition, the law also provides that the health care provider who certifies death shall not be involved in the removal or transplant of organs or tissues. The National Organ Transplant Act of 1984 prohibits selling or purchasing of organs and regulates this area of medical and nursing practice. Organ and tissue donation remains voluntary. Consent forms are available for this purpose.

AUTOPSIES An autopsy requires consent by the patient before his or her death or by a close family member at the time of the patient's death (Autopsy Consent, 1998). The priority for giving consent for autopsies is (1) the patient, in writing before death; (2) durable power of attorney; (3) surviving spouse; and (4) surviving child, parent, brother, or sister in the order named. State statutes specify that when there are reasonable grounds to believe that a patient died as a result of violence, homicide, suicide, accident, or death occurring in any unusual or suspicious manner, you need to notify the coroner. You also notify the coroner if a patient's death is unforeseen and sudden and a health care provider has not seen the patient in over 36 hours.

CONFIDENTIALITY The Health Insurance Portability and Accountability Act of 1996 (HIPAA) sets standards regarding the electronic exchange of private and sensitive health information. Known as the Privacy Standards (Carter, 2008), these rules create patient rights to consent to use and disclose protected health information, to inspect and copy one's medical record, and to amend mistaken or incomplete information. In addition, the standards require all hospitals and health agencies to have specific policies and procedures in place to ensure compliance with the standards. The policies and procedures need to provide reasonable safeguards to protect written and verbal communications about patients. Although HIPAA will not require such things as soundproof rooms in hospitals, it does mean that nurses and health care providers need to avoid discussing patients in public hallways and provide reasonable levels of privacy in communicating with and about patients in any matter. HIPAA violations have civil and criminal sanctions. Patient confidentiality is a right of the patient, and it is a privilege that the patient entrusts you with his or her personal health information. Dealing with deliberate violations of a patient's confidential personal health information by other staff members is a difficult situation. The best action to take is to advise the staff members to stop, inform the nursing supervisor, and complete an occurrence report.

Issues of disclosure, privacy, and confidentiality are an important concern when working with patients or peers infected with blood-borne illnesses such as human immunodeficiency virus (HIV) or acquired immunodeficiency virus (AIDS), hepatitis, and sexually transmitted illnesses. You will care for these patients in every segment of your nursing practice. Use standard precautions as a standard of care when caring for all patients. The ADA (1995) applies to persons with AIDS. This federal law protects the rights of disabled people and HIV-infected patients. Health care workers and other employees who refuse to work with HIV-infected people will leave companies open to indirect charges of discrimination if the employer does not monitor the work environment. Several cases have held that the health care provider is obligated to disclose the fact that he or she is infected with HIV. The ADA regulations protect the privacy of infected people by giving individuals the opportunity to decide whether to disclose their disability. As a health care worker, it is not a requirement for you to be tested for HIV as a condition of employment. If you are contaminated by a patient whose HIV status is unknown, you cannot check the patient's blood for HIV without the patient's consent.

OTHER LEGAL ISSUES IN NURSING PRACTICE

As a nurse, you will be faced with nursing issues that will become liability concerns. It is important for you to anticipate these issues so you are better prepared to deal with any problems that arise.

Physician or Health Care Provider Orders

The patient's physician or health care provider is responsible for directing the medical treatment of the patient. You are responsible for carrying out that medical treatment unless the order is in error, violates hospital policy, or is harmful to the patient. Therefore you will assess all physician or health care provider orders, and if you determine they are erroneous or harmful, obtain further clarification from that physician or health care provider (Figure 4-1). If the physician or health care provider confirms the order, but you still believe that it is inappropriate, inform the nurse manager or the nursing supervisor. Do not carry out the order if there is a risk that harm will come to your patient. Your supervisor will help resolve the questionable order. If you knowingly carry out the questionable order without obtaining any supporting consultation from your supervisor or ad-

ministrative staff, you are legally responsible for the harm suffered by your patient. In the case of Lynette Donovan, the nurses understood that the patient's cast was causing a decrease in adequate circulation to her leg. Mr. Ortiz, learning that the nursing staff was unable to contact Lynette's health care provider, should have immediately notified his nursing instructor. Together, the nursing instructor and the nursing staff should have then notified the hospital nursing supervisor. In this type of situation, it is always important to put the patient's interests first while attempting to maintain a collegial approach in providing the ordered health care treatments (Schmalenberg and others, 2005).

Make sure all physician or health care provider orders are in writing and dated and timed appropriately. Make sure that they are transcribed correctly. Verbal orders or telephone orders are not recommended because they leave possibilities for error. If a verbal or telephone order is necessary in an emergency, make sure the physician or health care provider writes and signs it as soon as possible, usually within 24 hours (TJC, 2008c).

Nursing Students

Nursing students are responsible for all of their actions that cause harm to patients (*Dimora v. Cleveland Clinics Foundation*, 1996). When a patient is injured as a direct result of your actions, you, your instructor, the staff nurses working with you, and the hospital or health care facility may all share the liability for the incorrect action. Faculty members are responsible for instructing and observing their students, but in some situations staff nurses also share these responsibilities. As a nursing student, no one should assign you to perform tasks for which you are unprepared. Your instructors should carefully supervise you as you learn new procedures. Every

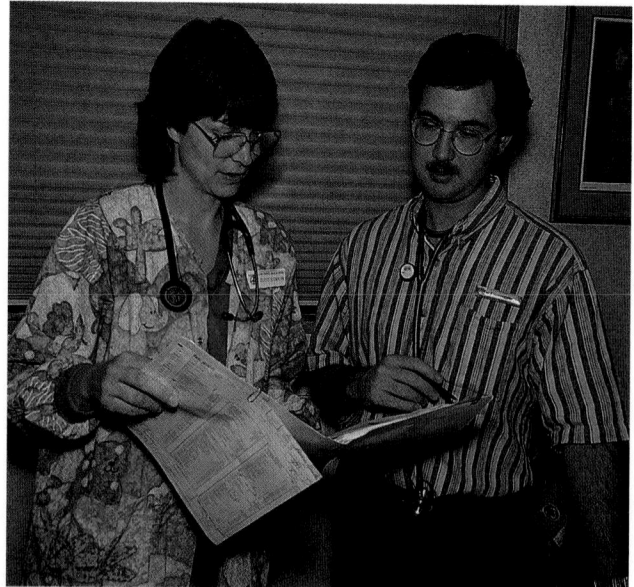

Figure 4-1 ■ If an order creates questions, the nurse clarifies it with the physician or health care provider.

nursing school should provide clear definitions of student responsibility. During the clinical rotation, generally the school's liability insurance covers you; however, always check with your school as to the specific coverage.

Sometimes you will be employed as a nursing assistant or a nurse's aide when you are not attending classes. During the time when you work as an employee of a health care facility, perform only tasks that appear in a job description for a nurse's aide or nursing assistant. For example, even if you have learned how to administer intramuscular medications as a nursing student, do not perform this task as a nurse's aide.

Patient Abandonment and Delegation Issues

You will encounter inadequate staffing during times of nursing shortages and staff downsizing periods in an effort to achieve cost containment. The Joint Commission (2008b) requires institutions to have guidelines for the number of staff needed to care for patients. Liability issues exist if a health care facility does not have enough registered nurses to provide competent and safe care and if a patient is injured as a result of negligent care by any personnel. If you are assigned to care for more patients than is reasonable for safe care, notify your nursing supervisor. If you are required to accept the assignment, document this information in writing and provide the document to nursing administrators. Although documentation does not relieve you of responsibility if patients suffer harm because of inattention, it shows that you attempted to act appropriately. Whenever you document information about short staffing, keep a copy of the document. Do not walk out when staffing is inadequate because this act could be regarded as patient abandonment. It is important to know your institution's policies and procedures on how to handle inadequate staffing before such a situation arises. Registered nurses are always responsible for making nursing care judgments based on the nursing process. Even when a registered nurse delegates care to nursing assistive personnel or licensed practical nurses, the nurse maintains responsibility for patient outcomes (Box 4-5).

Nurses within acute and long-term care facilities are often required to "float" from the area in which they normally practice to other nursing units. If you float, inform your supervisor if you lack experience in caring for the types of patients on the new nursing unit. Request an orientation to the unit. When you float to a nursing unit, you will be held to the same standard of care as nurses who regularly work in that area. A supervisor is liable if a staff nurse is assigned to a patient for whom he or she cannot safely care. In one case the court noted that if employers are going to float nurses out of their usual work area of practice, then the employers need to provide training and education to prepare the nurses to work in the other areas (*Winkelman v. Beloit Memorial Hospital,* 1992).

Controlled Substances

The Comprehensive Drug Abuse Prevention and Control Act (1970) was passed to control and regulate hospital drug distribution systems of narcotics, antidepressants, hypnotics, sedatives, stimulants, and hallucinogens. You administer controlled substances only under the direction of a licensed physician. However, several states allow advanced practice nurses to prescribe controlled substances.

Controlled substances are securely locked away, and only authorized personnel have access to them. Maintain precise records regarding the dispensing, wasting, and storage of controlled substances. There are criminal penalties for the misuse of controlled substances. There have been cases in which physicians have illegally prescribed and dispensed controlled substances. If you are employed by such a physician and fail to report these activities, you are legally accountable for aiding and abetting the physician.

Reporting Obligations

Health care providers are required to report incidents such as child, spousal, or elder abuse; rape; gunshot wounds; attempted suicide; and certain communicable diseases.

| BOX 4-5 | BEST PRACTICES |

SUMMARY OF EVIDENCE

Increases in health care costs coupled with decreases in health care reimbursements and the overall nursing shortage require nurses to more frequently delegate tasks to nursing assistive personnel (NAP). Ambiguous understanding of what is required in appropriate delegation will result in inadequate supervision of NAPs and lead to errors and negative patient outcomes.

Seventeen in-depth interviews with baccalaureate-prepared nurses from a variety of acute care settings were conducted to explore the nature and significance of delegation to NAPs. The average number of years of experience in nursing was 8.8 years. Results showed that nurses define delegation in different ways. A racial difference between groups has implications for both relationships and communication between nurses and NAPs. Lack of trust and respect among members of the work group can affect the group process.

APPLICATION TO NURSING PRACTICE

- Delegation is defined as the transfer of responsibility for the performance of an activity from one individual to another while retaining accountability for the outcome.
- Trust and respect are important for nurse-NAP communication.
- Communication in the nurse-NAP relationship affects the quality of patient care.

REFERENCE

Standing T, Anthony M: Delegation: what it means to acute care nurses, *Appl Nurs Res* 21:8, 2008.

To encourage reports of suspected cases, states provide legal immunity for the reporter if the person makes the report in good faith. Health care professionals who do not report suspected child abuse or neglect are liable for civil or criminal legal action. You are also required to report unsafe or impaired professionals. Because required reporting information varies among states, become familiar with the appropriate statutes in your state and the policies and procedures of your employing health care facility.

KEY POINTS

- Registered nurses are licensed by the state in which they practice.
- Under the law you are required to follow standards of care, which originate in Nurse Practice Acts, the guidelines of professional organizations, and written policies and procedures of employing institutions.
- You are responsible for performing procedures correctly and exercising professional judgment when you carry out physician or health care provider orders.
- All patients are entitled to confidential health care and freedom from unauthorized release of information.
- You will be liable for malpractice if the following are established: (1) you (defendant) owed a duty to the patient (plaintiff), (2) you did not carry out that duty or breached that duty, (3) the patient was injured, and (4) your failure to carry out that duty caused the patient's injury.
- Informed consent must meet the following criteria: (1) the person giving consent is competent and of legal age; (2) the consent is given voluntarily; (3) the person giving consent thoroughly understands the procedure, its risks and benefits, and alternative procedures; and (4) the person giving consent has a right to have all questions answered satisfactorily.
- You are obligated to follow the physician's or health care provider's order unless you believe that it is in error, violates hospital policy, or is possibly harmful to the patient, in which case you make a formal report explaining the refusal.
- You file an occurrence report in any unusual situation that will potentially cause harm to a patient; such reports are also for quality improvement and risk management.
- The civil law system is concerned with the protection of a person's private rights, and the criminal law system deals with the rights of individuals and society as defined by legislative statutes.
- Legal issues involving death include documenting all events surrounding the death, treating a deceased person with dignity, and obtaining timely consent for an autopsy from the decedent or close family member.
- A competent adult is able to legally give consent to donate specific organs, and nurses are sometimes able to serve as witnesses to this decision.
- You need to know the laws that apply to your specific area of practice.
- Depending on state laws, nurses are required to report possible criminal activities such as child abuse, as well as certain communicable diseases.

CRITICAL THINKING EXERCISES

Review the case study at the beginning of this chapter, and answer the following questions. Remember that Lynette Donovan is legally a minor. She is hurt and afraid and in an unfamiliar setting. She may not be comfortable speaking with the health care providers who are present, and her expressions of pain may be modified by the circumstances she is in.

1. Identify the elements of malpractice and how they apply to Lynette Donovan's case.
   a. Who owes a duty to Miss Donovan?
   b. Where would David Ortiz, the nursing student, look to determine whether he owes a duty to Lynette Donovan?
   c. What is the standard of care owed to Miss Donovan?
   d. Was the duty to Miss Donovan met?

Lynette Donovan developed gangrene in the right leg. She requires a right below-the-knee amputation.

2. Is Lynette Donovan capable of providing consent for this procedure? What things should be included in the discussion to provide informed consent?
3. David Ortiz is returning from escorting Miss Donovan to the operating room for her procedure. He gets on the elevator, where there are several visitors and two nursing supervisors who are talking about the health care provider who "made Donovan lose her leg."
   a. What are the liability issues here?
   b. Are any laws broken?
   c. What should David Ortiz do?

evolve   *Answers to Critical Thinking Questions can be found on the Evolve website.*

REVIEW QUESTIONS

1. The nurse understands that state law affects the way patient care is performed. Therefore he does an Internet search of which of the following on his state's website?
   1. HIPAA
   2. ADA
   3. Nurse Practice Act
   4. Uniform Anatomical Gift Act

2. When preparing an occurrence report, the nurse understands that:
   1. A copy should be put in the patient's record
   2. Subjective information should always be included
   3. Statements made by the patient should be included in the report
   4. If someone was at fault, that person should be blamed in the report

3. Even though you may witness the patient's signature on a form, obtaining informed consent is the responsibility of the:
   1. Patient
   2. Physician or health care provider
   3. Student nurse
   4. Supervising nurse

4. Your employer's malpractice insurance covers you for:
   1. Incidents that occur at your home
   2. Incidents that occur while you are driving to work
   3. Incidents that occur when you are driving home from work
   4. Incidents that occur while you are working within the scope of your employment

5. When you stop to help in an emergency at the scene of an accident, if the injured party files suit and your employing institution's insurance does not cover you, you will probably be covered by:
   1. Your automobile insurance
   2. Your home owner's insurance
   3. The *Patient Care Partnership,* which may grant immunity from suit if the injured party consents
   4. Good Samaritan laws, which grant immunity from suit if there is no gross negligence

6. You are obligated to follow a physician's or health care provider's order unless:
   1. The order is a verbal order
   2. The order is illegible
   3. The order has not been transcribed
   4. The order is in error, violates hospital policy, or would be detrimental to the patient

7. A 75-year-old Hispanic woman is scheduled for colon cancer surgery in the morning. You are the night nurse and discover that the patient has decided not to have the surgery even though the consent form has been signed. What is the best action for you to take?
   1. Remind the patient that the consent is a legal document and once signed, remains in effect for 24 hours.
   2. Report the situation to the health care provider, and record it in the nurses' notes.
   3. Attempt to convince the patient that the procedure is necessary.
   4. Point out that without the procedure, the patient may die of cancer.

8. One of the elements of negligence is a breach of the standard of care or duty. Standard of care may best be defined as which of the following? Select all that apply.
   1. Nursing competence as defined by the State Nurse Practice Act
   2. The degree of judgment and skill in nursing care given by a reasonable and prudent professional under similar circumstances
   3. Health services as prescribed by community ordinances
   4. Giving care to patients in good faith to the best of one's ability

9. The nurse suspects that an older adult patient newly admitted to the nursing division is a victim of abuse based on verbal statements and the patient's overall appearance and condition. Which of the following actions is the best action for the nurse to take?
   1. Do nothing at this time, but monitor the patient's changing condition.
   2. Contact the patient's family to report what the patient has stated.
   3. Provide the patient with the telephone number for the Department of Aging.
   4. Document the patient's statements along with the nursing assessment of the patient and contact the patient's health care provider and the nursing supervisor.

10. You are the night shift nurse for a hospital nursing division of 30 acutely ill patients. There are two nurse assistants assigned to work the night shift with you. Based on the staffing and end-of-shift reports, you have determined that there is insufficient staff to safely take care of the patients on this nursing division. What is the best action for you to take?
    1. Leave the nursing division immediately.
    2. Call your nursing supervisor, inform him or her of the situation, and leave the nursing division.
    3. Contact each patient's health care provider, and inform him or her of the situation.
    4. Call your nursing supervisor to inform him or her of the situation, and document.

Answers to Review Questions can be found on pages 1197-1198.

REFERENCES

American Nurses Association: *A new code of ethics*, Silver Spring, Md, 2001, The Association.

Atwood D: Impact of medical apology statutes and policies, *J Nurs Law* 12(1):43. 2008.

Bolin J: When nurses are reported to the national practitioner data, *J Nurs Law* 10(3):141, 2005.

Brown C and others: Litigation impact of never events, *Health Lawyer News* 12(2):26, 2008.

Cady R: Nurse executive's legal primer, *JONAS Healthc Law Ethics Regul* 7(1):10, 2005.

Carpenter D: Never land, *Hospitals and Health Networks, Health Forum,* November 2007, http://www.hhamag.com.

Carter P: *HIPAA compliance handbook*, Austin, Tex, 2008, Wolters Kluwer.

Chervenak J: Medical professionals and the law: our role as experts, defendants, and litigators, *J Nurs Law* 12(1):13, 2008.

Clifford R: Who can obtain a patient's consent? Answer elusive, *The Medical-Legal News*, Sun Rays Productions, September/October 2008.

Dachs R, Elias J: What you need to know when called upon to be a good Samaritan, *Fam Pract Manage* 15(4):38, 2008.

Evans K, Cotter V: Avoiding restraints in patients with dementia, *Am J Nurs* 108(3):40, 2008.

Garner B: *Black's law dictionary*, pocket ed 3, St. Paul, 2006, West Publishing.

Johnstone M, Kanitsaki O: Culture, language, and patient safety: making the link, *Int J Qual Health Care* 18(5):383, 2006.

Karno S: Defending your license, *J Nurs Law* 10(4):214, 2005.

Kohn L and others: *To err is human, building a safer health system,* Washington, DC, 2000, National Academies Press.

Kon A: When parents refuse treatment for their child, *JONAS Healthc Law Ethics Regul* 8(1):5, 2006.

Ludwick R and others: Safety work: initiating, maintaining, and terminating restraints, *Clin Nurse Spec* 22(2):81, 2008.

Martin E, Law J: *A dictionary of law*, ed 6, New York, 2006, Oxford University Press.

Missouri State Board of Nursing position statement: patient abandonment, *Missouri State Board of Nursing Newsletter* 8(3):19, 2006.

Monarch K: Documentation. I. Principles for self-protection, *Am J Nurs* 107(7):58, 2007.

Schmalenberg C and others: Excellence through evidence: securing collegial/collaborative nurse-physician relationships, *J Nurs Adm* 35(11):507, 2005.

Standing T, Anthony M: Delegation: what it means to acute care nurses, *Appl Nurs Res* 21:8, 2008.

The Joint Commission: *Comprehensive accreditation manual for behavioral health care*, http://www.jointcommision.org, accessed November 24, 2008a.

The Joint Commission: *Comprehensive accreditation manual for hospitals*, http://www.jointcommission.org, accessed November 24, 2008b.

The Joint Commission: *National patient safety goals*, 2008c, http://www.jointcommission.org.

Vukadinovich DM: Minors' rights to consent to treatment: navigating the complexity of state laws, *J Health Law* 37(4):667, 2004.

Wacks R: *Law: a very short introduction*, New York, 2008, Oxford University Press

STATUTES

Americans With Disabilities Act, 42 USC §121.010-12213 (1995).

Autopsy Consent, Mo Rev Stat §194.115 (1998).

Comprehensive Drug Abuse Prevention and Control Act, Pub L No 91-513, 84 Stat §1236 (1970).

Good Samaritan Law, Mo Rev Stat §537.037 (1998).

Health Insurance Portability and Accountability Act of 1996, Pub L No. 104 (1996).

National Organ Transplant Act, Pub L No. 98-507 (1984).

Patient Self-Determination Act, 42 CFR 417 (1991).

Resident's Rights, Medicaid Statute, 42 USCA §1396R (1988).

Uniform Anatomical Gift Act (1987).

Uniform Determination of Death Act (1980).

CASES

Cruzan v. Director Missouri Department of Health, 497 US 261 (1990).

Darling v. Charleston Community Memorial Hospital, 33 Ill2d 326, 331, 211 NE2d 253 (1965).

Dimora v. Cleveland Clinics Foundation, 1996.

In re Intracare Hospital, 2007 WL 2682268 (Tex App, September 13, 2007).

In re Schiller, 148 NJ Super 168 (1977).

Roe v. Wade, 410 US 113 (1973).

Winkelman v. Beloit Memorial Hospital, 484 NW2d 211 (1992).

Ethics 5

MEDIA RESOURCES

 CD COMPANION 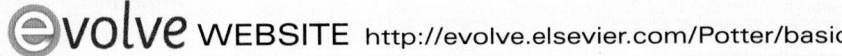 WEBSITE http://evolve.elsevier.com/Potter/basic

- Crossword Puzzle
- English/Spanish Audio Glossary

OBJECTIVES

- Explain the importance of accountability and responsibility in nursing practice.
- Discuss patient advocacy.
- Describe the role of ethics in nursing practice.

- Explain a process for analyzing an ethical dilemma.
- Describe ethical conflicts nurses experience in different clinical settings.

KEY TERMS

advocacy, p. 64
autonomy, p. 63
beneficence, p. 63
bioethics, p. 62
code of ethics, p. 63
competence, p. 64

confidentiality, p. 64
deontology, p. 66
ethical dilemma, p. 65
ethical principles, p. 63
ethics, p. 62

ethics of care, p. 66
feminist ethics, p. 66
fidelity, p. 63
institutional ethics
   committee, p. 67

justice, p. 63
morals, p. 62
nonmaleficence, p. 63
utilitarianism, p. 66
value, p. 62

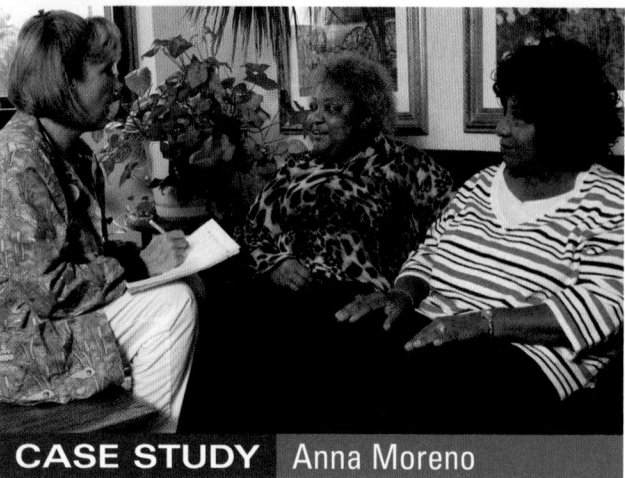

CASE STUDY   Anna Moreno

Anna Moreno, an 82-year-old African American widow and retired schoolteacher, lives with her 55-year-old daughter and three teenage grandchildren. Her daughter Lucille is a single mother and a full-time nurse. Anna Moreno assists with the care of her grandchildren when her daughter is at work. She also volunteers at the library and at her church. She has diabetes and high blood pressure, both controlled with diet and medication.

Anna's daughter accompanies her mother to the physician's office for a routine visit. When her mother steps out to have some laboratory work done, Lucille asks to speak privately to the nurse, Mary Ann, and reveals some serious concerns. Lucille had received a call from the manager of the library where her mother volunteers. The manager described finding Ms. Moreno in the janitor's closet the other day, confused and tearful. The manager expressed growing concern about Ms. Moreno's ability to finish tasks, such as reshelving books and taking phone messages. She recommended that Lucille get an evaluation of her mother's mental status. Lucille tells the nurse that she is not at all convinced that her mother is having mental problems. From Mary Ann's perspective, Lucille seems angry and defensive about the manager's report. She even accuses the manager of discrimination against older adults. She adamantly refuses offers of a physical or mental evaluation for her mother, or even to discuss the issues with her mother. Instead, she requests that the nurse write a letter that validates Anna Moreno's good health. After all, Lucille argues, her mother's blood pressure is normal, and her blood glucose levels are within normal limits. Mary Ann realizes that this situation is complex. She will need the help of others to sort out the best, most ethical response to Lucille's request.

ETHICS

As a nurse, you will play an important and intimate role in the lives of your patients. Your relationship with patients and with others on the health care team sometimes requires participation in difficult or controversial decisions. Because we live in a country of many cultures, you may face complicated situations arising from these differences. With the support of professional codes of practice and a commitment to critical thinking, you can contribute a vital and unique voice to the resolution of ethical dilemmas.

The study of ethics has occupied the attention of civilization for thousands of years. When human beings gather in community, they turn to concerns about right living. Whether you look to the ancient Chinese philosophers, the dialogues of the ancient Greeks, or traces of Mayan and Aztec culture, you will find evidence of a fundamental human effort to define right and wrong behavior. The term **ethics** refers to the consideration of standards of conduct or the study of philosophical ideals of right and wrong behavior (*American Heritage Dictionary*, 2006).

Basic Definitions

Ethical issues differ from legal issues. Systems of government determine the content of the law. Breaking a law usually results in a public consequence, such as a ticket for speeding or jail time for stealing. The law guides public behavior that will affect others and preserve community. In the case of Ms. Moreno, age discrimination laws guide the behavior of the librarians. If Ms. Moreno is in fact experiencing age discrimination, the librarians could suffer the consequences of breaking a law.

Ethics has a broader base of interest and includes personal behavior and issues of character, such as kindness, tolerance, and generosity. The terms *ethics* and *morals* sometimes are used interchangeably. **Morals** usually refer to judgment about behavior, and ethics is the study of the ideals of right and wrong behavior. Moral codes reflect the character of the social setting from which they come. In the case study, the nurse, Mary Ann, will use ethical standards of practice to guide her management of the complex health and social issues that this family currently faces.

A **value** is a personal belief about the worth you hold for an idea, a custom, or an object. The values you hold reflect cultural and social influences. For example, if your family makes a living in a rural place, you may value the environment differently from someone who visits rural areas for recreation. You use your values to shape your own point of view. Systems of ethics usually grow from shared values, negotiated and discussed over time by people who share values, such as religious groups, ethnic groups, or work groups. As you enter the nursing profession, you will undergo socialization into the profession. You will learn professional values that define your role as a nurse and that will influence your point of view. When you have a clear understanding of nursing values, as well as your personal values and own point of view, you will be able to work with the health care team in making effective ethical decisions.

The study of **bioethics** represents a particular branch of ethics, namely, the study of ethics within the field of health care. The bioethical field of study pertains to those who work in clinical settings, research, or education. Increasingly, the term

TABLE 5-1	Principles of Health Care Ethics
PRINCIPLE	**DEFINITION**
Autonomy	Independence; self-determination; self-reliance
Justice	Fairness or equity
Fidelity	Faithfulness; striving to keep promises
Beneficence	Actively seeking benefits; promotion of good
Nonmaleficence	Actively seeking to do no harm

clinical ethics is replacing the term bioethics (Chally and Hough, 2007). The field of bioethics is a prominent branch of the study of ethics, especially in the last 25 years. When researchers perfected kidney transplant technology in the early 1970s, the immediate ethical concern became the limited number of kidneys available compared with the greater number of patients in need of a transplant. The arrival of advanced medical technologies requires society to face difficult ethical questions. Who should get what resources? What is quality of life? Who should decide? In the study of bioethics, health care professionals agree to negotiate these difficult and important questions.

Nursing professionals play an important role in the practice of bioethics. Skill and confidence in one's own point of view as a participant in the interdisciplinary process of ethics is critical to the successful resolution of ethical issues. As Chally and Hough (2007) explain, "When an ethical decision is made, everyone must respect and value the perspectives held by others. Through respectful collaboration, the best decision can be reached in even the most difficult dilemma." Nurses participate in bioethical discussion in two distinct ways, as professionals and colleagues. As professionals, nurses construct a professional code of ethics that reflects and defines practice. As colleagues in the practice of health care delivery, nurses develop a specific point of view for contribution to ethical discussions about health care issues.

Ethical Principles

Practitioners in health care delivery agree to a set of ethical principles that guide professional practice and decision making. These principles are common to all professions in health care. You will find these principles especially useful because they guide nursing's commitment to advocacy, an important concept in caring for others (Table 5-1).

Autonomy refers to a person's independence. As a principle in bioethics, autonomy represents an agreement to respect a patient's right to determine a course of action. For example, before surgery, the patient is required to sign a consent form. The purpose of the consent is to ensure in writing that the health care team respects the patient's independence by obtaining permission to proceed. The consent process implies that if a patient refuses treatment, in most cases the health care team will agree to honor the patient's refusal.

Justice refers to the principle of fairness. You will often refer to this principle when discussing issues of health care resources. What constitutes a fair distribution of resources is not always clear. For example, approximately three times more candidates are on a waiting list for liver transplants than there are livers available for transplant in the United States. The just distribution of available organs is difficult to determine. In the United States a national multidisciplinary committee strives for fairness by ranking recipients according to need, rather than resorting to selling organs for profit or distributing them by lottery.

Fidelity refers to the agreement to keep promises. The principle of fidelity also promotes your obligation as a nurse to follow through with the care offered to patients. For example, if you assess a patient for pain and then offer a plan to manage the pain, the principle of fidelity encourages you to do your best to keep the promise to improve the patient's comfort.

The principle of **beneficence** promotes taking positive, active steps to help others. It encourages you to do good for the patient. Beneficence guides decisions in which the benefits of a treatment pose a risk to the patient's well-being or dignity. A child's immunization causes discomfort during administration, but the benefits of protection from disease, both for the individual and for society, outweigh the temporary discomforts. The agreement to act with beneficence requires that the best interest of the patient remains more important than self-interest. For example, you will not simply obey medical orders, but you also will act thoughtfully to understand patient needs and then work actively to help meet those needs.

Nonmaleficence refers to the fundamental agreement to do no harm. It is closely related to the principle of beneficence. This principle will be helpful in guiding your discussions about new or controversial technologies. For example, a bone marrow transplant procedure may promise a chance at cure, but the long-term prognosis is uncertain, or the procedure requires long periods of pain or suffering. You will consider these risks in relationship to the potential good that may come of the procedure. The principle of nonmaleficence promotes a continuing effort to consider the potential for harm even when it is necessary to promote health.

Codes of Ethics

A **code of ethics** is a set of **ethical principles** that all members of a profession generally accept. A profession's ethical code states the group's expectations and standards of behavior. Codes serve as guidelines to assist nurses and other professionals when conflict or disagreement arises about correct practice or behavior. The code of ethics for nursing sets forth ideals of nursing conduct and provides a common foundation for nursing education. The American Nurses Association (ANA) and the International Council of Nurses (ICN) have established widely accepted codes that you as a nurse will follow. Although these codes differ in specific emphasis, they

BOX 5-1   American Nurses Association Code of Ethics

1 The nurse, in all professional relationships, practices with compassion and respect for the inherent dignity, worth, and uniqueness of every individual, unrestricted by considerations of social or economic status, personal attributes, or the nature of health problems.

2 The nurse's primary commitment is to the patient, whether an individual, family, group, or community.

3 The nurse promotes, advocates for, and strives to protect the health, safety, and rights of the patient.

4 The nurse is responsible and accountable for individual nursing practice and determines the appropriate delegation of tasks consistent with the nurse's obligation to provide optimum patient care.

5 The nurse owes the same duties to self as to others, including the responsibility to preserve integrity and safety, to maintain competence, and to continue personal and professional growth.

6 The nurse participates in establishing, maintaining, and improving health care environments and conditions of employment conducive to the provision of high-quality health care and consistent with the values of the profession through individual and collective action.

7 The nurse participates in the advancement of the profession through contributions to practice, education, administration, and knowledge development.

8 The nurse collaborates with other health professionals and the public in promoting community, national, and international efforts to meet health needs.

9 The profession of nursing, as represented by associations and their members, is responsible for articulating nursing values, for maintaining the integrity of the profession and its practice, and for shaping social policy.

Reprinted with permission from American Nurses Association, *Code of ethics for nurses with interpretive statements,* © 2001 American Nurses Publishing, American Nurses Foundation/American Nurses Association, Washington, DC.

reflect the same underlying principles (Boxes 5-1 and 5-2), including responsibility, accountability, respect for confidentiality, competency, judgment, and advocacy.

A nurse assumes responsibility and accountability for all nursing care delivered. Responsibility refers to the execution of duties associated with a nurse's particular role. The responsible nurse demonstrates characteristics of reliability and dependability. For example, when administering a medication, you are responsible for assessing the patient's need for the drug, for giving it safely and correctly, and for evaluating the patient's response to it. By agreeing to responsibility, you will gain trust from patients, colleagues, and society.

When nurses perform care, they are accountable. Accountability refers to the ability to answer for your actions. You are accountable to yourself most of all. You also balance accountability to the patient, the profession, the employing institution, and society. *For example, in the case study, Mary Ann demonstrates accountability when she decides to organize a family conference. To best serve the interests of Ms. Moreno as well as her family, Mary Ann knows that she will need to do more than simply refuse to write a letter. The goal is the promotion of health and advocacy for the patient. The principle that guides Mary Ann is accountability.*

The concept of **confidentiality** in health care has widespread acceptance in the United States. Federal legislation known as HIPAA (Health Insurance Portability and Accountability Act of 1996) requires that those with access to personal health information not disclose the information to a third party without patient consent. HIPAA legislation defines the rights and privileges of patients for protection of privacy without diminishing access to quality care and sets fines for violations (U.S. Department of Health and Human Services [USDHHS], 2002). You cannot copy or forward medical records without a patient's consent. Health care workers are not allowed to share health care information with others without specific patient consent. This includes laboratory results, diagnosis, and prognosis. In addition, family members or friends of the patient are not permitted access to the patient's personal health information without the patient's consent. Conflicting obligations arise when a patient wants to keep information from insurance companies or from employers to preserve coverage or a job. The commitment to confidentiality is particularly challenging as medical records become computerized. Preservation of confidentiality is often in competition with the need to facilitate access to information. Health care institutions work to protect confidentiality by using special access codes that limit what certain employees are able to find on a computer system.

A responsible nurse is competent in knowledge and skills. **Competence** refers to specific knowledge and skills necessary to perform a task (*American Heritage Dictionary*, 2006). In the practice of nursing, competence ensures the provision of safe nursing care. Regulations that guide the documentation of competence vary from state to state, but the agreement to practice with competence is a common denominator for all states and is in the nursing code of ethics. For example, you make sure you know about a drug before you administer it. You understand the desired effect and possible side effects. Because you are competent, the patient is able to trust that the medications you offer are safe.

Judgment refers to the ability to form an opinion or draw sound conclusions (*American Heritage Dictionary*, 2006). In order to practice critical thinking, you will learn to practice good judgment in nursing school (see Chapter 7). You will improve your judgment skills continuously over your career.

Advocacy involves giving patients the information they need to make decisions and then supporting those decisions. It implies that caregivers try to understand and clearly state a

BOX 5-2   The ICN Code of Ethics for Nurses

PREAMBLE

Nurses have four fundamental responsibilities: to promote health, to prevent illness, to restore health, and to alleviate suffering. The need for nursing is universal.

Inherent in nursing is respect for human life, including the right to life, to dignity, and to be treated with respect. Considerations of age, color, creed, culture, disability or illness, gender, nationality, politics, race, and social status do not restrict nursing care.

Nurses render health services to the individual, the family, and the community and coordinate their services with those of related groups.

THE CODE

The *ICN Code of Ethics for Nurses* has four principal elements that outline the standards of ethical conduct.

ELEMENTS OF THE CODE

1 Nurses and People

The nurse's primary professional responsibility is to people requiring nursing care.

In providing care, the nurse promotes an environment in which the human rights, values, customs, and spiritual beliefs of the individual, family, and community are respected.

The nurse ensures that the individual receives sufficient information on which to base consent for care and related treatment.

The nurse holds in confidence personal information and uses judgment in sharing this information.

The nurse shares with society the responsibility for initiating and supporting action to meet the health and social needs of the public, in particular those of vulnerable populations.

The nurse also shares responsibility to sustain and protect the natural environment from depletion, pollution, degradation, and destruction.

2 Nurses and Practice

The nurse carries personal responsibility and accountability for nursing practice and for maintaining competence by continual learning.

The nurse maintains a standard of personal health such that the ability to provide care is not compromised.

The nurse uses judgment regarding individual competence when accepting and delegating responsibility.

The nurse at all times maintains standards of personal conduct that reflect well on the profession and enhance public confidence.

The nurse, in providing care, ensures that use of technology and scientific advances are compatible with the safety, dignity, and rights of people.

3 Nurses and the Profession

The nurse assumes the major role in determining and implementing acceptable standards of clinical nursing practice, management, research, and education.

The nurse is active in developing a core of research-based professional knowledge.

The nurse, acting through the professional organization, participates in creating and maintaining equitable social and economic working conditions in nursing.

4 Nurses and Co-workers

The nurses sustains a cooperative relationship with co-workers in nursing and other fields.

The nurse takes appropriate action to safeguard individuals when a co-worker or any other person endangers the patient's care.

Modified from International Council of Nurses: *ICN code of ethics for nurses,* Geneva, 2000, 3, place Jean-Marteau, CH-1201, The Association. *ICN,* International Council of Nurses.

patient's point of view to other health care providers. Within the health care system a multidisciplinary team delivers patient care. All members advocate for the patient. You are an important and unique part of that team. You get to know your patients through your assessments, while administering difficult or uncomfortable procedures, while teaching new skills, and preparing for discharge or home care. These activities allow you to witness important aspects of a patient's ability to cope, learn, and heal. Your ability to document, articulate, and contribute forms a key aspect of patient advocacy.

Developing a Personal Point of View

The ability to clarify and express your own point of view and then to assess and support the point of view of patients will help you to adhere to a professional code of ethics. An individual's point of view reflects cultural and social influences. Relationships with others and personal values influence point of view. Values vary among people and develop and change over time. Understanding your own values and recognizing the value systems of others will help reduce conflict during decision making.

An **ethical dilemma** exists when the right thing to do is not clear or when members of the health care team cannot agree on the right thing to do. Many ethical dilemmas require the negotiation of differing points of view. Once you understand and are able to clarify your own point of view, you will turn to the patient and begin to clarify the patient's point of view. Your goal is effective nurse-patient communication. As the patient becomes more willing to express problems and feelings, you will better establish an individualized plan of care. If ethical problems arise, a clear understanding of the patient's point of view will help you speak for the patient even if your own point of view differs.

In the case study, an ethical dilemma is taking shape. Ms. Moreno may be experiencing age discrimination at the library. But if declining health is the real cause of her problem, then the daughter's hostility will delay proper evaluation of the situation. Mary Ann is in a position to advocate for several competing points of view, including that of Anna Moreno herself. The action that she takes will require personal deliberation and perhaps the help of others to evaluate all of the options.

When the situation concerns issues of health, personal habits, and quality of life, all participants in a discussion will benefit from clarity of personal values and personal points of view. Your respect for patient differences and your skills in helping a patient clarify a point of view will promote your ability to teach and to heal. Ethics concerns itself with what people see as good and in that sense flows from values and personal points of view. Ethics is a disciplined reflection on good conduct, character, and motives that seeks to settle claims of what constitutes the "good" or valuable among people with differences. The use of ethics in decision making means going beyond personal preferences to establish standards on which individuals, professions, and societies can agree.

ETHICAL SYSTEMS

The traditional study of ethics is highly abstract and theoretical at times (Beauchamp and Childress, 2008; O'Neil, 1998). When health care providers struggle with ethical dilemmas, they need a concrete plan of action to resolve dilemmas. Traditional theories of ethics provide a foundation for devising strategies that settle ethical problems. These philosophies overlap in some areas and compete in others. Many health care providers use language from one or another of these philosophies when they discuss ethical issues. These philosophies will influence your point of view, but ultimately the choices you make about them are yours to make. Your personal values will influence which of these or what combination of them will work for you as you learn to navigate difficult ethical situations.

Deontology

This system of ethics is perhaps most familiar to health care practitioners. **Deontology** defines actions as right or wrong based on "right-making characteristics" like truth and justice (Beauchamp and Childress, 2008). You can determine the rightness or wrongness of an act according to deontology, by holding up the act to these basic principles. Deontology locates the essence of right or wrong, as opposed to looking to consequences of actions to determine right or wrong. The use of ethical principles such as justice, autonomy, and beneficence (see Table 5-1, p. 63) constitutes the practice of deontology.

Deontology proposes that to evaluate an ethical situation, we should determine the presence or absence of autonomy, justice, fidelity, beneficence, and nonmaleficence in a situation. We then use this determination as a guide for decisions about right action. If an act is just, respects autonomy, and provides good, then the act is ethical. Difficulty arises when a person must choose between conflicting principles. Conflicts can occur when people do not agree on definitions of the principles.

Utilitarianism

You use a utilitarian ethic when determining the value of something based primarily on its usefulness. The greatest good for the greatest number of people is the guiding principle for action in this system. As with deontology, utilitarianism relies on the application of the principles of "good" and "greatest." Difficulties arise when people have conflicting definitions of "greatest good." The fundamental difference between utilitarianism and deontology lies in the focus on consequences or outcomes. **Utilitarianism** guides us to measure the effect, or consequences, that an act will have. Deontology, by comparison, focuses less on consequences, and looks to the presence of pure principle.

Feminist Ethics

The foundation for feminist ethics grew from social changes that occurred as women entered the workplace during the twentieth century. Until the early 1980s, prominent thinkers held that men more commonly reached higher stages of moral development than women (Kohlberg, 1981). For Kohlberg, moral development occurs in measurable, predictable stages. The most complex stage incorporates a sense of justice, and by Kohlberg's measure, young girls do not reach this stage as often as young boys. Carol Gilligan's groundbreaking work (1993) argued that Kohlberg's definitions of moral development were gender biased. Gilligan attempted to respect gender differences without valuing one gender over the other. She maintained that young girls pay attention to community and specific circumstances, whereas young boys paid attention to abstract ideals or principles.

Feminist ethics proposes that we ask routinely how ethical decisions will affect women (Lindeman, 2005) as a way to repair a history of inequality. For example, in a discussion regarding the ethics of fetal surgery (surgical intervention before birth of the child), feminist ethics proposes that we remember to take into consideration the effect of the intervention on the mother as well as its effects on the fetus.

Ethics of Care

Proponents of ethics of care pay special attention to the nursing point of view and nursing practice (Fry, 1989). As Leininger (1988) notes, care is the "central and unifying domain for the body of knowledge and practices in nursing." Its principles, however, apply to all members of a health care community, not just nurses (see Chapter 18). Nurses base their work in caring: for the patient, for the patient's family, and for the maintenance of the institutions that provide health care services. **Ethics of care** suggest that health care workers will resolve ethical dilemmas by paying attention to relationships and stories of the participants and by the promotion of a fundamental act of caring. Attention to relationships distinguishes the ethics of care from other ethical viewpoints because it does not necessarily apply universal principles that are intellectual or analytical (Watson, 1994).

How to Process an Ethical Dilemma

Ethical problems are distressing for patients and caregivers. You do not obtain an ethical outcome, however, by considering only what people want and feel. A guide for processing ethical dilemmas serves to protect individual points of view while promoting resolution.

Most health care institutions have an **institutional ethics committee** to process ethical dilemmas. Such committees are generally multidisciplinary, with representatives from nursing, medicine, and other professional disciplines and from the community. Some institutions, especially hospitals, maintain a council specifically for nurses. Such a council educates nurses and others about the ethical process. A nursing ethics committee is especially helpful for the nurse who feels powerless or confused in the presence of an ethical dilemma. Ethics committees provide education, policy recommendation, and case consultation or review. Any involved person, including nurses or other health care providers, patients, and families of patients, can request access to an ethics committee.

Ethical issues are also processed in settings other than in a committee. Nurses provide insight about ethical problems at family conferences, staff meetings, or even in one-on-one meetings. Many ethical problems begin when people feel misled or are not aware of their options and do not know when to speak up about their concerns. Patients and health care workers address such concerns in a variety of constructive settings. Ethics committees serve to complement relationships and offer a valuable resource for strengthening them.

Whether you resolve an ethical dilemma in a committee setting, at the bedside, or in a family conference, you will apply a careful processing of the dilemma (Box 5-3). Resolving an ethical dilemma is similar to the nursing process because it requires deliberate, systematic thinking (Chally and Hough, 2007). The following offers details for processing an ethical dilemma.

Step 1: Is this an ethical dilemma?

The first step guides you to determine if the problem is an ethical one. Not all problems are ethical. You will learn to

---

BOX 5-3 How to Process an Ethical Dilemma: Ms. Moreno

Step 1. Is this an ethical dilemma?

If a review of scientific data does not resolve the question, the question is perplexing, and the answer will have profound relevance for several areas of human concern, then an ethical dilemma exists.

In the case study, Mary Ann is perplexed by her options. She cannot write a letter about Ms. Moreno's state of health without knowing more, but Ms. Moreno's daughter refuses to seek more information. For Mary Ann, an ethical dilemma exists.

Step 2. Gather all information relevant to the case.

Complete assessment of the facts of the case is critical to an effective decision. An overlooked fact sometimes provides quick resolution or deeply affects the options available. Patient, family, institutional, and social perspectives are important sources of relevant information.

In the case of Ms. Moreno, the medical record would provide important information. Other sources might include psychosocial information about Ms. Moreno's daughter and her children.

Step 3. Examine and determine your own values and opinions about the issues.

Values clarification provides a foundation for clarity and for confidence during discussions that are necessary for resolution of a dilemma. Taking this step ensures that you are able to distinguish between your personal values and those of the other participants and allows you to become a more open listener.

If you were the clinic nurse in the case study, how would you feel about elder care, child care, working mothers?

Step 4. State the problem clearly.

A clear, simple statement of the dilemma is not always easy, but it is essential for the next step to take place.

The immediate dilemma in the case study involves the request to validate Ms. Moreno's competence, without enough information to make an honest assessment.

Step 5. Consider possible courses of action.

To respect all sides of an issue, it is helpful to list potential actions, especially when the list will reflect opinions that conflict.

In the case study, actions might include consulting with a social worker and a gerontologist. Eventually, the course of action will likely involve decisions about Anna Moreno's ability to continue her work at the library.

Step 6. Negotiate the outcome.

Sometimes courses of action that seem unlikely at the beginning of the process take on new possibility as they are put to rational and respectful consideration. Negotiation requires a confidence in your own point of view and a deep respect for the opinions of others.

For Anna Moreno and her family, effective negotiation with Anna's daughter is critical to a positive outcome.

Step 7. Evaluate the action.

The last step in resolving an ethical dilemma involves evaluating the outcomes. Do the interventions provide for compromise that is acceptable to all? Have the actions taken helped to answer the questions that you identified at the beginning of the process? An ethical dilemma is often emotionally complicated, so it will be helpful to review the original issues to ensure that the process has worked.

For Anna Moreno, even though the dilemma arose around the request for a letter, other issues were identified and addressed during the process: Ms. Moreno's possible mental decline, child care issues for Ms. Moreno's grandchildren, and the fact that her daughter Lucille was refusing outside help. Because the nurse gathered all the facts and included others in the process, the resolution was effective and satisfying.

distinguish ethical problems from questions of procedure, legality, or medical diagnosis. Curtin and Flaherty (1988) suggest that a true ethical dilemma has one or more of the following characteristics:

1. Scientific data alone do not resolve the dilemma. To make this determination, you gather detailed information about the situation from medical records and health care literature and in consultation with colleagues or with the patient and family. For example, what at first appears to be a dilemma might resolve after you learn that a review of a diagnostic procedure reveals a different prognosis.
2. Dilemmas are perplexing. You cannot easily think logically or make a decision about the problem, or you may disagree with a decision that others are making, and the difference of opinion is perplexing.
3. The answer to the problem will have profound relevance for several areas of human concern.

In the case study, Mary Ann faces difficult decisions. She wants to secure a proper evaluation for Ms. Moreno, but the daughter seems adamantly against it at this point. Mary Ann may believe that the daughter is right about her perceptions of age discrimination at the library. Further information will help to determine a solution, but roadblocks such as Lucille's refusal to request an evaluation of her mother's cognitive skills will complicate this goal. The situation is frustrating, and the right course of action is not immediately clear.

Step 2: Gather all relevant information.

Accurate and complete information is essential for the ethical process to go forward.

For example, Mary Ann already knows quite a bit about the health and the social situation of Ms. Moreno, but what about the grandchildren? What about Lucille's job situation? What is Anna Moreno's cognitive skill level, at least so far as Mary Ann is able to determine? Perhaps most important of all, what does Ms. Moreno want?

Step 3: Examine and determine your own values and opinions about the issues.

A part of gathering information will include a determination of your own opinion about the issues. The distinction between personal opinion and the facts of the case or the opinions of others is essential to reach resolution. People come to different conclusions about the same situation with no malice intended toward other people. Remembering this will help you to be an effective moderator in conversation.

Considering the possibility that Lucille is correct in her accusations about the librarian is an important part of the process. More likely, Lucille is overreacting to the situation and is in denial about her mother's health, because the loss of her mother's child care support will profoundly affect Lucille's ability to keep her full-time job. What if Mary Ann has strong opinions against single motherhood? The ability to process any dilemma requires that personal values be clear and that you respect the values of others.

Step 4: State the problem clearly.

After reviewing relevant information, develop a clear statement of the problem in language that all involved in the ethical discussion will understand. The statement lays the groundwork for the negotiations that follow. Discussions are more likely to remain focused and constructive when all parties agree on the dilemma statement.

In the case of Ms. Moreno, what is wrong with her, if anything, and who will best make that determination? Is Anna Moreno the best person to decide about her own well-being, or is the daughter, Lucille, the right person? What about Mary Ann? Can she make independent decisions regarding the health of Ms. Moreno?

Step 5: Consider possible courses of action.

You facilitate a discussion of ethical dilemmas by listing possible courses of action as they occur to the group. Possibilities can occur at any time during the discussion.

A discussion with the librarian, Anna Moreno, Lucille, and Mary Ann will clarify the situation. Perhaps Mary Ann can bring in a social worker to evaluate the home setting, as well as to offer an independent opinion about Ms. Moreno's cognitive skills. The timing of the discussion is important because Lucille works nights. She will most likely function better if they schedule a meeting around her usual sleep times during the day. The grandchildren could participate in a part of the meeting, depending on their ages. Important questions remain: Is Ms. Moreno competent to give consent about her own health care, and is she competent to perform daily activities independently and responsibly?

Step 6: Negotiate the outcome.

Mary Ann consults with Ms. Moreno's health care provider. They create a plan that involves multidisciplinary action. Mary Ann organizes a family conference at which a nonthreatening discussion unfolds. Participants include a social worker with expertise in community resources and the pastor from the church Anna Moreno and her daughter attend. During the discussion Anna asks for her husband and becomes angry when Lucille reminds her that her husband died 5 years ago. As Lucille begins to realize that her mother's condition is worse than she realized, she begins crying. The team of people at the meeting recognizes that this family has suddenly become a vulnerable family, with issues of health and well-being at risk. They help Lucille take immediate action to obtain family leave from work, and they begin the long task of taking care of all the other issues that affect the situation: financial constraints, the care of the children, the care of Anna, confidentiality, and issues of consent (how much does Anna understand, and can she realistically consent to medical procedures?). The pastor helps to end the meeting with a prayer, which brings great comfort to the family.

Step 7: Evaluate the action.

Make decisions and evaluate them in an ongoing manner.

Documentation of the ethical process takes a variety of forms. Whenever the process involves a family conference or results in a change in the management plan, you will document the process in the medical record. Some institutions use a formal consultation format whenever a request for discussion comes to the ethics committee. If the ethical dilemma does not directly affect patient care, however, documentation occurs by means of minutes from a meeting or in a memorandum to affected parties.

COMMON ETHICAL PROBLEMS IN NURSING

In any practice setting you will be confronted with ethical issues unique to that practice. The following sections describe examples of ethical dilemmas common in health care settings today.

Allocation of Scarce Resources: The Nursing Shortage

The nursing shortage in the United States is a real and a growing problem. Buerhaus and others (2009) estimate that the shortage could reach as high as 500,000 by 2025. The American Hospital Association (2007) reported that in 2007 approximately 116,000 positions for nurses remained unfilled at hospitals around the United States, a vacancy rate over 8%. Contributing factors involve cultural, economic, and social elements. For example, nursing faculty shortages restrict the ability of schools to accept students. Over 40,000 applicants to baccalaureate and graduate nursing programs had to be turned away in 2007 because nursing programs did not have room for them, in large part due to insufficient number of teachers (American Association of Colleges of Nursing, 2008). Of nurses who remain in practice, the average age is increasing, up to 46.8 years in 2004, compared with 45.2 in 2000 (USDHHS, 2007).

The nursing shortage can result in difficult working conditions that affect patient outcomes. The Institute of Medicine's report on the magnitude of medication errors includes discussion on the role of the nurse, and the role of inadequate staffing as a source of medication error (Kohn, Corrigan, and Donaldson, 2000).

You can consider the shortage in terms of ethical concerns. How does a nurse decide what is the best course to take when a patient care assignment feels too large to be safe? California is the first state in the United States to pass mandated staffing ratios. Laws limit the number of patients assigned to a nurse. The law stipulates that if a hospital does not have enough nurses to fulfill staffing requirements, then the hospital must "close beds," restricting access to care. The nursing shortage and the mandated staffing ratios create ethical dilemmas. Professional issues of advocacy and patient abandonment compete with ethical concerns about beneficence, malfeasance, and justice. Political solutions, in addition to personal decisions, can play a role in the resolution of ethical dilemmas such as the nursing shortage.

Managed Care

In the acute care setting, managed care systems emphasize the value of decreasing hospitalization days. To safely accomplish a shorter hospitalization, patient education and discharge planning fall to the bedside nurse. An ethical dilemma arises if you determine that the patient and the patient's family have not mastered a skill needed to provide safe care in the home, yet the patient's insurance will not cover further days in the hospital.

Step 1: Is this an ethical dilemma?

The situation is perplexing because it seems that whether or not the patient remains in the hospital, unwanted consequences will result. A safe and affordable solution to this dilemma has relevance for the patient and for the acute care setting.

Step 2: Gather all the information relevant to the case.

Who pays for this patient's care, and who in this setting is responsible for negotiating with payers? What is the patient's prognosis, and how long will home care be necessary? What will be the financial impact of unsafe care in the home? How much more time do you think the patient needs to learn the needed skill? Can a home care service provide the care and further teaching?

Step 3: Examine and determine your own values and opinions on the issues.

You may have had a variety of experiences with managed care in the past, some positive and some negative. It will be important to separate personal responses in the past from this current situation. A professional evaluation of the patient's readiness for discharge will play a critical role in the negotiations, so make sure you clearly understand your own opinion and that you have an accurate assessment of the patient's situation.

Step 4: State the problem clearly.

What resources will provide the safest *and* most cost-effective care for this patient? How do you protect the principle of beneficence for this patient and yet remain accountable to the hospital and to the managed care plan?

Step 5: Consider possible courses of action.

You decide to take time to inform administrators and health care providers about the patient's lack of knowledge. You propose a solution by investigating the location and quality of home care services. You learn more from the patient about family resources.

Step 6: Negotiate the outcome.

Working with social workers, health care providers, and admission and utilization review personnel helps you develop a safe plan for discharge. Certainly, working within the guidelines of the managed care plan is essential for success. In addition, the patient responds to the dilemma by identifying other family members or community resources that facilitate a safe discharge. At the very least, you ensure that the health care provider and others become aware of the potential for unsafe conditions after discharge.

Step 7: Evaluate the action.

The nature of the outcome will depend on your ability to pursue an option that protects this patient during and after discharge.

End-of-Life Issues

Working with chronically ill or disabled patients involves decisions about quality of life, such as the patient's ability to maintain independence and functional status. You may also

BOX 5-4   BEST PRACTICES

Do Not Resuscitate Decisions

SUMMARY OF EVIDENCE

Discussions about end of life and "do not resuscitate" (DNR) orders are generally considered the obligation of physicians. Nurses often participate in and may even initiate the discussion with physicians, but nurses rarely if ever initiate DNR discussions with patients or families. Nurses may even be prohibited by policy from initiating such discussions. Surveys performed at several critical care units, however, reveal that nurses are more likely than physicians to believe that nurses should be able to conduct DNR discussions. Furthermore, 69% of physicians interviewed agreed. Nurses also expressed more comfort and satisfaction with end-of-life discussions than did the physician respondents. As the study authors comment, this comfort may flow from the greater amount of time that nurses spend with patients in critical care settings, compared with physicians. The surveys were administered to nurses, attending physicians, interns, and residents. Responses were evaluated statistically using standardized measures.

APPLICATION TO NURSING PRACTICE

The results of this investigation raise important issues about care delivered to patients who are dying. As the authors pose in this study, "Why are staff nurses not allowed, in most settings, to initiate DNR discussions?" Their findings raise "ethical questions about the proper division of responsibilities between physicians and nurses in caring for patients at the end of life, about which powers should be reserved for physicians, about the meaning of caring for patients as a team, and about what policy truly would best serve the patients whom all health care professionals have pledged to serve."

REFERENCE

Sulmasy DP and others: Beliefs and attitudes of nurses and physicians about do not resuscitate orders and who should speak to patients and families about them, *Crit Care Med* 36(6):1817, June 2008.

confront situations where decisions related to death and dying will be critical to the resolution of ethical dilemmas (Box 5-4). For example, a patient who is profoundly disabled by a recent stroke begins to suffer from aspiration problems during feedings. Would a gastrostomy tube serve to prevent aspiration, or would it represent a surgical intervention that prolongs suffering?

Step 1: Is this an ethical dilemma?

Scientific data help to predict improved nutrition and improved safety for this patient, but they do not help to address the ethical issues about quality of life. You are puzzled, as is the family, about the right decision. A decision that felt "right" to all parties would have profound relevance for this dilemma and influence similar clinical situations in a positive way.

Step 2: Gather all the information relevant to the case.

What is the prognosis for this patient? What are the surgical risks and benefits from placement of the gastrostomy tube? What is the medical risk for aspiration pneumonia in this patient before and after tube placement? Would pneumonia and the treatment represent an uncomfortable experience for the patient? Does the patient have a living will or advance directive or has the patient assigned medical power of attorney to another person (see Box 5-4)?

Step 3: Examine and determine your own values and opinions on the issues.

Begin by exploring your personal feelings about the quality of this patient's life. Is the patient able to express an opinion? If the answer is yes, you probably have personal opinions about the competence of the patient. These opinions are important to articulate. How do you feel about the competence of the family members and significant others? If the patient or health care workers made a decision with which you disagree, it is important to consider whether you could still participate in the care of the patient. Could you advocate for a position that was in conflict with your own values?

Step 4: State the problem clearly.

Will a gastrostomy tube improve the quality of this patient's life, or will a gastrostomy tube prolong suffering? How can the team best respect this patient's autonomy?

Step 5: Consider possible courses of action.

The patient could have the gastrostomy tube placed or perhaps have a nasogastric tube placed temporarily while the more difficult ethical issues are explored with the patient and the patient's family. The patient or the patient's significant others could decide against the insertion of a gastrostomy tube. If the patient decides against the gastrostomy tube, then you could make a referral to hospice care to ensure continued support for the patient and the family.

Step 6: Negotiate the outcome.

If the patient is a competent adult, the patient's decision will determine the outcome. If the patient is not competent, then the health care team will have to rely on family members, significant others, or even legal documents that identify legal guardians to make the decision. In this last case the decision is sometimes more difficult to obtain. Your role in the negotiations includes patient advocacy and the contribution of the nursing perspective on quality of life for this individual. You also need to be honest and truthful with the family (Clark and Volker, 2003).

Step 7: Evaluate the action.

Regardless of the decision in this case, it is possible to reverse the decision if conditions or feelings change. Continuing discussion with the patient and the family or significant others ensures a satisfactory conclusion to this dilemma.

Cultural and Religious Sensitivity

The professional standards of justice and beneficence require respect for cultural differences in the health care setting, regardless of personal opinion or feeling. Occasionally you will face a challenging situation in which cultural differences present an ethical dilemma. For example, a 15-year-old girl is admitted for management of her leukemia. You note that the adolescent's religious beliefs do not allow her to receive blood transfusions, yet her condition will soon require a blood transfusion to prevent harmful consequences. Her parents share her religious convictions but are willing to compromise. The 15-year-old refuses to compromise.

Step 1: Is this an ethical dilemma?

Further review of the clinical situation will not change the dilemma. Scientific data will not affect the strong feelings of the child or her parents. The case is perplexing because respecting the patient's autonomy conflicts with the health care team's wish to do no harm. The resolution of this dilemma will be difficult and will have profound relevance for several areas of concern, including the life of the patient.

Step 2: Gather all the information relevant to the case.

How soon does the patient need the transfusion? What are the legal definitions of "minor" in your state? Has the family agreed to transfusions in the past, and if so, how was the compromise reached? What are the specific religious constraints against blood transfusions that affect this case? Is the patient competent? Is she fully aware of the consequences of her decision to refuse the transfusion?

Step 3: Examine and determine your own values and opinions about the issues.

How do you feel about this patient's religious beliefs? How close or distant are the patient's beliefs from your personal beliefs? What is your personal opinion on the rights of minors to determine their medical course?

Step 4: State the problem clearly.

A patient, who is a minor, will refuse a lifesaving transfusion on the grounds of religious belief. If she is forced to receive the transfusion, she will consider herself violated in the eyes of her God. If she does not receive the transfusion, she will probably not survive.

Step 5: Consider possible courses of action.

The parents and health care team could force the patient to receive a transfusion, which will require restraints or use of physical force. You could respect the patient's wishes. You could encourage the patient and her family to explore this dilemma with the guidance of a religious leader from their faith.

Step 6: Negotiate the outcome.

In this case, your contribution consists of accurate documentation of the patient's state of mind. A patient care conference with the patient and her family is necessary. If the medical team decides to insist on the transfusion, then they will seek a court order. As advocate for the patient, even in the face of personal disagreement, you will ensure that the patient's voice is fairly represented to the judge.

Step 7: Evaluate the action.

The outcome will depend on the ability of the conference members to reach agreement. The goal will be the balancing of respect for autonomy with the principle of beneficence.

Delegation

Most health care delivery models involve nursing assistive personnel such as nurse assistants and technicians, and licensed practical nurses who work with registered nurses in providing patient care. The registered nurse uses delegation skills and the guidance of legal statutes to determine and assign work to others on the health care team. Occasionally this collaboration presents ethical dilemmas. Some dilemmas are especially troubling because the registered nurse is ultimately accountable for patient care. Furthermore, the issues are not always associated directly with patient care, but with behavior and work habits. For example, an unlicensed nurse assistant who is basically a reliable team member performs her work in a timely and accurate manner. But you notice that the assistant spends most of her time with one patient, ignoring the special needs of others.

Step 1: Is this an ethical dilemma?

Technically this situation constitutes a personnel issue rather than an ethical dilemma. However, professional standards of beneficence and justice suggest that nurses equally distribute care for patients. Because the assistant's behavior is otherwise meeting expectations, the situation is perplexing. A solution could have relevance for her work with others.

Step 2: Gather all information relevant to the situation.

If other nurses work with this nurse assistant, how do they describe their relationship with her? What is her job description officially? What was her training for this position? Who is her supervisor? How do patients describe her care? How does the law hold you accountable for the actions of others on the health care team?

Step 3: Examine and determine your own values and opinions on the issue.

What are your personal opinions about the team approach to nursing? Have you had training in delegation skills or supervision skills? How does the nurse assistant's behavior affect your work responsibilities?

Step 4: State the problem clearly.

Is this nurse assistant working in an appropriate or inappropriate way? If inappropriate, who is responsible for correcting the behavior?

Step 5: Consider possible courses of action.

You could meet privately with the assistant to talk about the reasons for the nurse assistant's behavior and determine resolutions. You could refer the situation to a supervisor. You could develop and provide classes on setting priorities for all assistants.

Step 6: Negotiate the outcome.

First consult with the nursing supervisor or unit manager. It is important to stay informed about institutional policies and to seek guidance from colleagues. What does the law dictate in regard to accountability for patient care? The ability to advocate for nursing standards, especially an ethic of care, will remain a professional obligation. The recognition and articulation of an ethical dilemma begin the process.

Step 7: Evaluate the action.

Monitoring patient satisfaction may be the best way to measure the outcome of this dilemma.

To resolve an ethical problem, learn to depend on a systematic process that helps all participants gain a common understanding of the problem and to plan a responsible course of action. Ethical dilemmas can present great challenges, but the challenges are almost always resolvable. As a nurse, you offer a unique, valuable voice to the process of resolution.

KEY POINTS

- Basic principles of ethics in health care include autonomy, justice, fidelity, beneficence, and nonmaleficence.
- A code of ethics provides a foundation for professional nursing.
- Professional nursing promotes accountability, responsibility, and advocacy.
- An ethical nurse maintains competence in practice and assumes responsibility for nursing judgments.
- The primary functions of advocacy are to inform and to support.
- Professional nurses have a commitment to patients, the profession, and society to provide high-quality health care.
- Ethical problems arise from differences in values, changing professional roles, technological advances, and uncertainty in decision making.
- Ethical dilemmas in nursing will occur in any segment of the health care delivery system.
- A standard process for critical thinking in the face of ethical dilemmas helps nurses resolve difficult situations.
- The nurse's point of view provides a unique and valuable voice in the resolution of ethical dilemmas.

CRITICAL THINKING EXERCISES

In the case study at the beginning of this chapter, the nurse Mary Ann had been asked by the patient's daughter to vouch for the patient's well-being, and yet the patient's daughter refused to allow an assessment of her mother's cognitive condition.

1. Mary Ann could have simply refused to write the letter, but she felt obligated to investigate further. Describe the professional characteristic illustrated by Mary Ann's decision to investigate further.
2. If you were responsible for organizing a patient care conference for Anna Moreno, what disciplines besides your own would you consider including? List at least two, and explain why you would include them.
3. Can you explain Mary Ann's actions in terms of the basic principles of ethics? Discuss how each principle helped to guide Mary Ann in her resolution of the dilemma.

ⓔvolve   *Answers to Critical Thinking Questions can be found on the Evolve website.*

REVIEW QUESTIONS

1. Ethical dilemmas often arise over a conflict of opinions. Each of the following steps constitutes a correct step to take toward resolution of an ethical dilemma. Which step occurs first?
   1. Clarify your own values about the issue.
   2. Call a meeting in which those involved in the dilemma can discuss (negotiate) the possible solutions to the dilemma.
   3. List the potential actions that you can take to resolve the dilemma.
   4. Gather all relevant information regarding the clinical, social, and spiritual aspects of the dilemma.
2. In the United States, access to health care usually depends on a patient's ability to pay for health care, either through insurance or by paying cash. You are caring for a patient who needs a liver transplant to survive. This patient has been out of work for several months and does not have insurance or enough cash to pay for the transplant. The primary principle at stake in a discussion about the ethics of this situation is:
   1. Accountability, because you as the nurse are accountable for the well-being of this patient
   2. Respect for autonomy, because this patient's autonomy will be violated if he does not receive the liver transplant
   3. Ethics of care, because the caring action would be to provide resources for a liver transplant
   4. Justice, because the first and greatest question in this situation is how to determine the just distribution of resources

3. The code of ethics for nurses is a set of ethical principles that all members of the profession generally accept. Elements within the code include:
   1. Continuing education requirements, staffing ratios, and compensation guidelines
   2. Principles including responsibility, accountability, competency, and advocacy
   3. Research about best practices in a variety of health care settings
   4. Historical foundations of nursing as defined by Florence Nightingale
4. In most ethical dilemmas the solution to the dilemma requires negotiation among members of the health care team. As the nurse, your point of view is valuable because:
   1. Nurses have a legal license that mandates their presence at ethical discussions
   2. The principle of autonomy guides all participants to respect their own self-worth
   3. Nurses develop a relationship with the patient that is unique among all care providers
   4. The nurses' code of ethics recommends that a nurse be present at any ethical discussion about patient care

5. The philosophy of utilitarianism proposes that:
   1. The value of something is determined by its usefulness to society
   2. The value of people is determined solely by leaders in the Unitarian church
   3. The decision to provide medical care depends on a measure of the moral life that the patient has led so far
   4. The best way to determine the solution to an ethical dilemma is to refer the case to the attending health care provider
6. The philosophy sometimes called the ethics of care suggests that you resolve an ethical dilemma best by attention to:
   1. Relationships
   2. Ethical principles
   3. Communication principles
   4. Code of ethics for nurses
7. Health care providers, including professional nurses, agree to "do no harm" to their patients. The point of this agreement is to reassure the public that in all ways the health care team will not only work to heal patients, but they agree to do this in the least painful and harmful way possible. The principle that describes this agreement is called:
   1. Beneficence
   2. Accountability
   3. Nonmaleficence
   4. Respect for autonomy
8. Nurses and other providers agree to be advocates for their patients. Practice of advocacy calls for the nurse to:
   1. Seek out graduate education as soon as possible
   2. Work to understand the law as it applies to the patient's clinical condition
   3. Assess the patient's point of view and prepare to articulate this point of view
   4. Document all clinical changes in the medical record in a timely and legible way

Answers to Review Questions can be found on pages 1197-1198.

REFERENCES

American Association of Colleges of Nursing: *2007-2008 enrollment and graduations in baccalaureate and graduate programs in nursing,* 2008, http://www.aacn.nche.edu/Media/factsheets/FacultyShortage.htm.

American heritage dictionary, ed 4, Boston, 2006, Houghton Mifflin.

American Hospital Association: *The 2007 state of America's hospitals: taking the pulse,* http://www.aha.org/aha/content/2007/PowerPoint/StateofHospitalsChartPack2007.ppt

American Nurses Association: *Code of ethics for nurses with interpretative statements,* Washington, DC, 2001, The Association.

Beauchamp T, Childress J: *Principles of biomedical ethics,* ed 5, New York, 2008, Oxford University Press.

Buerhaus P and others: *The future of the nursing workforce in the United States: data , trends and implications,* Boston, 2009, Jones & Bartlett.

Chally PS, Hough MC: Nursing ethics. In Chitty KK: *Professional nursing: concepts and challenges,* ed 4, St. Louis, 2007, Saunders.

Clark AP, Volker DL: Truthfulness, *Clin Nurse Spec* 17(1):17, 2003.

Curtin L, Flaherty MJ: *Nursing ethics: theories and pragmatics,* Bowie, Md, 1988, Brady.

Fry ST: The role of caring in a theory of nursing ethics, *Hypatia* 4(2):88, 1989.

Gilligan C: *In a different voice,* Cambridge, Mass, 1993, Harvard University Press.

International Council of Nurses: *ICN code of ethics for nurses,* Geneva, 2000, The Council.

Kohlberg L: *Essays on moral development,* vols 1-3, San Francisco, 1981, Harper & Row.

Kohn LT, Corrigan JM, Donaldson MS, editors: *To err is human,* Washington, DC, 2000, National Academies Press.

Leininger M: *Caring: an essential human need,* Detroit, 1988, Wayne State University Press.

Lindeman H: *An invitation to feminist ethics,* New York, 2005, McGraw-Hill Humanities.

O'Neil J: Ethical decision making and the role of nursing. In Deloughery G: *Issues and trends in nursing,* ed 3, St. Louis, 1998, Mosby.

Sulmasy DP and others: Beliefs and attitudes of nurses and physicians about do not resuscitate orders and who should speak to patients and families about them, *Crit Care Med* 36(6):1817, 2008.

U.S. Department of Health and Human Services: *HHS fact sheet: modifications to the standards for privacy of individually identifiable health information—final rule,* August 9, 2002, http://www.hhs.gov/news/press/2002pres/20020809.html.

U.S. Department of Health and Human Services, Federal Division of Nursing: *2004 National sample survey of registered nurses,* 2007, http://bhpr.hrsa.gov/healthworkforce/rnsurvey04/.

Watson J, editor: *Applying art and science of human caring.* New York, 1994, National League of Nursing Press.

6 Evidence-Based Practice

 CD COMPANION 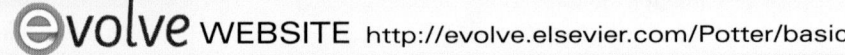 **WEBSITE** http://evolve.elsevier.com/Potter/basic

- Crossword Puzzle
- English/Spanish Audio Glossary

OBJECTIVES

- Describe the six steps of evidence-based practice.
- Develop a PICO or PICOT question.
- Discuss the levels of evidence in the literature.
- Explain why critiquing of the literature is a necessary step in evidence-based practice.
- Discuss ways to apply evidence in practice.

- Discuss factors to consider in the selection of outcome measures for an evidence-based practice change.
- Explain how nursing research improves nursing practice.
- Explain the relationship between evidence-based practice and performance improvement.

KEY TERMS

bias, p. 79
clinical guidelines, p. 77
evidence-based practice, p. 75
hypotheses, p. 80

nursing-sensitive outcome, p. 82
peer-reviewed, p. 77
performance improvement (PI), p. 84

PICO, p. 76
Plan, Do, Study, Act (PDSA), p. 84
quality improvement (QI), p. 84

reliable, p. 80
sentinel event, p. 84
valid, p. 80
variables, p. 80

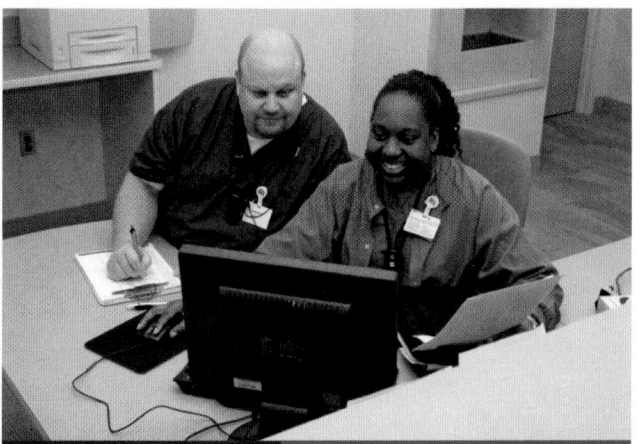

CASE STUDY Shana and Eric

Shana and Eric are two nurses who work in the surgical intensive care unit (ICU). They belong to their unit practice committee (UPC), which consists of a group of staff nurses, a pharmacist, an infection control practitioner, and a physician. The committee meets monthly to discuss practice issues on the unit and has received a copy of the monthly report on the quality indicators for their unit. Shana notes that the incidence of catheter-related bloodstream infections (CR-BSIs) has steadily increased during the last 3 months. Patients with central venous catheters (CVCs), used to deliver fluids and medications over extended periods of time (see Chapter 17), are becoming infected, but why? Is there a problem with the type of dressing placed over the catheter or the way the site is cleansed before insertion (see Chapter 13)?

Shana and Eric volunteer as part of their committee responsibilities to implement an evidence-based practice project. Their first step will be to develop a clinical question and then search the scientific literature. Their aim is to determine what evidence is available so that they can make an informed decision about the best approaches for reducing CR-BSIs in their patients.

Many nurses practice nursing according to what they learn in nursing school, their experiences in practice, and the policies and procedures of their institutions. When nurses fail to routinely question their practices and do not seek new scientific information, nursing practice becomes rapidly outdated and patient care suffers (Melnyk and Fineout-Overholt, 2005). When this occurs, nursing is then based more on tradition and not on up-to-date information. The use of best evidence when making decisions about patient care enhances clinical performance and enables nurses to help patients and families achieve best outcomes.

A CASE FOR EVIDENCE-BASED PRACTICE

Evidence-based practice (EBP) dates back to the founder of nursing, Florence Nightingale. She was an astute observer who asked questions, formed hypotheses (suggested explanations for observable phenomena), collected and analyzed data, and then used the information to improve the care of her patients. Today EBP is an important health care initiative. Nurses practice in an "age of accountability" in which quality and cost issues drive the direction of health care (Newhouse and others, 2005). The general public is more informed about their own health, the health care issues affecting society, and the incidence of medical errors within health care institutions. More people now question why certain health care approaches are used, which ones work, and which ones do not. Thus EBP is one response to this shift in thinking, which nurses and other health professionals cannot ignore (Newhouse and others, 2005). EBP is a guide for how nurses make accurate, timely, and appropriate clinical decisions.

Nurse clinicians regularly face important clinical decisions when caring for patients (e.g., Are there better ways of providing patient care? Is a change in nursing practice indicated?). It is very important to review available research findings, apply clinical judgment and expertise, and then translate the best evidence into best practices at a patient's bedside. For example, using a sliding board to transfer a patient from bed to stretcher instead of lifting and using the research-based Braden scale (see Chapter 36) to routinely assess a patient's risk for skin breakdown are examples of using evidence at the bedside. **Evidence-based practice** is a problem-solving approach to clinical practice that combines the conscientious use of best evidence in combination with a clinician's expertise, patient preferences and values, and available healthcare resources in making decisions about patient care (Melnyk and Fineout-Overholt, 2005; Sackett and others, 2000).

EBP is becoming a goal for all health care institutions, and thus staff nurses are being asked to integrate evidence into their daily practice (Phillips and others, 2006). Typically, new students will diligently read their textbooks and the assigned scientific articles. A good textbook incorporates current evidence into the practice guidelines and procedures it describes. However, a textbook relies on the scientific literature, and sometimes information on a particular topic is outdated by the time a book is published. Scientific articles from nursing and the health care literature are available on almost any topic involving nursing practice. However, although the scientific basis of nursing practice has grown, some practices are not "research based." This means that some nursing practices are not based on findings from well-designed research studies because findings are inconclusive or researchers have not yet studied the practices (Titler and others, 2001). The challenge is to obtain the very best, most current information at the right time, when you need it for patient care.

The best scientific evidence comes from well-designed, systematically conducted research studies, usually found in scientific journals. Unfortunately, much of that evidence never reaches the bedside. Nurses in practice settings, unlike educational settings, do not have easy access to databases for scientific literature. Instead, nurses often care for patients on the basis of tradition, convenience, or the standard, "It has always been done this way."

Other valuable sources of evidence are non–research based. They include the following:

- Performance improvement data
- Risk management data
- International and local clinical guidelines
- Infection control data
- Benchmarking
- Retrospective or concurrent chart reviews
- Clinicians' expertise

It is important for you to seek out research evidence rather than solely depending on non–research-based evidence. When you face a clinical problem, ask yourself where the best evidence is to help you find the best solution in caring for patients.

Even when you use the best evidence available, application and outcomes will differ based on your patients' values, preferences, concerns, and/or expectations (Oncology Nursing Society [ONS], 2005). EBP is not finding research evidence and blindly applying it without using good judgment. The correct application of EBP involves ethical and accountable professional nursing practice (Avis and Freshwater, 2006). In addition, EBP involves a participatory approach, with nurses working with other health care practitioners in seeking best evidence and ensuring it is relevant to their unique group of patients (Baumbusch and others, 2008). As a nurse, you will use critical thinking skills to determine what evidence is appropriate and related to your patients' clinical situations. For example, a single research article involving older adults shows that the use of therapeutic touch is effective in reducing patients' perceptions of abdominal pain. However, if your patients have cultural beliefs that discourage use of touch, you will likely need to search for a different evidence-based therapy that your patients will accept. Using your clinical expertise and considering patients' values and preferences ensure that you will apply the evidence available in practice both safely and appropriately.

Steps of Evidence-Based Practice

EBP is a systematic approach to determine the most current and relevant evidence upon which to base patient care decisions (Brancato, 2006). Melnyk and Fineout-Overholt (2005) recommend a six-step process for EBP:

- Ask a clinical question.
- Collect the most relevant and best evidence.
- Critically appraise the evidence you gather.
- Integrate all evidence with your clinical expertise and patient preferences and values in making a practice decision or change.
- Evaluate the practice decision or change.
- Communicate results of the change.

ASK THE CLINICAL QUESTION Always think about your practice when caring for patients. Question what does not make sense to you, and question what you think needs clarification. Think about a problem or area of interest that is time consuming, costly, or not logical (Callister and others, 2005). If you keep a clinical journal, your entries will be a rich

BOX 6-1	Developing a PICO or PICOT Question

P = Patient population of interest
Identify your patients by age, gender, ethnicity, disease, or health problem.

I = Intervention of interest
What is the intervention you want to use in practice (e.g., a treatment, diagnostic test, educational approach)?

C = Comparison of interest
What is the usual standard of care or current intervention you use now in practice?

O = Outcome
What result do you wish to achieve or observe as a result of an intervention (e.g., change in patient behavior, physical finding, patient perception)?

T = Type of study
What level of research study (e.g., systematic review or randomized controlled trial) do you wish to look for in the literature review?

source for clinical questions. Titler and others (2001) suggest using problem- and knowledge-focused triggers to think critically about clinical and operational nursing-unit issues. A problem-focused trigger is one you face while caring for a patient or a trend you see on a nursing unit. For example, Shana and Eric have identified from the quality indicator report that the trend in CR-BSIs has increased over each of the last 3 months. Both nurses want to identify a solution to reduce the infection rate in the ICU. Examples of problem-focused triggers resulting from patient care might include a patient injury or the inability to achieve a successful patient or family outcome. Such triggers lead to questions such as "What is the best approach to teach a family caregiver about a patient's expected side effects of medication?" or "How can I reduce falls among older adults on my unit?"

A knowledge-focused trigger is a question that arises as a result of new information available on a topic. For example, "What is the current evidence for the best way to educate patients with low health literacy?" Important sources of new scientific information are the standards and practice guidelines available from national agencies such as the Agency for Healthcare Research and Quality (AHRQ), the American Pain Society (APS), and the American Association of Critical-Care Nurses (AACN). Other sources of knowledge-focused triggers include recent research publications and nurse experts within an organization (Titler and others, 1994).

The questions you ask will lead you to the evidence for an answer. When you ask a question and then go to the scientific literature, you do not want to read 100 articles to find the handful that are most helpful. You want to be able to read the best four to six articles that specifically address your practice question. Melnyk and Fineout-Overholt (2005) suggest using a **PICO** format to state questions. Other educators suggest using a PICOT format (Box 6-1). A formatted question helps you to identify the key words that will then allow you to conduct a successful literature search. For example, Shana and Eric first went to the literature with a general background question: "What aseptic techniques affect CR-BSI in central venous catheters?" They were quickly frustrated when they found numerous articles about different factors that influence CR-BSI in CVCs. They decide to write a focused PICO question: "Does the use of 2% chlorhexidine (I) compared with alcohol (C) for cleansing CVC insertion sites of surgical patients (P) reduce the incidence of CR-BSI (O)?" Another PICO question is "Does the use of maximum sterile barrier techniques (I) compared with sterile gloving only (C) reduce the incidence of CR-BSI (O) in postoperative surgical patients (P)?" A well-designed PICO question does not have to follow the sequence of P, I, C, and O, but the aim is to ask a question that contains as many of the PICO elements as possible. If you ask a PICOT question, it allows you to focus on certain types of research studies that pertain to your question.

Inappropriately formed questions (e.g., What is the best way to reduce CR-BSI? What is the best way to measure blood pressure?) are background questions that will lead to many irrelevant sources of information, making it difficult to find the best evidence. However, it is sometimes necessary to begin with a background question if you do not have the knowledge needed to form a more specific PICO question. The PICO format allows you to ask questions that are intervention focused. Some questions that arise in nursing practice do not always contain all of the PICO elements. An example is a meaning-focused question such as "How do women with breast cancer (P) rate their quality of life (O)?" which contains only a P and an O.

The questions you ask in a PICO format identify knowledge gaps within a clinical situation. The type of evidence you do not have for clinical practice becomes clearer when you ask well–thought-out questions. Examples of different knowledge gaps include the following (ONS, 2005):

- *Diagnosis:* questions about the selection and interpretation of diagnostic tests. Example: Does the use of a disposable oral thermometer compared with an electronic oral thermometer measure body temperature accurately in a patient with an endotracheal tube?
- *Prognosis:* questions about the patient's likely clinical outcome from disease or treatment. Example: Is there a difference in the incidence of deep vein thrombosis in surgical patients receiving subcutaneous heparin compared with subcutaneous low-molecular-weight heparin?
- *Therapy:* questions about the selection of the most beneficial treatments. Example: What bowel regimen is most effective in relieving constipation caused by the administration of opioid therapy in patients with chronic pain?
- *Prevention:* questions about screening and preventive approaches to reduce the risk for disease. Example: Does a prostate specific antigen (PSA) test in an older man who is asymptomatic of prostate disease decrease his risk for death from prostate cancer?
- *Education:* questions about best teaching strategies for nurses, patients, or family members. Example: Does the use of visual aids compared with low-literacy teaching booklets improve adherence to therapeutic diets among adults with low literacy?

Remember, do not simply be satisfied with clinical routines. Do question and use critical thinking to consider better ways to provide patient care.

COLLECT THE BEST EVIDENCE Once you have a clear and concise PICO question, you are ready to search for evidence. There are thousands of resources available to search for evidence, including websites, agency procedure manuals, performance improvement data, existing clinical practice guidelines, and computerized bibliographical databases. Do not hesitate to ask for help to find appropriate evidence. Your faculty will of course always be a key resource. When you are assigned to a health care setting, consider using experts such as advanced practice nurses, staff educators, risk managers, and infection control nurses.

When you go to the scientific literature for evidence, it is wise to seek the assistance of a medical librarian. A medical librarian knows the various databases that are available to you (Box 6-2). The databases are repositories of published scientific studies, including peer-reviewed research. A **peer-reviewed** article is one submitted for publication and reviewed by a panel of experts familiar with the topic or subject matter of the article. The librarian is available to translate your PICO question into the language or key words that will yield the best evidence search. When conducting a search, you will enter and manipulate different key words until you get the combination that gives you the articles you want to read about your question. For example, Shana and Eric's PICO question includes the key words "catheter-related bloodstream infection," "surgical patients," "chlorhexidine," and "alcohol." When you enter a word to search into a database, be prepared for some confusion with the evidence you obtain. The vocabulary in published articles is often vague. The word you select sometimes has one meaning to one author and a very different meaning to another. A medical librarian can help you learn how to choose alternative words (e.g., "surgery" versus "surgical patients") or terms that identify your PICO question and thus ensures you obtain evidence about your question.

MEDLINE and CINAHL are among the best-known comprehensive databases and represent the scientific knowledge base of health care (Melnyk and Fineout-Overholt, 2005). Some databases are available through vendors at a cost, whereas others are free of charge. As a student, you will have access to a vendor paid by your school. Vendors such as OVID usually offer several different databases. There are also databases available free on the Internet. The Cochrane Database of Systematic Reviews is a valuable resource that contains high-quality, independent evidence for health care decision making. The Cochrane Database includes the full text of regularly updated systematic reviews. The AHRQ supports the National Guidelines Clearinghouse (NGC) database. It contains **clinical guidelines**, systematically developed statements about a plan of care for a specific set of clinical circumstances involving a

BOX 6-2   Searchable Scientific Literature Databases and Sources

CINAHL	Cumulative Index of Nursing and Allied Health Literature. Includes studies in nursing, allied health, and biomedicine. http://www.cinahl.com/
MEDLINE	Includes studies in medicine, nursing, dentistry, psychiatry, veterinary medicine, and allied health. http://www.ncbi.nim.nih.gov
PsycINFO	Psychology and related health care disciplines. http://www.apa.org/psycinfo/
Cochrane Database of Systematic Reviews	Full text of regularly updated systematic reviews prepared by the Cochrane Collaboration. Includes completed reviews and protocols. http://www.cochrane.org/reviews
National Guidelines Clearinghouse	Repository for structured abstracts (summaries) about clinical guidelines and their development. Also includes condensed version of guideline for viewing. http://www.guideline.gov/
PubMed	Health science library at the National Library of Medicine. Offers free access to journal articles. http://www.nlm.nih.gov
World Views on Evidence-Based Nursing	Electronic journal containing articles that provide a synthesis of research and an annotated bibliography for selected references.
Middlesex University	Provides a Web-based tutorial that teaches the basic steps of the EBP process. http://www.mdx.ac.uk/www/rctsh/ebp/main.htm

EBP, Evidence-based practice.

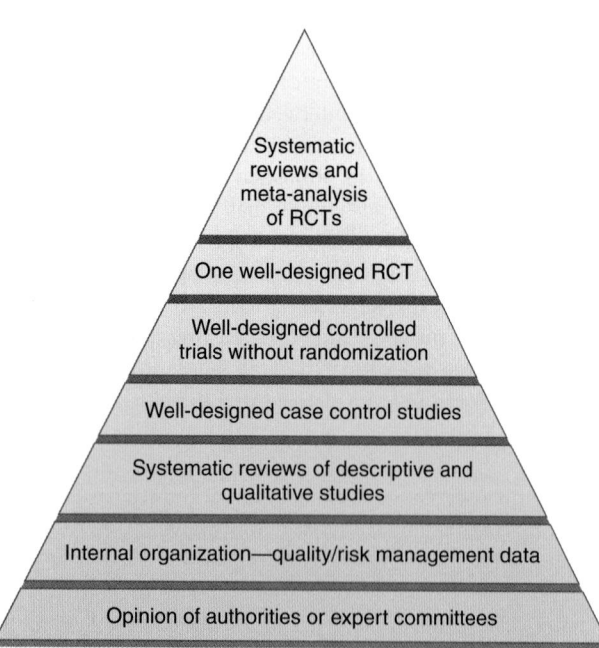

Figure 6-1 ■ Hierarchy of evidence. *RCTs,* Randomized controlled trials. (Modified from Guyatt G, Rennie D: *User's guide to the medical literature,* Chicago, 2002, American Medical Association; Melnyk BM, Fineout-Overholt E: *Evidence-based practice in nursing and healthcare: a guide to best practice,* Philadelphia, 2005, Lippincott Williams & Wilkins.)

specific patient population. Examples of clinical guidelines on NCG include care of children and adolescents with type 1 diabetes and practice guidelines for the treatment of adults with low back pain. The NGC is invaluable when you want to develop a plan of care for a patient (see Chapter 8).

The pyramid in Figure 6-1 represents one example of the hierarchy of available evidence. At this point in your nursing career, you cannot be an expert on all aspects of the types of research studies conducted. But you can learn enough about the types of studies to help you know which ones have the best scientific evidence. At the top of the pyramid are systematic reviews or meta-analyses, which are state-of-the-science summaries from an individual researcher or panel of experts. If you are lucky to find a systematic review on your PICO question, it means that a researcher has asked the same PICO question as yours, reviewed the highest level of evidence available (e.g., randomized controlled trials [RCTs]), and then reported on the state or level of evidence available. A good systematic review basically does a literature search on a topic for you and tells you what evidence exists about your question. In a systematic review the researcher will report on whether the evidence is conclusive and in favor of the intervention or whether further study is necessary, and why.

An RCT is the highest level of experimental research. In an experiment a researcher tests an intervention (e.g., method for intravenous site care or patient education) against the

BOX 6-3   Example of a Randomized Controlled Trial (RCT)

Research question: Will the use of simulation training compared with traditional lecture format improve nursing students' competency in physical examination techniques?

Subjects: 130 associate-degree students in first clinical semester.

Randomization: Students are randomly assigned to one of the two education groups.

Treatment group: 65 students attend a 3-hour simulation laboratory on physical examination techniques.

Control group: 65 students attend a 3-hour lecture on physical examination techniques.

Outcome measure: Both groups are tested 2 weeks after the class for their ability to demonstrate physical examination techniques on patients visiting an outpatient clinic.

Analysis: Statistical tests compare the competency test results for the two groups. Statistics will show if the treatment (simulation laboratory) has the predicted effect of improved competency.

usual standard of care (Box 6-3). Researchers assign subjects in an experiment to either a control or treatment group through random assignment. In other words, all of the subjects have an equal chance to be in either group. The treatment group receives the experimental intervention, and the control group receives the usual standard of care. The researchers measure both groups for the same outcomes to see if the experimental intervention made a difference. When an RCT is completed, the researcher will know if the intervention leads to better outcomes than the standard of care.

As you look at the hierarchy pyramid in Figure 6-1, the level of rigor or exactness in how researchers conduct studies moves down the pyramid. The RCT is the most precise form of experimental study. A single RCT is not as conclusive as a systematic review. However, a single RCT that tests the same intervention as your question will provide very useful evidence. Controlled trials without randomization are studies that test interventions, but researchers have not randomized the subjects into the control or treatment groups. For example, subjects might be selected by the convenience of the researcher (e.g., patients chosen in the order of admission to a hospital). Thus there is potential **bias** in how the study is designed, which can distort study findings. How subjects fall into the control or treatment group sometimes influences the results. Careful critique will allow you to identify if bias was in a study and whether or not it affected the findings or evidence. This will affect your decision to use the evidence.

In a well-designed case control study, researchers study one group of subjects with a certain condition (e.g., young women with cervical cancer) at the same time as another group of subjects who do not have the condition. A case control study determines if there is an association between one or more predictor variables and the condition (Melnyk and Fineout-Overholt, 2005). For example, is there an association between predictors such as health literacy level, socioeconomic status, or financial resources and the incidence of cervical cancer? Often a case control study is conducted retrospectively, or after the fact. Researchers look back in time and review available data (e.g., medical record reviews) about the two groups of subjects to understand what variables explain the condition. These studies usually involve a small number of subjects, but there is again a risk for bias. Sometimes the subjects in the two groups differ on certain other variables (e.g., education or access to a physician) that also influence the incidence of the condition, more so than the variables being studied.

Nonexperimental descriptive studies are common in nursing research. Such a study describes, explains, or predicts phenomena. Examples of descriptive studies include the following: What are factors that increase the occurrence of CR-BSIs? What factors contribute to falls by hospitalized patients with cancer? When a researcher wants to learn if there is a relationship between two variables (e.g., type of catheter dressing and CR-BSIs), a correlational descriptive study is appropriate. The researcher learns if the two variables are correlated or likely associated with one another. Often the findings from descriptive studies will lead researchers to design studies involving the testing of interventions. For example, if the researcher learns that CR-BSIs are associated with a type of catheter dressing, the researcher might test a new type of dressing or approach for application.

Many questions about nursing practice are not focused on selection of best interventions, but instead focus on a better understanding of the nature of patients' health problems. Nurses care for patients' responses to a disease or health problem. For example, we assist patients with problems such as knowledge deficits, symptom management, and coping with psychological distress. RCTs do not always address how patients experience these types of health problems.

Qualitative research offers answers when trying to understand patients' experiences with health problems and the contexts of their experiences. Patients have the chance to tell their stories and share their experiences in qualitative studies. The findings are in-depth because patients usually describe their experiences in detail. Examples of qualitative study topics include "family members' perceptions of nursing hospice care" and "the experience of living with chronic ulcerative colitis." Qualitative research is invaluable in identifying information about how patients cope or manage various health problems and their perceptions of illness.

Health care agencies routinely gather data about trends in clinical practice. Most hospitals, for example, keep monthly records on key quality indicators such as medication errors or infection rates. All Magnet-designated hospitals (see Chapter 2) maintain the National Database of Nursing Quality Indicators (NDNQI). The database includes information from all Magnet hospitals on falls, pressure ulcer incidence, and nurse satisfaction. Typically quality and risk management data will not give you evidence in finding a solution to a problem, but the data will inform you about the nature or severity of problems occurring within the health care setting. Access to quality data may help you refine or redirect your PICO question.

The use of clinical experts may be at the bottom of the evidence pyramid, but do not consider clinical experts as a poor source of evidence. Expert clinicians use evidence frequently as they build their own practice, and they are rich sources of information for clinical problems.

CRITIQUE THE EVIDENCE Perhaps the most difficult step in the EBP process is critiquing or analyzing the available evidence. Once you have conducted a literature search, you now have some scientific articles to read and review. During the review you will determine the value, feasibility, and utility of evidence for making a practice change (ONS, 2005). When you critique evidence, you evaluate the scientific worth and whether the findings apply to your clinical situation or area of interest. For example, Shana and Eric will review their articles on CR-BSIs and decide if there is convincing evidence for the use of chlorhexidine instead of alcohol in cleansing catheter sites. Some clinicians rate the level of evidence according to an evidence hierarchy similar to the one in Figure 6-1 (p. 78). For example, evidence from a systematic review would be rated a 1, whereas evidence from published clinical articles might be rated a lower level 6 (Oman, Duran, and Fink, 2008). After reviewing each study, you summarize the critiques so that you have a sense of what evidence is available to answer your PICO question. After critiquing the evidence you will be able to answer the following questions: Do the articles together offer evidence to answer my PICO question? Do the articles show the evidence is true, **reliable,** and **valid?** Can I use the evidence in practice?

As a student new to nursing, it will take time for you to acquire the skills to critique research evidence. When you read an article from the literature, do not let the statistics or technical wording cause you to put the article down and walk away. Know the elements of an article, and use a careful approach when reviewing each one. Evidence-based articles include the following elements:

- *Abstract:* An abstract is a brief summary of the article that quickly tells you if the article is research or clinically based. An abstract summarizes the purpose of the study or clinical review, the major themes or findings, and the implications for nursing practice.
- *Introduction:* The introduction of a scientific article describes its purpose and the importance of the topic for the audience who reads the article. There is usually brief supporting evidence as to why the topic is important from the author's point of view.

Together, the abstract and introduction tell you if you want to continue to read the entire article. You will know if the topic of the article is similar to your PICO question or related closely enough to provide you useful information. Continue to read the next elements of the article:

- *Literature review or background:* A good author offers a detailed background of previous studies and the level of

evidence, or clinical information, that exists about the topic of the article. The literature review explains what led the author to conduct a study or report on the clinical topic. This section of an article is very valuable. Perhaps the article itself does not address your specific PICO question the way you want, but it will possibly lead you to other more useful articles. Once you read the literature review, you should have a good idea of how past research led to the researcher's question. For example, a study designed to test the effects of aseptic practices on CR-BSI will review literature that describes the nature of CR-BSI and the patients most at risk, the type of factors shown previously in the literature to contribute to CR-BSI, and any previous interventions used to prevent CR-BSI.

- *Manuscript narrative:* The "middle section" or narrative of a manuscript differs according to the type of evidence-based article it is (Melnyk and Fineout-Overholt, 2005). A clinical article will describe a clinical topic, which often includes a description of a patient population, the nature of a certain disease or health alteration, how patients are affected, and the appropriate nursing therapies. An author sometimes writes a clinical article to explain how to use a therapy or new technology. A research article will contain several subsections within the narrative, including the following:

  - Purpose statement—explains the focus or intent of a study. It identifies what concepts will be researched. This includes research questions (what the researcher intends to learn from the study) or **hypotheses**—predictions made about the relationship between study **variables** (concepts, characteristics, or traits that vary among subjects). An example of a research question: Does the use of chlorhexidine 2% compared with povidone-iodine reduce catheter-related bloodstream infection in patients with CVCs?

  - Methods or design—explains how researchers organize and conduct studies in order to answer the research questions or to test the hypotheses. This is where you learn what type of study it is (e.g., RCT, case control, qualitative study). You also learn how many subjects or persons are in a study. In health care studies, subjects may include patients, family members, or health care staff. The language in the methods section is sometimes confusing when it explains how a researcher designs a study to minimize bias so as to obtain the most accurate results possible. Use your faculty member as a resource to help interpret this section.

- *Results or conclusions:* Clinical and research articles will have a summary section. In a clinical article, the author explains the clinical implications for the topic presented. In a research article, the author details the results of the study and explains whether a hypothesis is supported or how a research question is answered. This section will include either a statistical analysis or a very thorough summary of the descriptive themes and ideas that arise from the researcher's analysis of data. Do not let the statistics in an article stump you. Read carefully, and ask these questions: Does the researcher describe the results? Were the results significant (unlikely to have occurred by chance)? Were the results clinically relevant (pertinent or connected to your clinical situation)? Have a faculty member assist you in interpreting statistical results. A good author will also discuss any limitations to a study in the results section. This information on limitations will be valuable in helping you decide if you want to use the evidence with your patients.

- *Clinical implications:* A research article will include a section that explains if the findings from the study have clinical implications. The researcher will explain how to apply findings in a practice setting for the type of subjects studied.

After you have critiqued each article for your PICO question, combine the findings from all of the articles to determine the state of the evidence. Use critical thinking to consider the scientific rigor of the evidence and how well it answers your area of interest. Consider the evidence in light of your patients' concerns and preferences and available health care resources. Your review of articles offers a snapshot conclusion of the combined evidence on your PICO question. As a new nurse, you will learn to judge whether to use the evidence for a particular patient or group of patients, who usually have complex health care situations (Melnyk and Fineout-Overholt, 2005). Decide if the evidence is relevant and applicable to your setting of practice and if it has the potential for improving patient outcomes (Box 6-4). Ethically it is important to consider evidence that will benefit patients and do no harm.

In the case of Shana and Eric, they have critiqued several articles about the use of chlorhexidine and other antibiotic solutions for preventing CR-BSI. They now bring the summary to their UPC. The entire committee collaborates and applies their clinical expertise. They consider the types of patients they see in their intensive care unit and then determine if the evidence is strong enough for use in practice. The critique shows that chlorhexidine is safe to use with surgical ICU patients and should replace the use of alcohol.

INTEGRATE THE EVIDENCE Once you decide that the evidence is strong and applicable to your patients and clinical situation, incorporate the recommended evidence into practice. The easiest step is to take the evidence you find and apply it in your plan of care for a patient (see Chapter 8). Use the evidence as the scientific rationale for an intervention you plan to try. For instance, you are assigned to work in a nursing center, and you care for a patient who wanders. Your review of the literature offered evidence on techniques to reduce wandering. You decide to use the technique during your next clinical assignment. You use the technique with your assigned patient, or you work with a group of other students or nurses in revising a policy and procedure or developing a new clinical protocol for the nursing center.

A common approach used for integrating evidence into practice is to incorporate new evidence into policies and procedures. A key feature of a practice environment that supports the use of best evidence is requiring clinical practice policies and procedures to be evidence based (Oman and others, 2008). Many organizations involve staff nurses and research-prepared advanced practice nurses to review scientific articles relevant to policies and procedures and to then make appropriate revisions. Policies and procedures are important tools for supporting hospital-based nurses in using evidence in their everyday practice and promoting positive patient outcomes.

After reviewing the evidence on CR-BSI presented by Shana and Eric, the UPC decides to revise the policy and procedure for central catheter insertion and maintenance. The evidence shows the use of chlorhexidine and full barrier precautions are effective in reducing CR-BSI. Thus the evidence becomes part of the new guidelines for site cleansing, insertion, and dressing care. With the revision to policy, Shana, Eric, and the ICU nurses implement the new central catheter policy and procedure.

You can use evidence in a variety of other ways through teaching tools, clinical practice guidelines, and new assessment or documentation tools. Depending on the amount of change needed to apply evidence in practice, it becomes necessary to involve a number of staff from a given nursing unit. It is important to consider the setting in which you want to

---

BOX 6-4   BEST PRACTICES

SUMMARY OF EVIDENCE
Evidence-based practice (EBP) is still a relatively new concept in nursing school curriculums. In a descriptive study involving nursing students in Norway, faculty educated their students about the three steps of EBP: forming a question, searching the evidence, and critically appraising the evidence. Students were asked to review two scientific articles relating to their question. During classes the students discussed different sections of the articles to understand the most relevant information. At the end of the course the

students took an examination that required them to critically evaluate a new article. The study surveyed students at the end of the course. The majority of students reported that having learned steps of EBP they were better able to critically review scientific articles.

APPLICATION TO NURSING PRACTICE
Knowledge about the EBP process increases nursing students' critical thinking attitudes about evidence and their ability to use evidence in their practice.

REFERENCE
Smith-Strom H, Nortvedt MW: Evaluation of evidence-based methods used to teach nursing students to critically appraise evidence, *J Nurs Educ* 47(8):372, 2008.

apply the evidence. Is there support from all staff? Do(es) the practice change(s) fit with the scope of practice in the clinical setting? Are there resources (time, secretarial support, and staff) available to make a change?

As a nursing student integrating evidence, your focus will begin with searching for and applying best evidence to improve the care you directly provide your patients. Using an EBP approach will improve your skills and knowledge as a nurse and improve your patients' outcomes.

EVALUATE THE PRACTICE DECISION OR CHANGE

After applying evidence in your practice, your next step is to evaluate the effect. How does the intervention work? How effective was the clinical decision for your patient or practice setting? Sometimes your evaluation is as simple as determining if the expected outcome you set for a specific intervention is met (see Chapter 8). For example, when using a new approach to preoperative teaching, does the patient learn what to expect after surgery?

When an evidence-based practice change occurs on a larger scale, an evaluation will be more formal. For example, evidence of factors that place patients at risk for pressure ulcers leads a nursing unit to adopt a new skin care protocol. To evaluate the protocol, the nurses on the EBP team will track the outcome of incidence of pressure ulcers over a course of time (e.g., 6 months to a year). In addition, the nurses will collect data to describe both the patients who develop ulcers and those that do not. This comparative information is valuable in determining the effects of the protocol and whether modifications are necessary.

The evaluation of an EBP change determines if the practice change is desirable, if you need to modify your intervention, or if you need to discontinue the practice change. Unforeseen variables may lead to results that you do not anticipate. For example, the changes made in the protocol developed by Shana and Eric might lead to an increase in CR-BSIs. If this is not determined during evaluation, the practice would continue and patients would suffer. **Never** implement a practice change without evaluating its effect.

Outcomes Measurement   To be effective in evaluating the effects of an EBP change, you must measure outcomes. An outcome is an observable effect of an intervention (see Chapter 8). The use of outcome measures for evaluation is effective in determining if a patient progresses or if a practice change was beneficial or effective. It is important to know that an outcome is not a measure of a care provider

action. For example, if you implement the use of around-the-clock (ATC) administration of analgesics for postoperative pain instead of the usual approach to administration whenever there is a need (prn) (see Chapter 16), an outcome is not whether the nurses are successful in documenting patient pain scores. The documentation of patients' pain scores is a process indicator, not an outcome measure. Process indicators simply tell you if an intervention was completed. The outcome is the patients' actual ratings of pain on the pain scales. The pain ratings will tell you if the use of ATC analgesia effectively reduces patients' pain more so than the traditional prn approach.

It is important to be able to link a nursing intervention to a patient outcome. Usually a nursing intervention is just one element of many therapies for patient care. The more care providers that are involved in an intervention and the more complex the intervention, the more difficult it is to identify which action or care provider was responsible for the outcome. A **nursing-sensitive outcome** focuses on how nursing interventions affect patients and offers a measure of nursing's contribution to patient care (ONS, 2008). Nursing-sensitive outcomes look at the effects of interventions within the scope of nursing practice and integral to the processes of nursing care. Examples of nursing-sensitive outcomes include the following (ONS, 2008):

- Symptoms (e.g., pain, fatigue, nausea)
- Functional status (e.g., activity tolerance, ability to perform activities of daily living and instrumental activities of daily living)
- Safety (e.g., incidence of falls, infections, pressure ulcers)
- Psychological distress (e.g., anxiety, depression)

When selecting an outcome to evaluate a practice change, consider the type of measurement to use. Will you observe a patient behavior or collect a physiological measure (e.g., weight or blood pressure), conduct an interview, audit an existing medical record, or check results in a laboratory report? If you do not choose the correct measurement approach, you will not be certain if an outcome was met (Table 6-1). For example, if you administer analgesics and use relaxation techniques to reduce a patient's pain, your outcome of reduced pain will be measured by using a pain rating scale. In Shana and Eric's case, they will measure the incidence of CR-BSI among patients with central catheters.

TABLE 6-1 Outcome Measurement	
OUTCOME	**MEASUREMENT APPROACH**
Patient will lose 10 lb in 2 months	Weight
Patient will describe side effects of antihypertensive medication	Patient interview
Patient will be satisfied with nursing care	Patient satisfaction survey
Patient will express less fatigue after a 4-week exercise program	Self-report fatigue scale
Incidence of methicillin-resistant *Staphylococcus aureus* will drop among surgical patients	Medical record laboratory reports

The measurement will be review of laboratory reports for positive blood cultures of patients with central lines during a 1-month period.

An outcome measure should always be appropriate for your patients or families. When you implement an EBP change, will you observe patients or will you ask the patients to complete a survey or questionnaire? Consider if any outcome measure is too difficult for a patient to complete due to factors such as pain, fatigue, or level of consciousness. For example, there are scales designed for measuring dyspnea, a distressful sensation of uncomfortable breathing. Some of the scales involve observations by nurses, and some involve surveys completed by patients. Some of the scales are short (two to three items), whereas others are very lengthy. If you are measuring dyspnea in patients who are in palliative care, you will likely choose a scale that is short and easy to collect by an observer. If you are measuring dyspnea of patients in an exercise clinic, you might choose the more lengthy tool that a patient has time to complete.

You will be more successful in implementing EBP when outcome measurement plans are acceptable and important to the clinicians involved. This of course means including colleagues in any EBP project from the beginning when you select outcome measures. It is also important to be consistent and accurate when collecting outcome measures. Any clinicians who are involved in outcome measurement should receive proper training in data measurement and collection. For example, if outcome measurement involves a new device such as a pulse oximeter, each data collector must show competence in use of the oximeter. Those who collect outcome data must collect the data in the same way. For example, if you decide to use a new patient satisfaction survey, EBP team members should practice administering the tool and then use a single set of guidelines for administering the tool to patients. Competence and consistency in measurement help to ensure quality outcome data. Outcome measurement contributes to the body of evidence and strengthens the process of evidence-based practice. Showing how an EBP change affects outcomes builds on the knowledge we have about nursing practice.

COMMUNICATE THE RESULTS After collecting outcome measures and evaluating the effects of an EBP change, it becomes necessary to communicate results. If you implement an evidence-based intervention at an individual patient level, you let the patient know the results of your therapy. Is the patient's wound showing signs of healing? Has the patient correctly learned how to self-administer an injection? When your practice change occurs on a larger unit level, the first group to communicate results to is the clinical staff of a nursing unit. The EBP team should share results in a larger staff meeting or perhaps in a unit-based newsletter. Clinicians enjoy and appreciate seeing the results of a practice change. In addition, the practice change will more likely be sustainable, remaining in place, when staff are able to see that a change has been beneficial.

It is important for a health care agency to benefit as much as possible from EBP. When a nursing unit or clinical area makes an EBP change, you should communicate the results to the entire agency. Nurses and other clinicians from different units might choose to make the same type of practice change. They can achieve this through agency committees, grand rounds presentations, and EBP seminars.

As a professional nurse, it is critical for you to contribute to the growing knowledge of nursing practice. When you are involved in an EBP change, consider how you can communicate your results to the profession at large. Becoming involved in professional societies or organizations allows you to present EBP changes in scientific abstracts, poster presentations, or even in podium presentations.

NURSING RESEARCH

After completing a thorough review and critique of the scientific literature, you might not have strength of evidence to make a practice change. Instead you might find a gap in knowledge or that your PICO question is unanswered. When that occurs, the best way to answer your question is through the research process. At this time in your career you will not be conducting research, but it is important for you to understand the process. Research is a systematic process that asks and answers questions to generate new knowledge. The knowledge then provides a scientific basis for nursing practice and validates the effectiveness of nursing interventions. This chapter does not cover the details of how to conduct research.

Nursing research is a way to identify new knowledge, improve professional education and practice, and use resources effectively. In the past, much of the information used in nursing practice was borrowed from other disciplines such as biology, physiology, psychology, and sociology. Often this information was applied to nursing without testing or comparing ways of caring for patients. For example, nurses use several methods to help patients sleep. Interventions such as giving a patient a back rub, making sure that the bed is clean and comfortable, preparing the environment by dimming the lights, and talking to a worried or anxious patient are frequently used nursing measures and, in general, are logical, commonsense approaches. However, when you consider these measures in greater depth, questions arise about their applications. For example, are they the best methods to promote sleep? Do different patients in different situations require other interventions to promote sleep?

Research provides a way for nursing questions and problems to be studied in greater depth within the context of nursing. When a review of existing evidence fails to answer a question, nursing research becomes the next choice. Nursing interventions must be tested through research to determine the measures that work best with specific patients. Nursing research then creates the evidence for EBP. Nursing research improves nursing practice and raises the standards for the profession. Promoting EBP and research increases your scientific knowledge base for practice. The recipients of these improvements to practice are your patients, their families, and the communities in which they live.

QUALITY AND PERFORMANCE IMPROVEMENT

Near the bottom of the evidence pyramid (see Figure 6-1) you will find quality data. Every health care organization gathers data on a number of health outcome measures as a way to determine their quality of care. Examples of quality data include fall rates, number of medication errors, incidence of pressure ulcers, and infection rates. Health care organizations actively promote efforts for improving patient care and outcomes, particularly with respect to reducing medical errors and enhancing patient safety. Quality data are the outcome of both quality improvement and performance improvement initiatives. The Joint Commission (TJC) defines **quality improvement (QI)** as an approach to the continuous study and improvement of the processes of providing health care services to meet the needs of patients and others (TJC, 2008a). An institution's QI program focuses on improvement of health care–related processes (e.g., medication delivery and fall prevention). Performance measurement means what an institution does and how well it does it. In **performance improvement (PI)** an organization analyzes and evaluates current performance to use results to develop focused improvement actions. PI activities are typically clinical projects conceived in response to identified clinical problems and designed to use research findings to improve clinical practice (Melnyk and Fineout-Overholt, 2005).

EBP and QI go hand in hand. It is important when implementing an EBP project to review available QI data. The information is invaluable for understanding the extent of a problem within your organization. QI data offer information about how to focus EBP efforts. For example, if a nursing unit has experienced a rise in the fall rate over the last several months, the QI data can be valuable in identifying the type of patients who fall, time of day of falls, and possible precipitating factors (e.g., efforts to reach bathroom, multiple medications, or patient confusion). A thorough analysis of QI data then leads clinicians to identify the best evidence available for correcting quality problems. For example, QI data will help form a PICO question, such as, "Do surgical patients who develop confusion have increased fall rates compared with those without confusion?" Once the staff integrates the evidence into a fall prevention protocol, they will implement the protocol (in this case, focusing efforts on techniques for reducing confusion) and evaluate its results. Reliable, good-quality data improve the relevance and scope of an EBP project.

Quality Improvement Programs

A well-organized QI program focuses on processes or systems that significantly contribute to outcomes. Facilities need an organization-wide, systematic approach to ensure that every-one supports a continuous QI philosophy. This begins with the organizational culture, in which all staff members understand their responsibility toward maintaining and improving quality. Typically in health care, many persons are involved in single processes of care. For example, medication delivery involves the health care provider who prescribes medications, the secretary who communicates new orders being written, the pharmacist who prepares the dosage, the transporter who delivers medications, and the nurse who prepares and administers the drugs. Thus all members of the health care team collaborate together in QI activities. As a member of the nursing team, you will participate in recognizing trends in practice, identifying when recurrent problems develop, and initiating opportunities to improve the quality of care.

The QI process begins at the staff level, where all disciplines become involved in defining problems. This requires staff members to know the practice standards or guidelines that define quality. Unit QI committees review activities or services considered to be most important in providing quality care to patients. To identify the greatest opportunity for improving quality, the committees consider those activities that are high volume (greater than 50% of a unit's activity), high risk (potential for trauma or death), and problem areas for patients, staff, or the institution. For example, on an orthopedic nursing unit, hip surgery volume is high, older adults over 80 years of age have more postoperative complications, and family members are dissatisfied with patients' pain control. Any one of these factors could become the focus of a QI project. Another example is The Joint Commission's annual patient safety goals (2008b), which provide an excellent focus for QI initiatives (see Chapter 27). Sometimes a problem is presented to a committee in the form of a **sentinel event,** an unexpected occurrence involving death or serious physical or psychological injury. Once a committee defines the problem, it applies a formal model for exploring and resolving quality concerns. There are many models for QI and PI. One model is the PDSA cycle—plan, do, study, act:

Plan: Review available data to understand existing practice conditions or problems to identify the need for change.
Do: Select an intervention on the basis of the data reviewed, and implement the change.
Study: Study (evaluate) the results of the change.
Act: If the process change is successful with positive outcomes, act on the practices by incorporating them into daily unit performance.

In the following example, a QI committee applies the **Plan, Do, Study, Act (PDSA)** model for addressing a practice problem.

On the 32-bed medicine oncology unit there has been an increased incidence of patient falls. The number of falls has risen over the last 6 months. Added to the problem is the fact that the oncology patients receive chemotherapy, which lowers their platelet counts and increases their susceptibility to injury (bruising and serious bleeding internally) when they fall. One of The Joint Commission's patient safety goals for 2009 is reduc-

ing the risk for patient harm resulting from falls (TJC, 2008a). The nurse manager on the oncology unit brings together a QI committee consisting of nurses, a pharmacist, a physical therapist, a physician, and risk management staff. The QI committee conducts a root cause analysis in their planning. The members review all available data to find the real cause of the problem and then work on dealing with it. The committee learns that the majority of falls involve adults under the age of 60 years. The patients fall when trying to reach the bathroom or when they are trying to get up to a chair. Many patients have received intravenous Benadryl, a medication administered before blood transfusions that can cause dizziness as a side effect.

The committee members conduct a literature review on the evidence. They develop a PICO question: "Does Benadryl compared with no pretransfusion medication increase fall risk among cancer patients?" and a background question, "What interventions related to fall prevention have reduced falls among patients with cancer?" Based on a review and critique of the scientific evidence, the committee selects an intervention, an hourly nursing rounds protocol. The plan is to have registered nurses (RNs) check on patients on the even hours and nursing assistive personnel (NAP) check routinely on odd hours. During rounds the RNs and NAP apply approaches specific to their competencies to focus on key fall risk factors. The NAP offer patients the chance to toilet, provide timely comfort measures, and remove barriers around the patient's bedside. The RNs monitor patients' responses to analgesics and the effects of Benadryl (e.g., dizziness or sleepiness), and

discuss the patient's unique risks for falling. The outcome measure used to determine efficacy of the hourly rounds protocol is the monthly fall index in addition to a short data form on characteristics of patients who fall. After implementing the protocol, the nursing staff gathers data for 3 months to evaluate if falls have declined. The committee compiles the monthly fall index ratings and the data from the short data forms to determine if the rounding protocol was effective. The results showed that the incidence of falls decreased consistently over the 3 months. A fall did occur during a change-of-shift report. The committee decides to permanently implement the nursing rounds protocol. Discussion also involves how to adjust to making sure nurses conduct rounds even when staffing is low or involved in change-of-shift report.

QI combined with EBP is the foundation for excellent patient care and outcomes. Once a QI committee makes a practice change, it is important to communicate results to staff in all appropriate organizational departments. Practice changes will likely not last when QI committees fail to report findings and results of interventions. Regular discussions of QI activities through staff meetings, newsletters, and memos are good communication strategies. Often a QI study reveals information that will prompt organization-wide change. An organization must be responsible for responding to the problem with the appropriate resources. Revision of policies and procedures, modification of standards of care, and implementation of new support services are examples of ways an organization responds.

KEY POINTS

- Evidence-based practice involves the review of available research findings, application of clinical judgment and expertise, and then translation of the best evidence into best practices at a patient's bedside.
- The six steps of evidence-based practice provide a systematic approach to rational clinical decision making.
- The components of a PICO question are **P**atient or population of interest, **I**ntervention of interest, **C**omparative intervention, and **O**utcome.
- The correct application of EBP involves ethical and accountable professional nursing practice.
- Problem-focused or knowledge-focused triggers help in the identification of a concise clinical question.
- A concise PICO question consists of key words for conducting a literature search that will provide scientific articles to address your practice question.
- The hierarchy of available evidence offers a guide about the types of literature or information that offer the best scientific evidence
- Expert clinicians are a rich source of evidence because they use evidence frequently to build their own practice and solve clinical problems.

- The critiquing of evidence involves evaluation of the scientific worth and clinical applicability of each study's findings.
- By understanding the elements of a scientific article you will be able to better critique the information effectively for relevance and applicability to your PICO question.
- A key feature of a practice environment that supports the use of best evidence is requiring clinical practice policies and procedures to be evidence based.
- The evaluation of an evidence-based practice change determines if the practice change is desirable, if you need to modify your intervention, or if you need to discontinue the practice change.
- When selecting a nursing-sensitive outcome measure, be sure it is an outcome that is affected by nursing care, that it is appropriate for the group you are caring for, and that it is important to the other clinicians you work with.
- By communicating evidence-based practice changes to a nursing staff, it is more likely that the changes will remain in place.
- Outcome measurement contributes to the body of evidence and strengthens the process of evidence-based practice.

CRITICAL THINKING EXERCISES

The surgical intensive care unit (ICU) where Shana and Eric work has had an increased incidence of ventilator-associated pneumonia developing in their patients. Patients on ventilators are at risk for aspirating mucus from their oral cavity into their trachea and lungs, leading to pneumonia. The unit practice committee believes that it is a clinical problem that warrants an EBP project. A physician on the committee reports that the medical ICU has started to use an antiseptic mouthwash instead of a saline rinse for oral care. The committee believes that the development of a protocol for oral care might be the answer.

1. Write a PICO question for this clinical problem.

Among the articles obtained from the literature search, there is one that describes a study involving 45 patients in a cardiac intensive care unit. All patients were on ventilators and received chlorhexidine solution for mouth care that was administered every 2 hours during their entire length of stay in the ICU. At the time of discharge the researchers recorded the number of patients who had developed ventilator-associated pneumonia.

They also collected information about the characteristics of the patients. The findings showed that patients who developed ventilator-associated pneumonia were older and more likely to have a history of lung problems.

2. How would you describe this type of study?
3. If Shana and Eric were to find a randomized controlled trial that tested the use of chlorhexidine for preventing ventilator-associated pneumonia, explain how that study would be different from the one described in question 2.

During a UPC meeting, Shana is asked by a team member for help in identifying an outcome measure. The team member's clinical question is, "Does listening to music on an iPod improve the quality of sleep in ICU patients?"

4. What would be an outcome measure for this question? What factors should be considered in measuring the outcome?

⊜volve   *Answers to Critical Thinking Questions can be found on the Evolve website.*

REVIEW QUESTIONS

1. An operating room nurse is talking with colleagues during a meeting and asks, "The surgery floors have reported an increased incidence of wound infections. I wonder if we should be using chlorhexidine instead of povidone-iodine (Betadine) to clean the skin of our surgical patients?" In this clinical example, what would be the *I* in a PICO question?
   1. Betadine
   2. Chlorhexidine
   3. Operating room nurse
   4. Wound infection
2. Number the following steps of evidence-based practice in the appropriate order:
   —— Critically appraise the evidence you gather.
   —— Ask the burning clinical question.
   —— Evaluate the practice decision or change.
   —— Collect the most relevant and best evidence.
   —— Integrate the evidence.
   —— Communicate the results.
3. A nurse on an oncology unit decides to implement a practice change involving use of a DVD program to teach patients about chemotherapy side effects. The nurse will measure the outcome of the practice change using what type of measurement?
   1. Measure of the patient's pain
   2. Chart audit of teaching sessions
   3. Observation of patient reading information booklet
   4. Having patient complete a test on knowledge of chemotherapy side effects
4. A new nurse on an orthopedic unit is assigned to a patient in skeletal traction. The nurse asks a colleague, "What is the best practice for cleaning pin sites in skeletal traction?" This question is an example of a:
   1. Knowledge-focused trigger
   2. Problem-focused trigger

   3. PICO question
   4. Hypothesis
5. The nurses on a medicine unit have seen an increase in the number of pressure ulcers developing in their patients. The nurses decide to initiate a quality improvement project using the PDSA model. Which of the following is an example of "Do" from that model?
   1. Review the QI reports on the six patients who developed ulcers over the last 3 months.
   2. Implement the new skin care protocol on all medicine units.
   3. Review the incidence of pressure ulcers on patients cared for using the protocol.
   4. Based on findings from patients who developed ulcers, implement an evidence-based skin care protocol on all units.
6. After a review of the literature regarding health literacy, the nurses in an obstetrics/gynecology clinic decide that it is necessary to revise the instructional manual on cervical cancer screening to a lower reading level. Their patients are from a lower socioeconomic background and do not adhere to recommended screening. Their hope is that by using the instructional materials over time they will see more women come to the clinic for annual Pap smears. The outcome measure for this project would be:
   1. Patients' reading level
   2. Patients' adherence to annual Pap smears
   3. Patients' ability to identify risks for cervical cancer
   4. The number of patients who are given the new instructional manual

7. Consider the following PICO question: "Does the use of an automatic blood pressure device compared with a manual sphygmomanometer measure blood pressure accurately in a patient with hypertension?" What type of PICO question is this?
   1. Prognosis
   2. Prevention
   3. Diagnosis
   4. Therapy

8. During an evidence-based practice committee meeting, a nurse discusses the review of an article about the removal of nail polish before measuring pulse oximetry. The nurse reports there is no conclusive evidence from the study that it is necessary to remove nail polish. A colleague on the committee asks the nurse, "What level of evidence do you have?" The colleague's question is referring to:
   1. The scientific validity of the study findings
   2. The number of articles that the nurse reviewed on the topic
   3. Whether or not the pulse oximeter in the study is similar to the one used on the nurse's unit
   4. The level in the hierarchy of evidence for the article that was reviewed by the nurse

Answers to Review Questions can be found on pages 1197-1198.

REFERENCES

Avis M, Freshwater D: Evidence for practice, epistemology, and critical reflection, *Nurs Philos* 7(4):216, 2006.

Baumbusch JL and others: Pursuing common agendas: a collaborative model for knowledge translation between research and practice I clinical settings, *Res Nurs Health* 31(2):130, 2008.

Brancato VC: An innovative clinical practicum to teach evidence-based practice, *Nurs Educ* 31(5):195, 2006.

Callister LC and others: Inquiry in baccalaureate nursing education: fostering evidence-based practice, *J Nurs Educ* 44(2):59, 2005.

Melnyk BM, Fineout-Overholt E: *Evidence-based practice in nursing and healthcare: a guide to best practice*, Philadelphia, 2005, Lippincott Williams & Wilkins.

Newhouse R and others: Evidence-based practice: a practical approach to implementation, *J Nurs Adm* 35(1):35, 2005.

Oman K, Duran C, Fink R: Evidence-based policy and procedures: an algorithm for success, *J Nurs Adm* 38(1):47, 2008.

Oncology Nursing Society: *Evidence based practice resource area*, http://onsopcontent.ons.org/toolkits/evidence/Definitions/index.shtml, accessed November, 2005.

Oncology Nursing Society: *Nursing-sensitive patient outcomes*, http://www.ons.org/outcomes/measures/outcomes.shtml, accessed June 26, 2008.

Phillips J and others: Where's the evidence? An innovative approach to teaching staff about evidence-based practice, *J Nurses Staff Dev* 22(6):296, 2006.

Sackett DL and others: *Evidence-based medicine: how to practice and teach EBM*, London, 2000, Churchill Livingstone.

Smith-Strom H, Nortvedt MW: Evaluation of evidence-based methods used to teach nursing students to critically appraise evidence, *J Nurs Educ* 47(8):372, 2008.

The Joint Commission: *Comprehensive accreditation manual for hospitals: the official handbook*, Chicago, 2008a, The Commission.

The Joint Commission: *National patient safety goals*, 2009 Hospital/Critical Access Hospital National Patient Safety Goals, http://www.jointcommission.org/PatientSafety, accessed July 5, 2008b.

Titler MG and others: Infusing research into practice to promote quality care, *Nurs Res* 43(5):307, 1994.

Titler MG and others: The Iowa Model of Evidence-Based Practice to Promote Quality Care, *Crit Care Nurs Clin North Am* 13(4):497, 2001.

7 Critical Thinking

MEDIA RESOURCES

 CD COMPANION 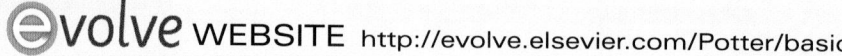 **WEBSITE** http://evolve.elsevier.com/Potter/basic

- Crossword Puzzle
- English/Spanish Audio Glossary

OBJECTIVES

- Describe characteristics of a critical thinker.
- Discuss the nurse's responsibility in making clinical decisions.
- Describe the components of a critical thinking model for clinical decision making.
- Discuss critical thinking skills used in nursing practice.
- Explain the relationship between clinical experience and critical thinking.

- Discuss the effect attitudes for critical thinking have on clinical decision making.
- Explain how professional standards influence a nurse's clinical decisions.
- Discuss how reflection improves a nurse's clinical practice.
- Discuss the relationship of the nursing process to critical thinking.

KEY TERMS

clinical decision making, p. 95

clinical inference, p. 95

critical thinking, p. 89

decision making, p. 93

diagnostic reasoning p. 93

intuition, p. 91

nursing process, p. 96

problem solving, p. 93

reflection, p. 90

scientific method, p. 93

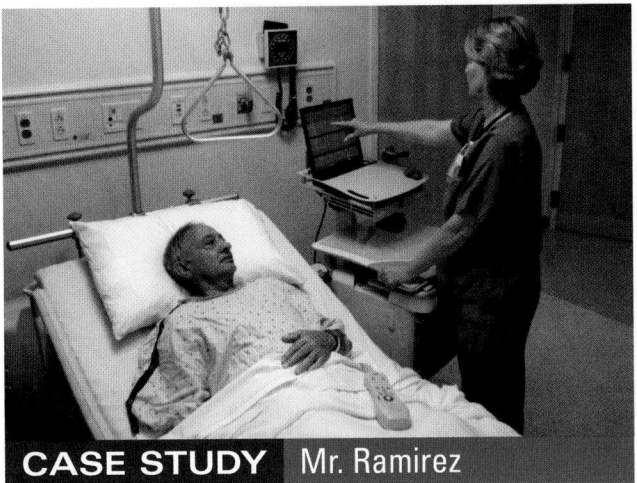

CASE STUDY Mr. Ramirez

Carla is a third-year nursing student assigned to a surgical nursing unit. Mr. Javier Ramirez is a 55-year-old construction worker, admitted to the unit after falling off scaffolding on a construction site. His x-ray films revealed a right fractured femur and right wrist fracture. An abdominal computed tomography (CT) scan shows bruising of the liver. Mr Ramirez has not been hospitalized in the past. When he first meets Carla, he is very quiet and asks few questions. His leg is in skeletal traction, and his right arm is in a soft cast. Carla decides she needs to begin her care by assessing Mr. Ramirez and determining his health status. She begins by reviewing his medical history. She learns he has a history of smoking and was diagnosed with type 2 diabetes just 5 years ago.

As a professional nurse, you will care for patients with uniquely different types of health care problems. Each situation will require critical thinking so that you can make the necessary decisions for your patient to receive the very best nursing care. Being a good critical thinker means that you organize and analyze information, recognize patterns, and make good decisions when you face any clinical situation. Critical thinking skills allow you to make high-quality judgments about patient care. For example, when Carla notices that Mr. Ramirez is slow to respond to her questions, grimaces when shifting weight on his back, and is reluctant to have a bed bath, her critical thinking leads to the inference that Mr. Ramirez is in pain. Carla decides to assess the situation more thoroughly by asking Mr. Ramirez specific questions about his comfort, such as "Tell me if you are hurting," "Show me where the pain is located," and "Is this pain you have felt before?" Applying clinical judgment will allow Carla to act and provide appropriate pain therapies. Critical thinking is a process that nurses acquire through hard work, commitment, and an active curiosity about learning. This chapter introduces you to a model for critical thinking that will better prepare you to face patient situations and determine the type of nursing care each patient requires.

CLINICAL DECISIONS IN NURSING PRACTICE

When caring for patients, you are responsible for making accurate and appropriate clinical decisions. Clinical decision making is a skill that separates professional nurses from nursing assistive personnel (NAP). To help patients maintain, regain, or improve their health you must think critically to problem solve and find solutions for patients' health problems. Many patients have health care alterations that present clinical pictures that are not immediately clear and thus do not quickly reveal the actions you should take. Instead, you must learn to question, wonder, and explore different interpretations. Then you try to find the set of actions that best help your patients.

No two patients have identical health problems. Because each patient is unique, nurses face challenges in making clinical decisions. You will observe each patient closely, search for and examine ideas, then make inferences or draw conclusions about patient problems. Then you will consider scientific principles relating to the problems, recognize the problems, and provide appropriate nursing care. You will learn to creatively seek new knowledge as needed, act quickly when events change, and make decisions that promote the patient's well-being. Although the responsibility for making clinical decisions seems challenging, it is what makes nursing a rewarding profession.

CRITICAL THINKING DEFINED

Thinking and learning are interrelated processes. The longer you practice as a nurse, the more your knowledge and practical experiences broaden your ability to make thoughtful observations, judgments, and decisions. **Critical thinking** is a process and a set of skills (Cirocco, 2007; Profetto-McGrath and others, 2003). Chaffee (2002) defined critical thinking as the active, organized, cognitive process used to carefully examine one's thinking and the thinking of others. It involves recognizing that an issue (e.g., patient problem) exists, analyzing information related to the issue (e.g., clinical data about a patient), evaluating information (including assumptions and evidence), and drawing conclusions (Settersten and Lauver, 2004). When you care for a patient, critical thinking begins by asking these questions: What do I really know about this nursing care situation? How do I know it? What are the options available to me? (Paul and Heaslip, 1995). For example, Carla knows that Mr. Ramirez is likely to be in pain because he is reluctant to move and take part in any activity. Her options are to conduct a thorough pain assessment and learn how Mr. Ramirez feels about his pain. She must also be culturally sensitive and consider how Mr. Ramirez's Hispanic heritage may influence his response to pain. Carla will then take what she learns and use pain control therapies that Mr. Ramirez will likely accept.

Nurses begin to learn critical thinking early in their practice. For example, when Carla first learned about administer-

---

TABLE 7-1 Critical Thinking Skills

SKILL	NURSING PRACTICE APPLICATION
Interpretation	Be orderly in data collection. For example, use a systematic approach to assess all characteristics of a patient's pain. Look for patterns to categorize data (e.g., defining characteristics of a nursing diagnoses [see Chapter 8]).
Analysis	Be open-minded as you look at information about a patient. Do not make careless assumptions. Do the data reveal what you believe is true, or are there other options?
Inference	Look at the meaning and significance of findings. Are there relationships between findings? Do the data about the patient help you see that a problem exists?
Evaluation	Look at all situations objectively. Use criteria (e.g., expected outcomes, learning objectives) to determine results of nursing actions (see Chapter 8). Reflect on your own behavior and how it affects the evaluation process.
Explanation	Support your findings and conclusions. Use scientific and experiential knowledge to select strategies you use in the care of patients.
Self-regulation	Reflect on your experiences. Identify how you will improve your own performance.

Modified from Facione P: *Critical thinking: a statement of expert consensus for purposes of educational assessment and instruction. The Delphi report: research findings and recommendations prepared for the American Philosophical Association,* ERIC Doc No. ED 315-423, Washington, DC, 1990, ERIC.

TABLE 7-2 Concepts for a Critical Thinker

CONCEPT	COMPONENT
Truth seeking	Seek the truth; be courageous about asking questions; be honest and objective about pursuing questions.
Open-mindedness	Be tolerant of different views; be sensitive to the possibility of your own biases; respect the right of others to have different opinions.
Analyticity	Be alert to potentially problematic situations; anticipate possible results or consequences; value reason; use evidence-based knowledge.
Systematicity	Be organized; focus; work hard in any inquiry.
Self-confidence	Trust in your own reasoning processes.
Inquisitiveness	Be eager to acquire knowledge and learn explanations even when applications of the knowledge are not immediately clear. Value learning for learning's sake.
Maturity	Multiple solutions are acceptable. Reflect on your own judgments; have cognitive maturity.

Modified from Facione N, Facione P: Externalizing the critical thinking in knowledge development and clinical judgement, *Nurs Outlook* 44:129, 1996.

---

ing hygiene measures to patients, she read the nursing literature to learn more about the concept of comfort. What are the criteria for comfort? How do patients from other cultures perceive comfort? What are the different factors that contribute to comfort? The use of evidence-based knowledge (see Chapter 6), or knowledge based on research or clinical expertise, makes nurses more informed critical thinkers. Thinking critically and learning about the concept of comfort prepares Carla to better anticipate her patients' needs. She will also identify problems more quickly and provide appropriate care. Critical thinking is a commitment to think clearly, precisely, and accurately and to act on what you know about a situation. When you think about understanding and assisting patients in finding solutions to their health problems, the process becomes purposeful and goal oriented.

Critical thinking requires cognitive skills and the tendency to ask questions and to remain well informed. There are core critical thinking skills that, when applied to nursing, show the complex nature of clinical decision making (Table 7-1). Applying these skills takes practice. You will need to have a sound knowledge base and thoughtfully consider the knowledge you gain during experiences with patients.

Critical thinking is not memorizing information or a list of steps to take (Cirocco, 2007). Instead, it is a reflective, purposeful, and self-regulating process (Facione and Facione, 1996). Learning to think critically helps you to care for patients as their advocate and to make informed choices about their care. Facione and Facione (1996) identified concepts for thinking critically (Table 7-2). Without these concepts, critical thinking skills are difficult to use. Critical thinking is more than just problem solving. It is an attempt to continually improve how you apply yourself when faced with patient care problems.

Reflection

When you care for patients, critical thinking begins by thinking about previous situations and considering relevant issues: How did I act? What could I have done differently? or What should I do if I have the same opportunity in the future? **Reflection** is a part of critical thinking that involves the process of purposefully thinking back or recalling a situation to

BOX 7-1   Tips on Facilitating Reflection

- Stop and think about what is going on with your patient. What do your assessment findings mean? What physical or behavioral changes are occurring? How do these changes compare with normal or baseline findings for the patient?
- Reflect carefully on any critical incidents (e.g., safety episodes, cardiac arrests, central events in the progression of a patient's disease, complex-care patients) (Bittner and Tobin, 1998). What occurred? What actions did you take? How did the patient respond? Were there any other options you thought of taking?
- At the end of each day after caring for a patient, take time to reflect. Ask yourself whether you achieved your original plan of care. If you did, why were you successful? If you did not, what were the barriers or problems? What would you do differently or the same?
- Keep a journal of your patient care experiences. A record of your experience will help you develop an awareness of how you use clinical decision-making skills (Kessler and Lund, 2004). Be sure to include the following: identification, description, significance, and implications. Telling a story and drawing a picture are two ways to identify the experience you wish to reflect on. Describe in detail what you felt, thought, and did. Analyze experience by considering feelings, thoughts, and possible meanings. It helps to look for themes in your entries. For example, if you have cared for several patients with cardiac problems, what common themes do you see that will better prepare you for the next patient? Challenge any preconceived ideas you have when you look at actual situations. Describe the implications of the experience in terms of your own clinical practice or self-perceptions as a learner. Refer to the journal often when you care for patients who have similar situations.
- Talk with a close friend who works with you and has observed your clinical work. Ask if the friend's observations are the same as yours.
- Keep all written care plans or clinical papers. Use them frequently as a resource for care of future patients.
- Take time to reflect, both after having cared for a patient and before caring for new patients with similar conditions. How is your current patient similar to or different from previous patients?

discover its purpose or meaning. For example, before beginning care for Mr. Ramirez, Carla thinks to herself about a recent experience she had with a patient who suffered chronic pain from a bone tumor. Although the condition is different from that of Mr. Ramirez, the experience of caring for the patient is invaluable. Carla goes through introspection or self-questioning to consider the approaches she used for her patient with a bone tumor. What might she have done differently when the patient reported little benefit from using relaxation exercises? Was her response appropriate when the patient said, "I don't know, I feel like I will never get any relief." How does this experience influence her ability to care for Mr. Ramirez? It is helpful for you as a nurse to think back on a patient situation to explore the factors that influenced how you handled the situation. Reflection is like rewinding a videotape. It involves playing back a situation in your head and taking time to honestly review everything you remember about the situation. Reflection requires adequate knowledge, and it is the ability to recreate ideas and experiences (Sewell, 2008). By reviewing your actions you see successes and opportunities for improvement. Always be cautious in using reflection. Too much emphasis on reflection can block thinking in the here and now, because it often creates second-guessing.

Reflection helps you to seek and understand the relationships between concepts learned in class and real-life clinical situations. It is learning through investigational discovery (Kessler and Lund, 2004). Through reflection, you judge your personal performance and how well you followed standards of nursing practice in your care. Reflection helps make sense out of an experience so that the next time a similar experience happens, you will use approaches that were successful or change an approach to achieve better patient outcomes.

Reflection is different for each individual. Learning to be reflective takes practice because it involves connecting clinical content with thought processes and self-awareness. It is not simply describing what you observed or did for a patient (Kessler and Lund, 2004). When you reflect on a clinical experience, be open to new information and look at the patient's perspective, as well as your own. Reflection will assist you with identifying areas of strength and areas you may wish to develop further so as to improve your clinical practice (Cirocco, 2007). Learning from experience with patients can create an "aha" feeling, because reflection reveals an awareness of how well you are performing as a professional. Box 7-1 lists tips on how to use reflection in your practice.

Language and Intuition

Use of language is another important aspect of critical thinking. Critical thinkers use language precisely and clearly. When language is unclear and inaccurate, it reflects sloppy thinking. It is important to communicate clearly with patients, their families, and health care professionals. When you use incorrect terminology and jargon or vague descriptions, communication is ineffective. If you do not obtain a professional interpreter when communicating with patients who speak a different language, you are taking the risk for miscommunicating important information. When you are vague or unclear with your patient and the nursing team, then your patient may be unable to cooperate with nursing therapies, and members of the nursing team will have difficulty following through on your recommendations because your communication was unclear. Critical thinking requires you to carefully frame your thoughts and to send a message that is clear.

Intuition is the inner sensing or "gut feeling" that something is so. For example, you walk into a patient's room and, by

BOX 7-2   BEST PRACTICES

Thinking During Medication Administration

SUMMARY OF EVIDENCE

A study involving interviews with 40 nurses practicing in inpatient units in a teaching hospital found 10 different categories of nurses' thinking during medication administration. Nurses think beyond just rules and procedures. Instead, even a common procedure such as medication administration involves critical thinking and good use of clinical judgment. The 10 categories of thinking are communication, dose-time, checking, assessment, evaluation, teaching, side effects, workarounds, anticipating problem solving, and drug administration.

APPLICATION TO NURSING PRACTICE

- Nursing care involves thinking processes that are based on patient information and professional knowledge.
- Thinking becomes even more focused when nurses must make judgments about dosage, timing, or selection of specific medications (e.g., pain management, adjusting insulin doses).
- Nurses must be constantly vigilant to ensure patients receive appropriate medication safely.

REFERENCE

Eisenhauer LA, Hurley AC, Dolan N: Nurses' reported thinking during medication administration, *J Nurs Scholarsh* 39(1):82, 2007.

looking at the patient's appearance without the benefit of a thorough assessment, sense that he or she has worsened physically. Intuition is a common experience that many people have when interacting with their environments. Mothers develop an intuition about their children's behavior, especially after having had more than one child. Intuition is a component of clinical judgment and decision making, and it develops through clinical experience (Rew and Barrow, 2007). For example, Carla has extensive clinical experience from her home care rotation. She now intuitively knows to suspect that a patient is depressed by looking at the patient's expression, seeing disorder in the home environment, and making a quick assessment of the patient's mood. Intuition acts as a trigger, leading the nurse to consciously search for data that confirm the sense of a change in a patient's status (King and Clark, 2002).

Quality nursing practice does not depend solely on intuition. Just as it is critical to know what knowledge you have, it is even more critical to know the knowledge you lack. Trust your intuition as a red flag that something is not quite right, but do not take your intuition as an automatic fact. Always combine intuition with objective, scientific evidence (Rew and Barrow, 2007). Whenever you have an intuitive thought, look further to assess a patient's situation and consult with other professional colleagues. If you do not recognize what you do not know about patients, there is a risk for malpractice and even harming your patients. Thoughtful analysis of what you know, plus a review of the most current clinical data, allows you to make accurate and sound clinical decisions.

Thinking and Learning

Learning is a lifelong process. Intellectual and emotional growth involves gaining new knowledge and refining the ability to think, problem solve, and make judgments. To learn, you must be flexible and always open to new information. The science of nursing is growing rapidly, and there will always be new evidence for nurses to apply in practice (see Chapter 6). As you have new experiences and apply the knowledge gained, you will learn to form assumptions, present ideas, and make valid conclusions.

Thinking about your practice as a nurse requires vigilance, which involves remaining alert and attentive to whatever activity or task you are conducting. Even routine procedures such as medication administration require vigilant thinking (Box 7-2). When you care for a patient, always think ahead and ask, What is the patient's status now? How might it change and why? What do I know to improve the patient's condition? In what way will a specific therapy affect the patient? How do I evaluate if the patient benefited? Do not allow your thinking to become routine or standardized. Instead, learn to look beyond the obvious and explore each patient's response to health alterations, and recognize what actions are needed to benefit the patient. After caring for many patients you will learn to recognize patterns of behavior, see commonalities in signs and symptoms, and anticipate reactions to therapies. Thinking about each experience allows you to anticipate each patient's needs and recognize the patient's problems.

LEVELS OF CRITICAL THINKING IN NURSING

Your ability to think critically grows as you gain new knowledge and experience in nursing practice. Kataoka-Yahiro and Saylor (1994) developed a critical thinking model (Figure 7-1) that includes three levels of critical thinking in nursing: basic, complex, and commitment.

Basic Critical Thinking

At the basic level of critical thinking a learner trusts that experts have the right answers for every problem. Thinking is concrete and based on a set of rules or principles. For example, a nursing student uses a hospital procedure manual to confirm how to insert a feeding tube. The student follows the procedure step-by-step without adjusting the procedure to meet a patient's unique needs (e.g., positioning limitations or difficulty swallowing). At this level, answers to complex problems are either right or wrong (e.g., the tube will not advance

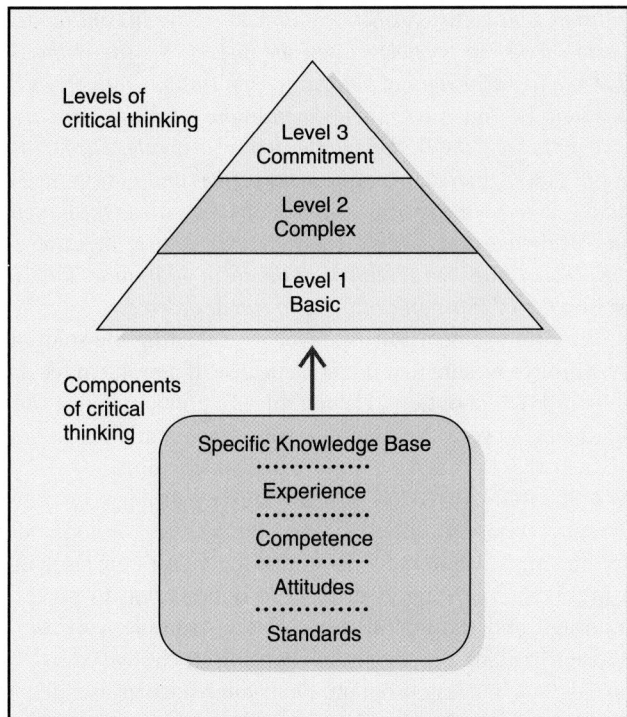

Figure 7-1 ▦ Critical thinking model for nursing judgment. (Redrawn from Kataoka-Yahiro M, Saylor C: A critical thinking model for nursing judgment, *J Nurs Educ* 33(8):351, 1994. Modified from Glaser E: *An experiment in the development of critical thinking*, New York, 1941, Bureau of Publications, Teachers College, Columbia University; Miller J, Malcolm N: Critical thinking in the nursing curriculum, *Nurs Health Care* 11:67, 1990; Paul R: The art of redesigning instruction. In Willsen J, Blinker AJA, editors: *Critical thinking how to prepare students for a rapidly changing world*, Santa Rosa, Calif, 1993, Foundation for Critical Thinking.)

because it is coiled in the throat), and one right answer usually exists for each problem. Basic critical thinking is an early step in the development of reasoning (Kataoka-Yahiro and Saylor, 1994). A basic critical thinker learns to accept the diverse opinions and values of experts (e.g., instructors and staff nurses). However, weak competencies and inflexible attitudes slow a person's ability to move to the next level of critical thinking.

Complex Critical Thinking

Complex critical thinkers begin to separate themselves from authorities. They analyze and examine choices more independently. The person's thinking abilities and initiative to look beyond expert opinion begin to change. A nurse learns that alternative and perhaps conflicting solutions do exist.

Consider Mr. Ramirez, who continues to experience pain in his leg. He rates his pain at a level of a 6 on a scale of 0 to 10. The physician increased his dosage of morphine sulfate yesterday evening, which the patient self-administers through use of patient-controlled analgesia (PCA). Carla wonders if perhaps

something else is contributing to the pain other than the trauma from his leg fracture. She has read that cultural ethnicity can influence how patients perceive pain (see Chapter 31). She decides she needs to understand what the injury and pain mean to Mr. Ramirez and whether that is influencing how he expresses the pain and whether he is using the PCA correctly.

In complex critical thinking, you learn to synthesize knowledge. This means you develop a new thought or idea based on your experience and knowledge over time. When you choose therapies for patients, each option has benefits and risks that you weigh in making a decision. Thinking becomes more creative and innovative. At this level, you are more willing to consider deviations from standard protocols or procedures and to provide more individualized care.

Commitment

The third level of critical thinking is commitment (Kataoka-Yahiro and Saylor, 1994). A person anticipates the need to make choices without assistance from others. A person accepts accountability for whatever decision he or she makes. A nurse does more than consider the complex alternatives a problem poses. At the commitment level, a nurse chooses an action or belief based on the alternatives available and stands by it. Consider the situation of a 53-year-old woman recently diagnosed with breast cancer. At first she delayed seeking treatment because of her fear of hospitals and her family history of breast cancer. She skipped her last clinic appointment. Her nurse learns that the woman's daughter has been helpful in the past in aiding her mother to sort out decisions. The nurse discusses the woman's concerns and asks to involve the daughter in a discussion. Then the nurse helps the mother sort out her worries with the daughter to make a decision about her treatment. She learns that the woman had a concern for her family and perceived that she would become a burden. The daughter and mother are able to sort out worries and misconceptions, and the woman decides to begin therapy.

CRITICAL THINKING COMPETENCIES

Another component of Kataoka-Yahiro and Saylor's model (1994) (see Figure 7-1) is critical thinking competencies, the cognitive processes a nurse uses to make judgments about patients' clinical care. There are three competencies: general critical thinking, specific critical thinking in clinical situations, and specific critical thinking in nursing (Kataoka-Yahiro and Saylor, 1994). General critical thinking processes are not unique to the nursing profession. They include the **scientific method, problem solving,** and **decision making.** Specific critical thinking competencies in clinical situations include clinical inference, **diagnostic reasoning,** and clinical decision making. The specific critical thinking competency in nursing is the nursing process (see Chapter 8), which involves each of the other three specific critical thinking competencies.

General Critical Thinking Processes

SCIENTIFIC METHOD The scientific method is a way to solve problems using reasoning. It is the systematic, ordered approach to gathering data and solving problems. The scientific method is used in nursing, medicine, and a variety of other disciplines. It is the foundation for research in nursing practice. The steps of the scientific method are as follows:

- Problem identification
- Collection of data
- Formulation of a question or hypothesis
- Testing the question or hypothesis
- Evaluating results of the study

The scientific method is one formal way to approach a problem, plan a solution, test the solution, and come to a conclusion. Table 7-3 provides an example of a nursing practice question solved using the scientific method.

PROBLEM SOLVING We all face problems every day, whether it is how to help a friend who has lost his or her job or how to operate a DVD player correctly. Nurses face problems routinely, such as determining why an intravenous (IV) infusion is not functioning, dealing with a patient's unwillingness to follow a treatment plan, or selecting the right type of dressing to cover a wound. Problem solving represents a higher level of cognitive function. A traditional approach for solving problems is to clarify the problem, analyze possible causes, identify alternatives, assess each alternative, choose one, implement it, and evaluate whether the problem was solved. A systematic approach to problem solving makes it more likely that you will find an appropriate solution.

In the case of Mr. Ramirez, Carla comes into his room because the IV pump alarm is sounding. She finds that the patient's IV medication is not infusing at the desired rate. The IV infusion is necessary for Mr. Ramirez to receive his antibiotics. Carla checks out possible causes: she inspects the site of the IV line and looks for signs of phlebitis or infiltration, both of which can slow IV flow rates. Then she positions Mr. Ramirez's arm straight to see if the IV flows at the desired drip rate. The IV rate is still slower than desired. She looks further and notices the IV tubing is under the patient's left hip. She repositions the patient and straightens the tubing. The flow immediately increases to the ordered rate. Carla returns to the room 30 minutes later to be sure the IV infusion continues to run as ordered.

Effective problem solving involves evaluating the solution over time to be sure that it is still effective. If a problem recurs, you try different options. Having solved a problem in one situation adds to your experience in your practice and allows you to apply that knowledge in future patient situations.

DECISION MAKING When you face a problem or situation and choose a course of action from several options, you are making a decision. Decision making focuses on resolving a problem. Following a set of criteria helps you to make a thorough and thoughtful decision. For example, you use a decision-making process when choosing an elective course to take in your nursing program. First, you recognize and define the problem or situation (need to select a course that meets program requirements). Then you assess all the options (consider courses recommended by faculty and colleagues or choose one that is scheduled for a convenient time). Next, you weigh each option against a set of criteria (reputation of faculty, value of course for your career goals), and test possible options (talk directly with the faculty). Finally, you consider the consequences of the decision (examine pros and cons of selecting one course over another), and then make a final decision. Although the set of criteria seems to follow a sequence of steps, decision making involves moving back and forth in considering all criteria. The decision-making process leads to informed

---

TABLE 7-3   Using the Scientific Method to Solve Nursing Practice Questions

Clinical Problem: The incidence of a health care–associated infection, *Clostridium difficile infection,* has increased on a hospital's general medicine unit. The nursing staff have met to discuss factors that may be influencing the problem. They note that visitors are inconsistent in the use of antiseptic hand rubs. A staff member questions if use of hand rubs is the best approach for this type of infection.

Problem identification	The incidence of *C. difficile* has increased among patients on a general medicine unit.
Data collection	Review the literature about the nature of *C. difficile* infection and the hand antiseptic techniques that have been used to prevent the infection. Review any studies that have investigated hand-hygiene practices of visitors of hospital patients. Talk with infection control specialists for the hospital.
Form a research question to study the problem	Does visitor use of antiseptic hand rub with chlorhexidine versus hand washing with soap and water reduce incidence of *C. difficile* infection in medical patients?
Answer the question	Plan a 2-month study whereby patients' visitors are asked to use chlorhexidine to rub their hands before entering and leaving patient rooms. During the 2 months track the incidence of *C. difficile* infection among patients. Discontinue use of chlorhexidine, and have visitors perform hand washing with soap and water. Continue this practice for 2 months, and track the incidence of *C. difficile* infection.
Evaluate the results of the study. Is the research question answered?	Compare the incidence of *C. difficile* infection over 2 months for each of the two hand-hygiene methods.

conclusions that are supported by evidence and by reason (Bandman and Bandman, 1995). In a clinical setting you learn to make sound decisions by approaching each clinical situation thoughtfully and systematically by using each step of the decision-making process mentioned earlier. Decision making goes hand in hand with problem solving.

Specific Critical Thinking Competencies

CLINICAL INFERENCE As a nurse you are constantly making patient observations, conducting measurements, talking with patients, and reviewing information about patients from family members, other health care providers, and the medical record. **Clinical inference** is a critical thinking skill in which you make tentative conclusions based on observed data or cues existing in patient situations (Wolf, Serembus, and Farley, 2001). As you review data about patients, you learn to see patterns in the information. For example, when a patient tells a nurse he is reluctant to go to a test, has never had the test before, and adamantly requests information from his doctor, the nurse may begin to infer there is a problem regarding the patient's knowledge about the test or perhaps the patient is anxious or angry. Your ability to make a clinical inference will lead you to forming nursing diagnoses.

DIAGNOSTIC REASONING The process of collecting information about a patient and coming to a conclusion about his or her health problems involves diagnostic reasoning. Diagnostic reasoning involves the use of cognitive thinking, metacognition (thinking about thinking), and assessment skills to structure situations so you can apply knowledge (Kuiper, 2008). Expert nurses make diagnostic conclusions in the form of nursing diagnoses (see Chapter 8). Nurses do not make medical diagnoses, but they do assess and monitor patients' medical conditions to determine their level of progress. A nurse's diagnostic conclusions helps a health care provider pinpoint the nature of a patient's problem more quickly and select proper therapies.

Because you are a new nurse, it will take time to make accurate diagnostic decisions. However, with more experience and knowledge, and the recognition of how diagnostic conclusions are formed, you will gain the necessary expertise. In nursing the formation of nursing diagnoses is part of the nursing process (see Chapter 8). The accuracy of diagnostic reasoning depends on how well a nurse attends to a patient's signs and symptoms, identifies tentative patterns in the data by making inferences, gathers additional data to rule out possible diagnoses, and finally forms a diagnostic conclusion. A methodical approach to diagnostic reasoning provides a clear perspective of a patient's health status and whether or not the patient is progressing.

In nursing, diagnostic reasoning is a process of using the data you gather, forming inferences, and then logically explaining a clinical judgment. *For example, after Carla repositions Mr. Ramirez, she observes an area of redness over his left heel. Redness could be due to inflammation or pressure on the skin. She explores for more information and palpates the area, noting it is tender to touch and warm. She asks Mr. Ramirez if he has been moving his leg much, and he says, "No, I just haven't moved it too much; I*

am afraid I will hurt my other leg." These initial findings imply that excess pressure is being applied to the heel. Carla gently applies pressure to the area with her finger and notes that after releasing pressure the area does not blanch or turn white, a key sign of excess pressure. She thinks about what she knows about normal skin integrity, the effects of immobility, and the effects of pressure on the skin. The information she collects leads her to determine Mr. Ramirez has an early-stage pressure ulcer. The nursing diagnosis would be "impaired skin integrity."

CLINICAL DECISION MAKING Clinical decision making is a problem-solving activity that focuses on selecting appropriate treatment after forming diagnostic conclusions. When you face a clinical problem, such as a patient who has an area of redness over the heel, you make a decision that identifies the problem (a pressure ulcer), and then you choose the best nursing interventions (skin care and turning). Nurses make clinical decisions all the time in an attempt to improve a patient's health or to maintain wellness. This means minimizing the severity of the problem or resolving the problem completely. **Clinical decision making** requires careful reasoning so that you choose the options for the best patient outcomes on the basis of the patient's condition and priority of the problem.

You improve your clinical decision making by knowing your patients. Nurse researchers have found that expert nurses develop a level of knowing that leads to pattern recognition of patient symptoms and responses (White, 2003). For example, an expert nurse who has worked on a general surgery unit for many years is more likely able to detect internal hemorrhage (fall in blood pressure, rapid pulse, change in consciousness) than a new nurse. Over time, a combination of experience, time spent in a specific clinical area, and the quality of relationships formed with patients allow nurses to know clinical situations and to quickly anticipate and select the right course of action. Spending more time during initial patient assessments to observe and measure normal and abnormal findings is a way to improve knowing your patients. Also, consistently monitoring patients as problems develop helps you to see how clinical changes evolve over time.

Strader (1992) offered a set of decision-making criteria to help nurses make appropriate clinical decisions. Those criteria are still useful today:

- What needs to be achieved (healing of the skin, removal of pressure)?
- What needs to be preserved (mobility, nutrition, comfort)?
- What needs to be avoided (further tissue injury, infection)?

Clinical decision-making criteria assist you in setting clinical care priorities (see Chapter 8). Because different patients bring different variables to a situation, an activity may be more of a priority in one situation and less of a priority in another. For example, if a patient is physically dependent, unable to eat, and incontinent of urine, skin integrity is a greater priority than if the patient is immobile but continent of urine and able to eat a normal diet. Do not assume that a certain condition is an automatic priority. For example, you expect a patient immediately out of surgery will experience a certain level of pain, which is often a priority of nursing care. However, if the patient is experiencing anxiety that heightens pain perception, it becomes necessary to focus on ways to relieve anxiety before pain-relief measures can be effective.

After you determine a patient's nursing care priorities, choose the nursing therapies most likely to relieve each problem. A wide range of choices may be available, from nurse-administered to patient self-care therapies. Collaborate with the patient, and then select, test, and evaluate each approach. Try to anticipate what might go wrong, and consider different approaches to minimize or prevent problems.

You will make decisions about individual patients and about groups of patients. When you care for several patients at one time, you will need to use decision-making criteria. These criteria include the clinical conditions of the patients, Maslow's hierarchy of needs (see Chapter 1), risks involved in treatment delays, and the patients' expectations of care to determine which patients have the greatest priorities for care. For example, a patient whose blood pressure drops suddenly and who faints requires attention immediately in contrast to the patient who needs assistance walking down the hallway. Visit the patient who has had no visitors and has recently been given a diagnosis of cancer before checking on the recovering surgical patient whose family has just arrived.

THE NURSING PROCESS AS A COMPETENCY The critical thinking competency unique to nurses is the application of the nursing process (Kataoka-Yahiro and Saylor, 1994). The **nursing process** is a systematic process that incorporates diagnostic reasoning and clinical decision making through five steps: assessment, diagnosis, planning, imple-

mentation, and evaluation. The purpose of the process is to diagnose and treat human responses to actual or potential health problems (American Nurses Association, 2003). Use of the process allows nurses to identify patient problems accurately and to then meet agreed-upon outcomes for better health. The format for the nursing process is unique to the discipline of nursing and offers a common language and way for nurses to "think through" patients' clinical problems (Kataoka-Yahiro and Saylor, 1994).

The nursing process is often called a blueprint or plan for patient care. It is flexible enough for you to use in all settings and with all patients. When you use the nursing process, you collect information about a patient, identify the patient's health care needs, determine priorities, and establish goals and expected outcomes of care. Then you develop and communicate a patient-centered plan of care, deliver nursing interventions, and evaluate the effectiveness of your care (Table 7-4). When you are competent in using the nursing process, you will be able to focus not only on a single patient problem but on multiple problems. As a nurse, always think about and recognize what step of the process you are using. Within each step of the process you will apply critical thinking to provide the very best professional care to your patients. A detailed description of the nursing process is in Chapter 8.

A CRITICAL THINKING MODEL

Models help explain concepts. Because critical thinking is complex, a model helps explain what is involved as you make clinical decisions and judgments about your patients.

TABLE 7-4 Summary of Nursing Process

COMPONENT	PURPOSE	STEPS
Assessment	To gather, verify, and communicate data about patient so that database is established	Collect nursing health history. Perform physical examination. Collect laboratory data. Validate or confirm data are correct. Cluster data by common themes or problem areas. Document data.
Nursing diagnosis	To examine patient data to identify their health care needs to formulate nursing diagnoses	Analyze and interpret data. Identify patient problems. Form nursing diagnoses. Document nursing diagnoses.
Planning	To identify patient's goals; to determine priorities of care; to determine expected outcomes; to design nursing strategies to achieve goals of care	Identify patient goals. Establish expected outcomes. Select nursing actions. Delegate interventions. Write nursing care plan. Collaborate with other health care providers.
Implementation	To carry out nursing actions necessary for accomplishing plan of care	Perform nursing interventions. Reassess patient. Review and modify existing care plan.
Evaluation	To determine extent to which interventions helped achieve goals of care	Compare patient response with expected outcomes. Analyze reasons for results and conclusions. Modify care plan.

Kataoka-Yahiro and Saylor (1994) developed a model of critical thinking for nursing judgment based in part on previous work by Paul (1993), Glaser (1941), and Miller and Malcolm (1990) (see Figure 7-1, p. 93). The model defines the outcome of critical thinking: nursing judgment that is relevant to nursing problems in a variety of settings. According to the model, there are five elements of critical thinking: knowledge base, experience, competence (e.g., problem solving or clinical decision making), attitudes, and standards. Nurses perform critical thinking within the competency of the nursing process. The elements of the model combine to explain how nurses make clinical decisions that are necessary for safe, effective nursing care (Box 7-3).

Specific Knowledge Base

The first element of critical thinking is a nurse's specific knowledge base. This varies according to your educational experience, including basic nursing education, continuing education courses, and additional college degrees. In addition, it includes reading the nursing literature to remain current in nursing science. Your knowledge base includes information and theory from the basic sciences, humanities, behavioral sciences, and nursing. You use your knowledge base in a different way from other health care professionals in regard to how you think about patient problems. The broad knowledge base gives you a holistic view of patients and their health care needs. The depth and extent of knowledge influence your ability to think critically about nursing problems. In the case study, Carla is just starting her third year of study in nursing. Before she entered nursing, Carla completed 12 college credit hours in psychology. She changed her major and chose nursing as her focus. Carla has successfully completed basic science courses, pharmacology, an informatics elective, introduction to nursing, and health assessment courses. Although she is new to nursing, her preparation and knowledge base will help her make the clinical decisions necessary to care for Mr. Ramirez.

Experience

The second component of the critical thinking model is experience in nursing. Nursing is a practice discipline (Borbasi, Jackson, and Wilkes, 2005). This means that you develop knowledge of nursing through practice, or the care of patients. Clinical learning experiences are necessary for you to acquire clinical decision making skills. You will learn from your experiences in observing, sensing, and talking with patients and then reflecting actively on your experiences alone and with faculty and fellow students. Clinical experience is the laboratory for testing nursing knowledge. "Textbook" approaches lay important groundwork for practice, but you must adapt your practice to each setting, the unique qualities of each patient, and the experiences you have gained from caring for previous patients. Benner (1984) notes that the expert nurse understands the context of a clinical situation, recognizes signs suggesting patterns, and interprets them as relevant or irrelevant. This level of competency comes with experience and a commitment to learning. Perhaps the best lesson you can learn is to value all patient experiences. Each clinical experience becomes a stepping stone to build new knowledge and stimulate innovative thinking.

Attitudes for Critical Thinking

The fourth component of the critical thinking model is attitudes. Paul (1993) identifies 11 attitudes that are central features of a critical thinker (see Box 7-3). These attitudes define how a successful critical thinker approaches a problem. For example, Carla cares for Mr. Ramirez, who faces many weeks of rehabilitation following his injuries. Carla must persevere to under-

---

BOX 7-3	Components of Critical Thinking in Nursing

I. Specific knowledge base in nursing
II. Experience in nursing
III. Critical thinking competencies
   A. General critical thinking competencies
   B. Specific critical thinking competencies in clinical situations
   C. Specific critical thinking competency in nursing—the nursing process
IV. Attitudes for critical thinking
   A. Confidence
   B. Independence
   C. Fairness
   D. Responsibility
   E. Risk taking
   F. Discipline
   G. Perseverance
   H. Creativity
   I. Curiosity
   J. Integrity
   K. Humility
V. Standards for critical thinking
   A. Intellectual standards
      1. Clear
      2. Precise
      3. Specific
      4. Accurate
      5. Relevant
      6. Plausible
      7. Consistent
      8. Logical
      9. Deep
      10. Broad
      11. Complete
      12. Significant
      13. Adequate (for purpose)
      14. Fair
   B. Professional standards
      1. Ethical criteria for nursing judgment
      2. Criteria for evaluation
      3. Professional responsibility

Modified from Kataoka-Yahiro M, Saylor C: A critical thinking model for nursing judgment, *J Nurs Educ* 33(8):351, 1994. Data from Paul RW: The art of redesigning instruction. In Willsen J, Blinker AJA, editors: *Critical thinking: how to prepare students for a rapidly changing world,* Santa Rosa, 1993, Calif, Foundation for Critical Thinking.

stand how the patient feels about this disruption in his life. She must also think independently to find interventions that will help Mr. Ramirez communicate his concerns with other health care providers. Carla will apply the attitude of integrity when she recognizes that problems exist and accepts the need for evidence to support what she thinks is the best approach to care for Mr. Ramirez. Critical thinking attitudes are guidelines for how to solve a problem or make a decision. You must have cognitive skills to think critically, but it is also important to use these skills fairly and responsibly. Table 7-5 summarizes how nurses use critical thinking attitudes in practice situations. A summary of each critical thinking attitude follows.

CONFIDENCE To be confident is to feel certain in your ability to accomplish a task or goal, such as performing a nursing procedure or making a nursing diagnosis. Confidence grows with experience in recognizing your strengths and limitations. You gradually shift your focus from your own needs (e.g., remembering the steps to perform a procedure) to the patient's needs (White, 2003). When you lack confidence in your ability to complete a nursing skill, you focus on your feelings of anxiety in not knowing what to do. This prevents you from attending to a patient. Confidence is not a feeling of superiority. Instead, confident critical thinkers are aware of the balance between what they know and what they do not know. When you are confident, your patients recognize it by how you communicate and the way you perform nursing care. Confidence builds trust between you and your patients and conveys a sense of caring.

THINKING INDEPENDENTLY As you gain new knowledge, you learn to consider a wide range of ideas and concepts before forming an opinion or making a judgment. This does not mean you ignore other people's ideas. Instead, you learn to consider all sides of a situation. However, a critical thinker does not accept another person's ideas without question. When thinking independently, you challenge the ways others think and look for rational and logical answers to problems. An independent thinker applies evidence-based practice (see Chapter 6) when facing clinical decisions. Independent thinking and reasoning are essential to the improvement and expansion of nursing knowledge and practice.

TABLE 7-5   Critical Thinking Attitudes and Applications in Nursing Practice

CRITICAL THINKING ATTITUDE	APPLICATION IN PRACTICE
Confidence	Learn how to introduce yourself to a patient: "Mrs. Tyms, I am Chuck Lord, your nurse for this shift. I will be responsible for your nursing care and will work with your doctor to make sure you are comfortable." Speak with conviction when you begin a treatment or procedure. Do not let a patient think you are unsure of performing care safely. Always be prepared (e.g., equipment organized, other patient needs met) before performing a nursing activity.
Thinking independently	Read the nursing literature, especially when there are different views on the same subject. Talk with colleagues and expert staff nurses to share ideas about nursing interventions.
Fairness	Listen to both sides in any discussion. If a patient or family member complains about a colleague, listen to the story and then speak with the colleague as well. Weigh all the facts.
Responsibility and accountability	Ask for help if you are not sure about how to perform an aspect of patient care. Report any problems immediately. Follow standards of practice in your care.
Risk taking	If your knowledge causes you to question a health care provider's order, do so. Offer alternative approaches to nursing care when colleagues are having little success with patients.
Discipline	Be thorough in whatever you do. Use known criteria for activities such as assessment and evaluation. Take time to be thorough.
Perseverance	Be wary of an easy answer. If colleagues give you information about a patient and some facts are missing, clarify information or talk to the patient directly. If the same problems continue to occur on a nursing division, bring colleagues together, look for a pattern, and find a solution.
Creativity	Look for different approaches if interventions are not working. For example, a patient may need a different positioning technique or a different instructional approach that will suit his or her unique needs.
Curiosity	Always ask why. A clinical sign or symptom can indicate a variety of problems. Explore and learn more about the patient to make the right clinical judgments.
Integrity	Recognize when your opinions may conflict with those of a patient; review your position, and decide how best to proceed to reach mutually beneficial outcomes.
Humility	Recognize when you need more information to make a decision. When you are new to a clinical division and unfamiliar with the patients, ask for an orientation to the area. Ask nurses regularly assigned to the area for assistance. Read the professional journals regularly to keep updated on new approaches to care.

FAIRNESS A critical thinker deals with situations in a just manner. This means that bias or prejudice does not enter into a decision. For example, regardless of how you feel about obesity, you should not allow personal attitudes to influence the way you deliver care to a patient who is overweight. If you are fair, you look at a situation objectively and analyze all viewpoints to understand the situation completely before arriving at a decision. Having a sense of imagination aids in the development of fairness. Imagining what it is like to be in the situation your patients face helps you to see situations with new eyes and appreciate their complexity.

RESPONSIBILITY AND ACCOUNTABILITY When caring for patients, you are responsible for correctly performing nursing care activities based on standards of practice. The standards are the minimum level of performance accepted to ensure high-quality care. For example, do not take shortcuts when you administer medications to a patient. You are responsible for following the "six rights" of medication administration. It is your responsibility to be competent while performing nursing therapies. When you are competent, you become better at making clinical decisions about and with patients. When you care for a patient, you are answerable, or accountable, for the results of your nursing actions. As an accountable nurse, you are reliable and willing to recognize when nursing care is effective or ineffective. Ultimately, you assume accountability for your decisions and the results of your actions made on the patient's behalf.

RISK TAKING People often associate taking risks with danger. Using your cell phone while driving 60 miles an hour down a highway is a risk that might result in injury to you as well as drivers around you. However, taking risks is not always negative. Risk taking is desirable, particularly when the result is a positive outcome. A critical thinker is willing to take certain risks in trying different ways to solve problems. The willingness to take risks comes from experience with similar problems. In nursing, risk taking frequently results in patient care innovations. Nurses in the past have taken risks in trying different approaches to skin and wound care and pain management, to name a few. As a result, the nurses used more effective interventions than traditional approaches. When taking a risk, you consider all options, analyze any potential danger to a patient, and then act in a well-reasoned, logical, and thoughtful manner. In the end, the evaluation of patient outcomes is critical.

DISCIPLINE A good critical thinker uses discipline. A disciplined thinker misses few details and follows an orderly approach when making decisions or taking action. For example, you have a patient who is in pain. Instead of only asking the patient, "How severe is your pain on a scale of 0 to 10?" you ask more specific questions. A disciplined thinker will ask, "What makes the pain worse? Where does it hurt, and how often does it hurt?" Being disciplined will help you select more appropriate nursing interventions. Disciplined thinking does not lessen your creativity, but instead ensures that your decision making is systematic, accurate, and comprehensive.

PERSEVERANCE A critical thinker is determined to find effective solutions to patient care problems. This is especially important when problems remain unresolved or when they re-

occur. You must learn as much as possible about a problem and try various approaches to care. Perseverance means to continue to seek additional resources until you find a successful approach. A critical thinker who perseveres is not satisfied with minimal effort, but constantly tries to achieve the highest level of quality care. *Carla has assessed that Mr. Ramirez is still uncomfortable. Although his pain score has fallen to a 4, he still appears restless and tells Carla, "I just have trouble with my leg feeling right. It still aches." Rather than being satisfied with Mr. Ramirez using the PCA, Carla decides to ask Mr. Ramirez more about what he does to help himself relax when he is at home. He tells her that he likes to listen to Mexican music on his iPod. Carla has Mr. Ramirez's wife bring his iPod to the hospital and helps him position the earpiece. She also instructs the patient in simple relaxation exercises. An hour later Carla finds Mr. Ramirez sleeping comfortably; her perseverance successfully led to the patient's pain relief.*

CREATIVITY Creativity involves original thinking. This means you find solutions outside of the standard routines of care. Creativity is a great motivator that helps you to think of options and unique approaches. A patient's clinical problems, social support systems, and living environment are just a few examples of factors that can make the simplest nursing procedure more complicated. Because of these, you need to consider a creative approach for the patient's unique situation.

CURIOSITY Probably the favorite question of a critical thinker is, "Why?" In any clinical situation you will learn a great deal of information about a patient. As you analyze patient information, data patterns emerge. Often the data are unclear. Being curious motivates you to question further, investigate a clinical situation, and obtain all of the information needed to make a decision.

INTEGRITY Critical thinkers question and test their own knowledge and beliefs. Your personal integrity as a nurse builds trust from peers and subordinates. A person of integrity is honest and willing to admit to any mistakes or inconsistencies in his or her own behavior, ideas, and beliefs. There are few of us who have not made mistakes in our practice. To be a strong professional you must follow high practice standards even in difficult times.

HUMILITY It is important for you to admit to your limitations in knowledge and skill. Critical thinkers admit what they do not know and try to find the knowledge they need to make a proper decision. It is very common for you to be an expert in one area of clinical practice but a novice in another area. A patient's safety and welfare are at risk if you cannot admit your inability to deal with a practice problem. You must rethink a situation, learn additional knowledge, and then use the information to form an opinion and draw a conclusion.

Standards for Critical Thinking

The fifth component of the critical thinking model includes intellectual and professional standards (Kataoka-Yahiro and Saylor, 1994). Paul (1993) identified the 14 intellectual standards (see Box 7-3, p. 97) universal for critical thinking. An intellectual standard is a guideline or principle for rational thought. When you consider any patient problem or situation, it is important to apply the standards such as accuracy, consistency, and relevance to make sure that clinical decisions are just. For example, when Carla examines the condition of Mr. Ramirez's skin where the skeletal pin is inserted, she will consistently inspect the site and note if there is any foul odor from the wound. She will provide an accurate description of the wound in the nurses' notes and include relevant information such as the condition and position of the pin itself. The use of intellectual standards involves a rigorous approach to clinical practice and demonstrates that critical thinking is not random.

There are professional standards for critical thinking. These standards are based on ethical criteria (see Chapter 5), evidence-based criteria used for evaluation, and criteria for professional responsibility. To apply professional standards correctly, nurses must use critical thinking for the good of individuals or groups (Kataoka-Yahiro and Saylor, 1994). Professional standards also help maintain a high level of quality. For example, Carla knows that by practicing the ethical standard of autonomy, she allows Mr. Ramirez to be involved in decisions about all aspects of his care.

You will also use evidence-based criteria to make clinical judgments. These criteria come from research or from standards developed by clinical experts. The clinical practice guidelines developed for intravenous infusions by the Infusion Nurses Society (2006) is one example of this. A clinical practice guideline includes standards for the treatment of select clinical conditions. The standards set the minimum requirements, or criteria, necessary to make sure patients receive quality care. Evaluation criteria are another type of standard for evaluating patients' clinical progress. When you plan care for a patient, you identify outcomes to achieve (see Chapter 8). You then use evaluation criteria to determine if a patient reaches those outcomes. Clinical staff use the criteria to make sound and consistent clinical judgments. Evaluation criteria also include norms found through nursing research that you apply to determine the clinical status of a patient. Box 7-4 summarizes types of evaluation criteria available for use in your daily practice.

The standards of professional responsibility include those standards you find from Nurse Practice Acts, institutional practice guidelines, policies and procedures, and professional organizations' standards of practice. Each institution you work in will have a manual of policies and procedures, explaining how to perform nursing procedures. The American Nurses Association Standards of Care (see Chapter 4) is one example of a professional organization's standards of practice. Standards "raise the bar" for the responsibilities and accountabilities that a nurse undertakes to guarantee quality health care to the public.

BOX 7-4	Examples of Outcomes and Corresponding Evaluation Criteria

OUTCOME: PAIN RELIEF

Evaluation Criteria: *Character of pain, including the following:* Onset (When did it first start?), duration (How long does it last during an episode? How long has the pain been bothering the patient?), location (What area of body is involved?), severity (How intense is the pain based on objective measure using a visual analog scale?), type or description of pain (Is it aching, burning, cramping?), precipitating factors (What causes the pain to begin?), relieving factors (What helps to reduce or eliminate the pain?), other related symptoms (e.g., nausea, dizziness, blurred vision).

OUTCOME: IMPROVED PHYSICAL FUNCTION

Evaluation Criteria: *Ability to perform activities of daily living* (e.g., bathing, grooming, toileting) *or instrumental activities of daily living* (e.g., check writing, buying groceries, cleaning home).

OUTCOME: PATIENT LEARNING

Evaluation Criteria: *Patient recall of information* (e.g., can patient describe how to perform a skill or discuss when to notify a health care provider about health changes?), *Patient's ability to perform learned skill correctly* (can patient demonstrate the skill learned?), *Patient's success in adapting knowledge or skill in the home* (while visiting the home, does the patient apply knowledge correctly?).

DEVELOPING CRITICAL THINKING SKILLS

You will develop critical thinking skills by learning how to connect knowledge and theory with practice. It is a challenge to see the relationship between what you learn in a classroom, from reading, having dialogue with instructors and students, and then applying knowledge during patient care. Reflective journaling and concept maps are two approaches for developing critical thinking.

Reflective Journaling

As described earlier, reflection is an important aspect of critical thinking. Purposeful reflection leads to a deeper understanding of issues and to the development of judgment and skill (Cirocco, 2007). One activity that will help you develop into a critical thinker is reflective journaling. Kok and Chabeli (2002) conducted a focus group with six fourth-year nursing students who had used reflective journaling during their psychiatric clinical experience. The students' positive perception was that reflection promoted the development of problem-solving skills and self-evaluation leads to intellectual growth and self awareness.

Reflective writing requires you to record your whole clinical experience in your own words in a personal journal. It is not simply a focus on nursing skills. Returning to the journal as a resource gives you the chance to explore personal perceptions you had during patient care and to develop the ability to apply theory in practice. Use of a journal also improves your observation and descriptive skills. Writing skills also improve through the development of conceptual clarity. Sewell (2008) recommends that you answer the following questions in a journal entry:

- Did I respond appropriately? How should I have responded?
- Were there consequences to my actions, What were they, and whom did they affect?
- Why did I react like that? What was I thinking at that moment?
- Should I have reacted differently?
- What was I trying to achieve?
- Was I working from just instinct or evidence-based practice?
- How did I feel about the experience when it occurred? When it ended, did I feel differently?

Keeping a journal of your patient care experiences will help you become aware of how you use clinical decision-making skills (Kessler and Lund, 2004).

Concept Mapping

As a nurse, you will care for patients who have multiple health problems. You will learn how to assess those problems and develop nursing diagnoses. A concept map is a visual representation of patient problems and interventions that shows their relationship to one another (Schuster, 2003). The primary purpose of a concept map is to synthesize relevant data about a patient, including assessment data, nursing diagnoses, health needs, nursing interventions, and evaluation measures (Hill, 2006). It is a strategy for developing reflective thinking skills. Through a concept map you learn to organize or link

information about a patient in a unique and meaningful way, so that diverse sources of information connect into new wholes (Ferrario, 2004). You will learn to recognize how a patient's multiple problems are interrelated and that often a single nursing intervention is effective for more than one problem. Similarly, by focusing on a particular patient problem, this tool often assists you in resolving associated problems. Concept maps take on many visual forms. Most students use a model that makes the concept map a working document. As a student, you will write and develop a map during your care for a patient. Chapter 8 offers actual examples of concept maps and provides details on their development.

CRITICAL THINKING SYNTHESIS

Critical thinking is a reasoning process by which you reflect on and analyze your own thoughts, actions, and knowledge and then make decisions about patient care. To be a good critical thinker requires dedication and a desire to grow intellectually. As a beginning nurse, it is important to learn the steps of the nursing process and to incorporate the elements of critical thinking (Figure 7-2). The two processes go hand in hand in making clinical decisions. This text provides a model to show you how important critical thinking is in nursing practice. Throughout the clinical chapters of this text, the components of critical thinking are emphasized to help you better understand their relationship to the nursing process.

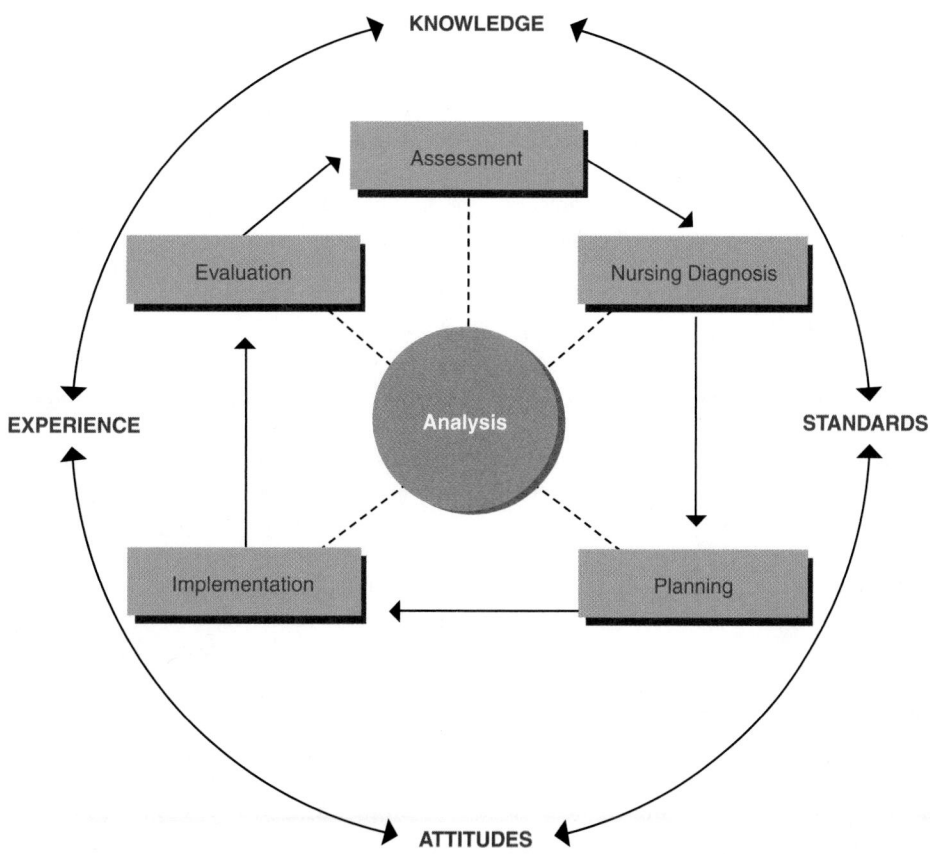

Figure 7-2 ■ Synthesis of critical thinking with the nursing process competency.

KEY POINTS

- Critical thinking is a process that involves recognizing that a patient problem exists, analyzing information related to the problem, evaluating assumptions and evidence, and drawing conclusions.
- Reflection is a process of purposefully thinking back on a situation to self-evaluate and review successes or opportunities for improvement.
- Intuition develops through clinical experience and acts as a trigger, leading the nurse to consciously search for data that confirm the sense of a change in a patient's status.
- Thinking about your practice, even routine procedures, requires vigilance, and always remaining alert and attentive to whatever activity or task you are conducting.
- There are three levels of critical thinking in nursing: basic, complex, and commitment.
- In complex critical thinking you learn to analyze and examine alternatives more independently and take initiative to solve problems.
- The specific critical thinking competency in nursing is the nursing process, which involves clinical inference, diagnostic reasoning, and clinical decision making.
- When you face a problem or situation and choose a course of action from several options, you are making a decision, which also involves asking what needs to be achieved, preserved, and avoided.
- The accuracy of diagnostic reasoning depends on how well you attend to the patient's signs and symptoms, identify patterns in the data, gather additional data to rule out possible diagnoses, and finally form a diagnostic conclusion.
- The model of critical thinking for nursing judgment consists of five elements: knowledge, experience, critical thinking competencies (e.g., nursing process), attitudes, and intellectual and professional standards.
- You will learn from your experiences in observing, sensing, and talking with patients and then reflecting actively on your experiences alone and with health care colleagues.
- Use critical thinking attitudes such as fairness and risk taking to guide problem solving and decision making.
- The nursing process is the competency used by nurses in performing critical thinking.
- Reflective writing requires you to record your whole clinical experience and to then use the journal as a resource that gives you the chance to explore personal perceptions you had during patient care.

CRITICAL THINKING EXERCISES

Mr. Ramirez asks Carla to come to his room. He tells Carla that he began to feel a different pain in his stomach. Carla asks him to place his hand over the area of discomfort. Mr. Ramirez places his hand over the right lower quadrant of his abdomen. On a scale of 0 to 10, Mr. Ramirez rates his pain at a 7. Carla inspects the area more closely and palpates gently over the abdomen for presence of tenderness. She also notes the abdomen feels very tight. The increased pain and tightness suggests something is causing pressure in the abdomen. It could mean the patient is having bleeding from his bruised liver. Carla decides to call Mr. Ramirez's physician immediately. She does what she can to position him more comfortably and makes sure his leg discomfort is under control.

1. Describe the critical thinking attitudes Carla used to assess Mr. Ramirez's pain.
2. Carla's thought that Mr. Ramirez has pressure developing in his abdomen is an example of what critical thinking competency? Explain.
3. Describe the intellectual standards that Carla applied with asking Mr. Ramirez to rate his pain.
4. What knowledge did Carla apply in this clinical situation?

ⓔvolve   *Answers to Critical Thinking Questions can be found on the Evolve website.*

REVIEW QUESTIONS

1. A nurse uses an institution's policy and procedure manual to confirm how to apply a surgical dressing. The level of critical thinking the nurse is using is:
   1. Commitment
   2. Complex critical thinking
   3. Scientific method
   4. Basic critical thinking
2. The nurse enters the room of a patient with diabetes and heart disease. The nurse notes that the patient's color and facial expression suggest something is not right. An assessment of vital signs, the patient's blood glucose level, and a review of the patient's diet intake this morning help the nurse to verify the patient has a low blood glucose level.

   The nurse's reaction to the patient's color and expression is best described as:
   1. Diagnostic reasoning
   2. Intuition
   3. Thinking independently
   4. Clinical inference
3. A patient in hospice care has worsened over the course of the last 4 hours. The nurse knows how close the patient is to his daughter. The daughter has been out of town on an important work assignment. The patient asks the nurse to not call the daughter for fear it would interfere with her work. The nurse decides to call the daughter to notify her of her father's condition. She tells the patient of her action. This is an example of which critical thinking attitude?

1. Curiosity
2. Discipline
3. Integrity
4. Risk taking

4. The nurse cares for a patient receiving tube feedings. The nurse tries to irrigate the tube but is not successful. The nurse checks the medical record to see if other nurses have had difficulty with the tube. The nurse checks the tube and finds no kinking. The nurse's actions are an example of what critical thinking competency?
1. Responsibility
2. Clinical inference
3. Problem solving
4. Preciseness

5. The nurse has a patient with a peripheral IV infusion. Last week the nurse cared for a patient whose IV site developed the complication of phlebitis. The nurse is more prepared to observe for developing problems with this newly assigned patient because of:
1. Reflection
2. Curiosity
3. Experience
4. Knowledge

6. The nurse completes his clinical day and discusses his experience with his best friend. The nurse is concerned about an error he made in setting up an IV infusion. He recalls being distracted when the charge nurse asked a question in the medication room. He states, "You know, so much was happening at the time, I should have stopped to answer the question and then double-checked my IV infusion tubing." This is an example of:

1. Risk taking
2. Humility
3. Reflection
4. Problem solving

7. A nurse is about to begin her morning rounds, but before doing so, reads in one patient's chart that a diagnosis of ovarian cancer had just been made. The nurse plans to do her routine physical check of the patient when she first enters the room but then plans to also talk with the patient about her feelings regarding her diagnosis. The nurse's decision to assess her patient's feelings is an example of what critical thinking standard?
1. Relevant
2. Precise
3. Deep
4. Logical

8. A newly oriented nurse has been caring for a patient with a deep pressure ulcer for 2 days. The patient has an order for the application of a negative pressure wound vacuum system. The nurse has not yet had the opportunity to use the wound vacuum system. The nurse approaches the charge nurse and asks for assistance in applying the treatment. This is an example of the critical thinking attitude of:
1. Responsibility
2. Inference
3. Creativity
4. Humility

Answers to Review Questions can be found on pages 1197-1198.

REFERENCES

American Nurses Association: *Nursing's social policy statement*, Washington, DC, 2003, The Association.

Bandman EL, Bandman B: *Critical thinking in nursing*, ed 2, Norwalk, Conn, 1995, Appleton & Lange.

Benner P: *From novice to expert*, Menlo Park, Calif, 1984, Addison Wesley.

Bittner NP, Tobin E: Critical thinking: strategies for clinical practice, *J Nurs Staff Dev* 14(6):267, 1998.

Borbasi S, Jackson D, Wilkes L: Fieldwork in nursing research: positionality, practicalities and predicaments, *J Adv Nurs* 51(5):493, 2005.

Chaffee J: *Thinking critically*, ed 7, Boston, 2002, Houghton Mifflin.

Cirocco M: How reflective practice improves nurses' critical thinking ability, *Gastroenterol Nurs* 30(6):405, 2007.

Eisenhauer LA, Hurley AC, Dolan N: Nurses' reported thinking during medication administration, *J Nurs Scholarsh* 39(1):82, 2007.

Facione N, Facione P: Externalizing the critical thinking in knowledge development and clinical judgment, *Nurs Outlook* 44:129, 1996.

Facione P: *Critical thinking: a statement of expert consensus for purposes of educational assessment and instruction. The Delphi report: research findings and recommendations prepared for the American Philosophical Association*, ERIC Doc No. ED 315-423, Washington, DC, 1990, ERIC.

Ferrario CG: Developing nurses' critical thinking skills with concept mapping, *J Nurses Staff Develop* 20(6):261, 2004.

Glaser E: *An experiment in the development of critical thinking*, New York, 1941, Bureau of Publications, Teachers College, Columbia University.

Hill C: Integrating clinical experiences into the concept mapping process, *Nurs Educ* 31(1):36, 2006.

Infusion Nurses Society: Infusion nursing standards of practice, *J Intraven Nurs* 29(1S):S1, 2006.

Kataoka-Yahiro M, Saylor C: A critical thinking model for nursing judgment, *J Nurs Educ* 33(8):351, 1994.

Kessler PD, Lund CH: Reflective journaling: developing an online journal for distance education, *Nurse Educ* 29(1):20, 2004.

King L, Clark JM: Intuition and the development of expertise in surgical ward and intensive care nurses, *J Adv Nurs* 37(4):322, 2002.

Kok J, Chabeli MM: Reflective journal writing: how it promotes reflective thinking in clinical nursing education: a students' perspective, *Curationis* 25(3):35, 2002.

Kuiper R: Use of personal digital assistants to support clinical reasoning in undergraduate baccalaureate nursing students, *Comput Inform Nur* 26(2):90, 2008.

Miller M, Malcolm N: Critical thinking in the nursing curriculum, *Nurs Health Care* 11:67, 1990.

Paul R: The art of redesigning instruction. In Willsen J, Blinker AJA, editors: *Critical thinking: how to prepare students for a rapidly changing world*, Santa Rosa, Calif, 1993, Foundation for Critical Thinking.

Paul RW, Heaslip P: Critical thinking and intuitive nursing practice, *J Adv Nurs* 22: 40, 1995.

Profetto-McGrath J and others: A study of critical thinking and research utilization among nurses, *West J Nurs Res* 25(3):322, 2003.

Rew L, Barrow EM: State of the science: intuition in nursing, a generation of studying the phenomenon, *ANS Adv Nurs Sci* 30(1):E15, 2007.

Schuster PM: *Concept mapping: a critical thinking approach to care planning*, St. Louis, 2003, Mosby.

Settersten L, Lauver DR: Critical thinking, perceived health status, and participation in health behaviors, *Nurs Res* 53(1):11, 2004.

Sewell EA: Journaling as a mechanism to facilitate graduate nurses' role transition, *J Nurses Staff Dev* 24(2):49, 2008.

Strader M: Critical thinking. In Sullivan EJ, Decker PJ: *Effective management in nursing*, ed 3, Redwood City, Calif, 1992, Addison-Wesley Nursing.

White AH: Clinical decision making among fourth year nursing students: an interpretive study, *J Nurs Educ* 42(3):113, 2003.

Wolf ZR, Serembus JF, Beitz J: Clinical inference of nursing students concerning harmful outcomes after medication errors, *Nurse Educ* 26(6):268, 2001.

Nursing Process

MEDIA RESOURCES

 CD COMPANION 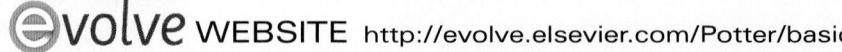 WEBSITE http://evolve.elsevier.com/Potter/basic

- Crossword Puzzle
- English/Spanish Audio Glossary

OBJECTIVES

- Describe each step of the nursing process.
- Explain the relationship between critical thinking and steps of the nursing process.
- Discuss approaches to data collection in nursing assessment.
- Differentiate between subjective and objective data.
- Explain the type of conclusions that result from data analysis.
- List the steps of the nursing diagnostic process.
- Describe the way in which defining characteristics and the etiological process individualize a nursing diagnosis.

- Discuss the process of priority setting.
- Describe goal setting.
- Discuss the difference between a goal and an expected outcome.
- Identify examples of nursing-sensitive outcomes.
- Develop a plan of care from a nursing assessment.
- Discuss the process of selecting nursing interventions.
- Describe how to evaluate nursing interventions selected for a patient.
- Describe how evaluation leads to revision or modification of a plan of care.

KEY TERMS

KEY TERMS, CONT.

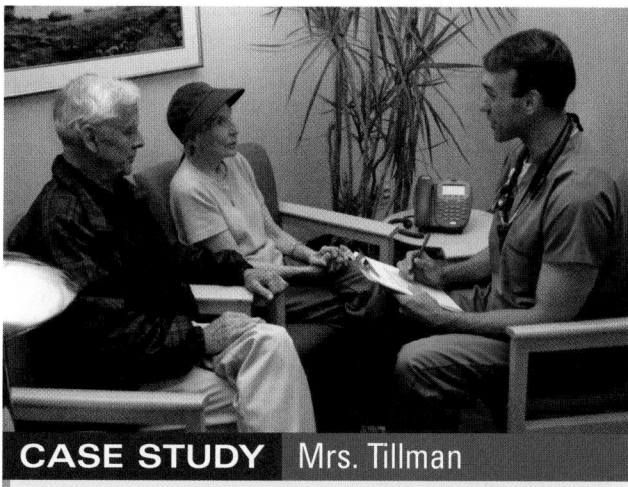

CASE STUDY   Mrs. Tillman

Rich is a nursing student who is assigned to care for Mrs. Jane Tillman, a 63-year-old woman with metastatic breast cancer. Mrs. Tillman recently retired after being a schoolteacher for 35 years. She had chemotherapy and radiation for her cancer, but now x-ray films show the tumor has spread to her lungs. Rich sees Mrs. Tillman and her husband, Greg, during the patient's visit to the outpatient cancer clinic. Rich observes the patient sighing deeply and looking down as she talks with her husband. Rich knows from reading the medical record that the couple was told about Mrs. Tillman's prognosis during their last visit. Rich also reviewed information about chemotherapy and radiation therapy to learn about the various complications and health problems these therapies can cause. He prepares to use the nursing process to determine Mrs. Tillman's current health status and to plan nursing therapies. His first step will be a thorough assessment, involving an interview with the patient and her husband and a health examination of the patient.

The **nursing process** is a professional nurse's approach to identifying, diagnosing, and treating human responses to health and illness (American Nurses Association, 2003). It is the basic nursing competency for critical thinking and fundamental to how nurses practice. As a nurse, you will learn to integrate elements of critical thinking to form judgments and make safe and effective clinical decisions through the nursing process. The process includes five steps: assessment, nursing diagnosis, planning, implementation,

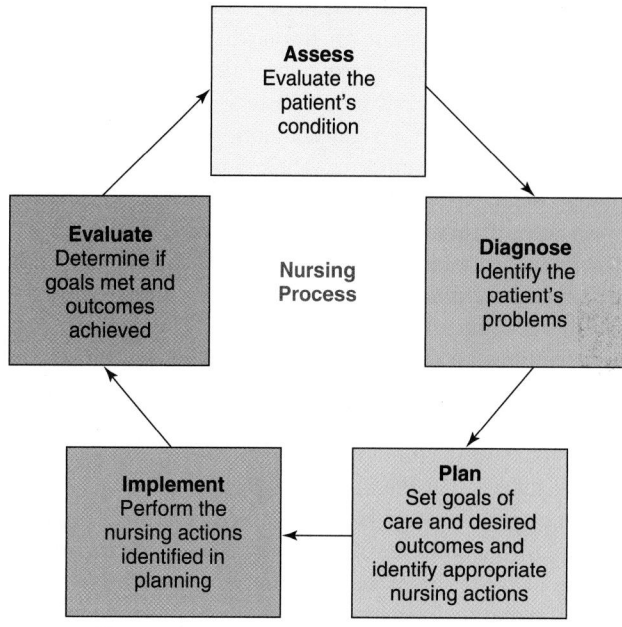

Figure 8-1 ▇ Five-step nursing process.

and evaluation (Figure 8-1). Initially you will learn how to apply the process step-by-step. However, as you gain more clinical experience and care for more than one patient, you will learn to move back and forth through the steps of the process, critically making judgments about your patients' clinical situations and individualizing your approaches to care. The nursing process is central to your ability to provide timely and appropriate care to your patients.

ASSESSMENT

Assessment is the deliberate and systematic collection of data about a patient. The data will reveal a patient's current and past health status, functional status, and present and past coping patterns (Carpenito-Moyet, 2008). Assessment requires you to apply critical thinking so that in the end, you have a clear picture of a patient's condition. There are two steps in nursing assessment:

• Collection and verification of data from a primary source (the patient) and secondary sources (e.g., family, friends, health professionals, medical record)

- Analysis of all data as a basis for the second step of the nursing process, developing nursing diagnoses and identifying collaborative problems

The purpose of the assessment is to establish a thorough **database** about a patient. Thus you first apply knowledge that helps you identify what to assess. For example, your knowledge from the physical, biological, and social sciences allows you to ask relevant questions about a patient's health status and response to illness. You use this knowledge to collect relevant physical assessment data related to a patient's clinical condition. Critical thinking attitudes and intellectual standards allow you to direct questions expertly, clarify data, and gather further data for validation. Then you will see the data patterns that reflect problems. Your experience allows you to recognize and anticipate what and how to assess correctly. Experience will lead you to ask the right questions, choosing only those that will give you the most relevant and useful information.

An assessment database includes a patient's comprehensive **health history,** which includes information about a patient's physical and developmental status, emotional health, social practices and resources, goals, values, lifestyle, and expectations about the health care system. The database also includes physical examination findings and a summary of results from laboratory and diagnostic testing. The knowledge you gather about the patient's medical diagnosis and treatment from the literature and medical record is also part of the database that then leads you to fully understand your patient's condition and health care needs. Critical thinking applied throughout the assessment process allows you to form conclusions or make decisions about a patient's health condition and to direct assessment activities in a meaningful and purposeful way (see Chapter 7).

Rich introduces himself to Mrs. and Mr. Tillman and explains his role in the clinic. "I am a nursing student assigned to you today. I want to take some time to talk with you and ask you a few questions to see how you are doing. Then I will want to examine you by taking your blood pressure, listening to your lungs, and performing some other measures to get a good idea of your condition. I will be sharing what I find with your doctor. Then I want to work with you to put a plan together for your care. Is that okay with you?" Mrs. Tillman responds hesitantly, "Well, I guess so, I'm just not sure what to expect." Rich responds, "Well, let's start there. Tell me what you have been told by your doctor." Mrs. Tillman answers, "My breast cancer has spread; it is in my lungs." Rich notes, "I noticed you were sighing a minute ago. You look a bit down." Mrs. Tillman responds, "I am so tired, and I have gone through two different courses of chemo and then radiation; nothing has worked. Lately I just haven't had the energy to do what I like to do around the house. My husband and I are worn out." Mr. Tillman responds, "Yes, cancer is just exhausting." Rich replies, "It sounds as though this has been difficult for both of you. Mrs. Tillman, you say you are tired. Tell me how you spend a typical day. I want to learn about the symptoms you are having from your cancer and treatment." Rich reflects to himself and considers the physical examination techniques he will want to use later to explore each symptom.

Rich has set the stage to begin an initial nursing assessment. He knows that a terminal disease can cause considerable grief as well as numerous physical changes. He wants to explore Mrs. Tillman's symptom experience and also learn her feelings about cancer so that he can get a clearer sense of her emotional reaction. He applies critical thinking by asking relevant questions that will help reveal a clear picture of how cancer is affecting the patient on a daily basis. His knowledge base also leads him to direct the assessment of Mrs. Tillman's symptoms, because cancer and cancer treatment can cause a variety of physical and psychological changes. Good communication skills and critical thinking allow Rich to begin to gather information for a complete, accurate, and relevant database.

Prior clinical experience contributes to assessment skills. For example, if you cared for a patient with heart disease in the past, you will know the type of factors that precipitate or signal chest pain. Thus you would assess thoroughly the types of factors that typically precede a patient's chest pain. You become competent in assessment through validation of abnormal assessment findings and personal observation of assessments performed by skilled nurses. You also learn to apply standards of practice and accepted standards of "normal" physical assessment data when assessing a patient. These standards help you to collect the right kind of information and ensure that you have a standard against which to compare your findings. The use of attributes such as curiosity, perseverance, and risk taking then ensures that your database is thorough and complete.

Data Collection

When you assess a patient, think critically about what to assess. Determine what questions or measurements are appropriate based on your clinical knowledge and experience. Once you start, select questions and measurements based on your patient's responses. When you first meet a patient, make a quick observational overview or screening. Usually you will base your overview on the treatment situation. For example, a community health nurse assesses the neighborhood and the community of the patient, or an emergency department nurse uses the ABC (airway-breathing-circulation) approach. Another example is a home care nurse focusing on the patient's environment and approaches to coping with illness. You need to differentiate important data from all of the information you collect. A **cue** is information that you obtain through use of the senses. An **inference** is your judgment or interpretation of those cues (Figure 8-2). For example, the cue of Mrs. Tillman

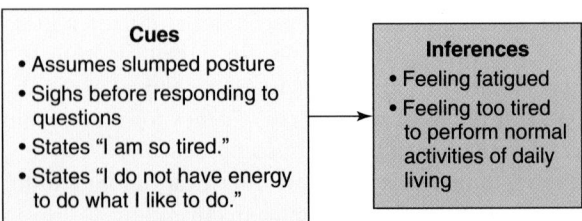

Figure 8-2 ■ Observational overview using cues and forming inferences.

expressing a sense of feeling tired and not having energy for daily routines lead you to infer a problem with activity. Anything a patient says and any behaviors you observe are important cues. It is possible to miss cues when you conduct your initial overview. However, always be observant and try to interpret cues from the patient to know how in-depth your eventual assessment needs to be.

After your observational overview, you will begin to focus on assessment cues and patterns of information that suggest problem areas. However, it is essential to conduct a comprehensive assessment when you can. There are two approaches for a comprehensive assessment. One involves use of a structured database format, based upon an accepted theoretical framework or practice standard. Gordon's 11 **functional health patterns** (1994) and Pender's health promotion model (Pender, Murdaugh, and Parsons, 2006) are examples. The theory or practice standard provides categories of information for you to assess. Gordon's functional health pattern assessment model provides a holistic framework for assessment of the patient's health history, from which you will derive a broad range of nursing diagnoses (Gordon, 1994). Box 8-1 offers examples of the types of assessment data you would collect using Gordon's functional health pattern model. An assessment moves from the general to the specific. For example, you assess all of Gordon's 11 functional health patterns to determine if any problems exist. The premise is that the categories will lead you to perform the most comprehensive assessment of the patient's health care problems.

The second approach for conducting a comprehensive assessment is the problem-focused approach. You focus on the patient's situation and begin with problematic areas, such as a patient's report of feeling tired. Then you ask the patient follow-up questions to clarify and expand. For example, in the case of Mrs. Tillman, Rich asks how her lack of energy affects her ability to perform routine tasks and the extent to which it affects her physically (Table 8-1). Once Rich completes his initial assessment, he thoroughly analyzes the extent and nature of Mrs. Tillman's sense of feeling tired. This allows him to correctly identify her health problem so as to develop a comprehensive treatment plan.

BOX 8-1   Typology of 11 Functional Health Patterns

Health perception–health management pattern: Describes the patient's self-report of health and well-being; how health is managed (e.g., frequency of physician visits, adherence to prescribed therapies at home); knowledge of preventive health practices

Nutritional-metabolic pattern: Describes the patient's daily/weekly pattern of food and fluid intake (e.g., food preferences, special diet, food restrictions, appetite); actual weight, weight loss or gain

Elimination pattern: Describes patterns of excretory function (bowel, bladder, and skin)

Activity-exercise pattern: Describes patterns of exercise, activity, leisure, and recreation; ability to perform activities of daily living

Sleep-rest pattern: Describes patterns of sleep, rest, and relaxation

Cognitive-perceptual pattern: Describes sensory-perceptual patterns; language adequacy, memory, decision-making ability

Self-perception–self-concept pattern: Describes the patient's self-concept pattern and perceptions of self (e.g., self-concept/worth, emotional patterns, body image)

Role-relationship pattern: Describes the patient's pattern of role engagements and relationships

Sexuality-reproductive pattern: Describes the patient's patterns of satisfaction and dissatisfaction with sexuality pattern; patient's reproductive pattern; premenopausal and postmenopausal problems

Coping–stress-tolerance pattern: Describes the patient's ability to manage stress; sources of support; effectiveness of the pattern in terms of stress tolerance

Value-belief pattern: Describes patterns of values, beliefs (including spiritual practices), and goals that guide the patient's choices or decisions

Data from Gordon M: *Nursing diagnosis: process and application,* ed 3, St. Louis, 1994, Mosby; Carpenito-Moyet LJ: *Nursing diagnosis: application to clinical practice,* ed 12, Philadelphia, 2008, Lippincott Williams & Wilkins.

TABLE 8-1   FOCUSED PATIENT ASSESSMENT

FACTORS TO ASSESS	QUESTIONS	PHYSICAL ASSESSMENT
Ability to perform routine tasks	Tell me how your feeling tired affects the way you are able to do household chores. Describe for me what you did in a typical day before you got cancer. How has this changed?	Observe how quickly patient responds to questions. Observe posture and body movements.
Extent the lack of energy affects her physically	Tell me how your feeling tired affects your interest in sexual activity. Do you feel you have more energy after you sleep or rest?	

Whatever approach you use for assessment, you will begin to cluster cues, make inferences, and identify emerging patterns and potential problems. To do this well, you anticipate critically, which means you always try to stay a step ahead of the assessment. For example, if you suspect a patient has a certain type of health problem (e.g., fatigue), you pose questions that deal with responses typically seen with fatigue. Remember to always have supporting cues before you make an inference. Inferences will lead you to further questions. Once you ask a question or make an observation of a patient, the information branches to an additional series of questions or observations (Figure 8-3). You take a risk when you do not anticipate assessment questions. This can cause an incomplete assessment, or you might fail to recognize cues and dismiss relevant problems. Knowing how to probe and frame questions is a skill that will grow with experience. You will learn to decide which questions are relevant to a situation while at the same time being sure the assessment is complete.

TYPES OF DATA   There are two primary sources of data, subjective and objective. **Subjective data** are your patients' verbal descriptions of their health problems. Only patients provide subjective data. For example, Mrs. Tillman's statements about being worn out and dealing with a difficult experience are subjective findings. Subjective data usually include feelings of anxiety, physical discomfort, or mental stress. Although only patients provide subjective data relevant to their health condition, be aware that these problems sometimes result in physiological changes, which you can further explore through objective data collection.

Objective data are observations or measurements of a patient's health status. Inspection of the condition of a wound or observation of a patient's posture and gait are examples of objective data. You base your measurements of objective data on an accepted standard, such as the Fahrenheit or Celsius measure on a thermometer, centimeters on a measuring tape, or known characteristics of behaviors. When you collect objective data, apply critical thinking intellectual standards (e.g., clear, precise, and consistent). Do not include your personal interpretive statements.

SOURCES OF DATA   As a nurse, you will obtain data from a variety of sources. Each source of data provides information about the patient's level of wellness, risk factors, health practices and goals, and patterns of health and illness.

Patient   A patient is usually your best source of information. A patient who is alert and answers questions appropriately provides the most accurate information about health care needs, lifestyle patterns, present and past illnesses, perception of symptoms, and changes in activities of daily living (ADLs). Always consider the setting for your assessment. A patient experiencing acute pain in an emergency department will not offer the same depth of information as one who comes to an outpatient clinic for a routine checkup. Always be attentive and show a caring presence with the patient (see Chapter 18). Patients are less likely to fully reveal the nature of their health care problems when nurses show little interest or are easily distracted by activities around them.

Family and Significant Others   Family members and significant others are primary sources of information for infants, children, critically ill adults, patients with mental handicaps, or patients who are unconscious or have reduced cognitive function. In cases of severe illness or emergencies, families are often the only available sources of information for nurses and other health care providers. The family and significant others are also good secondary sources of information. They confirm information a patient provides (e.g., whether a patient takes medications regularly at home or how well the patient eats). Include the family when appropriate. Remember, a patient does not always want you to question the family. Often spouses or close friends will sit in during an assessment and provide their view of the patient's health problems or needs. Not only do they supply information about the patient's current health status, but they are

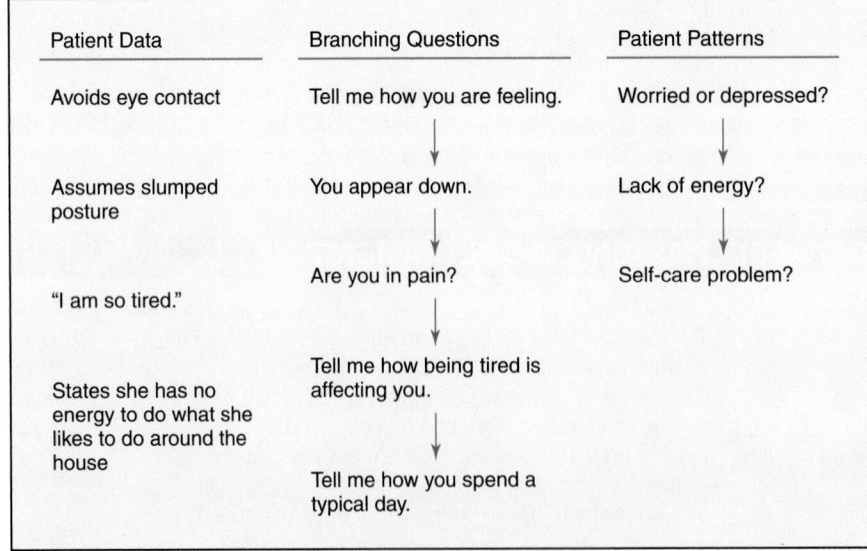

Patient Data	Branching Questions	Patient Patterns
Avoids eye contact	Tell me how you are feeling. ↓	Worried or depressed? ↓
Assumes slumped posture	You appear down. ↓	Lack of energy? ↓
"I am so tired."	Are you in pain? ↓	Self-care problem?
States she has no energy to do what she likes to do around the house	Tell me how being tired is affecting you. ↓ Tell me how you spend a typical day.	

Figure 8-3 ■ Example of branching logic for selecting assessment questions.

also able to tell when changes in the patient's status occurred. Family members are often very well informed because of their experiences living with the patient and observing how health problems affect daily living activities. For example, Mr. Tillman is an excellent resource for describing how his wife's lack of energy affects her day to day.

Health Care Team   You will frequently communicate with other health care team members when gathering information about patients. In the acute care setting the change-of-shift report is the way for nurses on one shift to communicate information to nurses on the oncoming shift (see Chapter 9). Typically, when nurses and other health care providers consult on a patient's condition, each contributes information about the patient. This includes how the patient is interacting within the health care environment, the patient's reactions to treatment, the results of diagnostic procedures or therapies, and how the patient responds to visitors. Every member of the health care team is a source of information for identifying and verifying information about the patient.

Medical Records   The medical record is a source for the patient's medical history, laboratory and diagnostic test results, current physical findings, and the health care provider's treatment plan. Data in the records offer a baseline and ongoing information about the patient's response to illness and progress to date. The Health Insurance Portability and Accountability Act (HIPAA) of 1996 has a privacy rule that came into effect in 2003 to set standards for the protection of health information (HIPAAdvisory, 2003). Information in a patient's record is confidential. Each health care agency has policies governing how health care providers can share information. A nurse can review a patient's medical record for assessment data, but needs to know the agency policies governing how to share the information with other staff. The medical record is a valuable tool to check the consistency and similarities of your personal observations.

Other Records and the Literature   Educational, military, and employment records often contain pertinent health care information (e.g., immunizations or prior illnesses). If a patient received services at a community clinic or different hospital, the nurse first obtains written permission from the patient or guardian before seeing the records. New HIPAA regulations dictate specifically how to obtain an information release (HIPAAdvisory, 2003). Consult your agency's policies.

Reviewing nursing, medical, and pharmacological literature about a patient's illness completes your assessment database. This review increases your knowledge about expected signs and symptoms, treatment, prognosis of specific illnesses and established standards of therapeutic practice. Always be sure to review the most current evidence in the literature as it applies to your patient (see Chapter 6). A knowledgeable nurse obtains pertinent, accurate, and complete information for the assessment database.

Methods of Data Collection

As a nurse, you will use the patient interview as the tool for assessing a patient's health history. Once you have collected data, you will then proceed to a physical examination.

Interview and Health History   The first step in establishing a database is to collect subjective information while interviewing a patient. An interview is an organized conversation with the patient (see Chapter 10). The initial interview involves assessing the patient's health history and obtaining information about the current illness. During the initial interview you have the opportunity to:

1. Introduce yourself to the patient, explain your role, and explain the role of others during care
2. Establish a caring therapeutic relationship with the patient
3. Gain insight about the patient's concerns and worries
4. Determine the patient's goals and expectations of the health care delivery system
5. Obtain cues about which parts of the data collection phase require in-depth investigation

Later interviews allow you to assess more about a patient's situation and to focus on specific problem areas. An interview helps patients to explain their own interpretations and understandings of their conditions. Therefore you and the patient will be partners during the interview; you do not control the interview. An interview consists of three phases: orientation, working, and termination.

Always prepare for an interview. Collect any available information about the patient, and then create a favorable environment for the interview. For example, review the information you learn during change-of-shift report, and then plan to interview the patient during rounds and before you begin to deliver patient care. In a hospital setting, you may have to provide measures for symptom relief before the patient is able to talk comfortably with you. In the home, choose a location that is quiet and as free of interruptions as is possible.

Orientation Phase   The orientation phase begins with introducing yourself and your position and explaining the purpose of the interview. Explain to patients why you are collecting data, and assure the patient that the information will remain confidential and will be used only by health care professionals who provide his or her care. HIPAA regulations require patients to sign an authorization before you collect personal health data (HIPAAdvisory, 2003). This usually occurs in admitting or screening areas before you meet the patient. Chapter 9 reviews protected health information.

During orientation you establish trust and confidence with a patient. One important goal for the initial interview is to lay the groundwork for understanding the patient's needs. In the initial discussion between Rich and Mrs. Tillman, Rich explains that he wants to put a plan together and in order to do so he wants to understand more about how Mrs. Tillman's cancer affects her during a typical day. He also tells the patient that he wants to learn more about the symptoms she is having.

Another goal for the interview is to begin a relationship that allows the patient to become an active partner in decisions about care. As the orientation phase proceeds, the patient should begin to feel more comfortable speaking with you. Initially you might gather demographic data (e.g., date of birth, gender, address, family members' names and addresses), as specified by the facility. Because this information is the least personal, it helps initiate development of the therapeutic relationship and eases transition into the working portion of the interview.

Working Phase During the working phase you gather information about the patient's health status. Remember to stay focused, orderly, and unhurried. You will begin by obtaining the patient's health history (Box 8-2). Use a variety of communication strategies such as active listening, paraphrasing, and summarizing to promote a clear interaction (see Chapter 10) and to construct a thorough database. The use of open-ended questions in particular encourages patients to tell their story in detail.

Rich begins the working phase of his interview by focusing on Mrs. Tillman's sense of "feeling worn out." Rich attends to Mrs. Tillman's concerns, immediately making her a partner in the interview, and then focuses on details that will reveal the extent to which cancer is affecting her life.

BOX 8-2   Basic Components for a Nursing Health History

Reasons for seeking health care: Goals of care, expectation of the services and care delivered, and expectations of the health care system

Present illness or health concern: Onset, symptoms, nature of symptoms (e.g., sudden or gradual), duration, precipitating factors, relief measures, and weight loss or gain

Health history: Prior illnesses throughout development, injuries and hospitalizations, surgeries, blood transfusions, allergies, immunizations, habits (e.g., smoking, caffeine intake, alcohol or drug abuse), prescribed and self-prescribed medications, work habits, relaxation activities, and sleep, exercise, and eating or nutritional patterns

Family history: Health status of the immediate family and living relatives, cause of death of relatives, and risk factor analyses for cancer, heart disease, diabetes mellitus, kidney disease, hypertension, or mental disorders

Environmental history: Hazards, pollutants, and physical safety

Psychosocial and cultural history: Primary language, cultural group, community resources, mood, attention span, and developmental stage

Review of systems: Head-to-toe review of all major body systems, as well as the patient's knowledge of and compliance with health care (e.g., frequency of breast or testicular self-examination or last visual acuity examination). Another option for an approach is to use *functional health patterns* as the method for organizing assessment data

---

Rich: "You say you are worn out; tell me how you spend a typical day."

Mrs. Tillman: "When I first wake up, I actually feel pretty good. I am able to get through breakfast and most of my bath before I start to feel tired."

Rich: "Uh-huh, go on." (active listening and probing)

Mrs. Tillman: "I used to do my errands midmorning, but I seem to lose energy. My husband has decided to retire early along with me. He helps me a great deal."

Rich: "You say you lose energy; tell me how you feel." (paraphrase and open-ended question)

Mrs. Tillman: "I just feel this sensation that I cannot do any more. I am too weak to move. I often have to take a nap midmorning. Isn't that ridiculous? The cancer has just weakened me so much."

Rich: "How you feel is not ridiculous; tell me how you feel after you nap." (open-ended question)

Rich explores in depth how Mrs. Tillman is physically affected by her cancer. He also gathers information from Mr. Tillman. The information will ultimately direct him in identifying the patient's health problems and choosing appropriate nursing therapies.

The first interview with a patient is often the most extensive of all interviews. Ongoing interviews, which occur each time you interact with your patient, do not need to be as extensive. They update the patient's status and focus more on changes in previously identified ongoing and new problems.

Termination Phase As in the other phases of the interview, the termination phase requires skill on the part of the interviewer. Give your patient a clue that the interview is coming to an end. For example, you say, "There are just two more questions" or "We'll be finished in 5 to 6 minutes." This helps the patient maintain direct attention without being distracted by wondering when the interview will end. This approach also gives the patient a chance to ask questions. When ending the interview, summarize the important points and ask your patient if the summary is accurate. End the interview in a friendly manner, telling the patient when you will return to provide care. For example, "Thanks, Mrs. Tillman. You have given me a good picture of your health and how you have been affected. It is important for you to understand how we expect the cancer will affect you and how we can help you manage your symptoms. Is that correct? I hope to develop a plan of care that will manage your difficulty breathing and sense of fatigue. Do you have any questions?"

INTERVIEW TECHNIQUES The way in which you conduct an interview is just as important as the questions you ask. Pay attention to the environment, patient comfort, and communication techniques (see Chapter 10) to be successful. During the interview, direct the flow of conversation so that you obtain adequate information and the patient has the chance to contribute freely. Ideally you want patients to tell their stories about their health problems so that you can obtain as many details as possible.

Some interviews will be focused, whereas others will be comprehensive. Listen and consider the information shared. This helps you direct the patient to give more detail or to discuss a topic that might reveal a possible problem. Because a patient's report will include subjective information, validate data from the interview later with objective data. For example, Mrs. Tillman reports she often feels too weak to move. Rich will later measure her muscle strength and tolerance to walking.

Remember that patients also obtain information during interviews. If you establish a positive nurse-patient relationship, the patient will feel comfortable asking you questions about planned treatments, diagnostic procedures, and need for resources. Patients need this information to make decisions about their health care.

A good interview environment is free of distractions, unnecessary noise, and interruptions. The patient is more likely to be candid if the interview is private, out of earshot of other patients, visitors, and staff. Timing is important in avoiding interruptions. If possible, set aside a 15- to 30-minute period when no other activities are planned. Another option in a busy hospital setting is to set aside two 15-minute periods during your shift. Help the patient to feel relaxed and unhurried. Before you begin the interview, be sure the patient is comfortable. Comfort factors include adequate light, warmth, and positioning. Sit facing the patient to facilitate eye contact. During the interview, observe your patient for signs of discomfort or fatigue.

When the interview involves a health history, try to find out, in the patient's own words, what the health problem is and what is likely causing it. Remember, patients are usually the best resources in explaining their health history. Begin by asking the patient a question to elicit his or her story. For example, say, "Tell me the reason you came to the hospital today" or "Tell me about the problems you are having." The use of **open-ended questions** prompts patients to describe a situation in more than one or two words. This technique leads to a discussion in which patients actively describe their health status. The use of open-ended questions strengthens the nurse-patient relationship because it shows that you want to invest time in hearing the patient's thoughts. Encourage the patient to tell the story all the way through. Reinforce your interest by using good eye contact and listening skills. Use **back-channeling,** which is the practice of giving positive comments such as "all right," "go on," or "uh-huh" to the speaker. These indicate that you have heard what the patient says and are attentive to hear the full story.

Once patients tell their story, use a problem-seeking interview technique. This approach takes the information provided in the patient's story and then more fully describes and identifies specific problem areas. For example, focus on the symptoms the patient identifies, and ask **closed-ended questions** that limit the patient's answers to one or two words such as "yes" or "no" or a number or frequency of a symptom. For example, ask "How often do you feel really tired or fatigued?" or "After taking a nap, do you feel more rested?" As closed-ended questions reveal more information, you have the patient discuss historical information in more detail. A good interviewer leaves with a complete story that contains enough detail for understanding the patient's perceptions of his or her health status, as well as the information needed to help identify nursing diagnoses and/or collaborative health problems. Always clarify or validate any information that is unclear.

PHYSICAL EXAMINATION A physical examination allows a nurse to examine the patient's body to determine his or her state of health. A physical examination involves use of the techniques of inspection, palpation, percussion, auscultation, and smell. A complete examination includes a patient's height, weight, vital signs (see Chapter 14), general appearance and behavior, and a head-to-toe examination of all body systems (see Chapter 15).

OBSERVATION OF PATIENT'S BEHAVIOR During an interview and physical examination it is important for you to closely observe a patient's verbal and nonverbal behaviors. This information adds depth to the objective database. You learn to determine whether data obtained by observation match what the patient states verbally. For example, if a patient expresses no concern about an upcoming diagnostic test but appears anxious and irritable, verbal and nonverbal data conflict. Observations lead you to gather the additional objective information to form accurate conclusions about a patient's condition.

An important aspect of observation includes a patient's level of function: the physical, developmental, psychological, and social aspects of everyday living. Observation of the level of function is different from what you learn about function during the interview. You observe what you see the patient doing, such as self-feeding or making a decision, rather than what the patient says he or she can do. Level of function differs from a physical assessment. The level of function involves a person's ability to perform during everyday activities. The hands-on physical examination measures the extent of function through measures such as range of motion and muscle strength.

DIAGNOSTIC AND LABORATORY DATA The results of diagnostic and laboratory tests identify or verify alterations questioned or identified during the nursing health history and physical examination. For example, during the health history the patient reports having had a bad cold for 6 days and at present has a productive cough with brown sputum and mild shortness of breath. On physical examination, you notice an elevated temperature, increased respirations, and decreased breath sounds in the right lower lobe. You review the results of an ordered complete blood count (CBC) and note the white blood cell count is elevated (indicating an infection). In addition, the radiologist's report of a chest x-ray examination shows the presence of a right lower lobe infiltrate. Such findings combined suggest the patient has the medical diagnosis of pneumonia and the associated nursing diagnosis of *impaired gas exchange*. When a patient collects and monitors laboratory data at home, such as with routine blood glucose monitoring for diabetes, ask the patient about the routine results to determine the patient's response to illness and the effects of treatment measures.

Compare laboratory data with the established norms for a particular test, age-group, and gender.

Cultural Considerations in Assessment

Good assessment techniques are important, especially when caring for patients from cultures different from your own. Communication and culture are interrelated in the way individuals express feelings verbally and nonverbally. When you learn the variations in how people of different cultures communicate, you will likely gather more accurate information from patients. For example, patients of Spanish and French heritage use firm eye contact when speaking. However, this is considered rude among Asian and Middle Eastern cultures. Americans tend to let the eyes wander (Seidel and others, 2006). Using the right approach with eye contact will show respect for your patient and likely result in the patient sharing more information. When you assess patients, consider the many factors that will influence their health because of their cultural background. Chapter 19 covers the process to use in conducting a thorough cultural assessment. To start an assessment, Seidel and others (2006) offer useful questions to begin to explore a patient's illness or health care problem in context of the patient's culture:

* What do you call your problem?
* What do you think caused your problem?
* What does your sickness do to you?
* Why did you come to me for treatment?
* What are the most important problems your sickness has caused for you?
* What worries you and frightens you the most about your sickness?

Data Validation

The ability to make accurate judgments on the basis of an assessment requires critical thinking. Once you have collected your data, validate the data you have. This will help you to more accurately analyze and interpret the patient's clinical picture. **Validation** of assessment data is the comparison of data with another source to confirm their accuracy. For example, Rich observes Mrs. Tillman crying and logically infers it is related to her cancer diagnosis. Making such an initial inference is not wrong, but problems result if you do not validate the inference with the patient. Rich should ask, "I notice that you have been crying, can you tell me about it?" By doing so, Rich will discover the real reason for Mrs. Tillman's crying.

Ask your patient to validate the information you gather during the interview and health history. Validate findings from physical examination and observation of patient behavior by comparing data in the medical record and by consulting with other health team members or even family members. Validation often will lead you to gather more assessment data because it clarifies vague or ambiguous data. Occasionally you will need to reassess previously covered areas of the nursing history or gather further physical examination data. A nurse continually analyzes and thinks about a patient's database, enabling one to fully understand the problems, judge their extent, and discover possible relationships between the problems.

Rich gathers initial data about Mrs. Tillman's physical health, having focused on her lack of energy and "feeling tired" and the effects it has on her ability to conduct daily activities. He applied critical thinking in his assessment to consider what he knew about the effects of cancer and the therapies Mrs. Tillman has received, such as chemotherapy. The patient takes more frequent naps and reports little energy to do routine chores or engage in any social activities. Rich also learns a great deal about Mrs. Tillman's feelings about having advanced-stage cancer. He uses intellectual standards, being precise (specific feelings about prognosis), consistent, and accurate (use of a self-report scale to measure her perceptions of her quality of life), and complete (probing to determine how her feelings affect her relationship with her husband). Rich learns that Mrs. Tillman worries about her husband. She tells Rich, "He means so much to me. The doctor has told me what to expect. I know this is going to be very hard for him." Rich could make several inferences from this comment, but he applies the critical thinking attitude of discipline and validates his inferences, "You sound worried about your husband. Describe what is bothering you." Mrs. Tillman confirms Rich's assessment, "I am worried about Greg because he tries so hard to help me. I am worried he will get worn out too."

Data Documentation and Communication

Communication of assessment findings, either verbally or through documentation, is the last step of a complete assessment. The timely, thorough, and accurate communication of facts is necessary in order to ensure continuity and appropriateness of patient care. If you do not report or record an assessment finding or problem interpretation, it is lost and unavailable to anyone else caring for the patient (see Chapter 9). If you do not give specific information, you will leave another health care team member uninformed and often with only general impressions. Observation, reporting, and recording of a patient's status is a legal and professional responsibility. The Nurse Practice Acts in all states and the American Nurses Association policy statement (2003) mandate, or require, accurate data collection and recording as independent functions essential to the role of a professional nurse.

NURSING DIAGNOSIS

After reviewing and validating a patient's assessment, the next step of the nursing process is to form diagnostic conclusions to determine the patient's problems and level of care required. If a nurse forms an accurate diagnostic conclusion, nursing therapies will then be appropriate and relevant. A nurse will make a diagnostic conclusion either in the form of a nursing diagnosis or a collaborative problem. A **nursing diagnosis** is a clinical judgment about individual, family, or community responses to actual and potential health problems or life processes. A nursing diagnosis provides the basis selection of nursing interventions to achieve outcomes for which the nurse is accountable (NANDA International, 2009). It is a statement that describes a patient's actual or potential response to a health problem that the nurse is licensed and competent to treat. Never confuse a medical diagnosis with a nursing diagnosis. A **medical diagnosis** is the identification of a disease condition based on an evaluation of physical signs, symptoms, history, and diagnostic tests and procedures. Physicians and certified advanced practice nurses make medical diagnoses. Physicians are licensed to treat diseases or pathological processes described in medical diagnostic statements. For example, a physician will treat a patient with the medical diagnosis of cancer through medications, radiation, and surgery. An advanced practice nurse can also treat medical diagnoses but does not perform surgery. In contrast, a patient's responses to cancer, such as symptoms of pain and nausea and insufficient knowledge about treatment, are nursing diagnoses that nurses manage.

A **collaborative problem** is an actual or potential physiological complication that nurses monitor to detect the onset of changes in a patient's status (Carpenito-Moyet, 2008). When collaborative problems develop, nurses intervene in collaboration with personnel from other health care disciplines, such as social workers and dietitians. Nurses manage collaborative problems such as hemorrhage or infection using both physician-prescribed and nursing-prescribed interventions. For example, a patient who has a surgical wound is at risk for developing an infection, so a physician prescribes antibiotics. The nurse monitors the patient for signs of infection, provides meticulous wound care, and administers the prescribed antibiotics.

Nurses use scientific and nursing knowledge and previous experience to analyze and interpret assessment data in identifying nursing diagnoses and collaborative problems unique for their patients. The remainder of this section will focus on the reasoning process for making a nursing diagnosis.

Critical Thinking and the Nursing Diagnostic Process

Diagnostic reasoning involves logically analyzing and interpreting assessment data about a patient to form a clinical judgment, in this case a nursing diagnosis. The **nursing diagnostic process** flows from the assessment process and includes data clustering, interpretation and analysis, identifying patient needs, and formulating the nursing diagnosis or collaborative problem (Figure 8-4).

When you correctly analyze assessment data, you will be able to identify patients' problems and make clinical decisions about their care. Analysis begins by organizing all of your data into meaningful and usable **data clusters,** keeping in mind the patient's response to illness. During clustering, a cue or an individual sign, symptom, or finding will alert your thinking more than others. You begin to see how different data relate together. For example, Mrs. Tillman talks about not having any energy, taking frequent naps, and not being able to do usual activities such as preparing meals. These cues show a pattern. **Data analysis** and interpretation involves recognizing patterns or trends in the clustered data, comparing them with standards, and then coming to a reasoned conclusion about the patient's response to a health problem. Rich compares Mrs. Tillman's signs and symptoms with nor-

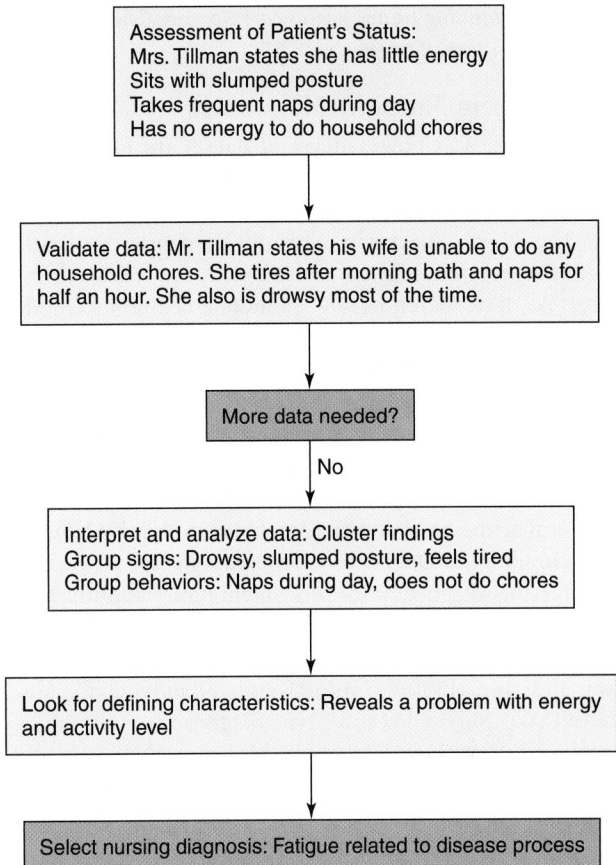

Figure 8-4 ■ Nursing diagnostic process for Mrs. Tillman.

mal standards for a woman her age, such as feeling rested, sleeping through the night, and being able to perform daily routines. Mrs. Tillman's clinical picture suggests that as a response to her cancer, Mrs. Tillman is experiencing a pattern of fatigue that affects her activity level.

Through reasoning and judgment a nurse decides what assessment information explains a patient's health status. Often a patient will present multiple cues, suggesting more than one type of health problem or need. At times you will have to gather additional data for clarification of your interpretation. For example, *Mrs. Tillman tells Rich that she has many unanswered questions, even though her doctor has talked about how her cancer will progress. She says, "I hope I can just not wake up one morning." Rich infers that Mrs. Tillman dreads how the cancer will affect her. He seeks further information, "Let's talk about what your doctor said about the cancer." Mrs. Tillman relates, "He says that further chemotherapy will likely not be effective. I can expect to have trouble breathing and possibly pain, but he said he will be sure to give me what I need." Rich clarifies, "You sound a bit uncertain. Are you concerned that you will suffer?" Mrs. Tillman begins to cry, "Yes, oh yes, that is my greatest fear. I really do not know what to expect." Rich further clarifies, "Have you received an explanation about palliative care?" Mrs. Tillman replies, "No, I haven't. What does that mean?" In looking for additional patterns of data, Rich decides Mrs. Tillman is having a difficult time anticipating her impending death and has insuffi-*

cient understanding of her health care options. These problems add to her pattern of fatigue.

Forming the Nursing Diagnosis

Once a nurse sees how patterns of data point to a patient's health problems, it becomes important to identify those problems in a way that will be clear to all health care providers. The North American Nursing Diagnosis Association (NANDA) was established in 1982 with the following purpose: "To develop, refine, and promote a taxonomy (model) of nursing diagnostic terms of general use for professional nurses" (Kim, McFarland, and McLean, 1984). Nursing professionals wanted to create a listing of nursing diagnoses similar to the list of medical diagnoses used by physicians. It was NANDA's intent to create a common language for nurses to be able to identify patient health problems and thus provide similar therapies for each problem. Today, **NANDA International (NANDA-I)** has developed a model for organizing nursing diagnoses for documentation, auditing, and communication purposes. The model includes 13 domains (e.g., health promotion and comfort), 47 classes (e.g., health awareness and physical comfort), and 188 nursing diagnoses (NANDA-I, 2009) (Box 8-3). New diagnoses are continually developed through research and added to the NANDA-I listing. The use of standard formal nursing diagnoses serves several purposes:

* Provides a precise definition that gives all members of the health care team a common language for understanding patient needs
* Allows nurses to communicate what they do among themselves, with other health care professionals, and with the public
* Distinguishes the nurse's role from that of physicians and other health care providers
* Helps nurses to focus on the scope of nursing practice
* Fosters the development of nursing knowledge

As a nurse reviews all assessment data, he or she compares the clusters and patterns of data with the clinical criteria for making a nursing diagnosis. **Defining characteristics** are the clinical criteria or assessment findings that support an actual nursing diagnosis. NANDA-I–approved nursing diagnoses have identified sets of defining characteristics that support identification of each nursing diagnosis (NANDA-I, 2009). Over time you will begin to become familiar with the defining characteristics for the more common nursing diagnoses in your practice. This will make recognition of nursing diagnoses easier. Box 8-4 shows an example of an approved nursing diagnosis and its associated defining characteristics and related factors. As you analyze clusters of data, you begin to consider various diagnoses that might apply to your patient. For example, Rich reviews findings pertaining to Mrs. Tillman, who reported feeling tired and having a lack of energy. The defining characteristics of being tired and lacking energy could apply to the nursing diagnoses of fatigue and activity intolerance. However, Rich's assessment probed further to reveal Mrs. Tillman's

inability to maintain usual levels of activity or routines, pointing his diagnostic conclusion toward fatigue. It is important to learn that the absence of certain defining characteristics suggests that you reject a diagnosis under consideration. Carefully examine defining characteristics that support or eliminate a nursing diagnosis. To be more accurate, review all characteristics, eliminate nonrelevant ones, and confirm relevant ones.

While focusing on patterns of defining characteristics, you also compare a patient's pattern of data with data that are consistent with normal, healthful patterns. Use accepted norms as the basis for comparison and judgment. This includes using laboratory and diagnostic test values, professional standards, and normal anatomical or physiological limits. When comparing patterns, judge whether the grouped signs and symptoms are normal for the patient and whether they are within the range of healthful responses. As you isolate the defining characteristics that are not within healthy norms, you will identify a patient need or problem. In the example of Mrs. Tillman, Rich assessed a verbal report of feeling tired and lacking energy. These symptoms are not common for a 63-year-old and indicate a basic problem involving the patient's ability to participate in normal activity. He also learned that Mrs. Tillman has difficulty completing routine chores at times and requires frequent naps during the day. Rich recognized that Mrs. Tillman had a problem, but he reviewed the NANDA-I classifications to define her problem more specifically. He looked first at the domain of activity/rest. NANDA-I has a variety of nursing diagnoses that can apply to activity/rest (e.g., *activity intolerance, risk for activity intolerance, fatigue,* and *impaired walking*). After carefully reviewing Mrs. Tillman's presenting symptoms, Rich selected *fatigue.* The key to Rich's diagnosis was assessing how the patient's lack of energy affected her daily activities.

It is critical for a nurse to eventually arrive at the correct diagnostic label for a patient's need. A nurse usually moves from general to specific. It helps to think of the problem identification phase as the general health care problem and the formulation of the nursing diagnosis as the specific health problem. When you begin to identify a problem, review the NANDA-I domains to help you focus on nursing diagnoses pertinent to a particular domain.

TYPES OF NURSING DIAGNOSES NANDA-I has identified five types of nursing diagnoses: actual, health promotion, risk, syndrome, and wellness, diagnoses (NANDA-I, 2009). An actual nursing diagnosis describes human responses to health conditions or life processes that exist in an individual, family, or community. These types of diagnoses require a nurse's active interventions. The selection of an actual diagnosis means that sufficient assessment data are available to establish existence of the nursing diagnosis. In the case of Mrs. Tillman, *fatigue* and *death anxiety* are actual nursing diagnoses.

A health promotion nursing diagnosis is a clinical judgment of a person's, family's, or community's motivation and desire to increase well-being and actualize human health potential as expressed in the readiness to enhance specific health behaviors,

BOX 8-3   NANDA International Nursing Diagnoses

Activity intolerance
Risk for Activity intolerance
Ineffective Activity planning
Ineffective Airway clearance
Latex Allergy response
Risk for latex Allergy response
Anxiety
Death Anxiety
Risk for Aspiration
Risk for impaired Attachment
Autonomic dysreflexia
Risk for Autonomic dysreflexia
Risk-prone health Behavior
Risk for Bleeding
Disturbed Body image
Risk for imbalanced Body temperature
Bowel incontinence
Effective Breastfeeding
Ineffective Breastfeeding
Interrupted Breastfeeding
Ineffective Breathing pattern
Decreased Cardiac output
Caregiver role strain
Risk for Caregiver role strain
Readiness for enhanced Childbearing process
Readiness for enhanced Comfort
Impaired Comfort
Impaired verbal Communication
Readiness for enhanced Communication
Decisional Conflict
Parental role Conflict
Acute Confusion
Chronic Confusion
Risk for Acute Confusion
Constipation
Perceived Constipation
Risk for Constipation
Contamination
Risk for Contamination
Compromised family Coping
Defensive Coping
Disabled family Coping
Ineffective Coping
Ineffective community Coping
Readiness for enhanced Coping
Readiness for enhanced community Coping
Readiness for enhanced family Coping
Risk for sudden infant Death syndrome
Readiness for enhanced Decision-Making
Ineffective Denial
Impaired Dentition
Risk for delayed Development
Diarrhea
Risk for compromised human Dignity
Moral Distress
Risk for Disuse syndrome
Deficient Diversional activity
Risk for Electrolyte imbalance
Disturbed Energy field

Impaired Environmental interpretation syndrome
Adult Failure to thrive
Risk for Falls
Dysfunctional Family processes
Interrupted Family processes
Readiness for enhanced Family processes
Fatigue
Fear
Ineffective infant Feeding pattern
Readiness for enhanced Fluid balance
Deficient Fluid volume
Excess Fluid volume
Risk for deficient Fluid volume
Risk for imbalanced Fluid volume
Impaired Gas exchange
Risk for unstable blood Glucose level
Grieving
Complicated Grieving
Risk for complicated Grieving
Delayed Growth and development
Risk for disproportionate Growth
Ineffective Health maintenance
Ineffective self Health management
Impaired Home maintenance
Readiness for enhanced Hope
Hopelessness
Hyperthermia
Hypothermia
Disturbed personal Identity
Readiness for enhanced Immunization status
Functional urinary Incontinence
Overflow urinary Incontinence
Reflex urinary Incontinence
Stress urinary Incontinence
Urge urinary Incontinence
Risk for urge urinary Incontinence
Risk for Ineffective Renal Perfusion
Disorganized Infant behavior
Risk for disorganized Infant behavior
Readiness for enhanced organized Infant behavior
Risk for Infection
Risk for Injury
Risk for perioperative-positioning Injury
Insomnia
Decreased Intracranial adaptive capacity
Neonatal Jaundice
Deficient Knowledge
Readiness for enhanced Knowledge
Sedentary Lifestyle
Risk for impaired Liver function
Risk for Loneliness
Risk for disturbed Maternal/Fetal dyad
Impaired Memory
Impaired bed Mobility
Impaired physical Mobility
Impaired wheelchair Mobility
Dysfunctional gastrointestinal Motility
Risk for dysfunctional gastrointestinal Motility
Nausea

Continued

BOX 8-3 NANDA International Nursing Diagnoses—cont'd

Self-**Neglect**
Unilateral **Neglect**
Noncompliance
Imbalanced **Nutrition**: less than body requirements
Imbalanced **Nutrition**: more than body requirements
Readiness for enhanced **Nutrition**
Risk for imbalanced **Nutrition**: more than body requirements
Impaired **Oral** mucous membrane
Acute **Pain**
Chronic **Pain**
Readiness for enhanced **Parenting**
Impaired **Parenting**
Risk for impaired **Parenting**
Risk for decreased cardiac tissue **Perfusion**
Risk for ineffective cerebral tissue **Perfusion**
Risk for ineffective gastrointestinal **Perfusion**
Ineffective peripheral tissue **Perfusion**
Risk for **Peripheral** neurovascular dysfunction
Risk for **Poisoning**
Post-Trauma syndrome
Risk for **Post-Trauma** syndrome
Readiness for enhanced **Power**
Powerlessness
Risk for **Powerlessness**
Ineffective **Protection**
Rape-Trauma syndrome
Readiness for enhanced **Relationship**
Impaired **Religiosity**
Readiness for enhanced **Religiosity**
Risk for impaired **Religiosity**
Relocation stress syndrome
Risk for **Relocation** stress syndrome
Risk for compromised **Resilience**
Readiness for enhanced **Resilience**
Impaired individual **Resilience**
Ineffective **Role** performance
Readiness for enhanced **Self-Care**
Bathing **Self-Care** deficit
Dressing **Self-Care** deficit
Feeding **Self-Care** deficit
Toileting **Self-Care** deficit
Readiness for enhanced **Self-Concept**

Chronic low **Self-Esteem**
Situational low **Self-Esteem**
Risk for situational low **Self-Esteem**
Readiness for enhanced **Self Health** management
Self-Mutilation
Risk for **Self-Mutilation**
Disturbed **Sensory** perception
Sexual dysfunction
Ineffective **Sexuality** pattern
Risk for **Shock**
Impaired **Skin** integrity
Risk for impaired **Skin** integrity
Sleep deprivation
Readiness for enhanced **Sleep**
Disturbed **Sleep** pattern
Impaired **Social** interaction
Social isolation
Chronic **Sorrow**
Spiritual distress
Risk for **Spiritual** distress
Readiness for enhanced **Spiritual** well-being
Stress overload
Risk for **Suffocation**
Risk for **Suicide**
Delayed **Surgical** recovery
Impaired **Swallowing**
Ineffective family **Therapeutic** regimen management
Ineffective **Thermoregulation**
Impaired **Tissue** integrity
Impaired **Transfer** ability
Risk for **Trauma**
Risk for vascular **Trauma**
Impaired **Urinary** elimination
Readiness for enhanced **Urinary** elimination
Urinary retention
Impaired spontaneous **Ventilation**
Dysfunctional **Ventilatory** weaning response
Risk for other-directed **Violence**
Risk for self-directed **Violence**
Impaired **Walking**
Wandering

Nursing Diagnoses—Definitions and Classification 2009-2011 © 2009, 2007, 2003, 2001, 1998, 1996, 1994 NANDA International. Used by arrangement with Wiley-Blackwell Publishing, a company of John Wiley & Sons, Inc. In order to make safe and effective judgments using NANDA-I nursing diagnoses it is essential that nurses refer to the definitions and defining characteristics of the diagnoses listed in this work.

BOX 8-4 Example of a NANDA International–Approved Nursing Diagnosis With Defining Characteristics and Related Factors

DIAGNOSIS: FATIGUE

DEFINING CHARACTERISTICS

Inability to maintain usual level of physical activity
Inability to maintain usual routines
Lack of energy
Lethargy
Increase in rest requirements

RELATED FACTORS (EXAMPLES)

Psychological: Anxiety, stress, depression
Physiological: Anemia, disease states, malnutrition
Environmental: Humidity, lights, noise
Situational: Negative life events, occupation

Used with permission from NANDA International: *NANDA-I nursing diagnoses: definitions and classification 2009-2011,* Oxford, UK, 2009, Wiley-Blackwell.

such as nutrition and exercise. Health promotion diagnoses can be used in any health state and do not require a patient to have a high level of wellness. This readiness is supported by defining characteristics (NANDA-I, 2009). *Readiness for enhanced comfort* is an example of a health promotion diagnosis.

A risk nursing diagnosis describes human responses to health conditions or life processes that have a chance of developing in a vulnerable individual, family, or community. It is supported by risk factors that contribute to increased vulnerability (NANDA-I, 2009). The key assessment for this type of diagnosis is the data that support the patient's vulnerability or risk. Such data include physiological, psychosocial, familial, lifestyle, and environmental factors that increase the patient's vulnerability to, or likelihood of developing, the condition. For example, with Mrs. Tillman having symptoms of fatigue, Rich would assess further for risk diagnoses such as *risk for falls.*

A syndrome diagnosis is a cluster or group of signs and symptoms that almost always occur together. Together, these clusters represent a distinct clinical picture (NANDA-I, 2009).

A wellness nursing diagnosis describes human responses to levels of wellness in an individual, group, or community. It is supported by defining characteristics (manifestations, signs, and symptoms) that cluster in patterns of related cues and or inferences (NANDA-I, 2009). It is a clinical judgment about an individual, group, or community in transition from a specific level of wellness to a higher level of wellness. You will select this type of diagnosis when a patient wishes to or has achieved an optimal level of health. One example is *readiness for enhanced spiritual well-being.* When this diagnosis applies, your patient is able to experience and integrate meaning and purpose in life. Thus you would introduce the use of art, music, or perhaps literature to help the patient connect with self or a higher being.

COMPONENTS OF A NURSING DIAGNOSIS The identification of a nursing diagnosis flows from the assessment and diagnostic process. Throughout this book, nursing diagnoses are worded in a two-part format: the diagnostic label followed by a statement of a related factor (Table 8-2). It is this two-part form that provides a diagnosis with meaning and relevance for a particular patient.

Diagnostic Label The diagnostic label is the name of the nursing diagnosis within the NANDA-I taxonomy (see Box 8-3, p. 115). It describes the essence of a patient's response to a health condition in as few words as possible. Diagnostic labels include descriptors that give additional meaning to the diagnosis. For example, the diagnosis *impaired physical mobility* includes the descriptor *impaired.* The term *impaired* describes the nature of or change in mobility that best describes the patient's response. Examples of other descriptors are *compromised, decreased, delayed,* or *effective.*

Related Factor The **related factor** is a condition or etiologic factor that appears to show some type of patterned relationship with the nursing diagnosis (NANDA-I, 2009). It comes from the patient's assessment data, and for this reason assessment data need to be accurate. A related factor provides context for the defining characteristics. It is a condition associated with or contributing to the diagnosis. For example, a nursing diagnostic statement applicable to Mrs. Tillman includes the diagnostic label (e.g., *fatigue*) and the related factor (e.g., *the disease process of cancer*). Related factors include four categories: pathophysiological (biological or psychological), treatment-related, situational (environmental or personal), and maturational (Carpenito-Moyet, 2008). The "related to" phrase is not a cause-and-effect statement; rather, it indicates that the etiology contributes to or is associated with the problem (Figure 8-5). The "related to" phrase requires you to use critical thinking skills to individualize the nursing diagnosis and subsequent interventions.

The **etiology** is always within the domain of nursing practice and a condition that responds to nursing interventions. Sometimes nurses record medical diagnoses as the etiologies of nursing diagnoses. This is incorrect. Nursing interventions cannot

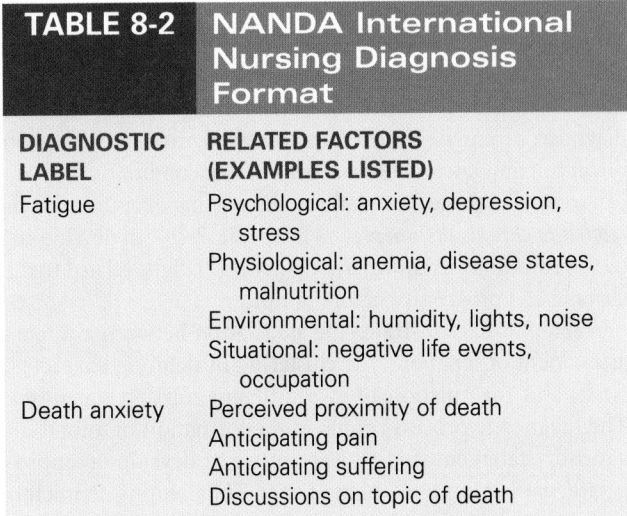

TABLE 8-2	NANDA International Nursing Diagnosis Format
DIAGNOSTIC LABEL	**RELATED FACTORS (EXAMPLES LISTED)**
Fatigue	Psychological: anxiety, depression, stress
	Physiological: anemia, disease states, malnutrition
	Environmental: humidity, lights, noise
	Situational: negative life events, occupation
Death anxiety	Perceived proximity of death
	Anticipating pain
	Anticipating suffering
	Discussions on topic of death

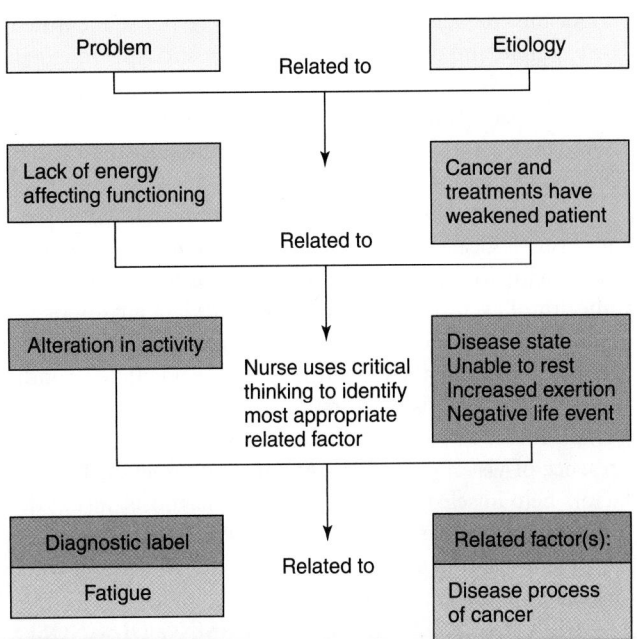

Figure 8-5 ■ Relationship between diagnostic label and etiology (related factor). (Redrawn from Hickey P: *Nursing process handbook,* St. Louis, 1990, Mosby.)

TABLE 8-3   Formulation of Nursing Diagnoses

ASSESSMENT ACTIVITIES	DEFINING CHARACTERISTICS (CLUSTERING CUES)	NURSING DIAGNOSIS	ETIOLOGIES ("RELATED TO")
Ask patient to describe usual physical activity performed during the day	Inability to maintain usual level of physical activity	Fatigue	Disease process of cancer
Observe patient during care activites	Lethargic		
	Drowsy		
Question patient about frequency of rest periods	Increase in rest requirements		
Ask patient to talk about any concerns or worries related to diagnosis of cancer	Reports fear of suffering related to dying	Death anxiety	Anticipating suffering
Have patient describe her emotions	Reports deep sadness		
Ask patient to discuss how she feels her illness will affect her relationship with her husband	Reports worry about the impact of her own death on significant others		

change a medical diagnosis. For example, in the case of Mrs. Tillman, nursing interventions cannot change cancer. Thus the diagnosis of *fatigue related to cancer* is incorrect. Instead, you direct nursing interventions at behavior or conditions that you can treat or manage. For example, the nursing diagnosis *fatigue related to chronic disease process* is correct. Rich can develop interventions that are known to help manage fatigue related to the chronic and progressive nature of cancer.

Table 8-3 demonstrates the association between a nurse's assessment of a patient, the clustering of defining characteristics, and formulation of two different nursing diagnoses. The diagnostic process results in the formation of a total diagnostic statement that allows a nurse to develop an appropriate, patient-centered plan of care. The defining characteristics and relevant etiologies are from NANDA-I (2009).

Definition NANDA-I approves a definition for each diagnosis following clinical use and testing. The definition describes the characteristics of the human response identified. For example, the definition of the diagnostic label *fatigue* is an "overwhelming sustained sense of exhaustion and decreased capacity for physical and mental work at usual level" (NANDA-I, 2009). Always refer to a definition to assist you in identifying a patient's diagnosis.

Risk Factors Risk factors are environmental, physiological, psychological, genetic, or chemical elements that increase the vulnerability of an individual, family, or community to an unhealthful event (NANDA-I, 2009). They are a component of all risk nursing diagnoses. The risk factors are cues to indicate that a risk nursing diagnosis applies to a patient's condition. Examples of risk factors for the nursing diagnosis *risk for falls* include a history of falls, age 65 or over, lives alone, presence of visual limitations, and urinary urgency. The risk factors help in selecting the correct risk diagnosis, just as defining characteristics help in the formulation of actual nursing diagnoses. In addition, risk factors are also useful when you plan nursing interventions.

CULTURAL RELEVANCE OF NURSING DIAGNOSES

When you select nursing diagnoses, always consider your patient's culture. Similarly, consider your own cultural back-

ground. A patient's culture influences the type of health care problems he or she experiences. When making a diagnosis, consider how culture influences the related factor for your diagnostic statement. For example, *impaired verbal communication related to cultural differences* or *noncompliance related to patient's value system* reflect diagnostic conclusions that consider a patient's unique cultural needs.

Wieck (1996) studied how cultural differences among nurses influenced the choice of defining characteristics in making nursing diagnoses. The researchers studied the diagnosis of pain within six different cultural groups of nurses. Generally, the nurses were consistent in selecting defining characteristics. However, when diagnosing pain, some nurses did not select restlessness or grimace as defining characteristics. The nurses were not familiar with these characteristics because people in their culture did not exhibit restlessness or grimace when in pain. Being culturally aware will improve your diagnostic accuracy.

SOURCES OF DIAGNOSTIC ERRORS Errors occur in the diagnostic process during data collection, data interpretation, clustering, and statement of the nursing diagnosis. Apply methodical critical thinking for an accurate nursing diagnostic process.

Errors in Data Collection To avoid errors in data collection, be knowledgeable and skilled in all assessment techniques. Avoid inaccurate or missing data, and collect data in an organized way. The following practice tips are essential to avoid data collection errors:

- Review your level of comfort and competence with interview and physical assessment skills before you begin data collection.
- Approach assessment in steps. Focus on completing a patient interview before starting an examination. Perhaps focus on only one body system to learn how to gather a complete assessment. Then move to a more complex head-to-toe examination.
- Review your clinical assessments in clinical or classroom settings, giving you a constructive learning opportunity

to determine how to revise an assessment or to gather additional information.

- Organize the examination. Properly prepare the patient and environment for the examination (see Chapter 15).

Errors in Interpretation and Analysis   After data collection, review your database to decide if it is accurate and complete. Review data to validate that measurable, objective physical findings support subjective data. For example, when a patient reports "difficulty breathing," you want to also listen to lung sounds and assess respiratory rate and rhythm. When data are not validated, the result is an inaccurate match between clinical cues and the nursing diagnosis. Be careful to consider any conflicting cues or decide if there are insufficient cues to form a diagnosis. Also, it is important to consider a patient's cultural background or developmental stage when you interpret the meaning of cues. For example, a patient from the Middle East may express pain very differently than a patient from an Asian country. Misinterpreting how patients express pain could easily lead to an inaccurate diagnosis.

Errors in Data Clustering   Errors will result when you cluster data prematurely, incorrectly, or not at all. Premature clustering occurs when you make the nursing diagnosis before grouping all data. For example, a patient has urinary incontinence and states he has urgency and nocturia. You cluster the available data and identify *impaired urinary elimination* as a probable nursing diagnosis. Incorrect clustering occurs when you try to make the nursing diagnosis fit the signs and symptoms obtained. In this example, further assessment reveals the patient also has bladder distention and dribbling; thus the correct diagnosis is *urinary retention*. The nursing diagnosis comes from the data, not the other way around. An incorrect nursing diagnosis will affect the quality of nursing care.

Errors in the Diagnostic Statement   The correct selection of a diagnostic statement is more likely to result in the appropriate selection of nursing interventions and outcomes (Dochterman and Jones, 2003). To reduce errors, word the diagnostic statement in appropriate, concise, and precise language. Use correct terminology reflecting the patient's response to the illness or condition. Use of standardized nursing language from NANDA-I ensures accuracy. Follow these guidelines:

1. Be sure the etiology portion of the diagnosis is within the scope of nursing practice.
2. Identify the patient's response, not the medical diagnosis (Carpenito-Moyet, 2008). Because the medical diagnosis requires medical interventions, it is legally inadvisable to include it in the nursing diagnosis. Change the diagnosis *fatigue related to cancer* to *fatigue related to chronic disease process*.
3. Identify a NANDA-I diagnostic statement, not a symptom. Identify nursing diagnoses from a cluster of defining characteristics that apply to a patient; one symptom is insufficient for problem identification. For example, shortness of breath alone does not identify a diagnosis.

In contrast, shortness of breath, pain on inspiration, and productive cough in a postoperative patient form the cluster for *ineffective breathing pattern related to increased airway secretions*.

4. Identify a treatable etiology, not a clinical sign or chronic problem. You will select interventions to correct the etiology of the problem. A diagnostic test or chronic dysfunction is not an etiology that a nursing intervention is able to treat. A patient with cancer often develops anemia, reflected in low red blood cell counts. The diagnosis *fatigue related to low red blood cell counts* is an incorrect diagnostic statement. Fatigue related to the chronic disease process is appropriate, because it allows you to focus interventions on the physical responses common in chronic progressive disease.
5. Identify the problem caused by the treatment or diagnostic study rather than the treatment or study itself. Patients respond to diagnostic tests and medical treatment in many ways. These responses are the area of nursing concern. The patient who has severe chest pain and is scheduled for a cardiac catheterization may have a nursing diagnosis of *anxiety related to lack of knowledge about cardiac catheterization*.
6. Identify the patient response to the equipment rather than the equipment itself. Change the diagnosis *anxiety related to cardiac monitor* to *deficient knowledge regarding the need for cardiac monitoring*.
7. Identify the patient's problems rather than your problems with nursing care. Nursing diagnoses are always patient centered and form the basis for goal-directed care. The statement "potential intravenous complications related to poor vascular access" indicates a nursing problem in initiating intravenous therapy. The diagnosis *risk for infection related to presence of invasive lines* properly centers attention on patient needs.
8. Identify the patient problem rather than the nursing intervention. You will identify nursing interventions later when you plan care to alleviate patient problems. The statement "offer bedpan frequently because of altered elimination patterns" changes to the diagnosis *diarrhea related to food intolerance*. This corrects the misstatement and allows proper implementation of the nursing process.
9. Identify the patient problem rather than the goal. You will set goals during the planning step of the nursing process. Goals serve as a basis to decide if you achieve resolution of a health problem, not to identify the problem. Change the statement "patient needs high-protein diet related to potential alteration in nutrition" to *imbalanced nutrition: less than body requirements related to inadequate protein intake*. This diagnosis would allow you to then plan on the basis of the correct etiology.
10. Make professional rather than prejudicial judgments. Base nursing diagnoses on subjective and objective patient data, and do not include your personal beliefs and values. Remove your judgment from *risk for impaired skin integrity related to poor hygiene habits* by changing

the nursing diagnosis to *risk for impaired skin integrity related to lack of knowledge about perineal care.*

11. Avoid legally inadvisable statements that imply blame, negligence, or malpractice (Carpenito-Moyet, 2008). The diagnosis *chronic pain related to insufficient pain medication* implies that the health care provider gave an inadequate prescription. The correct way to identify the problem is to write *chronic pain related to improper use of medications.*

12. Identify the problem and etiology so as to avoid a circular statement. Such statements are vague and give no direction to nursing care. Change the diagnosis *acute pain related to alteration in comfort* to the specific patient problem and cause: *acute pain related to incisional trauma.*

13. Identify only one patient problem in a diagnostic statement. Every problem has different specific expected outcomes. Confusion during the planning step occurs when you include multiple problems in a nursing diagnosis. It is, however, permissible to include multiple etiologies contributing to one patient problem. Restate *pain and anxiety related to difficulty in ambulating* as two nursing diagnoses, such as *impaired physical mobility related to pain in right knee* and *anxiety related to fear of fall.*

DOCUMENTATION After identifying a patient's nursing diagnoses, list them on the plan of care, whether this is in the form of computerized care plans or a problem list on a nursing Kardex (see Chapter 9). In a clinical facility, list nursing diagnoses chronologically as you identify them. When initiating an original care plan, always place the highest priority nursing diagnoses first. Then add additional nursing diagnoses to the list. Date a nursing diagnosis at the time of entry. When caring for a patient, always review the list and identify those nursing diagnoses with the greatest priority regardless of chronological order.

PLANNING

After you identify a patient's nursing diagnoses and collaborative problems, you begin the planning step of the nursing process. **Planning** involves setting priorities, identifying patient-centered goals and expected outcomes, and prescribing nursing interventions. Perhaps the most important principle to learn about planning is the individualization of a plan of care for each patient's unique needs. The nursing diagnoses and problems you identify direct your selection of nursing interventions and the goals and outcomes you hope to achieve.

Establishing Priorities

A single patient often has multiple diagnoses and collaborative problems. Eventually you will care for groups of patients. Being able to carefully and wisely set priorities for a single patient or group of patients ensures the most timely and ef-

fective care. Priority setting is the ordering of nursing diagnoses or patient problems using notions of urgency and importance to establish a preferential order for nursing actions. In other words, as you care for patients, there are aspects of care that you need to deal with before others. By ranking nursing diagnoses in order of importance, you attend to your patient's most important needs and better organize ongoing care activities. Priorities help you to anticipate and sequence nursing interventions when a patient has multiple problems. Together with your patients, you will select mutually agreed-on priorities based on the urgency of the problem, the patient's safety and desires, the nature of the treatment indicated, and the relationship among the diagnoses. Establishing priorities is not just a matter of numbering the nursing diagnosis on the basis of severity or physiological importance.

In regard to importance, classify priorities as high, intermediate, or low. Nursing diagnoses that, if untreated, result in harm to the patient or others have the highest priority. One way to consider diagnoses of high priority is to consider Maslow's hierarchy of needs. For example, you will want to attend to a patient's oxygen, fluid, and nutrition needs before you focus on shelter or sexual needs. However, it is always important to consider each patient's unique case. High priorities are sometimes both psychological and physiological. Avoid classifying only physiological nursing diagnoses as high priority. Consider Mrs. Tillman's case study. The nursing diagnosis of *death anxiety* is a high-priority diagnosis because it has the potential for impacting Mrs. Tillman's ability to become a participant in her own care and to maintain a healthy relationship with her husband.

Intermediate-priority nursing diagnoses involve the non-emergent, non–life-threatening needs of a patient. In Mrs. Tillman's case, *fatigue* is an intermediate diagnosis. Mrs. Tillman's activity problem is linked with the progressive nature of her cancer and will be an ongoing challenge. Energy conservation and management therapies are important but not a life-threatening issue.

Low-priority nursing diagnoses are patient needs that are usually directly related to a specific illness or prognosis but may affect the patient's future well-being. Mrs. Tillman's nurse, Rich, knows that as her disease progresses, Mrs. Tillman will have more health care needs. Her husband may assume even more responsibility for in-home care. *Deficient knowledge regarding palliative care related to inexperience* is a relevant diagnosis, but of lower priority at this time compared with the other diagnoses. Rich will plan in future clinic visits when to begin discussion about palliative care with the Tillman family.

The order of priorities changes as a patient's condition changes. Each time you begin a sequence of care such as the beginning of a hospital shift or during a clinic visit, it is important to reorder priorities. Ongoing patient assessment is needed to determine the status of the patient's nursing diagnoses. The proper order of priorities ensures that you meet patients' needs in a timely and effective way.

Priority setting also involves prioritizing specific interventions that you plan to use for a patient. For example, as Rich considers the high-priority diagnosis of *death anxiety,* he will decide whether to complete individual counseling with Mrs. Tillman first or conduct a care conference with the patient, her husband, and the clinic nurse practitioner. Rich needs to prioritize interventions so as to be most effective in meeting desired goals and outcomes. It is always important to involve the patient in priority setting. In some situations you and the patient will assign different priority rankings to nursing diagnoses and collaborative problems. If you each place a different value on health care needs and treatments, resolve these differences through open communication. However, when the patient's physiological and emotional needs are at stake, you need to assume primary responsibility for setting priorities.

Critical Thinking in Setting Goals and Expected Outcomes

Once you identify a nursing diagnosis for a patient, ask yourself, What is the best approach to address and resolve the problem? What do you plan to achieve? Goals and expected outcomes are specific statements of patient behavior or physiological responses that you set to resolve a nursing diagnosis or collaborative problem. Goals and expected outcomes serve two purposes: to provide clear direction for the selection and use of nursing interventions and to provide focus for evaluating the effectiveness of the interventions.

GOALS OF CARE A goal is a broad statement that describes a desired change in a patient's condition or behavior. In the case of Mrs. Tillman, who has a diagnosis of *fatigue related to chronic disease process,* a goal of care would be "Patient achieves improved energy level within 2 weeks." A patient-centered **goal** is a specific and measurable behavior or response that reflects the patient's highest possible level of wellness and independence in function. A goal is realistic and based on patient needs and resources. A patient goal represents predicted resolution of a problem, evidence of progress toward problem resolution, progress toward improved health status, or continued maintenance of good health or function (Carpenito-Moyet, 2008). A goal contains singular behaviors or responses. A goal written as "Patient will follow an exercise plan and understand exercise benefits" is incorrect because the statement includes two different patient behaviors, follow and understand. Instead, word the goal as "Patient will understand exercise benefits." The outcome statements are the specific criteria for measuring success of the goal. For example, "Patient will describe three benefits from progressive exercise."

Each goal is time limited so that the health care team has a common time frame for problem resolution. The time frame depends on the nature of the problem, etiology, overall condition of the patient, and treatment setting. A *short-term goal* is an objective behavior or response that you expect the patient to achieve in a short time, usually less than a week. In an acute care setting, you may set goals for over a course of just a few hours. For example, "Patient will maintain a balanced fluid status within the next 12 hours." A *long-term goal* is an objective behavior or response that you expect the patient to achieve over a longer period, usually over several days, weeks, or months. Goal setting establishes the framework for the nursing care plan. Table 8-4 shows the progression from nursing diagnoses to goals and expected outcomes, which you individualize to meet patient needs.

Goals are often based on standards of care or clinical guidelines established for minimal safe practice. For example, the Infusion Nurses Society (INS) has standards of care for prevention of the intravenous (IV) complication of phlebitis. When a nurse cares for a patient with a peripheral IV catheter, the goal "The IV site will remain free of phlebitis" is established on the basis of sound nursing practice standards.

ROLE OF THE PATIENT IN GOAL SETTING Always partner with your patients when setting goals. Mutual goal setting involves the patient and family (when appropriate) in prioritizing the goals of care and in developing a plan of action to achieve those goals. Unless goals are mutually set and there is a clear plan of action, patients will fail to participate in the plan of care. Patients need to understand and see the value of nursing therapies, even though they are oftentimes totally dependent on you as the nurse. When developing goals, you act as an advocate or supporter for the patient to develop nursing interventions that promote the patient's return to health or prevent further deterioration when possible.

EXPECTED OUTCOMES In order for Rich to evaluate if Mrs. Tillman progresses and achieves the goal of an improved energy level within 2 weeks, expected outcomes are necessary. **Expected outcomes** are observable effects (e.g., change in patient's physical condition or behavior) that are the result of an intervention. In Mrs. Tillman's case, a measurable outcome for the goal of improved energy level would include

TABLE 8-4 Examples of Goal Setting With Expected Outcomes for Mrs. Tillman

NURSING DIAGNOSES	GOALS	EXPECTED OUTCOMES
Fatigue related to chronic disease process	Mrs. Tillman achieves an improved energy level within 2 weeks.	Patient's self-report of fatigue will be 3 or less on a scale of 0 to 10 in 2 weeks. Patient is able to perform some household chores in 1 week.
Death anxiety related to anticipation of suffering	Mrs. Tillman will express belief that she will achieve a comfortable death in 3 weeks.	Patient seeks information about palliative care treatment in 1 week. Patient reports acceptable comfort level in 2 weeks. Patient participates in health care decisions in 1 week.

TABLE 8-5	Examples of NANDA International Nursing Diagnoses and Suggested NOC Linkages	
NURSING DIAGNOSIS	**SUGGESTED NOC OUTCOMES (EXAMPLES)**	**OUTCOME INDICATORS (EXAMPLES)**
Fatigue	Activity tolerance	Walking pace
		Ease of performing activities of daily living
		Pulse rate with activity
		Ease of breathing with activity
	Energy conservation	Balances activity and rest
		Uses naps to restore energy
		Adapts lifestyle to energy level
Deficient knowledge regarding palliative care	Knowledge of treatment regimen	Rationale for treatment
		Self-care responsibilities for ongoing treatment
		Expected effects of treatment

NOC, Nursing Outcomes Classification.

"Patient's self-report of fatigue will be 3 or less on a scale of 0 to 10" and "Patient will be able to complete bathing without taking rest periods." The outcomes will gauge Rich's success in selecting interventions that effectively lessen Mrs. Tillman's fatigue. An outcome includes measurable criteria (e.g., 3 or less on a scale of 0 to 10, completes bathing without taking rest) to evaluate goal achievement (Table 8-5). Achieving outcomes means a goal has been met. Expected outcomes provide a focus or direction for nursing care because they are the desired physical, psychological, social, emotional, developmental, or spiritual responses that show resolution of a patient's health problems.

Typically all health care providers contribute to affecting patient outcomes. A **nursing-sensitive outcome** is a measurable patient or family state, behavior, or perception largely influenced by and sensitive to nursing interventions (Moorhead, Johnson, and Maas, 2008). Examples of nursing-sensitive outcomes include reduction in pain severity, incidence of pressure ulcers, and incidence of falls. In comparison, outcomes largely influenced by medical interventions include patient mortality and hospital readmission.

Outcomes should be measurable, reliable, valid, suited to the patient, and sensitive to change (Melnyk and Fineout-Overholt, 2005). Consider the example of Mrs. Tillman's problem of fatigue. An outcome measure is a self-report fatigue scale. The scale provides a measurable way to objectively assess the patient's level of fatigue. Self-report scales have been shown to be reliable (consistently measures the outcome) and valid (accuracy of a measure). A self-report scale is easy for a patient to complete without causing anxiety or physical distress as in the case of an exercise test. The patient's perceptions of fatigue can change over time and be reflected by differences in the fatigue scale.

You will normally develop several expected outcomes for each nursing diagnosis and goal. The reason for multiple outcomes is that sometimes one nursing action is not enough to resolve a patient problem. The listing of the step-by-step expected outcomes gives you practical guidance in planning interventions. Always write expected outcomes sequentially with time frames. Time frames give you progressive steps in which to move a patient toward recovery. They also give an order for when to perform nursing interventions. In addition, time frames set limits for problem resolution.

Nursing Outcomes Classification   There is much attention in the current health care environment to measuring outcomes sensitive to nursing interventions. The Iowa Intervention Project has published the *Nursing Outcomes Classification (NOC)* and has linked the outcomes to NANDA-I nursing diagnoses (Moorhead and others, 2008). For any given NANDA-I nursing diagnosis there are multiple NOC-suggested outcomes. These outcomes have labels for describing the focus of nursing care and then include indicators for use in measuring success with interventions (see Table 8-5). The NOC contains outcomes for individuals, family caregivers, the family, and the community for all types of health care settings. Outcome measurement captures the changes in the status of patients over time and allows nurses to improve patient care quality and to add to nursing knowledge (Moorhead and others, 2008). The use of a common set of outcomes allows nurses to study the effects of nursing interventions over time and across settings. The 2008 edition of NOC includes 385 outcomes with definitions, indicators, and measurement scales. Use of NOC outcomes in planning care for patients provides a common nursing language for all nurses to use in measuring the success of their interventions. The NOC system is a classification system of nursing-sensitive outcomes. One of the purposes of NOC is to identify, label, validate, and classify nursing-sensitive patient outcomes (Moorhead and others, 2008).

COMBINING GOALS AND OUTCOME STATEMENTS
Many schools of nursing use a format for stating goals and outcomes as one statement. Staff in health care agencies often refer to the terms *goals* and *outcomes* interchangeably. This is acceptable as long as the criteria for writing goals and outcomes are met. The statement "Patient will experience an improved energy level as evidenced by a self-report of fatigue at 3 or less on a scale of 0 to 10 within 2 weeks" is acceptable. The goal portion of the statement broadly describes the desired

patient status (improved energy level), and the outcome portion contains an observable criterion (3 on a scale of 0 to 10) to measure success. The documentation format used by health care agencies guides how nurses write goals and outcomes.

GUIDELINES FOR WRITING GOALS AND EXPECTED OUTCOMES Follow these seven guidelines when writing goals and expected outcomes.

Patient centered: Outcomes and goals reflect the patient behaviors or responses expected as a result of nursing interventions. Write the goal to reflect this, not to reflect your goals or interventions. A correct outcome statement is "Patient will ambulate in the hall 3 times a day." A common error is to write "Ambulate patient in the hall 3 times a day."

Singular goal or outcome: To ensure precise evaluation of care, each goal and outcome addresses only one behavior or response. If an outcome reads "Patient's lungs will be clear to auscultation and respiratory rate will be 22 breaths per minute by 8/22," consider the outcome when you evaluate that the lungs are clear but the respiratory rate is 28 breaths per minute. It will be difficult to determine whether the expected outcome has been achieved. By splitting the statement into two parts, "Lungs will be clear to auscultation by 8/22" and "Respiratory rate will be 22 breaths per minute by 8/22," you determine specifically if the patient achieves each outcome. Singularity allows you to decide if there is a need to modify the plan of care.

Observable: You must be able to observe if change takes place in a patient's status. Observable changes occur in physiological findings and the patient's knowledge, perceptions, and behaviors. For example, you observe the goal "Patient achieves improved activity tolerance" through the outcome of "Patient's heart rate remains within 10% of baseline following exercise." The outcome statement "Patient will appear less short of breath" is not a correct statement because there is no specific observable behavior for "will appear less short of breath."

Measurable: You will learn to write goals and expected outcomes that set standards against which to measure the patient's response to nursing care. Examples such as "Body temperature will remain 98.6° F" and "Apical pulse will remain between 60 and 100 beats per minute" allow you to objectively measure changes in the patient's status. Do not use vague qualifiers such as "normal," "acceptable," "stable," or "sufficient" in the expected outcome statement. Vague terms result in guesswork in determining a patient's response to care. Terms describing quality, quantity, frequency, length, or weight allow you to accurately evaluate if outcomes are met.

Time limited: The time frame for each goal and expected outcome indicates when you expect the response to occur. Time frames assist you and the patient in determining if progress is being made at a reasonable rate. If not, revision of the plan of care will be necessary. Time frames also promote accountability in the delivery and management of nursing care.

Mutual factors: Mutually set goals and expected outcomes ensure that the patient and nurse agree on the direction and time limits of care. Mutual goal setting increases the patient's motivation and cooperation. As a patient advocate, you will apply standards of practice, patient safety, and basic human needs when assisting patients with setting goals.

Realistic: Set goals and expected outcomes that the patient is able to reach. Achievable goals give patients a sense of accomplishment. In turn, this sense of accomplishment further increases the patient's motivation and cooperation. When establishing realistic goals, be sure to know the resources of the health care facility, family, and patient. For example, will a patient's cultural beliefs affect the goal you set? Does the patient have the necessary resources in the home to successfully meet goals?

Critical Thinking in Planning Nursing Care

Nursing interventions are treatments, based upon clinical judgment and knowledge, that nurses perform to enhance patient outcomes (Bulechek, Butcher, and Dochterman, 2008). During planning you make clinical decisions by choosing the interventions most appropriate to your patient's nursing diagnoses and collaborative problems. The actual implementation of these interventions occurs during the implementation phase of the nursing process. Choosing suitable nursing interventions involves critical thinking applied in decision making. To select interventions you need to be competent in three areas: (1) knowing the **scientific rationale,** or reason, for the interventions; (2) possessing the necessary psychomotor and interpersonal skills to perform the interventions; and (3) being able to function within a particular setting to use the available health care resources effectively (Bulechek and others, 2008).

TYPES OF INTERVENTIONS There are three categories of nursing interventions: nurse-initiated, physician-initiated, and collaborative interventions. Nurse-initiated interventions are the **independent nursing interventions** that nurses initiate on their own to act on a patient's behalf. These do not require direction or an order from another health care professional. Examples include elevating an edematous extremity, offering counseling on coping, and instructing patients about medication side effects. Independent nursing interventions are autonomous actions based on scientific rationale. These interventions benefit the patient in a predicted way related to nursing diagnoses and patient goals (Bulechek and others, 2008). Independent interventions require no supervision or direction from others. Each state within the United States has developed Nurse Practice Acts that define the legal scope of nursing practice (see Chapter 4). According to State Nurse Practice Acts, independent nursing interventions pertain to ADLs, health education and promotion, and counseling.

Physician-initiated interventions are **dependent nursing interventions** or actions that require an order from a physician or another health care professional. Such interventions are based on the health care provider's response to treat or manage a medical diagnosis. Nurse practitioners working in collaborative

BOX 8-5   Selecting Nursing Interventions

CHARACTERISTICS OF THE NURSING DIAGNOSIS

- Interventions should alter the etiological (related to) factor associated with the diagnostic label.
- When an etiological factor cannot change, direct interventions toward treating the signs and symptoms (e.g., NANDA-I defining characteristics).
- For potential or high-risk diagnoses, direct interventions at altering or eliminating risk factors for the nursing diagnoses.

EXPECTED OUTCOMES

- Specify expected outcomes before choosing interventions.
- Identify for each patient the outcomes that can be reasonably expected and attained as the result of nursing care.
- Use the Nursing Outcomes Classification to specify outcomes.

EVIDENCE BASE

- Know the research base for an intervention.
- Research will indicate the effectiveness of using an intervention with certain types of patients.
- When research is not available, use scientific principles (e.g., safety) or consult experts.

FEASIBILITY OF THE INTERVENTION

- A specific intervention has the potential for interacting with other interventions.
- Consider cost: Is the intervention clinically effective and cost efficient?
- Consider time: Are time and personnel resources available?

ACCEPTABILITY TO THE PATIENT

- An intervention must be acceptable to the patient and family and match a patient's goals, health care values, and culture.
- Promote informed choice; help a patient know how he or she is expected to participate.

CAPABILITY

- Be prepared to carry out the intervention.
- Be competent in knowing the scientific rationale for the intervention, possessing necessary psychomotor and interpersonal skills and being able to function in the particular setting.

Modified from Bulechek GM, Butcher HK, Dochterman JM: *Nursing interventions classification (NIC)*, ed 5, St. Louis, 2008, Mosby.

agreements with physicians or who are licensed independently by state practice acts also write such interventions. As a nurse, you intervene by carrying out the independent provider's written and/or verbal orders. Administering a medication, implementing an invasive procedure, and preparing a patient for diagnostic tests are examples of such interventions.

Each dependent nursing intervention involves specific nursing responsibilities and technical nursing knowledge. For example, when administering medications, you are responsible for knowing the classification of the drug, its physiological action, normal dosage, side effects, and nursing interventions related to its action or side effects (see Chapter 16). When a physician orders diagnostic testing, you are responsible for scheduling the test, preparing the patient, and knowing the normal findings and associated nursing implications.

Collaborative interventions, or interdependent nursing interventions, are therapies that require the combined knowledge, skill, and expertise of multiple health care professionals. Typically when you plan care for a patient, you will review the necessary interventions and determine if collaboration from other health care professionals is necessary. For example, in the case study, Rich decides to have an interdisciplinary health care team conference to discuss a palliative care plan for Mrs. Tillman. Interdisciplinary conferences bring professionals from all disciplines involved in the patient's care to the table so that together they can establish and execute the most appropriate plan of care.

SELECTION OF INTERVENTIONS Never select interventions for a patient randomly. Patients with the diagnosis of

anxiety, for example, do not always need care in the same way with the same interventions. You treat *anxiety* related to the uncertainty of results from a diagnostic test differently from *anxiety* related to a threat to loss of a loved one. When choosing interventions, consider six factors: (1) characteristics of the nursing diagnosis, (2) expected outcomes and goals, (3) evidence base (research or clinical practice guidelines) for the intervention, (4) feasibility of the intervention, (5) acceptability to the patient, and (6) your own competency (Bulechek and others, 2008) (Box 8-5). Review resources such as evidence in the literature, standard protocols or guidelines, the Nursing Interventions Classification (NIC), critical pathways, and current textbooks when choosing interventions. Collaboration with other health care professionals is also useful. As you select interventions, review your patient's needs, values, priorities, and previous experiences to select those nursing interventions that have the best potential for achieving the expected outcomes.

Nursing Interventions Classification   The Iowa Intervention Project developed a set of nursing interventions that provides a level of standardization to enhance communication of nursing care across all health care settings and to compare outcomes (Bulechek and others, 2008; Iowa Intervention Project, 1993). The NIC model includes three levels: 7 domains, 30 classes, and 542 interventions for ease of use. The domains (Level 1) are the highest level, using broad terms (e.g., safety and basic physiological) to organize the more specific classes and interventions (Table 8-6). The second level of the model includes 30 classes, which offer useful clinical categories to refer to when selecting interventions

TABLE 8-6   Nursing Interventions Classification (NIC) Taxonomy

DOMAIN 1
LEVEL 1 DOMAINS
1. Physiological: Basic
Care that supports physical functioning

Level 2 Classes

A *Activity and Exercise Management:* Interventions to organize or assist with physical activity and energy conservation and expenditure

B *Elimination Management:* Interventions to establish and maintain regular bowel and urinary elimination patterns and manage complications due to altered patterns

C *Immobility Management:* Interventions to manage restricted body movement and the sequelae

D *Nutrition Support:* Interventions to modify or maintain nutritional status

E *Physical Comfort Promotion:* Interventions to promote comfort using physical techniques

F *Self-Care Facilitation:* Interventions to provide or assist with routine activities of daily living

G *Electrolyte and Acid-Base Management:* Interventions to regulate electrolyte/acid-base balance and prevent complications

DOMAIN 2
2. Physiological: Complex
Care that supports homeostatic regulation

H *Drug Management:* Interventions to facilitate desired effects of pharmacological agents

I *Neurologic Management:* Interventions to optimize neurologic functions

J *Perioperative Care:* Interventions to provide care before, during, and immediately after surgery

K *Respiratory Management:* Interventions to promote airway patency and gas exchange

L *Skin/Wound Management:* Interventions to maintain or restore tissue integrity

M *Thermoregulation:* Interventions to maintain body temperature within a normal range

N *Tissue Perfusion Management:* Interventions to optimize circulation of blood and fluids to the tissue

DOMAIN 3
3. Behavioral
Care that supports psychosocial functioning and facilitates life-style changes

O *Behavior Therapy:* Interventions to reinforce or promote desirable behaviors or alter undesirable behaviors

P *Cognitive Therapy:* Interventions to reinforce or promote desirable cognitive functioning or alter undesirable cognitive functioning

Q *Communication Enhancement:* Interventions to facilitate delivering and receiving verbal and nonverbal messages

R *Coping Assistance:* Interventions to assist another to build on own strengths, to adapt to a change in function, or to achieve a higher level of function

S *Patient Education:* Interventions to facilitate learning

T *Psychological Comfort Promotion:* Interventions to promote comfort using psychological techniques

DOMAIN 4
4. Safety
Care that supports protection against harm

U *Crisis Management:* Interventions to provide immediate short-term help in both psychological and physiological crises

V *Risk Management:* Interventions to initiate risk-reduction activities and continue monitoring risks over time

DOMAIN 5
5. Family
Care that supports the family unit

W *Childbearing Care:* Interventions to assist in understanding and coping with the psychological and physiological changes during the childbearing period

Z *Childrearing Care:* Interventions to assist in rearing children

X *Lifespan Care:* Interventions to facilitate family unit functioning and promote the health and welfare of family members throughout the lifespan

DOMAIN 6
6. Health System
Care that supports effective use of the health care delivery system

Y *Health System Mediation:* Interventions to facilitate the interface between patient/family and the health care system

a *Health System Management:* Interventions to provide and enhance support services for the delivery of care

b *Information Management:* Interventions to facilitate communication among health care providers

DOMAIN 7
7. Community
Care that supports the health of the community

c *Community Health Promotion:* Interventions that promote the health of the whole community

d *Community Risk Management:* Interventions that assist in detecting or preventing health risks to the whole community

From Bulechek GM, Butcher HK, Dochterman JM: *Nursing interventions classification (NIC),* ed 5, St. Louis, 2008, Mosby.

(Box 8-6). Each intervention then has a variety of nursing activities from which to choose (Box 8-7). The NIC interventions link with NANDA-I nursing diagnoses. For example, Mrs. Tillman has the problem of *fatigue,* which falls under the domain of Physiologic: Basic, and the class of activity and exercise management. Under the class of activity and exercise management, there are a variety of interventions from which to choose (e.g., energy management, exercise therapy: ambulation). When you then refer to an intervention within NIC, such as energy management, there are numerous nursing activities or interventions to choose from (see Mrs. Tillman's care plan). NIC is a valuable resource for you to select interventions for your unique patients.

Systems for Planning Nursing Care

In any health care setting, a nurse is responsible for providing a plan of nursing care for each patient. The plan of care sometimes takes several forms (e.g., nursing Kardex, standardized care plans, and computerized plans). More hospitals today are

adopting electronic health records (EHRs) and a documentation system that includes software programs for nursing care plans (Moody and others, 2004). Generally a nursing care plan includes nursing diagnoses, goals and/or expected outcomes, and specific nursing interventions so that any nurse is able to quickly identify a patient's needs and situation. Electronic care plans often follow a standardized format, but you can individualize each plan to a unique patient's needs. In hospitals and community-based settings, patients receive care from more than one nurse, physician, or allied health professional. Thus there are more institutions that are developing **interdisciplinary care plans**. An interdisciplinary care plan includes contributions from all disciplines involved in patient care. It improves the coordination of all patient therapies.

A nursing care plan reduces the risk for incomplete, incorrect, or inaccurate care. The plan is a guideline for coordinating nursing care, promoting continuity of care, and listing outcome criteria for the evaluation of care. The care plan communicates nursing care priorities to other health care professionals and identifies and coordinates resources for delivering nursing care. For example, a plan might list the specific equipment and supplies necessary for nursing treatments (e.g., dressing change).

The nursing care plan enhances the continuity of nursing care by listing specific nursing actions necessary to achieve the goals of care. Nurses who care for the patient will carry out the interventions throughout a given shift of care during a patient's length of stay. A correctly formulated nursing care plan makes it easy to continue care from one nurse to another. Care plans organize information exchanged by nurses in change-of-shift reports (see Chapter 9). You will learn to focus your reports on the nursing care and treatments and expected outcomes documented in your care plans. At the end of a shift, you will discuss the care plan and the patient's overall progress with the next caregiver. Thus all nurses are able to discuss current and relevant information about the patient's plan of care.

The care plan includes the patient's long-term needs. Incorporating the goals of the care plan into discharge planning is important. This is especially true for a patient undergoing long-term rehabilitation in the community who will require ongoing home care. Same-day surgeries and earlier discharges from hospitals require you as the nurse to begin planning discharge needs from the moment the patient enters a health care agency. The adaptation of the care plan enhances the continuity of nursing care between nurses working in hospital settings and those working in community agencies. Figure 8-6 provides

---

BOX 8-6   Examples of Level 3 Interventions for Activity and Exercise Management

A. ACTIVITY AND EXERCISE MANAGEMENT
Interventions to organize or assist with physical activity and energy conservation and expenditure.

Level 3 Interventions
Body Mechanics Promotion
Energy Management
Exercise Promotion
Exercise Promotion: Strength Training
Exercise Therapy: Ambulation
Exercise Therapy: Balance
Teaching Prescribed Activity/Exercise

Examples of Linked Nursing Diagnoses:
Activity Intolerance
Fatigue
Mobility, Impaired Physical

From Bulechek GM, Butcher HK, Dochterman JM: *Nursing interventions classification (NIC),* ed 5, St. Louis, 2008, Mosby.

BOX 8-7   Examples of Nursing Activities for Level 3 Interventions

LEVEL 3 INTERVENTION—BODY MECHANICS PROMOTION
Instruct to use a firm mattress
Assist to demonstrate appropriate sleeping positions
Assist to avoid sitting in the same position for prolonged periods
Assist patient to identify appropriate posture exercises

LEVEL 3 INTERVENTION—EXERCISE THERAPY: JOINT MOBILITY
Initiate pain control measures before beginning joint exercise
Encourage active range-of-motion (ROM) exercises, according to regular planned schedule
Encourage patient to visualize body motion before beginning movement
Encourage ambulation, if appropriate

From Bulechek GM, Butcher HK, Dochterman JM: *Nursing interventions classification (NIC),* ed 5, St. Louis, 2008, Mosby.

CARE PLAN   Death Anxiety

 ASSESSMENT

Rich learns in his initial discussions with Mrs. Tillman that she feels a sense of dread and uncertainty about the course of cancer. Mrs. Tillman shares her emotions through crying and sadness in the way she looks down and has difficulty talking about her condition. She has admitted to Rich that her greatest fear is not knowing if she might suffer from her disease. Rich knows from his review of pathophysiology the probable course of the patient's disease and the type of palliative care treatments her physician will recommend. He decides to assess further the extent of her death anxiety.

ASSESSMENT ACTIVITIES	FINDINGS/DEFINING CHARACTERISTICS*
Ask Mrs. Tillman to discuss her concerns about the effect her illness will have on her husband.	Patient is **concerned that husband will work too hard** and begin to have more physical problems.
Have Mrs. Tillman explain what she fears most about having a terminal illness.	Patient states that she **worries** she will have **difficulty getting her breath for a prolonged time.**
Question Mrs. Tillman about her desire to be able to make decisions regarding palliative care.	Patient expresses **concern about having little control** over what will happen.

NURSING DIAGNOSIS: Death anxiety related to anticipation of suffering.

PLANNING

GOAL	EXPECTED OUTCOMES (NOC)†
	Anxiety Level
Mrs. Tillman expresses belief that she will achieve a comfortable death within 3 weeks.	• Patient will verbalize feeling less anxious about the course of her disease in 1 week.
	• Patient uses relaxation techniques when anxiety heightens by 2 weeks.
	Participation in Health Care Decisions
	• Patient is able to specify her priorities in palliative care plan in 2 weeks.
	• Patient and husband establish end-of-life care plan in 3 weeks.

INTERVENTIONS (NIC)‡	RATIONALE
Anxiety Reduction	
• Plan a palliative care conference with patient, husband, and health care team and provide factual information on treatment options and availability of respite care for husband.	Information that helps patients understand their condition, disease course, and the benefits and burdens of treatment options, preserves their autonomy and lessens uncertainty (Weiner and Roth, 2006).
• Instruct patient in guided imagery and passive relaxation exercises.	Patients with advanced disease such as cancer require a moderate expenditure of energy to perform active progressive relaxation exercise. This can increase a person's existing fatigue. Passive relaxation and guided imagery are more appropriate options (Kilkus, 2008).
• Explain specifically how palliative care measures will reduce symptoms patient is most anxious about.	You can lessen anxiety in patients with a terminal illness by addressing the underlying cause of the anxiety (Whitecar, Maxwell, and Douglas, 2004).

*Defining characteristics** are shown in **bold** type.
†Outcomes classification labels from Moorhead S, and others, editors: *Nursing outcomes classification (NOC)*, ed 4, St. Louis, 2008, Mosby.
‡Intervention classification labels from Bulechek GM and others, editors: *Nursing interventions classification (NIC)*, ed 5, St. Louis, 2008.

Figure 8-6 ■ Care plan for Mrs. Tillman.

Continued

CARE PLAN   Death Anxiety—cont'd

INTERVENTIONS (NIC)‡

Decision-Making Support

- Provide information requested by patient, and help to identify advantages and disadvantages of all alternatives.

- Facilitate a discussion between patient and husband about end-of-life treatment preferences regarding life-extending treatment.

RATIONALE

Respect for a patient's autonomy involves a commitment to support a patient's ability to make decisions in a well-informed way.

Difficult end-of-life decisions complicate the survivor's grief and create family divisions. When these decisions are handled well, participants experience a meaningful conclusion to the loved one's death (Doka, 2005).

EVALUATION

NURSING ACTIONS	PATIENT RESPONSE/FINDING	ACHIEVMENT OF OUTCOME
• Question Mrs. Tillman about level of anxiety she feels.	Patient states she feels less worried about suffering. "I know what I'm facing, and I know what they can give me when I have trouble breathing."	Patient obtaining control over anxiety, accepting course of her disease.
• Ask Mr. Tillman if Mrs. Tillman practices guided imagery at home.	Husband reports patient uses guided imagery each afternoon for a period of 20 minutes.	Patient is applying anxiety control technique effectively in the home.
• Have Mrs. Tillman discuss her feelings about an end-of-life care plan.	Patient is planning to discuss feelings with husband. Has not finalized plan yet. Wants to know more about respite care for husband.	Further discussion and support necessary to help patient and husband finalize an end-of-life care plan.

Figure 8-6 ■ cont'd.

an example of the care plan format used throughout this text.

STUDENT CARE PLANS Student care plans are useful for learning the problem-solving technique, the nursing process, skills of written communication, and organizational skills needed for nursing care. Most important, a student care plan helps you apply knowledge gained from the nursing and medical literature and the classroom to a practice situation. Students typically write care plans for each nursing diagnosis, using a columnar format that includes assessment findings, goals, expected outcomes, nursing interventions with supporting rationales, and evaluative outcome criteria. The student care plan is more elaborate than a care plan in a hospital or community health care agency because its purpose is to teach the process of planning care. Each nursing school uses a different format for student care plans. Some schools model the student care plan on what their related health care agencies use.

CONCEPT MAPPING When you care for patients, it is a challenge to think about all of their needs and problems. This is especially true because of a nurse's holistic view of patients. Few patients have only a single nursing diagnosis. Usually you will care for patients with multiple nursing diagnoses. Then, when you care for multiple patients, it becomes even more challenging to prioritize and focus on all patients' diagnoses. There is a learning approach, concept mapping, that helps you organize and link data about a patient's multiple diagnoses in a logical way. Concept mapping is a way to graphically represent the connections between concepts (e.g., nursing diagnoses) that relate to a central subject (e.g., a patient's health problems). It is a method that encourages nursing students to think critically, organize information, understand complex relationships between nursing diagnoses and nursing interventions, and integrate theoretical knowledge into practice (Harpaz, Balik, and Ehrenfeld, 2004). A concept map forms a picture of each patient's diagnoses and the interconnections between the assessment data and nursing interventions associated with the patient problems. The use of concept maps is a way for students to synthesize clinical experiences and prepare for preclinical and postclinical conferences (Hill, 2006).

Concept mapping is a way to develop reflective thinking skills (Box 8-8). If you consider what happens in the context of patient care, patient information, nursing diagnoses, interdisciplinary interventions, and patient outcomes are all interrelated and ordered to produce a plan of care (Ferrario, 2004). A **concept map** provides a visual representation of the complex

Critical Thinking in Use of Concept Maps

SUMMARY OF EVIDENCE

Concept maps are a strategy for facilitating critical thinking. A concept map has the potential to promote the development of self-appraisal and individual thinking processes. However, research has been limited in being able to show a relationship between concept mapping and critical thinking competencies. Students in their second year of baccalaureate studies developed concept map care plans for patients assigned during their clinical rotations. Faculty scored all concept maps using an evaluation tool based on six critical thinking competencies: interpretation, analysis, evaluation, inference, explanation, and self-regulation. In addition, a group of the students also participated in a focus session to discuss the experience of developing and using concept maps in the clinical setting. The students' concept maps were scored, showing evidence of critical thinking. The students accurately interpreted and analyzed patient information, identified relevant patient problems, and made accurate conclusions. Students expressed that developing concept maps helped them look at the whole picture and to identify links and multiple concerns affecting patients.

APPLICATION TO NURSING PRACTICE
- The use of concept maps improves students' preparedness for their clinical experience.
- Repeated practice and discussion with faculty facilitates the level of critical thinking in concept maps.
- Use of concept maps fosters a holistic view of patients and better understanding of multiple concerns.

REFERENCE

Hicks-Moore SL, Pastirik PJ: Evaluating critical thinking in clinical concept maps: a pilot study, *Int J Nurs Educ Scholarsh* 3(1):Article27, 2006.

---

level of thinking that nursing care requires. By using a concept map you create a visual representation of your patient's medical problems, nursing assessment data, nursing diagnoses, and their relationship to one another. As you proceed in applying each step of the nursing process, your concept map expands with more detail about planned interventions. Figure 8-7 shows a concept map for Mrs. Tillman that includes the patient's assessment and four nursing diagnoses. As Rich forms his concept map, he will begin to see relationships between the nursing diagnoses. For example, Mrs. Tillman's *death anxiety* makes it more difficult for her to sleep. The disturbance in sleep aggravates her chronic fatigue. The diagnoses of *deficient knowledge* and *death anxiety* are also interrelated. Having a poor understanding of her condition heightens her anxiety. Rich's next step is to begin to plan interventions for each nursing diagnosis while recognizing how the interventions can apply to more than one diagnosis (Figure 8-8). Here are tips to help you develop a concept map:

1. Begin by collecting the patient's clinical assessment data.
2. Review all information about the patient's health problems, treatments, and medications in course textbooks, scientific literature, and other related resources.
3. Review any standardized nursing care plans, clinical pathways, protocols, or patient education materials developed for patients on the nursing unit.
4. Prepare the concept map by first developing a skeleton diagram of the patient's health problems. Write the patient's major medical diagnoses in the middle of the map and key assessment priorities. Next, add boxes for the patient's nursing care needs like spokes on a wheel.
5. In each box, identify and group clinical assessment data that seem to form patterns. Do not worry if you have difficulty labeling nursing diagnoses at first. It is important to first recognize the major nursing care focus for the patient. Remember, sometimes symptoms apply to more than one nursing diagnosis. Repeat symptoms under different categories when appropriate.
6. Analyze relationships among the nursing diagnoses. Draw lines between nursing diagnoses to show relationships. The links must be accurate, meaningful, and complete. You must be able to explain why nursing diagnoses are related.
7. List on the map the nursing interventions you select to attain the outcomes for each nursing diagnosis.
8. While caring for your patient, write down the patient's responses to each nursing activity. Also write your clinical impressions and inferences regarding the patient's progress toward expected outcomes and the effectiveness of interventions. You can use the map as a working tool and revise as needed.

CRITICAL PATHWAYS **Critical pathways** are patient care management plans that provide the multidisciplinary health team with the activities and tasks to be put into practice sequentially; their main purpose is to deliver timely care at each phase of the care process for a specific type of patient (Espinosa-Aguilar and others, 2008). A critical pathway clearly defines transition points in patient progress and draws a coordinated map of activities by which the health team can help to make these transitions as efficient as possible. A pathway allows staff from all disciplines, such as medicine, nursing, and pharmacy, to develop integrated care plans for a projected length of stay or number of visits. For example, a pathway for a surgical procedure will recommend on a day-by-day basis the patient's activities, consultation, procedures, discharge planning activities, and educational topics expected for the patient's progression to discharge. It will also include outcomes such as the patient's ability to begin ambulation or to describe postoperative

CONCEPT MAP

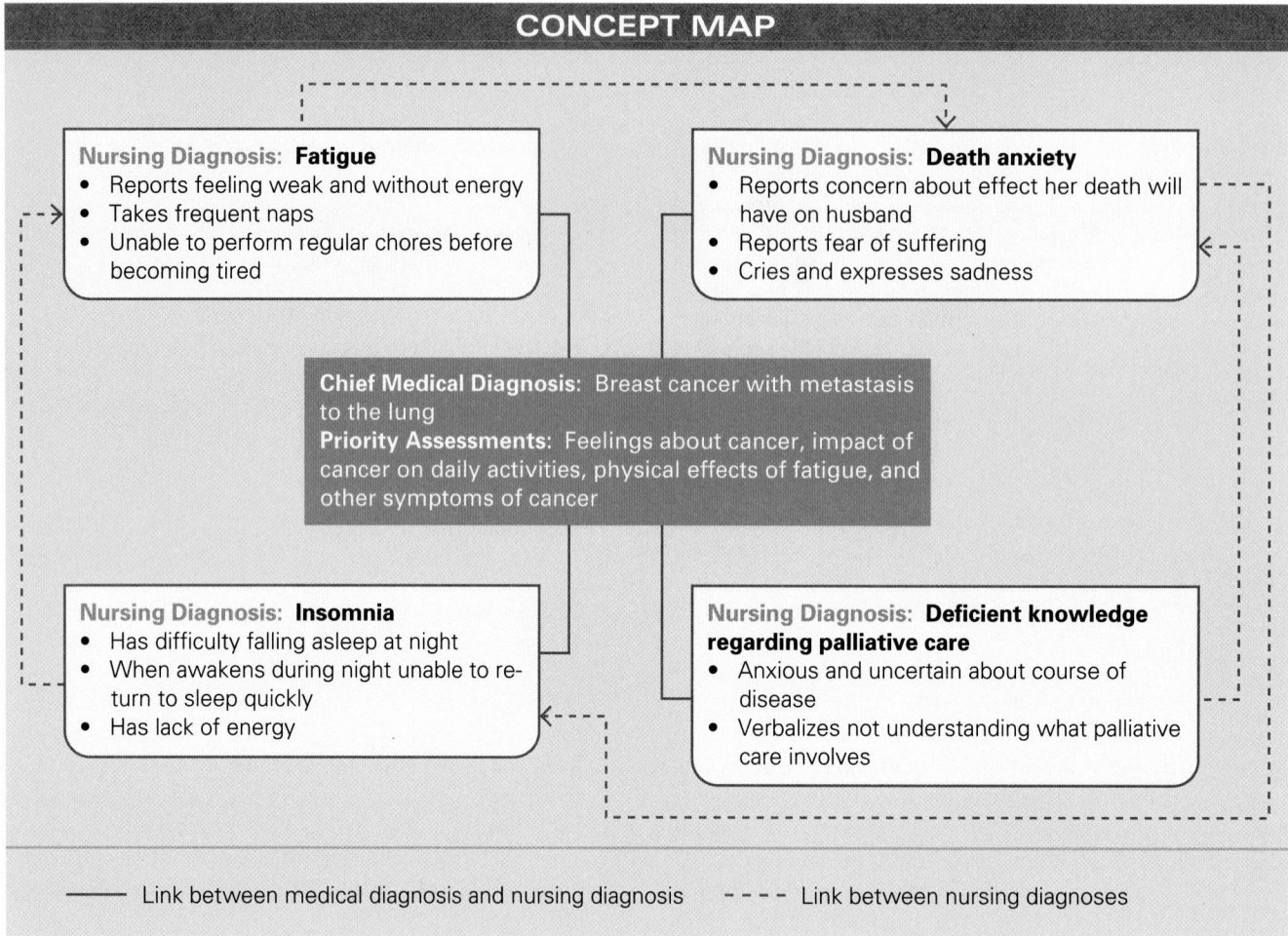

Nursing Diagnosis: Fatigue
- Reports feeling weak and without energy
- Takes frequent naps
- Unable to perform regular chores before becoming tired

Nursing Diagnosis: Death anxiety
- Reports concern about effect her death will have on husband
- Reports fear of suffering
- Cries and expresses sadness

Chief Medical Diagnosis: Breast cancer with metastasis to the lung
Priority Assessments: Feelings about cancer, impact of cancer on daily activities, physical effects of fatigue, and other symptoms of cancer

Nursing Diagnosis: Insomnia
- Has difficulty falling asleep at night
- When awakens during night unable to return to sleep quickly
- Has lack of energy

Nursing Diagnosis: Deficient knowledge regarding palliative care
- Anxious and uncertain about course of disease
- Verbalizes not understanding what palliative care involves

—— Link between medical diagnosis and nursing diagnosis   - - - - Link between nursing diagnoses

Figure 8-7 ▓ Concept Map with nursing diagnoses.

restrictions. A pathway ensures continuity of care because it maps out clearly the responsibility of each health care discipline. Well-developed pathways incorporate evidence-based protocols used in the care of the specific case type. You can use the pathway to monitor a patient's progress and as a documentation tool.

Consulting Other Health Care Professionals

Planning involves consultation with members of the health care team. Consultation occurs at any step in the nursing process, but you will consult most often during planning and implementation. During these times you are more likely to identify a problem requiring additional knowledge, skills, or community or agency resources. **Consultation** is a process in which you seek the expertise of a specialist, such as your nursing instructor or a clinical nurse specialist, to identify ways to handle problems in patient care management or in the planning and implementation of therapies. Consultation is based on the problem-solving approach, and the consultant is the stimulus for change. Oftentimes an experienced nurse is a valuable consultant when you face an unfamiliar patient care situation. Through consultation and collabora-

tion you are able to use the best resources to individualize nursing actions to meet expected outcomes.

WHEN TO CONSULT Consultation occurs when you identify a problem that you cannot solve using personal knowledge, skills, and resources. Consultation with other care providers increases your knowledge about the patient's problem and helps you to learn skills and obtain resources. A good time to consult with another health care professional is when the exact problem remains unclear. An objective consultant enters a situation and more clearly assesses and identifies the nature of a problem.

HOW TO CONSULT Begin with your own understanding of a patient's clinical problems. The first step in making a consultation is to identify the general problem area. Second, direct the consultation to the appropriate professional, such as another nurse, a social worker, or a dietitian. Third, provide the consultant with relevant information and resources about the problem area. Include a relevant, brief summary of the problem, methods used to resolve the problem so far, and outcomes of those methods. Share information from the patient's medical record and conversations with nurses, other members of the health team, and the patient's family.

CONCEPT MAP

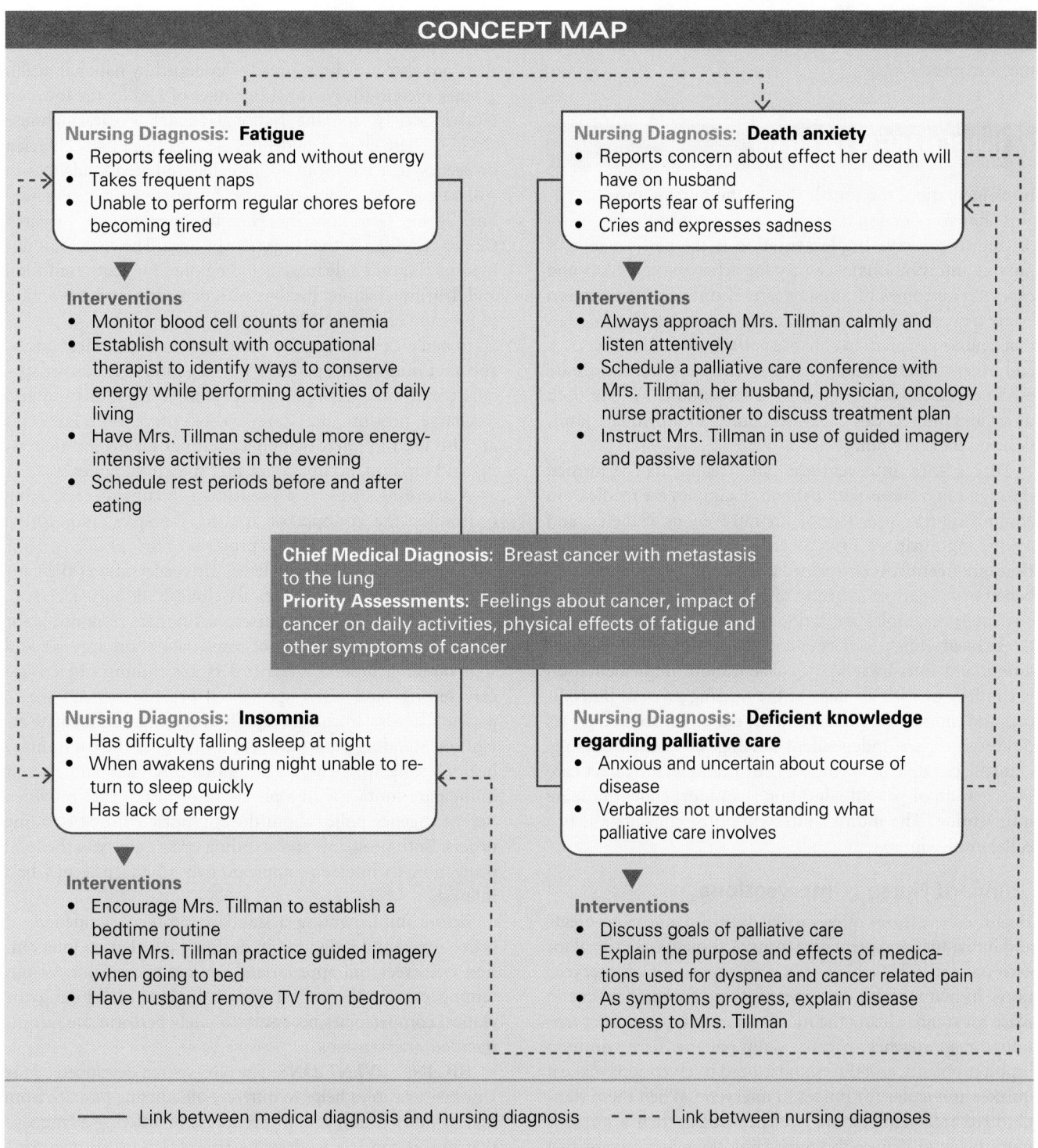

Nursing Diagnosis: Fatigue
- Reports feeling weak and without energy
- Takes frequent naps
- Unable to perform regular chores before becoming tired

Interventions
- Monitor blood cell counts for anemia
- Establish consult with occupational therapist to identify ways to conserve energy while performing activities of daily living
- Have Mrs. Tillman schedule more energy-intensive activities in the evening
- Schedule rest periods before and after eating

Nursing Diagnosis: Death anxiety
- Reports concern about effect her death will have on husband
- Reports fear of suffering
- Cries and expresses sadness

Interventions
- Always approach Mrs. Tillman calmly and listen attentively
- Schedule a palliative care conference with Mrs. Tillman, her husband, physician, oncology nurse practitioner to discuss treatment plan
- Instruct Mrs. Tillman in use of guided imagery and passive relaxation

Chief Medical Diagnosis: Breast cancer with metastasis to the lung
Priority Assessments: Feelings about cancer, impact of cancer on daily activities, physical effects of fatigue and other symptoms of cancer

Nursing Diagnosis: Insomnia
- Has difficulty falling asleep at night
- When awakens during night unable to return to sleep quickly
- Has lack of energy

Interventions
- Encourage Mrs. Tillman to establish a bedtime routine
- Have Mrs. Tillman practice guided imagery when going to bed
- Have husband remove TV from bedroom

Nursing Diagnosis: Deficient knowledge regarding palliative care
- Anxious and uncertain about course of disease
- Verbalizes not understanding what palliative care involves

Interventions
- Discuss goals of palliative care
- Explain the purpose and effects of medications used for dyspnea and cancer related pain
- As symptoms progress, explain disease process to Mrs. Tillman

——— Link between medical diagnosis and nursing diagnosis   - - - - Link between nursing diagnoses

Figure 8-8 ■ Concept Map with interventions. *ADLs,* Activities of daily living.

Fourth, do not prejudice or influence consultants. Consultants are in the clinical setting to help identify and resolve a nursing problem, and biasing or prejudicing them can block problem resolution. Avoid bias by not overloading consultants with subjective and emotional conclusions about the patient and problem. Fifth, be available to discuss the consultant's findings and recommendations. When you request a consultation, provide a private, comfortable atmosphere for the consultant and the patient. However, this does not mean that you leave the environment. A common mistake is turning the whole problem over to the consultant. The consultant is not there to take over the problem but to assist you in resolving it. When possible, request the consultation for a day when both you and the consultant are working and during a time when there are few distractions. Finally, include the consultant's recommendations in the care plan. The success of the advice depends on the implementation of the problem-solving strategies. Always give the consultant feedback about the outcomes.

IMPLEMENTATION

Implementation, the fourth step of the nursing process, begins after you develop the care plan. It involves the provision of care to patients. **Implementation** is the performance of nursing interventions necessary for achieving the goals and expected outcomes of nursing care. A **nursing intervention** is any treatment, based on clinical judgment and knowledge, that a nurse performs to enhance patient outcomes (Bulechek and others, 2008). Ideally the interventions a nurse uses are evidence based (see Chapter 6). Interventions include both direct and indirect care measures, aimed at individuals, families, and the community.

Direct care interventions are treatments performed through interactions with patients. Examples are medication administration, insertion of an intravenous catheter, and counseling during a time of grief. **Indirect care interventions** are treatments performed away from the patient but on behalf of the patient or group of patients (Bulechek and others, 2008). Examples are action aimed at managing the patient's environment (safety and infection control), documentation, and interdisciplinary collaboration. Implementation is continuous with all steps of the nursing process. Both direct and indirect care interventions fall under the categories discussed earlier: independent nursing, dependent nursing, and collaborative interventions. For example, the direct care intervention of patient education is an independent nursing intervention. The indirect intervention of consultation is a collaborative intervention.

Standard Nursing Interventions

Health care settings offer various ways for nurses to create and individualize patient care plans. Although it is critical for each patient to have his or her own unique set of interventions, in many health care systems there are mechanisms in place for standardizing the more common types of interventions or approaches to care. Many patients have common health problems, and thus standardized interventions make it quicker and easier for nurses to intervene. When these standardized interventions are evidence based, then a nurse is more likely to deliver the most clinically effective care that will result in the best patient outcomes.

CLINICAL PRACTICE GUIDELINES AND PROTOCOLS
A **clinical guideline** or protocol is a document that guides decisions and interventions for specific health care problems or conditions, such as the treatment for a patient who has had a stroke or the administration of chemotherapy. Ideally the guideline or protocol is developed on the basis of an authoritative examination of current scientific evidence and assists health care providers in making decisions about appropriate health care for specific clinical circumstances (National Guideline Clearinghouse, 2009). Often clinicians within a health care agency will review the scientific literature and their own standard of practice to create a clinical practice guideline. However, there are also guidelines already developed by national health groups, such as the National Institutes of Health, the Infusion Nurses Society, and the National Guideline Clearinghouse (NGC). These clinical guidelines are available to any clinician or agency that wishes to adopt evidence-based guidelines in patient care. One valuable source for nursing practice guidelines is the Gerontological Nursing Interventions Research Center (GNIRC) at the University of Iowa. The center has numerous clinical guidelines, including ones for acute confusion and delirium, bathing persons with dementia, and prevention of pressure ulcers (GNIRC, 2008).

In acute care settings it is common to find clinical protocols that outline independent nursing interventions for specific conditions. Examples are protocols for admission and discharge, pressure ulcer care, and fall prevention. Protocols are also used in interdisciplinary settings for diagnostic testing and physical, occupational, and speech therapies.

A **standing order** is a preprinted document containing orders for the conduct of routine therapies, monitoring guidelines, and/or diagnostic procedures for specific patients with identified clinical problems. The orders direct the conduct of patient care in various clinical settings. Licensed, prescribing physicians or nurse practitioners responsible for a patient's care at the time of implementation approve and sign standing orders. These orders are common in critical care settings and other specialized practice settings where patients' needs can change rapidly and require immediate attention. Standing orders are also common in the community health setting, where nurses face situations that do not permit immediate contact with a physician or health care provider. Refer to agency policy about the appropriate use of standing orders. Both protocols and standing orders give you the legal protection to intervene appropriately in the patient's best interest.

Before implementing a standard protocol, guideline, or order, use sound judgment in deciding whether an intervention is correct and appropriate. You are responsible for obtaining correct theoretical knowledge and developing the clinical competencies necessary to safely perform the recommended interventions.

NIC INTERVENTIONS
The NIC system developed by the University of Iowa helps to differentiate nursing practice from that of other health care professionals by offering a language that nurses can use to describe sets of actions in delivering nursing care. The NIC interventions offer a level of standardization to enhance communication of nursing care across settings and to compare outcomes. The NIC system has been incorporated into many health care information systems. By using NIC, nurses learn the common interventions recommended for the various NANDA-I nursing diagnoses.

Critical Thinking in Implementation

The selection of nursing interventions for a patient is part of clinical decision making. The critical thinking model discussed in Chapter 6 provides a framework for how to make decisions when implementing nursing care. Your knowledge about a patient's health problems will lead you to select appropriate therapies. For example, knowledge of the disease course of metastatic cancer will allow Rich to select interventions for pain relief, fatigue, and breathing alterations. His knowledge of the NIC classification will direct him to select specific care activities for each of Mrs. Tillman's nursing diagnoses.

You will also apply prior clinical experiences in performing specific interventions. Consider what interventions have worked before and what have not worked in previous clinical situations. Be aware of both professional and agency standards of practice. Standards of practice offer guidelines for selection of interventions, their frequency, and the determination of whether the procedures may be delegated. In Mrs. Tillman's case the NGC has a guideline for cancer pain management that would be very helpful. As you perform any nursing intervention, apply intellectual standards. For example, when teaching patients, be relevant, clear, and logical to promote patient learning (see Chapter 11). All critical thinking attitudes, such as confidence, creativity, and discipline, apply to implementation. A beginning student will need supervision from an instructor or experienced nurse to guide the decision-making process for implementation.

Implementation Process

Preparation for implementation ensures efficient, safe, and effective nursing care. Follow these five preparatory activities: reassess the patient, review and revise the existing nursing care plan, organize resources and care delivery, anticipate and prevent complications, and implement nursing interventions.

REASSESSING THE PATIENT Patient assessment is a continuous process that occurs each time you interact with a patient. When you gather new data and identify a new patient need, you modify the care plan. You also modify a plan when you resolve a patient's health care need. Just before implementing a nursing activity, reassess the patient. This is a partial assessment and sometimes focuses on one dimension of the patient, such as level of comfort, or on one system, such as the cardiovascular system. The reassessment helps you to decide if the proposed nursing activity is still appropriate for the patient's level of wellness. For example, you planned to assist a patient with ambulation following lunch; however, a reassessment reveals shortness of breath and increased fatigue, which require you to assist the patient back to bed.

REVIEWING AND REVISING THE CARE PLAN After reassessing a patient, review the care plan, and compare assessment data to validate the nursing diagnoses. Then determine whether the nursing interventions are the most appropriate. If the patient's status has changed and the nursing diagnosis and related interventions are no longer appropriate, modify the nursing care plan. An out-of-date or incorrect care plan compromises the quality of nursing care. Review and modification enable you to provide timely nursing interventions to best meet a patient's needs. There are four steps to modifying the written care plan:

1. Revise data in the assessment section to reflect the patient's current status. Date any new data to inform other health team members of the time that the change occurred.
2. Revise nursing diagnoses. Delete diagnoses that are no longer relevant, and add and date any new diagnoses. It is necessary to revise related factors, as well as the patient's goals, outcomes, and priorities.
3. Revise specific interventions that correspond to the new nursing diagnoses and goals. This revision should reflect the patient's present status.
4. Determine the method of evaluation to achieve outcomes.

Rich prepares to have a discussion with Mrs. Tillman and her husband about palliative care. Before he begins, Rich reassesses Mrs. Tillman's level of anxiety to learn more specifically about what is contributing to her worry about suffering. She explains that she has a general sense of dread and does not want to have a lot of pain. Her worries keep her from sleeping at night on a regular basis. Rich probes this further and with new information identifies the nursing diagnosis of disturbed sleep pattern. *He revises his plan to focus instruction on planned comfort measures.*

ORGANIZING RESOURCES AND CARE DELIVERY A facility's resources include equipment and skilled personnel. Organization of equipment and personnel makes timely, efficient, and skilled patient care possible. Preparation for care delivery also involves preparing the environment and patient for nursing interventions.

Equipment Most nursing procedures require some equipment or supplies. Decide what supplies are necessary, and determine their availability before you start implementation. Equipment should be in working order to ensure safe use. Place supplies in a convenient location to provide easy access during a procedure. Have extra supplies available in case of errors or accidents, but do not open extra supplies unless they are needed. This controls health care costs. After a procedure, return any unopened supplies.

Personnel Nursing care delivery models vary among facilities (see Chapter 12). The model by which nursing is organized determines how nursing personnel deliver patient care. For example, a registered nurse's (RN's) accountabilities differ in a team nursing model from those in a primary nursing model. A primary nurse is accountable for the nursing care a patient receives during his or her length of stay or course of visits. A team nurse is accountable for the specific shift in which he or she works. As a nurse, you are responsible for determining whether to perform an intervention or to delegate it to another member of the nursing team. Your assessment of a patient directs the decision about delegation and not the intervention alone. For example, you know nursing assistive personnel (NAP) can competently ambulate patients. However, you learn that a patient experienced an increased pulse rate after walking during the previous shift, so you decide to personally assist the patient with ambulation and evaluate the patient's cardiac status. In this case, you redirect the NAP to perform an intervention for a more stable patient.

Nursing staff work together as patients' needs demand it. If a patient makes a request, such as for use of a bedpan, position the patient on the pan if you have time rather than trying to find the NAP who is in a different room. When interventions are complex or physically difficult, you may need assistance from colleagues. You will be more effective in performing procedures, for example, when NAP assist you with patient positioning and in handing you supplies during the procedure.

Environment A patient's care environment needs to be safe and conducive for implementing therapies. Patient safety is your first concern. If the patient has sensory deficits, physical disability, or an alteration in level of consciousness, arrange the environment to prevent injury. As examples, provide assistive devices (e.g., walkers or eyeglasses), rearrange furniture and equipment, and make rooms free of clutter. Patients benefit most from nursing interventions when surroundings are compatible with care activities. When you need to expose a patient's body parts, do so privately because the patient will be more relaxed. Reduce distractions to enhance learning opportunities. Make sure the lighting is adequate to perform procedures correctly.

Patient Before you deliver interventions, be sure the patient is as physically and psychologically comfortable as possible. For example, symptoms such as nausea or pain interfere with a patient's full concentration and cooperation. Offer comfort measures before initiating interventions to help the patient participate more fully. If you need a patient to be alert, give a dose of pain medication to relieve discomfort but not impair mental faculties (e.g., ability to follow instruction, reasoning, and communication). If a patient is fatigued, delay ambulation until after the patient has had a chance to rest. Even if symptoms are not a factor, make the patient physically comfortable during interventions. Start any intervention by controlling environmental factors, positioning, and taking care of other physical needs (e.g., elimination). Also consider the patient's level of endurance, and plan only the amount of activity the patient can comfortably tolerate.

Awareness of the patient's psychosocial needs helps you create a favorable emotional climate. Some patients feel reassured by having a significant other present for encouragement and moral support. Other strategies include planning sufficient time or multiple opportunities for the patient to work through and vent feelings and anxieties. Adequate preparation allows the patient to obtain maximal benefit from each intervention.

ANTICIPATING AND PREVENTING COMPLICATIONS Risks to patients come from both illness and treatment. As a nurse, look for and recognize these risks, adapt your choice of interventions to the situation, evaluate the relative benefit of the treatment versus the risk, and take risk prevention measures. Many conditions place patients at risk for complications. For example, a patient who had a stroke has limited mobility and is at risk for developing pressure ulcers. Nurses are often the first ones to detect changes in patients' conditions. Your knowledge of pathophysiology and previous patient care experiences help to identify possible complications that can occur. A thorough assessment reveals the level of the patient's current risk. Scientific rationales for how certain interventions (e.g., turning and use of pressure-relief devices) prevent or minimize complications help you to select the preventive measures that will likely be most useful. Some nursing procedures pose risks for patients. Be aware of potential complications, and take precautions. For instance, the patient who is to have a urinary catheter inserted is at risk for infection. In this situation, thorough cleansing of the urethra before insertion reduces infection risk.

Identifying Areas of Assistance Certain nursing situations require you to obtain assistance by seeking additional personnel, knowledge, and/or nursing skills. Before beginning care, review the plan to determine the need for assistance and the type required. Sometimes you will need assistance in performing a procedure, providing comfort measures, or preparing the patient for a procedure. For example, when you care for a patient who is overweight and immobilized, you will require additional personnel and transfer equipment to turn and position the patient safely. Be sure to determine the number of additional personnel in advance and when you need them. Discuss your need for assistance with potential resources, such as other nurses or NAP.

You will require additional knowledge and skills in situations in which you are less familiar or experienced. For example, seek additional knowledge when you give a new medication or implement a new procedure. You will find such information in a hospital's formulary or procedure book. If you are still uncertain about the new medication or procedure, ask other members of the health care team.

Because of the continual growth in health care technology, you may lack the skills needed to perform a new procedure. When this occurs, first locate information about the procedure in the literature and the agency's procedures book. Next, collect all equipment necessary for the procedure. Finally, ask another nurse who is experienced in performing the procedure to provide assistance and guidance. The assistance can come from another staff nurse, a supervisor, educator, or a nurse specialist. Requesting assistance occurs frequently in practice and is a learning process that continues throughout educational experiences and into professional development.

IMPLEMENTATION SKILLS Nursing practice includes cognitive, interpersonal, and psychomotor (technical) skills. You need each type of skill to implement direct and indirect nursing interventions. You are responsible for knowing when one type of implementation skill is preferred over another and for having the necessary knowledge and skill to perform each.

Cognitive Skills Cognitive skills involve the application of critical thinking in the nursing process. Always use good judgment and sound clinical decision making when performing any intervention. This ensures that no nursing action is automatic. Always think and anticipate so that you individualize patient care appropriately. Know the rationale for therapeutic interventions, and understand normal and abnormal physiological and psychological responses. Know the evidence in nursing science to ensure that you deliver the most current and relevant nursing interventions.

Interpersonal Skills Interpersonal skills are essential for effective nursing action. Develop a trusting relationship, express a level of caring, and communicate clearly with the patient and family (see Chapter 10). Good communication is critical for keeping patients informed, providing effective teaching, and effectively supporting patients who have challenging emotional needs. Proper use of interpersonal skills enables you to perceive a patient's verbal and nonverbal communication accurately. As a member of the health care team, you communicate patient problems and needs clearly, intelligently and in a timely manner.

Psychomotor Skills Psychomotor skills require the integration of cognitive and motor activities. For example, when taking a pulse, you need to understand anatomy and physiology (cognitive) and assume the proper positioning and use of touch to detect the pulse correctly (motor). With time and practice you will learn to perform skills correctly, smoothly, and confidently. This is critical in establishing patient trust. You are responsible for acquiring necessary psychomotor skills. In the case of a new skill, assess your level of competency and obtain the necessary resources to ensure the patient receives safe treatment.

Direct Care

Nurses provide a wide variety of direct care measures, those activities that nurses perform through patient interaction. How a nurse interacts affects the success of any direct care activity. Remain sensitive to a patient's clinical condition, values and beliefs, expectations, and cultural views. All direct care measures require competent, safe practice. Show a caring approach when you provide direct care.

ACTIVITIES OF DAILY LIVING ADLs are activities usually performed during a normal day; including ambulation, eating, dressing, bathing, and grooming. A patient's need for assistance with ADLs may be temporary, as in the case of an acute illness, or permanent. A patient with impaired mobility because of bilateral arm casts has a temporary need for assistance. After the casts are removed, the patient will gradually regain the strength and range of motion needed to perform ADLs. A patient with an irreversible injury to the cervical spinal cord is paralyzed and thus has a permanent need for assistance. Rehabilitation would not be realistic for such a patient. Instead, through restorative care, the patient will learn new ways to perform ADLs so as to be less dependent on others.

When an assessment reveals a patient is experiencing fatigue, a limitation in mobility, confusion, and/or pain, assistance with ADLs is likely needed. Assistance can range from partial to complete care. Always consider a patient's preferences when assisting with ADLs. Consultation with physical or occupational therapy is also helpful. Involve the patient in planning the timing and types of interventions to enhance self-esteem and the willingness to become more independent.

INSTRUMENTAL ACTIVITIES OF DAILY LIVING Illness or disability sometimes alters a patient's ability to be independent in society. **Instrumental activities of daily living (IADLs)** include skills such as shopping, preparing meals, writing checks, and taking medications. Nurses in home care and community nursing frequently assist patients in adapting ways to perform IADLs. Often family and friends are excellent resources for assisting patients. In acute care it is important for you to anticipate how patients' illnesses affect their ability to perform IADLs so that you make the appropriate referrals.

PHYSICAL CARE TECHNIQUES You will routinely use a variety of physical care techniques when caring for patients. Physical care techniques involve the safe and competent administration of nursing procedures (e.g., inserting a urinary catheter, performing range-of-motion exercises). The specific knowledge and skills needed to perform these procedures are in subsequent clinical chapters of this text. Common methods for administering physical care techniques appropriately include protecting you and the patient from injury, using proper infection control practices, staying organized, and positioning patients correctly. When you apply physical care during a procedure, know the clinical practice guidelines and how to perform the procedure, the standard frequency, and the expected outcomes.

LIFESAVING MEASURES A lifesaving measure is a physical care technique that you use when a patient's physiological or psychological state is threatened. The purpose of lifesaving measures is to restore physiological and psychological balance. Such measures include administering emergency medications, performing cardiopulmonary resuscitation, and protecting a violent patient. When an inexperienced nurse faces a situation requiring emergency measures, it is critical to get the assistance of an experienced professional.

COUNSELING **Counseling** is a direct care method that helps patients use a problem-solving process to recognize and manage stress and to facilitate interpersonal relationships. As a nurse, you will counsel patients to accept actual or impending changes resulting from stress. Counseling involves emotional, intellectual, spiritual, and psychological support (see Chapters 24 and 25). Examples of counseling strategies are behavior modification, bereavement counseling, biofeedback, and crisis intervention. A patient and family who need nursing counseling have normal adjustment difficulties and are upset or frustrated, but they are not necessarily psychologically disabled. A good example is the case of Mr. Tillman, who faces normal grief and the uncertainty of how cancer will affect his wife and his relationship with her. Nurse counseling encourages patients to examine available alternatives and decide which choices are useful and appropriate. When patients are able to examine alternatives, they develop a sense of control and are able to better manage stress. When patients have psychiatric diagnoses such as severe depression or schizophrenia, they require specialized therapy by mental health nurses or social workers, psychologists, or psychiatrists.

TEACHING Teaching is an important nursing responsibility. In teaching, the focus of change is intellectual growth or the acquisition of new knowledge or psychomotor skills (Redman, 2005). As a nurse, you teach correct principles, procedures, and techniques of health care to inform patients about their health status and to prepare them for self-care (see Chapter 11).

When patients are unable to assume self-care, nurses then focus teaching efforts on family caregivers. Teaching takes place in all health care settings. As a nurse, you are responsible for assessing the learning needs and readiness of patients and family caregivers and you are accountable for the quality of education you deliver. Know your patients; be aware of the cultural and social factors that influence their willingness and ability to learn. It is also important to know your patient's health literacy level. Can he or she read directions or make calculations that are necessary with self-care skills? The teaching-learning process is an active interaction between the teacher and learner in which you, the teacher, address specific learning objectives. This process offers an organizational structure and framework for patient education.

CONTROLLING FOR ADVERSE REACTIONS An adverse reaction is a harmful or unintended effect of a medication, diagnostic test, or therapeutic intervention. Adverse reactions can possibly follow any nursing intervention, so learn to anticipate them and know the adverse reactions to expect. Nursing actions that control for adverse reactions reduce or counteract the reaction. For example, when applying a moist heat compress, you want to prevent burning the patient's skin. First assess the area requiring the compress. After application of the compress, check the area every 5 minutes for any adverse reaction, such as excessive reddening of the skin from the heat. When administering a medication, understand the known and potential side effects of the drug. After administration of the medication, evaluate the patient's response for adverse effects. Also know the drugs available to counteract any side effects. Although adverse reactions are not common, they do occur. It is important that you recognize the signs and symptoms of an adverse reaction and intervene in a timely manner.

PREVENTIVE MEASURES Preventive nursing actions promote health and prevent illness to avoid the need for acute or rehabilitative health care. Prevention includes promotion of the patient's health potential, application of prescribed measures (e.g., immunizations), health teaching, and identification of risks for illness and/or trauma. Consider the situation of Mrs. Tillman. Rich worries that with her fatigue and the progressive nature of her cancer, she is likely to become weaker and less mobile. Rich recommends preventive measures to make the Tillmans' home setting safer. Rich assesses the Tillman's home environment and chooses the interventions (i.e., installing grab bars in the bath and rearranging furniture) that will improve Mrs. Tillman's safety and ability to move about comfortably in her home. All patients need preventive nursing interventions aimed at promoting health and preventing illness. As changes in the health care system continue, there is and will be greater emphasis on health promotion and illness prevention.

Indirect Care

Indirect care measures are actions that support the effectiveness of direct care measures (Bulechek and others, 2008). Many indirect measures are managerial in nature, such as documentation and medical order transcription. Others are environmental, such as specimen and supply management. A good amount of a nurse's time is spent in indirect care activities. For example, communication of information about patients (e.g., change-of-shift report and consultation) is critical to ensure that direct care activities are planned and coordinated with proper resources. Delegation of care to nursing assistive personnel is another indirect care activity. Proper delegation ensures that the right care providers perform the right tasks so that an RN and NAP work most efficiently for the patient.

DELEGATING, SUPERVISING, AND EVALUATING THE WORK OF OTHER STAFF MEMBERS Depending on the system of health care delivery, the nurse who develops the care plan frequently does not perform all of the nursing interventions. Some activities you will coordinate and delegate to other members of the health care team (see Chapter 12). Remember, an RN delegates components of care but not the nursing process itself (American Nurses Association, 2008). Noninvasive and frequently repetitive interventions such as skin care, ambulation, grooming, and hygiene measures are examples of care activities that you will assign to NAP such as certified nurse assistants. Licensed practical nurses perform these measures in addition to medication administration and many invasive tasks (e.g., dressing care and catheterization). The nursing tasks or activities that members of the nursing team perform under the direction of an RN are identified according to legal parameters defined by each state in its Nurse Practice Act and by the scope of practice and standards established by professional nursing organizations (ANA, 2008).When you delegate aspects of care to another staff member, you are responsible for assigning the task and making sure the staff member completes the task according to the standard of care. You are also responsible for delegating direct care interventions to personnel competent to provide the care.

EVALUATION

After a patient diagnosed with pneumonia has completed a 5-day dose pack of antibiotics, the health care provider has the patient return to the office to have a chest x-ray examination to determine if the pneumonia has cleared. When a nurse on a surgical unit provides wound care, he or she first assesses the appearance of the wound, applies the appropriate dressing, and then returns later to inspect the wound to see if it has healed. These two scenarios depict the process of evaluation, the last step of the nursing process. The health care provider orders a chest x-ray examination and the nurse reinspects the wound. Evaluation is the critical step of the nursing process that involves an examination of a condition or situation and then a judgment as to whether change has occurred.

Evaluation is crucial to deciding whether, after interventions have been delivered, a patient's condition or well-being improves (see Care Plan, p. 127). You apply all that you know about a patient and the patient's condition, as well as experience with previous patients, to evaluate if nursing care was effective. **You conduct evaluation to determine if expected**

outcomes are met, not if nursing interventions were completed. For example, in Rich's plan of care for Mrs. Tillman he has established the outcome of "The patient will verbalize feeling less anxious about the course of her disease." Rich implements educational interventions to improve Mrs. Tillman's knowledge and anxiety reduction exercises. Evaluation *does* involve questioning Mrs. Tillman about her feelings toward her disease. Evaluation *does not* involve observation of her performing anxiety reduction exercises. Expected outcomes are the standards against which you judge if goals have been met and if care is successful.

Critical Thinking and Evaluation

Evaluation is an ongoing process you conduct while caring for a patient. Once you deliver an intervention, you gather subjective and objective data from the patient, family, and health care team members. This includes reviewing knowledge about the patient's current condition, treatment, and resources available for recovery. By referring to previous experiences caring for similar patients, you are in a better position to know how to evaluate your patient. You then apply critical thinking attitudes and standards to determine whether outcomes of care are achieved. If outcomes are met, the overall goals for the patient are also met. You compare patient behavior and responses assessed before delivering nursing interventions with behavior and responses that occur after administering nursing care. For example, Rich's initial assessment revealed Mrs. Tillman's sense of anxiety about her impending death and uncertainty about her course of illness. On a subsequent clinic visit, he considers the following questions: Has the patient's condition improved? Can the patient improve, or are there physical or psychological factors preventing recovery? To what degree does the patient's emotional health influence response to therapies? To evaluate Mrs. Tillman's progress, he asks her how she now feels about the cancer and its anticipated effects. Mrs. Tillman is able to talk about her cancer without crying. She also tells Rich, "I think I have a better idea of what to expect, but more important, I know my doctor will do all he can to make me comfortable." The evaluation shows the patient has accepted her prognosis and has a better sense of control over her condition.

In evaluation you make clinical decisions and continually redirect nursing care. For example, when evaluating a patient for a change in pain severity, you apply knowledge of disease processes, physiological responses to interventions, and the correct procedure for measuring pain severity to interpret whether a change has occurred and whether the change is desirable. If the patient continues to report pain at a higher level on a pain scale than expected, you might consult with the health care provider to increase an analgesic dose or try different noninvasive approaches to help the patient relax and concentrate less on the pain. You will continue to evaluate until the patient achieves pain relief.

Positive evaluations occur when you achieve expected outcomes that lead you to conclude that the nursing interventions effectively met the patient's goals. Negative evaluations or undesired results indicate that the interventions were not effective in minimizing or resolving the actual problem or avoiding a potential problem. Sometimes new data reveal a patient's condition altered the patient's ability to meet the expected outcome. As a result, change the care plan and try different therapies or a different approach in administering existing therapies.

This sequence of critically evaluating and revising therapies continues until you and the patient appropriately resolve the problems. Outcomes must be realistic and adjusted based on the patient's prognosis and nursing diagnoses. Remember that evaluation is dynamic and ever changing, depending on the patient's nursing diagnoses and condition. A patient whose health status continuously changes requires more frequent evaluation. In addition, priority diagnoses are usually evaluated first. For example, you evaluate a patient's *acute pain* before evaluating the status of *deficient knowledge*.

The Evaluation Process

The evaluation process includes five elements: (1) identifying evaluative criteria and standards, (2) collecting data to determine if you met the criteria or standards, (3) interpreting and summarizing findings, (4) documenting findings, and (5) terminating, continuing, or revising the care plan.

IDENTIFYING CRITERIA AND STANDARDS Your evaluative criteria include the goals and expected outcomes established during planning. Thus evaluation is most effective when you know what to observe or measure. During evaluation you compare your findings with the goals and expected outcomes set for your patient. Proper evaluation allows you to determine whether each patient reaches a level of wellness or recovery that is reflected in the goals of care.

COLLECTING DATA Evaluating a patient's response to nursing care requires the use of evaluative measures, which are simply assessment skills and techniques (e.g., auscultation of lung sounds, observation of a patient's skill performance, or discussion of the patient's feelings). In fact, evaluative measures are the same as assessment measures, but you perform them at the point of care when you make decisions about the patient's status and progress. The intent of assessment is to identify what if any problem exists. The intent of evaluation is to determine if the known problems have remained the same, improved, worsened, or otherwise changed.

In many clinical situations it is important to collect evaluative measures over a period of time to determine if a pattern of improvement or change exists. For example, a one-time observation of a pressure ulcer is insufficient to determine that the ulcer is healing. You want to see a consistency in change. For example, over a period of 2 days is the pressure ulcer decreasing in size? Is the amount of drainage declining? Recognizing a pattern of improvement or decline allows you to reason and decide if the patient's problems are resolved.

The primary source of data for evaluation is the patient. However, you will also use input from the family and other caregivers. For example, you ask a family member to report on the amount of food the patient eats during a meal or how well the patient is able to sleep during the night. You will sometimes consult with colleagues about how the patient responded to therapies (e.g., pain medication) during a previous shift. In addition to outcomes, it is also important to evaluate if you met the patient's expectations of care. You will evaluate patients about their perceptions of care, such as "Did you receive the type of pain relief you expected?" This level of evaluation is important to determine the patient's satisfaction with care and to strengthen partnering between you and the patient.

INTERPRETING AND SUMMARIZING FINDINGS An expert nurse recognizes relevant evidence, even evidence that does not match clinical expectations, and makes judgments about a patient's condition. To develop clinical judgment you learn to match the results of evaluative measures with expected outcomes to determine if a patient's status is improving or not. When interpreting findings, you compare the patient's behavioral responses and physiological signs and symptoms you expect to see with those actually seen during evaluation. To objectively evaluate the degree of success in achieving outcomes of care, use the following steps:

1. Examine the outcome criteria to identify the exact desired patient behavior or response.
2. Measure the patient's actual behavior or response.
3. Compare the established outcome criteria with the actual behavior or response.
4. Judge the degree of agreement between outcome criteria and the actual behavior or response.
5. If there is no agreement (or only partial agreement) between outcome criteria and patient response, why did they not agree? Identify any barriers?

Evaluation is easier to perform after you care for a patient over a period of time. You can then make subtle comparisons of patient responses and behaviors. When you have not had the chance to care for a patient over an extended time, evaluation improves by referring to previous experiences and asking colleagues familiar with the patient to confirm evaluation findings.

Remember to evaluate each expected outcome and its place in the sequence of care. If not, it will be difficult to determine which outcome in the sequence was not met. This prevents you from revising and redirecting the plan of care at the most appropriate time.

DOCUMENTING FINDINGS Documentation and reporting are a part of evaluation. Accurate information needs to be present in a patient's medical record for nurses and other health care providers to make ongoing clinical decisions. When documenting the patient's response to interventions, always describe the same evaluative measures. Your aim is to present a clear argument from the evaluative data as to whether a patient is progressing or not. Communicate a patient's progress toward meeting outcomes and goals on assessment flow sheets and summary progress notes, and by sharing information between nurses during change-of-shift reports (see Chapter 9).

CARE PLAN REVISION The result of interpreting evaluative data allows you to decide if you need to revise the plan

of care. If you meet a goal successfully, discontinue that portion of the care plan. Unmet and partially met goals require you to continue intervention. After you evaluate a patient, you may want to modify or add nursing diagnoses with appropriate goals and expected outcomes and to establish interventions. You must also redefine priorities. This is an important step in critical thinking—knowing how the patient is progressing and how problems either resolve or worsen.

Careful monitoring and early detection of problems are a patient's first line of defense. Base clinical judgments on your observations of what is occurring with a specific patient and not merely what happens to patients in general. Frequently changes are not very obvious. Evaluations are patient specific, based on a close familiarity with each patient's behavior, physical status, and reaction to caregivers.

Discontinuing a Care Plan After you determine that expected outcomes and goals have been met, you confirm this evaluation with the patient when possible. If you and the patient agree, then you discontinue that portion of the care plan. Documentation of a discontinued plan ensures that other nurses will not unnecessarily continue interventions for that portion of the plan of care. Continuity of care assumes that care provided to patients is relevant and timely. You will waste much time when you do not communicate achieved goals.

Modifying a Care Plan When goals are not met, you identify the factors that interfere with goal achievement. Usually a change in the patient's condition, needs, or abilities makes alteration of the care plan necessary. For example, *While monitoring Mrs. Tillman's level of fatigue, Rich learns during a follow-up visit that Mrs. Tillman is now having difficulty breathing. Her breathing rate is elevated and more shallow than her last visit. She confirms that she experiences shortness of breath, especially when climbing stairs at home. Her breathing difficulty has also aggravated her sense of fatigue. Mrs. Tillman explains, "I sometimes do not have the energy just to dress and even eat." Rich knows the breathing problem is related to progression of the cancer and thus establishes a new diagnosis,* impaired gas exchange related to damaged alveolar capillary membrane.

At times a lack of goal achievement results from an error in nursing judgment or failure to follow each step of the nursing process. Patients often have multiple problems. Always remember the possibility of overlooking or misjudging something. When there is failure to achieve a goal, no matter what the reason, repeat the entire nursing process sequence for that nursing diagnosis to discover changes the plan needs. You then will reassess the patient, determine accuracy of the nursing diagnosis, establish new goals and expected outcomes, and select new interventions.

A complete reassessment of all patient factors relating to the nursing diagnosis and etiology is necessary when modifying a plan. Apply critical thinking as you compare new data about the patient's condition with previously assessed information. Knowledge from previous experiences helps you direct the reassessment process. Caring for patients who have had similar health problems gives you a strong background of knowledge to use for anticipating patient needs and knowing what to assess. Reassessment ensures that the database is accurate and relevant (standards for critical thinking). It will also reveal any missing link, or piece of information that was overlooked and perhaps responsible for preventing goal achievement. You sort, validate, and cluster all new data to analyze and interpret differences from the original database.

After reassessment, determine what nursing diagnoses are accurate for the situation. Ask yourself whether you selected the correct diagnosis and whether it and the etiological factor are current. Then revise the problem list to reflect the patient's changed status. You may make a new diagnosis. You base nursing care on an accurate list of nursing diagnoses. Accuracy is more important than the number of diagnoses selected. As the patient's condition changes, the diagnoses do as well.

When you modify a care plan, also review the goals and expected outcomes for needed changes. Examine the goals for unchanged nursing diagnoses. Are they still appropriate? A change in one diagnosis may affect others. For example, if Mrs. Tillman now has *impaired gas exchange*, it likely will require Rich to alter goals and outcomes with respect to her problem of *fatigue*. It is also important to determine that each goal and expected outcome is realistic for the problem, etiology, and time frame. Unrealistic expected outcomes and time frames make goal achievement difficult.

Clearly document goals and expected outcomes for new or revised nursing diagnoses so that all team members are aware of the revised care plan. When the goal is still appropriate but has not yet been met, you may change the evaluation date to allow more time. You may also decide at this time to change interventions. For example, when a patient's wound does not heal with a transparent dressing, you may choose a different dressing material such as a colloid dressing instead. All goals and expected outcomes are patient centered, with realistic expectations for patient achievement.

The evaluation of interventions examines two factors: the appropriateness of the interventions selected and the correct application of the intervention. The appropriateness of an intervention is based on the standard of care for a patient's health problem. A **standard of care** is the minimum level of care accepted to ensure high quality of care to patients. Standards of care define the types of therapies typically administered to patients with specific problems or needs. If the patient who is receiving chemotherapy for leukemia has the nursing diagnosis *nausea related to pharyngeal irritation*, the standard of care established by a nursing department for this problem includes pain-control measures, mouth-care guidelines, and diet therapy. The nurse reviews the standard of care to determine if the right interventions have been chosen or if additional ones are needed.

You may only need to increase or decrease the frequency of interventions when you revise a care plan. Use clinical judgment based on previous experience and the patient's actual response to therapy. For example, if a patient continues to have congested lung sounds, you increase the frequency of coughing and deep-breathing exercises to remove secretions.

During evaluation you may find that some planned interventions are designed for an inappropriate level of nursing care. If you need to change the level of care, substitute a different action verb, such as *assist* in place of *provide*, or *demonstrate* in place of *describe*. For example, assisting a patient with walking requires a nurse to be at the patient's side during ambulation, whereas providing an assistive device suggests the patient is more independent. Sometimes the level of care is appropriate, but the interventions are unsuitable because of a change in the expected outcome. In this case, discontinue the interventions and plan new ones.

Make any changes in the plan of care based on the nature of the patient's unfavorable response. Consulting with other health care providers often yields suggestions for improving the approach to care delivery. Practicing nurses are usually excellent resources because of their experience. Simply changing the care plan is not enough. Implement the new plan, and reevaluate the patient's response to the nursing actions. Remember, *evaluation is continuous*.

KEY POINTS

- The nursing process has five steps: assessment, nursing diagnosis, planning, implementation, and evaluation.
- Use of the nursing process is the foundation for clinical decision making.
- When you first meet a patient, you will conduct an initial assessment screening and then focus on cues and patterns of information to make a more comprehensive assessment.
- Attention to the environment, patient comfort, and communication techniques ensures a successful assessment interview.
- Data analysis involves recognizing patterns or trends, comparing data with standards, and then forming a reasoned conclusion about the data's meaning.

- Data clustering organizes assessment data into meaningful clusters of defining characteristics or sets of signs and symptoms.
- The diagnostic process includes analysis and interpretation of data, identification of patient and family needs, and formulation of nursing diagnoses and collaborative problems.
- Nursing diagnoses provide the basis for selection of nursing interventions to achieve outcomes for which a nurse is accountable.
- NANDA International defines five types of nursing diagnoses: actual, health promotion, risk, syndrome, and wellness.

- The absence of certain defining characteristics, following a patient assessment, suggests that you reject a nursing diagnosis under consideration.
- Nursing diagnostic errors may lead to inappropriate and/or inadequate nursing care.
- During the planning component, you determine patient goals, establish priorities, develop expected outcomes of nursing care, and write a nursing care plan.
- The Nursing Outcomes Classification (NOC) has labels for describing the focus of nursing care and then includes indicators for use in measuring success with interventions.
- The nurse begins a care plan by first addressing the nursing diagnoses that have the highest priority.
- The care plan is a guideline for patient care so that all members of the health care team can quickly understand the care given.
- A concept map organizes and links data about a patient's multiple diagnoses in a logical way.

- There are three types of nursing interventions: nurse-initiated, physician-initiated, and collaborative.
- The Nursing Interventions Classification (NIC) is a comprehensive standardized classification of the interventions that nurses use in the care of patients.
- Direct care interventions include activities of daily living, instrumental activities of daily living, physical care, counseling, teaching, controlling for adverse reactions, lifesaving measures, and preventive measures.
- Evaluation determines a patient's response to nursing actions and whether goals have been met.
- You evaluate by comparing the patient's response to nursing actions with expected outcomes established during planning.
- When goals of care are not met, you identify factors that interfere with goal achievement, reassess the patient's condition, revise existing or develop new nursing diagnoses, and select appropriate interventions.

CRITICAL THINKING EXERCISES

Rich takes time to talk with Mr. Tillman and learns that he has been experiencing headaches for over 2 weeks and has difficulty falling asleep at night. Since taking on more responsibility for household chores, Mr. Tillman has little time for playing golf with friends. Mr. Tillman worries about whether he will be able to support his wife as her cancer progresses. Rich notices frustration in Mr. Tillman's tone of voice. Mr. Tillman tells Rich, "I love my wife very much. I just think she will need a lot of care".

1. Identify the cues from which Rich infers that Mr. Tillman has a problem related to stress.
2. Identify a nursing diagnostic label appropriate to Mr. Tillman's situation and data that support this diagnosis.
3. What additional information do you need to determine the related factor for the diagnosis?
4. Is there any indication there might be another nursing diagnosis applicable to Mr. Tillman? Explain.

⊖volve   *Answers to Critical Thinking Questions can be found on the Evolve website.*

REVIEW QUESTIONS

1. A patient tells the nurse, "I have had this dull ache in my side now for 4 days; it really hurts when I bend over." The nurse responds, "Uh-huh—go on." The nurse's response is an example of:
   1. Inference
   2. A cue
   3. Back-channeling
   4. Open-ended question
2. A patient has a pressure ulcer resulting from urine incontinence and sustained pressure over her coccyx. The nursing plan of care includes a goal of "Pressure ulcer will heal in 3 weeks." Which of the following is an evaluative measure for this goal?
   1. Turn patient every 90 minutes.
   2. Measure the diameter of the ulcer.
   3. Measure the color of the patient's urine.
   4. Determine patient's report of discomfort during turning.
3. A nurse has been interviewing a newly assigned patient. The cues from the assessment suggest that the patient has

had a problem with breathing. The nurse does not validate the findings by doing a physical examination. This is an example of what type of error?
   1. Error in data clustering
   2. Error in data collection
   3. Error in diagnostic statement
   4. Error in interpretation and analysis
4. Roberta is a nursing student reporting off at the end of her shift to John, an RN. Roberta tells John that her patient has a priority nursing diagnosis of pain. She tells John that the last time the ordered analgesic was given was 2 hours ago. The patient continues to report pain at a level of 4. Roberta also tried repositioning and distraction to reduce the patient's discomfort. Roberta has observed her patient grimace while turning. What expected outcome measure did Roberta report to John?
   1. Administration of the analgesic as ordered
   2. The use of distraction as a pain-relief measure
   3. The reported pain level of 4 on a scale of 0 to 10
   4. Observation of the patient grimacing during turning

5. The nurse prepares to administer care to a patient by first positioning him more comfortably. She inspects his surgical wound and reinforces the dressing with extra tape. The nurse explains the procedure she will use for insertion of a urinary catheter. She prepares the patient and inserts the catheter. Which of the following steps was a dependent nursing intervention?

   1. Insertion of the urinary catheter
   2. Reinforcement of dressing with tape
   3. Instruction about the procedure for insertion of the urinary catheter
   4. Positioning the patient for comfort.

6. A nursing student completes an assessment of a patient who just returned from a diagnostic procedure. The patient's blood pressure is 92/70 mm Hg, and the patient reports feeling dizzy. The student goes to the medical record to learn what the patient's blood pressure and symptoms were before the diagnostic test. The nursing student's review of the medical record for data is an example of:

   1. Validation
   2. Data analysis
   3. Consultation
   4. Outcome measurement

7. Mrs. Weber is a 52-year-old patient who is facing reconstructive breast surgery. She has not had surgery in the past and is asking questions of the nurses in the outpatient surgery center. Mrs. Weber tells the nurse she would like to know more about what to expect. The nurse identifies the nursing diagnosis of *readiness for enhanced knowledge related to planned surgery*. An example of a goal for this diagnosis would be:

   1. Provide instruction on routine postoperative monitoring
   2. Perform vital sign measurement every hour following surgery
   3. Patient identifies reason for vital sign monitoring following surgery
   4. By day of surgery, patient understands the routine monitoring protocol following surgery

Answers to Review Questions can be found on pages 1197-1198.

REFERENCES

American Nurses Association: *Nursing: a social policy statement*, ed 2, Washington, DC, 2003, The Association.

American Nurses Association: *Principles for delegation*, http://www.safestaffingsaveslives.org//WhatisSafeStaffing/SafeStaffingPrinciples/PrinciplesforDelegationhtml.aspx, accessed September 13, 2008.

Bulechek GM and others, editors: *Nursing interventions classification (NIC)*, ed 5, St. Louis, 2008, Mosby.

Carpenito-Moyet LJ: *Nursing diagnosis: application to clinical practice*, ed 12, Philadelphia, 2008, Lippincott Williams & Wilkins.

Dochterman JM, Jones, DA: *Unifying nursing languages: the harmonization of NANDA, NIC, NOC*, Washington, DC, 2003, American Nurses Association.

Doka K: Ethics, end-of-life decisions and grief, *Mortality* 10(1):83, 2005.

Espinosa-Aguilar A and others: Design and validation of a critical pathway for hospital management of patients with severe traumatic brain injury, *J Trauma* 64(5):1327, 2008.

Ferrario C: Developing clinical reasoning strategies: cognitive shortcuts, *J Nurses Staff Dev* 20(5):229, 2004.

Gerontological Nursing Intervention Research Center: *Evidence-based guidelines*, University of Iowa, http://www.nursing.uiowa.edu/excellence/nursing_intervention, accessed September 5, 2008.

Gordon M: *Nursing diagnosis: process and application*, ed 3, St. Louis, 1994, Mosby.

Harpaz I, Balik C, Ehrenfeld M: Concept mapping: an educational strategy for advancing nursing education, *Nurs Forum* 39(2):27, 2004.

Hickey P: *Nursing process handbook*, St. Louis, 1990, Mosby.

Hicks-Moore SL, Pastirik PJ: Evaluating critical thinking in clinical concept maps: a pilot study, *Int J Nurs Educ Scholarsh* 3(1):Article 27, 2006.

Hill CM: Integrating clinical experiences into the concept mapping process, *Nurse Educ* 31(1):36, 2006.

HIPAAdvisory: *OCR guidance explaining significant aspects of the privacy rule*, 2003, http://www.hipaadvisory.com/regs/finalprivacymod/guidance.htm.

Iowa Intervention Project: The NIC taxonomy structure, *Image J Nurs Sch* 25:1816, 1993.

Kilkus S: Complementary and alternative therapies. In Potter PA, Perry AG: *Fundamental of Nursing*, ed 7, St. Louis, 2009, Mosby.

Kim MJ, McFarland GK, McLean AM, editors: *Classification of nursing diagnoses: proceedings of the fifth conference (NANDA)*, St. Louis, 1984, Mosby.

Melnyk BM, Fineout-Overholt E: *Evidence-based practice in nursing and healthcare*, Philadelphia, 2005, Lippincott Williams & Wilkins.

Moody LE and others: Electronic health records documentation in nursing, *Comput Nurs* 22(6):337, 2004.

Moorhead S and others, editors: *Nursing outcomes classification (NOC)*, ed 4, St. Louis, 2008, Mosby.

NANDA International: *NANDA International nursing diagnoses: definitions and classifications, 2009-2011*, Oxford, UK, 2009, Wiley-Blackwell.

National Guideline Clearinghouse: *NGC-Clinical practice guidelines*, Agency for Healthcare Research and Quality, last modified May 18, 2009, http://www.guideline.gov, accessed May 23, 2009.

Pender NJ, Murdaugh CL, Parsons MA: *Health promotion in nursing practice*, ed 6, Upper Saddle River, NJ, 2006, Pearson Prentice-Hall.

Redman BK: *The practice of patient education*, ed 10, St. Louis, 2005, Mosby.

Seidel HM and others: *Mosby's guide to physical examination*, ed 6, St. Louis, 2006, Mosby.

Weiner J, Roth J: Avoiding iatrogenic harm to patient and family while discussing goals of care near end of life, *J Palliat Med* 9(2):451, 2006.

Whitecar P, Maxwell T, Douglas A: Principles of palliative care medicine. II. Pain and symptom management, *Adv Studies Med* 4(2):88, 2004.

Wieck KL: Diagnostic language consistency among multicultural English-speaking nurses, *Nurs Diagn* 7(2):70, 1996.

Informatics and Documentation

MEDIA RESOURCES

CD COMPANION   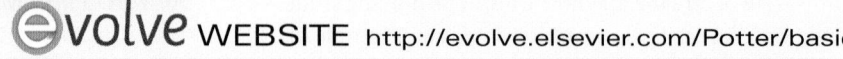 **WEBSITE** http://evolve.elsevier.com/Potter/basic

- Crossword Puzzle
- English/Spanish Audio Glossary

OBJECTIVES

- Identify key reasons for reporting and recording patient care.
- Describe guidelines for effective documentation and reporting in a variety of health care settings.
- Describe methods for multidisciplinary communication within the health care team.
- Compare different methods used in documentation.
- Discuss the advantages of using a critical path as a documentation tool.

- Identify common record-keeping forms.
- Discuss advantages and disadvantages of standardized documentation forms.
- Discuss advantages of computerized documentation.
- Discuss the relationship between informatics and quality health care.

KEY TERMS

accreditation, p. 144
acuity recording, p. 151
case management plan, p. 150
change-of-shift report, p. 153
charting by exception (CBE), p. 150
computerized provider order entry (CPOE), p. 160

diagnosis-related groups (DRGs), p. 146
documentation, p. 143
electronic health record (EHR), p. 160
firewall, p. 159
flow sheets, p. 151
focus charting, p. 150
graphic records, p. 151
hand-off report, p. 153
health care information system (HIS), p. 156

incident (occurrence) report, p. 155
informatics, p. 155
information technology (IT), p. 156
interdisciplinary care plan, p. 149
Kardex, p. 151
nursing informatics, p. 156

password, p. 159
PIE note, p. 150
problem-oriented medical record (POMR), p. 148
record, p. 144
reports, p. 144
SOAP note, p. 149
transfer report, p. 154
variances, p. 151

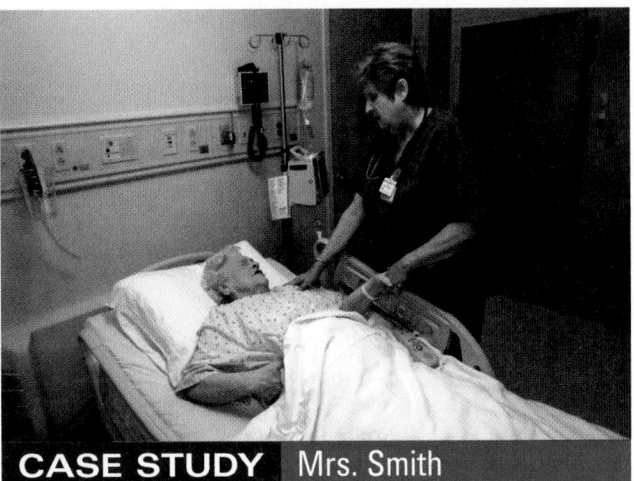

CASE STUDY Mrs. Smith

Mrs. Smith is a 93-year-old patient with a history of heart disease and chronic back pain. She lives alone and cares for her own needs around the house. She typically deals with her back pain by going to a chiropractor. However, recently the pain has gotten more severe and not resolved with the usual treatments. Today she awoke unable to get out of bed. She called the local ambulance, which took her to the emergency department. After receiving intravenous pain medication, she was admitted to the medical unit for further evaluation of her back pain, which she rated a 10 on scale of 0 to 10. After undergoing some diagnostic tests, it was determined she had fractures in her lower spine that were the result of severe osteoarthritis and could be treated with surgery. While completing Mrs. Smith's admission history, you find out that she had a total knee replacement 3 years ago and pain was not well controlled at that time. She returned to the medical unit after the operation. Both physical therapy and nursing were active in establishing a plan of care that would promote the same level of independence she had before this hospitalization.

Documentation is a vital aspect of nursing practice. It is defined as anything written or printed within a patient record, which may be either paper, electronic, or a combination of both formats. The information you communicate about patient care reflects the quality of your care and provides accountability for each health care team member's care. The patient record provides evidence for credentialing, research, and reimbursement, as well as providing a database for planning health care (American Nurses Association [ANA], 2005). You document in the medical record the expected outcomes and the nursing care you provide for a patient (e.g., assessments and interventions).

The health care environment creates many challenges for accurately documenting and reporting the care delivered to patients. The quality of nursing care depends on your ability to communicate effectively verbally and in writing, and you are held accountable for the accuracy of documentation you enter into the patient's record. Regulations from agencies such as The Joint Commission and the Centers for Medicare and Medicaid Services (CMS) require health care institutions to monitor and evaluate the quality and appropriateness of patient care (ANA, 2005) (see Chapters 2 and 6). Typically, such monitoring and evaluation occur through the auditing of information health care providers document in patient records. As of October 1, 2008, Medicare no longer reimburses hospitals for certain preventable conditions, such as hospital-acquired infections, such as a urinary tract infection from catheterization (Arias, 2008). Thus it becomes even more important that your documentation accurately reflect the current status of the patient, especially upon admission, transfer, or discharge.

CONFIDENTIALITY

Do not disclose information about patients' status to other patients, family members (unless granted by the patient), or to health care staff not involved in their care. Legal and ethical obligations require you to keep information about patients strictly confidential. In 2003 legislation to protect patient privacy for health information in the form of the Health Insurance Portability and Accountability Act (HIPAA) was finalized (U.S. Department of Health and Human Services [USDHHS], 2003). This legislation governs all areas of health information management, including reimbursement, medical record coding, security, and patient record management. Previously the rule required written consent for disclosure of all patient information. Under new regulations, in order to eliminate barriers that could delay access to care, providers are required only to notify patients of their privacy policy and to make a reasonable effort to get written acknowledgment of this notification. As a result, patients have more control over their personal health care information and who has access to this information (USDHHS, 2003).

Sometimes you have a reason for using health care records for data gathering, research, or continuing education. This is permitted if you use the records as specified and permission is granted. When you are a student in a clinical setting, confidentiality and compliance with HIPAA legislation are part of professional practice. You may review the medical record only for information needed to provide safe, efficient care. For example, when you are assigned to provide complete care for a patient, you need to review the current medical record and plan of care. However, you do not share this information with other classmates. In addition, never access the medical records of other patients on the specific clinical care area. Access to electronic health records is traced through the user login information. Not only is it unethical to view medical records of other patients, but breaches of confidentiality can lead to disciplinary action by employers and even possible dismissal from work. To further maintain confidentiality and protect patient privacy, make sure written materials used in your student clinical practice do not have patient identifiers, such as room number, date of birth, medical record number, or other identifiable demographic information (Wimberley and others, 2005). Never print material from the electronic health record for personal use.

STANDARDS

Within a health care organization there are standards that govern the type of information you document and to which you are accountable. Institutional standards or policies often dictate the frequency of documentation, such as how often you record a nursing assessment or a patient's level of pain. Know the standards of your health care organization to ensure complete and accurate documentation. Nurses are expected to meet the standard of care for every nursing task they perform. Patient records can be used as evidence in a court of law if standards are not met (ANA, 2005).

In addition, your documentation needs to conform to the standards of the National Committee for Quality Assurance (NCQA) and accrediting bodies such as The Joint Commission to maintain institutional **accreditation** to minimize liability. Usually an organization incorporates accreditation standards into its policies and revises documentation forms to suit those standards. Current documentation standards require that all patients admitted to a health care facility have an assessment of physical, psychosocial, environmental, self-care, knowledge level, and discharge planning needs. The Joint Commission standards require that your documentation be within the context of the nursing process, including evidence of patient and family teaching and discharge planning (The Joint Commission [TJC], 2008b). Other standards, such as HIPAA, include those directed by state and federal regulatory agencies and are enforced through the Department of Justice, and the CMS (ANA, 2005).

MULTIDISCIPLINARY COMMUNICATION WITHIN THE HEALTH CARE TEAM

Patient care requires effective communication among all members of the health care team. The typical patient has many caregivers, including nurses, physicians, nursing assistive personnel, and therapists. A documentation system that reflects multidisciplinary plans of care for a patient provides continuity of care. Because large multidisciplinary teams usually care for patients, accurate documentation is needed to protect patients from fragmented and possibly dangerous care (Mosby, 2006). Thus the overall purpose of the medical record is to ensure all health team members are working toward a common goal of providing safe, effective, continuity of care.

Effective communication takes place along two approaches, the patient's record and reports. A patient's **record** or chart is a confidential, permanent legal documentation of information relevant to that patient's health care. Information about the patient's health care is recorded after each patient contact. The record is a continuing account of the patient's health care status and is available to all members of the health care team.

Each patient record includes the following:

- Patient identification and demographic data
- Admission data
- A signed consent for treatment
- Physician's or health care provider's orders
- Medical history and physical examination
- Nurses' documentation of ongoing assessments, a plan of care, interventions, and evaluation
- Medication records
- Progress notes from health care provider's, such as physicians, advanced practice nurses, respiratory therapists and physical therapists
- Results of diagnostic and therapeutic tests and procedures
- Advance directives, as needed
- Discharge plan and summary information (TJC, 2008b)

Reports are oral, written, or audiotaped exchanges of information between members of the health care team. Common reports given by nurses include change-of-shift reports, telephone reports, transfer reports, and incident reports. A physician or health care provider may call a nursing unit to receive a verbal report on a patient's condition and progress. The laboratory submits a written report providing the results of diagnostic tests. A transfer report informs the staff of a receiving health care setting about the type of care a patient will require.

PURPOSE OF RECORDS

The medical record is the only permanent record documenting patient care from admission to discharge. Documentation serves multiple purposes, including communication, legal documentation, reimbursement, education, research, and auditing and monitoring (ANA, 2005). The patient is the focus of all documentation (Hafernick, 2007).

Communication

The record is a way for health care team members to provide continuity of care and to communicate patient needs and progress toward meeting desired patient outcomes. The record includes the patient's responses to interventions and changes made in the plan of care. The record is the most current and accurate source of information about a patient's health care status. The information communicated in a record prepares you to know a patient thoroughly so that you can make timely and appropriate care decisions. Base your communication on your assessment findings. It is best to document at the same time as the intervention or as close to it as possible (Austin, 2006).

Legal Documentation

Because jurors usually rely on information documented in the medical record to determine what patient care was provided, effective documentation is one of the best defenses for legal claims associated with health care (Table 9-1) (Mosby,

TABLE 9-1 Legal Guidelines for Recording

GUIDELINES	RATIONALE	CORRECT ACTION
Do not erase, apply correction fluid, or scratch out errors made while recording.	Charting becomes illegible: it may appear as if you were attempting to hide information or deface record.	Draw single line through error, write word *error* above it, and sign your name or initials. Then record note correctly. Check agency policy (Monarch, 2007).
Do not write retaliatory or critical comments about patient or care by other health care professionals.	Statements can be used as evidence for nonprofessional behavior or poor quality of care.	Enter only objective descriptions of patient's behavior; patient comments should be quoted (Monarch, 2007).
Need to add additional patient information.	New information is acquired.	If additional information is to be added to an existing entry, write the date and time of the new entry on the next available space and include "Addendum to note of [date and time of prior note]" (Mosby, 2006).
	Forgot to chart during a shift.	Write the current date and time in the next available space, and write "Late entry for [date and time/shift missed]" (Mosby, 2006).
Correct all errors promptly.	Errors in recording can lead to errors in treatment.	Avoid rushing to complete charting; be sure information is accurate.
Record all facts.	Record must be accurate and reliable.	Be certain entry is factual; do not speculate or guess (Monarch, 2007).
Do not leave blank spaces in nurses' notes.	Another person can add incorrect information in space.	Chart consecutively, line by line; if space is left, draw line horizontally through it and sign your name at end.
Record all entries legibly and in black ink.	Illegible entries can be misinterpreted, causing errors and lawsuits; ink cannot be erased; black ink is more legible when records are photocopied or transferred to microfilm.	Never erase entries or use correction fluid, and never use pencil or pens with erasable ink.
If order is questioned, record that clarification was sought.	If you perform an order known to be incorrect, you are just as liable for prosecution as the physician or health care provider is.	Do not record "physician made error." Instead, chart that "Dr. Smith was called to clarify order for analgesic" (Monarch, 2007).
Chart only for yourself.	You are accountable for information you enter into chart.	Never chart for someone else. **Exception:** If caregiver has left unit for day and calls with information that needs to be documented, include the name of the source of information in the entry and include that the information was provided via telephone.
Avoid using generalized, empty phrases such as "status unchanged" or "had good day."	Specific information about patient's condition or case can be accidentally deleted if information is too generalized.	Use complete, concise descriptions of care.
Begin each entry with date and time, and end with your signature and title.	This guideline ensures that correct sequence of events is recorded; signature documents who is accountable for care delivered.	Do not wait until end of shift to record important changes that occurred several hours earlier; be sure to sign each entry (McGeehan, 2007).
For computer documentation keep your password to yourself.	Maintains security and confidentiality.	Once logged onto the computer, do not leave the computer screen unattended and log out when you are done charting (Mosby, 2006).

2006). To limit nursing liability, your documentation must follow organizational standards for documentation, which include a clear indication of the individualized and goal-directed nursing care you provide (ANA, 2005). The best way to ensure documentation meets legal standards is to record information as you provide care. This increases the likelihood that your documentation is accurate and most current. It is important to avoid recording information that is routine, superficial, or not relevant.

Reimbursement

Charting also determines the amount of reimbursement a health care agency receives. **Diagnosis-related groups (DRGs)** are the basis for establishing reimbursement for patient care. A DRG is a classification based on patients' medical diagnoses. Under the prospective payment system, Medicare reimburses hospitals a set dollar amount for each DRG (see Chapter 2). Your nursing documentation verifies specific nursing care provided and thus supports the reimbursement your health care agency receives (ANA, 2005).

The patient's medical record is also audited to review financial charges of equipment and services used in the patient's care. Private insurance carriers and auditors from federal agencies review records to determine the reimbursement that a patient or a health care agency receives. Insurance companies do not reimburse for unskilled nursing care. They pay only for skilled medical and nursing care. Timely and accurate documentation of supplies and equipment used helps determine the patient's financial charges.

Education

A patient's record contains a variety of information (e.g., medical and nursing diagnoses, signs and symptoms of disease, successful and unsuccessful therapies, diagnostic findings, and patient behaviors). Reading the patient care record is an effective way to learn the nature of an illness and the patient's response to the illness. Review of patients with similar medical problems allows you to identify patterns and trends. Such information builds your clinical knowledge. As you identify patterns associated with specific diseases and conditions, you are able to anticipate the type of care your patient will require.

Research

Statistical data are important elements of patient records, including the frequency of clinical disorders, complications, use of specific medical and nursing therapies, recoveries from illness, and mortality. After obtaining appropriate agency approvals, a nurse researcher review patients' records in a research study to collect information on a particular health problem. Analysis of the data collected contributes to evidence-based nursing practice and quality health care (ANA, 2005). For example, if a nurse researcher suspects that early ambulation decreases the complication rate in postoperative patients, the researcher reviews the records of select surgical patients to compare the rates of postoperative complications with early versus late ambulation.

Auditing and Monitoring

The Joint Commission (2008b) requires hospitals to establish performance improvement programs to conduct objective, ongoing reviews of patient care and asks institutions to establish standards for quality care. Audits help to determine whether standards of care are met. Audits assess the standard of records and identify areas for improvement and staff development (McGeehan, 2007). For example, nurses may monitor records to determine their success in documenting institution of fall precautions or evaluation of pain measures. The nurses then share any deficiencies identified during monitoring with all members of the nursing staff so that corrections in policy or practice can be made. Performance improvement programs keep you informed of the extent to which you meet standards of nursing practice (ANA, 2005) (see Chapter 2).

GUIDELINES FOR QUALITY DOCUMENTATION AND REPORTING

High-quality documentation and reporting are necessary to enhance efficient, safe, individualized patient care. Documentation systems must ensure the security and confidentiality of patient information at all times (ANA, 2005). Accurate, consistent, and complete documentation is one of the best defenses of legal claims associated with nursing care. Documentation must reflect patient responses and outcomes related to nursing care received, be timely and sequential, be retrievable on a permanent basis, and have the ability to be audited (ANA, 2005; Austin, 2006; Ferrell, 2007; Monarch, 2007). Problems arise when a record is reviewed in a malpractice suit and there are time gaps, information is squeezed between lines or crossed out, or key facts were omitted (Austin, 2006).

In some settings, agency policy requires a registered nurse to cosign documentation completed by licensed practical or vocational nurses, students, or assistive personnel. A cosignature indicates that the supervising nurse reviewed the record entry and was aware of the care and patient status even though others delivered the care. Nurses must assess the patient themselves and read medical record entries before cosigning another health care provider's assessment record (Monarch, 2007).

To limit liability, nursing documentation must clearly indicate that individualized, goal-directed nursing care was provided to a patient based on the nursing assessment. The record must be specific in its documentation of who did what, when, and how (Ferrell, 2007). The recorded information in the patient's record must describe exactly what happened to a patient. The best way to ensure documentation meets legal standards is to record information as you provide care (Austin, 2006; McGeehan, 2007). This increases the likelihood of your documentation being accurate and most current. Never use the record for complaining, finger-pointing, or commenting on other non–patient care issues. Only information relevant to patient care belongs in the record. High-quality documentation and reporting has five important characteristics: it is factual, accurate, complete, current, and organized.

Factual

A record contains descriptive, objective information about what you see, hear, feel, and smell. Objective data are data that are measurable and observable, such as a patient's report of pain severity on a scale of 0 to 10, the size of a wound, or a patient's pulse oximetry reading. To be factual, avoid words such as *appears, seems,* or *apparently* because they are vague and lead to conclusions that you cannot support by objective information.

The only subjective data included in a record are what the patient says. Write subjective information with quotation marks, using the patient's own words. For example, a patient's statement *"My lower back hurts"* is subjective and acceptable documentation. Another example is stated as follows: *Reports feeling a pressure in chest.* It is acceptable not to use quotation marks when you paraphrase the patient's words. When documenting subjective information, it is also important to include complementary objective findings so that your database is as descriptive as possible.

Accurate

The use of precise measurements makes documentation more accurate. For example, documenting "Voided 450 mL clear urine" is more accurate than "Voided an adequate amount." To avoid misunderstandings and promote patient safety, write out any abbreviations that are possibly confusing. The 2009 National Patient Safety Goals (NPSGs) require that health care institutions standardize abbreviations, acronyms, symbols, and dose designations throughout their system. The NPSGs also require institutions to identify a "do not use" list of abbreviations, acronyms, symbols, and dose designations (TJC, 2008c) (see Chapter 16). It is important for you to know an institution's acceptable and unacceptable abbreviation list to keep your documentation accurate and compliant with requirements. For example, the abbreviation for every day (qd) **should no longer be used.** If a treatment or medication is needed daily, the written order or care plan should use the term "daily" or "every day." The abbreviation qd (every day) can be misinterpreted to mean O.D. (right eye).

Correct spelling demonstrates a level of competency and attention to detail. Misspelled words lead to confusion. For example, often words sound the same but have different meanings, such as *accept* and *except* or *dysphagia* and *dysphasia.* Incorrect use of terms alters the intended meaning.

The Joint Commission (2008b) requires that all entries in medical records be dated and that there is a method to identify all authors of entries. Therefore any descriptive entry in a patient's record ends with the caregiver's full name and status. Occasionally you will include observations reported to another caregiver or interventions performed by someone else—for example, "Patient suctioned by Judith Hill, RN." As a nursing student, you need to enter your full name, and student nurse abbreviation, such as "Marianne Smith, SN [student nurse]." The abbreviation for *student nurse* often differs regionally, being either *NS,* which stands for *nursing student,* or *SN,* which stands for *student nurse.* The signature holds this person accountable for information recorded.

Complete

The information within a recorded entry or a report needs to be complete, containing appropriate and essential information. Criteria for thorough communication exist for certain health problems or nursing activities (Table 9-2). Make written entries in the patient's medical record, describing nursing care that you administer and the patient's response. For example:

0845 Reports continuous throbbing pain on lateral aspect of left fractured femur increased with movement of the leg with a severity of 8 (scale 0-10). B/P = 132/74, T = 37°, P = 92, R = 18. Morphine sulfate 5 mg IV given for pain. Sue Jacobs, RN.

0915 Reports pain at 2 (scale 0-10) and able to turn in bed independently. Sue Jacobs, RN.

Include routine activities such as daily hygiene measures, vital signs, and pain assessment in flow sheets or graphic records. Describe these activities in greater detail when it is relevant because of a change in functional ability or status. For example, you have a patient who has previously required a total bath and now the patient has improved and is able to wash his or her face, hands, and upper body. This warrants additional documentation.

Current

Making entries promptly is essential in effective documentation (TJC, 2008b). Delays in documentation result in serious omissions and untimely delays in patient care. To increase currency and decrease unnecessary duplication, many health care agencies keep records near the patient's bedside to facilitate immediate documentation of care activities. You need to communicate the following nursing care at the time of occurrence:

1. Vital signs
2. Pain assessment, also referred to as the fifth vital sign
3. Administration of medications and treatments
4. Preparation for diagnostic tests or surgery
5. Change in patient status and who was notified
6. Treatment for sudden changes in patient status
7. Patient response to intervention
8. Preoperative checklist
9. Admission, transfer, discharge, or death of patient

Many agencies use military time, a 24-hour time cycle. The military clock begins at 1 minute after midnight as 0001 and ends with midnight at 2400. For example, 10:22 AM is 1022 military time; 1:00 PM is 1300 military time. Figure 9-1 shows military time on a clockface.

Organized

Written communication is easier to understand when written in a logical order. For example, an organized note describes your assessment, interventions, and the patient's response in

TABLE 9-2 Examples of Criteria for Documentation and Reporting

TOPIC	CRITERIA TO DOCUMENT OR REPORT
ASSESSMENT	
Subjective data (patient behavior [e.g., anxiety, confusion, hostility])	• Description of episode in quotation marks • Onset, location, description of condition (severity, duration, frequency; precipitating, aggravating, and relieving factors) • Onset, behaviors exhibited, precipitating factors
Objective data (e.g., rash, tenderness, breath sounds)	• Onset, location, description of condition (severity, duration, frequency; precipitating, aggravating, and relieving factors)
NURSING INTERVENTIONS AND EVALUATION	
Treatments (e.g., enema, bath, dressing change)	• Time administered, equipment used (if appropriate), patient's response (objective and subjective changes) compared with previous treatment; for example, "rated pain 0 on a scale of 0 to 10 during dressing change" or "reported severe abdominal cramping during enema"

Medication administration	• Immediately after administration, document time medication given, dose, route, any preliminary assessments (e.g., pain level, vital signs), patient response or effect of medication; for example:
	  • 1500 Pain reported at 6 (scale 0-10). Tylenol 500 mg given PO
	    1530: Patient reports pain level 2 (scale 0-10)
	  • 1000: Pruritus and hives developed over lower abdomen 1 hour after penicillin was given

Patient teaching	• Information presented, method of instruction (e.g., discussion, demonstration, videotape, booklet), patient response, including questions and evidence of understanding such as return demonstration or change in behavior
Discharge planning	• Measurable patient goals or expected outcomes, progress toward goals, need for referrals

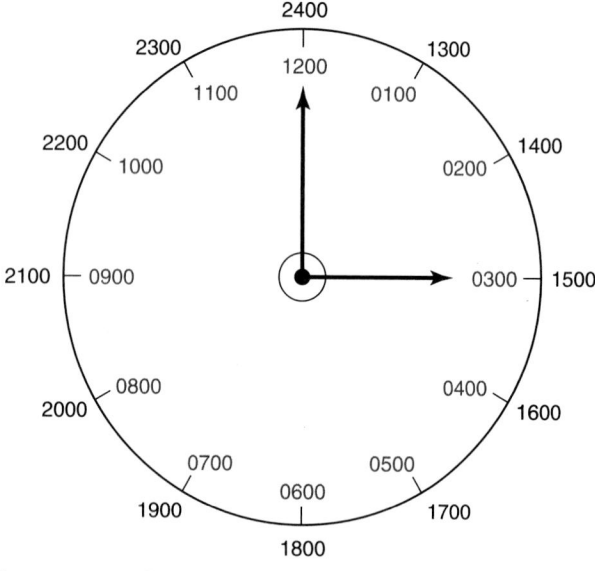

Figure 9-1 ■ Comparison of 24 hours of military time with the hourly positions on the clockface for civilian time.

a sequence. It is also more effective when notes are concise, clear, and to the point. To make clear and organized entries it is often helpful to make a list of what you need to include before beginning to write in the permanent legal record. Organizing your information into categories minimizes frustration in trying to recall patient care activities provided. Suggested categories include what the patient tells you directly or from indirect sources if the patient is incapacitated; what you

assess; what you do, including interventions performed in response to assessment findings; and what you teach to the patient and family (Mosby, 2006). Applying the nursing process gives logic and order to nursing documentation.

METHODS OF DOCUMENTATION

The documentation system selected by a nursing service reflects the philosophy of the department. Staff use the same documentation system throughout an agency. There are several acceptable methods for recording health care information (Table 9-3).

Problem-Oriented Medical Records

The **problem-oriented medical record (POMR)** is a structured method of documentation that emphasizes the patient's problems. The method is organized in a way to correspond to the nursing process and facilitates communication of patient needs. Organization of data is by problem or diagnosis. Ideally, each member of the health care team contributes to a single list of identified patient problems. The POMR has the following major sections: database, problem list, initial care plan, discharge summary, and progress notes.

DATABASE The database contains all available assessment information pertaining to the patient. This section is the foundation for identifying patient problems and planning care. The database remains active and current, and you make revisions as new data are available.

PROBLEM LIST The problem list is developed after a review of the patient data. You identify priority problems, and

TABLE 9-3 Formats for Documenting

Case study continuation: You need to record the information obtained from Mrs. Smith during the admission process. The following shows examples of various formats.

Narrative note	Stated: "I'm dreading surgery. Last time I had such pain when I got out of bed." Discussed alternatives for pain control and importance of postoperative activity. Encouraged to ask for pain medication before pain is severe. Stated: "I feel better prepared now." Able to verbalize that activity enhances circulation and healing.
SOAP	*S* (subjective data): "I'm dreading surgery. Last time I had such pain when I got out of bed." *O* (objective data): Noted muscle tension and loud voice. *A* (assessment/analysis): Fear of postoperative pain. *P* (plan): Assess pain level every 2 hours. Provide comfort measures, and give analgesics as needed.
PIE charting	*P* (problem): "I'm dreading surgery. Last time I had such pain when I got out of bed." *I* (intervention): Discussed alternatives for pain control and importance of postoperative activity. Encouraged to ask for pain medication before pain is severe. *E* (evaluation): "I feel better prepared now." Able to verbalize that activity enhances circulation and healing.
Focus charting	*D* (data): "I'm dreading surgery. Last time I had such pain when I got out of bed." *A* (action): Discussed alternatives for pain control and importance of postoperative activity. Encouraged to ask for pain medication before pain is severe. *R* (response): "I feel better prepared now." Able to verbalize that activity enhances circulation and healing. NOTE: Some agencies add *P* (plan). Example: *P* (plan): Assess pain level every 2 hours. Provide comfort measures, and give analgesics as needed.

list all problems in chronological order to serve as an organizing guide for the patient's care. Add new problems to the list as you identify them on the basis of your ongoing nursing assessment. After you have resolved a problem, record the data, and draw a line through the problem and its number.

CARE PLAN The Joint Commission standards (2008b) require that a care plan, also called a "plan of care," be developed for all patients on admission to acute, subacute, rehabilitation, or extended care agencies. Disciplines involved in the patient's care develop a care plan, sometimes referred to as an **interdisciplinary care plan,** for each problem listed. For example, a physical therapist communicates a plan for increasing a patient's ambulation, while a speech therapist communicates a plan to improve the patient's swallowing. Nurses document a plan of care in a variety of formats. Generally these plans of care include nursing diagnoses, expected outcomes, and interventions (see Chapter 8).

PROGRESS NOTES Health care team members use progress notes to monitor and record the progress of a patient's problems. Narrative notes, flow sheets, discharge summaries, and structured notes are formats you use to document the patient's progress.

Narrative Documentation Narrative documentation is the traditional method for recording nursing care. However, in many settings other methods have replaced narrative charting. Narrative charting uses a storylike format to document information specific to patient conditions and nursing care. Narrative charting is beneficial in emergency situations in which a chronological order of events is important. However, narrative charting does have some disadvantages, including the tendency to be repetitive and time consuming, and it requires the reader to sort through much information to locate the desired patient information (Hafernick, 2007) (see Table 9-3).

Discharge Summary Forms There is much emphasis placed on preparing a patient for a timely discharge from a health care institution. Ideally, you begin discharge planning on admission and in some cases even before admission, as is necessary with same-day surgery admissions and childbirth. When doing discharge planning, be responsive to changes in the patient's condition and involve the patient and family in the discharge planning process (see Chapter 2).

The primary goal of a discharge summary is to ensure the continuity of care, whether the patient is going home or transferring to another institution. A nursing discharge note needs to cover the care delivered and changes in patient status while in the hospital, the patient status at discharge, and recommendations for continuing care (Helleso, 2006). The Joint Commission specifies what is to be included in a concise discharge summary note. You will need to include the reason for hospitalization; the care, treatment, and services provided; the patient's condition at discharge; and information provided to the patient and family, such as discharge instructions or referrals made (TJC, 2008b). Discharge summary forms make the summary concise and instructive. Many forms include copies that you give to the patient, family members, or home care nurses. Discharge summaries involve multiple disciplines and help to ensure that your patient leaves the hospital in a timely manner with the appropriate health care resources (Box 9-1).

SOAP Documentation One format for entering a progress note is the **SOAP note.** SOAP is an acronym for the following:

S: Subjective data (verbalizations of the patient)
O: Objective data (data that are measured and observed)
A: Assessment (diagnosis based on the subjective and objective data)
P: Plan (what the caregiver plans to do)

An *I* and *E* are sometimes added (i.e., SOAPIE) in various institutions. The *I* stands for *intervention,* and the *E* represents *evaluation.* The logic for SOAP(IE) notes is similar to

BOX 9-1 Discharge Summary Information

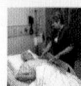
Mrs. Smith has been discharged by her physician. The following are some of the key points that you will want to consider in providing discharge information.

- Use clear, concise descriptions using words Mrs. Smith understands.
- Provide step-by-step description of how to perform a procedure (e.g., home medication administration).
- Reinforce explanation with printed instructions.
- Identify precautions to follow when performing self-care or administering medications.
- Review signs and symptoms of complications the patient needs to report to her health care provider.
- Obtain feedback from Mrs. Smith regarding discharge instructions.
- List names and phone numbers of health care providers and community resources for Mrs. Smith to contact.
- Identify any unresolved problem, including plans for follow-up and continuous treatment.
- List actual time of discharge, mode of transportation, and who accompanied Mrs. Smith.
- Document the patient encounter accordingly.

Example of a sample discharge note: Instructed when to return to the physician for follow-up care, restrictions on how much to lift at home (no more than 10 lb), and how to best manage her pain at home. Verbalized understanding of the need to be watchful of lifting techniques, as well as the prescribed pain medication action, side effects, and how often she could take the medication. Informed to notify the doctor if the pain does not subside with the prescribed pain medication dosage. Discharged via wheelchair at 1440 accompanied by daughter-in-law.

---

that of the nursing process: Collect data about each of your patient's problems, draw conclusions, and develop a plan of care. Number each SOAP note, and title it according to the problem on the list (see Table 9-3).

PIE Documentation The **PIE note** documentation format is similar to SOAP charting in its problem-oriented nature. However, it differs from the SOAP method in that PIE charting has a nursing origin, whereas SOAP originated from the medical model. PIE is an acronym for *problem, interventions, evaluation* as follows (see Table 9-3, p. 149):

P: Problem or nursing diagnosis applicable to patient
I: Interventions or actions taken
E: Evaluation of the outcomes of nursing interventions

The PIE format simplifies documentation by unifying the care plan and progress notes into a complete record. The PIE format also differs from SOAP because the narrative note does not include assessment information. Your daily assessment data appear on special flow sheets, thus preventing duplication of information. You number or label the PIE notes according to the patient's problems. Then, once a patient's problem becomes resolved, you drop the problem from daily documentation. Continuing problems are documented daily.

Focus Charting A third narrative format is **focus charting.** It is a unique narrative format in that it places less emphasis on patient problems and instead focuses on patient concerns such as a sign or symptom, a condition, a behavior, or a significant event. Each entry includes data, actions, and patient response (DAR) for the particular patient situation. Focus charting combines a shorthand approach to documenting normal assessments and routine care with a concise longhand method for documenting exceptions to predetermined norms. In addition, focus charting saves time because it is easy for multiple caregivers to understand, it is adaptable to most health care settings, and it enables all caregivers to track the patient's condition and progress toward the outcomes of care. A disadvantage of focus charting is that it can be challenging to write accurate logical notes (Mosby, 2006) (see Table 9-3, p. 149).

Charting by Exception

Charting by exception (CBE) is an innovative approach to reduce the time required to complete documentation. In a CBE system, an agency defines criteria for nursing assessments and standards of practice for nursing interventions. Thus CBE simply involves completing a flow sheet that incorporates those standard assessment criteria and interventions. As a result, you use a check mark on the flow sheet to indicate normal findings or routine interventions. You write narrative information only if abnormal findings, or variances in the use of interventions occur (Childers, 2005). You can create problems if you chart normal findings along with the exceptions (Austin, 2006). Therefore, by following the agency standards for charting in the CBE system, when you see any entries in the chart, you know that something out of the ordinary has occurred. This makes it easier to track unexpected changes in a patient's condition as they develop.

Case Management Plan and Critical Pathways

The **case management plan** of delivering care uses a multidisciplinary approach to documenting patient care and focuses on providing quality care in a cost-effective manner (Hafernick, 2007). Critical pathways have multiple aims, including standardizing practice and improving multidisciplinary coordination (Hunter and Segrott, 2008). The concept refers to specific guidelines for care that describe patient treatment goals and outline the sequence and timing of interventions for meeting the goals efficiently (El Baz and others, 2007). They are usually organized according to categories, such as activity, diet, treatments, protocols, and discharge planning. Critical pathways are also referred to as clinical pathways, integrated care pathways, care maps, or care paths (El Baz and others, 2007). Whatever the label, the pathway provides a summary of the standardized plan of care within a case management plan.

Advantages of case management plans include the ability for various health care team members to note variances in care, to establish outcomes, to identify potential problems, to specify standards from the patient perspective, and to know what to expect. Disadvantages focus on the need for acceptance of the recording form by all health care providers and individuals knowledgeable in the process to develop pathways (Hafernick, 2007).

Because of the nature of human response, there are **variances** in patient outcomes when the patient deviates from the critical path plan. These variances are deviations or detours from the pathway and refer to either positive or negative changes, depending on the clinical situation. A positive variance occurs when a patient progresses more rapidly than the case management plan expected (e.g., discontinuation of a nasogastric tube a day early). A negative variance occurs when the activities on the clinical pathway do not occur as predicted or the patient does not meet the expected outcomes. An example of a negative variance is the addition of oxygen therapy for a patient experiencing breathing problems following surgery. Your responsibility is to determine why the problem arose and to implement changes to eliminate the variance or to justify the actions taken to manage the critical path deviation.

COMMON RECORD-KEEPING FORMS

The patient chart includes a variety of forms to make documentation easy, quick, and comprehensive. When possible, avoid duplication within the record.

Admission Nursing History Forms

Admission nursing history forms provide baseline data for later comparisons with changes in the patient's condition. The form allows the admitting nurse to make a thorough assessment (e.g., biographical data, physical and psychosocial/cultural assessment, and review of health risk factors) and to identify relevant nursing diagnoses or problems for the patient's care plan. Each institution designs nursing history forms based on its standards of practice and philosophy of nursing care.

Flow Sheets and Graphic Records

Flow sheets and **graphic records** allow documentation of certain routine observations or specific measurements made repeatedly, such as height and weight and activities of daily living such as the bath, vital signs, pain assessment, and intake and output. Flow sheets provide a quick and easy reference for assessing changes in a patient's status. Critical care units commonly use flow sheets for many types of data. Flow sheets are an effective way to record information so that you are able to observe trends over time. Flow sheets are part of the permanent record. Figure 9-2 is an example of a nursing assessment flow sheet.

When documenting a significant change on a flow sheet, you describe the change in the progress notes and describe nursing measures implemented in response to the change. For example, if a patient's blood pressure becomes dangerously high, record in the progress note the blood pressure; related assessments, such as flushing and headache; and the medication administered to lower the pressure. Also, include evaluation of the interventions, for example, serial blood pressure and other pertinent evaluation measures.

Patient Care Summary or Kardex

Many hospitals now have computerized systems that provide certain basic information in the form of a patient care summary. This summary prints for each patient during each shift. Data automatically update as orders enter the system and as nurses make decisions. In some settings a **Kardex** (flip-over card file) kept at the nurses' station provides information for the daily care of a patient. It often has two parts: an activity and treatment section and a nursing care plan section. The updated information in the Kardex eliminates the need for you to refer repeatedly to the patient's chart. Information commonly found in the Kardex or patient care summary includes the following:

1. Basic demographic data (name, age, sex)
2. Primary medical diagnosis and significant medical history
3. Current health care provider's orders (e.g., diet, activity, vital signs, blood tests, diagnostic tests)
4. A nursing care plan or plan of care
5. Nursing orders or nursing interventions (e.g., intake and output, positioning, comfort measures, fall prevention, teaching)
6. Scheduled tests and procedures
7. Safety precautions used in the patient's care
8. Factors related to activities of daily living
9. Nearest relative/guardian or person to contact in an emergency
10. Emergency code status (e.g., "do not resuscitate" order)
11. Allergies

Acuity Recording

An **acuity recording** system determines the hours of care for a nursing unit and the number of staff required to care for a given group of patients. Each morning staff nurses are typically required to enter the acuity scores of each of their patients into a computerized documentation system. Managerial and administrative staff gather the acuity data electronically to make staffing decisions. For example, an acuity system rates a patient's activity from 1 to 5 (1 requires the most time, 5 requires the least amount of time). A patient returning from surgery who requires many assessments and interventions rates as an acuity level 2. On the same continuum, another patient awaiting discharge after a very successful recovery from surgery rates as an acuity level 5. Managers then determine staffing assignments by examining the total acuity points of the patients on a particular nursing unit. For example, more experienced nurses may care for patients with higher acuity.

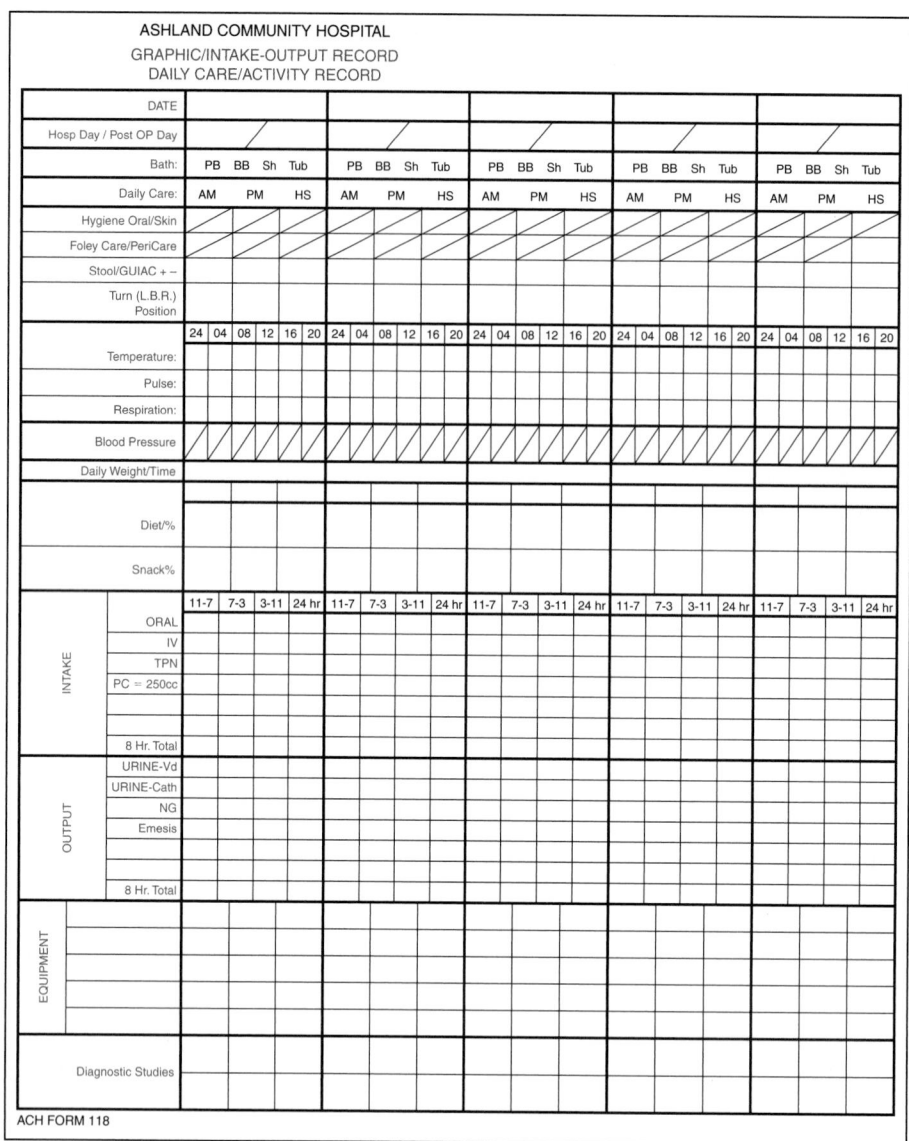

Figure 9-2 ■ Nursing assessment flow sheet. (Courtesy Ashland Community Hospital, Ashland, Ore.)

Standardized Care Plans

Some institutions use standardized care plans to make documentation more efficient. The plans, based on the institution's standards of nursing practice, are preprinted established guidelines used to care for patients with similar health problems. After completing a nursing assessment, place the appropriate standard care plans in your patient's record. It is very important that you make necessary modifications to individualize each care plan. Most standardized plans also allow the addition of specific desired outcomes and the target dates of achievement of these outcomes (see Chapter 8).

HOME CARE DOCUMENTATION

Home care continues to grow as increasing numbers of older adults use home care services. Medicare has specific guidelines for establishing eligibility for home care reimbursement. When

you provide home care, your documentation must specifically address the category of care and your patient's response to care. Documentation in the home care system has different implications than in other areas of nursing. The documentation is both the quality control and the justification for reimbursement from Medicare, Medicaid, or private insurance companies (USDHHS, 2003). Home care agencies are evaluated for accurate, complete charting; adherence to standards that govern their reimbursement; and quality of care. Document all of your services for payment (e.g., direct skilled care, patient instructions, skilled observation, and evaluation visits) (TJC, 2008a). Home care documentation includes the following: resource numbers in case of emergency; the ability of the patient or caregiver to perform needed home care procedures as well as ability to troubleshoot equipment needs, and ability to recognize potential complications. Documentation also needs to show evidence that the home environment is safe for the treatment being received.

LONG-TERM CARE DOCUMENTATION

Increasing numbers of older adults and people with disabilities in the United States require care in long-term health care facilities. Nursing personnel often face documentation challenges much different from those in the acute care setting. CMS released new guidelines effective August 2007 related to accidents and supervision of residents of long-term care facilities. This change requires careful documentation (Senft, 2008). Changes in the Medicare program in the form of the prospective payment system determine the standards and policies for reimbursement and documentation in long-term health care. Assess each resident in a long-term care agency receiving funding from Medicare and Medicaid programs using the Resident Assessment Instrument/Minimum Data Set (RAI/MDS). This documentation tool was mandated by the Omnibus Budget Reconciliation Act of 1987 and updated in 1995. It provides standardized protocols for assessment and care planning, as well as a minimum data set to promote quality improvement within and across facilities (Dellefield, 2007). When you review residents' records for reimbursement, there is an expectation that these protocols, such as skin assessments, wound care, and assisted ambulation, are carried out. Documentation supports a multidisciplinary approach to the assessment and planning process for patients. Communication among nurses, social workers, recreational therapists, and dietitians is essential in the regulated documentation process. The fiscal support for long-term care residents hinges on the justification of nursing care as demonstrated in sound documentation of the services rendered (Dellefield, 2007).

REPORTING

Reports are an exchange of information among health care team members. A report reflects a summary of activities or observations seen, performed, or heard by the health care provider. The types of reports most commonly used by nurses include the hand-off report, telephone report, and incident (occurrence) report.

Hand-Off Report

A **hand-off report** happens any time one health care provider transfers care of a patient to another health care provider. The purpose of hand-off reports is to provide better continuity and individualized care for patients. For example, if you find that a patient breathes better in a certain position, you relay that information to the next nurse caring for the patient. Examples of hand-off reports include change-of-shift reports and transfer reports.

Standardizing communication during hand-off reports is one of the 2009 National Patient Safety Goals (NPSGs). Hand-off communications includes up-to-date information about the patient's condition, required care, treatments, medications, services, and any recent or anticipated changes (TJC, 2008c). Information during patient hand-off can be given face-to-face, in writing, or verbally, such as over the telephone or via audiorecording.

Regardless of the way hand-off reports are given, the NPSGs state it is essential for staff to have an opportunity for last-minute updates, to clarify information, or to receive information on care events or changes in the patient's condition. Properly performed, a hand-off report provides an opportunity to share essential information to provide for patient safety and continuity of care (Schroeder, 2006).

An effective hand-off report is quick and efficient. A good report provides a baseline for comparisons and indicates the kind of care anticipated for the next nurse who will be caring for the patient. An organized and concise approach helps you set goals and anticipate patient needs and lessens the chance of overlooking important information. A sample format is as follows: background information (name, age, and medical diagnosis); primary health problem; unusual occurrences; discharge planning issues; identification of significant changes in measurable terms (e.g., pain scale); observations; findings; time when new, STAT, or prn medications were given; care required, such as medications that need to be started, when to assess the effectiveness of STAT/prn medications, or when a dressing needs to be changed next; progress with teaching; interventions; and family involvement. It is especially important to report any recent changes or priority situations concerning the patient's condition. Report elements should not include normal findings or routine information retrievable from other sources or derogatory or inappropriate comments about the patient or family, which could possibly lead to legal charges if overheard by the patient or family (Benson and others, 2007). This kind of language will contribute to prejudicial opinions about the patient.

CHANGE-OF-SHIFT REPORT The **change-of-shift report** is one type of hand-off report that occurs at the end of each shift. This report provides the transfer of relevant information from nurses who have completed a shift of care to nurses about to begin a shift of care. Shift reports happen in a variety of ways.

Sometimes nurses walk with each other from one patient's room to the next. This is called walking rounds. Walking reports given in person or during rounds allow you to obtain immediate feedback when questions arise about a patient's care. When you make rounds, the patient and family members also have the opportunity to participate in any discussions and care decisions. However, be careful about mentioning information that the patient should not hear, for example, new laboratory or diagnostic reports not yet explained by the health care provider.

Shift reports can also be given orally. Oral reports can occur in person, with staff members from both shifts participating. Oral reports can also be audiotaped before the end of the shift by the nurse going off duty; the incoming staff then listens to the report before assuming patient care. Recording reports often enhances efficiency and minimizes social interactions.

TRANSFER REPORTS Patients frequently transfer from one unit to another or to another facility to receive different levels of care. For example, patients transfer from intensive care units to general nursing units when the level of care no longer requires intense monitoring. A **transfer report** is another type of hand-off report that involves communication of information about patients from the nurse on the sending unit to the nurse on the receiving unit. Transfer reports are usually completed by phone or in person. When giving a transfer report, include the following information:

1. Patient's name, age, health care provider(s), and medical diagnosis
2. Summary of medical progress up to the time of transfer
3. Current health status (physical and psychosocial)
4. Allergies
5. Emergency code status
6. Family support
7. Current nursing diagnoses or problems and care plan
8. Any critical assessments or interventions to be completed shortly after transfer (helps receiving nurse to establish priorities of care)
9. Up-to-date reconciled medication list (TJC, 2008b)
10. Need for any special equipment, such as isolation equipment, suction equipment, or traction

At the completion of the transfer report the receiving nurse clarifies information by asking questions about the patient's status. Some institutions require a written transfer report sheet that includes information communicated in the transfer report.

Telephone Reports and Orders

TELEPHONE REPORTS A registered nurse makes a telephone report when significant events or changes in a patient's condition have occurred. A telephone report needs to include clear, accurate, and concise information. About 60% of the worst type of medical errors, called sentinel events, relate to communication problems that often arise during telephone reports (Hemmila, 2006). Thus some institutions use SBAR, an acronym that stands for *situation-background-assessment-recommendation*. SBAR standardizes telephone communication of significant events or changes in the patient's condition. Therefore it is a communication strategy designed to improve patient safety. For example, when describing the *situation*, you include the admitting and secondary diagnoses as well as the problem your patient is having as the current issue. *Background* information includes pertinent medical history, previous laboratory tests and treatments, psychosocial issues, allergies, and current code status. For *assessment* data, include significant findings in your head-to-toe physical assessment, recent vital signs, current treatment measures, restrictions, recent laboratory results and diagnostics, and pain status. Then provide your *recommendation*, in which you suggest a plan of care and what needs to be addressed (Hemmila, 2006).

Document every phone call you make to a health care provider. Your documentation includes when the call was made, who made it (if you did not make the call), who was called, to whom information was given, what information was given, what information was received, and verification of the information with the provider. The 2009 NPSGs require that health care institutions identify a process for a verification "read-back" when receiving information or critical test results. An example follows: "Laboratory technician J. Ignacio reported a potassium level of 5.9. Information was transcribed and read back for verification. Dr. Wade notified at 2030. D. Markle, RN, read back."

TELEPHONE ORDERS AND VERBAL ORDERS A telephone order (TO) involves a health care provider stating a prescribed therapy over the phone to a registered nurse, whereas a verbal order (VO) involves the health care provider giving orders to a nurse while they are standing near each other. Telephone and verbal orders frequently occur at night or during an emergency and frequently cause medical errors (Bombard, 2008). As part of the 2009 NPSGs, the person receiving a verbal or telephone order must write down the complete order or enter it into the computer as it is being given. Then the nurse must read it back, called "read-back," and receive confirmation from the person who gave the order (Bombard, 2008; TJC, 2008c). An example follows: "10/16/2007: 0815, Tylenol 3, 2 tablets, every 6 hours for incisional pain. TO Dr. Knight/J. Woods, RN, read back." The health care provider later verifies the telephone or verbal order legally by signing it within a set time (e.g., 24 hours) as set by hospital policy. Telephone and verbal orders are used only when absolutely necessary and not for the sake of convenience. In some situations it is prudent to have a second person listen to telephone orders. Check agency policy. Box 9-2 provides guidelines that promote accuracy when receiving telephone orders.

Incident or Occurrence Reports

An incident is any event not consistent with the routine operation of a health care unit or routine care of a patient. Examples include patient falls, needle-stick injuries, a visitor

BOX 9-2	Guidelines for Telephone Orders and Verbal Orders

Clearly identify the patient's name, room number, and diagnosis.

Read back all orders to the health care provider (TJC, 2008b).

Use clarification questions to avoid misunderstandings.

Write "TO" (telephone order) or "VO" (verbal order), including date and time, name of patient, complete order; sign the name of the health care provider and nurse.

Follow agency policies; some institutions require documentation of the "read-back" or require two nurses to review and sign telephone (and verbal) orders.

The health care provider cosigns the order within the time frame required by the institution (usually 24 hours—check agency policy).

becoming ill, and medication errors. Completion of an **incident report,** also called an **occurrence report,** occurs when there is an actual or potential injury; this report is not a part of the patient record (see Chapter 4).

Always contact the patient's health care provider to examine the patient at the time of the event. It is important not to state that an error occurred in the patient's medical record. Instead, you document an objective description of what happened, what you observed, and what follow-up actions were taken in the patient's medical record. It is also important to evaluate and document the patient's response to the error or incident.

Follow agency policy when making an incident report. Incident reports are an important part of quality improvement. The overall goal is to identify changes needed to prevent future reoccurrence. Note that you do not include mention the incident report in the patient's medical record. File the report with the appropriate risk management department of the institution. Analysis of incident (or occurrence) reports helps identify trends within an organization that provide justification for changes in policies and procedures or for in-service programs. (See Chapter 4 for other examples and further discussion.)

NURSING INFORMATICS

Although many agencies still use paper/handwritten formats for documentation of the continuity of care, as described in the previous section, there is an increasing trend toward computerization of health care records in acute care settings, outpatient settings, and home care, as well as long-term care setting (Box 9-3). Experts estimate that much of your knowledge will be obsolete in 5 years or less (Thede, 2003). You cannot be expected to know everything. Computerization of health care records provides a mechanism for identification, acquisition, manipulation, storage, and presentation of data so they can be transformed into information. The federal directive to have computer-based health care records by 2014 will necessitate nurses of the twenty-first century to have broadened skill sets to deliver quality patient care (National League for Nursing [NLN], 2008). Today's nurses need to be knowledgeable in the science of nursing informatics.

Informatics is the science and art of turning data into information. Informatics focuses on information and knowledge acquisition, rather than the tool, the computer. All nurses deal with data, information, and knowledge (Hebda and others, 2009). The previous section on documentation explains the importance of knowing how to record and report data and information as well as to critically think and apply knowledge to use information for patient care. Informatics describes the study of the retrieval, storage, presentation, and sharing of data, information, and knowledge to provide quality, safe patient care.

Information is the structure on which health care is built. Informatics uses data and information to convert to new knowledge. Informatics includes four key concepts. *Data,* the first concept of the informatics continuum, include numbers, characters, or facts that are collected according to a perceived

BOX 9-3   BEST PRACTICES

Comparison of Time Spent Documenting in Paper-Based Records and Electronic Medical Record

SUMMARY OF EVIDENCE

In an effort to determine the potential time saving of implementation of computerized provider order entry (CPOE), the documentation time spent by nurses before and after implementation of electronic medical record (EMR) was compared by several researchers. Some experts believe that using an EMR will reduce the time that nurses spend on documentation and free up more time for patient care. Previous studies suggest that on average nurses using a paper-based documentation system spend about 30% of their working time on documentation. In simpler terms, this means that nurses spend more than 3 hours out of each 12-hour shift on documentation. By comparison, some studies found that use of online documentation, as in an EMR, reduced that proportion by 50%. This amounted to freeing up an additional 1½ hours per nurse per 12-hour shift. However, changing to electronic documentation does not always change the amount of time nurses spend doing routine documentation. Some studies also show that the amount of time spent documenting depends upon the workload of the nurse and varies by hour of day. For example, one study showed that documenting the discharge of a patient going home took less time than documenting the discharge of a patient going to a nursing home, while another study showed most admission and discharge documentation in one study occurred between noon and 2 PM. Some factors that affect switching to electronic documentation include the reluctance of some nurses to accept technological advances. Successful implementation of EMR and CPOE requires the commitment of the entire nursing staff.

APPLICATION TO NURSING PRACTICE
- Adoption of CPOE may eliminate work and reduce documentation time.
- Transition from paper to online documentation systems presents both opportunities and challenges to nurses.

REFERENCES
Choi WH and others: Comparison of direct and indirect nursing-care times between physician order entry system and electronic medical records, *Stud Health Technol Inform* 122:288, 2006.
Hakes B, Whittington J: Assessing the impact of an electronic medical record on nurse documentation time, *Comput Inform Nurs* 26(4):234, 2008.
Smith K and others: Evaluating the impact of computerized clinical documentation, *Comput Inform Nurs* 23(3):132, 2005.

need for analysis and possible action. Data have no significance beyond their existence. For example, what does the number 180 mean? It could be a laboratory value, a street number, or a secret code. By itself, "180" means nothing. It represents data. *Information*, the second concept, is data that are interpreted, organized, or structured. Information provides the answers to "who, what, when, where" questions. If you take the blood pressure of a 57-year-old postoperative patient and the systolic blood pressure reading is 180 mm Hg and the diastolic blood pressure is 90 mm Hg, you have useful information. When the number 180 is combined with other data, it becomes meaningful. The data become information. The vital signs now have meaning when interpreted. *Knowledge* is the application of data and information. It answers the "how" question. You know the patient just had surgery and has a history of high blood pressure and did not receive the morning dose of antihypertensive medication. Using knowledge is essential in making decisions. You synthesized information (knowledge) from past experiences of caring for other postoperative patients with high blood pressure. Knowledge creates new questions and areas of research. You report the changes to the patient's health care provider (wisdom). *Wisdom* answers the "why" question and focuses on the appropriate application of that knowledge (ANA, 2008). Wisdom comes with experience. In the above scenario, using evidence found in the scientific literature, you apply knowledge of pharmacology and intervene to manage the patient's blood pressure.

It is a challenge in health care settings to easily access data and information about patients. This is especially the case when you record information manually on printed forms. For example, a nurse working in risk management who is interested in investigating patient falls has to review page by page the records of patients who have fallen to identify the common factors contributing to falls. Remember, three important purposes of medical records are communication, education, and research. When health care organizations rely on handwritten patient records, locating, summarizing, and comparing information is slow and difficult. Finding information for medical record purposes of health care education, research, audits, and reimbursement becomes cumbersome and inefficient. The Institute of Medicine (IOM) (2001) recognized that the only way to use data and information to improve care delivery, as well as for quality improvement, research, and education, is through information technology.

Information technology (IT) refers to the management and processing of information, generally with the assistance of computers (Hebda and others, 2009). IT includes not only the use of computers, but also the knowledge of *how* to use computer technology, such as databases, programming languages and tools, and communication protocols (Burke and Weill, 2005). Technology serves as the tool that allows transfer of the information that improves care. However, technology alone does not improve the efficiency and effectiveness of patient care. You will be expected to understand technology's capabilities and limitations. IT supports the process of synthesizing data and information into knowledge and wisdom,

which is at the center of NI (ANA, 2008). Information technologies hold the promise to transform health care practice and promote patient safety (IOM, 2001). IT is critical to all aspects of clinical decision making, consumer education, professional development, research, and the delivery of population-based care. IT offers tremendous opportunities to enhance clinical practice and appropriateness of care and to increase efficiency and effectiveness in health care organizations (Healthcare Information and Management Systems Society [HIMSS], 2006).

A **health care information system (HIS)** is a group of systems used within a health care enterprise that support and enhance health care (Hebda and others, 2009). The role of HIS has grown more important because the public has a heightened awareness of reports of medical errors through public media, as well as various initiatives implemented nationally, such as HIPAA, personal health records, and electronic medical records.

A HIS consists of two major types of information systems: clinical information systems and administrative information systems. From a historical standpoint, administrative health care information systems have been in existence longer. Administrative information systems comprise databases such as payroll, financial, and quality assurance systems. On the other hand, CIS support those activities used to plan, implement, and evaluate care. There are several types of clinical information systems, including nursing, pharmacy, office management systems, computerized provider order entry (CPOE) systems, and radiology to name a few. Together, the two systems operate to make the entry and communication of data and information more efficient. You will find that any single health care agency will use one or several of the clinical information systems and administrative information systems. For example, a small community hospital uses a nursing information system; an order entry system; and laboratory, radiology, and pharmacy systems to coordinate its core patient care services. A nurse working in such a hospital documents nursing care on a computer, locates and reviews laboratory test results, orders sterile supplies, and enters health care provider orders for x-ray films and patients' medications. The billing of patient care services and payroll occur through use of administrative information systems.

Nursing Information Systems

Nursing information systems are one of many subspecialties of clinical information systems. Many hospitals now have NIS that support the documentation of nursing process activities and offer resources for managing nursing care delivery (Figure 9-3). A reliable nursing information system is the product of nursing informatics. **Nursing informatics** is defined as a nursing specialty that manages and communicates data, information, knowledge, and wisdom by integrating nursing, computer, and information science (ANA, 2008). Nursing informatics facilitates the integration of data, information, and knowledge to support patients, nurses and other providers in decision making in all roles and settings. Nursing informatics supports new initiatives occurring within the

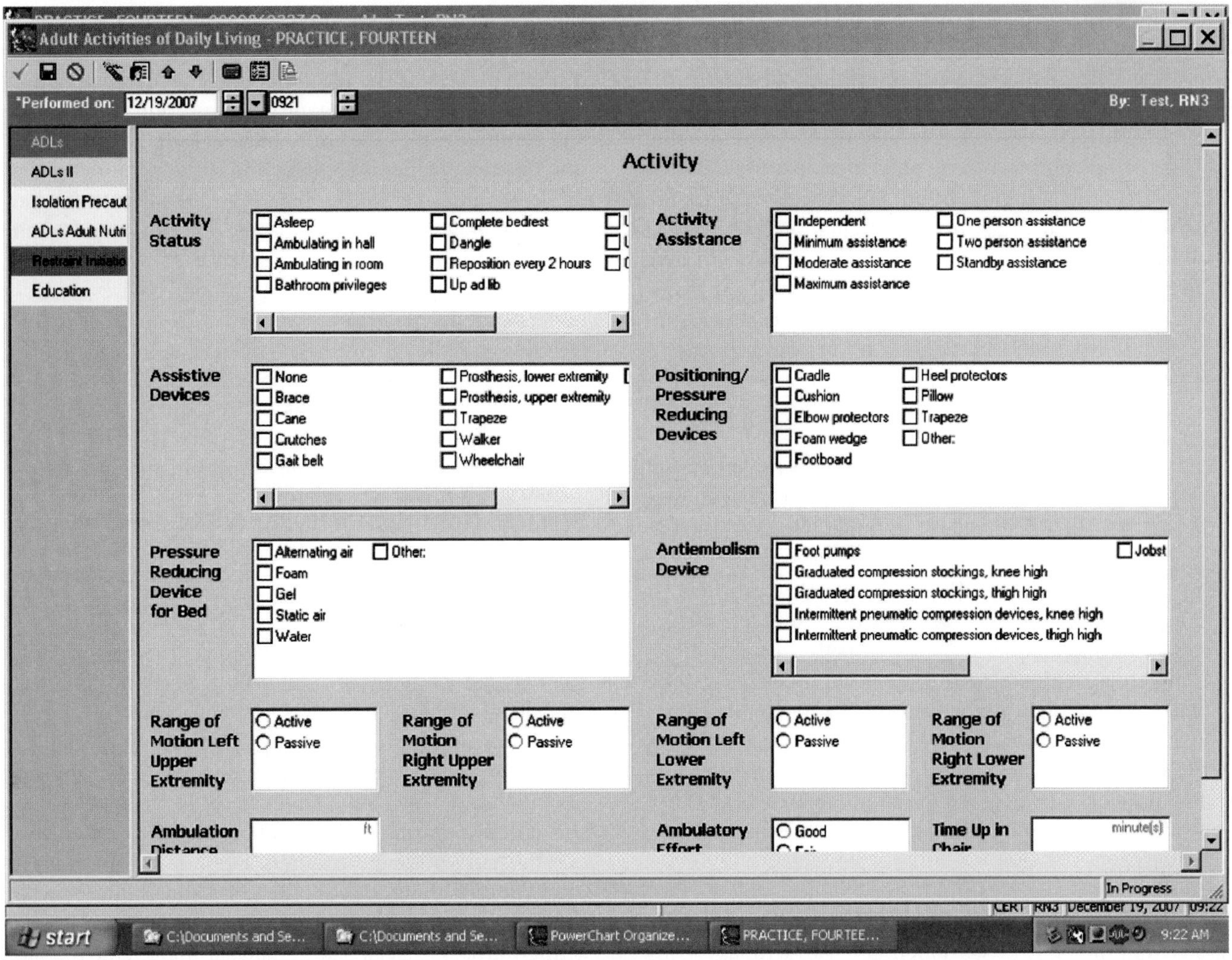

Figure 9-3 ■ Example of a screen for nursing assessment of activity, part of a clinical information system program.

health care arena, such as CPOE, electronic medication administration records, and clinical documentation (Malloch, 2007). The application of nursing informatics results in an efficient and effective nursing information system. Nursing informatics improves the health of individuals, families, communities, and populations by effectively managing information and enhancing communication (ANA, 2008). Because of rapidly advancing, emerging health care technologies, nursing practice of the future will not be the same as it is today. Nurses need knowledge and skills in computer literacy, information literacy, and use of information technologies (NLN, 2008). Nurses need knowledge of informatics.

Numerous organizations, including the National League for Nursing (NLN), the American Nurses Association (ANA), the Technology Informatics Guiding Education Reform, and the Robert Wood Johnson Foundation Quality and Safety Education for Nurses Initiative, have recommended all nurses acquire a minimal level of awareness and competence in informatics and use of information technology (NLN, 2008). Competence in informatics is not the same as computer competency. To become competent in informatics you need to be able to use evolving methods of discovering, retrieving, and using information in your practice (Hebda and others, 2009). This means that you learn to recognize when you need information, as well as having the skills to find, evaluate, and use needed clinical information effectively.

A good nursing information system incorporates principles of nursing informatics and supports the work you do. You want to be able to easily access a computer program, review the patient's medical history and orders, and then go to the patient's bedside to conduct a comprehensive assessment. Once you have completed the assessment, you enter data into the computer terminal at the patient's bedside and develop a plan of care from the information gathered. The plan of care incorporates evidence-based practice guidelines, which you have found using your information science skills. The computer allows you to quickly share the plan of care with the patient. Periodically you will return to the computer to check on laboratory test results and document the therapies you administer. The computer screens and optional pop-up windows make it easy to locate information, enter and compare data, and make changes. Nursing information systems have specific functions that support the nursing process from both clinical and managerial perspectives. Typically the components of a nursing information system include patient management, decision support, and documentation functions. The nursing information system can help you in determining diagnosis, preparing and implementing nursing care plans, and evaluating care provided.

Nursing information systems have two designs: nursing process design and protocol or critical pathway design (Hebda and others, 2009). The nursing process design is the most traditional. It organizes documentation within well-established formats, such as admission and postoperative assessments, problem lists, medication lists, care plans, physical assessments, discharge planning instructions, and intervention lists, such as routine care or complex patient care needs, or notes. Documentation of progress notes occurs through use of narrative notes, charting by exception, and flow sheet charting.

The second design model for a nursing information system is the protocol or critical pathway design (Hebda and others, 2009). This design offers a multidisciplinary format to managing information. All health care providers select one or more critical pathways to document care they provided. If several pathways are selected, then an advanced system merges protocols so that a master protocol or path is used to direct patient care activities. Standard physician order sets can be included, automatically processed by the system, and integrated into medication delivery. The NIS identifies variances to the attainment of anticipated outcomes. The information system provides all caregivers the ability to analyze variance and offers an accurate clinical picture of the patient's progress.

Advantages of a Nursing Information System

As stated in the previous section, health care settings are increasingly using computers for documentation purposes. Anecdotal reports and descriptive studies suggest that nursing information systems offer important advantages to nurses in practice. Some of the benefits of implementing nursing information systems include improved quality of data (usefulness and relevant), as well as documentation that is more complete, accurate, legible, and up-to-date with less noted redundancy (Oroviogoicoechea and others, 2007). Other advantages of NIS include increased direct patient care time, better access to information, reduced errors of omission, reduced hospital costs, increased job satisfaction, compliance with accrediting agency mandates, and development of a common clinical database (Hebda and others, 2009).

The transition from paper to online documentation systems presents both opportunities and challenges to nurses. Successful implementation of computer-based nursing process documentation requires a high level of acceptance of the nursing process, careful preparation of predefined care plans, organizational preparation, and inclusion of future users, including bedside nurses, in the development process. It is also essential to have sufficient technical equipment with integration into the hospital information system.

A barrier to the successful implementation of a clinical information system is the reluctance on the part of some nurses and other clinical staff to accept technological advances. Often clinicians fail to understand how technology can improve the way they deliver care and enhance clinical decision processes. The successful implementation of a nursing information system requires preparation, involvement, and commitment of the entire nursing staff. Integrating NIS into nursing practice is complex and includes more than just implementing a new technology. It also requires staff education, changing attitudes and cultures, as well as standardizing documentation and health care practices (Oroviogoicoechea and others, 2007). Successful integration requires nurses to understand the potential of informatics and information technology. Although promoters of nursing information systems suggest adoption of computerized charting provides a time saving for nursing workload, currently there is inconsistent evidence of time saved with use of electronic patient records (Choi and others, 2006; Smith and others, 2005).

Privacy, Confidentiality, and Security Mechanisms

The implementation of HIPAA regulations heightened awareness about information security and privacy practices. HIPAA was the first federal legislation to protect automated patient records and to provide uniform protection nationwide (Hebda and others, 2009). HIPAA regulations called for the establishment of an electronic patient records system and process to protect the privacy of individual health information (Steward, 2005). Electronic records facilitate efficient and effective sharing of information, but the ease of access raises concern among consumers. Eight in 10 Americans express concern about identity theft or fraud, and 77% report concern about their medical information being used for marketing purposes (Healthcare Financial Management, 2007). Computerized documentation has legal risks. Just as you need to understand how violations occur in a paper documentation system, you must also understand how information systems influence privacy, confidentiality, and security.

Privacy includes the right to determine what information shared with a health care worker will become known to others. When using a computerized documenting system, you must make sure the computer screen is not visible to anyone except the person doing the charting (Hebda and others, 2009).

Confidentiality of access to computerized records is a major issue with electronic records just as it is with paper records. Protecting privacy through confidentiality policies and technology is a critical component of quality health care. Standards within HIPAA address criteria for standardizing electronic transmission of health information by focusing on the need to protect security, integrity, and authenticity of health information. HIPAA also requires institutions to protect the confidentiality of medical information stored in electronic records against reasonable and anticipated threats (Steward, 2005). The first line of maintaining patient confidentiality is achieved with a login process authenticating that the person is granted access (Thede, 2003). Authentication of the user is through an access code accompanied by a password.

A **password** is a collection of alphanumeric characters that a user types into the computer before accessing a program. A user is usually required to enter a password after the entry and acceptance of an access code or user name. A password does not appear on the computer screen when it is typed, nor should it be known to anyone but the user and information systems administrators (Hebda and others, 2009). Strong passwords use combinations of letters, numbers, and symbols that are not easy to guess. When using a health care agency computer system, it is essential that you do not share your computer password, under any circumstances, with anyone. A good system requires frequent and random changes in personal passwords to prevent unauthorized persons from tampering with records. In addition, most staff have access only to patients in their work area. Select staff (e.g., administrators or risk managers) may be given authority to access all patient records. Most breaches of confidentiality come from inside the agency (Thede, 2003).

Data security has three aspects: ensuring accuracy of data, protection of the data from unauthorized eyes inside or outside of the agency, and protection from data loss (Thede, 2003). Data accuracy is ensured through mechanisms that check data during input and provide for correction of entries made in error. Accuracy of original data is the responsibility of the user.

Protection from inside intrusions occurs with audit trails. Audit trails are discoverable by a court of law. The trail reveals both unauthorized access and the identity of the person committing the violation. Another method to protect access to records from inside intrusions occurs with an automatic sign-off, a mechanism designed to log off a user from the computer system after a specified period of inactivity on the computer (Hebda and others, 2009). An automatic sign-off is often found in most patient care areas, as well as other departments that handle sensitive data.

Protection from outside intrusions occurs with installation of firewalls and antivirus and spy ware detection software. A **firewall** is a combination of hardware and software that protects private network resources (e.g., a hospital's information system) from outside hackers, network damage, and theft or misuse of information. Computer data need protection from data loss due to either a system problem or a disaster, natural or otherwise (Thede, 2003).

The data security process has taken on new meaning since the events of September 11, 2001. A disaster recovery plan must be in place. All agencies must routinely create back-up data and store the data off-site in a secure place (Thede, 2003). Other considerations to maintain the security of the health care data include placing computers or file servers in restricted areas. This form of security may have limited benefit, especially if an organization uses mobile wireless devices such as notebooks, tablet personal computers (PCs), and personal digital assistants (PDAs). These devices are easy to misplace or lose and can fall into the wrong hands. An organization may use motion detectors or alarms with these devices to help prevent theft.

HANDLING AND DISPOSAL OF INFORMATION The first section of this chapter has made clear how important it is to keep medical records confidential. However, it is equally important to safeguard the information that is printed from the electronic record or extracted for report purposes. For example, a nurse prints a copy of a nursing activities work list to use as a day planner while administering care to patients. The nurse refers to information on the list and add handwritten notes to enter later into the computer. Information on the list is considered personal health identifiers (PHIs), must be kept confidential, and not left out for view by unauthorized persons. The nurse destroys all printed information when it is no longer needed.

The printing and faxing of information from a patient's record is a primary source for the unauthorized release of information. All papers containing PHIs (e.g., Social Security number, date of birth or age, or patient's name or address) must be destroyed. Most agencies have shredders or locked receptacles for shredding and later incineration. Nurses also work in settings where they are responsible for erasing computer files from the hard drive containing calendars, surgery or diagnostic procedure schedules, or other daily records that contain PHIs (Hebda and others, 2009). Be sure you know the disposal policies for records in the institution where you work.

An institution needs to have sound policies for the use of fax machines, specifically what types of information you can send to which departments. Information that you send by fax should not exceed that requested or required for immediate clinical needs. There are some steps to take to enhance fax security (Hebda and others, 2009):

- Confirm that fax numbers are correct before sending to be sure you direct information properly.
- Use a cover sheet, especially if a fax machine serves a number of different users.
- Authenticate at both ends of the transmission before data transmission to verify the source and destination are correct.
- Use programmed speed-dial keys to eliminate the chance of a dialing error and misdirected information.
- Place fax machines in a secure area.
- Limit machine access to designated individuals.
- Log fax transmissions. This feature is often available electronically on the machine.

Clinical Information Systems

Any clinician, including nurses, physicians, pharmacists, social workers, and therapists will use programs available on a clinical information system. These programs include monitoring systems, order entry systems, and laboratory, radiology, and pharmacy systems. A monitoring system includes devices that automatically monitor and record biometric measurements (e.g., vital signs, oxygen saturation, cardiac index, and stroke volume) in critical care and specialty areas. The devices send measurements electronically, direct to the nursing documentation system. Two important features of clinical information systems include order entry systems and the electronic health record.

Order entry systems allow you to order supplies and services from another department. An example is the ability to order sterile supplies from the central supply processing department. This eliminates written order forms and expedites the delivery of needed supplies to a nursing unit. The **computerized provider order entry (CPOE)** is one type of order entry system gaining popularity in the larger medical centers across the country, particularly with medication orders. Advantages of CPOE include reduced use of resources, reduced length of stay, and an overall reduction in costs (Sengstack and Gugerty, 2004). More important, most CPOE systems have significant potential to reduce medication errors associated with illegibility and inappropriate drug use and dosing (Sengstack and Gugerty, 2004).

CPOE refers to a process by which the health care provider directly enters orders for patient care into the hospital information system. In advanced systems, CPOE has built-in reminders and alerts that help the patient's provider to select the most appropriate medication or diagnostic test. There are major initiatives from the IOM to improve the quality of care and reduce medication errors. Many believe CPOE is the answer. Such factors as difficult system sign-on procedures, limited system access or response time, lack of funding, inadequate access to clinical data to support the expert decision-making features, and the perception by physicians that CPOE offers them few benefits have slowed the implementation of CPOE (Sengstack and Gugerty, 2004).

The Electronic Health Record

The technology that exists for computerization in the health care delivery system is virtually unlimited and holds potential for improving the accuracy and efficiency of documentation. The need for patient safety has driven the increased usage of computerized documentation systems. The traditional paper medical record no longer meets the needs of today's health care industry. A paper record is episode oriented, with a separate record for each patient visit to a health care agency (Hebda and others, 2009). Key information, such as patient allergies, current medications, and complications from treatment may be lost from one episode of care (e.g., hospitalization or clinic visit) to the next, jeopardizing a patient's safety.

The **electronic health record (EHR)** is a longitudinal electronic record of patient health information generated by one or more encounters in any care delivery setting (HIMSS, 2006). It ensures coordination of care because all primary caregivers can view a common record of a patient's entire health care experience including inpatient, outpatient, and emergency care (Halamka, 2006). Computerized documentation systems minimize repetitive clerical and monitoring tasks and increase your time for direct patient care. The EHR provides a way to manage information in an integrated manner and to provide high-quality care in a cost-effective manner (IOM, 2003).

Using an EHR has many benefits. The record contains information from many health-related encounters. EHRs reflect the current health status and lifetime medical history of an individual and decrease the amount of time spent waiting for information when a patient is in one location and the chart is in another location. It also allows health care providers to get information in real time and share information between disciplines to facilitate quality patient-centered care (IOM, 2003; Thede, 2003). EHRs make hospitals more efficient, reduce medical errors by improved communication, reduce malpractice premiums, lower health care costs, and improve work performance (Halamka, 2006; Kossman and Scheidenhelm, 2008; Steward, 2005). An EHR also includes results of diagnostic studies that may include images and sound, as well as decision-support software programs. Because an unlimited number of patient records can be potentially stored within an EHR system, health care providers can access clinical data to identify quality issues, link interventions with positive outcomes, and make evidence-based decisions (Hebda and others, 2009).

Some of the risks associated with the electronic system are the same as mentioned in the above section on nursing information systems. Opponents believe that storing records electronically could result in major violations of patient privacy (Steward, 2005). Other issues focus on patient confidentiality, potential for hackers to attain confidential information, and the lack of adequate sanctions for such misuse. Although there typically are mechanisms in place to correct errors within the electronic documentation system, in some instances, errors may be transmitted before corrections are made. You must remember that charting guidelines pertaining to factual, accurate, complete, and current still pertain to the electronic document. Just as in a paper documentation system, "if it's not documented" within the electronic record, "it's not done."

Those who support the development of an EHR believe that it improves patient and clinician satisfaction because it improves continuity of health care from one episode of illness to another. A clinician can access relevant and timely information about a patient so as to focus on the priority problems of care and to make timely, well-informed clinical decisions. An EHR is a powerful tool because of the decision-support resources it contains. For example, in a hospital setting an EHR gathers data and performs checking to support regulatory and accreditation requirements. It also includes tools to guide and critique medication administration—right patient, right drug, right route, right dose, right time, and right documentation. An EHR also contains basic decision-support tools such as physician order sets, interdisciplinary treatment plans, and rules based on documentation templates. The evidence that comes from the clinical information in an EHR provides an excellent foundation for an organization to identify clinical problem areas and to initiate clinical research trials (IOM, 2003).

The ultimate development of an EHR for patients will affect the entire health care community. Currently the American Medical Association, American Nurses Association, the Healthcare Information and Management Systems Society (HIMSS), and the American Medical Informatics Association are just some of the organizations charged with the task of facilitating rapid input to support the adoption of EHR standards (Hebda and others, 2009). All disciplines and health care organizations will benefit. The key advantages for nursing include the following: providing a means to easily compare data from different health care encounters, maintaining an ongoing record of a patient's education and learning in all health care encounters, offering better quality and easily accessible data for research, automating critical and clinical pathways of care, and comparing ongoing clinical data about a patient with original baseline information.

Guidelines have been developed by the American Nurses Association, the American Medical Record Association, and the Canadian Nurses Association to assist you in safe computer charting (Moody and others, 2004):

1. Do not share the password used to enter and sign off computer files with other caregivers. A good system requires frequent changes in personal passwords to prevent unauthorized persons from accessing and tampering with records.
2. Avoid leaving the computer terminal unattended when logged on.
3. Follow the correct protocol for correcting errors according to agency policy.
4. Software systems have a system for backup files. If you inadvertently delete part of the permanent record, follow agency policy. It is necessary to type an explanation into the computer file with the date, time, and your initials and to submit an explanation in writing to your manager (Thede, 2003).
5. Avoid leaving information about a patient displayed on a monitor where others can see it. Keep a log that accounts for every copy of a computerized file that you have generated from the system.
6. Follow the agency's confidentiality procedures for documenting sensitive material, such as a diagnosis of human immune deficiency virus (HIV) infection.
7. Protection of printouts from computerized records is important. Shredding of printouts and the logging of the number of copies generated by each caregiver are ways to minimize duplicate records and protect the confidentiality of patient information.

KEY POINTS

- A patient's health care record is a confidential, written legal documentation of the care received.
- The record is a continuing account of the patient's health care status and is available to all members of the health care team. It facilitates communication with health care providers for continuity of patient care, maintains a legal and financial record of care, aids in clinical research, and guides professional and organizational performance improvement.
- Your full signature with title on an entry in a record designates accountability for the contents of that entry.
- Accurate and timely record keeping requires an objective interpretation of data with precise measurements, correct spelling, and proper use of abbreviations.
- Effective documentation verifies the specific nursing care provided, use of services and equipment, and medications and thus supports the reimbursement your health care agency receives.
- Document changes in a patient's condition and patient's responses to interventions as they happen to keep a record current.
- To limit liability, nursing documentation exactly describes what happened to a patient and must clearly indicate that individualized, goal-directed nursing care was provided based on the nursing assessment.
- Organize problem-oriented medical records by the patient's health care problems.
- Medicare guidelines for establishing a patient's home care reimbursement are the basis for documentation by home care nurses.
- Long-term care documentation is multidisciplinary and closely linked with fiscal requirements of outside agencies.
- Computerized information systems provide information about patients in an organized and easily accessible fashion.
- The major purpose of hand-off reports is to maintain continuity of care.
- When information relevant to care is communicated by telephone, verify the information by a "read-back" process.
- Incident (occurrence) reports objectively describe any event not consistent with the routine care of a patient.
- A hospital information system consists of two major types of information systems: clinical information systems and administrative information systems.
- Nursing informatics facilitates the integration of data, information, knowledge, and wisdom to support patients, nurses, and other providers in decision making in all roles and settings.
- Protection of the confidentiality of patient's health information and the security of computer systems must remain a top priority. Login processes, audit trails, firewalls, data recovery processes, and policies governing handling and disposal of information all work to protect patient information.
- The computerized health record improves continuity of health care by providing the ability to compare data from various health care encounters and offering easily accessible data for purposes of communication, reducing liability, reimbursement, education, research, and auditing and monitoring.

CRITICAL THINKING EXERCISES

Mrs. Smith continued to have pain during the course of her post-operative stay in the hospital. Initially she received pain medication through her intravenous line. Now she is nearing discharge and is receiving oral pain medication on an as-needed basis. While you were at lunch, her roommate, Mrs. Jones, requested pain medication. The nurse covering for you inadvertently administered the medication to Mrs. Smith instead of Mrs. Jones. When you return from lunch, you discover the medication error. Mrs. Smith also says she is experiencing constipation and is feeling uncomfortable. You check her medical record and notice that her last bowel movement was more than 3 days ago. During your assessment, you find that Mrs. Smith describes her abdominal discomfort as a feeling of "fullness" and she rates it as a 3 on a scale of 0 to 10. Her abdomen is slightly firm upon palpation.

1. You talk with the primary nurse about the current situation with Mrs. Jones. The nurse needs to contact Mrs. Jones' physician about the medication error and her constipation. You expect the nurse will receive an order from the physician at the end of their telephone conversation. When taking a telephone order from a health care provider, it is common for most organizations to require the nurse to:
   a. Photocopy the order for your records
   b. Write the order in its entirety and read it back to the health care provider for verification
   c. Write the order but do not implement until it has been signed by the health care provider
   d. Take the order from the health care provider but insist that the health care provider come to the patient care division to write the order himself or herself

2. What documentation do you need to put in Mrs. Smith's medical record about the medication error?
   a. A note describing the incident, Mrs. Smith's reaction, who was notified, and any actions taken
   b. A note about who made the error and why it occurred
   c. A note describing the incident, Mrs. Smith's reaction, who was notified, any actions taken, and that an incident report was completed
   d. A note that includes only Mrs. Smith's symptoms and what you did to relieve them

3. Mrs. Smith's constipation is also a current issue. Using the SBAR format, prepare the information that the nurse needs to provide to the physician to treat the constipation.

4. Although the medical record of Mrs. Smith fulfills many purposes, its primary purpose is to:
   a. Defend the caregivers in case of allegations of medical malpractice with the wrong medication administered
   b. Provide documentation for the performance improvement processes within the facility
   c. Support continuity of patient care
   d. Develop standards of care within the facility

evolve   Answers to Critical Thinking Questions can be found on the Evolve website.

REVIEW QUESTIONS

1. Which of the following statements is true?
   1. Oral reports are more accurate than written reports because they give a more complete picture of the patient's health.
   2. The health care provider should avoid reading previous patient assessments to prevent forming preconceived judgments about care.
   3. The health care provider should document as soon as possible after providing patient care.
   4. The advantage of CBE is that it originates from a nursing model rather than a medical model.

2. The advantage of focus charting is that:
   1. It focuses on tracking patient problems
   2. It enables all caregivers to track the patient's condition and progress toward the outcomes of care
   3. It uses check marks in a flow sheet
   4. It details the use of services and equipment on a spreadsheet

3. A secondary benefit of thorough documentation is that information gathered from a patient record can be used to:
   1. Protect the nurse in legal cases
   2. Show that the patient was unpleasant to staff
   3. Document the author's assessment of other health care providers
   4. Document opinions about the patient's family

4. When giving a change-of-shift report, you are expected to:
   1. Include community resources that the patient can contact
   2. Include a step-by-step description of how to perform procedures
   3. Provide an organized and concise description of patient status and anticipated needs
   4. Review signs and symptoms of complications that should be reported to the health care provider

5. When you receive telephone orders from a health care provider, you must:
   1. Make a photocopy of the order to avoid errors
   2. Read back the order to the prescriber
   3. Wait until the prescriber signs the order
   4. Include why the telephone order was needed

6. When documenting in the patient's record, which of the following should you avoid writing down?
   1. The patient's diagnosis
   2. Any patient's previous assessment
   3. What the next caregiver will need to know to better care for the patient.
   4. Your complaints about the patient.

7. A nurse makes the following documentation in the patient record: "0830 Patient appears to be in severe pain and refuses to ambulate. Blood pressure and pulse are elevated. Physician notified and analgesic administered as ordered with adequate response. J Cass, RN." The most significant statement about the documentation would be that it is:
   1. Acceptable because it includes assessment, interventions, and evaluation
   2. Good because it shows immediate responsiveness to the problem
   3. Inadequate because pain is not described on a scale of 0 to 10
   4. Unacceptable because it is vague subjective data

8. Documentation of assessment of a patient recovering from surgery includes the following information: complete bath; level of pain 6 (scale 0 to 10); turning in bed with assist of one; and dressing clean, dry, and intact. The least appropriate information is:
   1. Complete bath
   2. Level of pain
   3. Turning in bed with assistance
   4. Status of the dressing

9. A nurse documents an assessment completed at 5 PM. In military time this is:
   1. 0500
   2. 1500
   3. 1700
   4. 2100

10. A patient's race, weight, and marital or employment status are examples of:
    1. Data
    2. Information
    3. Knowledge
    4. Wisdom

Answers to Review Questions can be found on pages 1197-1198.

REFERENCES

American Nurses Association: *Principles for documentation, principles for practice: a resource package for registered nurses*, Silver Spring, Md, 2005, The Association.

American Nurses Association: *Nursing informatics scope and standards of practice*, Silver Spring, Md, 2008, The Association.

Arias K: Mandatory reporting and pay for performance: health care infections in the limelight, *AORN J* 87(4):750, 2008.

Austin S: Ladies and gentleman of the jury, I present the nursing documentation, *Nursing* 36(1):56, 2006.

Benson E and others: Improving nursing shift-to-shift report, *J Nurs Care Qual* 22(1):80, 2007.

Bombard C: Lines of communication, *Nurs Spectr (Gt Chic Ne Ill Nw Indiana Ed)* 21(4):24, 2008.

Burke L, Weill B: *Information technology for the health professions*, ed 2, Upper Saddle River, NJ, 2005, Pearson Prentice Hall.

Childers KP: Paying a price for poor documentation, *Nursing* 35(11):32hn4, 2005.

Choi WH and others: Comparison of direct and indirect nursing-care times between physician order entry system and electronic medical records, *Stud Health Technol Inform* 122:288, 2006.

Dellefield M: Implementation of the resident assessment instrument/minimum data set in the nursing home as organization: implications for quality improvement in RN clinical assessment *Geriatr Nurs* 28(6):377, 2007.

El Baz N and others: Are the outcomes of clinical pathways evidence-based? A critical appraisal of clinical pathway evaluation research, *J Eval Clin Pract* 13:920, 2007.

Ferrell KG: Documentation. II. The best evidence of care, *Am J Nurs* 107(7):61, 2007.

Hafernick D: *Charting the course for nursing: who benefits when documentation is complete?* American Journal of Nursing and Trinity Healthforce Learning, EDA 422-0002, 2007, http://www.twlk.com/healthcare/422-0002.pdf, accessed July, 2008.

Hakes B, Whittington J: Assessing the impact of an electronic medical record on nurse documentation time, *Comput Inform Nurs* 26(4):234, 2008.

Halamka J: The perfect storm for electronic health records, *J Healthc Inf Manag* 20(3):25, 2006.

Healthcare Financial Management: Americans concerned about safety, accuracy of electronic health records: survey, *Healthc Financ Manage* 61(2):14, 2007.

Healthcare Information and Management Systems Society: *Nursing informatics for the twenty-first century: an international look at practice, trends, and the future*, Chicago, 2006, The Society.

Hebda T and others: *Handbook of informatics for nurses and health care professionals*, ed 4, Upper Saddle River, NJ, 2009, Pearson Prentice Hall.

Helleso R: Information handling in the nursing discharge note, *J Clin Nurs* 15:11, 2006.

Hemmila D: Talking the talk: hospitals use SBAR to standardize communication, *NurseWeek* 7(17):26, 2006.

Hunter B, Segrott J: Re-mapping client journeys and professional identities: a review of the literature on clinical pathways, *Int J Nurs Stud* 45(4):608, 2008.

Institute of Medicine: *Crossing the quality chasm: a new health system for the twenty-first century*, Committee on Quality of Health Care in America, Washington, DC, 2001, National Academy Press, http://www.iom.edu/CMS/8089/5432.aspx.

Institute of Medicine: *Key capabilities of an electronic health record system: letter report*, Committee on Data Standards for Patient Safety, Washington, DC, 2003, National Academy Press, http://www.nap.edu/catalog/10781.html.

Kossman SP, Scheidenhelm S: Nurses' perceptions of the impact of electronic health records on work and patient outcomes, *Comput Inform Nurs* 26(2):69, 2008.

Malloch K: The electronic health record: an essential tool for advancing patient safety, *Nurs Outlook* 55(3):159, 2007.

McGeehan R: Best practice in record keeping, *Nurs Stand* 21(17):51, 2007.

Monarch K: Documentation. I. Principles for self-protection, *Am J Nurs* 107(7):58, 2007.

Moody LE and others: Electronic health records documentation in nursing, *Comput Inform Nurs* 22(6):337, 2004.

Mosby: *Mosby's surefire documentation: how, what, and when nurses need to document*, St. Louis, 2006, Elsevier.

National League for Nursing: *Position statement preparing the next generation of nurses to practice in a technology-rich environment: an informatics agenda*, May 9, 2008, National League for Nursing, http://www.nln.org/aboutnln/PositionStatements/index.htm, accessed July 2008.

Oroviogoicoechea C and others: Review: evaluating information systems in nursing, *J Clin Nurs* 17(5):567, 2007.

Schroeder S: Picking up the PACE: a new template for shift report, *Nursing* 36(10):22, 2006.

Senft D: Accidents and supervision: new CMS F-tag guidance, *Geriatr Nurs* 29(1):12, 2008.

Sengstack PP, Gugerty B: CPOE systems: success factors and implementation issues, *J Healthc Inf Manag* 18(1):36, 2004.

Smith K and others: Evaluating the impact of computerized clinical documentation, *Comput Inform Nurs* 23(3):132, 2005.

Steward M: Electronic medical records: privacy, confidentiality, liability, *J Leg Med* 26(4):491, 2005.

The Joint Commission: *2008 Standard improvement initiative: home care accreditation program: accreditation requirements*, effective January 2008, 2008a, The Commission, http://www.jointcommission.org/AccreditationPrograms/Homecare/Standards/09_FAQs/.

The Joint Commission: *2008 Standard improvement initiative: hospital accreditation program*, effective January 2009, 2008b, The Commission, http://www.joint-commission.org/AccreditationPrograms/Hospitals/.

The Joint Commission: *2009 National patient safety goals*, 2008c, The Joint Commission, http://www.jointcommission.org/PatientSafety/NationalPatientSafetyGoals/.

Thede LQ: *Informatics and nursing opportunities and challenges*, ed 2, Philadelphia, 2003, Lippincott Williams & Wilkins.

U.S. Department of Health and Human Services: *OCR privacy brief: summary of the HIPAA privacy rule*, May 2003, http://www.hhs.gov/ocr/privacysummary.pdf.

Wimberley P and others: HIPAA and nursing education: how to teach in a paranoid health care environment, *J Nurs Educ* 44(11):489, 2005.

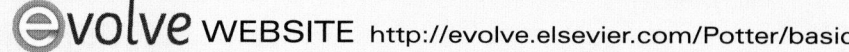
OBJECTIVES

- Describe the elements of the communication process.
- Describe the three levels of communication and their uses in nursing.
- Differentiate aspects of verbal and nonverbal communication.
- Identify features and expected outcomes of the nurse-patient helping relationship.
- Describe a nurse's focus within each phase of a therapeutic nurse-patient helping relationship.

- Describe behaviors and techniques that affect communication.
- Explain the focus of communication within each phase of the nursing process.
- Discuss effective communication for patients of varying developmental levels.
- Explain techniques used to assist patients with special communication needs.

KEY TERMS

active listening, p. 176
assertive communication, p. 179
channel, p. 167
communication, p. 166
connotative meaning, p. 168

denotative meaning, p. 168
empathy, p. 176
environment, p. 167
feedback, p. 167
interpersonal communication, p. 167
intrapersonal communication, p. 167

lateral violence, p. 171
message, p. 167
metacommunication, p. 170
nonverbal communication, p. 168
public communication, p. 167
receiver, p. 167

referent, p. 167
sender, p. 167
sympathy, p. 179
therapeutic communication, p. 170
touch, p. 180
verbal communication, p. 168

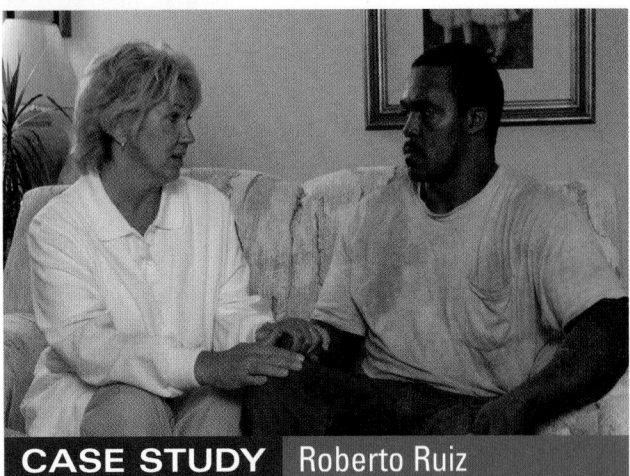

CASE STUDY Roberto Ruiz

Roberto Ruiz is a 44-year-old man of Puerto Rican descent referred to hospice because he suffers from human immune deficiency virus (HIV)/acquired immunodeficiency syndrome (AIDS). After being near death, Roberto has gotten better and is at home. He is weak and stays in most of the time because of his compromised immune system. He gave his beloved dog to a friend in case he did not survive his last hospitalization. Hospice goals were to support his medication regimen, manage his pain, and promote quality of life.

Roberto lives alone and has an extensive network of friends, having lived and worked in the community for over 10 years. His home is full of special art objects that he has collected. Roberto appears tired, speaks softly, and smiles frequently. He talks about how his quality of life is better now than it has ever been. His home is a haven or sanctuary, and he feels peaceful.

Suzanne is a 54-year-old nurse whose mother died 10 years ago and had received hospice care. This was a brief but significant experience that gave her a dedication to hospice and a commitment to maximizing quality of life in end-of-life care.

Communication in nursing is a journey to a destination of clear meaning. Nurses travel this road to help patients and families heal and to promote health and wholeness. Communication is at the heart of nursing and is essential in conveying caring and applying nursing skills and knowledge. Clear, caring communication takes a lifetime to master but develops one moment at a time. Start today to pay attention to communication in your life. Watch what you and others say, how it is said, the nonverbal messages, and what words people choose in written and electronic communication. Consider what is not said, but implied by posture or tone of voice or a "look."

You will learn from every interaction. Sometimes these treasures are lessons you learn from awkward moments or missed opportunities. Sometimes these treasures are when a patient shows gratitude for your gentle touch by comfortable silence and eye contact. Finch (2006) noted that in today's complex work environment it is more important than ever to communicate in order to provide optimal patient care. McGilton and others (2006) found that a program to enhance nurses' communication skills increased job satisfaction. When you focus on the patient, you can make a difference, learn from every interaction, and build competency in therapeutic, interpersonal communication.

You use nonverbal, verbal, and technological skills to communicate in both personal and impersonal situations. You send and receive information through many different channels. You communicate in person, in writing, over the telephone, through fax and electronic mail, through the Internet, and in ways we cannot yet imagine. Communication in all of these modes is an ongoing, dynamic, and often complex process.

THE POWER OF COMMUNICATION

As with any aspect of therapy, communication may result in both harm and good. Your posture, your expressions and gestures, every word you choose and phrase you speak can hurt or heal through the messages they send. Even techniques meant to be therapeutic can have unexpected negative effects. Failure to communicate leads to serious problems, increases liability, and threatens professional credibility. Inappropriate or missing communication causes delays in health care delivery, adding cost to the patient and agency. Respect communication for its potential power, and do not misuse it to manipulate or bully others. Good communication empowers others and enables people to know themselves and to make their own choices.

Self-awareness is important for effective communication (Jack and Smith, 2007). As you know more about yourself, you will be able to relate to others more effectively. Reflection on your interactions increases your understanding of the communication process and improves your ability to communicate with your patients. Reflect on interactions by asking yourself questions such as, What happened? Who was involved? What went wrong? and How did you feel about it? To interpret, you answer, What did I hope or expect to happen? What interfered with the outcome? What factors were involved? To learn, you reflect on what the story tells you about yourself and the lessons you learned.

In a team meeting Suzanne reflects on her concerns when she first worked with patients who had HIV/AIDS. Now Suzanne has a very different perspective and is able to see Roberto as a person and not as a fearful disease. He is one of her favorite patients. Roberto has introduced her to the healing power of music, and they chat about favorite movies. Seeing how Roberto savors moments of his day, she begins to pay more attention to appreciating her own life and adds music and art to her environment.

BASIC ELEMENTS OF THE COMMUNICATION PROCESS

Figure 10-1 outlines the basic elements of the communication process. This simple model helps you to identify essential components of communication. People in conversation rarely analyze the meaning of every gesture or word. In your professional role, you will learn to pay attention to each aspect so that interactions are purposeful and effective. Here is a summary of the elements of communication:

- The **referent** motivates one person to communicate with another. In a health care environment, sights, sounds, odors, time schedules, emotions, sensations, perceptions, and other cues initiate communication. Considering the referent during an interaction helps the sender develop and organize the message.
- The **sender** is the person who delivers the message. The roles of sender and receiver change back and forth as two persons interact.
- The **message** is the content of the conversation, including verbal and nonverbal information the sender expresses. The most effective message is clear, organized, and expressed in a manner familiar to both the sender and the receiver.
- The **channel** is the means of conveying and receiving the message through visual, auditory, and tactile senses. For example, your facial expression sends a visual message, and spoken words travel through auditory channels. Usually, the more channels the sender uses to convey a message, the more clearly the receiver will understand the message.
- You send the message to the **receiver.** The message acts as one of the receiver's referents, prompting a response. The more the sender and receiver have in common and the closer the relationship, the more likely the receiver will accurately perceive the sender's meaning and respond appropriately.
- The **environment** is the physical and emotional climate in which the interaction takes place. Make the environment comfortable and suitable to the participants' needs for effective communication. The more positive an environment, the more successful the communication exchange.
- The message the receiver returns to the sender is **feedback.** Feedback indicates whether the receiver understood the meaning of the sender's message. Your positive intent is not enough to ensure accurate reception of a message. Seek verbal and nonverbal feedback from the receiver to be sure the receiver understands the message.

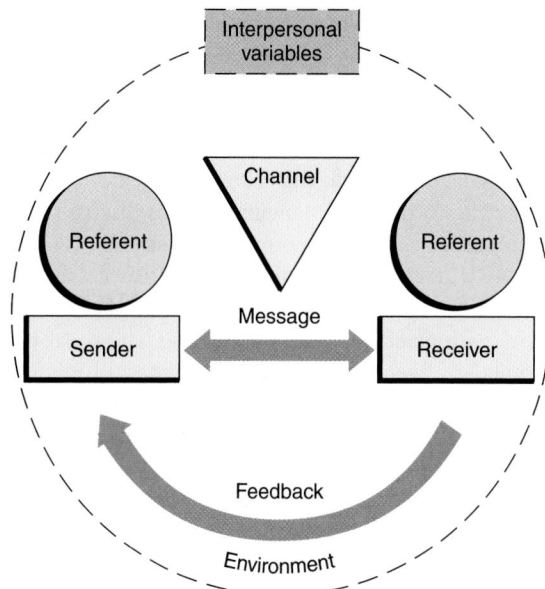

Figure 10-1 ■ Communication as active process between sender and receiver.

LEVELS OF COMMUNICATION

As a nurse, you communicate at different levels. You communicate with yourself, with other individuals, and with groups. Each level of communication is important and affects your nursing practice. **Intrapersonal communication,** also called self-talk, is a powerful form of communication that occurs within an individual. People "talk to themselves" by forming thoughts internally that strongly influence perceptions, feelings, behavior, self-concept, and performance. Self-talk is a mental rehearsal for difficult tasks or situations so individuals deal with them more effectively (Gibson and Foster, 2007). Be aware of the nature and content of your own thinking, and try to replace negative, self-defeating thoughts with positive ones. Use positive self-talk to overcome obstacles and boost your confidence (White, 2008). In forms such as imagery or meditation, you use it to enhance coping and reduce stress.

Interpersonal communication is interaction that occurs between two people or within a small group. It refers to nonverbal and verbal behavior within a social context and includes the use of symbols and cues to give and receive meaning. Because messages received are sometimes different from messages intended, validate or mutually negotiate the meaning between participants. Effective interpersonal communication includes idea sharing, problem solving, expressing feelings, decision making, goal accomplishment, team building, and personal growth.

Public communication is the interaction of one individual with large groups of people. You will have opportunities to speak with groups of patients or consumers about health-related topics. You will make special adaptations in eye contact, posture, gestures, voice inflection, and use of media materials to communicate messages effectively.

FORMS OF COMMUNICATION

You send messages in many different ways: verbally, nonverbally, concretely, and symbolically. People express themselves through language, movements, gestures, voice inflection, facial expressions, and use of space. Many forms of communication combine to create meaning in the sender's message.

Verbal Communication

Verbal communication involves the spoken or written word. Verbal language is a code that conveys specific meaning as you combine words. The following sections discuss the most important aspects of verbal communication.

VOCABULARY Communication is unsuccessful if the receiver cannot translate a sender's words and phrases. You will work with persons of various cultures who speak different languages. Even people who speak the same language use subcultural variations of words. For example, *dinner* means a midday meal for some, whereas others use *dinner* to mean the last meal of the day. Medical terms or jargon often sound like a foreign language. Children use special words to describe bodily functions or a favorite blanket or toy. Adolescents often use words in unique ways that are unfamiliar to adults.

DENOTATIVE AND CONNOTATIVE MEANING A single word sometimes has several meanings. Individuals who use a common language share the **denotative meaning** of a word. The word *baseball* has the same meaning for all individuals who speak English, but the word *code* denotes cardiac arrest primarily to health care providers. The **connotative meaning** is the shade or interpretation of a word's meaning influenced by the thoughts, feelings, or ideas people have about the word. Families who are told a loved one is in serious condition might believe that death is near, but to nurses the term *serious* may simply describe the nature of the illness.

PACING Talking rapidly, using awkward pauses, or speaking slowly and deliberately conveys an unintended message. Consider the following exchange:

Patient: "Do you know if the doctor found anything wrong?"
Nurse: "No . . . but I'm sure if he did . . . he would have come to explain things to you." (then very rapidly) "Now let's get back to where we were."

Long pauses and a rapid shift to another subject give the impression that you are hiding the truth. Speak slowly, enunciate clearly, and use pauses to accentuate or stress a particular point or to give the listener time to understand.

INTONATION Tone of voice dramatically affects a message's meaning, and emotions directly influence tone of voice. A simple question or statement can express enthusiasm, anger, or concern. Be aware of your intonation to avoid sending unintended messages. If the patient interprets your message as uncaring or condescending, communication is blocked. Pay attention to a patient's intonation for information about his or her emotional state or energy level.

CLARITY AND BREVITY Effective communication is simple, short, and to the point to minimize confusion. Avoid phrases such as "you know" or "OK?" at the end of every sentence. Give examples to clarify messages for the receiver. Use short sentences and words that express an idea simply and directly.

TIMING AND RELEVANCE Timing is critical in communication. Even if a message is clear, poor timing prevents it from being effective. Do not begin routine teaching when a patient is in severe pain or emotional distress. The best time for interaction is when a patient expresses an interest in communicating. Relevant messages are more effective. When a patient is facing emergency surgery, discussing the risks of smoking is less relevant than discussing what the staff will do to prepare the patient for surgery.

Nonverbal Communication

Nonverbal communication includes messages sent through the language of the body, without using words. Nonverbal forms of communication include facial expressions; vocal cues; eye contact; action cues, such as gestures; posture; touch; odor; physical appearance; dress; silence; and the use of time (Arnold and Boggs, 2007). Nonverbal communication often accurately reveals true feelings, because you have less control over nonverbal reactions. A patient who says he feels fine but frowns while moving and holds his body rigidly is probably in pain. Nonverbal cues add meaning to verbal communication and help you judge the reliability of verbal messages. Nonverbal behaviors vary in different cultures. Gestures or expressions that are acceptable in one culture may have a different meaning and be considered rude in another culture (Arnold and Boggs, 2007).

Because nonverbal messages are usually not as obvious as verbal messages, become an astute observer of nonverbal behavior. Be sure your nonverbal and verbal messages match. If you say a patient is getting better but wear an expression of doubt, you will not relieve a patient's anxiety.

PERSONAL APPEARANCE Physical characteristics, manner of dress and grooming, and jewelry are indicators of well-being, personality, social status, occupation, religion, culture, and self-concept. First impressions are largely based on appearance. Your physical appearance influences a patient's perception of care. You will wear uniforms, scrub suits, laboratory coats, business suits, or street clothes depending on your role. Although your dress may not reflect your abilities, it takes longer to establish trust if your clothing differs from a patient's preconceived image.

POSTURE AND GAIT The way people sit, stand, and move is a form of self-expression. Posture and gait reflect emotions, self-concept, and health status. An erect posture and a quick, purposeful gait communicate a sense of well-being and confidence. A slumped posture and slow, shuffling gait may indicate depression or fatigue. Leaning forward conveys attention. Leaning backward in a more relaxed manner shows less interest or indicates caution.

FACIAL EXPRESSION The face, the most expressive part of the body, reveals emotions such as surprise, fear, anger, happiness, and sadness. The sender's facial expressions often become the basis for judgments by the receiver. However, because of the diversity in facial expressions, meanings are often misunderstood. Facial expressions reveal, contradict, or suppress true emotions. People are often unaware of the messages their expressions send. When facial expressions are unclear, seek verbal feedback about the sender's intent. A patient who frowns after receiving information may be confused, angry, disapproving, or simply concentrating on a reply. In this case, say, "I notice you're frowning," and encourage clarification of the patient's response.

Patients watch nurses closely. Consider the effect your facial expression has on a patient who asks, "Am I going to die?" The slightest change in the eyes, lips, or face will reveal your true feelings. Learn to avoid showing overt shock, disgust, dismay, or other distressing reactions in the patient's presence.

EYE CONTACT Americans generally maintain eye contact to signal a readiness to communicate, regardless of social class. By maintaining eye contact during conversation, you communicate respect and a willingness to listen. Eye contact also allows you to observe another closely. Lack of eye contact indicates anxiety, defensiveness, discomfort, or a lack of confidence in communicating. However, some cultures, such as Asian and Indochinese, Native American, and Appalachian, consider eye contact to be intrusive, threatening, or harmful and minimize its use (Understanding Transcultural Nursing, 2005). Always consider the person's culture when interpreting the meaning of eye contact.

Eye movements communicate feelings and emotions. Wide eyes express frankness, terror, and innocence. Downward glances show modesty. Raised upper eyelids reveal displeasure, and a constant stare may be associated with hatred or coldness. Looking down on a person establishes authority, whereas interacting at the same eye level indicates equality in the relationship. You appear less dominant and less threatening when interacting at the patient's eye level. Rising to the same eye level of an angry person helps establish your independence.

GESTURES A salute, a thumbs-up, and a tapping foot are types of gestures. Hands and feet emphasize, punctuate, and clarify the spoken word. Gestures alone carry specific meanings, or they may create messages with other communication cues. A finger pointed toward a person may communicate several different meanings, but if you frown and have a stern tone of voice, the gesture becomes a sign of accusation or threat.

TERRITORIALITY AND SPACE Territoriality is the need to gain, maintain, and defend one's exclusive right to space. *Territory* is separated and made visible to others, such as a fence around a yard. *Personal space* is invisible, individual, and travels with the person. During interpersonal interaction, people consciously maintain varying distances between themselves, depending on the nature of the relationship and situation. When personal space is threatened, people respond defensively and communicate less effectively. Examples of nursing actions within the four zones of personal space are listed in Box 10-1 (Kneisl and Trigoboff, 2009).

You must frequently move into patients' territory and personal space because of the nature of caregiving. Convey confidence, gentleness, and respect for privacy, especially when actions require intimate contact. Knock before you enter a room. As you leave, ask if the patient wants the door open or closed. Ask if you can reposition the bed table and what items the patient wants close by.

BOX 10-1 Nursing Actions Within the Zones of Personal Space and Touch

ZONES OF PERSONAL SPACE

Intimate Zone (0 to 18 inches)
- Holding a crying infant
- Performing physical assessment
- Bathing, grooming, dressing, feeding, and toileting a patient
- Changing a patient's dressing

Personal Zone (18 inches to 4 feet)
- Sitting at a patient's bedside
- Taking the patient's nursing history
- Teaching an individual patient
- Exchanging information at change of shift

Social Zone (4 to 12 feet)
- Making rounds with a health care provider
- Sitting at the head of a conference table
- Teaching a class for patients with diabetes
- Conducting a family support group

Public Zone (12 feet and greater)
- Speaking at a community forum
- Testifying at a legislative hearing
- Lecturing to a class of students

ZONES OF TOUCH

Social Zone (Permission Not Needed)
- Hands
- Arms
- Shoulders
- Back

Consent Zone (Permission Needed)
- Mouth
- Wrists
- Feet

Vulnerable Zone (Special Care Needed)
- Face
- Neck
- Front of body

Intimate Zone (Great Sensitivity Needed)
- Genitalia

BOX 10-2 Contextual Factors Influencing Communication

PSYCHOPHYSIOLOGICAL CONTEXT—THE *INTERNAL FACTORS* INFLUENCING COMMUNICATION
- Physical health
- Emotional status
- Growth and development status
- Unmet needs
- Attitudes, values, and beliefs
- Perceptions and personality
- Self-concept and self-esteem

RELATIONAL CONTEXT—THE *NATURE OF THE RELATIONSHIP* BETWEEN THE PARTICIPANTS
- Social, helping, or working relationship
- Level of trust and self-disclosure between participants
- Shared history of participants
- Balance of power and control

SITUATIONAL CONTEXT—THE *REASON FOR* THE COMMUNICATION
Information exchange
- Goal achievement
- Problem resolution
- Expression of feelings

ENVIRONMENTAL CONTEXT—THE *PHYSICAL SURROUNDINGS* IN WHICH COMMUNICATION TAKES PLACE
- Degree of privacy
- Degree of comfort and safety
- Noise level
- Presence of distractions

CULTURAL CONTEXT—THE *SOCIOCULTURAL ELEMENTS* THAT AFFECT THE INTERACTION
- Educational level of participants
- Language and self-expression patterns
- Customs and expectations

FACTORS INFLUENCING COMMUNICATION

Contextual aspects that influence the nature of communication and interpersonal relationships are described in Box 10-2. Awareness of these factors helps you to make sound decisions during the communication process.

Metacommunication is exploration of all factors that influence communication. Awareness of influencing factors helps you better understand what is communicated (Arnold and Boggs, 2007). For example, the patient who has had facial surgery tells you, "This scar doesn't look as bad as I thought it would," but is teary and appears apprehensive. Your nursing experience with facial disfigurement teaches you how anxious people are about a part of the body that everyone can see. Awareness that the patient's verbal and nonverbal behaviors do not match prompts you to explore the patient's feelings and concerns. This analysis of all aspects of communication is metacommunication.

THE NURSE-PATIENT HELPING RELATIONSHIP

As Suzanne works with Roberto, she develops a helping relationship. They work together to manage his pain. Roberto says, "I can stand some pain. I don't want to be 'out of it.' I want to feel alive." Suzanne sees Roberto as a courageous man. His passion

for life is inspiring. From her coursework in end-of-life care (ELNEC, 2000), Suzanne knows that posing questions for the patient's reflection helps her assess his needs and support his self-care strategies. "What are your needs at this time?" "What are your concerns at this time and for the future?" Roberto talks about wanting to get strong enough to have his dog again. He wants to make a trip home to New York to visit his family and make peace.

A helping relationship between you and your patient does not just happen. You create it with care and skill, and build it on the patient's trust in you as a nurse. Through **therapeutic communication,** you develop a relationship with the patient to meet several purposes. Box 10-3 summarizes the four phases of the nurse-patient relationship. Imogene King (1971), a nurse theorist, calls the nurse-patient relationship "learning experiences whereby two people interact to face an immediate health problem, to share, if possible, in resolving it, and to discover ways to adapt to the situation." You help patients to clarify needs and goals, solve problems, and cope with situational or maturational crises. You also help patients explore the meaning of their illness experience and sort out responses to stressful situations to increase coping skills (Arnold and Boggs, 2007). Creating this therapeutic environment depends on your ability to communicate, provide comfort, and help the patient meet his or her needs. Comforting strategies include gentle humor, physical comfort measures, emotionally supportive statements, and comforting and connecting touch. You provide information, support patients' active decision making, and offer opportunities for patients to engage in social exchange.

BOX 10-3   Phases of the Helping Relationship

PREINTERACTION PHASE—BEFORE MEETING THE PATIENT, YOU:

- Review available data, including the medical and nursing histories
- Talk to other caregivers who may have information about the patient
- Anticipate health concerns or issues that may arise
- Identify a location and setting that will foster comfortable, private interaction
- Plan enough time for the initial interaction

ORIENTATION PHASE—WHEN YOU AND THE PATIENT MEET AND GET TO KNOW ONE ANOTHER, YOU:

- Set the tone for the relationship by adopting a warm, empathetic, caring manner
- Recognize that the initial relationship may be superficial, uncertain, and tentative
- Expect the patient to test your competence and commitment
- Closely observe the patient and expect to be closely observed by the patient
- Begin to make inferences and form judgments about patient messages and behavior
- Assess the patient's health status
- Prioritize patient problems and identify patient goals
- Clarify the patient's and your roles
- Form contracts with the patient to specify roles
- Let the patient know when you will terminate the relationship

WORKING PHASE—WHEN YOU AND THE PATIENT WORK TOGETHER TO SOLVE PROBLEMS AND ACCOMPLISH GOALS, YOU:

- Encourage and help the patient to express feelings about his or her health
- Encourage and help the patient with self-exploration
- Provide information needed to understand and change behavior
- Encourage and help the patient to set goals
- Take actions to meet the goals set with the patient
- Use therapeutic communication skills to facilitate successful interactions
- Use appropriate self-disclosure and confrontation

TERMINATION PHASE—DURING THE ENDING OF THE RELATIONSHIP, YOU:

- Remind the patient that termination is near
- Evaluate goal achievement with the patient
- Reminisce about the relationship with the patient
- Separate from the patient by relinquishing responsibility for his or her care
- Achieve a smooth transition for the patient to other caregivers as needed

Suzanne demonstrates caring for Roberto as she takes time to look at a picture of Roberto's dog dressed in a special sweater to celebrate the dog's homecoming.

NURSE–HEALTH TEAM MEMBER RELATIONSHIPS

Communication with other members of the health care team affects patient safety and the work environment. Breakdown in communication is the more frequent cause of serious injuries in health care settings (World Health Organization, 2007). When patients move from one nursing unit to another or from one provider to another, also known as hand-offs, there is a risk for miscommunication. Accurate communication is essential to prevent errors.

Use of common language when communicating critical information helps prevent misunderstandings. SBAR is a popular communication tool that helps standardize communication between health care providers. SBAR stands for *situation, background, assessment,* and *recommendation* (Pope, Rodzen, and Spross, 2008). In the case study, when Roberto's pain is no longer adequately controlled, Suzanne would communicate to Roberto's health care provider that he needs better pain control

(situation) and then give the health care provider brief information about his history, noting that Roberto does not want to be "out of it" (background). Suzanne would then give an accurate description of his pain (assessment) and request a modification of Roberto's pain regimen (recommendation). Research indicates that effective communication with the health care provider and other health team members ensures patient safety and promotes optimal patient outcomes (Box 10-4).

Nurses frequently work as a team. Effective communication and camaraderie between nurses in a work setting is essential for teamwork, which affects nurse recruitment and retention. Social, informational, and therapeutic interactions help team members build morale, accomplish goals, and strengthen working relationships. **Lateral violence** sometimes occurs in nurse-nurse interactions and includes behaviors such as withholding information, backbiting, making snide remarks, and nonverbal expressions of disapproval such as raising eyebrows or making faces. New graduates and nurses new to the unit are most likely to face problems with lateral violence. All nurses require skill in conflict management and assertive communication to help them deal with these situations (Patterson, 2007). Developing a support system with nurses on your units and other new graduates will help you positively address incidents of lateral violence.

BOX 10-4   BEST PRACTICES
Communication With the Health Care Team

SUMMARY OF EVIDENCE

Effective communication with the health care provider and other members of the health care team promotes optimal patient outcomes. The Joint Commission reported that breakdown in communication was the root cause of sentinel events between 1995 and 2006. Sentinel events are unexpected occurrences that result in death or serious injury. Communication when the patient is handed over from one provider to another or from one setting to another is especially a problem. Hand-over communication occurs during nurse change-of-shift report, transfer between units or facilities, report between departments such as from the emergency department to an inpatient unit, and between disciplines such as between physical therapy and nursing. Communication is also important when nurses are communicating changes in a patient's condition to other members of the health care team. Common language for communicating critical information can help prevent misunderstandings. Health care providers need to allow sufficient time to ask and respond to questions. Reading back of information also helps identify any miscommunication and ensures the information received is accurate. Intimidating and disruptive behaviors affect communication. Nurses are sometimes reluctant to communicate concerns or problems because they are afraid of the response.

APPLICATION TO NURSING PRACTICE

Develop common language for critical information for hand-over communications and to communicate changes in a patient's condition.

- Use a communication tool such as SBAR to standardize communication.
- Use a standardized format for shift-change report.
- Use a standardized format for report when patients are transferred to other units or facilities.
- Provide the opportunity for questions and confirmation of understanding of communication.
- Have face-to-face communication when possible.
- Read back all physician or health care provider orders or other pertinent information.
- Allow time for questions and clarification of information.
- Create a culture of patient safety that allows questions and open communication.
- Work in multidisciplinary teams to develop common language.
- Develop skills in assertive communication and conflict management.

REFERENCES

Leonard M, Graham S, Bonacum D: The human factor: the critical importance of effective teamwork and communication in providing safe care, *Qual Saf Health Care* 13:i85, 2004.

Markley J, Winbery S: Communication with physicians: how agencies can be heard, *Home Health Care Manage Pract* 20(2):161, 2008.

Rodgers KL: Using the SBAR communication technique to improve nurse-physician phone communication: a pilot study, *AAACN Viewpoint* 29(2):7, 2007.

The Joint Commission: Behaviors that undermine a culture of safety, *Sentinel Event Alert,* issue 40, July 9, 2008.

World Health Organization: Communication during patient hand-overs, *Patient Safety Solutions* 1:solution 3, May 2007, http://www.who.int/patientsafety/solutions/patientsafety/PS-Solution3.pdf.

COMMUNICATION WITHIN CARING RELATIONSHIPS

Therapeutic communication strengthens all caring relationships established within the professional role. You create caring and helping relationships with the qualities and behavior explained in this section.

Establishing a Therapeutic Relationship

PROFESSIONALISM The patient's acceptance of you as a professional often depends on the manner in which you present a professional and caring image. Verbal and nonverbal behaviors influence the helping relationship. Professional appearance, demeanor, and behavior are important in establishing trustworthiness and competence. When you act professionally, you communicate that you have assumed the professional helping role, are clinically skilled, and that your focus is on the patient. Inappropriate appearance and behavior in those who hold a professional role harm the image of nursing. Consider the level of trust a patient feels with each nurse in the following examples.

Annie Robbins is late for her shift. She left her stethoscope and notepad at home. She is chewing gum, she has a large chunky necklace and long dangling hair, and her underwear is visible beneath her uniform. She is wearing heavy makeup and perfume, has long painted fingernails, and there is smoke on her breath and clothing. She giggles, talks loudly, uses slang, rolls her eyes, grimaces, and writes vital signs on the skin of her hand. She reacts to problems by blaming others and behaving immaturely.

Mary Kline arrives at work on time and is organized, well prepared, and equipped for the responsibilities of her nursing role. She is clean, well-groomed, appropriately dressed, and scent- and odor-free. Her behavior reflects warmth, friendliness, confidence, and competence. She speaks clearly, uses good grammar, and listens to others. She helps and supports teammates, communicates effectively, and handles problems in a mature manner.

COURTESY Common courtesy is important to your role. It conveys respect for others and oneself. Courtesy techniques include saying hello and goodbye, knocking on doors before entering, introducing oneself, and stating one's purpose. Other aspects of courtesy are addressing people by name, saying "please" and "thank you" to team members, and apologizing for making an error or causing someone distress. These are all parts of good professional communication. When you are discourteous, patients and staff will perceive you as rude or insensitive. Discourtesy sets up barriers between you and the patient and causes friction or tension among team members.

Self-introduction is especially important. Failure to give your name, indicate your professional status, or acknowledge the patient creates uncertainty about the interaction and conveys an impersonal lack of commitment or caring. Make eye contact and smile. Acknowledge others by name to show your respect for the dignity and uniqueness of the other person. Begin initial interactions by using the patient's last name to show respect. Ask others how they would like you to address them, and let them know your personal preference as well. Using first names is appropriate for infants, young children, confused or unconscious patients, and close team members.

Avoid Terms of Endearment Calling the patient "honey," "dear," "Grandpa," or "sweetheart" rather than by a personal name is inappropriate. Such casual familiarity from caregivers offends most people. **Avoid referring to patients by diagnosis, room number, or other attribute.** When you refer to patients by attributes rather than their names, it is demeaning and sends the message that you do not care enough about the person to know him or her as an individual.

CONFIDENTIALITY Always safeguard a patient's right to privacy by carefully protecting information of a confidential nature. Reassure the person that you will keep information private, and then keep that promise. Resist the temptation to share exciting or shocking information. Do not share information with people who are genuinely interested and concerned but have no legal right to the information.

Patient: "What's wrong with my roommate? She seems so sick."
Nurse: "I know you're concerned about Mrs. Hoover, but I can't share any personal information about a patient..."

If you have to report information to others, tell the patient in advance, if possible. Sharing personal information or gossiping about others violates nursing's ethical code and practice standards. It sends the message that you are not trustworthy and damages interpersonal relationships.

TRUST Trust is an essential building block of the helping relationship. You foster trust when you communicate warmth and caring and demonstrate consistency, reliability, honesty, and competence. Trusting another person involves risk and vulnerability, but it also fosters open, therapeutic communication and enhances the expression of feelings, thoughts, and needs. Do not compromise trust by acting as if you are "too busy." Such a response becomes a protective excuse for not becoming involved with the patient.

Being untrustworthy or dishonest seriously damages relationships and violates legal and ethical standards of practice. Although it is not always easy, do not withhold key information, lie, or distort the truth. For example, a patient asks why the nurse is collecting his 24-hour urine sample again.

Nurse, lying: "The lab wants us to repeat the test, because their machine broke down during the analysis and they need a fresh specimen."
A better response is, "I'm sorry, Mr. Gottleib. One of the staff didn't save some of your urine by mistake. We will make every effort to make sure it is all saved this time."

ACCEPTANCE AND RESPECT Conveying acceptance means that you are nonjudgmental. As a nurse, you are expected to provide high-quality care regardless of social or economic status, personal attributes, or the nature of an illness. Acceptance is a willingness to hear a message or to acknowledge feelings. This does not mean that you agree or approve. Acceptance includes giving positive feedback, making sure verbal and nonverbal cues match, and using touch. Being empathetic, restating, and avoiding arguments also show acceptance and respect.

AVAILABILITY Availability means being present for the other person when needed and offering your presence even when the patient does not express the need verbally. You do this by showing a caring attitude, demonstrating your willingness to listen and talk, or by just being physically present. Do not avoid patients whose behavior is troublesome. Such avoidance often increases the patient's negative behavior. Being *task oriented*, or making a technical procedure (e.g., administration of a medication) the focus of an interaction, is another way of not being emotionally available. You miss opportunities to assess the patient, explore concerns, calm anxiety, demonstrate empathy, teach, or involve the patient in care. Patients will perceive you as cold, uncaring, and unapproachable when you are task oriented. As a student, it is difficult to integrate therapeutic communication when you perform technical skills because of the need to focus on the procedure. In time you learn to do both and promote more satisfactory interactions. Consider the quality of care given in each of the following scenarios.

Nurse A silently enters the patient's room: "It's time for your pain shot."
The patient, Mr. Stewart, is mildly startled and grimaces. As he starts to ask a question, Nurse A quickly reaches for his arm, gives the injection, then leaves.
Nurse B, calling the patient's name as she enters the room: "Mr. Stewart, I have your pain medication. Are you feeling as uncomfortable as you look?"
Patient: "Yes, my back feels like a knife went through it. Will the pain ever go away?"
Nurse B lays syringe down and sits by patient: "It's common to have some pain the first few days after surgery, but I'll work with you to keep you comfortable. This medicine should help. I'll give

the shot and then show you how to move in bed so the pain won't get worse. If you have breakthrough pain, I will call the doctor to see about adjusting your medicine."

Nurse B assessed the patient's need for a caring presence and provided caring by setting aside her own task and being available for the patient. Notice that this intervention was brief yet effective. Question the assumption that nurses do not "have time" for caring connections.

SOCIALIZING Socializing is an important component of your communication as a nurse. You use it as a tool to get to know one another and to help people relax. At the beginning of an interaction use social conversation that is easy and superficial to make connections. This helps the patient feel comfortable in sharing feelings and concerns. Consider Suzanne's friendly, informal, and warm communication style in establishing trust with Roberto:

Suzanne: "That's a beautiful piece of art, Roberto."
Roberto: "Yes, isn't it? I found it in a little shop in Italy."
Suzanne: "You traveled to Italy?"
Roberto: "Yes it was a great trip, and this painting reminds me of that wonderful time."

Avoid Inappropriate Socializing Move beyond social conversation to talk about issues or concerns affecting the patient's health.

COMMUNICATION WITHIN THE NURSING PROCESS

In the nursing process you use communication to gather information, develop the nursing diagnosis, plan your care, implement nursing interventions, and evaluate your care (see Chapter 8). You also may use the nursing process to address communication problems. Although the nursing process is a reliable framework for delivering comprehensive patient care, it will not work well unless you master the art of effective interpersonal communication. Successful communication occurs with knowledge acquired from books, experiences, and observation of others' communication skills. Communication techniques used within the nursing process are also applied during the problem-solving process with team members to resolve problems or accomplish goals within the clinical setting (Box 10-5).

■■■ASSESSMENT

Use communication during the assessment phase of the nursing process to gather information about a patient. The time you spend assessing patients is a good time to establish the rapport needed for good communication. For example, through therapeutic communication techniques, you collect data about the patient's medical history and current problem or concern. To learn more about Roberto's pain, Suzanne asks him, "How is your pain different than it was last week?" Systematically collect data and then organize the data you collect. Document information you obtain from the patient, family, and significant others.

PHYSICAL AND EMOTIONAL FACTORS Assess physical or psychological factors that influence communication. Many altered health states limit communication, including facial trauma, cancer of the larynx or trachea, aphasia after a stroke, breathing problems, Alzheimer's disease, high anxiety, and heavy sedation. Certain mental illnesses such as psychoses or depression cause patients to have flight of ideas, constant verbalization of the same words or phrases, or a slow speech pattern. Review the patient's medical record for relevant information. The record will describe any physical barriers to speech, neurological deficits, and pathophysiological conditions affecting hearing or vision. Also, review the medication record. Opiates, antidepressants, neuroleptics, hypnotics, or sedatives cause patients to slur words or use incom-

---

BOX 10-5   Communication Through the Nursing Process

ASSESSMENT
- Interviewing and history taking
- Physical examination (use of visual, auditory, and tactile channels)
- Observation of nonverbal behavior
- Review of medical records, literature, diagnostic tests

NURSING DIAGNOSIS
- Written analysis of assessment findings
- Discussion of health care needs and priorities with patient and family

PLANNING
- Written care plans
- Health team planning sessions
- Discussions with patient and family to determine methods of implementation
- Making referrals

IMPLEMENTATION
- Discussion with other health professionals
- Health teaching
- Provision of therapeutic support
- Contact with other health resources
- Record of patient's progress in care plan and nurses' notes

EVALUATION
- Acquisition of verbal and nonverbal feedback
- Written results of expected outcomes
- Update of written care plan
- Explanation of revisions to patient

plete sentences. Communicate directly with patients and family members to fully assess communication difficulties and build a plan to enhance communication.

DEVELOPMENTAL FACTORS Consider a patient's developmental level when assessing communication. An infant's self-expression is limited to crying, body movement, and facial expression. Older children express their needs more directly. Pay attention to your nonverbal behavior when working with children. Sudden movements, threatening gestures, and loud noises can be frightening. Include the parents as sources of information about the child's health.

Advancing age influences communication. Problems with hearing or speech are barriers to communication. Assess the hearing ability of older adults (see Chapter 15). Get an older adult's attention before you begin your assessment questions. Face the patient, and stand or sit on the same level so the patient can read your lips. Speak slowly and clearly. Give older adults enough time to ask questions. Do not assume an older adult has communication impairments.

SOCIOCULTURAL FACTORS When caring for patients from diverse cultures, recognize how to adapt your communication approach. Show respect for all persons whatever their age, gender, religion, socioeconomic group, sexual orientation, or ethnicity. Recognize and attend to any personal biases or prejudices that might interfere with patients' care. Take cultural issues into account, and work to be culturally sensitive. Accept patients' rights to adhere to cultural customs and norms. Persons of different cultures use different types of verbal and nonverbal cues to convey meaning. Make a conscious effort not to interpret messages through your own cultural perspective; instead consider the context of the other individual's background. Avoid stereotyping persons from other cultures or making jokes about them (see Chapter 19). Consider the cultural sensitivity the nurse demonstrates in our case study:

Suzanne, the hospice nurse, arrives at Roberto's home for a visit. He offers her a snack and a beverage. She knows that Roberto has limited resources but graciously accepts the food and drink because she understands that in the Puerto Rican culture it would be insulting to refuse. Suzanne learns that Roberto wants to travel to New York to see his family. With further investigation she learns that he has several siblings living nearby and that the family in New York consists of two uncles and several cousins. Her understanding of the importance of the extended family in the Puerto Rican culture helps her appreciate the importance of the trip to New York. Expressing an understanding of the importance of the trip, even though he is in poor health and it will be a difficult trip, demonstrates cultural sensitivity.

Cultural insensitivity in communication takes many forms, including making fun of another's culture, ethnicity, language, or dress. Telling jokes that make fun of specific cultures, stereotyping, patronizing, and incorrectly interpreting culturally based behavior are culturally insensitive. Do not behave in ways that offend the cultural practices of others. In the example above, Suzanne did not refuse her patient's offer of food and drink or question why he felt it important to see more distant relatives.

LANGUAGE There may be language barriers with foreign-born patients and those who speak English as a second language. It is essential that you assess the patient's understanding of all communication and obtain a professional interpreter as needed to ensure accurate communication.

GENDER Gender influences how we think, act, feel, and communicate. There are differences in male and female communication patterns. Males grow up using communication to achieve goals, establish individual status and authority, and compete for attention and power. Females grow up using communication to build connections and cooperate with others. Females also communicate to respond to, show interest in, and support others and are more likely to discuss feelings and personal issues. Men tend to communicate in a more task-oriented fashion and more directly express disagreements and what they want done. A male nurse might say to his colleague, "Help me turn Jeremy." A female nurse might say, "Jeremy needs to be turned," expecting her colleague to understand the implied request for help. Men use more banter, teasing, and playful "put-downs." They sometimes hesitate to ask questions for fear of appearing unknowledgeable, whereas women ask questions to elicit information. Men usually want others to know of their accomplishments; women tend to downplay their achievements. It is important for you to recognize a patient's gender communication pattern. Gender-insensitive communication means a nurse of one gender misinterprets or reacts to messages differently from that intended by the other gender. Being insensitive can block any attempt at forming a therapeutic nurse-patient relationship. Newer research studies the differences between male and female communication patterns (Arnold and Boggs, 2007). You need to assess communication patterns of each individual, and not make assumptions simply based on gender.

■■■NURSING DIAGNOSIS

After collecting assessment data from a patient, cluster pertinent defining characteristics for patterns and problems. Success in accurately identifying the patient's communication problem ensures the formulation of an accurate nursing diagnosis. Nursing diagnoses for patients with communication difficulties often include the following:

- *Anxiety*
- *Impaired verbal communication*
- *Compromised family coping*
- *Ineffective coping*
- *Readiness for enhanced family coping*
- *Powerlessness*
- *Impaired social interaction*

Impaired verbal communication is the nursing diagnostic label to describe the patient who has limited or no ability to communicate verbally. This diagnosis is useful for a wide variety of patients with special problems and needs related to communication. It is defined as "decreased, delayed, or absent ability to receive, process, transmit, and use a system of symbols" (Gulanick and Myers, 2007). A patient with this diagnosis will have defining characteristics such as the inability to articulate words, difficulty forming words, and difficulty in understanding. The related factor for a diagnosis should focus on the cause of the communication disorder. In the case of impaired verbal communication, a related factor might be physiological, mechanical, anatomical, psychological, cultural, or developmental. Be accurate in choosing a related factor so that the interventions you select will effectively resolve the patient's problem.

■■■PLANNING

Once you identify the nature of a patient's communication problem, you need to consider several factors to design a plan of care. For example, motivation improves communication. Patients often need encouragement to try different communication strategies. Also, select interventions and communication techniques appropriate for the patient's age, cultural beliefs, and practices. Plan to allow patients adequate time to practice new communication approaches. It also helps to plan practice sessions in a quiet, private environment. When possible, involve the family in selecting approaches that will foster communication with the patient.

GOALS AND OUTCOMES A plan of care supporting effective communication will have the ultimate goal of a patient being able to communicate his or her needs. Select expected outcomes that are specific and measurable. After you have implemented your interventions, outcomes allow you to determine if your goal was achieved. For example, the outcomes for Roberto include the following:

- Patient identifies two methods to maintain communication with family in New York.
- Patient verbalizes his concerns regarding his declining health.
- Patient initiates conversation about his preferences for care as he becomes weaker.

Sometimes you will care for patients who have difficulty in sending, receiving, and interpreting messages. This interferes with healthy interpersonal relationships. In this case, impaired communication is a contributing factor to other nursing diagnoses such as *impaired social interaction* or *ineffective coping*. Plan interventions in this case to help patients improve their communication skills. For example, role-play helps patients rehearse situations in which they have difficulty communicating.

SETTING PRIORITIES Always include the patient in setting goals and expected outcomes. You will not make any progress if the patient is not interested in achieving the goal you chose. You cannot address all problems at the same time, so consider which is most important. Always maintain an open line of communication so that the patient can express any immediate needs or problems. Keep a call light in reach for the patient restricted to bed, or provide appropriate alternative communication devices such as a message board or Braille computer. If you plan to have a lengthy discussion with a patient, be sure to take care of the patient's physical needs first to avoid interruptions. Make the patient comfortable by ensuring that any symptoms are under control.

CONTINUITY OF CARE Remember to include family caregivers during the planning and implementation phases of the nursing process. This collaboration supports the family and patient. When you use collaboration, patients are more likely to comply with plans. Collaboration also promotes communication among family members to facilitate positive patient-family relationships. Encourage collaboration by asking others for ideas and suggestions about how to reach goals. It gives others the opportunity to express themselves and strengthens problem-solving ability.

Also, collaborate with other health care providers who have expertise in communication strategies. Speech therapists help patients with aphasia. Professional interpreters are invaluable when a patient speaks a foreign language. Mental health clinical nurse specialists help in communicating with angry or highly anxious patients.

■■■IMPLEMENTATION

In carrying out any plan of care, nurses need to use communication techniques that are appropriate for the patient's individual needs. Before learning how to adapt communication methods to help patients with serious communication impairments, it is necessary to learn mental health clinical communication techniques that are the foundation of professional communication. It is also important to understand which communication techniques create barriers to effective interaction.

THERAPEUTIC COMMUNICATION TECHNIQUES Therapeutic communication techniques are specific responses that encourage the expression of feelings and ideas and convey acceptance and respect (Box 10-6). By learning therapeutic communication techniques you become aware of the variety of nursing responses possible in different situations. Although some of the techniques may seem artificial or unnatural at first, your skill and comfort will increase with practice and experience. Satisfaction will result as you achieve outcomes through the therapeutic relationships you form.

Sharing Empathy **Empathy** is the ability to understand and accept another person's perspective (Arnold and Boggs, 2007). You can never totally know another's experiences because you are not in that person's situation, but you can try to understand what the person is going through.

Empathetic statements reflect an understanding of what the patient communicated and tell the patient that you heard both the feeling and the factual content of the communication. This allows the patient to validate or clarify feelings and perceptions. Empathetic responses are neutral and nonjudgmental and foster shared respect. Use them to establish trust in very difficult situations. In the case study Roberto stated he did not want to be out of it, that he wanted to feel alive. An empathetic response from Suzanne is, "It sounds like you don't like to take much pain medication because feeling 'out of it' makes it hard to do the things you want to do. I'm concerned that too much pain might also make it difficult for you to do what you want to do."

Active Listening **Active listening** means being attentive to what the patient is saying both verbally and nonverbally. Active

BOX 10-6 Therapeutic Communication Techniques

 In the case study, Roberto now expresses the desire to visit his family in New York and make peace with them. In one conversation about his relationship with his family, Suzanne demonstrates the use of several communication techniques.

USING SILENCE
• Suzanne sits quietly with Roberto and allows him time to collect his thoughts.

PARAPHRASING
• *Roberto:* "I have some stuff I need to work out with my uncle so I need to go see him."
• *Suzanne:* "You feel it is important to go visit your uncle to address some unresolved issues."

CLARIFYING
• *Roberto:* "Yeah, and I can't deal with the problems with my uncle when I'm out of it."
• *Suzanne:* "When you say 'out of it,' do you mean the medication makes it hard to think straight?"

SHARING HOPE
• *Roberto:* "I just don't know if I'll be able to make the trip to see my uncle, and it's really important to work things out with him."
• *Suzanne:* "I believe you will find a way to make peace with your uncle."

listening facilitates patient communication. The ancient Greek philosopher Epictetus stated, "We have two ears and one mouth so we may listen more and talk less." That is good advice for nurses. Active listening enhances trust because the nurse communicates acceptance and respect for the patient. Several nonverbal skills facilitate attentive listening. You identify them by the acronym SOLER (Townsend, 2006):

S—Sit facing the patient. This posture gives the message that you are there to listen and are interested in what the patient is saying.

O—Observe an open posture (e.g., keep arms and legs uncrossed). This posture suggests that you are "open" to what the patient says. A "closed" position conveys a defensive attitude, possibly provoking a similar response in the patient.

L—Lean toward the patient. This posture conveys that you are involved and interested in the interaction.

E—Establish and maintain eye contact. This behavior conveys your involvement in and willingness to listen to what the patient is saying. Absence of eye contact or shifting of the eyes gives the message that you are not interested in what the patient is saying. Be aware of cultural considerations regarding eye contact

R—Relax. It is important to communicate a sense of being relaxed and comfortable with the patient. Restlessness communicates a lack of interest and conveys a feeling of discomfort to the patient.

Sharing Observations Nurses make observations by commenting on how the other person looks, sounds, or acts. Stating observations often helps the patient communicate without the need for extensive questioning, focusing, or clarification. This technique helps start a conversation with quiet or withdrawn persons. Do not state observations that will embarrass or anger the patient, such as telling someone "You look a mess!" Even if such an observation is made with humor, the patient can become resentful.

Sharing observations differs from making assumptions, which means drawing unnecessary conclusions about the other person without validating them. Making assumptions puts the patient in the position of having to contradict the nurse. Examples include the nurse interpreting fatigue as depression and assuming that untouched food indicates lack of interest in meeting nutritional goals. Making observations is a gentler and safer technique: "I see you did not eat any breakfast...," "You look tense...," or a positive observation such as "I see you have been organizing your photos...."

Using Silence It takes time and experience to become comfortable with silence. Most people have a natural tendency to fill empty spaces with words, but sometimes what those spaces really need is time for the nurse and patient to observe one another, sort out feelings, and think how to say things. Silence is useful when people face decisions that require much thought. For example, if Roberto and Suzanne were discussing the possibility of his needing to move out of his home to get the care he needs, silence could give him time to collect his thoughts and consider the alternatives. Silence is especially therapeutic during times of sadness or grief.

Providing Information Providing relevant information helps your patients make decisions, experience less anxiety, and feel safe and secure. Speak in simple language, and translate medical terms. When offering options, stress that the patient has the right to make decisions. The nurse also provides information that enables others to understand what is happening and what to expect. For example, Suzanne explains, "Roberto, this pain medication may make you feel a little sleepy and groggy at first, but those side effects usually go away after 2 or 3 days."

Clarifying Clarifying validates whether the person interpreted the message correctly. Any time a message is unclear or ambiguous, try to restate it, or ask the other person to restate it, explain further, or give an example of what they mean. For example, Suzanne says, "I'm not sure what you mean; when you say 'out of it,' you mean the medication makes it difficult to think straight?"

Focusing Focusing directs conversation to a specific topic or issue when a discussion becomes unclear. Focusing limits the area to which the sender can respond. Use it when the sender rambles or introduces many unrelated topics in the same conversation. For example, if Roberto said, "I had a nice visit with my friend this morning. He's going to stop over tomorrow. I've been able to take care of my dog better. My medications are doing okay, but the pain's still there. I've been looking at my art collection today, and I'm not sure what I want to do with it when I'm gone. You like art—I could recommend a good gallery if you want to buy some." Suzanne focuses the conversation by replying, "You've been thinking about what to do with your special belongings?"

Paraphrasing Paraphrasing is restating the sender's message in the receiver's own words to make sure you have received information accurately. Be careful not to change the meaning when you paraphrase. Confirm the meaning with the patient. For example, Roberto states, "I've been walking more, and I'm able to do most of my household chores. I don't need as much help around here now." Suzanne replies, "You feel you're getting stronger and more independent. Is that correct?"

Summarizing Summarizing is a concise review of main ideas from a discussion. It brings a sense of satisfaction and closure to an individual conversation or during the termination phase of a nurse-patient relationship. By reviewing a conversation, you focus on key issues and obtain additional relevant information as needed. For example, after a session with much discussion about Roberto's plans and progress, Suzanne summarizes, "Today we talked about your plans to visit your family in New York and some things you can do to help increase your strength. You seem to understand the importance of eating right. Let me know if there is any other information I can get you."

Self-Disclosure You may use self-disclosure during the working phase of a helping relationship. Self-disclosures are personal statements intentionally revealed to the other person. The purpose is to model and educate, foster a therapeutic alliance, validate reality, and encourage autonomy (Stuart and Laraia, 2005). Keep self-disclosures relevant and appropriate. Make these statements to benefit the patient, not you, and use them sparingly so that the patient remains the focus of the interaction. Roberto's brother comes to visit and expresses how hard it is to make time for everything. An inappropriate response from Suzanne would be, "My mother had cancer and was in hospice too. It was so long and drawn out. I was so sad for so long. Even taking care of the kids was hard." An appropriate response is, "When my mother was dying, I was torn between wanting to stay with her every moment and trying to meet the needs of my little kids. Is that how it is for you?"

Sharing Hope Nurses recognize that hope is essential for healing and learn to communicate a "sense of possibility" to others. You give hope by commenting on the positive aspects of the other person's behavior, performance, or response. Sharing a vision of the future and reminding others of their resources and strengths also strengthens hope. You can reassure patients that there are many kinds of hope and that meaning and personal growth can come from illness experiences.

NONTHERAPEUTIC COMMUNICATION TECHNIQUES Certain communication techniques hinder or damage professional relationships. These specific techniques are nontherapeutic or blocking and will often cause recipients to use defenses to avoid being hurt or negatively affected. Nontherapeutic techniques discourage further expression of feelings and ideas and engender negative responses or behaviors in others.

Inattentive Listening Behaviors and nonverbal expressions such as fidgeting, breaking eye contact, daydreaming during conversation, and "pseudolistening" (pretending to listen when one really is not) convey the message that what the sender has to say is not important. These behaviors discourage conversation and damage trust. Further examples are looking at your watch, tapping your foot impatiently, and gazing out the window as the patient talks.

Using Medical Vocabulary Technical words can cause confusion and anxiety. Avoid use of such terms, or translate them into lay terms.

Prying or Asking Personal Questions Asking irrelevant personal questions simply to satisfy your curiosity is inappropriate and invasive. If patients wish to share private information, they will.

Giving Approval or Disapproval Do not impose your own attitudes, values, beliefs, and moral standards on others while in the professional helping role. People have the right to be themselves and make their own decisions. Avoid using terms such as *should, ought, good, bad, right,* or *wrong.* Agreeing, disagreeing, or sharing your personal opinion sends the subtle message that you have the right to make value judgments about patient decisions. Instead, offer options and help the other person anticipate the consequences of decisions. The problem and its solution belong to the patient, not the nurse.

> *Roberto:* "I really want to go visit my uncles in New York, but I'm not sure I'm up for the trip."
> *Suzanne:* "I don't think it's a good idea to try to travel that far."

A better response is, "It sounds like you miss your family. Let's talk about your options for maintaining contact."

Changing the Subject Changing the subject is a common problem when you are uncomfortable with a topic, but it is insensitive and tends to block further communication.

Automatic Responses Clichés or stereotypical remarks such as, "You're never given more than you can handle," tend to belittle the patient's feelings and minimize the importance of his or her message. These automatic phrases communicate that you are not taking concerns seriously or responding thoughtfully.

False Reassurance When a patient is seriously ill or distressed, you may be tempted to offer hope to the patient with statements such as, "I'm sure everything will be okay." Although you may be trying to be kind, false reassurance discounts the patient's concerns or situation and tends to block communication.

Asking for Explanations Sometimes asking "why" implies an accusation and results in resentment, insecurity, and mistrust. Try to phrase questions without using "why." Rather than "Why are you not taking the medications the doctor prescribed?" you could say, "Tell me about the problems you are having with your medications."

Arguing Challenging or arguing with someone's perception of a situation denies that his or her perceptions are real and implies that they are lying, misinformed, or uneducated. If Roberto tells Suzanne he has no appetite and is not eating, her response of "You must be eating, you have not lost any weight" would block communication. Suzanne needs to present information or reality in a way that avoids argument. A better response is, "I see you have not lost any weight; tell me how you are meeting your nutritional needs since you don't have much of an appetite."

Being Defensive When patients express criticism, listen to what they have to say. Listening does not imply agreement. To discover reasons for the patient's anger or dissatisfaction, you need to listen uncritically. By avoiding defensiveness, you are able to defuse anger and uncover deeper concerns. Rather than saying, "None of the nurses would intentionally ignore you," you respond, "You feel the nurses are ignoring you."

Sympathy Sympathy is the concern, sorrow, or pity you feel for the patient when you personally identify with the patient's needs (Grover, 2005). Unlike empathy, which tries to understand the patient's experience, sympathy takes a subjective look at the patient's world. Sharing sympathy with another feels good, creates a bond, and minimizes differences, but it can prevent effective problem solving and impair good judgment. When you share the patient's needs, you are assuming the patient's feelings are similar to your own and you are unable to help the patient select realistic solutions for problems. For example, in the case study, if in response to Roberto's statement about his pain Suzanne had said, "Oh I know just what you mean, I hate feeling drugged up," Roberto would not have had a chance to clarify his feelings and Suzanne would miss an opportunity to get a deeper understanding of his perception of the situation.

DECISION MAKING AND COMMUNICATION As a nurse, you constantly make decisions about what, when, where, why, and how to send messages to others. Deciding which techniques best fit each unique nursing scenario is challenging. Situations that challenge your decision-making skills and call for careful use of therapeutic techniques often involve persons such as those described in Box 10-7. Practice helps, so take the initiative to discuss and role-play these scenarios before facing them in the clinical setting.

ASSERTIVENESS AND AUTONOMY Assertive communication is based on a philosophy of protecting individual rights and responsibilities. It includes the ability to be self-directive in acting to accomplish goals and advocate for others. An assertive response promotes self-esteem and upholds personal and professional rights. Feelings of security, competence, power, and professionalism characterize assertive responses. Assertive statements convey a message without resorting to sarcasm, whining, anger, blaming, or manipulation. Assertive responses are good tools to deal with criticism, change, negative conditions in personal or professional life, and conflict or stress in relationships.

Assertive responses often contain "I" messages, such as "I want," "I need," "I think," or "I feel." Simple assertive messages are usually stated in three parts, referencing the nurse, the other individual's behavior, and its effect.

Nurse to nurse: "When you are late for work, I have to stay late and that makes me late picking up my children from the babysitter."

BOX 10-7   Challenging Communication Situations

DIFFICULT DIAGNOSES OR CLINICAL SITUATION
- The *grieving* mother whose baby has died
- A *frantic* man who was just told his wife was in a serious accident

PATIENTS AND FAMILIES EXPERIENCING STRONG EMOTIONS
- The *anxious, nervous* person who cannot cope with what is happening
- The *angry, hostile* person newly diagnosed with cancer who does not listen to explanations
- The *ranting and raving* person who blames nursing staff unfairly

COPING WITH PERSONAL FEELINGS WHILE STILL NEEDING TO CARE FOR PATIENTS
- Feeling helpless when cancer has progressed
- Grief over the death of a long-term patient

From Sheldon LK, Barrett R, Ellington L: Difficult communication in nursing, *J Nurs Scholarsh* 38(2):141, 2006.

You can state a more complex assertive message by using the ASSERT formula (Berko and others, 1997):

Action: Describe the action that prompted the need for the message.
Subjective: Express a subjective interpretation of the action.
Sensations: Express sensations related to the action.
Effects: Indicate the effects of the action.
Request: Make a request of the other person.
Tell: Tell your intentions if the request is not met.

Nurse to supervisor: "When you say I'm not performing well, that sounds serious. I feel surprised and confused, because I had a sense that I was doing a good job. Please give me some examples of what you mean. If there are none, I'll discuss this evaluation with the director of nursing."

Avoid Passive Responses Passive responses avoid issues or conflict. Some characteristics are feelings of sadness, depression, anxiety, and hopelessness.

Nurse to co-worker, hopelessly: "I guess there's nothing we can do about it."
Nurse to spouse during argument: "Whatever you say."
A better response is, "What can we do to make things better?"

Avoid Aggressive Responses Aggressive responses provoke confrontation at the other person's expense. Some characteristics of aggression are feelings of anger, frustration, resentment, and stress.

Nurse to angry patient: "Who do you think you are? You can't talk to me that way."
A better response is, "I want to hear your concerns and help you have a positive experience. Can we take a deep breath and talk about them now, or should I come back later?"

HUMOR Humor is a coping strategy that adds perspective and helps you and the patient adjust to stress. The Association for Applied and Therapeutic Humor (2008) defines therapeutic humor as "any intervention that promotes health and wellness by stimulating a playful discovery, expression or appreciation of the absurdity or incongruity of life's situations." Laughter is a diversion from stress-related tension. It provides a sense of well-being and more of a feeling of control or mastery. Humor helps provide emotional support to patients and humanizes the illness experience. Laughter provides both a psychological and physical release for you and the patient; promotes open, relaxed interaction; and illustrates our shared experience in being human.

You assess whether humor is appropriate by noticing if patients use humor in their conversations. Start with small doses to see if this is helpful. To offer positive humor, share humorous incidents or situations, offer a clown nose to someone who could use a laugh, or share puns or simple jokes that are not offensive. Positive humor is associated with hope, love, and joy with the intent to bring people closer. Avoid negative humor, which is inappropriate. Ethnic, religious, sexist, ageist, or put-down humor creates distance. Realize that humor sometimes backfires; not everyone will appreciate a humorous approach because of negative moods, stress, or physical discomfort. Humor is often a signal for closer attention. When a patient preparing for surgery quips, "Well, I won't die from it," gently explore concerns of the patient.

Sometimes health care providers use dark, negative humor after difficult or traumatic situations to survive a situation intact and to relieve tension and stress. This "coping humor" may seem callous or uncaring by those not involved in the situation. Avoid using "coping humor" within earshot of patients or their loved ones. Understand that humor is a release, but timing, content, and receptivity are important in the use of therapeutic humor (Arnold and Boggs, 2007).

TOUCH **Touch** is one of the nurse's most potent forms of communication. Nurses are privileged to experience more of this intimate form of personal contact than almost any other professional. Touch conveys many messages, such as affection, emotional support, encouragement, and personal attention (Figure 10-2). Comfort touch, such as holding a hand, is important for vulnerable patients who are experiencing severe illness with its accompanying physical and emotional losses.

Benner (2004) wrote about a colleague's experience as a critical care patient. A nurse rubbed her shoulders to soothe and comfort her. The nurse enjoyed providing this comfort and savored this moment of caring connection. She valued this as part of the art of nursing, which is sometimes left out due to the emphasis on the high-tech nature of our work. Sometimes touch is misinterpreted. Always be sensitive to the patient's response to touch. Following are examples of inappropriate and appropriate use of touch:

Inappropriate touch: In a cancer support group, the wife of a patient had her arms wrapped around herself as if she were "holding herself together." The nurse moved too quickly and tried to hug the wife without permission. The wife backed off and struggled to hold back tears.

Appropriate touch: The nurse says, "I see you are distressed. Would a hug help?" The woman is then free to decline this well-intended act that might trigger tears that would embarrass this very private person.

Another concern is the confusion about the use of touch with culturally diverse patients (Box 10-8). Some risk is involved. You must look for cues that a patient would welcome touch. We use touch to awaken patients, to get their attention, or to add emphasis to explanations. Touch may also convey understanding better than words or gestures. Therapeutic

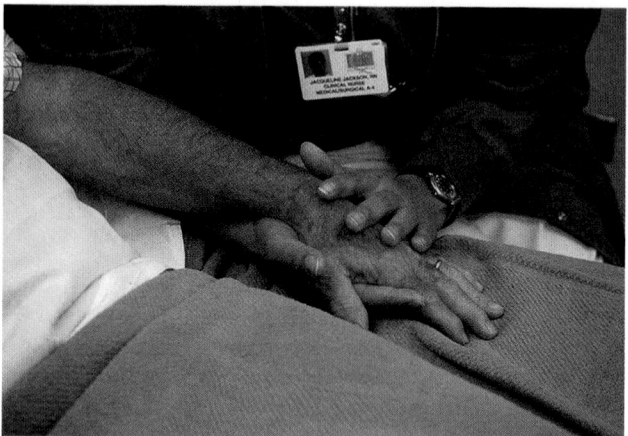

Figure 10-2 ■ The nurse uses touch to communicate.

BOX 10-8   CULTURAL FOCUS

 Suzanne works with patients from a variety of cultures. She likes to use touch to communicate caring and compassion, but finds some patients are uncomfortable with her touch. When she holds their hand or puts her arm around their shoulder, some patients become very quiet or pull back. Suzanne explores how different cultures perceive touch in order to provide more culturally sensitive care. She learns that among people from Africa and Southeast Asia the head is considered the seat of life and should not be touched except by close kin (Miller, 1995) and that touching the head of a patient by a nonrelative may predispose to loss of one's spirit and power. She also learned that Amish patients consider touching taboo between unrelated males and females.

IMPLICATIONS FOR PRACTICE
- Ask permission before touching a patient of another culture.
- Use same-gender caregivers for female and older patients from Asian, Middle Eastern, Hispanic, African, and Amish cultures, especially when touch is involved.
- Avoid touching the head of a patient from Africa or Southeast Asia.

touch is a special form of alternative touch therapy used by specially educated nurses for health assessment, pain reduction, and relaxation by influencing a patient's body energy fields. In therapeutic touch, specially educated nurses pass their hands over the body without actually touching to balance the energy fields and provide an environment for optimal health (Hawranik, Johnston, and Deatrich, 2008).

Because much of what you do involves touching, learn to use touch wisely. The zones of touch are described in Box 10-1 (p. 169). Touch delivered in the social or consent zones is less anxiety producing than touch delivered in the vulnerable or intimate zones. Students initially find giving intimate care stressful, especially with patients of the opposite sex. Shift your focus from personal discomfort to your role as a caregiver with the intent to provide sensitive nursing care. Trust that you will become more comfortable with experience. Remember that the patient who is ill and dependent must permit closer physical contact than is normally tolerated and may be uncomfortable with touch. Remain sensitive to your own responses and to patients' feelings. If a patient refuses to hold your hand while in pain or pulls away from physical contact, this signals that the patient is uncomfortable with being touched. People perceive touch negatively when it is given without consent; used within a hostile or mistrusting relationship; and delivered to a vulnerable, intimate, or painful area of the body. Your touch should never be angry, rough, violent, overly stimulating, threatening, overly tentative, sexual, or unnecessarily painful.

COMMUNICATING WITH PATIENTS WITH SPECIAL NEEDS Many health problems and human responses contribute to impaired communication. This includes the infant whose self-expression is limited to crying, body movement, and facial expression. Others with special needs are patients who are hearing and visually impaired, persons suffering from a stroke or late-stage Alzheimer's disease, and persons with autism or schizophrenia who respond to internal stimuli and misinterpret external stimuli. The person who does not speak or understand English and the patient with learning disabilities and limited vocal skills who uses gaze and body orientation to display a readiness to communicate will challenge you to accommodate their special needs. In addition, unresponsive or heavily sedated patients are sometimes unable to send or receive verbal messages.

The patient who cannot communicate effectively has difficulty expressing needs and responding appropriately to the environment and requires special thought and sensitivity. Such persons benefit greatly when you adapt communication techniques to their circumstances (Box 10-9). When caring for a patient with *impaired verbal communication related to a language barrier,* you may provide a table of simple words in the patient's language. The patient's use of the table will meet the expected outcome of the patient communicating basic needs such as food, water, toileting, rest, and pain relief. Collaborate with team members to design the best communication strategies.

Good communication improves the quality of your patient's interpersonal relationships and well-being. If the patient uses ineffective communication techniques that interfere with coping or interpersonal relationships, intervene to help your patient send, receive, and interpret messages more effectively. Be a communication role model and teacher to help patients express needs, feelings, and concerns. Help patients develop social interaction skills and communicate thoughts and feelings clearly. This will help them interpret messages sent from others, increasing their autonomy and assertiveness. Methods such as role-playing allow patients to practice situations in which they have difficulty communicating.

Providing Alternative Communication Methods Patients with physical communication barriers (e.g., those with a laryngectomy or endotracheal tube) may be unable to speak, or the clarity of speech may be so poor that they need alternative methods of communication (see Box 10-9). To decrease frustration, provide simple communication methods and allow the patient time to respond. The patient must be physically able to use the method you provide (e.g., communication boards or pencil and pad). Patients who are unable to speak are at risk for injury unless they are able to communicate personal needs quickly.

Communicating With Children Communication with a child requires special considerations to develop a working relationship with the child and family. Because contact between parent and child is usually close, assume the information communicated by parents is reliable, although some parents may exaggerate. Offer a child toys or materials so the parent gives full attention to your information gathering. Give periodic attention to infants and younger children as they play to include them. An older child can be actively involved in communication. Consider the influence of development on language and thought processes.

Children, particularly the young, are especially responsive to nonverbal messages. Sudden movements or gestures can be frightening. Remain calm and gentle, and, if possible, let the child make the first move. Use a quiet, friendly, confident tone of voice. The child feels helpless in most situations involving health care personnel. When it is necessary to give explanations or directions, use simple, direct language and be honest. To minimize fear and anxiety, prepare the child by explaining what to expect. Avoid staring, and meet the child at eye level.

Drawing and playing with young children allows the child to communicate nonverbally (making the drawing) and verbally (explaining the picture) (Figure 10-3). Use a child's drawing as a basis for beginning a conversation.

Communicating With Older Adult Patients The majority of older adults experience some loss of sensory function (Hartford Institute, 2005). Sensory alterations prevent receiving messages clearly. Many older adults adapt to sensory losses and learn to communicate effectively. When obvious deficits exist, maximize existing motor and sensory function to help the patient communicate more effectively (see Box 10-9). You can make some simple modifications in

BOX 10-9 Communicating With Patients Who Have Special Needs

PATIENTS WITH DIFFICULTY HEARING
- Avoid shouting.
- Use simple sentences.
- Punctuate speech with facial expression and gestures.

PATIENTS WITH DIFFICULTY SEEING
- Communicate verbally before touching the patient.
- Orient the patient to sounds in the environment.
- Inform the patient when the conversation is over and when you are leaving the room.

PATIENTS WHO ARE MUTE OR CANNOT SPEAK CLEARLY
- Place a sign by unit call system to answer call light in person.
- Listen attentively, be patient, and do not interrupt.
- Do not finish patients' sentences for them.
- Ask simple questions that require "yes" or "no" answers.
- Allow time for understanding and responses.
- Use visual cues (e.g., words, pictures, objects) when possible.
- Allow only one person to speak at a time.
- Do not shout or speak too loudly.
- Encourage the patient to converse.
- Let the patient know if you do not understand.
- Use communication aids as needed:
  - Pad and felt-tipped pen or Magic Slate
  - Flash cards
  - Communication board with words, letters, or pictures denoting basic needs
  - Computer toy ("speak and spell" type)
  - Call bells or alarms
  - Sign language
  - Use of eye blinks or movement of fingers for simple responses ("yes" or "no")

PATIENTS WHO ARE COGNITIVELY IMPAIRED
- Reduce environmental distractions while conversing.
- Get the patient's attention before speaking.
- Use simple sentences, and avoid long explanations.
- Avoid shifting from subject to subject.
- Ask one question at a time.
- Allow time for the patient to respond.
- Include family and friends in conversations, especially in subjects known to the patient.

PATIENTS WHO ARE UNRESPONSIVE
- Call the patient by name during interactions.
- Communicate both verbally and by touch.
- Speak to the patient as though he or she could hear.
- Explain all procedures and sensations.

PATIENTS WHO DO NOT SPEAK ENGLISH
- Speak to the patient in a normal tone of voice (shouting may be interpreted as anger).
- Establish a method for the patient to signal the desire to communicate (call light or bell).
- Provide a professional interpreter/translator as needed:
  - Use a person familiar with the patient's culture and with biomedicine if possible.
  - Allow plenty of time for the interpreter to transmit messages.
  - Communicate directly to the patient and family rather than the interpreter.
  - Ask one question at a time.
  - Avoid making comments to the interpreter about the patient or family (they may understand some English).
- Develop a communication board, pictures, or cards using words translated into English for the patient to make basic requests (e.g., pain medication, water, elimination).
- Have a dictionary (e.g., English/Spanish) available if the patient can read.

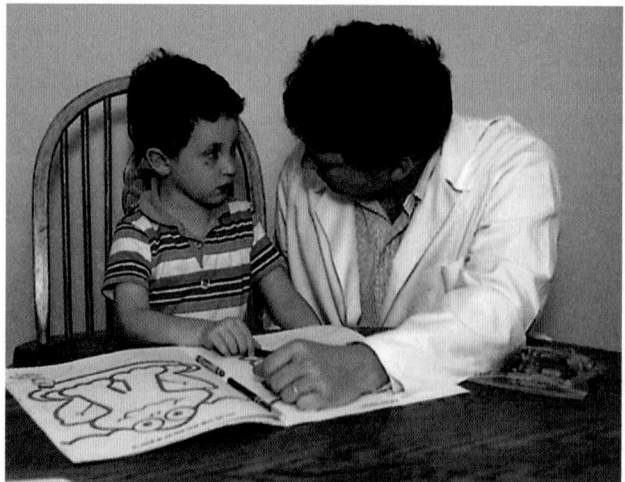

Figure 10-3 ■ Drawing helps children communicate.

BOX 10-10   CARE OF THE OLDER ADULT

Improving Communication

In communicating with older adults, the primary goal is to establish a reliable communication system that all health care team members easily understand. Ideally, an interdisciplinary model delivers effective care for older adults. Communication with older adults requires special attention. Be aware of the physical, psychological, and social changes of aging.

Use the following interventions to assist with impaired communication with older adults:

- During conversation, maintain a quiet environment that is free from background noise.
- Avoid shifting from subject to subject; allow time for conversation.
- Be an attentive listener. Use explorative questions to facilitate conversation (e.g., "How do you feel?").

- Avoid long sentences to explain the subject. Try to keep it short, simple, and to the point.
- Allow the older adult the opportunity to reminisce. Reminiscing has therapeutic properties that increase the sense of well-being.
- If you are experiencing problems understanding the patient (e.g., dysarthria), let the patient know and facilitate methods that help the patient speak more clearly. Consult with a speech therapist if necessary.
- Include the patient's family and friends in conversations, particularly in subjects known to the patient.
- Be aware of cultural differences among patients.

---

your approach and the environment to improve communication with older adults (Box 10-10). Identify these challenges, and work with the patient to enhance effective communication. Attend to the wisdom these patients have to offer you, and think of them as teachers about living.

■■■EVALUATION

Together, you and the patient determine the success of the plan of care by evaluating patient communication outcomes. Ask yourself if you understood what your patient communicated, if your patient had the opportunity to express feelings and concerns, and if your patient has unresolved needs.

PATIENT CARE Evaluate whether communication interventions were effective. Compare the expected outcomes you established in the plan of care with the actual outcomes you observe when interacting with patients. If you meet your outcomes, you have resolved the goals of care and the nursing diagnosis. When outcomes remain unmet, you may revise the existing plan with new goals, outcomes, and/or interventions. For example, if using a pen and paper proves frustrating for a nonverbal patient whose handwriting is shaky, you revise the care plan to include use of a picture board instead. In this case, observing the patient's handwriting and asking other caregivers about the patient's success in communicating needs would be your evaluation measures. Remember, careful evaluation requires you to make observations similar to those in your original assessment. For example, after initially assessing the extent of a patient's ability to hear the spoken word and providing various interventions to promote hearing, you then return

to evaluate the patient's ability to hear any interaction or instruction. It is also helpful to question the patient about whether needs were adequately met.

You can evaluate the effectiveness of your own communication by making process recordings, or written records of your verbal and nonverbal interactions with patients. These recordings are useful in reflecting about how your communication style might improve.

PATIENT EXPECTATIONS Review the patient's expectations of care and determine if the patient achieved expectations. This is an important part of the evaluation process. Ask patients and their families for input about goal achievement, factors that affected outcomes, and suggestions for changes in the plan of care. Suzanne consistently asked Roberto if the pain medications were relieving his discomfort. He was pleased that she was open to working with him to balance pain management with the clarity of his thinking.

Avoiding patient input during evaluation and care plan modification will lead to a task-oriented rather than a critical thinking, patient-centered approach to nursing. It denies the patient's right to see the total picture of care and to be involved in all phases of the nursing process. A goal of total pain relief for Roberto was incompatible with his own goals of being alert enough to care for his dog and work with his art collection. Suzanne's willingness to consistently reevaluate the plan of care affected Roberto's quality of life. She used her therapeutic communication skills to engage the team in holistic care to address his goals for body, mind, and spiritual well-being. They focused on helping Roberto live every moment of his life the way he wanted to live it.

KEY POINTS

- Communication is a powerful therapeutic tool and an essential nursing skill used to influence others and achieve positive health outcomes.
- Nurses consider many contexts and factors influencing communication when making decisions about what, when, where, how, why, and with whom to communicate.
- Communication is most effective when the receiver and sender accurately perceive the meaning of one another's messages.
- Effective verbal communication requires appropriate intonation, clear and concise phrasing, proper pacing of statements, and proper timing and relevance of a message.
- Effective nonverbal communication complements and strengthens the message conveyed by verbal communication.
- Strengthen helping relationships by establishing trust, empathy, autonomy, confidentiality, and professional competence.
- Effective communication techniques are facilitative and tend to encourage the other person to openly express ideas, feelings, or concerns.
- Ineffective communication techniques are inhibiting and tend to block the other person's willingness to openly express ideas, feelings, or concerns.
- The nurse blends social and informational interactions with therapeutic communication techniques so that others explore feelings and manage health issues.
- When using therapeutic humor, consider timing, receptivity, and content of the humorous intervention.
- Methods that facilitate communication with children include sitting at eye level; interacting with parents; using simple, direct language; and incorporating play activities.
- Older adult patients with sensory, motor, or cognitive impairments require the adaptation of communication techniques to make up for their loss of function and special needs.
- Desired outcomes for patients with impaired verbal communication include increased satisfaction with interpersonal interactions, the ability to send and receive clear messages, and attendance to and accurate interpretation of verbal and nonverbal cues.

CRITICAL THINKING EXERCISES

Roberto Ruiz developed pneumonia and became very weak. You are filling in for Suzanne while she is on vacation and come to check on him. You find him in bed, and he has not eaten since the evening before because he is too weak to fix a meal, his oxygen level is low, and he is having pain with frequent coughing. It is apparent he is not able to care for himself.

1. You believe Roberto needs either hospitalization or inpatient hospice. Roberto is adamant that he will not leave his home. What communication techniques would you use to address this concern?

2. You approach Roberto and put your hand on his shoulder. He responds angrily and tells you to leave him alone. What should you do?

3. What factors are influencing Roberto's communication?

4. Roberto has called a good friend, and the friend is going to stay with him for a couple days. Roberto wants his pneumonia treated, but he does not want extraordinary measures taken. You call Roberto's physician, give an update on his condition, and determine the medical plan of care. How could you best communicate with the physician?

ⓔvolve   *Answers to Critical Thinking Questions can be found on the Evolve website.*

REVIEW QUESTIONS

1. The nurse summarizes the conversation with a patient to determine if the patient has been understood. This is what element of the communication process?
   1. Referent
   2. Channel
   3. Environment
   4. Feedback

2. Mr. Sakda's parents immigrated from Thailand. When taking care of him, you note he looks relaxed and smiles but seldom looks at you directly. How should you respond?
   1. Use therapeutic communication to assess for increased anxiety.
   2. Sit down, and move closer so you are at eye level.
   3. Deflect your eyes downward show respect.
   4. Continue to maintain eye contact.

3. Mrs. Jones states she gets anxious when she thinks about giving herself insulin. How could you use your understanding of intrapersonal communication to help with this?
   1. Provide her the opportunity to practice drawing up insulin.
   2. Coach her to give herself positive messages about her ability to do this.
   3. Bring her written material that clearly describes the steps of insulin administration.
   4. Use therapeutic communication to help her express her feeling about giving herself an injection.

4. The nurse has a patient who has become short of breath, and the nurse calls the physician using SBAR to help with the communication. What would the nurse first address?
   1. The respiratory rate is 28 breaths per minute.
   2. The patient has a history of lung cancer.
   3. The patient has become short of breath.
   4. The nurse requests an order for a breathing treatment.

5. Which of the following actions establishes a therapeutic relationship?
   1. Call all patients by first name unless they request otherwise.
   2. Tell your patient when you will be back, and follow through on that promise.
   3. Do all care as quickly as possible, and leave the room so the patient can rest.
   4. Visit with other members of the health care team while providing care.

6. You are caring for a patient who is facing amputation of his leg. During the orientation phase of the relationship, what would you do?
   1. Summarize what you have talked about in the previous sessions.
   2. Review the medical record, and talk to other nurses about how the patient is reacting.
   3. Explore the patient's feelings about losing his leg.
   4. Visit with the patient about his favorite baseball team.

7. The nurse states, "When you tell me you're having a hard time living up to expectations, are you talking about what your family expects you to do?" The nurse is using which therapeutic communication technique?
   1. Providing information
   2. Clarifying
   3. Focusing
   4. Paraphrasing

8. Which of the following statements would be most likely to block communication?
   1. "You look kind of tired today."
   2. "Why do you always put so much salt on your food?"
   3. "It sounds like this has been a hard time for you."
   4. "If you use your oxygen when you walk, you may be able to walk farther."

9. You are caring for an 80-year-old woman, and you ask her a question while you are across the room washing your hands. She does not answer. What should you do next?
   1. Leave the room quietly because she evidently does not want to be bothered right now.
   2. Repeat the question in a loud voice, speaking very slowly.
   3. Move to her bedside, get her attention, and repeat the question while facing her.
   4. Bring her a communication board so she can express her needs.

10. You ask another nurse how to collect a specific laboratory specimen. The nurse raises her eyebrows and states, "Why don't you figure it out?" What would be the best response?
   1. Say nothing and walk away. Find a different nurse to help you.
   2. "When you brush me off like that, it takes me even longer to do my job."
   3. "Why do you always put me down like that?"
   4. "I guess I just enjoy having you make fun of me."

Answers to Review Questions can be found on pages 1197-1198.

REFERENCES

Arnold EC, Boggs KU: *Interpersonal relationships: professional communication skills for nurses*, ed 5, St. Louis, 2007, Saunders.

Association for Applied and Therapeutic Humor, 2008, http://www.aath.org/.

Benner P: Relational ethics of comfort, touch, and solace: endangered arts? *Am J Crit Care* 13(4):346, 2004.

Berko MR and others: *Connecting: a culture-sensitive approach to interpersonal communication competency*, ed 2, Philadelphia, 1997, Harcourt Brace.

ELNEC: Module 6, Communication, *End –of Life Nursing Education Consortium Training Program*, 2000, Washington, DC, 2003, American Association of Colleges of Nursing and Duarte, Calif, City of Hope.

Finch LP: Patients' communication with nurses: relational communication and preferred nurse behaviors, *Int J Human Caring* 10(4):14, 2006.

Gibson AS, Foster C: The role of self-talk in the awareness of physiological state and physical performance, *Sports Med* 37(12):1029, 2007.

Grover S: Shaping effective communication skills and therapeutic relationships at work: the foundation of collaboration, *AAOHN J* 53(4):177, 2005.

Gulanick M, Myers J: *Nursing care plans*, ed 6, St. Louis, 2007, Mosby.

Hartford Institute for Geriatric Nursing *Sensory change*, 2005, http://www.consultgerirn.org/topics/sensory_changes/want_to_know_more.

Hawranik P, Johnston P, Deatrich J: Therapeutic touch and agitation in individuals with Alzheimer's disease, *West J Nurs Res* 30(4):417, 2008.

Jack K, Smith A: Promoting self-awareness in nurses to improve nursing practice, *Nurs Stand* 21(32):47, 2007.

King I: *Toward a theory for nursing*, New York, 1971, John Wiley & Sons.

Kneisl CR, Trigoboff E: *Contemporary psychiatric-mental health nursing*, ed 2, Upper Saddle River, NJ, 2009, Pearson Education Inc.

Leonard M, Graham S, Bonacum D: The human factor: the critical importance of effective teamwork and communication in providing safe care, *Qual Saf Health Care* 13:i85, 2004.

Markley J, Winbery S: Communication with physicians: how agencies can be heard, *Home Health Care Manage Pract* 20(2):161, 2008.

McGilton K and others: Communication enhancement: nurse and patient satisfaction in a complex continuing care facility, *J Adv Nurs* 54(1):35, 2006.

Miller JA: Caring for Cambodian refugees in the emergency department, *J Emerg Nurs* 21(6):498, 1995.

Patterson P: Lateral violence: why it's serious and what OR managers can do, *OR Manager* 23(12):12, 2007.

Pope B, Rodzen L, Spross G: Raising the SBAR: how better communication improves patient outcomes, *Nursing* 38(3):41, 2008.

Rodgers KL: Using the SBAR communication technique to improve nurse-physician phone communication: a pilot study, *AAACN Viewpoint* 29(2):7, 2007.

Sheldon LK, Barrett R, Ellington L: Difficult communication in nursing, *J Nurs Scholarsh* 38(2):141, 2006.

Stuart GW, Laraia MT: *Principles and practice of psychiatric nursing*, ed 8, St. Louis, 2005, Mosby.

The Joint Commission: Behaviors that undermine a culture of safety, *Sentinel Event Alert*, issue 40, July 9, 2008, http://www.jointcommission.org/SentinelEvents/SentinelEventAlert/sea_40.htm.

Townsend MC: *Psychiatric mental health nursing: concepts of care in evidence-based practice*, ed 5, Philadelphia, 2006, FA Davis.

Understanding transcultural nursing, *Nursing* 35(Suppl Career):14, 2005.

White SJ: Using self-talk to embrace career satisfaction and performance, *Am J Health Syst Pharm* 65(6):514, 2008.

World Health Organization: Communication during patient hand-overs, *Patient Safety Solutions* 1:solution 3, May 2007, http://www.who.int/patientsafety/solutions/patientsafety/PS-Solution3.pdf.

11 Patient Education

MEDIA RESOURCES

 CD COMPANION 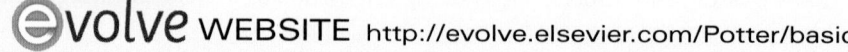 **WEBSITE** http://evolve.elsevier.com/Potter/basic

- Crossword Puzzle
- English/Spanish Audio Glossary

OBJECTIVES

- Identify appropriate topics for a patient's health education needs.
- Describe the similarities and differences between teaching and learning.
- Identify the purposes of patient education.
- Compare the communication and teaching processes.
- Describe the domains of learning.
- Differentiate factors that determine readiness to learn from those that determine ability to learn.
- Compare the nursing and teaching processes.
- Write learning objectives for a teaching plan.

- Describe the characteristics of an environment that promotes learning.
- Identify the principles of effective teaching.
- Describe ways to adapt teaching for patients with different learning needs.
- Use the nursing process to make a teaching plan of care.
- Describe ways to incorporate teaching with routine nursing care.
- Identify methods for evaluating learning.
- Describe appropriate documentation of teaching.

KEY TERMS

affective learning, p. 190
analogies, p. 202
attentional set, p. 190
cognitive learning, p. 190

functional illiteracy, p. 196
health literacy, p. 196
learning, p. 188

learning objective, p. 188
motivation, p. 190
psychomotor learning, p. 190

reinforcement, p. 201
return demonstration, p. 202
teaching, p. 189

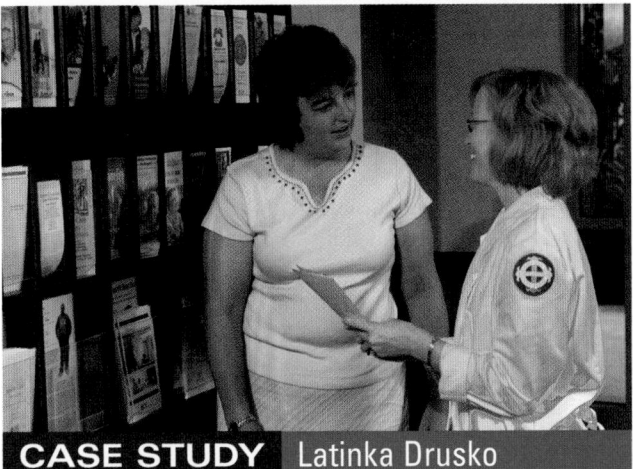

CASE STUDY Latinka Drusko

Latinka Drusko is a 55-year-old accountant. She immigrated to the United States from Bosnia in 1991 and has two grown sons who live close to her. Latinka's husband recently died. Latinka is overweight and smokes 1 to 1½ packs of cigarettes a day. She is visiting her advanced practice nurse for her yearly physical.

Ashley is a 23-year-old nursing student assigned to care for Latinka. During their first visit, Latinka states, "I am interested in getting some information to help me become healthier. I would like to stop smoking and lose some weight. Do you think you can help me?" Ashley gives Latinka some written material and sets up a time when they can meet later.

Being a patient educator is one of the most important professional nursing roles. Factors such as shorter hospital stays and the increased demand on nurses' time complicate the ability to provide quality patient education. As nurses try to find the most effective way to educate patients, health care consumers have become more assertive in seeking information, understanding health, and finding resources available within the health care system. Providing patients with self-care information is necessary to ensure continuity of care from the hospital to the home. Patient education is important because the patient has a right to know and to be informed about diagnosis and prognosis of illness, treatment options, how to perform care activities in the home, and risks associated with treatments. Patient education is the responsibility of the professional nurse. Therefore nurses cannot delegate patient education. A well-designed, comprehensive teaching plan that fits your patients' unique learning needs reduces health care costs and improves the quality of care. Ultimately, patient education helps patients make informed decisions about their health care and to become healthier and more independent (Edelman and Mandle, 2006).

STANDARDS FOR PATIENT EDUCATION

All State Nurse Practice Acts recognize that patient education is a professional responsibility of the nurse (Bastable, 2008). In addition, several accrediting agencies set guidelines for providing patient education in health care institutions. These guidelines ensure that patients and their families receive information necessary to maintain the patient's optimal level of health. In the United States, The Joint Commission (TJC) (2008b) sets standards for patient and family education and includes patient education in its National Patient Safety Goals. These standards require you and the health care team to provide patient education about topics affecting patients' health, such as medications, nutrition, and how to be involved in the plan of care. Consider patients' psychosocial, spiritual, and cultural values when providing education, and document education you provide in your patient's medical record.

PURPOSES OF PATIENT EDUCATION

The goal of patient education is to assist individuals, families, or communities in achieving optimal levels of health (Edelman and Mandle, 2006). In today's health care arena, patients know more about health and want to be involved in health maintenance. To meet this need, provide education to patients in convenient and familiar places (e.g., in their homes, churches, or schools). Comprehensive patient education includes three important purposes, each involving a separate phase of health care.

Maintenance and Promotion of Health and Illness Prevention

As a nurse, you are a resource for people who want to know more about their health. People participate in healthy activities such as regular exercise and health screening programs to maintain or improve their health. You provide patient education in many places such as schools, homes, clinics, and the workplace to help patients adopt healthy behaviors (Box 11-1). For example, in childbearing classes, expectant parents learn about physical and psychological changes in the woman and about fetal development. After learning about normal childbearing, the mother is more likely to engage in physical exercise, and the father is more likely to support the mother during her pregnancy. When patients become more conscious about their health, they are more likely to seek early diagnosis of health problems (Redman, 2007).

Restoration of Health

Injured or ill patients need information or skills to help improve or restore their level of health (see Box 11-1). Patients recovering from or adapting to illness or injury typically seek information about their condition. However, patients who find it difficult to adapt to illness may become passive and uninterested in learning. As a nurse, you need to identify the patient's readiness to learn and motivate the patient to learn (Redman, 2007).

Family or friends often positively contribute to a patient's return to health and need to know as much as the patient. If you exclude these individuals from the patient's teaching

BOX 11-1	**Topics for Health Education**

HEALTH MAINTENANCE AND PROMOTION AND ILLNESS PREVENTION
- First aid
- Avoidance of risk factors (e.g., smoking, alcohol)
- Growth and development
- Hygiene
- Immunizations
- Prenatal care and normal childbearing
- Nutrition
- Exercise
- Safety (e.g., in home, car, workplace, hospital)
- Screening (e.g., blood pressure, vision, cholesterol level)
- Lifestyle changes to reduce risk factors (e.g., smoking cessation, substance abuse treatment)

RESTORATION OF HEALTH
- Patient's disease or condition
  - Anatomy and physiology of body system affected
  - Cause of disease
  - Origin of symptoms
  - Expected effects on other body systems
  - Prognosis
  - Limitations on function
  - Rationale for treatment
  - Medications
  - Tests and therapies
  - Nursing measures
  - Surgical intervention
  - Expected duration of care
  - Hospital or clinic environment
  - Hospital or clinic staff
  - Long-term care
  - How patient can participate in care

COPING WITH IMPAIRED FUNCTION
- Home care
  - Medications
  - Diet
  - Activity
  - Self-help devices
- Rehabilitation of remaining function
  - Physical therapy
  - Occupational therapy
  - Speech therapy
- Prevention of complications
  - Knowledge of risk factors
  - Implications of noncompliance with therapy

plan, conflicts may arise. However, do not assume that you should involve the family. Assess the patient-family relationship before including the family in patient education.

Coping With Impaired Functioning

Not all patients fully recover from illness or injury. Many learn to cope with permanent health changes. In these cases, patients need new knowledge and skills to continue activities of daily living (see Box 11-1). For example, the patient who loses the ability to speak after surgery of the larynx learns new ways of communicating. The patient with heart disease learns about diet, medication, and exercise to reduce further heart damage.

Changes in function can be physical or psychosocial. In the case of serious illness or injury, such as a heart attack or spinal cord injury, the patient's family often partners with the patient and learns how to help the patient manage health care needs. In these cases, you need to include the family when appropriate in patient education. Begin teaching as soon as you identify the patient's needs and determine that the family is willing to help. Provide information that helps families cope with and adapt to emotional effects when your patients have long-term psychosocial problems, such as alcoholism or drug dependence. To be most effective, compare the desired level of health with your patient's actual state of health when providing patient education.

TEACHING AND LEARNING

It is impossible to separate teaching from learning. **Teaching** is an interactive process that promotes learning. It consists of a conscious and deliberate set of actions that helps individuals gain new knowledge, change attitudes, adopt new behaviors, or perform new skills (Bastable, 2008; Redman, 2007). A teacher provides information that encourages the learner to engage in activities that lead to a desired change.

Learning is the purposeful acquisition of new knowledge, attitudes, behaviors, or skills (Bastable, 2008). Learning is a complex process, especially if the patient is learning new skills, changing existing attitudes, transferring knowledge to new situations, or solving problems (Redman, 2007). Generally teaching and learning begin when a person identifies a need for knowing or acquiring an ability to do something. Teaching is most effective when it responds to a learner's immediate needs. The teacher identifies these needs by asking questions and determining the learner's interests. After you identify what you need to teach, develop specific learning objectives. A **learning objective** describes what the patient will be able to do after successful instruction. Interpersonal communication is essential for successful teaching (Redman, 2007) (see Chapter 10).

Role of the Nurse in Teaching and Learning

You have an ethical responsibility to teach your patients. This responsibility is outlined in the *Code of Ethics for Nurses* (ANA, 2001) and in the *Patient Care Partnership* (American Hospital Association, 2003). Both of these documents indicate that patients have the right to make informed decisions about their care, which requires accurate, complete, and relevant information. Furthermore, The Joint Commission's Speak Up Initiatives (2008a) help patients become more involved in their care and help ensure that patients are aware of their right to know about the care they will receive in a language they can understand. You enhance patient safety by teaching patients about the part they can play in their care to prevent medical errors.

Your responsibility is to provide information your patients and their families need. To be successful, you need to do the following:

- Answer patient's questions
- Provide information based on patient's health needs or treatment plans
- Clarify information from a variety of sources (e.g., health care providers, newspapers, television, the Internet)

To be an effective educator, engage your patients as partners in learning. Do not merely pass on facts. For example, when Ashley considers her approaches for teaching Latinka, she will individualize her educational approach based on Latinka's desire and interest in making a behavior change, her existing knowledge about the effects of smoking, and her preferences for ways to learn. By engaging Latinka in the teaching and learning experience, Ashley will achieve greater success in making her teaching relevant and meaningful to Latinka. Always carefully determine what your patients need to know, and provide education when they are ready to learn. Then, always be sure to evaluate the outcomes of teaching, did the patient learn? When you value and tailor educational approaches, patients are better prepared to assume health care responsibilities. The evaluation of patient outcomes following patient education is an important nursing issue (Bastable, 2008; Redman, 2007).

TEACHING AS COMMUNICATION

The **teaching** process closely parallels the communication process (see Chapter 10). Effective teaching depends in part on the effectiveness of your communication skills. A teacher applies each element of the communication process while giving information to learners. Thus the teacher and learner become involved in a teaching process that increases the learner's knowledge and skills.

Compare the steps of the teaching process with those of the communication process (Table 11-1). You are the sender

TABLE 11-1 Comparison of the Communication and Teaching Process

COMMUNICATION	TEACHING
REFERENT Idea that initiates reason for communication	Perceived need to provide a person with information, establishment of relevant learning objectives by teacher
SENDER Person who conveys message to another	Teacher who performs activities aimed at assisting other person to learn
INTRAPERSONAL VARIABLES (SENDER) Knowledge, values, emotions, and sociocultural influences that affect sender's thoughts	Teacher's philosophy of education (based on learning theory), knowledge of teaching content, teaching approach, experiences in teaching, emotions, and values
MESSAGE Information expressed or transmitted by sender	Content or information taught
CHANNELS Methods used to transmit message (visual, auditory, touch)	Methods used to present content (visual and auditory materials, touch, taste, smell)
RECEIVER Person to whom message is sent	Learner
INTRAPERSONAL VARIABLES (RECEIVER) Knowledge, values, emotions, and sociocultural influences that affect receiver's thoughts	Willingness and ability to learn (physical and emotional health, education, experience, developmental level)
FEEDBACK Information revealing that true meaning of message was received	Determination of whether the learner achieved learning objectives

who wants to communicate a message to the patient. Promote learning by communicating in a language recognized by the patient. Many interpersonal variables influence your style and approach. Attitudes, values, cultural preferences, emotions, and knowledge influence the way you send messages. Evaluating past experiences with teaching will help you choose the best way to present information (Bastable, 2008).

The receiver in the teaching-learning process is the learner. Interpersonal variables affect your patient's readiness and ability to learn. Language, attitudes, literacy level, cultural preferences, and values influence the ability to understand a message. The ability to learn depends on emotional and physical health, stage of development, and previous knowledge.

To be an effective teacher, have a method to evaluate the success of a teaching plan and provide positive reinforcement to your patient (Bastable, 2008; Redman, 2007). Examples of evaluating the effectiveness of your teaching include having your patients show you how to perform a newly learned skill (e.g., self-catheterization) and asking your patients to explain how they will incorporate newly ordered medications into their daily routines.

DOMAINS OF LEARNING

Learning occurs in three domains or areas: (1) cognitive (understanding), (2) affective (attitudes), and (3) psychomotor (motor skills).

Cognitive learning includes what the patient actually knows and understands. All intellectual behaviors are in the cognitive domain. This includes the following:

- Acquisition of knowledge
- Comprehension (ability to understand)
- Application (using abstract ideas in concrete situations)
- Analysis (relating ideas in an organized way)
- Synthesis (recognizing parts of information as a whole)
- Evaluation (judging the worth of a body of information)

Affective learning includes the patient's feelings, attitudes, opinions, and values. Although the affective domain is sometimes hard to identify, it greatly affects the success of education, either positively or negatively. Affective learning includes active listening and responding with a consistent value system.

Psychomotor learning occurs when patients acquire skills that require the integration of knowledge and physical skills. Examples of psychomotor learning are learning to walk with a walker and giving an insulin injection. As patients are able to complete psychomotor skills with more confidence, they are able to perform the behaviors in more complex or different situations. Adaptation occurs when your patient changes a response when unexpected problems arise. This results in originating, which involves creating new patterns of behavior.

Some topics involve all domains, whereas others involve only one. Patients often need to learn in each domain. For example, patients diagnosed with high blood pressure need to understand how their blood pressure affects the body and what they can do to lower their blood pressure (cognitive domain). Patients begin to accept the chronic nature of high blood pressure by learning positive ways to cope with their illness (affective domain). Many patients learn to take their blood pressure at home. This requires them to learn how to use a sphygmomanometer for home use (psychomotor domain). When you understand each learning domain, you are better prepared to use appropriate teaching techniques and apply the basic principles of learning.

BASIC LEARNING PRINCIPLES

To teach effectively and efficiently, you first need to understand how people learn. Learning depends on the motivation to learn, the ability to learn, and the learning environment. The ability to learn depends on physical and cognitive characteristics, one's developmental level, physical wellness, and intellectual thought processes. Remember that people have different preferences for learning and that they learn information in different ways and at different speeds. Therefore, to be most effective, include a combination of teaching approaches that meet multiple learning preferences (Felder, 2008).

Motivation to Learn

Motivation is an internal impulse (e.g., an idea, an emotion, or a physical need) that causes a person to take action and addresses a person's desire to learn (Redman, 2007). Previous knowledge, attitudes, and sociocultural factors influence motivation. If a person does not want to learn, it is unlikely that learning will occur. Often patient motives are physical. Some patients are motivated to learn so they can return to a previous level of functioning. For example, a patient with a lower limb amputation is motivated to learn to walk with a prosthesis. Motivation to learn is often dependent on the patient's situation and needs. For example, patients who need knowledge for survival have a stronger motivation to learn than patients who need knowledge for promoting health (Bastable, 2008).

An **attentional set** is the mental state that allows the learner to focus on and understand the material. Before learning anything, patients must be able to pay attention to or concentrate on the information they will learn. Physical discomfort, anxiety, and environmental distractions make it more difficult for the patient to concentrate. Any physical condition that impairs your patient's ability to concentrate (e.g., pain, nausea, fatigue, or hunger) interferes with learning. Therefore determine your patient's level of comfort by assessing verbal and nonverbal cues before beginning a teaching plan. Teach only when the patient is able to focus on the information.

As anxiety increases, the patient's ability to pay attention decreases. Anxiety is uneasiness or uncertainty resulting from anticipating a threat or danger. Patients feel anxious when faced with change or the need to act differently. Learning requires a change in behavior and thus produces anxiety. A mild level of anxiety may motivate learning. However, a high level of anxiety prevents learning from taking place. It disables a person, creating an inability to attend to anything other than relieving the anxiety. Be sure to manage your patient's anxiety before providing education to improve comprehension and understanding of the information given (Stephenson, 2006).

Health education often involves changing attitudes and values that are not easy to change simply by teaching facts. Knowing your patient's culture (see Chapter 19) and health beliefs (see Chapter 1) will help you determine the factors that will motivate learning (Box 11-2). Do not assume that you know what your patient believes; your patient's view of health may not match your view of health (Li, Stotts, and Froelicher, 2007). Include health beliefs that motivate your patient to learn in the teaching plan. For example, if your patient is a busy executive with high blood pressure, use the patient's desire to succeed and the concern that illness will impair work to motivate behavioral change. To facilitate successful teaching, encourage the motivating factor for several months after the initial teaching intervention.

You enhance learning by actively involving patients in the educational session (Edelman and Mandle, 2006). A patient's involvement in learning implies an eagerness to acquire knowledge or skills and allows the patient to make decisions during teaching sessions. For example, to help a patient with diabetes learn to monitor blood glucose levels, you assist the patient in choosing a blood glucose meter and have the patient use the meter under your supervision. You also incorporate the patient's lifestyle into a schedule for blood glucose testing (Figure 11-1).

READINESS TO LEARN Many factors affect readiness to learn. For example, your patients cannot learn when they are unwilling or unable to accept the reality of illness. A loss of

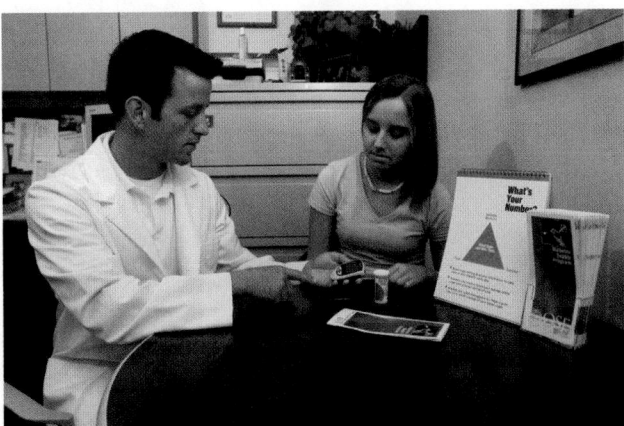

Figure 11-1 ■ **Nurse instructing a patient with a glucose meter.**

BOX 11-2   CULTURAL FOCUS

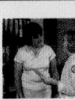 Ashley recognizes that she knows very little about Bosnian culture. Therefore, before she meets with Latinka, Ashley takes some time to read about the Bosnian culture. Ashley finds that during the 1990s about 300,000 people from Bosnia immigrated to the United States as a result of the Balkan wars. The immigrants were older and experienced significant trauma related to the war. Many women experienced personal violence or witnessed violence toward their family and friends. Thus they have a higher incidence of mental illnesses. People from Bosnia tend to have strong ties with their families and communities. Common values include hospitality, spontaneity, owning a home, and telling stories. Bosnians have unique health concerns. There is a high prevalence of smoking that increased during and after the war. In Bosnia walking and bicycling are common, but in the United States this type of exercise is less common because places are further apart from each other and there is more traffic. Folk and family remedies are often passed down from mother to daughter. Common treatments include using herbal teas for colds or the flu. Bosnians also came from a society that provided universal insurance coverage. They are often disappointed with health care in America, and many do not comply with medical prescriptions. Ashley uses this information about Bosnian culture to develop a culturally competent plan that focuses on helping Latinka lose weight and stop smoking.

IMPLICATIONS FOR PRACTICE

- Ashley has a better understanding of Bosnian culture, but she recognizes that not all Bosnian people are the same. Therefore Ashley assesses Latinka's values and her beliefs about the American health care system.
- Ashley asks Latinka about her experiences with the war in Bosnia and is prepared to deal with sensitive issues related to mental health.
- Ashley asks Latinka to describe the coping strategies she used to deal with the war and immigration to the United States.
- Ashley helps Latinka develop healthy coping strategies to deal with her feelings and fears.
- Latinka shares that she is very close to her children and her neighbors. Many times, people who are successful at sticking to an exercise plan exercise with other people. Therefore Ashley helps Latinka develop an exercise routine that includes her children and friends.

Data from Berman H, Girón ERI, Marroquin AP: A narrative study of refugee women who have experienced violence in the context of war, *Can J Nurs Res* 38(4):33, 2006; Corvo K, Peterson J: Posttraumatic stress symptoms, language acquisition, and self-sufficiency: a study of Bosnian refugees, *J Soc Work* 5(2):205, 2005; Das J and others: Mental health and poverty in developing countries: revisiting the relationship, *Soc Sci Med* 65(3):467, 2007; Lipson JG and others: Bosnian and Soviet refugees' experiences with health care, *West J Nurs Res* 25(7):854, 2003; MapZones: *Bosnia Hercegovina: culture,* 2008, http://www.mapzones.com/world/europe/bosnia_hercegovina/cultureindex.php; Snyder CS and others: Social work with Bosnian Muslim refugee children and families: a review of the literature, *Child Welfare* 84(5):607, 2005.

health is usually very difficult for patients to accept. The stages of grieving (see Chapter 25) encompass a series of responses patients experience during illness and affect readiness to learn. People experience these stages at different rates. It is important to properly time patient teaching to ease your patient's adjustment to illness or disability (Table 11-2). Introduce the teaching plan when your patient enters the stage of acceptance, which is most compatible with learning. Continue to teach as long as the patient remains in a stage conductive to learning. If patients are not ready to learn, include family members in your teaching when appropriate and consider referring the patient to a home care nurse to ensure patient needs are met.

Ability to Learn

Your patient's developmental level and cognitive and physical capabilities influence the ability to learn. Consider these important factors while developing a teaching plan.

DEVELOPMENTAL CAPABILITY Learning, like developmental growth, is an evolving process. Therefore consider your patient's stage of development and intellectual abilities so your teaching will be successful. Learning occurs more readily when new information complements existing knowledge. Assess the patient's level of knowledge, intellectual skills and literacy level before beginning a teaching plan. For example, before reviewing a teaching booklet about healthy food choices, determine your patient's understanding of nutrition, as well as reading and comprehension skills.

AGE-GROUP Age often reflects the developmental capability for learning and learning behaviors that the patient is able to acquire. Without proper biological, motor, language, and personal-social development, many types of learning cannot take place (see Chapter 21). Adapt your teaching approach based on the patient's developmental level (Box 11-3). When teaching children, it is very important to ensure that the information you provide is appropriate to the child's developmental stage. As people mature into adulthood, they often become more self-directed and are able to identify their own learning needs. Enhance learning by encouraging the adult learner to reflect on personal and life experiences. Assess what the adult patient knows, teach what the patient wants to know, and set mutual goals to improve educational outcomes (Bastable, 2006). Consider generational differences as well. For example, many baby boomers prefer visual aids and focusing on one topic at a time, whereas younger patients prefer using computers.

TABLE 11-2	Relationship Between Psychosocial Adaptation to Illness and Learning		
STAGE	**PATIENT'S BEHAVIOR**	**LEARNING IMPLICATIONS**	**RATIONALE**
Denial or disbelief	Patient avoids discussion of illness ("There's nothing wrong with me") and disregards physical restrictions. Patient suppresses and distorts information that has not been presented clearly.	Provide support, empathy, and careful explanations of all procedures while they are being done. Let patient know you are available for discussion. Explain situation to family. Teach in present tense (explain current therapy).	Patient is not prepared to deal with problem. Any attempt to convince or tell patient about illness will result in further anger or withdrawal. Provide only information patient pursues or absolutely requires.
Anger	Patient blames and complains and often directs anger at nurse.	Do not argue with patient, but listen to concerns. Teach in present tense. Reassure family of patient's normality.	Patient needs opportunity to express feelings and anger. Patient is still not prepared to face future.
Bargaining	Patient offers to live better life in exchange for promise of better health ("If God lets me live, I promise to be more careful").	Continue to introduce only reality. Teach only in present tense.	Patient is still unwilling to accept limitations.
Resolution	Patient begins to express emotions openly, realizes that illness has created changes, and begins to ask questions.	Encourage expression of feelings. Begin to share information needed for future, and set aside formal times for discussion.	Patient begins to perceive need for assistance and is ready to accept responsibility for learning.
Acceptance	Patient recognizes reality of condition, actively pursues information, and strives for independence.	Focus teaching on future skills and knowledge required. Continue to teach about present occurrences. Involve family in teaching information for discharge.	Patient is more easily motivated to learn. Acceptance of illness reflects willingness to deal with its implications.

PHYSICAL CAPABILITY The ability to learn often depends on a person's level of physical development and overall physical health. To learn psychomotor skills, your patient needs to have the necessary level of strength, coordination, and sensory acuity. For example, it is unrealistic for you to teach your patient to transfer from a bed to a wheelchair if the patient has insufficient upper body strength. Do not overestimate or underestimate the patient's physical abilities. To learn psychomotor skills, your patient requires the following characteristics:

1. Size (height and weight sufficient for the task to be performed or the equipment to be used [e.g., crutch walking])
2. Strength (ability of the patient to follow strenuous exercise program)
3. Coordination (dexterity needed for complicated motor skills such as using utensils or changing a bandage)
4. Sensory acuity (visual, auditory, tactile, gustatory, and olfactory: sensory resources needed to receive and respond to messages taught)

Any condition (e.g., fatigue, breathing difficulty, or depression) that drains a person's energy will impair the ability to learn. Postpone teaching when an illness becomes aggravated by complications such as pain, fever, or respiratory difficulty. After working with your patient, assess the patient's energy level by noting the patient's willingness to communicate, amount of activity initiated, and responsiveness toward questions. Stop teaching if your patient tires; resume teaching when your patient feels rested.

Learning Environment

Factors in the physical environment where teaching takes place make learning a pleasant or difficult experience. Choose settings that help your patients focus attention on their learning task. Consider the number of people you are teaching, need for privacy, room temperature and ventilation, room lighting, noise, and room furniture when choosing the setting.

The ideal environment that promotes learning is a room that has good lighting and ventilation, appropriate furniture, and a comfortable temperature (Figure 11-2). A darkened room interferes with the patient's ability to see the demonstration of a skill or visual aids such as posters or pamphlets. A room that is too cold, hot, or stuffy will make the patient too uncomfortable to pay attention to you. Comfortable furniture eliminates distractions such as the need to change position or shift body weight. It is also important to choose a quiet setting that offers privacy and where interruptions are infrequent. If your patient desires, include family members in discussions. However, remember that some patients are reluctant to engage in discussions about their illnesses when family members are present.

Teaching a group of patients requires a room that allows everyone to be seated comfortably and within hearing distance of the teacher. The room needs to comfortably hold all members of the group. If the room is too large, participants

---

BOX 11-3 Teaching Methods Based on Patient's Developmental Capacity

INFANT
- Keep routines (e.g., feeding, bathing) consistent.
- Hold infant firmly while smiling and speaking softly to convey sense of trust.
- Have infant touch different textures (e.g., soft fabric, hard plastic).

TODDLER
- Use play to teach procedure or activity (e.g., handling examination equipment, applying bandage to doll).
- Offer picture books that describe story of children in hospital or clinic.
- Use simple words such as *cut* instead of *laceration* to promote understanding.

PRESCHOOLER
- Use role-playing, imitation, and play to make it fun for preschoolers to learn.
- Encourage questions and offer explanations. Use simple explanations and demonstrations.
- Encourage children to learn together through pictures and short stories about how to perform hygiene.

SCHOOL-AGE CHILD
- Teach psychomotor skills needed to maintain health. (Complicated skills, such as learning to use a syringe, take considerable practice.)
- Offer opportunities to discuss health problems and answer questions.

ADOLESCENT
- Help adolescent learn about feelings and need for self-expression.
- Use teaching as collaborative activity.
- Allow adolescents to make decisions about health and health promotion (safety, sex education, substance abuse).
- Use problem solving to help adolescents make choices.

YOUNG OR MIDDLE ADULT
- Encourage participation in teaching plan by setting mutual goals.
- Encourage independent learning.
- Offer information so that adult understands effects of health problem.

OLDER ADULT
- Teach when patient is alert and rested.
- Involve adult in discussion or activity.
- Focus on wellness and the person's strength.
- Use approaches that enhance reception of stimuli for patients with sensory alterations (see Chapter 37).
- Keep teaching sessions short.

are often tempted to sit outside the group along the perimeter. Arranging the group to allow participants to observe one another (e.g., in a circle) further enhances learning. More effective communication occurs as learners observe the verbal and nonverbal interactions of others.

INTEGRATING THE NURSING AND TEACHING PROCESSES

There are distinct similarities between the nursing process (see Chapter 8) and the teaching process. Both processes require critical thinking (Box 11-4). When using the nursing process, assessment reveals your patient's health care needs.

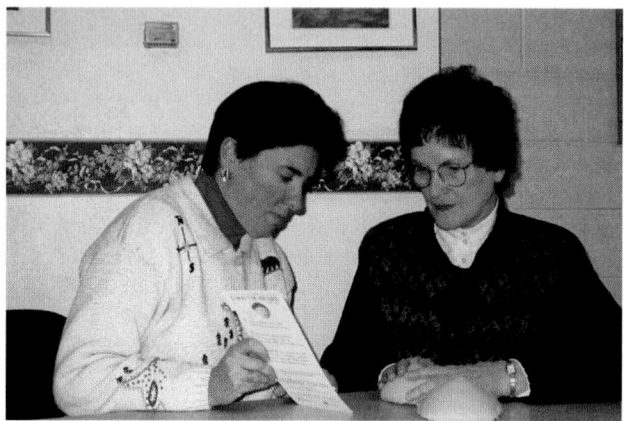

Figure 11-2 ■ Choosing a comfortable, pleasant environment enhances the learning experience. The nurse is explaining the breast self-examination procedure to the patient.

Use assessment data to determine the nursing diagnoses unique to your patient's situation. Then develop and implement an individualized plan of care with appropriate interventions and evaluate the level of success in meeting the goals of care.

While determining your patients' nursing diagnoses, you often identify educational needs. When education becomes a part of the care plan, the teaching process begins. The teaching process requires you to analyze the patient's needs, motivation, and ability to learn (Table 11-3). Learning needs specify the information or skills your patient requires. You set specific learning objectives and implement the teaching plan, using teaching and learning principles to ensure that your patient acquires knowledge and skills. Finally, the teaching process requires an evaluation of learning based on learning objectives.

■■■ASSESSMENT

An effective assessment provides the basis for individualized patient teaching (Wingard, 2005). Assess the patient's learning needs to determine what you need to teach and the patient's ability and willingness to learn. A thorough assessment will help you identify available learning resources and choose the best teaching methods. Assessment also ensures a more individualized approach toward patient education (Table 11-4).

PATIENT EXPECTATIONS   Together, you and your patient identify critical information the patient needs to know. It is also essential to understand what your patient expects to learn. For example, if your patient is newly diagnosed with type 1 diabetes mellitus, ask what your patient expects to learn regarding diabetes self-management. Does the patient expect to self-administer the insulin, or is the expectation that a spouse will give the injection? Assess your patient's expectations in all three learning domains. Questions such as

BOX 11-4   SYNTHESIS IN PRACTICE

 Ashley decides to continue to care for Latinka during the rest of her clinical rotation. As Ashley begins to assess Latinka's educational needs, she reviews Latinka's health concerns and requests for information. Ashley knows that people learn best when you provide the information they want. Ashley also wants to provide culturally competent patient education. Therefore, Ashley knows that assessing Latinka's perceptions of the American health care system and concerns related to immigrating to the United States is a priority before she begins teaching about losing weight and smoking cessation.

Ashley's parents decided to stop smoking and have not smoked for 6 months. Ashley talks with her parents to find out what strategies helped them best to quit smoking. Ashley recalls that her mother gained about 10 pounds when she quit smoking. Ashley also remembers reading a research article that found that several women in the study gained weight after they quit smoking. Because Latinka expressed an interest in losing weight and quitting smoking, Ashley decides she needs to help Latinka develop healthy strategies that do not involve food to cope with nicotine withdrawal symptoms.

Ashley knows that she has the ethical responsibility to provide culturally sensitive patient teaching. She needs to accept Latinka and respect her culture when providing patient teaching. Ashley found some patient education handouts about smoking cessation, but the handouts were designed for whites and African Americans, not for Bosnians. Therefore Ashley decides to take the printed information home with her and makes revisions so the information reflects Latinka's cultural preferences. Ashley also makes sure that the information is written in words that are easy to understand. She realizes that if Latinka cannot read English well, she will need the printed information translated into Bosnian. Ashley is excited to learn more about Latinka and her culture. After establishing a caring relationship with Latinka, Ashley begins to assess Latinka's health needs and learning styles so she can put together an effective individualized teaching plan.

"What do you think is important for you to know to take care of yourself?" allow the patient to be an active participant in planning self-care. Learning needs change depending on your patient's health status. Assessment of learning needs is an ongoing activity. Examples of key areas of assessment are (1) questions raised by the patient or family about health issues; (2) the patient's understanding of current health status, implications of illness, types of therapy, and prognosis; (3) information or skills needed to perform self-care; (4) experiences that influence the patient's need to learn; and (5) information necessary for family members to meet the patient's needs.

MOTIVATION TO LEARN Ask questions that identify your patient's motivation to learn. These questions help determine whether the patient is prepared and willing to learn. Ask questions that relate to the patient's learning behaviors, health beliefs, attitudes about health care providers, knowledge of information to be learned, physical symptoms that interfere with learning (e.g., fatigue, pain, or dizziness), sociocultural background, and learning-style preference.

ABILITY TO LEARN Determine the patient's physical and cognitive ability to learn. Many factors impair the ability to learn. You need to assess the patient's physical strength and coordination, presence of sensory deficits, the patient's reading and developmental level (see Box 11-3, p. 193), and the patient's level of cognitive functioning (see Chapter 21). Also assess for pain, fatigue, anxiety, or any other symptoms that interfere with your patient's ability to pay attention to and participate in their learning.

TEACHING ENVIRONMENT Create an environment for a teaching session that is favorable to learning. Assess for distractions, noise, the patient's comfort level (e.g., sitting or

TABLE 11-3 Comparison of the Nursing and Teaching Processes

BASIC STEPS	NURSING PROCESS	TEACHING PROCESS
Assessment	Collect data about patient's physical, psychological, social, cultural, developmental, and spiritual needs from patient, family, and all databases, medical record, nursing history, and literature.	Gather data about patient's learning needs, literacy level, motivation, ability to learn, and teaching resources from patient, family, learning environment, and all databases.
Nursing diagnosis	Identify appropriate nursing diagnoses.	Identify patient's learning needs on basis of three domains of learning.
Planning	Develop individualized care plan. Set diagnosis priorities based on patient's immediate needs.	Establish learning objectives, stated in behavioral terms. Identify priorities regarding learning needs. Collaborate with patient on teaching plan.
Implementation	Collaborate with patient on care plan. Perform nursing care therapies. Include patient as active participant in care. Involve family in care as appropriate.	Identify type of teaching method to use. Implement teaching methods. Actively involve patient in learning activities. Include family participation as appropriate.
Evaluation	Identify success in meeting desired outcomes and goals of nursing care.	Determine outcomes of teaching-learning process. Measure patient's ability to achieve learning objectives. Reteach as needed.

TABLE 11-4 FOCUSED PATIENT ASSESSMENT

FACTORS TO ASSESS	QUESTIONS	PHYSICAL ASSESSMENT
Learning needs	Tell me what you know about your illness and its treatment. What information do you need to know that would help you better manage your disease?	Observe for a puzzled expression on the patient's face.
Resources for learning	Is there someone who can help you at home? Will you have any trouble getting to the local health department to obtain teaching materials?	Observe for signs of anxiety when discussing home and transportation issues.
Ability to learn	Do you wear glasses or contacts? Do you have trouble seeing words printed in the newspaper? Do you have any difficulties hearing when someone speaks you?	Observe where the patient holds the reading material and for squinting of eyes when reading. Observe whether the patient turns the head when attempting to listen.

lying, the need to toilet), and the availability of rooms and equipment. In the home setting, lighting, space, and the availability of equipment are especially important to assess.

RESOURCES FOR LEARNING Identify resources for learning, which often include the support of family members or significant others. If you include family or significant others, assess how ready family and friends are to learn how to help care for the patient. Determine the family perceptions of the patient's illness, the patient's willingness to involve family members in care, and the family's willingness to help provide care. Also determine the resources available in the home and the teaching tools needed. Ensure that available teaching resources such as brochures, audiovisual materials, and posters are available when needed. Select the most appropriate teaching tool for the patient's needs and ability to learn. Any teaching material you use needs to be current, presented logically, and written or presented in words your learner can understand (Atack, Luke, and Chien, 2008; Koniak-Griffin and others, 2008).

CULTURAL CONSIDERATIONS Assess the language the patient most commonly uses. Make sure informational brochures are in your patient's native language, if possible. Some institutions have translators that can help with this. Determine the patient's role in the family and how the patient's culture influences the patient's perception of illness (Chang and Kelly, 2007). Explore the significance of prescribed medications and therapies in the patient's culture, and explore alternative therapies the patient uses. Teaching that does not include cultural considerations is ineffective (Koniak-Griffin and others, 2008; Matsuyama and others, 2007).

HEALTH LITERACY Current evidence shows that health literacy is a strong predictor of health status and patient outcomes (Attwood, 2008; Kendig, 2006). Therefore you need to assess your patients' health literacy before providing instruction. **Health literacy** includes patients' reading and math skills, comprehension, the ability to make health-related decisions, and successful functioning as a consumer of health care (Speros, 2005). **Functional illiteracy,** the inability to read above a fifth-grade level, is a major problem in America today. The National Adult Literacy Survey, conducted in the United States in 2003, found that more than 75 million Americans had basic or below-basic levels of health literacy. Approximately 14% of adults could not understand a basic patient education pamphlet, and 36% could not perform moderately difficult tasks, such as reading a chart that described childhood vaccinations. Older adults, men, people who did not speak English before entering school, people living below poverty level, and people without a high school education tended to have reduced health literacy. Although illiteracy existed among all races, white and Asian/Pacific Islander adults had higher literacy levels than those for African American, Native American/Alaska Native, Hispanic, and multiracial adults (Kutner and others, 2006).

Adding to the problems related to health literacy, the readability of health education material ranges from a sixth- to eighth-grade reading level or higher (Erlen, 2004). Currently,

printed and online materials often exceed the patient's reading level (Badarudeen and Sabharwal, 2008; Hoffman and McKenna, 2006; Shieh and Hosei, 2008). Removing medical terms from information lowers the reading level, but even this is not enough to bring the reading level of information to an acceptable level (Sand-Jecklin, 2007). Unfortunately, health care professionals do not always address the gap between patients' reading levels and the readability of educational materials (Attwood, 2008; Matsuyama and others, 2007). This results in unsafe patient care. To ensure patient safety, all health care providers need to make sure that information is presented clearly and in a culturally sensitive manner (TJC, 2007).

Although assessing patient's health literacy is sometimes challenging, you need to identify problems with health literacy and provide appropriate education to your patients who have special health literacy needs to ensure safe care (Institute of Medicine, 2004; TJC, 2007). Current evidence shows that many Americans read and understand information that is 3 to 5 years below their last level of formal education. In addition, many people will say they are good readers even if they cannot read (Cutilli, 2005). There are a variety of screening tools you can use to assess your patient's health literacy. The Wide Range Achievement Test (WRAT 3) evaluates reading, spelling, and arithmetic skills for patients ranging in age from 5 to 74 years. The Rapid Estimate of Adult Literacy in Medicine (REALM) uses pronunciation of health care terms to determine approximate reading level. If you do not have an assessment tool readily available, you can ask your patients to read an educational pamphlet and then ask them to put the information into their own words. In addition to reading skills, you need to assess your patients' ability to use math skills effectively and make appropriate health care decisions. Be sure that you are sensitive and maintain a therapeutic relationship with your patients when you are assessing their health literacy. Functional illiteracy frequently decreases feelings of self-worth and self-respect. Thus patients who have problems with health literacy are often ashamed of not being able to understand you and will often try to mask their challenges in comprehending information (Erlen, 2004).

■■■NURSING DIAGNOSIS

After assessing information related to your patient's ability and need to learn, interpret data and cluster defining characteristics to form nursing diagnoses that reflect the patient's specific learning needs. This ensures that teaching will be goal directed and individualized. If a patient has several learning needs, the nursing diagnoses will guide priority setting.

Several NANDA International nursing diagnoses apply to learning needs. When the diagnosis is *deficient* knowledge, the diagnostic statement describes the specific type of learning need and the related factor, for example, *deficient knowledge regarding psychomotor learning related to newly ordered injectable medication.* Each diagnostic statement describes the specific type of learning need and its cause. Classifying diagnoses by the three learning domains helps you focus specifically on the subject matter and teaching methods. Examples of nursing diagnoses that indicate learning needs include the following:

- *Ineffective health maintenance*
- *Deficient knowledge (affective, cognitive, psychomotor)*
- *Noncompliance (with medications)*
- *Ineffective self-health management*
- *Impaired home maintenance*
- *Ineffective family therapeutic regimen management*

When the nurse can manage or eliminate health care problems through education, the related factor of the diagnostic statement is *deficient knowledge.* For example, when your older adult patient is not taking a medication at the appropriate time because she does not understand how the medication works (*noncompliance with medication schedule related to deficient knowledge*), focus on explaining the action of the medication and its purpose. Other nursing diagnoses (e.g., *acute pain* or *fatigue*) indicate that barriers to learning

exist.). Delay teaching until you resolve the priority nursing diagnosis in these cases.

■■■PLANNING

After determining nursing diagnoses, identify your patient's learning needs and develop a teaching care plan. For the plan to be effective, collaborate with the patient, family, and other members of the health care team. The plan should include topics for instruction, teaching resources (e.g., equipment or booklets), recommendations for involving family, and teaching objectives. The setting influences the complexity of the plan. No matter what the length, the teaching plan provides continuity of instruction, especially when several nurses or disciplines share teaching responsibilities.

GOALS AND OUTCOMES It is very important to set clear goals and measurable outcomes so you can effectively evaluate and change a teaching plan as needed. Include the patient if possible when establishing learning goals and outcomes (see Care Plan). Expected outcomes guide the choice

---

CARE PLAN | Readiness for Enhanced Knowledge

ASSESSMENT

Ashley knows that people who smoke are at risk for developing cancer. When Ashley met with Latinka last week, Latinka stated that she currently smokes 1-1½ packs of cigarettes a day, and her husband recently died of bladder cancer. Latinka mentioned that she was concerned about dying from cancer. After thinking about their previous meeting, Ashleys plans to assess Latinka's willingness to stop smoking and potential barriers Latinka might experience if she decides to stop smoking.

ASSESSMENT ACTIVITIES*	FINDINGS/DEFINING CHARACTERISTICS*
Assess how motivated Latinka is to stop smoking	Latinka tried to quit smoking once before, but she states, "When my husband was diagnosed with cancer, the stress was too much, so I started smoking again. **I want to now get control of my health. I just don't know how to do it."**
Assess Latinka's readiness to learn about smoking cessation	Latinka is **concerned about how smoking is affecting her health.** She knows that cigarette smoking is a risk factor for cancer and states **she is ready to quit smoking for good.**

NURSING DIAGNOSIS: Readiness for enhanced knowledge related to desire to learn about smoking cessation.

PLANNING

GOAL

- Latinka will understand the effects of smoking on her health within 3 weeks.

- Latinka will quit smoking through the use of a smoking cessation plan within 6 months.

EXPECTED OUTCOMES (NOC)†

Knowledge: Health Promotion
- Latinka will read information about smoking cessation and the unhealthy effects of tobacco within 2 weeks.
- Latinka will describe how smoking affects her health within 3 weeks.

Risk Control: Tobacco Use
- Latinka will attend a community smoking cessation class within 2 weeks.
- Latinka will describe strategies to use at home to quit smoking.
- Latinka will follow strategies for smoking cessation within a month.

CARE PLAN   Readiness for Enhanced Knowledge—cont'd

INTERVENTIONS (NIC)‡

Health Education

- Incorporate explanation of benefits of smoking cessation into Latinka's current knowledge and health beliefs.

- Develop and/or find educational materials about smoking cessation that are based on assessment of Latinka's learning needs and readiness and motivation to change.
- Use group discussions and role-playing to influence health beliefs, attitudes, and values.
- Plan long-term telephone follow-up to reinforce healthy behavior.

Self-Modification Assistance

- Encourage Latinka to identify small successes.

Smoking Cessation Assistance

- Help Latinka set a definite quit date within the next 2 weeks.
- Manage nicotine replacement therapy.

RATIONALE

Health care providers need to determine the, health beliefs, and perceived barriers to smoking cessation in order for teaching and smoking cessation interventions to be successful (Kerr and others, 2006).

Educational materials designed for the patient's unique needs and situations are effective in promoting smoking cessation (Lancaster and Stead, 2005).

Role-playing and having the patient perform behaviors enhances healthy behaviors (Bandura, 1997).

Long-term follow-up and calling patients on the telephone while they are in the process of smoking cessation promotes successful patient behaviors (Abdullah and others, 2005; Rice and Stead, 2008).

Relapses in smoking cessation are common. Helping patients see their successes encourages continued efforts to stop smoking and enhances the patient's self-efficacy beliefs (Hertel and others, 2008).

Setting a specific quit date boosts the commitment to quit smoking (Andrews, Heath, and Graham-Garcia, 2004).

Using nicotine replacement therapy, such as a transdermal nicotine patch, promotes success with smoking cessation (Ahijevych, 2005; Jonsdottir and others, 2004).

EVALUATION

NURSING ACTIONS	PATIENT RESPONSE/FINDING	ACHIEVEMENT OF OUTCOME
Ask Latinka to explain the effects of smoking on her health.	Latinka says she is almost embarrassed that she has not quit smoking sooner. She is able to explain how smoking affects breathing and the health of her lungs.	Latinka has a good working knowledge of the physical effects of smoking.
Ask Latinka to describe the strategies she has planned to quit smoking.	Latinka decided to quit smoking on her birthday. She states her children call her once a day to check on her progress and provide support. She is using nicotine patches, but she admits that she forgets to change the patch "every now and then."	Latinka has developed and is implementing her smoking cessation plan. She needs further help identifying strategies that will help her remember to use her nicotine patches as ordered.
Ask Latinka to describe what she does whenever she is tempted to start smoking again.	Latinka states she either chews sugar-free gum or calls one of her sons if she is tempted to smoke a cigarette.	Latinka implements healthy behaviors whenever she is tempted to smoke.

*Defining characteristics are shown in **bold** type.
†Outcomes classification labels from Moorhead S and others, editors: *Nursing outcomes classification (NOC)*, ed 4, St. Louis, 2008, Mosby.
‡Intervention classification labels from Bulechek GM and others, editors: *Nursing interventions classification (NIC)*, ed 5, St. Louis, 2008, Mosby.

of teaching strategies and who is involved in the plan. Learning objectives are either short term (relating to immediate learning needs) or long term (relating to permanent adaptation to a health problem). Each objective is a statement of a single behavior that identifies the patient's ability to do something after a learning experience. The objective contains an active verb describing what the learner will do after the objective is met, such as walk with crutches, administer an injection, or identify drug doses. Use a verb that has few interpretations, and state the verb in terms of how the patient is to demonstrate learning (Redman, 2007).

In some health care settings, you will develop written teaching plans. In these cases, include topics for instruction as well as resources, recommendations for involving family, and objectives of the teaching plan. Some plans are very detailed, whereas others are in an outline format (Box 11-5). Remember that the more specific your plan is, the easier it is to follow.

SETTING PRIORITIES Learning objectives identify the expected outcomes of a planned learning experience, which help establish priorities for learning. Prioritize learning needs with your patient by focusing on what the patient needs to know, his or her nursing diagnoses and previous knowledge (Figure 11-3). In most situations it is not appropriate to delegate educational interventions to nursing assistive personnel. As the nurse, you are ultimately responsible for ensuring that all teaching needs have been met.. Usually, teaching needs focused on patient safety issues are the most important. For example, a patient with newly diagnosed hypertension and angina needs to learn about newly prescribed medications, which typically include nitroglycerin spray for angina and a calcium channel blocker. In this situation, knowledge regarding the early identification of chest pain and appropriate use of the nitroglycerin spray is the learning priority.

Timing When is the right time to teach? When a patient first enters a clinic or hospital? At discharge? At home? Each is appropriate because patients have learning needs and opportunities as long as they stay in the health care system. There are times that are not appropriate for teaching. For example, it is not appropriate to teach a patient who just received bad results about a diagnostic test. Plan to teach when the patient is most attentive, receptive, and alert. The frequency of sessions depends on the learner's abilities and the complexity of the material (Bastable, 2006).

The length of teaching sessions also affects learning. Prolonged sessions cause patients to lose concentration and attentiveness, especially older adult patients. It is easier to maintain patients' interests when educational sessions are shorter (e.g., lasting 20 to 30 minutes) and more frequent. Nonverbal cues, such as poor eye contact or slumped posture, indicate a patient has lost concentration. If you note a loss of concentration, stop the session.

Organizing Teaching Material Give careful consideration to the order of information presented. An outline of content helps to organize information into a logical sequence. Material should progress from simple to complex because a person learns simple facts and concepts before learning how to make

---

BOX 11-5   PATIENT TEACHING

Healthy Food Choices

 Before planning educational sessions, Ashley assesses what Latinka expects to learn while they are together. Latinka asks Ashley to help her make healthier food choices. Ashley responds to this request for information and begins by determining what Latinka normally eats. The Bosnian diet is high in animal fats and has a Turkish influence. Meat, bread, vegetables, stews, cheese, legumes, fish, eggs, coffee, sweetened fruit juices, and sweet cakes are common in the Bosnian diet. Using this information, Ashley develops the following teaching plan for Latinka:

OUTCOME
At the end of the teaching session, Latinka will identify three ways to make her diet lower in fat and calories.

TEACHING STRATEGIES
- Complete a diet history to explore what Latinka commonly eats.
- Review Latinka's favorite recipes and meals, and make suggestions of food substitutions that will make meals healthier (e.g., eat fruit instead of drinking sweetened fruit juice; use ground turkey, low-fat cheese, margarine or vegetable oil, and decrease number of eggs used in recipes).
- Encourage Latinka to increase the number of legumes and fresh vegetables in her diet while decreasing the amount of sweet bread she eats.
- Provide Latinka with culturally sensitive teaching handouts on healthy food choices.
- Summarize what was taught.
- Make a follow-up appointment to reinforce teaching.

EVALUATION STRATEGIES
- Have Latinka complete a 3-day food diary, and evaluate her food choices on her follow-up appointment.
- Ask Latinka to describe what substitutions to make in her favorite recipes to make them healthier.
- Ask Latinka to make a healthy menu for 2 days.

Data from Flowers DL: Culturally competent nursing care: a challenge for the twenty-first century, *Crit Care Nurse* 24(4):48, 2004; Jonsson IM and others: Choice of food and food traditions in pre-war Bosnia-Herzegovina: focus group interviews with immigrant women in Sweden, *Ethn Health* 7(3):149, 2002; Lipson JG and others: Bosnian and Soviet refugees' experiences with health care, *West J Nurs Res* 25(7):854, 2003; Mukeshimana C: Health assessment of Bosnian refugees in Black Hawk County, Iowa, *Int J Global Health* 1(2):24, 2001.

---

associations or complex interpretations of ideas. For example, to teach a woman how to feed her husband who has a gastric tube, first teach the wife how to measure the tube feeding and how to manipulate the equipment. Once you accomplish this, teach her how to administer the feeding.

Because patients are more likely to remember information taught in the beginning of a teaching session, present essential information first. Informative but less critical content

CONCEPT MAP

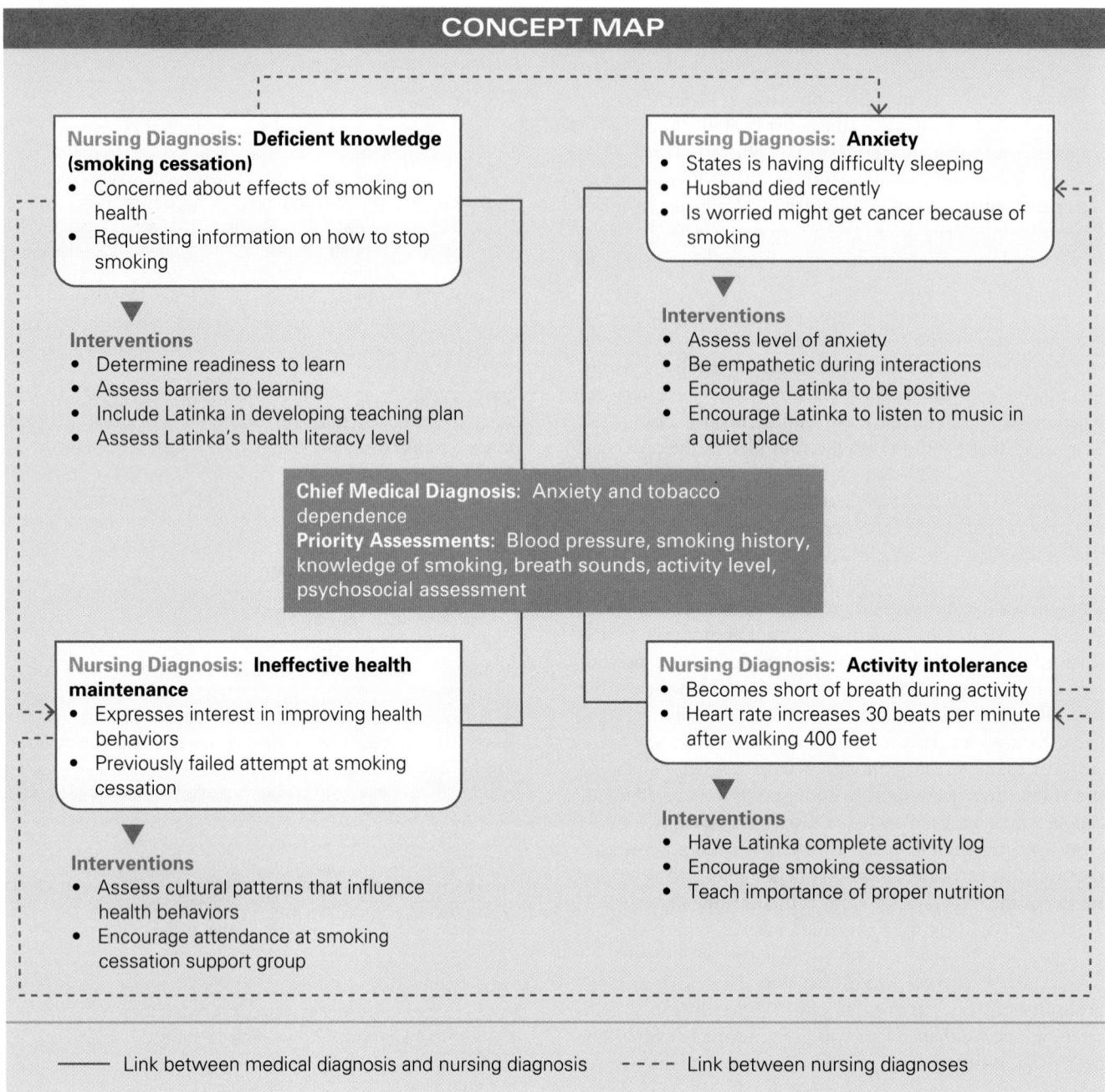

Nursing Diagnosis: Deficient knowledge (smoking cessation)
- Concerned about effects of smoking on health
- Requesting information on how to stop smoking

Interventions
- Determine readiness to learn
- Assess barriers to learning
- Include Latinka in developing teaching plan
- Assess Latinka's health literacy level

Nursing Diagnosis: Anxiety
- States is having difficulty sleeping
- Husband died recently
- Is worried might get cancer because of smoking

Interventions
- Assess level of anxiety
- Be empathetic during interactions
- Encourage Latinka to be positive
- Encourage Latinka to listen to music in a quiet place

Chief Medical Diagnosis: Anxiety and tobacco dependence
Priority Assessments: Blood pressure, smoking history, knowledge of smoking, breath sounds, activity level, psychosocial assessment

Nursing Diagnosis: Ineffective health maintenance
- Expresses interest in improving health behaviors
- Previously failed attempt at smoking cessation

Interventions
- Assess cultural patterns that influence health behaviors
- Encourage attendance at smoking cessation support group

Nursing Diagnosis: Activity intolerance
- Becomes short of breath during activity
- Heart rate increases 30 beats per minute after walking 400 feet

Interventions
- Have Latinka complete activity log
- Encourage smoking cessation
- Teach importance of proper nutrition

——— Link between medical diagnosis and nursing diagnosis   - - - - Link between nursing diagnoses

Figure 11-3 ■ Concept Map.

follows the essential information. Other interventions that reinforce learning include using repetition and summarizing key points (Bastable, 2006).

COLLABORATIVE CARE Patients receive education in almost every health care setting. Although you are the primary member of the health care team responsible for patient education, often your patients' educational needs are highly complex. To successfully meet your patients' needs, collaboration with other health care professionals is required. Refer patients to appropriate multidisciplinary health care providers if indicated. For example, you refer a patient with a new diagnosis of chronic renal failure to a dietitian for dietary teaching. Patients in acute care settings often require assistance from discharge planners, case managers, and commu-

nity agencies to be successfully discharged to home. It is your responsibility to collaborate with and include these multidisciplinary health care team members in the teaching plan. A variety of educational resources is available in the community, including diabetes education clinics, prenatal classes, and support groups. Be aware of potential resources, and obtain consults for your patients when needed. Encourage your patients to use these resources, and reinforce information provided.

■■■IMPLEMENTATION

Implementation of a teaching plan requires you to use critical thinking while you analyze assessment data and apply teaching and learning principles. Implementation involves believing that each interaction with a patient is an opportunity to teach. Use evidence-based interventions to create an effective and active learning environment, and maximize opportunities for learning. Because learning situations vary, there is no single correct way to teach. The principles of teaching are in effect techniques that incorporate the principles of learning.

TEACHING APPROACHES You will teach your patients in a variety of ways. To be a successful teacher, choose a teaching approach that matches your patient's needs. A patient's learning needs change over time. Therefore modify your teaching approach as you care for a patient over time.

Telling The telling approach is useful when teaching limited information, such as when you are preparing the patient for an emergent diagnostic procedure. Outline the task the patient needs to do, and give explicit instructions. There is no time for feedback with this method.

Participating When using the participating approach, you and the patient set objectives and participate in the learning process together. The patient helps decide content, and you guide and counsel the patient. For example, a parent with a child diagnosed with sickle cell disease works with you to manage the child's pain. At the end of each teaching session, you review the objectives with the parent and child and plan or revise what you will cover the next time you meet.

Entrusting The entrusting approach provides the patient the opportunity to manage self-care. The patient accepts responsibilities and correctly performs the task while you observe the patient's progress and remain available for assistance. For example, a patient who is receiving continuous intravenous pain medication at home for end-stage cancer requires a higher dose of pain medication. The patient understands the dosage of the medication and how the medication pump works. You help the patient determine an appropriate new pain medication dosage and allow the patient to adjust the settings on the medication pump.

Reinforcing **Reinforcement** is using a stimulus that increases the probability of a response. A learner who receives reinforcement before or after a desired learning behavior will likely repeat the behavior. Feedback is a common form of reinforcement. Reinforcers are positive or negative. Positive reinforcement, such as a smile or praise and support, produces the desired responses. Although negative reinforcement (e.g., frowning) may work, people usually respond better to positive reinforcement.

Three types of reinforcers are social, material, and activity. Use social reinforcers (e.g., smiles, compliments, words of encouragement, or physical contact) to acknowledge a learned behavior. Examples of material reinforcers are food, toys, and music. These work best with young children. Activity reinforcers (e.g., physical therapy) rely on the principle that a person is motivated to engage in an activity if there is an opportunity to participate in more desirable activity upon completion of this first activity. Choosing an appropriate reinforcer involves careful thought and attention to individual preferences. Never use reinforcers as threats. Reinforcement is not effective with every patient.

INCORPORATING TEACHING WITH NURSING CARE As you gain confidence in your knowledge and clinical skills, you will find you are able to teach more effectively while you are providing care to your patients. For example, you educate your patient on the actions of medications while you are administering them. When you follow a teaching plan informally, your patient feels less pressure to perform and learning becomes more of a shared activity. Teaching during routine care is efficient and cost-effective.

TEACHING METHODS Active participation is a key to learning. By actively experiencing a learning event, your patient is more likely to retain knowledge. A teaching method is the way you deliver information and is based on the patient's learning needs (Box 11-6). The instructional method you choose depends on the time available for teaching, the setting, the resources available, and your comfort level with teaching. Skilled teachers are flexible and combine more than one method into a teaching plan.

One-on-One Discussion Whenever you teach a patient at the bedside, in a health care provider's office, or in the home, you share information through one-on-one discussion. You provide information informally, allowing the patient to ask questions or share concerns. Use various teaching aids during the discussion depending on the patient's learning needs.

Group Instruction Group instruction offers an economical way to teach a number of patients at one time, and often the experience of being part of a group may provide the support necessary for patients to meet learning objectives (Redman, 2007). Group instruction often involves both lecture and discussion. Lectures are efficient in helping groups of patients learn about a subject. After hearing information from a lecture, learners need the opportunity to share ideas and seek clarification. Group discussions allow patients and families to learn from each other as they share common experiences.

Preparatory Instruction Patients frequently face unfamiliar tests or procedures that create anxiety. Providing information about procedures helps patients feel less anxious because they understand what to expect during the procedure. When preparatory instructions accurately describe the actual experience, the patient is able to cope more effectively with the stress from procedures and therapies. The following are guidelines for giving preparatory explanations:

1. Describe physical sensations during the procedure, but do not evaluate them. For example, when drawing a blood specimen, explain that the patient will feel a sticking sensation as the needle punctures the skin.
2. Describe the cause of the sensation, preventing false impressions of the experience. For example, explain that a needle insertion burns because alcohol used to cleanse the skin enters the puncture site.
3. Prepare patients only for aspects of the experience that have commonly been noticed by other patients. For example, explain that it is normal for a tight tourniquet to cause a person's hand to tingle and feel numb.

| BOX 11-6 | Teaching Methods Based on Patient's Learning Needs |

COGNITIVE

Discussion (One-on-One or Group)
- Involves nurse and patient or nurse with several patients
- Promotes active participation and focuses on topics of interest to patient
- Allows peer support
- Enhances application and analysis of new information

Lecture
- More formal method of instruction because teacher controls it
- Helps learner acquire new knowledge and gain comprehension

Question-and-Answer Session
- Designed specifically to address patient's concerns
- Assists patient in applying knowledge

Role-Play, Discovery
- Allows patient to actively apply knowledge in controlled situation
- Promotes synthesis of information and problem solving

Independent Project (Computer-Assisted Instruction), Field Experience
- Allows patient to assume responsibility for completing learning activities at own pace
- Promotes analysis, synthesis, and evaluation of new information and skills

AFFECTIVE

Role Play
- Allows expression of values, feelings, and attitudes

Discussion (Group)
- Allows patient to acquire support from others in group
- Permits patient to learn from others' experiences
- Promotes responding, valuing, and organization

Discussion (One-on-One)
- Allows discussion of personal, sensitive topics of interest or concern

PSYCHOMOTOR

Demonstration
- Provides presentation of procedures or skills by nurse
- Permits patient to incorporate modeling of nurse's behavior
- Allows nurse to control questioning during demonstration

Practice
- Gives patient opportunity to perform skills using equipment
- Provides repetition

Return Demonstration
- Permits patient to perform skills as nurse observes
- Is excellent source of feedback and reinforcement

Independent Project, Game
- Requires teaching method that promotes adaptation and origination of psychomotor learning
- Permits learner to use new skills

Demonstrations Demonstrations are useful methods for teaching psychomotor skills. An effective demonstration requires advance planning. When using a demonstration, include the following steps:

1. Assemble and organize equipment.
2. Perform each step in sequence while analyzing the knowledge and skills involved.
3. Determine when to give explanations, considering the patient's learning needs.
4. Judge the proper speed and timing of the demonstration, based on the patient's cognitive abilities and anxiety level.

Demonstrate the procedure or skill under the same conditions that the patient will experience at home and in the same order in which the patient will perform it. Encourage the patient to ask questions so that the patient clearly understands each step. To enable the patient to easily observe each step of the procedure, perform demonstrations slowly, and avoid rushing. Give the patient the opportunity to practice the procedure under supervision. At the end of the session,

have the patient perform a **return demonstration**. During a return demonstration, the patient completes the procedure independently to show competence.

Analogies Learning occurs when a teacher translates complex language or ideas into words or concepts that the patient understands. **Analogies** add to verbal instruction by providing familiar images that make complex information more real and understandable (Redman, 2007). For example, comparing arterial blood pressure to the flow of water through a hose is an analogy that is useful when explaining hypertension to a patient. When using analogies, know the concept, keep the analogy simple and clear, and be aware of the patient's background, experience, and culture.

Role-Play During role-play, you ask your patients to play themselves or someone else in the situation. Patients learn required skills and feel more confident in performing them independently following the role-play. For example, you are teaching a family caregiver effective communication strategies to use with an older, confused parent. You pretend to be the parent who is having difficulty getting dressed. The caregiver responds to you in this situation. At the end of the session, you help the caregiver evaluate the response and determine if an alternative approach would have been more effective.

Simulation   Simulation is a useful technique for teaching problem solving, application, and independent thinking. During individual or group discussion, you present a problem or situation pertaining to the patients' learning for patients to solve. For example, you ask patients with heart disease to plan a meal low in cholesterol.

MAINTAINING ATTENTION AND PARTICIPATION

All of the senses are channels for presenting information. Patients learn better when you stimulate multiple senses while you teach. In addition, your actions can increase learner attention and participation. When conducting a discussion with a patient, change the tone and intensity of your voice, make eye contact, and use gestures that accentuate key points of discussion. A learner remains interested in a teacher who is actively enthusiastic about the subject under discussion (Billings and Halstead, 2009).

ILLITERACY AND OTHER DISABILITIES

Medical terms are very confusing, so you need to provide information in words your patients are able to understand. People who have problems with illiteracy or other learning disabilities often have difficulty analyzing instructions and synthesizing information. They often also have limited problem-solving skills and will not ask questions to clarify information. Use a variety of interventions (e.g., audiotapes, videos, or drawing pictures) with patients who have low health literacy or other difficulties learning (Box 11-7).

Sometimes you will have to provide education to patients who have sensory alterations (see Chapter 37). When caring for patients who are deaf, you may need to include a sign language interpreter to help implement your interventions. Visual impairments also can affect the teaching strategy you use. Many times patients who are blind or have reduced vision have acute listening skills. To enhance communication and decrease anxiety, tell the patient you are there and do not shout during teaching sessions.

CULTURAL DIVERSITY

Health education materials often fail to recognize cultural beliefs, values, language, perceptions, and attitudes held by patients and families. Be aware of the patient's cultural background, beliefs, and ability to understand instructions not written in the patient's native language. Cultural diversity is widespread and poses a great challenge to provide culturally sensitive health care and patient education (Hatcher and Whittemore, 2007; Li and others, 2007). Effective educational strategies often require the use of different patterns of communication (TJC, 2007). When educating patients of different ethnic groups, do the following (Chang and Kelly, 2007):

1. Become aware of each culture's distinctive aspects.
2. If an interpreter is necessary, first determine your patient's beliefs about using an interpreter—in some cultures it is inappropriate to discuss private health-related issues with other people, people of other genders, or people who are younger. Always use a professional interpreter who understands medical terminology.

BOX 11-7   Patient Teaching Strategies for the Patient With Limited Health Literacy

- Make time for one-on-one educational sessions.
- Individualize teaching materials to meet the patient's needs and match the patient's reading level; if you do not know the patient's reading level, provide information at a fifth-grade or lower level.
- Provide information in a variety of ways (e.g., written, on a computer, videotape, audiotape).
- Make teaching materials visually appealing.
- Use simple words the patient can understand (e.g., shot instead of injection, walk instead of ambulate).
- Use the active voice when providing instructions (e.g., tell patient to "take medicine before bedtime" instead of "medicine should be taken at bedtime").
- Use examples to keep the patient an active participant in learning.
- Present the most important information first, and summarize it at the end of the session.
- Space out information to decrease intimidation.
- Use pictures or illustrations when possible.
- Encourage patients to ask questions during the teaching session.
- Ask specific questions (e.g., "When will you take this medicine?"), and ask the patient to "teach back" or "show back" what you have taught to assess your patient's knowledge level.
- Observe the patient's ability to perform the desired behaviors.

Modified from Erlen JA: Functional health illiteracy: ethical concerns, *Orthop Nurs* 23(2):150, 2004; Schaefer CT: Integrated review of health literacy interventions, *Orthop Nurs* 27(5):302, 2008; The Joint Commission: *"What did the doctor say?" improving health literacy to protect patient safety,* 2007, http://www.jointcommission.org/NR/rdonlyres/D5248B2E-E7E6-4121-8874-99C7B4888301/0/improving_health_literacy.pdf.

---

3. Demonstrate respect for your patient and the family, and address them using their appropriate titles and pronounce their names correctly.
4. Use culturally relevant teaching resources and approaches.

SPECIAL NEEDS OF CHILDREN AND OLDER ADULTS

The choice of instructional methods and application of teaching-learning principles is based on a patient's age. Children, adults, and older adults learn differently. Adapt teaching strategies to each learner's abilities and developmental stage.

Children pass through several developmental stages (see Chapter 21). In each stage children gain new cognitive and psychomotor abilities that respond to different types of learning. You will need parental input and participation when providing health education to children.

Because the population of older adults continues to increase and the care of the older adult is becoming more complex, the effectiveness of nursing interventions used in teach-

BOX 11-8   BEST PRACTICES

Improving Medication Adherence in Older Adults

SUMMARY OF EVIDENCE

Many older adults take medications every day to control and prevent the progression of their chronic illnesses. Taking medications as prescribed is often difficult for older adults because of the cognitive and physical changes that are associated with aging. When older adults do not take their medications as prescribed, they are at risk for poor outcomes such as adverse drug reactions and declining health status. There are many reasons why older patients have trouble taking their medications correctly. Factors that affect medication adherence include previous experiences with medications, cultural preferences, personal beliefs, side effects of medications, and financial constraints. Patient education is one way to promote medication adherence in the older adult. Effective medication education often includes verbal and written information as well as information provided using technology (e.g., computers or telephone calls from nurses or automated computer voices). Effective education also occurs in a variety of inpatient and outpatient settings and includes information given to the patient at discharge. Nurses provide information about the patient's medications, side effects, and medication schedule. How-

ever, medication adherence requires more than just education. Use interventions that require patients' active involvement. Interventions such as allowing patients to administer their own medications under supervision, using psychosocial interventions that motivate patients to take their medications as prescribed, and having patients monitor and record their symptoms (e.g., taking their blood pressure or weighing themselves) enhance educational outcomes and promote adherence to medications.

APPLICATION TO NURSING PRACTICE

- You are responsible and accountable for providing medication education and addressing medication adherence with your patients.
- Individualize your teaching based on your patients' beliefs about medications, cultural factors, and functional status.
- Include your patients' family and significant others, as appropriate, when providing medication teaching.
- Implement interventions that encourage your patients to be actively involved in managing their care.

REFERENCE

Ruppar TM, Conn VS, Russell CL: Medication adherence interventions for older adults: literature review, *Res Theory Nurs Pract* 22(2):114, 2008.

BOX 11-9   CARE OF THE OLDER ADULT

Effective Teaching Strategies for the Older Adult

- Provide individualized information that is based on what the patient needs to know.
- Present information slowly in frequent sessions.
- Include family members when necessary.
- Repeat information frequently.
- Reinforce teaching with audiovisual material, written exercises, and practice.
- Emphasize the older adult's current concerns and past positive coping strategies.
- Allow more time for learners to express themselves, demonstrate learning, and ask questions.
- Establish measurable and realistic short-term goals.
- Establish follow-up sessions.
- Base new information on patients' previous level of learning.

Data from Ebersole P and others: *Toward healthy aging*, ed 7, St. Louis, 2008, Mosby; Edelman CL, Mandle CL: *Health promotion throughout the life span*, ed 6, St. Louis, 2006, Mosby.

ing older adults is frequently evaluated in nursing research (Box 11-8). Older adults experience numerous physical and psychological changes as they age. These changes sometimes create barriers to learning. Sensory changes require teaching methods that enhance the patient's functioning (Lubkin and

Larsen, 2009). For example, if your patient has changes in visual acuity, use large-print materials. Older adults learn and remember effectively if you pace the learning properly and if the material is relevant to the learner's needs and abilities (Ebersole and others, 2008). Educational strategies for gerontological nursing practice are highlighted in Box 11-9.

■■■ EVALUATION

PATIENT CARE Patient education is not complete until you evaluate the outcomes of the teaching-learning process (see Care Plan, p. 197). During evaluation, determine if your patient achieved learning objectives set during the planning stage (Box 11-10). Use return demonstrations, questions, observation of patient behaviors, role-playing, and discussions to evaluate your patient's learning. For example, to evaluate learning in the patient who was taught how to use a three-point crutch gait, ask the patient to demonstrate crutch-walking technique while walking to the end of the hall.

If evaluation indicates that a knowledge or skill deficit still exists, modify the teaching plan. Alternative teaching methods often help to clarify information or strengthen skills that the patient was unable to comprehend or perform originally. Evaluation also reveals new learning needs or new factors that may interfere with the patient's ability to learn. Use this information to update the teaching plan and make it relevant to patient needs. Like the nursing process, the teaching process is continuous and ever-changing.

PATIENT EXPECTATIONS After you educate patients to manage their health promotion activities, disease processes,

BOX 11-10 EVALUATION

After Ashley and Latinka met for the first time, Latinka decided to quit smoking on her birthday, which was in 1½ weeks. During that time Ashley made an appointment for Latinka to see the advanced practice nurse at the health department so Latinka could get a prescription for nicotine patches. Ashley and Latinka decided to meet together 2 weeks after Latinka started her smoking cessation plan. In the meantime Ashley called Latinka on her birthday to provide encouragement and support.

Today Ashley and Latinka meet to evaluate how the teaching plan is going. Ashley completes a physical assessment and asks Latinka questions about her progress to date. Latinka states she is less short of breath and has more energy now that she is not smoking. She feels better about herself and likes that her house does not smell like cigarette smoke as much any more. Latinka's sons, who also smoked, decided to quit with their mom as a birthday present. Latinka states, "If one of us feels like smoking, we call each other for help. It is really nice that we can support each other together." Ashley reinforces that having a good support system at home will help Latinka continue not to smoke. Latinka also relates that the nicotine patch is working well. She still suffers from nicotine withdrawal symptoms, but Latinka says, "They aren't that bad as long as I use my patches."

Because Ashley is also concerned about Latinka's weight management plan, she asks Latinka about her level of exercise and diet choices since the last time they met. Latinka says that she walks with her sons 2 days a week, and she walks with her neighbor another 2 days a week. She has been experimenting with her recipes also. She made her famous *burek*, which is a Bosnian meat pie. She used egg whites instead of egg yolks and ground sirloin instead of ground beef. She added more vegetables to her recipe and decreased the amount of butter she used. Latinka said, "I thought it was good, but I wasn't sure if it matched up to my old recipe. So, I served it to my boys, and they didn't even notice the difference."

Ashley reviews healthy coping strategies with Latinka and provides reinforcement for all the positive changes made so far. They decide to meet again in 3 weeks. Ashley asks Latinka if there is anything that Latinka would like to review at their next appointment. Latinka says, "I think I would like to review all the good things that will happen to me now that I am not smoking. I also want to talk about what I am going to do with all the money I am saving now that I don't smoke. I might even bring you a sample from my new stew recipe." Latinka tells Ashley she is so glad that Ashley is her nurse. Ashley feels a sense of satisfaction. She has helped Latinka make healthy changes, and she looks forward to learning more about Bosnian culture.

DOCUMENTATION NOTE

"Outcomes of education plan assessed. Reports quit smoking about 4 weeks ago on birthday. Sons have quit smoking also, providing support for each other. Has symptoms of nicotine withdrawal, but reports the nicotine replacement patch is helpful in minimizing symptoms. Verbalized increased feelings of energy and less shortness of breath. Walking 4 days a week with sons and neighbor. Is successfully experimenting with healthy substitutions in family recipes. Has requested to review short-term benefits associated with smoking cessation and will review diet information at next visit."

and physical and functional limitations, you send them back to their home and community. It is important to have a method for evaluating your patient's expectations regarding patient education. Did your patient and family receive the education they expected? Were the expectations regarding self-care met? Are there some education expectations remaining? Did the educational program increase your patients' comfort in managing their health status in their home? If your patients' expectations are not met, then you increase the risk is increased that your patients will not continue following the prescribed treatment plan, will be less independent, and perhaps will ignore signs and/or symptoms indicating a need to make an appointment with their health care provider.

DOCUMENTATION OF PATIENT TEACHING

Because patient teaching often occurs informally (e.g., during medication administration or physical examination), it is difficult to document patient education consistently. However, because you are professionally and legally responsible for providing accurate and timely information to patients, quality documentation is essential. Documentation also helps members of the health care team coordinate patient education. Document the following information about patient education:

1. *Assessment data and related nursing diagnoses:* Provide information and support for goals and outcomes.
2. *Interventions planned and used:* Planned education provides continuity of care. Specifically describe subject matter so that other nurses can follow up and reinforce teaching (e.g., "verbalized side effects of digoxin").
3. *Evaluation of learning:* Document evidence of learning (e.g., a return demonstration of coughing and deep breathing). This informs staff about the patient's progress and determines material that you still need to teach.
4. *Ability of patient and/or family to manage care:* Identify needs for outpatient or home care follow-up after discharge. Appropriate referrals better meet the patient's needs.

KEY POINTS

- Health education is aimed at the promotion, restoration, and maintenance of health.
- Teaching is most effective when it is responsive to the learner's needs and requires the learner's active involvement.
- Teaching is a form of interpersonal communication, with teacher and student actively involved in a process that increases the student's knowledge and skills.
- Teaching a patient a specific behavior involves incorporation of behaviors from all three learning domains.
- A person's health beliefs influence the willingness to gain the knowledge and skills necessary to maintain health.
- Patients of different age-groups require different teaching strategies as a result of developmental capabilities.
- Presentation of teaching content progresses from simple to more complex ideas.
- Assess the reading ability and the ability of the patient to understand health information before providing patient education.

- Patient teaching is culturally sensitive and individualized to meet the needs of the patient.
- The patient is an active participant in a teaching plan, agreeing to the plan, helping to choose instructional methods, and recommending times for instruction.
- A combination of teaching methods improves the learner's attentiveness and involvement.
- Teaching methodologies match the patient's learning need.
- Learning objectives describe what a person is to learn in behavioral terms.
- Evaluate a patient's learning by observing the performance of expected learning behaviors under desired conditions.

CRITICAL THINKING EXERCISES

Latinka and Ashley continue to meet to monitor Latinka's success with her smoking cessation plan. Overall, Latinka is doing well with her plan, but she continues to forget to change her nicotine patch. As a result, Latinka's nurse practitioner decides to discontinue the nicotine patch and starts Latinka on a nonnicotine prescription medication used to help people stop smoking.

1. After assessing Latinka, Ashley enters the following nursing diagnoses on the care plan. Which of these nursing diagnoses is the priority at this time? Explain your answer.
   a. *Readiness for enhanced knowledge* (new medication) related to inexperience with new medicine
   b. *Anxiety* related to change in medications
   c. *Ineffective health maintenance* related to difficulty adhering to medication schedule
2. When Ashley teaches Latinka about smoking cessation and her new medication schedule, which of the domains of learning are involved?
   a. Cognitive learning
   b. Psychomotor learning
   c. Affective learning
   d. All the above
3. As Ashley teaches Latinka about her new medication, Ashley suspects that Latinka is experiencing difficulty understanding the written medication information provided by the manufacturer. Why do you think Latinka cannot

understand the material? Describe the educational interventions Ashley needs to use at this time.

4. Latinka is diagnosed with high blood pressure. She is having a hard time dealing with her diagnosis. Ashley determines she is in the anger stage of adaptation to illness. Ashley knows it is important to match your timing of education with how the patient adapts to an illness. Match the stages of adaptation listed below with the appropriate nursing interventions.

Stage	Nursing Intervention
1. Denial or disbelief	a. Focus on what Latinka will need to know in the future, and involve the family in learning.
2. Anger	b. Encourage Latinka to express feelings, and set aside times for teaching sessions.
3. Bargaining	c. Let Latinka know you are ready to talk whenever she is ready to talk, and provide emotional support.
4. Resolution	d. Do not argue with Latinka, and assure the family that this is a normal response.
5. Acceptance	e. Teach in present tense, and discuss the reality of the illness.

ⓔvolve   *Answers to Critical Thinking Questions can be found on the Evolve website.*

REVIEW QUESTIONS

1. A patient has been started on a diuretic for hypertension and needs to learn about the medication's side effects. Understanding this information will require learning in the:
   1. Cognitive domain
   2. Affective domain
   3. Psychomotor domain
   4. Attentional domain

2. Which of the following are effective teaching-learning principles a nurse uses when teaching a new mother how to breast-feed her baby? Select all that apply.
   1. Provide patient education when there are visitors in the room.
   2. Time teaching sessions to coincide with times when the patient's baby is hungry.
   3. Provide patient teaching when the patient is well rested and the baby is not crying.
   4. Include the patient's spouse in educational sessions if it is okay with her.
   5. Assess the patient's feelings about being a new mom and beliefs about breast-feeding at the end of the teaching session.

3. A nursing student is preparing to teach third-grade students about the importance of exercise. To achieve the best learning outcomes, the nursing student:
   1. Provides information using a lecture
   2. Provides several teaching handouts the children can take home
   3. Develops activities that encourage the children to make a plan to exercise daily
   4. Completes an extensive literature search focusing on prevention of childhood obesity

4. An 86-year-old woman's priority nursing diagnosis is *disturbed sleep pattern related to anxiety and lack of understanding of upcoming surgery.* The nurse teaches the patient what to expect before, during, and after surgery. The nurse knows the patient understands the procedures to expect after surgery when the patient:
   1. Demonstrates how she will get out of bed following her surgery
   2. States that she needs to ask her daughter to be at the hospital the day of her surgery
   3. Needs reinforcement of information regarding pain management and activity following surgery
   4. Calls her friends to tell them about the day of her surgery and how long she will be in the hospital

5. A patient is being discharged in 2 days and will need to self-administer a medication subcutaneously. The patient has not had to take this medication in the past. The nurse allows the patient to prepare and administer her own injections. The teaching approach used in this situation is the:
   1. Telling approach
   2. Selling approach
   3. Entrusting approach
   4. Participating approach

6. A 68-year-old man needs to learn how to do self-catheterization. In teaching the patient about this, you need to:
   1. Speak loudly and clearly
   2. Demonstrate the skill quickly and efficiently
   3. Expect the patient to understand the information the first time you present it
   4. Allow the patient time to express his feelings about catheterizing himself and ask questions

7. A nurse is a preceptor for a nursing student who is caring for a 10-year-old boy with asthma. The nursing student needs to teach the child how to use an inhaler. The nurse intervenes when the student:
   1. Gives the child time to ask questions
   2. Demonstrates how to use the inhaler step by step
   3. Encourages the child to learn how to use the inhaler on his own
   4. Assesses the child's hand strength and ability to administer the medication

8. A nurse is preparing to teach a patient with poor health literacy about a new medication. What does the nurse do first?
   1. Schedules frequent teaching sessions
   2. Establishes a therapeutic relationship with the patient
   3. Asks the patient to explain what was taught and provide a return demonstration of skills learned
   4. Includes the most important information about the medication at the beginning of the teaching session

9. A nurse plans to use individualized computer instruction with a group of low-income mothers at the public health department. Which of the following will the nurse do before beginning instruction?
   1. Determines the patients' psychomotor skills
   2. Makes sure that the most important information is presented last
   3. Assesses the reading level of the information provided on the computer
   4. Ensures there are photographs included in the computer program

10. Which of the following interventions implemented by the nurse when caring for a patient who recently had a stroke indicates that the nurse is incorporating teaching with nursing care?
    1. The nurse speaks clearly and develops alternative communication methods if needed.
    2. The nurse describes the importance of changing positions while turning the patient onto the side.
    3. The nurse determines the patient's reading level and ensures that teaching materials are written at the appropriate level.
    4. The nurse assesses the patient's culture and ensures that food delivered by the kitchen is consistent with the patient's cultural preferences.

Answers to Review Questions can be found on pages 1197-1198.

REFERENCES

Abdullah AS and others: Smoking cessation intervention in parents of young children: a randomized controlled trial, *Addiction* 100(11):1731, 2005.

Ahijevych K: Review: all forms of nicotine replacement therapy are effective for smoking cessation, *Evid Based Nurs* 8(1):13, 2005.

American Hospital Association: *The patient care partnership*, 2003, http://www.aha.org/aha/issues/Communicating-With-Patients/pt-care-partnership.html.

American Nurses Association: *Code of ethics for nurses*, 2001, http://nursingworld.org/MainMenuCategories/ThePracticeofProfessionalNursing/EthicsStandards/CodeofEthics.aspx.

Andrews JO, Heath J, Graham-Garcia J: Management of tobacco dependence in older adults: using evidence-based strategies, *J Gerontol Nurs* 30(12):13, 2004.

Atack L, Luke R, Chien E: Evaluation of patient satisfaction with tailored online patient education information, *Comput Inform Nurs* 26(5):258, 2008.

Attwood CA: Health literacy: do your patients really understand? *AACN Viewpoint* 30(2):3, 2008.

Badarudeen S, Sabharwal S: Readability of patient education materials from the American Academy of Orthopaedic Surgeons and Pediatric Orthopaedic Society of North America web sites, *J Bone Joint Surg Am* 90(1):199, 2008.

Bandura A: *Self-efficacy: the exercise of control*, New York, 1997, WH Freeman.

Bastable S: *Essentials of patient education*, Sudbury, Mass, 2006, Jones & Bartlett.

Bastable S: *Nurse as educator: principles of teaching and learning for nursing practice*, ed 3, Sudbury, Mass, 2008, Jones & Bartlett.

Berman H, Girón ERI, Marroquin AP: A narrative study of refugee women who have experienced violence in the context of war, *Can J Nurs Res* 38(4):33, 2006.

Billings DM, Halstead, JA: *Teaching in nursing: a guide for faculty*, ed 3, St. Louis, 2009, Saunders.

Bulechek GM and others, editors: *Nursing interventions classification (NIC)*, ed 5, St. Louis, 2008, Mosby.

Chang M, Kelly AF: Patient education: addressing cultural diversity and health literacy issues, *Urol Nurs* 27(5):411, 2007.

Corvo K, Peterson J: Post-traumatic stress symptoms, language acquisition, and self-sufficiency: a study of Bosnian refugees, *J Soc Work* 5(2):205, 2005.

Cutilli CC: Do your patients understand? Determining your patients' health literacy skills, *Orthop Nurs* 24(5):372, 2005.

Das J and others: Mental health and poverty in developing countries: revisiting the relationship, *Soc Sci Med* 65(3):467, 2007.

Ebersole P and others: *Toward healthy aging*, ed 7, St. Louis, 2008, Mosby.

Edelman CL, Mandle CL: *Health promotion throughout the life span*, ed 6, St. Louis, 2006, Mosby.

Erlen JA: Functional health illiteracy: ethical concerns, *Orthop Nurs* 23(2):150, 2004.

Felder R: *Learning styles*, 2008, http://www4.ncsu.edu/unity/lockers/users/f/felder/public/Learning_Styles.html.

Flowers DL: Culturally competent nursing care: a challenge for the twenty-first century, *Crit Care Nurse* 24(4):48, 2004.

Hatcher E, Whittemore R: Hispanic adults' beliefs about type 2 diabetes: clinical implications, *J Am Acad Nurse Pract* 19:536, 2007.

Hertel AW and others: The impact of expectations and satisfaction on the initiation and maintenance of smoking cessation: an experimental test, *Health Psychol* 27(3):S197, 2008.

Hoffman T, McKenna K: Analysis of stroke patients' and carers' reading ability and the content and design of written materials: recommendations for improving written stroke information, *Patient Educ Couns* 60(3):286, 2006.

Institute of Medicine: *Health literacy: a prescription to end confusion*, 2004, http://www.iom.edu/CMS/3775/3827/19723.aspx.

Jonsdottir H and others: Multicomponent individualized smoking cessation intervention for patients with lung disease, *J Adv Nurs* 48(6):594, 2004.

Jonsson IM and others: Choice of food and food traditions in pre-war Bosnia-Herzegovina: focus group interviews with immigrant women in Sweden, *Ethn Health* 7(3):149, 2002.

Kendig S: Word power: the effect of literacy on health outcomes, *AWHONN Lifelines* 10(4):327, 2006.

Kerr S and others: Smoking after the age of 65 years: a qualitative exploration of older current and former smokers' views on smoking, stopping smoking, and smoking cessation resources and services, *Health Soc Care Community* 14(6):572, 2006.

Koniak-Griffin D and others: HIV prevention for Latino adolescent mothers and their partners *West J Nurs Res* 30(6):724, 2008.

Kutner M and others: *The health literacy of America's adults: results from the 2003 National Assessment of Adult Literacy* (NCES 2006-483), Washington, DC, 2006, US Department of Education, National Center for Education Statistics, http://nces.ed.gov/pubsearch/pubsinfo.asp?pubid52006483.

Lancaster T, Stead LF: Self-help interventions for smoking cessation, *Cochrane Database Syst Rev* 2005(3):CD001118.

Li WW, Stotts NA, Froelicher ES: Compliance with antihypertensive medication in Chinese immigrants: cultural specific issues and theoretical application, *Res Theory Nurs Pract* 21(4):236, 2007.

Lipson JG and others: Bosnian and Soviet refugees' experiences with health care, *West J Nurs Res* 25(7):854, 2003.

Lubkin IM, Larsen PD: *Chronic illness: impact and interventions*, ed 7, Sudbury, Mass, 2009, Jones & Bartlett.

MapZones: *Bosnia Herzegovina: culture*, 2008, http://www.mapzones.com/world/europe/bosnia_hercegovina/cultureindex.php.

Matsuyama RK and others: Cultural perceptions in cancer care among African American and Caucasian patients, *J Natl Med Assoc* 99(10):1113, 2007.

Moorhead S and others editors: *Nursing outcomes classification (NOC)*, ed 4, St. Louis, 2008, Mosby.

Mukeshimana C: Health assessment of Bosnian refugees in Black Hawk County, Iowa, *Int J Global Health* 1(2):24, 2001.

Redman BK: *The practice of patient education*, ed 10, St. Louis, 2007, Mosby.

Rice VH, Stead LF: Nursing interventions for smoking cessation, *Cochrane Database Syst Rev* 2008(1):CD001188.

Ruppar TM, Conn VS, Russell CL: Medication adherence interventions for older adults: literature review, *Res Theory Nurs Pract* 22(2):114, 2008.

Sand-Jecklin K: The impact of medical terminology on readability of patient education materials, *J Community Health Nurs* 24(7):119, 2007.

Schaefer CT: Integrated review of health literacy interventions, *Orthop Nurs* 27(5):302, 2008.

Shieh C, Hosei B: Printed health information materials: evaluation of readability and suitability, *J Community Health Nurs* 25(2):73, 2008.

Snyder CS and others: Social work with Bosnian Muslim refugee children and families: a review of the literature, *Child Welfare* 84(5):607, 2005.

Speros C: Health literacy: concept analysis, *J Adv Nurs* 50(6):633, 2005.

Stephenson PL: Before the teaching begins: managing patient anxiety prior to providing education, *Clin J Oncol Nurs* 10(2):241, 2006.

The Joint Commission: *"What did the doctor say?"* Improving health literacy to protect patient safety, 2007, http://www.jointcommission.org/NR/rdonlyres/D5248B2E-E7E6-4121-8874-99C7B4888301/0/improving_health_literacy.pdf.

The Joint Commission: *Speak up initiatives*, 2008a, http://www.jointcommission.org/PatientSafety/SpeakUp/.

The Joint Commission: *2009 National patient safety goals*, 2008b, http://www.jointcommission.org/PatientSafety/NationalPatientSafetyGoals/.

Wingard R: Patient education and the nursing process: meeting the patient's needs, *Nephrol Nurs J* 32(2):211, 2005.

Managing Patient Care

MEDIA RESOURCES

 CD COMPANION 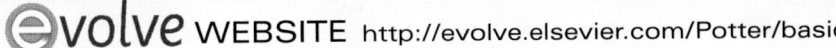 WEBSITE http://evolve.elsevier.com/Potter/basic

- Crossword Puzzle
- English/Spanish Audio Glossary

OBJECTIVES

- Discuss the importance of education in professional nursing practice.
- Describe the purpose of professional standards of nursing practice.
- Differentiate among the types of nursing care delivery models.
- Describe the elements of decentralized decision making.

- Discuss the ways in which a nurse manager supports staff involvement in a decentralized decision-making model.
- Discuss ways to apply clinical care coordination skills in nursing practice.
- Discuss principles to follow in the appropriate delegation of patient care activities.

KEY TERMS

accountability, p. 217
authority, p. 217
code of ethics, p. 211
decentralized management, p. 217

delegation, p. 212
functional nursing, p. 215
licensed practical nurse (LPN), p. 210

licensed vocational nurse (LVN), p. 210
primary nursing, p. 216
registered nurse (RN), p. 211

responsibility, p. 217
team nursing, p. 216
total patient care, p. 216

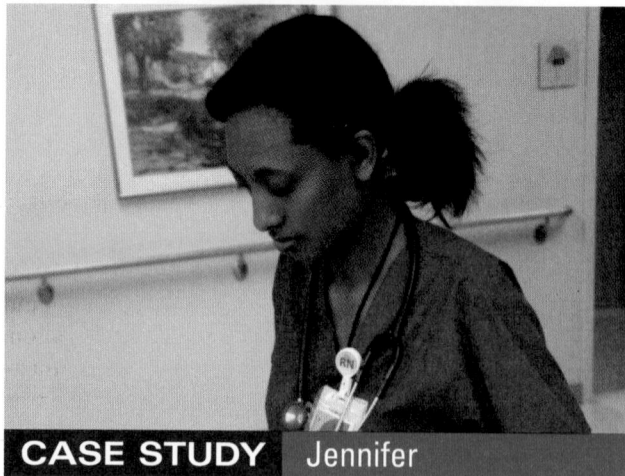

CASE STUDY   Jennifer

Jennifer is a nursing student assigned to care for three patients as part of her final clinical experience. Her first patient is Mrs. Sinclair, who will have surgery at 1 PM to repair her fractured right hip. It is the first time she has had surgery. It is now 11:30 AM. The operating room (OR) has notified Jennifer that OR staff will pick up Mrs. Sinclair in 30 minutes. Jennifer enters Mrs. Sinclair's room to complete the preoperative checklist and to make final preparations for surgery. She finds Mrs. Sinclair moving about restlessly in bed and reluctant to talk. At the same time, the call light system at the bedside comes on and the unit clerk notifies Jennifer that her second patient, Mr. Timmons, has finished his lunch and is ready for his pain medication so he can ambulate down the hall. Mr. Timmons had abdominal surgery 2 days ago for removal of a colon tumor. Her third patient, Mr. Dodson, has a postoperative wound infection. He is due for his next dose of antibiotic medication. Jennifer also recognizes that his wet-to-dry abdominal dressing is due to be changed.

As a nursing student, it is important for you to acquire the necessary knowledge and competencies that ultimately allow you to practice as an entry-level nurse (Box 12-1). Regardless of the type of setting you eventually choose to work in as a nurse, you will be responsible for practicing professional standards of care, using organizational resources, and participating in organizational routines. While doing this you will provide direct patient care, use your time productively, collaborate with all members of the health care team, and use certain leadership characteristics to manage others on the nursing team (Wywialowski, 2004). The delivery of nursing care within the health care system is a challenge because of the changes that are influencing health professionals, patients, and health care organizations (see Chapter 2). However, change offers opportunities. As you develop the knowledge and skills to become a nurse, you will learn what it takes to effectively manage the patients you care for and to take the initiative in becoming a leader among your professional colleagues.

BOX 12-1   Entry-Level Staff Nurse Competencies

- Develop a knowledge base relevant to nursing practice.
- Include a code of conduct in practice that commits the nurse to provide care based on assessed patient needs.
- Use the nursing process to make clinical decisions.
- View patients holistically.
- Use oral and written communication skills effectively in interactions with patients, families, nursing staff, and interdisciplinary groups.
- Exhibit a sense of professionalism.
- Accept responsibility to follow an ethical code of conduct.
- Show self-respect and respect for others.
- Interpret legal issues involved in health care.
- Comply with state licensure laws and nurse practice acts, American Nurses Association standards of practice, and institutional policies and procedures.
- Defend one's own decisions.
- Participate in life-long learning to remain competent in a changing practice environment.
- Serve as a role model.
- Show accountability for own nursing actions.
- Delegate care activities appropriately.

Modified from Wywialowski EF: *Managing client care,* ed 3, St. Louis, 2004, Mosby.

PROFESSIONALISM

Nursing is a profession. A person who acts professionally is conscientious in actions, knowledgeable in the subject, and responsible to self and others. Professions possess the following characteristics:

- An extended education of members and a basic liberal education foundation
- A theoretical body of knowledge leading to defined skills, abilities, and norms
- Provision of a specific service
- Autonomy in decision making and practice
- A code of ethics for practice

Nursing shares each of these characteristics, offering an opportunity for the growth and enrichment of all of its members.

Licensed Practical Nurse/Licensed Vocational Nurse Education

A licensed practical or vocational nurse is educated in basic nursing techniques and direct patient care. The **licensed practical nurse (LPN)** or **licensed vocational nurse (LVN)** is a nurse who has completed a practical nursing program and passed a licensure examination (NCLEX-PN®). The LPN/LVN practices under the supervision of a registered nurse

(RN) or other licensed person. The responsibilities and scope of practice are set by each state board of nursing. An LPN/LVN, or in Canada a registered nurse's assistant (RNA), generally receives 1 year of education and clinical preparation in a community college or other agency. There are some RN programs that allow an LPN to enter the program at an advanced level.

Registered Nurse Education

As a profession, nursing requires that its members possess a significant amount of education. There are various educational routes for becoming a **registered nurse (RN).** Currently in the United States an individual becomes an RN by completion of an associate degree, diploma, or baccalaureate degree program in nursing. In Canada there are currently only diploma and baccalaureate degrees. The Canadian Nurses Association (2004) has identified the baccalaureate degree as the entry to practice standard for RNs. Nursing education provides the solid foundation for practice, and it responds to changes in health care created by scientific and technological advances.

After completion of the professional education program, RN candidates in the United States must pass the National Council Licensure Examination for Registered Nurses (NCLEX-RN), which the individual state boards of nursing administer. Regardless of candidates' educational preparation, the examination for RN licensure is the same in every state, ensuring a standardized minimum knowledge base for the patient population nurses serve. In all Canadian provinces except Quebec, new graduates must pass the Canadian Registered Nurse Examination (CRNE) to become an RN. Whether nurses are able to practice in a state or province other than their own depends on the agreement between the states or provinces involved.

The opportunities in the nursing profession are limitless, but often they require a professional nurse to pursue additional education. A nurse has the opportunity to choose to work toward certification in a specific area of clinical nursing practice. Minimum practice requirements are set based on the certification the nurse is seeking, such as in critical care, oncology, or gerontology. National nursing organizations, such as the American Nurses Association (ANA), have many types of certifications for nurses to work toward. After passing the initial examination, the nurse maintains certification by ongoing continuing education and clinical practice.

Advanced Education

There are roles for registered nurses in nursing that require advanced educational degrees. A master's degree in nursing (e.g., master of arts in nursing [MA], master of nursing [MN], or master of science in nursing [MSN]) is for RNs with a bachelor of science in nursing (BSN) seeking roles as nurse educator, clinical nurse specialist, nurse administrator, or nurse practitioner. The degree provides the advanced clinician with strong skills in nursing science and theory with emphasis in the basic sciences and research-based clinical practice related to a specialty. There are also roles within nursing that require doctoral degrees. There are two doctorate degree options for nurses. The doctor of philosophy (PhD) has a focus on research, and the doctor of nursing practice (DNP) has a focus on advanced clinical practice. Expanding clinical and research roles, new areas of nursing, such as nursing informatics, and the influential presence of nursing in public policy and health care planning are just a few reasons for increasing the number of nurses with doctoral degrees. The health care industry needs nurses prepared at the doctorate level to educate nursing students and those seeking advanced academic and clinical preparation. Nurses with doctorates advance the profession by conducting and disseminating research and developing and testing theory.

Theory

The practice of professional nursing and nursing knowledge have been developed in part through nursing theories, global views that help to describe, predict, or prescribe activities for the practice of nursing. Theoretical models provide frameworks for how nurses practice. Typically a nursing school's curriculum integrates a theoretical model. Examples of theories used in education and practice are Orem's self-care deficit theory, Benner's primacy of caring, and Roy's adaptation theory. There are also nursing organizations that adopt a nursing theory as the foundation for the organization's standards of nursing care. The ongoing development of nursing theory or nursing science involves generating knowledge to advance and support nursing practice and health care (Alligood and Marriner Tomey, 2006).

Service

Nursing is a service profession and a vital and indispensable part of the health care delivery system. Nurses in practice today maintain a consumer and service-based focus. Patients are more aware and knowledgeable about their health care problems, their options, and their rights. As a nurse you will work with the patient and family, individualizing care while incorporating their preferences and expectations. Show respect for patients by providing care on time, displaying a caring attitude, and considering patients' cultural and social differences. Collaborating with necessary health care providers ensures a smooth continuation of care from one setting to the next.

Autonomy

Autonomy is essential to professional nursing. Autonomy means that a person is reasonably independent and self-governing in decision making and practice. You reach autonomy through experience, advanced education, and the support of an organization that values the independent role of the nurse. With increased autonomy comes greater responsibility and accountability for the performance of nursing care activities.

Code of Ethics

Nursing has a **code of ethics** that defines the principles by which nurses function (see Chapter 5). In addition, nurses incorporate their own values and ethics into practice. The

ANA's *Code of Ethics for Nurses With Interpretive Statements* (2001) provides a guide for carrying out nursing responsibilities to ensure high-quality nursing care and to provide for the ethical obligations of the profession.

STANDARDS OF NURSING PRACTICE

Nursing is a helping, independent profession that provides services that contribute to the health of people. Three essential components of professional nursing are care, cure, and coordination. The *care* aspect is more than "to take care of"; it is also "caring about." Caring is relational and requires you as a nurse to understand the patient's needs so you can individualize nursing therapies (see Chapter 18). When you promote health and healing, you are practicing the *cure* aspect of professional nursing. To cure is to assist patients in under-

standing their health problems and to help them to cope. The cure aspect involves the administration of treatments and the use of clinical nursing judgment in determining, on the basis of patient outcomes, whether the plan of care is effective. *Coordination* of care involves organizing and timing medical and other professional and technical services to meet the holistic needs of a patient. Often a patient requires many services simultaneously for care to be effective. A professional nurse also supervises, teaches, and directs all of those involved in nursing care.

As an independent profession, nursing has increasingly set its own standards for practice. These standards are guidelines for how nurses perform professionally and how they exercise the care, cure, and coordination aspects of nursing. Clinical, academic, and administrative nurse experts have developed standards of nursing practice. As an example, the ANA has published *Nursing: Scope and Standards of Practice* (2004). Within this document are Standards of Professional Performance (Table 12-1) and Standards of Practice (Table 12-2).

TABLE 12-1 ANA Standards of Professional Performance

STANDARD	DEFINITION	MEASUREMENT CRITERIA*
7: Quality of practice	The registered nurse systematically enhances the quality and effectiveness of nursing practice.	Participates in quality improvement activities Practice changes are a result of quality-of-care activities Uses quality improvement activities to initiate changes in nursing practice and the health care delivery system Uses creativity and innovation in nursing practice to improve care delivery
8: Education	The registered nurse attains knowledge and competency that reflects current nursing practice.	Participates in ongoing educational activities related to appropriate knowledge bases and professional issues Demonstrates commitment to lifelong learning Seeks experiences to maintain clinical skills Seeks knowledge and skills appropriate to the practice setting
9: Professional practice evaluation	The registered nurse evaluates one's own nursing practice in relation to professional practice standards and guidelines, relevant statutes, rules, and regulations.	Engages in self-evaluation on a regular basis Seeks constructive feedback regarding one's own practice Takes action to achieve goals identified during the evaluation process Participates in systematic peer review as appropriate Practice reflects knowledge of current professional practice standards, laws, and regulations Provides age-appropriate care in culturally and ethnically sensitive manner
10: Collegiality	The registered nurse interacts with and contributes to the professional development of peers and colleagues.	Shares knowledge and skills with peers and colleagues Provides peers with feedback regarding their practice Interacts with peers and colleagues to enhance one's own professional nursing practice Maintains compassionate and caring relationships with peers and colleagues Contributes to an environment that is conducive to the education of health care professionals Contributes to a supportive and healthy work environment

Modified from American Nurses Association: *Nursing: scope and standards of practice*, Washington, DC, 2004, The Association.
ANA, American Nurses Association.
*For a complete list of measurement criteria, consult *Nursing: scope and standards of practice.*

TABLE 12-1	ANA Standards of Professional Performance—cont'd	
STANDARD	DEFINITION	MEASUREMENT CRITERIA*
11: Collaboration	The registered nurse collaborates with patient, family, and others in the conduct of nursing practice.	Communicates with the patient, family, and health care providers regarding patient care and the nurse's role in the provision of care Collaborates with the patient, family, and other health care providers in the formulation of overall goals and the plan of care and in the decisions related to care and delivery of services Partners with others to effect change and generate positive outcomes Documents referrals, including provisions for continuity of care
12: Ethics	The registered nurse integrates ethical provisions in all areas of practice.	Practice is guided by the *Code of Ethics for Nurses With Interpretive Statements* Maintains patient confidentiality Serves as a patient advocate Maintains therapeutic and professional patient-nurse relationship Delivers care in a manner that preserves patient autonomy, dignity, and rights Seeks available resources in formulating ethical decisions Reports illegal, incompetent, or impaired practices

13: Research	The registered nurse integrates research findings into practice.	Utilizes best available evidence including research findings to guide practice decisions
		Participates in research activities as appropriate to the nurse's education and position, such as the following:
		  Identifying clinical problems suitable for nursing research
		  Participating in data collection
		  Participating in a formal committee or program
		  Sharing research activities with others
		  Conducting research
		  Critiquing research for application to practice
		  Uses research findings in the development of policies, procedures, and practice guidelines for patient care
		  Incorporates research as a basis for learning

14: Resource utilization	The registered nurse considers factors related to safety, effectiveness, cost, and impact on practice in the planning and delivery of nursing services.	Evaluates factors related to safety, effectiveness, availability, and cost when practice options would result in the same expected patient outcome Assists the patient and family in identifying and securing appropriate and available services to address health-related needs Assigns or delegates tasks based on the needs and condition of the patient, the potential for harm, the stability of the patient's condition, the complexity of the task, and the predictability of the outcome Assists the patient and family in becoming informed consumers about the cost, risks, and benefits of treatment and care
15: Leadership	The registered nurse provides leadership in the professional practice setting and the profession.	Engages in teamwork Works to create and maintain healthy work environments Teaches others to succeed by mentoring and other strategies Exhibits creativity and flexibility during change Directs coordination of care across settings and caregivers Serves in key roles in the work setting Promotes advancement of the profession

TABLE 12-2   ANA Standards of Practice

STANDARD	MEASUREMENT CRITERIA
1. ASSESSMENT The registered nurse collects comprehensive data pertinent to the patient's health or the situation.	Data collection involves the patient, significant others, and health care providers, when appropriate. The patient's immediate condition or needs determine the priority of data collection. Collects pertinent data using appropriate assessment techniques. Documents relevant data in a retrievable form. Collects data in a systematic and ongoing process.
2. DIAGNOSIS The registered nurse analyzes the assessment data to determine the diagnoses or issues.	Derives the diagnoses or issues from the assessment data. Validates the diagnoses with the patient, family, and other health care providers, when possible and appropriate. Documents diagnoses in a manner that facilitates the determination of expected outcomes and plan of care.
3. OUTCOMES IDENTIFICATION The registered nurse identifies expected outcomes for a plan individualized to the patient or the situation.	Derives outcomes from the diagnoses. Formulates outcomes mutually with the patient and health care providers, when possible. Outcomes are culturally appropriate and realistic in relation to the patient's present and potential capabilities. Outcomes are attainable in relation to resources available to the patient. Includes a time estimate for attainment of expected outcomes. Outcomes provide direction for continuity of care. Documents expected outcomes as measurable goals.
4. PLANNING The registered nurse develops a plan that prescribes strategies and alternatives to attain expected outcomes.	The plan is individualized to the patient and patient's condition or needs. Develops the plan with the patient, significant others, and health care providers, when appropriate. The plan reflects current nursing practice. Provides for continuity within the plan. Considers economic impact of the plan. Establishes the plan priorities. Documents the plan.
5. IMPLEMENTATION The registered nurse implements the identified plan.	Utilizes evidence-based interventions and treatments specific to the diagnosis or problem. Implements the plan in a safe and timely manner. Documents implementation and any modifications. Collaborates with nursing colleagues to implement the plan. Utilizes community resources and systems to implement the plan.
6. EVALUATION The registered nurse evaluates progress toward attainment of outcomes.	Evaluation is systematic, ongoing, and criterion-based. Involves the patient and others involved in the care or situation in the evaluative process. Uses ongoing assessment data to revise diagnoses, outcomes, the plan, and the implementation as needed. Documents revisions in diagnoses, outcomes, and the plan of care. Evaluates the effectiveness of interventions in relation to outcomes. Documents the results of the evaluation.

Modified from American Nurses Association: *Nursing: scope and standards of practice,* Washington, DC, 2004, The Association.
ANA, American Nurses Association.

Standards of Care

In the practice setting it is important to have objective guidelines for providing and evaluating nursing care. Standards of nursing care are developed and established on the basis of strong scientific research and the work of clinical nurse experts. The purpose of a standard of care is to describe the common level of professional nursing care in order to judge the quality of nursing practice (Thompson and others, 2007). An organization sometimes adopts a general set of standards for nursing care, such as organizational protocols, policies, or procedures. For example, an organization has a written nasogastric tube protocol based on research findings. This protocol spells out the expected nursing care for patients with nasogastric tubes in that organization. Individual nursing units or work groups also establish standards of care to address the unique needs of patients for whom they care. For example, an oncology nursing unit develops standards of care for pain management and palliative care for patients with cancer. Standards of care are important if a legal dispute arises over whether a nurse practiced appropriately in a particular case (see Chapter 4). More important, standards of care establish the guidelines for nursing excellence within an organization.

BUILDING A NURSING TEAM

Nurses want to work within an institutional culture that promotes autonomy and quality (Wywialowski, 2004). Your education and the commitment you make in practicing within established standards and guidelines will ensure a rewarding professional career. It is also important to work as a member of a cohesive and strong nursing team that values mentoring, integrity, and respect for teamwork. An empowering work environment brings out the best in a professional. It concentrates on effective patient care systems (e.g., patient assessment, referral mechanisms, and collaboration between nurses and health care providers), supports risk taking and innovation, focuses on results and rewards, and offers professional opportunities for growth and advancement. Effective team development requires team building, respectful negotiation, conflict management, and a workplace that facilitates collaboration (Lindeke and Sieckert, 2005).

One way of creating an empowering work environment is through the Magnet Recognition Program. The American Nurses Credentialing Center developed the Magnet Recognition Program in the early 1990s. The Magnet Recognition Program recognizes nursing services that build programs of excellence for the delivery of nursing care, promote quality in environments that support professional nursing practice, and promote achievement of positive patient outcomes (American Nurses Credentialing Center, 2008). A Magnet hospital has a culture that is dynamic and positive for nurses. Typically a Magnet hospital has a system to recognize and reward nurses for clinical performance, has research programs, and uses evidence-based practice. The nurses have professional autonomy over their practice and control over the practice environment (Wolf, Triolo, and Reid Ponte, 2008). A Magnet hospital empowers the nursing team to make changes and be innovative. This culture produces a strong collaborative relationship among team members and improves patient quality outcomes (see Chapter 2).

The Institute of Medicine (IOM) (2004) called for health care to transform the work environment to focus on keeping patients safe. Nurses, because of their focus on patient assessment and evaluation, are key team members to participate in transforming the health care environment. As a part of this transformation, the IOM (2001) called for all health care professionals to be educated to deliver patient-centered care using evidence-based practice, quality improvement approaches, and informatics. Nurses need to deliver safe, effective quality patient care through collaboration as a member of an interdisciplinary team (IOM, 2001).

It takes an excellent nurse manager and an excellent nursing staff to achieve an enriching work culture and environment. Together a manager and the nursing staff share a philosophy of care for their work unit. A philosophy of care incorporates the professional nursing staff's values and concerns for the way that they view and care for patients. For example, a philosophy addresses the nursing unit's purpose, how staff will work with patients and families, and the standards of care for the work unit. A philosophy is a vision for how to practice nursing. Integral to the philosophy of care is the selection of a nursing care delivery model and management structure that support professional nursing practice.

Nursing Care Delivery Models

A nursing care delivery model allows you as a nurse to help your patients achieve desirable outcomes. Economic issues, political issues, the focus on quality and patient satisfaction, and the social environment have contributed to the development of models of nursing care delivery (Tiedeman and Lookinland, 2004). There are a variety of nursing care delivery models. Team nursing, primary nursing, and total patient care models are most common in acute care settings. Case management and primary nursing are the common nursing care delivery models used in the home care setting.

FUNCTIONAL NURSING **Functional nursing** is a model of care that evolved in the 1940s and is task focused, not patient focused. In this model different tasks are divided into functional categories, with one nurse assuming responsibility for specific tasks. For example, one nurse does the hygiene and dressing changes, whereas another nurse assumes responsibility for medication administration. Typically a lead nurse responsible for a specific shift assigns available nursing staff members according to their qualifications, their particular abilities, and tasks to be completed. Nurses become highly competent with tasks that are repeatedly assigned to them. The major disadvantages of functional nursing are problems with continuity of care, fragmentation of care, absence of a holistic view of patients, and the possibility that care will become mechanical (Tiedeman and Lookinland, 2004). In other words, a task-focused approach does not ensure that patient care needs are met shift to shift. Communication is not always clear, because a single nurse is not responsible for the overall care of the patient. This model places more emphasis on nurses' following rules, regulations, and policies and does not promote nurses' decision making, autonomy, or professional development.

TEAM NURSING Team nursing was developed during the 1950s. In **team nursing** an RN leads a team composed of other RNs, LPN/LVNs, and nursing assistive personnel or technicians. The team members provide direct patient care to groups of patients, under the direction of the RN team leader. In this model the RN gives the nurse assistants patient assignments rather than assigning particular nursing tasks. The team leader provides strong leadership and communicates clearly (Tiedeman and Lookinland, 2004). When team nursing is used, there are generally fewer RNs than LPN/LVNs and other staff.

The team leader develops patient care plans and coordinates care delivered by the nursing team. The team leader also provides care requiring complex nursing skills, problem solves with physicians and members of other disciplines, and assists the team in evaluating the effectiveness of their care (Wywialowski, 2004). Limitations to the model include the task orientation of the model, which leads to fragmentation of patient care, and the lack of time the team leader spends with patients. Depending on the mix of staff members, this sometimes means that patients see an RN infrequently. Risks exist if an RN is unable to do necessary patient assessments and be involved in important clinical decision making. Nurses are not always assigned to the same patients each day, which potentially causes lack of continuity of care. Another disadvantage is that the model is expensive because of the increased number of personnel needed (Tiedeman and Lookinland, 2004). An advantage of team nursing is the collaborative style that encourages each member of the team to help the other members.

TOTAL PATIENT CARE **Total patient care** was the original care delivery model developed during Florence Nightingale's time. The model disappeared in the 1930s but gained popularity again in the 1980s (Tiedeman and Lookinland, 2004). An RN is responsible for all aspects of care for one or more patients during an assigned shift. The RN delegates aspects of care to an LPN or nursing assistive personnel but is accountable for care of all assigned patients. The nurse works directly with the patient, family, health care provider, and health care team members. The model has a shift-based focus. The same nurse does not necessarily care for the same patient over successive days or visits. Continuity and coordination of care from shift to shift or day to day is a problem if staff members do not clearly communicate patient needs to one another. Patient satisfaction with this model tends to be high, but the model is not cost-effective because it requires a high number of RNs to deliver care (Tiedeman and Lookinland, 2004).

PRIMARY NURSING The **primary nursing** model of care delivery was developed in the 1960s with the aim of placing RNs at the bedside and improving the professional relationships among staff members (Tiedeman and Lookinland,

2004). The model became more popular in the 1970s and early 1980s as hospitals began to employ more RNs. Primary nursing supports a philosophy regarding nurse and patient relationships. Primary nursing is a model of care delivery whereby an RN assumes responsibility for a caseload of patients over time (e.g., a length of stay in a hospital or a series of home care visits). Typically the RN selects the patients for his or her caseload and cares for the same patients during their hospitalization or stay in the health care setting. The RN assesses patient needs, develops a care plan, and ensures that the designated caregiver delivers the appropriate nursing interventions to the patient.

Primary nursing maintains continuity of care across shifts, days, or visits. The model increases nursing autonomy and improves collaboration between nurses and health care providers. It is applied in any health care setting. When a primary nurse is off-duty, associate nurses, including LPN/LVNs or other RNs, follow through with the developed plan of care. If there are differences in opinion as to patient needs, associates and primary nurses collaborate to redefine the plan as needed.

Although primary nursing requires the presence of more professional staff members, this does not mean that the model is more costly. Care consistently managed by a single professional minimizes delays in therapies, improves collaboration with other professionals, and improves the patient-nurse relationship.

CASE MANAGEMENT Case management is a delivery of care approach that emerged in the 1980s as health care institutions needed to provide complex cost-effective care. Case management coordinates and links health care services to patients and their families (see Chapter 2). Case management requires an RN to maintain responsibility for patient care from admission to after discharge (Wywialowski, 2004). What is unique about case management is that clinicians, either as individuals or as part of a collaborative group, oversee the management of patients with specific case types, focusing on length of stay and improving clinical outcomes (e.g., patients with specific diagnoses presenting complex nursing and medical problems) (Thomas, 2008). They are usually held accountable for some standard of cost management and quality. A case manager coordinates a patient's acute care in the hospital, for example, and then follows the patient after discharge home. For example, the case manager calls a meeting of the patient, family, social services, dietitian, and physical therapist to plan the discharge of a patient following a stroke. Case managers do not always provide direct care. Instead, they collaborate with and supervise the care other staff members deliver and actively coordinate patient discharge planning. Many organizations use critical pathways, which are multidisciplinary treatment plans, in a case management delivery system as a mechanism to improve patient and institutional outcomes (Thomas, 2008) (see Chapter 2). Advantages of case management include cost-effectiveness, focus on patients' complex health needs, efficiency in planning discharge, and multidisciplinary collaboration (Wywialowski, 2004).

Decentralized Decision Making

Decentralized management, in which decision making is made at the staff level, is very common within health care organizations. It is clear that progressive health care organizations achieve more when they actively involve employees at all levels. Advantages of decentralization include increased morale and improved interpersonal relationships among staff. Staff members feel more important and are more willing to contribute. Decentralization also promotes creativity in problem solving (Marriner Tomey, 2009). As a result, the role of a nurse manager has become critical in the management of effective nursing units or groups. Box 12-2 highlights the diverse responsibilities assumed by nursing managers. To make decentralized decision making work, managers need to move decision making down to the staff level. On a nursing unit, it is important for all staff members (RNs, LPNs, and LVNs), nursing assistive personnel, and unit secretaries to feel involved, particularly with issues affecting their ability to care for patients. Key elements of the decentralized decision making are responsibility, authority, and accountability (Marriner Tomey, 2009).

Responsibility refers to the duties and activities that an individual is employed to perform. For professional nurses, a position description outlines the nurse's responsibilities in patient care and in level of participation as a member of the nursing unit. Responsibility reflects ownership and obligation; the individual who oversees the employee gives responsibility, and the employee accepts it. For example, a primary

nurse is responsible for completing a nursing assessment of all assigned patients and for developing a plan of care that addresses each of the patient's nursing diagnoses. The nurse is also responsible for making sure that other staff members know what care they are responsible for performing. As the staff delivers the plan of care, the primary nurse is responsible for evaluating whether the plan is successful and what to do when it is not successful. This responsibility becomes a work ethic for the nurse in delivering excellent patient care.

Authority refers to the official power to act in areas in which an individual has been given and accepts responsibility (Marriner Tomey, 2009). It provides the nurse power to make final decisions and give instructions related to the decisions. For example, a primary nurse, managing a caseload of patients, discovers that members of the nursing team did not follow through on a discharge teaching plan for an assigned patient. The primary nurse has the authority to consult other nurses to learn why they did not follow recommendations on the plan of care and to choose appropriate teaching strategies for the patient that all members of the team will follow. The primary nurse has the final authority in selecting the best course of action for the patient's care.

Accountability refers to liability or individuals being answerable for their actions. It involves follow-up and a reflective analysis of your decisions to evaluate their effectiveness. A primary nurse delegates responsibility but is accountable for his or her patients' outcomes (Marriner Tomey, 2009). As an example, a primary nurse is accountable for ensuring that a patient learns the information necessary to improve self-care. By using authority in bringing the nursing team together, the primary nurse determines if collaboration was successful, if continuity in teaching occurred, and if the patient and family understood the information.

A successful decentralized nursing unit exercises these three elements on an ongoing basis. An effective manager sets the same expectations for the staff in how to make decisions. Staff members must feel comfortable in expressing differences of opinion and in challenging ways in which the team functions. Staff members do this while recognizing their own responsibility, authority, and accountability. Ultimately, decentralized decision making allows a nursing unit to achieve its vision of what professional nursing care should be.

STAFF INVOLVEMENT With decentralized decision making on a nursing unit, all staff members actively participate in unit activities (Figure 12-1). Because the work environment promotes participation, all staff members benefit from the knowledge and skills of the entire work group. If the staff members learn to value knowledge and the contributions of colleagues, better patient care will be an outcome. The nursing manager supports staff involvement through a variety of ways:

1. *Establishment of nursing practice or problem-solving committees:* Staff committees establish and maintain professional nursing practice on a unit. Practice committees become involved in activities such as the review and revision of standards of care, development of policy and pro-

---

BOX 12-2 Responsibilities of the Nurse Manager

- Assist staff in establishing yearly goals for the unit and the systems needed to accomplish goals.
- Monitor professional nursing standards of practice on the unit.
- Develop an ongoing staff development plan, including one for new employees.
- Recruit new employees (interview and hire).
- Conduct routine staff evaluations.
- Establish self as a role model for positive customer service (customers include patients, families, and other health care team members).
- Serve as an advocate for the nursing staff to the administration of the institution.
- Submit staffing schedules for the unit.
- Conduct regular patient rounds and help to solve patient or family complaints.
- Establish and implement a quality improvement (QI) plan for the unit.
- Review and recommend new equipment needs for the unit.
- Conduct regular staff meetings.
- Conduct rounds with health care provider.
- Establish and support necessary staff and interdisciplinary committees.

cedure, and resolution of repeated patient satisfaction issues. These activities ensure the delivery of quality care on the unit. A senior staff member usually chairs a committee. Managers do not always sit on the committee, but they receive regular reports of committee progress. The nature of work on the nursing unit determines committee membership. At times, members of other disciplines, for example, pharmacy, respiratory therapy, or clinical nutrition, participate on practice committees.

2. *Encouraging collaboration between nurses and health care providers:* The collaboration between nurses and health

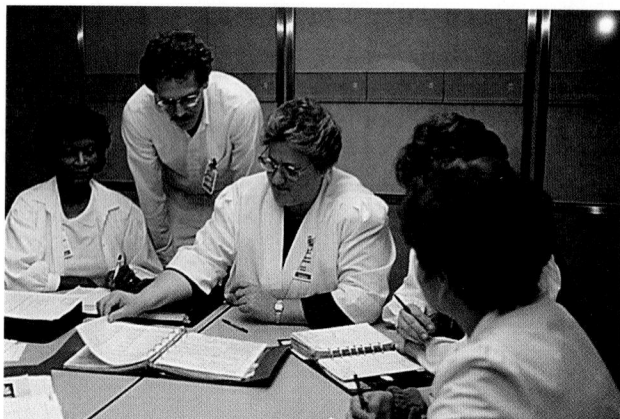

Figure 12-1 ■ Nursing staff collaborating on practice issues.

care providers is influenced by the unit's delivery of care model. If the unit practices team nursing, it is important for team leaders to regularly participate in rounds with the patient's health care providers. If the unit practices primary nursing, the health care provider communicates either with each primary nurse or the associate nurse who is assuming care for the patient on that day. The manager avoids taking care of problems for the staff. Instead, staff members learn to keep health care providers informed on important information about their patients. Open communication, trust, and mutual respect are critical for successful nurse-physician collaboration (Lindeke and Sieckert, 2005) (Box 12-3).

3. *Interdisciplinary collaboration:* The emphasis on efficiency in health care delivery brings all members of the health care team together. The staff recognizes the importance of prompt referrals and timely communication. Interdisciplinary collaboration involves bringing representatives of the various disciplines together in practice projects, in-services, conferences, and staff meetings. This brings different points of view to the table to identify, clarify, and solve complex patient problems (Gardner, 2005). When all members of the interdisciplinary team are interested, collaboration is an effective strategy to manage conflict (Arford, 2005; Seago, 2008).

4. *Staff communication:* In the present health care environment, it is difficult for a manager to get a clear, accurate, and timely message to all members of a nursing staff.

BOX 12-3 **BEST PRACTICES**

Nurse-Physician Collaboration

SUMMARY OF EVIDENCE

Collaboration comes from the Latin words *col*, meaning with or together, and *laborare*, meaning work (Dougherty and Larson, 2005). In health care, nurse-physician collaboration is a partnership, relationship, or process of ongoing interactions (Schmalenberg and others, 2005; Tschannen, 2004). The health care organization is a key factor in creating an environment and culture that values and promotes collaboration (Tschannen, 2004). There is a positive relationship between the degree of nurse-physician collaboration and positive patient outcomes and satisfaction (Dougherty and Larson, 2005; Seago, 2008). When structured team rounds were conducted on an adult unit, there was an average shortened length of stay, improved staff satisfaction, and increased perception of good communication and teamwork (Zwarenstein and Bryant, 2000). Nurse-physician collaboration has been shown to be an effective communication tool to reduce errors (Dougherty and Larson, 2005; Seago, 2008). The foundation of nurse-physician collaboration is trust, respect, and good communication. This leads to joint decision making and adaptation of care to meet patient needs (Schmalenberg and others, 2005; Zwarenstein and Bryant, 2000).

APPLICATION TO NURSING PRACTICE
- Open communication that focuses on the patient is foundational to the collaborative process.
- Choose an organization whose culture promotes nurse-physician collaboration.
- Promoting an environment of trust and respect fosters the development of collaborative relationships.
- Effective collaboration moves beyond the nurse and physician to include other health care team members.

REFERENCES

Dougherty MB, Larson E: A review of instruments measuring nurse-physician collaboration, *J Nurs Adm* 35(5):224, 2005.
Schmalenberg C and others: Excellence through evidence: securing collegial/collaborative nurse-physician relationships, part I, *J Nurs Adm* 35(10):450, 2005.
Seago JA: Professional communication. In Agency for Healthcare Research and Quality: *Patient safety and quality: an evidence-based handbook for nurses*, AHRQ Pub No. 08-0043, Rockville, Md, 2008, The Agency.
Tschannen D: The effect of individual characteristics on perceptions of collaboration in the work environment, *Medsurg Nurs* 13(15):312, 2004.
Zwarenstein M, Bryant W: Interventions to promote collaboration between nurses and doctors, *Cochrane Database Syst Rev* 2000(2):CD000072, DOI:10.1002/14651858.CD000072.

Staff members may become uneasy and distrusting if they fail to hear about planned changes on their unit. However, a manager does not assume total responsibility for all communication. Instead, the manager establishes a variety of approaches to ensure the quick and accurate communication of information to all staff members. For example, many managers distribute biweekly or monthly newsletters of ongoing unit or health care agency activities. They also post minutes of staff and practice committee meetings in an accessible location for all staff members to read. When the manager needs to discuss important issues regarding the operations of the unit or the organization with the staff, the manager conducts staff meetings. When the unit has practice or quality improvement committees, the manager assigns each member responsibility to communicate directly to a select number of staff members. In that way all staff members are contacted and have the opportunity to comment.

5. *Staff education:* A professional nursing staff always grows in knowledge. It is impossible to remain knowledgeable of current medical and nursing practice trends without ongoing education. The nurse manager is responsible for giving staff members the necessary opportunities to remain competent in their practice. This involves planning in-service training sessions, sending staff members to professional conferences, and having staff members present case studies or practice issues during staff meetings.

Leadership Skills for Nursing Students

As you begin to assume clinical assignments, it is important for you not only to learn how to care for patients but also to become a responsible and productive team member. Start by always being responsible and accountable for the care you provide your patients. Learn to become a leader by making good clinical decisions and by learning from your mistakes. Seek help, collaborate closely with professional nurses, and strive to improve your performance during each patient interaction. Use the following skills to become a competent professional. These skills require you to think critically and solve problems in the clinical setting. Critically thinking allows nurses to provide higher quality care, meet the needs of patients while considering the preferences, consider alternatives to problems, understand the rationale for performing nursing interventions, and evaluate the effectiveness of interventions (Benner, Hughes, and Sutphen, 2008). Clinical experiences help to develop these critical thinking skills (Toofany, 2008).

CLINICAL CARE COORDINATION Learn to acquire the skills necessary to deliver patient care competently and in a timely and effective manner. In the beginning you may care for only one patient, but eventually you will care for groups of patients. Clinical care coordination includes clinical decision making, priority setting, organizational skills, use of resources, time management, and evaluation. These activities of clinical care coordination require use of critical reflection, critical reasoning, and clinical judgment (Benner and others, 2008).

Clinical Decisions When you begin a patient assignment, always conduct a focused but complete assessment of the patient's condition and ask what outcomes the patient expects in his or her care. This will allow you to know the patient so that you understand the patient's situation, helping you to recognize the patient's responses and patterns during care. Your assessment will also direct you in making accurate clinical decisions about your patient's needs (see Chapter 8). Failing to make accurate clinical judgments about a patient has undesirable outcomes. The patient's condition will worsen or remain the same when the potential for improvement is lost. An important lesson in clinical care is being thorough. Always attend to the patient, look for any cues (obvious or subtle) that point to a pattern of findings, and direct your assessment to explore the pattern further. Accurate clinical decision making keeps you focused on the proper course of action. Never hesitate to ask for assistance when a patient's assessment reveals a changing clinical condition.

Priority Setting As you begin to make clinical judgments (including nursing diagnoses), a picture of the patient's total needs begins to form. While planning care, decide what patient needs or problems to address first (see Chapter 8). It is important to prioritize in all caregiving situations because it allows you to see relationships between patient problems and to avoid delays in action (Hendry and Walker, 2004). To make this decision, use Maslow's hierarchy of needs. According to Maslow, meet the patient's physiological needs such as oxygen, food, water, sleep, and elimination first. After meeting the physiological needs, meet the patient's higher-level needs of safety, security, belonging, esteem, and self-actualization (Marriner Tomey, 2009). Hendry and Walker (2004) classify patient problems in three priority levels:

- *High priority:* An immediate threat to a patient's survival or safety, such as a physiological episode of obstructed airway, loss of consciousness, or a psychological episode of an anxiety attack.
- *Intermediate priority:* Nonemergency, non–life-threatening actual or potential needs that the patient and family are experiencing. Anticipating teaching needs of patients related to a new drug or taking measures to decrease postoperative complications are examples of intermediate priorities.
- *Low priority:* Actual or potential problems that may not be directly related to the patient's illness or disease. These problems are often related to the patient's developmental needs and/or long-term health care needs. An example of a low-priority problem is teaching for self-care in the home before discharge of a patient who has just been admitted to the hospital.

Many patients have all three types of priorities, requiring you to make careful judgments in choosing your course of action. Obviously, high-priority needs demand your immediate attention. When a patient has diverse priority needs, sometimes it helps to focus on the patient's basic needs. For example, you have a patient in traction who reports being uncomfortable from being in the same position. The dietary assistant arrives in the room to deliver a meal tray. Instead of immediately assisting the patient with the meal, you reposition the patient and offer basic hygiene measures. The patient will likely become more interested in eating after you make him or her feel comfortable. The patient will also then be more receptive to any instruction you provide.

Over time you will also be required to meet the priority needs of a group of patients. This requires you to know the priority needs of each patient within the group; assess each patient's needs as soon as possible while addressing high and intermediate needs in a timely manner. To identify which patients require assessment first, you rely on information from the change-of-shift report, the agency's classification system that identifies patient acuity, and information from the patient's medical record. Over time you will learn to spontaneously rank patients' needs by priority or urgency. Remember to think about the resources you have available, be flexible in recognizing that priority needs change, and consider how you will use your time wisely. The case study provides an example of how to prioritize your patient care (Box 12-4).

You must also set priorities on the basis of patient expectations. Sometimes you have an excellent plan of care established, but if your patient is resistant to certain therapies or disagrees with your approach, you will gain very little success. Working closely with the patient and family is important.

BOX 12-4   Case Study: Priority Setting—Jennifer

 In setting her priorities, Jennifer remembers the categories of priority needs she learned in school and prioritizes her care according to these. Jennifer asks the unit clerk to send John, another nursing student, to Mr. Timmons' room to check on him and tell him that Jennifer is preparing a patient for surgery and will be with Mr. Timmons as soon as she finishes. Jennifer stays with Mrs. Sinclair and begins an assessment of her to determine the cause of the restlessness. She also asks Mrs. Sinclair if she has any questions or concerns about surgery. Mrs. Sinclair voices her concerns about pain after surgery. Jennifer reinforces the earlier teaching she did on patient-controlled analgesia pumps. This seems to relax Mrs. Sinclair. Jennifer completes her preoperative preparation and checklist. She tells Mrs. Sinclair that the operating room staff will be here in 15 minutes to get her. Jennifer then goes to assess Mr. Timmons' pain. She prepares and administers the prescribed pain medication for Mr. Timmons. Jennifer asks Tina, the nursing assistant, to assist Mr. Timmons with his walk. Jennifer obtains and verifies the antibiotic for Mr. Dodson. On the way to the room, she gathers the supplies for the dressing change. In Mr. Dodson's room, she first verifies Mr. Dodson's identification using two acceptable identifiers and administers the antibiotic. After Mr. Dodson takes his antibiotic, Jennifer sets up and then completes the dressing change. She finishes caring for Mr. Dodson by documenting the care she performed.

Share the priorities you define with the patient to establish a level of agreement and cooperation.

Organizational Skills Implementing a plan of care requires you to be effective and efficient. Effective use of time entails doing the right things, whereas efficient use of time entails doing things right (Wywialowski, 2004). As you address your patient's priorities, certain organizational skills will ensure that you become more efficient. Efficient care conserves effort and minimizes interruptions. One way to be efficient is by combining various nursing activities, in other words, doing more than one thing at a time. This of course takes practice. For example, during medication administration or while obtaining a specimen, combine therapeutic communication skills, teaching interventions, and assessment and evaluation. Always try to establish and strengthen relationships with patients and use any patient contact as an opportunity to teach or give important information. Always attend to the patient's behaviors and responses to therapies to assess if any new problems are developing and to evaluate responses to interventions.

A nursing procedure is easier to perform if you are well organized. Prepare in advance by having all necessary equipment and supplies available and making sure to prepare the patient. Be sure the patient is comfortable, positioned correctly for the procedure, and well informed to increase the likelihood the procedure will go smoothly. Sometimes you will need the assistance of colleagues to perform or complete a procedure (e.g., helping to turn a patient for an enema or handing supplies during a dressing change). It is always wise to have the work area organized and preliminary steps completed before asking colleagues for assistance.

When you try to deliver care based on established priorities, events sometimes occur that interfere with your plans. For example, just as you begin to provide a patient's bath, the x-ray technician enters to obtain a portable chest film. Once the technician completes the x-ray procedure, the phlebotomist arrives to draw a sample of blood. Your priorities seem to conflict with the priorities of other health care personnel. It is important to always keep the patient's needs as the center of attention. The patient experienced symptoms earlier that required a chest film and laboratory work. In such a case it is important to be sure to complete the diagnostic tests. In another example, a patient is waiting to visit family and the chest film was a routine order from 2 days ago. The patient's condition has since stabilized, and the x-ray technician is willing to return later to shoot the film. Attending to the patient's hygiene and comfort so that the family is able to visit is more of a priority at this time.

Use of Resources Another important aspect of clinical care coordination is appropriate use of resources. Resources in this case include members of the health care team. In any setting the administration of patient care occurs more smoothly when staff members work together. As a student, always look for opportunities to help other staff members. For example, answer a call light, help a staff member make a bed, or offer to sit and talk with another nurse's patient. Also, never hesitate to ask staff members to help you, especially when there is the opportunity to make a procedure or activity more comfortable and safer for the patient. For example, assistance in turning, positioning, and ambulating patients is frequently necessary when patients experience impaired mobility. Have a staff member assist with handing you equipment and supplies during a more complicated procedure, such as catheter insertion or a dressing change, to make the procedure more efficient. This is an excellent way for you to learn how to delegate aspects of care activities and to work with nursing assistive personnel.

There are also times when you will recognize personal limitations and use professional resources for assistance. For example, you assess a patient and find relevant clinical signs and symptoms but are unfamiliar with the patient's underlying physical condition. You then consult with an RN who confirms your findings and helps you take the proper course of action for the patient. Throughout your professional career there are always new experiences. A leader knows his or her limitations and seeks professional colleagues for guidance and support.

Time Management. A nurse's attitude and how a nurse values time affect time management (Wywialowski, 2004). Changes in health care and increasing complexity of patients create stress for nurses as they work to meet patient needs (Marriner Tomey, 2009). One way to manage this stress is through the use of time management skills. These skills involve learning how, where, and when to use your time. Managing yourself better leads to better management of your time (Hackworth, 2008). Because you have a limited amount of time with patients, it is essential to remain goal oriented and focused on your patients' priorities. For example, priorities of care help you determine what procedures you will perform first, patient assessments that you will do on an ongoing basis, and the anticipated response of your patient to care activities.

One useful time management skill involves making a priority to-do list (Hackworth, 2008). When you first begin working with a patient or group of patients, make a list that sequences the nursing activities you will perform. The change-of-shift report will help you prioritize activities based on what you learn about your patients' conditions and the care provided before your arrival to the unit. Consider activities that have specific time limits in terms of addressing patient needs, such as administering a pain medication before a scheduled procedure or instructing a patient before discharge home. Also, analyze the items on your list that agency policies or routines will schedule. Note which activities need to be done on time and which activities you are able to do at your discretion (Wywialowski, 2004). For instance, you need to administer medications within a specific schedule, but you can also perform other activities while you are in the patient's room. Finally, estimate the amount of time needed to complete the various activities. Activities requiring the assistance of other staff members usually take longer because you will plan around their schedule.

Good time management also involves setting goals to help you complete one task before starting another (Hackworth,

2008). Complete the activities you begin with one patient before moving on to the next if possible. Your care will then become less fragmented, and you will better focus on what you are doing for each patient. As a result, it is less likely that you will make errors in your care. Other strategies to help you manage your time are keeping your work area clean and clutter free, delegating tasks as possible, and trying to decrease interruptions as you are completing tasks (Pearce, 2007).

Evaluation   One of the most important aspects of clinical care coordination is evaluation (see Chapter 8). It is a mistake to think that evaluation occurs at the end of an activity. Evaluation is an ongoing process. Once you assess a patient's needs and begin therapies directed at a specific problem area, immediately evaluate if therapies are effective and the patient's response. The process of evaluation compares actual patient outcomes with expected outcomes. When expected outcomes are not being met, evaluation reveals the need to continue current therapies for a longer period, revise approaches to care, or introduce new therapies. Throughout the day as you care for a patient, anticipate when you need to return to the bedside to evaluate your care. For example, you decide to return 30 minutes after you administered a medication, 15 minutes after an intravenous (IV) line has begun infusing, or 60 minutes after discussing discharge instructions with the patient and family.

Keeping a focus on evaluation of the patient's progress lessens the chance of becoming distracted by the tasks of care. It is common to assume that staying focused on planned activities ensures that you perform care appropriately. However, task orientation does not ensure good patient outcomes. The competent nurse learns that at the heart of good organizational skills is the constant inquiry into the patient's condition and progress toward an improved level of health.

TEAM COMMUNICATION   As a part of a nursing team, each nurse is responsible for open and professional verbal and electronic communication (Lindeke and Sieckert, 2005). Many health care institutions are using standardized communication methods such as SBAR (situation, background, assessment, recommendation) to decrease errors and improve teamwork and communication (see Chapter 9) (Leonard, Graham, and Bonacum, 2004). Regardless of the setting, nurses learn that an enriching, professional environment is one in which staff members respect one another's ideas, share information, and keep one another informed. On a busy nursing unit this means keeping the nurse in charge of the unit and colleagues informed about patients with emerging problems (Box 12-5). This also includes informing health care providers who have been called for consultation. In a clinic setting it means sharing unusual diagnostic findings or conveying important information regarding a patient's source of family support. One way of fostering good team communication is by setting expectations of one another. Always treat colleagues with respect. Listen to the ideas of other staff members without interruption. Be honest and direct in what you say. Clarify what others are saying, and build on the merits of co-workers' ideas (Marriner Tomey, 2009). When using electronic communication, be open and courteous, summa-

BOX 12-5   SBAR as Communication Tool

 Thirty minutes after Jennifer administered 1 tablet of Percodan 20 mg PO to Mr. Timmons she evaluates its effect. Mr. Timmons tells her that that his pain is still an 8 on the 0 to 10 pain scale. Jennifer prepares an SBAR to contact the health care provider.

Situation: Thirty minutes after Mr. Timmons received his pain medication, he continues to rate his pain as an 8 on the 0 to 10 pain scale.

Background: Mr. Timmons had abdominal surgery 2 days ago for removal of a colon tumor. He had his patient-controlled analgesia (PCA) pump with intravenous (IV) morphine removed 4 hours ago. He has one tablet of Percodan 20 mg PO ordered every 6 hours. This is the first dose of the oral medication that was administered.

Assessment: One tablet of Percodan 20 mg PO is not sufficient to manage Mr. Timmons' pain on the second postoperative day. He does not want to walk with the level of pain he is experiencing.

Recommendation: Request a change of the pain medication order to an increase in dose or a different medication every 4 hours for Mr. Timmons.

---

rize issues, and send messages with only needed details (Lindeke and Sieckert, 2005). An efficient team counts on all members when needs arise. Sharing expectations of what, when, and how to communicate is a step toward establishing a strong work team.

DELEGATION The art of effective delegation is a skill you as a student need to observe and practice to improve your management skills. Delegation is the process of assigning part of one person's responsibility to another qualified person in a specific situation (National Council of State Boards of Nursing [NCSBN], 1995). One purpose of delegation is to improve efficiency. For example, asking a staff member to obtain an ordered specimen while you attend to a patient's pain medication request effectively prevents a delay in the patient's gaining pain relief. Delegation also provides job enrichment. A nurse shows trust in colleagues by delegating tasks to them and showing staff members that they are important players in the delivery of care. Never delegate a task that you dislike doing or would not do yourself, because this creates negative feelings and poor working relationships. Remember that even though the delegation of a task transfers the responsibility and authority to another person, you are still accountable for the delegated tasks.

Professional nurses are finding themselves in situations in which they need more support to do the daily, repetitive tasks of care, such as basic hygiene, specimen collection, and feeding patients. The RN needs time to coordinate care delivery for groups of patients, to conduct individual assessments, and to make professional judgments about a patient's health and therapeutic needs. The RN also needs time to deliver complex therapies and to provide patient counseling and

education. An LPN/LVN in acute care benefits from acquiring support to deliver care to a group of patients whose needs are complex. In long-term care settings the LPN/LVN directs care and relies on nursing assistive personnel to provide basic care measures. A nurse is simply not able to do all the work necessary to care for groups of patients.

To be able to perform your professional responsibilities as a nurse, learn how to work effectively with other staff members. Each health care team member has a set of job responsibilities that contribute to the overall care of patients. As a nurse, your job will be to help the care team work efficiently. Because you will oversee the care of groups of patients, it will become necessary at times for you to delegate work to others.

The American Nurses Association (1997) defines **delegation** as transferring responsibility for the performance of an activity or task while retaining accountability for the outcome. For example, you delegate catheter care to competent and trained nursing assistive personnel after you have assessed the condition of the patient's catheter and perineal tissues. However, you are ultimately accountable for having the patient receive catheter care. As the RN, you remain accountable for the overall nursing care of the patient when you delegate responsibilities to a competent individual (Marriner Tomey, 2009). Because the steps of the nursing process of assessment, diagnosis, planning, and evaluation require you to use nursing judgment, you will not delegate these activities (ANA and NCSBN, 2006). Thus exercise good judgment at all times in deciding what tasks to delegate and in what situations. The National Council of State Boards of Nursing offers guidelines for delegation of tasks in accordance with an RN's legal scope of practice (Box 12-6).

It is important to recognize that in regard to delegation to nursing assistive personnel, you delegate tasks, not patients. Further, do not automatically delegate a task because it is a task but because it is appropriate for someone else to perform the task. For example, as the nurse you are always responsible for the assessment of a patient's ongoing status, but if a patient is stable, you delegate vital sign monitoring to nursing assistive personnel. It is important for you to collaborate with nursing assistive personnel and ask them to take on tasks that you determine are safe and appropriate for them to provide.

Effective delegation requires constant communication. Know how to give clear instructions, effectively prioritize patient needs and therapies, and be able to give staff members timely and meaningful feedback. Make sure to listen so that all participants understand expectations regarding patient care. You need to communicate when and what information to report, such as expected observations and specific patient outcomes (NCSBN, 2005). During delegation, communication is a two-way process. Therefore allow nursing assistive personnel the chance to ask questions and have your expectations made clear (ANA and NCSBN, 2006).

The final step in delegation is evaluation of the staff member's performance, achievement of the patient's outcomes, the communication process used, and any problems or concerns that occurred (NCSBN, 2005). Provide praise

BOX 12-6 — The Five Rights of Delegation

RIGHT TASK
The right task is one that you can delegate for a specific patient, such as tasks that are repetitive, require little supervision, are relatively noninvasive, have results that are predictable, and have minimal potential risk.

RIGHT CIRCUMSTANCES
Consider the patient setting, available resources, and other relevant factors before delegating. In an acute care setting, patients' conditions can change quickly. Good clinical decision making and critical thinking are needed to ensure that the nursing assistive personnel has the appropriate resources, equipment, and supervision to provide safe and effective care.

RIGHT PERSON
The right person is delegating the right tasks to the right person to be performed on the right person.

RIGHT DIRECTION/COMMUNICATION
Give a clear, concise description of the task, including its objective, limits, and expectations. Communication must be ongoing between the nurse and nursing assistive personnel during a shift of care.

RIGHT SUPERVISION
Provide appropriate monitoring, evaluation, intervention as needed, and feedback. Nursing assistive personnel should feel comfortable asking questions and seeking assistance.

Modified from Hudspeth R: Understanding delegation is a critical competency for nurses in the new millennium, *Nurse Admin Q* 31(2):183, 2007; National Council of State Boards of Nursing: *Delegation: concepts and decision-making process*, Chicago, 1995, The Council; National Council of State Boards of Nursing, *The five rights of delegation*, Chicago, 1997, The Council; American Nurses Association (ANA) and National Council of State Boards of Nursing (NCSBN): *Joint statement on delegation*, http://www.ncsbn.org/pdfs/joint_statement.pdf, 2006.

and recognition when the staff member performs the task correctly and does a good job. If the staff member's performance is not satisfactory, give constructive and appropriate feedback. Feedback given should be specific in regard to any mistakes that the staff members make, explaining how to avoid the mistake or a better way to handle the situation. Give feedback in private to preserve the staff member's dignity. When you give feedback, make sure to focus on things that are changeable, choose only one issue at a time, and give specific details (Case, 2004).

Here are a few tips on appropriate delegation (McEnroe Ayers and Montgomery, 2008):

- *Assess the knowledge and skills of the person you are delegating to:* Determine what nursing assistive personnel know and what they are able to do by asking open-ended questions that will elicit conversation and details on what the person knows. For example, ask, "How do you usually put the cuff on when you measure a blood pressure?" or "Tell me how you prepare the tubing before you give an enema."
- *Match tasks to the assistant's skills:* Know what skills the training program includes for nursing assistive personnel at your facility. Determine if personnel have learned critical thinking skills, such as knowing when a patient is in danger or knowing what changes to report.
- *Communicate clearly:* Always provide complete, accurate, and clear directions by describing a task, the desired outcome, and the time period within which the person is to complete the task. Never give instructions through another staff member. Make the person feel as though he or she is part of the team. For example, "I'd like you to help me by getting Mr. Floyd up to ambulate before lunch. Be sure to check his blood pressure before he stands, and write your finding on the graphic sheet. OK?"
- *Listen attentively:* Listen to the response of nursing assistive personnel after you provide directions. Do they feel comfortable in asking questions or requesting clarification? If you encourage a response, listen to what the person has to say. Be especially attentive if the staff member has been given a deadline to meet by another nurse. Help sort out priorities.
- *Provide feedback:* Always give nursing assistive personnel feedback regarding performance, regardless of outcome. Let them know when a job was well done. If an outcome is undesirable, find a private place to discuss what occurred, any miscommunication, and how to achieve a better outcome in the future.

KEY POINTS

- A profession possesses the characteristics of extended education, theory, service, autonomy, and a code of ethics.
- The essential components of professional nursing are care, cure, and coordination.
- Standards of care offer objective guidelines for nurses to provide care and to evaluate care.
- A manager sets a philosophy for a work unit, ensures appropriate staffing, and mobilizes staff and institutional resources to achieve objectives. A manager also motivates staff members to carry out their work, sets standards of performance, and makes the right decisions to achieve objectives.
- Empowering staff members brings out the best in a manager and allows him or her to concentrate on effective patient care systems, to support risk taking and innovation, and to focus on results and rewards.
- Nursing care delivery models vary by the responsibility of the RN in coordinating care delivery and the roles other staff members play in assisting with care.

- Critical to the success of decentralized decision making is making staff members aware that they have the responsibility, authority, and accountability for the care they give and the decisions they make.
- A nurse manager fosters decentralized decision making by establishing nursing practice committees and supporting interdisciplinary collaboration between nurses and health care providers.
- Clinical care coordination involves accurate clinical decision making, establishing priorities, efficient organizational skills, appropriate use of resources and time management skills, and an ongoing evaluation of care activities.
- Each member of a nursing work team is responsible for open, professional communication.
- When done correctly, delegation improves job efficiency and job enrichment.
- Exercise good judgment at all times in deciding what tasks to delegate and in what situations.

CRITICAL THINKING EXERCISES

During her second week on clinical, Jennifer is assigned to Mr. Ambrose and Mrs. Harris. Mr. Ambrose, who was admitted 2 days ago for gastrointestinal bleeding, is ready to ambulate down the hall for his evening walk. Mr. Ambrose's physician has ordered a stool specimen. Mrs. Harris had a colostomy created during abdominal surgery earlier in the morning. Jennifer finds that Mr. Ambrose is resting comfortably and visiting with his daughter. He is eager to go for his walk. Mrs. Harris is very restless and experiencing discomfort from her nasogastric tube and incision. Jennifer checks her Foley catheter and finds that she has voided 20 mL of urine in the last 2 hours.

1. As Jennifer assesses Mr. Ambrose and Mrs. Harris, she identifies multiple needs for both patients. Which patient does Jennifer need to focus on first? Identify three priority needs of this patient. Explain your answer.

2. Which tasks are appropriate for Jennifer to delegate to the nurse technician, Linda? Explain your answer.

3. Jennifer observed Sally, another nurse, delegating the task of taking Mrs. Millman, one of Sally's patients, to the bathroom. Which activities by Sally indicate to Linda that she practiced appropriate delegation when delegating the task of taking Mrs. Millman to the bathroom? Select all that apply.

a. Sally mentally reviewed Mrs. Millman's condition and determined that she could ambulate to the bathroom with the assistance of one person.

b. Sally instructed Linda to take Mrs. Millman to the bathroom as soon as possible.

c. Sally told Linda she would answer her question about whether Mrs. Millman has activity limitations later because she had to administer a STAT medication.

d. Sally asked Linda if she thought that she could get Mrs. Millman out of bed on her own and walk her to the bathroom.

e. Sally told Linda in the break room that she did not save Mrs. Millman's urine for the 12-hour urine collection that was in progress.

f. Sally told Linda she would come in and see if she needed assistance with Mrs. Millman right after she administered a medication.

4. Jennifer tells her nursing instructor that it is hard for her to delegate to the nursing assistive personnel. Jennifer's instructor gives her helpful tips on how to improve her delegation skills. Explain the five rights of delegation that Jennifer's nursing instructor should review with Jennifer. Provide an example for each of the rights.

⊖volve   *Answers to Critical Thinking Questions can be found on the Evolve website.*

REVIEW QUESTIONS

1. While administering medications, the nurse realizes that the wrong dose of a medication was given to the patient. The nurse completes an occurrence report and notifies the patient's health care provider. This is an example of the nurse exercising:
   1. Authority
   2. Responsibility
   3. Accountability
   4. Decision making

2. During morning rounds the nurse assesses the condition of a patient who had major heart surgery 2 days ago. His vital signs are stable. The nurse finds the incision is clean and healing well. The patient complains of pain in his lower leg where a vein graft for the heart surgery was removed. The IV solution is infusing at 100 mL/hr but only 150 mL remains before the infusion runs out. An order exists for the patient to ambulate twice a day. What action should the nurse do first?
   1. Replace the IV bag with a new one.
   2. Administer an analgesic for the patient's leg pain.
   3. Provide instruction on complications of wound healing.
   4. Ambulate the patient 50 feet in the hall.

3. The nurse checks her patient, a 62-year-old man admitted to the hospital with pneumonia. The patient has been coughing profusely and has required nasotracheal suctioning. He also has an IV infusion of antibiotics. The patient is febrile with a temperature of 101° F (38.3° C). He asks the nurse if he can have a bed bath because he has been perspiring profusely. The task for the nurse to delegate to the nurse assistant working with her today is:
   1. Teaching the use of incentive spirometer
   2. Changing the IV dressing
   3. Nasotracheal suctioning
   4. Administering a bed bath

4. The nurse has completed morning rounds on her assigned patients and is giving the nursing assistant directions for what he needs to do for the next hour. An example of an appropriate way to communicate directions when delegating nursing care is:
   1. "Please go to room 20A and see what the patient needs."
   2. "I would like you to take all the vital signs for rooms 12 and 13 and let me know if there are any problems."
   3. "Would you start the patient's bath while I check on the IV line in room 14? I will help you with turning her so I can assess her skin and decide on the turning schedule we will need to follow."
   4. "I want you to help the patient in room 16B off the bedpan, and while you are at it, get a specimen if he passed any stool. I don't think I can go in his room one more time, so I would appreciate your help."

5. You are caring for a patient who was started on insulin for newly diagnosed diabetes mellitus. You need to teach the patient and family about insulin administration. You recognize that this is classified as what type of priority?
   1. High
   2. Immediate

3. Intermediate
4. Low

6. You are an RN providing care to an assigned group of patients. You are responsible for developing the patient care plan, working directly with the patient and family, and interacting with other members of the health care team. What type of nursing care delivery model are you participating in?
   1. Total patient care
   2. Functional nursing
   3. Primary nursing
   4. Team nursing

7. The nurse asks the nursing assistant to walk the patient 100 feet in the hall. The nurse tells the nursing assistant to take the patient's pulse before and after the walk and to notify him what the pulse rates are. The nurse's interaction with the nursing assistant is an example of which of the five rights of delegation?
   1. Right supervision
   2. Right task
   3. Right direction
   4. Right circumstances

8. Which task is appropriate for the RN to delegate to the nursing assistant?
   1. Assessing the vital signs on a patient who had a total knee replacement 2 days ago.
   2. Explaining to a patient about the colonoscopy that is scheduled for tomorrow morning.
   3. Completing the documentation of the patient teaching done on a newly prescribed medication.
   4. Administering the contrast medium to a patient who is having an abdominal computed tomography (CT) scan later in the morning.

9. Which activity has the highest priority and should be completed first by the nurse?
   1. Collect a culture and sensitivity specimen from the patient's infected foot ulcer.
   2. Administer morphine sulfate for the patient's incision pain rated as a 6 on a 0 to 10 pain scale.
   3. Irrigate the patient's nasogastric tube for the complaint of nausea.
   4. Provide teaching on insulin administration to the patient on his new diagnosis of diabetes mellitus.

10. Which activity by the nursing student shows a strategy for effective time management?
    1. The student makes two trips to the supply room to gather materials for a dressing change.
    2. The student stopped twice while setting up her medications to help another student.
    3. The student commented on how unorganized she felt and stated that she would do better next week.
    4. After listening to the change-of-shift report, the student revises the schedule she developed last night for the clinical day.

Answers to Review Questions can be found on pages 1197-1198.

REFERENCES

Alligood MR, Marriner Tomey A: *Nursing theory: utilization and application*, ed 3, St. Louis, 2006, Mosby.

American Nurses Association: *Definitions related to ANA 1992 position statement on unlicensed assistive personnel*, 1997, http://www. nursingworld.org/readroom/position/uap/uapuse.htm.

American Nurses Association: *Code of ethics for nurses with interpretive statements*, Washington, DC, 2001, The Association.

American Nurses Association: *Nursing: scope and standards of practice*, Washington, DC, 2004, The Association.

American Nurses Association (ANA) and National Council of State Boards of Nursing (NCSBN): *Joint statement on delegation*, http://www.ncsbn.org/pdfs/joint_statement.pdf, 2006.

American Nurses Credentialing Center: *ANCC Magnet recognition program*, 2008, http://www.nursecredentialing.org/magnet/index.html.

Arford PH: Nurse-physician communication: an organizational accountability, *Nurs Econ* 23(2):72, 2005.

Benner P, Hughes RG, Sutphen M: Clinical reasoning, decision making, and action: thinking critically and clinically. In Agency for Healthcare Research and Quality: *Patient safety and quality: an evidence-based handbook for nurses*, AHRQ Pub No. 08-0043, Rockville, Md, 2008, The Agency.

Canadian Nurses Association: *Education preparation for entry into practice*, Ottawa, 2004, The Association, http://www.cna-nurses.ca/frames/policies/policiesmainframe.htm.

Case B: Delegation skills: critical-thinking strategies you can apply to the challenges of delegating, *Greater Chicago/Wisconsin/Indiana Advance for Nurses* 19(July 19), 2004.

Dougherty MB, Larson E: A review of instruments measuring nurse-physician collaboration, *J Nurs Adm* 35(5):224, 2005.

Gardner DB: Ten lessons in collaboration, *Online J Issues Nurs* 10(1):Manuscript 1, 2005, http://www.nursingworld.org/ojin/topic26/tpc26_1.htm.

Hackworth T: Time management for the nurse leader, *Nursing 2008 Critical Care*, 3(2):10, 2008.

Hendry C, Walker A: Priority setting in clinical nursing practice: literature review, *J Adv Nurs* 47(4):427, 2004.

Hudspeth R: Understanding delegation is a critical competency for nurses in the new millennium, *Nurse Admin Q* 31(2):183, 2007.

Institute of Medicine: *Crossing the quality chasm: a new health system for the twenty-first century*, Washington, DC, National Academies Press, 2001.

Institute of Medicine: *Keeping patients safe: transforming the work environment*, Washington, DC, National Academies Press, 2004.

Leonard M, Graham S, Bonacum D: The human factor: the critical importance of effective teamwork and communication in providing safe care, *Qual Saf Health Care* 13(Suppl 1):i85, 2004.

Lindeke LL, Sieckert AM: Nurse-physician workplace collaboration, *Online J Issues Nurs* 10(1):Manuscript 4, 2005, http://www.nursingworld.org/ojin/topic26/tpc26_4.htm.

Marriner Tomey A: *Guide to nursing management and leadership*, ed 8, St. Louis, 2009, Mosby.

McEnroe Ayers DM, Montgomery M: Delegating the "right" way, *Nursing* 38(4):56hnl, 2008.

National Council of State Boards of Nursing: *Delegation: concepts and decision-making process*, Chicago, 1995, The Council.

National Council of State Boards of Nursing: *The five rights of delegation*, Chicago, 1997, The Council.

National Council of State Boards of Nursing: *Working with others: a position paper*, Chicago, 2005, The Council.

Pearce C: Ten steps to managing time, *Nurs Manage* 14(1):23, 2007.

Schmalenberg C and others: Excellence through evidence: securing collegial/collaborative nurse-physician relationships, part I, *J Nurs Adm* 35(10):450, 2005.

Seago JA: Professional communication. In Agency for Healthcare Research and Quality: *Patient safety and quality: an evidence-based handbook for nurses*, AHRQ Pub No. 08-0043, Rockville, Md, 2008, The Agency.

Thomas PL: Case manager role definitions: do they make an organizational impact? *Prof Case Manage* 13(2):61, 2008.

Thompson P and others: Contemporary issues in healthcare workplace. In Mason DJ and others: *Policy and politics in nursing and healthcare*, ed 5, St. Louis, 2007, Mosby.

Tiedeman ME, Lookinland S: Traditional models of care delivery: what have we learned? *J Nurs Adm* 34(6):291, 2004.

Toofany S: Critical thinking among nurses, *Nurs Manage* 14(9):28, 2008.

Tschannen D: The effect of individual characteristics on perceptions of collaboration in the work environment, *Medsurg Nurs* 13(15):312, 2004.

Wolf G, Triolo P, Reid Ponte P: Magnet recognition program: the next generation, *J Nurs Adm* 38(4):200, 2008.

Wywialowski E: *Managing patient care*, ed 3, St. Louis, 2004, Mosby.

Zwarenstein M, Bryant W: Interventions to promote collaboration between nurses and doctors, *Cochrane Database Syst Rev* 2000(2):CD000072, DOI:10.1002/14651858.CD000072.

Infection Prevention and Control

MEDIA RESOURCES

 CD COMPANION 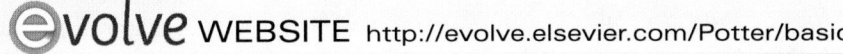 **WEBSITE** http://evolve.elsevier.com/Potter/basic

- Crossword Puzzle
- English/Spanish Audio Glossary

OBJECTIVES

- Identify the body's normal defenses against infection.
- Discuss the events of the inflammatory response.
- Describe the signs and symptoms of a localized and a systemic infection.
- Describe characteristics of each link of the infection chain.
- Assess patients at risk for acquiring an infection.
- Explain conditions that promote development of health care–associated infections.

- Describe strategies for standard precautions.
- Identify principles of medical and surgical asepsis.
- Describe nursing interventions designed to break each link in the infection chain.
- Perform proper barrier isolation techniques.
- Perform proper procedures for hand hygiene.
- Apply and remove a surgical mask and gloves using correct technique.

KEY TERMS

airborne precautions, p. 246
antibody, p. 230
antigen, p. 231
asepsis, p. 232
aseptic technique, p. 232
asymptomatic, p. 228
carriers, p. 228
colonization, p. 228
communicable disease, p. 228

contact precautions, p. 246
disinfection, p. 238
droplet precautions, p. 246
endogenous infection, p. 231
exogenous infection, p. 231
flora, p. 230

health care–acquired infection (HAI), p. 231
immunity, p. 230
infection, p. 228
inflammation, p. 231
inflammatory response, p. 230
medical asepsis, p. 232
microorganisms, p. 228
necrotic, p. 231
pathogenicity, p. 230

pathogens, p. 228
reservoir, p. 228
standard precautions, p. 237
sterilization, p. 238
suprainfection, p. 231
surgical asepsis, p. 233
symptomatic, p. 228
transmission-based precautions, p. 237
virulence, p. 228

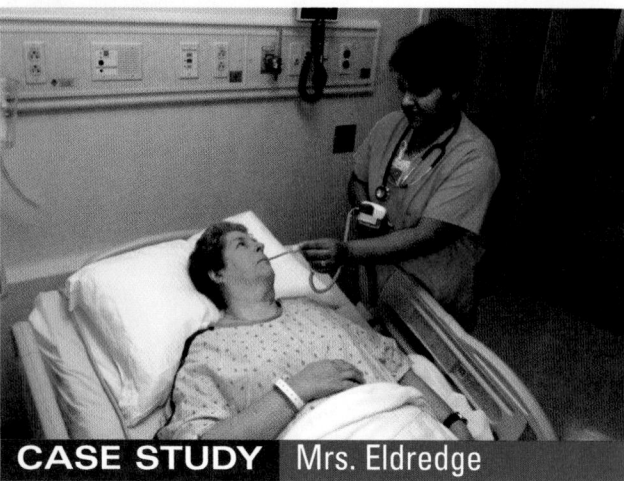

CASE STUDY   Mrs. Eldredge

Mrs. Eldredge is a 63-year-old woman with diabetes who underwent a total hip replacement. She did well after surgery, and the plan is to discharge her on the afternoon of her fourth postoperative day. Her blood glucose levels are well controlled with medication and diet. She lives alone and enjoys an active social life.

Kathy Jackson is a nursing student doing a home health clinical rotation. She visited Mrs. Eldredge in the hospital, and she saw her immediately after she returned home and 1 week later. Now 2 weeks after surgery she complains to Kathy that she is having increased pain in her hip. Kathy observes the incision and notes that it is red, swollen, and warm. Mrs. Eldredge also has a low-grade fever with a temperature of 99.8° F. Kathy phones Mrs. Eldredge's care provider and schedules a follow-up appointment for the next day.

Current trends, public awareness, and rising costs of health care have increased the importance of infection prevention and control. Increases in drug-resistant microorganisms and concern about occupational exposure to tuberculosis (TB), human immune deficiency virus (HIV), and hepatitis have increased concern about transmission of infections. As a nurse, you will participate in cost-effective quality health care by using strategies that prevent or reduce the risk for infections. This chapter emphasizes techniques for prevention and control of infections and the critical thinking skills necessary to achieve these goals.

SCIENTIFIC KNOWLEDGE BASE

Nature of Infection

An **infection** is the invasion of a susceptible host (e.g. a patient) by potentially harmful **microorganisms** (pathogens), resulting in disease. The principal infecting agents are bacteria, viruses, fungi, and protozoa (Table 13-1). It is important to know the difference between an infection and colonization. **Colonization** is the presence and growth of microorganisms within a host but without tissue invasion or damage (Tweeten, 2005). All persons have microorganisms on their skin, but usually no disease results. Disease or infection re-

sults only if the **pathogens** grow or multiply and alter normal tissue function. An infectious disease transmitted directly from one person to another is considered a contagious or **communicable disease** (Tweeten, 2005). If the pathogens multiply and cause clinical signs and symptoms, the infection is **symptomatic.** If clinical signs and symptoms are not present, the illness is termed **asymptomatic.** Hepatitis C is a communicable disease that is often asymptomatic. It is most efficiently transmitted through the direct entry of blood into the skin through a percutaneous exposure, even if the source (patient) is asymptomatic (Centers for Disease Control and Prevention [CDC], 2001).

Chain of Infection

The presence of a pathogen does not mean that an infection will begin. The process resulting in an infection is referred to as the chain of infection. Components of the chain include the infectious agent or pathogen, reservoir or place for pathogen growth, portal of exit from the reservoir, mode of transmission or vehicle, portal of entry into the reservoir, and a susceptible host (Figure 13-1). Infection develops if the links in this chain remain intact. Preventing infections involves breaking the chain of infection.

INFECTIOUS AGENT The development of an infection depends on the number of microorganisms present; their **virulence,** or the ability to produce disease; their ability to enter and survive in the host; and the susceptibility of the host. Resident skin microorganisms are not virulent. However, they can cause serious infection when surgery or an invasive procedure allows them to enter deep inside tissues or when a patient is severely immunocompromised. This occurs when the patient's immune system is impaired, which may result from cancer chemotherapy, organ antirejection medication, or acquired immunodeficiency syndrome (AIDS).

RESERVOIR A place where microorganisms survive, multiply, and wait to transfer to a susceptible host is called a **reservoir.** Common reservoirs are humans and animals (hosts), insects, food, water, and organic matter on inanimate surfaces (fomites). Frequent reservoirs for health care–associated infections (HAIs) include health care workers (especially their hands), patients' body excretions and secretions, equipment, and the health care environment. There are two types of human reservoirs: those with acute or symptomatic disease and those who show no signs of disease but are **carriers** of the disease. Humans can transmit microorganisms in either case.

PORTAL OF EXIT After microorganisms find a site in which to grow and multiply, they must find a portal of exit if they are to enter another host and cause disease. Microorganisms exit through a variety of sites such as skin and mucous membranes, respiratory tract, gastrointestinal tract, urinary tract, and reproductive tract and in blood.

MODES OF TRANSMISSION Many times there is little that you are able to do about the infectious agent or the susceptible host, but by practicing infection prevention and control techniques, such as hand hygiene, you interrupt the mode of transmission (Box 13-1). The same microorganism

TABLE 13-1 Common Pathogens and Some Infections or Diseases They Produce

ORGANISM	MAJOR RESERVOIR(S)	MAJOR DISEASES/INFECTIONS
BACTERIA		
Escherichia coli	Colon	Gastroenteritis, urinary tract infection
Staphylococcus aureus	Skin, hair, upper respiratory tract	Wound infection, abscess, cellulitis, osteomyelitis, bacteremia, pneumonia, food poisoning, toxic shock syndrome
Streptococcus (beta hemolytic group A) organisms	Oropharynx, skin, perianal area	"Strep throat," rheumatic fever, scarlet fever, impetigo, wound infection
Streptococcus (beta hemolytic group B) organisms	Adult genitalia	Urinary tract infection, wound infection, postpartum sepsis, neonatal sepsis
Mycobacterium tuberculosis	Droplet nuclei from lungs	Tuberculosis
Neisseria gonorrhoeae	Genitourinary tract, rectum, mouth	Sexually transmitted infection, pelvic inflammatory disease, septic arthritis, newborn ophthalmitis
Rickettsia rickettsii	Wood tick	Rocky Mountain spotted fever
Staphylococcus epidermidis	Skin	Wound infection, bacteremia
VIRUSES		
Hepatitis A virus	Feces	Hepatitis A
Hepatitis B virus	Blood, certain body fluids, tissues involved in sexual contact	Hepatitis B
Hepatitis C virus	Blood, certain body fluids, tissues involved in sexual contact	Hepatitis C
Herpes simplex virus (type I)	Lesions of mouth, skin, genitals	Cold sores, herpetic whitlow, sexually transmitted disease
Human immune deficiency virus (HIV)	Blood, semen, vaginal secretions via sexual contact	Acquired immunodeficiency syndrome (AIDS)
FUNGI		
Aspergillus organisms	Soil, dust, mouth, skin, colon, genital tract	Aspergillosis, pneumonia, sepsis
Candida albicans	Skin, mouth, genital tract	Candidiasis, pneumonia, sepsis
PROTOZOA		
Plasmodium falciparum	Blood	Malaria

Modified from Ritter H: Clinical microbiology. In Carrico R, editor: *APIC text of infection control and epidemiology,* Washington, DC, 2005, Association for Professionals in Infection Control and Epidemiology, Inc.

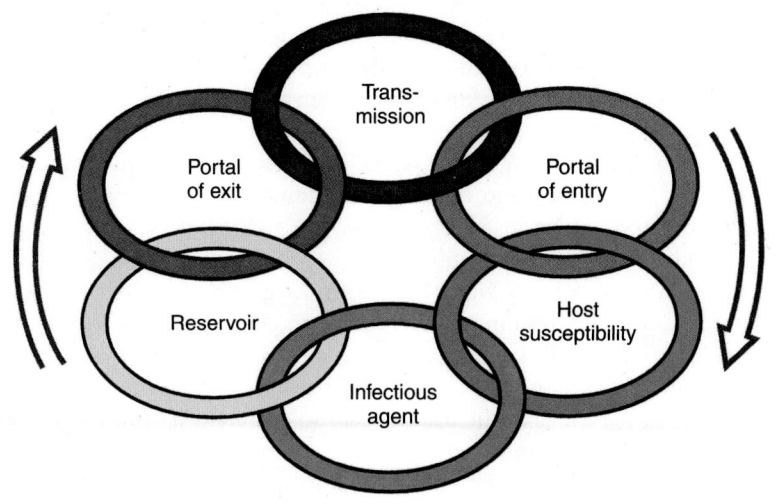

Figure 13-1 ■ Chain of infection.

ROUTES AND MEANS

Contact
- *Direct:* Person-to-person or physical contact between source and susceptible host (e.g., touching patient feces and then touching own face or mouth or consuming contaminated food)
- *Indirect:* Personal contact of susceptible host with contaminated inanimate object (e.g., needles or sharps, dressings)
- *Droplet:* Large particles that travel up to 3 feet and come in contact with susceptible host (e.g., from coughing, sneezing, talking)

Airborne
- Droplet nuclei, residue or evaporated droplets suspended in air (e.g., from coughing, sneezing, talking)

Vehicles
- Contaminated items
- Water
- Drugs, solutions
- Blood
- Food (improperly handled, stored, cooked; fresh or thawed meats)

Vector
- External mechanical transfer (flies)
- Internal transmission such as with parasitic conditions between vector and host, for example:
  - Mosquito
  - Louse
  - Tick
  - Flea

Modified from Tweeten S: General principles of epidemiology. In Carrico R, editor: *APIC text of infection control and epidemiology,* Washington, DC, 2005, Association for Professionals in Infection Control and Epidemiology, Inc.

is sometimes transmitted by more than one route. For example, the virus that causes chickenpox spreads by airborne route in droplet nuclei and also by direct contact with vesicle fluid. Hands of health care workers often transmit microorganisms. This mode of transmission is called direct transmission. Indirect transmission occurs when microorganisms are transmitted from contaminated equipment that is being used on the patient, such as a blood pressure cuff or a contaminated bed rail (CDC, 2002; Cipriano, 2007).

PORTAL OF ENTRY   Organisms are able to enter the body through the same routes they use for exiting. Common portals of entry include broken skin, mucous membranes, genitourinary (GU) tract, gastrointestinal (GI) tract, and respiratory tract. For example, obstruction to the flow of urine due to the presence of a blocked urinary catheter allows organisms to ascend the urethra.

SUSCEPTIBLE HOST   Susceptibility to an infection depends on the individual's degree of resistance to pathogens.

Although everyone is constantly in contact with large numbers of microorganisms, an infection does not develop until an individual becomes susceptible to the strength and numbers of those microorganisms. The more virulent an organism, the greater the dose, the more likely a person will develop an infection. Some of the factors that influence a person's susceptibility (degree of resistance) include age, nutritional status, presence of chronic disease, trauma, and smoking. Organisms with resistance to key antibiotics are becoming more common in all health care settings, but especially acute care. This is associated with the frequent and sometimes inappropriate use of antibiotics over the years in all settings (i.e., acute care, ambulatory care, clinics, and long-term care). A person's natural defenses against infection and certain risk factors affect susceptibility (see Assessment section).

A host is no longer considered susceptible if it has acquired **immunity** through either a natural or an artificially induced event. Natural active immunity results from having a certain disease, such as measles, and mounting an immune response that usually lasts a lifetime. Active immunity also results from the administration of a vaccine (Haiduven and Poland, 2005). Natural passive immunity is the acquisition of an **antibody** by one person from another, such as a baby born with its mother's antibodies. The baby acquires these antibodies through the placenta during the last months of pregnancy. This type of immunity is of short duration, usually lasting only a few weeks to months.

Course of Infection

Infections follow a progressive course (Figure 13-2). The severity depends on the extent of the infection, the **pathogenicity** and virulence of the causative microorganism, and the host's susceptibility. If the infection is localized, such as in a wound, antibiotic therapy and proper wound care control the infection's spread and minimize the illness. The patient usually experiences only localized symptoms such as pain, tenderness, and swelling at the wound site. An infection that affects the entire body instead of just a single organ or part is systemic, characterized by a fever and increase in white blood cells. Often systemic infections are fatal.

Defenses Against Infection

The body has normal defenses against infection, including normal flora, body system defenses, and the immune system. Intact skin protects from pathogens, and linings of the nasal passages act to prevent organisms from entering the lungs. Each organ system has defense mechanisms to prevent exposure to infection. In addition, the body's **inflammatory response** is a protective reaction that neutralizes pathogens and repairs body cells.

NORMAL FLORA   Large numbers of microorganisms residing on the surface and deep layers of the skin, in the saliva and oral mucosa, and in the intestinal walls make up the body's normal **flora**. Normal flora usually do not cause disease but instead help to maintain health. For example, the skin's flora reduce multiplication of organisms landing on the skin. The number and variety of flora maintain a sensitive

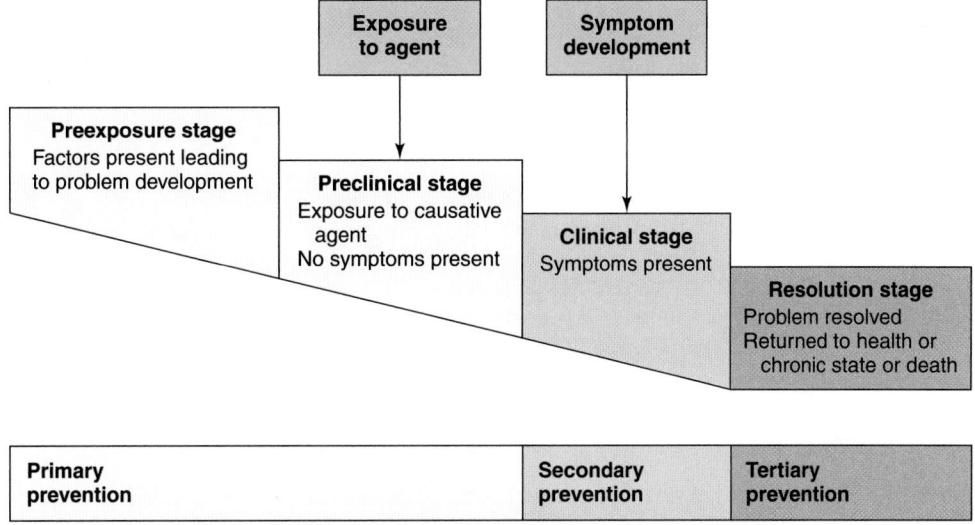

Figure 13-2 ■ Stages of the natural history of a condition and their relationship to primary, secondary, and tertiary levels of prevention. (From Clark MJ: *Community health nursing: caring for populations,* ed 4, Upper Saddle River, NJ, 2003, Pearson Education.)

balance with other microorganisms to prevent infection. Any factor that disrupts this balance places a person at increased risk for infection. For example, the use of broad-spectrum antibiotics for the treatment of infection eliminates or changes normal bacterial flora, leading to **suprainfection.** Microorganisms resistant to antibiotics then cause serious infection (Arnold and McDonald, 2005).

BODY SYSTEM DEFENSES Microorganisms are able to easily enter the skin, respiratory tract, and gastrointestinal tract. However, these body systems also have unique defenses against infection, physiologically suited to their structure and function (Table 13-2). Any condition that impairs an organ's specialized defenses increases susceptibility to infection. When a person ages, normal physiological changes occur that influence susceptibility to infection (Box 13-2).

INFLAMMATION The body's cellular response to injury or infection is **inflammation.** Inflammation is a protective vascular reaction that delivers fluid, blood products, and nutrients to interstitial tissues in an area of injury. This process neutralizes and eliminates pathogens or **necrotic** tissues and establishes a means of repairing body cells and tissues (Table 13-3, p. 234). Signs of inflammation include swelling, redness, heat, pain or tenderness, and loss of function in the affected body part. When inflammation becomes systemic, signs and symptoms can include fever, leukocytosis (increased number of white blood cells), malaise, anorexia, nausea, vomiting, and lymph node enlargement. Many physical agents (e.g., temperature extremes and radiation), chemical agents (e.g., gastric acid or poisons), and microorganisms trigger the inflammatory response.

IMMUNE RESPONSE When a foreign material (**antigen**) enters the body, a series of responses changes the body's biological makeup. The next time that antigen enters the body, antibodies bind to the antigens they find and neutralize, destroy, or eliminate them.

Health Care–Acquired Infection

Patients in health care settings, especially hospitals and long-term care facilities, are at a higher risk for infection than those patients seen in the home. Patients in health care settings often have multiple illnesses, are older adults, and are often poorly nourished. These factors make them more susceptible to infection. In addition, many patients have a lowered resistance to infection because of underlying medical conditions (e.g., HIV, diabetes mellitus, autoimmune disorders, or malignancies) that impair or damage the body's immune response. Invasive treatment devices such as intravenous (IV) catheters or indwelling urinary catheters impair or bypass the body's natural defenses against microorganisms. Treatments with multiple antibiotics for long periods of time are also associated with an increased risk for certain infections (Arnold and McDonald, 2005; Stricof, 2005).

When a patient develops an infection that was not present or incubating at the time of admission to a health care setting, it is called a **health care–acquired infection (HAI).** A community-acquired infection is one that was present at the time of admission to a health care setting. The conscientious practice of hand hygiene and aseptic technique reduces the risk for HAIs. The Joint Commission listed the reduction of HAIs as one of the National Patient Safety Goals in 2009.

HAIs may be exogenous or endogenous. An **exogenous infection** comes from microorganisms found outside the individual, such as *Salmonella, Clostridium tetani,* and *Aspergillus.* They do not exist as normal flora. **Endogenous infection** occurs when part of the patient's flora becomes altered and an overgrowth results (e.g., staphylococci, enterococci, yeasts, and streptococci). This often happens when a patient receives broad-spectrum antibiotics that alter normal flora. When sufficient numbers of microorganisms normally found in one body site move to another site, an endogenous infection devel-

TABLE 13-2 Normal Body System Defense Mechanisms Against Infection

DEFENSE MECHANISMS	ACTION	FACTORS THAT MAY ALTER DEFENSE
SKIN		
Intact multilayered surface, body's first line of defense against infection	Provides mechanical barrier to microorganisms and antibacterial activity	Cuts, abrasions, puncture wounds, areas of maceration
Shedding of outer layer of skin cells	Removes organisms that adhere to skin's outer layers	Failure to bathe regularly, improper hand-hygiene techniques
Sebum	Contains fatty acid that kills some bacteria	Excessive bathing
MOUTH		
Intact multilayered mucosa	Provides mechanical barrier to microorganisms	Lacerations, trauma, extracted teeth
Saliva	Washes away particles containing microorganisms	Poor oral hygiene, dehydration
	Contains microbial inhibitors (e.g., lysozyme)	
EYE		
Tearing and blinking	Provides mechanisms to reduce entry (blinking) or to assist in washing away (tearing) particles containing pathogens	Injury, exposure-splash, splatter of blood or other potentially infectious material into the eye
RESPIRATORY TRACT		
Cilia lining upper airways, coated by mucus	Trap inhaled microbes and sweep them outward in mucus to be expectorated or swallowed	Smoking, high concentration of oxygen and carbon dioxide, decreased humidity, cold air
Macrophages	Engulf and destroy microorganisms that reach lung's alveoli	Smoking Immunosuppression
URINARY TRACT		
Flushing action of urine flow	Washes away microorganisms on lining of bladder and urethra	Obstruction to normal flow by urinary catheter placement, obstruction from growth or tumor, or delayed micturition
Intact multilayered epithelium	Provides barrier to microorganisms	Introduction of urinary catheter, continual movement of catheter in urethra
GASTROINTESTINAL TRACT		
Acidity of gastric secretions	Chemically destroys microorganisms incapable of surviving low pH	Administration of antacids Histamine-2 blockers
Rapid peristalsis in small intestine	Prevents retention of bacterial contents	Delayed motility from impaction of fecal contents in large bowel or mechanical obstruction by masses
VAGINA		
At puberty, normal flora cause vaginal secretions to achieve low pH	Inhibits growth of many microorganisms	Antibiotics and birth control pills that disrupt normal flora

ops. The number of microorganisms needed to cause an HAI depends on the virulence of the organism, the host's susceptibility, and the body site affected (Box 13-3, p. 234).

ASEPSIS Efforts to minimize the onset and spread of infection are based on the principles of aseptic technique. **Aseptic technique** is an effort to keep the patient as free from exposure to infection-causing pathogens as possible. The term **asepsis** means the absence of disease-producing microorganisms. The two types of aseptic technique are medical asepsis and surgical asepsis.

Medical asepsis, or clean techniques, includes procedures used to reduce the number of and prevent the spread of

BOX 13-2   CARE OF THE OLDER ADULT

Infection Control Considerations

Older adults experience a number of age-associated physiological changes that influence susceptibility to infection. These changes include the following:

- Fewer tears to flush and remove debris from the eye and a decrease in lysozymes that affect certain microorganisms. A decreased blink reflex leads to corneal dryness. Caution patients and families to observe for eye infections and use artificial tears when necessary.
- Drying of the oral mucosa and recession and weakening of gingival tissues require frequent oral hygiene and regular dental care.
- Increased chest diameter and rigidity, weakened cough, decreased ability to swallow, and decreased elastic tissue surrounding alveoli predispose older adults to ventilatory problems. Aspiration and postoperative pneumonia are common complications.
- When caring for older adult patients, elevate the head of the bed and encourage the patient to ambulate as soon as possible (unless contraindicated). Instruct and assist patient in deep breathing and coughing techniques.
- Decreased production of digestive juices and a reduction in intestinal motility affect removal of potential pathogens in the bowel. Patients and families should learn about safe food preparation and eat foods that are nutritionally good and easy to digest. Provide smaller meals more frequently.
- Thinning of the dermal and epidermal skin layers, along with a decrease in skin elasticity, predisposes older adults to skin tearing. Meticulous nursing care is necessary to prevent pressure ulcers in bedridden patients (see Chapter 35).
- Decreased production of T lymphocytes and B lymphocytes. With reduced immunity it is important for older adults to receive regular immunizations and medical checkups.

Modified from Gantz M: Geriatrics. In Carrico R, editor: *APIC text of infection control and epidemiology,* Washington, DC, 2005, Association for Professionals in Infection Control and Epidemiology, Inc.

microorganisms. Hand hygiene, barrier techniques, and routine environmental cleaning are examples of medical asepsis.

Surgical asepsis, or sterile technique, includes procedures to eliminate all microorganisms from an area. Sterilization destroys all microorganisms and their spores (CDC, 2008b; Rutala and Weber, 2005). Nurses in the operating room, labor and delivery, and at the bedside practice sterile technique when using sterile instruments and supplies for patient care. Surgical asepsis demands the highest level of aseptic technique and requires that all areas be kept free of infectious microorganisms (Association of periOperative Registered Nurses [AORN], 2009).

Health care workers are responsible for providing a safe environment for the patient. It is easy to forget key procedural steps or to take shortcuts that break aseptic procedures when hurried. Failure to follow proper technique places patients at risk for an infection that can seriously impair their recovery and may even lead to death.

NURSING KNOWLEDGE BASE

Body substances such as feces, urine, and wound drainage contain potentially infectious microorganisms. For this reason, health care workers are at risk for exposure to microorganisms in the hospital, long-term care, and home settings (Fauerbach, 2005). Nursing science has contributed to identifying specific infection prevention practices for health care workers. These practices reduce the risk for cross contamination and transmission to other patients when caring for a patient with a known or suspected infection (CDC, 2007).

The experience of having a serious infection creates feelings of anxiety, frustration, loneliness, and anger in patients and/or their families (Catalano and others, 2003; Maunder, 2003). These feelings worsen when patients are isolated to prevent transmission of a microorganism to other patients or health care staff. Isolation disrupts normal social relationships with visitors and caregivers. Patient safety may be an additional risk for the patient on isolation precautions (Murphy, 2005). For example, an older adult patient with dementia is at increased risk for falling when confined in a room with the door closed. Family members sometimes fear the possibility of developing the infection and may avoid contact with the patient. Some patients perceive the simple procedures of proper hand hygiene and gown and glove use as evidence of rejection. Help patients and families reduce some of these feelings by discussing the disease process, explaining isolation procedures, and maintaining a friendly, understanding manner.

Cultural, religious, or social beliefs influence how a patient reacts to an infectious disease and also influence infection prevention. Use extra caution to make certain the patient and family understand the therapeutic purpose of isolation. For example, the isolation of a loved one is considered disrespectful and uncaring behavior in many cultures (Hispanics, Africans, and Asians) (Mashaba, 2002). Social support for patients promotes their adherence to treatment. Russell and Henderson (2003) reported that, even though health care providers recommend annual vaccination against influenza, beliefs about disease and vaccination influence a health care worker's decision to be vaccinated.

How a patient reacts to an infection or infectious disease is important for you to know in establishing a plan of care. The challenge is to identify and support those behaviors that maintain human health or prevent infection.

NURSING PROCESS

■■■ASSESSMENT

Assess all risk factors for a patient's susceptibility to infection and their current clinical status (Box 13-4). A review of the medical history with the patient and family sometimes re-

TABLE 13-3   Inflammation

PHYSIOLOGICAL RESPONSE	SIGNS AND SYMPTOMS
VASCULAR AND CELLULAR RESPONSE	
Arterioles supplying infected or injured area dilate, delivering blood and leukocytes.	Redness
Tissue necrosis causes release of histamine, bradykinin, prostaglandin, and serotonin, which increase blood vessel permeability.	Warmth
	Edema
Fluid, protein, and cells enter interstitial spaces to cause swelling.	Pain
White blood cells (WBCs) enter tissues and phagocytose microorganisms. More WBCs are released into bloodstream.	WBC count normally 5000-10,000/mm^3; value is increased with infection, inflammation, stress, trauma
Phagocytic release of pyrogens from bacteria occurs.	Fever
INFLAMMATORY EXUDATE	
Fluid, dead cells, and WBCs form exudate at inflammatory site that later clears with lymphatic drainage.	Purulent drainage
	Serous or sanguineous exudates
TISSUE REPAIR	
Healthy new cells replace damaged cells. Cells mature to take on structural characteristics and appearance of injured cells.	Tissue defects heal and close

BOX 13-3   Examples of Sites for and Causes of Health Care–Acquired Infections

Improperly performing hand hygiene increases patient risk for all types of health care–acquired infections.

URINARY TRACT
- Unsterile insertion of urinary catheter
- Improper positioning of the drainage tubing
- Open drainage system
- Disconnection of catheter and tube
- Contact between drainage bag port and contaminated surface
- Improper specimen collection technique
- Obstruction or interference with urinary drainage
- Urine in catheter or drainage tube being allowed to reenter bladder (reflux)
- Repeated catheter irrigations

SURGICAL OR TRAUMATIC WOUNDS
- Improper skin preparation before surgery (i.e., shaving versus clipping hair; not performing a preoperative bath or shower)
- Failure to cleanse skin surface properly

- Failure to use aseptic technique during dressing changes
- Use of contaminated antiseptic solutions

RESPIRATORY TRACT
- Contaminated respiratory therapy equipment
- Failure to use aseptic technique while suctioning airway
- Improper disposal of secretions

BLOODSTREAM
- Contamination of IV fluids by tubing
- Insertion of drug additives to IV fluid
- Addition of connecting tube or stopcocks to IV system
- Improper care of needle insertion site
- Contaminated needles or catheters
- Failure to change IV access site when inflammation first appears
- Improper technique during administration of multiple blood products
- Improper care of peritoneal or hemodialysis shunts
- Improperly accessing an IV port

IV, Intravenous.

veals a recent exposure to a communicable disease. By assessing existing signs and symptoms (such as the condition of a wound, the presence of fever), you will determine whether a patient's clinical condition indicates the onset or extension of an infection. During the interview process, assess the patient's and family's knowledge of a known infection or disease to determine the course of the condition and their level of knowledge of infection control practices.

Because a patient's nutritional health directly influences susceptibility to infection, a thorough diet history is neces-

sary. Determine a patient's normal daily nutrient intake and whether preexisting problems such as impaired swallowing or oral pain alter food intake.

Review laboratory data as soon as they are available (Table 13-4). Laboratory values such as increased white blood cells (WBCs) and/or a positive blood culture often indicate infection. When assessing laboratory data, consider the age of the patient. For example, in the older adult, bacterial growth in urine without clinical symptoms does not always indicate the presence of a urinary tract infection (Gantz, 2005).

BOX 13-4 Factors Affecting Susceptibility to Infection

AGE
- Infants have immature immune systems.
- Children acquire more immunity but are susceptible to infectious diseases such as mumps and measles if unvaccinated.
- Young and middle-age adults have refined body system defenses and immunity.
- Older adults' immune responses decline, and the structure and function of major organs change (see Box 13-2, p. 233).

HEREDITY
- Certain congenital and genetic chromosomal disorders sometimes have an effect on humoral or cellular immunity.
- Patients with diabetes, and those with a hereditary predisposition to diabetes, are at increased risk for infections and delayed wound healing.

CULTURAL PRACTICES
- Various cultural or religious beliefs or practices influence patients' decisions to seek treatment for an infection or to use methods to prevent infections. For example, a Native American or Latino patient may seek treatment from a "healer" rather than a health care provider, or a patient may not use a condom because of religious beliefs.

NUTRITIONAL STATUS
- A reduction in protein, carbohydrates, and fats as a result of illness, inadequate diet, or debility increases a patient's susceptibility to infection and delays wound repair.

STRESS
- Increased stress elevates cortisone levels, causing decreased resistance to infection.
- Continuous stress exhausts energy stores.

REST AND EXERCISE
- Inadequate rest and exercise increase stress and decrease body functions such as elimination and circulation.

INADEQUATE DEFENSES
- Primary and secondary defenses are altered (e.g., broken skin or mucosa, traumatized tissue, suppressed immune response).

PERSONAL HABITS
- Smoking reduces respiratory ciliary action and decreases resistance to respiratory infections.
- Alcohol ingestion impairs the effect of antibiotics.
- Risky sexual behavior, such as multiple sex partners, increases the chance for exposure to HIV and agents of other sexually transmitted diseases.

ENVIRONMENTAL FACTORS
- Crowded living conditions and adequacy and safety of water supply influence the patient's susceptibility to infections.
- Inadequate refrigeration and cooking facilities increase a patient's exposure to food-borne illness such as salmonellosis or campylobacteriosis.

IMMUNIZATION/DISEASE HISTORY
- Patients who have not received recommended immunizations are at risk for vaccine-preventable diseases such as measles, mumps, and rubella.
- Older adults with underlying medical conditions decrease their susceptibility to influenza and pneumococcal pneumonia through immunizations.

MEDICAL THERAPIES
- Certain drugs, such as cortisone, and certain invasive therapies, such as intravenous catheters or surgeries, increase the risk for infection.

CLINICAL APPEARANCE AND DATA
- Localized infections usually present with redness, swelling, and pain or tenderness. There is sometimes a purulent drainage from wounds or lesions.
- Systemic infections present with fever, chills, nausea and vomiting, loss of appetite, or lymph node enlargement.
- Clinical data may show an increase in white blood cells (WBCs), a positive culture, or an abnormal x-ray examination.

HIV, Human immune deficiency virus.

The early recognition of infection assists you in making the correct nursing diagnosis and establishing a treatment plan. In addition, alert other members of the health care team to the need for further investigation of the patient's condition, facilitating initiation of prompt therapy and barrier protection. Because of increased attention to the prevention of infection, the Centers for Disease Control and Prevention (CDC) (2007) and the Occupational Safety and Health Administration (OSHA) (1991) have stressed the importance of barrier protection.

Also assess the effects an infection has on the patient and family. Patients with chronic or serious infection such as tuberculosis or AIDS experience psychological and social problems from self-imposed isolation or rejection by friends and family. Ask the patient how the infection is affecting his or her ability to maintain relationships and perform activities of daily living. Determine whether chronic infection has drained the patient's financial resources.

PATIENT EXPECTATIONS Identify patients' expectations about their care, and involve them in planning their

TABLE 13-4 Laboratory Tests to Screen for Infection

LABORATORY VALUE	NORMAL (ADULT) VALUES	INDICATION OF INFECTION
White blood cell (WBC) count	5,000-10,000/mm³	Increased in acute infection, decreased in certain viral or overwhelming infections
Erythrocyte sedimentation rate	Up to 15 mm/hr for men and 20 mm/hr for women	Elevated in presence of inflammatory process
Iron level	Male 80-180 mcg/dL; female 60-160 mcg/dL	Decreased in chronic infection
Cultures of blood	Normally sterile, without microorganism growth	Presence of microorganism; growth may indicate infection
Cultures of wound, sputum, and throat	Possible normal flora	Presence of microorganism growth may indicate infection
Urinalysis	Nitrite and leukocyte negative	Nitrite and leukocyte positive, WBC greater than 20/mm³
DIFFERENTIAL COUNT (PERCENTAGE OF EACH TYPE OF WBC)		
Neutrophils	55%-70%	Increased in acute infection, may be decreased in overwhelming bacterial infection (older adult)
Lymphocytes	20%-40%	Increased in chronic bacterial and viral infection, decreased in sepsis
Monocytes	2%-8%	Increased in protozoal, rickettsial, and tuberculosis infections
Eosinophils	1%-4%	Increased in parasitic infection
Basophils	0.5%-1%	Normal during infection

care. Some patients and their families wish to know more about the disease process, whereas others only want to know the interventions necessary to treat the infection and prevent future infections. Encourage patients to verbalize their expectations so that you are able to establish interventions to meet patients' priorities.

■■■NURSING DIAGNOSIS

Following assessment, review all of your findings, analyze clusters of defining characteristics, and select accurate and relevant nursing diagnoses. For the nursing diagnosis *risk for infection*, defining characteristics include risk factors such as inadequate primary defenses (e.g., broken skin or stasis of body fluids), inadequate secondary defenses (e.g., decreased hemoglobin and white blood cells), and chronic disease.

Clusters of defining characteristics lead to the selection of a nursing diagnosis. The related factors, revealed in the assessment, ensure individualization of the diagnosis. For example, you have a patient with a decreased WBC count, multiple intravenous catheters, and inflammation around a single catheter site. You diagnose the patient as being at *risk for infection related to intravenous catheter placement*. The related factor, *intravenous catheter placement*, will direct you to change the catheter regularly and take measures to minimize microorganism transfer through the intravenous system, such as scrubbing the hub of the catheter before accessing the intravenous line to give medication (Marschall and others, 2008). An accurate related factor ensures a more thorough care plan.

Infection or its associated treatment is the related factor for a number of nursing diagnoses. In the case of the diagnosis *social isolation*, the related factor is sometimes the isolation precautions used. Direct nursing interventions in these situations at minimizing the effect isolation has on the patient's ability to socialize. Nursing diagnoses you might use with patients susceptible to or affected by infection include the following:

- *Disturbed body image*
- *Risk for falls*
- *Risk for infection*
- *Imbalanced nutrition: less than body requirements*
- *Acute pain*
- *Impaired skin integrity*
- *Social isolation*
- *Impaired tissue integrity*

The presence of an actual infection poses a collaborative problem requiring your intervention. Objective data such as an elevated temperature, open draining wound, inflammation of a wound site, and laboratory values revealing an increased WBC count indicate an actual infection. Subjective findings include the patient's complaint of chills, malaise, or tenderness at the wound site. Work with health care providers, registered dietitians, and other team members in monitoring the infection, providing therapies such as antibiotic administration and wound care and implementing appropriate infection prevention and control measures.

■■■PLANNING

Develop the patient's care plan based on each nursing diagnosis. For each diagnosis identify specific goals and outcomes, set priorities, and plan for continuing care after discharge.

GOALS AND OUTCOMES Select achievable goals in collaboration with the patient, family, and other health care team members. For example, in an acute care setting your goal for the diagnosis *risk for infection* is "to control or decrease the progression of infection." An outcome is "Patient's wound drainage decreases in 3 days." In this plan you involve other members of the health care team such as the infection prevention and control nurse or the wound care nurse as necessary.

SETTING PRIORITIES Set the priorities for care based on the patient's nursing diagnoses. Give special attention to any urgent needs the infection creates. For example, if the patient's infection becomes systemic, you will need to manage fever and prevent dehydration. Once the infection begins to resolve, focus priorities on patient education and emotional support.

COLLABORATIVE CARE It is important that the patient's required level of care be maintained after discharge. Assess the patient, family, and other caregivers for their ability to provide care at home. For example, assess whether the patient or a family member is able to perform necessary dressing changes. Involve other members of the health care team such as the discharge planner or social services if necessary.

■■■IMPLEMENTATION

Your nursing interventions will control and prevent infection. These interventions are applicable for all types of health care settings, including the patient's home.

HEALTH PROMOTION Prevention is key to reducing infections in all health care settings. Review with and teach patients and their families measures that strengthen the host's defenses, such as nutrition, recommended immunizations, personal hygiene, and regular rest and exercise (Box 13-5). In addition, explain infection prevention and control principles, such as hand hygiene and methods for disposing of medical waste, designed to prevent infections from occurring. Based on your assessment of the patient's cultural views and preferences integrate infection prevention and control measures into the patient's daily lifestyle and cultural practices.

Nutrition Nutrition has a major influence on resistance to infection. Nutritional requirements vary depending on age, health status, and other variables. A proper diet helps the immune system function and consists of a variety of foods from all food groups (see Chapter 32). In collaboration with registered dietitians or alone, design education programs specific to patients' learning needs. Cultural considerations such as food selection and method of preparation are critical in influencing a patient's nutritional status. Teach the patient the importance a proper diet plays in maintaining immunity and preventing infection. Incorporate the patient's food preferences when possible.

Hygiene One infection prevention and control goal of personal hygiene is to reduce microorganisms on the skin and maintain the well-being of mucous membranes such as the mouth and vagina (Fauerbach, 2005). Patients need to understand the techniques for cleansing the skin and how to avoid spread of microorganisms in body secretions or excretions. For example, teach the patient to wash the perineum from clean to dirty, from the urethra down toward the rectum, using a clean washcloth (see Chapter 28). Also encourage the patient to maintain good oral hygiene.

Immunization Immunization programs for infants and children have decreased the occurrence of many childhood diseases such as diphtheria, whooping cough, and measles. More recently developed vaccines for hepatitis A and chickenpox (varicella) provide immunity to both adults and children for highly communicable diseases (Haiduvian and Poland, 2005). In addition, specific vaccines such as influenza and pneumococcal vaccines have decreased the mortality and morbidity previously seen in older adults or patients with underlying medical problems such as chronic lung disease (CLD). Advise patients about the advantages of immunizations, but also make them aware of the contraindications for certain vaccines, especially in pregnant or lactating women.

Adequate Rest and Regular Exercise Adequate rest (see Chapter 30) and regular exercise help prevent infection. Physical exercise increases lung capacity, circulation, energy, and endurance. It also decreases stress and improves appetite, sleeping, and elimination. Balance the need for regular exercise with the need for rest and sleep. Some patients need education stressing the importance of sleep and rest for infection prevention.

ACUTE CARE A patient with an infection has many needs. By monitoring the course of the infection carefully, you choose the most appropriate measures to maintain or restore the patient's health. Disinfection and sterilization of supplies and good hand hygiene are examples of aseptic methods used to control the spread of microorganisms.

When a patient develops an infection, continue preventive care to reduce the risk for transmission to health care workers and other patients. Good hand hygiene and use of barriers, such as gloves or masks, minimize everyone's exposure to infection (Hilburn and others, 2003). These measures are known as **standard precautions,** which are used routinely with every patient regardless of diagnosis. Patients with communicable diseases and infections that are easily transmissible to others require special precaution called **transmission-based precautions** (CDC, 2007). Isolation precautions involve control of a patient's environment by forming barriers against bacterial spread.

Treatment of an infection includes identification and elimination of the organism and support of the patient's defenses. Nurses collect specimens of body fluids or drainage from infected body sites and send the specimens to the laboratory for cultures. When the causative organism is identified, the health care provider may prescribe an antibiotic. Administer antibiotics carefully, watching for allergic reactions and assessing the effect on the patient's infection. If the patient is discharged

BOX 13-5   PATIENT TEACHING

Infection Prevention and Control

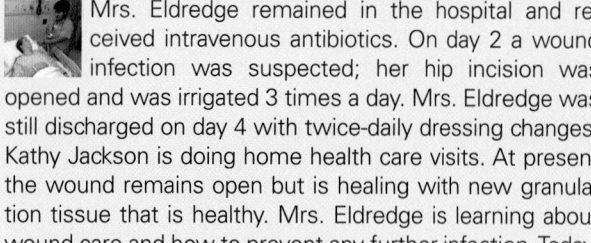 Mrs. Eldredge remained in the hospital and received intravenous antibiotics. On day 2 a wound infection was suspected; her hip incision was opened and was irrigated 3 times a day. Mrs. Eldredge was still discharged on day 4 with twice-daily dressing changes. Kathy Jackson is doing home health care visits. At present the wound remains open but is healing with new granulation tissue that is healthy. Mrs. Eldredge is learning about wound care and how to prevent any further infection. Today, Kathy is visiting Mrs. Eldredge and is teaching her about infection prevention and control practices

OUTCOME
- Patient will assume self-care using proper infection prevention and control techniques.

TEACHING STRATEGIES
- Instruct patient about proper hand-hygiene practices before and after wound care.
- Demonstrate proper hand hygiene, explaining that the patient should perform before and after all wound care and when infected body fluids are contacted.
- Instruct patient about the signs and symptoms of wound infection and when to notify the physician.
- Instruct patient to place contaminated dressings and other disposable items containing infectious body fluids in impervious plastic or brown paper bags. Place needles in metal containers such as soda cans or coffee cans and tape the openings shut. **Some states have specific requirements for sharps disposal. Check local regulations.**
- Instruct patient to clean noticeably soiled linen separate from other laundry. Wash in warm water with detergent. No special recommendations for setting dryer temperature.

EVALUATION STRATEGIES
- Ask patient to describe techniques used to reduce transmission of infection.
- Have patient demonstrate hand hygiene and disposal of contaminated dressings.
- Ask patient to identify signs of recurring wound infection.

home while receiving antibiotics, educate the patient on the importance of completing the antibiotic as prescribed.

Systemic infections, those that affect the body as a whole, require measures to manage or prevent the complications of fever (see Chapter 14). Drinking fluids regularly prevents dehydration resulting from diaphoresis. Increased metabolism requires an adequate nutritional intake. Rest preserves energy for the healing process.

Localized infections often require measures to facilitate removal of infectious organisms such as using moist-to-dry dressings or irrigating wounds (see Chapter 36) to remove infected drainage from wound sites. Applying warm compresses helps blood flow to an infected site, thus delivering components of the blood needed to fight an infection. Use medical and surgical aseptic techniques to manage wounds and handle infected drainage or body fluids correctly.

During any infection you support the patient's body defense mechanisms. For example, when a patient has diarrhea, cleanse the skin promptly and dry it thoroughly to prevent breakdown.

Medical Asepsis Basic medical aseptic techniques break the infection chain. You will use these techniques for all patients, even when there is not an infection diagnosed. Aggressive preventive measures are highly effective in reducing HAIs.

Control or Elimination of Infectious Agents. With the increased use of disposable equipment, nurses are sometimes less aware of disinfection and sterilization procedures. The proper cleaning, disinfection, and sterilization of contaminated objects significantly reduces and/or eliminates microorganisms (CDC, 2008b; Rutala and Weber, 2005).

Cleaning. Cleaning involves removing organic material such as blood or inorganic material such as soil from objects. Generally this involves the use of water, a detergent/disinfectant, and proper mechanical scrubbing action. Cleaning occurs before disinfection and sterilization procedures (CDC, 2008b; Rutala and Weber, 2005). Check the policy of the health care facility before cleaning. In most institutions technicians will clean equipment. When cleaning objects soiled with blood or body fluids, apply personal protective equipment (PPE) such as gloves, goggles, and mask to protect yourself from splashing fluids.

Disinfection and Sterilization. Disinfection and sterilization use both physical and chemical processes. Both processes disrupt the internal functioning of microorganisms by destroying cell proteins. **Disinfection** eliminates almost all pathogenic organisms, with the exception of bacterial spores. **Sterilization** eliminates or destroys all forms of microbial life, including spores (Rutala and Weber, 2005). Sterilization methods include processing items using steam, dry heat, hydrogen peroxide plasma, or ethylene oxide (ETO). The level of disinfection and sterilization required depends on the type and use of the contaminated item (Box 13-6). You have the responsibility of checking for package integrity and/or expiration dates before using an object designated as sterile. Dispose of items not meeting the criteria for being sterile, or return them to the sterilization-processing department (CDC, 2008b).

Control or Elimination of Reservoirs To control or eliminate infection in reservoir sites, eliminate sources of body fluids, drainage, or solutions that possibly harbor microorganisms. In addition, carefully discard disposable articles that become contaminated with infectious material (Box 13-7).

Control of Portals of Exit To control organisms exiting through the respiratory tract, avoid talking, sneezing, or coughing directly over a surgical wound or sterile dressing field. Also teach patients to protect others when they sneeze or cough, and give patients disposable wipes or tissues to control spread of microorganisms. Try not to work with

BOX 13-6   Categories of Items Requiring Sterilization, Disinfection, and Cleaning

CRITICAL ITEMS

Items that enter sterile tissue or the vascular system present a high risk for infection if the items are contaminated with microorganisms, especially bacterial spores. *Critical items* must be *sterile*. Some of these items follow:

- Surgical instruments
- Cardiac or intravascular catheters
- Urinary catheters
- Implants

SEMICRITICAL ITEMS

Items that come in contact with mucous membranes or nonintact skin also present a risk. These objects must be free of all microorganisms (except bacterial spores). *Semicritical items* must be *high-level disinfected (HLD)* or *sterilized*. Some of these items follow:

- Respiratory and anesthesia equipment
- Endoscopes
- Endotracheal tubes
- Gastrointestinal endoscopes
- Diaphragm fitting rings
  After rinsing, items must be dried and stored in a manner to protect from damage and contamination.

NONCRITICAL ITEMS

Items that come in contact with intact skin but not mucous membranes must be clean. *Noncritical items* must be *disinfected*. Some of these items follow:

- Bedpans
- Blood pressure cuffs
- Bed rails
- Linens
- Stethoscopes
- Bedside trays and patient furniture
- Food utensils

BOX 13-7   Infection Prevention and Control to Reduce Reservoirs of Infection

BATHING

- Use soap and water to remove drainage, dried secretions, or excess perspiration.

DRESSING CHANGES

- Change dressings that become wet and/or soiled (see Chapter 36).

CONTAMINATED ARTICLES

- Place tissues, soiled dressings, or soiled linen in fluid-resistant bags for proper disposal.

CONTAMINATED SHARPS

- Place all needles—safety needles and needleless systems—into puncture-proof containers, which should be located at the site of use. Federal law requires the use of needle safety technology. Blood tube holders are single use only (OSHA, 2001).

BEDSIDE UNIT

- Keep table surfaces clean and dry.

BOTTLED SOLUTIONS

- Do not leave bottled solutions open.
- Keep solutions tightly capped.
- Date bottles when opened, and discard in 24 hours.

SURGICAL WOUNDS

Keep drainage tubes and collection bags patent to prevent accumulation of serous fluid under the skin surface.

DRAINAGE BOTTLES AND BAGS

- Wear gloves and protective eyewear if splashing or spraying with contaminated blood or body fluids is anticipated.
- Empty and dispose of drainage suction bottles according to facility policy.
- Empty all drainage systems on each shift unless otherwise ordered by a physician.
- Never raise a drainage system (e.g., urinary drainage bag) above the level of the site being drained unless it is clamped off.

---

patients who are highly susceptible to infection if you have a cold or other communicable infection.

Another way of controlling the exit of microorganisms is by using standard precautions when handling body fluids such as urine, feces, and wound drainage. Wear clean gloves if there is a chance of contact with any blood or body fluids, and perform hand hygiene after providing care. Be sure to bag contaminated items appropriately.

Control of Transmission Effective infection prevention and control requires that you know the modes of transmission of microorganisms and the methods of control. In any health care setting a patient usually has a personal set of care items. Sharing graduated containers for measuring urine, bath basins, and eating utensils easily readily to transmission of infection. When using a stethoscope, always wipe off the bell, diaphragm, and ear tips with a disinfectant (such as an alcohol wipe) before proceeding to the next patient. Ear tips

are a common location for staphylococcal organisms (Guinto and others, 2002).

Because certain microorganisms travel easily through the air, do not shake linens or bedclothes. Dust with a treated or dampened cloth to prevent dust particles from entering the air.

To prevent transmission of microorganisms through indirect contact, do not allow soiled items and equipment to touch your clothing. A common error is to carry dirty linen in the arms against the uniform. Use special linen bags, or carry soiled linen with the hands held out from the body. Never put clean or soiled linens on the floor.

Hand Hygiene. The most important and most basic technique in preventing and controlling transmission of infection is hand hygiene (Box 13-8). Hand hygiene (Box 13-9) is a general term that applies to hand washing, antiseptic handwash, antiseptic hand rub, or surgical hand antisepsis. Hand washing refers to washing hands with plain soap and water. An antiseptic handwash means washing hands with water and soap or other detergents containing an antiseptic agent. An antiseptic hand rub means an antiseptic hand rub prod-

uct, such as alcohol, applied to all surfaces of the hands to reduce the number of microorganisms present. Surgical hand antisepsis is an antiseptic handwash or antiseptic hand rub technique that surgical personnel perform preoperatively to eliminate transient and reduce resident hand flora. Antiseptic detergent preparations have persistent antimicrobial activity (CDC, 2008a).

When hands are visibly dirty or contaminated with proteinaceous material or visibly soiled with blood or other body fluids, wash them with either a plain soap or an antimicrobial soap and water. Hand washing is also indicated before eating, after using the restroom, and if you become exposed to spore-forming organisms (e.g., *Clostridium difficile*) (Underwood, 2005). You may use an alcohol-based hand rub for routinely decontaminating hands in the following situations:

1. Before, after and between direct patient contact (e.g., taking a pulse, lifting a patient, performing a procedure).
2. Before putting on sterile gloves and before inserting indwelling urinary catheters, peripheral vascular catheters, or other invasive devices
3. After contact with body fluids or excretions, mucous membranes, nonintact skin and wound dressings *if hands are not visibly soiled*
4. When moving from a contaminated body site to a clean body site during care
5. After contact with surfaces or objects in the patient's room (e.g., overbed table, bed linen, IV pump).
6. After removing gloves (CDC, 2008a)

You may also wash hands with an antimicrobial soap and water in these situations.

Isolation and Barrier Protection. In 2007 the CDC published revised guidelines for isolation precautions. Facilities modify these guidelines according to need and as dictated by state or local regulations (Seigel and others, 2007). The CDC recommendations contain two tiers of precautions (Table 13-5, p. 243). The first and most important tier is called standard precautions, and the CDC designed it to be used for care of all patients, in all settings, regardless of diagnosis. Standard precautions apply to contact with blood, body fluid, nonintact skin, and mucous membranes from all patients. These precautions protect the patient and provide protection for the health care worker as directed by the Occupational Safety and Health Administration (Box 13-10, p. 244).

Assess the need for barrier precautions based on potential transmission of infection, regardless of the patient's diagnosis. For example, because droplet nuclei transmit TB, you need only a special mask or respirator as a barrier protection. When suctioning a patient with a tracheostomy, wearing gloves, eyewear, and a mask is appropriate protection.

The second tier of precautions the CDC designed is for care of patients with specific types of infection. The precautions apply to patients known or suspected to be infected or colonized with microorganisms transmitted by droplets, by

---

BOX 13-8   BEST PRACTICES

Factors Promoting Hand and Fingernail Hygiene Practices

SUMMARY OF EVIDENCE

Health care workers' hands are a potential source of contaminants. Contaminated hands and fingernails have the potential to pass microorganisms from one patient to the next. Evidence supports the use of specific products for routine hand hygiene. A research study compared products to determine the effect of an alcohol gel hand sanitizer by caregivers on infection types and rates in an acute care facility (Hilburn and others, 2003). Researchers collected data during a 13-month period when an orthopedic unit used alcohol gel hand sanitizers. The researchers compared the findings with data from the same unit during a baseline period when they did not use the sanitizers. The study demonstrated a 36.1% decrease in infection rates during the time when they used the hand sanitizer, indicating that use of an alcohol hand sanitizer decreased infection rates and provided a valuable tool for infection prevention and control.

In addition, there is strong evidence to support the fact that artificial nails, long nails, and nails with nail polish harbor an increased number of microorganisms. Boyce and Pittet (2008) analyzed multiple research studies documenting the presence of increased microorganisms in health care workers with artificial and long nails. In addition, long nails also carried more pathogens than short, well-manicured nails. Last, nail polish, especially cracked nail polish, was another area on the nails with increased microorganisms.

APPLICATION TO NURSING PRACTICE
- Use the hand gel correctly to ensure maximum antibacterial effect.
- Proper hand hygiene, including the use of alcohol hand gels, helps to prevent transmission of infections to health care workers' patients.
- Do not wear long, polished, or artificial nails in patient care settings.
- Keep nails well manicured, and free of rough edges, hangnails, or cuticle cuts.

Data from Hilburn J and others: Use of alcohol hand sanitizer as an infection control strategy in an acute care facility, *Am J Infect Control* 31:119, 2003; Boyce JM, Petit D: *HICPAC/SHEA/APIC/IDSA Hand Hygiene Task Force and the CDC Healthcare Control Practices Advisory Committee guidelines for hand hygiene in health care settings,* Atlanta, 2008, Centers for Disease Control and Prevention.

Text continued on p. 246.

BOX 13-9   PROCEDURAL GUIDELINES

Hand Hygiene

DELEGATION CONSIDERATIONS: The skill of hand hygiene is performed by all caregivers. *Hand hygiene is not optional.*

EQUIPMENT: Alcohol-based waterless antiseptic containing emollients, easy-to-reach sink with warm running water, antimicrobial or nonantimicrobial soap, paper towels or air dryer, and disposable nail cleaner *(optional)*

1 Inspect surface of hands for breaks or cuts in skin or cuticles.

2 Note condition of nails. Nail tips should be less than ¼ inch long and free of artificial nails or extenders or polish, especially cracked polish. Avoid artificial nails and long or unkempt nails, which harbor microbial loads (CDC, 2008a). Your agency may ban these depending upon their policy. Report and cover any skin lesions before providing patient care.

3 Inspect hands for visible soiling.

4 Push wristwatch and long uniform sleeves above wrists. Avoid wearing rings. If worn, remove during washing. Be sure fingernails are short, filed, and smooth.

5 Hand antisepsis using an instant alcohol waterless antiseptic rub:

   a **Following manufacturer's directions,** dispense ample amount of product into palm of one hand (see illustration).

   b Rub hands together, covering all surfaces of hands and fingers with antiseptic (see illustration).

   c Rub hands together until the alcohol is dry. Allow hands to completely dry before applying gloves.

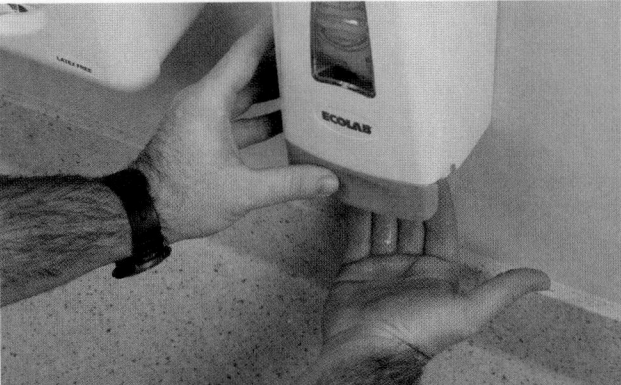

Step 5a ■ Apply waterless antiseptic to hands.

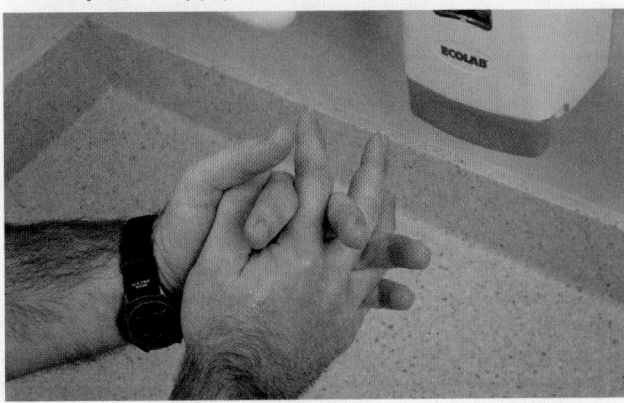

Step 5b ■ Rub hands thoroughly.

6 Hand washing using regular lotion soap or antimicrobial soap and water:

   a Stand in front of sink, keeping hands and uniform away from sink surface. (If hands touch sink during hand washing, repeat.)

   b Turn faucet on or push knee pedals laterally or press pedals with foot to regulate flow and temperature (see illustration).

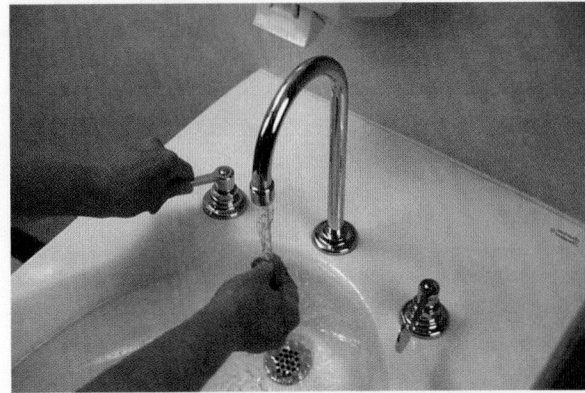

Step 6b ■ Regulate flow of water.

   c Avoid splashing water against uniform.

   d Regulate flow of water so that temperature is warm.

   e Wet hands and wrists thoroughly under running water. Keep hands and forearms lower than elbows during washing.

   f Apply 3 to 5 mL of antiseptic soap, and rub hands together, lathering thoroughly (see illustration, p. 242). Soap granules and leaflet preparations may be used.

Critical Decision Point: The decision whether to use an antiseptic soap or alcohol-based hand sanitizer is dependent on the procedure you will perform and the patient's immune status.

   g Wash hands using plenty of lather and friction for at least 15 seconds. A tip is to sing the Happy Birthday song twice. Interlace fingers, and rub palms and back of hands with circular motion at least 5 times each. Keep fingertips down to facilitate removal of microorganisms.

   h Areas under fingernails are often soiled. Clean them with the fingernails of other hand and additional soap, or clean with a disposable nail cleaner.

   i Rinse hands and wrists thoroughly, keeping hands down and elbows up (see illustration, p. 242).

   j Dry hands thoroughly from fingers to wrists and forearms with paper towel, single-use cloth, or warm air dryer.

   k If used, discard paper towel in proper receptacle.

   l To turn off hand faucet, use clean, dry paper towel. Avoid touching handles with hands (see illustration, p. 242). Turn off water with foot or knee pedals (if applicable).

BOX 13-9   PROCEDURAL GUIDELINES—cont'd

Hand Hygiene—cont'd

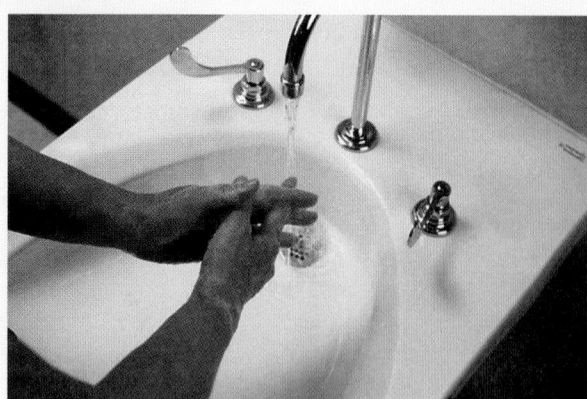

Step 6f ■ Lather hands thoroughly.

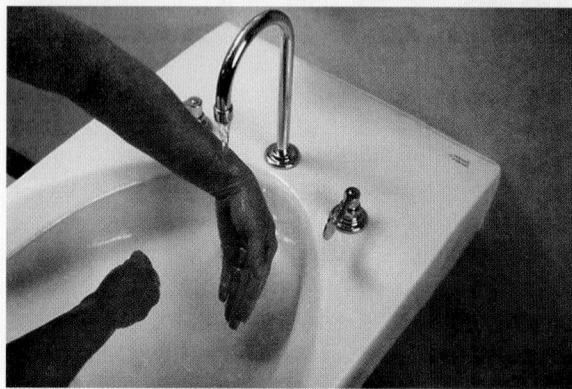

Step 6i ■ Rinsing hands.

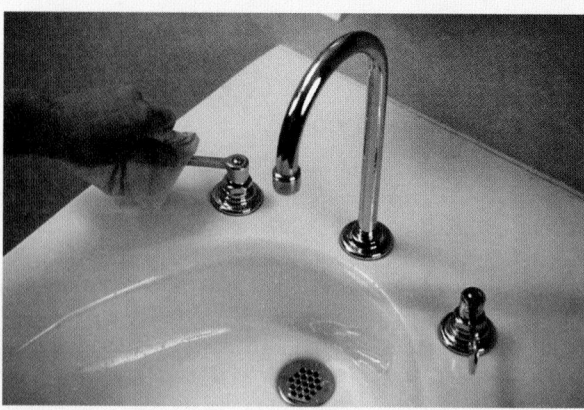

Step 6l ■ Turning off faucet with clean, dry paper towel.

7 Apply lotion to hands. Use the facility-provided lotion if available. Avoid petroleum-based lotions.

TABLE 13-5　Centers for Disease Control and Prevention Isolation Guidelines

STANDARD PRECAUTIONS (TIER 1) FOR USE WITH ALL PATIENTS

- Standard precautions apply to blood, blood products, all body fluids, secretions, excretions (except sweat), nonintact skin, and mucous membranes.
- Perform hand hygiene before, after, and between direct contact with patients. (Example of between contact – cleaning hands after a patient care activity, moving to a non patient care activity, then cleaning hands again before returning to perform patient contact).
- Perform hand hygiene after contact with blood, body fluids, secretions, and excretions and after contact with surfaces or articles in a patient room; and immediately after gloves are removed.
- When hands are visibly soiled or contaminated with blood or body fluids, wash them with either a nonantimicrobial soap or an antimicrobial soap and water.
- When hands are not visibly soiled or contaminated with blood or body fluids, use an alcohol-based hand rub to perform hand hygiene.
- Wash hands with nonantimicrobial soap and water if contact with spores (e.g., *Clostridium difficile*) is likely to have occurred.
- Do not wear artificial fingernails or extenders if duties include direct contact with patients at high risk for infection and associated adverse outcomes.
- Wear gloves when touching blood, body fluids, secretions, excretions, nonintact skin, mucous membranes, or contaminated items or surfaces is likely. Remove gloves and perform hand hygiene between patient care encounters and when going from a contaminated to a clean body site.
- Wear PPE when the anticipated patient interaction indicates that contact with blood or body fluids may occur.
- A private room is unnecessary unless the patient's hygiene is unacceptable (e.g. uncontained secretions, excretions or wound drainage).
- Discard all contaminated sharp instruments and needles in a puncture-resistant container. Health care facilities must make available needleless devices. Any needles should be disposed of uncapped or a mechanical safety device is activated for recapping.
- Respiratory hygiene/cough etiquette: Have patients cover the nose/mouth when coughing or sneezing; use tissues to contain respiratory secretions, and dispose of in nearest waste container; perform hand hygiene after contacting respiratory secretions and contaminated object/materials; contain respiratory secretions with procedure or surgical masks; sit at least 3 feet away from others if coughing.

TRANSMISSION-BASED PRECAUTIONS (TIER TWO) FOR USE WITH SPECIFIC TYPES OF PATIENTS

CATEGORY	INFECTION/CONDITION	BARRIER PROTECTION
Airborne precautions (Droplet nuclei smaller than 5 microns)	Measles, chickenpox (varicella), disseminated varicella zoster, pulmonary or laryngeal tuberculosis	Private room, negative-pressure airflow of at least 6 to 12 exchanges per hour via HEPA filtration. Mask or respiratory protection device, n95 respirator (depending on condition)
Droplet precautions (Droplets larger than 5 microns; being with 3 feet of the patient)	Diphtheria (pharyngeal), rubella, streptococcal pharyngitis, pneumonia or scarlet fever in infants and young children, pertussis, mumps, *Mycoplasma* pneumonia, meningococcal pneumonia or sepsis, pneumonic plague	Private room or cohort patients. Mask or respirator is required (depending on condition) (refer to agency policy)
Contact precautions (Direct patient or environmental contact)	Colonization or infection with multidrug-resistant organisms such as VRE and MRSA, *Clostridium difficile*, shigella and other enteric pathogens; major wound infections; herpes simplex; scabies; varicella zoster (disseminated); respiratory syncytial virus in infants, young children or immunocompromised adults	Private room or cohort patients (see agency policy), gloves, gowns
Protective environment	Allogeneic hematopoietic stem cell transplants	Private room; positive airflow with 12 or more air exchanges per hour; HEPA filtration for incoming air. Mask to be worn by patient when out of room during times of construction in area.

HEPA, High efficiency particulate air; *MRSA,* methicillin-resistant *Staphylococcus aureus*; *TB,* tuberculosis; *VRE,* vancomycin-resistant enterococci.

Modified from Centers for Disease Control and Prevention, Hospital Infection Control Practice Advisory Committee: Guidelines for isolation precautions in hospitals, *MMWR Morb Mortal Wkly Rep* 57/RR-16:39, 2007.

BOX 13-10 PROCEDURAL GUIDELINES

Caring for a Patient on Isolation Precautions

DELEGATION CONSIDERATIONS: The skill of caring for patients on isolation precautions can be delegated to nursing assistive personnel (NAP). However, it is the nurse who assesses the patient's status and isolation indications. Instruct NAP about:

- Reason patient is on isolation precautions
- Special precautions regarding individual patient needs, such as transportation to diagnostic tests

EQUIPMENT: Personal protective equipment (PPE) determined by type of isolation: gowns, gloves, mask, protective eyewear or face shield; supplies necessary for procedures performed in room—soiled linen and trash receptacles, sharps container, disposable blood pressure (BP) cuff

1 Assess isolation indications (e.g., patient's medical history for exposure, laboratory tests, wound drainage).

2 Review laboratory test results to identify type of microorganism for which patient is isolated and if patient is immunosuppressed.

3 Review agency policies and precautions necessary for the specific isolation system, and consider care measures you will perform while in patient's room.

4 Review nurses' notes or speak with colleagues regarding patient's emotional state and adjustment to isolation.

5 Assess whether patient has a known latex allergy so as to avoid sensitivity or allergic reaction.

6 Perform hand hygiene, and prepare all equipment you will need to take into patient's room. In some cases, equipment may remain in the room (stethoscope or BP cuff). Decide which isolation equipment is necessary before entering the patient's room. For example, decide whether you will need a gown and gloves for a patient on contact precautions or if you will need a special respirator mask for a patient on airborne precautions.

7 Prepare for entrance into isolation room:

   a Apply cover gown, being sure it covers all outer garments. Pull sleeves down to wrist. Tie securely at neck and waist (see illustration).

   b Apply either surgical mask or fitted respirator around mouth and nose. (Type and fit-testing will depend on type of precautions and facility policy.) The nurse must have a medical evaluation and be fit tested before using a respirator (OSHA, 1995).

   c If needed, apply eyewear or goggles snugly around face and eyes. If prescription glasses are worn, side shield may be used.

   d Apply clean gloves. (NOTE: Wear unpowdered, latex-free gloves.) If gloves are worn with gown, bring glove cuffs over edge of gown sleeves (see illustration).

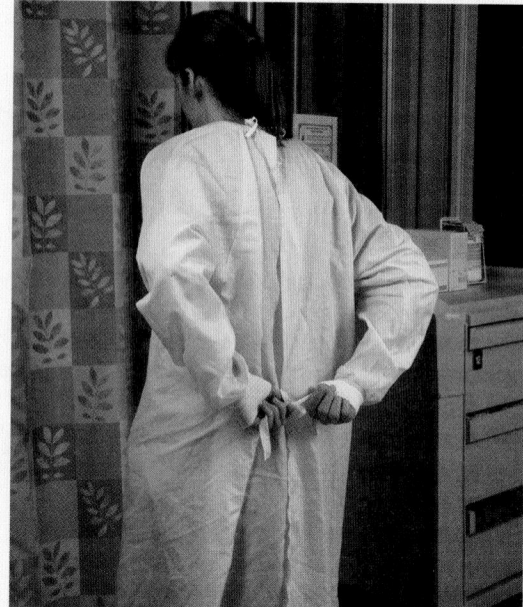

Step 7a ▪ Tying gown at waist.

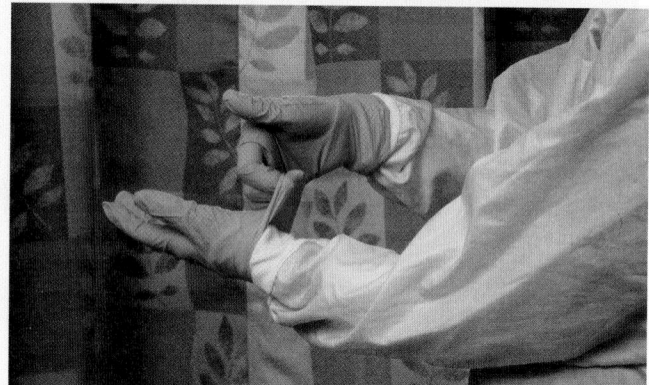

Step 7d ▪ Applying gloves over gown sleeves.

8 Enter patient's room. Arrange supplies and equipment. (If equipment will be removed from room for reuse, place on clean paper towel.)

9 Explain purpose of isolation and necessary precautions to patient and family. Offer opportunity to ask questions. Assess for evidence of emotional problems that can occur from isolation.

BOX 13-10	PROCEDURAL GUIDELINES

Caring for a Patient on Isolation Precautions—cont'd

10 Assess vital signs.

  a If patient is infected or colonized with a resistant organism (e.g., vancomycin-resistant enterococci [VRE], methicillin-resistant *Staphylococcus aureus* [MRSA]), equipment remains in room. This includes the stethoscope and blood pressure cuff.

  b If stethoscope is to be reused, clean diaphragm or bell with alcohol. Set aside on clean surface.

  c Use individual electronic or disposable thermometer.

Critical Decision Point: If disposable thermometers indicate a fever, assess for other signs/symptoms. Confirm fever using an electronic thermometer (Potter and others, 2003).

---

11 Administer medications (see Chapter 16):

  a Give oral medication in wrapper or cup.

  b Dispose of wrapper or cup in plastic-lined receptacle.

  c Administer injection, being sure to wear gloves.

  d Discard safety needle and syringe or uncapped needle into the sharps container.

  e Place a reusable syringe (e.g., Carpuject) on clean towel for eventual removal and disinfection.

  f If you are not wearing gloves and hands come into contact with contaminated article or body fluids, perform hand hygiene as soon as possible.

12 Administer hygiene, encouraging the patient to discuss questions or concerns about isolation. Use informal teaching at this time.

  a Avoid allowing gown to become wet. Carry washbasin out away from gown, avoid leaning against any wet surface.

  b Remove linen from bed; avoid contact with gown. Place in leakproof linen bag.

  c Change gloves and perform hand hygiene if they become excessively soiled and further care is necessary.

13 Collect specimens:

  a Place specimen containers on clean paper towel in patient's bathroom. Follow procedure for collecting specimen of body fluids.

  b Transfer specimen to container without soiling outside of container. Place container in plastic bag, and place label on outside of bag or as per facility policy.

  c Perform hand hygiene and reglove if additional procedures are needed.

  d Check label on specimen for accuracy. Send to laboratory. Label containers with a biohazard label (see illustration).

14 Dispose of linen and trash bags as they become full:

  a Use sturdy, moisture-resistant single bags to contain soiled articles. Use double bag if outside of bag is contaminated.

  b Tie bags securely at top in knot (see illustration).

15 Remove all reusable equipment. Clean any contaminated surfaces (check health care facility or agency policy).

16 Resupply room as needed. Have a staff member outside the isolation room hand you new supplies.

17 Explain to patient when you plan to return to room. Ask whether patient requires any personal care items, books, or magazines.

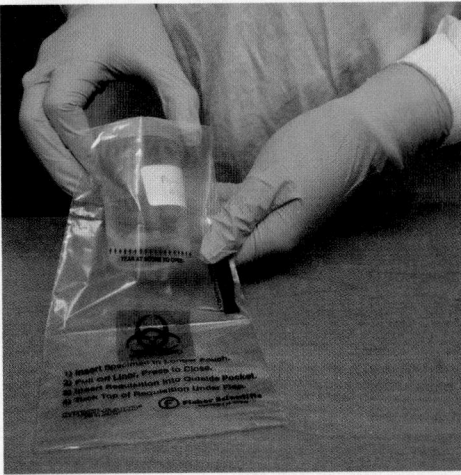

Step 13d ■ Specimen container placed in biohazard bag.

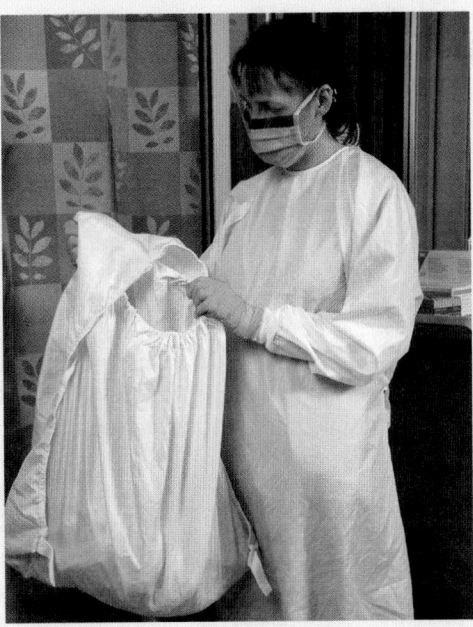

Step 14b ■ Tie trash bag securely.

BOX 13-10   PROCEDURAL GUIDELINES
Caring for a Patient on Isolation Precautions—cont'd

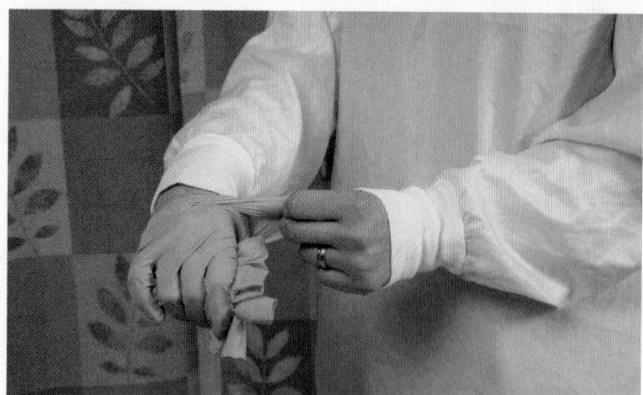

Step 18a ■ Removing gloves.

18 Leave isolation room. The order for removing PPE depends on what was needed for the type of isolation. The sequence listed is based on full PPE being required.
   a Remove gloves. Remove one glove by grasping cuff and pulling glove inside out over hand. Hold removed glove in glove hand. With ungloved hand, slide finger inside cuff of remaining glove at wrist. Pull glove off over first glove. Discard gloves in proper container (see illustration).
   b Remove eyewear/face shield or goggles by handling at headband or earpieces. Discard in proper container.
   c Untie neck strings and then back strings of gown. Allow gown to fall from shoulders (see illustration). Remove hands from sleeves without touching outside of gown. Hold gown inside at shoulder seams and fold inside out. Discard in laundry bag if gown is made of fabric or in trash can if gown is disposable.

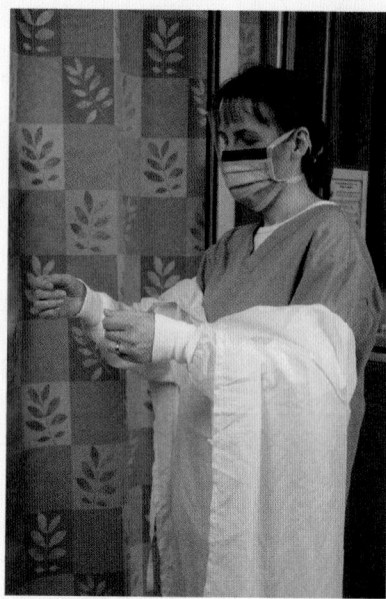

Step 18c ■ Remove gown by allowing it to fall from shoulders.

   d Remove mask—If mask loops over your ears, remove from ears and pull away from face. For a tie-on mask, untie *bottom* mask strings and then top strings. Hold top strings and pull mask away from face, and drop into trash receptacle. Do not touch outer surface of mask.
   e Perform hand hygiene.
   f Leave room and close door, if necessary. (Make sure door is closed if patient is on airborne precautions.)
   g Dispose of all contaminated supplies and equipment in a manner that prevents spread of microorganisms to other persons (check health care facility or agency policy).

the airborne route, or by contact with contaminated surfaces or dry skin. There are three types of transmission-based precautions: **airborne, droplet,** and **contact precautions.** They are used singly or in combination for diseases (e.g., chickenpox) that have multiple routes of transmission. Use them in addition to standard precautions.

Because of the resurgence of TB, the CDC (2005) has developed guidelines to prevent the transmission of TB in the health care worker and stresses the importance of isolation for the patient with known or suspected TB in a special negative-pressure room. Close the doors to the patient's room to control direction of airflow. Wear a special high-filtration particulate respirator on entering a respiratory isolation room. Make sure respirators are able to fit health care workers with different facial sizes and characteristics. When

worn correctly, particulate respirators and masks (Figures 13-3 and 13-4) have a tighter face seal and filter at a higher level than routine surgical masks (OSHA, 1995).

In 2007 the CDC issued guidelines for prevention of transmission of certain drug-resistant organisms, primarily vancomycin-resistant enterococci (VRE) and methicillin-resistant *Staphylococcus aureus* (MRSA). These guidelines included reducing inappropriate antimicrobial use and following procedures to reduce spread of the organisms within health care institutions.

Regardless of the type of isolation or barrier protection used, follow certain basic principles when delivering care in a patient's room. Understand how certain diseases are transmitted and what barriers you need to prevent transmission. For example, you do not routinely need to wear a gown or gloves when giving oral medications, but you do need these barriers when changing a dressing from a draining wound. However, gloves are appropriate when assisting a patient with an oral medication if the patient needs assistance putting the medication in the mouth.

Take care to avoid exposing an article brought into a patient's room to any infectious material. Bag or decontaminate any contaminated article (e.g., blood pressure cuff) according to agency policy. Decontaminate equipment that must be shared among patients.

Before you institute isolation measures, explain to the patient and family the nature of the patient's condition, the purpose of the isolation barriers, and ways to carry out specific precautions. Teach the patient and family the proper way to perform hand hygiene and apply gloves, masks, or gowns. Demonstrate each procedure, and give the patient and family an opportunity to practice.

Explain methods of transmission of infectious organisms so that the patient and family members understand the difference between contaminated and clean objects. Provide for the patient's sensory stimulation during isolation. Encourage the family to bring the patient reading materials, puzzle books, and similar items. Take the opportunity to listen to the patient's concerns or interests. If you rush care or show a lack of interest in the patient's needs, the patient will feel rejected and even more isolated. Explain the patient's potential risk for depression or loneliness to family members. Encourage visitors to avoid negative expressions or actions concerning isolation. Advise family members on ways to provide meaningful stimulation.

Protective Environment. In some situations you will use special rooms for highly susceptible patients, such as transplant recipients and patients with neutropenia (low white blood cell count). When a private room is recommended, post a card on the patient's room door, listing the precautions in use (check agency policy). The card is a handy reference for health care workers and visitors and alerts all who enter the room of any special precautions in use. Each facility is different, so make sure you follow the facility's policies on isolation practice (Seigel and others, 2007).

The isolation room or an adjoining anteroom, if present, will need to contain hand-hygiene supplies, bathing, and toilet facilities. Personnel and visitors need to perform hand hygiene before entering a patient's room and upon exiting the room. If toilet facilities are unavailable, there are special procedures for handling portable commodes, bedpans, or urinals (check agency policy). Store PPE in an anteroom between the room and hallway or in a convenient location close to the point of use. Resupply PPE as needed.

Each patient care room, including those used for isolation, contains a trash container with plastic liners. Rooms used for isolation also contain a soiled linen hamper. These containers prevent transmission of microorganisms by preventing leakage and waste from contaminating the outside surface. Have a disposable, rigid container available in the room to discard used needles, sharps, and syringes.

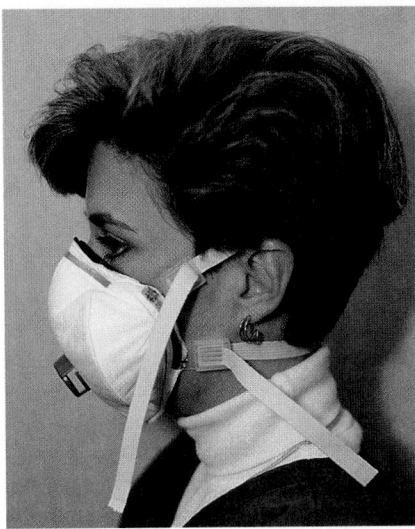

Figure 13-3 ■ Disposable high efficiency particulate air (HEPA)-purifying respirator.

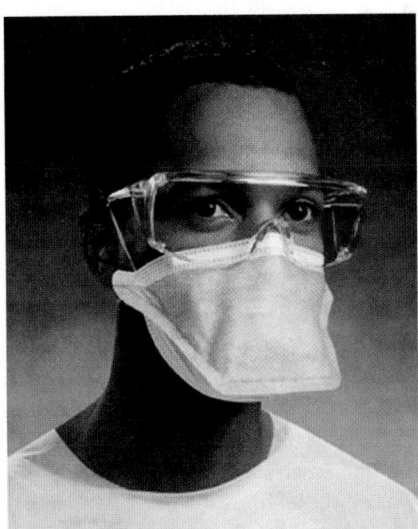

Figure 13-4 ■ N95 respirator mask with protective eyewear (Courtesy Kimberly-Clark Healthcare, Roswell, Ga.)

Depending on the microorganisms identified and the mode of transmission, critically evaluate what articles or equipment to take into an isolation room. For example, the Hospital Infection Control Practices Advisory Committee (HICPAC) of the CDC recommends taking only dedicated articles into an isolation room of a patient infected or colonized with VRE (CDC, 2007).

Personal Protective Equipment. Gowns or cover-ups protect health care workers from coming in contact with infected blood and body fluids or materials. Gowns used for barrier protection are made of a fluid-resistant material, and you need to change the gown immediately if it is damaged or heavily contaminated.

Gowns should be worn if soiling of the skin or clothing is likely from contact with blood, body fluids or if patient has uncontained secretions. Isolation gowns usually open at the back and have ties or snaps at the neck and waist to keep the gown closed and secure. A gown is long enough to cover all outer garments. Long sleeves with tight-fitting cuffs provide added protection.

Wear a mask or respirator if you anticipate splashing or spraying of blood or body fluids. The mask also protects you from inhaling microorganisms from a patient's respiratory tract and prevents the transmission of pathogens from your respiratory tract. Occasionally a patient who is susceptible to infection will wear a mask to prevent inhalation of pathogens. Patients requiring respiratory precautions wear surgical masks when ambulating or being transported outside of their room to protect other patients and personnel.

Masks prevent the transmission of infections caused by direct contact with mucous membranes. A mask discourages the wearer from touching the nose or mouth. A properly applied mask fits snugly over the mouth and nose so that the pathogens and body fluids cannot enter or escape through the sides (Box 13-11). If the person wears glasses, the top edge of the mask fits below the glasses so they will not cloud over as the person exhales. Keep talking to a minimum while wearing a mask. Discard a mask that has become moist, because it is ineffective. Discard the mask when leaving the patient's room. Warn patients and family members that a mask may cause a sensation of smothering. If family members become uncomfortable, have them leave the room and discard the mask.

Apply disposable gloves when there is a risk for exposing the hands to blood, body fluids, mucous membranes, nonintact skin, or potentially infectious material on objects or surfaces. In addition, use gloves when you have scratches or breaks in the skin and when performing venipuncture or finger or heel sticks. You may wear gloves alone or in combination with other PPE. When other PPE is necessary, first put on a mask and eyewear (if required), apply a gown (if required), and then apply gloves. Pull the glove cuffs up over the wrists or cuffs of a gown.

After contacting infectious material, change gloves and perform hand hygiene even if you have not finished caring for the patient. If your actions do not involve more patient contact, it is unnecessary to reapply gloves. Teach patients and their families the reasons for wearing gloves and the correct method for applying gloves.

Many gloves used for barrier protection or surgical asepsis are made of latex. Before applying latex gloves, assess the patient's potential for having a latex allergy. Individuals most at risk include those with a history of spina bifida, congenital or urogenital defects, indwelling urinary catheterization, use of condom catheters, multiple childhood surgeries, and food allergies. If the patient has a history of occupational exposure to latex, that too is a risk. The symptoms of latex allergy range

---

BOX 13-11　PROCEDURAL GUIDELINES

Applying a Surgical Type of Mask

DELEGATION CONSIDERATIONS: The skill of applying a surgical mask may be delegated when personnel are trained in required sterile procedure.

EQUIPMENT: Disposable mask

1 Find top edge of mask (usually has thin metal strip along edge). Pliable metal fits snugly against bridge of nose.
2 Hold mask by top two strings or loops. Tie two top ties at top of back of head (see illustration), with ties above ears. (*Alternative:* Slip loops over each ear.)

3 Tie two lower ties snugly around neck with mask well under chin (see illustration).
4 Gently pinch upper metal band around bridge of nose. NOTE: Change mask if wet, moist, or contaminated.

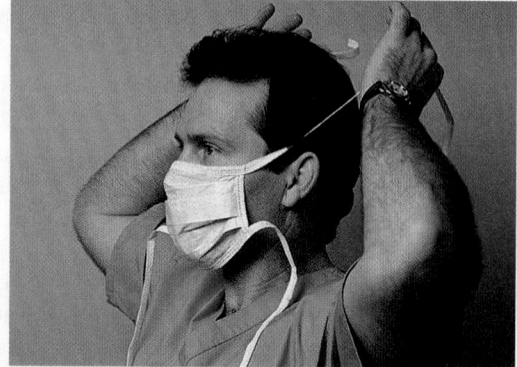

Step 2 ■ Attaching top two ties of a tie-on mask.

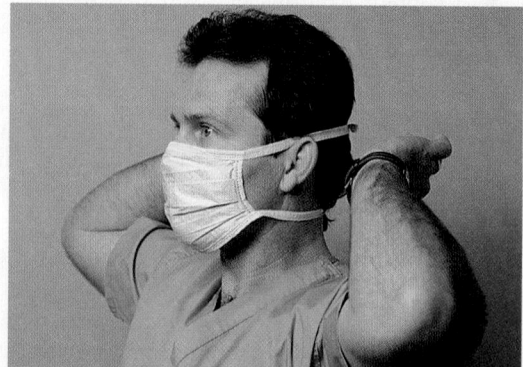

Step 3 ■ Securing the bottom two ties of a tie-on mask.

from mild dermatitis to severe anaphylactic shock. Latex sensitivity results from repeated contact or by inhaling aerosolized latex allergens contained in the glove powder.

The Association of periOperative Registered Nurses (2009) provides the following suggestions for nurses to avoid becoming latex allergic:

1. Whenever possible, wear powder-free gloves (they are lower in protein allergens).
2. Wear gloves only when indicated.
3. Wash with a pH-balanced soap immediately after removing gloves.
4. Apply only non–oil-based hand care products (oil-based products break down latex allergens).
5. If a reaction or dermatitis occurs, report to employee health service and/or seek medical treatment immediately.

Wear eyewear and face shields, properly fitted, during procedures where it is possible to splatter the eyes or face with blood or other infectious material (see Figure 13-4, p. 247). In many instances caregivers purchase their own eyewear with prescription lenses. Regular glasses are insufficient. Glasses need to have side shields to prevent material from entering the eye between the glasses and face.

Specimen Collection. A patient with a suspected or actual infectious disease sometimes undergoes many laboratory studies. Body fluids and materials suspected of containing infectious organisms are collected for culture and sensitivity tests. In the laboratory the specimen is placed in a special medium that promotes the growth of organisms. A laboratory technologist then identifies the type of microorganisms growing in the culture. Additional sensitivity test results indicate the antibiotics to which the organisms are resistant or sensitive. This helps the health care providers choose the proper medications to use in the patient's treatment.

Obtain all culture specimens with sterile equipment. Collecting fresh material from the site of infection, as in the case of wound drainage, ensures that resident flora do not contaminate the specimen. Seal all specimen containers tightly to prevent spillage and contamination of the outside of the container (Box 13-12). After you transfer the specimens to containers, label each specimen properly with the patient's name, patient identifier, date and time, and type of specimen. Label specimens in the presence of the patient (The Joint Commission [TJC], 2009). Place the specimen containers in labeled leak-proof biohazard bags before transporting them to the laboratory. Follow facility policy.

Bagging. Bagging articles generally is the same for all patients regardless of whether the patient is on isolation or not. Bagging articles prevents accidental exposure of personnel to contaminated articles and prevents contamination of the surrounding environment. Specific procedures for specimen transport are institution dependent (Ritter, 2005).

Place all soiled linen in a designated waterproof impervious bag in the patient's room. Do not overfill the bag. Handle,

transport, and process linen soiled with blood or body fluids in a way that will prevent exposure of skin or mucous membrane and/or contamination of the health care worker's clothing. Some hospitals still require double bagging. A standard-size linen bag, not overfilled, tied securely and intact is adequate to prevent infection transmission. Consult agency policy and any applicable regulations for the proper procedure.

Biohazardous waste includes both infectious and medical waste that must be disposed of in special red bags. These disposal procedures are a high expense for health care facilities. Consider the following waste materials as infectious or medical waste (Hedrick and Wideman, 2005):

- Cultures, including discarded cultures of infectious organisms
- Pathological waste, such as discarded human tissue, organs, and body parts
- Blood and blood products, including discarded serum or plasma and materials containing free-flowing blood
- Sharps, including discarded needles, syringes, scalpels, blood vials, broken or unbroken glass, and pipettes
- Selected isolation material, discarded waste material from patients with highly communicable diseases

Removal of Protective Equipment. The method of removing protective clothing, gloves, eyewear, gown, and mask before leaving an isolation room depends on the protective equipment worn at the time. If you wear all four protective items, first remove the gloves, because they are most likely to be contaminated. If you untie a gown with gloves still on, there is a chance of contaminating your hair or a portion of your uniform. The procedural guidelines for isolation precautions review steps for removing PPE (see Box 13-10, p. 244).

Transporting Patients. Patients infected with highly communicable organisms, such as the TB bacillus, may leave their rooms only for essential purposes such as diagnostic procedures or surgery. Before transferring the patient to a wheelchair or stretcher, give the patient the appropriate barrier protection. For example, a patient infected by an organism transmitted by the respiratory tract needs to wear a surgical mask. Personnel transporting the patient practice the appropriate precautions while in the patient's room and remove PPE upon leaving the patient's room. Notify personnel in diagnostic areas or the operating room that the patient is on isolation precautions. Record the type of isolation on the patient's chart, and explain ways to avoid transmitting infection during transport (Seigel and others, 2007).

Control of Portals of Entry Many measures that control the exit of microorganisms also control the entrance of pathogens. Evaluate the patient, and provide interventions to control and prevent organisms from gaining a portal of entry (Box 13-13).

Protection of the Susceptible Host A patient's resistance to infection improves by initiating measures that protect normal body defense mechanisms. In the acute care setting, many of the interventions either promote existing body de-

BOX 13-12	Specimen Collection Techniques*

Ensure that all specimen containers used have the biohazard symbol on the outside.

WOUND SPECIMEN

Clean site with sterile water or saline prior to wound specimen collection (see Chapter 36). Apply gloves and use cotton-tipped swab or syringe to collect as much drainage as possible. Have clean test tube or culture tube ready on clean paper towel. After swabbing center of wound site, grasp collection tube with a paper towel. Carefully insert swab without touching outside of tube. After securing tube's top, transfer tube into biohazard bag for transport and perform hand hygiene.

BLOOD SPECIMEN (This procedure is usually performed by the laboratory technician.)

Wearing gloves, use a needle safe syringe and culture media bottles to collect up to 10 mL of blood per culture bottle (check health care facility or agency policy). After prepping, perform venipuncture at two different sites to decrease likelihood of both specimens being contaminated with skin flora. Place blood culture bottles on a clean paper towel on bedside table or other surface; swab off bottle tops with alcohol. Inject appropriate amount of blood into each bottle. Transfer specimen into clean, labeled biohazard bag for transport. Remove gloves and perform hand hygiene.

STOOL SPECIMEN

Wearing gloves, use clean cup with seal top (need not be sterile) and tongue blade to collect small amount of stool, approximately 2 to 3 cm. Place cup on clean paper towel in patient's bathroom. Using tongue blade, collect needed amount of feces from patient's bedpan. Transfer feces to cup without touching cup's outside surface. Dispose of tongue blade, and place seal on cup. Transfer specimen into clean biohazard bag for transport. Remove gloves and perform hand hygiene.

URINE SPECIMEN

Apply gloves and use needle safe syringe and sterile cup to collect 1 to 5 mL of urine. Place cup or tube on clean towel in patient's bathroom. If patient has a urinary catheter, use a needleless safety syringe to collect specimen from the sampling port on the catheter (see manufacturer's instructions). Have patient follow procedure to obtain a clean voided specimen (see Chapter 33) if not catheterized. Secure top of transfer container, label for transport, and place in a biohazard bag. Remove gloves and perform hand hygiene.

From Pagana KD, Pagana TJ: *Mosby's diagnostic and laboratory test reference*, ed 9, St. Louis, 2009, Mosby.

*Health care facility or agency policies may differ on type of containers and amount of specimen material required.

BOX 13-13	Infection Control of Portals of Entry

INTACT SKIN AND MUCOSA
- Keep skin clean and well lubricated.
- Avoid positioning patients on tubes or objects that might cause breaks in skin.
- Use dry, wrinkle-free linen.
- Offer frequent oral hygiene (see Chapter 28).
- Provide frequent position changes for patients with impaired mobility.
- Clean skin of incontinent patients with nonabrasive agent; avoid drying with abrasive towel or tissue.

URINARY TRACT
- Teach women to clean rectum and perineum by wiping from area of least contamination (urinary meatus) toward area of most contamination (rectum).
- Do not allow urine in drainage bags and tubes to flow back into the bladder. Never raise a drainage system above the level of the bladder.
- Keep points of connection between catheter or drain and tubing closed.

INVASIVE TUBES AND LINES
- When obtaining specimens from drainage tubes or inserting needles into intravenous lines, disinfect tubes and ports by wiping them liberally with a disinfectant solution before entering the system. Scrub the hub before accessing the site.

WOUND CARE
- Keep draining wounds covered to contain drainage.
- Clean outward from a wound site using a clean swab for each application (see Chapter 36).

fense mechanisms or control exposure to microorganisms. For example, regular bathing removes transient microorganisms from the skin. Lubrication helps to keep the skin hydrated and intact. Regular oral hygiene removes proteins in the saliva that attract microorganisms. Flossing removes tartar and plaque that cause infection. An adequate fluid intake promotes normal urine formation and a resultant outflow of urine to flush the bladder and urethra of microorganisms. For immobilized or dependent patients, regular coughing and deep breathing exercises remove mucus from lower airways.

Role of the Infection Prevention and Control Department Most health care facilities employ health professionals who are specially trained in the area of infection prevention and control. Their responsibilities include collection and analysis of data on HAIs, surveillance of multidrug-resistant organisms, and providing consultation and education to staff and others on infection prevention and control.

Health Promotion in Health Care Workers and Patients A health care worker who becomes ill exposes susceptible patients to infectious diseases. An institution's employee health service provides programs to assist in infection prevention and control, such as immunization programs, recommendations for work restrictions, and protocols for management of job-related exposures to infectious diseases.

Surgical Asepsis Surgical asepsis, or aseptic technique, is designed to eliminate all microorganisms, including spores and pathogens, from an object and to protect an area from these microorganisms. Surgical asepsis requires more precautions than medical asepsis. Breaks in technique will result in contamination, thus increasing the patient's risk for infection (Church, 2005).

Although you commonly practice surgical asepsis in the operating room, labor and delivery area, and major diagnostic or procedural areas, you will also use surgical aseptic techniques at the patient's bedside (e.g., when inserting intravenous catheters). Use surgical asepsis during procedures that require intentional perforation of the patient's skin (e.g., surgical incision), when the skin's integrity is broken related to trauma or burns, and during procedures that involve insertion of a catheter or surgical instruments into sterile body cavities (AORN, 2009; Church, 2005).

Multiple steps involving sterile technique are used in the operating room, such as applying a mask, protective eyewear, and a cap; performing a surgical scrub; and applying a sterile gown and gloves. In contrast, performing a sterile dressing change at a patient's bedside requires only hand hygiene and putting on sterile gloves (Box 13-14). Regardless of the procedures followed in different settings, the use of surgical asepsis depends on developing an aseptic conscience. Always recognize the importance of strict adherence to aseptic principles. Also, be an excellent role model and patient advocate, reinforcing proper practice for other caregivers (AORN, 2009).

Preparation for Sterile Procedures In treatment rooms and at the bedside it is important to have a patient's full cooperation in maintaining aseptic technique. Therefore assess the patient's understanding of sterile procedure and the reasons for not moving or interfering with the procedure. Special precautions, such as masking the patient or changing the patient's position, are sometimes necessary to prevent contamination during procedures. Determine whether a patient has undergone a sterile procedure in the past. Explain how you will perform the procedure and what the patient can do to avoid contaminating sterile objects:

1. Avoid sudden movements of body parts covered by sterile drapes.
2. Do not touch sterile supplies, drapes, or your sterile gloves and gown.
3. Avoid coughing, sneezing, or talking over a sterile area.

Certain sterile procedures last for an extended time. Assess the patient's needs (e.g., pain control or elimination) in advance, and anticipate factors that will disrupt a procedure. If a patient is in pain, try to administer analgesics no more than 30 minutes before a sterile procedure begins. Patients often are placed in relatively uncomfortable positions during sterile procedures. Help the patient to assume the most comfortable position possible. Finally, the patient's condition sometimes results in events that contaminate a sterile field. For example, a patient with a respiratory infection coughs, transmitting organisms that contaminate the sterile field. Anticipate such a problem and have a solution ready, such as offering a mask to the patient before the procedure begins.

Principles of Surgical Asepsis Principles of surgical asepsis include the following:

1. *A sterile object remains sterile only when touched by another sterile object.* The following principles guide you in placement and handling of sterile objects:
   - Sterile touching sterile remains sterile; for example, wear sterile gloves to handle objects on a sterile field.
   - Sterile touching clean becomes contaminated; for example, if the sterile tip of a syringe touches the surface of a clean disposable glove, the syringe is contaminated.
   - Sterile touching contaminated becomes contaminated; for example, when you touch a sterile object with an ungloved hand, the object is contaminated.
   - Sterile touching questionable is contaminated; for example, when you find a tear or break in the covering of a sterile object, discard or reprocess it regardless of whether the object appears untouched.
2. *Place only sterile objects on a sterile field.* Be sure item is sterile before use. The package or container holding a sterile object must be intact and dry. A package that is torn, punctured, wet, or open is unsterile. When placing sterile items on sterile field (e.g., sterile drape), do not reach over the field (Figure 13-5).
3. *A sterile object or field out of the range of vision or an object held below a person's waist is contaminated.* Never turn your back on a sterile tray or leave it unattended. Any object held below waist level is considered contaminated because you cannot view it at all times. Keep sterile objects either on or out over the sterile field.
4. *A sterile object or field becomes contaminated by prolonged exposure to the air.* Avoid activities that create air currents, such as excessive movements or rearranging linen after a sterile object or field becomes exposed. When opening sterile packages, minimize the number of people walking into the area. Microorganisms also travel by droplet through the air. No one should talk, laugh, sneeze, or cough over a sterile field or when gathering and using sterile equipment. When opening a tray and adding sterile equipment, wear a mask. Microorganisms traveling through the air can fall on sterile items or fields if you reach over the work area (Box 13-15, p. 254).
5. *A sterile object or field becomes contaminated by capillary action when a sterile surface comes in contact with a wet contaminated surface.* Moisture seeps through a sterile package's protective covering, allowing microorganisms to travel to the sterile object. When stored sterile packages become wet, discard the objects immediately or send

BOX 13-14 PROCEDURAL GUIDELINES

Putting on Sterile Gloves

DELEGATION CONSIDERATIONS: The skill of sterile glove application may be delegated if personnel are qualified to perform sterile glove procedure.

EQUIPMENT: Pair of sterile gloves

1 Consider the procedure you will perform, and consult agency policy on use of gloves.

2 Inspect hands for cuts, open lesions, or abrasions. Cover with an occlusive dressing before gloving.

3 Assess whether the patient or health care worker has a known allergy to latex.

4 Determine correct glove size and type of glove material you will use.

5 Examine glove package to ensure package is not wet, torn, or discolored.

6 **Apply Sterile Gloves**

   a Perform thorough hand hygiene.

   b Remove outer glove package wrapper by carefully separating and peeling apart sides.

   c Grasp inner package, and lay it on clean, flat surface just above waist level. Open package, keeping gloves on wrapper's inside surface.

   d Identify right and left glove. Each glove has a cuff approximately 5 cm (2 inches) wide. Glove dominant hand first. In the illustrations, the left hand is dominant.

   e With thumb and first two fingers of nondominant hand, grasp edge of cuff of the glove for the dominant hand. Touch only glove's inside surface.

   f Carefully pull glove over dominant hand (see illustration 1), leaving a cuff and being sure the cuff does not roll up wrist. Be sure thumb and fingers are in proper spaces (see illustration 2).

   g With gloved dominant hand, slip fingers underneath second glove's cuff (see illustration).

   h Carefully pull second glove over nondominant hand (see illustration). Do not allow fingers and thumb of gloved dominant hand to touch any part of exposed nondominant hand. Keep thumb of dominant hand abducted.

   i After second glove is on, interlock hands and keep above waist level (see illustration). Cuffs usually fall down after application. Be sure to touch only sterile sides.

7 Dispose of gloves

   a Follow steps for glove removal (see Box 13-10, step 18a, p. 244).

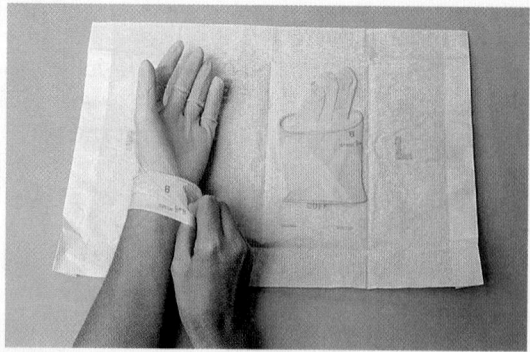

Step 6f(2) ■ Ensure thumb and fingers are in proper spaces.

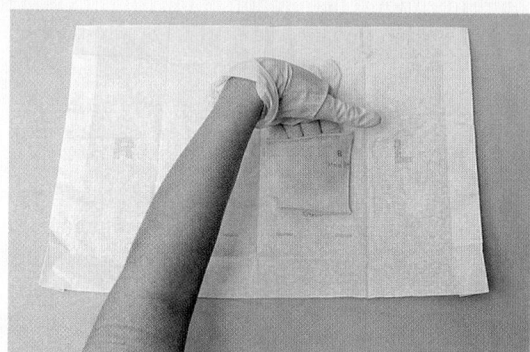

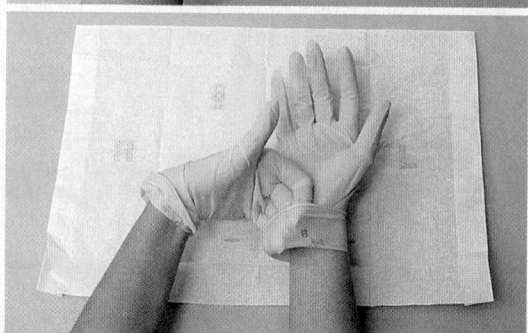

Steps 6g and h ■ Using gloved dominant hand to pull glove onto nondominant hand.

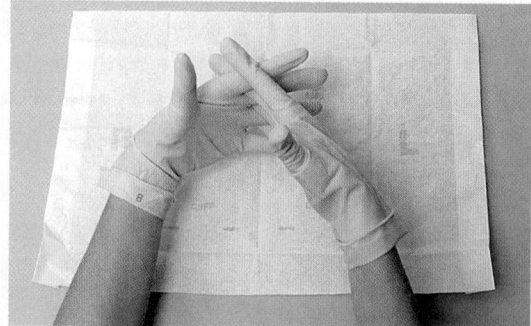

Step 6i ■ Interlock hands, touching only sterile sides.

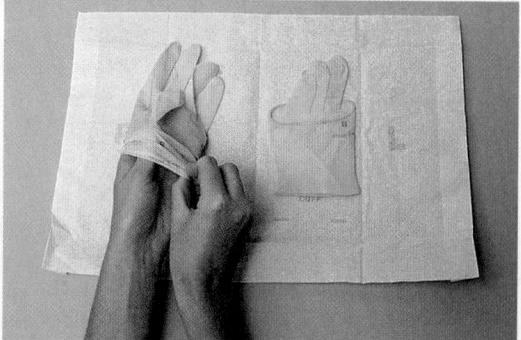

Step 6f(1) ■ Pulling glove over dominant hand.

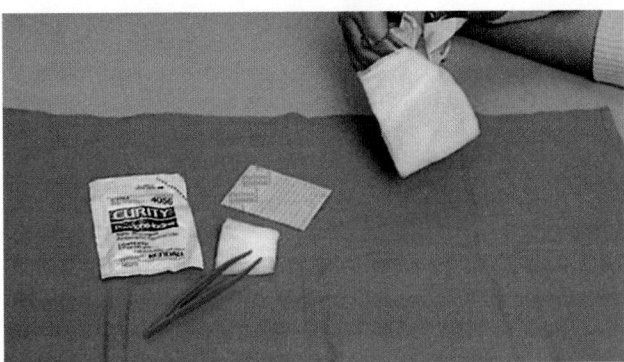

Figure 13-5 ■ Adding item to a sterile field.

the equipment for resterilization. Spilling solution over a sterile drape contaminates the field unless the drape cannot be penetrated by moisture.

6. *Because fluid flows in the direction of gravity, a sterile object becomes contaminated if gravity causes a contaminated liquid to flow over the object's surface.* To avoid contamination during a surgical hand scrub, hold your hands above the elbows. This allows water to flow downward without contaminating your hands and fingers. Because gravity makes water flow downward, this is also the reason for drying from fingers to elbows with the hands held up, after the scrub.

7. *The edges of a sterile field or container are contaminated.* A 2.5-cm (1-inch) border around a sterile towel or drape is considered contaminated (Box 13-16). The edges of sterile containers become exposed to air after they are open and are thus contaminated. After you remove a sterile needle from its protective cap or after you remove forceps from a container, the objects must not touch the container's edge. The lip of an opened bottle of solution also becomes contaminated after it is exposed to air. When pouring a sterile liquid, first pour a small amount of solution and discard it. The solution washes away any microorganisms on the bottle lip. Then pour the liquid a second time to fill a sterile container with the amount of solution you need.

RESTORATIVE CARE The need for infection prevention and control is also present when patients are in the restorative phase of their care. Nurses in long-term care settings contribute to high-quality health care by practicing skills and techniques necessary to prevent infections.

Long-Term Care Some of the same risks for infections that are present in acute care apply in long-term care facilities, such as skilled nursing homes (Rosenbaum and others, 2005). Risks for HAIs increase because of the usual age of patients seen in long-term care facilities. For example, in

older adults several age-associated physical changes alter the natural barriers to infections (see Box 13-2, p. 233).

Pneumonia, urinary tract infections, and pressure ulcer infections are the three most common infections in long-term care facilities. You will play an important role in the control of these infections by using critical thinking skills and knowledge of how to prevent these infections. See Chapters 29, 33, and 36 for additional information on approaches for preventing and managing these infections.

■ ■ ■ EVALUATION

PATIENT CARE The evaluation of patients' status is important in preventing infection or caring for a local infection or infectious process. Measure the success of infection prevention and control techniques by determining whether you achieved the goals for preventing or reducing infection. Compare a patient's response such as a decline in fever or decreased wound drainage. In some situations you will evaluate the patient's response to proposed environmental changes. For example, when a patient is discharged home with a draining wound, medical asepsis in the home is important. The patient and family members need to practice proper hand-hygiene techniques when interacting with the patient or any care-related equipment. You evaluate their ability to follow medical asepsis through direct observation. Another example is observing if items in the patient's living area (e.g., bed linen, nightstand, or personal bathroom) are properly cleaned.

Patients with wounds, either surgical or traumatic wounds, require extensive management (see Chapter 36). Infection control practices are designed to either prevent or control spread of wound infection. Accordingly, evaluate the patient response to nursing interventions by noting fever, wound pain or drainage, swelling around the wound, decreased energy, and increasing fatigue. Evaluation of wound status and patient response to wound healing is a priority. You cannot always use fever as a sole measure because a fever may appear later in the wound infection process, especially with chronic wounds.

PATIENT EXPECTATIONS When providing patient care routinely review whether you are meeting the patients' expectations. Ask your patient if the infected wound feels better after wound care and if the wound pain is controlled. If your patient is going to be discharged home with an open wound, help the patient identify concerns and determine what the patient needs to ease the transition.

Attentive listening to your patients and their families assists you in determining their level of satisfaction with care and if the plan of care met their expectations. Maintain open communication, and give your patients an opportunity to express new expectations, their satisfaction, and care concerns as they transition from your care to their home or another care setting.

BOX 13-15   PROCEDURAL GUIDELINES

Opening Wrapped Sterile Items

DELEGATION CONSIDERATIONS: The skill of opening wrapped sterile items may be delegated if personnel are qualified to perform the procedure.

EQUIPMENT: Sterile kit or package

1 Place sterile kit or package containing sterile items on clean, dry, flat work surface above waist level.
2 Open outside cover, and remove kit from dust cover. Place on work surface.
3 Grasp outer surface of tip of top outermost flap.
4 Open outermost flap away from body, keeping arm outstretched and away from sterile field (see illustration).
5 Grasp outside surface of edge of first side flap.

6 Open side flap, pulling to side, allowing it to lie flat on table surface. Keep your arm to the side and not over sterile surface (see illustration). Do not allow flaps to spring back over sterile contents.
7 Repeat steps for second side flap (see illustration).
8 Grasp outside border of last and innermost flap.
9 Stand away from sterile package, and pull flap back, allowing it to fall flat on table (see illustration).
10 Use the inner surface of the package (except for the 1-inch border around the edges) as a field to add additional items, because it is sterile. Grasp the 1-inch border to move the field over the work surface.

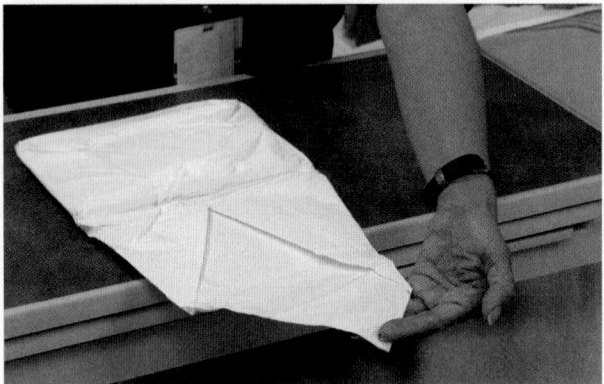

Step 4 ■ Open top flap away from body.

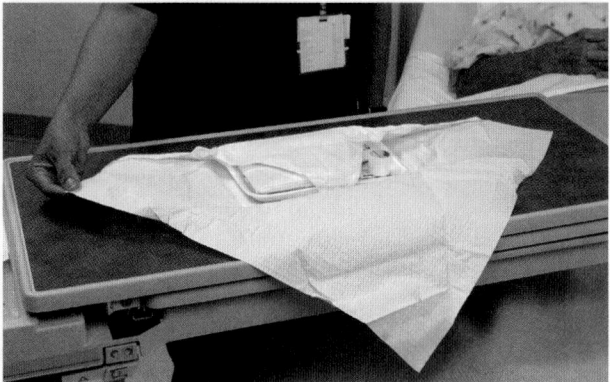

Step 7 ■ Open second side flap.

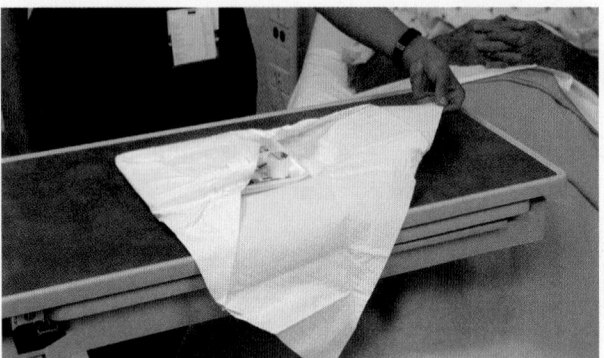

Step 6 ■ The nurse's arm is kept out away from the sterile field while opening a side flap.

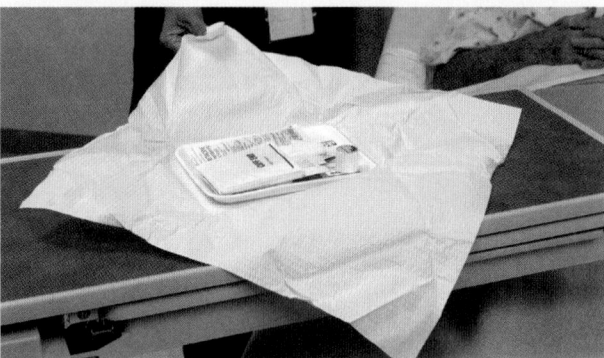

Step 9 ■ Open back flap.

BOX 13-16 PROCEDURAL GUIDELINES

Preparation of a Sterile Field

DELEGATION CONSIDERATIONS: The skill of preparing a sterile field may be delegated to personnel qualified to perform the procedure.

EQUIPMENT: Sterile pack, sterile gloves *(optional)*

1 Perform hand hygiene.
2 Place pack containing sterile drape on work surface, and open as described in "Opening Wrapped Sterile Items," Box 13-15.
3 Apply sterile gloves *(optional; check agency policy)*.
4 With fingertips of one hand, pick up the folded top edge of the sterile drape along the 1-inch border.
5 Gently lift the drape up from its outer cover, and let it unfold by itself without touching any object. Keep it above the waist. Discard the outer cover with the other hand.

6 With the other hand, grasp an adjacent corner of the drape and hold it straight up and away from the body (see illustration).
7 Holding the drape, first position and lay the bottom half over the intended work surface (see illustration).
8 Allow the top half of the drape to be placed over the work surface last (see illustration).
9 Grasp the 1-inch border around the edge to position as needed.

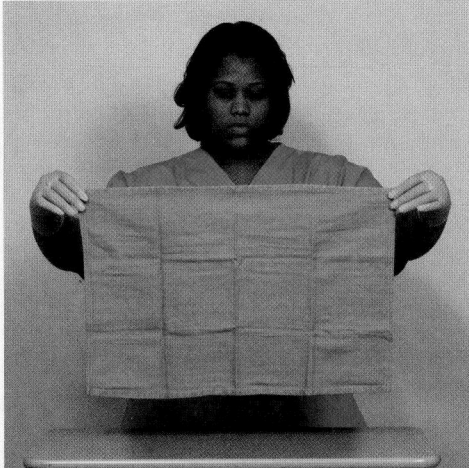

Step 6 ■ Hold corners of sterile drape up and away from body.

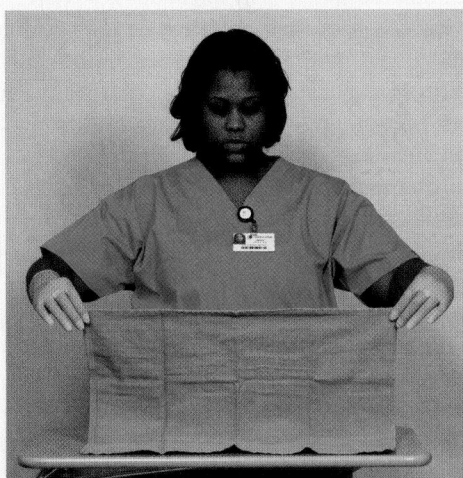

Step 7 ■ Position bottom half of sterile drape over top half of work surface.

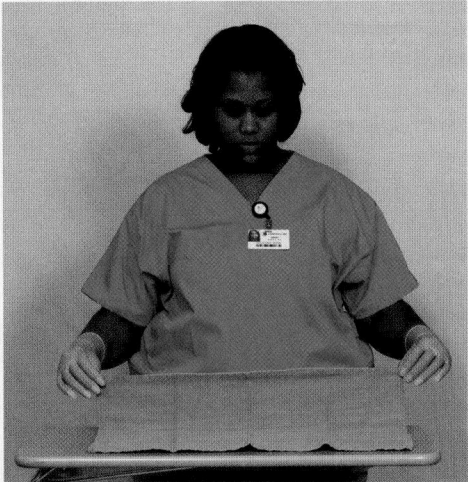

Step 8 ■ Allow top half of drape to be placed over bottom half of work surface.

KEY POINTS

- Normal body flora help the body resist infection by reducing the reproduction of pathogenic microorganisms.
- Immunity to infection depends on the capacity to produce antibodies in response to exposure to an antigen.
- An infection can develop if the six elements of the infection chain are present and uninterrupted.
- A microorganism's virulence depends on its ability to resist attack by the body's normal defenses.
- Increasing age, poor nutrition, stress, inherited conditions, chronic disease, and treatments or conditions that compromise the immune response increase susceptibility to infection.
- Wear gloves when in contact with blood or potentially infectious material. Wear a gown and mask in combination with an eye protection device such as goggles or glasses with solid side shields whenever you anticipate splashes or spray of blood or potentially infectious material.
- Invasive procedures, medical therapies, long hospitalization, and contact with health care personnel increase a hospitalized patient's risk for acquiring a health care–associated infection.
- Surgical asepsis requires more stringent techniques than medical asepsis.

- The CDC recommends that you consider all patients as potentially infected with HIV and other blood-borne pathogens; therefore health care workers reduce the risk for exposure to blood and body fluids by following standard precautions.
- Standard precautions involve using appropriate barrier protection with all patients
- Following aseptic principles is the key to your success in preventing patients from acquiring infections.
- A patient on isolation precautions is subject to sensory deprivation because of the restricted environment.
- Nonadherence with hand hygiene is the main cause of health care–associated infections.
- An infection prevention and control professional provides educational and consultative services to maintain aseptic practices.
- If the skin is broken or if you perform an invasive procedure into a body cavity normally free of microorganisms, use surgical aseptic practices.
- A sterile object becomes contaminated by direct contact with a clean or contaminated object, by exposure to airborne microorganisms, or by contact with a wet surface.

CRITICAL THINKING EXERCISES

Mrs. Eldredge was rehospitalized for a surgical site infection. Kathy is not able to care for Mrs. Eldredge, but one of her classmates, Carman Hernandez, assumes care. Carman assesses Mrs. Eldredge's incision and observes warmth, swelling, and redness, with a small amount of yellow drainage coming from the incision. She also has a fever with temperature of 102° F, a pulse of 104, and blood pressure and respirations within normal ranges. Carman and the registered dietitian do a nutritional assessment on Mrs. Eldredge and note that she had poor nutritional intake 1 month before her surgery because of hip pain and an inability to stand to prepare meals. In addition, when she was home and her incisional pain increased and she developed a fever, she did not feel like eating. Her weight loss is minimal, 3 lb. However, her nutritional laboratory test results note that she is anemic and her serum protein levels are decreased. In addition, her blood glucose is also slightly elevated. Mrs. Eldredge's health care provider orders a wound culture. In

addition Mrs. Eldredge is receiving wound care, antibiotic therapy, and supportive care, including nutrition and progressive exercise.

1. List three assessment findings that indicate Mrs. Eldredge's surgical site infection.
2. Mrs. Eldredge's wound culture grew a resistant strain of *S. aureus*. Carman checked the facility's policy for isolation precautions and found that Mrs. Eldredge needed to be on contact precautions. What are Carman's next steps?
3. Carman are preparing to change Mrs. Eldredge's dressing. What personal protective equipment does she wear to perform this procedure? Explain your answer.
4. Explain why Mrs. Eldredge's nutritional assessment is important for infection control.

⊝volve   *Answers to Critical Thinking Questions can be found on the Evolve website.*

REVIEW QUESTIONS

1. The **most** effective way to break the chain of infection is by:
   1. Performing hand hygiene
   2. Wearing gloves
   3. Placing patients in isolation
   4. Providing private rooms for all patients

2. A patient's surgical wound has become swollen, red, and tender. You note that the patient has a new fever and leukocytosis. Your best immediate intervention is to:
   1. Use surgical technique to change the dressing
   2. Reassure the patient and recheck the wound later
   3. Notify the health care provider and support the patient's fluid and nutritional needs
   4. Alert the patient and caregivers to the presence of an infection to ensure care after discharge

3. A patient has an indwelling urinary catheter. You recognize that the catheter represents a risk for urinary tract infection because:
   1. It keeps an incontinent patient's skin dry
   2. It can get caught in the linens or equipment
   3. It obstructs the normal flushing action of urine flow
   4. It allows the patient to remain hydrated without having to urinate

4. You have redressed a patient's wound and now plan to administer a medication to the patient. It is important to:
   1. Remove gloves and perform hand hygiene before leaving the room
   2. Remove gloves and perform hand hygiene before administering the medication
   3. Leave the gloves on to administer the medication
   4. Leave the medication on the bedside table to avoid having to remove gloves

5. You need to wear a gown when working with a patient:
   1. If the patient's hygiene is poor
   2. If the patient has AIDS or hepatitis
   3. If you are assisting with medication administration
   4. If blood or body fluids may get on your clothing from a task you plan to perform

6. Identify when the nurse should remove gloves and perform hand hygiene. Select all that apply:
   1. Only after wound care
   2. When leaving the room
   3. When you have completed all tasks for the patient
   4. When the specific task you put them on for is completed

7. The most likely means of transmitting infection between patients is:
   1. Exposure to another patient's cough
   2. Sharing equipment among patients
   3. Disposing of soiled linen in a shared linen bag
   4. Contact with a health care worker's hands

8. Your ungloved hands come in contact with the drainage from the patient's wound. To clean your hands you should:
   1. Wash them with soap and water
   2. Use an alcohol-based hand cleaner
   3. Rinse them and use the alcohol-based hand cleaner
   4. Wipe them with a paper towel

9. A patient is placed on contact precautions for an infection with a resistant organism. You notice the patient seems to be depressed and withdrawn. The best intervention is to:
   1. Lower the lighting and reduce noise to calm the patient
   2. Reduce the level of precautions to permit greater interaction with the patient
   3. Explain the reason for contact precautions and answer the patient's questions
   4. Limit family and other caregiver visits to reduce the risk for spreading the infection

10. After coming in contact with a patient on isolation, visitors are encouraged to:
   1. Wear gloves before eating or handling food
   2. Leave the facility to prevent contamination of others
   3. Perform hand hygiene upon leaving the patient's room
   4. Use an empty room to talk with family members.

Answers to Review Questions can be found on pages 1197-1198.

REFERENCES

Association of periOperative Nurses (AORN): *Perioperative standards and recommended practices*, Denver, 2009, The Association.

Arnold F, McDonald LC: Antimicrobials and resistance. In Carrico R, editor: *APIC text of infection control and epidemiology*, Washington, DC, 2005, Association for Professionals in Infection Control and Epidemiology, Inc.

Boyce JM, Petit D: *HICPAC/SHEA/APIC/IDSA Hand Hygiene Task Force and the CDC Healthcare Control Practices Advisory Committee guidelines for hand hygiene in health care settings*, Atlanta, 2008, Centers for Disease Control and Prevention.

Catalano G and others: Anxiety and depression in hospitalized patients in resistant organism isolation, *South Med J*, 96(2):141-145, 2003.

Centers for Disease Control and Prevention: *Guidelines for the prevention and transmission of hepatitis B, hepatitis C and human immunodeficiency virus in health care personnel*, Atlanta, June 29, 2001, Centers for Disease Control and Prevention.

Centers for Disease Control and Prevention: Guidelines for preventing the transmission of *Mycobacterium tuberculosis* in health-care facilities, *MMWR Recomm Rep* 54:RR-17, 2005.

Centers for Disease Control and Prevention, Hospital Infection Control Practice Advisory Committee and the HICPAC/SHEA/APIC/IDSA Hand Hygiene Task Force: Guidelines for hand hygiene in health care setting, *MMWR Recomm Rep* 51(No RR-16), 2002.

Centers for Disease Control and Prevention, Hospital Infection Control Practice Advisory Committee: Guidelines for isolation precautions in hospitals, *MMWR Recomm Rep* 57(RR-16):39, 2007.

Centers for Disease Control and Prevention, Hospital Infection Control Practice Advisory Committee and the HICPAC/SHEA/APIC/IDSA Hand Hygiene Task Force: *Guideline for hand hygiene in health-care settings*, Atlanta, 2008a, Centers for Disease Control and Prevention.

Centers for Disease Control and Prevention and the Hospital Infection Control Practice Advisory Committee, Rutala W, Weber D, and the Healthcare Infection Control Practices and Advisory Committee: *Guidelines for disinfection and sterilization in healthcare facilities,* 2008b, http://www.cdc.gov/ncidod/eid/vol7no2/rutala.htm, accessed February 2009.

Church NB: Surgical services. In Carrico R, editor: *APIC text of infection control and epidemiology,* Washington, DC, 2005, Association for Professionals in Infection Control and Epidemiology, Inc.

Cipriano P: Save a life—wash your hands, *Am Nurse Today* 2(1):10, 2007, http://www.AmericanNurseToday.com.

Clark MJ: *Community health nursing: caring for populations,* ed 4, Upper Saddle River, NJ, 2003, Pearson Education.

Fauerbach L: Risk factors for infection transmission. In Carrico R, editor: *APIC text of infection control and epidemiology,* Washington, DC, 2005, Association for Professionals in Infection Control and Epidemiology, Inc.

Gantz M: Geriatrics. In Carrico R, editor: *APIC text of infection control and epidemiology,* Washington, DC, 2005, Association for Professionals in Infection Control and Epidemiology, Inc.

Guinto CH and others: Evaluation of dedicated stethoscopes as a potential source of nosocomial pathogens, *Am J Infect Control* 30(8):499, 2002.

Haiduven D, Poland G: Immunization in the healthcare worker. In Carrico R, editor: *APIC text of infection control and epidemiology,* Washington, DC, 2005, Association for Professionals in Infection Control and Epidemiology, Inc.

Hedrick E, Wideman JM: Waste management. In Carrico R, editor: *APIC text of infection control and epidemiology,* Washington, DC, 2005, Association for Professionals in Infection Control and Epidemiology, Inc.

Hilburn J and others: Use of alcohol hand sanitizer as an infection control strategy in an acute care facility, *Am J Infect Control* 31:119, 2003.

Marschall J and others: Strategies to prevent central-line associated bloodstream infections in acute care hospitals, *Infect Control Hosp Epidemiol* 29(1):S22, 2008.

Mashaba G: South African culturally based health-illness patterns and humanistic care practices. In Leininger M, McFarland M: *Transcultural nursing,* New York, 2002, McGraw-Hill.

Maunder R and others: The immediate psychological and occupational impact of the 2003 SARS outbreak in a teaching hospital, *Can Med Assoc J,* 168:1245-1251, 2003.

Murphy D: Patient safety. In Carrico R, editor: *APIC text of infection control and epidemiology,* Washington, DC, 2005, Association for Professionals in Infection Control and Epidemiology, Inc.

Occupational Safety and Health Administration: Occupational exposure to blood borne pathogens: final rule, 29 CFR 1919:1130, *Federal Register* 56:64175, 1991.

Occupational Safety and Health Administration: Respiratory protective devices: final rules and notice, *Federal Register* 60:30336, 1995.

Occupational Safety and Health Administration: Needlestick Safety Prevention Act of 2000, 29CFR part 1910, *Federal Register* 66:5317, 2001, updated April 2007, http://www.osha.gov/SLTC/bloodbornepathogens/index.html.

Pagana KD, Pagana TJ: *Mosby's diagnostic and laboratory test reference,* ed 9, St. Louis, 2009, Mosby.

Potter P and others: Evaluation of chemical dot thermometers for measuring body temperature of orally intubated patients, *Am J Crit Care* 12(5):403, 2003.

Ritter H: Clinical microbiology. In Carrico R, editor: *APIC text of infection control and epidemiology,* Washington, DC, 2005, Association for Professionals in Infection Control and Epidemiology, Inc.

Rosenbaum P and others: Long-term care. In Carrico R, editor: *APIC text of infection control and epidemiology,* Washington, DC, 2005, Association for Professionals in Infection Control and Epidemiology, Inc.

Russell ML, Henderson EA: The measurement of influenza vaccine coverage among health care workers, *Am J Infect Control* 31:457, 2003.

Rutala WA, Weber DJ: Cleaning, disinfection, and sterilization in healthcare facilities. In Carrico R, editor: *APIC text of infection control and epidemiology,* Washington, DC, 2005, Association for Professionals in Infection Control and Epidemiology, Inc.

Seigel JD and others: *2007 Guideline for isolation precautions: preventing transmission of infectious agents in healthcare settings,* June 2007, Centers for Disease Control and Prevention, http://www.cdc.gov/ncidod/dhqp/pdf/guidelines/Isolation2007.pdf, accessed February 2009.

Stricof RL: Endoscopy. In Carrico R, editor: *APIC text of infection control and epidemiology,* Washington, DC, 2005, Association for Professionals in Infection Control and Epidemiology, Inc.

The Joint Commission Resources, Inc: *2009 patient safety goals,* Chicago, 2008, The Joint Commission.

Tweeten S: General principles of epidemiology. In Carrico R, editor: *APIC text of infection control and epidemiology,* Washington, DC, 2005, Association for Professionals in Infection Control and Epidemiology, Inc.

Underwood M: Hand hygiene. In Carrico R, editor: *APIC text of infection control and epidemiology,* Washington, DC, 2005, Association for Professionals in Infection Control and Epidemiology.

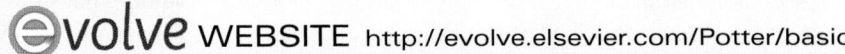
OBJECTIVES

- Explain the principles and mechanisms of thermo-regulation.
- Describe nursing interventions that promote heat loss and heat conservation.
- Discuss physiological changes associated with fever.
- Accurately assess body temperature, pulse, respiration, oxygen saturation, and blood pressure.

- Describe factors that cause variations in vital signs.
- Identify ranges of acceptable vital sign values for an adult, child, and infant.
- Explain variations in techniques used to assess vital signs in an infant, a child, and an adult.
- Correctly delegate vital sign measurement to nursing assistive personnel.

KEY TERMS

afebrile, p. 263
antipyretic, p. 264
apical pulse, p. 269
apnea, p. 278
auscultatory gap, p. 275
bradycardia, p. 270
bradypnea, p. 278
core temperature, p. 261
diaphoresis, p. 261
diastolic pressure, p. 270
digital thermometers, p. 266

dysrhythmia, p. 270
eupnea, p. 278
febrile, p. 261
fever, p. 261
heat stroke, p. 264
hematocrit, p. 300
hemoglobin, p. 300
hypertension, p. 271
hyperthermia, p. 264
hypotension, p. 272
hypothermia, p. 264

infrared thermometer, p. 266
Korotkoff sound, p. 274
nonshivering thermo-genesis, p. 261
orthostatic hypotension, p. 273
oxygen saturation, p. 279
perfusion, p. 278
pulse deficit, p. 270
pulse pressure, p. 270
pyrexia, p. 261

red blood cell count, p. 300
sphygmomanometer, p. 273
systolic pressure, p. 270
tachycardia, p. 270
tachypnea, p. 278
vasoconstriction, p. 262
vasodilation, p. 261
ventilation, p. 278
vital signs, p. 260

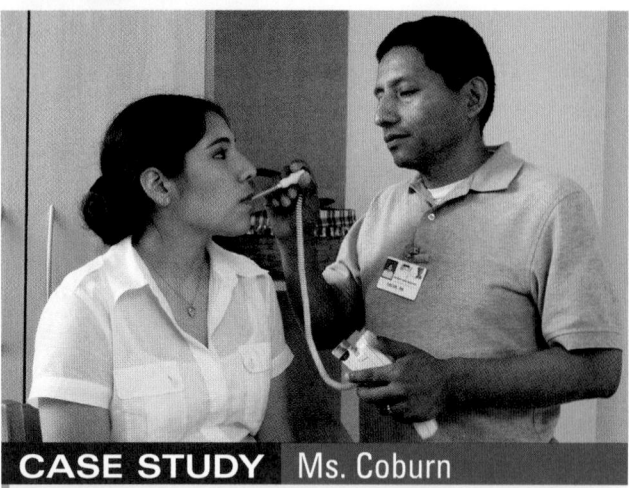

CASE STUDY   Ms. Coburn

Ms. Coburn is a 26-year-old schoolteacher. Her maternal grandparents immigrated to America from Brazil. She lives alone in an apartment building. She smokes one pack of cigarettes a day. She has smoked since she was 16 years old, and she is 20 lb overweight. She made an appointment at the neighborhood clinic because she started having headaches and frequently felt tired.

Miguel is a 42-year-old Hispanic nurse who works in the neighborhood clinic. He enjoys providing health-related teaching to the patients at the clinic and has provided nursing care for Ms. Coburn for the past 2 years. During Ms. Coburn's office visit, Miguel assesses Ms. Coburn's symptoms. He asks her about her headache and her fatigue. After interviewing Ms. Coburn, Miguel takes her vital signs. Her temperature is 98° F, her respiratory rate is 14 breaths per minute, her pulse is 86 beats per minute, and her blood pressure is 164/98 mm Hg. Ms. Coburn asks Miguel, "So, does this mean I am healthy?" Miguel responds, "Ms. Coburn, your blood pressure is pretty high right now. After you see the nurse practitioner today, I am going to take your blood pressure again. We are also going to talk about the changes you can begin to make to help you be healthier and feel better."

The cardinal **vital signs** are temperature, pulse, respiration, blood pressure (BP), and oxygen saturation. Assessment of a sixth vital sign, pain, is a standard of care in health care settings (see Chapter 31). Frequently pain and discomfort are the problems that lead a patient to seek health care. Therefore assessing your patient for pain helps you understand the patient's clinical status and progress.

Many factors such as the temperature of the environment, physical exertion, and the effects of illness cause vital signs to change, sometimes outside the acceptable range. Measurement of vital signs and the assessment of pain provide data to determine a patient's usual state of health (baseline data) and response to physical and psychological stress and to medical and nursing therapies (see Chapter 31). A change in vital signs indicates a change in physiological functioning or a change in comfort, signaling the need for medical or nursing intervention.

Measurement of vital signs is a quick and efficient way of monitoring a patient's condition or identifying problems and evaluating the patient's response to intervention. The basic skills required to measure vital signs are simple, but do not take them for granted. Vital signs and other physiological measurements are the basis for clinical problem solving.

GUIDELINES FOR MEASURING VITAL SIGNS

You assess vital signs whenever a patient enters a health care agency. A complete set of vital signs is included in a complete physical assessment (see Chapter 15), or vital signs are obtained individually to assess a patient's condition. A patient's needs and condition determine when, where, how, and by whom vital signs are measured. It is important that you are able to measure vital signs correctly, understand and interpret the values, communicate findings appropriately, and begin interventions as needed. Use the following guidelines to help you incorporate vital sign measurements into nursing practice:

1. When caring for the patient, you are responsible for vital sign measurement. You may delegate the measurement of selected vital signs (e.g., in stable patients) to nursing assistive personnel (NAP). However, it is your responsibility to review vital sign measurements, interpret their significance, and make decisions about interventions.
2. Make sure equipment is in working order and appropriate to ensure accurate findings.
3. Select equipment based on the patient's condition and characteristics (e.g., do not use a regular adult-size blood pressure cuff for an obese patient).
4. Know the patient's usual range of vital signs. A patient's usual values sometimes differ from the standard range for that age or physical state. Use the patient's usual values as a baseline for comparison with findings taken later.
5. Know the patient's medical history, therapies, and prescribed medications. Some illnesses or treatments cause predictable vital sign changes.
6. Control or minimize environmental factors that affect vital signs. Measuring the pulse after the patient exercises will yield a value that is not a true indicator of the patient's condition.
7. Use an organized, systematic approach when measuring vital signs.
8. Based on a patient's condition, collaborate with the health care provider to decide the frequency of vital sign assessment. In the hospital the health care provider orders a minimum frequency of vital sign measurements for each patient. After surgery or treatment intervention, you obtain vital signs frequently to detect complications. As a patient's physical condition worsens, it is

often necessary to monitor vital signs as often as every 5 to 10 minutes. You will use vital sign assessment during medication administration as well. For example, the health care provider may order certain cardiac drugs to be given within a range of pulse or blood pressure values. Outside of the hospital, vital sign assessment occurs whenever the patient seeks care from a health care provider. In either environment you are responsible for judging whether your patients need more frequent assessments (Box 14-1).

9. Analyze the results of vital sign measurement. Do not interpret vital sign findings without knowing your patient's other physical signs or symptoms and ongoing health status.

10. Verify and communicate significant changes in vital signs. Baseline measurements allow you to identify and interpret changes in vital signs. When vital signs appear abnormal, have another nurse or health care provider repeat the measurement. Inform the nurse in charge or health care provider of abnormal vital signs immediately, document findings in the patient's record, and report vital sign changes to nurses working the next shift.

BODY TEMPERATURE

Body temperature is the difference between the amount of heat produced by body processes and the amount of heat lost to the external environment.

$$\text{Heat produced} - \text{Heat lost} = \text{Body temperature}$$

Despite environmental temperature extremes and physical activity, temperature-control mechanisms of human beings

keep the body's **core temperature,** or temperature of deep tissues, relatively constant during sleep, during exposure to cold, and during strenuous exercise. However, surface temperature fluctuates, depending on blood flow to the skin and the amount of heat lost to the external environment. The body's tissues and cells function best within a relatively narrow temperature range, from 36° to 38° C (96.8° to 100.4° F), but no single temperature is normal for all people. For healthy young adults the average oral temperature is 37° C (98.6° F). Time of day affects body temperature with the lowest temperature at 6 AM and the highest body temperature at 4 PM in healthy volunteers (Henker and Carlson, 2007). The circadian rhythm alters body temperature about 0.5° C (0.9° F) throughout each day. An acceptable temperature range for adults depends on age, gender, range of physical activity, and state of health.

Women generally experience greater fluctuations in body temperature than men. Hormonal variations during the menstrual cycle cause body temperature fluctuations. Progesterone levels rise and fall cyclically during menstruation. When progesterone levels are low, the body temperature is a few tenths of a degree below baseline. The lower temperature persists until ovulation occurs. During ovulation, greater amounts of progesterone enter the circulation and raise the body temperature to previous baseline levels or higher. These temperature variations help to predict a woman's most fertile time to become pregnant. Body temperature changes also occur during menopause. Women who have stopped menstruating often experience periods of intense body heat and sweating lasting from 30 seconds to 5 minutes. During these periods there are often intermittent increases in skin temperatures of up to 4° C (7.2° F).

Temperatures vary depending on the measurement site. Sites reflecting core temperature, such as the pulmonary artery, are more reliable indicators of body temperature than sites reflecting surface temperature, such as the armpit or axilla. The pulmonary artery offers accurate readings because of the blood mix from all regions of the body and is the standard used in determining the accuracy of all other sites used to measure body temperature.

Body Temperature Regulation

Physiological and behavioral mechanisms precisely regulate and control body temperature mechanisms. For the body temperature to stay constant and within an acceptable range, the body has to maintain the relationship between heat production and heat loss.

NEURAL AND VASCULAR CONTROL The hypothalamus, located between the cerebral hemispheres of the brain, controls body temperature by attempting to maintain a comfortable temperature or "set point." When the hypothalamus senses an increase in body temperature, it sends impulses out to reduce body temperature by sweating and **vasodilation** (widening of blood vessels). The increased blood flow to the skin enables heat loss through radiation. If the hypothalamus senses the body's temperature is lower than the set point, it sends signals out to increase heat production by muscle shivering or heat conservation by **vasoconstriction** (narrowing of surface blood vessels). Disease or trauma to the hypothalamus or spinal cord, which carries hypothalamic messages, decreases the body's ability to control body temperature.

HEAT PRODUCTION Temperature regulation relies on normal heat production processes. Heat is produced as a by-product of metabolism. As metabolism increases, the body produces additional heat. When metabolism decreases, the body produces less heat. Heat production occurs during rest, voluntary movement, involuntary shivering, and **nonshivering thermogenesis.** The voluntary movement of muscular activity during exercise requires additional energy. Metabolism increases during activity, sometimes causing heat production to increase up to 50 times normal. Shivering is an involuntary body response to temperature differences in the body. Shivering can increases heat production 4 to 5 times greater than normal. Because neonates cannot shiver, a limited amount of vascular brown adipose tissue, present at birth, is metabolized for heat production, or nonshivering thermogenesis.

HEAT LOSS Heat loss and heat production occur at the same time. The skin's exposure to the environment results in constant, normal heat loss through radiation, conduction, convection, and evaporation. Infants and young children, who have a larger ratio of surface area to body weight, lose more heat to the environment than adults.

Radiation is the transfer of heat between two objects without physical contact. Heat radiates from the skin to any surrounding cooler object. Up to 85% of the human body's surface area radiates heat to the environment. During surgery a patient can lose heat by radiation in the cool environment of the operating room.

Conduction is the transfer of heat from one object to another with direct contact. When the warm skin touches a cooler object, heat transfers from the skin to the object until their temperatures are similar. Heat conducts through solids, gases, and liquids. Conduction normally results in a small amount of heat loss. You can increase a patient's conductive heat loss by applying an ice pack or bathing a patient with tepid water. Applying several layers of clothing reduces conductive loss. The body gains heat by conduction when it contacts materials warmer than skin temperature, such as prewarmed blankets.

Convection is the transfer of heat away from the body by air movement. A fan promotes heat loss through convection. Convective heat loss increases when moistened skin comes into contact with slightly moving air.

Evaporation is the transfer of heat energy when a liquid is changed to a gas. The body continuously loses heat by evaporation. About 600 to 900 mL of water a day evaporates from the skin and lungs, resulting in water and heat loss. By regulating perspiration or sweating, the body promotes additional evaporative heat loss. **Diaphoresis** is visually evident perspiration, usually on the forehead, upper chest, and arms. Body temperature lowers with diaphoresis.

SKIN IN TEMPERATURE REGULATION The skin regulates temperature through insulation of the body. The skin, subcutaneous tissue, and fat keep heat inside the body. Persons with more body fat have more natural insulation than do slim and muscular people. The way the skin (along with neural control) regulates body temperature is similar to the way a car radiator controls engine temperature. The car engine generates a great deal of heat. Water pumps through the engine to collect the heat and carry it to the radiator, where a fan transfers the heat from the water to the outside air. In our body the internal organs produce heat, and during exercise or increased sympathetic stimulation, the amount of heat produced is greater than the usual core temperature. Blood flows from the internal organs, carrying heat to the body surface. There blood passing through the vascular areas of the hands and feet varies from minimal flow to as much as 30% of the blood pumped from the heart. Heat transfers from the blood, through vessel walls, to the skin's surface and is lost to the environment through heat loss mechanisms.

BEHAVIORAL CONTROL When the environmental temperature falls, a person adds clothing, moves to a warmer place, raises the thermostat setting on a furnace, increases muscular activity by running in place, or sits with arms and legs tightly wrapped together. In contrast, when the temperature becomes hot, a person removes clothing, stops activity, lowers the thermostat setting on an air conditioner, seeks a cooler place, or takes a cool shower. Infants and older adults sometimes need help in maintaining a comfortable body temperature. Illness or impaired thought processes result in an inability to recognize the need to change behavior for temperature control.

Temperature Alterations

Changes in body temperature are related to excess heat production, heat loss, too little heat production, or any combination of these alterations. The nature of the change affects the type of clinical problems experienced by a patient.

FEVER The condition of **pyrexia,** or **fever,** occurs because heat loss mechanisms are unable to keep pace with excess heat production, resulting in an abnormal rise in body temperature. A temperature elevation greater than 1° C above usual diurnal body temperature is considered a fever (Thompson, 2005). A fever is usually not harmful if it stays below 39° C (102.2° F) in adults or 40° C (104° F) in children. A single temperature reading does not always indicate a fever. You determine if a patient has a fever by taking several temperature readings at different times of the day and comparing these with the usual value for that patient at that time.

A true fever results from an alteration in the hypothalamic set point. Substances that trigger the immune system, such as bacteria or viruses, stimulate the release of hormones in an effort to promote the body's defense against infection. These hormones also trigger the hypothalamus to raise the set point, inducing a **febrile** episode. To reach the new set point, the body produces and conserves heat. The patient experiences chills, shivers, and feels cold, even though the body temperature is rising. If the set point has been "overshot" or the immune triggers are removed, the skin becomes warm and flushed because of vasodilation. Diaphoresis results in evaporative heat loss. When the fever "breaks," the temperature returns to an acceptable range and the patient becomes **afebrile.** A fever pattern is present when a febrile episode reoccurs (Box 14-2).

Fever, or pyrexia, is an important defense mechanism. Therefore most health care providers will not treat an adult's fever until it is over 39° C (102.2° F). Mild temperature elevations enhance the body's immune system by stimulating white blood cell production. Increased temperature reduces the concentration of iron in the blood plasma, causing the growth of bacteria to slow. Fever also fights viral infections by stimulating interferon, the body's natural virus-fighting substance.

Fevers also serve a diagnostic purpose. Fever patterns differ depending on the causative pyrogen (substance, such as bacteria, that causes the fever). The duration and degree of fever depend on the pyrogen's strength and the ability of the individual to respond. The term *fever of unknown origin* (FUO) refers to a fever whose cause health care providers cannot determine.

Treatment for a fever depends on its cause, any adverse effects, and the strength, intensity, and duration of the elevated temperature. You play a key role in assessing fever and implementing temperature-reducing strategies (Box 14-3). The goal is a "safe" rather than a "low" temperature. The health care provider determines the cause of the fever by isolating the causative bacterium or virus. In this case you will get the necessary culture specimens for laboratory analysis, such as urine, blood, sputum, and wound drainage. The health care provider will order appropriate antibiotics to be given after obtaining the cultures. Antibiotics destroy bacteria and eliminate the body's stimulus for fever.

Most fevers in children are of a viral origin, last only briefly, and have limited effects (Walsh and others, 2005). However, children have immature temperature control mechanisms, so temperatures can rise rapidly. Dehydration and febrile seizures occur during rising temperatures in children between 6 months and 3 years of age. Febrile seizures are unusual in children over 5 years of age. The extent of the temperature change, often exceeding 38.8° C (102° F), seems to be a more important factor than the rapidity of the temperature increase. Interventions for children's fevers are based on their response to the illness and not on the temperature level itself (Walsh and others, 2005).

Sometimes a fever results from a hypersensitivity response to a medication, especially when the medication is taken for the first time. These fevers are often accompanied by other allergy symptoms such as rash or itching. Treatment involves stopping the medication.

The objective of fever therapy is to increase heat loss, reduce heat production, and prevent complications. Nondrug therapies (e.g., using nursing strategies) for fever increase

---

BOX 14-2 Patterns of Fever

Sustained A constant body temperature continuously above 38° C (100.4° F) that demonstrates little fluctuation

Intermittent Fever spikes mixed with usual temperature levels; temperature returns to acceptable value at least once in 24 hours

Remittent Fever spikes and falls without a return to acceptable temperature levels

Relapsing Periods of febrile episodes mixed with acceptable temperature values; febrile episodes and periods of normothermia are sometimes longer than 24 hours

---

BOX 14-3 Nursing Management of Patients With a Fever

ASSESSMENT
- Obtain frequent temperature readings (i.e., temporal, tympanic, rectal) during a fever.
- Assess for contributing factors such as dehydration, infection, or environmental temperature.
- Identify physiological response to fever (e.g., diaphoresis, tachycardia, hypotension).
- Obtain all vital signs.
- Assess skin color and temperature, presence of thirst, anorexia, and malaise; observe for shivering and diaphoresis.
- Assess patient comfort and well-being.

INTERVENTIONS (UNLESS CONTRAINDICATED)
- Obtain blood cultures when ordered (see Chapter 13). Obtain blood specimens at the same time as a temperature spike, when the causative organism is most prevalent.
- Minimize heat production: reduce the frequency of activities that increase oxygen demand such as excessive turning and ambulation; allow rest periods; limit physical activity.
- Maximize heat loss: reduce external covering on patient's body without causing shivering; keep clothing and bed linen dry.
- Satisfy requirements for increased metabolic rate: provide supplemental oxygen therapy as ordered to improve oxygen delivery to body cells; provide measures to stimulate appetite, and offer well-balanced meals; provide fluids (at least 3 L/day for a patient with normal cardiac and renal function) to replace fluids lost through insensible water loss and sweating.
- Promote patient comfort: encourage oral hygiene because oral mucous membranes dry easily from dehydration; control temperature of the environment without inducing shivering; apply cool, damp cloth to patient forehead.
- Identify onset and duration of febrile episode phases: examine previous temperature measurements for trends.
- Initiate health teaching as indicated.
- Maintain environmental temperature at 21° to 27° C (70° to 80° F).

heat loss by evaporation, conduction, convection, or radiation. Use caution when implementing nursing measures, and think about heat production and heat loss mechanisms. For example, when you use nursing measures to enhance body cooling, make sure to avoid stimulating shivering. Shivering is counterproductive because of the heat produced by muscle activity. Physical cooling, including the use of water-cooled blankets, is appropriate when the patient's own thermoregulation fails or in patients with neurological damage (e.g., spinal cord injury).

Antipyretics are drugs that reduce fever. Nonsteroidal drugs such as acetaminophen, salicylates, indomethacin, ibuprofen, and ketorolac reduce fever by increasing heat loss. Health care providers generally order antipyretics if a fever is over 39° C (102.2° F). Corticosteroids reduce heat production by interfering with the hypothalamic response. These drugs mask signs of infection by suppressing the immune system. Thus patients on steroids need to be observed closely, especially if they are at risk for infection. Corticosteroids are not used to treat a fever. However, it is important to be aware of their effect on suppressing the ability of the patient to develop a fever in response to bacterial or viral infections.

HYPERTHERMIA An elevated body temperature related to the body's inability to promote heat loss or reduce heat production is **hyperthermia.** Whereas fever (pyrexia) is an upward shift in the set point, hyperthermia is due to an overload on the temperature release mechanisms (Thompson, 2005). Any disease of or trauma to the hypothalamus impairs heat loss mechanisms. Educate patients at risk for hyperthermia to do the following:

- Avoid strenuous exercise in hot, humid weather
- Avoid exercising in areas with poor ventilation
- Drink fluids such as water and clear fruit juices before, during, and after exercise
- Wear light, loose-fitting, light-colored clothing
- Wear a protective covering over the head when outdoors
- Expose themselves to hot climates gradually

Prolonged exposure to the sun or high environmental temperatures overwhelms the body's heat loss mechanisms. Heat also depresses hypothalamic function. These conditions cause **heat stroke,** a dangerous heat emergency, defined as a body temperature of 40° C (104° F) or more (Lewis, 2007). Signs and symptoms of heat stroke include giddiness, confusion, delirium, excess thirst, nausea, muscle cramps, visual disturbances, and even incontinence. The most important sign of heat stroke is hot, dry skin. A heat stroke can be fatal. **Call 9-1-1** for emergency assistance as you begin cooling the person:

- Move the person out of the sun to the shade or a shelter.
- Cool the person quickly. Ways to cool include placing wet towels over the skin, placing the person in a tub of tepid water or into a tepid shower, spraying the person with cool water from a garden hose, and placing oscillating fans in the room.

- If the person can drink, give cool nonalcoholic liquids.
- Continue to take the temperature until it drops to 38.3° to 38.8° C (101° to 102° F).

Emergency medical treatment includes applying hypothermia blankets, giving intravenous (IV) fluids, and irrigating the stomach and lower bowel with cool solutions.

HYPOTHERMIA Heat loss during prolonged exposure to cold overwhelms the body's ability to produce heat, causing **hypothermia.** Hypothermia is classified by core temperature measurements as mild, moderate, or severe (Table 14-1). Hypothermia is either intentional or accidental. During prolonged neurological or cardiac surgery, surgeons use intentional hypothermia to reduce the body's needs for oxygenated blood.

Accidental hypothermia usually develops gradually and may go unnoticed for several hours. The hypothermic patient suffers from uncontrolled shivering, loss of memory, depression, and poor judgment. As the body temperature falls below 34° C (93.2° F), heart and respiratory rates and blood pressure decrease.

The priority treatment for hypothermia is to prevent a further decrease in body temperature. Removing wet clothes, replacing them with dry ones, and wrapping the patient in blankets are key nursing interventions. In emergencies, away from a health care setting, the patient can lie under blankets next to a warm person. A conscious patient benefits from drinking hot liquids such as soup, while avoiding alcohol and caffeinated fluids. Keeping the head covered, placing the patient near a fire or in a warm room, or placing heating pads next to areas of the body (head and neck) that lose heat the quickest helps.

Prevention is the key for patients at risk for hypothermia. Prevention involves educating patients, family members, and friends. Patients most at risk include the very young and the very old and persons debilitated by trauma, stroke, diabetes, drug or alcohol intoxication, sepsis, and Raynaud's disease. Patients with mental illness or handicaps often fall victim to hypothermia because they are unaware of the dangers of cold conditions. Persons without adequate home heating, shelter, diet, or clothing are also at risk.

Measurement of Temperature

Assessment of temperature regulation requires you to make judgments about the site for temperature measurement, type of thermometer, and frequency of measurement.

SITES You measure body temperature using core or body surface sites. The core temperatures of the pulmonary artery,

TABLE 14-1	Classification of Hypothermia	
	C	F
Mild	34°-36°	93.2°-96.8°
Moderate	30°-34°	86.0°-93.2°
Severe	<30°	<86.0°

esophagus, and urinary bladder are often used in intensive care settings and require continuous invasive monitoring devices placed in body cavities or organs. You obtain intermittent temperature measurements at surface sites, routinely from the tympanic membrane, temporal artery, mouth, rectum, and axilla. You can also apply noninvasive chemically prepared thermometer patches to the skin.

To ensure accurate temperature readings, measure each site correctly (Skill 14-1). Depending on the site you use, temperatures will normally vary between 36.0° C (96.8° F) and 38.0° C (100.4° F). It is generally accepted that rectal temperatures are usually 0.5° C (0.9° F) higher than oral temperatures, and tympanic and axillary temperatures are usu-

ally 0.5° C (0.9° F) lower than oral temperatures. Sites reflecting core temperatures are more reliable than sites reflecting surface temperature. Each temperature measurement site has advantages and disadvantages (Box 14-4). Choose the safest and most accurate site for the patient. When possible use the same site when repeated measurements are needed.

THERMOMETERS Four types of thermometers are commonly available for measuring body temperature: electronic, infrared, digital, and disposable chemical dot. The mercury-in-glass thermometer was once the standard device found in the clinical setting but has been eliminated from health care facilities because of the environmental hazards of mercury. However, some patients still use mercury-in-glass

---

BOX 14-4 Advantages and Limitations of Select Temperature Measurement Sites

SITE ADVANTAGES

ORAL
Easily accessible—requires no position change.
Comfortable for patient.
Provides accurate surface temperature reading.
Reflects rapid change in core temperature.
Shown to be a reliable route to measure temperature for intubated patients.

TYMPANIC MEMBRANE
Easily accessible site.
Minimal patient repositioning required.
Can be obtained without disturbing or waking the patient.
Used for patients with tachypnea without affecting breathing.
Provides accurate core reading because eardrum is close to hypothalamus; sensitive to core temperature changes.
Very rapid measurement (2 to 5 seconds).
Unaffected by oral intake of food or fluids or by smoking.
Best to use in children age 2 and older.

RECTAL
Argued to be more reliable than alternative sites when oral temperature is difficult or impossible to obtain.

SITE LIMITATIONS

Causes delay in measurement if patient recently ingested hot/cold fluids or foods, smoked, or chewed gum.
Not used with patients who have had oral surgery, trauma, shaking or chills, or history of seizures.
Not used with infants, small children, or confused, unconscious, or uncooperative patients.
Risk for body fluid exposure.

More variability of measurement than with other core temperature devices (Lawson, Bridges, and Ballou, 2007).
Requires removal of hearing aids before measurement.
Requires disposable sensor cover with only one size available.
Otitis media and cerumen impaction distort readings (Lawson and others, 2007).
Not used with patients who have had surgery of the ear or tympanic membrane.
Does not accurately measure core temperature changes during and after exercise.
Affected by ambient temperature devices such as incubators, radiant warmers, and facial fans.
Anatomy of ear canal makes it difficult to position correctly in neonates, infants, and children younger than 3 years old.
Inaccuracies reported because of incorrect positioning of handheld unit (Farnell and others, 2005).

Lags behind core temperature during rapid temperature changes (Henker and Carlson, 2007).
Not used for patients with diarrhea or patients who have had rectal surgery, rectal disorders, bleeding tendencies, or neutropenia.
Requires positioning and is a source of patient embarrassment and anxiety.
Risk for body fluid exposure.
Requires lubrication.
Not used for routine vital signs in newborns.
Readings sometimes influenced by impacted stool (Maxton, Justin, and Gilles, 2004).

Continued

BOX 14-4   Advantages and Limitations of Select Temperature Measurement Sites—cont'd

SITE ADVANTAGES

AXILLA
Safe and inexpensive.
Used with newborns, children of any age, and unconscious patients.

SKIN
Inexpensive.
Provides continuous reading.
Safe and noninvasive.

TEMPORAL ARTERY
Easy to access without position change.
Very rapid measurement.
No risk for injury to patient or nurse.
Eliminates need to disrobe or unbundle.
Comfortable for patient.
Used in premature infants, newborns, and children.
Reflects rapid change in core temperature.
Sensor cover not required.

SITE LIMITATIONS

Long measurement time.
Requires continuous positioning.
Measurement lags behind core temperature during rapid temperature changes.
Not recommended to detect fever in infants and young children.
Requires exposure of thorax, which results in temperature loss, especially in newborns.
Affected by exposure to the environment, including time to place thermometer (Maxton and others, 2004).
Underestimates core temperature (Lawson and others, 2007).

Measurement lags behind those obtained at other sites during temperature changes, especially during hyperthermia.
Diaphoresis or sweat impairs adhesion.
Affected by environmental temperature.
Cannot be used on patients with adhesive allergy.

Inaccurate with head covering or hair on forehead.
Affected by skin moisture such as diaphoresis or sweating.

---

thermometers at home. When you find a mercury-in-glass thermometer in the home, teach the patient about safer temperature devices and encourage the disposal of mercury products at appropriate neighborhood hazardous disposal locations.

Each device measures temperature in either the Celsius or Fahrenheit scale. Electronic thermometers allow you to convert scales by activating a switch. When it is necessary to manually convert temperature readings, use the following formulas:

To convert Fahrenheit to Celsius, subtract 32 from the Fahrenheit reading and multiply the result by $5/9$.

$$\text{Example: } (104° \text{ F} - 32° \text{ F}) \times 5/9 = 40° \text{ C}$$

To convert Celsius to Fahrenheit, multiply the Celsius reading by $9/5$ and add 32 to the product.

$$\text{Example: } (9/5 \times 40° \text{ C}) + 32 = 104° \text{ F}$$

Electronic Thermometers   Electronic thermometers consist of a rechargeable battery–powered display unit, a thin wire cord, and a temperature-processing probe or sensor covered by a disposable probe cover (Figure 14-1). Separate probes are available for oral (blue tip) and rectal (red tip) use.

You obtain axillary temperatures with the oral probe. Electronic thermometers provide two modes of operation, 4-second predictive temperatures and 3-minute standard temperatures. In day-to-day clinical situations the 4-second predictive is more common.

Infrared thermometers rely on thermal radiation from the ear canal, tympanic membrane, axilla, and temporal artery to measure body temperature. The tympanic membrane thermometer has an otoscope-like speculum with an infrared sensor tip that detects heat radiated from the tympanic membrane of the ear (Figure 14-2). Within seconds after placement in the ear canal and pressing the scan button, a sound signals when the peak temperature has been measured and a reading appears on the display unit. The temporal artery thermometer measures blood flow through the superficial temporal artery. You sweep an infrared handheld scanner across the forehead or just behind the ear (Figure 14-3). After scanning is complete, a reading appears on the display unit. Tympanic and temporal artery temperatures are considered reliable noninvasive measures of core temperature (see Box 14-4).

Digital thermometers contain a probe connected to a microprocessor chip, which translates signals into degrees

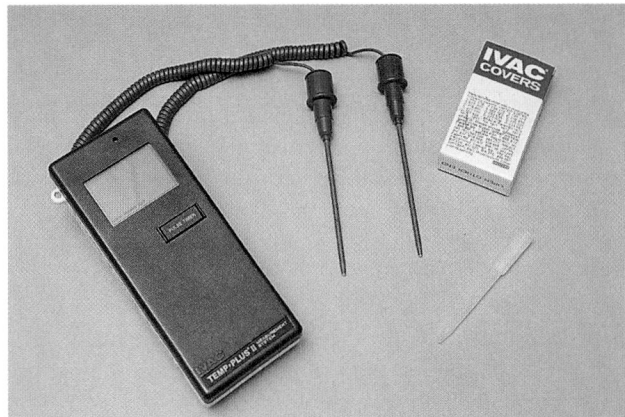

Figure 14-1 ■ Electronic thermometer used for oral, rectal, and axillary measurements.

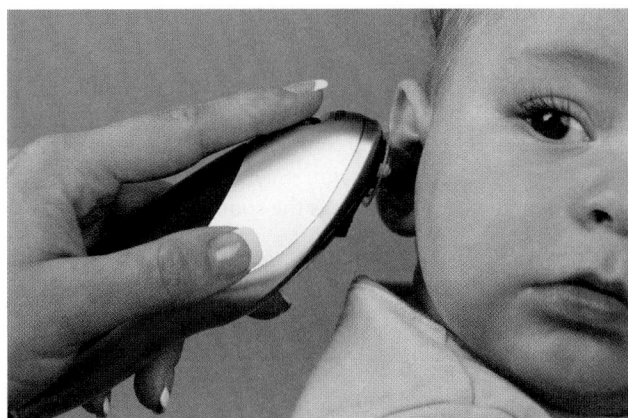

Figure 14-2 ■ Tympanic membrane thermometer. (Courtesy Welch Allyn.)

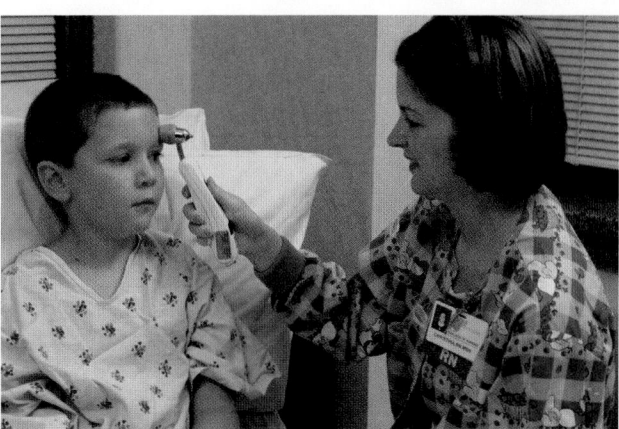

Figure 14-3 ■ Temporal artery thermometer scanning forehead.

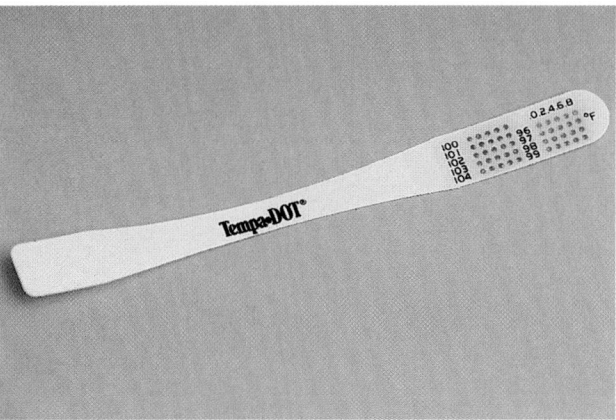

Figure 14-4 ■ Disposable, single-use thermometer strip.

and sends a temperature measurement to a digital display. A digital thermometer can be used for oral, rectal, and axillary measurements.

Chemical Dot Thermometers Single-use or reusable chemical dot thermometers are thin strips of plastic with a temperature sensor at one end. The sensor consists of chemically impregnated dots that change color at different temperatures. In the Celsius version, there are 50 dots, each representing temperature increments of 0.1° C over a range of 35.5° C to 40.4° C. The Fahrenheit version has 45 dots with increments of 0.2° F over a range of 96.0° F to 104.8° F. Chemical dots on the thermometer change color to reflect temperature reading, usually within 60 seconds. Most are designed for single use (Figure 14-4). Therefore they are useful in caring for patients on protective isolation (see Chapter 13). In one brand that you can reuse on the same patient, the chemical dots return to the original color within a few seconds. You usually use the chemical dots for oral temperatures. You also use them at axillary or rectal sites, covered by a plastic sheath at the latter site, with a placement time of 3 minutes (Farnell and others, 2005). Chemical dot ther-

mometers are useful for screening temperatures, especially in infants and young children. Use electronic thermometers to confirm measurements made with a chemical dot thermometer when treatment decisions are involved (Fallis and others, 2006).

Another form of disposable thermometer is a temperature-sensitive patch or tape. Applied to the forehead or abdomen, temperature-sensitive areas of the patch change color at different temperatures.

PULSE

The pulse is the palpable bounding of the blood flow in a peripheral artery. The ejection of blood from the heart distends the walls of the aorta. Approximately 60 to 70 mL of blood enters the aorta with each heart contraction. Because of the force of the blood exiting the heart, aortic distention creates a pulse wave that travels rapidly toward the extremities. When the pulse wave reaches a peripheral artery (e.g., in the wrist), it feels like a tap when the artery is lightly palpated against underlying bone or muscle. The number of pulsing sensations occurring in 1 minute is the pulse rate.

Locating a Peripheral Pulse

You assess any accessible artery for pulse rate (Figure 14-5), but you will most often use the radial or carotid artery because they are easy to locate and palpate. When a patient's condition suddenly deteriorates, use the carotid site to quickly find a pulse.

The radial and apical locations are the most common sites for pulse rate assessment. Use the radial or carotid pulse when teaching patients how to monitor their own heart rates (e.g.,

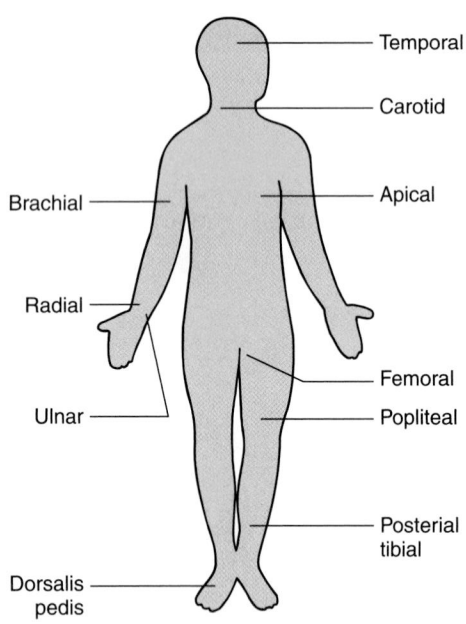

Figure 14-5 ■ Location of peripheral pulses.

athletes or patients using heart medications). If the radial pulse is abnormal, difficult to palpate, or inaccessible because of a dressing or cast, assess the apical pulse. When a patient takes a medication that affects the heart rate, the apical pulse provides a more accurate assessment of heart rate. Table 14-2 summarizes pulse sites and criteria for measurement. Skill 14-2 outlines radial and apical pulse rate assessment.

Using a Stethoscope

You will need a stethoscope to auscultate the sound waves that create an apical pulse (Figure 14-6). The five major parts of the stethoscope are the earpieces, binaurals, tubing, bell chestpiece, and diaphragm chestpiece.

Make sure the plastic or rubber earpieces fit snugly and comfortably in your ears. Also, make sure the binaurals are angled and strong enough so the earpieces stay firmly in place without causing discomfort. The earpieces follow the contour of the ear canal, pointing toward the face when the stethoscope is in place.

The polyvinyl tubing is flexible and 30 to 45 cm (12 to 18 inches) in length. Longer tubing decreases sound wave transmission. The tubing is thick-walled and moderately rigid to eliminate transmission of environmental noise and prevent kinking, which distorts the sound. Stethoscopes have one or two tubes.

The chestpiece consists of a bell and a diaphragm that rotates into position depending on which part you chose to use. To test, lightly tap to determine which side is functioning. The diaphragm is the circular, flat-surfaced portion of the chestpiece covered with a thin plastic disk. It transmits high-pitched sounds created by the high-velocity movement of air and blood. You auscultate bowel, lung, and heart

TABLE 14-2	**Pulse Sites**	
SITE	**LOCATION**	**ASSESSMENT CRITERIA**
Temporal	Over temporal bone of head, above and lateral to eye	Easily accessible site used to assess pulse in children
Carotid	Along medial edge of sternocleidomastoid muscle in neck	Easily accessible site used in patient with physiological shock or during adult CPR when other sites are not palpable; site to assess character of peripheral pulse
Apical	Fifth intercostal space at left midclavicular line	Site used to auscultate for apical pulse
Brachial	Groove between biceps and triceps muscles at antecubital fossa	Site used to assess upper extremity blood pressure; used during infant CPR
Radial	Radial or thumb side of forearm at the wrist	Common site used to assess character of pulse peripherally; assesses status of circulation to hand
Ulnar	Ulnar side of forearm at wrist	Site used to assess status of circulation to ulnar side of hand; used to perform Allen's test
Femoral	Below inguinal ligament, midway between symphysis pubis and anterior superior iliac spine	Site used to assess character of pulse in patient with physiological shock or during CPR when other pulses are not palpable; assesses status of circulation to the leg
Popliteal	Behind knee in popliteal fossa	Site used to auscultate lower extremity blood pressure; assesses status of circulation to the lower leg
Posterior tibial	Inner side of ankle, below medial malleolus	Site used to assess status of circulation to the foot
Dorsalis pedis	Along top of foot, between extension tendons of great and first toe	Site used to assess status of circulation to the foot

CPR, Cardiopulmonary resuscitation.

sounds using the diaphragm. Always place the stethoscope directly on the skin, because clothing obscures the sound. Position the diaphragm to make a tight seal against the patient's skin (Figure 14-7). Exert enough pressure on the diaphragm to leave a temporary red ring on the patient's skin when the diaphragm is removed.

The bell is the cone-shaped chestpiece usually surrounded by a rubber ring to avoid chilling the patient. The bell transmits low-pitched sounds created by the low-velocity movement of blood. You auscultate heart and vascular sounds using the bell. Apply the bell lightly, resting the chestpiece on the skin (Figure 14-8). Compressing the bell against the skin reduces low-pitched sounds.

Some stethoscopes have one chestpiece that combines features of the bell and diaphragm. When you use light pressure, the chestpiece is a bell; when you exert more pressure, the bell converts to a diaphragm. The size of the stethoscope chestpiece varies from small, used for infants and young children, to large. You determine the appropriate-size chestpiece by assessing the surface area you will auscultate.

The stethoscope is a delicate instrument and requires proper care for optimal function. Remove the earpieces regularly, and clean them of cerumen (earwax). Inspect the bell and diaphragm for dust, lint, and body oils, and clean with either alcohol or mild soap and water between patients. There is currently no evidence suggesting the ideal frequency for cleansing; however, there is evidence that the bell and diaphragm become contaminated with microorganisms. Fabric stethoscope covers have been shown to present a potential infection control problem because they are used for prolonged periods, are infrequently laundered, and are contaminated with bacteria (Milam and others, 2001).

Assessment of Pulse

PULSE RATE Before measuring a pulse, review your patient's record to obtain a baseline rate for comparison. Pulse rate varies with the patient's age. You compare the patient's actual pulse rate with the expected usual values (Table 14-3). When assessing the pulse, consider the variety of factors influencing pulse rate (Table 14-4). A combination of these factors often causes significant changes. If you detect an abnormal rate while palpating a peripheral pulse, the next step is to assess the apical rate. The apical rate requires auscultation of the heart sounds, which provides a more accurate assessment of cardiac contraction.

You assess the **apical pulse** by listening for heart sounds (see Chapter 15). After properly positioning the bell or the diaphragm of the stethoscope on the chest, try to identify the first and second heart sounds (S_1 and S_2). At normal slow rates, S_1 is low pitched and dull, sounding like a "lub." S_2 is a higher pitched and shorter sound and creates the sound "dub." Count each set of "lub-dub" as one heartbeat. Count the number of "lub-dubs" occurring in 1 minute.

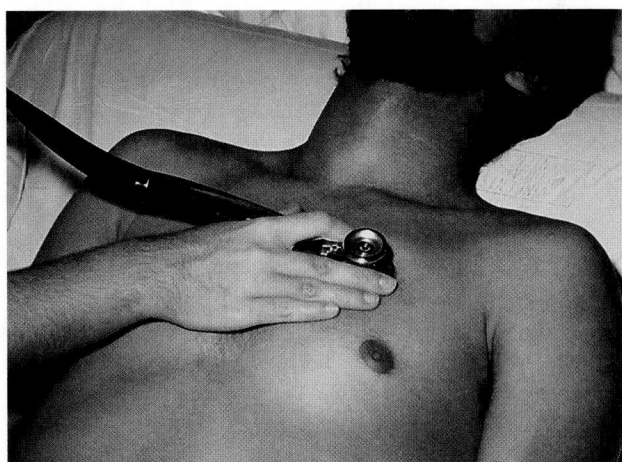

Figure 14-7 ■ Positioning the diaphragm of the stethoscope.

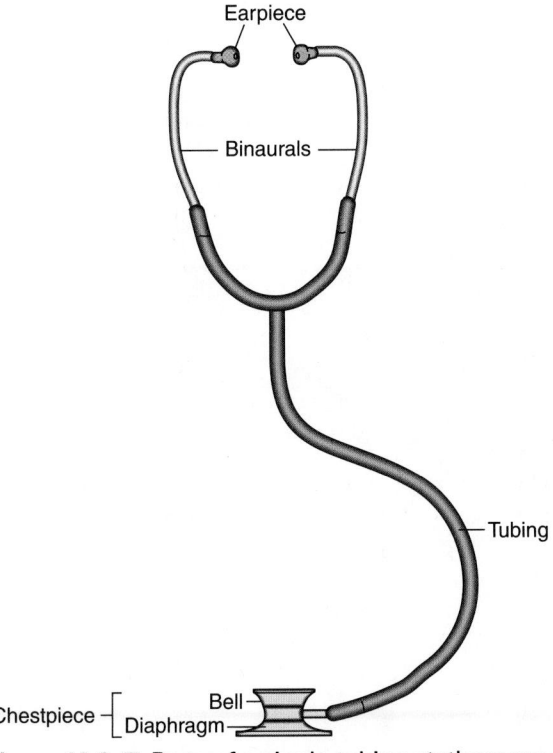

Figure 14-6 ■ Parts of a single-tubing stethoscope.

Earpiece

Binaurals

Tubing

Chestpiece — Bell / Diaphragm

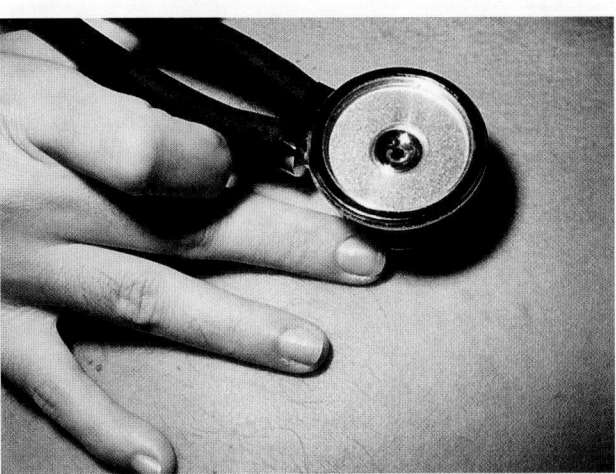

Figure 14-8 ■ Positioning the bell of the stethoscope.

Pulse rate assessment often reveals variations in heart rate. Two common abnormalities in heart rate are **tachycardia** and **bradycardia.** Tachycardia is an abnormally elevated heart rate, more than 100 beats per minute in adults. Bradycardia is a slow rate, less than 60 beats per minute in adults.

PULSE RHYTHM Normally a regular interval of time occurs between each pulse or heartbeat. A regular interval interrupted by an early beat, late beat, or a missed beat indicates an abnormal rhythm or **dysrhythmia.** A dysrhythmia alters cardiac function, particularly if it occurs repetitively. If a dysrhythmia is present, you need to assess the regularity of its occurrence. Dysrhythmias are regularly irregular or irregularly irregular. The health care provider sometimes orders additional tests to evaluate the occurrence of dysrhythmias (see Chapter 26).

An inefficient contraction of the heart that fails to transmit a pulse wave to the peripheral pulse site creates a **pulse deficit.** To assess a pulse deficit, ask a colleague to assess the radial pulse rate while you assess the apical rate. When you compare rates and find a difference between the apical and radial pulse rates, a pulse deficit exists. Pulse deficits are frequently associated with dysrhythmias.

STRENGTH AND EQUALITY The strength or amplitude of a pulse reflects the volume and pressure of the blood ejected against the arterial wall with each heart contraction and the condition of the arterial vascular system leading to the pulse site. Normally the pulse strength remains the same with each heartbeat. Assess both radial pulses to compare the characteristics of each. Pulse strength or amplitude is assigned a number grade and described as increased, full, or bounding (+3); normal, easily palpable (+2); thready, weak, barely palpable (+1); or absent (0) (Jarvis, 2008). You evaluate pulse strength and equality during assessment of the vascular system (see Chapter 15).

BLOOD PRESSURE

Blood pressure is the force exerted on the walls of an artery created by the pulsing blood under pressure from the heart. Blood flows throughout the circulatory system because of pressure changes, moving from an area of high pressure to an area of low pressure. The heart's contraction ejects blood under high pressure into the aorta. The peak pressure (**systolic pressure**) occurs when the heart's ventricular contraction, or systole, forces blood under high pressure into the aorta. When the ventricles relax, the blood remaining in the arteries exerts a minimum or **diastolic pressure.** Diastolic pressure is the minimal pressure exerted against the arterial wall at all times.

The standard unit for measuring blood pressure is millimeters of mercury (mm Hg). The measurement indicates the height to which the blood pressure raises a column of mercury. You record blood pressure as a ratio with the systolic reading before the diastolic (e.g., 120/80 mm Hg). The difference between systolic and diastolic pressure is the **pulse pressure.** For a BP of 120/80 mm Hg, the pulse pressure is 40.

Physiology of Arterial Blood Pressure

Blood pressure depends on the interrelationships of cardiac output, peripheral vascular resistance, blood volume, blood viscosity, and artery elasticity. An increase in cardiac output is sometimes the result of greater heart muscle contractility, an increase in heart rate, or an increase in blood volume. An increase in cardiac output increases blood pressure. When periph-

TABLE 14-3	Acceptable Ranges of Heart Rate for Age	
AGE		**HEART RATE (beats/min)**
Infant		120-160
Toddler		90-140
Preschooler		80-110
School-ager		75-100
Adolescent		60-90
Adult		60-100

TABLE 14-4	Factors Influencing Pulse Rates	
FACTOR	**INCREASE PULSE RATE**	**DECREASE PULSE RATE**
Exercise	Short-term exercise	Long-term exercise conditions the heart, resulting in lower rate at rest and quicker return to resting level after exercise
Temperature	Fever, heat, hyperthermia	Hypothermia
Emotions	Acute pain and anxiety increase sympathetic stimulation, affecting heart rate	Unrelieved severe pain increases parasympathetic stimulation, affecting heart rate; relaxation
Drugs	Positive chronotropic drugs such as epinephrine	Negative chronotropic drugs such as digitalis, beta-adrenergic blockers
Hemorrhage	Loss of blood increases sympathetic stimulation	
Postural changes	Standing or sitting	Lying down
Pulmonary conditions	Diseases causing poor oxygenation, such as asthma and chronic obstructive pulmonary disease (COPD)	

eral arteries constrict, such as during periods of stress, peripheral vascular resistance increases, which results in an increase in BP. As vessels dilate and resistance falls, blood pressure drops. When blood is forced through the rigid arteries, blood pressure rises. If the blood volume decreases, such as during dehydration or hemorrhage, there is less pressure exerted against arterial walls and blood pressure falls. When the hematocrit rises, the percentage of red blood cells in the blood increases, causing an increase in blood viscosity. The heart then contracts more forcefully to move the viscous blood through the circulatory system, resulting in an increased blood pressure.

Blood Pressure Variations

Many factors during the day continually influence blood pressure. A single measurement does not adequately reflect a patient's blood pressure. Blood pressure trends, not individual measurements, guide nursing interventions. Your understanding of the factors that influence blood pressure results in a more accurate interpretation of blood pressure measurements. Box 14-5 summarizes factors affecting blood pressure.

HYPERTENSION The most common alteration in blood pressure is **hypertension,** an often asymptomatic disorder

BOX 14-5 Factors Influencing Blood Pressure

AGE

Blood pressure (BP) tends to rise with advancing age:

AGE	ARTERIAL PRESSURE (mm Hg)
Newborn (3000 g [6.6 lb])	40 (mean)
1 month	85/54
1 year	95/65
6 years	105/65
10-13 years	110/65
14-17 years	119/75

You assess the level of a child's or adolescent's BP with respect to body size and age. Larger children have higher BPs than smaller children of the same age. Older adults have a rise in systolic pressure related to decreased elasticity of blood used.

GENDER
* There is no clinically significant difference in BP levels between boys and girls before puberty.
* After puberty, males have higher readings.
* During and after menopause, women have higher BPs than men of the same age.

ETHNICITY
* The incidence of hypertension is higher in African Americans than in European Americans.
* African Americans tend to develop more severe hypertension at an earlier age and have twice the risk for complications of hypertension such as stroke and heart attack (Appel, Brands, and Daniels, 2006). Hypertension-related deaths are also higher among African Americans.

SYMPATHETIC STIMULATION
* Pain, anxiety, and fear stimulate the sympathetic nervous system, causing BP to rise. A full bladder can increase sympathetic stimulation, elevating BP (Pickering and others, 2005). Anxiety raises BP as much as 30 mm Hg.

DAILY VARIATION
* BP varies throughout the day with lower blood pressure during sleep, increasing during the day (Redon, 2004).
* BP can drop 10% to 20% during nighttime sleep (Giles, 2006).

MEDICATION
* Some medications directly or indirectly affect BP. Antihypertensive medications and narcotic analgesics lower BP. Vasoconstrictors increase BP.

ACTIVITY
* Older adults often experience a 5- to 10-mm Hg fall in blood pressure about 1 hour after eating.
* BP falls as a person moves from lying to sitting or standing position; normal postural variations are minimal.
* Increase in oxygen demand by the body during activity increases BP.

Continued

BOX 14-5   Factors Influencing Blood Pressure—cont'd

WEIGHT

Obesity is a risk factor for hypertension (Appel and others, 2006).

Diet

A diet low in sodium and high in potassium can reduce BP. Vegetarian diets, as well as limited alcohol consumption (fewer than two drinks per day for men and one per day for women), are associated with low BP (Appel and others, 2006). BP reductions are greater among older adults implementing dietary modifications.

SMOKING

Smoking results in vasoconstriction, a narrowing of blood vessels. BP rises when a person smokes and returns to baseline in about 15 minutes after stopping smoking (NHBPEP, 2003).

Data from National High Blood Pressure Education Program; National Heart, Lung, and Blood Institute; National Institutes of Health: The seventh report of the Joint National Committee on Detection, Evaluation, and Treatment of High Blood Pressure, *JAMA* 289(19):560, 2003; Brashers VL: *Clinical application of pathophysiology,* ed 3, St. Louis, 2006, Mosby; Hockenberry MJ, Wilson D: *Wong's nursing care of infants and children,* ed 8, St. Louis, 2008, Mosby.

TABLE 14-5   Classification of Blood Pressure for Adults 18 Years and Older

CATEGORY	SYSTOLIC (mm Hg)*		DIASTOLIC (mm Hg)*
Normal	<120		<80
Prehypertension†	120-139	or	80-89
Stage 1 hypertension	140-159	or	90-99
Stage 2 hypertension	≥160	or	≥100

Data from National High Blood Pressure Education Program; National Heart, Lung, and Blood Institute; National Institutes of Health: The seventh report of the Joint National Committee on Detection, Evaluation and Treatment of High Blood Pressure, *JAMA* 289(19):2560, 2003.
*Based on the average of two or more readings taken at each of two or more visits after an initial screening. Patient should not be taking antihypertensive drugs and not be acutely ill. When systolic and diastolic blood pressures fall into different categories, select the higher category to classify the individual's blood pressure status. For example, classify 160/92 mm Hg as stage 2 hypertension.
†Based on average of two or more readings.

TABLE 14-6   Recommendations for Blood Pressure Follow-up

INITIAL BLOOD PRESSURE	FOLLOW-UP RECOMMENDED*
Normal	Recheck in 2 years.
Prehypertension	Recheck in 1 year.†
Stage 1 hypertension	Confirm within 2 months.†
Stage 2 hypertension	Evaluate or refer to source of care within 1 month. For those with higher pressure (e.g., >180/110 mm Hg), evaluate and treat immediately or within 1 week depending on clinical situation and complications.

Data from National High Blood Pressure Education Program; National Heart, Lung, and Blood Institute; National Institutes of Health: The seventh report of the Joint National Committee on Detection, Evaluation and Treatment of High Blood Pressure, *JAMA* 289(19):2560, 2003.
*Modify the scheduling of follow-up according to reliable information about past blood pressure measurements, other cardiovascular risk factors, or target organ damage.
†Provide advice about lifestyle modifications.

characterized by persistently elevated BP. The Joint National Committee on Prevention, Detection, Evaluation, and Treatment of High Blood Pressure (JNC) (National High Blood Pressure Education Program [NHBPEP], 2003) has set criteria for determining categories of hypertension (Table 14-5). Prehypertension is a designation for patients at high risk for developing hypertension. In these patients, early intervention by adopting healthy lifestyles reduces the risk or prevents hypertension. Persons with a family history of hypertension are at significant risk. Obesity, cigarette smoking, heavy alcohol consumption, high blood cholesterol levels, and continued exposure to stress are also linked to hypertension.

Hypertension is defined as systolic blood pressure of 140 mm Hg or greater, diastolic blood pressure of 90 mm Hg or greater or the need for antihypertensive medication (NHBPEP, 2003). The diagnosis of hypertension in adults is made on the average of two or more readings taken at each of two or more visits after an initial screening. One blood pressure recording revealing a high systolic blood pressure or diastolic blood pressure does not qualify as a diagnosis of hypertension. However, if you assess a high reading (for example, 150/90 mm Hg), encourage the patient to return for another checkup within 2 months (Table 14-6).

HYPOTENSION Hypotension is present when the systolic blood pressure drops to 90 mm Hg or below. Although some adults have low blood pressure normally, for a majority of people hypotension is an abnormal finding associated with an illness (e.g., hemorrhage or myocardial infarction). Hypotension occurs when arteries dilate, the peripheral vascular

BOX 14-6   PROCEDURAL GUIDELINES

Measuring Orthostatic Blood Pressure

DELEGATION CONSIDERATIONS: The skill of measuring orthostatic blood pressure (BP) cannot be delegated to nursing assistive personnel.

EQUIPMENT: Sphygmomanometer, stethoscope

1 With patient supine, take BP reading in each arm. Select arm with highest systolic reading for subsequent measurements.

2 Leaving BP cuff in place, help patient to sitting position. After 1 to 3 minutes with patient in sitting position, take BP reading. If orthostatic signs or symptoms occur such as dizziness, weakness, light-headedness, feeling faint, or sudden pallor, stop BP measurement and return patient to a supine position.

3 Leaving BP cuff in place, help patient to standing position. After 1 to 3 minutes with patient in standing position, take BP. If orthostatic signs or symptoms occur (as noted), stop BP measurement and help patient to a supine position. In most cases, you will detect orthostatic hypotension within 1 minute of standing.

4 Record patient's BP in each position; for example: "140/80 supine, 132/72 sitting, 108/60 standing." Note any additional symptoms or complaints.

5 Report findings of orthostatic hypotension or orthostatic signs or symptoms to nurse in charge or health care provider. Instruct patient to ask for assistance when getting out of bed if orthostatic hypotension is present or orthostatic signs or symptoms occur.

---

resistance decreases, the circulating blood volume decreases, or the heart fails to provide adequate cardiac output. Signs and symptoms associated with hypotension include pallor, skin mottling, clamminess, confusion, dizziness, chest pain, increased heart rate, and decreased urine output. Hypotension is usually life threatening and needs to be reported immediately to the patient's healthcare provider.

Orthostatic hypotension, also referred to as postural hypotension, is a reduction of systolic blood pressure of at least 20 mm Hg or reduction of diastolic blood pressure of at least 10 mm Hg within 3 minutes of quiet standing (Pickering and others, 2005). It occurs with the drop in blood pressure seen in patients with normal blood pressure on rising to an upright position and is associated with symptoms of light-headedness or dizziness. In severe cases, loss of consciousness occurs. When a healthy person changes from a lying to sitting to standing position, the peripheral blood vessels in the legs constrict, preventing the pooling of blood in the legs caused by gravity. Orthostatic hypotension occurs when the peripheral blood vessels in the legs are already constricted or are unable to constrict in response to a change in position. Fluid volume deficit from decreased blood volume, dehydration, or recent blood loss, as well as prolonged bed rest, anemia, or antihypertensive medications, place patients at risk for orthostatic hypotension. Assess for orthostatic hypotension by obtaining pulse and blood pressure readings with the patient supine, sitting, and standing (Box 14-6).

Measurement of Blood Pressure

You measure arterial blood pressure either directly (invasively) or indirectly (noninvasively). The direct method requires the insertion of a thin catheter into an artery. The risks of continuous invasive blood pressure monitoring require use in an intensive care setting. The more common noninvasive method requires use of the **sphygmomanometer** and stethoscope. You measure blood pressure indirectly by auscultation or palpation. Most use the auscultation technique (Skill 14-3).

BLOOD PRESSURE EQUIPMENT Before assessing blood pressure, you need to be comfortable using a sphygmomanometer and stethoscope. A sphygmomanometer includes a pressure manometer, an occlusive cloth or disposable vinyl cuff that encloses an inflatable rubber bladder, and a pressure bulb with a release valve that inflates the bladder. The aneroid manometer has a glass-enclosed circular gauge containing a needle that registers millimeter calibrations. Aneroid manometers are safe, lightweight, portable, and compact (Figure 14-9). Before using the manometer, be sure that the needle points to zero. Metal parts in the aneroid manometer are subject to temperature variations and need to be checked every 6 months to verify their accuracy. Mercury manometers, once the standard device for blood pressure measurement, have been prohibited in health care settings because of the hazard of mercury. Most municipalities have also prohibited the sale or use of mercury-containing devices.

The release valves of the sphygmomanometer must be clean and freely movable in either direction. The valve, when closed, should hold the pressure constant. Frequent calibration is needed to ensure accurate measurements. A sticky valve makes pressure cuff deflation hard to regulate. The pressure bulb and tubing should be airtight.

Cloth or disposable vinyl compression cuffs contain an inflatable bladder and come in several different sizes. The size selected is proportional to the circumference of the limb being assessed. Ideally you select a cuff that is 40% of the circumference (or 20% wider than the diameter) of the midpoint of the limb that you use to measure the blood pressure. The bladder, enclosed by the cuff, encircles at least 80% of the arm of an adult and the entire arm of a child (NHBPEP, 2003). Many adults require a large adult cuff. The lower edge of the cuff is above the antecubital fossa, allowing room for placement of the stethoscope. An improperly placed or fitting cuff causes inaccurate blood pressure measurement (Table 14-7).

AUSCULTATION The best environment for blood pressure measurement by auscultation is in a quiet room at a

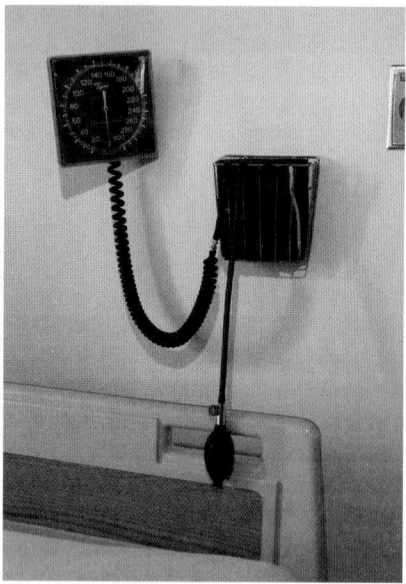

Figure 14-9 ■ Wall-mounted aneroid sphygmomanometer.

TABLE 14-7	Common Mistakes in Blood Pressure Assessment
ERROR	**EFFECT**
Bladder or cuff too wide	False-low reading
Bladder or cuff too narrow too short	False-high reading
Cuff wrapped too loosely or unevenly	False-high reading
Deflating cuff too slowly	False-high diastolic reading
Deflating cuff too quickly	False-low systolic and false-high diastolic reading
Arm below heart level	False-high reading
Arm above heart level	False-low reading
Arm not supported	False-high reading
Stethoscope that fits poorly or impairment of the examiner's hearing, causing sounds to be muffled	False-low systolic and false-high diastolic reading
Stethoscope applied too firmly against antecubital fossa	False-low diastolic reading
Inflating too slowly	False-high diastolic reading
Repeating assessments too quickly	False-high systolic reading
Inadequate inflation level	False-low systolic reading
Multiple examiners using different Korotkoff sounds for diastolic readings	False-high systolic and false-low diastolic reading

comfortable temperature. Although the patient is able to lie or stand, sitting is the best position. Have a patient assume the same position during each blood pressure measurement to permit a meaningful comparison of values. Before assessment, control factors responsible for artificially high readings such as pain, anxiety, or exertion. *As an example, in the case study, Ms. Coburn was obviously anxious when first entering the examination room. After Ms. Coburn sees the nurse practitioner, Miguel retakes her blood pressure. Ms. Coburn's blood pressure this time is 146/94 mm Hg, compared with the first reading of 164/98 mm Hg.*

The patient's perception that the physical or interpersonal environment is stressful will affect the blood pressure. Measurements taken at home are sometimes different from those taken at the patient's place of employment or health care provider's office.

During the initial assessment, obtain and record the blood pressure in both arms. Normally there is a difference of 5 to 10 mm Hg between the right and left arms. In subsequent assessments, measure the blood pressure in the arm with the higher pressure. Pressure differences between extremities greater than 20 mm Hg indicate vascular problems. You need to report these differences to the nurse in charge or health care provider.

Indirect measurement of arterial blood pressure works on a basic principle of pressure. Blood flows freely through an artery until an inflated cuff applies pressure to tissues and causes the artery to collapse. When the cuff slowly deflates, the point at which blood flow returns and sound appears through auscultation is the systolic pressure.

In 1905, Nikolai Korotkoff, a Russian surgeon, first described the sounds heard over an artery during cuff deflation. The first **Korotkoff sound** is a clear, rhythmic tapping series that corresponds to the pulse rate and gradually increases in intensity. Onset of the sound corresponds to the systolic pressure. A murmur or swishing sound appears as the cuff continues to deflate, which is the second Korotkoff sound. As the artery distends, blood flow becomes turbulent. The third Korotkoff sound is a crisper and more intense tapping. The fourth Korotkoff sound becomes muffled and low pitched as the cuff is further deflated. The onset of the fourth Korotkoff sound is the diastolic pressure in infants and children, pregnant women, and patients with elevated cardiac output or peripheral vasodilation. The fifth Korotkoff sound is the disappearance of sound; in adolescents and most adults, this sound corresponds with the diastolic pressure (Figure 14-10). In some patients the sounds are clear and distinct. In other patients you hear only the beginning and the ending sounds.

The American Heart Association recommends recording two numbers for a blood pressure measurement: the point on the manometer when you hear the first sound for systolic and the point on the manometer when you hear the fifth sound (disappearance of sound) for diastolic (NHBPEP, 2003). Some institutions recommend recording the point when you hear the fourth sound as well, especially for patients with hypertension. You divide the numbers by slashed lines (e.g., 120/80, 120/100/80), note the arm used to measure the blood pressure (e.g., RA 130/70), and record the patient's position (e.g., LA 158/78, sitting).

You will make many decisions about a patient's care and implement nursing interventions on the basis of blood pressure measurements in conjunction with other findings. Obtaining an accurate blood pressure is critical (Box 14-7). There are several possibilities for error if you do not follow the auscultation procedure correctly (see Table 14-7). If you are unsure of a reading, ask a colleague to reassess the blood pressure.

ULTRASONIC STETHOSCOPE If you are unable to auscultate Korotkoff sounds because of a weakened arterial pulse, use an ultrasonic stethoscope (see Chapter 15). This stethoscope allows you to hear low-frequency systolic sounds and is commonly used in measuring the blood pressure of infants and children, and for investigating low blood pressure in adults.

PALPATION Indirect measurement of blood pressure by palpation is useful for patients whose arterial pulsations are too weak to create Korotkoff sounds. Severe blood loss and weakened heart contractility are examples of conditions that result in blood pressures too low to auscultate accurately. In this case, you assess the systolic blood pressure by palpation (Box 14-8). The diastolic pressure is difficult to determine by palpation. When you use the palpation technique, you record the systolic value and the manner in which you measured it (e.g., RA 78/−, palpated).

You can use the palpation technique along with auscultation. In some hypertensive patients the sounds usually heard over the brachial artery when the cuff pressure is high disappear as pressure is reduced and then reappear at a lower level. This temporary disappearance of sound is the **auscultatory gap.** It typically occurs between the first and second Korotkoff sounds. The gap in sound sometimes covers a range of 40 mm Hg, possibly causing an underestimation of systolic

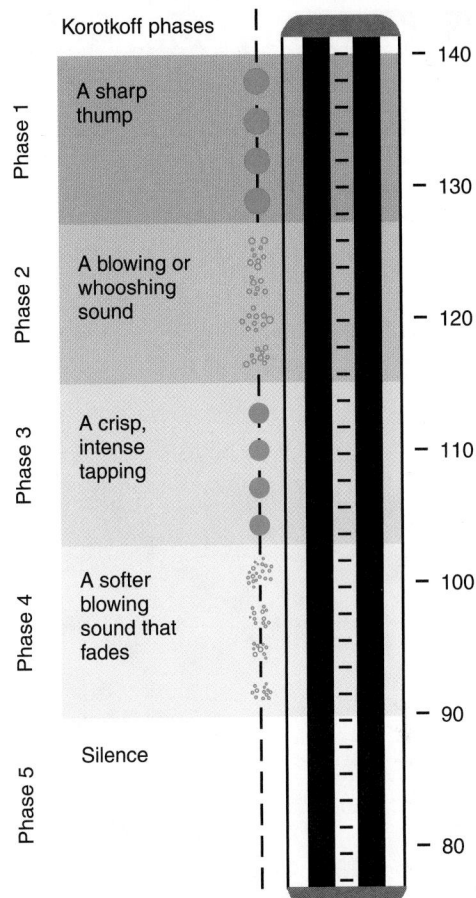

Figure 14-10 ▓ The sounds auscultated during blood pressure measurement can be differentiated into five Korotkoff phases. In this example, the blood pressure is 140/90.

BOX 14-7   BEST PRACTICES

SUMMARY OF EVIDENCE

The size and placement of blood pressure (BP) cuffs are critical for obtaining accurate BP measurements. Traditionally the BP cuff is applied to the upper arm, between the shoulder and the elbow. In some patients when the upper arm is not accessible or when the arm is too large for the BP cuff, health care providers will apply the cuff to the forearm, between the elbow and the wrist. Research on the accuracy of forearm BP measurements includes studies using stethoscope and sphygmomanometers as well as automatic BP devices. Findings have differed among researchers, with some reporting similar BP measurements between upper and lower arms, and others reporting values as much as 10 mm Hg lower in the forearm. Schell and others (2005) compared upper and forearm measurements using automatic BP devices in medical-surgical patients. The patients

were able to assume a supine position with the head of bed elevated. The researchers concluded that the measurement sites are not interchangeable and that measurements can differ by as much as 20 mm Hg.

APPLICATION TO NURSING PRACTICE

- Noninvasive measurement of BP in the forearm should not be substituted for measurement in the upper arm in medical-surgical patients who are supine or lying with the head of the bed elevated 45 degrees, unless there is no other option.
- Proper cuff size is critical for accurate BP measurements.
- When repeating BP values, be aware of the site of the measurement in order to determine trends.
- Document the location of BP measurement when recording values.

REFERENCE

Schell K and others: Clinical comparison of automatic noninvasive measurements of blood pressure in the forearm and upper arm, *Am J Crit Care* 14(3):232, 2005.

BOX 14-8 PROCEDURAL GUIDELINES

Palpating the Systolic Blood Pressure

DELEGATION CONSIDERATIONS The skill of obtaining blood pressure (BP) by palpation cannot be delegated to nursing assistive personnel.

EQUIPMENT Sphygmomanometer

1 Perform hand hygiene.
2 Apply BP cuff to the extremity selected for measurement.
3 Continually palpate the brachial, radial, or popliteal artery of the selected extremity with fingertips of one hand.

4 Inflate the BP cuff 30 mm Hg above the point at which you no longer palpate the pulse.
5 Slowly release valve and deflate cuff, allowing manometer needle to fall at rate of 2 mm Hg per second.
6 Note point on manometer when pulse is again palpable; this is the systolic BP.
7 Deflate cuff rapidly and completely. Remove cuff from patient's extremity unless you need to repeat the measurement.
8 Perform hand hygiene.

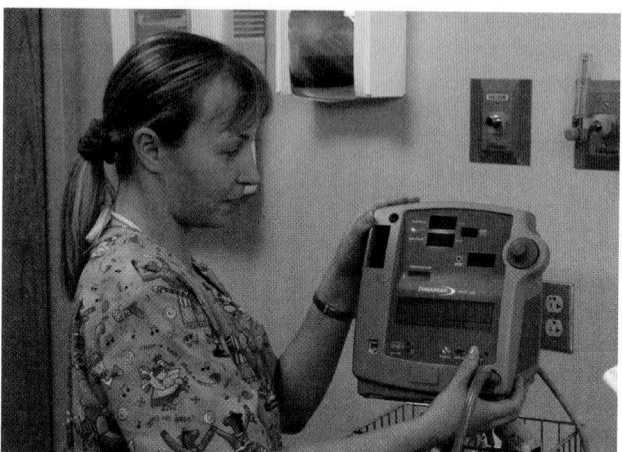

Figure 14-11 ■ Electronic blood pressure machines vary in appearance.

BOX 14-9 Advantages and Limitations of Automatic Blood Pressure Machines

ADVANTAGES
- Ease of use.
- Efficient when frequent repeated measurements are indicated.
- Ability to use a stethoscope not required.
- Allows you to record blood pressure (BP) more frequently, as often as every 15 seconds with accuracy.

LIMITATIONS
- Expensive.
- Requires source of electricity.
- Requires space to position machine.
- Sensitive to outside motion interference; not used in patients with seizures, tremors, or shivers or patients unable to cooperate.
- Not accurate for hypotensive patients or in conditions with reduced blood flow (e.g., hypothermia) (Bern and others, 2007).
- Adherence to accuracy standards for electronic BP machine manufacturers is voluntary.
- Vulnerable to error in patients with irregular heart rate and obese extremities.
- Systolic BP may be overestimated (Bern and others, 2007).

pressure or an overestimation of diastolic pressure. Be certain to inflate the cuff high enough to hear the true systolic pressure before the auscultatory gap. Palpation of the radial artery helps to determine how high to inflate the cuff. You inflate the cuff 30 mm Hg above the pressure at which you palpate the radial pulse. You then record the range of pressures in which the auscultatory gap occurs (e.g., "BP RA 180/94 with an auscultatory gap from 180 to 160").

ELECTRONIC BLOOD PRESSURE MACHINES Many different styles of electronic blood pressure machines are available to determine blood pressure automatically (Figure 14-11). Electronic blood pressure machines rely on an electronic sensor to detect the vibrations caused by the rush of blood through an artery. When the cuff deflates, one style of blood pressure machine determines the initial burst of oscillations and translates the information to a systolic pressure reading. The machine records a diastolic measurement when the oscillations are lowest, just before they stop. Although electronic blood pressure machines are fast and free the care provider for other activities, you must consider the advantages and limitations of electronic blood pressure machines (Box 14-9). Use the devices when you need frequent assessments, such as in critically ill or potentially unstable patients, during or after invasive procedures, or when therapies require frequent monitoring (Box 14-10).

BLOOD PRESSURE ASSESSMENT IN LOWER EXTREMITIES If the patient has dressings, casts, intravenous catheters, or arteriovenous fistulas or shunts in the upper extremities, measure blood pressure in a lower extremity. Comparing upper extremity blood pressure with the blood pressure in the legs is also necessary for patients with certain cardiac and blood pressure abnormalities. The popli-

BOX 14-10   PROCEDURAL GUIDELINES

Automatic Blood Pressure Measurement

DELEGATION CONSIDERATIONS: The skill of blood pressure (BP) measurement using an electronic BP machine can be delegated to nursing assistive personnel (NAP) unless the patient is considered unstable. The nurse instructs the NAP to:

- Obtain BP measurements at appropriate times as determined by agency policy, health care provider's order, or patient condition such as frequent postoperative measurements
- Consider patient-specific factors that affect the patient's usual values
- Select appropriate limb for BP measurement
- Select appropriate-size BP cuff for designated extremity and appropriate cuff for the machine
- Immediately report any abnormalities, which you will confirm

EQUIPMENT: Electronic BP machine, BP cuff of appropriate size as recommended by manufacturer, source of electricity

1 Determine the appropriateness of using electronic BP measurement. Patients with irregular heart rate, peripheral vascular disease, seizures, tremors, and shivering are not candidates for this device.

2 Determine best site for cuff placement (see Skill 14-3, Assessment Step 3).

3 Assist patient to comfortable position, either lying or sitting. Plug in device, and place device near patient, ensuring that connector hose, between cuff and machine, will reach.

4 Locate on/off switch, and turn on machine to enable device to self-test computer systems.

5 Select appropriate cuff size for patient extremity and appropriate cuff for machine. Electronic BP cuff and machine are matched by manufacturer and are not interchangeable.

6 Expose extremity for measurement by removing constricting clothing to ensure proper cuff application. Do not place BP cuff over clothing.

7 Prepare BP cuff by manually squeezing all the air out of the cuff and connecting cuff to connector hose.

8 Wrap flattened cuff snugly around extremity, verifying that only one finger fits between cuff and patient's skin. Make sure the "artery" arrow marked on the outside of the cuff is correctly placed (see illustration for Skill 14-3, Implementation Step 3, illustration *B*).

9 Verify that connector hose between cuff and machine is not kinked. Kinking prevents proper inflation and deflation of cuff.

10 Following manufacturer's directions, set the frequency control of automatic or manual, then press start button. The first BP measurement will pump the cuff to a peak pressure of about 180 mm Hg. After this pressure is reached, the machine begins a deflation sequence that determines the BP. The first reading determines the peak pressure inflation for additional measurements.

11 When deflation is complete, digital display will provide the most recent values and flash time in minutes that has elapsed since the measurement occurred.

Critical Decision Point: If unable to obtain BP with electronic device, verify machine connections (e.g., plugged into working electrical outlet, hose-cuff connections tight, machine on, correct cuff). Repeat electronic BP; if unable to obtain, use auscultatory technique (see Skill 14-3).

12 Set frequency of BP measurements, upper and lower alarm limits for systolic, diastolic, and mean BP readings. Intervals between BP measurements are set from 1 to 90 minutes. The nurse determines frequency and alarm limits based on patient's acceptable range of BP, nursing judgment, facility standards, or health care provider's order.

13 You are able to obtain additional readings at any time by pressing the start button. (Sometimes you will need these for unstable patients.) Pressing the cancel button immediately deflates the cuff.

14 If frequent BP measurements are required, leave the cuff in place. Remove cuff every 2 hours to assess underlying skin integrity and if possible, alternate BP sites. Patients with abnormal bleeding tendencies are at risk for microvascular rupture from repeated inflations. When you are finished using the electronic BP machine, clean BP cuff according to facility policy to reduce transmission of microorganisms.

15 Compare electronic BP readings with auscultatory BP measurements to verify accuracy of electronic BP device.

16 Record BP and site assessed on vital sign flow sheet, nurses' notes, or electronic medical record. Record any signs of BP alterations in nurses' notes. Report abnormal findings to nurse in charge or health care provider.

---

teal artery, palpable behind the knee in the popliteal space, is the site for auscultation. Position the cuff with the bladder over the posterior aspect of the midthigh, 2.5 cm (1 inch) above the popliteal artery. Make sure the cuff is wide enough and long enough to allow for the larger girth of the thigh. For most measurements, place the patient in a prone position. If such a position is impossible, flex the knee slightly for easier access to the artery (Figure 14-12). The procedure is identical to brachial artery auscultation. Systolic pressure in the legs is usually higher by 10 to 40 mm Hg than in the brachial artery, but the diastolic pressure is the same.

ASSESSMENT OF BLOOD PRESSURE IN CHILDREN

All children 3 years of age through adolescence should have blood pressure checked at least yearly. Blood pressure in children changes with growth and development (Falkner and Daniels, 2004). Help parents understand the importance of this routine screening to detect children who are at risk for hypertension. The measurement of blood pressure in infants and children is difficult for several reasons:

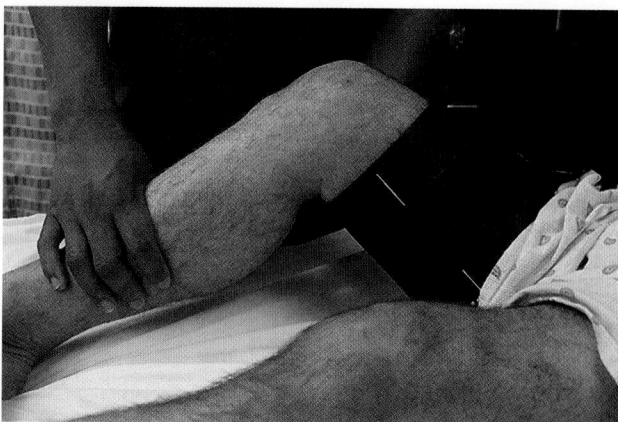

Figure 14-12 ■ Lower extremity blood pressure cuff positioned above popliteal artery at midthigh with knee flexed.

1. Different arm size requires careful and appropriate cuff size selection.
2. Readings are difficult to obtain in restless or anxious infants and children.
3. Placing stethoscope too firmly on the antecubital fossa causes errors in auscultation.
4. Korotkoff sounds are difficult to hear in children because of low frequency and amplitude; a pediatric stethoscope bell is helpful.

The same auscultation method used with adults is appropriate for children. An infant or child younger than 5 years of age lies supine with the arm supported at heart level. Older children sit. It is important for the child to be relaxed and calm. Allow at least 15 minutes for children to recover from recent activity or excitement before taking a reading. Use these 15 minutes for other quiet nursing activities. It helps to have a parent nearby. You prepare the child for the blood pressure cuff's unusual sensation during inflation. Most children understand the analogy of a "tight hug on your arm" and will be more cooperative. Do not choose a cuff based on the name of the cuff (e.g., "infant"). Average width of a cuff bladder for an infant is 2½ to 3¼ inches; average width of a cuff bladder for a child is 4¾ to 5½ inches.

RESPIRATION

Respiration is the mechanism the body uses to exchange gases between the atmosphere, the blood, and the cells. Respiration involves three processes: **ventilation** (the mechanical movement of gases into and out of the lungs), diffusion (the movement of oxygen [O_2] and carbon dioxide [CO_2] between the alveoli and the red blood cells), and **perfusion** (the distribution of red blood cells to and from the pulmonary capillaries). Analyzing respiratory ability requires integrating assessment data from all three processes. You assess ventilation by determining respiratory rate, respiratory depth,

and respiratory rhythm, and you assess diffusion and perfusion by determining oxygen saturation.

Assessment of Ventilation

Adults normally breathe in a smooth, uninterrupted pattern of 12 to 20 breaths per minute. Levels of CO_2 in the arterial blood normally regulate ventilation. The normal rate and depth of ventilation, **eupnea,** is interrupted by sighing. The sigh, a prolonged deeper breath, is a protective physiological mechanism for expanding small airways and alveoli not ventilated during a normal breath.

Accurate assessment of ventilation depends on recognizing normal thoracic and abdominal movements. During quiet breathing, the chest wall gently rises and falls. When breathing requires greater effort, the intercostal and accessory muscles work actively to move air in and out. The shoulders sometimes rise and fall and the accessory muscles of ventilation in the neck visibly contract. Diaphragmatic movement becomes less noticeable as costal breathing increases.

Measurement of Respiration

Accurate measurement of respiration requires observation and palpation of chest wall movement. A sudden change in the character of respirations is an important assessment finding. For example, slow respirations in a patient with head trauma can indicate injury to the brain stem.

When assessing respiration, keep in mind the patient's usual respiratory rate and pattern and the influence any disease or illness has on respiratory function. Also consider the relationship between respiratory and cardiovascular function and the influence of therapies on respiration. Box 14-11 summarizes factors influencing respiration. The objective measurement of respiration includes the rate and depth of breathing and the rhythm of ventilatory movements (Skill 14-4).

RESPIRATORY RATE Observe a full inspiration and expiration when counting ventilations or respiratory rate. The respiratory rate varies with age (Table 14-8). A respiratory rate less than 12 per minute or lower than acceptable limits is **bradypnea,** whereas a rate over 20 or greater than the acceptable limits is **tachypnea. Apnea** is the lack of respiratory movements. A respiratory monitoring device that helps assess respiratory rate is the apnea monitor. This noninvasive device uses electrodes attached to the patient's chest wall to sense movement. An absence of chest wall movement triggers the apnea alarm. Apnea monitoring is used frequently in the hospital and home to observe for prolonged apneic events in infants.

VENTILATORY DEPTH You assess the depth of respirations by observing the degree of movement in the chest wall. Ventilatory movements are deep, normal, or shallow. A deep respiration involves a full expansion of the lungs with obvious movement of the rib cage and full exhalation. A normal respiration is relaxed, automatic, and silent. Respirations are shallow when only a small quantity of air passes through the lungs and ventilatory movement is difficult to see. Use more objective techniques (such as lung excursion) if you observe

BOX 14-11   Factors Influencing Character of Respirations

EXERCISE
- Exercise increases respiration rate and depth to meet the body's need for additional oxygen and to rid the body of CO_2.

ACUTE PAIN
- Pain alters rate and rhythm of respirations; breathing becomes shallow.
- Patient inhibits or splints chest wall movement when pain is in area of chest or abdomen.

ANXIETY
- Anxiety increases respiration rate and depth as a result of sympathetic stimulation.

SMOKING
- Chronic smoking changes pulmonary airways, resulting in increased respiratory rate at rest when not smoking.

BODY POSITION
- Standing or sitting erect promotes full ventilatory movement and lung expansion; stooped or slumped position impairs ventilatory movement; lying flat prevents full chest expansion.

MEDICATIONS
- General anesthetics, sedative-hypnotics, and excessive doses of opioid analgesics depress respiration rate and depth.
- Amphetamines and cocaine may increase rate and depth; bronchodilators cause airway dilation that can ultimately slow respiratory rate.

NEUROLOGICAL INJURY
- Damage to the brain stem impairs the respiratory center and inhibits respiratory rate and rhythm.

HEMOGLOBIN FUNCTION
- Decreased hemoglobin levels (anemia) reduce oxygen-carrying capacity of the blood, which increases respiratory rate.
- Increased altitude lowers the amount of saturated hemoglobin, which increases respiratory rate and depth.
- Abnormal blood cell function (e.g., sickle cell disease) reduces ability of hemoglobin to carry oxygen, which increases respiratory rate and depth.

TABLE 14-8   Acceptable Range of Respiratory Rates for Age

AGE	RATE (breaths/min)
Newborn	35-40
Infant (6 months)	30-50
Toddler (2 years)	25-32
Child	20-30
Adolescent	16-20
Adult	12-20

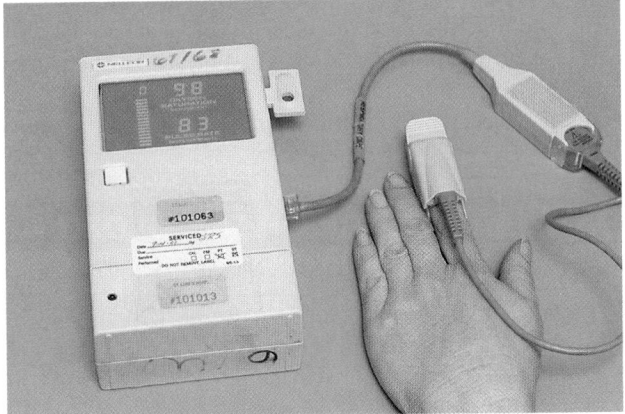

Figure 14-13 ■ Pulse oximeter connected to finger sensor.

that chest movement is unusually shallow or not symmetrical (see Chapter 15).

VENTILATORY RHYTHM Respiratory rhythm or breathing pattern is either regular or irregular. While assessing respiration, observe the interval between each respiratory cycle. With normal breathing, a regular interval occurs between each respiratory cycle. If you observe an irregular ventilatory rhythm, such as periods of apnea with shallow or deep breathing, you need a more detailed physical assessment (see Chapter 29). Infants tend to breathe less regularly. Young children sometimes breathe slowly for a few seconds and then suddenly breathe more rapidly.

MEASUREMENT OF OXYGEN SATURATION (PULSE OXIMETRY)

Pulse oximetry is the indirect measurement of **oxygen saturation** for a patient's vital sign database (Skill 14-5). The oximeter is a photosensor with a light-emitting diode (LED) connected by a cable to an oximeter (Figure 14-13). The LED emits light wavelengths that oxygenated and deoxygenated hemoglobin molecules absorb differently. Oximeters measure the different absorption spectra of oxygenated and deoxygenated hemoglobin. Based on electronic measures of oxygenation at the peak of the pulse, oxygen saturation is computed and displayed of the arterial blood almost instantly. The more hemoglobin saturated by oxygen, the higher the oxygen saturation. Normally SpO_2 is greater than 90%.

The measurement of SpO_2 is simple and painless and carries fewer risks than those associated with invasive measurements of SaO_2 such as arterial blood gas sampling. A vascular, pulsatile area (e.g., fingertip or earlobe) is needed to detect the degree of change in the transmitted light. Factors that affect light transmission (such as sensor movement) or peripheral arterial pulsations (such as hypotension or anemia) also affect the measurement of SpO_2. An awareness of these factors will allow you to interpret abnormal SpO_2 measurements accurately. You can measure SpO_2 intermittently or continuously. You will use continuous SpO_2 monitoring to assess ongoing therapies. You can program alarm limits to alert you if the patient's SpO_2 drops to an unacceptable level.

SPECIAL CONSIDERATIONS

Physiological changes due to aging influence the measurement and interpretation of older adults' vital signs (Box 14-12). After you obtain vital signs and inform the patient of the results, patient teaching may be required (Box 14-13). For example, teach patients with hypothermia to avoid factors that contribute to heat loss. Teach patients with hyperthermia ways to improve comfort. Patients with hypertension require education on risk factor modification. Teach patients taking cardiac medications affecting pulse rate how to obtain their own heart rate.

DOCUMENTING VITAL SIGNS

Specific graphic flow sheets exist for recording vital signs (see Chapter 9). Vital signs are also entered directly in electronic medical records at the patient's bedside. Identify and use the agency's policy for documenting vital signs. In a community-based setting, you record vital signs in the progress notes for that particular clinic or home visit. Record any patient teaching regarding vital signs. When a vital sign is above or below the expected value, enter a note in the patient's database regarding the finding and related interventions.

BOX 14-12 CARE OF THE OLDER ADULT
Considerations When Obtaining Vital Sign Measurements

TEMPERATURE
- The normal temperature of older adults is at the lower end of the acceptable temperature range, 36° C (96.8° F). Therefore temperatures considered normal for an adult may represent a fever in an older adult.
- Older adults are very sensitive to slight changes in environmental temperature because their thermoregulatory systems are not as efficient (Ebersole and others, 2004).
- A decrease in sweat gland reactivity in the older adult results in a higher threshold for sweating at high temperatures, which leads to hyperthermia and heatstroke.
- With aging, loss of subcutaneous fat reduces the insulating capacity of the skin; older men are at especially high risk for hypothermia.

PULSE RATE
- It is often difficult to palpate the pulse of an older adult. A Doppler device will provide a more accurate reading.
- The older adult has a decreased heart rate at rest (Ebersole and others, 2004).
- It takes longer for the heart rate to rise in the older adult to meet sudden increased demands that result from stress, illness, or excitement. Once elevated, the pulse rate of an older adult takes longer to return to normal resting rate (Ebersole and others, 2004).
- When assessing the apical rate of an older woman, lift the breast tissue gently and place the stethoscope at the fifth intercostal space (ICS) or the lower edge of the breast.
- Heart sounds are sometimes muffled or difficult to hear in older adults because of an increase in air space in the lungs.

BLOOD PRESSURE
- The normal range for blood pressure is the same for older adults and younger people (NHBPEP, 2003).
- Older adults often have decreased upper arm mass, which requires special attention to selection of blood pressure cuff size.
- Skin of older adults is more fragile and susceptible to cuff pressure injury when blood pressure measurements are frequent.
- Older adults sometimes have an increase in systolic pressure related to decreased vessel elasticity, whereas the diastolic pressure remains the same, resulting in a wider pulse pressure.
- Instruct older adults to change position slowly and wait after each change to avoid orthostatic hypotension and prevent injuries.

RESPIRATION
- Aging causes ossification of costal cartilage and downward slant of ribs, resulting in a more rigid rib cage, which reduces chest wall expansion. Kyphosis and scoliosis, which may occur in older adults, also restrict chest expansion and decrease tidal volume.
- The respiratory system matures by the time a person reaches 20 years of age and begins to decline in healthy people after the age of 25. Despite this decline, older adults are able to breathe effortlessly as long as they are healthy. However, sudden events that require an increased demand for oxygen (e.g., exercise, stress, illness) can create shortness of breath in the older adult (Ebersole and others, 2004).
- Identifying an acceptable pulse oximeter sensor site is difficult with older adults because of the likelihood of peripheral vascular disease, decreased cardiac output, cold-induced vasoconstriction, and anemia, which decrease pulsatile flow.

BOX 14-13   Vital Sign Patient Teaching Considerations

After caring for Ms. Coburn, Miguel sees the need to educate Ms. Coburn about the different types of vital signs. Based on Ms. Coburn's current problems, Miguel determines the priority is to focus on hypertension and ways to prevent or control elevated blood pressure (BP). Miguel states, "We need to watch your blood pressure closely over the next few weeks. In the meantime, remember you decided that you are going to walk for at least 15 minutes 3 days a week, try to eat foods with less salt, and think about not smoking anymore. To maintain your overall health, you also need to know information about temperature, pulse, and respirations as well as blood pressure." Miguel then implements a teaching plan.

Outcome: Ms. Coburn will verbalize understanding of how temperature, pulse, BP, and respirations relate to her health status.

Teaching Strategies: When educating Ms. Coburn about vital sign measurement, Miguel considers the following issues and implements appropriate teaching strategies:

TEMPERATURE

- Identify Ms. Coburn's ability to initiate preventive health measures and recognize alteration in body temperature. Educate Ms. Coburn and her family about measures to prevent body temperature alterations.
- Explain the risk factors for hypothermia: fatigue; malnutrition; cold, wet clothing; alcohol intoxication.
- Educate about the risk factors for heat stroke: strenuous exercise in hot, humid weather; tight-fitting clothing in hot environments; exercising in poorly ventilated areas; sudden exposure to hot climates; poor fluid intake before, during, and after exercise.
- Educate Ms. Coburn about the importance of taking and continuing antibiotics as directed until course of treatment is completed if she needs antibiotic therapy.

PULSE RATE

- Teach Ms. Coburn how to take her carotid pulse. Patients taking certain cardiac and antihypertensive medications need to learn to assess their own pulse rates to detect side effects and the safety of taking these medications.
- Explain the need to take pulse before, during, and after exercise. Patients who exercise or are in cardiac rehabilitation programs need to learn to assess their own pulse to determine their response to the exercise.

BLOOD PRESSURE

- Educate Ms. Coburn about the risk factors for hypertension. People with family history of hypertension are at significant risk. Obesity, cigarette smoking, heavy alcohol consumption, high blood cholesterol and triglyceride levels, and continued exposure to stress are factors linked to hypertension (NHBPEP, 2003).
- Ensure Ms. Coburn understands her own blood BP values, long-term follow-up care and therapy, the usual lack of symptoms, therapy's ability to control but not cure hypertension, and benefits of a consistently followed treatment plan.
- Explain the importance of an appropriate-size BP cuff for home use and demonstrate how to use the BP cuff.
- Instruct the patient or the caregiver to take BP readings at the same time each day and after patient has had a brief rest. Instruct to take measurements while patient is sitting or lying down and to use same position and arm each time BP is taken.
- Describe how to determine the size of BP cuff needed. If the BP is difficult to hear, it is possible that the BP cuff is too loose, not big enough, or too narrow. Other possible problems include the stethoscope is not over the arterial pulse, the BP cuff was deflated too quickly or too slowly, or BP cuff was not pumped high enough for systolic readings.

RESPIRATION

- Explain the effect of high-risk behaviors such as cigarette smoking on oxygen saturation.
- Teach deep breathing and coughing exercises if Ms. Coburn experiences decreased ventilation.
- Instruct Ms. Coburn or her family to contact home care nurse or health care provider if unusual fluctuations in respiratory rate or rhythm occur.
- Educate Ms. Coburn about the signs and symptoms of hypoxemia: headache, somnolence, confusion, dusky color, shortness of breath, dyspnea.

Evaluation Strategies:
- Have Ms. Coburn describe her normal vital sign values.
- Ask Ms. Coburn to state three risk factors for hypertension.
- Observe Ms. Coburn take her temperature and BP with the equipment she will use at home. Evaluate her technique and provide guidance as needed.
- Have Ms. Coburn take her carotid pulse while you take her radial pulse. Determine her accuracy in pulse taking by comparing the pulse rate she measured with the one you obtained.

SAFETY GUIDELINES FOR NURSING SKILLS

Ensuring patient safety is an essential role of the professional nurse. To ensure patient safety, communicate clearly with members of the health care team, assess and incorporate the patient's priorities of care and preferences, and use the best evidence when making decisions about your patient's care. When performing the skills in this chapter, remember the following points to ensure safe, individualized patient care:

- Vital sign measurement devices are often shared among patients. Cleaning each device carefully between patients will decrease the patients' risk for infection.
- Blood pressure cuffs and pulse oximetry sensors can apply excessive pressure on fragile skin. Rotating sites during repeated measurements decreases risk for skin breakdown.
- Analyze the trends of vital sign measurement, and report abnormal findings to the health care provider.
- Determine vital sign frequency based on the patient's condition.

SKILL 14-1   MEASURING BODY TEMPERATURE

View Video!

DELEGATION CONSIDERATIONS

The skill of temperature measurement can be delegated to nursing assistive personnel (NAP). The nurse instructs the NAP to:

- Select the appropriate route and device to measure temperature
- Take appropriate precautions when properly positioning the patient for rectal temperature measurement
- Consider patient-specific factors that will falsely raise or lower temperature
- Obtain temperature measurements at appropriate times as determined by agency policy or health care provider's orders or patient condition, such as when a patient is shivering or feels warm
- Know the usual temperature values for the patient
- Immediately report any abnormal temperatures, which you will need to confirm

EQUIPMENT

- Appropriate thermometer
- Soft tissue or wipe
- Alcohol swab
- Water-soluble lubricant (for rectal measurements only)
- Pen, vital sign flow sheet or record or patient's electronic medical record
- Clean gloves, plastic thermometer sleeve, disposable probe or sensor cover
- Towel

STEP	RATIONALE

ASSESSMENT

1 Assess for signs and symptoms that accompany temperature alterations.
   Hyperthermia: Decreased skin turgor; tachycardia; hypotension; concentrated urine.
   Heatstroke: Hot, dry skin; tachycardia; hypotension; excessive thirst; muscle cramps; visual disturbances; confusion or delirium.
   Hypothermia: Pale skin; skin cool or cold to touch; bradycardia and dysrhythmias; uncontrollable shivering; reduced level of consciousness; shallow respirations.

Physical signs and symptoms indicate abnormal temperature, indicating need for temperature measurement. You accurately assess nature of variations.

2 Determine any activity that will interfere with accuracy of temperature measurement. When taking oral temperature, wait 15 minutes before measuring temperature if patient has smoked, chewed gum, or ingested hot or cold liquid or food.

Smoking, chewing gum, and ingesting hot or cold substances may cause false temperature readings in oral cavity.

3 Determine appropriate site and measurement device you will use.

Chosen on basis of preferred site for temperature measurement and any patient contraindications (see Box 14-4).

4 Determine previous baseline temperature and measurement site from patient's record.

Allows for assessment of change in patient's condition with future measurements.

PLANNING

1 Explain route by which you will take temperature and importance of maintaining proper position until reading is complete.

Patients are often curious about such measurements and may prematurely remove thermometer to read results.

STEP	RATIONALE

IMPLEMENTATION

1 Perform hand hygiene.

2 Assist patient to a comfortable position that provides easy access to temperature measurement site.

3 Obtain temperature reading.

    A Oral Temperature Measurement With Electronic Thermometer:

        (1) Apply clean gloves *(optional)*.

        (2) Remove thermometer pack from charging unit. Attach oral thermometer probe stem (blue tip) to thermometer unit. Grasp top of probe stem, being careful not to apply pressure on the ejection button.

        (3) Slide disposable plastic probe cover over thermometer probe stem until cover locks in place (see illustrations).

Reduces transmission of microorganisms.

Ensures patient comfort and accuracy of temperature reading.

Use of oral probe cover, which is removable without physical contact, minimizes need to wear gloves.

Charging provides battery power. Ejection button releases plastic cover from probe stem.

Soft plastic cover will not break in patient's mouth and prevents transmission of microorganisms between patients.

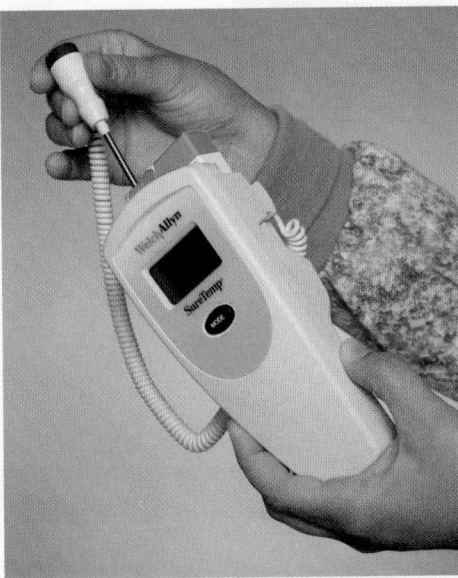 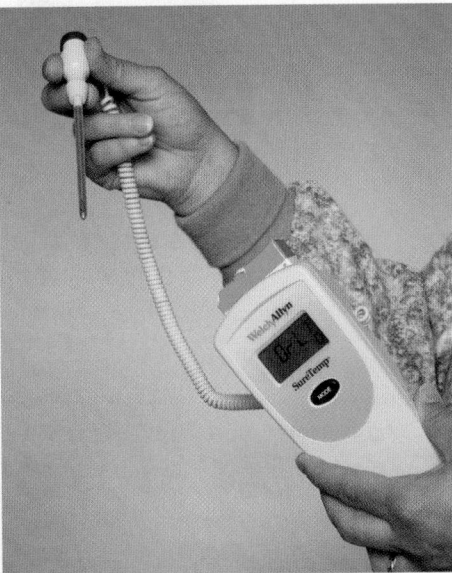

Step 3A(3) ▪ Disposable plastic cover is placed over the probe.

SKILL 14-1   MEASURING BODY TEMPERATURE—cont'd

STEP	RATIONALE
(4) Ask patient to open mouth; then gently place thermometer probe under tongue in posterior sublingual pocket lateral to center of lower jaw (see illustration).	Heat from superficial blood vessels in sublingual pocket produces temperature reading. With electronic thermometer, temperatures in right and left posterior sublingual pocket are significantly higher than in area under front of tongue.

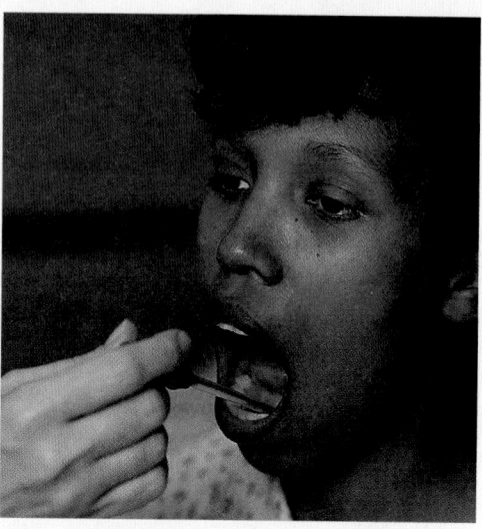

Step 3A(4) ■ Probe under tongue in posterior sublingual pocket.

(5) Ask patient to hold thermometer probe with lips closed.	Maintains proper position of thermometer during recording.
(6) Leave thermometer probe in place until audible signal indicates completion and patient's temperature appears on digital display; remove thermometer probe from under patient's tongue.	Makes sure probe stays in place until signal occurs to ensure accurate reading.
(7) Push ejection button on thermometer probe stem to discard plastic probe cover into appropriate receptacle.	Reduces transmission of microorganisms.
(8) Return thermometer probe stem to storage position of recording unit.	Returning probe stem automatically causes digital reading to disappear. Storage position protects stem.
(9) If gloves worn, remove and dispose of in appropriate receptacle. Perform hand hygiene.	Reduces transmission of microorganisms.
(10) Return thermometer to charger.	Maintains battery charge of thermometer unit.
B Rectal Temperature Measurement With Electronic Thermometer:	
(1) Draw curtain around bed, and/or close room door. Assist patient to side-lying or Sims' position with upper leg flexed. Move aside bed linen to expose only anal area. Keep patient's upper body and lower extremities covered with sheet or blanket.	Maintains patient's privacy, minimizes embarrassment, and promotes comfort.
(2) Apply clean gloves.	Maintains standard precautions when exposed to items soiled with body fluids (e.g., feces).
(3) Remove thermometer pack from charging unit. Attach rectal thermometer probe stem (red tip) to thermometer unit. Grasp top of probe stem, being careful not to apply pressure on the ejection button.	Charging provides battery power. Ejection button releases plastic cover from probe stem.
(4) Slide disposable plastic probe cover over thermometer probe stem until cover locks in place.	Probe cover prevents transmission of microorganisms between patients.
(5) Squeeze liberal portion of lubricant onto tissue. Dip thermometer probe's blunt end into lubricant, covering 2.5 to 3.5 cm (1 to 1½ inch) for adult.	Lubrication minimizes trauma to rectal mucosa during insertion. Tissue avoids contamination of remaining lubricant in container.

STEP	RATIONALE
(6) With nondominant hand, separate patient's buttocks to expose anus. Ask patient to breathe slowly and relax.	Fully exposes anus for thermometer insertion. Relaxes anal sphincter for easier thermometer insertion.
(7) Gently insert thermometer probe into anus in direction of umbilicus 2.5 to 3.5 cm (1 to 1½ inch) for adult. If resistance is felt during insertion, withdraw immediately. Do not force thermometer.	Ensures adequate exposure against blood vessels in rectal wall.

• *Critical Decision Point:* If you cannot adequately insert thermometer into rectum, remove thermometer and consider alternative method for obtaining temperature.

STEP	RATIONALE
(8) Once positioned, hold thermometer probe in place until audible signal indicates completion and patient's temperature appears on digital display; remove thermometer probe from anus (see illustration).	Probe needs to stay in place until signal occurs to ensure accurate reading.

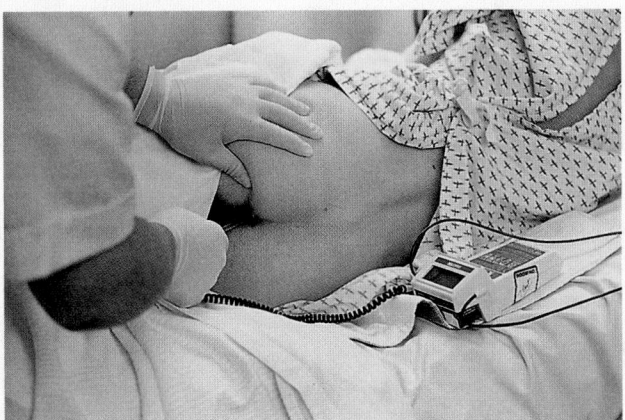

Step 3B(8) ■ **Probe removed smoothly from anus.**

STEP	RATIONALE
(9) Push ejection button on thermometer stem to discard plastic probe cover into an appropriate receptacle. Wipe probe stem with alcohol swab, paying particular attention to ridges where probe stem connects to probe.	Reduces transmission of microorganisms.
(10) Return thermometer stem to storage position of recording unit.	Returning thermometer stem to storage position automatically causes digital reading to disappear. Storage position protects stem.
(11) Wipe patient's anal area with tissue or soft wipe to remove lubricant or feces, and discard tissue. Assist patient in assuming a comfortable position.	Provides for comfort and hygiene.
(12) Remove and dispose of gloves in appropriate receptacle. Perform hand hygiene.	Reduces transmission of microorganisms.
(13) Return thermometer to charger.	Maintains battery charge of thermometer unit.
C Axillary Temperature Measurement With Electronic Thermometer:	
(1) Draw curtain around bed, and/or close room door. Assist patient to supine or sitting position. Move clothing or gown away from shoulder and arm.	Maintains patient's privacy, minimizes embarrassment, and promotes comfort. Exposes axilla for correct thermometer probe placement.
(2) Remove thermometer pack from charging unit. Attach oral thermometer probe stem (blue tip) to thermometer unit. Grasp top of thermometer probe stem, being careful not to apply pressure on ejection button.	Ejection button releases plastic cover from probe.

SKILL 14-1	MEASURING BODY TEMPERATURE—cont'd

STEP	RATIONALE
(3) Slide disposable plastic probe cover over thermometer stem until cover locks in place.	Probe cover prevents transmission of microorganisms between patients.
(4) Raise patient's arm away from torso. Inspect for skin lesions and excessive perspiration. Insert thermometer probe into center of axilla, lower arm over probe, and place arm across patient's chest.	Maintains proper position of probe against blood vessels in axilla.

• *Critical Decision Point:* Do not use axilla if skin lesions are present because local temperature may be altered and area may be painful to touch.

STEP	RATIONALE
(5) Once positioned, hold thermometer probe in place until audible signal indicates completion and patient's temperature appears on digital display; remove thermometer probe from axilla.	Thermometer probe needs to stay in place until signal occurs to ensure accurate reading.
(6) Push ejection button on thermometer stem to discard plastic probe cover into appropriate receptacle.	Reduces transmission of microorganisms.
(7) Return thermometer stem to storage position of recording unit.	Returning thermometer stem to storage position automatically causes digital reading to disappear. Storage position protects stem.
(8) Assist patient in assuming a comfortable position, replacing linen or gown.	Restores comfort and sense of well-being.
(9) Perform hand hygiene.	Reduces transmission of microorganisms.
(10) Return thermometer to charger.	Maintains battery charge of thermometer unit.
D Tympanic Membrane Temperature Measurement With Infrared Thermometer:	
(1) Assist patient in assuming comfortable position with head turned toward side, away from you. If patient has been lying on one side, use upper ear. Obtain temperature from patient's right ear if you are right handed. Obtain temperature from patient's left ear if you are left handed.	Ensures comfort and exposes auditory canal for accurate temperature measurement. Heat trapped in ear facing down will cause falsely high temperature readings. Using the appropriate hand will reduce the angle of approach. The less acute the angle, the better is the probe seal.
(2) Note if there is obvious earwax present in the patient's ear canal.	Earwax on the lens cover of speculum will block a clear optical pathway. Switch to other ear, or select alternative measurement site.
(3) Remove thermometer handheld unit from charging base, being careful not to apply pressure to the ejection button.	Base provides battery power. Removal of handheld unit from base prepares it to measure temperature. Ejection button releases plastic probe cover from thermometer tip.
(4) Slide disposable speculum cover over otoscope-like tip until it locks into place. Be careful not to touch lens cover.	Soft plastic probe cover prevents transmission of microorganisms between patients. Lens cover must be free of dust, fingerprints, and earwax to ensure clear optical path. Earwax can lower tympanic temperature by 0.3° C (0.6° F) (Farnell and others, 2005).

STEP	RATIONALE

(5) Insert infrared speculum into ear canal following manufacturer's instructions for tympanic probe positioning (see illustration):

Correct positioning of the speculum probe tip with respect to ear canal allows maximum exposure of tympanic membrane.

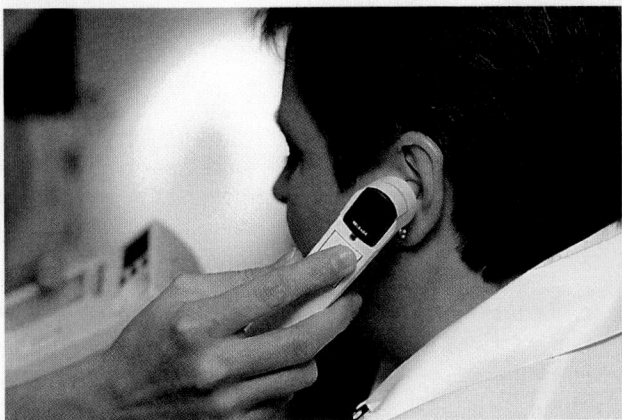

Step 3D(5) ■ Tympanic membrane thermometer with probe cover placed in patient's ear.

(a) Pull ear pinna backward, up, and out for an adult. For children younger than 3 years of age, point covered probe toward midpoint between eyebrow and sideburns.

The ear tug straightens the external auditory canal, allowing maximum exposure of the tympanic membrane.

(b) Move thermometer in a figure-eight pattern.

Some manufacturers recommend movement of the speculum tip in a figure-eight pattern that allows the sensor to detect maximum tympanic membrane heat radiation.

(c) Fit speculum tip snugly into canal and do not move, pointing speculum tip toward nose.

Gentle pressure seals ear canal from ambient air temperature, which alters readings as much as 2.8° C (5° F). Operator error will lead to falsely low temperature readings.

(6) Once positioned, press scan button on handheld unit. Leave speculum in place until audible signal indicates completion and patient's temperature appears on digital display.

Pressing scan button causes detection of infrared energy. Speculum probe tip needs to stay in place until signal indicating device has detected infrared energy.

(7) Carefully remove speculum from auditory canal.

Prevents rubbing of sensitive outer ear lining.

(8) Push ejection button on handheld unit to discard speculum cover into appropriate receptacle.

Reduces transmission of microorganisms. Automatically causes digital reading to disappear.

(9) If temperature is abnormal or a second reading is necessary, replace speculum cover and wait 2 to 3 minutes before repeating the measurement in the same ear or repeat measurement in other ear. Consider trying an alternative temperature site or instrument.

Time allows ear canal to regain usual temperature readings.

(10) Return handheld unit to thermometer base.

Protects sensor tip from damage.

(11) Assist patient in assuming a comfortable position.

Restores comfort and sense of well-being.

(12) Perform hand hygiene.

Reduces transmission of microorganisms.

E Temporal Artery Temperature Measurement With Infrared Thermometer:

(1) Ensure that forehead is dry; wipe with towel if needed.

Thermometer sensor is distorted by moist skin.

(2) Place sensor flush on patient's forehead.

Contact avoids measurement of ambient temperature.

(3) Press red scan button with your thumb. Slowly slide thermometer straight across forehead while keeping sensor flush on skin (see Figure 14-3, p. 267).

Continuous scanning for the highest temperature will continue until you release the scan button.

SKILL 14-1	MEASURING BODY TEMPERATURE—cont'd

STEP	RATIONALE
(4) Keeping the scan button pressed, lift sensor from forehead and touch sensor to skin on the neck, just behind the earlobe. Peak temperature occurs when clicking sound during scanning stops. Read digital display, then release scan button.	Sensor confirms highest temperature behind earlobe.
(5) Clean sensor with alcohol swab.	Prevents transmission of microorganisms.
(6) Perform hand hygiene.	Reduces transmission of microorganisms.
4 Inform patient of temperature reading and document measurement.	Promotes participation in care and understanding of health status.

EVALUATION

1 If you are assessing temperature for the first time, establish temperature as baseline if it is within acceptable range.	Used to compare future temperature measurements.
2 Compare temperature reading with patient's previous temperature and acceptable temperature range for patient's age-group.	Body temperature fluctuates within narrow range; comparison reveals presence of abnormality. Improper placement or movement of thermometer causes inaccuracies.
3 If patient has fever, take temperature approximately 30 minutes after administering antipyretics, and every 4 hours until temperature stabilizes.	Will determine if temperature begins to fall in response to therapy.

RECORDING AND REPORTING

- Record temperature and route in nurses' notes, vital sign flow sheet, or electronic medical record. Record in nurses' notes any signs or symptoms of temperature alterations.
- Document measurement of temperature after administration of specific therapies in narrative form in nurses' notes.

- Report abnormal findings to nurse in charge or health care provider immediately.

UNEXPECTED OUTCOMES AND RELATED INTERVENTIONS

- Temperature is 1° C or more *above* usual range.
  - Assess possible sites for localized infection and for related data suggesting systemic infection.
  - Follow interventions listed in Box 14-3, p. 263.
  - If fever persists or reaches unacceptable level as defined by health care provider, administer antipyretics as ordered.

- Temperature is 1° C or more *below* usual range.
  - Initiate measures to increase body temperature.
  - Remove any wet clothing or linen, and cover patient with warm blankets.
  - Close room doors to eliminate drafts.
  - Encourage warm liquids.
  - Monitor apical pulse rate and rhythm (see Skill 14-2) because hypothermia causes bradycardia and dysrhythmias.

SKILL 14-2	ASSESSING THE RADIAL AND APICAL PULSES

DELEGATION CONSIDERATIONS

The skill of pulse measurement can be delegated to nursing assistive personnel (NAP) if the patient is stable and not at high risk for acute or serious cardiac problems. The nurse instructs the NAP to:

- Consider factors related to the patient's history, usual values, or risk for abnormally slow or irregular pulse
- Obtain appropriate pulse measurement frequency at appropriate times as determined by agency policy, health care provider's orders, or patient condition, such as the presence of chest pain or dizziness
- Immediately report any abnormalities, which the nurse will confirm

EQUIPMENT

- Wristwatch with second hand or digital display
- Pen, pencil, vital sign flow sheet or record or patient's electronic medical record
- Stethoscope (apical pulse only)
- Alcohol swab

STEP	**RATIONALE**

ASSESSMENT

1 Determine need to obtain radial and/or apical pulse:

   a Assess risk factors for pulse alterations.
     • History of heart disease
     • Cardiac dysrhythmia
     • Onset of sudden chest pain or acute pain from any site
     • Invasive cardiovascular diagnostic tests
     • Surgery
     • Sudden infusion of large volume of IV fluid
     • Internal or external hemorrhage, dehydration
     • Administration of medications that alter cardiac function.

These conditions place patients at risk for pulse alterations. A history of peripheral vascular disease often alters pulse rate and quality.

   b Assess for signs and symptoms of altered cardiac function such as dyspnea, fatigue, chest pain, orthopnea, syncope, palpitations (person's unpleasant awareness of heartbeat), edema of dependent body parts, cyanosis or pallor of skin (see Chapter 29).

Physical signs and symptoms indicate alteration in cardiac function, which affects pulse rate and rhythm.

   c Assess for signs and symptoms of peripheral vascular disease such as pale, cool extremities; thin, shiny skin with decreased hair growth; thickened nails.

Physical signs and symptoms indicate alteration in local arterial blood flow.

2 Assess for factors that influence pulse rate and rhythm: age, exercise, position changes, fluid balance, medications, temperature, sympathetic stimulation.

Allows you to accurately assess presence and significance of pulse alterations. Acceptable range of pulse rate changes with age (see Table 14-3, p. 270).

3 Determine patient's previous baseline pulse rate (if available) from patient's record.

Allows you to assess for change in condition. Provides comparison with future pulse measurements.

4 Determine if patient has a latex allergy.

If patient has a latex allergy, verify that stethoscope is latex-free.

PLANNING

1 Explain to patient that you will assess pulse or heart rate. Encourage patient to relax and not speak. If patient has been active, wait 5 to 10 minutes before assessing pulse.

Activity and anxiety elevate heart rate. Patient's voice interferes with your ability to hear sound when measuring apical pulse. Obtaining pulse rates at rest allows for objective comparison of values.

SKILL 14-2	ASSESSING THE RADIAL AND APICAL PULSES—cont'd

STEP	RATIONALE

IMPLEMENTATION

1 Perform hand hygiene.

Reduces transmission of microorganisms.

2 If necessary, draw curtain around bed and/or close door.

Maintains privacy.

3 Obtain pulse measurement.

   A **Radial Pulse:**

      (1) Assist patient with assuming a supine or sitting position.

Provides easy access to pulse sites.

      (2) If supine, place patient's forearm straight alongside or across lower chest or upper abdomen with wrist extended straight (see illustration). If sitting, bend patient's elbow 90 degrees and support lower arm on chair or on your arm.

Relaxed position of lower arm and extension of wrist permit full exposure of artery to palpation.

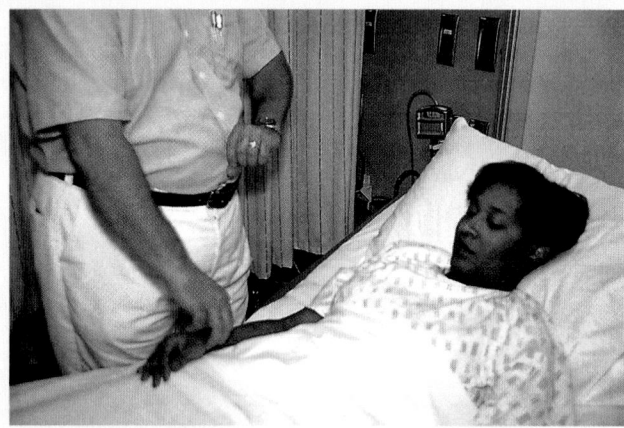

Step 3A(2) ■ Pulse check with patient's forearm at side with wrist extended.

      (3) Place tips of first two or middle three fingers of your hand over groove along radial or thumb side of patient's inner wrist (see illustration). Slightly extend the wrist with palm down until you note the strongest pulse.

Fingertips are most sensitive parts of your hand to palpate arterial pulsation. Your thumb has a pulsation that will interfere with accuracy.

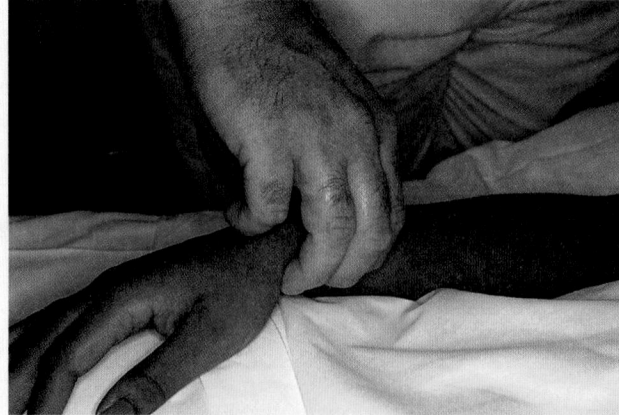

Step 3A(3) ■ Hand placement for pulse checks.

STEP	RATIONALE
(4) Lightly compress against radius, obliterate pulse initially, and then relax pressure so pulse becomes easily palpable.	Pulse is more accurate with moderate pressure. Too much pressure occludes pulse and impairs blood flow.
(5) Determine strength of pulse. Note whether thrust of vessel against fingertips is full or bounding (+4); normal, easily palpable (+2); thready, weak, barely palpable (+1); or absent (0).	Strength reflects volume of blood ejected against arterial wall with each heart contraction. Accurate description of strength improves communication among nurses and other health care providers.
(6) After you feel the pulse regularly, look at watch's second hand and begin to count rate: when sweep hand hits number on dial, start counting with zero, then one, two, and so on.	Rate is accurate only after you are sure pulse can be palpated. Timing begins with zero. Count of one is first beat palpated after timing begins.
(7) If pulse is regular, count rate for 30 seconds and multiply total by 2.	A 30-second count is accurate for rapid, slow, or regular pulse rates.
(8) If pulse is irregular, count rate for 60 seconds. Assess frequency and pattern of irregularity.	Inefficient contraction of heart fails to transmit pulse wave resulting in irregular pulse. Longer time period promotes accurate count.
(9) When pulse is irregular, compare radial pulses bilaterally.	A marked inequality indicates compromised arterial flow to one extremity, and you need to take action.

- ***Critical Decision Point:*** If pulse is irregular, assess for pulse deficit. Count apical pulse (Step 3B) while a colleague counts radial pulse. Begin pulse count by calling out loud simultaneously when to begin measuring pulses. If pulse count differs by more than 2, a pulse deficit exists, which sometimes indicates alterations in cardiac function.

B Apical Pulse:

(1) Clean earpieces and diaphragm of stethoscope with alcohol swab. Perform hand hygiene.	Reduces transmission of microorganisms.
(2) Draw curtain around bed, and/or close door.	Maintains privacy and minimizes embarrassment.
(3) Assist patient to supine or sitting position. Move bed linen and gown to uncover sternum and left side of chest.	Exposes portion of chest wall for selection of auscultatory site.
(4) Locate anatomical landmarks to identify the apical impulse, also called the point of maximal impulse (PMI) (see illustration for Step 3B[4]A to D). The heart is located behind and to left of sternum with base at top and apex at bottom. Find the angle of Louis just below the suprasternal notch between the sternal body and manubrium; feels like a bony prominence. Slip fingers down each side of the angle to find the second intercostal space (ICS). Carefully move fingers down the left side of the sternum to the fifth ICS and laterally to the left midclavicular line (MCL). A light tap felt within an area 1 to 2 cm (½ to 1 inch) of the apical impulse is reflected from the apex of the heart.	Use of anatomical landmarks allows correct placement of stethoscope over apex of heart. This position enhances ability to hear heart sounds clearly. If unable to palpate the apical impulse, reposition patient on left side. In the presence of serious heart disease, locate the apical impulse to the left of the MCL or at the sixth ICS.

SKILL 14-2   ASSESSING THE RADIAL AND APICAL PULSES—cont'd

STEP	RATIONALE

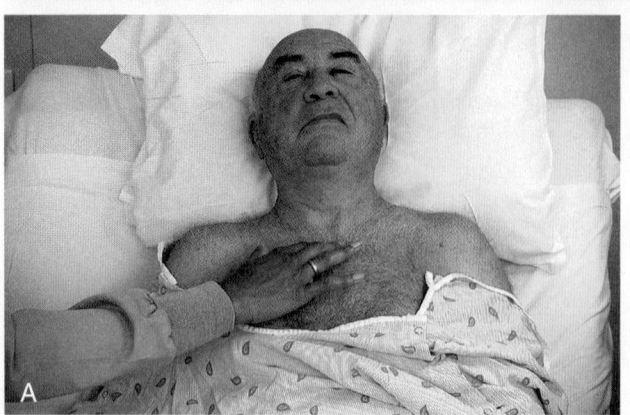

Step 3B(4)A ■ Locating the angle of Louis.

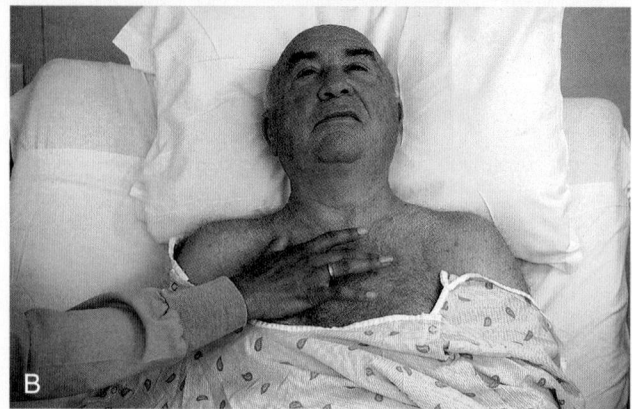

Step 3B(4)B ■ Locating the left second intercostal space (2ICS).

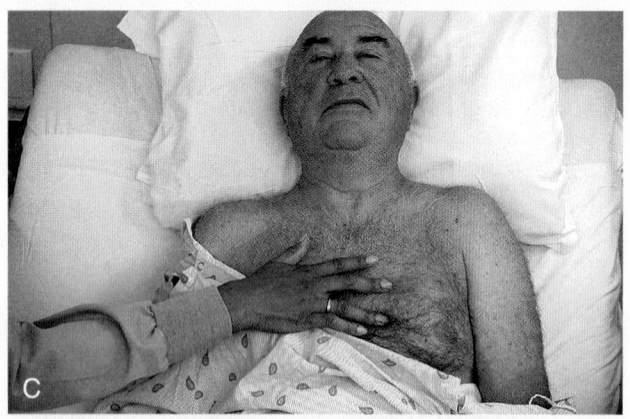

Step 3B(4)C ■ Moving down the left side of the sternum to fifth intercostal space (5ICS).

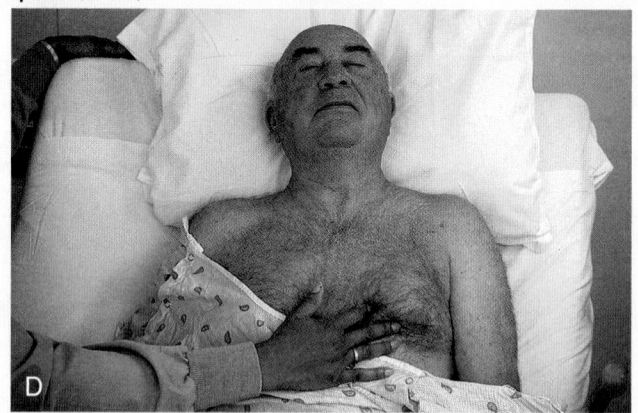

Step 3B(4)D ■ Locating the apical impulse.

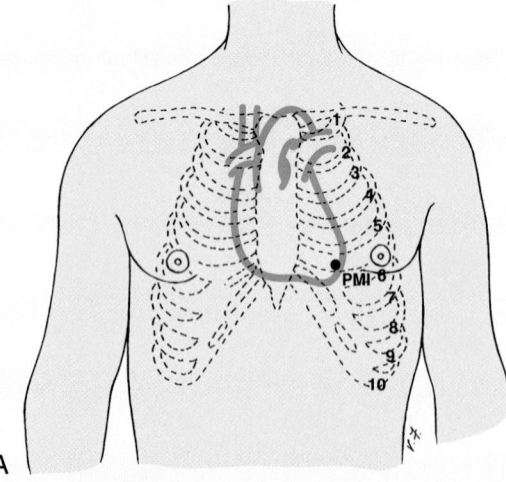

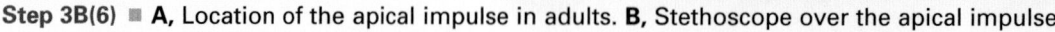

Step 3B(6) ■ **A,** Location of the apical impulse in adults. **B,** Stethoscope over the apical impulse.

(5) Place diaphragm of stethoscope in palm of hand for 5 to 10 seconds.

Warming of metal or plastic diaphragm prevents patient from being startled and promotes comfort.

(6) Place diaphragm of stethoscope over the apical impulse at the fifth ICS, at left MCL, and auscultate for normal S_1 and S_2 heart sounds (heard as "lub-dub") (see illustrations).

Allow stethoscope tubing to extend straight without kinks so it does not distort sound transmission. Normal sounds S_1 and S_2 are high pitched and best heard with the diaphragm.

STEP	**RATIONALE**
(7) When you hear S_1 and S_2 with regularity, use watch's second hand or digital display and begin to count rate: when sweep hand hits number on dial, start counting with zero, then one, two, and so on.	Apical rate is accurate only after you are able to hear sounds clearly. Timing begins with zero. Count of one is first sound auscultated after timing begins.
(8) If apical rate is regular, count for 30 seconds and multiply by 2.	You assess regular apical rate for 30 seconds.

• **Critical Decision Point:** If heart rate is irregular or patient is receiving cardiovascular medication, count for 1 minute (60 seconds). Irregular rate is more accurately assessed when measured over longer interval (Evans and others, 2004).

(9) Note if heart rate is irregular, and describe pattern of irregularity (S_1 and S_2 occurring early or later after previous sequence of sounds; for example, every third or every fourth beat is skipped).	Irregular heart rate indicates dysrhythmia. Regular occurrence of dysrhythmia within 1 minute indicates inefficient contraction of heart and alteration in cardiac function.
(10) Replace patient's gown and bed linen; assist patient in returning to comfortable position.	Restores comfort and promotes sense of well-being.
(11) Perform hand hygiene.	Reduces transmission of microorganisms.
(12) Clean earpieces and diaphragm of stethoscope with alcohol swab routinely after each use.	Stethoscopes are frequently contaminated with microorganisms. Regular disinfection controls health care–acquired infections.
(13) Discuss findings with patient as needed, and document measurement.	Promotes participation in care and understanding of health status.

EVALUATION

1 Compare readings with previous baseline and/or acceptable range of heart rate for patient's age (see Table 14-3, p. 270).	Evaluates for change in condition and presence of cardiac alterations.
2 Compare peripheral pulse rate with apical rate, and note any discrepancy.	Differences between measurements indicate pulse deficit and warn of cardiovascular compromise. Some abnormalities require therapy.
3 Compare radial pulse equality, and note any discrepancy.	Differences between radial arteries indicate compromised peripheral vascular system.
4 Correlate pulse rate with data obtained from blood pressure and related signs and symptoms (palpitations, dizziness).	Pulse rate and blood pressure are interrelated.

RECORDING AND REPORTING

- Record pulse rate and assessment site in nurses' notes, vital signs flow sheet, or electronic medical record.
- Record pulse rate after administration of specific therapies, and document in narrative in nurses' notes.

- Record any signs and symptoms of alteration in cardiac function in nurses' notes.
- Report abnormal findings to nurse in charge or health care provider immediately.

UNEXPECTED OUTCOMES AND RELATED INTERVENTIONS

- Radial pulse is weak, thready, or difficult to palpate.
  - Assess both radial pulses, and compare findings. Local obstruction to one extremity (e.g., blood clot, edema) decreases peripheral blood flow.
  - Assess for swelling in surrounding tissues or any encumbrance (e.g., dressing or cast) that impedes blood flow.
  - Perform complete assessment of all peripheral pulses (see Chapter 15).
  - Obtain Doppler or ultrasound stethoscope to detect low-velocity blood flow.
  - Observe for signs and symptoms associated with altered tissue perfusion, including pallor and cool skin temperature of tissue distal to the weak pulse.
  - Auscultate apical pulse to determine pulse rate, and identify pulse deficit.
  - Have a second nurse assess pulses.

- Apical pulse is greater than expected normal value. (See Table 14-3, p. 270 for expected values, e.g., heart rate greater than 100 beats per minute [tachycardia] in an adult patient.)
  - Identify related data, including pain, fear, anxiety, recent exercise, hypotension, blood loss, fever, or inadequate oxygenation.
  - Observe for signs and symptoms of inadequate cardiac output, including fatigue, chest pain, orthopnea, cyanosis.
- Apical pulse is less than expected normal value. (See Table 14-3 for expected values, e.g., heart rate less than 60 beats per minute [bradycardia] in an adult patient.)
  - Observe for factors that alter heart rate such as digoxin, beta-blockers, and antidysrhythmics; it is sometimes necessary to withhold prescribed medications until the health care provider is able to evaluate the need to adjust the dosage.
  - Observe for signs and symptoms of inadequate cardiac function, including fatigue, chest pain, orthopnea, cyanosis.

DELEGATION CONSIDERATIONS

The skill of blood pressure measurement can be delegated to nursing assistive personnel (NAP) unless the patient is considered unstable. The nurse instructs the NAP to:

- Obtain blood pressure measurements at appropriate times as determined by agency policy, health care provider's order, or patient condition
- Consider patient-specific factors related to patient's usual values and risk for orthostatic hypotension
- Select appropriate limb for blood pressure measurement
- Select appropriate-size blood pressure cuff for designated extremity
- Immediately report any abnormalities, which the nurse will confirm

EQUIPMENT

- Aneroid sphygmomanometer
- Cloth or disposable vinyl pressure cuff of appropriate size for patient's extremity
- Stethoscope
- Alcohol swab
- Pen, vital sign flow sheet or record or patient's electronic medical record

STEP	RATIONALE

ASSESSMENT

1 Determine need to assess patient's BP:
  a Assess for risk factors:

Conditions place patients at risk for BP alterations.

- History of cardiovascular disease
- Renal disease
- Diabetes
- Circulatory shock (hypovolemic, septic, cardiogenic, or neurogenic)
- Acute pain
- Rapid IV infusion of fluids or blood products
- Increased intracranial pressure
- Postoperative conditions
- Toxemia of pregnancy

STEP	RATIONALE
b Assess for signs and symptoms of BP alterations:	Physical signs and symptoms sometimes indicate alterations in BP.
(1) High BP (hypertension) is often asymptomatic until pressure is very high. Assess for headache (usually occipital), flushing of face, nosebleed, and fatigue in older adults.	Hypertension is often asymptomatic.
(2) Low BP (hypotension) is associated with dizziness; confusion; restlessness; pale, dusky, or cyanotic skin and mucous membranes; cool, mottled skin over extremities.	
2 Assess for factors that influence BP (see Box 14-5, p. 271).	Allows nurse to control for factors so as to measure BP accurately.
3 Determine best site for BP assessment. Avoid applying cuff to extremity when intravenous fluids are infusing; an arteriovenous shunt or fistula is present; breast or axillary surgery has been performed on that side; extremity has been traumatized or diseased or requires a cast or bulky bandage. Use the lower extremities when the brachial arteries are inaccessible.	Inappropriate site selection results in poor amplification of sounds, causing inaccurate readings. Application of pressure from inflated bladder temporarily impairs blood flow and will further compromise circulation in extremity that already has impaired blood flow.
4 Determine previous baseline BP (if available) from patient's record. Determine if patient has a latex allergy.	Allows you to assess for change in condition. Provides comparison with future BP measurements. If patient has a latex allergy, verify that stethoscope and BP cuff are latex-free.

PLANNING

1 Explain to patient that you will assess BP. Have patient rest at least 5 minutes before measuring lying or sitting BP and 1 minute when standing (NHBPEP, 2003). Ask patient not to speak while measuring BP (NHBPEP, 2003).	Reduces anxiety, which falsely elevates readings. BP readings taken at different times are more objective to compare when assessed with patient at rest. Exercise causes false elevations in BP. Talking to a patient when assessing the BP increases readings 10% to 40%.
2 Be sure patient has not ingested caffeine or smoked for 30 minutes before BP assessment (NHBPEP, 2003).	Caffeine or nicotine causes false elevations in BP. Smoking increases BP immediately and lasts up to 15 minutes. Caffeine increases BP up to 3 hours.
3 Have patient assume sitting position. Be sure room is warm, quiet, and relaxing.	Maintains patient's comfort during measurement. Sitting is preferred to lying. Diastolic pressure measured with the sitting is approximately 5 mm Hg higher than when measured supine (Pickering and others, 2005). The patient's perceptions that the physical or interpersonal environment is stressful affect the BP measurement. Talking and background noise result in inaccurate readings (Pickering and others, 2005).
4 Select cuff of appropriate size.	Improper cuff size results in inaccurate readings (see Table 14-7, p. 274). If cuff is too small, it tends to come loose as inflated or results in false-high readings. If the cuff is too large, false-low readings result.
5 Clean stethoscope earpieces and diaphragm with alcohol swab. Perform hand hygiene.	Reduces transmission of microorganisms.

SKILL 14-3	BLOOD PRESSURE MEASUREMENT—cont'd

STEP	RATIONALE

IMPLEMENTATION

1 Assess BP by auscultation. With patient sitting or lying, position patient's forearm, supported if needed at heart level, with palm turned up (see illustration); for thigh, position with knee slightly flexed. If sitting, instruct patient to keep feet flat on floor without legs crossed. If supine, support the patient's arm with a pillow so that the cuff is at the level of the right atrium.

If arm is extended and not supported, patient will perform isometric exercise that increases diastolic pressure (Adiyaman and others, 2006). Placement of arm above the level of the heart causes false-low reading 2 mm Hg for each inch above heart level (Pickering and others, 2005). Even in the supine position a diastolic pressure effect up to 3 to 4 mm Hg occurs for each 5 cm change in heart level. Leg crossing falsely increases systolic BP by 2 to 8 mm Hg (Pickering and others, 2005).

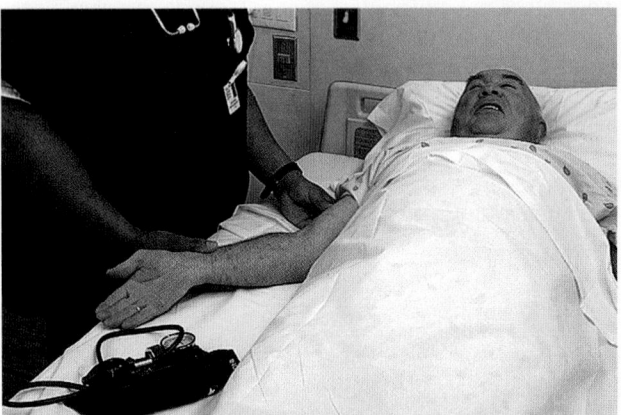

Step 1 ■ Patient's forearm supported in bed.

2 Expose extremity (arm or leg) fully by removing constricting clothing.

3 Palpate brachial artery (arm) or popliteal artery (leg). With cuff fully deflated, apply bladder of cuff above artery by centering arrows marked on cuff over artery. If there are no center arrows on cuff, estimate the center of the bladder and place this center over artery. Position cuff 2.5 cm (1 inch) above site of pulsation (antecubital or popliteal space). With cuff fully deflated, wrap cuff evenly and snugly around extremity (see illustrations).

Ensures proper cuff application. Do not place BP cuff over clothing.

Inflating bladder directly over artery ensures proper pressure is applied during inflation. Loose-fitting cuff causes false-high readings.

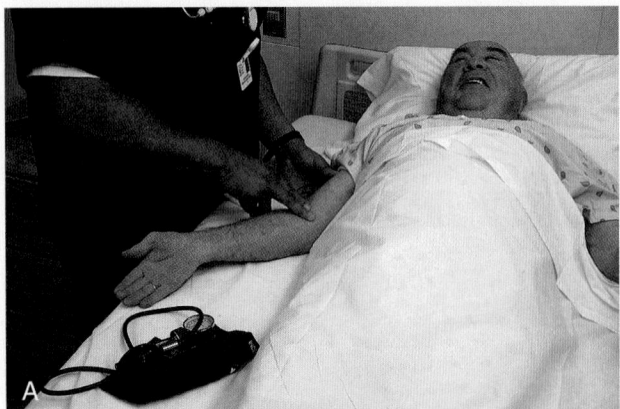

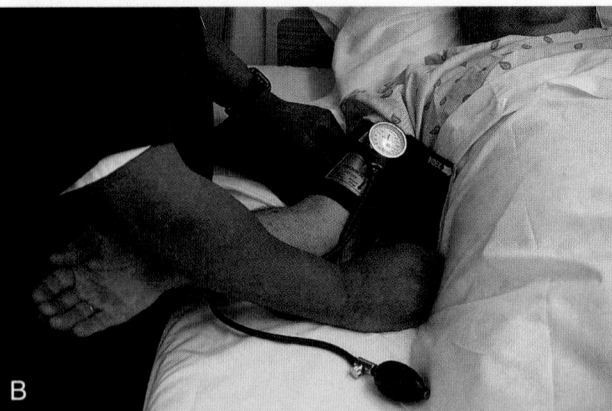

Step 3 ■ **A,** Nurse palpating patient's brachial artery. **B,** Center bladder of cuff above artery.

STEP	RATIONALE

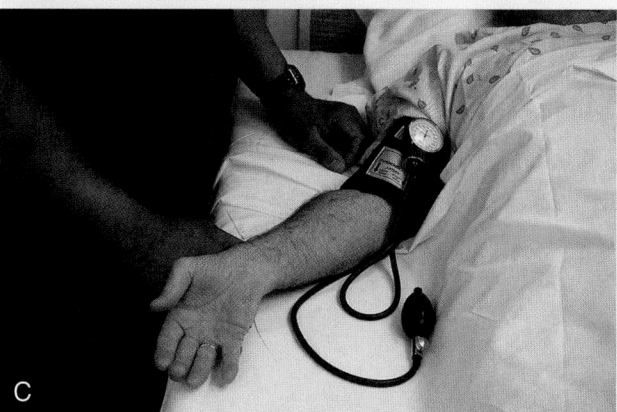

Step 3C ■ Blood pressure cuff wrapped around upper arm.

4 Position manometer vertically at eye level. Make sure observer is no farther than 1 m (approximately 1 yard) away.

Looking up or down at the scale results in inaccurate readings.

5 Measure BP.

  A Two-Step Method:

    (1) Relocate pulse. Palpate the artery distal to the cuff with fingertips of nondominant hand while inflating cuff rapidly to a pressure 30 mm Hg above point at which pulse disappears. Slowly deflate cuff, and note point when pulse reappears. Deflate cuff fully and wait 30 seconds.

Estimating systolic pressure prevents false-low readings, which result in the presence of an auscultatory gap. Palpation determines maximal inflation point for accurate reading. If unable to palpate artery because of weakened pulse, use an ultrasonic stethoscope (see Chapter 15). Completely deflating cuff prevents venous congestion and false-high readings.

    (2) Place stethoscope earpieces in ears, and be sure sounds are clear, not muffled.

Ensures each earpiece follows angle of ear canal to facilitate hearing.

    (3) Relocate artery, and place bell or diaphragm of stethoscope over it. Do not allow chestpiece to touch cuff or clothing (see illustration).

Proper stethoscope placement ensures the best sound reception. The bell provides better sound reproduction, while the diaphragm is easier to secure with fingers and covers a larger area. Stethoscope improperly positioned causes muffled sounds that often result in false-low systolic and false-high diastolic readings.

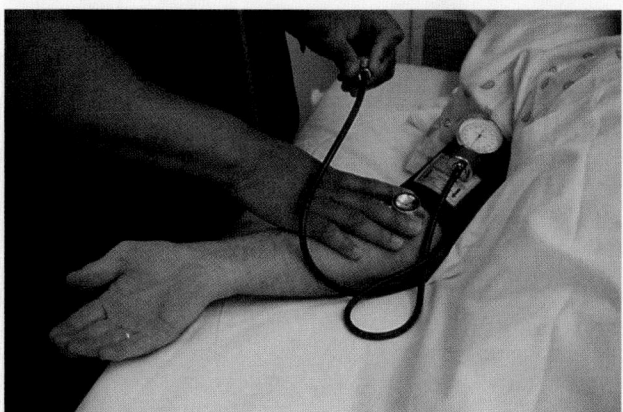

Step 5A(3) ■ Stethoscope placed over brachial artery to measure blood pressure.

SKILL 14-3   BLOOD PRESSURE MEASUREMENT—cont'd

STEP	RATIONALE
(4) Close valve of pressure bulb clockwise until tight.	Tightening of valve prevents air leak during inflation.
(5) Quickly inflate cuff to 30 mm Hg above patient's estimated systolic pressure (see illustration).	Rapid inflation ensures accurate measurement of systolic pressure.

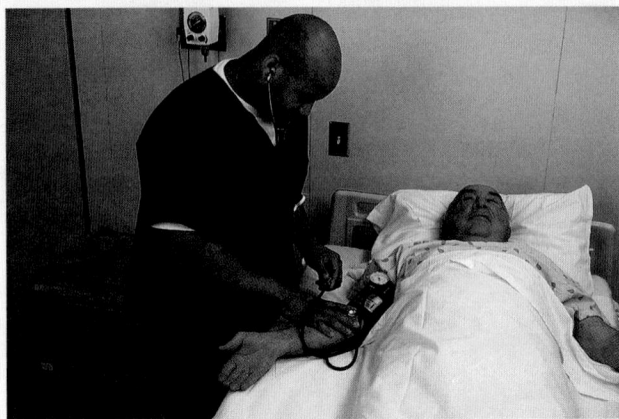

Step 5A(5) ■ Inflating the BP cuff.

(6) Slowly release pressure bulb valve, and allow manometer needle gauge to fall at rate of 2 to 3 mm Hg per second.	Too-rapid or too-slow a decline in pressure release causes inaccurate readings.
(7) Note point on manometer when you hear the first clear sound. The sound will slowly increase in intensity.	First Korotkoff sound reflects systolic BP.
(8) Continue to deflate cuff gradually, noting point at which sound disappears in adults. Note pressure to nearest 2 mm Hg. Listen for 20 to 30 mm Hg after the last sound, and then allow remaining air to escape quickly.	Beginning of the fifth Korotkoff sound is an indication of diastolic pressure in adults (NHBPEP, 2003). The fourth Korotkoff sound involves distinct muffling and is an indication of diastolic pressure in children (NHBPEP, 2003).

B One-Step Method:

(1) Place stethoscope earpieces in ears, and be sure sounds are clear, not muffled.	Earpiece should follow the angle of ear canal to facilitate hearing.
(2) Relocate artery, and place diaphragm of stethoscope over it. Do not allow chestpiece to touch cuff or clothing.	Proper stethoscope placement ensures optimal sound reception.
(3) Close valve of pressure bulb clockwise until tight.	Tightening of valve prevents air leak during inflation.
(4) Quickly inflate cuff to 30 mm Hg above patient's usual systolic pressure.	Inflation above systolic level ensures accurate measurement of systolic pressure.
(5) Slowly release pressure bulb valve, and allow manometer needle to fall at rate of 2 to 3 mm Hg per second. Note point on manometer when you hear the first clear sound. The sound will slowly increase in intensity.	Too rapid or slow a decline in pressure release causes inaccurate readings. The first Korotkoff sounds reflect systolic pressure.
(6) Continue to deflate cuff gradually, noting point at which sound disappears in adults. Note pressure to nearest 2 mm Hg. Listen for 20 to 30 mm Hg after the last sound, and then allow remaining air to escape quickly.	Beginning of the fifth Korotkoff sound is an indication of diastolic pressure in adults (NHBPEP, 2003). The fourth Korotkoff sound involves distinct muffling of sounds and is an indication of diastolic pressure in children (NHBPEP, 2003).
6 The American Heart Association recommends the average of two sets of BP measurements, 2 minutes apart. Use the second set of BP measurements as the patient's baseline.	Two sets of BP measurements help to prevent false positives based on a patient's sympathetic response (alert reaction). Averaging minimizes the effect of anxiety, which often causes a first reading to be higher than subsequent measurements (NHBPEP, 2003).
7 Remove cuff from patient's extremity unless you need to repeat measurement. If this is the first assessment of patient, repeat procedure on the other extremity.	Comparison of BP in both extremities detects circulatory problems. (Normal difference of 5 to 10 mm Hg exists between extremities.)
8 Assist patient in returning to comfortable position, and cover arm or leg if previously clothed.	Restores comfort and promotes sense of well-being.

STEP	RATIONALE
9 Discuss findings with patient as needed.	Promotes participation in care and understanding of health status. Makes patient accountable for follow-up assessment.
10 Perform hand hygiene. Clean earpieces, bell, and diaphragm of stethoscope with alcohol swab.	Reduces transmission of microorganisms from patient to patient.

EVALUATION

1 Compare reading with previous baseline and/or acceptable value of BP for patient's age.	Evaluates for change in condition and alterations.
2 Compare BP in both arms or both legs.	If using upper extremities, use the arm with higher pressure for subsequent assessments unless contraindicated.
3 Correlate BP with data obtained from pulse assessment and related cardiovascular signs and symptoms.	BP and heart rate are interrelated.

RECORDING AND REPORTING

- Record BP and site assessed on vital sign flow sheet, nurses' notes, or patient's electronic medical record.
- Record any signs and symptoms of BP alterations in narrative form in nurses' notes.

- Document measurement of BP after administration of specific therapies in narrative form in nurses' notes.
- Report abnormal findings to nurse in charge or health care provider immediately.

UNEXPECTED OUTCOMES AND RELATED INTERVENTIONS

- Unable to obtain BP reading.
  - Determine that no immediate crisis is present by assessing pulse and respiratory rate.
  - Assess for signs and symptoms of altered cardiac function; if present, notify nurse in charge or health care provider immediately.
  - Use alternative sites or procedures to obtain BP: auscultate BP in different extremity, use an ultrasonic stethoscope, implement palpation method to obtain systolic BP.
  - Repeat any electronic BP measurement with sphygmomanometer. Electronic BP measurements are less accurate in low blood flow conditions.
- Blood pressure is above acceptable range.
  - Repeat BP measurement in other extremity, and compare findings.
  - Verify correct selection and placement of cuff; with cuff below the right atrium when BP is obtained.
  - Ask nurse colleague to repeat measurement in 1 to 2 minutes.
  - Observe for related symptoms, though symptoms are sometimes not apparent until BP is extremely elevated.
  - Report elevated BP to nurse in charge, or health care provider to initiate appropriate evaluation and treatment.
  - Administer antihypertensive medications as ordered.

- BP is not sufficient for adequate perfusion and oxygenation of tissues.
  - Compare BP value to baseline. A systolic reading of 90 mm Hg is an acceptable value for some patients.
  - Place patient in supine position to enhance circulation, and restrict activity that may decrease BP further.
  - Assess for signs and symptoms associated with hypotension, including tachycardia; weak, thready pulse; weakness; dizziness; confusion; cool, pale dusky or cyanotic skin.
  - Assess for factors that would contribute to a low BP, including hemorrhage and dilation of blood vessels resulting from hypothermia, anesthesia, or medication side effects.
  - Notify nurse in charge or health care provider immediately.
  - Increase rate of IV infusion, or administer vasoconstricting drugs if ordered.
- Patient has a difference of more than 20 mm Hg systolic or diastolic when comparing BP measurements on upper extremities.
  - Report abnormal findings to nurse in charge or health care provider.

SKILL 14-4	ASSESSING RESPIRATION

DELEGATION CONSIDERATIONS

The skill of respiration assessment can be delegated to nursing assistive personnel (NAP) unless the patient is considered unstable. The nurse instructs the NAP to:

- Obtain respiration measurements at appropriate times as determined by agency policy, health care provider's order, or patient condition such as onset of labored breathing or complaints of breathing difficulty
- Consider specific patient factors related to history or risk for increased or decreased respiratory rate or irregular respiration.

- Immediately report any abnormalities in respiratory rate or rhythm, which you will confirm

EQUIPMENT

- Wristwatch with second hand or digital display
- Pen, pencil, vital sign flow sheet or patient's medical record

STEP	RATIONALE

ASSESSMENT

1 Determine need to assess patient's respiration:
  a Assess for risk factors:
  - Fever
  - Pain and anxiety
  - Diseases of chest wall or muscles
  - Constrictive chest or abdominal dressings
  - Presence of abdominal incisions
  - Gastric distention
  - Chronic pulmonary disease (emphysema, bronchitis, asthma)
  - Traumatic injury to chest wall
  - Presence of a chest tube
  - Respiratory infection (pneumonia, acute bronchitis)
  - Pulmonary edema and emboli

  Conditions that place patient at risk for ventilatory alterations are detected by changes in respiratory rate, depth, and rhythm, head injury with damage to brain stem, and anemia.

  b Assess for signs and symptoms of respiratory alterations, such as bluish or cyanotic appearance of nail beds, lips, mucous membranes, and skin; restlessness, irritability, confusion, reduced level of consciousness; pain during inspiration; labored or difficult breathing; orthopnea; use of accessory muscles; adventitious breath sounds (see Chapter 15), inability to breathe spontaneously; thick, frothy, blood-tinged, or large amounts of sputum produced on coughing.

  Physical signs and symptoms sometimes indicate alterations in respiratory status related to ventilation.

2 Assess pertinent laboratory values:
  a Arterial blood gases (ABGs) (values vary slightly within institutions). Normal values are:
  pH 7.35 to 7.45
  $PaCO_2$ 35 to 45 mm Hg
  Hg PaO_2 80 to 100 mm Hg
  SaO_2 95% to 100%

  Arterial blood gases measure arterial blood pH, partial pressure of O_2 and CO_2, and arterial O_2 saturation, which reflect patient's oxygenation status.

  b Pulse oximetry (SpO_2): Usual value of SpO_2 95% to 100%; a value less than 90% is considered hypoxemia; values below 90% are acceptable only in certain chronic disease conditions.

  SpO_2 less than 90% is often accompanied by changes in respiratory rate, depth, and rhythm.

  c Complete blood count (CBC): Normal CBC for adults (values may vary within institutions): **hemoglobin:** 14 to 18 g/100 mL, males; 12 to 16 g/100 mL, females; **hematocrit:** 42% to 52%, males; 37% to 47%, females; **red blood cell count:** 4.7 to 6.1 million/mm³, males; 4.2 to 5.4 million/mm³, females (Pagana and Pagana, 2009).

  Complete blood count measures red blood cell count, volume of red blood cells, and concentration of hemoglobin, which reflects patient's blood capacity to carry O_2.

3 Assess for factors that influence respirations (see Box 14-11, p. 279).

  Allows you to control for factors that might alter findings.

STEP	RATIONALE

4 Determine previous baseline respiratory rate (if available) from patient's record.

5 Assess respirations after measuring the pulse in an adult.

Allows you to assess for change in condition. Provides value for comparison with future respiratory measurements.

Inconspicuous assessment of respirations immediately after pulse assessment prevents patient from consciously or unintentionally altering rate and depth of breathing.

PLANNING

1 Be sure patient is in comfortable position, preferably sitting or lying with the head of the bed elevated 45 to 60 degrees. If patient has been active, wait 5 to 10 minutes before assessing respirations.

Sitting erect promotes full ventilatory movement. Position of discomfort causes patient to breathe more rapidly. Exercise increases respiratory rate and depth. Assessing respirations while patient rests allows for objective comparison of values.

- **Critical Decision Point:** Assess patients with difficulty breathing (dyspnea), such as those with heart failure or abdominal ascites or in late stages of pregnancy, in the position of greatest comfort. Repositioning will increase the work of breathing, which will increase respiratory rate.

IMPLEMENTATION

1 Draw curtain around bed, and/or close door. Perform hand hygiene.

2 Be sure patient's chest is visible. If necessary, move bed linen or gown.

3 Place patient's arm in relaxed position across the abdomen or lower chest, or place your hand directly over patient's upper abdomen (see illustration).

Maintains privacy. Prevents transmission of microorganisms.

Ensures clear view of chest wall and abdominal movements.

A similar position used during pulse assessment allows you to assess respiratory rate subtly. Patient's hand or your hand rises and falls during respiratory cycle.

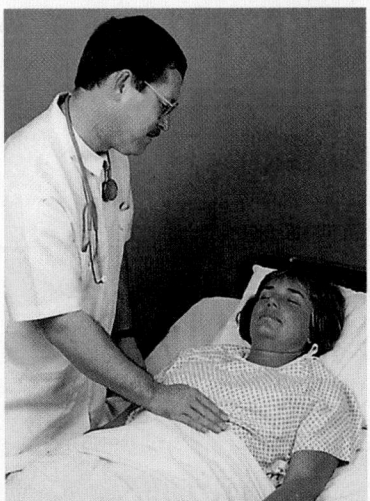

Step 3 ■ Nurse's hand placed over patient's abdomen to check respiratory rate.

4 Observe complete respiratory cycle (one inspiration and one expiration).

5 After observing cycle, look at watch's second hand and begin to count rate: when sweep hand hits number on dial, begin time frame, counting one with first full respiratory cycle.

6 If rhythm is regular, count number of respirations in 30 seconds and multiply by 2. If rhythm is irregular, less than 12, or greater than 20, count for 1 full minute.

You determine an accurate rate only after viewing the entire respiratory cycle.

Timing begins with count of one. Respirations occur more slowly than pulse; thus timing does not begin with zero.

Respiratory rate is equivalent to number of respirations per minute. Suspected irregularities require assessment for at least 1 minute.

SKILL 14-4	ASSESSING RESPIRATION—cont'd

STEP	RATIONALE
7 Note depth of respirations, subjectively assessed by observing degree of chest wall movement while counting rate. Also assess depth by palpating chest wall excursion or auscultating the posterior thorax (see Chapter 15) after you have counted the rate. Describe depth as shallow, normal, or deep.	Character of ventilatory movement reveals specific disease state restricting volume of air moving into and out of the lungs.
8 Note rhythm of ventilatory cycle. Normal breathing is regular and uninterrupted. Do not confuse sighing with abnormal rhythm.	Character of ventilations reveals specific types of alterations. Periodically people unconsciously take single deep breaths or sighs to expand small airways prone to collapse.

- *Critical Decision Point:* An irregular respiratory pattern or occurrence of periods of apnea (cessation of respiration for several seconds) is a symptom of underlying disease in the adult and must be reported to the nurse in charge or health care provider. The patient may require further assessment (see Chapter 29) and need immediate intervention. An irregular respiratory rate and short apneic spells are normal for newborns.

9 Replace bed linen and patient's gown.	Restores comfort and promotes sense of well-being.
10 Perform hand hygiene.	Reduces transmission of microorganisms.
11 Discuss findings with patient as needed.	Promotes participation in care and understanding of health status.

EVALUATION

1 If you are assessing respiration for the first time, establish rate, rhythm, and depth as baseline if within acceptable range.	Used to compare future respiratory assessment.
2 Compare respiration with patient's previous baseline and usual rate, rhythm, and depth.	Allows you to assess for changes in patient's condition and for presence of respiratory alterations.
3 Correlate respiratory rate, depth, and rhythm with data obtained from pulse oximetry (Skill 14-5) and arterial blood gas measurements if available.	Ventilation, perfusion, and diffusion are interrelated.

RECORDING AND REPORTING

- Record respiratory rate and character in nurses' notes, vital sign flow sheet, or electronic medical record.
- Record abnormal depth and rhythm in narrative form in nurses' notes.
- Document measurement of respiratory rate after administration of specific therapies in narrative form in nurses' notes.

- Document type and amount of oxygen therapy if used by patient during assessment.
- Report abnormal findings to nurse in charge or health care provider immediately.

UNEXPECTED OUTCOMES AND RELATED INTERVENTIONS

- Respiratory rate is below 12 (bradypnea) or above 20 (tachypnea). Breathing pattern is irregular. Depth of respirations may be increased or decreased; patient complains of feeling short of breath.
  - Observe for related factors, including obstructed airway, noisy respirations, cyanosis, restlessness, irritability, confusion, productive cough, use of accessory muscles, and abnormal breath sounds (see Chapter 15).

- Assist patient to supported sitting position (semi-Fowler's or high-Fowler's) unless contraindicated.
- Provide oxygen as ordered (see Chapter 29).
- Assess for environmental factors that influence patient's respiratory rate such as secondhand smoke, poor ventilation, or gas fumes.

SKILL 14-5   MEASURING OXYGEN SATURATION (PULSE OXIMETRY)

DELEGATION CONSIDERATIONS

The skill of oxygen saturation measurement can be delegated to nursing assistive personnel (NAP) unless patient is unstable. The nurse instructs the NAP to:

• Obtain oxygen saturation measurements at appropriate times as determined by agency policy, health care provider's order, or patient condition such as onset of labored breathing or cyanosis

• Select appropriate sensor site, probe, and patient position for measurement of oxygen saturation

• Immediately report any reading lower than 90%, which the nurse will need to confirm

• Refrain from using pulse oximetry as an assessment of heart rate because the oximeter will not detect an irregular pulse

EQUIPMENT

• Oximeter
• Oximeter probe appropriate for patient and recommended by oximeter manufacturer
• Acetone or nail polish remover if needed
• Pen, vital sign flow sheet or record or patient's medical record

STEP	RATIONALE

ASSESSMENT

1 Determine need to measure patient's oxygen saturation:

a Assess risk factors for decreased oxygen saturation, including acute or chronic compromised respiratory function, recovery from general anesthesia or conscious sedation, traumatic injury to chest wall with or without collapse of underlying lung tissue, ventilator dependence, and changes in supplemental oxygen therapy or activity intolerance.

Certain conditions place patients at risk for decreased oxygen saturation.

b Assess for signs and symptoms of alterations in oxygen saturation such as altered respiratory rate, depth, or rhythm; adventitious breath sounds (see Chapter 15); cyanotic appearance of nail beds, lips, mucous membranes, skin; restlessness, irritability, confusion; reduced level of consciousness; labored or difficult breathing.

Physical signs and symptoms indicate abnormal oxygen saturation. SpO_2 generally must fall below 85% before any changes in skin color are noted (Giuliano and Higgins, 2005).

2 Assess for factors that normally influence measurement of SpO_2 such as oxygen therapy, respiratory therapy such as postural drainage and percussion, hypotension, hemoglobin level, body temperature, and medications such as bronchodilators.

Allows you to control for factors that might alter findings and to accurately assess oxygen saturation variations. Peripheral vasoconstriction related to hypothermia interferes with SpO_2 determination (Giuliano and Higgins, 2005).

3 Determine previous baseline SpO_2 (if available) from patient's record.

Baseline information provides basis for comparison and assists in assessment of current status and evaluation of interventions.

4 Determine most appropriate patient-specific site (e.g., finger, earlobe, bridge of nose, forehead) for sensor probe placement by measuring capillary refill (see Chapter 15). If capillary refill time is more than 3 seconds, select alternative site.

Changes in SpO_2 are reflected in the circulation of the finger capillary bed within 30 seconds and the earlobe capillary bed within 5 to 10 seconds.

a Site must have adequate local circulation and be free of moisture.

Finger and earlobe sensors require pulsating vascular bed to identify hemoglobin molecules that absorb emitted light. Moisture impedes ability of the sensor to detect SpO_2 levels.

b A finger free of polish is preferred.

Research on the influence of nail polish is contradictory. Brown and blue nail polish can falsely lower SpO_2 but is not clinically significant (Rodden and others, 2007).

c If patient has tremors or is likely to move, use earlobe or forehead.

Motion artifact is the most common cause of inaccurate readings (Giuliano and Liu, 2006). Second-generation pulse oximeters are more motion tolerant.

d If patient is obese, clip-on probe may not fit properly; obtain a disposable (tape-on) sensor.

5 Determine if patient has latex allergy.

If patient has latex sensitivity or a latex allergy, do not use adhesive sensors.

SKILL 14-5	MEASURING OXYGEN SATURATION (PULSE OXIMETRY)—cont'd

STEP	RATIONALE

PLANNING

1 Obtain oximeter and appropriate probe for patient, and place at bedside.

2 Explain purpose of procedure to patient and how you will measure oxygen saturation. Instruct patient to breathe normally.

Mixing probes from different manufacturers will result in burn injury to patient.

Promotes patient cooperation and increases compliance. Prevents large fluctuations in minute ventilation and possible error in SpO_2 readings.

IMPLEMENTATION

1 Perform hand hygiene.

2 Position patient comfortably. If finger monitoring site is chosen, support lower arm.

3 If finger to be used, remove fingernail polish from digit with acetone or polish remover. Acrylic nails without polish do not interfere with SpO_2 determination.

4 Attach sensor to monitoring site. Instruct patient that clip-on sensor will feel like tight elastic band on the finger or ear but will not hurt.

Reduces transmission of microorganisms.

Ensures probe positioning and decreases motion artifact that interferes with SpO_2 determination.

Opaque coatings can decrease light transmission. Nail polish containing blue pigment absorbs light emissions and may falsely alter saturation.

Patient may not expect pressure of sensor's spring tension on finger or earlobe. Select sensor site based on peripheral circulation and extremity temperature. Peripheral vasoconstriction alters SpO_2.

- *Critical Decision Point:* Do not attach sensor to finger, ear, or bridge of nose if area is edematous or skin integrity is compromised. Do not attach sensor to hypothermic finger. Select ear or bridge of nose if adult patient has a history of peripheral vascular disease. Do not place sensor on same extremity as used for electronic BP cuff because blood flow to finger will be temporarily interrupted when cuff inflates, resulting in inaccurate reading that triggers alarms. Do not use earlobe and bridge of nose sensors for infants and toddlers because their skin is fragile.

5 Once sensor is in place, turn on oximeter by activating power. Observe pulse waveform/intensity display and audible beep. Correlate oximeter pulse rate with patient's radial pulse.

Pulse waveform/intensity display enables detection of valid pulse or presence of interfering signal. Pitch of audible beep is proportional to SpO_2 value. Double-checking pulse rate ensures oximeter accuracy. Oximeter pulse rate, patient's radial pulse, and apical pulse rate should be the same.

- *Critical Decision Point:* If oximeter pulse rate, patient's radial pulse, and apical pulse are different, reevaluate oximeter probe placement and reassess pulse rates.

6 Inform patient that oximeter will alarm if sensor falls off or if patient moves sensor.

7 Leave sensor in place until oximeter readout reaches constant value and pulse display reaches full strength during each cardiac cycle. Read SpO_2 on digital display.

8 If patient requires continuous SpO_2 monitoring, verify SpO_2 alarm limits and alarm volume, which are preset by the manufacturer at a low of 85% and a high of 100%. You determine the limits for SpO_2 and pulse rate alarms based on each patient's condition. Verify that alarms are on. Assess skin integrity under sensor every 2 hours. Relocate sensor at least every 24 hours or more frequently if skin integrity is altered or tissue perfusion compromised.

9 Discuss findings with patient as needed.

Readings take 10 to 30 seconds, depending on site selected.

Ensures alarms are set at appropriate limits and volumes to avoid frightening patients and visitors. Spring tension of sensor or sensitivity to disposable sensor adhesive causes skin irritation and leads to disruption of skin integrity.

Promotes participation in care and understanding of health status.

STEP	RATIONALE
10 If intermittent or spot-checking SpO$_2$ measurements are planned, remove sensor and turn oximeter power off. Store sensor in appropriate location.	Batteries will drain if oximeter is left on. Oximeter sensors are expensive and vulnerable to damage.
11 Assist patient in returning to comfortable position.	Restores comfort and promotes sense of well-being.
12 Perform hand hygiene.	Reduces transmission of microorganisms.

EVALUATION

1 Compare SpO$_2$ readings with patient baseline and acceptable values.	Comparison reveals presence of abnormality.
2 Compare SpO$_2$ with SaO$_2$ obtained from ABG measurements (see Chapter 29) if available.	Documents reliability of noninvasive assessment. Pulse oximetry only warns of dangerous low levels of oxygen saturation. Values are not accurate under 80%.
3 Correlate SpO$_2$ reading with data obtained from respiratory rate, depth, and rhythm assessment (see Skill 14-4). Note use of oxygen therapy.	Measurements assessing ventilation, perfusion, and diffusion are interrelated.
4 During continuous monitoring, assess skin integrity underneath probe at least every 2 hours, based on patient's peripheral circulation.	Prevents tissue ischemia.

RECORDING AND REPORTING

- Record SpO$_2$ value on nurses' notes, vital sign flow sheet, or electronic medical record.
- Record type and amount of oxygen therapy used by patient during assessment.
- Record any signs and symptoms of reduced oxygen saturation in narrative form in nurses' notes.

- Document measurement of SpO$_2$ after administration of specific therapies in narrative form in nurses' notes.
- Report abnormal findings to nurse in charge or health care provider immediately.

UNEXPECTED OUTCOMES AND RELATED INTERVENTIONS

- SpO$_2$ is less than 90%.
  - Verify that oximeter sensor is intact and not influenced by outside light transmission.
  - Assess for signs and symptoms of decreased oxygenation, including anxiety, cyanosis, restlessness, and tachycardia.
  - Verify that supplemental oxygen is delivered as ordered and is functioning properly.

- Minimize factors that decrease SpO$_2$ such as lung secretions, increased activity, and hyperthermia.
- Assist patient to a position that maximizes ventilatory effort; for example, place an obese patient in a high-Fowler's position.
- Notify nurse in charge or health care provider.

KEY POINTS

- Vital sign measurement includes the physiological measurements of temperature, pulse, blood pressure, respiration, and oxygen saturation.
- You measure vital signs as part of a complete physical examination or in a review of a patient's condition.
- Measure vital signs when the patient is at rest and the environment is controlled for comfort.
- You evaluate vital sign changes with other physical assessment findings using clinical judgment to determine measurement frequency.
- Knowledge of the factors influencing vital signs assists in determining and evaluating abnormal values.
- Changes related to aging influence the vital sign measurement and nursing interventions for older adults.
- Vital signs provide a basis for evaluating response to nursing interventions.
- Changes in one vital sign often influence characteristics of the other vital signs.

- Help the patient maintain body temperature by initiating interventions that promote heat loss, production, or conservation.
- Measurement of temperature using the temporal artery is the least invasive, most accurate method of obtaining core temperature.
- Respiratory assessment includes determining the effectiveness of ventilation, perfusion, and diffusion.
- Assessment of respiration involves observing ventilatory movements throughout the respiratory cycle.
- Hypertension is diagnosed only after an average of readings made during two or more subsequent visits reveals an elevated blood pressure.
- Selecting and applying the blood pressure measurement cuff improperly will result in errors in blood pressure measurement.

CRITICAL THINKING EXERCISES

Ms. Coburn, the 26-year-old schoolteacher, lives alone on the eighth floor of an apartment building. On a hot August day, she calls 911, unable to breathe. She is taken to your emergency department, where upon arrival her skin is warm and dry to touch. Her face is flushed, and she appears to have labored breathing. She states that she has not been drinking much lately because she has become nauseated from the heat. Her apartment is not air-conditioned, and one of her two windows will not open. She complains of being tired and irritable. During her recent clinic visit Ms. Coburn's blood pressure was elevated (164/98 first reading, 146/94 second reading). After starting an IV line in the left antecubital space, you receive Ms. Coburn on your medical unit.

1. **a.** List the vital signs you will obtain in order of priority.
   b. Which vital signs do you delegate to the nursing assistant after you first assess Ms. Coburn?
   c. What instructions do you give the nursing assistant?
   d. How often do you ask the nursing assistant to obtain vital signs?
2. Ms. Coburn's vital signs are as follows: blood pressure right arm 116/92 mm Hg; left arm 112/64 mm Hg lying in bed; right radial pulse 128 beats per minute, +4 strength; respiratory rate 26 breaths per minute and regular; SpO₂ 98% on room air.; temporal artery temperature 39.2 ° C (102.6° F).

   a. What is your priority action?
   b. Which vital sign do you evaluate next?
   c. What directions do you give the nursing assistant related to vital sign measurement?
   d. Explain the difference between hyperthermia and pyrexia.
3. You are caring for Ms. Coburn the day after her admission. During shift report you learn that she has complained of shortness of breath and a productive cough of thick brown secretions.
   a. What is your priority action?
   b. What is the priority vital sign you need to obtain?
   c. What directions do you give the nursing assistant related to vital sign measurement?
4. The nursing assistant reports Ms. Coburn's most recent blood pressure to you as 150/94 mm Hg. Because Ms. Coburn has received her discharge orders, she will be picked up by a friend in about an hour.
   a. What is your priority action?
   b. What patient education do you need to evaluate before Ms. Coburn is discharged?

℮volve   *Answers to Critical Thinking Questions can be found on the Evolve website.*

REVIEW QUESTIONS

1. A 68-year-old woman whose husband died last year walks into the wellness clinic of the assisted living facility. She reports that she feels depressed and tired all the time. She provides you with a list of medications, one of which her health care provider altered in the last 3 weeks, atenolol, a beta-adrenergic blocker. Knowing that beta-adrenergic blockers have the potential to cause hypotension and bradycardia, which vital signs can you delegate to the clinic's nursing assistant? Select all that apply.
   1. Blood pressure
   2. Temperature and respiratory rate
   3. Oxygen saturation
   4. Heart rate

2. A patient's blood pressure is 102/58 mm Hg in the right arm. On the patient's last visit, the blood pressure was 142/60 mm Hg in the left arm. What is your priority nursing action?
   1. Repeat the blood pressure in the right arm.
   2. Obtain the blood pressure in the left arm.
   3. Allow the patient to relax for 15 minutes.
   4. Notify the health care provider.

3. A 53-year-old man has just returned from the postanesthesia care unit (PACU) following a small bowel resection. He has smoked 2 packs per day since he was 18 years old. His admission vital signs obtained by the nursing assistant are heart rate 114 beats per minute, BP 118/72 mm Hg, tympanic temperature 97.8° F, respiratory rate 8 breaths per minute, and SpO_2 94% using 3 L of oxygen via nasal cannula. How do you describe his vital signs?
   1. Bradycardia with apnea
   2. Tachycardia with hypoxia
   3. Bradycardia and bradypnea
   4. Tachycardia and bradypnea

4. Thirty minutes after returning from the PACU your patient's pulse oximeter alarms, and you note the SpO_2 is 89%. While she was sleeping, the oxygen cannula fell out of her nose. What is your priority nursing action?
   1. Reposition the oximeter probe.
   2. Reposition the nasal cannula.
   3. Obtain the patient's respiratory rate while asleep.
   4. Shake the patient to see if she wakes.

5. Poor oxygenation of the blood ordinarily will affect the pulse rate and cause it to become:
   1. Bounding
   2. Irregular
   3. Tachycardic
   4. Bradycardic

6. You dangle your patient on the side of the bed 6 hours after surgery. The nursing assistant obtains a blood pressure of 92/58 mm Hg while he is sitting. The difference between his postoperative BP of 118/58 mm Hg and the sitting blood pressure is described as:
   1. Hypotensive response to surgery
   2. Normal response to repositioning
   3. Orthostatic hypotension
   4. Side effect of fluid shift

7. You help your patient get out of bed 1 day after surgery for a bowel obstruction. He complains of dizziness and nausea. Your immediate action is to:
   1. Assist him to a supine position
   2. Assess blood pressure
   3. Report findings to the nurse in charge
   4. Question the patient about palpitations

8. Following surgery, your patient's systolic blood pressure drops 25 mm Hg when you are helping him out of bed. What is the likely cause for the change in blood pressure?
   1. Pain caused by movement
   2. Blood loss during surgery
   3. Increase in heart rate as a result of stress
   4. Movement too soon after surgery

9. You have assigned routine vital signs to a new nursing assistant recently hired by your clinic manager. You notice that the nursing assistant's last three patients have had unusually low blood pressures that you have had to reconfirm. What is the most likely reason for the low blood pressures that the nursing assistant is obtaining?
   1. BP cuff was too wide for arm circumference.
   2. Bladder was inflated and deflated too slowly.
   3. Patient's arm was not supported during measurement.
   4. BP cuff was not wrapped evenly around arm.

10. An experienced nursing assistant complains about the vital signs that a newly hired nursing assistant has obtained. The experienced nursing assistant has been asked to retake a BP that the newly hired nursing assistant has taken 3 times this week. As the RN, what action do you take?
    1. Do not delegate vital signs to the newly hired nursing assistant.
    2. Delegate only temperature and respiratory rate to the newly hired nursing assistant.
    3. Report the newly hired nursing assistant to your supervisor.
    4. Observe the newly hired nursing assistant as she obtains a blood pressure and pulse on a patient.

Answers to Review Questions can be found on pages 1197-1198.

REFERENCES

Adiyaman A and others: The position of the arm during blood pressure measurement in sitting position, *Blood Press Monit* 11(6):309, 2006.

Appel LJ, Brands MW, Daniels SR: Dietary approaches to prevent and treat hypertension, *Hypertension* 47:296, 2006.

Bern L and others: Differences in blood pressure values obtained with automated and manual methods in medical inpatients, *Medsurg Nurs* 16(6):356, 2007.

Brashers VL: *Clinical application of pathophysiology*, ed 3, St. Louis, 2006, Mosby.

Ebersole P and others: *Toward healthy aging: human needs and nursing response*, ed 6, St. Louis, 2004, Mosby.

Evans D and others: *Vital signs: a systematic review*, Adelaide, South Australia, 2004, Joanna Briggs Institute for Evidence Based Nursing and Midwifery.

Falkner B, Daniels SR: Summary of the Fourth Report on the Diagnosis, Evaluation and Treatment of High Blood Pressure in Children and Adolescents, *Hypertension* 44:387, 2004.

Fallis WM and others: A multimethod approach to evaluate chemical dot thermometers for oral temperature measurement, *J Nurs Meas* 14(3):151, 2006.

Farnell S and others: Temperature measurement: comparison of non-invasive methods used in adult critical care, *J Clin Nurs* 14:632, 2005.

Giles TD: Circadian rhythm of blood pressure and the relation to cardiovascular events, *J Hypertens* 24(Suppl 2):S11, 2006.

Giuliano KK, Higgins TL: New generation pulse oximetry in the care of critically ill patients, *Am J Crit Care* 14(1):26, 2005.

Giuliano KK, Liu LM: Knowledge of pulse oximetry among critical care nurses, *Dimens Crit Care* 25(1):44, 2006.

Henker R, Carlson KK: Fever: applying research to bedside practice, *AACN Adv Crit Care* 18(1):76, 2007.

Hockenberry MJ, Wilson D: *Wong's nursing care of infants and children*, ed 8, St. Louis, 2007, Mosby.

Jarvis C: *Physical examination and health assessment*, ed 5, St. Louis, 2008, Saunders.

Lawson L, Bridges EJ, Ballou I: Accuracy and precision of noninvasive core temperature measurement in adult intensive care patients, *Am J Crit Care* (16):485, 2007.

Lewis M: Heatstroke in older adults, *Am J Nurs* 107(6):52, 2007.

Maxton FJ, Justin L, Gilles D: Estimating core temperature in infants and children after cardiac surgery: a comparison of six methods, *J Adv Nurs* 45(2):214, 2004.

Milam MW and others: Bacterial contamination of fabric stethoscope covers: the velveteen rabbit of healthcare? *Infect Control Hosp Epidemiol* 22(10):653, 2001.

National High Blood Pressure Education Program; National Heart, Lung, and Blood Institute; National Institutes of Health: The seventh report of the Joint National Committee on Detection, Evaluation, and Treatment of High Blood Pressure, *JAMA* 289(19):2560, 2003.

Pagana KD, Pagana TK: *Mosby's diagnostic and laboratory test reference*, ed 9, St. Louis, 2009, Mosby.

Pickering TG and others: Recommendations for blood pressure measurement in humans and experimental animals. I. Blood pressure measurement in humans, *Hypertension* 45:142, 2005.

Redon J: The normal circadian pattern of blood pressure: implications for treatment, *Int J Clin Pract* 58(Suppl 145):3, 2004.

Rodden A and others: Does fingernail polish affect pulse oximeter readings? *Intensive Crit Care Nurs* 23(1):51, 2007.

Schell K and others: Clinical comparison of automatic noninvasive measurements of blood pressure in the forearm and upper arm, *Am J Crit Care* 14(3):232, 2005.

Thompson HJ: Fever: a concept analysis, *J Adv Nurs* 51(5):484, 2005.

Walsh AM and others: Fever management: paediatric nurses' knowledge, attitudes and influencing factors, *J Adv Nurs* 49(5):453, 2005.

CHAPTER 15

Health Assessment and Physical Examination

MEDIA RESOURCES

CD COMPANION 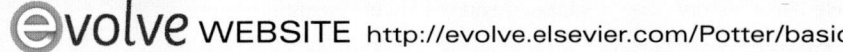 **WEBSITE** http://evolve.elsevier.com/Potter/basic

- Crossword Puzzle
- English/Spanish Audio Glossary

OBJECTIVES

- Discuss the purposes of physical assessment.
- Describe the techniques used with each assessment skill.
- Discuss how cultural diversity influences health assessment.
- Describe proper positioning for the patient during each phase of the examination.
- List techniques to promote the patient's physical and psychological comfort during an examination.
- Make environmental preparations before an examination.
- Describe interview techniques used to enhance communication during history taking.

- Identify data to collect from the nursing history before an examination.
- Discuss ways to incorporate health promotion and health teaching into an assessment.
- Discuss normal physical findings for patients across the life span.
- Identify self-screening assessments commonly performed by patients.
- Use physical assessment techniques and skills during routine nursing care.
- Document assessment findings on appropriate forms.
- Communicate abnormal findings to appropriate personnel.

KEY TERMS

adventitious sounds, p. 337
atrophy, p. 323
auscultation, p. 312
bruit, p. 343
cerumen, p. 329
costovertebral angle (CVA), p. 353

crackles, p. 337
cyanosis, p. 320
dorsum, p. 322
dyspnea, p. 335
edema, p. 320
erythema, p. 321
indurated, p. 322

inspection, p. 311
integument, p. 319
intercostal space, p. 335
jaundice, p. 321
olfaction, p. 312
orthopnea, p. 335

pallor, p. 321
palpation, p. 311
percussion, p. 312
petechiae, p. 322
phlebitis, p. 348
thrill, p. 343
turgor, p. 322

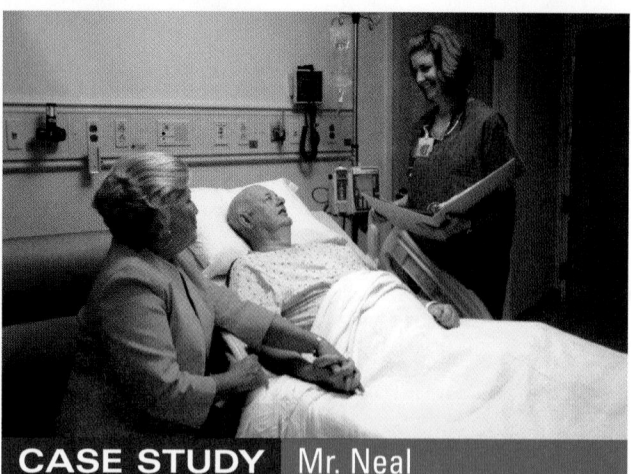

CASE STUDY Mr. Neal

Mr. Neal, a 76-year-old retired college professor, has a history of rectal bleeding and change in bowel habits. He has a history of a high-fat diet and mild hypertension and smokes 2 packs of cigarettes a day. He denies any family history of colon cancer. Mr. Neal is being admitted to the surgical floor for bowel surgery. His wife is with him when he is admitted.

Jane is the nursing student assigned to care for Mr. Neal during the day shift. Jane begins her assessments with a review of Mr. Neal's chart and health care provider's orders.

While working in a variety of settings, nurses seek information about patients' health status. You will possibly conduct health assessments at health fairs, at screening clinics, in health care providers' offices, in a patient's home, or in acute care settings. Health screenings focus on a specific physical problem. For example, blood pressure screenings detect the risk for high blood pressure. If a screening determines that a patient has a risk for a disease, you refer the patient for a more complete physical examination.

A complete health assessment involves a nursing history and behavioral and physical examination. The health history involves a lengthy patient interview to gather subjective data about the patient's condition. A physical examination is a head-to-toe review of body systems that offers objective information about the patient. Physical assessment skills are used during an examination to make clinical judgments. The patient's condition and response affect the extent of the examination. The accuracy of the physical assessment will influence the choice of therapies a patient receives and the evaluation of response to those therapies. Continuity in health care improves when you make ongoing, objective, and comprehensive assessments.

PURPOSES OF PHYSICAL EXAMINATION

An examination is designed for the patient's needs. In the acutely ill patient you assess only the involved body system(s). You then conduct a more comprehensive examination when the patient feels more at ease, so that you then are able to learn about the patient's total health status. You perform a complete physical examination for routine screening to promote wellness behaviors and preventive health care measures; to determine eligibility for health insurance, military service, or a new job; and to admit a patient to a hospital setting or long-term care facility. Use physical examination to do the following:

1. Gather baseline data about the patient's health status
2. Supplement, confirm, or refute data obtained in the history
3. Confirm and identify nursing diagnoses
4. Make clinical judgments about a patient's changing health status and management
5. Evaluate the outcomes of care

Developing a Database

Gather information about the patient's health status from the health history. A subsequent physical examination can reveal information that refutes, confirms, or supplements the history. Think critically about the information the patient provides, apply knowledge from previous clinical care, and methodically conduct the examination to create a clear picture of the patient's status. A complete assessment is necessary to form a nursing diagnosis. Learn to group significant findings into patterns of data that reveal actual or "risk for" nursing diagnoses (see Chapter 8). Gather information obtained during the initial physical examination to provide a baseline of the patient's functional abilities. Use this baseline as a comparison for future assessment findings.

CULTURAL SENSITIVITY

Respect the cultural differences of patients when completing an examination (see Chapter 19). It is important to remember that cultural differences influence a patient's behavior. Consider the patient's health beliefs, use of alternative therapies, nutritional habits, relationships with family, and comfort with your physical closeness during the examination and history taking.

Be culturally aware, and avoid stereotyping on the basis of gender or race. There is a difference between cultural and physical characteristics. Learn to recognize common disorders for those ethnic populations within the community. Recognition of cultural diversity helps to respect a patient's uniqueness and to provide higher-quality care. Improved patient outcomes result from recognition of and respect for cultural diversity (Giger and others, 2007).

INTEGRATION OF PHYSICAL ASSESSMENT WITH NURSING CARE

Learn to integrate an examination during routine patient care. For example, assess the condition of the skin during a bed bath, or observe a patient's gait, range of motion (ROM), or muscle strength as the patient ambulates. This practice makes more efficient use of time.

SKILLS OF PHYSICAL ASSESSMENT

A comprehensive physical assessment involves the use of five skills: inspection, palpation, percussion, auscultation, and olfaction.

Inspection

Inspection is the use of vision and hearing to distinguish normal from abnormal findings. It is important to know what to consider normal for patients of different age-groups. You will need experience to recognize normal variations among patients. Inspection is a simple technique, and the quality of an inspection depends upon your willingness to be thorough and systematic. To inspect body parts accurately, follow these principles:

1. Make sure adequate lighting is available.
2. Position and expose body parts so you can view all surfaces.
3. Inspect each area for size, shape, color, symmetry, position, and abnormalities.
4. When possible, compare each area inspected with the same area on the opposite side of the body.
5. Use additional light (e.g., a penlight) to inspect body cavities.
6. Do not hurry inspection. Pay attention to detail.

After inspection of a body part, findings sometimes indicate the need for further examination. Use palpation with or after visual inspection.

Palpation

Palpation involves the use of the hands to touch body parts to make sensitive assessments. It typically occurs right after inspection. The exception is when examining the abdomen. Then palpation occurs after auscultation. Use palpation to examine all accessible parts of the body. For example, palpate the skin for temperature, moisture, texture, turgor, tenderness, and thickness. Palpate the abdomen for tenderness, distention, or masses. Use different parts of the hand to detect characteristics such as texture, temperature, and perception of movement.

Assist the patient with relaxing and positioning comfortably because muscle tension during palpation impairs the

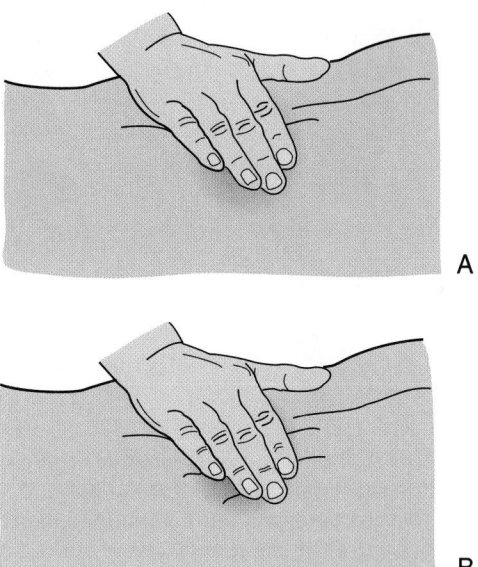

Figure 15-1 ■ **A,** During light palpation, gentle pressure against underlying skin and tissues can detect areas of irregularity and tenderness. **B,** During deep palpation, depress tissue to assess condition of underlying organs.

ability to palpate correctly. Asking the patient to take slow, deep breaths enhances muscle relaxation. *Palpate tender areas last.* Be sure to ask the patient to point out the more sensitive areas, and note any nonverbal signs of discomfort.

You need warm hands, short fingernails, and a gentle approach for this technique. Perform palpation slowly, gently, and deliberately. Light palpation of structures such as the abdomen determines areas of tenderness (Figure 15-1, *A*). Place your hand on the part you are examining, and depress about 1 cm (½ inch). Examine tender areas further for potentially serious abnormalities. Light, intermittent pressure is best when palpating; heavy, prolonged pressure causes loss of sensitivity in the hand.

After light palpation, use deeper palpation to examine the condition of organs (Figure 15-1, *B*). Depress the area you are examining deeply and evenly (Seidel and others, 2006). Caution is the rule. To avoid injuring a patient, do not try deep palpation without clinical supervision. Apply deep palpation with one hand or both hands (bimanually). Bimanual palpation involves one hand placed over the other while applying pressure. The upper hand exerts downward pressure as the other hand feels the subtle characteristics of underlying organs and masses. Seek the assistance of a qualified instructor before attempting deep palpation.

Use the most sensitive parts of the hand, the palmar surface of the fingers and finger pads, to determine position, texture, size, consistency, masses, fluid, and pulsation (Figure 15-2, *A*). Measure temperature using the dorsal surface, or back, of the hand (Figure 15-2, *B*). The palm of the hand (Figure 15-2, *C*) is more sensitive to vibration. Measure position, consistency, and turgor by lightly grasping the body part with the fingertips (Figure 15-2, *D*).

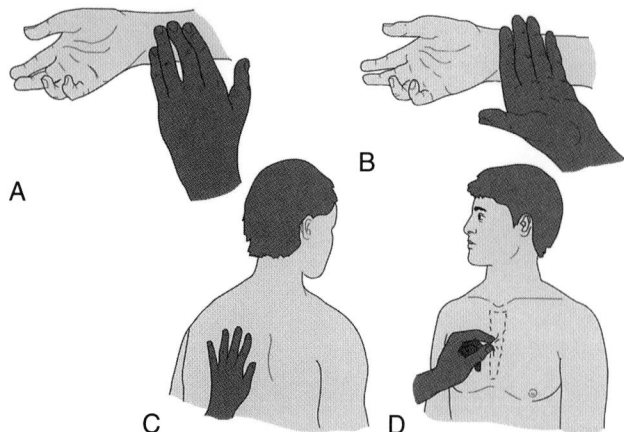

Figure 15-2 ■ **A,** Radial pulse is detected with pads of fingertips, the most sensitive part of the hand. **B,** Dorsum of hand detects temperature variations in skin. **C,** The bony part of the palm at the base of the fingers detects vibrations. **D,** Skin is grasped with fingertips to assess turgor.

Do not palpate without considering the patient's condition. For example, if the patient has a fractured rib, use extra care to locate the painful area. Do not palpate a vital artery with pressure that obstructs blood flow.

Percussion

Percussion involves tapping the body with the fingertips to produce a vibration that travels through body tissues. The character of the sound determines the location, size, and density of underlying structures to verify abnormalities assessed by palpation and auscultation. This vibration is transmitted through the body tissues, and the character of the sound heard depends on the density of the underlying tissue. By knowing the way various densities influence sound, you locate organs or masses, map their boundaries, and determine their size. An abnormal sound suggests a mass or substance such as air or fluid within an organ or body cavity. The skill of percussion requires dexterity and is usually reserved for advanced practitioners.

Auscultation

Auscultation is listening with a stethoscope to sounds produced by the body. First learn the normal sounds the cardiovascular, respiratory, and gastrointestinal (GI) systems make, such as movement of air through the lungs. Recognize abnormal sounds after learning normal variations. Becoming more proficient at auscultation occurs by knowing the type of sounds each body structure makes and the location in which you hear the sounds best. Also learn which areas do not normally emit sounds.

To auscultate, you need good hearing acuity, a good stethoscope, and knowledge of how to use the stethoscope properly. If you have a hearing disorder, use a stethoscope with greater sound amplification. It is essential to place the stethoscope directly on a patient's skin because clothing ob-

scures and changes sound. Chapter 14 describes the parts of the stethoscope and its general use. The bell is best for low-pitched sounds, such as vascular and certain heart sounds, and the diaphragm is best for high-pitched sounds, such as bowel and lung sounds.

Be familiar with the stethoscope before attempting to use it. Practice using the stethoscope. Extraneous sounds created by movement of the tubing or chestpiece interfere with auscultation of body organ sounds. By deliberately producing these sounds, you learn to recognize and disregard them during the actual examination (Box 15-1). Learn to recognize the following characteristics of sounds:

* *Frequency:* Number of sound wave cycles generated per second by a vibrating object. The higher the frequency, the higher the pitch of a sound and vice versa.
* *Loudness:* Amplitude of a sound wave. Auscultated sounds are described as loud or soft.
* *Quality:* Sounds of similar frequency and loudness from different sources. Terms such as blowing or gurgling describe quality of sound.
* *Duration:* Length of time that sound vibrations last. Duration of sound is short, medium, or long. Layers of soft tissue dampen the duration of sounds from deep internal organs.

Auscultation requires concentration and practice. Always consider the part of the body auscultated and the cause of the sounds. For example, the sounds heard over the abdomen are caused by intestinal peristalsis. Learn where you hear the sound best. You hear peristalsis over all four abdominal quadrants as intermittent "tinkling" sounds. After understanding the cause and character of normal auscultated sounds, it becomes easier to recognize abnormal sounds and their origins.

Olfaction

While assessing a patient, become familiar with the nature and source of body odors (Table 15-1). **Olfaction** helps to detect abnormalities not recognized by other means. For example, if a patient's cast has a sweet, heavy, thick odor, this indicates an underlying infection. Findings from olfaction allows detection of serious abnormalities.

PREPARATION FOR ASSESSMENT

Proper preparation of the environment, equipment, and patient ensures a smooth examination with few interruptions. A disorganized approach when preparing for a physical examination causes errors and incomplete findings. Always use standard precautions throughout the examination (see Chapter 13). It is necessary to wear gloves during palpation and percussion when there is a possibility of coming in contact with body fluids to reduce contact with microorganisms.

BOX 15-1   Using a Stethoscope

1 Place earpieces in both ears with tips of earpieces turned toward the face. *Lightly* blow into the diaphragm. Again place earpieces in your ears, this time with ends turned toward the back of the head. *Lightly* blow into the stethoscope's diaphragm. You will find that you hear clearer sounds with the earpiece turned toward the face. After you have learned the right fit for the loudest sound, wear the stethoscope the same way each time.

2 Put the stethoscope on, and *lightly* blow into the diaphragm. If sound is barely audible, *lightly* blow into the bell. Sound is carried through only one part of the chest piece at a time. If the sound is greatly amplified through the diaphragm, the diaphragm is in position for use. If sound is barely audible through the diaphragm, the bell is in position for use.

3 Place the diaphragm over the anterior part of your chest. Ask a friend to speak in a normal conversational tone. Environmental noise seriously detracts from hearing the noise created by body organs. When using a stethoscope, the patient and the examiner need to remain quiet.

4 Put the stethoscope on, and gently tap the tubing. It is often difficult to avoid stretching or moving the stethoscope's tubing. Position yourself so that the tubing hangs free. Moving or touching the tubing creates extraneous sounds.

5 *Care of the stethoscope:* Remove earpieces regularly, and clean or remove cerumen (earwax). Keep the bell and diaphragm free of dust, lint, and body oils. Keep the tubing away from your body oils. Avoid draping the stethoscope around the neck next to the skin. To clean, wipe the entire stethoscope (diaphragm, tubing, etc.) with alcohol or soapy water. Be sure to dry all parts thoroughly. Follow the manufacturer's recommendations.

6 *Infection control:* Harmful bacteria, even antibiotic-resistant microorganisms, transfer from patient to patient when using portable equipment such as stethoscopes (Truscott, 2005). Follow institution infection control guidelines, especially contact precautions to decrease this risk. Clean the stethoscope (diaphragm/bell) with a disinfectant before reuse on another patient. Using a disinfectant such as isopropyl alcohol (with or without chlorhexidine), benzalkonium, and sodium hypochlorite are effective in reducing the number of bacterial colonies. Earpieces of stethoscopes are sources of transferable bacteria as well when you inadvertently touch your ears and then care for the patient. Potential pathogens could contaminate earpieces. Using hand hygiene, before and after patient contact, decreases the risk for transmitting microorganisms from your ear to your patient. Do not use cloth stethoscope covers because these have been shown to become easily contaminated.

TABLE 15-1   Assessment of Characteristic Odors

ODOR	SITE OR SOURCE	POTENTIAL CAUSES
Alcohol	Oral cavity	Ingestion of alcohol, diabetes
Ammonia	Urine	Urinary tract infection, renal failure
Body odor	Skin, particularly in areas where body parts rub together (e.g., under arms and breasts)	Poor hygiene, excess perspiration (hyperhidrosis), foul-smelling perspiration (bromhidrosis)
	Wound site	Wound abscess
	Vomitus	Abdominal irritation, contaminated food
Feces	Vomitus/oral cavity (fecal odor)	Bowel obstruction
	Rectal area	Fecal incontinence
Foul-smelling stools in infant	Stool	Malabsorption syndrome
Halitosis	Oral cavity	Poor dental and oral hygiene, gum disease
Sweet, fruity ketones	Oral cavity	Diabetic ketoacidosis
Stale urine	Skin	Uremic acidosis
Sweet, heavy, thick odor	Draining wound	*Pseudomonas* (bacterial) infection
Musty odor	Casted body part	Infection inside cast
Fetid, sweet odor	Tracheostomy or mucus secretions	Infection of bronchial tree (*Pseudomonas* bacteria)

Environment

A physical examination requires privacy. A well-equipped examination room is preferable, but often the examination occurs in the patient's room. In the home you may perform the examination in the patient's bedroom. Adequate lighting is necessary for proper illumination of body parts. Ideally an examination room is soundproof, so patients feel comfortable discussing their conditions. Be sure to eliminate sources of noise, take precautions to prevent interruptions, and make sure the room is warm enough to maintain comfort.

Sometimes it is difficult to perform a complete examination when patients are in beds or on stretchers. Special examination tables make patients easily accessible and help them assume special positions. Carefully assist patients so they do not fall while getting on and off the table. Do not leave a confused, combative, or uncooperative patient unsupervised on an examination table.

Examination tables are often hard and uncomfortable. When the patient lies supine, raise the head of the table about 30 degrees. Also, give the patient a small pillow to use. When examining a patient in bed, raise the bed to reach the patient's body parts more easily.

Equipment

Perform hand hygiene thoroughly before equipment preparation and the examination. Set up equipment so it is readily available and arranged in order for easy use (Box 15-2). Keep equipment as warm as appropriate. Rub the diaphragm of the stethoscope briskly between the hands before applying it to the skin. Check all equipment to ensure that it functions properly. The ophthalmoscope and otoscope require good batteries and light bulbs.

Physical Preparation of the Patient

The patient's physical comfort is vital for a successful examination. Before starting, ask if the patient needs to use the restroom. An empty bladder and bowel facilitate examination of the abdomen, genitalia, and rectum. If needed, collect urine or fecal specimens at this time. Be sure to explain the proper method for collecting specimens, and make sure to label each specimen properly.

Physical preparation involves being sure the patient is dressed and draped properly. The patient in the hospital will be wearing a simple gown. An outpatient will have to undress and wear a light cover gown. If the examination is limited to certain body systems, it is not always necessary for the patient to undress completely. Provide the patient privacy and plenty of time during undressing. Walking into the room as the patient undresses causes embarrassment. Drapes and gowns are made of linen or disposable paper. After patients have undressed and put on a gown, they sit or lie down on the examination table with the drape over the lap or lower trunk. Make sure the patient stays warm by eliminating drafts, controlling room temperature, and providing warm blankets. Routinely ask if the patient is comfortable.

POSITIONING During the examination, ask the patient to assume proper positions so body parts are accessible and patients stay comfortable. Table 15-2 lists the preferred positions for each part of the examination and contains figures illustrating these positions. Patients' abilities to assume positions will depend on their physical strength, mobility, ease of breathing, age, and degree of wellness. Explain the positions, and assist patients in assuming them. Adjust the drapes so the area examined is accessible, making sure not to unnecessarily expose a body part. A patient may assume more than one position. To decrease the number of times the patient changes positions, organize the examination so that you perform all techniques requiring a sitting position first, then perform those that require a supine position next, and so forth. Use extra care when positioning older adults, because they are more prone to having disabilities and limitations.

PSYCHOLOGICAL PREPARATION OF THE PATIENT
Many patients find an examination tiring or stressful, or they

---

BOX 15-2 Equipment and Supplies for Physical Assessment

- Cervical brush or broom (if needed)
- Cotton applicators
- Disposable pad/paper towels
- Drapes
- Eye chart (e.g., Snellen chart)
- Flashlight and spotlight
- Forms (e.g., physical, laboratory)
- Gloves (sterile or clean)
- Gown for patient
- Ophthalmoscope
- Otoscope
- Papanicolaou (Pap) liquid prep (if needed)
- Percussion (reflex) hammer
- Pulse oximeter
- Ruler
- Scale with height measurement rod
- Specimen containers, slides, wooden or plastic spatula, and cytologic fixative (if needed)
- Sphygmomanometer and cuff
- Sterile swabs
- Stethoscope
- Tape measure
- Thermometer
- Tissues
- Tongue depressors
- Tuning fork
- Vaginal speculum (if needed)
- Water-soluble lubricant
- Wristwatch with second hand or digital display

---

experience anxiety about possible findings. A thorough explanation of the purpose and steps of each assessment lets patients know what to expect and what to do so that they can cooperate. Keep explanations simple and clear. Help patients feel free to ask questions and mention any discomfort. As you examine each body system, give a more detailed explanation. Convey an open, professional and relaxed approach. A stiff, formal approach will inhibit the patient's ability to communicate, but being too casual will not give the patient confidence in your ability (Seidel and others, 2006).

When the patient and nurse are of opposite gender, it helps to have a third person of the patient's gender in the room. The presence of a third person assures the patient that you will behave ethically. This person is also a witness to the conduct of the examiner and the patient.

During the examination, watch the patient's emotional responses. Observe whether the patient's facial expression shows fear or concern and if body movements show anxiety. Remain calm, and explain each step clearly. It is sometimes necessary to stop the examination and ask how the patient feels. Do not force a patient to continue. Postponing the examination is advantageous because the findings will be more accurate when the patient can cooperate and relax. If the patient's fears result from misconceptions, clarify the purpose of the examination and how you will perform it.

Assessment of Age-Groups

Different interview styles and approaches are needed to perform a health history and examine patients of different age-groups. When assessing children, be sensitive and anticipate

TABLE 15-2   Positions for Examination

POSITION	AREAS ASSESSED	RATIONALE	LIMITATIONS
Sitting	Head and neck, back, posterior thorax and lungs, anterior thorax and lungs, breasts, axillae, heart, vital signs, and upper extremities	Sitting upright provides full expansion of lungs and provides better visualization of symmetry of upper body parts.	Physically weakened patient is sometimes unable to sit. Use supine position with head of bed elevated instead.
Supine	Head and neck, anterior thorax and lungs, breasts, axillae, heart, abdomen, extremities, pulses	This is most normally relaxed position. It provides easy access to pulse sites.	If patient becomes short of breath easily, raise head of bed.
Dorsal recumbent	Head and neck, anterior thorax and lungs, breasts, axillae, heart, abdomen	This position is for abdominal assessment because it promotes relaxation of abdominal muscles.	Patients with painful disorders are more comfortable with knees flexed.
Lithotomy*	Female genitalia and genital tract	This position provides maximal exposure of genitalia and facilitates insertion of vaginal speculum.	Lithotomy position is embarrassing and uncomfortable, so examiner minimizes time that the patient spends in it. Keep patient well draped.
Sims'*	Rectum and vagina	Flexion of hip and knee improves exposure of rectal area.	Joint deformities hinder patient's ability to bend hip and knee.
Prone	Musculoskeletal system	This position is only for assessing extension of hip joint, skin, buttocks.	Patients with respiratory difficulties do not tolerate this position well.
Lateral recumbent	Heart	This position aids in detecting murmurs.	Patients with respiratory difficulties do not tolerate this position well.
Knee-chest*	Rectum	This position provides maximal exposure of rectal area.	This position is embarrassing and uncomfortable.

*Patients with arthritis or other joint deformities may be unable to assume this position.

the child's reaction to the examination as a strange and unfamiliar experience. Routine pediatric examinations focus on health promotion and illness prevention, particularly for the care of well children who receive competent parenting and have no serious health problems (Hockenberry and Wilson, 2007). This examination focuses on growth and development, sensory screening, dental examination, and behavioral assessment. Children who are chronically ill or disabled, foster children, foreign-born, or adopted sometimes require additional assessments because of their unique health risks. When examining children, the following tips assist in data collection:

1. It is helpful to gain a child's trust before doing any type of an examination. Talk and play with the child first. It also helps to perform parts of the examination that you can do visually before actually touching the child.
2. Children will feel safer during an examination if it is initiated from the periphery and then moves to the central. For example, examine the extremities before moving to the chest.
3. When obtaining histories of infants and children, gather all or part of the information from parents or guardians.
4. Because parents sometimes think they are being tested or judged by the examiner, offer support during examination, and do not pass judgment.

5. Call children by their preferred name, and address parents formally (e.g., as "Mr. and Mrs. Brown") rather than by first names.
6. Open-ended questions often allow parents to share more information and to describe more of the child's problems.
7. Older children and adolescents tend to respond best when treated as adults and individuals and often can provide details about their health history and severity of symptoms.
8. Remember, the adolescent has a right to confidentiality. After talking with parents about historical information, arrange to speak privately with the adolescent.

A comprehensive health assessment and examination of older adults includes physical data, developmental stage, family relationships, group involvement, and religious and occupational pursuits (Ebersole and others, 2008). An important part of health assessment involves analysis of basic activities of daily living (ADLs) (e.g., dressing, bathing, toileting, feeding, and continence) that are fundamental to independent living. In addition, you assess the more complex instrumental ADLs (e.g., using the telephone, preparing meals, and managing money). Any examination of an older adult also includes an evaluation of mental status.

During the examination, recognize that with advancing age the body does not respond vigorously to injury or disease. Therefore older persons do not always exhibit the expected signs and symptoms (Ebersole and others, 2008; Meiner and Lueckenotte, 2006). Characteristically, older adults have more blunted or atypical signs and symptoms. Principles to follow during examination of an older adult include the following:

1. Do not assume that aging is always accompanied by illness or disability. Older adults are able to adapt to change and maintain functional independence (Meiner and Lueckenotte, 2006).
2. Allow extra time and be patient, relaxed, and unhurried with older adults.
3. Provide adequate space for an examination, particularly if the patient uses a mobility aid.
4. Plan the history and examination, taking into account the older adult's energy level, physical limitations, pace, and adaptability. More than one session is sometimes necessary to complete the assessment (Meiner and Lueckenotte, 2006).
5. Measure performance under the most favorable conditions. Take advantage of natural opportunities for assessment (e.g., during bathing, grooming, mealtime) (Meiner and Lueckenotte, 2006).
6. Sequence an examination to keep position changes to a minimum. Be efficient throughout the examination to limit patient movement.
7. Be sure an examination of an older adult includes review of mental status.

ORGANIZATION OF THE EXAMINATION

A complete health assessment follows the format of the health history (see Chapter 8). Obtain information from the history to focus attention on specific parts of the examination. For example, if the history shows that the patient experiences difficulty in breathing, conduct an examination of the thorax and lungs more carefully. The examination supplements information from the history to confirm or refute the data.

Be systematic and well organized about the examination so you do not miss important assessments. A head-to-toe approach includes all body systems and helps to anticipate each step. In an adult begin by assessing the head and neck, progressing methodically down the body to include all body systems. Compare both sides of the body for symmetry. If a patient is seriously ill, examine the body system most at risk for being abnormal. If a patient becomes fatigued, provide rest periods. Perform any painful procedures near the end of the examination. Use common and accepted medical abbreviations to keep notes brief and concise. A physical assessment form allows you to record information in the same sequence it was gathered.

General Survey

Assessment begins when you first meet the patient. Determine the patient's reasons for seeking health care. Initial information from the general survey begins with a review of the patient's primary health problems. Make mental notes of the patient's behavior and appearance. Begin the examination with the general survey. The survey provides information about characteristics of an illness; a patient's hygiene, skin condition, and body image; emotional state; recent changes in weight; and developmental status. The survey reveals important information about the patient's behavior that influences how you will communicate instructions to the patient and continue the assessment.

GENERAL APPEARANCE AND BEHAVIOR Assess appearance and behavior while preparing the patient for the examination. The review of general appearance and behavior includes the following:

1. *Gender and race:* A person's gender affects the type of examination performed and the manner in which you make assessments. Different physical features are related to gender and race. Certain illnesses are more likely to affect a specific gender or race; for example, skin cancer is more common in white patients, and prostate cancer is higher in African Americans (American Cancer Society [ACS], 2009a).
2. *Age:* Age influences normal physical characteristics and a person's ability to participate in some parts of the examination.
3. *Signs of distress:* Sometimes there are obvious signs or symptoms indicating pain (grimacing, splinting painful area) or difficulty in breathing (shortness of breath,

sternal retraction) or anxiety. These signs help to establish priorities regarding what to examine first.

4. *Body type:* Observe if a patient appears trim and muscular, obese, or excessively thin. Body type reflects level of health, age, and lifestyle.

5. *Posture:* Normal standing posture is an upright stance with parallel alignment of hips and shoulders. Normal sitting posture involves some degree of rounding of the shoulders. Observe whether the patient has a slumped, erect, or bent posture. Posture often reflects mood or pain. Many older adults have a stooped, forward-bent posture, with hips and knees somewhat flexed and arms bent at the elbows, raising the level of the arms.

6. *Gait:* Observe the patient walking into the room or along the bedside (if ambulatory). Note whether movements are coordinated or uncoordinated. A person normally walks with arms swinging freely at the sides, with the head and face leading the body.

7. *Body movements:* Observe whether movements are purposeful. Note any tremors involving the extremities. Determine if any body parts are immobile.

8. *Hygiene and grooming:* Note the patient's level of cleanliness by observing the appearance of the hair, skin, and fingernails. Note if the patient's clothes are clean. Grooming depends on the activities being performed just before the examination, as well as the patient's occupation. Also note the amount and type of cosmetics used. Socioeconomic level may influence a patient's level of hygiene and grooming if the person does not have adequate bathing facilities or hygiene products.

9. *Dress:* Culture, lifestyle, socioeconomic level, and personal preference affect the type of clothes worn. Note if the type of clothing worn is appropriate for temperature and weather conditions. Depressed or mentally ill persons are often unable to choose proper clothing. An older adult tends to wear extra clothing because of sensitivity to cold.

10. *Body odor:* An unpleasant body odor results from physical exercise, poor hygiene, or certain disease states.

11. *Affect and mood:* Affect is a person's feelings as they appear to others. Patients express mood or emotional state verbally and nonverbally. Note if verbal expressions match nonverbal behavior. Observe if mood is appropriate for the situation. Observe facial expressions while asking questions.

12. *Speech:* Normal speech is understandable and moderately paced. It shows an association with the person's thoughts. Note if the patient talks rapidly or slowly. Emotions or neurological impairment may cause an abnormal speech pace. Observe if the patient speaks in a normal tone with clear inflection of words.

13. *Patient abuse.* Abuse of children, women, and older adults is a growing health problem. Obvious physical injury or neglect (e.g., evidence of malnutrition or presence of bruising on the extremities or trunk) are signs of possible abuse (Cattaneo and others, 2007; Cooper and others, 2008; Read and others, 2007). Assess for the patient's fear of the spouse or partner, caregiver, parent, or adult child.

Note if the partner or caregiver has a history of violence, alcoholism, or drug abuse. Is the person unemployed, ill, or frustrated in caring for the patient? *If you assess a pattern of findings indicating abuse, most states mandate a report to a social service center (refer to state guidelines). Obtain immediate consultation with a health care provider, social worker, and other support staff to facilitate placement in a safer environment.* Interview the patient privately. Patients are more likely to reveal problems to you when the suspected abuser is not present in the room. Table 15-3 summarizes clinical indicators of abuse.

14. *Substance abuse:* Substance abuse affects all socioeconomic groups. A single visit to a clinic does not always reveal the problem. Several visits often reveal behaviors that you can confirm with a well-focused history and physical examination. Approach the patient in a caring and nonjudgmental way because substance abuse involves both emotional and lifestyle issues. Box 15-3 lists patients to suspect for substance abuse. When you suspect abuse, ask the following CAGE questions (CAGE is an acronym for the following): Have you ever felt the need to *Cut down* on your drinking or drug use? Have people *Annoyed* you by criticizing your drinking or drug use? Have you ever felt bad or *Guilty* about your drinking or drug use? Have you ever used or had a drink first thing in the morning as an *Eye-opener* to steady your nerves or feel normal? If two or more of the CAGE questions are positive, strongly suspect substance abuse and consider how to motivate the patient to seek treatment (Feldstein and Miller, 2007; Van Hook and others, 2007).

VITAL SIGNS Assessment of vital signs (see Chapter 14) is the first part of the physical examination. Positioning or moving the patient can interfere with obtaining accurate values. You can also measure specific vital signs during assessment of individual body systems. Be sure to recheck and report any vital signs outside of normal ranges to the primary health care provider.

HEIGHT AND WEIGHT Height and weight reflect a person's general level of health. Weight is a routine measure during health screenings and visits to health care providers' offices or clinics. Both measures are routine when patients are admitted to a health care setting. Measuring an infant's or child's height and weight provides data about his or her growth and development. In older adults, height and weight coupled with a nutritional assessment determine the cause and treatment for chronic disease and help to identify feeding difficulty and other functional activities. Be sure to look for overall trends in height and weight changes.

A patient's weight will normally vary daily because of fluid loss or retention. Assessments screen for abnormal weight changes. The nursing history helps to focus on possible causes for weight changes. Determine the patient's current height and weight, noting weight gains or losses. Assess changes in diet habits, appetite, prescription or over-the-counter drugs, or physical symptoms. Standardized tables provide normal expected weights for a patient at a given height.

TABLE 15-3 Clinical Indicators of Abuse

PHYSICAL FINDINGS	BEHAVIORAL FINDINGS
CHILD SEXUAL ABUSE	
Vaginal or penile discharge	Problem in sleeping or eating
Blood on underclothing	Fear of certain people or places
Pain, itching, or unusual odor in genital area	Play activities recreate the abuse situation
Genital injuries	Regressed behavior
Difficulty sitting or walking	Sexual acting out
Pain while urinating; recurrent urinary tract infections	Knowledge of explicit sexual matters
Foreign bodies in rectum, urethra, or vagina	Preoccupation with others' or own genitals
Sexually transmitted diseases	Profound and rapid personality changes
Pregnancy in young adolescent	Rapidly declining school performance
	Poor relationship with peers
DOMESTIC ABUSE	
Injuries and trauma are inconsistent with reported cause	Attempted suicide
Multiple injuries involving head, face, neck, breasts, abdomen, and genitalia (black eyes, orbital fractures, broken nose, fractured skull, lip lacerations, broken teeth, strangulation marks)	Eating or sleeping disorders
	Anxiety
	Panic attacks
X-ray films show old and new fractures in different stages of healing	Pattern of substance abuse (follows physical abuse)
	Low self-esteem
Abrasions, lacerations, bruises, welts	Depression
Burns	Sense of helplessness
Human bites	Guilt
	Increased forgetfulness
	Stress-related complaints (headache, anxiety)
OLDER ADULT ABUSE	
Injuries and trauma are inconsistent with reported cause (e.g., cigarette burn, scratch, bruise, bite)	Dependent on caregiver
	Physically and/or cognitively impaired
Hematomas	Combative
Bruises at various stages of resolution	Wandering
Bruises, chafing, excoriation on wrist or legs (restraints)	Verbally belligerent
Burns	Minimal social support
Fractures inconsistent with cause described	Prolonged interval between injury and medical treatment
Dried blood	

Data from Cattaneo L and others: Intimate partner violence victims' accuracy in assessing their risk of re-abuse, *J Fam Violence* 22(6):429, 2007; Cooper C and others: The prevalence of elder abuse and neglect: a systematic review, *Age Aging* 37(2):151, 2008; Hockenberry MJ, Wilson D: *Wong's nursing care of infants and children,* ed 8, 2007, Mosby; Read J and others: Why, when and how to ask about childhood abuse, *Adv Psychiatr Treatment* 13:101, 2007.

Weigh patients at the same time of day, on the same scale, and in the same clothes to allow for an objective comparison of subsequent weights. Accuracy of measuring weight is important because health care providers often use weight to make medical and nursing decisions (e.g., drug dose determinations or positioning). Patients capable of bearing their own weight use a standing scale. Calibrate a standard platform scale by moving the large and small weights to zero. Make the balance beam level and steady by adjusting the calibrating knob. The patient stands on the scale platform and remains still. Move the largest weight to the 50-pound or 22.5-kg increment under the patient's weight. Then adjust the smaller weight to balance the scale at the nearest ¼ pound or 0.1 kg (Seidel and others, 2006). Electronic scales automatically display weight within sec-

onds. Electronic scales are automatically calibrated each time they are used.

Stretcher and chair scales are available for patients unable to bear weight. After you transfer the patient to the scale, a hydraulic device lifts the patient above the bed and measures the weight on a balance beam or digital display. Use caution when transferring patients to and from the scales.

Always weigh infants in baskets or on platform scales. Remove the infant's clothing, and weigh the infant naked (Hockenberry and Wilson, 2007). Keep the room warm to prevent chills. A light cloth or paper placed on the scale's surface prevents contamination from urine or feces. When weighing infants, hold a hand lightly above them to prevent accidental falls. Measure the weight of an infant in ounces, grams, and kilograms.

BOX 15-3 Red Flags for Suspicion of Substance Abuse

- Patients who frequently miss appointments
- Patients who frequently request written excuses for absence from work
- Patients who have chief complaints of insomnia, "bad nerves," or pain that does not fit a particular pattern
- Patients who often report lost prescriptions (e.g., tranquilizers, pain medications) or ask for frequent refills
- Patients who make frequent emergency department visits
- Patients who have a history of changing health care providers or who bring in medication bottles prescribed by several different providers
- Patients with histories of gastrointestinal bleeds, peptic ulcers, pancreatitis, cellulitis, or frequent pulmonary infections
- Patients with frequent sexually transmitted diseases, complicated pregnancies, multiple abortions, or sexual dysfunction
- Patients who complain of chest pains or palpitations or who have a history of admissions to rule out myocardial infarctions
- Patients who give histories of activities that place them at risk for human immune deficiency virus (HIV) infections (multiple partners, multiple rapes)
- Patients with family history of addiction; history of childhood sexual, physical, or emotional abuse; or social and financial or marital problems

Data from American Psychiatric Association: *Diagnostic and statistical manual of mental disorders*, ed 4, Washington, DC, 2000, The Association; Ries R, Wilford B: *Principles of addiction medicine*, ed 4, Chevy Chase, Md, 2009, Lippincott Williams & Wilkins.

To measure the height of a weight-bearing patient, have the patient remove his or her shoes. Place a paper towel on the scale platform so the patient's feet remain clean. The platform scale has a metal rod attached to the back of the scale; this swings out and over the crown of the patient's head. Have the patient stand erect. Measure the patient's height in inches or centimeters.

Remove the shoes of a non–weight-bearing patient (such as an infant), and position the patient supine on a firm surface (Figure 15-3). Portable devices are available that provide a reliable means to measure height. Place the infant on the device, having the caregiver hold the infant's head against the headboard. With the infant's legs straight at the knees, place the footboard against the bottom of the infant's feet. Record the infant's length to the nearest 0.5 cm or ¼ inch.

SKIN, HAIR, AND NAILS

The **integument** consists of the skin, hair, scalp, and nails. First inspect all skin surfaces, or assess the skin gradually while examining other body systems. Use the skills of inspection, palpation, and olfaction to assess the integument's function and integrity.

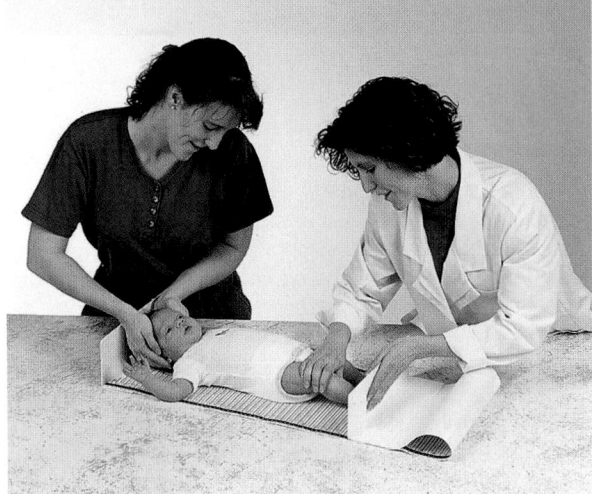

Figure 15-3 ■ Measuring infant length. (From Seidel HM and others: *Mosby's guide to physical examination*, ed 6, St. Louis, 2006, Mosby.)

Skin

Assessment of the skin reveals changes in oxygenation, circulation, nutrition, local tissue damage, and hydration. In a hospital setting the majority of patients are older adults, debilitated patients, or young but seriously ill patients. There are significant risks for skin lesions resulting from trauma to the skin during administration of care, from prolonged pressure during immobilization, or from reaction to medications used in treatment. Patients at high risk are the neurologically impaired, chronically ill, and orthopedic patients. Others at risk are patients with diminished mental status, poor tissue oxygenation, low cardiac output, or inadequate nutrition. In nursing homes and extended care facilities, patients are often at risk for many of the same problems, depending on their level of mobility and the presence of chronic illness. Routinely assess the skin to look for primary or initial lesions that develop. Without proper care, primary lesions can deteriorate to become secondary lesions that require more extensive nursing care.

Melanoma, an aggressive form of skin cancer, occurs primarily in light-pigmented people (ACS, 2007). Approximately 69,000 new cases of melanoma and 1.25 million cases of the highly curable basal cell and squamous cell cancers are diagnosed every year (Skin Cancer Foundation, 2009). Cutaneous malignancies are the most common neoplasms seen in patients. Make sure to perform a thorough skin assessment for all patients and educate them about self-examination (Box 15-4).

The condition of the patient's skin reveals the need for nursing intervention. Use assessment findings to determine the type of hygiene measures required to maintain integrity of the integument (Voegeli, 2008) (see Chapter 28). Adequate nutrition and hydration become goals of therapy if you identify an alteration in the status of the integument.

You need adequate lighting to accurately observe the skin. The recommended choice is natural or halogen lighting. For detecting skin changes in the dark-skinned patient, sunlight is the best choice (Newson, 2008). Room temperature also

BOX 15-4   BEST PRACTICES

Skin Cancer Prevention

SUMMARY OF EVIDENCE

The American Cancer Society (ACS) estimates there were 11,500 deaths from skin cancers in 2009 (ACS, 2009a). A melanoma is a cancerous (malignant) tumor that begins in the cells that produce the skin coloring (melanocytes). Melanoma is almost always curable in its early stages. However, it is likely to spread, and once it has spread to other parts of the body the chances for a cure are much less. There are several risk factors for melanoma: major factors are positive family history of melanoma, a prior melanoma, and multiple or unusual moles (nevi). Other factors include fair skin, freckling, and light hair; immune suppression; age under 30; excessive exposure to the sun (especially before age 18); and the use of tanning beds/booths (Goldberg and others, 2007).

The ACS (2009a) outlines the warning signs of skin cancer using the ABCD mnemonic: A is for **A**symmetry—look for uneven shape; B is for **B**order irregularity—look for edges that are blurred, notched, or ragged; C is for **C**olor—pigmentation is not uniform; blue, black, brown variegated, tan, or areas of unusual colors such as pink, white, gray, blue, or red are abnormal; and D is for **D**iameter, greater than the size of a typical pencil eraser.

Research has indicated that skin cancer, when detected early and treated properly, is highly curable. Overall survival rates for melanoma at the 5-year mark are 92%, with 99% for localized melanoma; when grouped in regional and distant stages, the survival rates dramatically decrease (ACS, 2009a). Therefore early intervention is of utmost importance.

The results from the research studies have made it a nursing responsibility to provide skin screening and intervention for all patients and families, especially those that have been identified as melanoma-prone (Loescher and others, 2009). Research has shown that educating children about sun-protective behaviors is difficult because children seem to possess strong attitudes against sun protection (DeMarco, 2008).

APPLICATION TO NURSING PRACTICE

- Instruct patients to conduct a complete monthly self-examination of the skin and scalp, noting moles, blemishes, and birthmarks.
- Perform the examination after a bath or shower, including a head-to-toe check.
- Use a well-lit room and mirrors to examine all skin surfaces. If necessary, have the patient ask a family member/significant other to aid in the investigation.
- Teach your patients to contact their health care provider if a skin lesion or mole starts to bleed or ooze or feels different (swollen, hard, lumpy, itchy, or tender to the touch). Especially instruct older adults, who tend to have delayed wound healing.
- Inform your patients of ways to prevent skin cancer by avoiding overexposure to the sun:
  - Wear sunglasses, wide-brimmed hats, and long sleeves and long pants.
  - Apply broad-spectrum sunscreens with SPF of 15 or greater to protect against ultraviolet B (UVB) and ultraviolet A (UVA) rays approximately 15 minutes before going into the sun and after swimming, perspiring, or bathing.
  - Avoid tanning under the direct sun at midday (10 AM to 4 PM).
  - Do not use indoor sunlamps, tanning parlors, or tanning pills.
- Inform patients who are on medications that make the skin more sensitive to the sun (e.g., oral contraceptives, statins, antiinflammatories, antihypertensives, immunosuppressives) to take extra precautions when spending time in the sun.
- Provide children with a sun protection educational program with a diversified curriculum, taught over an extended period of time (DeMarco, 2008).
- Inform patients to protect their children from the sun. Severe sunburns in childhood greatly increase melanoma risk later in life (ACS, 2009a).

REFERENCES

American Cancer Society: *Cancer facts and figures 2009,* New York, 2009a, The Society.
DeMarco R: Primary prevention of skin cancer in children and adolescents: a review of the literature, *J Pediatr Oncol Nurs* 25(2):67, 2008.
Goldberg MS and others: Risk factors for presumptive melanoma in skin cancer screening, *J Am Acad Dermatol* 57(1):60, 2007.
Loescher L and others: Perceptions of melanoma risk communications and risk control behaviors in melanoma prone families, *Oncol Nurs Forum* 34(1):169, 2007.

affects skin assessment. A room that is too warm causes superficial vasodilation, resulting in an increased redness of the skin. A cool environment causes the sensitive patient to develop **cyanosis** (bluish color) around the lips and nail beds (Anderson and others, 2007).

Use clean gloves for palpation if open, moist, or draining skin lesions are present. You will inspect all skin surfaces during an examination; begin with a brief overall visual review of the entire body. The examination includes inspecting the skin's color, moisture, temperature, texture, and turgor, vas-

cular changes, **edema,** and lesions. Carefully palpate any abnormalities. Skin odors are usually noted in skin folds, such as the axillae or under the female patient's breasts.

NURSING HISTORY Ask the patient about history of skin changes, including dryness, pruritus, sores, rashes, lumps, color, odor, and nonhealing lesions. Localized changes in skin color are sometimes the first indicators of skin cancer. Determine patient's history of sun exposure, use of sunscreen, and predisposition to develop skin cancer (fair, freckled, light-colored hair or eyes). Assess for use of topical

TABLE 15-4 Skin Color Variations

COLOR	CONDITION	CAUSES	ASSESSMENT LOCATIONS
Bluish (cyanosis)	Increased amount of deoxygenated hemoglobin (associated with hypoxia)	Heart or lung disease, cold environment	Nail beds, lips, base of tongue, skin (severe cases)
Pallor (decrease in color)	Reduced amount of oxyhemoglobin	Anemia	Face, conjunctivae, nail beds, palms of hands
	Reduced visibility of oxyhemoglobin resulting from decreased blood flow	Shock	Skin, nail beds, conjunctivae, lips
Loss of pigmentation	Vitiligo	Congenital or autoimmune condition causing lack of pigment	Patchy areas on skin over face, hands, arms
Yellow-orange (jaundice)	Increased deposit of bilirubin in tissues	Liver disease, destruction of red blood cells	Sclera, mucous membranes, skin
Red (erythema)	Increased visibility of oxyhemoglobin caused by dilation or increased blood flow	Fever, direct trauma, blushing, alcohol intake	Face, area of trauma, sacrum, shoulders, other common sites for pressure ulcers
Tan-brown	Increased amount of melanin	Suntan, pregnancy	Areas exposed to sun: face, arms; areolae, nipples

medications, sun lamps or tanning beds, and exposure to creosote, coal, tar, or radium.

COLOR   Skin color varies by body part and person. Despite individual variations, skin color is usually uniform over the body. Table 15-4 lists common variations in skin color. Normal skin pigmentation ranges from ivory or light pink to ruddy pink in light skin and from light to deep brown or olive in dark skin. In older adults, pigmentation increases unevenly, causing discolored skin. While inspecting the skin, be aware that cosmetics or tanning agents sometimes mask color.

The assessment of color first involves areas of the skin not exposed to the sun. Usually you see color hues best on the palms of the hands, soles of the feet, lips, tongue, and nail beds. Note if the skin is unusually pale or dark. Areas of increased color (hyperpigmentation) and decreased color (hypopigmentation) are common. Skin creases and folds are darker than the rest of the body in the dark-skinned patient.

Inspect sites where you can more easily identify abnormalities. For example, you can see **pallor** (unusual paleness) more easily in the face, buccal mucosa (mouth), conjunctivae, and nail beds. Observe for cyanosis (bluish discoloration) in the lips, nail beds, palpebral conjunctivae, and palms. It is more difficult to note changes such as pallor or cyanosis in patients with dark skin tones. In recognizing pallor in the dark-skinned patient, observe that normal brown skin appears to be yellow-brown and normal black skin appears to be ashen gray. Also assess the lips, nail beds, and mucous membranes for generalized pallor; if pallor is present, the mucous membranes will be ashen gray. Assessment of cyanosis in the dark-skinned patient requires that you observe areas where pigmentation occurs the least (conjunctivae, sclera, buccal mucosa, tongue, lips, nail beds, and palms and soles). In addition, verify these findings with clinical manifestations (Newson, 2008). A bluish-tint of the lips and gums may be a normal finding in dark-skinned patients (Seidel and others, 2006).

The best site to inspect for **jaundice** (yellow-orange discoloration) is the patient's sclera. You can see normal reactive

TABLE 15-5 Physical Findings of the Skin Indicative of Substance Abuse

PHYSICAL FINDING	COMMONLY ASSOCIATED DRUG
Diaphoresis	Sedative-hypnotic (including alcohol)
Spider angiomas	Alcohol, stimulants
Burns (especially fingers)	Alcohol
Needle marks	Opioids
Contusions, abrasions, cuts, scars	Alcohol, other sedative hypnotics
"Homemade" tattoos	Cocaine, intravenous opioids (prevents detection of injection sites)
Increased vascularity of face	Alcohol
Red, dry skin	Phencyclidine (PCP)

Modified from McHenry L and others: *Mosby's pharmacology in nursing*, ed 22, St. Louis, 2006, Mosby; Ries R, Wilford B: *Principles of addiction medicine*, ed 4, Chevy Chase, Md, 2009, Lippincott Williams & Wilkins.

hyperemia, or redness, most often in regions exposed to pressure such as the sacrum, heels, and greater trochanter (see Chapter 36). Inspect for any patches or areas of skin color variation. Localized skin changes, such as pallor or **erythema** (red discoloration), often indicate circulatory changes. For example, an area of erythema is due to localized vasodilation resulting from sunburn or fever. It is difficult to observe erythema in the dark-skinned patient, so palpate the area for heat and warmth to note the presence of skin inflammation. An area of an extremity that appears unusually pale results from an arterial occlusion or edema. Be sure to ask if the patient has noticed any changes in skin coloring.

There is a pattern of findings associated with patients who are chemically dependent and are intravenous (IV) drug abusers (Table 15-5). It is sometimes difficult to recognize signs and symptoms after one examination. Edematous, reddened, and warm areas along the arms and legs suggest a pattern of recent repeated IV injections. Evidence of old injection sites appears as hyperpigmented and shiny or scarred areas.

MOISTURE The hydration of skin and mucous membranes helps to reveal body fluid imbalances, changes in the skin's environment, and regulation of body temperature. Moisture refers to wetness and oiliness. The skin is normally smooth and dry. Skin folds such as the axillae are normally moist. Minimal perspiration or oiliness is present (Seidel and others, 2006). Increased perspiration is associated with activity, warm environments, obesity, anxiety, or excitement. Use ungloved fingertips to palpate skin surfaces and observe for dullness, dryness, crusting, and flaking. Flaking is the appearance of dandruff when the skin surface is lightly rubbed. Scaling involves fishlike scales that are easily rubbed off the skin's surface. Both flaking and scaling indicate abnormally dry skin. Excessively dry skin is common in older adults and persons who use excessive amounts of soap during bathing (Meiner and Lueckenotte, 2006). Other factors causing dry skin include lack of humidity, exposure to sun, smoking, stress, excessive perspiration, and dehydration (Bermann, 2007). Excessive dryness worsens existing skin conditions.

TEMPERATURE The temperature of the skin depends on the amount of blood circulating through the dermis. Increased or decreased skin temperature reflects an increase or decrease in blood flow. An increase in skin temperature often accompanies localized erythema or redness of the skin. A reduction in skin temperature reflects a decrease in blood flow. It is important to remember that a cold examination room affects the patient's skin temperature and color.

Accurately assess temperature by palpating the skin with the **dorsum**, or back, of the hand. Compare symmetrical body parts. Normally the skin temperature is warm. Skin temperature is the same throughout the body, and there are times it varies in one area. Always assess skin temperature for patients at risk for impaired circulation, such as after a cast application or vascular surgery. You can identify a stage I pressure ulcer early by noting warmth and erythema on an area of the skin (see Chapter 36).

TEXTURE The character of the skin's surface and the feel of deeper portions are its texture. Determine whether the patient's skin is smooth or rough, thin or thick, tight or supple, and **indurated** (hardened) or soft by stroking it lightly with the fingertips. The texture of the skin is normally smooth, soft, and flexible in children and adults. However, the texture is usually not uniform. The palms of the hands and soles of the feet tend to be thicker. In older adults the skin becomes wrinkled and leathery because of a decrease in collagen, subcutaneous fat, and sweat glands.

Localized changes result from trauma, surgical wounds, or lesions. When finding irregularities in texture such as scars or induration, ask the patient if there has been recent skin injury. Deeper palpation sometimes reveals irregularities such as tenderness or localized areas of induration commonly caused by repeated injections.

TURGOR **Turgor** is the skin's elasticity. Edema or dehydration diminishes turgor. Normally the skin loses its elasticity with age. To assess skin turgor, grasp a fold of skin on the back of the forearm or sternal area with the fingertips and release (Figure 15-4). Normally the skin lifts easily and snaps back immediately to its resting position. The skin stays pinched or tented when turgor is poor. The patient with poor turgor does not have resilience to the normal wear and tear on the skin. A decrease in turgor predisposes a patient to skin breakdown.

VASCULARITY The circulation of the skin affects color in localized areas and the appearance of superficial blood vessels. With aging, capillaries become fragile. Localized pressure areas, found after a patient has remained in one position, appear reddened, pink, or pale (see Chapter 36). **Petechiae** are pinpoint-size, red or purple spots on the skin caused by small hemorrhages in the skin layers. Petechiae do not blanch but may indicate serious blood-clotting disorders, drug reactions, or liver disease.

EDEMA Areas of the skin become swollen or edematous from fluid buildup in the tissues. Direct trauma and impairment of venous return are two common causes of edema. Inspect edematous areas for location, color, and shape. The formation of edema separates the skin's surface from the pigmented and vascular layers, masking skin color. Edematous skin also appears stretched and shiny. Palpate edematous areas to determine mobility, consistency, and tenderness. When pressure from your finger leaves an indentation in the edematous area, it is called *pitting edema*. To assess pitting edema, press the edematous area firmly with the thumb for several seconds and release. The depth of pitting, recorded in millimeters, determines the degree of edema (Seidel and others, 2006). For example, +1 edema equals 2 mm depth, and +2 edema equals 4 mm (see Figure 15-41, p. 347).

LESIONS The skin is normally free of lesions, except for common freckles or age-related changes such as skin tags or senile keratosis (thickening of skin), cherry angiomas (ruby red papules), and atrophic warts. Lesions are primary (occurring as initial spontaneous manifestations of a pathological process), such as an insect bite, or secondary (resulting from later formation of trauma to a primary lesion), such as a pressure ulcer. When you detect a lesion, inspect it for color, location, texture,

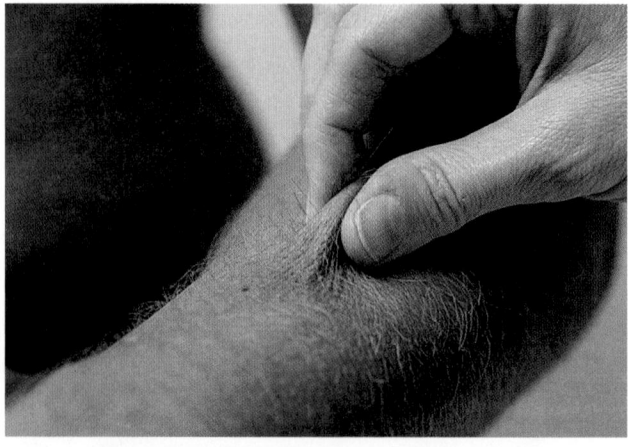

Figure 15-4 ■ Assessment of skin turgor.

size, shape, type (Box 15-5), grouping (e.g., clustered or linear), and distribution (localized or generalized). Observe any exudate for color, odor, amount, and consistency. Measure the size of the lesion by using a small, clear, flexible ruler, divided in centimeters. Measure lesions in height, width, and depth.

Palpation determines the lesion's mobility, contour (flat, raised, or depressed), and consistency (soft or indurated). Palpate gently, covering the entire area of the lesion. If the lesion is moist or has draining fluid, wear clean gloves during palpation. Note if the patient complains of tenderness during palpation. Cancerous lesions frequently undergo changes in color and size. Report abnormal lesions that have changed in character (e.g., color or size) to a health care provider for further examination.

Hair and Scalp

Inspecting the condition and distribution of body hair and integrity of the scalp requires good lighting. Assessment of the hair occurs during all portions of the examination. Assess the distribution, thickness, texture, and lubrication of hair.

NURSING HISTORY Determine if the patient wears a wig or hairpiece, and ask for it to be removed. Assess if the patient has noted change in growth or loss of hair or change in texture. Determine if the patient is on any medication that might alter hair texture or growth (e.g., chemotherapy or vasodilator).

During inspection explain that it is necessary to separate parts of the hair to detect abnormalities. Wear clean gloves to avoid possible infection from lesions or lice. First inspect the color, distribution, quantity, thickness, texture, and lubrication of body hair. Hair is normally distributed evenly, is neither excessively dry nor oily, and is pliant or flexible. While separating sections of scalp hair, observe for characteristics of color and coarseness. Normal terminal hair (long, coarse, thick hair on the scalp, axillae, and pubic areas) varies in color from light blond to black to gray. In older adults the hair becomes dull gray, white, or yellow. The hair also thins over the scalp, axillae, and pubic areas. Older men lose facial hair, whereas older women sometimes develop hair on the chin and upper lip.

BOX 15-5 Types of Primary Skin Lesions

Macule: Flat, nonpalpable change in skin color, smaller than 1.0 cm (e.g., freckle, petechia)

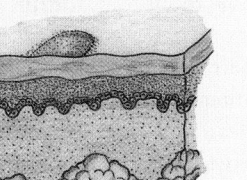

Tumor: Solid mass that extends deep through subcutaneous tissue, larger than 1.0 to 2.0 cm (e.g., epithelioma)

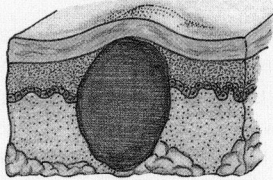

Pustule: Circumscribed elevation of skin similar to vesicle but filled with pus, varies in size (e.g., acne, staphylococcal infection)

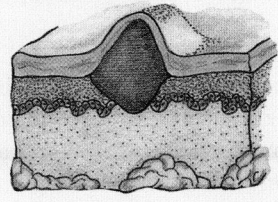

Papule: Palpable, circumscribed, solid elevation in skin, smaller than 0.5 cm (e.g., elevated nevus)

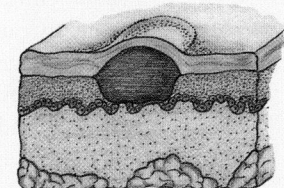

Wheal: Irregularly shaped, elevated area or superficial localized edema, varies in size (e.g., hive, mosquito bite)

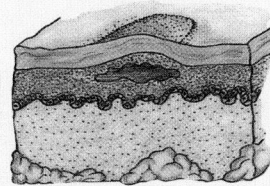

Ulcer: Deep loss of skin surface that sometimes extends to dermis and frequently bleeds and scars, varies in size (e.g., venous stasis ulcer)

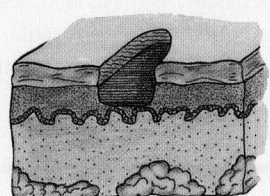

Nodule: Elevated solid mass, deeper and firmer than papule, 0.5 to 2.0 cm (e.g., wart)

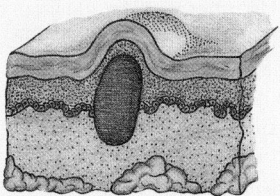

Vesicle: Circumscribed elevation of skin filled with serous fluid, smaller than 1.0 cm (e.g., herpes simplex, chickenpox)

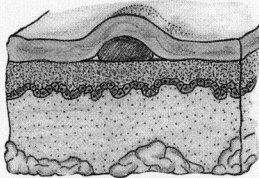

Atrophy: Thinning of skin with loss of normal skin furrow with skin appearing shiny and translucent, varies in size (e.g., arterial insufficiency)

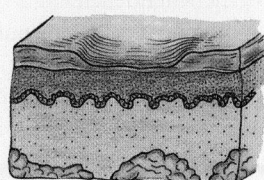

BOX 15-6 PATIENT TEACHING

Hair and Scalp Assessment

OUTCOME
- Patient will perform proper hygiene practices for care of the hair and scalp.

TEACHING STRATEGIES
- Instruct in basic hygiene practices for care of the hair and scalp (see Chapter 28).
- Instruct patients who have head lice to shampoo thoroughly with pediculicide (shampoo available at drug stores) in cold water, comb thoroughly with fine-tooth comb (following product directions), and discard comb. Caution against use of products containing lindane, a toxic ingredient known to cause adverse reactions. Repeat shampoo treatment 12 to 24 hours later.
- After combing, remove any detachable nits or nit cases with tweezers or between the fingernails. A dilute solution of vinegar and water helps loosen nits.
- Instruct patients and parents about ways to reduce transmission of lice:
  - Do not share personal care items with others.
  - Vacuum all rugs, car seats, pillows, furniture, and flooring thoroughly, and discard vacuum bag.
  - Seal nonwashable items in plastic bags for 14 days if parents are unable dry-clean or vacuum.
  - Use thorough hand-hygiene practices.
  - Launder all clothing, linen, and bedding in hot soap and water, and dry in a hot dryer for at least 20 minutes. Dry-clean nonwashable items.
  - Do not use insecticide.
- Instruct the patient to notify his or her partner if lice were sexually transmitted.
- Avoid physical contact with infested individuals and their belongings, especially clothing and bedding.
- Soak combs, brushes, and hair accessories in lice-killing products for 1 hour or in boiling water for 10 minutes.

EVALUATION STRATEGIES
- Have patient describe methods used to care for the hair and scalp.
- Have patient explain the steps to reduce lice transmission.

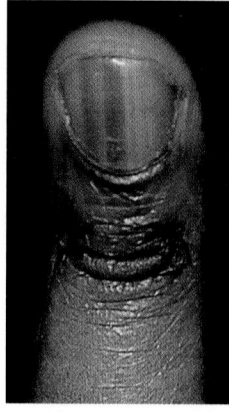

Figure 15-5 ■ Pigmented bands in nail of patient with dark skin. (From Seidel HM and others: *Mosby's guide to physical examination,* ed 6, St. Louis, 2006, Mosby.)

common over the lower extremities. In women, do not confuse a loss of hair with shaven legs.

Inspect the scalp for lesions, which are not easily noticed in thick hair. The scalp is normally smooth and inelastic, with even coloration. By carefully separating strands of hair, thoroughly examine the scalp for lesions. Note the characteristics of any scalp lesions. If you find lumps or bruises, ask if the patient has experienced recent head trauma. Moles on the scalp are common. Warn the patient that combing or brushing sometimes causes a mole to bleed. Dandruff or psoriasis frequently causes scaliness or dryness.

Careful inspection of hair follicles on the scalp and pubic areas may reveal lice or other parasites. There are head lice, body lice, and crab lice. Head and crab lice attach their eggs to hair. Lice eggs look like oval particles of dandruff. The lice themselves are difficult to see. Observe for bites or pustular eruptions in the follicles and in areas where skin surfaces meet, such as behind the ears and in the groin. The discovery of lice requires immediate treatment and family education (Box 15-6).

Nails

The condition of the nails reflects general health, state of nutrition, a person's occupation, and level of self-care. The most visible portion of the nails is the nail plate, the transparent layer of epithelial cells covering the nail bed. The vascularity of the nail bed creates the nail's underlying color. The semilunar, whitish area at the base of the nail bed is called the lunula, from which the nail plate develops.

NURSING HISTORY Ask the patient if there have been any recent changes in the nails (e.g., splitting, breaking, or thickening) or recent trauma. Determine the patient's nail care practices, such as acrylic nails. Determine if there are any risk factors for nail problems (e.g., diabetes mellitus, peripheral vascular disease, or older age).

Inspect the nail bed color, cleanliness, and length; the thickness and shape of the nail, the texture of the nail; the angle between the nail and the nail bed; and the condition of tissue around the nail. The nails are normally transparent, smooth, well rounded, and convex, with surrounding cuticles smooth, intact, and without inflammation. In whites, nail

Changes occur in the thickness, texture, and lubrication of scalp hair. Disturbances such as a febrile illness or scalp disease sometimes result in hair loss. Conditions such as thyroid disease alter the condition of the hair, making it fine and brittle. Hair loss (alopecia) or thinning of the hair is usually related to genetic tendencies and endocrine disorders such as diabetes and menopause. Poor nutrition causes stringy, dull, dry, and thin hair. The hair is lubricated from the oil of sebaceous glands. Excessively oily hair is associated with androgen hormone stimulation. Dry, brittle hair occurs with aging and excessive use of chemical agents.

The amount of hair covering the extremities is sometimes reduced as a result of aging. Arterial insufficiency is most

BOX 15-7   Abnormalities of the Nail Bed

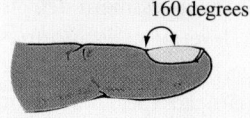

160 degrees **Normal nail:** Approximately 160-degree angle between nail plate and nail

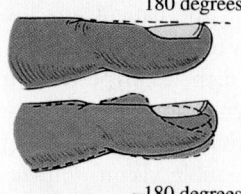

180 degrees

180 degrees

Clubbing: Change in angle between nail and nail base (eventually greater than 180 degrees); nail bed softening, with nail flattening; often, enlargement of fingertips
Causes: Chronic lack of oxygen: heart or pulmonary disease

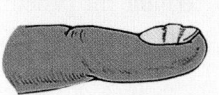

Beau's lines: Transverse depressions in nails indicating temporary disturbance of nail growth (nail grows out over several months)
Causes: Systemic illness such as severe infection; nail injury

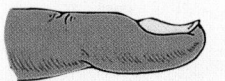

Koilonychia (spoon nail): Concave curves
Causes: Iron deficiency anemia, syphilis, use of strong detergents

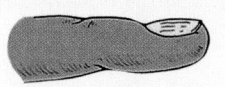

Splinter hemorrhages: Red or brown linear streaks in nail bed
Causes: Minor trauma, subacute bacterial endocarditis, trichinosis

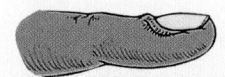

Paronychia: Inflammation of skin at base of nail
Causes: Local infection, trauma

BOX 15-8   PATIENT TEACHING

Nail Assessment

OUTCOME
- Patient properly cares for fingernails, feet, and toenails.

TEACHING STRATEGIES
- Instruct patient to cut nails only after soaking them about 10 minutes in warm water. (Exception: Patients with diabetes are warned against soaking nails because this dries the hands and feet; dry skin leads to infection.)
- Caution patient to avoid using over-the-counter preparations to treat corns, calluses, or ingrown toenails.
- Tell the patient to cut nails straight across and even with the tops of the fingers or toes. If the patient has diabetes, tell the patient to file rather than cut the nails (see Chapter 28).
- Instruct the patient to shape nails with a file or emery board.
- If patient has diabetes:
  - Wash feet daily in warm water, and carefully dry them, especially between the toes. Inspect feet each day in good lighting, looking for dry places and cracks in the skin. Soften dry feet by applying a cream or lotion such as Nivea, Eucerin, or Alpha Keri.
  - Do not put lotion between the toes; moisture between the toes promotes the growth of microorganisms, leading to infection.
  - Caution patient against using sharp objects to poke or dig under toenail or around the cuticle.
  - Have patient see a podiatrist for treatment of ingrown toenails and nails that are thick or tend to split.

EVALUATION STRATEGIES
- Inspect nails during next home visit.
- Have patient explain steps to avoid injury to the fingernails, feet, and toenails.

---

beds are pink and nails have translucent white tips. In dark-skinned patients, nail beds are darkly pigmented with a blue or reddish hue. A brown or black pigmentation is normal with longitudinal streaks (Figure 15-5). Trauma, cirrhosis, diabetes mellitus, and hypertension cause splinter hemorrhages. Vitamin, protein, and electrolyte changes cause various lines or bands to form on nail beds.

Nails normally grow at a constant rate, but direct injury or generalized disease impairs growth. With aging, the nails of the fingers and toes become harder and thicker. Longitudinal striations develop, and the rate of nail growth slows. Nails become more brittle, dull, and opaque and turn yellow in older adults because of insufficient calcium. Also with age, the cuticle becomes less thick and wide.

Inspection of the angle between the nail and nail bed normally reveals an angle of 160 degrees (Box 15-7). A larger angle and softening of the nail bed indicate chronic oxygenation problems. Palpate the nail base to determine firmness and condition of circulation. The nail base is normally firm.

To palpate, gently grasp the patient's finger and observe the color of the nail bed. Next, apply gentle, firm, quick pressure with the thumb to the nail bed and release and observe capillary refill. As you apply pressure, the nail bed appears white or blanched; however, the pink color should return immediately on release of pressure. You measure capillary pressure in seconds; less than 2 seconds is brisk, whereas greater than 4 seconds is sluggish. Failure of the pink color to return promptly indicates circulatory insufficiency. An ongoing bluish or purplish cast to the nail bed occurs with cyanosis. A white cast or pallor results from anemia.

Calluses and corns often occur on the toes or fingers. A callus is flat and painless, resulting from thickening of the epidermis. Friction and pressure from shoes causes corns, usually over bony prominences. During the examination instruct the patient in proper nail care (Box 15-8).

HEAD AND NECK

An examination of the head and neck includes assessment of the head, eyes, ears, nose, mouth, pharynx, and neck (lymph nodes, carotid arteries, thyroid gland, and trachea). During assessment of peripheral arteries also assess the carotid arteries. Assessment of the head and neck uses inspection, palpation, and auscultation.

Head

NURSING HISTORY Determine if the patient has a recent history of head trauma or neurological symptoms such as headache, dizziness, seizures, poor vision, or loss of consciousness. Review the patient's occupation, participation in contact sports, and use of protective head gear.

Inspect the patient's head, noting the position, size, shape, and contour. The head is normally held upright and midline to the trunk. Holding the head tilted to one side is an indication of unilateral hearing or visual loss. A horizontal jerking or bobbing indicates a tremor.

Note the patient's facial features, looking at the eyelids, eyebrows, nasolabial folds, and mouth for shape and symmetry. It is normal for slight asymmetry to exist. If there is facial asymmetry, note if all features on one side of the face are affected or if only a portion of the face is involved. Various neurological disorders such as a facial nerve paralysis affect different nerves that innervate muscles of the face.

Examine the size, shape, and contour of the skull. The skull is generally round with prominences in the frontal area anteriorly and the occipital area posteriorly. Trauma typically causes local skull deformities. In infants, a large head results from congenital anomalies or the accumulation of cerebrospinal fluid in the ventricles (hydrocephalus). Adults may have enlarged jaws and facial bones resulting from acromegaly. Palpate the skull for nodules or masses. Gently rotate the fingertips down the midline of the scalp and then along the sides of the head to identify abnormalities.

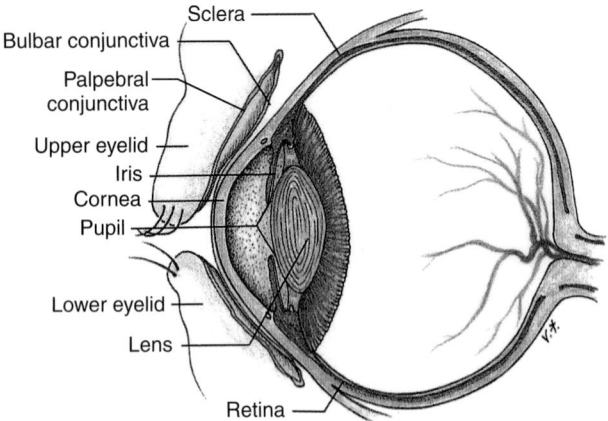

Figure 15-6 ■ Cross section of eye.

Labels: Sclera, Bulbar conjunctiva, Palpebral conjunctiva, Upper eyelid, Iris, Cornea, Pupil, Lower eyelid, Lens, Retina

Eyes

Examination of the eye includes assessment of visual acuity, visual fields, and external and internal eye structures. Figure 15-6 shows a cross section of the eye. The assessment detects visual alterations and determines the level of assistance patients require when ambulating or performing self-care activities. Patients with visual problems need special aids for reading educational materials or instructions.

NURSING HISTORY Review with the patient any history of partial or complete visual loss from eye disease (e.g., glaucoma or cataracts), eye trauma, diabetes, hypertension, or eye surgery. Assess for common symptoms of eye disease such as eye pain, photophobia (sensitivity to light), burning, itching, excessive tearing, diplopia (double vision), blurred vision, or visual disturbances (e.g., flashing lights, halos, or "film" over vision field). Review the patient's occupational history, use of glasses or contact lenses, use of safety glasses, and visits to optometrist (Box 15-9). Determine the patient's current medication use, including any eye medication.

BOX 15-9   PATIENT TEACHING

Eye Assessment

OUTCOMES
- Patient follows recommendations for regular eye examinations.
- Patient recognizes warning signs and symptoms of eye disease.
- Patient takes appropriate safety precautions to protect eyes and for visual deficits.

TEACHING STRATEGIES
- Tell patient that persons under age 40 need to have a complete eye examination every 3 to 5 years (or more often if family histories reveal risks such as diabetes or hypertension).
- Tell patients that persons over age 40 need to have a complete eye examination every 2 years to screen for conditions that may develop without patient awareness (e.g., glaucoma).
- Tell patients that persons over age 65 should have a yearly eye examination.
- Describe the typical symptoms of eye disease (see Chapter 37).
- Instruct older adults to take the following precautions because of normal visual changes: avoid or use caution while driving at night, increase lighting in the home to reduce risk for falls, and paint the first and last steps of a staircase and the edge of each step in between a bright color to aid in depth perception.

EVALUATION STRATEGIES
- Ask the patient and family member to report the most recent ophthalmologist visit.
- Have patient describe when to have eye examination.
- Ask patient to describe common symptoms of eye disease.
- Observe the home environment of a patient with visual deficits for safety hazards.

VISUAL ACUITY The assessment of visual acuity, the ability to see small details, tests central vision. The easiest way to assess visual acuity is to ask the patient to read printed material (Snellen chart) under adequate lighting. If patients use glasses or contact lenses, they should wear them during the assessment. Know the language the patient speaks and reading ability. Asking the patient to read aloud helps determine literacy. Position the patient 6 m (20 feet) away from the chart. Test each eye separately by covering one eye with a card or gauze square, careful to avoid pressure on the eye. A patient who has difficulty reading related to vision needs to consult an ophthalmologist or optometrist for further evaluation.

VISUAL FIELDS Objects in the periphery can normally be seen when a person looks straight ahead. To assess visual fields, have the patient stand or sit 60 cm (2 feet) away, facing you at eye level. The patient gently closes or covers one eye (e.g., the left) and looks at your eye directly opposite. Close the opposite eye so that the field of vision is superimposed on that of the patient. Move a finger equidistant at arm's length from you and the patient outside the field of vision, and then slowly bring it back into the visual field. Ask the patient to tell you when the finger is visible. If you see the finger before the patient does, this reveals that a portion of the patient's visual field is reduced.

EXTERNAL EYE STRUCTURES To inspect external eye structures, stand directly in front of the patient at eye level and ask the patient to look at your face.

Position and Alignment Assess the position of the eyes in relation to one another. Normally they are parallel to each other. Bulging eyes (exophthalmos) usually indicate hyperthyroidism. The crossing of eyes (strabismus) results from neuromuscular injury or inherited abnormalities. Tumors or inflammation of the orbit causes abnormal eye protrusion.

Eyebrows For the remainder of the examination the patient removes contact lenses. Inspect the eyebrows for size, extension, texture of hair, alignment, and movement. Coarseness of hair and failure to extend beyond the temporal canthus may reveal hypothyroidism. If the brows are thinned, this may indicate that the patient plucks or waxes the hair. Aging causes loss of the lateral third of the eyebrows. Have the patient raise and lower the eyebrows. The brows normally raise and lower symmetrically. An inability to move the eyebrows indicates a facial nerve paralysis (cranial nerve VII).

Eyelids Inspect the eyelids for position; color; condition and direction of lashes; and the patient's ability to open, close, and blink. When the eyes are open in a normal position, the lids do not cover the pupil, and you cannot see the sclera above the iris. The lids are also close to the eyeball. An abnormal drooping of the lid over the pupil is called ptosis, caused by edema or impairment of the third cranial nerve. In the older adult, ptosis results from a loss of elasticity that accompanies aging. Observe for defects in the position of the lid margins. An older adult frequently has lid margins that turn out (ectropion) or in (entropion). An entropion sometimes leads to the lashes of the lid irritating the conjunctiva and cornea, increasing risk for infection. The eyelashes are normally distributed evenly and curved outward away from the eye.

The lids normally close symmetrically. Failure of lids to close exposes the cornea to drying. This condition is common in unconscious patients or those with facial nerve paralysis. Ask the patient to open the eyes and observe the blink reflex. Normally a patient blinks involuntarily and bilaterally as many as 20 times a minute. The blink reflex lubricates the cornea. Report absent or infrequent, rapid, or monocular (one-eyed) blinking.

Lacrimal Apparatus The lacrimal gland (Figure 15-7), located in the upper, outer wall of the anterior part of the orbit, is responsible for tear production. Tears flow from the gland across the eye's surface to the lacrimal duct, which is in the nasal corner or inner canthus of the eye. Inspect the lacrimal gland for edema and redness. Palpate the gland area gently to detect tenderness. Normally the gland cannot be felt. The nasolacrimal duct may become obstructed, blocking the flow of tears. Observe for evidence of excess tearing or edema in the inner canthus. Gentle palpation of the duct at the lower eyelid just inside the orbital rim causes a regurgitation of tears.

Conjunctivae and Sclerae The bulbar conjunctiva covers the exposed surface of the eyeball up to the outer edge of the cornea. Observe the sclera under the bulbar conjunctiva; it normally has the color of white porcelain in whites and light yellow in dark-skinned patients. To view both structures, gently retract both lids simultaneously with thumb and index finger pressed against the lower and upper bony orbits. For adequate exposure retract the eyelids without placing pressure directly on the eyeball. Ask the patient to look up, down, and side to side. Inspect for color, texture, and the presence of edema or lesions.

Normally the conjunctivae are free of erythema. The presence of redness indicates allergic or infectious conjunctivitis. Conjunctivitis is a highly contagious infection, and the crusty drainage that collects on eyelid margins easily spreads from one eye to the other. Perform proper hand hygiene (see Chapter 13) before and after the examination. Wear clean gloves during the examination.

Corneas The cornea is the transparent, colorless portion of the eye covering the pupil and iris. From a side view, it looks like the crystal of a wristwatch. While the patient looks straight ahead, inspect the cornea for clarity and texture while shining

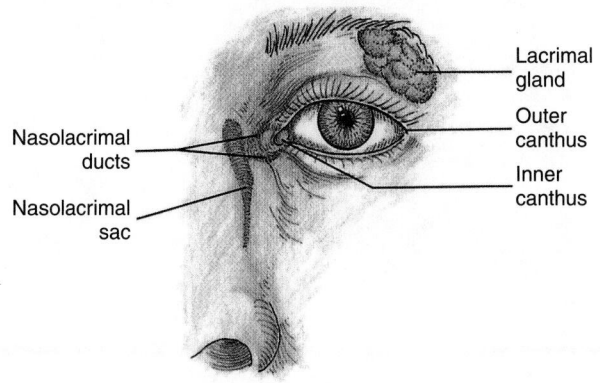

Figure 15-7 ■ Lacrimal apparatus.

a penlight obliquely across the cornea's surface. The cornea is normally shiny, transparent, and smooth. In older adults the cornea loses its luster. Any irregularity in the surface indicates an abrasion or tear that requires further examination by a health care provider. Both conditions are very painful. In an older adult the iris becomes faded. To test for the corneal blink reflex, see the cranial nerve function section of this chapter.

Pupils and Irises Observe the pupils for size, shape, equality, accommodation, and reaction to light. The pupils are normally black, round, regular, and equal in size (3 to 7 mm in diameter) (Figure 15-8). The iris should be clearly visible. Note the color and details of the iris.

Cloudy pupils indicate cataracts. Dilated pupils result from neurological disorders, glaucoma, trauma, eye medication, or withdrawal from opioids. Pinpoint pupils are a common sign of opioid intoxication. When shining a beam of light through the pupil and onto the retina, this stimulates the third cranial nerve and causes the muscles of the iris to constrict. Any abnormality along the nerve pathways from the retina to the iris alters the ability of the pupils to react to light. Changes in intracranial pressure, lesions along the nerve pathways, locally applied ophthalmic medications, and direct trauma to the eye alter pupillary reaction.

Test pupillary reflexes (to light and accommodation) in a dimly lit room. While the patient looks straight ahead, bring a penlight from the side of the patient's face, directing the light onto the pupil (Figure 15-9). If the patient looks at the light, there will be a false reaction to accommodation. A directly illuminated pupil constricts, and the opposite pupil constricts consensually. Observe the quickness and equality of the reflex. Repeat the examination for the opposite eye.

To test accommodation, ask the patient to gaze at a distant object (the far wall) and then at a test object (finger or pencil) held approximately 10 cm (4 inches) from the bridge of the

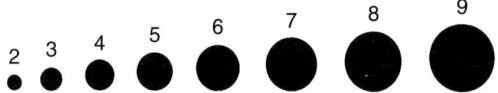

Figure 15-8 ■ Chart depicting pupillary size in millimeters.

patient's nose. The pupils normally converge and accommodate by constricting when looking at close objects. The pupil responses are equal. If assessment of pupillary reaction is normal in all tests, record the abbreviation PERRLA (pupils equal, round, reactive to light and accommodation).

INTERNAL EYE STRUCTURES An advanced nurse practitioner usually performs examination of the internal eye structures through the use of an ophthalmoscope. Patients in greatest need of the examination are those with diabetes, hypertension, and intracranial disorders.

Ears

The ear assessment determines the integrity of ear structures and hearing acuity. Inspect and palpate external ear structures, inspect middle ear structures with the otoscope, and test the inner ear by measuring the patient's hearing acuity. Assessment of patients with hearing impairment provides useful data in planning effective communication techniques.

NURSING HISTORY Review with the patient risk factors for hearing problems (e.g., intake of aspirin or noise exposure) and a history of ear trauma or surgery. Determine if the patient has ear pain, itching, discharge, tinnitus (ringing in ears), vertigo (loss of balance), or change in hearing. Note behavior that indicates a hearing loss, such as leaning forward to hear, inattentiveness to speech, and requests to repeat comments. Determine the onset and contributing factors to the hearing problem. Assess if the patient wears a hearing aid and how the patient normally cleans the ears.

AURICLES With the patient sitting, inspect the auricle's size, shape, symmetry, landmarks, position, and color. The auricles are normally of equal size and level with each other. The upper point of attachment to the head is normally in a straight line with the outer canthus, or corner of the eye. Ears that are low set or at an unusual angle are a sign of chromosome abnormality (e.g., Down syndrome). Ear color is the same as the face without moles, cysts, deformities, or nodules. Redness is a sign of inflammation or fever.

Palpate the auricles for texture, tenderness, swelling, and skin lesions. Auricles are normally smooth, firm, mobile, and without lesions. If the patient complains of pain, gently pull

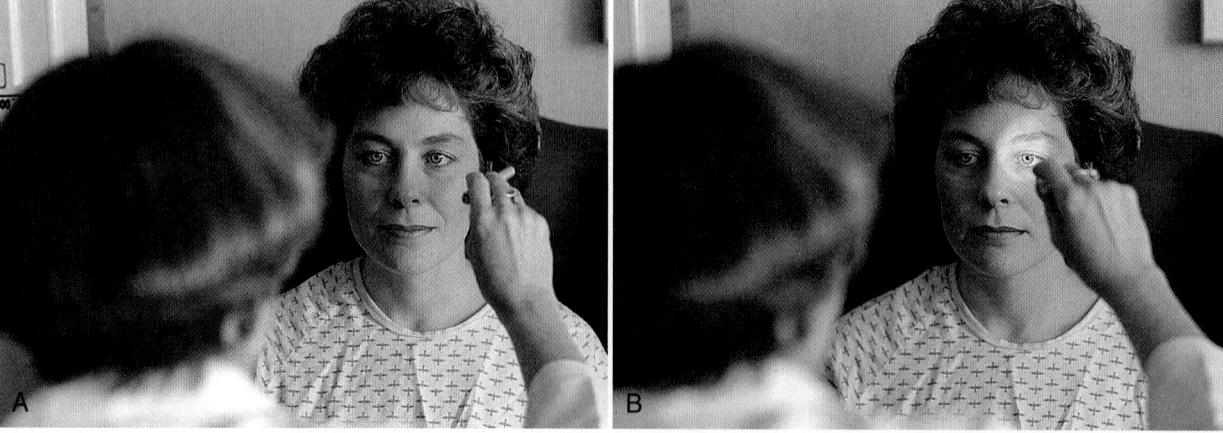

Figure 15-9 ■ **A,** To check pupillary reflexes, the nurse first holds the penlight to the side of patient's face. **B,** Illumination of pupil causes pupillary constriction.

the auricle and press on the tragus and palpate behind the ear over the mastoid process. If palpating the external ear increases the pain, an external ear infection is likely. If palpation of the auricle and tragus does not influence the pain, the patient may have a middle ear infection. Tenderness in the mastoid area indicates mastoiditis.

Inspect the opening of the ear canal for size and presence of discharge. If discharge is present, wear clean gloves during the examination. A swollen or occluded meatus is not normal. A yellow, waxy substance called **cerumen** is common. Yellow or green foul-smelling discharge indicates infection or a foreign body in the canal.

EAR CANALS AND EARDRUMS Observe the deeper structures of the external and middle ear with the use of an otoscope. A special ear speculum attaches to the handle of the ophthalmoscope. For best visualization select the largest speculum that fits comfortably in the patient's ear. Before inserting the speculum, check for foreign bodies in the opening of the auditory canal.

Make sure the patient avoids moving the head during the examination to avoid damage to the canal and tympanic membrane. Infants and young children often need to be restrained. Lie infants supine with their heads turned to one side and their arms held securely at their sides. Have young children sit on their parents' laps with their legs held between the parents' knees.

Turn on the otoscope by rotating the dial at the top of the handle. To insert the speculum properly, ask the patient to tip the head slightly to the opposite shoulder. Hold the handle of the otoscope in the space between the thumb and index finger, supported on the middle finger. This leaves the ulnar side of your hand to rest against the patient's head, stabilizing the otoscope as it is inserted into the canal (Seidel and others, 2006). Insert the scope while pulling the auricle upward and backward in the adult and older child (Figure 15-10). This maneuver straightens the ear canal. In children under 3 years of age, pull the auricle down and back.

Insert the speculum slightly down and forward, 1.0 to 1.5 cm (½ to ¾ inch) into the ear canal. Take care not to scrape the sensitive lining of the ear canal, which is painful. The ear canal normally has little cerumen and is uniformly pink with tiny hairs in the outer third of the canal. Observe for color, discharge, scaling, lesions, foreign bodies, and cerumen. Normally cerumen is dry (light brown to gray and flaky) or moist (dark yellow or brown) and sticky. Dry cerumen occurs in Asians and Native Americans about 85% of the time (Seidel and others, 2006). A reddened canal with discharge is a sign of inflammation or infection. In older adults, accumulated cerumen is a common problem. Buildup of cerumen creates a mild hearing loss. During the examination ask the patient how he or she normally cleans the ear canal (Box 15-10). Caution the patient on the danger of inserting pointed objects into the canal. Avoid the use of cotton-tipped applicators to clean the ears because this causes impaction of cerumen deep in the ear canal.

The light from the otoscope allows visualization of the eardrum (tympanic membrane). Know the common anatomical landmarks and their appearance (Figure 15-11).

Move the auricle to see the entire drum and its periphery. Because the eardrum is angled away from the ear canal, the light from the otoscope appears as a cone shape rather than a circle. The umbo is near the center of the drum, behind which is the attachment of the malleus. The underlying short

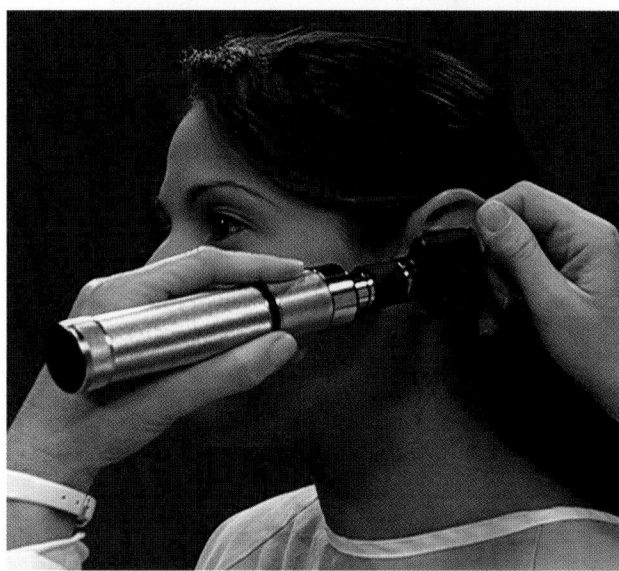

Figure 15-10 ■ Otoscopic examination. (From Seidel HM and others: *Mosby's guide to physical examination,* ed 6, St. Louis, 2006, Mosby.)

BOX 15-10   PATIENT TEACHING

Ear Assessment

OUTCOMES
- Patient uses proper technique for cleansing the ears.
- Patient follows preventive guidelines for screening of hearing loss.
- Patient with hearing loss communicates effectively.

TEACHING STRATEGIES
- Instruct the patient in the proper way to clean the outer ear (see Chapter 28), avoiding use of cotton-tipped applicators and sharp objects such as hairpins, which cause impaction of cerumen deep in ear canal or cause trauma.
- Tell the patient to avoid inserting pointed objects into the ear canal.
- Encourage patients over age 65 to have regular hearing checks. Explain that a reduction in hearing is a normal part of aging (see Chapter 37).
- Instruct family members of patients with hearing losses to avoid shouting and instead speak in low tones and to be sure the patient sees the speaker's face.

EVALUATION STRATEGIES
- Ask patient to explain the proper technique for cleansing the ears.
- In future visits, question patient about frequency of hearing checks.
- Observe patient with hearing loss interacting with family members.

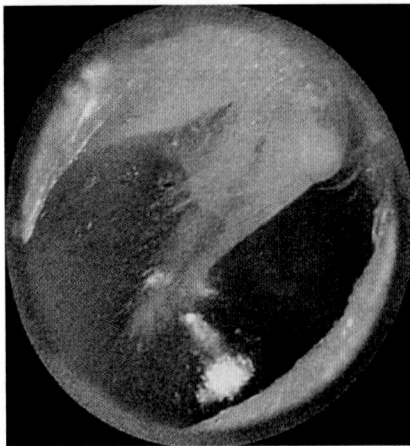

Figure 15-11 ■ Normal tympanic membrane. (Courtesy Dr. Richard A. Buckingham, Abraham Lincoln School of Medicine, University of Illinois, Chicago.)

process of the malleus creates a knoblike structure at the top of the drum. Check carefully to be sure there are no tears or breaks in the membrane of the eardrum. The normal eardrum is translucent, shiny, and pearly gray. It is free from tears or breaks. A pink or red bulging membrane indicates inflammation. A white color reveals pus behind it. The membrane is taut, except for the small triangular pars flaccida near the top. If cerumen is blocking the tympanic membrane, warm water irrigation will safely remove the wax.

HEARING ACUITY   The patient with a hearing loss often fails to respond to conversation. The three types of hearing loss are conduction, sensorineural, and mixed. A conduction loss interrupts sound waves as they travel from the outer ear to the cochlea of the inner ear because they are not transmitted through the outer and middle ear structures. A sensorineural loss involves the inner ear, auditory nerve, or hearing center of the brain. You conduct sound through the outer and middle ear structures, but the continued transmission of sound becomes interrupted at some point beyond the bony ossicles. A mixed loss involves a combination of conduction and sensorineural loss.

Patients working or living around loud noises are at risk for hearing loss. Adolescents are at risk for premature hearing loss from continued exposure to loud music from concerts or use of iPods and MP3 players. Older adults experience an inability to hear high-frequency sounds and consonants (e.g., *s, z, t,* and *g*). Deterioration of the cochlea and thickening of the tympanic membrane cause older adults to gradually lose hearing acuity. They are especially at risk for hearing loss caused by ototoxicity resulting from high maintenance doses of antibiotics (e.g., aminoglycosides).

To conduct a hearing assessment, have the patient remove any hearing aid if worn. Note the patient's response to questions. Normally the patient responds without excess requests to have the questions repeated. If you suspect a hearing loss, check the patient's response to the whispered voice. Test one ear at a time while the patient occludes the other ear with a finger. Ask the patient to gently move the finger up and down during the test. While standing 30 cm to 60 cm (1 to 2 feet)

BOX 15-11   PATIENT TEACHING

Nose and Sinus Assessment

OUTCOMES
- Patient will safely use over-the-counter nasal sprays.
- Parents will take proper measures to stop a child's nosebleed.
- Older adult will take safety precautions with loss of olfaction.

TEACHING STRATEGIES
- Caution patients against overuse of over-the-counter nasal sprays, which can lead to "rebound" effect, causing excess nasal congestion.
- Instruct parents in care of children with nosebleeds: have child sit up and lean forward to avoid aspiration of blood; apply pressure to anterior nose with thumb and forefinger as child breathes through mouth; and apply ice or a cold cloth to bridge of nose if pressure fails to stop bleeding.
- Instruct older adults to install smoke detectors on each floor of their home.
- Instruct older adults to always check dated labels on food to ensure against spoilage.

EVALUATION STRATEGIES
- Have patient explain proper use of over-the-counter nasal sprays.
- Have parents demonstrate and describe technique for stopping a nosebleed.
- Inspect patient's home during visit, and look for smoke detectors. Ask to check food items in the refrigerator.

---

from the testing ear, cover your mouth so the patient is unable to read lips. After exhaling fully, whisper softly toward the unoccluded ear, reciting random numbers with equally accented syllables such as *nine-four-ten*. If necessary, gradually increase voice intensity until the patient correctly repeats the numbers. Then test the other ear for comparison. Seidel and others (2006) report that patients normally hear numbers clearly when whispered, responding correctly 50% of the time. If a hearing loss is present, there are tests that experienced practitioners perform using a tuning fork or audiometry.

Nose and Sinuses

Assess the integrity of the nose and sinuses by inspection and palpation. The patient sits during the examination. A penlight allows for gross examination of each naris. A more detailed examination requires using a nasal speculum to inspect deeper nasal turbinates. Do not use a speculum unless a qualified practitioner is present.

NURSING HISTORY   Determine if the patient has a history of exposure to dust or pollutants, allergies, nasal obstruction, recent trauma, discharge, frequent infections, headaches, or postnasal drip. Assess for any history of nosebleed (epistaxis) or use of nasal sprays, including frequency and duration (Box 15-11). Ask if there are any breathing difficulties or snoring.

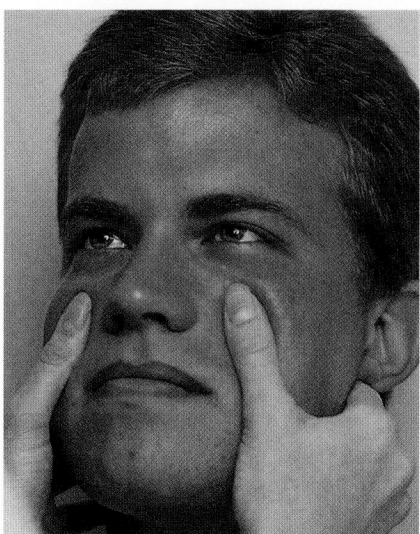

Figure 15-12 ■ Palpation of maxillary sinuses.

NOSE When inspecting the external nose, observe the shape, size, skin color, and presence of deformity or inflammation. The nose is normally smooth and symmetrical, with the same color as the face. Recent trauma causes edema and discoloration. If swelling or deformities exist, gently palpate the ridge and soft tissue of the nose by placing one finger on each side of the nasal arch and gently moving fingers from the nasal bridge to the tip. Note any tenderness, masses, and underlying deviations. Nasal structures are usually firm and stable.

When a person breathes, air normally passes freely through the nose. To assess patency of the nares, place a finger on the side of the patient's nose and occlude one naris. Ask the patient to breathe with the mouth closed. Repeat the procedure for the other naris.

While illuminating the anterior nares, inspect the mucosa for color, lesions, discharge, swelling, and evidence of bleeding. If discharge is present, apply clean gloves. Normal mucosa is pink and moist without lesions. Pale mucosa with clear discharge indicates allergy. A mucoid discharge indicates rhinitis. A sinus infection results in yellowish or greenish discharge. Habitual use of intranasal cocaine and opioids causes puffiness and increased vascularity of the nasal mucosa. For the patient with a nasogastric tube, check for local skin breakdown (excoriation) of the naris, characterized by redness and skin sloughing.

To view the septum and turbinates, have the patient tip the head back slightly to provide a clear view. Illuminate the septum and look for alignment, perforation, or bleeding. Normally the septum is close to the midline, and thicker anteriorly than posteriorly. Normal mucosa is pink and moist, without lesions. A deviated septum obstructs breathing and interferes with passage of an enteral nasal tube. Perforation of the septum often occurs after repeated use of intranasal cocaine. Note any polyps (tumorlike growths) or purulent drainage.

SINUSES Examination of the sinuses involves palpation. In cases of allergies or infection, the interior of the sinuses becomes inflamed and swollen. The most effective way to assess for tenderness is by externally palpating the frontal and maxillary facial areas (Figure 15-12). Palpate the frontal sinus by exerting pressure with the thumb up and under the patient's eyebrow. Gentle, upward pressure easily elicits tenderness if sinus irritation is present. Do not apply pressure to the eyes. If tenderness of sinuses is present, transilluminate the sinuses. This procedure requires advanced experience.

Mouth and Pharynx

Assess the mouth and pharynx to detect signs of overall health, determine oral hygiene needs, and develop therapies for patients with dehydration, restricted intake, oral trauma, or oral airway obstruction. To assess the oral cavity use a penlight and tongue depressor or single gauze square. Wear clean gloves during the examination. Have the patient sit or lie during the examination. Assess the oral cavity while administering oral hygiene.

NURSING HISTORY Determine if the patient wears dentures or retainers and if they fit comfortably. Assess for any recent changes in appetite or weight, which indicate problems with chewing and swallowing. Assess the patient's dental hygiene practices. To identify cancer risks, determine if the patient smokes, chews tobacco, or consumes alcohol. Identify if the patient still has his or her tonsils and adenoids.

LIPS Inspect the lips for color, texture, hydration, contour, and lesions. With the patient's mouth closed, view the lips from end to end. Normally they are pink, moist, symmetrical, smooth, and without lesions. Lip color in the dark-skinned patient varies from pink to plum. Have female patients remove their lipstick before the examination. Anemia causes pallor of the lips, with cyanosis caused by respiratory or cardiovascular problems. Any lesions such as nodules or ulcerations can be related to infection, irritation, or skin cancer.

BUCCAL MUCOSA, GUMS, AND TEETH Ask the patient to clench the teeth and smile to observe teeth occlusion. The upper molars normally rest directly on the lower molars, and the upper incisors slightly override the lower incisors. A symmetrical smile reveals normal facial nerve function.

Inspect the teeth to determine the quality of a patient's dental hygiene (Box 15-12). Note the position and alignment of the teeth. To examine the posterior surface of the teeth, have the patient open the mouth with lips relaxed. Use a tongue depressor to retract the lips and cheeks, especially when viewing the molars. Note the color of teeth and the presence of dental caries, tartar, and extraction sites. Normal healthy teeth are smooth, white, and shiny. A chalky white discoloration of the enamel is an early indication of caries formation. Brown or black discolorations indicate the formation of caries. An older adult's teeth often feel rough when tooth enamel calcifies and there may be loose or missing teeth because of increased bone resorption. Yellow and darkened teeth are also common in the older adult because of general wear and tear that exposes the darker, underlying dentin.

To view the inner oral mucosa, ask the patient to remove any dental appliance. View the inner oral mucosa by having the patient open the mouth slightly, and gently pull the lower lip away from the teeth (Figure 15-13, *A*). Repeat this process for the upper lip. Inspect the mucosa for color, hydration, texture, and lesions such as ulcers, abrasions, or cysts. Normally the mucosa is a glistening pink, smooth, and moist. Palpate any lesions with a gloved hand for tenderness, size, and consistency.

BOX 15-12   PATIENT TEACHING

Mouth and Pharyngeal Assessment

OUTCOMES
- Patient will practice proper oral hygiene measures and dental care.
- Patient will describe warning signs of oral cancer.
- Older adult will maintain normal intake of solid food.

TEACHING STRATEGIES
- Discuss proper techniques for oral hygiene, including brushing and flossing (see Chapter 28).
- Explain the early warning signs of oral cavity and pharynx cancer, including a sore that bleeds easily and does not heel, a lump or thickening, and red or white patch on the mucosa that persists. Difficulty chewing, swallowing, and moving the tongue or jaw are late symptoms (ACS, 2009a).
- Encourage regular dental examinations every 6 months for children, adults, and older adults.
- Identify older patients who have difficulty in chewing and changes in the teeth. Teach patients to eat soft foods, cut food into small pieces, and eat more frequent, smaller meals.

EVALUATION STRATEGIES
- Ask the patient to demonstrate brushing.
- Have patient identify when to have regular dental checkups.
- Have patient identify the warning signs of oral cavity and pharynx cancer.
- Ask the older adult to keep a diet record for 3 days.

To inspect the buccal mucosa, ask the patient to open the mouth and then gently retract the cheeks with a tongue depressor or gloved finger covered with gauze (Figure 15-13, *B*). View the surface of the mucosa from right to left and top to bottom. A penlight illuminates the most posterior portion of the mucosa. For patients with normal pigmentation, the buccal mucosa is a good site to inspect for jaundice and pallor. In older adults, the mucosa is normally dry because of reduced salivation. Thick white patches (leukoplakia) are often a precancerous lesion seen in heavy smokers and alcoholics. Palpate for any buccal lesions by placing the gloved index finger within the buccal cavity and the thumb on the outer surface of the cheek.

Examine the gums (gingivae) for color, edema, retraction, bleeding, and lesions while retracting the cheeks. Healthy gums are pink, moist, smooth, and tightly fit around each tooth. Dark-skinned patients often have patchy pigmentation. In older adults the gums are usually pale. Using clean gloves, palpate the gums to assess for lesions, thickening, or masses. Normally there is no tenderness. Spongy gums that bleed easily indicate periodontal disease or vitamin C deficiency.

TONGUE AND FLOOR OF MOUTH Carefully inspect the tongue on all sides, as well as the floor of the mouth. Have the patient relax the mouth and stick the tongue out halfway. If the patient protrudes the tongue too far, this will elicit the gag reflex. Using the penlight, examine the tongue for color, size, position, texture, movement, and coating or lesions. A normal tongue appears medium or dull red in color, moist, slightly rough on the top surface, and smooth along the lateral margins. When the tongue protrudes, it remains at midline. To test the tongue for mobility, ask the patient to raise the tongue and move it from side to side. The tongue should move freely.

The undersurface of the tongue and floor of the mouth are highly vascular. Take extra care to inspect this area, a common site of origin for oral cancer lesions. The patient lifts the tongue by placing its tip on the palate behind the upper incisors. Inspect for color, swelling, and lesions such as cysts. The ventral surface of the tongue is pink and smooth, with large veins between the frenulum folds.

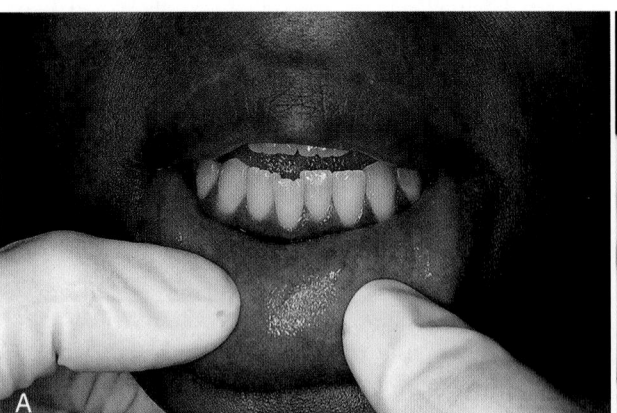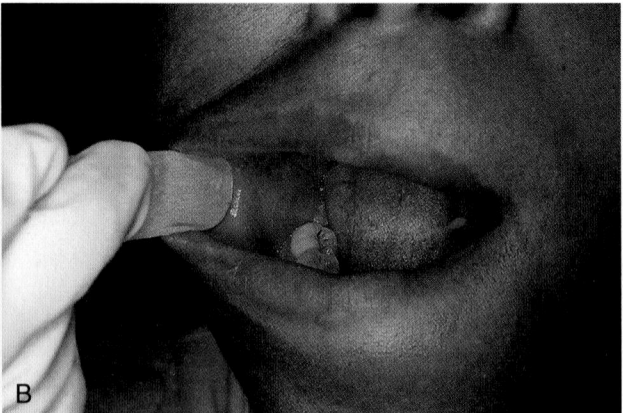

Figure 15-13 ■ **A,** Inspection of inner oral mucosa of lower lip. **B,** Retraction of the buccal mucosa allows for clear visualization.

PALATE Have the patient extend the head backward, holding the mouth open to allow you to inspect the hard and soft palates. The hard palate, or roof of the mouth, is located anteriorly. The whitish hard palate is dome shaped. The soft palate extends posteriorly toward the pharynx. It is normally light pink and smooth. Observe the palates for color, shape, texture, and extra bony prominences or defects.

PHARYNX Perform an examination of the pharyngeal structures to rule out infection, inflammation, or lesions. Have the patient tip the head back slightly, open the mouth wide, and say "Ah" while you place the tip of a tongue depressor on the middle third of the tongue. Take care not to press the lower lip against the teeth (Figure 15-14). By placing the tongue depressor too far anteriorly, the posterior part of the tongue mounds up, obstructing the view. Placing the tongue depressor on the posterior tongue elicits the gag reflex.

With a penlight, first inspect the uvula and soft palate. Both structures, which are innervated by the tenth cranial nerve (vagus), rise centrally as the patient says "Ah." Examine the anterior and posterior tonsillar pillars, and note the presence or absence of tonsillar tissue. The posterior pharynx is behind the pillars. Normally, pharyngeal structures are smooth, pink, and well hydrated. Small irregular spots of lymphatic tissue and small blood vessels are normal. Note edema, petechiae, lesions, or exudate. Patients with chronic sinus problems frequently exhibit a clear exudate that drains along the wall of the posterior pharynx. Yellow or green exudate indicates infection. A patient with a typical sore throat has a reddened and edematous uvula and tonsillar pillars with possible presence of yellow exudate.

Neck

Assessment of the neck includes assessing the neck muscles, lymph nodes of the head and neck, carotid arteries, jugular veins, thyroid gland, and trachea (Figure 15-15). Postpone the examination of the carotid arteries and jugular veins until the vascular system assessment. Inspect and palpate the neck to determine the integrity of neck structures and to examine the lymphatic system. An abnormality of superficial lymph nodes sometimes reveals the presence of infection or malignancy. Examination of the thyroid gland and trachea also aids in ruling out malignancies. Perform this examination with the patient sitting.

NURSING HISTORY Determine if the patient has had a recent cold or infection or enlarged lymph notes, exposure to radiation or toxic chemicals. If there are enlarged lymph nodes, consider reviewing history of intravenous drug use, hemophilia, and risk factors for human immune deficiency virus (HIV) infection. Ask if the patient has a history of hypothyroidism or hyperthyroidism, takes thyroid medication, or has a family history of thyroid disease. Ask the patient to describe any head or neck injury or pain of head and neck structures.

NECK MUSCLES First inspect the gross neck structures with the neck in the usual anatomical position. Observe for symmetry of neck muscles. Ask the patient to flex the neck with the chin to the chest, hyperextend the neck backward, and move the head laterally to each side and then sideways with the ear moving toward the shoulder. This tests the sternocleidomastoid and trapezius muscles. The neck normally moves freely without discomfort.

LYMPH NODES An extensive system of lymph nodes collects lymph from the head, ears, nose, cheeks, and lips (Figure 15-16). With the patient's chin raised and head tilted slightly back, first inspect the area where lymph nodes are distributed and compare both sides. This position stretches the skin slightly over any possible enlarged nodes. Inspect visible nodes for edema, erythema, or red streaks. Nodes are not normally visible.

Use a methodical approach to palpate the lymph nodes to avoid overlooking any single node or chain. The patient relaxes with the neck flexed slightly forward. Inspect and palpate both sides of the neck for comparison. During palpation either face or stand to the side of the patient for easy access to all nodes. Using the pads of the middle three fingers of each hand, gently palpate in a rotary motion over the nodes. Check each node methodically in the following sequence: occipital

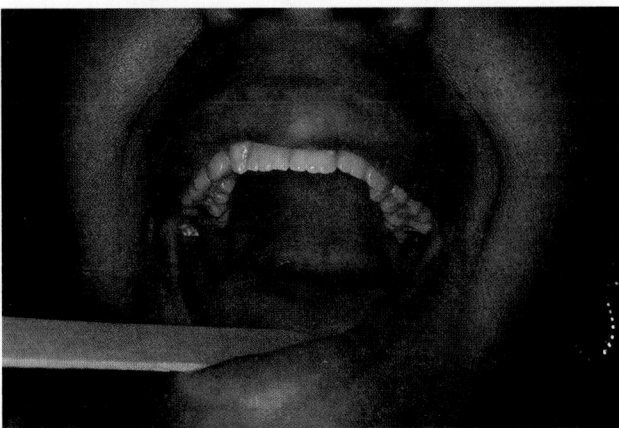

Figure 15-14 ■ A penlight and tongue depressor allow the visualization of the uvula and posterior soft palate.

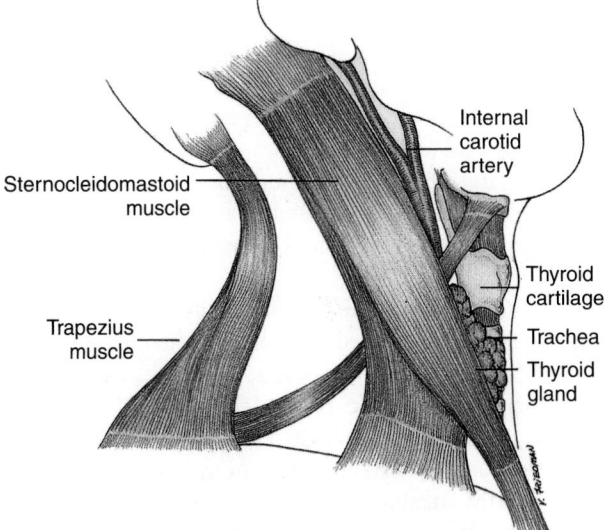

Figure 15-15 ■ Anatomical position of major neck structures. Note the triangles formed by the muscles.

Sternocleidomastoid muscle

Trapezius muscle

Internal carotid artery

Thyroid cartilage

Trachea

Thyroid gland

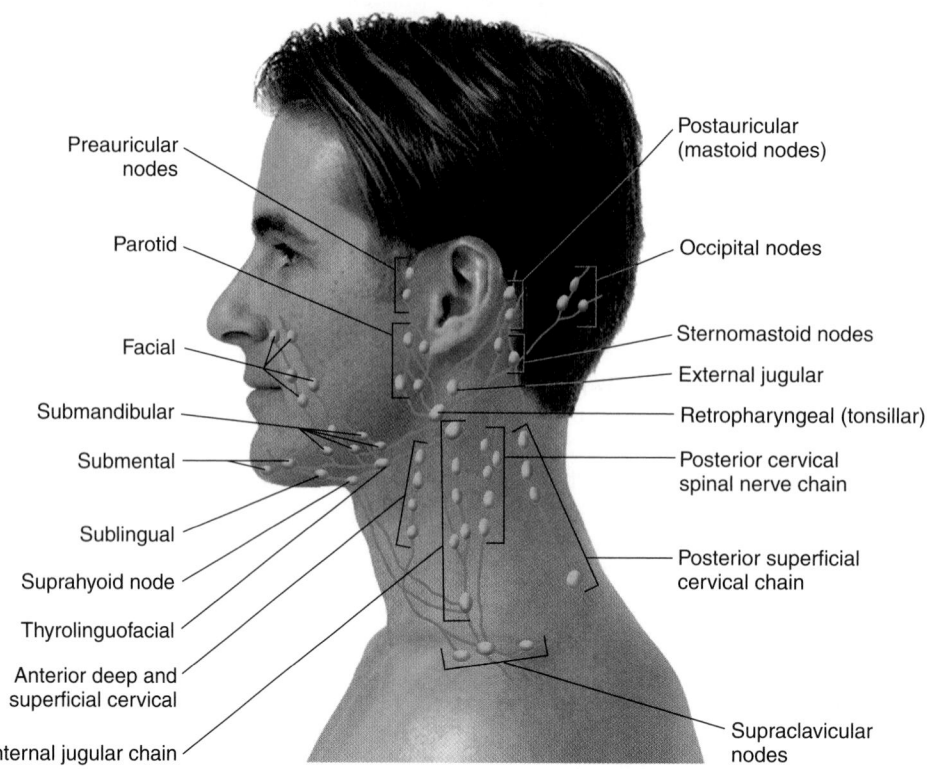

Figure 15-16 ■ Palpable lymph nodes in the head and neck. (From Seidel HM and others: *Mosby's guide to physical examination,* ed 6, St. Louis, 2006, Mosby.)

nodes at the base of the skull, postauricular nodes over the mastoid, preauricular nodes just in front of the ear, retropharyngeal nodes at the angle of the mandible, submandibular nodes, and submental nodes in the midline behind the mandibular tip. Try to detect enlargement, and note the location, size, shape, surface characteristics, consistency, mobility, tenderness, and warmth of the nodes. If the skin is mobile, move the skin over the area of the nodes (Figure 15-17) (Seidel and others, 2006). It is important to press underlying tissue in each area and not simply move the fingers over the skin. However, if you apply excessive pressure, you will miss small nodes and make it difficult to palpate the lymph nodes.

To palpate supraclavicular nodes ask the patient to bend the head forward and relax the shoulders. Palpate these nodes by hooking the index and third finger over the clavicle, lateral to the sternocleidomastoid muscle. Palpate the deep cervical nodes only with the fingers hooked around the sternocleidomastoid muscle.

Normally lymph nodes are not easily palpable. Lymph nodes that are large, fixed, inflamed, or tender indicate a problem such as local infection, systemic disease, or neoplasm (Seidel and others, 2006). Tenderness almost always indicates inflammation (Box 15-13). A problem involving a lymph node of the head and neck means an abnormality in the mouth, throat, abdomen, breasts, thorax, or arms. These are the areas drained by the head and neck nodes.

THYROID GLAND The thyroid gland lies in the anterior lower neck, in front of and to both sides of the trachea. The

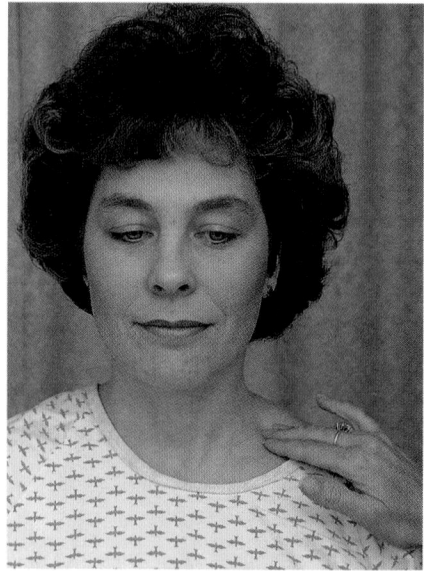

Figure 15-17 ■ Lymph node palpation.

gland is fixed to the trachea with the isthmus overlying the trachea and connecting the two irregular, cone-shaped lobes (Figure 15-18). Inspect the lower neck overlying the thyroid gland for obvious masses, symmetry, and any subtle fullness at the base of the neck. Offer the patient a glass of water, and, while observing the neck, have the patient swallow. This maneuver helps to visualize an abnormally enlarged thyroid

BOX 15-13   PATIENT TEACHING

Neck Assessment

OUTCOME
- Patient takes proper preventive action if a mass is noticed in the neck.

TEACHING STRATEGIES
- Stress the importance of regular compliance with medication schedule to patients with thyroid disease.
- Instruct patients about the lymph nodes and how infection commonly causes node tenderness.
- Instruct patients to call a health care provider when they notice a lump or mass in the neck.

EVALUATION STRATEGIES
- Have patient explain when to notify health care provider about a neck mass.

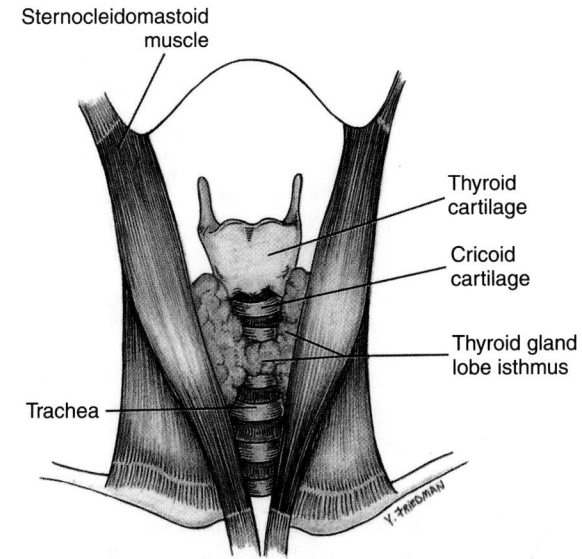

Figure 15-18 ▪ Anatomical position of the thyroid gland.

gland. More experienced nurses examine the thyroid by palpating for more subtle masses.

CAROTID ARTERY AND JUGULAR VEIN Examination of these vessels is discussed under examination of the vascular system.

TRACHEA The trachea is a part of the upper respiratory system that requires direct palpation. It is normally located in the midline above the suprasternal notch. Masses in the neck or mediastinum and pulmonary abnormalities cause lateral displacement. Have the patient sit or lie down during palpation. Determine the position of the trachea by palpating at the suprasternal notch, slipping the thumb and index fingers to each side. Note if your finger and thumb shift laterally. Do not apply forceful pressure to the trachea because this elicits coughing.

THORAX AND LUNGS

Physical assessment of the thorax and lungs requires an in-depth review of the ventilatory and respiratory functions of the lungs. If disease is affecting the lungs, it will affect other body systems as well. For example, reduced oxygenation causes changes in mental alertness because of the brain's sensitivity to lowered oxygen levels. You will use data from all body systems to determine the nature of pulmonary alterations.

Before assessing the thorax and lungs, be familiar with the landmarks of the chest (Figure 15-19). These landmarks help you locate findings and use assessment skills correctly. The patient's nipples, angle of Louis, suprasternal notch, costal angle, clavicles, and vertebrae are key landmarks that provide a series of imaginary lines for sign and symptom identification. Keep a mental image of the location of the lobes of the lung and the position of each rib (Figure 15-20). The proper orientation to anatomical structures ensures a thorough assessment of the anterior, lateral, and posterior thorax.

Locating the position of each rib is critical to visualizing the lobe of the lung being assessed. To begin, locate the angle of Louis, at the junction between the manubrium and the body of the sternum. Knowing that the second rib extends from the angle makes it easy to locate and palpate the **intercostal spaces** (between the ribs) in succession. The spinous process of the third thoracic vertebra and the fourth, fifth, and sixth ribs serve to locate the lobes of the lung laterally (Figure 15-21). The lower lobes project laterally and anteriorly.

Posteriorly the tip or inferior margin of the scapula lies approximately at the level of the seventh rib. Identify the seventh rib, count upward to locate the third thoracic vertebra, and align it with the inner borders of the scapula to locate the posterior lobes (Figure 15-22).

Examination of the lungs and thorax is most effective when the patient is undressed to the waist. Begin with the patient sitting for assessment of the posterior and lateral chest and sitting or lying down for examination of the anterior chest. A female patient may keep a gown draped loosely over her chest while you examine the posterior chest.

Nursing History

Assess for a history of tobacco or marijuana use, including type of tobacco, duration and amount (pack-years = number of years smoking × number of packs per day), age started, and efforts to quit and length of time since smoking stopped. Ask the patient about *persistent cough* (productive or nonproductive), *blood-streaked sputum*, *voice change*, *chest pain*, shortness of breath, **orthopnea** (must be in upright position to breathe), **dyspnea** (breathlessness) during exertion or at rest, poor activity tolerance, or *recurrent pneumonia or bronchitis*. This reveals cardiopulmonary problems and warning signs for lung cancer (symptoms in italics). Cigarette smoking accounts for 87% of all lung cancer deaths in the United States (National Cancer Institute, 2009). Determine if your

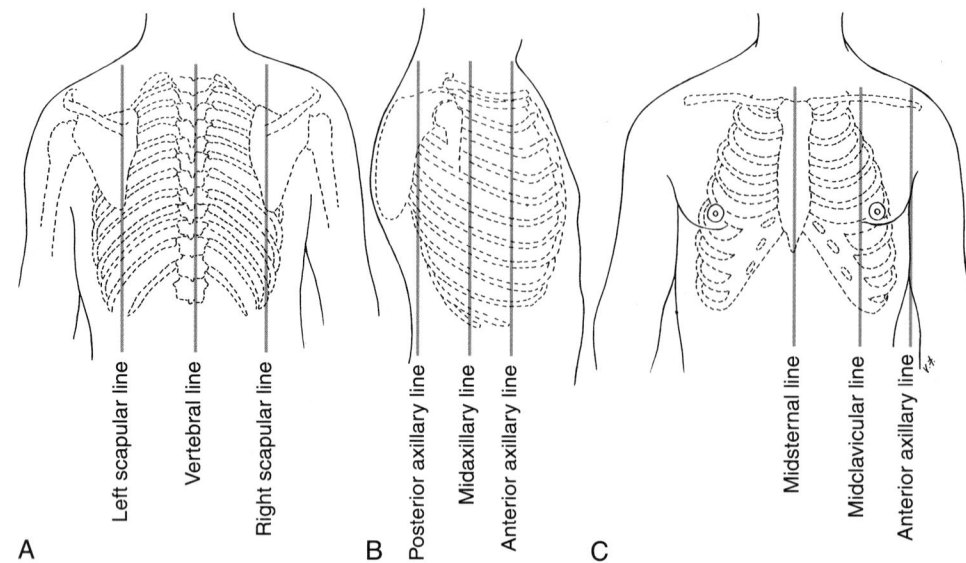

Figure 15-19 ■ Anatomical chest wall landmarks. **A,** Posterior chest. **B,** Lateral chest. **C,** Anterior chest.

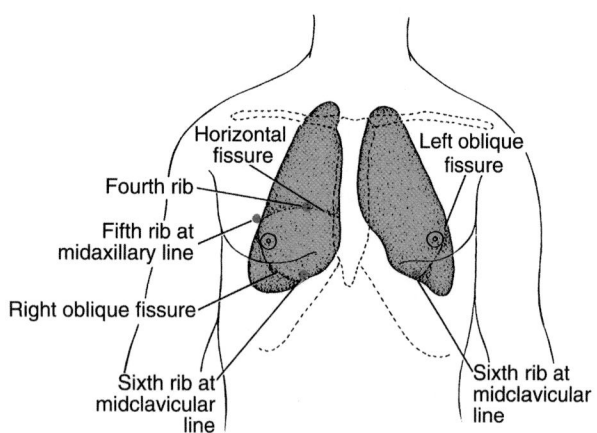

Figure 15-20 ■ Anterior position of lung lobes in relation to anatomical landmarks.

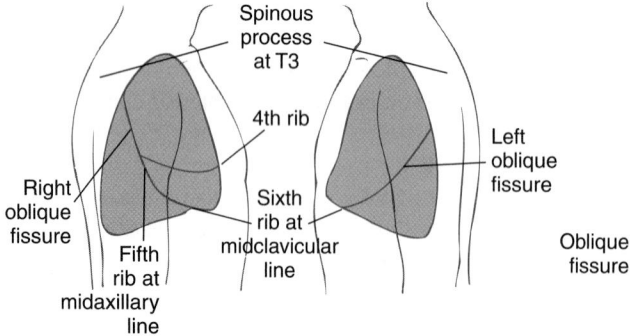

Figure 15-21 ■ Lateral position of lung lobes in relation to anatomical landmarks. T_3 Third thoracic vertebra.

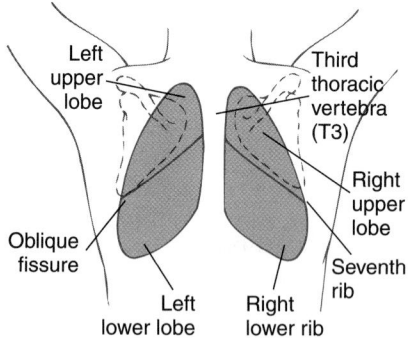

Figure 15-22 ■ Posterior position of lung lobes in relation to anatomical landmarks.

sweats, and fever. Assess history of allergies to airborne irritants, foods, drugs, or chemical substances. Ask if the patient has had pneumonia or influenza vaccine and a TB test. Review the patient's family history for cancer, tuberculosis, allergies, or chronic obstructive pulmonary disease.

Posterior Thorax

Begin examination of the posterior thorax by observing for any signs or symptoms in other body systems that indicate pulmonary problems. Reduced mental alertness, nasal flaring, somnolence (sleepiness), and cyanosis are examples of symptoms or findings that indicate oxygenation problems. Inspect the posterior thorax by observing the shape and symmetry of the chest from the patient's back and front. Note the anteroposterior diameter. Body shape or posture significantly impairs ventilatory movement. Normally the chest contour is symmetrical, with the anteroposterior diameter one third to one half the size of the transverse or side-to-side diameter. A barrel-shaped chest (anteroposterior diameter equals transverse) characterizes aging and chronic lung disease. Infants have an almost round shape. Congenital and postural altera-

patient works in an environment containing pollutants (e.g., asbestos or coal dust) or exposure to radiation.

Review risk factors for tuberculosis (TB) and/or HIV infection and assess for symptoms, including persistent cough, hemoptysis, unexplained weight loss, fatigue, anorexia, night

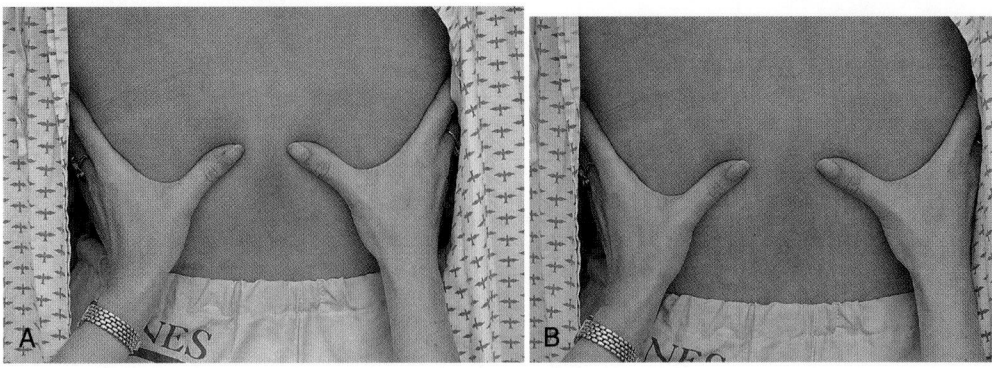

Figure 15-23 ■ **A,** Hand position for palpation of posterior thorax excursion. **B,** As the patient inhales, movement of chest (excursion) separates the thumbs.

tions cause abnormal contours. Some patients may lean over a table or splint the side of the chest because of a breathing problem. Splinting or holding the chest wall because of pain causes a patient to bend toward the affected side, which impairs ventilatory movement.

Standing at a midline position behind the patient, look for deformities, position of the spine, slope of the ribs, retraction of the intercostal spaces during inspiration, and bulging of the intercostal spaces during expiration. The scapulae are normally symmetrical and closely attached to the thoracic wall. The normal spine is straight without lateral deviation. Posteriorly, the ribs tend to slope across and down. The ribs and intercostal spaces are easier to see in a thin person. Normally no bulging or active movement occurs within the intercostal spaces during breathing. Bulging or retraction indicates that the patient is using great effort to breathe.

Also assess the rate and rhythm of breathing at this time (see Chapter 14). Observe the thorax as a whole. The thorax normally expands and relaxes with equality (symmetry) of movement bilaterally. In healthy adults the normal respiratory rate varies from 12 to 20 respirations per minute.

Palpate the posterior thorax beginning with the thoracic muscles and skeleton for lumps, masses, pulsations, and unusual movement. Avoid deep palpation if you note pain or tenderness. Fractured rib fragments could be displaced against vital organs. Normally the chest wall is not tender. If you find a suspicious mass or swollen area, lightly palpate it for size, shape, and typical qualities of a lesion.

To measure chest excursion or depth of breathing, stand behind the patient and place the thumbs along the spinal processes at the tenth rib, with the palms lightly contacting the posterior lateral surfaces. Place thumbs about 5 cm (2 inches) apart, pointing toward the spine and fingers pointing laterally (Figure 15-23, *A*). Press the hands toward the spine so that a small skin fold appears between the thumbs. Do not slide the hands over the skin. Instruct the patient to take a deep breath after exhaling. Note movement of the thumbs (Figure 15-23, *B*). Chest excursion should be symmetrical, separating the thumbs 3 to 5 cm (1¼ to 2 inches). Reduced chest excursion is caused by pain, postural deformity, or fatigue. In older adults, chest excursion normally declines because of costal cartilage calcification and respiratory muscle atrophy.

Auscultation assesses the movement of air through the tracheobronchial tree and detects mucus or obstructed airways. Normally air flows through the airways in an unobstructed pattern. Recognizing the sounds created by normal air flow allows for detection of sounds caused by airway obstruction.

Place the diaphragm of the stethoscope firmly on the skin, over the posterior chest wall between the ribs. The patient folds the arms in front of the chest and keeps the head bent forward while taking slow, deep breaths with the mouth slightly open. Listen to an entire inspiration and expiration at each position of the stethoscope (Figure 15-24, *A*). If sounds are faint, as in an obese patient, ask the patient to breathe harder and faster temporarily. Breath sounds are much louder in children because of their thin chest walls. In children the bell works best because of their small chest. Use a systematic pattern comparing the sounds in one region on one side of the body with sounds in the same region on the opposite side.

Auscultate for normal breath sounds and abnormal or **adventitious sounds.** Normal breath sounds differ in character, depending on the area you auscultate. Bronchovesicular and vesicular sounds are normally heard over the posterior thorax. Bronchovesicular sounds are medium-pitched blowing sounds normally heard between the scapulae. The sounds have equal inspiratory and expiratory phases. The character of bronchovesicular sounds is created by air moving through large airways. Vesicular sounds are normally heard over the periphery of the lungs. Air moving through the smaller airways creates these sounds. Vesicular sounds are soft, breezy, and low pitched, and the inspiratory phase is about three times longer than the expiratory phase.

Abnormal sounds result from air passing through moisture, mucus, or narrowed airways. They also result from alveoli suddenly reinflating or from an inflammation between the pleural linings of the lung. Adventitious sounds often occur superimposed over normal sounds. The four types of adventitious sounds are **crackles,** rhonchi, wheezes, and pleural friction rub. Each sound has its own cause and is characterized by typical auditory features (Table 15-6). Dur-

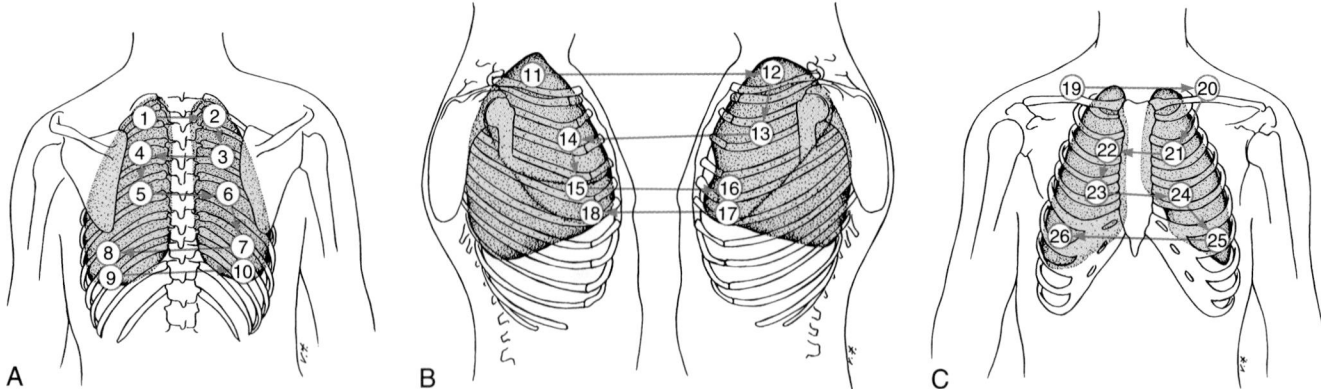

Figure 15-24 ■ **A** to **C,** A systematic pattern (posterior-lateral-anterior) is followed for palpating and auscultating the thorax.

TABLE 15-6   Adventitious Breath Sounds

SOUND	SITE AUSCULTATED	CAUSE	CHARACTER
Crackles	Most common in dependent lobes: right and left lung bases	Random, sudden reinflation of groups of alveoli; disruptive passage of air through small airways	Fine crackles are high-pitched fine, short, interrupted crackling sounds heard during end of inspiration, usually not cleared with coughing Moist crackles are lower, more moist sounds heard during middle of inspiration; not cleared with coughing Coarse crackles are loud, bubbly sounds heard during inspiration; not cleared with coughing
Rhonchi (sonorous wheeze)	Primarily heard over trachea and bronchi; if loud enough, can be heard over most lung fields	Muscular spasm, fluid, or mucus in larger airways, new growth or external pressure causing turbulence	Loud, low-pitched, rumbling coarse sounds heard either during inspiration or expiration; may be cleared by coughing
Wheezes (sibilant wheeze)	Heard over all lung fields	High-velocity airflow through severely narrowed or obstructed airway	High-pitched, continuous musical sounds like a squeak heard continuously during inspiration or expiration; usually louder on expiration
Pleural friction rub	Heard over anterior lateral lung field (if patient is sitting upright)	Inflamed pleura, parietal pleura rubbing against visceral pleura	Has dry, grating quality heard during inspiration; does not clear with coughing; heard loudest over lower lateral anterior surface

Data from Seidel HM and others: *Mosby's guide to physical examination,* ed 6, St. Louis, 2006, Mosby.

ing auscultation note the location and characteristics of the sounds, and listen for the absence of breath sounds (found in patients with collapsed or surgically removed lobes).

Lateral Thorax

Extend the assessment of the posterior thorax to the lateral sides of the chest (Figure 15-24, *B*). The patient sits during examination of the lateral chest. Have the patient raise the arms, to improve access to lateral thoracic structures. Use inspection, pal-

---

BOX 15-14 PATIENT TEACHING

Lung Assessment

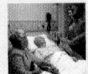

OUTCOMES
- Mr. Neal describes warning signs of lung disease.
- Mr. Neal and his wife receive annual influenza and pneumonia vaccines.
- Patient with chronic obstructive pulmonary disease (COPD) clears airways more effectively and reports shortness of breath.

TEACHING STRATEGIES
- Explain to Mr. Neal the risk factors for chronic lung disease and lung cancer, including cigarette smoking, history of smoking for over 20 years, exposure to environmental pollution, and radiation exposure from occupational, medical, and environmental sources. Exposure to residential radon and asbestos also increases risk, especially for cigarette smokers. Other risk factors include certain metals (arsenic, cadmium), some organic chemicals, and tuberculosis. Exposure to second-hand cigarette smoke increases risk for nonsmokers (ACS, 2009a).
- Share brochures on lung cancer from the American Cancer Society with Mr. Neal and family. Mr. Neal could benefit from this information before discharge from the hospital (see Case Study).
- Discuss with Mr. Neal the warning signs of lung cancer, such as a persistent cough, blood-streaked sputum, chest pains, and recurrent attacks of pneumonia or bronchitis.
- Counsel Mr. Neal and his wife on benefits of receiving influenza and pneumonia vaccinations as appropriate because of a greater susceptibility to respiratory infection.
- Instruct patients with COPD in coughing and pursed-lip–breathing exercises (see Chapter 29).
- Refer persons at risk for tuberculosis who visit clinics or health care centers for skin testing.

EVALUATION STRATEGIES
- Have Mr. Neal describe risk factors for lung disease and cancer.
- Ask Mr. Neal to identify any known risks for cancer.
- Ask Mr. Neal to list warning signs for cancer.
- In future visits, review Mr. Neal's immunization record.
- Observe Mr. Neal performing breathing and coughing exercises.

---

pation, and auscultation skills to examine the lateral thorax. Normally the breath sounds you hear are vesicular.

Anterior Thorax

Inspect the anterior thorax for the same features as the posterior thorax. The patient sits or lies down with the head elevated. Observe the accessory muscles of breathing: sternocleidomastoid, trapezius, and abdominal muscles. The accessory muscles move minimally with normal passive breathing. The accessory muscles and abdominal muscles contract when a patient requires effort to breathe as a result of strenuous exercise or disease (Box 15-14). Some patients produce a grunting sound.

Observe the width of the costal angle. It is usually larger than 90 degrees between the two costal margins. Observe the breathing pattern. Assess respiratory rate and rhythm anteriorly (see Chapter 14). The male patient's respirations are usually diaphragmatic, whereas the female's are more costal.

Palpate the anterior thoracic muscles and skeleton for lumps, masses, tenderness, or unusual movement. The sternum and xiphoid are relatively inflexible. To measure chest excursion anteriorly, place the thumbs parallel along the costal margin 6 cm (2½ inches) apart with the palms touching the anterolateral chest. Push the thumbs toward the midline to create a skin fold. As the patient inhales deeply, the thumbs normally separate approximately 3 to 5 cm (1¼ to 2 inches), with each side expanding equally. Chest excursion can be measured posteriorly from the lower lung border if breast tissue or a patient's large abdomen make anterior measurement difficult.

Auscultation of the anterior thorax follows a systematic pattern (Figure 15-24, *C*). Have the patient sit, if possible, to maximize chest expansion. Pay special attention to the lower lobes, where mucous secretions commonly gather. Listen for bronchovesicular and vesicular sounds above and below the clavicles and along the lung periphery. Auscultate for bronchial sounds, which are loud, high pitched, and hollow sounding, with expiration lasting longer than inspiration (3:2 ratio). You normally hear this sound over the trachea.

HEART

Compare your assessment of heart function with findings from the vascular assessment. Alterations in either system sometimes manifest as changes in the other. Some patients with signs and symptoms of heart (cardiac) problems have a life-threatening condition requiring immediate attention. In this case, act quickly and conduct only the portions of the examination that are absolutely necessary. When a patient is more stable, conduct a more thorough assessment.

Assess cardiac function through the anterior thorax. Form a mental image of the heart's exact location (Figure 15-25). In the adult the heart is located in the center of the chest (precordium) behind and to the left of the sternum, with a small section of the right atrium extending to the right of the sternum. The base of the heart is the upper portion, and the apex is the bottom tip. The surface of the right ventricle consti-

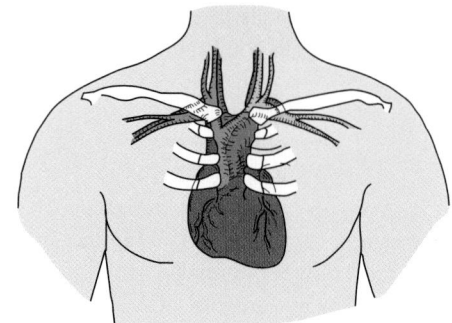

Figure 15-25 ■ Anatomical position of the heart.

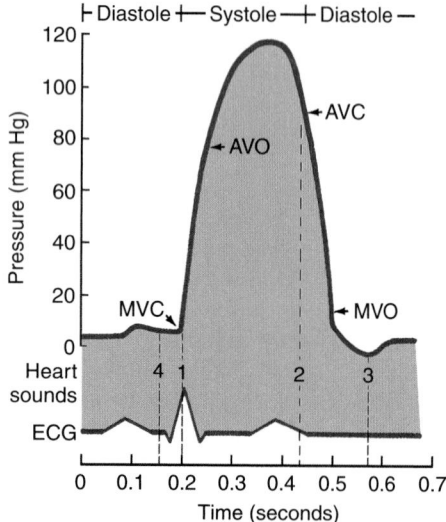

Figure 15-26 ■ Cardiac cycle. *MVC,* Mitral valve closes; *AVO,* aortic valve opens; *AVC,* aortic valve closes, *ECG,* electrocardiogram; *MVO,* mitral valve opens.

tutes most of the heart's anterior surface. A section of the left ventricle shapes the left anterior side of the apex. The point of maximal impulse (PMI) is palpable at the fifth intercostal space at the left midclavicular line in adults and children older than 7 years of age. In children younger than age 7 the PMI is at the fourth intercostal space at the left midclavicular line (Hockenberry and Wilson, 2007).

To assess heart function, you need to understand the cardiac cycle and associated physiological events (Figure 15-26). The heart normally pumps blood through its four chambers in a methodical, even sequence. Events on the left side occur just before those on the right. As the blood flows through each chamber, valves open and close, pressures within chambers rise and fall, and chambers contract. Each event creates a physiological sign. Both sides of the heart function in a coordinated fashion.

There are two phases to the cardiac cycle: systole and diastole. During systole the ventricles contract and eject blood from the left ventricle into the aorta and from the right ventricle into the pulmonary artery. During diastole the ventricles relax and the atria contract to move blood into the ventricles and fill the coronary arteries.

Heart sounds occur in relation to physiological events in the cardiac cycle. As systole begins, ventricular pressure rises and closes the mitral and tricuspid valves. Valve closure causes the first heart sound (S_1), often described as "lub." The ventricles then contract, and blood flows through the aorta and pulmonary circulation. After the ventricles empty, ventricular pressure falls below that in the aorta and pulmonary artery. This allows the aortic and pulmonic valves to close, causing the second heart sound (S_2), described as "dub." As ventricular pressure continues to fall, it drops below that of the atria. The mitral and tricuspid valves reopen to allow ventricular filling. Rapid ventricular filling may create a third heart sound (S_3), heard more often in children and young adults. An S_3 is an abnormal finding in adults over 30 years of age. A fourth heart sound (S_4) occurs when the atria contract to enhance ventricular filling. An S_4 may be heard in healthy older adults, children, and athletes, but it is not normal in adults. An S_4 needs to be reported to a health care provider.

Nursing History

The nursing history focuses on risk factors for cardiovascular disease (Box 15-15). Determine the patient's history of smoking, alcohol intake, caffeine intake, use of prescriptive and recreational drugs, exercise habits, and dietary patterns including fat and sodium intake. Determine if the patient is taking medications for cardiovascular function (e.g., antidysrhythmics or antihypertensives) and if the patient knows their purpose, dosage, and side effects. Assess for chest pain or discomfort, palpitations, excess fatigue, cough, dyspnea, edema of the feet, cyanosis, fainting, or orthopnea. These are key symptoms of heart disease. If the patient reports chest pain, determine if it is cardiac in nature; anginal pain is usually a deep pressure or ache that is substernal and diffuse, radiating to one or both arms, the neck, or the jaw. Determine if the patient has a stressful lifestyle. Assess for personal or family history of heart disease, diabetes, high cholesterol, hypertension, stroke, or rheumatic heart disease.

Inspection and Palpation

Ensure that the patient is comfortable and not anxious. Anxiety and discomfort may cause tachycardia, which will produce inaccurate findings. Use the skills of inspection and palpation simultaneously. The examination begins with the patient supine and the upper body elevated 45 degrees, because patients with heart disease frequently suffer shortness of breath while lying flat. Stand at the patient's right side. Do not let the patient talk, especially when auscultating heart sounds. Good lighting in the room is essential.

Direct your attention to the anatomical sites best suited for assessment of cardiac function. Inspect the angle of Louis; feel the ridge in the sternum approximately 5 cm (2 inches) below the sternal notch. Slip the fingers along the angle on each side of the sternum to feel the adjacent ribs. The intercostal spaces are just below each rib. The second intercostal space allows for identification of each of the six anatomical landmarks (Figure 15-27). The second intercostal space on the right is the aortic area, and the left second intercostal

BOX 15-15   PATIENT TEACHING

Heart Assessment

OUTCOMES
- Mr. Neal will describe risk factors for heart disease and take appropriate steps to reduce lifestyle risks.
- Mr. Neal will seek caregiver support with decreasing his risk for heart disease.

TEACHING STRATEGIES
- Explain to Mr. Neal the risk factors for heart disease, including high dietary intake of saturated fat or cholesterol, lack of regular aerobic exercise, smoking, excess weight, stressful lifestyle, hypertension, and family history of heart disease.
- Refer Mr. Neal to appropriate available resources for controlling or reducing risks (e.g., nutritional counseling, exercise class, stress-reduction programs).
- Explain to Mr. Neal that research shows clinical benefit from reducing dietary intake of cholesterol and saturated fats. Tell Mr. Neal that about 70% to 75% of saturated fatty acids come from meats, poultry, fish, and dairy products. The American Heart Association recommends a diet that includes an intake of total fat less than 35% of calories, saturated fatty acids less than 10% of calories, and cholesterol level less than 200 mg/dL (Moore, 2009).
- Encourage Mr. Neal to have regular measurement of total blood cholesterol levels and triglycerides. Desirable

levels are less than 200 mg/dL. You need more than one cholesterol measurement to assess the blood cholesterol level accurately. Low-density lipoprotein (LDL) cholesterol is the major component of atherosclerotic plaques. Separate measurement of LDL cholesterol is wise in a patient with high total blood cholesterol levels. An LDL cholesterol level of 160 mg/dL or higher is high risk (Moore, 2009).
- Encourage Mr. Neal to discuss with his health care provider the need for periodic C-reactive protein (CRP) testing. CRP levels assess a patient's cardiovascular disease risk.
- Advise Mr. Neal to avoid second-hand cigarette smoke because nicotine causes vasoconstriction.
- Advise Mr. Neal to quit smoking because this lowers the risk for coronary heart disease and coronary vascular disease (ACS, 2009a).
- Have Mr. Neal consult with his health care provider regarding the benefit of taking a daily low dose of aspirin.

EVALUATION STRATEGIES
- Ask Mr. Neal to identify risk factors for heart disease.
- Have Mr. Neal develop a meal plan low in saturated fat and cholesterol.
- Check Mr. Neal's cholesterol level during follow-up appointments.

---

space is the pulmonic area. You will need deeper palpation to feel the spaces in obese or heavily muscled patients. After locating the pulmonic area, move the fingers down the patient's left sternal border to the third intercostal space, called the second pulmonic area. The tricuspid area is located at the fourth or fifth intercostal space along the sternum. To find the apical area or mitral area, locate the fifth intercostal space just to the left of the sternum and move the fingers laterally, to the left midclavicular line. Locate the apical area with the palm of the hand or the fingertips. Normally you feel the apical impulse as a light tap in an area 1 to 2 cm (½ to ¾ inch) in diameter at the apex. Another landmark is the epigastric area at the tip of the sternum. You typically use it to palpate for aortic abnormalities.

Locate the six anatomical landmarks of the heart; inspect and palpate each area. Look for the appearance of pulsations, viewing each area over the chest at an angle to the side. Normally you will not see pulsations, except perhaps at the PMI in thin patients or at the epigastric area as a result of abdominal aortic pulsation. Use the proximal halves of the four fingers together, and then alternate with the ball of the hand to palpate for pulsations. Touch the areas gently to allow movements to lift the hand. Normally you will not feel any pulsations or vibrations in the second, third, or fourth intercostal spaces. Loud murmurs cause a vibration. Time palpated pulsations or vibrations and their occurrence in relation to systole or diastole by auscultating heart sounds simultaneously.

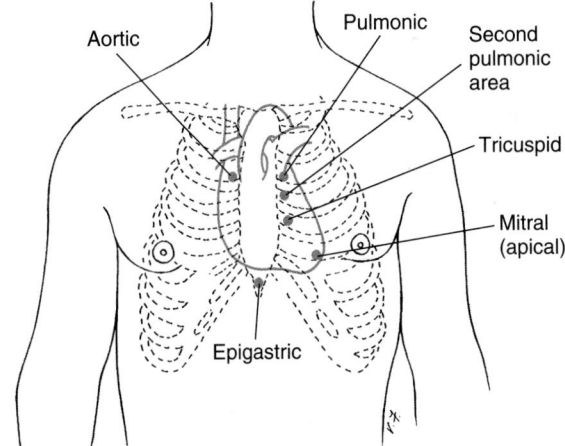

Figure 15-27 ■ Anatomical sites for assessment of cardiac function.

You should feel the apical impulse or PMI easily. If not, have the patient turn onto the left side, moving the heart closer to the chest wall. Estimate the size of the heart by noting the diameter of the PMI and its position relative to the midclavicular line. In cases of serious heart disease, the cardiac muscle enlarges, with the PMI found to the left of the midclavicular line. The PMI is sometimes difficult to find in older adults because the chest deepens in its anteroposterior diameter. It is also difficult to find in muscular or overweight patients. You usually find an infant's PMI at the third or fourth intercostal space. It is easy to palpate because of the child's thin chest wall.

Auscultation

Auscultation of the heart detects normal heart sounds, extra heart sounds, and murmurs. Concentrate on detecting low-intensity sounds caused by valve closure. To begin auscultation, eliminate all sources of room noise and explain the procedure to reduce the patient's anxiety. Follow a systematic pattern beginning at the aortic area and inching the stethoscope across each of the anatomical sites. Listen for the complete cycle ("lub-dub") of heart sounds clearly at each location. If you suspect a problem, repeat the sequence using the bell of the stethoscope. Sometimes the patient will assume three different positions during the examination (Figure 15-28):

- Sitting up and leaning forward (good for all areas and to hear high-pitched murmurs)
- Supine (good for all areas)
- Left lateral recumbent (good for all areas; best position to hear low-pitched sounds in diastole)

Learn to identify the first (S_1) and second (S_2) heart sounds. At normal rates, S_1 occurs after the long diastolic pause and preceding the short systolic pause. S_1 is high-pitched, dull in quality, and heard best at the apex. If it is difficult to hear S_1, time it in relation to the carotid pulse. S_2 follows the short systolic pause and precedes the long diastolic pause; you hear it best at the aortic area.

Auscultate for rate and rhythm after hearing both sounds clearly. Each combination of S_1 and S_2 or "lub-dub" counts as one heartbeat. Count the rate for 1 minute, and listen for the interval between S_1 and S_2, and then the time between S_2 and the next S_1. A regular rhythm involves regular intervals of time between each sequence of beats. There is a distinct silent pause between S_1 and S_2. Failure of the heart to beat at regular successive intervals is a dysrhythmia. Some dysrhythmias are life threatening.

When assessing an irregular heart rhythm, compare apical and radial pulse rates simultaneously to determine if a pulse deficit exists. Auscultate the apical pulse first, and then immediately assess the radial pulse (one-examiner technique). Assess the apical and radial rates at the same time when two examiners are present. When a patient has a pulse deficit, the radial pulse is slower than the apical because ineffective contractions fail to send pulse waves to the periphery. Report a difference in pulse rates to the health care provider immediately.

Assess extra heart sounds and murmurs at each auscultatory site. Use the bell of the stethoscope, and listen for low-pitched extra heart sounds such as S_3 and S_4 gallops, clicks, and rubs. Presence of extra heart sounds or murmurs sometimes indicates a pathological condition, so such sounds should be reported to the health care provider immediately. Typically, advanced practice nurses perform this portion of the examination.

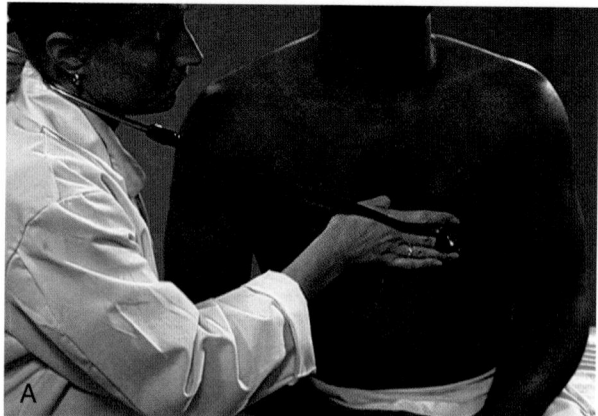

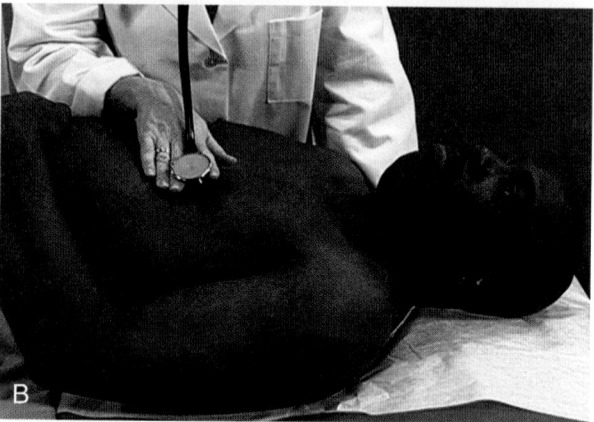

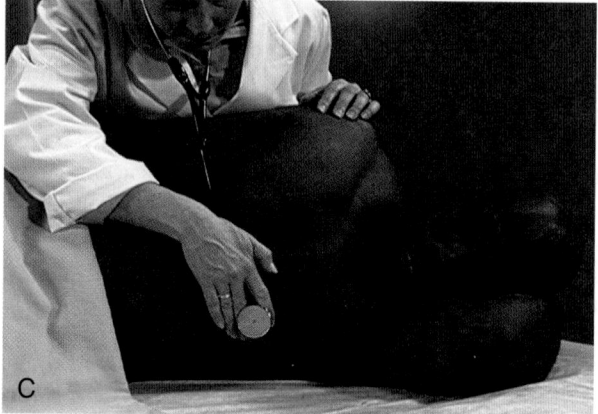

Figure 15-28 ■ Sequence of patient positions for heart auscultation. **A,** Sitting. **B,** Supine. **C,** Left lateral recumbent. (From Seidel HM and others: *Mosby's guide to physical examination,* ed 6, St. Louis, 2006, Mosby.)

VASCULAR SYSTEM

Examination of the vascular system includes measuring the blood pressure (see Chapter 14) and assessing the integrity of the peripheral vascular system. Use the skills of inspection, palpation, and auscultation. Perform portions of the vascular examination during other body system assessments. For example, check the carotid pulse after palpating the cervical lymph nodes.

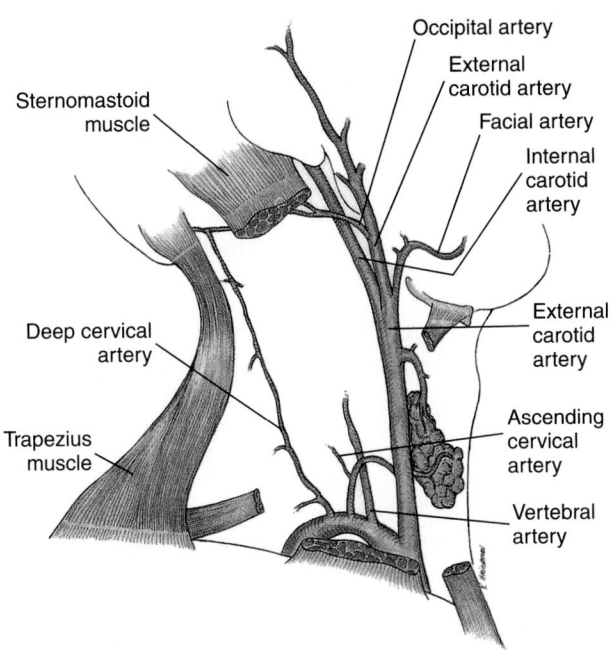

Figure 15-29 ■ Anatomical position of carotid artery.

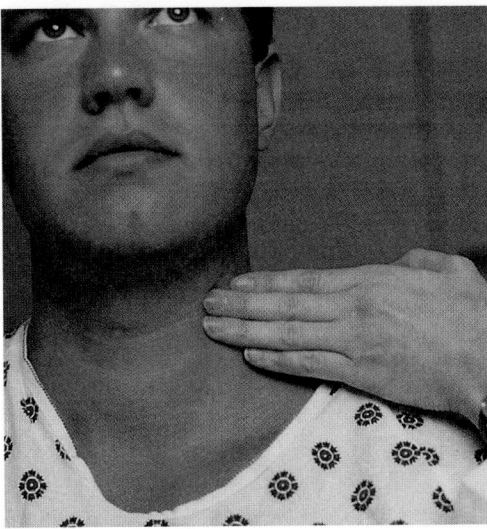

Figure 15-30 ■ Palpation of the internal carotid artery along the margin of the sternocleidomastoid muscle.

Health History

Determine if the patient has leg cramps, numbness or tingling in the extremities, sensation of cold hands or feet, pain in the legs, or swelling or cyanosis of the feet, ankles, or hands. These signs and symptoms may indicate vascular disease. If the patient has leg pain or cramping in the lower extremities, ask if walking or standing for long periods or during sleep aggravates or relieves the symptoms. This question helps to clarify if the problem is musculoskeletal or vascular. Ask patients if they wear tight-fitting garters or hosiery and sit or lie in bed with their legs crossed. These activities impair venous return. Consider previous cardiac risk factors that may predispose to vascular disease (e.g., smoking or nutritional problems). Assess the patient's medical history for heart disease, hypertension, phlebitis, diabetes, or varicose veins.

Carotid Arteries

When the left ventricle pumps blood into the aorta, the arterial system transmits pressure waves. The carotid artery reflects heart function better than peripheral arteries, because their pressure correlates with that of the aorta. The carotid artery supplies oxygenated blood to the head and neck (Figure 15-29). The overlying sternocleidomastoid muscle protects it.

To examine the carotid arteries, have the patient sit or lie supine with the head of the bed elevated 30 degrees. Examine one carotid artery at a time. If both arteries are simultaneously occluded during palpation, the patient will lose consciousness as a result of inadequate circulation to the brain. Do not palpate or massage the carotid arteries vigorously because the carotid sinus is in the upper third of the neck. The sinus sends impulses along the vagus nerve. Its stimulation causes a reflex drop in heart rate and blood pressure,

which causes syncope (light-headedness) or circulatory arrest. This is a particular problem for older adults.

Begin inspection of the neck for obvious pulsation of the artery. Have the patient turn the head slightly away from the artery being examined. Sometimes the wave of the pulse is visible. Absence of a pulse wave may indicate arterial occlusion (blockage) or stenosis (narrowing).

To palpate the pulse, ask the patient to look straight ahead or turn the head slightly toward the side being examined. Turning relaxes the sternocleidomastoid muscle. Slide the tips of your index and middle fingers around the medial edge of the sternocleidomastoid muscle. Gently palpate to avoid occlusion of circulation (Figure 15-30).

The normal carotid pulse is localized rather than diffuse. As a strong pulse, the carotid has a thrusting quality. As the patient breathes, no change occurs. Rotation of the neck or a shift from a sitting to a supine position does not change the carotid artery's quality. Both carotid arteries are normally equal in pulse rate, rhythm, and strength and are equally elastic. Diminished or unequal carotid pulsations indicate atherosclerosis (plaque buildup in arteries) or other forms of arterial disease.

The carotid is the most commonly auscultated pulse. Auscultation is especially important for middle-age or older adults or patients suspected of having cerebrovascular disease. When the lumen of a blood vessel is narrowed, blood flow is disturbed. As blood passes through the narrowed section, this creates turbulence, causing a blowing or swishing sound. The blowing sound is called a **bruit** (pronounced "brew-ee"). Place the bell of the stethoscope over the carotid artery at the base of the neck, and move it gradually toward the jaw. Ask the patient to hold his or her breath for a few heartbeats so that respiratory sounds will not interfere with auscultation (Seidel and others, 2006). Normally you do not hear any sound during carotid auscultation. Palpate the artery lightly for a **thrill** (palpable bruit) if you hear a bruit.

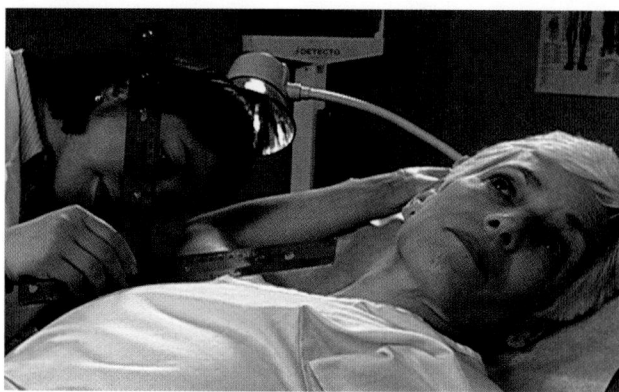

Figure 15-31 ■ Position of patient to assess jugular vein distention. (From Seidel HM and others: *Mosby's guide to physical examination,* ed 6, St. Louis, 2006, Mosby.)

Jugular Veins

The most accessible veins for examination are the internal and external jugular veins in the neck. Both veins drain bilaterally from the head and neck into the superior vena cava. The external jugular lies superficially and is just above the clavicle. The internal jugular lies deeper, along the carotid artery. Normally when a patient lies in the supine position, the external jugular distends and becomes easily visible. In contrast, the jugular veins normally flatten when the patient is in a sitting or standing position. Some patients with heart disease, however, have distended jugular veins when sitting.

To measure venous pressure inspect the jugular veins with the patient in the supine position (normally veins protrude), when standing (normally veins are flat), and when sitting at a 45-degree angle (jugular veins are distended only if patient has right-sided heart failure). An advanced practice nurse completes the specific measurement of jugular venous pressure (Figure 15-31).

Peripheral Arteries and Veins

To examine the peripheral vascular system, begin by assessing the adequacy of blood flow to the extremities by measuring arterial pulses and inspecting the skin and nails. Then assess the integrity of the venous system. Assess the arterial pulses in the extremities to determine sufficiency of the entire arterial circulation. Factors such as coagulation disorders, local trauma or surgery, constricting casts or bandages, and systemic diseases impair circulation to the extremities. Discuss risk factors for circulatory problems with the patient (Box 15-16).

PERIPHERAL ARTERIES Examine each peripheral artery using the distal pads of the second and third fingers. The thumb helps anchor the brachial and femoral arteries. Apply firm pressure, but avoid occluding a pulse. When a pulse is difficult to find, it helps to vary pressure and feel all around the pulse site. Be sure not to palpate your own pulse.

Routine vital signs usually include assessment of the rate and rhythm of the radial artery because it is easily accessible (see Chapter 14). Count the pulse for either 30 seconds or a full minute, depending on the character of the pulse. Always

---

---

count an irregular pulse for 60 seconds. With palpation, you normally feel the pulse wave at regular intervals. When an interval is interrupted by an early, late, or missed beat, the pulse rhythm is irregular. In emergencies health care providers usually assess the carotid artery because it is accessible and most useful in evaluating heart activity. To check local circulatory status of tissues, palpate the peripheral arteries long enough to note that a pulse is present.

Assess each peripheral artery for elasticity of the vessel wall, strength, and equality. The arterial wall is normally elastic, making it easily palpable. After depressing the artery, it will spring back to shape when pressure is released. An abnormal artery is described as hard, inelastic, or calcified.

The strength of a pulse is a measurement of the force with which blood is ejected against the arterial wall. Some examiners use a rating from 0 (absent) to 4 (full, bounding) (Seidel, 2006).

Measure all peripheral pulses for equality and symmetry. Compare pulses on each side of the body. Lack of symmetry indicates impaired circulation such as a localized obstruction or an abnormally positioned artery.

In the upper extremities the brachial artery channels blood to the radial and ulnar arteries of the forearm and hand. If circulation in this artery becomes blocked, the hands will not receive adequate blood flow. If circulation in the ra-

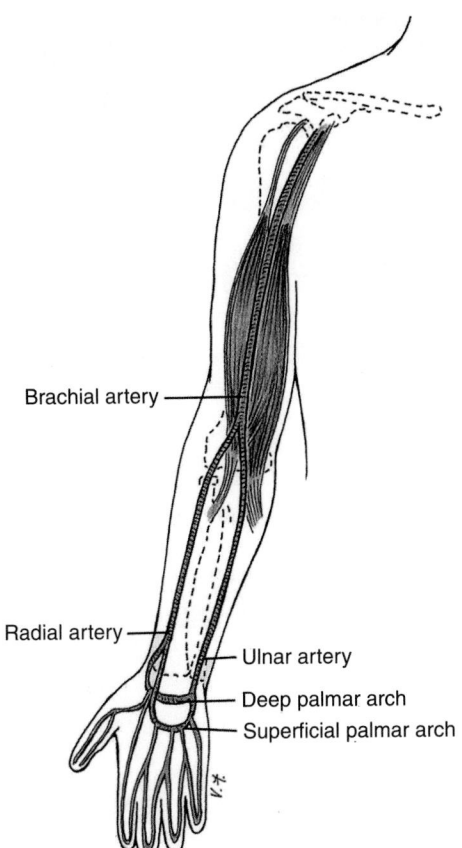

Figure 15-32 ■ Anatomical positions of brachial, radial, and ulnar arteries.

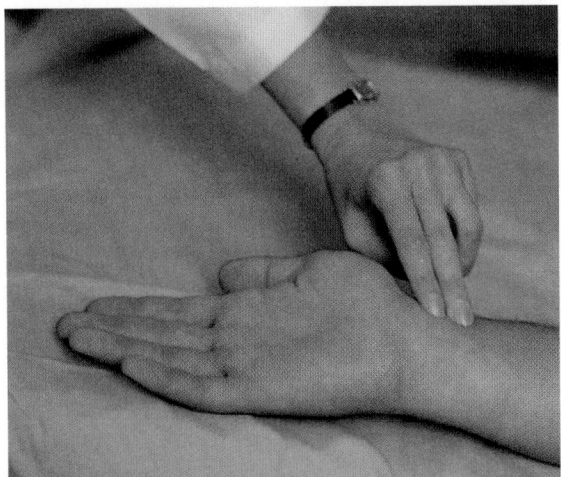

Figure 15-33 ■ Palpation of radial pulse.

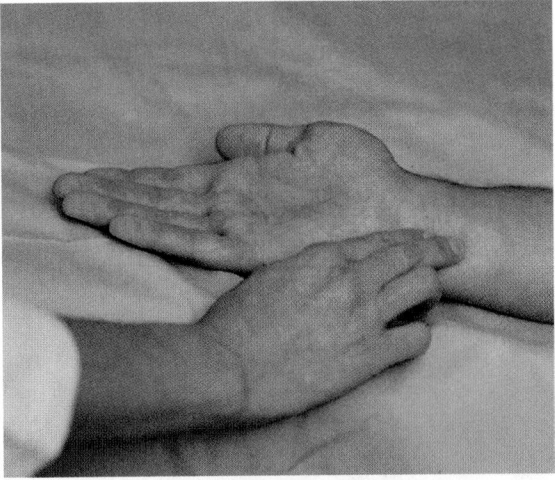

Figure 15-34 ■ Palpation of ulnar pulse.

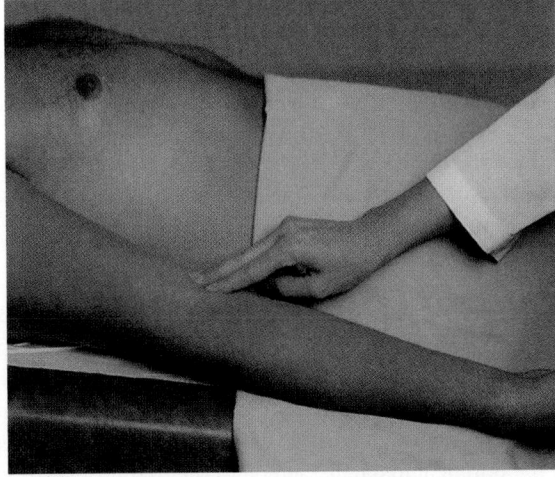

Figure 15-35 ■ Palpation of brachial pulse.

dial or ulnar artery becomes impaired, the hand will still receive adequate perfusion. An interconnection between the radial and ulnar arteries guards against arterial occlusion (Figure 15-32).

To locate pulses in the arm, have the patient sit or lie down. Find the radial pulse along the radial side of the forearm at the wrist. Thin individuals have a groove lateral to the flexor tendon of the wrist. Feel the radial pulse with light palpation in the groove (Figure 15-33). The ulnar pulse is on the opposite side of the wrist and feels less prominent (Figure 15-34). Palpate the ulnar pulse only when evaluating arterial insufficiency to the hand.

To palpate the brachial pulse, find the groove between the biceps and triceps muscle above the elbow at the antecubital fossa (Figure 15-35). The artery runs along the medial side of the extended arm. Palpate the artery with the fingertips of the first three fingers in the muscle groove.

The femoral artery is the primary artery in the leg, delivering blood to the popliteal, posterior tibial, and dorsalis pedis arteries (Figure 15-36). An interconnection between the posterior tibial and dorsalis pedis arteries guards against local arterial occlusion. Wearing disposable gloves, find the femoral pulse with the patient lying down with the inguinal area exposed (Figure 15-37). The femoral artery runs below the inguinal ligament, midway between the symphysis pubis and the anterosuperior iliac spine. Sometimes you will use deep palpation to feel the pulse. Bimanual palpation is effective in obese patients. Place the fingertips of both hands on opposite sides of the pulse site. Feel a pulsatile sensation when the arterial pulsation pushes the fingertips apart.

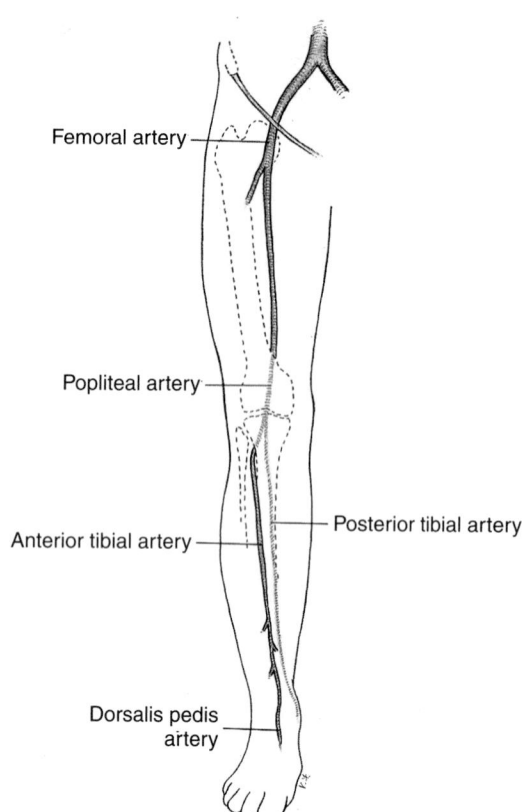

Figure 15-36 ■ Anatomical position of femoral, popliteal, dorsalis pedis, anterior tibial, and posterior tibial arteries.

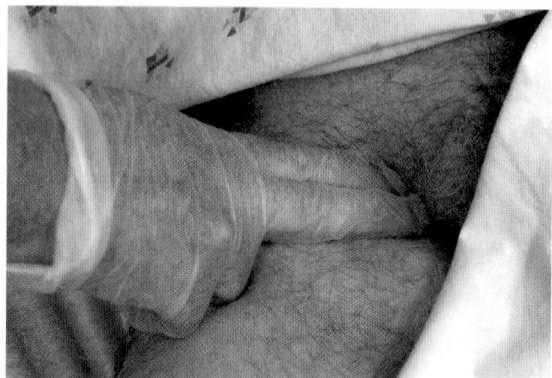

Figure 15-37 ■ Palpation of femoral pulse.

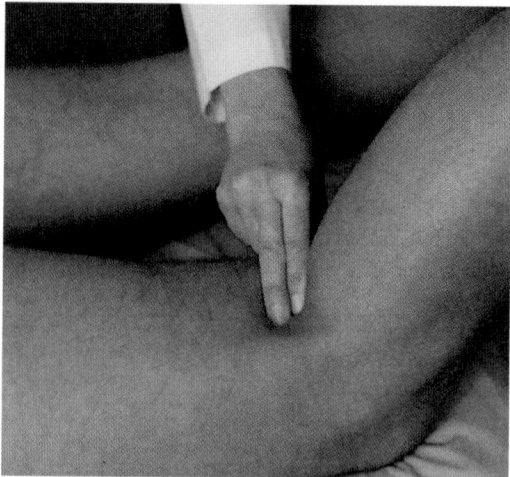

Figure 15-38 ■ Palpation of popliteal pulse.

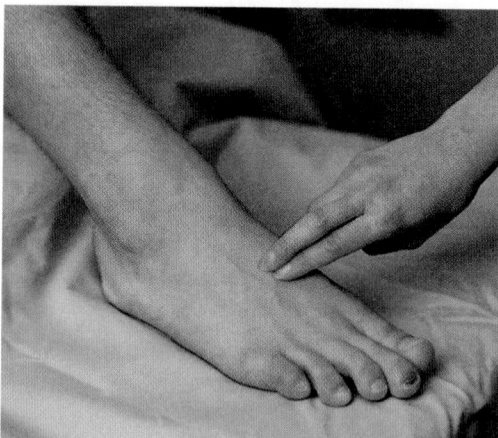

Figure 15-39 ■ Palpation of dorsalis pedis pulse.

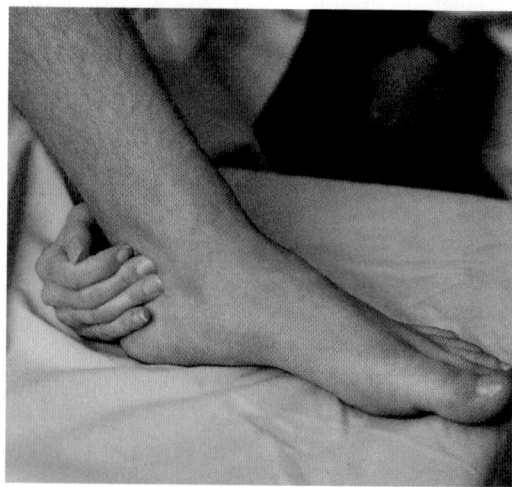

Figure 15-40 ■ Palpation of posterior tibial pulse.

The popliteal pulse runs behind the knee (Figure 15-38). Have the patient slightly flex the knee, with the foot resting on the examination table, or assume a prone position with the knee slightly flexed. Instruct the patient to keep leg muscles relaxed. Palpate with the fingers of both hands deeply into the popliteal fossa, just lateral to the midline. The popliteal pulse is difficult to locate.

With the patient's foot relaxed, locate the dorsalis pedis pulse. The artery runs along the top of the foot in a line with the groove between the extensor tendons of the great toe and first toe (Figure 15-39). To find the pulse, place the fingertips between the great and first toe and slowly move up the dorsum of the foot. This pulse is sometimes congenitally absent.

Find the posterior tibial pulse on the inner side of each ankle (Figure 15-40). Place the fingers behind and below the patient's medial malleolus (ankle bone). With the patient's foot relaxed and slightly extended, palpate the artery.

ULTRASOUND STETHOSCOPES If a pulse is difficult to palpate, an ultrasound (Doppler) stethoscope is a useful tool

TABLE 15-7 Signs of Venous and Arterial Insufficiency

ASSESSMENT CRITERION	VENOUS	ARTERIAL
Color	Normal or cyanotic	Pale; worsened by elevation of extremity; dusky red when extremity lowered
Temperature	Normal	Cool (blood flow blocked to extremity)
Pulse	Normal	Decreased or absent
Edema	Often marked	Absent or mild
Skin changes	Brown pigmentation around ankles	Thin, shiny skin; decreased hair growth; thickened nails

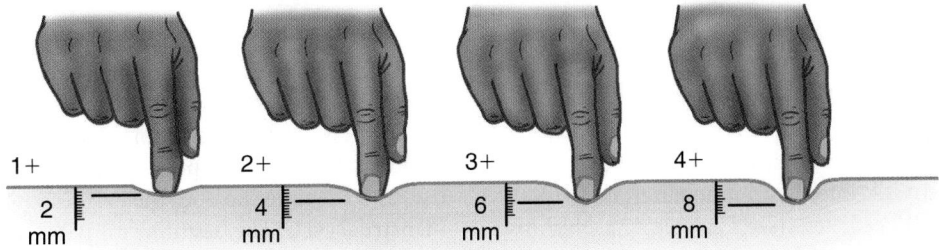

Figure 15-41 ■ Assessing for pitting edema. (From Seidel HM and others: *Mosby's guide to physical examination,* ed 6, St. Louis, 2006, Mosby.)

that amplifies sounds of a pulse wave. Apply a thin layer of transmission gel to the patient's skin at the pulse site or directly onto the transducer tip of the probe. Turn on the volume control, and place the tip of the probe at a 45- to 90-degree angle on the skin. Move the transducer until you hear a pulsating "whooshing" sound, which indicates that arterial blood flow is present.

Tissue Perfusion

The condition of the skin, mucosa, and nail beds offers useful data about the status of circulatory blood flow. Examine the face and upper extremities, looking at the color of skin, mucosa, and nail beds. The presence of cyanosis requires special attention. Heart disease sometimes causes central cyanosis (bluish discoloration of the lips, mouth, and conjunctivae), which indicates poor arterial oxygenation. Blue lips, earlobes, and nail beds are signs of peripheral cyanosis, which indicates peripheral vasoconstriction. When cyanosis is present, consult with a health care provider to have laboratory testing of oxygen saturation to determine severity of the problem. Examination of the nails involves inspection for clubbing (a bulging of the tissues at the nail base), resulting from insufficient oxygenation at the periphery from conditions such as congenital heart disease and chronic emphysema.

Inspect the lower extremities for changes in color, temperature, and condition of the skin indicating either arterial or venous alterations (Table 15-7). This is a good time to ask the patient about history of pain in the legs. If an arterial occlusion is present, the patient has signs resulting from absence of blood flow. Pain will be distal to the occlusion. The *5 Ps* characterize an occlusion: *pain, pallor, pulselessness, paresthesias,* and *paralysis.* Venous congestion causes tissue changes indicating inadequate circulatory flow back to the heart.

During examination of the lower extremities, also inspect skin and nail texture; hair distribution on the lower legs, feet, and toes; venous pattern; and scars, pigmentation, or ulcers. Palpate the legs for color and temperature. Assess for capillary refill.

The absence of hair growth over the legs indicates circulatory insufficiency. Remember, do not confuse an absence of hair on the legs with shaven legs. Also, many men have less hair around the calves because of tight-fitting dress socks or jeans. Chronic recurring ulcers of the feet or lower legs are a serious sign of circulatory insufficiency and require a health care provider's intervention.

Peripheral Veins

Assess the status of the peripheral veins by asking the patient to assume sitting and standing positions. Assessment includes inspection and palpation for varicosities, peripheral edema, and phlebitis. Varicosities are superficial veins that become dilated, especially when legs are in a dependent position. They are common in older adults because the veins normally fibrose, dilate, and stretch. They are also common in people who stand for prolonged periods. Varicosities in the anterior or medial part of the thigh and the posterolateral part of the calf are abnormal.

Dependent edema around the feet and ankles is a sign of venous insufficiency or right-sided heart failure. Dependent edema is common in older adults and persons who spend a lot of time standing (e.g., nurses, waitresses, and security guards). To assess for pitting edema, use your thumb to press firmly for several seconds over the medial malleolus or the shins and then release. A depression left in the skin indicates edema. Grading +1 through +4 characterizes the severity of the edema (Figure 15-41).

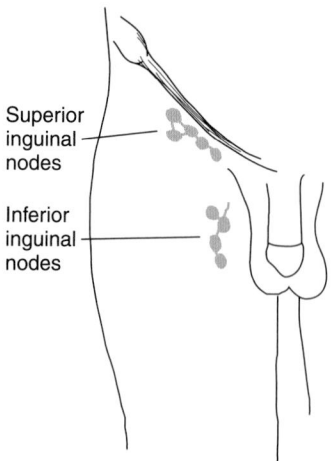

Superior inguinal nodes

Inferior inguinal nodes

Figure 15-42 ■ Inguinal lymph nodes.

Phlebitis (inflammation of a vein) occurs commonly after trauma to the vessel wall, infection, immobilization, or prolonged insertion of IV catheters (see Chapter 17). Phlebitis promotes clot formation, a potentially dangerous situation because a clot within a deep vein of the leg can become dislodged and travel through the heart, causing a pulmonary embolus. To assess for phlebitis inspect the calves for localized redness, tenderness, and swelling over vein sites. Gentle palpation of calf muscles reveals warmth, tenderness, and firmness of the muscle. Unilateral edema of the affected leg is one of the most reliable findings of phlebitis. A Doppler study is a noninvasive test that examines venous blood flow and is commonly done if deep vein thrombosis is suspected. Determine if dorsiflexion of the foot (Homans' sign) causes pain in the calf. However, Homans' sign is not always a reliable indicator for the presence or absence of phlebitis (Gorski, 2007). Performing the Homans' sign test is contraindicated in patients with known deep vein thrombosis. If a clot is present, it may become dislodged from its original site during this test, resulting in a pulmonary embolism.

Lymphatic System

Assess the lymphatic drainage of the lower extremities during examination of the vascular system or during the female or male genital examination. Superficial and deep lymph nodes drain the legs, but only two groups of superficial nodes are palpable. With the patient supine, palpate the area of the superior superficial inguinal nodes in the groin area (Figure 15-42). Then move your fingertips toward the inner thigh, feeling for any palpable inferior nodes. Use a firm but gentle pressure when palpating over each lymphatic chain. Multiple nodes are not normally palpable, although a few soft, nontender nodes are not unusual. Enlarged, hardened, tender nodes reveal potential sites of infection or metastatic disease.

BREASTS

It is important to examine the breasts of female and male patients. Males have a small amount of glandular tissue, a potential site for the growth of cancer cells, in the breast.

In contrast, the majority of the female breast is glandular tissue.

Female Breasts

Researchers predict that new cases of invasive breast cancer will affect more than 192,000 women and about 1900 men every year in the United States. Additionally, more than 62,000 cases of in situ breast cancer will be diagnosed (ACS, 2009). Breast cancer is second to lung cancer as the leading cause of death in women with cancer. Early detection is the key to cure. A responsibility for you is to teach patients health behaviors such as breast self-examination (BSE) (Box 15-17).

Breast self-examinations, once thought essential for early breast cancer detection, are now considered optional (ACS, 2009). The key is for women to know how their breasts usually look and feel and to report changes to a health care professional. If the patient performs BSE, assess the method she uses and the time she does the examination in relation to her menstrual cycle. The best time for BSE is when the breasts are not tender or swollen, usually a few days after a menstrual period ends. If the woman is postmenopausal, advise her to check her breasts on the same day each month. The pregnant woman should also check her breasts on a monthly basis.

Older women require special attention when reviewing the need for BSE. Fixed incomes limit many older women, and thus they fail to pursue regular clinical breast examination and mammography. Unfortunately, many older women ignore changes in their breasts, assuming they are a part of aging. In addition, physiological factors affect the ease with which older women can perform BSE. Musculoskeletal limitations, diminished peripheral sensation, reduced eyesight, and changes in joint range of motion limit palpation and inspection abilities. Find resources for older women, including free screening programs. Teach family members to perform the patient's examination.

The American Cancer Society (2009b) recommends the following guidelines for the early detection of breast cancer:

1. Monthly BSE is an option for women in their 20s.
2. Women 20 years of age and older need to report any breast changes to a health care provider immediately.
3. Women need a clinical breast examination by a health care provider every 3 years from ages 20 to 40, and yearly for women over age 40.
4. Women with a family history of breast cancer need a yearly examination by a health care provider.
5. Asymptomatic women need a screening mammogram by age 40; women age 40 and over need an annual mammogram.
6. For women with an increased risk, the ACS recommends discussion of screening options and additional testing with a health care provider.

The patient's history reveals normal development changes, as well as signs of breast disease. Because of this glandular structure, the breast undergoes changes during a woman's

BOX 15-17   PATIENT TEACHING

Female Breast Assessment

OUTCOME

- Patient will perform breast self-examination (BSE)
- Patient will have screening mammography performed at regular intervals, beginning at age 40.
- Patient will identify signs and symptoms of breast cancer.
- Patient will eat a low-fat diet.

TEACHING STRATEGIES

- Provide the following information about BSE:
  1. A woman has the option of performing breast self-examination (BSE) once a month to become familiar with the usual appearance and feel of her breasts. Familiarity makes it easier to notice any changes in the breast from one month to another. Early discovery of a change from what is "normal" is the main idea behind BSE.
  2. If you menstruate, the best time to do BSE is a few days after your period ends, when your breasts are least likely to be tender or swollen. If you no longer menstruate, pick a day, such as the first day of the month, to remind yourself it is time to do BSE.
- Teach the steps for performing BSE:
  1. Stand before a mirror. Inspect both breasts for anything unusual, such as any discharge from the nipples, puckering, dimpling, or scaling of the skin.

  The next two steps are designed to emphasize any change in the shape or contour of your breasts. As you do them, you will be able to feel your chest muscles tighten.

  2. Watching closely in the mirror, clasp your hands behind your head and swing elbows forward.
  3. Next, press hands firmly on hips and bow slightly toward your mirror as you pull your shoulders and elbows forward.

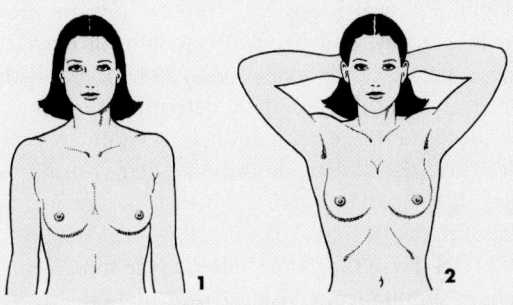

Some women do the next part of the examination in the shower. Fingers glide over soapy skin, making it easy to appreciate the texture underneath.

4. Raise your left arm over your head. Use three or four fingers of your right hand to explore your left breast firmly, carefully, and thoroughly. Beginning at the outer edge, press the flat part of your fingers in small circles, moving the circles slowly around the breast. Gradually work toward the nipple. Be sure to cover the entire breast. Pay special attention to the area between the breast and the armpit (upper outer quadrant), including the armpit itself. Feel for any unusual lump or mass under the skin.
5. Gently squeeze the nipple, and look for a discharge.
6. Repeat Steps 4 and 5 lying down. Lie flat on your back, with your left arm raised back and hand behind your neck and a pillow or folded towel under your left shoulder. This position flattens the breast and makes it easier to examine. Use the same circular motion described earlier.
7. Repeat on your right breast.

- Have the patient perform return demonstration of BSE, and offer the opportunity to ask questions.
- Explain recommended frequency of mammography and assessment by a health care provider.
- Discuss signs and symptoms of breast cancer.
- Discuss signs and symptoms of benign (fibrocystic) disease.
- Inform a woman who is obese or who has a family history of breast cancer that she is at higher risk for the disease (ACS, 2009a). Encourage following low-fat diet, including limiting meat consumption to well-trimmed, lean beef, pork, or lamb; removing skin from cooked chicken before eating it; selecting tuna and salmon packed in water and not oil; and using low-fat dairy products.
- Encourage the patient to reduce intake of caffeine. Although this is controversial, many believe decreasing caffeine intake reduces symptoms of benign (fibrocystic) breast disease.

EVALUATION STRATEGIES

- Observe patient demonstrate BSE.
- During future visits, determine if patient has had screening mammography.
- Have patient describe signs and symptoms of breast cancer compared with benign (fibrocystic) breast disease.

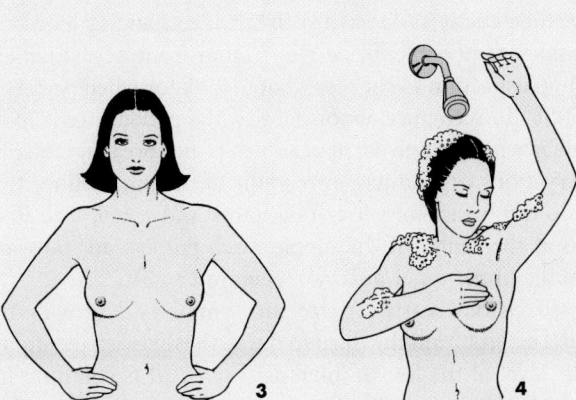
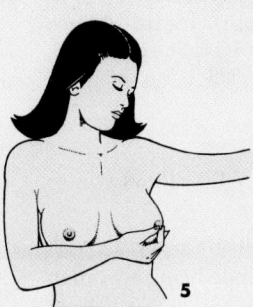
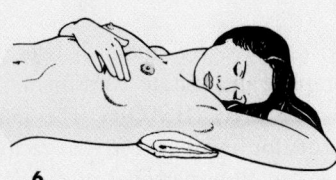

BOX 15-18   Normal Changes in the Breast During a Woman's Life Span

PUBERTY (8 TO 20 YEARS)*
Breasts mature in five stages. One breast may grow more rapidly than the other. The ages at which changes occur and rate of developmental progression vary.

Stage 1 (Preadolescent)
This stage involves elevation of the nipple only.

Stage 2
The breast and nipple elevate as a small mound, and the areolar diameters enlarge.

Stage 3
There is further enlargement and elevation of the breast and areola, with no separation of contour.

Stage 4
The areola and nipple project into the secondary mound above the level of the breast (does not occur in all girls).

Stage 5 (Mature Breast)
Only the nipple projects, and the areola recedes (varies in some women).

YOUNG ADULTHOOD (20 TO 30 YEARS)
Breasts reach full (nonpregnant) size. Shape is generally symmetrical. Breasts are sometimes unequal in size.

PREGNANCY
Breast size gradually enlarges to two to three times the previous size. Nipples enlarge and become erect. Areolae darken, and diameters increase. Superficial veins become prominent. The nipples expel a yellowish fluid (colostrum).

MENOPAUSE
Breasts shrink. Tissue becomes softer, sometimes flabby.

OLDER ADULTHOOD
Breasts become elongated, pendulous, and flaccid as a result of glandular tissue atrophy. The skin of the breasts tends to wrinkle, appearing loose and flabby.

Nipples become smaller, flatter, and lose erectile ability.† Nipples invert because of shrinkage and fibrotic changes.‡

Data from *Hockenberry MJ, Wilson D: *Wong's nursing care of infants and children,* ed 8, St. Louis, 2007, Mosby; †Seidel HM and others: *Mosby's guide to physical examination,* ed 6, St. Louis, 2006, Mosby; ‡Ebersole P and others: *Toward healthy aging,* ed 7, St. Louis, 2008, Mosby.

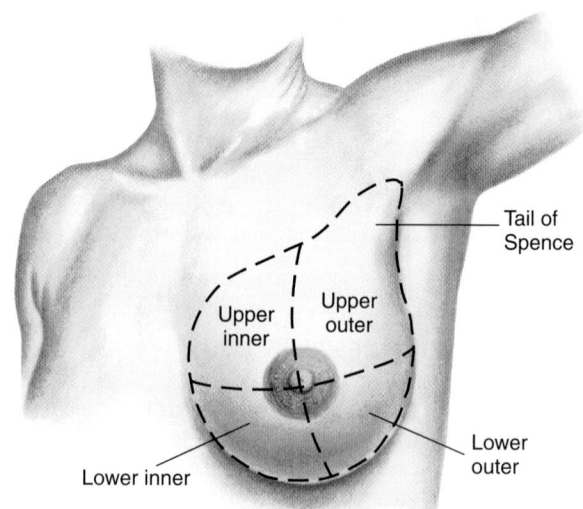

Figure 15-43 ■ Quadrants of the left breast and axillary tail of Spence. (From Seidel HM and others: *Mosby's guide to physical examination,* ed 6, St. Louis, 2006, Mosby.)

early-onset menarche (before age 13), or late-age menopause (after age 50). Other risk factors include never having children, giving birth to the first child after age 30, and a recent use of oral contraceptives. Ask if the patient (both sexes) has noticed a lump, thickening, pain, or tenderness of the breast; discharge, distortion, retraction, or scaling of the nipple; or change in breast size. Determine the patient's use of medications that increase risk (oral contraceptives, digitalis, diuretics, steroids, or estrogen). Determine the patient's caffeine intake to review risk factors for fibrocystic breast changes. Determine the patient's activity level, alcohol intake, and current weight. Physical inactivity, drinking one or more alcoholic drinks a day, and being overweight all correlate with increased breast cancer rates (ACS, 2009a). Ask if the patient performs monthly BSE. If so, determine the time of month she performs the examination in relation to menstrual cycle. Have the patient describe or demonstrate the method used. If the patient reports a breast mass, assess for related symptoms.

INSPECTION Have the patient remove the top gown or drape to allow simultaneous visualization of both breasts. Have the patient stand or sit with her arms hanging loosely at her sides. If possible, place a mirror in front of the patient during inspection so she sees what to look for when performing BSE. To recognize abnormalities, the patient needs to be familiar with the normal appearance of her breasts. Describe observations or findings in relation to imaginary lines that divide the breast into four quadrants and a tail. The lines cross at the center of the nipple. Each tail extends outward from the upper outer quadrant (Figure 15-43).

Inspect the breasts for size and symmetry. Normally the breasts extend from the third to the sixth ribs, with the nipple at the level of the fourth intercostal space. It is common for one breast to be smaller. However, inflammation or a mass

life. Knowledge of these changes (Box 15-18) allows you to complete an accurate assessment.

NURSING HISTORY The nursing history reveals risk factors for breast cancer. Risk factors include being a woman over age 40, a personal or family history of breast cancer,

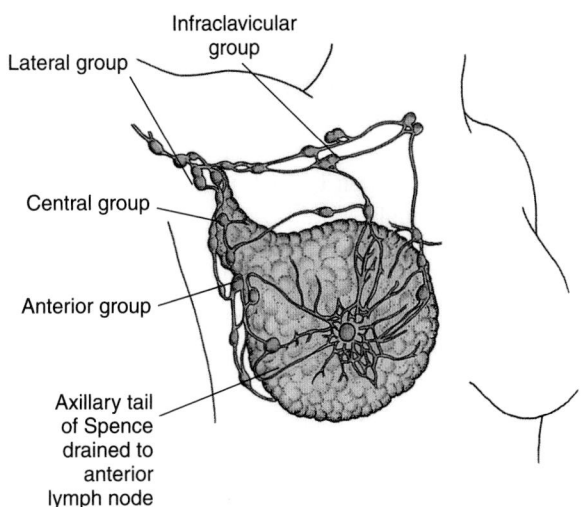

Figure 15-44 ■ Anatomical position of axillary and clavicular lymph nodes.

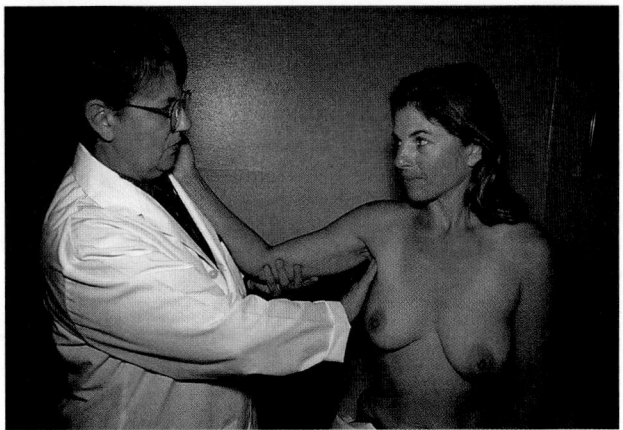

Figure 15-45 ■ Support the patient's arm and palpate axillary lymph nodes.

can cause a difference in size. With age, the ligaments supporting the breast tissue weaken, causing the breasts to sag and the nipples to lower.

Observe the contour or shape of the breasts, and note masses, flattening, retraction, or dimpling. Breasts vary in shape from convex to pendulous or conical. Retraction or dimpling results from invasion of underlying ligaments by tumors. The ligaments fibrose and pull the overlying skin inward toward the tumor. Edema also changes the contour of the breasts. To bring out the presence of retraction or changes in the shape of the breasts, ask the patient to assume three positions: raise arms above the head, press hands against the hips, and extend arms straight ahead while sitting and leaning forward. Each maneuver causes a contraction of the pectoral muscles, which will accentuate the presence of any retraction.

Carefully inspect the skin for color; venous pattern; and presence of edema, lesions, or inflammation. Lift each breast when necessary to observe lower and lateral aspects for color and texture changes. The breasts are the color of neighboring skin, and venous patterns are the same bilaterally. Venous patterns are easily visible in thin or pregnant women. Women with large breasts often have redness and excoriation of the undersurface caused by rubbing of skin surfaces.

Inspect the nipple and areola for size, color, shape, discharge, and the direction the nipples point. The normal areolae are round or oval and nearly equal bilaterally. Color ranges from pink to brown. In light-skinned women the areola turns brown during pregnancy and remains dark. In dark-skinned women the areola is brown before pregnancy (Seidel and others, 2006). Normally the nipples point in symmetrical directions, are everted, and have no drainage. If the nipples are inverted, ask if this has been present since birth. A recent inversion or inward turning of the nipple indicates an underlying growth. Rashes or ulcerations are not normal on the breast or nipples. Note any bleeding or discharge from the nipple. Clear yellow discharge 2 days after childbirth is common. While inspecting the breasts, explain the characteristics you see. Teach the patient the significance of abnormal signs or symptoms.

PALPATION Palpation assesses the condition of underlying breast tissue and lymph nodes. Breast tissue consists of glandular tissue, fibrous supportive ligaments, and fat. Glandular tissue is organized into lobes that end in ducts opening onto the nipple's surface. The largest portion of glandular tissue is in the upper outer quadrant and tail of each breast. Suspensory ligaments connect to skin and fascia underlying the breast to support the breast and maintain its upright position. Fatty tissue is located superficially and to the sides of the breast.

A large proportion of lymph from the breasts drains into axillary lymph nodes. Learn the location of supraclavicular, infraclavicular, and axillary nodes (Figure 15-44). The axillary nodes drain lymph from the chest wall, breasts, arms, and hands. A tumor of one breast sometimes involves nodes on both sides of the body.

To palpate lymph nodes have the patient sit with arms at her sides and muscles relaxed. While facing the patient and standing on the side you are examining, support the patient's arm in a flexed position and abduct the arm from the chest wall. Place the free hand against the patient's chest wall and high in the axillary hollow (Figure 15-45). With your fingertips press gently down over the surface of the ribs and muscles. Palpate the axillary nodes with the fingertips gently rolling soft tissue. Palpate four areas of the axilla: at the edge of the pectoralis major muscle along the anterior axillary line, the chest wall in the midaxillary area, the upper part of the humerus, and the anterior edge of the latissimus dorsi muscle along the posterior axillary line. Normally lymph nodes are not palpable. Note the number, consistency, mobility, and size of palpable nodes. A palpable node feels like a small mass that is hard, tender, and immobile. Also palpate along the upper and lower clavicular ridges. Reverse the procedure for the patient's other side.

Perform palpation of breast tissue with the patient lying supine and one arm behind the head (alternating with each breast). The supine position allows the breast tissue to flatten evenly against the chest wall. The patient raises her hand and places it behind the neck to further stretch and position breast tissue evenly. Place a small pillow or towel under the patient's shoulder blade to further position breast tissue.

If the patient complains of a mass, examine the opposite breast first to ensure an objective comparison of normal and abnormal tissue. Use the pads of the first three fingers to compress breast tissue gently against the chest wall, noting tissue consistency (Figure 15-46). Perform palpation systematically in one of three ways: (1) using a vertical technique with the fingers moving up and down each quadrant; (2) clockwise or counterclockwise, forming small circles with the fingers along each quadrant and the tail; or (3) palpating from center of the breast in a radial fashion, returning to the areola to begin each spoke (Figure 15-47). Whatever approach you use, be sure to cover the entire breast and tail, directing attention to any areas of tenderness. When palpating large, pendulous breasts, use a bimanual technique. Support the inferior portion of the breast in one hand while using the other hand to palpate breast tissue against the supporting hand.

During palpation note the consistency of breast tissue, which varies widely. The breasts of a young patient are firm and elastic. In an older patient the tissue may feel stringy and nodular. The patient's familiarity with the texture of her own breasts is most important. The lobular feel of glandular tissue is normal. The lower edge of each breast feels firm and hard. This is the normal inframammary ridge and is not a tumor.

It helps to move the patient's hand so she feels normal tissue variations. Palpate abnormal masses to determine location in relation to quadrants, diameter in centimeters, shape (e.g., round or discoid), consistency (soft, firm, or hard), tenderness, mobility, and discreteness (clear or unclear borders). Cancerous lesions are hard, fixed, nontender, irregular in shape, and usually unilateral.

Give special attention when palpating the nipple and areola. Palpate the entire surface gently. Use the thumb and index finger to compress the nipple, and note any discharge. During the examination of the nipple and areola, the nipple may become erect with wrinkling of the areola. These changes are normal.

After completing the examination, have the patient demonstrate self-palpation. Observe the patient's technique, and emphasize the importance of a systematic approach. Urge the patient to see her health care provider if she discovers an abnormal mass during monthly self-examination (see Box 15-17, p. 349).

Male Breasts

Examination of the male breast is relatively easy. Inspect the nipple and areola for nodules, edema, and ulceration. An enlarged male breast results from obesity or glandular enlargement. Breast enlargement in young males results from steroid use. Fatty tissue feels soft, whereas glandular tissue is firm. Use the same techniques to palpate for masses used in examination of the female breast. Because male breast cancer is relatively rare, routine self-examinations are unnecessary. However, men with a first-degree relative (e.g., mother) with breast cancer are at increased risk for the development of breast cancer and should perform regular breast self-examinations.

ABDOMEN

The abdominal examination is complex because of the number of organs located within and near the abdominal cavity. The examination includes an assessment of structures of the lower GI tract in addition to the liver, stomach, uterus, ovaries, kidneys, and bladder. Abdominal pain is one of the most common symptoms patients will report when seeking medical care. An accurate assessment requires matching patient history data with a careful assessment of the location of physical symptoms.

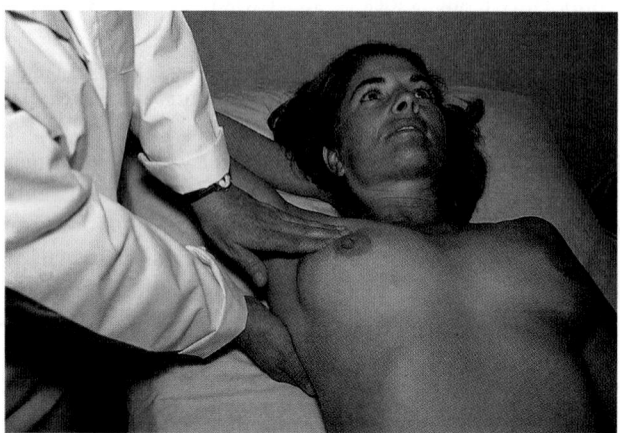

Figure 15-46 ■ The patient lies flat with arm abducted and hand under head to help flatten breast tissue evenly over the chest wall. Palpate each breast in systematic fashion.

Figure 15-47 ■ Various methods for breast palpation. **A,** Palpate from top to bottom in vertical strips. **B,** Palpate in concentric circles. **C,** Palpate out from the center in wedge sections. (From Seidel HM and others: *Mosby's guide to physical examination,* ed 6, St. Louis, 2006, Mosby.)

Vertical strip

Circular

Wedge

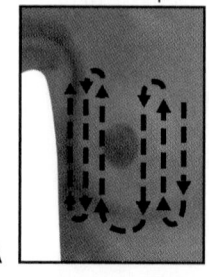
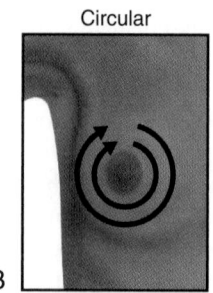
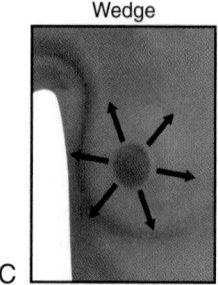

A   B   C

Assess the organs anteriorly and posteriorly. A system of landmarks helps to map out the abdominal region. The xiphoid process (tip of the sternum) is the upper boundary of the anterior abdominal region. The symphysis pubis is the lower boundary. By dividing the abdomen into four imaginary quadrants (Figure 15-48, *A*), refer to assessment findings and record them in relation to each quadrant. Posteriorly, the lower ribs and heavy back muscles protect the kidneys, which are located from the T12 to L3 vertebrae (Figure 15-48, *B*). The **costovertebral angle** formed by the last rib and vertebral column is a landmark used during palpation of the kidney.

During the abdominal examination, the patient needs to relax. Tight abdominal muscles make palpation difficult. Ask the patient to void before beginning. Be sure the room is warm, and drape the patient's upper chest and legs. The patient lies supine or in a dorsal recumbent position with the arms at the sides and knees slightly bent. Place small pillows beneath the knees. If the patient places the arms under the head, the abdominal muscles tighten. Proceed calmly and slowly, being sure there is adequate lighting. Expose the abdomen from just above the xiphoid process down to the symphysis pubis. Warm hands and stethoscope promote relax-

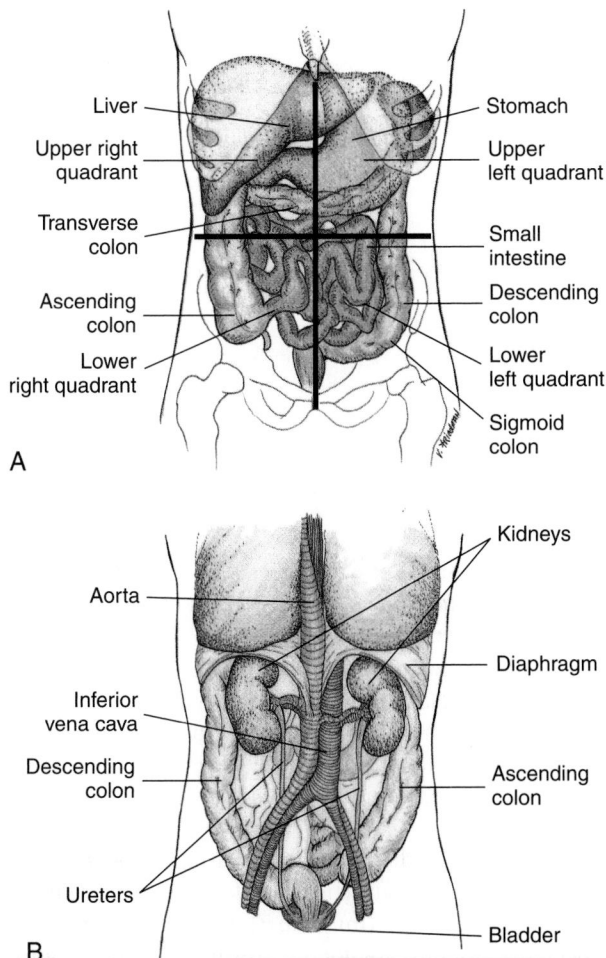

Figure 15-48 ■ **A,** Anterior view of abdomen divided by quadrants. **B,** Posterior view of abdominal sections.

ation. Ask the patient to report pain and point out areas of tenderness. Assess tender areas last.

The order for an abdominal examination differs slightly from that for previous assessments. Begin with inspection and then auscultation. By using auscultation before palpation, there is less chance of altering the frequency and character of bowel sounds. Have a tape measure and marking pen available during the examination.

Nursing History

Ask whether the patient has abdominal or low back pain, and assess the character of the pain in detail (see Chapter 31). Also review the patient's normal bowel habits and stool character, including use of laxatives. Determine if the patient has had abdominal surgery, trauma, or diagnostic tests of the GI tract. Assess for difficulty swallowing, belching, flatulence (gas), bloody emesis (hematemesis), black or tarry stools (melena), heartburn, diarrhea, or constipation. Assess if the patient has had a recent weight change or intolerance to diet (e.g., nausea, vomiting, or cramping). If the patient takes antiinflammatory drugs (e.g., aspirin, ibuprofen, or steroids) and antibiotics, there is risk for GI upset or bleeding. Inquire about a family history of cancer, kidney disease, alcoholism, hypertension, or heart disease. Assess the patient's usual intake of alcohol. Also determine if the female patient is pregnant, and note the date of her last menstrual period. Review the patient's history for risk factors for hepatitis B virus (HBV) exposure (e.g., hemodialysis or intravenous drug use). Finally, ask the patient to locate tender areas before beginning the examination.

Inspection

Always observe the patient during routine care activities. Note the patient's posture, and look for evidence of abdominal splinting, lying with the knees drawn up, or moving restlessly in bed. A patient free from abdominal pain will not guard or splint the abdomen. To inspect the abdomen for abnormal movement or shadows, stand on the patient's right side and inspect the abdomen from above. By sitting down to look across the abdomen, you assess abdominal contour. Direct the examination light over the abdomen.

SKIN Inspect the skin over the abdomen for color, scars, venous patterns, lesions, and striae (stretch marks). The skin is subject to the same color variations as the rest of the body. Venous patterns are normally faint, except in thin patients. Artificial openings indicate drainage sites resulting from surgery (see Chapter 38) or an ostomy (see Chapters 33 and 34). Scars reveal evidence of past trauma or surgery that created permanent changes in underlying organ anatomy. Bruising indicates accidental injury, physical abuse, or a type of bleeding disorder. Ask if the patient self-administers injections (e.g., insulin or low-molecular-weight heparin). Unexpected findings include generalized skin color changes such as jaundice or cyanosis. A glistening taut (tight) appearance indicates ascites.

UMBILICUS Note the position; shape; color; and presence of inflammation, discharge, or protruding masses. A normal umbilicus is flat or concave with the color the same as surrounding skin. Underlying masses cause displacement of the umbilicus.

CONTOUR AND SYMMETRY Inspect for contour, symmetry, and surface motion of the abdomen, noting any masses, bulging, or distention. A flat abdomen forms a horizontal plane from the xiphoid process to the symphysis pubis. A round abdomen protrudes in a convex sphere from a horizontal plane. A concave abdomen appears to sink into the muscular wall. Each of these findings is normal if the shape of the abdomen is symmetrical. In older adults there is often an overall increased distribution of adipose tissue. The presence of masses on only one side, or asymmetry, indicates an underlying pathological condition.

Intestinal gas, tumor, or fluid in the abdominal cavity causes distention (swelling). When distention is generalized, the entire abdomen protrudes. The skin often appears taut, as if it were stretched over the abdomen. When gas causes distention, the flanks do not bulge. However, if fluid is the source of the problem, such as in ascites, the flanks bulge. Ask the patient to roll onto one side. A protuberance forms on the dependent side if fluid is the cause of the distention. Ask the patient if the abdomen feels unusually tight. Be careful not to confuse distention with obesity. In obesity the abdomen is large, rolls of adipose tissue are often present along the flanks, and the patient does not complain of tightness in the abdomen. If abdominal distention is expected, measure the abdomen by placing a tape measure around the abdomen at the level of the umbilicus. Consecutive measurements will show any increase or decrease in distention. Use a marking pen to indicate where you applied the tape measure.

ENLARGED ORGANS OR MASSES Observe the contour of the abdomen while asking the patient to take a deep breath and hold it. Normally the contour remains smooth and symmetrical. To evaluate abdominal musculature, have the patient raise his or her head. This position causes superficial abdominal wall masses, hernias, and muscle separations to become more apparent.

MOVEMENT OR PULSATIONS Inspect for movement. Normally men breathe abdominally and women breathe more costally. A patient with severe pain has diminished respiratory movement and tightens abdominal muscles to guard against the pain. Observe for peristaltic movement and aortic pulsation by looking across the abdomen from side to side. These movements are visible in thin patients; otherwise no movement is present.

Auscultation

The abdominal examination is one exception when you auscultate before palpation to reduce the risk for altering the frequency and intensity of bowel sounds. Ask the patient not to speak. Patients with GI tubes connected to suction need them temporarily turned off before beginning the examination.

BOWEL MOTILITY Bowel sounds are the audible passage of air and fluid that normal intestinal contractions (peristalsis) create. Place the warmed diaphragm of the stethoscope lightly over each of the four quadrants. Normally air and fluid move through the intestines, creating soft gurgling

---

BOX 15-19   PATIENT TEACHING
Abdominal Assessment

OUTCOMES
- Patient will maintain normal bowel elimination.
- Patient will achieve pain relief.
- Patient at high risk for hepatitis B virus (HBV) will receive immunization.
- Patient will identify signs and symptoms of colon cancer.

TEACHING STRATEGIES
- Explain factors that promote normal bowel elimination, such as diet, regular exercise, limited use of over-the-counter drugs causing constipation, establishment of a regular elimination schedule, and a good fluid intake (see Chapter 34). Stress importance for older adults such as Mr. Neal (see Case Study).
- Caution patients about dangers of excessive use of laxatives or enemas.
- Instruct patients to have acute abdominal pain evaluated by a health care provider.
- If the patient has chronic pain, explain measures used for pain relief (e.g., relaxation exercises, positioning) (see Chapter 31).
- Instruct the patient about warning signs of colon cancer, including rectal bleeding, cramping pain in lower abdomen, black or tarry stools, blood in the stool, and a change in bowel habits (constipation or diarrhea).
- If patient is a health care worker or has contact with blood or body fluids of affected persons, encourage patient to receive series of three hepatitis B vaccine doses.

EVALUATION STRATEGIES
- Reassess patient's bowel elimination pattern and stool characteristics after therapy begins.
- Observe patient use pain-relief measures, and reassess character of pain.
- During future visits, check patient's compliance with HBV vaccine schedule.
- Ask patient to state signs and symptoms of colon cancer.

---

or clicking sounds that occur irregularly 5 to 35 times per minute (Seidel and others, 2006). Sounds may last ½ second to several seconds. It normally takes 5 to 20 seconds to hear a bowel sound. However, it takes 5 minutes of continuous listening before determining bowel sounds are absent. Auscultate all four quadrants to be sure you do not miss any sounds. The best time to auscultate is between meals. Sounds are generally described as normal, audible, absent, hyperactive, or hypoactive.

Absent sounds indicate a lack of peristalsis, possibly due to a bowel obstruction, paralytic ileus (decreased or absent peristalsis), or peritonitis (inflammation of the peritoneum). Hyperactive sounds are loud, "growling" sounds (borborygmi), which indicate increased GI motility. Inflammation of the bowel, anxiety, bleeding, excess ingestion of laxatives,

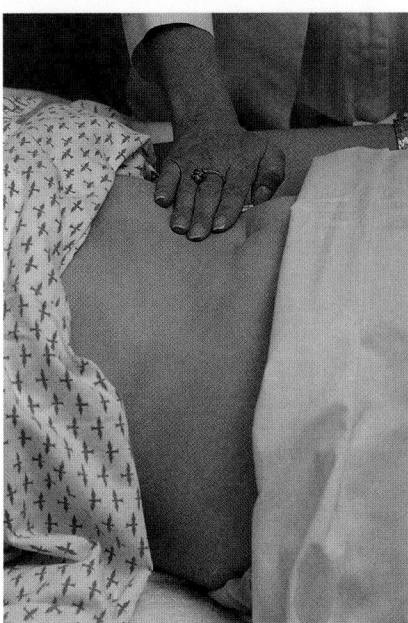

Figure 15-49 ■ Light palpation of the abdomen.

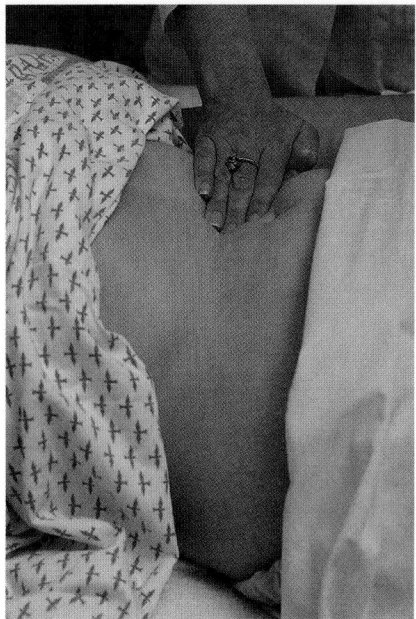

Figure 15-50 ■ Deep palpation of the abdomen.

and reaction of the intestines to certain foods cause increased motility (Box 15-19).

VASCULAR SOUNDS Bruits auscultated in affected blood vessels indicate narrowing of the blood vessels and turbulent disrupted blood flow. Presence of bruits in the abdominal area reveals aneurysms or stenotic vessels. Use the bell of the stethoscope to auscultate in the epigastric region and each of the four quadrants. Normally there are no vascular sounds over the aorta (midline through the abdomen) or femoral arteries (lower quadrants). Report a bruit immediately to a health care provider.

Palpation

Palpation primarily detects areas of abdominal tenderness, distention, or masses. As assessment skills improve, learn to palpate for specific organs such as the liver, using light and deep palpation.

Use light palpation over each abdominal quadrant. Initially avoid areas previously identified as problem spots. Lay the palm of the hand with fingers extended and approximated lightly on the abdomen. Explain the maneuver to the patient, and then with the palmar surface of the fingers depress 1.3 cm (½ inch) in a gentle dipping motion (Figure 15-49). Avoid quick jabs, and use smooth, coordinated movements. For ticklish patients, first place the patient's hand on the abdomen with your hand on the patient's hand; continue until the patient tolerates palpation. Assess for muscular resistance, tenderness, distention, and superficial organs or masses. Observe the patient's face for signs of discomfort. The abdomen is normally smooth with consistent softness and nontender without masses. The older adult often lacks abdominal tone.

With experience perform deep palpation (Figure 15-50) to assess abdominal organs and to detect less obvious masses. You will need short fingernails. It is important for the patient

to be relaxed while the hands depress approximately 2.5 to 7.5 cm (1 to 3 inches) into the abdomen. Never use deep palpation over a surgical incision or over extremely tender organs. It is also unwise to use deep palpation on abnormal masses. Deep pressure causes tenderness in the healthy patient over the cecum, sigmoid colon, and aorta and in the midline near the xiphoid process (Seidel and others, 2006).

Survey each quadrant systematically. Palpate masses for size, location, shape, consistency, tenderness, pulsation, and mobility. Test for rebound tenderness by pressing a hand slowly and deeply into the involved area and then letting go quickly. The test is positive if the patient feels pain when the hand is released. Rebound tenderness occurs in patients with peritoneal irritation such as in appendicitis; pancreatitis; or any peritoneal injury causing bile, blood, or enzymes to enter the peritoneal cavity.

AORTIC PULSATION To assess aortic pulsation, palpate with the thumb and forefinger of one hand deeply into the upper abdomen just left of the midline. Normally a pulsation is transmitted forward. If there is enlargement of the aorta from an aneurysm (localized dilation of a vessel wall), the pulsation expands laterally. Do not palpate a pulsating abdominal mass. In obese patients it is often necessary to palpate with both hands, one on each side of the aorta.

FEMALE GENITALIA AND REPRODUCTIVE TRACT

Examination of the female genitalia is embarrassing to the patient unless you use a calm, relaxed approach. The gynecological examination is one of the most difficult experiences for adolescents. Cultural background further adds to apprehension. For example, in some cultural groups, women will

BOX 15-20   PATIENT TEACHING

Female Genital and Reproductive Tract Assessment

OUTCOMES

- Patient will develop a routine gynecological examination schedule based on individual risk factors.
- Patient will follow safe sex practices.

TEACHING STRATEGIES

- Instruct the patient in the purpose and recommended frequency of Papanicolaou (Pap) smears and gynecological examinations. Explain that the Pap smear is needed annually for women who are sexually active or who are over age 21. Patients are screened more often if certain risk factors exist such as a weak immune system, multiple sex partners, smoking, and a history of infections (e.g., human papillomavirus [HPV]).
- Counsel females about genital HPV infection and the need to receive the HPV vaccine before becoming sexually active. The vaccine is ideally recommended for 11- and 12-year-old girls. Females who are already sexually active may benefit from the vaccine, but it may not be as effective if already exposed to HPV. It is also recommended for females age 13 through 26 who have not yet been vaccinated.
- Counsel patients with sexually transmitted illnesses (STIs) about diagnosis and treatment.
- Instruct in genital self-examination: Using a mirror, position self to examine the area covered by the pubic hair. Spread the hair apart, looking for bumps, sores, or blis-

ters, Also look for any warts, which appear as small, bumpy spots and enlarge to fleshy, cauliflower-like lesions. Next, spread the outer vaginal lips apart and look at the clitoris for bumps, blisters, sores, or warts. Also look at both sides of the inner vaginal lips. Inspect the area around the urinary and vaginal openings for bumps, blisters, sores, or warts.

- Explain warning signs of STIs: pain or burning on urination, pain during sex, pain in the pelvic area, bleeding between menstrual periods, an itchy rash around the vagina, and vaginal discharge.
- Teach measures to prevent STIs: male partner's use of condoms, restricting number of sexual partners, avoiding sex with persons who have several other partners, and perineal hygiene measures.
- Tell patients with STIs to inform their sexual partner(s) of the need for an examination.
- Reinforce the importance of perineal hygiene (as appropriate).

EVALUATION STRATEGIES

- Ask patient to explain the need for routine gynecological examination and Pap test.
- Have patient describe ways to prevent transmission of STIs.
- Ask patient to describe safe sex practices.

---

allow only a female health care provider to perform a physical assessment. Other cultures have a strong social value for modesty. Provide a thorough explanation as to the reason for the procedures used in the examination. Offer the patient the option of a chaperone during the examination (Edelman and others, 2007). The lithotomy position assumed during the examination is often a source of embarrassment. Make the patient feel comfortable by correctly positioning and draping her. Be sure to explain each portion of the examination in advance so that patients will anticipate each action. Adolescents sometimes choose to have parents present in the examination room.

Sometimes a patient requires a complete examination, including assessing external genitalia and performing a vaginal examination. The nurse will examine external genitalia while performing routine hygiene measures or preparing to insert a urinary catheter. An examination is a part of each woman's preventive health care, because ovarian cancer causes more deaths than any other cancer of the female reproductive system (ACS, 2009a).

Adolescents and young adults are examined because of the growing incidence of sexually transmitted infections (STIs). The average age of menarche among young girls has declined, and the majority of male and female teenagers are sexually active by age 19 (Hockenberry and Wilson, 2007). Rectal and anal assessments are combined with this examination because the patient assumes a lithotomy or dorsal recumbent position.

Nursing History

The nursing history reviews the patient's previous illness or surgeries involving reproductive organs, including STIs. A review of the menstrual history includes age at menarche, frequency and duration of menstrual cycle, character of flow, presence of dysmenorrhea (painful menstruation), pelvic pain, dates of last two menstrual periods, and premenstrual symptoms. Ask if the patient has had signs of bleeding, vaginal discharge, or pain outside the normal menstrual period or after menopause. Ask if the patient has symptoms or history of genitourinary problems such as burning during urination, frequency, urgency, nocturia, hematuria, incontinence, or stress incontinence.

Ask the patient to describe her obstetrical history, including each pregnancy and history of abortions or miscarriages. Also question the patient about current and past contraceptive practices and problems encountered. It is important to determine if the patient uses safe sex practices. Discuss risks of STIs and HIV infection. Also review a patient's risk for developing cervical, endometrial, or ovarian cancer (Box 15-20).

Preparation of the Patient

As a nursing student, your responsibility will be assisting the patient's primary health care provider with the examination. For a complete examination, you will need the following special equipment: examination table with stirrups, vaginal speculum of correct size, adjustable light source, sink, clean gloves, glass slides, plastic or wooden spatula, cervical brush or broom device, cytologic fixative, and culture plates or media (Seidel and others, 2006).

Make sure equipment is ready before the examination begins. Ask the patient to empty her bladder so that you can palpate the uterus and ovaries. Often it is necessary to collect a urine specimen. Assist the patient to the lithotomy position, in bed or on an examination table, for an external genitalia assessment. Assist the patient into stirrups for a speculum examination. Have the woman stabilize each foot in a stirrup, and then have her slide the buttocks down to the edge of the examining table. Place a hand at the edge of the table and instruct the patient to move until touching the hand. The patient's arms should be at her sides or folded across the chest to prevent tightening of abdominal muscles.

Provide a square drape or sheet to the patient. She holds one corner over her sternum, the adjacent corners fall over each knee, and the fourth corner falls over the perineum. After the examination begins, lift the drape over the perineum. The male examiner always needs to have a female in attendance during the examination. A female examiner may prefer to work alone but should have a female attendant if the patient is particularly anxious, is emotionally unstable, or has requested one (Edelman and others, 2007).

External Genitalia

Make sure the perineal area is well illuminated. Apply clean gloves on both hands. The perineum is extremely sensitive and tender; do not touch the area suddenly without warning the patient. It is best to touch the neighboring thigh first before advancing to the perineum.

While sitting at the end of the examination table or bed, inspect the quantity and distribution of hair growth. Preadolescents have no pubic hair. During adolescence hair grows along the labia, becoming darker, coarser, and curlier. In an adult, hair grows in a triangle over the female perineum and along the medial surface of the thighs. Hair is normally free of nits and lice.

Inspect surface characteristics of the labia majora. The skin of the perineum is smooth, clean, and slightly darker than other skin. The mucous membranes appear dark pink and moist. The labia majora are gaping or closed and appear dry or moist. They are usually symmetrical. After childbirth the labia majora separate, causing the labia minora to become more prominent. When a woman reaches menopause, the labia majora become thinned. With advancing age they become atrophied (decrease in size). The labia majora are normally without inflammation, edema, lesions, or lacerations.

To inspect the remaining external structures, use your nondominant hand and gently place the thumb and index finger inside the labia minora and retract the tissues outward (Figure 15-51). Be sure to have a firm hold to avoid repeated retraction against the sensitive tissues. Use the other hand to palpate the labia minora between the thumb and second fin-

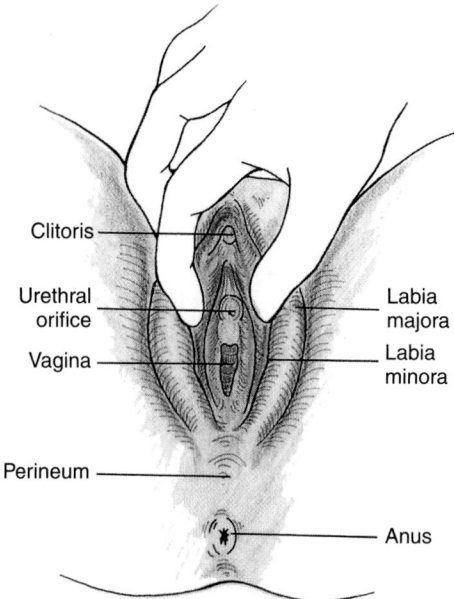

Figure 15-51 ■ Female external genitalia.

Labels: Clitoris, Urethral orifice, Vagina, Perineum, Labia majora, Labia minora, Anus

ger. On inspection, the labia minora are normally thinner than the labia majora, and one side is sometimes larger. The tissue feels soft on palpation and without tenderness. The size of the clitoris is variable, but it normally does not exceed 2 cm in length and 0.5 cm in diameter. Look for atrophy, inflammation, or adhesions. If inflamed, the clitoris will be a bright cherry red. In young women it is a common site for syphilitic lesions or chancres, which appear as small open ulcers that drain serous material. Older women may have malignant changes that result in dry, scaly, nodular lesions.

Inspect the urethral orifice carefully for color and position. It is normally intact and without inflammation. The urethral meatus is anterior to the vaginal orifice and is pink. It appears as a small slit or pinhole opening just above the vaginal canal. Note any discharge, polyps, or fistulas.

Inspect the vaginal orifice (introitus) for inflammation, edema, discoloration, discharge, and lesions. Normally the introitus is a thin vertical slit or a large orifice. The tissue is moist. While inspecting the vaginal orifice or introitus, notice the condition of the hymen, which is just inside the introitus. In the virgin the hymen restricts the opening of the vagina. Only remnants of the hymen remain after sexual intercourse.

Inspect the anus looking for lesions and hemorrhoids (see rectal examination). After completion of the external examination, dispose of examination gloves, offer the patient perineal hygiene, and perform hand hygiene.

Patients who are at risk for contracting STIs need to learn to perform a genital self-examination (see Box 15-20). The purpose of the examination is to detect any signs or symptoms of STIs. Many persons do not know they have an STI (e.g., chlamydial infection), and some STIs (e.g., syphilis) can remain undetected for years. Therefore it is essential to stress the importance of regular screening for STIs in sexually active individuals.

Speculum Examination of Internal Genitalia

An examination of internal genitalia requires much skill and practice. Advanced practice nurses and primary care providers will perform this examination. Beginning students will more than likely only observe the procedure or assist the examiner by helping the patient with positioning, handing off specimen supplies, and comforting the patient.

The examination involves use of a plastic or metal speculum, consisting of two blades and an adjustable thumbscrew. The examiner inserts the speculum into the vagina to assess the vaginal walls and cervix for cancerous lesions and other abnormalities. During the examination the examiner will collect a Papanicolaou (Pap) smear to test for cervical and vaginal cancer.

MALE GENITALIA

An examination of the male genitalia assesses the integrity of the external genitalia, inguinal ring, and canal. Because the incidence of STIs in adolescents and young adults is high, an assessment of the genitalia needs to be a routine part of any health maintenance examination for this age-group. Use a calm, gentle approach to lessen the patient's anxiety. Offer the patient the option of a chaperone during the examination. Have the patient void. Have the patient lie supine with the chest, abdomen, and lower legs draped or stand during the examination. Apply clean gloves.

Nursing History

Review the patient's normal urinary elimination pattern, including frequency of voiding; history of nocturia: character and volume of urine; daily fluid intake; and symptoms of burning, urgency and frequency, difficulty starting stream, and hematuria. The history also includes a review of previous surgery or illness involving urinary or reproductive organs, including STIs. The patient's sexual history and use of safe sex habits will identify any risks for HIV infection or other STIs. Patients at risk require extensive education. Ask if the patient has difficulty achieving erection or ejaculation, and review medications that influence sexual performance, including diuretics, sedatives, antihypertensives, and tranquilizers. Ask if the patient has noted penile pain or swelling, genital lesions, or urethral discharge, which indicate signs and symptoms of STIs. The patient's knowledge of testicular self-examination will provide a guide for health teaching (Box 15-21). Determine if the patient has noticed heaviness or painless enlargement of a testis or irregular lumps (warning signs of testicular cancer). If the patient reports an enlargement in the inguinal area, assess if it is intermittent or constant; associated with straining or lifting; painful; and whether coughing, lifting, or straining at stool increases the pain. These are all signs and symptoms that indicate an inguinal hernia.

Sexual Maturity

First, note the sexual maturity of the patient by observing the size and shape of the penis and testes; the size, color, and texture of scrotal skin; and the character and distribution of pubic hair. The testes first increase in size in preadolescence. During this time there is no pubic hair. By the end of puberty, the testes and penis enlarge to adult size and shape and scrotal skin darkens and becomes wrinkled. With puberty, hair becomes coarse and abundant in the pubic area. The penis has no hair, and the scrotum has very little hair. Also inspect the skin covering the genitalia for lice, rashes, excoriations, or lesions. Normally the skin is clear, without lesions.

Penis

To inspect penile surfaces thoroughly, manipulate the genitalia or have the patient assist. Inspect the corona, prepuce (foreskin), glans, urethral meatus, and shaft (Figure 15-52). In uncircumcised males retract the foreskin to reveal the glans and urethral meatus. The foreskin usually retracts easily. A small amount of white, thick smegma sometimes collects under this foreskin. In the circumcised male, the glans is exposed; in either case, the glans should look smooth and pink along all surfaces. The urethral meatus is slitlike and normally positioned at the tip of the glans. In some congenital conditions the meatus is displaced along the penile shaft. The area between the foreskin and glans is a common site for venereal lesions.

Gently compress the glans between your thumb and index finger; this opens the urethral meatus for inspection of discharge, lesions, and edema. Normally the opening is glistening and pink without discharge. Palpate any lesion gently to note tenderness, size, consistency, and shape. When inspection and palpation of the glans is complete, pull the foreskin down to its original position. Continue by inspecting the entire shaft of the penis, including the undersurface, looking for any lesions, scars, or edema. Palpate the shaft between the thumb and first two fingers to detect localized areas of hardness or tenderness. A patient who has lain in bed for a prolonged time may develop dependent edema in the penile shaft.

It is important for any male patient to learn to perform a genital self-examination to detect signs and symptoms of STIs. Many people who have an STI do not know it. Self-examination is a routine part of self-care (see Box 15-21).

Scrotum

Be especially cautious while inspecting and palpating the scrotum because the structures that lie within the scrotal sac are very sensitive. The scrotum is divided internally into two halves. Each half contains a testicle, epididymis, and the vas deferens, which travels upward into the inguinal ring. Normally the left testicle is lower than the right. Inspect the size, color, shape, and symmetry of the scrotum while observing for lesions or edema.

Gently lift the scrotum to view the posterior surface. The scrotal skin is usually loose, and the surface is coarse. The skin

BOX 15-21   PATIENT TEACHING

Male Genitalia Assessment

OUTCOMES

- Patient will perform genital self-examination and testicular self-examination.
- Patient will describe methods to prevent sexually transmitted infections (STIs).
- Patient will follow safe sex practices.

TEACHING STRATEGIES

- **Provide the following information about genital self-examination to all male patients 15 years and older:**
  - Perform the examination monthly, after a warm bath or shower, when the scrotal sac is relaxed and less thick.
  - Stand naked in front of a mirror, hold the penis in your hand, and examine the head. Pull back the foreskin if uncircumcised to expose the glans.
  - Inspect and palpate the entire head of the penis in a clockwise motion, looking carefully for any bumps, sores, blisters, or unusual discharge. Blisters and bumps may be light colored or red and resemble pimples.
  - Look for genital warts.
  - Look at the opening (urethral meatus) at the end of the penis for discharge.
  - Look along the entire shaft of the penis for the same signs.
  - Be sure to separate pubic hair at the base of the penis and carefully examine the skin underneath.
- **Provide the following information about testicular self-examination (TSE) to all men 15 years and older:**
  - Look for swelling or lumps in the skin of the scrotum while looking in the mirror.
  - Use both hands, placing the index and middle fingers under the testicles and the thumb on top (see the illustration).
  - Gently roll the testicle, feeling for lumps, swelling, soreness, or change in consistency (hardening).
  - Find the epididymis (a cordlike structure on the top and back of the testicle; it is not a lump).
  - Feel for small, pea-size lumps on the front and side of the testicle. The lumps are usually painless and are abnormal.
  - Call your health care provider about abnormal findings.
- Counsel patients with STIs about diagnosis and treatment.

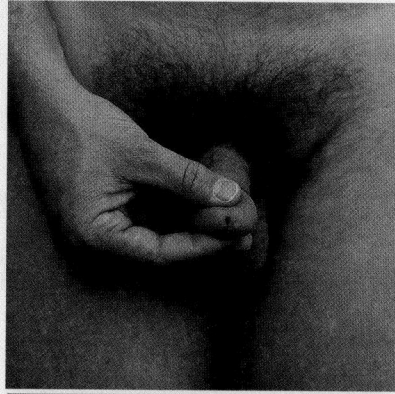
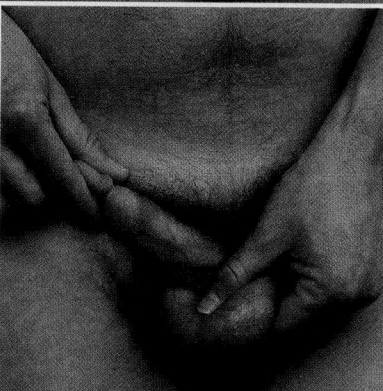

- Explain warning signs of STIs: Pain on urination and during sex, abnormal penile discharge (different from usual), swollen lymph nodes, or rash or ulcer on skin or genitalia.
- Teach measures to prevent STIs: Use of condoms, avoiding sex with infected partners, restricting number of sexual partners, avoiding sex with persons who have multiple partners, using regular perineal hygiene.
- Tell patients with an STI to inform sexual partner(s) of the need to have an examination.
- Instruct patient to seek treatment as soon as possible if partner becomes infected with an STI.

EVALUATION STRATEGIES

- Observe patient demonstrate genital self-examination and testicular self-examination.
- Ask patient to describe methods for preventing and treating STIs.

Illustrations from Seidel HM and others: *Mosby's guide to physical examination*, ed 6, St. Louis, 2006, Mosby.

---

color is often more deeply pigmented than body skin. Tightening or loss of wrinkling reveals edema. The size of the scrotum normally changes with temperature variations because its dartos muscle contracts in cold and relaxes in warm temperature. Lumps in the scrotal skin are commonly sebaceous cysts.

Testicular cancer is a solid tumor commonly found in young men ages 18 to 34 years. Early detection is critical.

Explain testicular self-examination while examining the patient. The testes are normally sensitive but not tender. The underlying testicles are normally ovoid and approximately 2 by 4 cm (⅘ by 1⅗ inches) in size. While the patient retracts the penis upward, gently palpate the testes and epididymis between the thumb and first two fingers (Figure 15-53). Note the size, shape, and consistency of tissue, and ask if the pa-

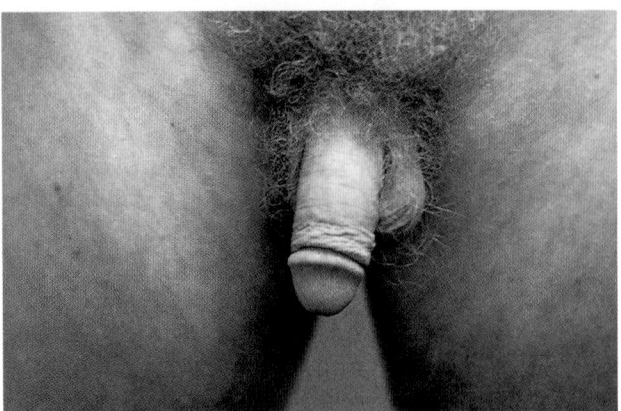

Figure 15-52 ■ Normal male genitalia (circumcised). (From Seidel HM and others: *Mosby's guide to physical examination,* ed 6, St. Louis, 2006, Mosby.)

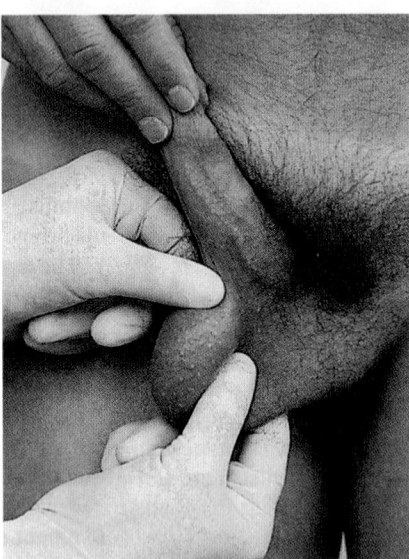

Figure 15-53 ■ Palpating contents of scrotal sac. (From Seidel HM and others: *Mosby's guide to physical examination,* ed 6, St. Louis, 2006. Mosby.)

tient feels any tenderness. The testes feel smooth and rubbery and are free from nodules. The epididymis is resilient. In the older adult the testicles decrease in size and are less firm during palpation. The most common symptoms of testicular cancer are a painless enlargement of one testis and appearance of a palpable small, hard lump about the size of a pea on the front or side of the testicle. Continue to palpate the vas deferens separately as it forms the spermatic cord toward the inguinal ring, noting nodules or swelling. It normally feels smooth and discrete.

Inguinal Ring and Canal

The external inguinal ring provides the opening for the spermatic cord to pass into the inguinal canal. The canal forms a passage through the abdominal wall, a potential site for hernia formation. A hernia is a protrusion of a portion of intestine through the inguinal wall or canal. Sometimes an intestinal loop enters the scrotum. The patient stands during this portion of the examination.

During inspection ask the patient to strain or bear down. The maneuver will help to make a hernia more visible. Look for obvious bulging in the inguinal area. Complete the examination by palpating for inguinal lymph nodes. Normally, small, nontender, mobile horizontal nodes are palpable. Any abnormality indicates local or systemic infection or malignant disease.

RECTUM AND ANUS

A good time to perform the rectal examination is after the genital examination. Usually you do not perform the examination in young children or adolescents. The examination detects colorectal cancer in its early stages. In men the rectal examination also detects prostatic tumors. The rectal examination is uncomfortable, so explaining all steps helps the patient relax.

Nursing History

The nursing history reviews the patient's personal and family history of colorectal cancer, polyps, or inflammatory bowel disease. Determine whether the patient has experienced bleeding from the rectum, black or tarry stools (melena), rectal pain, or change in bowel habits, all of which are warning signs of colorectal cancer. Assess the patient's dietary habits, including intake of high-fat foods, diet high in processed or red meats, or deficient fiber content, which are linked to colon cancer. Determine whether the patient has undergone screening for colorectal cancer (digital examination, fecal occult blood test, flexible sigmoidoscopy, and colonoscopy). Ask male patients if they have experienced weak or interrupted urine flow, an inability to urinate, or difficulty in starting or stopping the urine flow. In addition, ask if they have had polyuria; nocturia; hematuria; dysuria; or continuing pain in the lower back, pelvis, or upper thighs. These all are warning signs of prostate cancer. Also review the patient's use of laxatives, cathartics, codeine, or iron preparations, which can cause elimination problems (Box 15-22).

Inspection

Female patients remain in the dorsal recumbent position following genitalia examination, or they assume a side-lying (Sims') position. The best way to examine men is to have the patient stand and bend over forward with the hips flexed and upper body resting across the examination table. Examine a nonambulatory patient in Sims' position.

Using the nondominant hand, gently retract the buttocks to view the perianal and sacrococcygeal areas. Perianal skin is smooth and more pigmented and coarser than skin overlying the buttocks. Inspect anal tissue for skin characteristics, lesions, external hemorrhoids (dilated veins that appear as reddened skin protrusions), ulcers, inflammation, rashes, or excoriation. Anal tissues are moist and hairless, and the anus is held closed by the voluntary external sphincter. Next, ask the patient to bear down as though having a bowel movement. Any internal hemorrhoids or fissures will appear at this time. Use clock referents (e.g., 12 o'clock or 5 o'clock) to describe the location of findings. There normally is no protrusion of tissue.

BOX 15-22   PATIENT TEACHING

Rectal and Anal Assessment

OUTCOMES
- Patient will have a regular digital rectal examination performed appropriate to age.
- Patient will be able to identify symptoms of colorectal and prostatic cancer.

TEACHING STRATEGIES
- Discuss the American Cancer Society's (ACS's) guidelines (2009b) for early detection of colorectal cancer. Beginning at age 50, both men and women at average risk should use one of these screening tests:
  - Fecal occult blood test (FOBT) or fecal immunochemical test (FIT) yearly
  - Flexible sigmoidoscopy (FSIG): Visual inspection of the rectum and lower colon with a hollow, lighted tube performed by a health care provider every 5 years
  - Annual FOBT and FSIG every 5 years (preferred)
  - Double-contrast barium enema every 5 years
  - Colonoscopy every 10 years
  - CT colonoscopy every 5 years
- Individuals at increased risk need to discuss options with their health care provider
- Discuss warning signs of colorectal cancer.
- Discuss dietary planning and healthy lifestyle choices to maintain or improve colon health.
- Warn patients about problems caused by overuse of laxatives, cathartic medications, codeine, or enemas.

- Discuss with male patients the ACS's guidelines (2009b) for early detection of prostatic cancer:
  - The ACS does not support routine testing at this time.
  - Health care professionals should discuss potential benefits and limitations of prostate cancer early detection testing with men before any testing begins. This discussion should include an offer for testing with the prostate specific antigen (PSA) blood test and digital rectal examination yearly, beginning at age 50.
  - This discussion should start at age 45 for men at high risk. This includes African American men and men who have a first-degree relative diagnosed with prostate cancer at an early age (before 65).
- Discuss with male patients the warning signs of prostate cancer.

EVALUATION STRATEGIES
- During future visits, determine whether patient has had a rectal examination performed.
- Have patient explain warning signs of colorectal and prostate cancer.
- Ask the patient to describe lifestyle and food choices that maintain colon health.

Digital Palpation

Examine the anal canal and sphincters with digital palpation. In male patients, palpate the prostate gland to rule out enlargement. Usually advanced practitioners perform this portion of the examination.

MUSCULOSKELETAL SYSTEM

Conduct the musculoskeletal assessment as a separate examination, or integrate it into other parts of the total physical examination. Assess this system while performing other nursing care measures such as bathing or positioning. The assessment of the musculoskeletal system focuses on determining range of joint motion, muscle strength and tone, and joint and muscle condition. Frequently, muscular disorders are the result of neurological disease. For this reason health care providers often conduct a neurological assessment simultaneously.

While examining the patient's musculoskeletal function, visualize the anatomy of bone and muscle placement and joint structure (see Chapter 35). Joints vary in their degree of mobility. Some, as in the knee, are freely movable. The spinal vertebrae are examples of slightly movable joints. For a complete examination expose the muscles and joints so that they are free to move. Have the patient assume a sitting, supine, prone, or standing position while assessing muscle groups.

Nursing History

Determine the patient's involvement in competitive sports that may lead to a sports injury. Review the patient's history for osteoporosis risk factors, including the following: use of alcohol/caffeine; cigarette smoking; constant dieting; calcium intake less than 500 mg daily; thin and light body frame; nulliparous status; menopause before age 45; estrogen deficiency; postmenopause status; family history of osteoporosis; white, Asian, or Native American, or Northern European ancestry; advanced age; history of fractures/falls; sedentary lifestyle; chronic diseases (e.g., Cushing's disease, hyperthyroidism and hypothyroidism, malabsorption/malnutrition disorders, and neoplasms); long-term use of corticosteroids, methotrexate, phenytoin, and aluminum-containing antacids; lack of exposure to sunlight (Holcomb, 2006).

The nursing history includes the patient's description of any problems with bone, muscle, or joint function, including history of recent falls, trauma, lifting heavy objects, fractures, and bone or joint disease. It is useful to assess the patient's normal activity pattern, including the type of exercise routinely performed (Box 15-23). Also assess the nature and extent of pain or stiffness, and determine if alterations affect the patient's ability to perform ADLs and participate in social activities.

General Inspection

Observe the patient's gait and posture when entering the examination room. When a patient is unaware that he or she is

BOX 15-23   PATIENT TEACHING

Musculoskeletal Assessment

OUTCOMES
- Patient will follow measures to prevent or minimize osteoporosis.
- Patient will maintain proper body posture.

TEACHING STRATEGIES
- Instruct the patient in correct postural alignment. Consult with a physical therapist to provide the patient with exercises for improving posture.
- For women age 65 and older recommend routine screening for osteoporosis (Prihar and Katz, 2008). Recommend men for screening as well; they are equally at risk for development of osteoporosis as they age.
- To reduce bone demineralization, instruct older adults in a proper exercise program (e.g., weight-bearing, muscle-strengthening exercise) to be followed 3 or more times a week.
- Encourage intake of calcium and vitamin D to meet the recommended daily allowance. Increased vitamin D will aid calcium absorption.
- Recommendation for calcium supplements for adults over age 25 is 1000 to 1500 mg/day. For vitamin D supplements, instruct patients to take no more than 500 mg of calcium at one time.
- Explain to patients with low back pain that they will benefit from modification of worker risk factors (e.g., lifting heavy weights, use of protective equipment), regular aerobic exercise, exercises that strengthen the back and increase trunk flexibility, and learning how to lift properly.
- Instruct patient in use of assistive devices (e.g., zippers on clothing instead of buttons, elevation of chairs to minimize bending of knees and hips) when patient is unable to perform activities of daily living.
- Instruct older adults and those with osteoporosis in proper body mechanics and range-of-motion and moderate weight-bearing exercises (e.g., swimming, walking) to minimize trauma and subsequent bone fractures.
- Instruct older patients to pace activities to compensate for loss in muscle strength.

EVALUATION STRATEGIES
- Observe patient's posture.
- Ask patient to describe methods to prevent osteoporosis.
- Observe patient perform range-of-motion exercises.
- Have patient or family member describe use of self-care aids.

being observed, gait is more natural. Later a more formal test has the patient walk in a straight line away, turn, and return to the origin point. Note how the patient walks, sits, and rises from a sitting position. Normally patients walk with arms swinging freely at the sides and the head leading the body. Older adults walk with smaller steps and a wider base of sup-

port. Note foot dragging, limping, shuffling, and the position of the trunk in relation to the legs.

Observe the patient from the side in a standing position. The normal standing posture is an upright stance with parallel alignment of the hips and shoulders (Figure 15-54). There should be an even contour of the shoulders, level scapulae and iliac crests, alignment of the head over the gluteal folds, and symmetry of extremities. Looking sideways at the patient, note the normal cervical, thoracic, and lumbar curves. Holding the head erect is normal. As the patient sits, some degree of rounding of the shoulders is normal. Older adults tend to assume a stooped, forward-bent posture, with hips and knees somewhat flexed and arms bent at the elbows, raising the level of the arms.

Common postural abnormalities include kyphosis, lordosis, and scoliosis. Kyphosis, or hunchback, is an exaggeration of the posterior curvature of the thoracic spine. This postural abnormality is common in the older adult. Lordosis, or swayback, is an increased lumbar curvature. A lateral spinal curvature is called scoliosis. Loss of height is frequently the first clinical sign of osteoporosis, in which height loss occurs in the trunk as a result of vertebral fracture and collapse. Osteoporosis is a metabolic bone disease that causes a decrease in quality and quantity of bone. Osteoporosis affects 10 million Americans, and another 34 million are diagnosed with osteopenia, the majority of which are women (Silverman, 2008). This disease now affects 1 to 2 million men, and it will affect another 6 million women (Liu and others, 2008). Although a small amount of height loss is expected with aging, if the amount of loss is great, osteoporosis is likely. As men and women age, they are more likely to have osteoporotic fractures of the forearm/wrists, hips, and vertebrae (Holcomb, 2006).

During general inspection look at the extremities for overall size, gross deformity, bony enlargement, alignment, and symmetry. Normally there is bilateral symmetry in length, circumference, alignment, and position and number of skin folds (Seidel and others, 2006). A general review pinpoints areas requiring specialized assessment.

Palpation

Apply gentle palpation to all bones, joints, and surrounding muscles during a complete examination. In the case of a focused assessment, examine only the involved area. Note any heat, tenderness, edema, or resistance to pressure. The patient should feel no discomfort when you apply palpation. Muscles should be firm.

Range of Joint Motion

The examination includes comparison of both active and passive full ROM. Ask the patient to put each major joint and its muscle groups through full ROM. Learn the terminology for each joint movement (Table 15-8), and instruct the patient in how to move through each range of motion. To assess passive ROM, ask the patient to relax and then passively move the joints through their ROM. Compare the same body parts for equality in movement. Do not force a joint into a painful position. Know the normal range of each joint and the extent

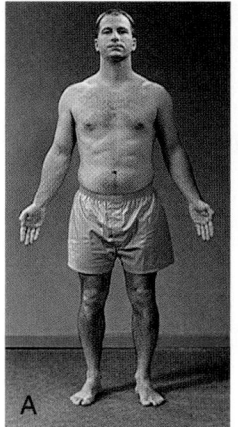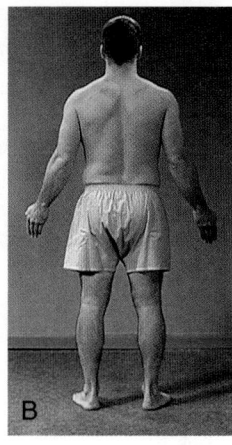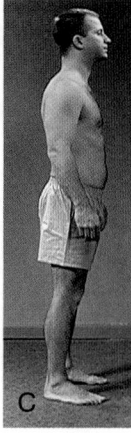

Figure 15-54 ■ Inspection of overall body posture. **A,** Anterior view. **B,** Posterior view. **C,** Lateral view. (From Seidel HM and others: *Mosby's guide to physical examination,* ed 6, St. Louis, 2006, Mosby.)

TABLE 15-8	Terminology for Normal Range-of-Motion Positions	
TERM	**RANGE OF MOTION**	**EXAMPLES OF JOINTS**
Flexion	Movement decreasing angle between two adjoining bones; bending of limb	Elbow, fingers, knee
Extension	Movement increasing angle between two adjoining bones	Elbow, fingers, knee
Hyper-extension	Movement of body part beyond its normal resting extended position	Head
Pronation	Movement of body part so that front or ventral surface faces downward	Hand, forearm
Supination	Movement of body part so that front or ventral surface faces upward	Hand, forearm
Abduction	Movement of extremity away from midline of body	Leg, arm, fingers
Adduction	Movement of extremity toward midline of body	Leg, arm, fingers
Internal rotation	Rotation of joint inward	Knee, hip
External rotation	Rotation of joint outward	Knee, hip
Eversion	Turning of body part away from midline	Foot
Inversion	Turning of body part toward midline	Foot
Dorsiflexion	Flexion of toes and foot upward	Foot
Plantar flexion	Bending of toes and foot downward	Foot

to which you can move the patient's joints. Ideally, assess the patient's normal range to determine a baseline for assessing later change. Joints are typically free from stiffness, instability, swelling, or inflammation. There should be no discomfort when applying pressure to bones and joints. In older adults, joints often become swollen and stiff, with reduced ROM resulting from cartilage erosion and fibrosis of synovial membranes. If a joint appears swollen and inflamed, palpate it for warmth.

Muscle Tone and Strength

Assess muscle strength and tone during ROM measurement. Note muscle tone, the slight muscular resistance felt as you move the relaxed extremity passively through its range of motion. Ask the patient to allow an extremity to relax or hang limp. This is often difficult, particularly if the patient feels pain in the extremity. Support the extremity and grasp each limb, moving it through the normal ROM (Figure 15-55). Normal tone causes a mild, even resistance to passive movement through the entire range.

If a muscle has increased tone, or hypertonicity, you will meet considerable resistance with sudden passive movement of a joint. Continued movement eventually causes the muscle to relax. A muscle that has little tone (hypotonicity) feels flabby. The involved extremity hangs loosely in a position determined by gravity.

For assessment of muscle strength the patient assumes a stable position. The patient performs maneuvers demonstrating strength of major muscle groups (Table 15-9). Compare symmetrical muscle pairs for strength, based on a grading scale of 0 to 5 (Table 15-10). The arm on the dominant side is normally stronger than the arm on the nondominant side. In the older adult a loss of muscle mass causes bilateral weakness, but muscle strength remains greater in the dominant arm or leg.

Examine each muscle group. Ask the patient first to flex the muscle to be examined and then to resist when you apply opposing force against that flexion. It is important to not allow the patient to move the joint. Gradually increase pressure to a muscle group (e.g., elbow extension). Have the patient resist the pressure applied by attempting to move against resistance (e.g., elbow flexion). The patient resists until instructed to stop. Vary the amount of pressure applied, and then observe the joint move. If you identify a weakness, compare the size of the muscle with its opposite counterpart by measuring the circumference of the muscle body with a tape measure. A muscle that has atrophied (reduced in size) feels soft and baggy when palpated.

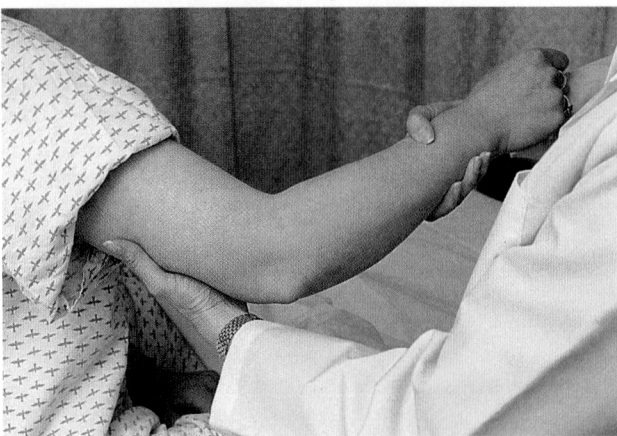

Figure 15-55 ■ Assess muscle tone.

TABLE 15-9 Maneuvers to Assess Muscle Strength

MUSCLE GROUP	MANEUVER
Neck (sterno-cleidomastoid)	Place hand firmly against patient's upper jaw. Ask patient to turn head laterally against resistance.
Shoulder (trapezius)	Place hand over midline of patient's shoulder, exerting firm pressure. Have patient raise shoulders against resistance.
Elbow	
Biceps	Pull down on forearm as patient attempts to flex arm.
Triceps	As you flex patient's arm, apply pressure against forearm. Ask patient to straighten arm.
Hip	
Quadriceps	When patient is sitting, apply downward pressure to thigh. Ask patient to raise leg up from table.
Gastrocnemius	Patient sits while examiner holds shin of flexed leg. Ask patient to straighten leg against resistance.

TABLE 15-10 Muscle Strength

MUSCLE FUNCTION LEVEL	SCALES	
	GRADE	% NORMAL
No evidence of contractility	0	0
Trace of movement	1	10
Full range of motion, not against gravity*	2	25
Full range of motion against gravity but not against resistance	3	50
Full range of motion against gravity and some resistance, but weak	4	75
Full range of motion against gravity, full resistance	5	100

From Seidel HM and others: *Mosby's guide to physical examination,* ed 6, St. Louis, 2006, Mosby.
*Passive movement.

NEUROLOGICAL SYSTEM

An assessment of neurological function alone is quite time consuming. For efficiency, integrate neurological measurements with other parts of the physical examination. For example, test cranial nerve function during the survey of the head and neck. Observe mental and emotional status during the initial interview.

Consider many variables when deciding the extent of the examination. A patient's level of consciousness influences the ability to follow directions. General physical status influences tolerance to assessment. The patient's chief complaint also helps to determine the need for a thorough neurological assessment. If the patient complains of headache or a recent loss of function in an extremity, the patient will need a complete neurological assessment. For a complete examination, you will need the following special equipment:

- Reading material
- Vials of aromatic substances (e.g., vanilla extract and coffee)
- Opposite tip of cotton swab or tongue blade broken in half
- Snellen eye chart
- Penlight
- Vials containing sugar or salt
- Tongue blade
- Two test tubes, one containing hot water, the other containing cold
- Cotton balls or cotton-tipped applicators
- Tuning fork
- Reflex hammer

Nursing History

Review the patient's use of analgesics, alcohol, sedative-hypnotics, antipsychotics, antidepressants, nervous system stimulants, or recreational drugs. Determine if the patient has a recent history of seizures/convulsions, and screen the patient for symptoms of headache, tremors, dizziness, vertigo, numbness or tingling of body parts, visual changes, weakness, pain, or changes in speech. The presence of any symptom then requires a more detailed review (e.g., onset, severity, precipitating factors, or sequence of events). Discuss with the patient's family any recent changes in the patient's behavior (e.g., increased irritability, mood swings, memory loss, or change in energy level). Ask the patient for a history of changes in vision, hearing, smell, taste, and touch. A history of head or spinal cord trauma, meningitis, congenital anomalies, neurological disease, or psychiatric counseling will focus your assessment of select findings. If an older adult patient displays sudden acute confusion (delirium), review history for drug toxicity, serious infections, metabolic disturbances, heart failure, and severe anemia.

Mental and Emotional Status

You learn about mental capacities and emotional state by interacting with the patient. Ask questions during an examination to gather data and observe the appropriateness of emotions and thoughts. There are special assessment tools designed to assess a patient's mental status. For example, the Mini-Mental State Examination (MMSE) measures patient's orientation and cognitive function. The MMSE asks questions such as "What is the date?"

To ensure an objective assessment, consider the patient's cultural and educational background, values, beliefs, and previous experiences. An alteration in mental or emotional status reflects a disturbance in cerebral functioning. The cerebral cortex controls and integrates intellectual and emotional functioning. Primary brain disorders, medications, and metabolic changes are examples of factors that change cerebral function.

Level of Consciousness

A person's level of consciousness exists along a continuum from being fully awake, alert, and cooperative to unresponsiveness to any form of external stimuli. Talk with the patient, asking questions about events involving the patient or concerns about any health problem. A fully conscious patient responds to questions quickly and expresses ideas logically. As the patient's consciousness lowers, use the Glasgow Coma Scale (GCS) for an objective measurement of consciousness on a numerical scale (Table 15-11). The patient needs to be as alert as possible before testing. Use caution when using the scale if a patient has sensory losses (e.g., vision or hearing). The GCS allows evaluation of a patient's neurological status over time. The higher the score, the better the patient's neurological function. Ask short, simple questions, such as "What is your name?" or "Where are you?" Also ask the patient to follow simple commands, such as "Move your toes."

If a patient is not conscious enough to follow commands, try to elicit a pain response. Apply firm pressure with the thumb over the root of the patient's fingernail. The normal response to painful stimuli is withdrawal of the body part from the stimulus.

Behavior and Appearance

Behaviors, moods, hygiene, grooming, and choice of dress reveal pertinent information about mental status. Remain perceptive of the patient's mannerisms and actions during the entire physical assessment. Note both nonverbal and verbal behaviors. Does the patient respond appropriately to directions? Does the patient's mood vary with no apparent cause? Does the patient show concern about appearance? Is the patient's hair clean and neatly groomed, and are the nails

ACTION	RESPONSE	SCORE
Eyes open	Spontaneously	4
	To speech	3
	To pain	2
	None	1
Best verbal response	Oriented	5
	Confused	4
	Inappropriate words	3
	Incomprehensible sounds	2
	None	1
Best motor response	Obeys commands	6
	Localized pain	5
	Flexion withdrawal	4
	Abnormal flexion	3
	Abnormal extension	2
	Flaccid	1
Patient's total score ranges from 3 to 15		

TABLE 15-11 Glasgow Coma Scale

trimmed and clean? The patient should behave in a manner expressing concern and interest in the examination. The patient should make eye contact and express appropriate feelings that correspond to the situation. Normally the patient's appearance will show some degree of personal hygiene.

Choice and fit of clothing reflect socioeconomic background or personal taste rather than deficiency in self-concept or self-care. Avoid being judgmental, and focus assessments on the appropriateness of clothing for the weather. Older adults sometimes neglect their appearance because of a lack of energy, finances, or reduced vision.

Language

Normal cerebral function allows a person to understand spoken or written words and to express the self through written words or gestures. Assess the patient's voice inflection, tone, and manner of speech. Normally the patient's voice has inflections, is clear and strong, and increases in volume appropriately. Speech is fluent. When communication is clearly ineffective (e.g., omission or addition of letters and words, misuse of words, or hesitations), assess the patient for aphasia. Injury to the cerebral cortex results in aphasia.

The two types of aphasia are sensory (or receptive) and motor (or expressive). With receptive aphasia a person cannot understand written or verbal speech. With expressive aphasia a person understands written and verbal speech but cannot write or speak appropriately when attempting to communicate. A patient sometimes suffers from a combination of receptive and expressive aphasia. When communication is ineffective, assess language capabilities with simple assessment techniques. Ask the patient to name familiar objects when pointing at them. Ask the patient to respond to simple verbal commands, such as "Stand up." Finally, ask the patient to read a simple sentence out loud. Normally a patient names objects correctly, follows commands, and reads sentences correctly.

Intellectual Function

Intellectual function includes memory, knowledge, abstract thinking, and judgment. Testing each aspect of function involves a specific technique. However, because cultural and educational background influences the ability to respond to test questions, do not ask questions related to concepts or ideas with which the patient is unfamiliar.

MEMORY Assess immediate recall and recent and remote memory. Patients demonstrate immediate recall by repeating a series of numbers in the order they are presented or in reverse order. Patients normally recall five to eight digits forward or four to six digits backward.

First ask to test the patient's memory. Then state clearly and slowly the names of three unrelated objects. After stating all three, ask the patient to repeat each. Continue until the patient is successful. Then, later in the assessment, ask the patient to repeat the three words again. The patient should be able to identify the three words. Another test for recent memory involves asking the patient to recall events occurring during the same day (e.g., what was eaten for breakfast). Validate information with a family member.

To assess past memory, ask the patient to recall the maiden name of the patient's mother, a birthday, or a special date in history. It is best to ask open-ended questions rather than simple yes/no questions. A patient usually has immediate recall of such information. With older adults do not interpret a hearing loss as confusion. Good communication techniques are necessary throughout the examination to ensure the patient clearly understands all the directions and testing.

KNOWLEDGE Assess knowledge by asking how much the patient knows about his or her illness or the reason for hospitalization. You can also ask the patient questions about basic facts (e.g., who is the president?). By assessing a patient's knowledge, you can determine the patient's ability to learn or understand. If there is an opportunity to teach, test the patient's mental status by asking for feedback during a follow-up visit.

ABSTRACT THINKING Interpreting abstract ideas or concepts reflects the capacity for abstract thinking. For an individual to explain common sayings such as "A stitch in time saves nine" or "Don't count your chickens before they're hatched," requires a higher level of intellectual functioning. Note whether the patient's explanations are relevant and concrete. The patient with altered mental state will probably interpret the phrase literally or will merely rephrase the words.

JUDGMENT Judgment requires a comparison and evaluation of facts and ideas to understand their relationships and to form appropriate conclusions. Attempt to measure the patient's ability to make logical decisions with questions such as "Why did you decide to seek health care?" or "What would you do if you suddenly became ill at home?" Normally a patient makes logical decisions.

Cranial Nerve Function

To assess cranial nerve function, you may test all 12 cranial nerves or a single nerve or related group of nerves. A dysfunction in one nerve reflects an alteration at some point along the distribution of the cranial nerve. Measurements used to assess the integrity of organs within the head and neck also assess cranial nerve function. A complete assessment involves testing the 12 cranial nerves in order of their numbers. To remember the order of the nerves, use this simple phrase: "On old Olympus' towering tops a Finn and German viewed some hops." The first letter of each word in the phrase is the same as the first letter of the names of the cranial nerves listed in order (Table 15-12).

Sensory Function

The sensory pathways of the central nervous system conduct the sensations of pain, temperature, position, vibration, and crude and finely localized touch. Different nerve pathways relay the sensations. Most patients require only a quick screening of sensory function, unless there are symptoms of reduced sensation, motor impairment, or paralysis.

Normally a patient has sensory responses to all stimuli tested. A patient feels sensations equally on both sides of the body in all areas. Perform all sensory testing with the patient's eyes closed so that the patient is unable to see when or where a stimulus strikes the skin (Table 15-13). Then apply stimuli in a random, unpredictable order to maintain the patient's attention and to prevent detection of a predictable pattern. Ask the patient to describe when, what, and where each stimulus is felt. Compare symmetrical areas of the body while applying stimuli to the arms, trunk, and legs.

Motor Function

An assessment of motor function includes measurements made during the musculoskeletal examination. In addition, you assess cerebellar function. The cerebellum coordinates muscular activity, maintains balance and equilibrium, and helps to control posture. Patients with any degree of motor dysfunction are at risk for injury (Box 15-24).

COORDINATION To avoid confusion, demonstrate each maneuver and then have the patient repeat it while you observe for smoothness and balance in the patient's movement. In older adults normally slow reaction time causes movements to be less rhythmical.

To assess fine motor function, have the patient extend the arms out to the sides and touch each forefinger alternately to the nose (first with eyes open, then with eyes closed). Normally the patient alternately touches the nose smoothly. Performing rapid, rhythmical, alternating movements demonstrates coordination in the upper extremities. While sitting, the patient begins by patting the knees with both hands. Then the patient alternately turns up the palm and back of the hands while continuously patting the knees. Patients should do the maneuver smoothly and regularly with increasing speed.

TABLE 15-12 Cranial Nerve Function and Assessment

CRANIAL NERVE	NAME	TYPE	FUNCTION	ASSESSMENT METHOD
I	Olfactory	Sensory	Sense of smell	Ask patient to identify different aromas in each nostril such as coffee and vanilla.
II	Optic	Sensory	Visual acuity and visual fields	Use Snellen chart, or ask patient to read printed material while wearing glasses.
III	Oculomotor	Motor	Pupil constriction and dilation Extraocular eye movement	Assess directions of gaze. Measure pupil reaction to light reflex and accommodation.
IV	Trochlear	Motor	Upward and downward movement of eyeball	Assess directions of gaze
V	Trigeminal	Sensory and motor	Sensory nerve to skin of face	Lightly touch cornea with wisp of cotton. Assess corneal reflex. Measure sensation of light pain and touch across skin of face.
			Motor nerve to muscles of jaw	Palpate temples as patient clenches teeth, observe chewing
VI	Abducens	Motor	Lateral movement of eyeballs	Assess directions of gaze.
VII	Facial	Motor and sensory	Facial expression	Look for asymmetry as patient smiles, frowns, puffs out cheeks, and raises and lowers eyebrows.
			Taste	Have patient identify salty or sweet taste on front of tongue.
VIII	Auditory	Sensory	Hearing and equilibrium	Assess ability to hear spoken word.
IX	Glossopharyngeal	Sensory and motor	Taste	Ask patient to identify sour or sweet taste on back of tongue.
			Ability to swallow and speak	Use tongue blade to elicit gag reflex, have person swallow
X	Vagus	Sensory and motor	Sensation of pharynx and behind ear	Ask patient to say "Ah." Observe movement of palate and pharynx.
			Movement of vocal cords	Assess speech for hoarseness.
XI	Spinal accessory	Motor	Movement of head and shoulders	Ask patient to shrug shoulders and turn head against passive resistance.
XII	Hypoglossal	Motor	Position of tongue	Ask patient to stick out tongue to midline and move it from side to side.

Test lower extremity coordination with the patient lying supine, legs extended. Place your hand at the ball of the patient's foot. The patient taps the hand with the foot as quickly as possible. Test each foot for speed and smoothness. The feet do not normally move as rapidly or evenly as the hands.

BALANCE Assess balance and gross motor function by asking the patient to stand with feet together, arms at the sides, both with eyes open and closed. Protect the patient's safety by standing at the side, and observe for swaying. Expect slight swaying of the body in the Romberg's test. A loss of balance (positive Romberg) causes a patient to fall to the side.

REFLEXES Eliciting reflexes demonstrates integrity of sensory and motor pathways. There are deep tendon reflexes, elicited by mildly stretching a muscle and tapping a tendon, and cutaneous reflexes elicited by stimulating the skin superficially.

AFTER THE EXAMINATION

Record findings from the physical assessment during the examination or at the end. Special forms are available to record data. Review all findings before assisting the patient with dressing in case of a need to recheck any information or gather additional data. Integrate physical assessment findings into the plan of care. Be sure to record a complete assessment.

After completing the assessment, give the patient time to dress. The hospitalized patient sometimes needs help with hygiene and returning to bed. When the patient is comfortable, it helps to share a summary of the assessment findings. If the findings have revealed serious abnormalities, such as an irregular heart rate, consult the patient's health care provider before revealing any findings. It is the health care provider's responsibility to make definitive medical diagnoses. Explain the type of abnormality found and the need for the health care provider to conduct an additional examination.

Delegate the cleaning of the examination area to support staff if needed. Use infection control practices in removing materials or instruments soiled with potentially infectious wastes. If the patient's bedside was the site for the examination, clear away soiled items from the bedside table and make sure the bed linen is dry and clean. The patient will appreciate a clean gown and the opportunity to wash the face and hands. Afterward, be sure to perform hand hygiene.

The patient often needs a number of ancillary examinations such as x-ray examinations, laboratory tests, or ultrasonography after a physical examination. The tests provide additional screening information to rule out and to help diagnose specific abnormalities found during the examination. Explain the purpose of these tests and the sensations that the patient will experience.

TABLE 15-13   Assessment of Sensory Nerve Function

FUNCTION	EQUIPMENT	METHOD	PRECAUTIONS
Pain	End of paper clip or wooden end of cotton applicator	Ask patient to voice when he or she feels dull or sharp sensation. Alternately apply sharp and blunt ends of paper clip to skin's surface. Note areas of numbness or increased sensitivity.	Remember that areas where skin is thickened, such as heel or sole of foot, are less sensitive to pain.
Temperature	Two test tubes, one filled with hot water; one with cold	Touch skin with tube. Ask patient to identify hot or cold sensation.	Omit test if pain sensation is normal.
Light touch	Cotton ball or cotton-tipped applicator	Apply light wisp of cotton to different points along skin's surface. Ask patient to voice when he or she feels sensation.	Apply at areas where skin is thin or more sensitive (e.g., face, neck, inner aspect of arms, top of feet and hands).
Vibration	Tuning fork	Apply stem of vibrating fork to distal interphalangeal joint of fingers and interphalangeal joint of great toe, elbow, and wrist. Have patient voice when and where he or she feels vibration.	Be sure patient feels vibration and not merely pressure.
Position		Grasp finger or toe, holding it by its sides with thumb and index finger. Alternate moving finger or toe up and down. Ask patient to state when finger is up or down. Repeat with toes.	Avoid rubbing adjacent appendages as you move finger or toe. Do not move joint laterally; return to neutral position before moving again.
Two-point discrimination	Two ends of paper clip	Lightly apply one or both ends of paper clip simultaneously to skin's surface. Ask patient whether he or she feels one or two pricks. Find the distance at which patient can no longer distinguish two points.	Apply paper clip tips to same anatomical site (e.g., fingertips, palm of hand, upper arms). Minimum distance at which patient discriminates two points varies (2 to 8 mm on fingertips).

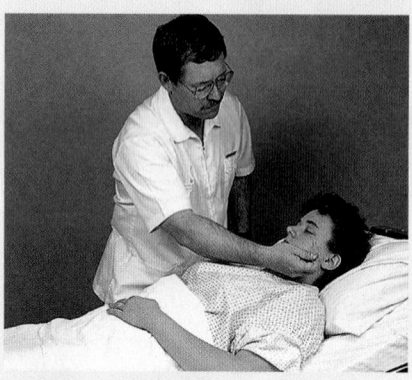

BOX 15-24 PATIENT TEACHING

Neurological Assessment

OUTCOMES

- Patient's family will understand the relationship of patient's behavioral and mental changes to physical status.
- Patient with sensory or motor impairment will select safety measure to use for self-care.
- Older adults will do routine skin inspection for injuries.

TEACHING STRATEGIES

- Teach patients that with any sudden weakness in their extremities or change in speech they need to seek emergency medical care to rule out stroke.
- Explain to family or friends the implications of any behavioral or mental impairment shown by the patient.
- If patient has sensory or motor impairments, explain measures to ensure safety (e.g., use of ambulation aids, use of safety bars in bathrooms or on stairways).

- Teach older adults to plan enough time to complete tasks because their reaction time is slow.
- Teach older adults to observe skin surface for areas of trauma because their perception of pain is reduced.

EVALUATION STRATEGIES

- Ask family to discuss patient behaviors that result from neurological impairments.
- Have patient explain safety measures used to prevent injury from sensory or motor limitations.
- Have older patient explain rationale for routine skin inspection.

KEY POINTS

- Baseline assessment findings reflect the patient's functional abilities and serve as the basis for comparison with subsequent assessment findings.
- Physical assessment of a child or infant requires the application of the principles of growth and development.
- Recognize that the normal process of aging affects physical findings collected from an older adult.
- Integrate patient teaching throughout the examination to help patients learn about health promotion and disease prevention.
- Inspection requires good lighting, full exposure of the body part, and a careful comparison of the part with its counterpart on the opposite side of the body.
- Palpation involves the use of parts of the hand to detect different types of physical characteristics.
- Use auscultation to assess the character of sounds created in various body organs.
- Perform a physical examination only after proper preparation of the environment and equipment and after preparing the patient physically and psychologically.
- Throughout the examination keep the patient warm, comfortable, and informed of each step of the assessment process.
- A competent examiner learns to be systematic while combining assessments of different body systems simultaneously.

- Information from the history helps to focus on body systems likely to be affected.
- Creating a mental image of internal organs in relation to external anatomical landmarks enhances accuracy in assessing the thorax, heart, and abdomen.
- When assessing heart sounds, imagine events occurring during the cardiac cycle.
- Never palpate the carotid arteries simultaneously.
- When examining a woman's breasts, explain the techniques for breast self-examination.
- The abdominal assessment differs from other portions of the examination in that auscultation follows inspection.
- During assessment of the genitalia, explain the technique for genital self-examination.
- Conduct an assessment of musculoskeletal function when observing the patient ambulate or participate in other active movements.
- Assess mental and emotional status by interacting with the patient throughout the examination.
- At the end of the examination provide for the patient's comfort, and then document a detailed summary of physical assessment findings.

CRITICAL THINKING EXERCISES

Jane continues to care for Mr. Neal. He had a colon resection for cancer 2 days ago. The morning shift has just started, and the night nurse reported that he had an "uneventful" night. Mr. Neal is allowed nothing by mouth (NPO) and has an IV line for parenteral fluids, a nasogastric (NG) tube connected to low intermittent suction, an abdominal dressing, and a urethral (Foley) catheter with gravity drainage.

1. **a.** What focused systems assessments does Jane need to complete?
   b. Describe the key elements in these assessments.

2. Upon entrance into Mr. Neal's room, Jane observes that he appears agitated and confused. How would Jane further evaluate his mental status? What condition may these symptoms indicate?

3. After Jane reorients Mr. Neal, he allows her to continue with the assessment. Upon auscultation of the lateral and posterior lung fields, Jane hears a crackling noise upon inspiration. What is this sound, and what does it indicate?

4. Jane next assesses Mr. Neal's cardiac status. His apical heart rate is 84 beats per minute, rhythm regular. Jane interprets this finding as:
   a. Abnormal
   b. Bradycardia
   c. Normal
   d. Tachycardia

5. Mr. Neal complains of abdominal incision pain. After evaluation of his pain status, Jane administers pain-relief medication. Following completion of this task, she inspects and then auscultates his abdomen. Before auscultation Jane would first (1) _____. After completion of the above task (1), Jane listens for 30 seconds at a site below and to the left of the umbilicus. She is unable to hear bowel sounds. The assessment indicates that:
   a. Jane is not listening in the correct place
   b. Jane needs to listen longer
   c. Jane's patient has a partial bowel obstruction
   d. Jane's patient has peritonitis

6. When Jane is examining Mr. Neal's lower extremities, he tells her that his left calf is tender to the touch. Jane notes unilateral leg swelling, and the area is reddened and warm to the touch. The assessment indicates that the patient:
   a. Has developed a phlebitis
   b. Has muscle fatigue
   c. Should not be concerned—all patients have these symptoms after major surgery
   d. Should have a Homans' sign test performed

evolve   *Answers to Critical Thinking Questions can be found on the Evolve website.*

REVIEW QUESTIONS

1. The nurse conducts a patient assessment on a 72-year-old woman and finds a capillary refill time of 4 seconds, a nailbed angle of 160 degrees, hardened nails, and splinter hemorrhages. Which findings are abnormal? Select all that apply.
   1. Capillary refill
   2. Nailbed angle
   3. Hardened nails
   4. Splinter hemorhages

2. To correctly palpate the patient's skin for temperature, the nurse uses the:
   1. Base of the hand
   2. Fingertips of the hand
   3. Dorsal surface of the hand
   4. Palmar surface of the hand

3. The patient's respiratory assessment reveals bilateral high pitched, continuous musical sounds heard loudest upon expiration. The nurse interprets these sounds as:
   1. Normal
   2. Crackles
   3. Rhonchi
   4. Wheezes

4. While auscultating heart sounds, the nurse documents that S_1 is heard best at the apex. This sound (S_1) correlates with closure of the:
   1. Aortic and mitral valves
   2. Mitral and tricuspid valves
   3. Aortic and pulmonic valves
   4. Tricuspid and pulmonic valves

5. To assess the patient's posterior tibial pulse, the nurse palpates:
   1. Behind the knee
   2. Over the lateral malleolus
   3. In the groove behind the medial malleolus
   4. Lateral to the extensor tendon of the great toe

6. To spread the breast tissue evenly over the chest wall during an examination, the nurse asks the patient to lie supine with:
   1. Hands clasped just above the umbilicus
   2. Both arms overhead with palms upward
   3. The dominant arm straight alongside the body
   4. The ipsilateral arm overhead with a small pillow under the shoulder

7. Assessment of which body system requires you to perform auscultation before palpation?
   1. Head and neck
   2. Lungs
   3. Abdomen
   4. Heart

8. The nurse is teaching a patient how to perform a testicular self-examination. The nurse instructs the patient:
   1. "Contact your health care provider if you feel a painless pea-size nodule."
   2. "The testes are normally round and movable and have a lumpy consistency."
   3. "The best time to do a testicular self-examination is before your bath or shower."
   4. "Perform a testicular self-examination every week to detect signs of testicular cancer."

9. The patient is being assessed for range of joint movement. The nurse asks the patient to move the arm away from the body, evaluating the movement of:
   1. Flexion
   2. Extension
   3. Abduction
   4. Adduction

10. The nurse asks the patient to smile, frown, and raise and lower the eyebrows; these actions evaluate cranial nerve number:
    1. VII—facial
    2. V—trigeminal
    3. III—oculomotor
    4. XII—hypoglossal

Answers to Review Questions can be found on pages 1197-1198.

REFERENCES

American Cancer Society: *Cancer facts and figures 2009*, http://www.cancer.org/docroot/STT/STT_0.asp, 2009a, accessed 7/28/09.

American Cancer Society: American Cancer Society guidelines for the early detection of cancer, retrieved 10/24/09 at http://www, 2009b.

American Psychiatric Association: *Diagnostic and statistical manual of mental disorders*, ed 4, Washington, DC, 2000, The Association.

Anderson J and others: What can you learn from a comprehensive skin assessment, *Nursing* 37(4):65, 2007.

Bermann P: Aging skin: causes, treatment, and prevention, *Nurs Clin North Am* 42(3):485, 2007.

Cattaneo L and others: Intimate partner violence victims' accuracy in assessing their risk of re-abuse, *J Fam Violence* 22(6):429, 2007.

Cooper C and others: The prevalence of elder abuse and neglect: a systematic review, *Age Aging* 37(2):151, 2008.

DeMarco R: Primary prevention of skin cancer in children and adolescents: a review of the literature, *J Pediatr Oncol Nurs* 25(2):67, 2008.

Ebersole P and others: *Toward healthy aging*, ed 7, St. Louis, 2008, Mosby.

Edelman A and others: Pelvic examination, *N Engl J Med* 356(26):e26, 2007.

Feldstein S, Miller W: Does subtle screening for substance abuse work? A review of the Substance Abuse Subtle Screening Inventory (SASSI), *Addiction* 102(1):41, 2007.

Giger J and others: Developing cultural competence to eliminate health disparities in ethnic minorities and other vulnerable populations, *J Transcult Nurs* 18(2):95, 2007.

Goldberg MS and others: Risk factors for presumptive melanoma in skin cancer screening, *J Am Acad Dermatol* 57(1):60, 2007.

Gorski, L: Venous thromboembolism: a common and preventable condition—implications for the home care nurse, *Home Healthc Nurse* 25(2):94, 2007.

Hockenberry MJ, Wilson D: *Wong's nursing care of infants and children*, ed 8, 2007, Mosby.

Holcomb SM: Osteoporosis, *Nursing* 36(4):48, 2006.

Jarvis C: *Physical examination & health assessment*, ed 5, St. Louis, 2008, Mosby.

Liu H and others: Screening for osteoporosis in men: a systematic review for an American College of Physicians Guideline, *Ann Intern Med* 148(9):685, 2008.

Loescher L and others: Perceptions of melanoma risk communications and risk control behaviors in melanoma prone families, *Oncol Nurs Forum* 34(1):169, 2007.

McHenry L and others: *Mosby's pharmacology in nursing*, ed 22, St. Louis, 2006, Mosby.

Meiner SE, Lueckenotte A: *Gerontologic nursing*, ed 3, St. Louis, 2006, Mosby.

Moore MC: *Pocket guide to nutritional care*, ed 6, St. Louis, 2009, Elsevier Mosby.

National Cancer Institute: National Cancer Institute face sheet: cigarette smoking and cancer, retrieved 10/24/09 at http://www.cancer.gov/cancertopics/factsheet/tobacco/cancer.

Newson P: Knowledge for practice: observations and assessment, *Nurs Residential Care* 10(4):165, 2008.

Prihar B, Katz S: Patient education as a tool to increase screening for osteoporosis, *J Am Geriatr Soc* 56(5):961, 2008.

Read J and others: Why, when and how to ask about childhood abuse, *Adv Psychiatr Treatment* 13:101, 2007.

Ries R, Wilford B: *Principles of addiction medicine*, ed 4, Chevy Chase, Md, 2009, Lippincott Williams & Wilkins.

Seidel HM and others: *Mosby's guide to physical examination*, ed 6, St. Louis, 2006, Mosby.

Silverman S: Osteoporosis and the new absolute risk algorithm, *Future Rheumatol* 3(1):15, 2008.

Skin Cancer Foundation: *Skin cancer facts*, retrieved 7/20/09 at http://www.skincancer.org/skin-cancer-facts/, 2009.

Truscott W: The role of PPE in contact transfer, *Infect Control Today* 9(10):18, 2005.

Van Hook S and others: The "six T's": barriers to screening teens for substance abuse in primary care, *J Adolesc Health* 40(5):456, 2007.

Voegeli D: Care or harm: exploring components in skin care regimens, *Br J Nurs* 17(1):24, 2008.

Administering Medications

MEDIA RESOURCES

 CD COMPANION 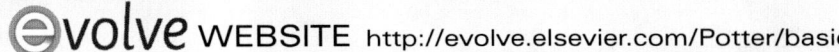 eVolve WEBSITE http://evolve.elsevier.com/Potter/basic

- Video Clips
- Crossword Puzzle
- English/Spanish Audio Glossary

OBJECTIVES

- Discuss legal responsibilities in medication prescription and administration.
- Describe the physiological mechanisms of medication action.
- Differentiate the types of adverse effects of medications.
- Discuss developmental factors that influence pharmacokinetics.
- Discuss factors that influence medication actions.
- Discuss methods used to teach a patient about prescribed medications.
- Describe the roles of the pharmacist, physician, health care provider, and nurse in medication administration.

- Describe factors to consider when choosing routes of medication administration.
- Correctly calculate a prescribed medication dosage.
- Discuss factors to include in assessing a patient's needs for and response to medication therapy.
- List the six rights of medication administration.
- Describe approaches used to reduce transmission of infection when administering medications.
- Correctly prepare and administer subcutaneous, intramuscular, and intradermal injections; intravenous medications; oral and topical skin preparations; eye, ear, and nose drops; vaginal instillations; rectal suppositories; and inhalants.

KEY TERMS

KEY TERMS, CONT.

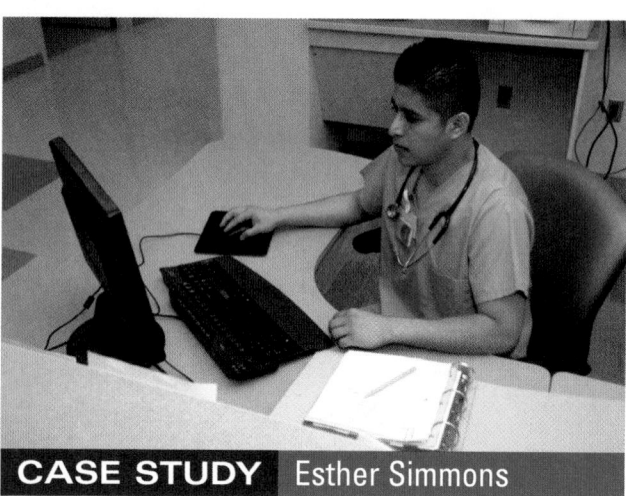

CASE STUDY   Esther Simmons

Esther Simmons is an 85-year-old African American woman who lives in her home. Esther is on a skilled care floor in a hospital following hip replacement surgery. Her strength and mobility are improving, and she is planning to return home with home care nursing within the week.

Emilio Fernandez is a 31-year-old nursing student who is assigned to care for Esther today. While reviewing the medical record, Emilio finds that Esther has several chronic illnesses, including diabetes, heart disease, hypertension, and arthritis. To manage these illnesses successfully, Esther needs to take many medications on a routine basis. Several of Esther's medications have changed, and several have been added since she was admitted. Based on this assessment, Emilio determines that Esther needs to learn how to administer her medications safely at home.

Patients with acute or chronic health problems often use a variety of medications. A medication is a substance used in the diagnosis, treatment, relief, or prevention of health alterations. No matter where patients receive their health care, you as the nurse will play an essential role in medication administration and teaching. You will also evaluate the effectiveness of medications in restoring or maintaining health. Your role in medication administration will differ based on the health care setting in which you practice.

In the primary care setting, patients often self-administer medications. In this setting you are responsible for evaluating the effects of the medications on the patient's health status and teaching the patient about medications and their side effects. You are also responsible for ensuring that patients follow medication regimens and for evaluating the patients' medication administration techniques. In the acute care setting, you will spend much time administering medications to patients. Before discharge you make sure that patients are adequately prepared to administer their medications. In the home, patients usually administer their own medications. When patients cannot administer their own medications, family caregivers are sometimes responsible for medication administration. In this situation, provide continued education to the patient, family, and/or caregiver in all aspects of medication administration.

SCIENTIFIC KNOWLEDGE BASE

Because medication administration is essential to nursing practice, you need to be knowledgeable about the actions and effects of the medications you give to patients. To safely and accurately administer medications, you need to have an understanding of pharmacokinetics (the movement of drugs in the human body), growth and development, nutrition, and mathematics.

Pharmacological Concepts

MEDICATION NAMES A medication sometimes has as many as three different names. A medication's chemical name is an exact description of the medication's composition and molecular structure. In clinical practice, health care workers rarely use chemical names. An example of a chemical name is *N*-acetyl-*para*-aminophenol, which is commonly known as Tylenol. The manufacturer who first develops the medication gives the generic or nonproprietary name, with United States Adopted Names Council (USANC) approval. Acetaminophen is an example of a generic name. It is the generic name for Tylenol. The generic name becomes the official name that is listed in publications such as the *United States Pharmacopeia* (USP). The trade or brand name (e.g., Tylenol) is the name under which a manufacturer markets a medication. The trade name has the symbol ® at the upper right of the name, indicating that the manufacturer has registered the medication's name. You will find medications under a variety of different names. Some medications often have similar spellings and may sound similar (e.g., Celebrex and Celexa). Medication errors often occur with medications that look alike and sound alike. Therefore hospitals and other health care organizations implement safety plans to prevent errors associated with medica-

BOX 16-1   Ways to Prevent Medication Errors Associated With Look-Alike Drugs

- Ensure medication is ordered by generic name (e.g., when brand names look alike/sound alike).
- Know the patient's medical diagnosis when reviewing prescriptions.
- Repeat verbal orders back to the prescriber and spell the name of the drug.
- Discuss with patient the name of the drug, indication, and instructions for use.
- Reinforce the prescriber's instructions at the time of patient counseling—a critical step in identifying errors.
- Advise patients to check the labels on their medications before taking them.

- Before administering a medication, review the name and indication with the patient if possible, and check that the patient's diagnosis matches the drug's indication.
- Have patients report any changes in medication appearance (e.g., size, color, smell) to their nurse, pharmacist, prescriber, and/or health care professional.
- Separate the look-alike sound-alike or easily confused medications in storage and medication dispensing areas.
- Place stickers with "Tall Man" letters near the similar named products (e.g., HydrALAzine Hydrochloride and HydrOXYzine Hydrochloride).
- Alert all staff to the potential for error and any actual errors that have occurred.

Modified from United States Pharmacopeia: *Similar drug names continue to be reported*, 2003, http://www.usp.org/patientSafety/newsletters/ practitionerReportingNews/prn1082003-10-23.html.

tions that are often confused with each other (Institute of Safe Medication Practices [ISMP], 2008a). One of the National Patient Safety Goals requires health care organizations to develop a list of at least 10 look-alike/sound-alike medications commonly used and set specific safety strategies for these medications (The Joint Commission [TJC], 2008b). Box 16-1 lists examples of strategies that help prevent medication errors caused by look-alike drugs.

CLASSIFICATION Medications with similar characteristics are grouped into classifications. Medication classification indicates the effect of the medication on a body system, the symptoms the medication relieves, or the medication's desired effect. Usually each class contains more than one medication that health care providers can prescribe for a type of health problem. For example, patients who have type 2 diabetes often take oral medications to lower their blood glucose level. These oral medications are called oral agents. There are five different classifications of oral agents: sulfonylureas, biguanides, thiazolidinedione derivatives, α-glucosidase inhibitors, and meglitinides. There are more than 20 different oral medications that fall within these five classifications (McKenry, Tessier, and Hogan, 2006). The physical and chemical compositions of medications within a class are sometimes slightly different. A prescriber chooses a particular oral agent based on patient characteristics, cost, efficacy, dosing frequency, or experience with the medication. A medication may also be part of more than one class. For example, aspirin is an analgesic, an antipyretic, and an antiinflammatory medication.

MEDICATION FORMS Medications are available in a variety of forms or preparations. The form of the medication determines its route of administration. Manufacturers make many medications in several forms, such as tablets, capsules, elixirs, and suppositories. When administering a medication, be certain to use the proper form (Table 16-1).

Medication Legislation and Standards

GOVERNMENTAL REGULATION OF MEDICATIONS The role of the U.S. government in regulation of the pharmaceutical industry is to protect the health of the people by ensuring that medications are safe and effective. The Pure Food and Drug Act requires all medications to be free of impure products. Subsequent legislation sets standards related to safety, potency, and effectiveness. Enforcement of medication laws rests with the U.S. Food and Drug Administration (FDA). The FDA ensures that all medications on the market undergo vigorous review before allowing manufacturers to distribute them to the public. State and local medication laws must comply with federal laws. Some individual states have stricter controls than the federal government.

In 1993 the FDA instituted the MedWatch program. This voluntary program encourages nurses and other health care professionals to report when a medication, product, or medical event causes serious harm to a patient. Mandatory reporting is required for medication manufacturers, distributors, and packers. MedWatch forms are available to report such events (USFDA, 2009).

HEALTH CARE INSTITUTIONS AND MEDICATION LAWS Health care institutions establish individual policies to meet federal, state, and local regulations. The size of an institution, the types of services it provides, and the types of personnel it employs influence these policies. Institutional policies are often more restrictive than governmental controls. An institution is concerned primarily with preventing health problems resulting from medication use. A common institutional policy is the automatic discontinuation of opioid analgesics after a set number of days. Although a prescriber may reorder the medication, this policy helps to control unnecessarily prolonged medication therapy.

MEDICATION REGULATIONS AND NURSING PRACTICE State Nurse Practice Acts have the most influence over nursing practice by defining the scope of nurses' professional functions and responsibilities. In general, most practice acts are purposefully broad so as not to limit nurses' professional responsibilities. Institutions and agencies interpret specific actions allowed under the acts, but they are not able to modify, expand, or restrict the act's intent. The primary intent of state Nurse Practice Acts is to protect the public from unskilled, undereducated, and unlicensed nurses.

TABLE 16-1   Forms of Medication by Route of Administration

MEDICATION FORMS COMMONLY PREPARED FOR ADMINISTRATION BY ORAL ROUTE

Solid Forms

Caplet	Solid dosage form for oral use; shaped like a capsule and coated for ease of swallowing.
Capsule	Medication encased in a gelatin shell.
Tablet	Powdered medication compressed into hard disk or cylinder.
Enteric coated	Tablet that is coated so that it does not dissolve in stomach; meant for intestinal absorption.

Liquid Forms

Elixir	Clear fluid containing water and alcohol; designed for oral use; usually has sweetener added.
Extract	Concentrated medication form made by removing the active portion of medication from its other components.
Aqueous solution	Substance dissolved in water and syrups.
Aqueous suspension	Finely dissolved particles in a liquid medium; when left standing, particles settle to bottom of container.
Syrup	Medication dissolved in a concentrated sugar solution.

OTHER ORAL FORMS AND TERMS ASSOCIATED WITH ORAL PREPARATIONS

Troche (lozenge)	Flat, round dosage form containing medication that dissolves in mouth; not meant for ingestion.
Aerosol	Aqueous medication sprayed and absorbed in the mouth and upper airway; not meant for ingestion.
Sustained release	Tablet or capsule that contains small particles of a medication coated with material that requires a varying amount of time to dissolve.

MEDICATION FORMS COMMONLY PREPARED FOR ADMINISTRATION BY TOPICAL ROUTE

Ointment (salve or cream)	Semisolid, externally applied preparation, usually containing one or more medications.
Liniment	Usually contains alcohol, oil, or soapy emollient.
Lotion	Semiliquid suspension often used to cool, protect, or clean skin.
Paste	Thick ointment; absorbed through the skin more slowly than ointment; often used for skin protection.
Transdermal patch	Medicated disk or patch; medication is absorbed through the skin over a designated period of time (e.g., 24 hours).

MEDICATION FORMS COMMONLY PREPARED FOR ADMINISTRATION BY PARENTERAL ROUTE

Solution	Sterile preparation that contains water with one or more dissolved compounds.
Powder	Sterile particles of medication that are dissolved in a sterile solution (e.g., water, normal saline) before administration.

MEDICATION FORMS COMMONLY PREPARED FOR INSTILLATION INTO BODY CAVITIES

Intraocular disk	Medicated disk (similar to a contact lens) that is inserted into the patient's eye. The medication is absorbed over a designated period of time.
Suppository	Solid dosage form mixed with gelatin and shaped in the form of a pellet for insertion into a body cavity (rectum or vagina). Melts when it reaches body temperature, allowing medication to be absorbed.

You are responsible for following legal provisions when administering controlled substances such as **opioids,** which are controlled through federal and state guidelines. Nurses who violate the Controlled Substances Act face fines, imprisonment, and loss of nurse licensure. Hospitals and other health care institutions have policies for the proper storage and distribution of narcotics (Box 16-2).

NONTHERAPEUTIC MEDICATION USE Medication misuse includes overuse, underuse, erratic use, and contraindicated use of medications. Patients of all ages misuse medications. Some people use medications for purposes other than their intended effect. Factors such as peer pressure, curiosity, and the pursuit of pleasure are some motivators for nontherapeutic medication use. Problems with medication use are not limited to heroin, cocaine, and other illegal drugs. The incidence of prescription and over-the-counter (OTC) drug misuse and abuse is also on the rise. The most commonly abused prescription medications include opioids, stimulants, tranquilizers, and sedatives. Common OTC medications patients misuse or abuse include cough syrup and cold medication (U.S. Department of Health and Human Services Substance Abuse and Mental Health Services Ad-

BOX 16-2 Guidelines for Safe Opiate Administration and Control

- Keep all opioids in a locked, secure place (e.g., cabinet or computerized medication cart).
- Keep a running count of opioids by counting them whenever dispensing them. If you find a discrepancy, correct and report the discrepancy immediately.
- Keep a record each time someone dispenses an opioid. The record includes the patient's name, date, time of drug administration, name of drug, and dosage. If the facility keeps a paper record, the nurse dispensing the drug signs the record. If the facility uses a computerized system, the computer records the nurse's name.
- Keep an ongoing record of opioids used and opioids remaining in the facility.
- If you have to waste part of a controlled substance, a second nurse witnesses the disposal of the unused portion. Both nurses record their names on the controlled substance record.

BOX 16-3 Nursing Interventions to Improve Adherence With Medications

- Involve the patient in deciding dosage schedule and regimen for drug preparation.
- Simplify the medication regimen as much as possible.
- Explain medication instructions using simple, easy-to-understand words.
- Provide memory aids (e.g., medication containers, charts) to reinforce teaching.
- Educate patients so they make informed decisions about medications.
- Educate patients about expected side effects of medications and how to reduce, eliminate, or manage the side effects.
- Encourage patients to use only one pharmacy if possible.
- Review the patient's medications regularly, and consult with the prescriber if unnecessary or duplicate medications are prescribed or if discrepancies exist between what the patient should be taking and what the patient is actually taking.
- Evaluate the effectiveness of communication between you and the patient and the effectiveness of medication education.
- Call patients who miss appointments with their health care providers to keep the patients involved with their care.

Data from Ebersole P and others: *Toward healthy aging: human needs and nursing response*, ed 7, St. Louis, 2008, Mosby; Haynes RB and others: Interventions for enhancing medication adherence, *Cochrane Database Syst Review* 2:2008.

ministration [USDHHS SAMHSA], 2008). Because the number of medications that are used in outpatient and home settings continues to increase, the number of fatal medication errors occurring in these settings has greatly increased. The risk is especially high in patients who use alcohol and/or street drugs (Phillips, Barker, and Eguchi, 2008).

You are ethically and legally responsible for understanding the problems of people who use medications improperly. **Medication abuse** happens when patients repeatedly use an addictive substance (e.g., opioids or alcohol). **Medication dependence** happens when a patient experiences withdrawal symptoms when the medication is stopped abruptly. When caring for patients with medication abuse or dependence, be aware of your values and attitudes about the willful use of potentially harmful substances. Therapeutic relationships develop when your personal values do not interfere with the acceptance or understanding of your patients' needs. Knowing the physical, psychological, and social changes resulting from medication abuse allows you to identify patients with medication problems.

Health professionals also misuse medications. Stress in the workplace, personal problems, and the strong desire to perform well are some factors that cause nurses to misuse medications. Recognize and understand the problems of colleagues who abuse medications. Many programs are available to assist these nurses toward recovery. These programs are offered through the institution's employees' assistance program (EAP), the State Board of Nursing, or community agencies.

Nonadherence Research shows that approximately 50% of patients do not adhere to taking their medications as prescribed (Haynes and others, 2008). Ethically, you need to understand why this happens. Poor patient education, fear of addiction, or the perception that a medication is not needed cause **nonadherence**. Nonadherence with medications affects the health and safety of all patients and is commonly found in older adults (Ebersole and others, 2008). Many factors contribute to nonadherence in older adult populations, such as depression, problems with cognitive or functional abilities, dislike for the side effects, a busy and active lifestyle, and inability to afford medications. Carefully assess the medications your patients take, and compare what your patients tell you they take with what their health care provider prescribed. If you suspect nonadherence, investigate contributing factors and work with the patient to develop a medication regimen the patient will follow. Implement interventions that help promote medication adherence (Box 16-3). Because of the negative outcomes associated with nonadherence, determining how to better help patients comply with medication schedules and other associated therapies has recently been a major focus of nursing research (Box 16-4).

Pharmacokinetics as the Basis of Medication Actions

For a medication to be therapeutically useful, it is taken into a patient's body; is absorbed and distributed to cells, tissues, or a specific organ; and alters physiological functions. **Pharmacokinetics** is the study of how medications enter the body, reach their site of action, metabolize, and exit the body

---

BOX 16-4   BEST PRACTICES

Promoting Medication Adherence in Patients With Schizophrenia

SUMMARY OF EVIDENCE

Promoting medication adherence in patients with mental illnesses such as schizophrenia is very difficult. These patients require several medications that have many adverse effects. Patients with schizophrenia often have difficulty managing their medications, and there is little research on how nurses can help patients with schizophrenia adhere to their medication schedule. When patients who have schizophrenia do not adhere to their medication schedule, they experience a variety of symptoms, including difficulties in thinking, speaking, and making rational decisions. These symptoms put the patient at great risk for injury. One nursing intervention used to promote medication adherence is called adherence therapy (AT). Nurses who use AT help their patients solve problems about their medications, work with their patients to develop a medication schedule, discuss how the patient feels about having to take medications, explore concerns the patient has about the medications, and talk about taking medications in the future. When nurses use AT, their patients tend to adhere to their medication schedule better for a variety of reasons. Patients experience fewer adverse effects from their medications and are more satisfied with their medications. They have more positive beliefs about their medications, and the symptoms of schizophrenia are better managed.

APPLICATION TO NURSING PRACTICE

- Encourage patients to participate in decisions about their medications with the health care team.
- Spend time and establish a trusting relationship with your patients to enhance adherence.
- Include patients when developing medication schedules. Take factors such as their daily routines and their beliefs and feelings about the medications into consideration.
- Ensure that patients understand their medication schedule as well as what can happen if they fail to follow their schedule.

REFERENCE

Maneesakorn S and others: An RCT of adherence therapy for people with schizophrenia in Chiang Mai, Thailand, *J Clin Nurs* 16(7):1302, 2007.

(McKenry and others, 2006). You will use knowledge of pharmacokinetics to time medication administration, select the route of administration, predict the patient's risk for alterations in medication action, and evaluate the patient's response to the medication.

ABSORPTION **Absorption** refers to passage of medication molecules into the blood from the site of administration. Factors that influence medication absorption are the route of administration, ability of the medication to dissolve, blood flow to the site of administration, body surface area, and lipid solubility of the medication.

Route of Administration You will administer medications by various routes. Each route has a different rate of absorption. When you place medications on the skin, absorption is slow because of the physical makeup of the skin. The body sometimes absorbs oral medications at a slow rate because they have to pass through the gastrointestinal (GI) tract to be absorbed. The body absorbs medications through the mucous membranes and respiratory airways quickly because these tissues contain many blood vessels. Intravenous (IV) injection produces the most rapid absorption because medications given in this route are immediately absorbed into the systemic circulation.

Ability of the Medication to Dissolve The ability of an oral medication to dissolve depends largely on its form of preparation. Solutions and suspensions are already in a liquid state and are easier for the body to absorb than tablets or capsules. Acidic medications are absorbed in the gastric mucosa rapidly, whereas medications that are alkaline are not absorbed until reaching the small intestine.

Blood Flow to the Area of Absorption The blood supply to the site of administration determines how quickly the body absorbs a drug. Sites with rich blood supplies absorb medications more quickly. For example, the body absorbs a medication administered in the muscle (intramuscular [IM] route) faster than a medication administered in the subcutaneous tissue (subcutaneous route). This is because the blood supply to muscle is richer than the blood supply to subcutaneous tissue.

Body Surface Area The size of the surface the medication comes in contact with affects how quickly the body absorbs the medication. If the surface area is large, the medication will be absorbed more quickly; thus the medication's effects will occur more quickly. This explains why many medications are absorbed more quickly and take effect faster when they are absorbed in the small intestine rather than the stomach (McKenry and others, 2006).

Lipid Solubility of the Medication Medications that are highly lipid soluble are easier for the body to absorb because they readily cross the cell membrane, which is made of a lipid layer. Another factor that affects absorption of a medication is the presence of food in the stomach. Some oral medications are absorbed more quickly on an empty stomach, whereas other medications are unaffected by gastric contents. In addition, some medications interfere with the absorption of each other if given at the same time. Use your knowledge about the factors that alter or impair absorption of medications to develop a medication administration schedule that ensures optimal absorption of your patients' drugs.

DISTRIBUTION After a medication is absorbed, it is distributed within the body to tissues and organs and ultimately to its specific site of action. The rate and extent of distribution depend on the physical and chemical properties of medications and the physiology of the person taking the medication.

Circulation Once a medication enters the bloodstream, the blood carries it throughout the tissues and organs of the body. How fast it gets there depends on the vascularity of the various tissues and organs. The distribution of a medication is inhibited when medical conditions limit blood flow or intended sites of action have a poor blood supply. For example, solid tumors have poor blood supply and sometimes do not respond to therapy intended to destroy them.

Membrane Permeability To be distributed to an organ, a medication needs to pass through all the biological membranes of that organ. Some membranes serve as barriers to the passage of medications. For example, the blood-brain barrier allows only lipid-soluble medications to pass into the brain and cerebrospinal fluid. Therefore central nervous system (CNS) infections sometimes require treatment with antibiotics injected directly into the subarachnoid space in the spinal cord. Older patients often experience adverse effects (e.g., confusion) as a result of the change in the permeability of the blood-brain barrier, with easier passage of fat-soluble medications. The placental membrane is a nonselective barrier to medications. Lipid-soluble and non–lipid-soluble agents cross the placenta and produce fetal deformities and respiratory depression.

Protein Binding The degree to which medications bind to serum proteins, such as albumin, affects medication distribution. Most medications bind to protein to some extent. When medications bind to albumin, they do not exert pharmacological activity. The unbound, or "free," medication is the active form of a medication. Older adults or patients with liver disease or malnutrition have decreased albumin in the bloodstream. Because more medication is unbound in these patients, they are at risk for an increase in medication activity, toxicity, or both.

METABOLISM After a medication reaches its site of action, it becomes metabolized. **Biotransformation** occurs when enzymes **detoxify** (remove toxic qualities), degrade (break down), and remove biologically active chemicals. Most biotransformation occurs within the liver, although the lungs, kidneys, blood, and intestines also metabolize medications. The liver is especially important because its specialized structure oxidizes and transforms many toxic substances. The liver degrades many harmful chemicals before they become distributed to the tissues. If a decrease in liver function occurs, such as with aging or liver disease, the body slowly eliminates a medication, resulting in a buildup of the medication. When organs that metabolize medications do not function correctly, patients are at risk for medication toxicity.

EXCRETION After medications are metabolized, they exit the body through the kidneys, liver, bowel, lungs, and exocrine glands. The chemical makeup of a medication determines which organ excretes the medication.

The kidneys are the main organs that excrete medications. Some medications escape extensive metabolism and exit unchanged in the urine. Other medications undergo biotransformation in the liver before the kidneys excrete them. If renal function declines, a patient is at risk for medication toxicity. If the kidney cannot adequately excrete a medica-tion, it is necessary to reduce the dose. Maintenance of an adequate fluid intake (50 mL/kg/day) promotes proper elimination of medications for the average adult.

Gaseous and volatile compounds, such as nitrous oxide and alcohol, exit through the lungs. Deep breathing and coughing (see Chapter 38) help a patient eliminate anesthetic gases more quickly following surgery. The exocrine glands excrete lipid-soluble medications. When medications exit through sweat glands, the skin sometimes becomes irritated. The nurse assists the patient in good hygiene practices (see Chapter 28) to promote cleanliness and skin integrity.

The GI tract is another route for medication excretion. Many medications enter the hepatic circulation to be broken down by the liver and excreted into the bile. After medications enter the intestines through the biliary tract, the intestines reabsorb them. Factors that increase peristalsis (e.g., laxatives or enemas) accelerate medication excretion through the feces, whereas factors that slow peristalsis (e.g., inactivity or improper diet) prolong a medication's effects.

Medications are often excreted through the mammary glands. In these cases there is a risk that a nursing infant will ingest the chemicals. Teach mothers to check on the safety of any medication used while breast-feeding.

Types of Medication Action

Medications vary considerably in the way they act. A patient does not always respond in the same way to each successive dose of a medication. Sometimes the same medication dosage causes very different responses in different patients. Box 16-5 lists important variables that influence medication action.

THERAPEUTIC EFFECTS Each medication has a **therapeutic effect,** the intended or desired physiological response of a medication. For example, you administer nitroglycerin to reduce cardiac workload and increase myocardial oxygen supply, which eliminates chest pain. Sometimes a single medication has many therapeutic effects. For example, aspirin is an analgesic, antipyretic, and antiinflammatory, and it reduces platelet aggregation (clumping of blood platelets). It is important to know what is wrong with your patient and the expected therapeutic effect for each medication your patient receives. This knowledge allows you to teach the patient about each medication's intended effect and to evaluate the effectiveness of the medication.

SIDE EFFECTS/ADVERSE REACTIONS Medications can react in the body to produce unpredictable and sometimes unexplainable response (McKenry and others, 2006). A **side effect** is a predictable and often unavoidable secondary effect produced at a usual therapeutic dose. For example, some antihypertensive medications and antidepressants often cause impotence in male patients. Some side effects are harmless, and some cause injury. If the side effects are serious enough to cancel the beneficial effects of a medication's therapeutic action, health care providers usually discontinue the medication. Patients often stop taking medications because of side effects. The most common side effects are anorexia, nausea, vomiting, constipation, drowsiness, and diarrhea.

BOX 16-5   Factors Influencing Drug Actions

GENETIC DIFFERENCES

- A person's genetic makeup influences drug metabolism. Members of a family sometimes have similar reactions to the same medication.

PHYSIOLOGICAL VARIABLES

- Gender, age, body weight, nutritional status, and illnesses all affect drug actions.
- Hormonal differences between men and women affect drug metabolism.
- Children usually require lower drug doses than adults. However, sometimes they need larger doses depending on the medication. The changes accompanying aging alter the influence of drugs.
- There is a direct relationship between the concentration of the medication administered and how quickly the medication is absorbed by body tissues.
- Diseases that impair the function of an organ responsible for normal pharmacokinetics also impair drug action (e.g., if a patient has liver failure, the metabolism of medications will be slower).

ENVIRONMENTAL CONDITIONS

- Stress and the exposure to heat and cold affect drug actions. For example, patients receiving vasodilators require lower drug dosages in warm weather.
- The setting in which a person takes a drug influences a patient's reaction. When patients are alone or isolated, they may need more pain medication than if they were in a room with other patients or if their families frequently visit them.

PSYCHOLOGICAL FACTORS

- A patient's attitude, reaction to the meaning of a drug, and the nurse's behavior affect drug actions. To enhance a medication's effect, ensure the patient understands and accepts the need for the drug, and administer it with supportive behavior.

DIET

- Medication and nutrient interactions alter a drug's action or the effect of a nutrient. For example, mineral oil decreases the absorption of fat-soluble vitamins.
- Proper drug metabolism requires healthy nutritional levels.

Adverse Effects Undesired, unintended, and often unpredictable responses to medication are referred to as **adverse effects.** For example, a patient becomes comatose after taking a drug. Some adverse effects are unexpected effects that researchers did not discover during drug testing. When this situation occurs, health care providers have to report the adverse effect to the FDA. Be alert, and assess unusual individual responses to drugs, especially with newly released medications. There is a continuum of adverse drug effects ranging from mild to severe. Patients most at risk for adverse medication reactions include the very young and older adults, women, patients taking multiple medications, patients extremely underweight or overweight, and patients with renal or liver disease. If adverse effects are mild and tolerable, patients often remain on the medications. However, if adverse effects are not tolerated and are potentially harmful, stop giving the medication immediately. Report all adverse reactions to the patient's health care provider, and record the adverse effects in the patient's medical record.

Toxic Effects Effects of medications that are capable of causing injury or death are referred to as **toxic effects.** They often develop after prolonged intake of a medication or when a medication accumulates in the blood because of impaired metabolism or excretion. Excess amounts of a medication within the body have lethal effects, depending on the medication's action. Do not give the medication if the patient experiences toxic effects, and report the effects to the patient's health care provider immediately. Sometimes antidotes are available to treat specific types of medication toxicity. For example, a patient experiencing toxic effects of morphine has severe respiratory depression. In this case naloxone (Narcan) is given to reverse the toxic effects of the morphine.

Idiosyncratic Reactions Some medications cause unpredictable effects, such as an **idiosyncratic reaction,** in which a patient overreacts or underreacts to a medication or has a reaction different from what is expected. For example, a child receiving an antihistamine (e.g., Benadryl) becomes extremely agitated or excited instead of drowsy. Stop giving the patient the medication if idiosyncratic reactions occur, and consult with the health care provider to determine if the patient needs to stop taking the drug.

Allergic Reactions When patients become immunologically sensitized to a medication after taking at least one dose of the medication **allergic reactions** occur. With repeated administration, the patient develops an allergic response to the medication, its chemical preservatives, or a metabolite. The medication or chemical acts as an antigen, triggering the release of the body's antibodies. When a patient's immune system causes abnormal reactions to a medication, the patient has a **medication allergy.** Allergic symptoms vary, depending on the individual and the medication and range from mild to severe. Table 16-2 summarizes common, mild allergy symptoms. Sudden constriction of bronchiolar muscles, edema of the pharynx and larynx, and severe wheezing and shortness of breath all characterize severe or **anaphylactic reactions.** In anaphylaxis a patient becomes severely hypotensive, necessitating emergency resuscitation measures. A patient with a known history of an allergy to a medication should not take the medication again. The patient also needs to wear a medical identification bracelet or medal (Figure 16-1) that alerts health care providers to the allergy in case the patient is unconscious when receiving medical care. Notify the patient's health care provider immediately if you

TABLE 16-2 Mild Allergic Reactions

SYMPTOM	DESCRIPTION
Urticaria (hives)	Raised, irregularly shaped skin eruptions with varying sizes and shapes; have reddened margins and pale centers.
Eczema (rash)	Small, raised vesicles that are usually reddened; often distributed over entire body
Pruritus	Itching of skin; accompanies most rashes
Rhinitis	Inflammation of mucous membranes lining nose; causes swelling and clear, watery discharge
Wheezing	Constriction of smooth muscles that surround bronchioles; occurs mainly on inspiration and can lead to airway obstruction
Angioedema	Short-term subcutaneous or submucosal swellings of the face, neck, lips, larynx, hands, feet, genitalia, or viscera

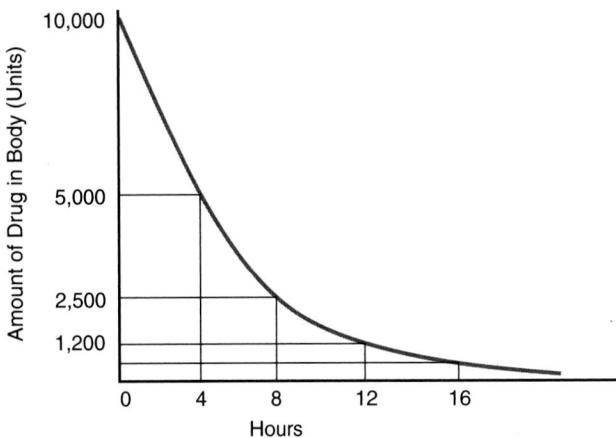

Figure 16-2 ■ Biological half-life ($t_{1/2}$). (McKenry L, Tessier E, Hogan M: *Mosby's pharmacology in nursing,* ed 22, St. Louis, 2006, Mosby.)

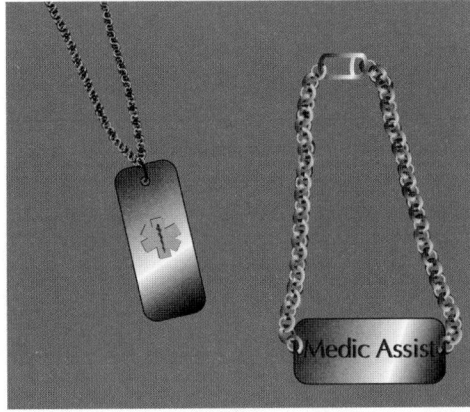

Figure 16-1 ■ Identification bracelet and medal.

suspect your patient is having an allergic reaction to a medication. Antihistamines, epinephrine, and bronchodilators are prescribed to treat anaphylactic reactions. Document medication allergies in the patient's medical record.

MEDICATION INTERACTIONS A **medication interaction** occurs when one medication modifies the action of another medication. A medication sometimes enhances or diminishes the action of other medications and alters the way in which the body absorbs, metabolizes, or eliminates another medication. Know the medications your patients take, and be aware of and assess for potential medication interactions. When two medications have a **synergistic effect,** the effect of the two medications combined is greater than the effects of the medications when given separately. For example, alcohol is a CNS depressant that has a synergistic effect on antihistamines, antidepressants, barbiturates, and opioids.

Sometimes a medication interaction is desirable. Often a health care provider orders combination medication therapy to create a medication interaction for the patient's benefit. For example, a patient with moderate hypertension typically receives several medications, such as diuretics and vasodilators, that act together to control blood pressure. Consult with your patient's health care provider when medication interactions are undesirable. Sometimes the timing of the medications needs to be changed, whereas other times one or both of the medications need to be changed or stopped.

MEDICATION DOSE RESPONSES A medication undergoes absorption, distribution, metabolism, and excretion after it enters the body. Except when administered intravenously, medications take time to enter the bloodstream.

All medications have a **biological half-life,** which is the time it takes for the body to lower the amount of unchanged medication by half. A drug with a short half-life (e.g., 2 to 3 hours) needs to be given more frequently than a drug with a longer half-life (e.g., 10 to 12 hours). A medication's half-life does not change with the dose of the medication; its half-life is always the same no matter how much medication is administered. For example, if you give 10,000 units of a medication, and the medication has a half-life of 4 hours, your patient will excrete 5000 units of the medication in 4 hours. In the next 4 hours, your patient will eliminate 2500 units. This process continues until the medication is totally eliminated from the patient's body (Figure 16-2). The goal of medication administration is to achieve a therapeutic plateau, a point when the blood level of a medication remains consistent. To maintain a therapeutic plateau, a patient receives regular fixed doses at specific intervals that correspond with their half-life. For example, research has shown that pain medications are most effective when they are given "around the clock" rather than when the patient intermittently complains of pain. This results in a constant serum level of pain medication. After an initial medication dose, the patient receives each successive dose when the previous dose reaches its half-life.

TABLE 16-3 Common Dosage Administration Schedules

ABBREVIATION	MEANING
AC, ac	Before meals
ad lib	As desired
BID, bid	Twice each day
Daily	Every day
PC, pc	After meals
prn	Whenever there is a need
qAM	Every morning, every AM
h, hr	Hour
qh	Every hour
q2h	Every 2 hours
q4h	Every 4 hours
q6h	Every 6 hours
q8h	Every 8 hours
QID, qid	4 times per day
STAT	Give immediately
TID, tid	3 times per day

TABLE 16-4 Terms Associated With Medication Actions

TERM	MEANING
Onset	Time it takes after you administer a drug for it to produce a response
Peak	Time it takes for a drug to reach its highest effective concentration
Trough	Minimum blood serum concentration of a drug reached just before the next scheduled dose
Duration	Time during which the drug is present in a concentration great enough to produce a response
Plateau	Blood serum concentration of a drug reached and maintained after repeated fixed doses

You and the patient will follow prescribed doses and dosage intervals. Table 16-3 lists common dosage schedules used in acute care settings. When you teach patients about dosage schedules, use language that is familiar to the patient. For example, when teaching a patient about twice-daily medication dosing, instruct the patient to take the medication in the morning and again in the evening. Knowledge of the time intervals of medication action will help you anticipate a medication's effect. With this knowledge, instruct the patient when to expect a response. Table 16-4 lists common terms associated with medication actions.

Routes of Administration

The route prescribed for administering a medication depends on the medication's properties and its desired effect. The route also depends on the patient's physical and mental con-

dition (Table 16-5). Collaborate with the prescriber in determining the best route for a patient's medication. For example, you are caring for a patient who has 650 mg of acetaminophen ordered by mouth every 4 hours as needed for a temperature greater than 38.0° C (100.4° F). Your patient has a temperature of 38.5° C (101.2° F), is vomiting, and is unable to tolerate oral fluids. You consult with the prescriber and have the medication changed to a rectal suppository because you know your patient cannot tolerate oral medications at this time.

ORAL ROUTES The oral route is the easiest and the most commonly used. Medications are given by mouth and swallowed with fluid. Oral medications have a slower onset of action and a more prolonged effect than parenteral medications. Patients generally prefer the oral route.

Sublingual Administration Some medications are readily absorbed after being placed under the tongue to dissolve (Figure 16-3). A medication given by the **sublingual** route should not be swallowed or chewed, or the desired effect will not be achieved. Nitroglycerin is commonly given by the sublingual route. Do not have the patient take a drink, eat, or chew gum until the medication is completely dissolved.

Buccal Administration Administration of a medication by the **buccal** route involves placing the solid medication in the mouth and against the mucous membranes of the cheek until the medication dissolves (Figure 16-4). Teach patients to alternate cheeks with each dose to avoid mucosal irritation. Also teach patients not to chew or swallow the medication or to take any liquids with it. A buccal medication acts locally on the mucosa or systemically as it is swallowed in a person's saliva.

PARENTERAL ROUTES **Parenteral administration** involves injecting a medication into body tissues. The four major parenteral routes are as follows:

1. **Subcutaneous:** Injection into tissues just below the dermis of the skin
2. **Intramuscular (IM):** Injection into a muscle
3. **Intravenous (IV):** Injection into a vein
4. **Intradermal (ID):** Injection into the dermis just under the epidermis

You administer some medications into body cavities through other routes, including epidural, intraperitoneal, intrathecal or intraspinal, intracardiac, intrapleural, intraarterial, intraosseous, and intraarticular routes. Nurses with advanced education or in advanced practice administer medications by these routes. Medication routes such as intracardiac or intraarticular are usually limited to physician administration. Regardless of who actually administers the medication by these routes, you are responsible for monitoring the integrity of the system of medication delivery, understanding the therapeutic value of the medication, and evaluating the patient's response to the therapy.

TOPICAL ADMINISTRATION Medications applied to the skin and mucous and respiratory membranes generally have local effects. Topical medication is applied to the skin

TABLE 16-5 Factors Influencing Choice of Administration Routes

ADVANTAGES BY ROUTE	DISADVANTAGES/CONTRAINDICATIONS
ORAL, BUCCAL, SUBLINGUAL ROUTES Convenient and comfortable. Economical. Sometimes produce local or systemic effects. Rarely cause anxiety.	Avoided when patient has alterations in GI function (e.g., nausea, vomiting), reduced GI motility (after general anesthesia or bowel inflammation), gastric suction, surgical resection of portion of GI tract, and reduced ability to swallow. Sometimes irritate lining of GI tract, discolor teeth, or have unpleasant tastes.
PARENTERAL (SUBCUTANEOUS, IM, IV, ID, EPIDURAL) Can be used when oral drugs are contraindicated. More rapid absorption occurs than with topical or oral routes. IV infusion provides drug delivery for critically ill patients. If peripheral perfusion is poor, IV route is preferred over injections. Epidural provides excellent pain control.	Risk for introducing infection. Some medications are more expensive. Risk for tissue damage. Subcutaneous, IM, and ID are not used in patients with bleeding tendencies. IM and IV are absorbed quickly, increasing risk for drug reactions. Sometimes cause considerable anxiety in many patients, especially children. Some patients experience pain with repeated needle sticks.
SKIN Primarily provides local effect. Painless. Limited side effects.	Absorption is too rapid if applied over skin abrasions, increasing systemic effects. Medications slowly absorbed through the skin.
Transdermal Prolonged systemic effects, with limited side effects.	Leaves oily or pasty substance on skin and soils clothing.
MUCOUS MEMBRANES* Local application to involved sites provides therapeutic effects. Aqueous solutions readily absorbed and capable of causing systemic effects. Potential route of administration when oral drugs are contraindicated.	Mucous membranes are highly sensitive to some drug concentrations. Insertion of rectal and vaginal medication often causes embarrassment. Patient with ruptured eardrum cannot receive irrigations. Rectal suppositories contraindicated if patient has active rectal bleeding or history of rectal surgery.
Inhalation Provides rapid relief for local respiratory problems. Easily used for introduction of general anesthetic gases.	Some local agents cause serious systemic effects.
Intraocular Disk Route is advantageous in that it does not require frequent administration like eye drops.	Local reactions can occur. Patient must be taught how to insert and remove disk. Expensive. Contraindicated with eye infections.

*Includes eyes, ears, nose, vagina, rectum, and ostomy.
GI, Gastrointestinal; *ID*, intradermal; *IM*, intramuscular; *IV*, intravenous.

by spreading it over an area, applying moist dressings, soaking body parts in a solution, or giving medicated baths. Systemic effects occur if a patient's skin is thin, if the medication concentration is high, or if contact with the skin is prolonged.

Some medications (e.g., nitroglycerin, Catapres, estrogens) have systemic effects because you give them topically by a **transdermal disk** or patch. The disk firmly holds the medicated ointment to the skin. Patients wear these topical applications for as little as 12 hours or as long as 7 days.

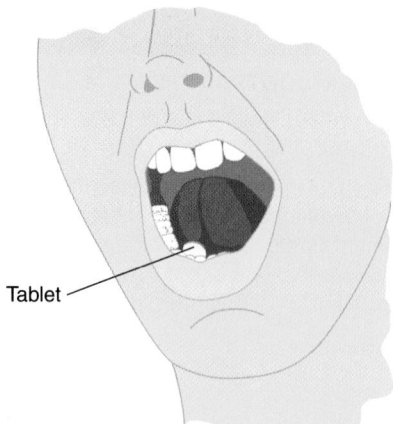

Figure 16-3 ■ Sublingual administration of a tablet.

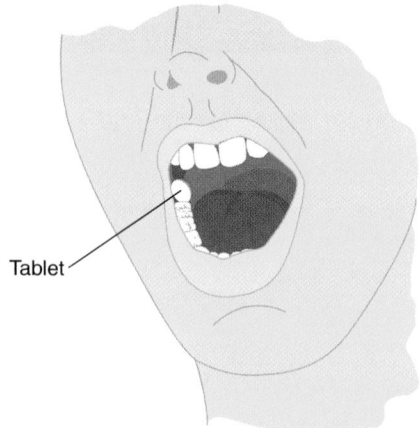

Figure 16-4 ■ Buccal administration of a tablet.

You can apply topical medications to mucous membranes in a variety of other ways, including the following:

1. By directly applying a liquid or ointment (e.g., eye drops, gargling, swabbing the throat)
2. By inserting a medication into a body cavity (e.g., placing a suppository in rectum or vagina, inserting medicated packing into vagina)
3. By instilling fluid into a body part or cavity (e.g., ear drops, nose drops, bladder or rectal instillation [fluid is retained])
4. By irrigating a body cavity (e.g., flushing eye, ear, vagina, bladder, or rectum with medicated fluid [fluid is not retained])
5. By spraying a medication into a body cavity (e.g., instillation into nose and throat)

Inhalation Route The deeper passages of the respiratory tract provide a large surface area for medication absorption. You administer medications through the **inhalation** route when you give medications into nasal passages, oral passages, or tubes that go from the patient's mouth to the trachea. Medications given by the inhalation route are readily absorbed and work quickly because of the rich vascular alveolar-capillary network in the pulmonary tissue. Inhaled medications have local or systemic effects.

Intraocular Route **Intraocular** medication delivery involves administering medication into the eye. One kind of intraocular route involves inserting a medication disk similar to a contact lens into the patient's eye. The eye medication disk has two soft outer layers that have medication enclosed in them. You insert the disk into the patient's eye, much like a contact lens. The disk remains in the patient's eye for up to 1 week (Alvarez-Lorenzo, Hiratani, and Concheiro, 2006). Pilocarpine, a medication used to treat glaucoma, is the most common medication disk used.

Systems of Medication Measurement

The proper administration of a medication requires the ability to compute medication doses accurately and measure medications correctly. A careless mistake in placing a decimal

point or adding a zero to a dose can lead to a fatal error. Check every dose carefully before giving a medication.

The health care industry uses the metric, apothecary, and household systems of measurement for medication therapy. Globally, most nations use the metric system as their standard of measurement. Although the U.S. Congress has not officially adopted the metric system, most health professionals in the United States use it. Health care providers usually write **prescriptions,** or orders for medications, that are to be self-administered at home by patients in household measures. Prescribers rarely use the **apothecary system,** a measurement system that includes ounces, pounds, and pints.

METRIC SYSTEM As a decimal system, the **metric system** is the most logically organized. Metric units are easy to convert and calculate using simple multiplication and division. Each basic unit of measurement is organized into units of 10. Multiplying or dividing by 10 forms secondary units. In multiplication the decimal point moves to the right; in division the decimal moves to the left. For example:

$$10.0 \text{ mg} \times 10 = 100.0 \text{ mg}$$
$$10.0 \text{ mg} \div 10 = 1.0 \text{ mg}$$

The basic units of measurement in the metric system are the meter (length), liter (volume), and gram (weight). For medication calculations use only the volume and weight units, and use lowercase or upper-case letters to designate units:

$$\text{Gram} = \text{g or Gm}$$
$$\text{Liter} = \text{l or L}$$
$$\text{Milligram} = \text{mg}$$
$$\text{Milliliter} = \text{mL}$$

A system of Latin prefixes designates subdivision of the basic units: deci- (1/10 or 0.1), centi- (1/100 or 0.01), and milli- (1/1000 or 0.001). Greek prefixes designate multiples of the basic units: deka- (10), hecto- (100), and kilo- (1000). Use fractions or multiples of a unit when writing medication doses in metric units. Always give fractions in decimal form:

$$500 \text{ mg or } 0.5 \text{ g, not } \frac{1}{2} \text{ g}$$
$$10 \text{ mL or } 0.01 \text{ L, not } \frac{1}{100} \text{ L}$$

TABLE 16-6	Equivalents of Measurement	
METRIC	**APOTHECARY**	**HOUSEHOLD**
1 mL	15-16 minims (m)	15 drops (gtt)
5 mL	1 fluidram (f℈)	1 teaspoon (tsp)
15 mL	4 fluidrams (f℈)	1 tablespoon (tbsp)
30 mL	1 fluid ounce (f℥)	2 tablespoons (tbsp)
240 mL	8 fluid ounces (f℥)	1 cup (c)
480 mL (approximately 500 mL)	1 pint (pt)	1 pint (pt)
960 mL (approximately 1 L)	1 quart (qt)	1 quart (qt)
3840 mL (approximately 5 L)	1 gallon (gal)	1 gallon (gal)

Many actual and potential medication errors occur with the use of fractions. Follow practice standards when medications are ordered in fractions to prevent medication errors. For example, to make the decimal point more visible, a leading zero is always placed in front of a decimal (e.g., use 0.5, not .5). On the other hand, do not use a trailing zero, a zero after a decimal point, because if a health care worker does not see the decimal point, the patient may end up receiving 10 times more medication than what is prescribed (e.g., use 5 not 5.0) (TJC, 2008b).

HOUSEHOLD MEASUREMENTS Household units of measurement are familiar to most people. The disadvantage with household measures is their inaccuracy. Household utensils, such as teaspoons and cups, often vary in size. Scales to measure pints or quarts are often not well calibrated. Household measures include drops, teaspoons, tablespoons, and cups for volume and pints and quarts for weight. Although pints and quarts are considered household measures, they are also used in the apothecary system.

The advantages of household measurements are their convenience and familiarity. When the accuracy of a medication dose is not critical, it is safe to use household measures. For example, you can safely measure many OTC medications by this method. Table 16-6 gives common equivalents from each measurement unit.

SOLUTIONS Solutions of various concentrations are used for **injections,** irrigations, and **infusions.** A **solution** is a given mass of solid substance dissolved in a known volume of fluid or a given volume of liquid dissolved in a known volume of another fluid. When a solid is dissolved in a fluid, the concentration is in units of mass per units of volume (e.g., g/mL, g/L, or mg/mL). You also express a concentration of a solution as a percentage. For example, a 10% solution is 10 g of solid dissolved in 100 mL of solution. A proportion also expresses concentrations. A $\frac{1}{1000}$ solution represents a solution containing 1 g of solid in 1000 mL of liquid or 1 mL of liquid mixed with 1000 mL of another liquid.

NURSING KNOWLEDGE BASE

The Institute of Medicine (IOM) (2003) published the book *To Err Is Human: Building a Safer Health System.* This book created national awareness about the effect of medical errors within the health care system. For example, about 98,000 people die in any given year as a result of medical errors that happen in hospitals. This means that more people die from medical errors than from motor vehicle accidents, breast cancer, acquired immunodeficiency syndrome (AIDS), and workplace injuries.

Nurses play an important role in patient safety, especially when it comes to medication administration. To safely administer medications to patients, you need to be able to calculate medication dosages accurately. You also need to understand the roles different health care providers play in the prescribing and administering of medications. Your previous learning is important. Apply what you know, and do not be afraid to ask questions when administering medications. Use the nursing process as a framework to organize your thoughts and actions.

Clinical Calculations

To administer medications safely, use your math skills to safely calculate medication dosages and to mix solutions. This is important because you will not always dispense medications in the unit of measure in which they are ordered. Medication companies package and bottle certain standard equivalents. For example, the patient's health care provider orders 250 mg of a medication that is available only in grams. You are responsible for converting available units of volume and weight to the desired doses. Therefore be aware of approximate equivalents in all major measurement systems.

CONVERSIONS WITHIN ONE SYSTEM Converting measurements within one system is relatively easy. In the metric system use division or multiplication. For example, to change milligrams to grams, divide by 1000 or move the decimal three points to the left:

$$1000 \text{ mg} = 1 \text{ g}$$
$$350 \text{ mg} = 0.35 \text{ g}$$

To convert liters to milliliters, multiply by 1000 or move the decimal three points to the right:

$$1 \text{ L} = 1000 \text{ mL}$$
$$0.25 \text{ L} = 250 \text{ mL}$$

To convert units of measurement within the apothecary or household system, you need to know the equivalent. For example, when converting fluid ounces to quarts, you know that 32 ounces is the equivalent of 1 quart. To convert 8 ounces to a quart measurement, divide 8 by 32 to get the equivalent, ¼ or 0.25 quart.

CONVERSION BETWEEN SYSTEMS Frequently you will determine the correct dose of a medication by converting weights or volumes from one system of measurement to another. For example, metric units are converted to equivalent household measures to ease medication administration at home. To convert from one measurement system to another, it is necessary to use equivalent measurements. Tables of equivalent measurements are available in all health care institutions. If a table is not available, the pharmacist is also a good resource for this information.

Before making a conversion, compare the measurement system available with what was ordered. For example, a health care provider orders 10 mL of Robitussin for your patient. To provide proper instruction to the patient, you will convert "mL" to a common household measurement. By referring to a table, such as Table 16-6 (p. 385), you determine that 10 mL = 2 teaspoons. Therefore you instruct the patient to take 2 teaspoons of Robitussin.

DOSAGE CALCULATIONS Methods used to calculate medications include the ratio and proportion method, the formula method, and dimensional analysis. Use the method that is the most logical to you. Before you begin any calculation, make a mental estimate of the approximate and reasonable dosage. If your estimate does not closely match the answer you calculate, you need to recheck your math before preparing and administering the medication. Many nursing students feel uncomfortable or anxious when they have to do medication calculations (Dopson, 2008; Greenfield, Whelan, and Cohn, 2006). To enhance accuracy and decrease your anxiety, choose a method of calculation that you are most comfortable with and use it consistently (Gray Morris, 2006).

Most health care agencies require a nurse to double-check calculations with another nurse before giving medications, especially when the risk for giving the wrong medication dose is high (e.g., heparin or insulin). **Always** have another nurse or health care professional double-check your work if the answer to a medication calculation seems unreasonable or inappropriate.

The Ratio and Proportion Method A ratio indicates the relationship between two numbers. The numbers in a ratio are separated by a colon (:). The colon in the ratio indicates you need to use division. Therefore you can think of a ratio as a fraction; the number to the left is the numerator and the number to the right is the denominator. For example, the ratio 1:2 is the same as ½. A proportion is an equation that has two ratios of equal value. You can write a proportion in one of three ways:

Example 1:   1:2 = 5:10
Example 2:   1:2 :: 5:10
Example 3:   ½ = ⁵⁄₁₀

In a proportion, the first and last numbers are called the extremes and the second and third numbers are called the means. If you multiply the extremes, you will get the same result as if you multiplied the means. For example, in the proportions above, if you multiply the means and extremes, you end up with the following equations: $1 \times 10 = 10$ and

$2 \times 5 = 10$. Because the numbers in a proportion are in a specific relationship with each other, if you know three of the numbers in the proportion, it is easy to calculate the unknown number. To use this method, you first need to make sure that all terms are in the same unit and system of measurement. After estimating the correct dose in your mind, set up the proportion, labeling all terms in the proportion. Place the ratio that you know (e.g., information on the drug label) first. Put the terms of the ratio in the same sequence (e.g., mg:mL = mg:mL). Cross multiply the means and the extremes and then divide both sides by the number before the x to obtain the dosage. Always remember to label your answer. If your answer is not close to your estimate, recheck your math.

Example: The patient's health care provider has ordered 100 mg of Dilantin to be administered in a gastric tube. The solution of Dilantin comes in a bottle labeled Dilantin 125 mg/5 mL. To determine how much Dilantin you need to give, you use the following steps:

1. Estimate the answer: The amount you have to give is a little less than the amount that is provided in the solution. Therefore the patient will need a little less than 5 mL of medication.
2. Set up the proportion:

$$\frac{125\ mg}{5\ mL} = \frac{100\ mg}{x\ mL}$$

3. Cross multiply the means and the extremes:

$$125x = 100 \times 5$$
$$125x = 500$$

4. Divide both sides by the number before x:

$$\frac{125x}{125} = \frac{500}{125}$$
$$x = \frac{500}{125}$$
$$x = 4\ mL$$

5. Compare your estimate from step 1 with your answer in step 4: The answer (4 mL) is close to the estimated amount (a little less than 5 mL). Therefore your answer is correct; prepare and administer 4 mL in the patient's gastric tube.

The Formula Method When you use the formula method to calculate medication dosages, you substitute information from the medication order into the formula. When using this method, first you need to memorize the formula. Estimate what you think the answer should be, then place all the information from the medication order into the formula and label all the parts in the formula. All measures in the formula need to be in the same units and system of measurement before calculating the dosage. If the measures are not in the same measurement system, convert the numbers to the same system before calculating the dosage. Calculate and label your answer. Compare your answer to your estimated answer; if your estimate is not similar to your answer, recheck your math. Use the following basic formula when using the formula method:

$$\frac{Dose\ Ordered}{Dose\ on\ Hand} \times Amount\ on\ Hand = Amount\ to\ Administer$$

The dose ordered is the amount of medication prescribed. The dose on hand is the weight or volume of medication available in units supplied by the pharmacy. It is expressed on the medication label as the contents of a tablet or capsule or as the amount of medication dissolved per unit volume of liquid. The amount on hand is the basic unit or quantity of the medication that contains the dose on hand. For solid medications, the amount on hand may be one capsule. The amount of liquid on hand may be 1 mL or 1 L. The amount to administer is the actual amount of available medication you will administer. The amount to administer is always expressed in the same unit as the amount on hand.

Example: Your patient needs to receive Demerol, 50 mg IM (dose ordered). The medication is available only in ampules containing 100 mg (dose on hand) in 1 mL (amount on hand). You apply the formula method as follows:

1. Estimate the answer: The medication is a liquid, so you will need to figure out the answer in mL. The amount that you need to give is ½ of what the dose is, so your answer is going to be about ½ mL.
2. Set up the formula:

$$\frac{Dose\ Ordered}{Dose\ on\ Hand} \times Amount\ on\ Hand = Amount\ to\ Administer$$

$$\frac{50\ mg}{100\ mg} \times 1\ mL = Amount\ to\ Administer$$

3. Calculate your answer:

$$\frac{50\ mg}{100\ mg} \times 1\ mL = 0.5\ mL$$

4. Compare your estimate from step 1 with your answer in step 3: both your estimate and your answer are the same; prepare 0.5 mL in a syringe and administer it to your patient.

Dimensional Analysis Dimensional analysis is also known as the factor-label method or the unit factor method. Because only one equation is needed and the same steps are used in solving every medication problem, you do not have to memorize formulas. Dimensional analysis requires you to use your critical thinking skills. Current evidence shows that nursing students who use dimensional analysis often calculate medications more accurately than when they use the formula method (Greenfield and others, 2006). Use the following steps to solve medication problems using dimensional analysis:

1. Identify the unit of measure that you need to administer. For example, if you are giving a pill, you will usually be giving a tablet or a capsule; for parenteral or oral medications, the unit is milliliters.
2. Estimate the answer in your mind.
3. Place the name or appropriate abbreviation for x on the left side of the equation (e.g., x tab, x mL).
4. Place available information from the problem in a fraction format on the right side of the equation. Place the abbreviation or unit that matches what you are going to administer (determined in step 1) in the numerator.
5. Look at the medication order and add other factors into the problem. Set up the numerator so that it matches the unit in the previous denominator.
6. Cancel out like units of measurement on the right side of the equation. You should end up with only one unit left in the equation, and it should match the unit on the left side of the equation.
7. Reduce to the lowest terms if possible, and solve the problem or solve for x. Label your answer.
8. Compare your estimate from step 1 with your answer in step 2.

Example: The patient's health care provider orders 0.5 g of ampicillin to be given IM q8h. You have a vial of ampicillin that says 250 mg/mL. Calculate the dose to administer using dimensional analysis by following these steps:

1. *Identify the unit of measure that you need to administer:* This medication will be given IM, which is a parenteral medication. Therefore your answer will be in milliliters.
2. *Estimate the answer in your mind:* The medication order of 0.5 g is larger than 250 mg. Because the medication is in a vial of 250 mg in 1 mL, you will need to give more than 1 mL. Based on your knowledge about converting in the metric system, you convert 0.5 g to milligrams by moving the decimal point three places to the right. Therefore 0.5 g is the same as 500 mg. The number 500 is two times 250, so the answer will be about 2 mL.
3. *Place the name or appropriate abbreviation for x on the left side of the equation:*

$$x\ mL =$$

4. *Place available information from the problem in a fraction format on the right side of the equation:* You are going to administer the medication in milliliters, so place the mL in the numerator.

$$x\ mL = \frac{1\ mL}{250\ mg}$$

5. *Look at the medication order, and add other factors into the problem. Set up the numerator so that it matches the unit in the previous denominator:* The order is for 0.5 g, and the medication is available in 250-mg vials. You know that 1 g = 1000 mg; add this conversion to your calculation.

$$x\ mL = \frac{1\ mL}{250\ mg} \times \frac{1000\ mg}{1\ g} \times \frac{0.5\ g}{1}$$

6. *Cancel out like units of measurement on the right side of the equation.*

$$x\ mL = \frac{1\ mL}{250\ \cancel{mg}} \times \frac{1000\ \cancel{mg}}{1\ \cancel{g}} \times \frac{0.5\ \cancel{g}}{1}$$

7. *Reduce to the lowest terms if possible, and solve the problem or solve for x. Label your answer.*

$$x = \frac{1000 \times 0.5}{250}$$

$$x = \frac{500}{250}$$

$$x = 2\ mL$$

8. *Compare your estimate from step 1 with your answer in step 2:* Your answer is 2 mL, which matches the estimate you made in step 2. Prepare and administer 2 mL of the medication as calculated.

PEDIATRIC DOSAGES Current evidence shows that children are three times more at risk for experiencing a medication error than adults. Most medication errors involving children occur because either the wrong dose or the wrong amount of the medication is given to the child (TJC, 2008a). The risk for medication errors in children is especially high because medications are ordered by weight, and many medications are packaged for adults.

Calculating children's medication dosages requires caution (Hockenberry and Wilson, 2009). Even small errors or discrepancies in medication amounts can negatively affect the child's health status (Gray Morris, 2006). A child's age, weight, and maturity of body systems affect the ability to metabolize and excrete medications. For example, premature infants have livers and kidneys that are not matured. Therefore they are especially susceptible to the harmful effects of medications. As children develop out of the newborn period, they metabolize drugs more quickly. This results in a need to give medications more frequently to achieve the desired effect of the medication. You will sometimes have difficulty evaluating the child's response to the medication, especially when the child cannot communicate with you verbally. For example, a side effect of vancomycin, an antibiotic, is ototoxicity. If a child who cannot talk yet is taking vancomycin, assessing for ototoxicity is challenging.

Remember the following guidelines whenever calculating pediatric dosages (Gray Morris, 2006):

1. Most pediatric medications are ordered in milligrams per kilogram (mg/kg). Therefore you need to ensure that the patient's weight is expressed in kilograms (kg). If you know the child's weight in pounds (lb), you will have to convert pounds to kilograms. Remember that 1 kg = 2.2 lb.
2. Pediatric doses are usually a lot smaller than adult doses for the same medication. You will frequently use micrograms and small syringes (e.g., tuberculin or 1 mL).

3. IM doses are very small and usually do not exceed 1 mL in small children or 0.5 mL in infants.
4. Subcutaneous dosages are also very small and do not usually exceed 0.5 mL.
5. Most medications are not rounded off to the nearest tenth. Instead, they are rounded to the nearest thousandth.
6. Measure dosages that are less than 1 mL in syringes that are marked in tenths of a milliliter if the dosage calculation comes out even and does not need to be rounded. If you need to round a medication to the nearest thousandth, use a tuberculin syringe for medication preparation.
7. Mentally estimate your patient's dose before beginning your calculation; label and compare your answer with your estimate before preparing the medication.
8. To determine if a dose is safe before you give the medication, compare and evaluate the amount of medication ordered over 24 hours with the recommended dosage.

There are different formulas and methods used to calculate drug dosages in children. The two most common methods of calculating pediatric dosages are based on a child's weight or body surface area (BSA). BSA is used in rare situations (e.g., determining chemotherapy doses). To estimate a child's BSA, use Mosteller's formula or the standard nomogram (e.g., the West nomogram). Refer to a pediatric or pharmacology resource, and consult with the patient's health care provider or the pharmacist if you have to calculate a medication based on BSA.

Most of the time you will calculate medications based on a child's weight. You can use the ratio and proportion method, the formula method, or dimensional analysis to calculate a pediatric dose using body weight. The example provided below explains how to use dimensional analysis to calculate pediatric doses. Refer to the sections above on ratio and proportion and the formula method if you decide those are the easier methods for you to use.

Example: You receive an order to give gentamicin sulfate 2.25 mg/kg q8h for a 5-year-old child who weighs 40 pounds (lb). The medication label says there is 10 mg of gentamicin sulfate in 1 mL of normal saline. How much gentamicin will you give?

1. *Identify the unit of measure that you need to administer:* This medication will be given IV piggyback, which is a parenteral medication. Therefore your answer will be in milliliters. The child's weight is in pounds, so convert the weight to kilograms.
2. *Estimate your answer in your mind:* Based on your knowledge about converting in the metric system, you know that 1 kg is about equal to 2 lb. If you know the patient's weight in pounds, you can divide the weight in half to estimate the patient's weight in kilograms. Half of 40 is 20, so the child is about 20 kg. The medication is ordered 2.25 mg/kg; if you multiply 20 (the approximate weight of the child in kg) by 2 (the approximate dosage of the medication ordered in mg), you get 40. In your estimates,

you have rounded down to the closest whole number; therefore you reason that you will need to give a little more than 40 mg of medication. Because the medication comes in a vial of 10 mg in 1 mL and 40 mg is 4 times larger than the medication's dosage of 10 mg, you will need to give a little more than 4 mL.

3. *Place the name or appropriate abbreviation for x on the left side of the equation:*

$$x \text{ mL} =$$

4. *Place available information from the problem and the medication in a fraction format on the right side of the equation.* Set up the numerator so that it matches the unit in the previous denominator: You are going to administer the medication in milliliters; therefore place the mL in the numerator.

$$x \text{ mL} = \frac{1 \, mL}{10 \, mg}$$

5. *Look at the medication order, and add other factors into the problem. Set up the numerator so that it matches the unit in the previous denominator:* You know that you need to give 2.25 mg/kg and that your patient weighs 40 lb. You also know that 1 kg = 2.2 lb.

$$x \text{ mL} = \frac{1 \, mL}{10 \, mg} \times \frac{2.25 \, mg}{1 \, kg} \times \frac{1 \, kg}{2.2 \, lb} \times \frac{40 \, lb}{1}$$

6. *Cancel out like units of measurement on the right side of the equation.*

$$x \text{ mL} = \frac{1 \, mL}{10 \, \cancel{mg}} \times \frac{2.25 \, \cancel{mg}}{1 \, \cancel{kg}} \times \frac{1 \, \cancel{kg}}{2.2 \, \cancel{lb}} \times \frac{40 \, \cancel{lb}}{1}$$

7. *Reduce to the lowest terms if possible, and solve the problem or solve for x. Label your answer.*

$$x \text{ mL} = \frac{2.25 \times 40}{10 \times 2.2}$$

$$x = \frac{90}{22}$$

$$x = 4.0909 \text{ mL}$$

8. *Compare your estimate from step 1 with your answer in step 2:* You round your answer to 4.091 mL, which is very close to the estimate you made in step 2. Your calculation is correct, and you can continue with medication preparation at this time.

Administering Medications

In addition to nurses, the prescriber and pharmacist also help to ensure the right medication gets to the right patient. However, as a nurse, you are accountable for knowing what medications are prescribed, their therapeutic and nontherapeutic effects, and the patient's needs and abilities related to medication administration. You also are responsible for evaluating the desired effects of the patient's medications.

PRESCRIBER'S ROLE The health care provider prescribes the patient's medications by writing an order on a form in the patient's medical record, in an order book, or on a legal prescription pad. Prescribers sometimes use computers or hand held electronic devices (e.g., personal digital assistants [PDAs]) when ordering medications. Telephone or verbal orders are given when written or electronic communication between the prescriber and the nurse is not possible.

It is your responsibility as a nurse to know which health care providers are able to prescribe medications. Examples of prescribers include physicians and advanced practice nurses (e.g., nurse practitioner, clinical nurse specialist, nurse midwife, nurse anesthetist). Practice acts vary by state, and policies vary by agency. Be sure that you are familiar with your Nurse Practice Act and agency policies when taking prescriptions and administering medications to protect your patient and yourself.

Written orders are signed by the prescriber. When a nurse receives a verbal order, such as a telephone order, the nurse writes the order and the name of the prescriber and then signs the order. The prescriber will countersign the order at a later time, usually within 24 hours after making the order. Box 16-6 provides guidelines for taking verbal orders for medications safely. Agency policies vary regarding who can take verbal orders and when they can be taken. Generally, nursing students cannot take medication orders, and verbal orders should be taken only in emergency situations. You cannot give any medication without an order. When a nurse takes a verbal order in person or over the telephone, he or she must read back the complete order to the prescriber (TJC, 2008b).

Common abbreviations are often used when writing orders. The abbreviations indicate dosage frequencies or times, routes of administration, and special information for giving the medication (see Table 16-3, p. 382). Many medication errors are related to the use of abbreviations. Table 16-7 lists abbreviations that are associated with a high incidence of medication errors. Do **not** use these abbreviations when documenting medication orders or when documenting other information about medications (ISMP, 2007b; National Coordinating Council for Medication Error Reporting and Prevention [NCCMERP], 2006; TJC, 2008b).

TYPES OF ORDERS IN ACUTE CARE AGENCIES You need to have an order for a medication before you can administer it to your patient. Five common types of medication orders are based on the frequency and/or urgency of medication administration.

Standing Orders You carry out a standing order until the health care provider cancels it by another order or until a prescribed number of days elapse. A standing order sometimes indicates a final date or number of dosages. Many institutions have policies for automatically discontinuing standing orders. The following are examples of standing orders:

Tetracycline, 500 mg PO q6h
Decadron, 5 mg PO daily for 5 days

BOX 16-6	Recommendations to Reduce Medication Errors Associated With Verbal Medication Orders and Prescriptions (NCCMERP, 2006)

PREAMBLE

Confusion over the similarity of drug names accounts for approximately 25% of all reports to the USP Medication Errors Reporting (MER) Program. To reduce confusion pertaining to verbal orders and to further support the Council's mission to minimize medication errors, the following recommendations have been developed.

In these recommendations, verbal orders are prescriptions or medication orders that are communicated as oral, spoken communications between senders and receivers face to face, by telephone, or by other auditory device.

RECOMMENDATIONS

1 Verbal communication of prescription or medication orders should be limited to urgent situations where immediate written or electronic communication is not feasible.

2 Health care organizations* should establish policies and procedures that:
   - Describe limitations or prohibitions on use of verbal orders
   - Provide a mechanism to ensure validity/authenticity of the prescriber
   - List the elements required for inclusion in a complete verbal order
   - Describe situations in which verbal orders may be used
   - List and define the individuals who may send and receive verbal orders
   - Provide guidelines for clear and effective communication of verbal orders

3 Leaders of health care organizations should promote a culture in which it is acceptable, and strongly encouraged, for staff to question prescribers when there are any questions or disagreements about verbal orders. Questions about verbal orders should be resolved prior to the preparation, dispensing, or administration of the medication.

4 Verbal orders for antineoplastic agents should **NOT** be permitted under any circumstances. These medications are not administered in emergency or urgent situations, and they have a narrow margin of safety.

5 Elements that should be included in a verbal order include:
   - Name of patient
   - Age and weight of patient, when appropriate

- Drug name
- Dosage form (e.g., tablets, capsules, inhalants)
- Exact strength or concentration
- Dose, frequency, and route
- Quantity and/or duration
- Purpose or indication (unless disclosure is considered inappropriate by the prescriber)
- Specific instructions for use
- Name of prescriber, and telephone number when appropriate
- Name of individual transmitting the order, if different from the prescriber.

6 The content of verbal orders should be clearly communicated:
   - The name of the drug should be confirmed by any of the following:
     - Spelling
     - Providing both the brand and generic names of the medication
     - Providing the indication for use
   - In order to avoid confusion with spoken numbers, a dose such as 50 mg should be dictated as "fifty milligrams...five zero milligrams" to distinguish from "fifteen milligrams...one five milligrams."
   - In order to avoid confusion with drug name modifiers, such as prefixes and suffixes, additional spelling-assistance methods should be used (i.e., S as in Sam, X as in x-ray).
   - Instructions for use should be provided without abbreviations. For example, "1 tab tid" should be communicated as "Take/give one tablet three times daily."
   - Whenever possible, the receiver of the order should **write** down the complete order to enter it into a computer, then **read** it back, and receive confirmation from the individual who gave the order or test result.

7 All verbal orders should be reduced immediately to writing and signed by the individual receiving the order.

8 Verbal orders should be documented in the patient's medical record, reviewed, and countersigned by the prescriber as soon as possible.

Adopted: February 20, 2001
Revised: February 24, 2006

*Health care organizations include community pharmacies, physicians' offices, hospitals, nursing homes, home care agencies, etc.
© 1998–2009 National Coordinating Council for Medication Error Reporting and Prevention. All Rights Reserved.
USP, U.S. Pharmacopeia.

prn Orders The health care provider sometimes orders a medication to be given only when a patient requires it. This is a prn order. You use objective and subjective assessment and nursing discretion to determine whether the patient needs the medication. Often the health care provider sets minimum intervals for the time of administration. This means you cannot give the medication any more frequently than when it is prescribed. Examples of prn orders include the following:

Morphine sulfate, 10 mg IM q4h prn for incisional pain
Maalox, 30 mL prn for heartburn

TABLE 16-7	**ISMP's List of Error-Prone Abbreviations, Symbols, and Dose Designations**

The abbreviations, symbols, and dose designations found in this table have been reported to ISMP through the USP-ISMP Medication Error Reporting Program as being frequently misinterpreted and involved in harmful medication errors. They should NEVER be used when communicating medical information. This includes internal communications, telephone/verbal prescriptions, computer-generated labels, labels for drug storage bins, medication administration records, as well as pharmacy and prescriber computer order entry screens.

The Joint Commission (TJC) has established a National Patient Safety Goal that specifies that certain abbreviations must appear on an accredited organization's do-not-use list; we have highlighted these items with a double asterisk (**). However, we hope that you will consider others beyond the minimum TJC requirements. By using and promoting safe practices and by educating one another about hazards, we can better protect our patients.

ABBREVIATIONS	INTENDED MEANING	MISINTERPRETATION	CORRECTION
µg	Microgram	Mistaken as "mg"	Use "mcg"
AD, AS, AU	Right ear, left ear, each ear	Mistaken as OD, OS, OU (right eye, left eye, each eye)	Use "right ear," "left ear," or "each ear"
OD, OS, OU	Right eye, left eye, each eye	Mistaken as AD, AS, AU (right ear, left ear, each ear)	Use "right eye," "left eye," or "each eye"
BT	Bedtime	Mistaken as "BID" (twice daily)	Use "bedtime"
cc	Cubic centimeters	Mistaken as "u" (units)	Use "mL"
D/C	Discharge or discontinue	Premature discontinuation of medications if D/C (intended to mean "discharge") has been misinterpreted as "discontinued" when followed by a list of discharge medications	Use "discharge" and "discontinue"
IJ	Injection	Mistaken as "IV" or "intrajugular"	Use "injection"
IN	Intranasal	Mistaken as "IM" or "IV"	Use "intranasal" or "NAS"
HS	Half-strength	Mistaken as bedtime (hour of sleep)	Use "half-strength"
hs	At bedtime, hour of sleep	Mistaken as half-strength	Use "bedtime"
IU**	International unit	Mistaken as IV (intravenous) or 10 (ten)	Use "units"
o.d. or OD	Once daily	Mistaken as "right eye" (OD—oculus dexter), leading to oral liquid medications administered in the eye	Use "daily"
OJ	Orange juice	Mistaken as OD or OS (right or left eye); drugs meant to be diluted in orange juice may be given in the eye	Use "orange juice"
Per os	By mouth, orally	The "os" can be mistaken as "left eye" (OS—oculus sinister)	Use "PO," "by mouth," or "orally"
q.d. or QD**	Every day	Mistaken as q.i.d., especially if the period after the "q" or the tail of the "q" is misunderstood as an "i"	Use "daily"
qhs	Nightly at bedtime	Mistaken as "qhr" or every hour	Use "nightly"
qn	Nightly or at bedtime	Mistaken as "qh" (every hour)	Use "nightly" or "at bedtime"
q.o.d. or QOD**	Every other day	Mistaken as "q.d." (daily) or "q.i.d." (four times daily) if the "o" is poorly written	Use "every other day"
q1d	Daily	Mistaken as q.i.d. (four times daily)	Use "daily"
q6PM, etc.	Every evening at 6 PM	Mistaken as every 6 hours	Use "6 PM nightly" or "6 PM daily"
SC, SQ, sub q	Subcutaneous	SC mistaken as SL (sublingual); SQ mistaken as "5 every;" the "q" in "sub q" has been mistaken as "every" (e.g., a heparin dose ordered "sub q 2 hours before surgery" misunderstood as every 2 hours before surgery)	Use "subcut" or "subcutaneously"
ss	Sliding scale (insulin) or ½ (apothecary)	Mistaken as "55"	Spell out "sliding scale;" use "one-half" or "½"

Continued

TABLE 16-7   ISMP's List of Error-Prone Abbreviations, Symbols, and Dose Designations—cont'd

ABBREVIATIONS	INTENDED MEANING	MISINTERPRETATION	CORRECTION
SSRI	Sliding scale regular insulin	Mistaken as selective-serotonin reuptake inhibitor	Spell out "sliding scale regular insulin"
SSI	Sliding scale insulin	Mistaken as Strong Solution of Iodine (Lugol's)	Spell out "sliding scale insulin"
ī/d	One daily	Mistaken as "tid"	Use "1 daily"
TIW or tiw	3 times a week	Mistaken as "3 times a day" or "twice in a week"	Use "3 times weekly"
U or u**	Unit	Mistaken as the number 0 or 4, causing a 10-fold overdose or greater (e.g., 4U seen as "40" or 4u seen as "44"); mistaken as "cc" so dose given in volume instead of units (e.g., 4u seen as 4cc)	Use "unit"

DOSE DESIGNATIONS AND OTHER INFORMATION	INTENDED MEANING	MISINTERPRETATION	CORRECTION
Trailing zero after decimal point (e.g., 1.0 mg)**	1 mg	Mistaken as 10 mg if the decimal point is not seen	Do not use trailing zeros for doses expressed in whole numbers
"Naked" decimal point (e.g., .5 mg)**	0.5 mg	Mistaken as 5 mg if the decimal point is not seen	Use zero before a decimal point when the dose is less than a whole unit
Drug name and dose run together (especially problematic for drug names that end in "l" such as Inderal40 mg; Tegretol300 mg)	Inderal 40 mg Tegretol 300 mg	Mistaken as Inderal 140 mg Mistaken as Tegretol 1300 mg	Place adequate space between the drug name, dose, and unit of measure
Numerical dose and unit of measure run together (e.g., 10mg, 100mL)	10 mg 100 mL	The "m" is sometimes mistaken as a zero or two zeros, risking a 10- to 100-fold overdose	Place adequate space between the dose and unit of measure
Abbreviations such as mg. or mL. with a period following the abbreviation	mg mL	The period is unnecessary and could be mistaken as the number 1 if written poorly	Use mg, mL, etc. without a terminal period
Large doses without properly placed commas (e.g., 100000 units; 1000000 units)	100,000 units 1,000,000 units	100000 has been mistaken as 10,000 or 1,000,000; 1000000 has been mistaken as 100,000	Use commas for dosing units at or above 1,000, or use words such as 100 "thousand" or 1 "million" to improve readability

DRUG NAME ABBREVIATIONS	INTENDED MEANING	MISINTERPRETATION	CORRECTION
ARA A	vidarabine	Mistaken as cytarabine (ARA C)	Use complete drug name
AZT	zidovudine (Retrovir)	Mistaken as azathioprine or aztreonam	Use complete drug name
CPZ	Compazine (prochlorperazine)	Mistaken as chlorpromazine	Use complete drug name
DPT	Demerol-Phenergan-Thorazine	Mistaken as diphtheria-pertussis-tetanus (vaccine)	Use complete drug name

TABLE 16-7   ISMP's List of Error-Prone Abbreviations, Symbols, and Dose Designations—cont'd

DRUG NAME ABBREVIATIONS	INTENDED MEANING	MISINTERPRETATION	CORRECTION
DTO	Diluted tincture of opium, or deodorized tincture of opium (Paregoric)	Mistaken as tincture of opium	Use complete drug name
HCl	hydrochloric acid or hydrochloride	Mistaken as potassium chloride (The "H" is misinterpreted as "K")	Use complete drug name unless expressed as a salt of a drug
HCT	hydrocortisone	Mistaken as hydrochlorothiazide	Use complete drug name
HCTZ	hydrochlorothiazide	Mistaken as hydrocortisone (seen as HCT250 mg)	Use complete drug name
MgSO4**	magnesium sulfate	Mistaken as morphine sulfate	Use complete drug name
MS, MSO4**	morphine sulfate	Mistaken as magnesium sulfate	Use complete drug name
MTX	methotrexate	Mistaken as mitoxantrone	Use complete drug name
PCA	procainamide	Mistaken as patient controlled analgesia	Use complete drug name
PTU	propylthiouracil	Mistaken as mercaptopurine	Use complete drug name
T3	Tylenol with codeine No. 3	Mistaken as liothyronine	Use complete drug name
TAC	triamcinolone	Mistaken as tetracaine, Adrenalin, cocaine	Use complete drug name
TNK	TNKase	Mistaken as "TPA"	Use complete drug name
ZnSO4	zinc sulfate	Mistaken as morphine sulfate	Use complete drug name

STEMMED DRUG NAMES	INTENDED MEANING	MISINTERPRETATION	CORRECTION
"Nitro" drip	nitroglycerin infusion	Mistaken as sodium nitroprusside infusion	Use complete drug name
"Norflox"	norfloxacin	Mistaken as Norflex	Use complete drug name
"IV Vanc"	intravenous vancomycin	Mistaken as Invanz	Use complete drug name

SYMBOLS	INTENDED MEANING	MISINTERPRETATION	CORRECTION
ʒ	Dram	Symbol for dram mistaken as "3"	Use the metric system
m	Minim	Symbol for minim mistaken as "mL"	Use "minim"
x3d	For three days	Mistaken as "3 doses"	Use "for three days"
> and <	Greater than and less than	Mistaken as opposite of intended; mistakenly use incorrect symbol; "< 10" mistaken as "40"	Use "greater than" or "less than"
/ (slash mark)	Separates two doses or indicates "per"	Mistaken as the number 1 (e.g., "25 units/10 units" misread as "25 units and 110" units)	Use "per" rather than a slash mark to separate doses
@	At	Mistaken as "2"	Use "at"
&	And	Mistaken as "2"	Use "and"
+	Plus or and	Mistaken as "4"	Use "and"
°	Hour	Mistaken as a zero (e.g., q2° seen as q 20)	Use "hr," "h," or "hour"

** These abbreviations are included on TJC's "minimum list" of dangerous abbreviations, acronyms, and symbols that must be included on an organization's "Do Not Use" list, effective January 1, 2004. Visit www.jointcommission.org for more information about this TJC requirement.
Permission is granted to reproduce material for internal newsletters or communications with proper attribution. Other reproduction is prohibited without written permission. Unless noted, reports were received through the USP-ISMP Medication Errors Reporting Program (MERP). Report actual and potential medication errors to the MERP via the web at www.ismp.org or by calling 1-800-FAIL-SAF(E). ISMP guarantees confidentiality of information received and respects reporters' wishes as to the level of detail included in publications.

When you administer prn medications, document the assessment data you used to decide to give the medication and the time of medication administration. Frequently evaluate the effectiveness of the medication, and record findings in the appropriate record.

The Joint Commission (2008b) discourages the use of range orders for prn medications because they are often unclear and have been a source of medication errors. An example of a range order is morphine sulfate 2-4 mg IV push q2-4h prn for pain. The Joint Commission recommends that health care agencies develop guidelines that define a safe way to implement range orders when they are needed. An example of a safer range order is increase morphine dosage 50% to 100% if pain is moderate to severe.

Single (One-Time) Orders A prescriber will often order a medication to be given only once at a specified time. This is common for preoperative medications or medications given before diagnostic examinations. For example:

Versed, 6 mg IM on call to OR

STAT Orders A STAT order means that you give a single dose of a medication immediately and only once. Health care providers usually write STAT orders for emergencies when the patient's condition changes suddenly. For example:

Give Apresoline, 10 mg IM STAT

Now Orders A now order is more specific than a one-time order and is used when a patient needs a medication quickly but not right away, as in a STAT order. When you receive a now order, you have up to 90 minutes to administer the medication. Only administer medications ordered now one time. For example:

Give vancomycin 1 g IV piggyback now

Some conditions change the status of a patient's medication orders. For example, surgery automatically cancels all the patient's preoperative medications (see Chapter 38). A transfer from a general medical unit to an intensive care unit also cancels all the patient's medication orders. Because the patient's condition changes after surgery or after transferring to an intensive care unit, the health care provider writes new orders. When a patient is transferred to another health care agency or to a different unit within a hospital or is discharged, the health care provider reviews the medications and writes new orders as indicated.

PRESCRIPTIONS Prescriptions are written for patients who are to take medications outside the hospital. The pre-scription includes more detailed information than a regular order because the patient needs to understand how to take the medication and when to refill the prescription if necessary. The parts of a prescription are included in Figure 16-5.

PHARMACIST'S ROLE The pharmacist prepares and distributes prescribed medications. Pharmacists also assess the medication plan and evaluate the patient's medication-related needs. The pharmacist is responsible for filling prescriptions accurately and for being sure that prescriptions are valid.

DISTRIBUTION SYSTEMS Systems for storing and distributing medications vary. Pharmacists provide the medications, but nurses distribute medications to patients. Institutions providing nursing care have special areas for stocking and dispensing medications, such as special medication rooms, portable locked carts, computerized medication cabinets, and individual storage units in patients' rooms. Medication storage areas need to be locked when unattended.

Unit Dose The unit-dose system uses portable carts containing a drawer with a 24-hour supply of medications for each patient. The unit dose is the ordered dose of medication the patient receives at one time. Each tablet or capsule is wrapped separately. At a designated time each day, the pharmacist refills the drawers in the cart with a fresh supply. The cart also contains limited amounts of prn and stock medications for special situations. The unit-dose system is designed to reduce the number of medication errors and saves steps in dispensing medications.

Automated Medication Dispensing Systems Automated medication dispensing systems (AMDSs) are used successfully throughout the United States (Figure 16-6). The systems within the health care agency are networked with each other and with other computer systems in the agency (e.g., the computerized medical record). AMDSs control the dispensing of all medications, including opioids. Each nurse has a security code, allowing access to the system. If your agency uses a system that requires bioidentification, you have to

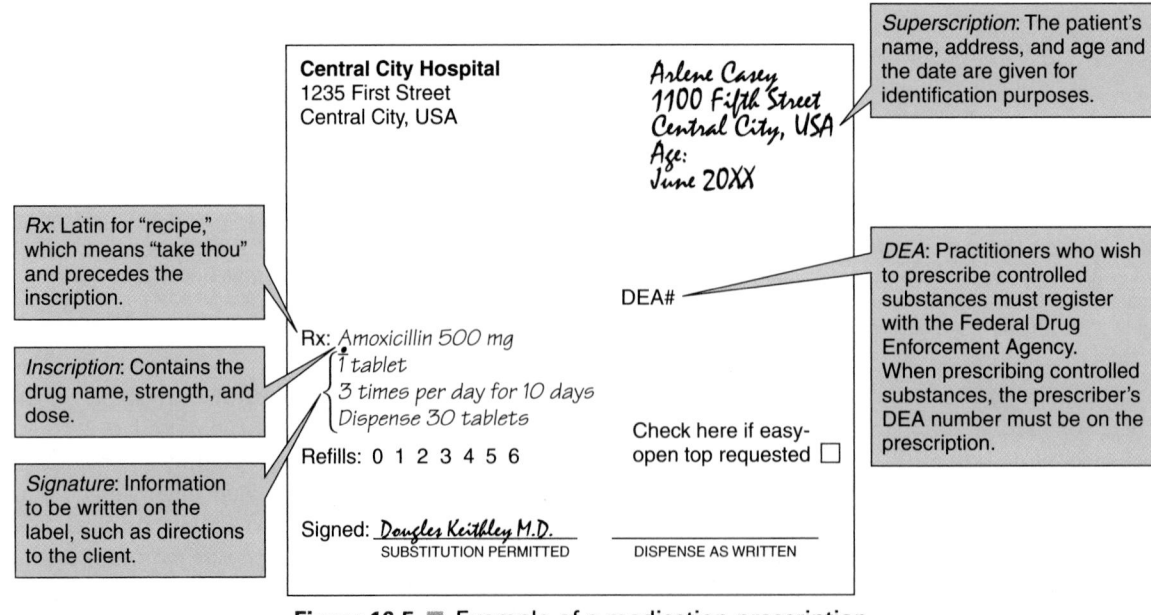

Figure 16-5 ■ Example of a medication prescription.

place your finger on a screen to access the computer. Once logged onto the AMDS, you select the patient's name and the patient's medication profile. Then you select the medication, dosage, and route from a list on the computer screen. The system opens the medication drawer or dispenses the medication to the nurse, records the event, and charges it to the patient. If the system is connected to the patient's medical record, information about the medication (e.g., name, dose, and time) and the name of the nurse who retrieved the medication from the AMDS are recorded in the patient's medical record. Some systems require nurses to scan bar codes before recording this information in the patient's computerized medical record (Figure 16-7). AMDS and bar code scanning often reduce the chance of medication errors (Foote and Coleman, 2008; Manno, 2006; Ross, 2008).

Nurse's Role The administration of medications to patients requires knowledge and a set of skills that are unique to nursing. Responsibilities of medication administration include administering medications correctly, monitoring their effects, assessing the patient's ability to self-administer medi-

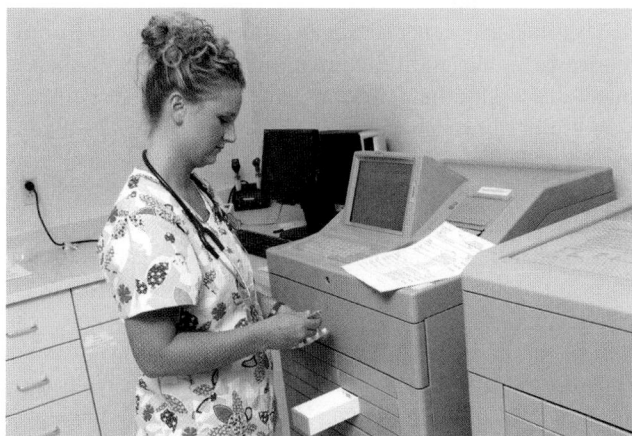

Figure 16-6 ■ Computer-controlled medication dispensing system.

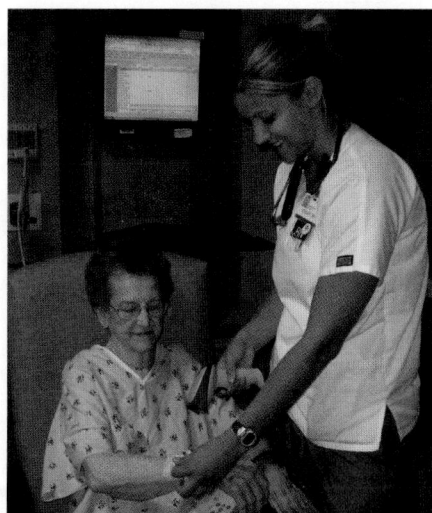

Figure 16-7 ■ Nurse using bar code scanner during medication administration.

cations, and determining whether a patient should receive a medication at a given time. Patient and family education about proper medication administration and monitoring is an integral part of the nurse's role. Never delegate this to nursing assistive personnel (NAP). Use the nursing process to integrate medication therapy into care.

Medication Errors

A **medication error** can cause or lead to inappropriate medication use or patient harm. Medication errors include inaccurate prescribing; administration of the wrong medication, route, and time interval; and administering extra doses or failing to administer a medication. Prevention of medication errors is a priority. The process of administering medications is very complex, which makes the process highly prone to errors. As a nurse, you play an essential role in the preparation and administration of medications. Therefore be vigilant in prevention of medication errors (Box 16-7). Advances in

BOX 16-7	Steps to Take in Preventing Medication Errors

- Prepare medications for only one patient at a time.
- Follow the six rights of medication administration.
- Be sure to read labels at least three times (comparing MAR with label) before administering the medication.
- Use at least two patient identifiers whenever administering a medication.
- Do not allow any other activity to interrupt your administration of medication to a patient (e.g., phone call, pager, discussions with other staff).
- Double-check all calculations, and verify with another nurse.
- Do not interpret illegible handwriting; clarify with prescriber.
- Question unusually large or small doses.
- Document all medications as soon as they are given.
- When you have made an error, reflect on what went wrong; ask how you could have prevented the error.
- Evaluate the context or situation in which a medication error occurred. This helps to determine if nurses have the necessary resources for safe medication administration.
- Attend in-service programs that focus on the medications you commonly administer.
- Ensure you are well rested when you are caring for patients. Current evidence shows that nurses make more errors when they are fatigued.
- Involve the patient when administering medications.
- Follow agency policies and protocols during medication administration; do not take short cuts.

Data from Alertness Solutions: *New survey uncovers how insomnia affects job performance and safety: first study uncovers how insomnia affects job performance and safety,* 2007, http://www.prnewswire.com/cgi-bin/stories.pl?ACCT=104&STORY=/www/story/06-12-2007/0004606266&EDATE; Dennison RD: A medication safety education program to reduce the risk of harm caused by medication errors, *J Contin Educ Nurs* 38(4):176, 2007; McIntyre LJ, Courey TJ: Safe medication administration, *J Nurs Care Qual* 22(1):40, 2007.

MAR, Medication administration record.

technology and informatics have helped decrease the occurrence of medication errors (Box 16-8).

Medication errors are often related to professional practice, health care product design, or procedures and systems such as product labeling and distribution. When an error occurs, the patient's safety and well-being become the top priority. As a nurse, assess and examine the patient's condition and notify the health care provider of the incident as soon as possible. Report the incident to the appropriate person in the institution (e.g., manager or supervisor) once the patient is stable.

When a medication error occurs and you are involved, you are responsible for preparing a written occurrence or incident report within 24 hours of the incident. The report includes patient identification information; the location and time of the incident; an accurate, factual description of what occurred and what was done; and the signature of the nurse involved. The incident report is not a permanent part of the medical record and should not be referred to in the patient's medical record (see Chapters 4 and 9). This legally protects the health care professional and agency. Agencies use occurrence reports to track incident patterns and to initiate quality improvement programs as needed.

Report all medication errors, including mistakes that do not cause obvious or immediate harm or near misses. You need to feel comfortable in reporting an error and not fear repercussions from managerial staff. Even when a patient suffers no harm from a medication error, the agency benefits from learning why the mistake occurred and what can be done to avoid similar errors in the future (Dennison, 2007).

Medication errors frequently occur when a patient is transferred (e.g., to another health care agency or to another unit within the hospital) or discharged. Therefore reconciling the patient's list of medications during the transfer or discharge process is a National Patient Safety Goal (TJC, 2008b). You will play an important role in **medication reconciliation** (Box 16-9). Medication reconciliation is a process in which you compare the medications your patient took in the previous setting (e.g., home or another nursing unit) with the current medication orders whenever you admit a patient to a new health care setting (Ptasinski, 2007).When the patient leaves that setting for another setting (e.g., skilled care facility or intensive care unit), you communicate your patient's current medications with the health care providers in the new setting. You also need to reconcile your patient's medications if your patient is discharged from the agency. Most health care agencies have computerized or written forms used to facilitate medication reconciliation (Carpi, 2008). Reconciling medications is challenging and requires a great deal of concentration and time. Eliminate distractions, and take your time when reconciling your patient's medications. Always clarify information whenever needed. You often will need to consult with your patient, the patient's caregivers, family members, physicians, advanced practice nurses, and pharmacists when reconciling a patient's medications (Beyea, 2007b).

BOX 16-8 Informatics and Medication Safety

Medication errors frequently happen when a nurse incorrectly administers medications at a patient's bedside. Innovations in technology and informatics have reduced the number of medication errors in nursing practice:
- Networked computers allow health care providers to see a current list of ordered and discontinued medications.
- Internet and intranet access allows nurses and other health care providers to access current information about medications (e.g., indications, desired effects, adverse effects) and specific agency policies that address medication administration (e.g., how fast to administer an intravenous push [IVP] medication).
- Some agencies have prescribers directly enter medication orders into a computer system or personal hand-held computer.
- Automated medication dispensing systems, bar coding technology, and electronic medication administration records (MARs) help with medication reconciliation, administration, and documentation (Carpi, 2008; Manno, 2006; Paoletti and others, 2007).

APPLICATION TO NURSING PRACTICE
- Actively participate in the evaluation and selection of advanced technologies. Also participate in the development of nursing policies and protocols used for medication administration.
- Always follow agency policies when administering medications.
- Implement agency policies when technology cannot be used (e.g., during downtime or power outages).
- Follow manufacturer's guidelines for care of electronic equipment, and report problems with technology immediately.

BOX 16-9 Process for Medication Reconciliation

1 **Verify:** Obtain a current list of the patient's medications.
2 **Clarify:** Make sure the list of medications, dosages, and frequencies is accurate; clarify the list with as many people as necessary (e.g., patient, caregiver, health care providers, pharmacists) to ensure list is accurate.
3 **Reconcile:** Compare new medication orders with the current list; investigate any discrepancies with the patient's health care provider.
4 **Transmit:** Communicate the updated and verified list to health care team members, caregivers, and the patient as appropriate.

Data from Beyea SC: Medication reconciliation: what every nurse needs to know, *AORN J* 85(1):193, 2007; Ptasinski C: Develop a medication reconciliation process, *Nurs Manage* 38(3):18, 2007.

CRITICAL THINKING

Synthesis

You will apply elements of critical thinking whenever you perform the nursing process with a patient. Consider the scientific knowledge you have learned, your experiences, critical thinking attitudes, and standards to ensure an individualized approach to patient care.

KNOWLEDGE You will use knowledge from many disciplines when administering medications. Knowledge of physiology and pathophysiology helps you understand why a particular medication has been prescribed for a patient and how this medication will alter the patient's physiology as it exerts its therapeutic effect. Your knowledge about medications is also important. The growing number of medications readily available to patients, the acute and complex nature of patient problems, higher acuity levels in acute care settings, and reductions in nursing and pharmacy staff contribute to the need for advanced knowledge about medications. Knowledge about growth and development principles is also useful in medication administration. For example, knowledge about child development indicates that children often perceive medication administration as a negative experience. Use principles from child development to ensure that the child cooperates with medication administration.

EXPERIENCE As a nursing student, you have limited experience with medication administration as it applies to professional practice. However, clinical experiences will provide you with the opportunity to apply the nursing process to medication administration. As you gain experience in medication administration, cognitive skills (e.g., medication calculations and recognizing side effects) and psychomotor skills (e.g., the preparation and actual administration of a medication) become more refined. As you acquire experience in observing patients' responses to medications, you will become more able to anticipate and evaluate the effects of medications.

ATTITUDES To administer medications safely to patients, several critical thinking attitudes are essential. For example, you show discipline when you take adequate time to prepare and administer medications. You take the time to read your patient's history and physical, review your patient's orders, look up medications you do not know in a medication reference book, and determine why your patient is taking each prescribed medication. Every step of safe medication administration requires a disciplined attitude and a comprehensive, systematic approach.

Responsibility is another critical thinking attitude that is essential to medication administration. When you administer a medication to a patient, you accept the responsibility that the medication or the nursing actions in administering it will not harm the patient in any way. You are responsible for knowing that the medication that is ordered for the patient is the correct medication and the correct dose. You are ultimately accountable for administering an ordered medication that is obviously inappropriate for the patient. Therefore be familiar with the therapeutic effect, usual dosage, anticipated changes in laboratory data, and side effects of all medications that you administer.

STANDARDS Professional standards guide medication administration. The American Nurses Association's (ANA's) *Standards of Nursing Practice* (see Chapters 4 and 12), based on the nursing process, apply to the activity of medication administration. Other professional nursing standards also apply. For example, the Association of periOperative Registered Nurses (AORN) has developed a guidance statement that helps maintain safe medication nursing practices in perioperative settings (AORN, 2008).

To ensure safe medication administration, be aware of the six rights of medication administration:

1. The right medication
2. The right dose
3. The right patient
4. The right route
5. The right time
6. The right documentation

Right Medication A medication order is required for any medication that you administer. Sometimes prescribers write orders by hand in the patient's chart. Alternatively, some agencies use computerized physician order entry (CPOE). CPOE allows the prescriber to electronically enter ordered medications. This eliminates the need for written orders. Regardless of how the order for the medication is received, you compare the written orders with the medication administration record (MAR) when health care providers first order medications. Also, verify medication information whenever new MARs are written or distributed or when patients transfer from one nursing unit or health care setting to another (TJC, 2008b).

Once you determine that the information on the MAR is accurate, use the MAR to prepare and administer medications. When preparing medications in bottles or containers, compare the label of the medication container with the medication administration order three times: (1) while removing the container from the drawer or shelf, (2) as you remove the amount of medication ordered from the container, and (3) at the bedside before administering the medication to the patient. Never prepare medications from unmarked containers or containers with illegible labels (TJC, 2008b). With unit-dose packaged medications, you check the medication's label and dosage when you take it out of the medication dispensing system. Finally, you verify all medications at the patient's bedside with the patient's MAR, using at least two patient identifiers before giving the patient any medications (TJC, 2008b).

Because the nurse who administers the medication is responsible for any errors related to that medication, only administer medications you prepare. If a patient questions a medication, it is important not to ignore these concerns. An alert patient will know whether a medication is different from those received before. In most cases the patient's medication order has been changed; however, the patient's questions sometimes reveal an error. Withhold the medication until you recheck it against the prescriber's orders. If a patient refuses a medication, discard it rather than returning it to the original container. You can save unit-dose medications if they are not opened.

At home, have patients keep medications in their original labeled containers. It helps to have patients use a written schedule to remember which medications they need to take.

Right Dose   The unit-dose system is designed to minimize errors. When you prepare a medication from a larger volume or strength than needed or when the health care provider orders a system of measurement different from what the pharmacist supplies, the chance for error increases. Have another nurse check your work when performing medication calculations or conversions.

After calculating dosages, prepare the medication using standard measurement devices. Use graduated cups, syringes, and scaled droppers to measure medications accurately. At home, have patients use kitchen measuring spoons or commercially available medication measuring devices rather than teaspoons and tablespoons, which vary in volume.

Medication errors often occur when pills need to be split. To promote patient safety in inpatient settings, pharmacists split the medications, label and package them, and then send them to the nurse for administration. If your patient has to split medications at home, provide clear instructions and ensure the patient has a pill-splitting device at home (ISMP, 2006).

Sometimes you crush a tablet so you can mix it in food. Make sure the crushing device is completely clean before crushing the tablet. Remnants of previously crushed medications increase a medication's concentration or result in the patient receiving a portion of an unprescribed medication. Mix crushed medications with very small amounts of food or liquid. Do not use the patient's favorite foods or liquids because medications alter their taste and decrease the patient's desire for them. This is especially a concern with pediatric patients.

You cannot crush all medications. Some medications, such as time-released or extended-release capsules, have special coatings to keep the medication from being absorbed too quickly. Refer to a medication reference, such as the "Do Not Crush List" published by ISMP (2008b), to ensure that you can safely crush the medication.

Right Patient   An important step in administering medications safely is being sure you give the medication to the right patient. It is difficult to remember every patient's name and face. Therefore, before giving a medication to a patient, you need to use at least two patient identifiers **every time** you administer medications, even if you know the patient (TJC, 2008b). Acceptable patient identifiers include the patient's name or an identification number assigned by a health care agency. Do not use the patient's room number as an identifier. To identify a patient correctly in an acute care setting, compare the patient identifiers on the MAR with the patient's identification bracelet while at the patient's bedside. If an identification bracelet becomes illegible or is missing, get a

new one for the patient. In health care settings that are not acute care settings, The Joint Commission (2008b) does not require the use of armbands for identification. However, you still need to use a system that verifies the patient's identification with at least two identifiers before administering medications.

The Joint Commission (2008b) does not require that patients state their names and other identifiers when administering medications. The required identification process mandates collecting patient identifiers reliably when the patient is admitted to a health care agency. Once the identifiers are assigned to the patient (e.g., putting identifiers on an armband and placing the armband on the patient), you use the identifiers to match the patient with the MAR, which lists the correct medications. Asking patients to state their full names and identification information provides you with a third way to verify that you are giving medications to the right person.

In addition to using two identifiers, some agencies use a wireless bar code scanner to help identify the right patient. This system requires you to scan a personal bar code that is commonly placed on your name tag first. Then you scan a bar code on the single-dose medication package. Finally, you scan the patient's armband (see Figure 16-7, p. 395). This information is then stored in a computer for documentation purposes. This system helps eliminate medication errors because it provides another step to ensure that the right patient receives the right medication (Mills and others, 2006; Paoletti and others, 2007; Skibinski and others, 2007).

Right Route   Always consult the prescriber when an order does not specify a route of administration. Likewise, if the specified route is not the recommended route or is not an appropriate route, alert the prescriber immediately.

Recent evidence shows that medication errors involving the wrong route are common. For example, enteral and parenteral medications are at risk for confusion in the pediatric population because liquid medications are frequently given orally. Therefore, when you prepare liquid medications, whether they are oral or parenteral, take precautions to ensure that you prepare and give the medications correctly. It is important to prepare injections only from preparations designed for parenteral use. The injection of a liquid designed for oral use produces local complications, such as sterile abscess or fatal systemic effects. Medication companies label parenteral medications "for injectable use only." Some agencies now use different syringes for enteral and parenteral medication administration. The enteral syringes are a different color than the parenteral syringes and are clearly labeled for oral or enteral use only. In addition, the syringe tips of these enteral syringes are incompatible with parenteral medication administration systems. Needles do not attach to the syringes, and the syringes cannot be inserted into any type of IV line (Bridge, 2007).

Right Time   Know why a medication is ordered for certain times of the day and whether you can alter the time schedule. For example, two medications are ordered, one q8h (every 8 hours) and the other 3 times a day. You will give both medications 3 times within a 24-hour period. The prescriber

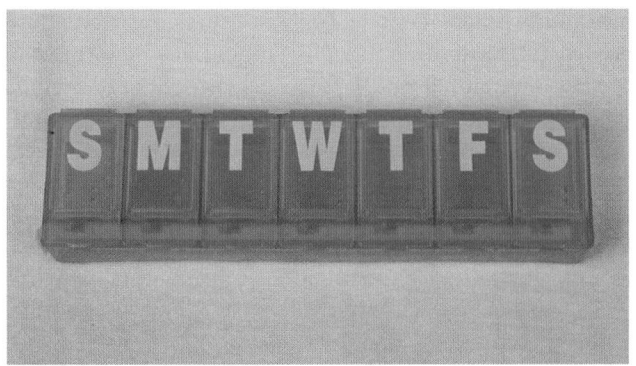

Figure 16-8 ■ Medication organization container to help patients remember to take medications.

intends for you to give the q8h medication every 8 hours around the clock to maintain therapeutic blood levels of the medication. In contrast, you give the 3 times per day medication at 3 different times during the waking hours. Each agency has a recommended time schedule for medications ordered at frequent intervals.

The prescriber often gives specific instructions about when to administer a medication. A preoperative medication to be given "on call" to surgery means that you will give the medication when the operating room staff members tell you they are coming to get the patient for surgery. You give a medication ordered pc (after meals) within 30 minutes after a meal when the patient has a full stomach. You give a STAT medication immediately.

Give priority to medications that must act at certain times. For example, you need to administer insulin at a precise interval before a meal. Give antibiotics on time around the clock to maintain therapeutic blood levels. Give all routinely ordered medications within 60 minutes of the time ordered (30 minutes before or after the prescribed time).

Some medications require your clinical judgment when determining the proper time for administration. Administer a prn sleeping medication when the patient is prepared for bed. Also, use nursing judgment when giving prn analgesics. For example, you sometimes need to obtain a STAT order from the health care provider if the patient requires a medication before the prn interval has elapsed. Document whenever you call the patient's health care provider to obtain a change in a medication's order.

At home some patients have to take many medications throughout the day. Help plan schedules based on recommended medication intervals and the patient's daily schedule. For patients who have difficulty remembering when to take medications, make a chart that lists the times when to take each medication or prepare a special container that organizes and stores medications according to when the patient needs to take them (Figure 16-8).

Right Documentation Nurses and other health care providers use accurate documentation to communicate with each other. Many medication errors result from inaccurate documentation. Therefore ensure that accurate and appropriate documentation exists before and after giving medications.

Before you administer medications, be sure the MAR indicates the patient's full name, the name of the ordered medications written out in full (no medication name abbreviations), the time the medication is to be administered, and the medication's dose, route, and frequency. Common problems with medication orders include incomplete information, inaccurate dosage form or strength, illegible orders or signature, incorrect placement of decimals, and nonstandard terminology. If you ever have questions about a medication order, contact the health care provider immediately to verify the order before giving your patient the medication. All prescribers need to provide accurate information about medication orders. If you are unable to contact the prescriber or resolve confusion about the medication, follow your agency's policy on whom you need to contact next. Often these policies are called "chain of command" policies. Follow your agency's chain of command policy until you resolve issues related to your patients' medications.

Some medications require you to assess the patient before giving them (e.g., you need to take the patient's blood pressure before administering an antihypertensive medication). Ensure that you document all preassessment data in the patient's medical record before administering the medication.

After you administer medications, record the administration of each medication on the MAR as soon as you give the medication. Never document that you have given a medication until you have actually given it. Inaccurate documentation, such as failing to document giving a medication or documenting an incorrect dose, leads to errors in subsequent decisions about your patient's care. Consider the following situation: A patient receives insulin before breakfast, but the nurse does not document the insulin dose. The nurse caring for the patient goes home, and the patient has a new nurse for the day. The new nurse notices that the insulin is not documented and assumes that the previous nurse did not give the insulin. Therefore the new nurse gives the patient another dose of insulin. About 2 hours later, the patient experiences low blood glucose levels, and this causes the patient to have seizures. Accurate documentation would have prevented this situation from happening.

You need to document the name of the medication, the dose, the time of administration, and the route on the MAR. Also document the site of any injections you give. Document the patient's responses to medications, either positive or negative, in the nursing notes. Notify the patient's health care provider of any negative responses to medications, and document the time, date, and name of the health care provider you notified in the patient's chart. The efforts you make in ensuring the right documentation will help you to provide safe care to your patients.

MAINTAINING PATIENTS' RIGHTS In accordance with *The Patient Care Partnership* (American Hospital Association [AHA], 2003) and because of the potential risks related to medication administration, a patient has the right to:

1. Be informed of medication name, purpose, action, and potential undesired effects
2. Refuse a medication regardless of the consequences

3. Have qualified nurses and other health care providers assess a medication history, including allergies and use of herbals
4. Be properly advised of the experimental nature of medication therapy and to give written consent for its use
5. Receive labeled medications safely without discomfort in accordance with the six rights of medication administration (see section on medication delivery)
6. Receive appropriate supportive therapy in relation to medication therapy
7. Not receive unnecessary medications
8. Be informed if prescribed medications are a part of a research study

NURSING PROCESS

■■■ ASSESSMENT

You will assess many factors to determine a patient's need for and potential response to medication therapy. Perform a thorough assessment on all your patients to help ensure safe medication administration.

HISTORY Before administering medications, obtain or review the patient's medical history. A patient's medical history will provide indications or contraindications for medication therapy. Disease or illness places patients at risk for adverse medication effects. For example, if a patient has a gastric ulcer, compounds containing aspirin will increase the likelihood of bleeding. Long-term health problems require specific medications. This knowledge will help you anticipate the medications your patient requires. A patient's surgical history indicates use of medications. For example, after a thyroidectomy a patient requires thyroid hormone replacement.

History of Allergies All members of the health care team need to know the patient's history of allergies to medications and foods. Many medications have ingredients found in food sources. For example, propofol, which is used for anesthesia and sedation, contains inactive ingredients of egg lecithin and soybean oil. Therefore patients who have an egg or soy allergy should not receive propofol (Wiesner and others, 2008). In an acute care setting, patients sometimes wear identification bands that list medication allergies. All allergies and the types of reactions are noted on the patient's admission notes, medication records, and history and physical.

Medication History When taking a medication history, assess what medications the patient takes, including prescription and nonprescription drugs and herbal supplements. Include the length of time the patient has taken each drug, current dosage schedule, whether the patient has experienced adverse effects to any of the medications, and if the patient takes medications correctly (e.g., count doses or have the patient keep a diary to track when medications are taken). In addition, review information about the medications, including action, purpose, normal dosages, routes, side effects, and nursing implications for administration and monitoring. Be sure that the prescriber has ordered a safe dose, especially when caring for older adults or children. Also, be aware of

medication interactions and special nursing interventions needed for medication administration. Often, you need to consult several references to gather needed information. Pharmacology textbooks and handbooks; electronic medication manuals available on a desktop, laptop, or handheld computer; nursing journals; the *Physicians' Desk Reference* (PDR); medication package inserts; and pharmacists are valuable resources. You are responsible for knowing as much as possible about each medication your patients receive.

Diet History A diet history describes the patient's normal eating patterns and food preferences. An effective dosage schedule is planned around normal eating patterns and food preferences. Some medications interact with food. In these cases, assess when patients take these medications to determine if they avoid foods that interact with their medications.

PATIENT'S PERCEPTUAL OR COORDINATION PROBLEMS For a patient with perceptual or coordination limitations, self-administration is sometimes difficult. Assess the patient's ability to prepare doses (e.g., open containers or fill syringes) and take medications (e.g., perform self-injection or instill eye drops) correctly. If the patient is unable to self-administer medications, you will need to assess whether family or friends will be available to assist.

PATIENT'S CURRENT CONDITION The ongoing physical or mental status of a patient affects whether you give a medication and how you administer it. Assess a patient carefully before giving any medication. For example, check the patient's blood pressure before giving an antihypertensive. If the blood pressure is unusually low (e.g., systolic pressure below 100 mm Hg), hold the medication and notify the patient's health care provider. Assessment findings serve as a baseline in evaluating the effects of medication therapy.

PATIENT'S ATTITUDE ABOUT MEDICATION USE Patients' attitudes about medications affect their adherence to their medication therapy. Sometimes patient attitudes reveal medication dependence or avoidance. Patients do not usually express their feelings about taking a medication, especially if dependence is a problem. Observe the patient's behavior for evidence of medication dependence or avoidance. Also assess the patient's cultural and personal beliefs about Western medicine to determine if the patient's beliefs interfere with medication compliance (Box 16-10 and Chapter 19).

PATIENT'S KNOWLEDGE AND UNDERSTANDING OF MEDICATION THERAPY The patient's knowledge and understanding of medication therapy influence the willingness or ability to follow a medication regimen. Unless a patient understands a medication's purpose, the importance of regular dosage schedules and proper administration methods, and the possible side effects, adherence is unlikely. If the patient cannot afford medications, discuss financial resources (Tseng and others, 2007). Questions used to assess the patient's knowledge of a medication include the following:

- What is it for?
- How is it taken?
- When is it taken?

BOX 16-10   CULTURAL FOCUS

Emilio is worried that Esther will have trouble managing her medications at home because she takes so many medications. He knows that to help Esther manage her medications at home, he needs to learn more about her culture. When compared with whites, people who are African American have a greater incidence of type 2 diabetes, and their diabetes often is not well controlled. In addition, they have poorer control of their blood pressure, their serum lipid levels are higher, and they are at increased risk for end-stage renal disease. Cost, transportation issues, and long wait times at the pharmacy often affect the ability of African Americans to adhere to their disease management plans. Although low socioeconomic status (SES) contributes to poorer health status, there are factors other than SES that negatively affect a person's health. In African Americans, being younger, being female, having more medications prescribed, and poor health status often contribute to a patient's difficulty in adhering to medication prescriptions at home. African American patients tend to manage their medications at home better when they understand their medication regimen and when they are able to afford their medications. Social support, a strong sense of spirituality, and belonging to a church are other factors that help African Americans successfully manage their medications.

IMPLICATIONS FOR PRACTICE

- Emilio knows that not all African American people are the same. To provide quality individualized care, he assesses Esther's cultural beliefs and determines what factors affected her ability to manage her medications before she entered the hospital.
- Emilio asks Esther about her relationships with family and friends and assesses her spiritual and religious preferences. He asks Esther to identify family and friends who can help her when she goes home.
- Because Esther had a hip replacement, Emilio anticipates that Esther will have difficulty getting her medications from the pharmacy. After discovering that Esther is active in her church, Emilio gets permission from Esther to contact the minister at her church. Emilio asks the minister to identify church members who are able to help Esther get to the pharmacy or go to the pharmacy for her so she can obtain her medications at home.
- Because she was so independent before her surgery, Emilio knows that Esther may become discouraged when she gets home because she will need help at home until she completely heals from her surgery. Emilio finds out that Esther has a strong sense of spirituality. Therefore he encourages Esther to use spirituality-based coping methods (e.g., praying, quiet reflection) when she goes home.

Data from Kripalani S and others: Medication use among inner-city patients after hospital discharge: patient-reported barriers and solutions, *Mayo Clin Proc* 83(5):529, 2008; Sunil TS, McGehee MA: Social and religious support on treatment adherence among HIV/AIDS patients by race/ethnicity, *Journal of HIV/AIDS & Social Services* 6(1-2):83, 2007; Sweet E and others: Relationships between skin color, income, and blood pressure among African Americans in the CARDIA study, *Am J Public Health* 97(12): 2253, 2007; Tang TS and others: Social support, quality of life, and self-care behaviors among African Americans with type 2 diabetes, *Diabetes Educ* 34(2):266, 2008; Tseng C and others: Race/ethnicity and economic differences in cost-related medication underuse among insured adults with diabetes, *Diabetes Care* 31(2):261, 2007.

- What side effects have there been?
- Have you ever stopped taking doses?
- Is there anything else you do not understand and would like to know about the medication?

PATIENT'S LEARNING NEEDS During assessment, you will discover that some patients do not understand their medications. When this happens, you need to determine your patient's readiness to learn, what the patient expects to learn, the patient's ability to learn, and what the patient understands about prescribed medications (see Chapter 11).

PATIENT EXPECTATIONS In assessing your patients' expectations about medication administration, determine your patients' perceptions about their illnesses and their medications. Your patients' expectations and beliefs about their medications, as well as their perceptions and preferences, influence their adherence to their medications. Do your patients believe their medications will be helpful? How do they feel about the medication's adverse effects? Do they believe that they will be able to afford their medications? It is your responsibility to monitor your patients' adherence to their medications. To facilitate adherence, develop a trusting relationship with your patients that is open, ongoing, and collaborative (Howland, 2007).

■■■NURSING DIAGNOSIS

Assessment provides data about the patient's condition, ability to self-administer medications, and medication adherence, which you will use to determine actual or potential problems with medication therapy. As you review your assessment data, you will see clusters or patterns that reveal defining characteristics for nursing diagnoses. For example, if a patient admits to missing a medication dose and states he or she is having trouble remembering when doses are due, these data often indicate the diagnosis of *ineffective therapeutic regimen management* regarding a medication schedule. Once you select the diagnosis, you need to identify the appropriate related factor. The related factors of inadequate resources versus lack of knowledge require different interventions. If the patient's ineffective medication management is related to inadequate finances, collaborate with family members, social workers, or community agencies to help the patient receive necessary medications. If the related factor is lack of knowledge, implement a teaching plan with follow-up. The following is a list of nursing diagnoses that you will use when administering medications to patients:

- *Anxiety*
- *Ineffective health maintenance*

- *Readiness for enhanced self-health management*
- *Deficient knowledge (medications)*
- *Noncompliance*
- *Effective therapeutic regimen management*
- *Ineffective family therapeutic regimen management*

Planning

During planning, organize nursing activities to ensure the safe administration of medications. Current evidence shows that distractions or hurrying during medication preparation and administration increase the risk for medication errors (Beyea, 2007a). Give yourself adequate time, and avoid interruptions and distractions when you prepare and administer medications. Some agencies have created quiet zones in medication rooms so nurses do not interrupt their colleagues when preparing medications. Another way to avoid medication errors is to have all the equipment you need available when you prepare medications. Diligent planning and following a safe routine every time you prepare and administer medications ensures safe medication administration.

GOALS AND OUTCOMES Goals of medication administration include better control of the patient's disease, improved health, and adherence to the medication regimen. Work closely with your patients to set goals, outcomes, and appropriate nursing interventions. Whether a patient attempts self-administration or you assume responsibility for administering medications, you set goals and expected outcomes to use time wisely during medication administration. For example, if you are caring for a patient with newly diagnosed hypertension, you establish the following goal and expected outcomes:

Goal: The patient will safely administer all medications before discharge.
Outcomes:

1. The patient will verbalize understanding of desired and adverse effects of medications before discharge.
2. The patient will describe doses and administration schedule for ordered medications before discharge.

SETTING PRIORITIES You will frequently need to set priorities during medication administration, especially when you care for multiple patients at the same time. It is important to assess your patient's clinical condition to determine which nursing diagnosis takes the greatest priority and which medications need to be administered first. Medications that are to be administered around the clock (e.g., antibiotics) need to be given in a timely manner to maintain therapeutic serum levels. Frequently medications given for pain or to prevent serious harm to the patient such as antihypertensives, cardiac medications, and antiseizure drugs are of a higher priority than other medications. The priorities for every patient will be different. It is your responsibility to know your patients and prioritize their needs appropriately.

In addition to administering medications, teaching patients about their medications is another priority. Plan to teach patients about their medications while you administer medications. Family members usually reinforce the importance of medication regimens. Therefore collaborate with the patient's family or friends when you provide instruction. When patients are hospitalized, begin teaching when the patient is admitted; do not postpone instruction until the day of discharge. In outpatient or community settings, ensure that patients know where and how to obtain medications and that they are able to read medication labels.

COLLABORATIVE CARE As patients move from one health care setting to another, it is essential to establish a plan for continuity of care. Make sure you reconcile your patients' medications every time you admit, transfer, or discharge them. Communicate the patients' medication lists to appropriate members of the health care team. Collaboration with other health care team members (e.g., health care providers, pharmacists, social workers, and dietitians) is essential in successful medication administration for your patients.

Implementation

HEALTH PROMOTION In promoting or maintaining the patient's health, remember that health beliefs, personal motivation, socioeconomic factors, and habits (e.g., excessive alcohol intake) influence the patient's adherence with the medication regimen. Several nursing interventions promote adherence to a medication regimen. These include teaching patients and their families about the benefits of medications and how and why to take them correctly. It is important to integrate the patient's health beliefs and cultural practices into the treatment plan. Make referrals to community resources if the patient is unable to afford or cannot arrange transportation to obtain necessary medications.

Patient and Family Teaching If you do not inform patients properly about medications or if your patients have problems with health literacy, it is possible that they will take their medications incorrectly or they will not take their medications at all. For patients with low health literacy, you need to adapt your approaches so patients will understand instruction. Provide information about the purpose of medications and their actions and effects. Many health care institutions offer easy-to-read patient education sheets on specific types of medications. A patient needs to know how to take a medication properly and what will happen if he or she fails to do so. For example, after receiving a prescription for an antibiotic, a patient needs to understand the importance of taking the full prescription. Failure to do this leads to a worsening of the condition, as well as the development of bacteria resistant to the medication. Also teach patients ways to change medication schedules to fit into their lifestyles. Patients who are placed on newly prescribed medications may need more involved instruction (Box 16-11). Ensure that everything you teach the patient and all teaching materials you provide match the patient's health literacy level (see Chapter 11).

When your patients depend on daily injections, they need to learn to prepare and administer an injection correctly using aseptic technique. Teach family members or friends to give injections in case the patient becomes ill or physically unable to handle a syringe. Provide specially designed equipment such as syringes with enlarged calibrated scales for

BOX 16-11   PATIENT TEACHING

Preparing for Home Medication Administration

 Emilio finds out that Esther will be going home at the end of the week. Before she can leave, she needs to learn how to self-administer her medications safely. Older adult patients often have difficulty with medication adherence because they have difficulty affording medications. Older adults also often take medications out of their normal containers, have difficulties opening medication packages, and often have problems related to health literacy. Based on this information, Emilio develops the following teaching plan for Esther:

OUTCOME

At the end of the teaching session, Esther will be able to self-administer her medications safely and correctly.

TEACHING STRATEGIES

- Sit with Esther at a table in a room that is well lit and has limited distractions (e.g., television off).
- Include Esther's caregivers in educational sessions.
- Have Esther's caregiver bring all of her medications from home to the hospital. Compare the medications Esther has at home with the medications she is going to take at home. Determine which medications Esther understands.
- Assess Esther's health literacy by determining her ability to understand what she reads and to do simple medica-

tion calculations. If she has poor health literacy, ensure that information is presented at a level Esther can understand, and arrange for help from family, friends, and/or home care nurses to help Esther when she goes home.
- Review information about medications, including desired effect, dose, frequency, and adverse effects with Esther. Show Esther how to use a medication organizer. Encourage Esther to leave medications not in the organizer in their original containers.
- Provide patient teaching materials that include helpful pictures to enhance Esther's understanding of prescribed medications. Ensure that the print and pictures on the teaching sheets are large enough for Esther to see.

EVALUATION STRATEGIES

- Ask Esther questions about her medications (e.g., "Why are you taking these medications?" "When do you take your medications?").
- Ask Esther to write out a medication schedule that includes how much of each medication she should take and when she should take it.
- Have Esther verbalize the symptoms related to the possible adverse effects of medications she is taking and identify what to report to her health care provider.
- Have Esther set up her own medications for one day, and evaluate her accuracy.

Data from Kairuz T and others: Identifying compliance issues with prescription medications among older people: a pilot study, *Drugs Aging* 25(2):153, 2008; Katz MG, Kripalani S, Weiss BD: Use of pictorial aids in medication instructions: a review of the literature, *Am J Health Syst Pharm* 63(1):2391, 2006; Yin HS and others: Association of low caregiver health literacy with reported use of nonstandardized dosing instruments and lack of knowledge of weight-based dosage, *Ambul Pediatr* 7(4):292, 2007.

BOX 16-12   Components of Medication Orders

A medication order needs to have the following:

Patient's full name: The patient's full name distinguishes the patient from other persons with the same last name.

Date and time that the order is written: Include the day, month, year, and time. Designating the time that an order is written clarifies when certain orders are to stop automatically. If an incident occurs involving a medication error, it is easier to document what happened when this information is available.

Drug name: The physician or advanced practice nurse will order a generic or trade-name drug. Correct spelling is essential in preventing confusion with drugs with similar spellings.

Dosage: Include the amount or the strength of the medication.

Route of administration: Drug route is important because you administer some drugs by more than one route. Be sure to clarify unsafe or illegible abbreviations with the prescriber to avoid medication errors.

Time and frequency of administration: You need to know when to initiate drug therapy. Orders for multiple doses establish a routine schedule for drug administration.

Signature of prescriber: The signature makes the order a legal request.

easier reading or braille-labeled medication vials for patients with visual alterations.

Patients need to be aware of the symptoms of medication side effects or toxicity. Inform family members of medication side effects, such as changes in behavior, because they often recognize these effects first. Your patients are better able to cope with problems caused by medications if they understand how and when to act. All patients need to learn the basic guidelines for medication safety. These guidelines ensure the proper use and storage of medications in the home.

ACUTE CARE ACTIVITIES In the acute care setting, expert nursing interventions, timely observation, and documentation of patient responses to medications are essential. Several nursing interventions are critical to providing safe and effective medication administration.

Receiving, Transcribing, and Communicating Medication Orders A medication order is required to administer any medication to a patient. The medication order needs to contain all the elements in Box 16-12. The process of verification of medications varies among health care agencies. During the transcription process the nurse and pharmacist check all medication orders for accuracy and thoroughness several times, and the prescriber's complete order is placed on the appropriate medication form, the MAR. The MAR includes the patient's name, room, and bed number, as well as the name, dosage, frequency, and route of administration for each medication. If the MAR is handwritten, you complete or update the MAR. Some agencies use a computer to generate the MAR (Figure 16-9). Use the MAR printout to record medications given. Sometimes the MAR is electronic and is viewed on a computer screen. Regardless of the type of MAR your agency uses, be sure you refer to the MAR each time you prepare a medication and have it available at the patient's bedside when administering medications. It is essential that you verify the accuracy of every medication you give to the patient with the patient's orders. If the medication order is incomplete, incorrect, or inappropriate or if there is a discrepancy between the written order and what is on the MAR, consult with the prescriber. Do not give the medication until you are certain that you are able to follow the six rights of medication administration. When you give the wrong medication or an incorrect dose, **you** are legally responsible for the error.

Accurate Dosage Calculation and Measurement You calculate each dose when preparing medications. To avoid calculation errors, pay close attention to the process of calculation, and avoid interruptions from other people or nursing activities. Ask another nurse to double-check your calculations against the prescriber's order if you are in doubt about the accuracy of your calculation or if you are calculating a new or unusual dose.

Correct Administration Before administering a medication to a patient, verify the patient's identity by using at least two patient identifiers (TJC, 2008b). Identifiers are usually on a patient's armband. Compare the two identifiers with the MAR to ensure that you are giving the medications to the correct patient. You also can ask the patient to state his or her name as a third identifier. Use aseptic technique and proper procedures when handling and giving medications. Some medications require an assessment before administration (e.g., assessing heart rate before giving a cardiac glycoside).

Recording Medication Administration After administering a medication, you record it immediately on the appropriate record form (see Figure 16-9). Never chart a medication before administering it. Recording immediately after administration prevents errors. The recording of a medication includes the name of the medication, dosage, route, and exact time of administration. Some agency policies also require that you record the location of an injection.

If a patient refuses a medication or is undergoing tests or procedures that result in a missed dose, explain why you did not give the medication in the nurses' notes. Some agencies require that you circle the prescribed administration time on the medication record when a patient misses a dose. Be sure to follow all agency policies when documenting medication administration.

RESTORATIVE AND CONTINUING CARE Because of the numerous types of restorative care settings, medication administration activities vary. In the home care and rehabilitation settings, patients usually administer their own medications. However, patients with functional limitations often need assistance from caregivers. Provide education to patients and/or caregivers to help them administer medications accurately and safely.

SPECIAL CONSIDERATIONS FOR ADMINISTERING MEDICATIONS TO SPECIFIC AGE-GROUPS A patient's developmental level affects how you administer medications. Knowledge of your patient's developmental needs helps you anticipate responses to medication therapy.

Infants and Children Children vary in age; weight; surface area; and the ability to absorb, metabolize, and excrete medications. Children's medication dosages are usually lower than those of adults, but with some medications, children require higher dosages than adults. Therefore take special caution when preparing medications for children. Medications are not always prepared and packaged in standardized dose ranges for children and often require careful calculations.

A child's parents often are valuable resources for determining the best way to give the child medications. Sometimes it is less traumatic for the child if a parent gives the medication while you supervise. Box 16-13 (p. 406) outlines tips for administering medications to children.

Older Adults Older adults also require special consideration during medication administration (Box 16-14, p. 406). In addition to physiological changes of aging (Figure 16-10, p. 407), behavioral and economic factors influence an older person's use of medications.

Polypharmacy. **Polypharmacy** happens when a patient uses two or more medications to treat the same illness, when a patient takes two or more medications from the same chemical class, or when the patient uses two or more medications with the same or similar actions to treat different illnesses (Ebersole and others, 2008; Sidhu and others, 2007). Polypharmacy also occurs when your patient mixes nutritional supplements or herbal products with medications. Because many older adults suffer chronic health problems, polypharmacy is common in older adults (Sidhu and others, 2007). When patients experience polypharmacy, there is a high risk for medication interactions with other medications and with foods that patients eat. There is also an increased risk for adverse reactions to the medications.

Sometimes polypharmacy happens when multiple drugs are needed to treat the patient's illnesses. For example, an older adult needs to take a diuretic, a beta-blocker, and an angiotensin-converting enzyme (ACE) inhibitor to control her blood pressure. However, polypharmacy becomes harmful when a patient takes more medications than needed. Many factors contribute to polypharmacy. Taking OTC medications frequently, lack of knowledge about medications, incorrect beliefs about medications, and visiting several health care providers to treat different illnesses increase the risk for polypharmacy (Sidhu and others, 2007). To decrease the risks associated with polypharmacy, work with your patient's prescribers to make sure that the patient's medication

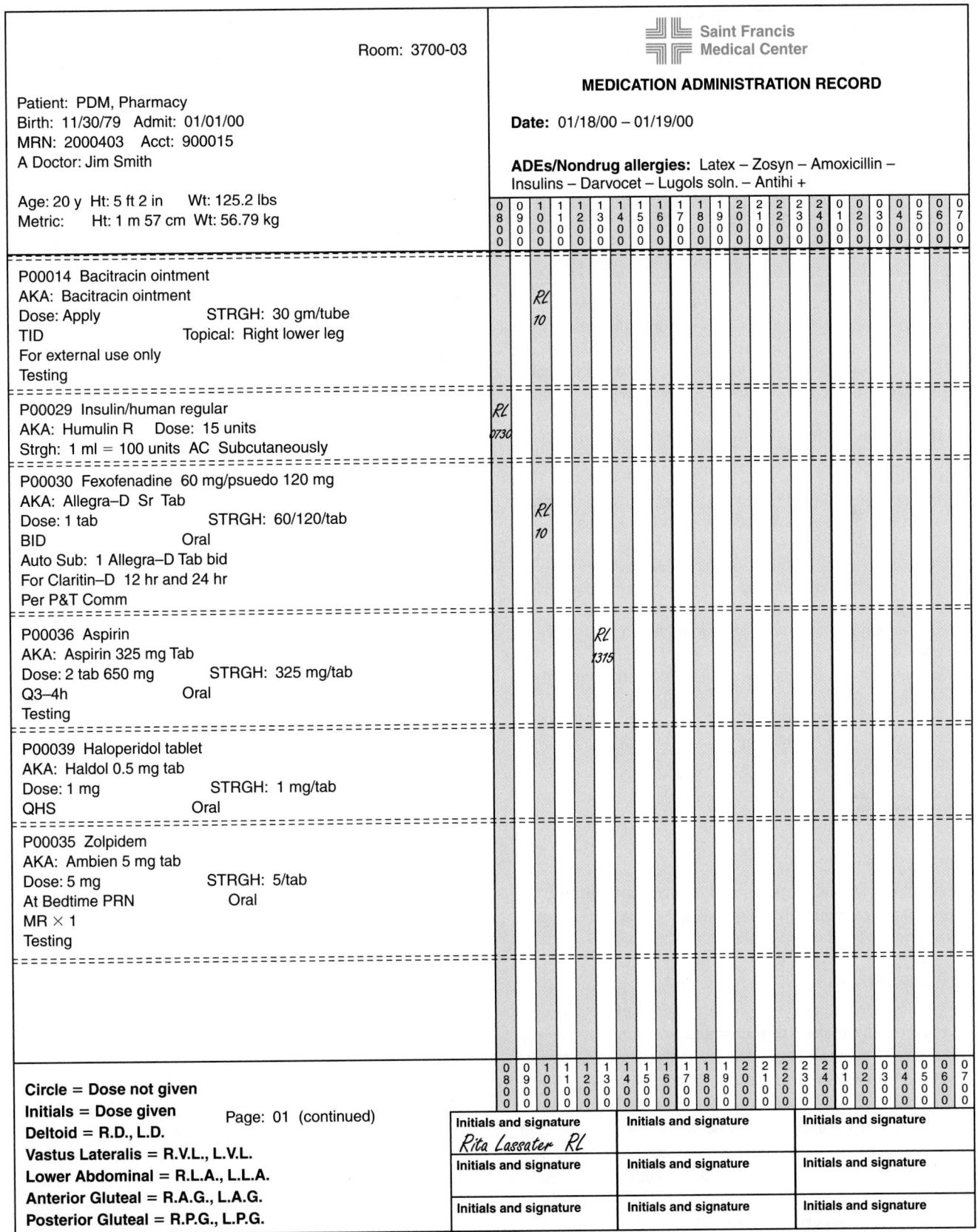

Figure 16-9 ■ Example of medication administration record (MAR). (Courtesy OSF Saint Francis Medical Center, Peoria, Ill.)

BOX 16-13 Tips for Administering Medications to Children

ORAL MEDICATIONS

- Liquids are safer and easier to swallow than pills to avoid aspiration.
- Offer juice, a soft drink, or a frozen juice bar after child swallows a drug.
- A carbonated beverage poured over finely crushed ice reduces nausea.
- When mixing drugs with palatable flavorings, such as syrup or honey, use only a small amount. Children sometimes refuse to take all of a larger mixture.
- Avoid mixing medications in foods or liquids the child enjoys because the child may then refuse them.
- Special medication cups, teaspoons, and droppers can be used to prepare liquid doses. However, a plastic disposable syringe without a needle is the most accurate device to measure liquid dosages.

INJECTIONS

- Be very careful when selecting IM injection sites. Infants and small children have underdeveloped muscles.
- Children can be unpredictable and uncooperative. Have someone available to hold a child if needed.
- Always awaken a sleeping child before giving the child an injection.
- Distracting the child with conversation or a toy reduces pain perception.
- Give the injection quickly, and do not fight with the child.
- Apply a lidocaine ointment to an injection site before the injection to reduce the pain perception during the injection.

IM, Intramuscular.

BOX 16-14 CARE OF THE OLDER ADULT

Special Considerations for Administering Medication to Older Adults

- Space medication times so they do not interfere with mealtimes.
- Have patient take medications in a comfortable setting that is free from distractions.
- Include a family member or caregiver when providing education about medications.
- If the patient has difficulty swallowing a large capsule or tablet, ask the health care provider to substitute a liquid medication if possible. Remember that crushing a tablet and placing it in applesauce or fruit juice will distort the action of some medications, reduce the dose, or cause choking or aspiration of particles of medication or applesauce.
- Provide memory aids in print large enough for the patient to see.
- Watch the patient remove the caps from pill bottles and prepare medications to ensure that the patient is preparing and taking medications accurately.
- Teach alternatives to medications if approved by the prescriber, such as proper diet instead of vitamins, exercise instead of laxatives, bedtime snacks instead of hypnotics, weight reduction, and limited salt or fats in diet instead of antihypertensive agents.

Modified from Ebersole P and others: *Toward healthy aging: human needs and nursing response,* ed 7, St. Louis, 2008, Mosby.

regimen is as simple as possible. Frequent communication among health care providers also helps decrease the effects of polypharmacy (Sidhu and others, 2007).

■■■■Evaluation

The goal of safe and effective medication administration involves careful evaluation of the patient's response to therapy and ability to assume responsibility for self-care. Use your knowledge of each of your patients' medications to evaluate their responses to medications on an ongoing basis. A change in your patient's condition can be related to a change in health status or may result from medications or both. Remember to evaluate your patients to determine if they have the desired effects of their medications. Also determine if your patients are experiencing any adverse effects from their medications.

You will use many different measures to evaluate patient responses to medications: direct observation of physiological measures (e.g., blood pressure or laboratory values), be-

havioral responses (e.g., level of agitation), and rating scales (e.g., pain scale). Also use patient statements and responses to questions you ask as evaluative measures (e.g., "I slept better last night"). Review your patients' goals, expected outcomes, and corresponding evaluative measures when determining effects of medication therapy. *For example, Esther, the patient in the case study in this chapter, is taking glyburide, which is an oral medication that is in the sulfonylurea classification and is taken by people who have type 2 diabetes to control their blood glucose levels. To evaluate the effectiveness of glyburide, Emilio first evaluates Esther's blood glucose levels. From Esther's medical record, Emilio determines that Esther's hemoglobin A_{1c} level is 6.8%. Emilio knows that the hemoglobin A_{1c} reflects a patient's average blood glucose level over the past 90 days. He also knows the target hemoglobin A_{1c} level for most adults who have type 2 diabetes is below 7% (American Diabetes Association [ADA], 2009). Because Esther's hemoglobin A_{1c} level is below 7%, Emilio concludes that Esther is experiencing the desired effect from her glyburide.*

From researching Esther's medications, Emilio finds out that the most common and potentially dangerous side effect of glyburide is hypoglycemia (blood glucose level less than 60 mg/dL). Because hypoglycemia can harm Esther, Emilio

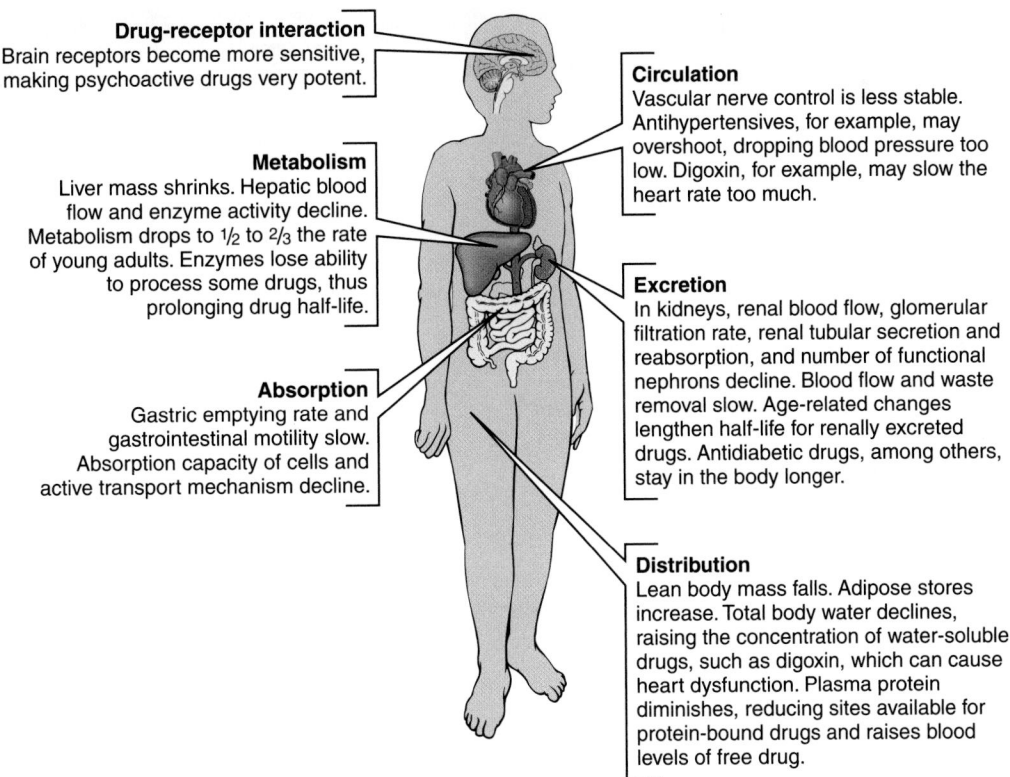

Drug-receptor interaction
Brain receptors become more sensitive, making psychoactive drugs very potent.

Metabolism
Liver mass shrinks. Hepatic blood flow and enzyme activity decline. Metabolism drops to 1/2 to 2/3 the rate of young adults. Enzymes lose ability to process some drugs, thus prolonging drug half-life.

Absorption
Gastric emptying rate and gastrointestinal motility slow. Absorption capacity of cells and active transport mechanism decline.

Circulation
Vascular nerve control is less stable. Antihypertensives, for example, may overshoot, dropping blood pressure too low. Digoxin, for example, may slow the heart rate too much.

Excretion
In kidneys, renal blood flow, glomerular filtration rate, renal tubular secretion and reabsorption, and number of functional nephrons decline. Blood flow and waste removal slow. Age-related changes lengthen half-life for renally excreted drugs. Antidiabetic drugs, among others, stay in the body longer.

Distribution
Lean body mass falls. Adipose stores increase. Total body water declines, raising the concentration of water-soluble drugs, such as digoxin, which can cause heart dysfunction. Plasma protein diminishes, reducing sites available for protein-bound drugs and raises blood levels of free drug.

Figure 16-10 ■ The effects of aging on drug metabolism. (From Lewis SL and others: *Medical-surgical nursing*, ed 7, St. Louis, 2007, Mosby.)

decides that he also needs to make sure Esther has not experienced hypoglycemia. After he reviews Esther's medical record, Emilio does not see any blood glucose levels that are below 60 mg/dL. Emilio wants to confirm this information, so he asks Esther if she ever experiences the symptoms of hypoglycemia such as shaking, dizziness, sweating, headaches, or increased heart rate. Esther states, "I was a little shaky yesterday just before dinner, but it wasn't too bad. Other than that, I can't remember any of those things happening to me." After questioning Esther about what happened yesterday afternoon, Emilio discovers that Esther was visiting with her family in the afternoon and did not eat her afternoon snack. Emilio provides patient education to Esther, enforcing the importance of eating her afternoon snack to prevent future hypoglycemic episodes. Because Esther has experienced only one recent episode of hypoglycemia that was caused by her not eating her snack, Emilio determines that Esther is experiencing the desired effect and is not experiencing any adverse effects from her glyburide.

In addition to the effectiveness of medications, you need to know if your patients are able to understand and safely administer their medications. The type of measurements you use varies with the action being evaluated, the reading skill and knowledge level of the patient, and the patient's cognitive and psychomotor ability. For example, if you are caring for a female patient who takes eye drops, it is important to watch the patient instill the drops into her eyes. When patients have to prepare and administer injections (e.g., insulin), you need to watch them prepare the medication in the syringe and administer the injection. To determine if your patients understand their medication schedules, ask them to verbalize when they take their medications and how much they take, or ask them to write out their schedule for you on a piece of paper.

You also need to determine your patients' ability to adhere to their medication routines. *Emilio, the nursing student in the case study, knows from the preparation he did before caring for Esther that older adult African American women often have trouble adhering to their medications when they are discharged from the hospital. He knows that issues related to poor knowledge about the medications, transportation, and cost often prohibit patients from taking their medications. Therefore he asks Esther to explain the purpose, dosage, and adverse effects of each medication. As Esther describes her medications, Emilio reinforces information as needed and gives Esther medication teaching sheets. He asks Esther if she thinks she is going to have any difficulty getting her medications. Esther tells Emilio that she knows she will be able to afford her medications, but she is worried because she is not going to be able to drive when she goes home. Together they decide that Emilio will call her pastor to see if there is anyone in her church who can help her get to the pharmacy.*

BOX 16-15   Interventions to Prevent Aspiration of Medications in Patients With Dysphagia

- Allow the patient to self-administer medications if possible.
- Position the patient in an upright, seated position with feet flat on the floor, hips and knees at 90 degrees, the head midline, and back erect if possible.
- When the patient puts the medication in the mouth, make sure the chin is tucked or tilted down slightly. When the patient swallows, the chin can be lifted and the head tilted back to help the medication get into the stomach.
- If the patient has unilateral weakness, place the medication in the stronger side of the mouth. Turning the head toward the weaker side helps the medication move down the stronger side of the esophagus.
- Administer medications one at a time, ensuring that the patient swallows each medication before introducing the next one.

- Thicker liquids are often easier to tolerate. Thicken regular liquids, or offer fruit nectars to enhance swallowing.
- You can crush some medications and place them into pureed foods if necessary. Refer to a medication reference to verify which medications are safe to crush.
- Straws decrease the amount of control the patient has over the amount of fluid taken into the mouth. Therefore do not have the patient use a straw.
- Time medications to coincide with meals if appropriate.
- Give medications at times when the patient is well rested and awake.
- Minimize distractions during medication administration times.
- If dysphagia is severe, explore alternative routes of administration (e.g., intravenous).

Evaluation of medication administration is an essential role of professional nursing that requires critical thinking skills and knowledge of medications, physiology, and pathophysiology. Thoroughly and accurately gather data, and complete a holistic evaluation of your patients. Your patients' clinical condition can change minute by minute. Compare expected and actual findings, and determine if predicted changes have occurred in your patients in response to their medications. When patients do not experience the expected outcomes of their medication therapy, investigate possible reasons and determine appropriate revision of the patient's care plan.

ORAL ADMINISTRATION

The easiest and most desirable way to administer medications is by mouth (see Skill 16-1). Patients usually are able to ingest or self-administer oral medications with a minimum of problems. Food delays stomach emptying, which often decreases the therapeutic effects of oral medications. Therefore most oral medications achieve their therapeutic action best if given 30 minutes to 1 hour before meals (McKenry and others, 2006). Most tablets and capsules need to be swallowed and administered with approximately 60 to 240 mL of fluid (as allowed). However, there are some situations that contraindicate the patient's ability to receive medications by mouth (see Table 16-5, p. 383). There are many medications that interact with food and herbal supplements. You are responsible for knowing about these interactions. Understanding how food and herbals affect medication absorption helps you determine the best time to give oral medications.

An important precaution to take when administering any oral preparation is to protect patients from aspiration.

Aspiration occurs when food, fluid, or medication intended for GI administration goes into the respiratory tract. Evaluate your patient's ability to swallow before administering oral medications. When there is a risk for aspiration, you will use certain interventions (Box 16-15). Properly positioning the patient is essential in preventing aspiration. When possible, place the patient in a seated or Fowler's position. If your patient has difficulty swallowing, consult appropriate personnel (e.g., speech therapist) for a swallow evaluation before administering oral medications, and use other routes of medication administration (e.g., intravenous or subcutaneous). Sometimes you will give medications through a nasogastric or feeding tube when the patient cannot swallow. Box 16-16 summarizes guidelines for administering medications through gastric tubes.

TOPICAL MEDICATION APPLICATIONS

Topical medications are medications applied locally, most often to intact skin. They come in the form of lotions, pastes, or ointments (see Table 16-1, p. 376). They are also applied to mucous membranes. Before and during any application, assess the skin thoroughly. Note the area applied and condition of skin in the patient's chart, and document the name and administration of the medication on the MAR.

Skin Applications

Because many locally applied medications, such as lotions, pastes, and ointments, create systemic and local effects, wear gloves and use applicators when administering them. Use sterile technique if the patient has an open wound. Skin encrustation and dead tissues harbor microorganisms

BOX 16-16 PROCEDURAL GUIDELINES

Administering Medications Through an NG Tube, G-Tube, J-Tube, or Small-Bore Feeding Tube

DELEGATION CONSIDERATIONS: The skill of administering medications through an enteral tube cannot be delegated to nursing assistive personnel (NAP). The nurse informs NAP to:

- Watch for the potential side effects of medications and report their occurrence

EQUIPMENT: 60-mL syringe (catheter tip for large-bore tubes; Luer-Lok tip for small-bore tubes), gastric pH test tape (scale of 0.0 to 11.0 or 14.0 preferred), graduated container, water, medication to be administered, pill crusher if medication is in tablet form, MAR, clean gloves

1. Check accuracy and completeness of each MAR with prescriber's written medication order. Check patient's name, drug name and dosage, route of administration, and time for administration.
2. Investigate and use alternative routes of medication administration if possible (e.g., transdermal, rectal, intravenous).
3. Avoid complicated medication schedules that frequently interrupt enteral feedings.
4. Prepare medication (see Skill 16-1, Implementation step 1). Check label of medication with MAR two times for accuracy. *This is the first and second accuracy check.*
5. Never add a medication directly to the tube feeding. Before administering the medication, determine if it needs to be given on an empty stomach or is compatible with the enteral feeding. If the medication needs to be given on an empty stomach or is not compatible with the feeding, the feeding needs to be held before and after medication administration. The amount of time to hold the feeding varies based on the medication. Usually you will hold the feeding 30 minutes to 1 hour before and after giving the medication. Verify the amount of time that you hold the feeding with your agency policy, a pharmacist, or a medication reference manual before administering the medication to maximize the medication's therapeutic effect.
6. Administer medications in a liquid form (suspension, elixir, solution) when possible to prevent obstruction of the tube.
7. Before crushing medications, be sure they can be crushed. Do not crush buccal, sublingual, enteric-coated, or sustained-release medications.
8. Take medications to patient at correct time, and perform hand hygiene.
9. Identify patient using two identifiers (e.g., name and birthday or name and account number, according to fa-

cility policy). Compare identifiers with information on patient's MAR or medical record.

10. Compare label of medications against MAR one more time at patient's bedside. *This is the third accuracy check.*
11. Explain procedure to patient, and educate patient about medications.
12. Dissolve each crushed tablet, gelatin capsule, and powder in a cup of 15 to 30 mL of warm water. Check with pharmacist whether any medications can be given together.
13. Do not give whole or undissolved medications through the feeding tube.
14. Put on clean gloves.
15. Verify placement of any tube that enters the mouth or nose using pH testing (see Chapter 32).
16. Assess gastric residual (see Chapter 32).
17. Flush tube with 30 mL warm water.
18. Draw up medication in syringe. Do **not** mix medications together unless approved by pharmacy.
19. Connect syringe with medication to NG tube, G-tube, J-tube, or small-bore feeding tube.
20. Administer medication either by pushing the medication through the tube with the syringe or by allowing medication to flow into body freely by using gravity. Administer each medication separately. If resistance is felt when pushing medication through the tube, stop medication administration and contact the patient's health care provider.
21. Flush tube with 15 to 30 mL of water between each medication. Unless contraindicated, the total amount of liquid volume administered to the patient for each medication is approximately 60 mL.
22. Once you have given all medications, flush tube once more with 30 to 60 mL warm water.
23. Clean area, and put supplies away.
24. Remove gloves, and perform hand hygiene.
25. Document name of medications, dose, route, and time on MAR.
26. Continually evaluate the patient's response to medication therapy. If the patient does not achieve the desired effect, a different medication or route of administration may be indicated because of problems with drug bioavailability when given by the enteral route. If patient self-administers medications, evaluate patient's ability to give medications and technique used. Provide and reinforce information as needed.

G-tube, Gastrostomy tube; *J-tube,* jejunostomy tube; *MAR,* medication administration record; *NG tube,* nasogastric tube.

and block contact of medications with the tissues to be treated. Therefore clean the skin thoroughly before applying topical medications.

Spread the medication evenly over the involved surface when applying ointments or pastes. In some cases you apply a gauze dressing over the medication to prevent soiling of clothes and wiping away of the medication. Apply each type of medication according to directions to ensure proper penetration and absorption. Spread lotions and creams lightly onto the skin's surface, because rubbing causes irritation. Apply a liniment by rubbing it gently but firmly into the skin. Dust a powder lightly to cover the affected area with a thin layer.

Some medications are given by a transdermal patch that delivers a timed-release dose for a significant amount of time (e.g., 12 hours or 24 hours). Before applying a new patch, remove the old one because medication remains on the patch even after its recommended duration of use. Harmful adverse effects often occur when a patch is not removed. For example, patients who use fentanyl patches for pain management sometimes experience respiratory depression, coma, and death when they are not removed. Transdermal patches are often transparent and are difficult to find. To remind nurses to remove the patch before applying a new one, many health care agencies include an order for removal of the patch on the MAR. When you apply a transdermal patch, document that you removed the old patch, and indicate where you placed the new one on the MAR. Additional safeguards include asking patients if they use transdermal patches, applying a visible label to the patch, and never assuming that an old patch has fallen off if you cannot find it; instead fully inspect the patient's skin before applying a new patch. Finally, because patients sometimes forget to mention topical medications, make sure you ask patients if they take any medications other than by the oral route (e.g., topical, transdermal, or cream) whenever taking a medication history (ISMP, 2008c).

Nasal Instillation

Patients with nasal sinus alterations often receive medications by spray, drops, or tampons (Box 16-17). The most commonly administered form of nasal instillation is decongestant spray or drops, used to relieve symptoms of sinus congestion and colds. Caution patients to avoid abuse of nose drops and sprays, because overuse leads to rebound nasal congestion. In addition, when patients swallow excess decon-

---

BOX 16-17   PROCEDURAL GUIDELINES

Administering Nasal Instillations

DELEGATION CONSIDERATIONS: The skill of administering nasal instillations cannot be delegated to nursing assistive personnel (NAP). The nurse informs NAP to:
- Watch for the potential side effects of medications and report their occurrence

EQUIPMENT: Prepared medication with clean dropper or spray container, facial tissue, small pillow *(optional)*, washcloth (optional), clean gloves (if patient has nasal drainage), MAR

1 Check accuracy and completeness of each MAR with prescriber's original medication order. Check patient's name, drug name and dosage, route of administration, and time for administration.
2 Determine which sinus is affected by referring to medical record if giving nasal drops.
3 Assess patient's medical history (e.g., history of hypertension, heart disease, diabetes mellitus, and hyperthyroidism) and allergies to medications and foods. Make sure patient's drug and food allergies are listed on the MAR and are prominently displayed on the patient's medical record per agency policy.
4 Perform hand hygiene. Using a penlight, inspect condition of nose and sinuses. Palpate sinuses for tenderness (see Chapter 15).
5 Assess patient's knowledge regarding use of nasal instillations and technique for instillation and willingness to learn self-administration.

6 Perform hand hygiene and prepare medication: See Skill 16-1, Implementation steps 1a-h, k-m. Be sure to compare label of medication against MAR at least two times while preparing medication for accuracy. *This is the first and second accuracy check.*
7 Take medications to patient at correct time, and perform hand hygiene.
8 Identify patient using two identifiers (e.g., name and birthday or name and account number, according to facility policy). Compare identifiers with information on patient's MAR or medical record.
9 Compare MAR with medication labels one more time at patient's bedside. *This is the third accuracy check.*
10 Explain procedure to patient regarding positioning and sensations to expect, such as burning or stinging of mucosa or choking sensation as medication trickles into throat.
11 Arrange supplies and medications at bedside. Apply clean gloves if patient has nasal drainage.
12 Gently roll or shake container.
13 Instruct patient to clear or blow nose gently unless contraindicated (e.g., risk for increased intracranial pressure or nosebleeds).

BOX 16-17   PROCEDURAL GUIDELINES—cont'd

Administering Nasal Instillations—cont'd

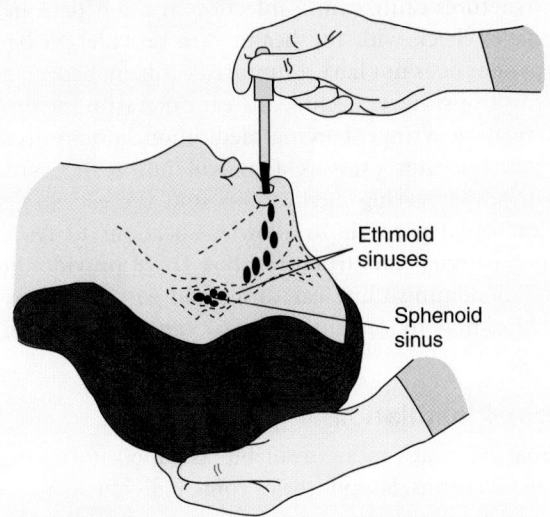

Step 14a(2) ■ Position for instilling nose drops into ethmoid or sphenoid sinus.

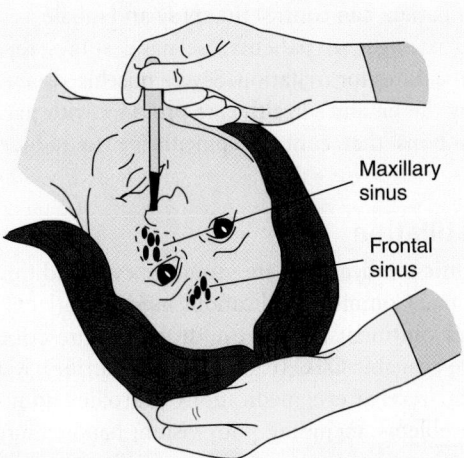

Step 14a(3) ■ Position for instilling nose drops into frontal and maxillary sinus.

14 *Administer nasal drops:*
  a Assist patient to supine position, and position head properly:
    (1) For access to posterior pharynx, tilt patient's head backward.
    (2) For access to ethmoid or sphenoid sinus, tilt head back over edge of bed or place small pillow under patient's shoulder and tilt head back (see illustration).
    (3) For access to frontal or maxillary sinus, tilt head back over edge of bed or pillow with head turned toward side to be treated (see illustration).
  b Support patient's head with nondominant hand.
  c Instruct patient to breathe through mouth.
  d Hold dropper 1 cm (½ inch) above nares, and instill prescribed number of drops toward midline of ethmoid bone.
  e Have patient remain in supine position 5 minutes.
  f Offer facial tissue to blot runny nose, but caution patient against blowing nose for several minutes.
15 *Administer nasal spray:*
  a Assist patient to supine position, and position head slightly tilted forward.
  b Help patient place spray nozzle into appropriate nares, pointing the nozzle to the side of the nose and away from the center of the nose.
  c Have patient spray medication into the nose while inhaling.
  d Help patient take nozzle out of nose, and instruct patient to breathe out through the mouth.
  e Offer facial tissue, but caution patient against blowing nose for several minutes.
16 Assist patient to a comfortable position after drug is absorbed.
17 Dispose of soiled supplies in proper container, and perform hand hygiene.
18 Document name of medication, dose, route, and time on MAR.
19 Observe patient for onset of side effects 15 to 30 minutes after administration. Ask if patient is able to breathe through nose after decongestant administration. May be necessary to have patient occlude one nostril at a time and breathe deeply.
20 Evaluate patient's response to medications at times that correlate with the medication's onset, peak, and duration. Evaluate patient for both desired effect and adverse effects. Determine patient's ability to self-administer medication, and provide appropriate teaching if needed.

gestant solution, serious systemic effects develop, especially in children. Saline drops are safer as a decongestant for children than nasal preparations that contain sympathomimetics (e.g., Afrin or Neo-Synephrine).

It is easier to have the patient self-administer sprays, because the patient can control the spray and inhale as it enters the nasal passages. If patients use nasal sprays repeatedly, observe the nares for irritation. Severe nosebleeds are usually treated by the patient's health care provider with packing or nasal tampons that contain epinephrine to reduce blood flow.

Eye Instillation

Ophthalmic medications are given for eye conditions such as glaucoma. Common medications used by patients are eye drops and ointments. Some eye drops are prescribed, and others are available OTC (e.g., Visine or Murine). Many patients who receive eye medications are older adults. Age-related problems, including poor vision, hand tremors, and difficulty grasping or manipulating small containers affect the ability of older adults to self-administer eye medications. Educate your patients and their family members about the proper techniques for administering eye medications (see Skill 16-2). Evaluate the patient's and family's ability to self-administer through a return demonstration of the procedure. Showing patients each step of the procedure for instilling eye drops will improve their adherence. Apply the following principles when administering eye medications:

1. Avoid instilling any form of eye medication directly onto the cornea. The cornea of the eye has many pain fibers and is thus very sensitive to anything applied to it.
2. Avoid touching the eyelids or other eye structures with eye droppers or ointment tubes. The risk for transmitting infection from one eye to the other is high.
3. Use eye medication only for the patient's affected eye.
4. Never allow a patient to use another patient's eye medications.

You will administer some medications using an intraocular disk (see Skill 16-2). Intraocular medicated disks resemble a contact lens. The medication is placed onto the conjunctival sac and is released over a period of time. The lens remains in place for up to 1 week (Alvarez-Lorenzo and others, 2006). Teach your patient receiving medications in this way to monitor for adverse reactions to the disk, as well as teaching methods of insertion and removal.

Ear Instillation

Internal ear structures are very sensitive to temperature extremes. Failure to instill ear drops or irrigating fluid at room temperature causes vertigo (severe dizziness) or nau-

sea. Although the structures of the outer ear are not sterile, you use sterile drops and solutions in case the eardrum is ruptured. The entrance of nonsterile solutions into middle ear structures can result in infection. If the patient has ear drainage, check with the health care provider to be sure the patient does not have a ruptured eardrum before instilling ear drops. Never occlude the ear canal with the dropper or irrigating syringe. Forcing medication into an occluded ear canal creates pressure that will injure the eardrum. When administering medications into the ear, straighten the ear canal properly to allow medications to reach the deeper, external ear structures. Box 16-18 provides guidelines for administering ear drops and ear irrigations and describes how to straighten the ear canal for children and for adults.

Vaginal Instillation

Vaginal medications are available as suppositories, foams, jellies, or creams. Suppositories come individually packaged and are stored in a refrigerator to prevent them from melting. After inserting a suppository into the vaginal cavity, body temperature causes it to melt and be distributed and absorbed. Administer foams, jellies, and creams with an applicator or inserter, and give a suppository with a gloved hand in accordance with standard precautions. Patients often prefer administering their own vaginal medications. Give the patient privacy to do this. After instillation of the medication, some patients wish to wear a perineal pad to collect drainage. Because you will often give vaginal medications to treat infection, discharge is usually foul smelling. Follow aseptic techniques, and offer your patient frequent opportunities to maintain perineal hygiene (see Chapter 28). Box 16-19 describes the steps to take when administering vaginal medications.

Rectal Instillation

Rectal suppositories are thinner and more bullet-shaped than vaginal suppositories. The rounded end prevents anal trauma during insertion. Rectal suppositories contain medications that exert local effects, such as promoting defecation, or systemic effects, such as reducing nausea. Rectal suppositories are often stored in the refrigerator until administered.

During administration, place the unwrapped suppository past the internal anal sphincter and against the rectal mucosa. Otherwise, the patient will expel the suppository before it dissolves and is absorbed into the mucosa. You will feel the sphincter relaxing around the finger when you administer the suppository. Do not force suppositories into a mass of fecal material. You will need to clear the rectum with a small cleansing enema before inserting a suppository. Box 16-20 (p. 415) describes the steps to use when administering rectal medications.

BOX 16-18   PROCEDURAL GUIDELINES

Administering Ear Medications

DELEGATION CONSIDERATIONS: The skill of administering ear medications cannot be delegated to nursing assistive personnel (NAP). The nurse informs NAP to:
- Watch for the potential side effects of medications and report their occurrence

EQUIPMENT: *Drops:* Medication bottle with dropper, cotton-tipped applicator, cotton ball (optional), clean gloves if patient has drainage from ear; *irrigation:* irrigating syringe, kidney basin, towel; MAR

1 Check accuracy and completeness of each MAR with prescriber's written medication order. Check patient's name, drug name and dosage, route of administration, and time for administration.
2 Assess patient's medical history (e.g., history of dizziness, hearing loss) and allergies to medications, food, and latex.
3 Perform hand hygiene and prepare medication (see Skill 16-1, Implementation steps 1a-h, k-m). Be sure to compare the label of the medication with the MAR at least two times during medication preparation. *This is the first and second accuracy check.*
4 Take medication to patient at correct time, and perform hand hygiene. Put on clean gloves if patient has ear drainage. NOTE: If patient has a latex allergy, use latex-free gloves.
5 Identify patient using two identifiers (e.g., name and birthday or name and account number, according to facility policy). Compare identifiers with information on patient's MAR or medical record.
6 Compare the label of the medication with the MAR one more time at the patient's bedside. *This is the third accuracy check.*
7 Explain procedure to patient regarding positioning and sensations to expect, such as hearing bubbling or feeling of water in ear as medication trickles into ear.
8 Teach patient about medication.
9 *Administer ear drops:*
  a Place patient in side-lying position if not contraindicated by patient's condition, with ear to be treated facing up. The patient may also sit in a chair or at the bedside.
  b Straighten ear canal by pulling auricle down and back for children less than 3 years or upward and outward for patients 3 years of age and older (Hockenberry and Wilson, 2009).
  c Instill prescribed drops holding dropper 1 cm (½ inch) above ear canal (see illustration).
  d Ask patient to remain in side-lying position for 2 to 3 minutes. Apply gentle massage or pressure to tragus of ear with finger.

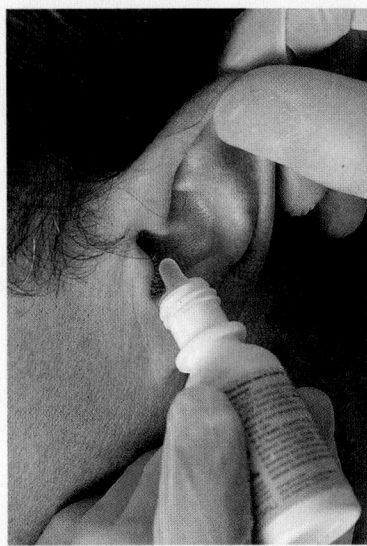

Step 9c ■ Instill prescribed drops holding dropper above ear canal.

  e If you place a cotton ball into the outermost part of ear canal, do not press cotton ball into the canal. Remove cotton after 15 minutes.
10 *Administer ear irrigations:*
  a Assess the tympanic membrane, or review medical record for history of eardrum perforation, which contraindicates ear irrigation.
  b Assist patient into sitting or lying position with head tilted or turned toward affected ear. Place towel under patient's head and shoulder, and have patient hold basin under affected ear.
  c Fill irrigating syringe with solution (approximately 50 mL) at room temperature.
  d Gently grasp auricle, and straighten ear by pulling it down and back for children less than 3 years or upward and outward for patients 3 years of age and older (Hockenberry and Wilson, 2009).
  e Slowly instill irrigating solution by holding tip of syringe 1 cm (½ inch) above opening of ear canal. Allow fluid to drain out during instillation. Continue until you cleanse the canal or use all solution.
11 Clean area, and put supplies away.
12 Remove gloves, and perform hand hygiene.
13 Document name of medication, dose, route, and time on MAR.
14 Evaluate patient's response to medication and ability to self-administer medication. Provide appropriate patient education as needed.

BOX 16-19   PROCEDURAL GUIDELINES

Administering Vaginal Medications

DELEGATION CONSIDERATIONS: The skill of administering vaginal medications cannot be delegated to nursing assistive personnel (NAP). The nurse informs NAP to:

- Watch for the potential side effects of medications and report their occurrence
- Offer to provide perineal care following medication administration

EQUIPMENT: Vaginal cream, foam, jelly, or suppository or irrigating solution with applicator (if required); clean gloves; towels and/or washcloth; perineal pad; drape or sheet; water-soluble lubricating jelly; MAR

1 Check accuracy and completeness of each MAR with prescriber's written medication order. Check patient's name, drug name and dosage, route of administration, and time for administration.
2 Assess patient's medical history (e.g., history of vaginal drainage) and allergies to medications, food, and latex.
3 Perform hand hygiene and prepare medication (see Skill 16-1, Implementation steps 1a-h, k-m). Compare the label of the medication with the MAR two times while preparing the medication. *This is the first and second accuracy check.*
4 Take medication to patient at the correct time, and perform hand hygiene.
5 Identify patient using two identifiers (e.g., name and birthday or name and account number, according to facility policy). Compare identifiers with information on patient's MAR or medical record.
6 Compare label of medication against the MAR one more time at the patient's bedside. *This is the third accuracy check.*
7 Explain procedure to patient regarding positioning and sensations to expect, such as feelings of moisture or wetness in the vaginal area. Be sure patient understands the procedure if she plans to self-administer medication. Teach patient about the medication.
8 Close room door or pull curtain to provide privacy.
9 Put on clean gloves. NOTE: If patient has a latex allergy, use latex-free gloves.

10 Be sure there is adequate lighting to visualize vaginal opening. Assess vaginal area, noting the appearance of any discharge and the condition of the external genitalia. Cleanse area with towel or washcloth if needed (see Chapters 15 and 28).
11 *Administer vaginal suppository:*
   a Remove suppository from wrapper, and apply liberal amount of sterile water-based lubricating jelly to smooth or rounded end. Lubricate gloved index finger of dominant hand.
   b With nondominant gloved hand, gently separate and hold labial folds.
   c With dominant gloved hand, gently insert rounded end of suppository along posterior wall of vaginal canal entire length of finger (7.5 to 10 cm or 3 to 4 inches) (see illustration).
   d Withdraw finger, and wipe away remaining lubricant from around vaginal opening and labia.
12 *Administer cream or foam:*
   a Fill cream or foam applicator following package directions.
   b With nondominant gloved hand, gently separate and hold labial folds.
   c With dominant gloved hand, gently insert applicator about 5 to 7.5 cm (2 to 3 inches). Push applicator plunger to deposit medication into vagina (see illustration).
   d Withdraw applicator, and place on paper towel. Wipe off residual cream from labia or vaginal opening.
13 Dispose of supplies, remove gloves, and perform hand hygiene.
14 Instruct patient to remain on back for at least 10 minutes.
15 Document name of medication, dose, route, and time on MAR.
16 If applicator is used, wearing gloves, wash with soap and warm water, rinse, and store for future use.
17 Offer perineal pad to patient when she begins to ambulate.
18 Evaluate patient's response to medication and ability to administer medication. Provide patient education as needed.

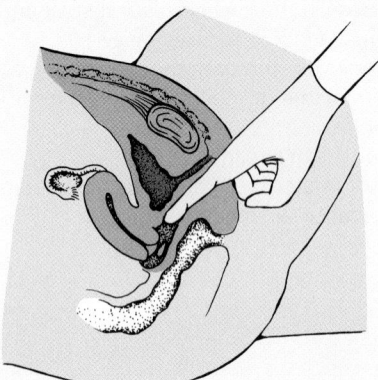

Step 11c ■ Insertion of a suppository into the vaginal canal.

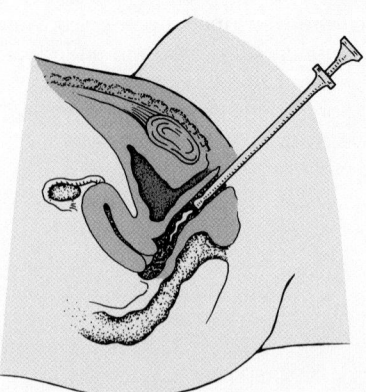

Step 12c ■ Instillation of medication in vaginal canal.

BOX 16-20 PROCEDURAL GUIDELINES

Administering Rectal Suppositories

DELEGATION CONSIDERATIONS: The skill of administering rectal medications cannot be delegated to nursing assistive personnel (NAP). The nurse informs NAP to:

- Watch for the potential side effects of medications and report their occurrence
- Offer to provide perineal care following medication administration

EQUIPMENT: Rectal suppository, clean gloves, drape or sheet, water-soluble lubricating jelly, tissue, MAR

1 Check accuracy and completeness of each MAR with prescriber's written medication order. Check patient's name, drug name and dosage, route of administration, and time for administration.

2 Assess patient's medical history (e.g., hemorrhoids, anal fissures) and allergies to medications, food, and latex.

3 Perform hand hygiene and prepare medication (see Skill 16-1, Implementation steps 1a-h, k-m). Be sure to compare the label of the medication with the MAR two times during medication preparation. *This is the first and second accuracy check.*

4 Take medication to patient at the correct time, and perform hand hygiene.

5 Identify patient using two identifiers (e.g., name and birthday or name and account number, according to facility policy). Compare identifiers with information on patient's MAR or medical record.

6 Compare the label of the medication with the MAR one more time at the patient's bedside. *This is the third accuracy check.*

7 Explain procedure to patient regarding positioning and sensations to expect, such as feelings of needing to defecate. Be sure patient understands the procedure if he or she plans to self-administer medication. Teach patient about the medication.

8 Close room door or pull curtain to provide privacy.

9 Put on clean gloves. NOTE: If patient has a latex allergy, use latex-free gloves.

10 Assist patient to the Sims' position. Keep patient draped with only anal area exposed. NOTE If patient has a latex allergy, use latex-free gloves.

11 Be sure there is adequate lighting to visualize anus. Assess external condition of anus, and palpate rectal walls as needed (see Chapters 15 and 34). Dispose of gloves in proper receptacle if soiled.

12 Apply new pair of clean gloves if gloves were discarded in previous step.

13 Remove suppository from wrapper, and lubricate rounded end with sterile water-soluble lubricating jelly (see illustration). Lubricate index finger of dominant hand with water-soluble jelly.

14 Ask patient to take slow deep breath through mouth and relax anal sphincter.

15 Retract buttocks with nondominant hand. Using dominant hand, insert suppository gently through anus, past internal sphincter and against rectal wall, 10 cm (4 inches)

in adults, or 5 cm (2 inches) in children and infants (see illustration). You may need to apply gentle pressure to hold buttocks together momentarily.

16 Withdraw finger, and wipe anal area with tissue.

17 Dispose of supplies, remove gloves, and perform hand hygiene.

18 Instruct patient to remain on side for at least 5 minutes.

19 If suppository is a laxative or stool softener, place call light within reach of the patient.

20 Document name of medication, dose, route, and time on MAR.

21 Evaluate patient's response to medication.

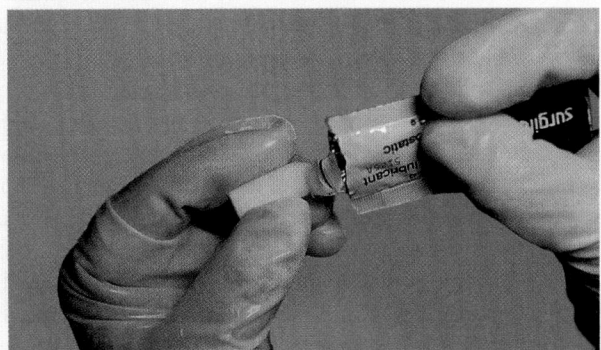

Step 13 ■ Lubricate tip of rectal suppository with water-soluble jelly.

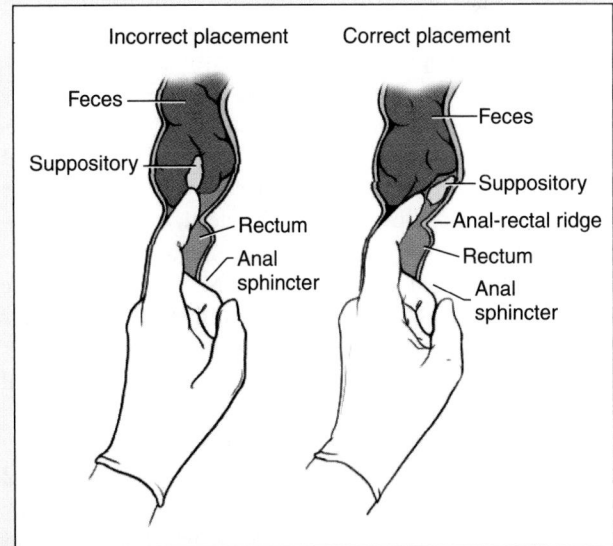

Step 15 ■ Inserting a rectal suppository. (From deWit S: *Fundamental concepts and skills for nursing*, ed 2, Philadelphia, 2005, WB Saunders.)

ADMINISTERING MEDICATIONS BY INHALATION

Medications administered with handheld inhalers are dispersed through an aerosol spray, mist, or powder that penetrates lung airways. The alveolar-capillary network absorbs medications rapidly. **Metered-dose inhalers (MDIs)**, also called **pressurized metered-dose inhalers (pMDIs),** and dry powder inhalers (DPIs) are devices used to deliver inhaled medications that usually produce local effects in the patient's airway, such as bronchodilation. Some medications create serious systemic side effects. MDIs use a chemical propellant to push the medicine out of the inhaler, whereas DPIs use energy created by the patient during inhalation to push the medication out of the inhaler (MayoClinic.com, 2008).

Patients who receive medications by inhalation frequently have a chronic respiratory disease, such as chronic asthma, emphysema, or bronchitis. Medications given by inhalation provide these patients with control of airway obstruction. Proper use of inhalers improves patient outcomes and decreases mortality associated with chronic airway diseases. However, current evidence shows that many patients do not use their inhalers correctly (Hess, 2008). Patient education is essential (see Skill 16-3).

MDIs are either squeeze-and-breathe inhalers or are activated by the patient's breath. The MDI consists of the canister, propellant, medication, metering valve, and actuator. The medication is usually in a suspension or a solution. To use a squeeze-and-breathe MDI a patient must use 5 to 10 lb of pressure to activate the aerosol. Assess if your patient has sufficient strength to correctly use the MDI by having the patient manipulate the device. Many patients who use MDIs are children or older adults with chronic respiratory disease. Because these two populations have diminished hand strength, it is especially important to assess if patients in these age-groups have enough strength to use the MDI. Breath-activated MDIs release the medication when the patient inhales. Release of the medication is dependent upon the patient's breath on inspiration (Capriotti, 2005). Your patient can use a spacer with the MDI. A spacer is a 4- to 8-inch–long tube that attaches to the MDI and allows the particles of medication to slow down and break into smaller pieces. This helps the medication get deeper into the lungs and enhances absorption (Hess, 2008). Spacers are helpful when the patient has difficulty coordinating the steps involved in self-administering inhaled medications.

DPIs hold dry, powdered medication and create an aerosol when the patient inhales through a reservoir to deliver the medication. Some DPIs are unit dosed, in which patients load a single dose of medication into the inhaler with each use, whereas other DPIs hold enough medication to be used in 1 month. DPIs require less manual dexterity. Because the patient activates the DPI when breathing, there is no need to coordinate puffs with inhalation, as when using an MDI. DPIs do not require a spacer. However, if the patient is in a humid climate, the medication can clump. The patient must be able to inhale fast enough to administer the entire dose of the medication.

Help your patients determine when inhalers are empty and need to be replaced. Do not float the MDI in water to determine how much medication is left because extra propellant in the MDI will allow the container to float even if it is empty (Hess, 2008). Devices are available that attach onto the MDI and count down the number of remaining doses. Some DPIs have an indicator that shows how many doses are left. However, these are not always accurate. Therefore the best way to calculate how long medication in an inhaler will last is to divide the number of doses in the container by the number of doses your patient takes per day. For example, your patient is to take albuterol, a beta-adrenergic agonist bronchodilator. The ordered dose is 2 puffs 4 times a day (qid). The canister has a total of 200 puffs. You complete the following calculations to determine how long the MDI will last:

$$2 \text{ puffs} \times 4 \text{ times a day} = 8 \text{ puffs per day}$$
$$200 \text{ puffs} \div 8 \text{ puffs per day} = 25 \text{ days}$$

Therefore the canister will last 25 days. To ensure that the patient does not run out of medication, teach your patient to refill the medication at least 7 to 10 days before it runs out.

ADMINISTERING MEDICATIONS BY IRRIGATION

You will use some medications to irrigate or wash out a body cavity. An irrigation delivers a stream of solution. Sterile water, saline, or antiseptic solution irrigations of the eye, ear, throat, vagina, and urinary tract are common. If there is a break in the skin or mucosa, use aseptic technique. When the cavity to be irrigated is not sterile, as is the case with the ear canal (see Box 16-18, p. 413) or vagina (see Box 16-19, p. 414), clean technique is acceptable. Irrigations cleanse an area, instill a medication, or apply hot or cold to injured tissue.

PARENTERAL ADMINISTRATION OF MEDICATIONS

Parenteral administration of medications is the administration of medications by injection. An injection is an invasive procedure that requires use of aseptic technique. After a needle pierces the skin, there is risk for infection. Use the following techniques to prevent an infection during an injection:

- Quickly draw the medication into the syringe to prevent contamination of solution in an ampule.
- Do not allow the ampule to stand open.
- Do not allow the needle to touch a contaminated surface (e.g., outer edges of ampule or vial, outer surface of needle cap, your hands, the countertop).

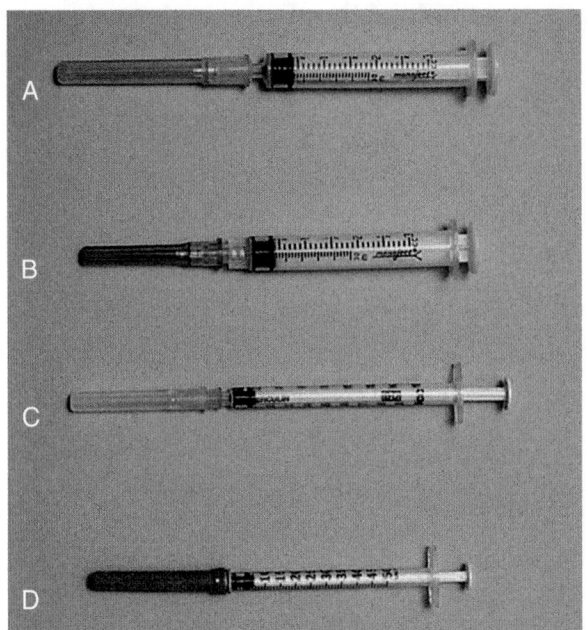

Figure 16-11 ■ Types of syringes. **A,** Plain tip marked in 0.1 (tenths). **B,** Luer-Lok marked in 0.01 (hundredths) for doses less than 1 mL. **C,** Tuberculin syringe marked in 0.01 (hundredths). **D,** Insulin syringe marked in units (50).

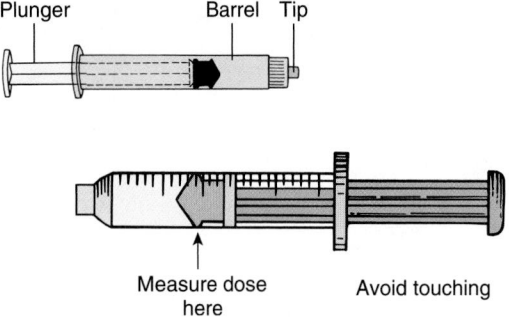

Figure 16-12 ■ Parts of a syringe.

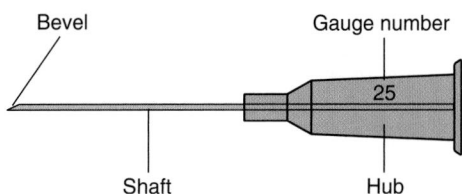

Figure 16-13 ■ Parts of a needle.

- Avoid touching the length of the plunger or inner part of the barrel. Keep tip of syringe covered with cap or needle.
- Wash skin soiled with dirt, drainage, or feces with soap and water. Use friction and a circular motion while cleaning with an antiseptic swab. Swab from center of site, and move outward in a 2-inch radius.

Each type of injection requires certain skills to ensure that the medication reaches the proper location. The effects of a parenterally administered medication develop rapidly, depending on the rate of medication absorption. Therefore you need to closely observe the patient's response to the medication.

Equipment

A variety of syringes and needles are available, each designed to deliver a certain volume of a medication to a specific type of tissue. Use nursing judgment when determining the syringe or needle that will be most appropriate.

SYRINGES Syringes have a cylindrical barrel with a close-fitting plunger and a tip designed to fit the hub of a hypodermic needle. Syringes are single use, disposable, and are classified as being Luer-Lok or non–Luer-Lok. Non–Luer-Lok syringes (Figure 16-11, *A*) have preattached needles or require needles that slip onto the tip. This name is based on the design on the syringe's tip. The needles twist onto Luer-Lok syringes (Figure 16-11, *B*) and lock themselves in place. This design prevents the inadvertent removal of the needle.

Syringes come in a number of sizes, ranging from 0.5 to 60 mL. It is unusual to use a syringe larger than 5 mL for an injection. A 1- to 3-mL syringe is usually adequate for IM and

subcutaneous injections (see Figure 16-11). You use large syringes to administer certain IV medications and irrigate wounds or drainage tubes. Some syringes are prepackaged with a needle attached. However, sometimes you need to change the needle based on the route of administration and the size of the patient.

Some syringes have two scales along the barrel; one is divided into minims and the other into tenths of a milliliter. The tuberculin syringe (see Figure 16-11, *C*) is calibrated in sixteenths of a minim and hundredths of a milliliter and has a capacity of 1 mL. You use tuberculin syringes to prepare small amounts of medications. You also use them for ID and subcutaneous injections.

Insulin syringes (see Figure 16-11, *D*) hold 0.3 to 1 mL and are calibrated in units. Most insulin syringes are U-100s, designed for use with U-100 strength insulin. Each milliliter of solution contains 100 units of insulin.

To fill a syringe, pull the plunger outward while the needle tip remains immersed in the prepared solution. To maintain sterility, touch the outside of the syringe barrel and the handle of the plunger, but do not touch the tip or inside of the barrel, the hub, the shaft of the plunger, and the needle (Figure 16-12).

NEEDLES Some needles come attached to syringes. Other needles come packaged individually to allow flexibility in selecting the right needle for a patient. Needles are disposable, and most are made of stainless steel. The needle has three parts: the hub, which fits onto the tip of a syringe; the shaft, which connects to the hub; and the bevel, or slanted tip (Figure 16-13). The tip of a needle, or the bevel, is always slanted. When injected into tissue, the bevel creates a narrow slit that quickly closes when you remove the needle. This prevents leakage of medication, blood, or serum. Long beveled tips are sharp and narrow, which minimizes discomfort when entering tissue used for subcutaneous or IM injections.

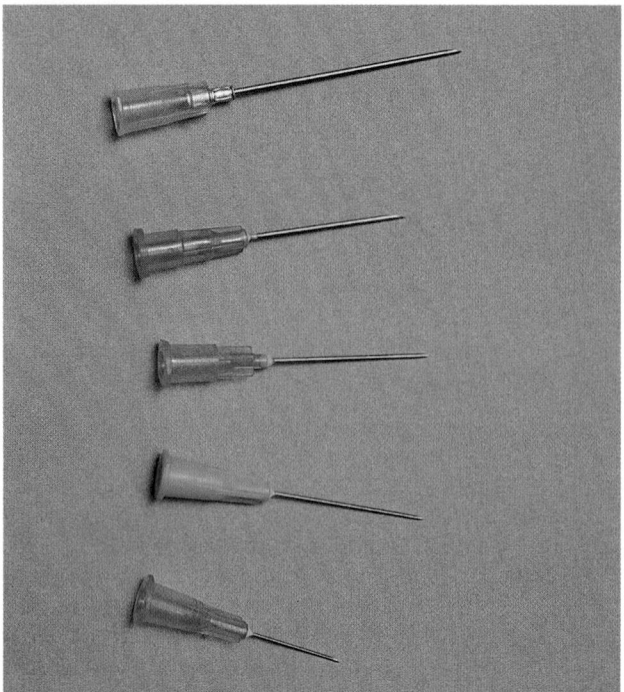

Figure 16-14 ■ Hypodermic needles *(top to bottom):* 19 gauge, 1½-inch length; 20 gauge, 1-inch length; 21 gauge, 1-inch length; 23 gauge, 1-inch length; and 25 gauge, ⅝-inch length.

Most needles vary in length from ¼ to 3½ inches (Figure 16-14). The needle length you choose depends on the patient's size and weight and the route of administration. A child or slender adult generally requires a shorter needle. Use longer needles (1 to 1½ inches) for IM injections and shorter needles (¼ to ⅝ inch) for subcutaneous injections. Needles also vary in gauge or circumference. As the needle gauge gets smaller, the needle diameter becomes larger (see Figure 16-14). The selection of a gauge depends on the length of the needle and the viscosity of fluid you will inject or infuse. The rationale for needle selection is included in each skill.

DISPOSABLE INJECTION UNITS Disposable, single-dose, prefilled syringes are available for some medications. With these syringes you do not need to prepare medication dosages, except perhaps to expel portions of unneeded medications.

Prefilled unit dose systems such as Tubex and Carpuject include reusable plastic syringe holders and disposable, pre-filled, sterile, glass cartridge units (Figure 16-15). When using this system, load the cartridge Luer tip first into the plastic syringe holder, and then secure it (following package directions) and check for air bubbles in the syringe. Advance the plunger to expel air and excess medication, as with a regular syringe. You can use the glass cartridge with needleless systems or safety needles. After giving the medication, dispose of the glass cartridge safely in a puncture-proof and leakproof receptacle.

Preparing an Injection From an Ampule

Ampules contain single doses of medication in a liquid. Ampules are available in many sizes, from 1 mL to 10 mL or more (Figure 16-16, *A*). An ampule is made of glass with a constricted, prescored neck that you snap off to allow access to the medication. A colored ring around the neck indicates where the ampule is prescored. Aspiration of the medication into a syringe occurs easily with a filter needle and syringe. You use filter needles when preparing medications from glass ampules to prevent glass particles from being drawn into the syringe with the medication (Preston and Hegadoren, 2004). Replace the filter needle with an appropriate-size needle or needleless access device before administering the medication.

Preparing an Injection From a Vial

A vial is a single-dose or multidose container with a rubber seal at the top (Figure 16-16, *B*). A metal cap protects the seal until it is ready to use. Vials contain liquid or dry forms of medications. Medications that are unstable in solution are packaged dry. The vial label specifies the solvent or diluent used to dissolve the medication and the amount of diluent needed to prepare a desired medication concentration. Normal saline and sterile distilled water are solutions commonly used to dissolve medications.

Unlike the ampule, the vial is a closed system. Inject air into it to withdraw the solution. A vacuum develops within the vial if you fail to inject air when withdrawing solution, making withdrawal of medication difficult (see Skill 16-4). Although not necessary, you may decide to use a filter needle when preparing medication from a vial, especially if you are concerned that you will draw parts of the rubber stopper or other particles into the syringe (Nicoll and Hesby, 2002).

To prepare a powdered medication, first draw up the amount and type of diluent or solvent recommended on the vial's label in a syringe. Inject the diluent into the vial in the same manner as injecting air into the vial. Most powdered medications dissolve easily. You have to withdraw the needle or the needleless access device from the vial when mixing the contents. Gently shake or roll the vial between your hands to thoroughly dissolve the powdered medication. Reinsert the needle or the needleless access device to draw up the dissolved medication. After mixing multidose vials, place a label that includes the date and time of mixing and the concentration of medication per milliliter on the vial. Multidose vials sometimes require refrigeration after they are diluted.

Mixing Medications

If two medications are compatible, it is possible to mix them in one injection. Most nursing units have charts that list common compatible medications. If you are uncertain about medication compatibilities, consult a pharmacist.

MIXING MEDICATIONS FROM A VIAL AND AN AMPULE When you mix two medications and one is in a vial and the other is in an ampule, prepare the medication from the vial first. Then withdraw the medication from the ampule using the same syringe and a filter needle.

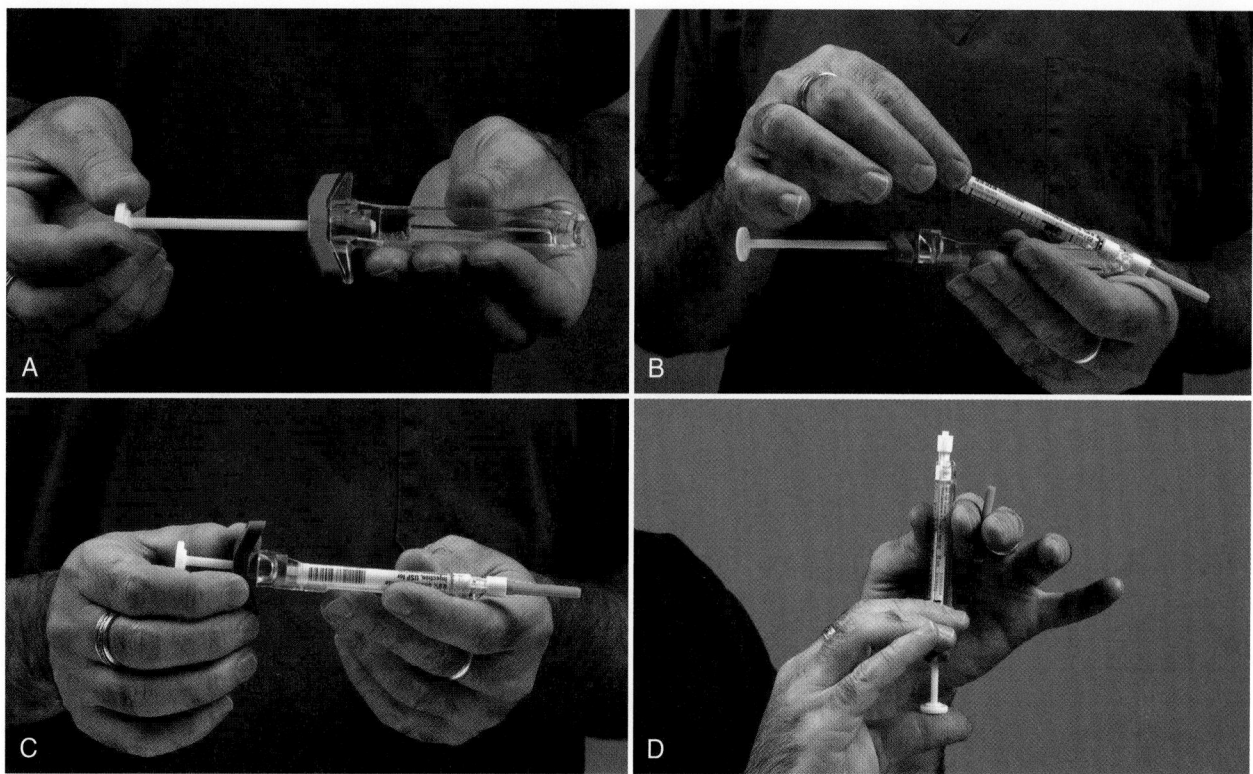

Figure 16-15 ▦ **A,** Carpuject syringe and prefilled sterile cartridge with needle. **B,** Assembling the Carpuject. **C,** The cartridge slides into the syringe barrel, turns, and locks at the needle end. The plunger then screws into the cartridge end. **D,** Expel excess medication to obtain accurate dose.

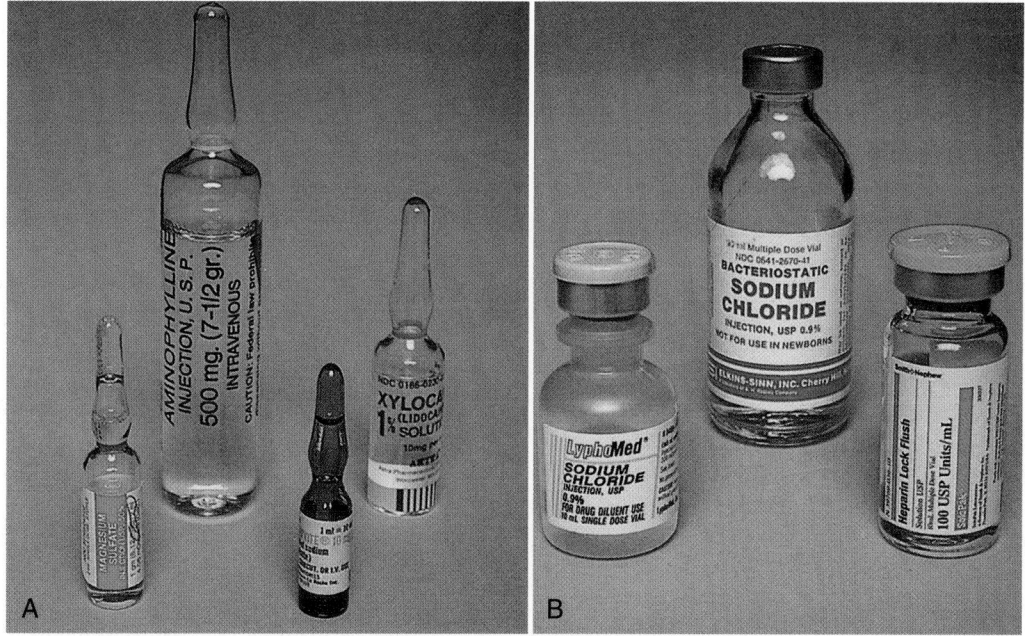

Figure 16-16 ▦ **A,** Medication in ampules. **B,** Medication in vials. Rubber top must be cleansed with alcohol when vial is opened or when it is reused.

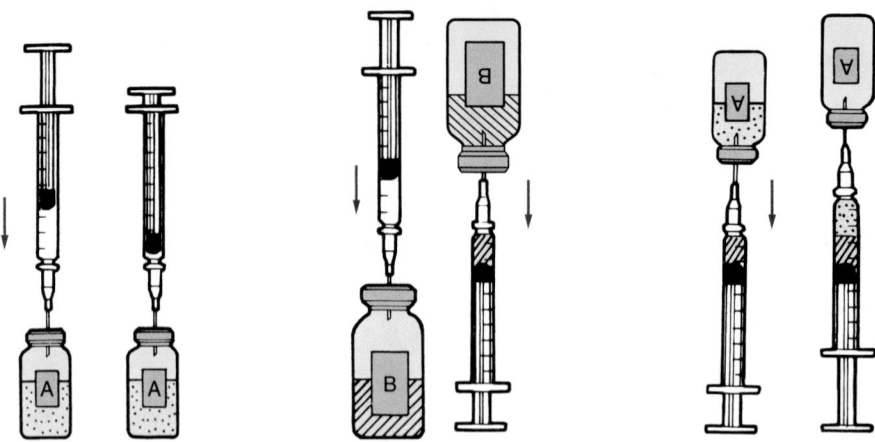

Figure 16-17 ■ Steps in mixing medications from two vials.

MIXING MEDICATIONS FROM TWO VIALS Use the following principles when mixing medications from two vials:

1. Do not contaminate one medication with another.
2. Ensure the final dosage is accurate.
3. Maintain aseptic technique.

You need only one syringe to mix medications from two vials (Figure 16-17). Aspirate the volume of air equivalent to the first medication's dose (vial A) into the syringe. Inject the air into vial A, making sure the needle does not touch the solution. Withdraw the needle or the needleless access device from vial A, and aspirate air that is equivalent to the second medication's dose (vial B) into the syringe. Inject the volume of air into vial B, and immediately withdraw the medication in vial B into the syringe. Then insert the needle or needleless access device into vial A, being careful not to push the plunger and expel the medication within the syringe into the vial. Withdraw the desired amount of medication from vial A into the syringe. After preparing the correct dose, withdraw the needle or needleless access device from vial A, and apply a new needle suitable for injection.

Insulin Preparation

Insulin is the hormone used to treat diabetes mellitus. You administer it by injection, because the GI tract will break down an oral form and destroy it. In the United States and Canada, health care providers usually prescribe insulin in concentrations of 100 units of insulin per milliliter of solution. This is called U-100 insulin. Insulin is also commercially available in concentrations of 500 units per milliliter, which is called U-500 insulin. When preparing insulin, you need to use the correct syringe; you use a 100-unit–scaled syringe to prepare 100-unit insulin. Because there is no insulin syringe currently designed to prepare U-500 insulin, many medication errors have resulted with use of this type of insulin. When ordering U-500 insulin, ensure prescribers specify units and volume (e.g., 150 units, 0.3 mL of U-500 insulin).

When preparing the dose, use tuberculin syringes to draw up the doses, and verify dosages with another nurse or a pharmacist before you administer it. Additional safeguards when using U-500 insulin include having the insulin listed as concentrated in computerized medication dispensing systems, making prescribers and pharmacists verify that the patient is to receive U-500 insulin when it is ordered, and only stocking it on patient care units when it is ordered for a specific patient (ISMP, 2007a).

Insulin is classified by rate of action, including rapid-acting, short-acting, intermediate-acting, and long-acting (Table 16-8). A patient with diabetes sometimes requires more than one type of insulin. In addition, a patient may receive several injections in a day. For example, in a two-dose protocol a combination of short- and intermediate-acting insulin is injected twice daily. Insulin protocols try to duplicate the normal pattern of a patient's insulin excretion from the pancreas.

Health care providers usually order insulin by specific dosages at select times or by a sliding scale. A sliding scale dictates a certain dosage based on the patient's blood glucose level. The American Diabetes Association (2009) does not recommend sliding scale orders. Reliance on sliding scale during a patient's hospitalization is unlikely to achieve glucose control. An example of a patient's sliding-scale insulin order reads as follows:

Give 5 units of regular insulin subcutaneously for blood glucose levels between 150 and 200 mg/dL.
Give 10 units of regular insulin for blood glucose levels between 201 and 275 mg/dL.
Call for blood glucose levels higher than 275 mg/dL.

Before drawing up insulin doses, gently roll all cloudy insulin preparations between the palms of the hands to resuspend the insulin. Do not shake insulin vials. Shaking causes bubbles to form; this takes up space in a syringe and alters the dosage.

If more than one type of insulin is required to manage the patient's diabetes, you can mix them in one syringe **if** they are

TABLE 16-8 Comparison of Insulin Preparations

INSULIN TYPE*	ONSET (HOURS)	PEAK EFFECT (HOURS)	DURATION OF ACTION (HOURS)
RAPID- AND SHORT-ACTING			
Insulin lispro (Humalog)	¼	1	4
Insulin aspart (NovoLog)	½	1-3	3-5
Regular insulin†	½-1	2-4	5-7
INTERMEDIATE-ACTING			
Insulin zinc suspension (Lente)	1-3	8-12	18-28
Isophane insulin suspension (NPH)	3-4	6-12	18-28
COMBINATION INSULINS			
Humulin 70/30 or Novolin 70/30 (70% NPH; 30% regular insulin)	½	4-8	24
Humulin 50/50 (50% NPH; 50% regular insulin)	½	3	22-24
Humalog mix 75/25 (75% lispro protamine suspension; 25% lispro insulin)	¼	½-6	24
NovoLog mix 70/30 (70% insulin aspart protamine; 30% insulin aspart)	¼	1-4	24
LONG-ACTING			
Extended insulin zinc suspension (Ultralente)	4-6	18-24	36
Insulin detemir (Levemir)‡	3-4	"Peakless"	24
Insulin glargine (Lantus)‡	1-5	Plateau	24

Modified from McKenry LM, Tessier E, Hogan M: *Pharmacology in nursing*, ed 22, St. Louis, 2006, Mosby.

*All above insulins are available in 100-unit strengths.
†This is the only insulin for IV or IM use; intravenously, the onset of action is within 10 to 30 minutes, peak effect within 20 to 30 minutes, and duration of action between 30 minutes and 1 hour.
‡Cannot be mixed with other insulins.

compatible (Box 16-21). If regular and intermediate-acting insulin are ordered, prepare the regular insulin first to prevent contamination with the intermediate-acting insulin. Use the following principles when mixing insulins (ADA, 2004; Novo Nordisk, 2008):

- Patients whose blood glucose levels are well controlled on a mixed-insulin dose need to maintain their individual routine when preparing and administering their insulin.
- Do not mix insulin with any other medications or diluents unless approved by the prescriber.
- Never mix insulin glargine (Lantus) or insulin detemir (Levemir) with other types of insulin.
- Inject rapid-acting insulins mixed with NPH, Lente, or Ultralente insulins within 15 minutes before a meal.
- Do not mix short-acting and Lente insulins unless the patient's blood glucose levels are currently under control with this mixture.
- Do not mix phosphate-buffered insulins (e.g., NPH) with Lente insulins.
- Verify insulin dosages with another nurse while you prepare them if required by agency policy.

Administering Injections

Each injection route differs based on the type of tissues the medication enters. The characteristics of the tissues influence the rate of medication absorption, which affects the onset of medication action. Before injecting a medication, know the volume of the medication to administer, the medication's characteristics and viscosity, and the location of anatomical structures underlying injection sites (see Skill 16-5).

Failure to select an injection site in relation to anatomical landmarks will result in nerve or bone damage during needle insertion. If you do not aspirate the syringe before injecting an IM medication, you may accidentally inject the medication directly into an artery or vein. Injecting too large a volume of medication for the site selected causes extreme pain and results in local tissue damage.

Many patients, particularly children, fear injections. You will give some patients with serious or chronic illnesses several injections daily. You are able to minimize the patient's discomfort in the following ways:

1. Use a sharp-beveled needle in the smallest suitable length and gauge.

2. Position the patient as comfortably as possible to reduce muscular tension.
3. Select the proper injection site, using anatomical landmarks.
4. Apply a vapocoolant spray (e.g., Fluori-Methane spray or ethyl chloride) or topical anesthetic (e.g., EMLA cream) to the injection site before giving the medication when possible.
5. Divert the patient's attention from the injection through conversation.
6. Insert the needle quickly and smoothly to minimize tissue pulling.
7. Hold the syringe steady while the needle remains in tissues.
8. Inject the medication slowly and steadily.

SUBCUTANEOUS INJECTIONS Subcutaneous injections involve injecting medications into the loose connective tissue under the dermis (see Skill 16-5). Because subcutaneous tissue is not as richly supplied with blood as the muscles, medication absorption is somewhat slower than with IM injections.

The best subcutaneous injection sites include the outer posterior aspect of the upper arms, the abdomen from below the costal margins to the iliac crests, and the anterior aspect of the thighs (Figure 16-18). The site most frequently recommended for heparin injections is the abdomen (Figure 16-19). The site used for enoxaparin (low-molecular-weight [LMW] heparin) is on the right or left side of the abdomen at least 2 inches from the umbilicus. This area is often called the patient's "love handles" (Sanofi-Aventis, 2007). It is also recommended that other types of heparin preparation be given in this site as well. Subcutaneous sites for other medications include the scapular areas of the upper back and the upper ventral or dorsal gluteal areas. Choose an injection site that is free of skin lesions, bony prominences, and large underlying muscles or nerves.

Recommended subcutaneous insulin injection sites include the upper arm, anterior and lateral portions of the thigh, buttocks, and abdomen. Rotating injections within the same body part for a sequence of injections provides more consistency in the absorption of insulin. For example, if you inject the morning insulin into the patient's arm, then give the next injection in a different place, about a finger width away, in the same arm. The rate of absorption is another factor in site selection for insulin administration. The abdomen has the quickest absorption rate, followed by the arms, thighs, and buttocks (ADA, 2004).

Small subcutaneous doses (0.5 to 1 mL) of water-soluble medications are preferred in adults because the subcutaneous tissue is sensitive to irritating solutions and large

BOX 16-21   PROCEDURAL GUIDELINES

Mixing Two Kinds of Insulin in One Syringe

DELEGATION CONSIDERATIONS: Do not delegate this skill. Instruct assistive personnel about the potential side effects of medications and the need to report their occurrence.

EQUIPMENT: Insulin vials, insulin syringe, alcohol swab, MAR
1 Check accuracy and completeness of each MAR or computer printout with prescriber's written medication order. Check patient's name, drug name and dosage, route of administration, and time for administration.
2 Verify insulin labels carefully against the MAR before preparing the dose to ensure that you give the correct type of insulin.
3 Perform hand hygiene.
4 If patient takes insulin that is cloudy, roll the bottle of insulin between the hands to resuspend the insulin preparation.
5 Wipe off tops of both insulin vials with alcohol swab.
6 Verify insulin dosages against MAR a second time.
7 If mixing rapid- or short-acting insulin with intermediate- or long-acting insulin, take insulin syringe and aspirate volume of air equivalent to dose to be withdrawn from intermediate- or long-acting insulin first. If two intermediate- or long-acting insulins are mixed, it makes no difference which vial you prepare first.

8 Insert needle, and inject air into vial of intermediate- or long-acting insulin. Do not let the tip of the needle touch the insulin.
9 Remove the syringe from the vial of insulin without aspirating medication.
10 With the same syringe, inject air, equal to the dose of rapid- or short-acting insulin, into the vial and withdraw the correct dose into the syringe.
11 Remove the syringe from the rapid- or short-acting insulin, and get rid of air bubbles to ensure accurate dosing.
12 After verifying insulin dosages with MAR a third time, determine which point on syringe scale combined units of insulin measure by adding the number of units of both insulins together (e.g., 5 units regular + 10 units NPH = 15 units total).
13 Place the needle of the syringe back into the vial of intermediate- or long-acting insulin. Be careful not to push plunger and inject insulin in syringe into the vial.
14 Invert the vial, and carefully withdraw the desired amount of insulin into syringe.
15 Withdraw needle, and check fluid level in syringe. Keep needle of prepared syringe sheathed or capped until ready to administer medication.
16 Dispose of soiled supplies in proper receptacle and perform hand hygiene.

Data from American Diabetes Association. From *Diabetes Care*, Vol. 27, 2004; S106–S109. Reprinted with permission from The American Diabetes Association, copyright © 2004.

volumes of medications. However, doses up to 2 mL may be given (Prettyman, 2005). In children, give smaller volumes, up to 0.5 mL (Hockenberry and Wilson, 2009). Collection of medications within the tissues causes sterile abscesses, which appear as hardened, painful lumps under the skin.

A patient's body weight indicates the depth of the subcutaneous layer. Therefore base the needle length and angle of insertion on the patient's weight. Generally a 25-gauge ⅝-inch needle inserted at a 45-degree angle (Figure 16-20) or a ½-inch needle inserted at a 90-degree angle deposits medications into the subcutaneous tissue of a normal-size patient. A child usually requires only a ½-inch (1.25 cm) needle (Shin and Kim, 2006). If the patient is obese, pinch the tissue and use a needle long enough to insert through fatty tissue at the base of the skinfold. Thin patients sometimes have insufficient tissue for subcutaneous injections. The upper abdomen is the best site for injection with this type of patient. To ensure a subcutaneous medication reaches the subcutaneous tissue, you use the following rule to determine the appropriate angle of injection: if you are able to grasp 2 inches (5 cm) of tissue, insert the needle at a 90-degree angle; if you are able to grasp 1 inch (2.5 cm), insert the needle at a 45-degree angle (Rushing, 2004).

INTRAMUSCULAR INJECTIONS The IM route provides faster medication absorption than the subcutaneous route because of a muscle's greater vascularity. However, IM injections are associated with many risks. Therefore, whenever administering a medication by the IM route, first verify that the injection is justified (Nicoll and Hesby, 2002; WHO, 2006). Some medications, such as influenza and pneumonia vaccinations, need to be given using the IM route. In these cases, ensure that you use the appropriate technique to inject the medication as safely as possible.

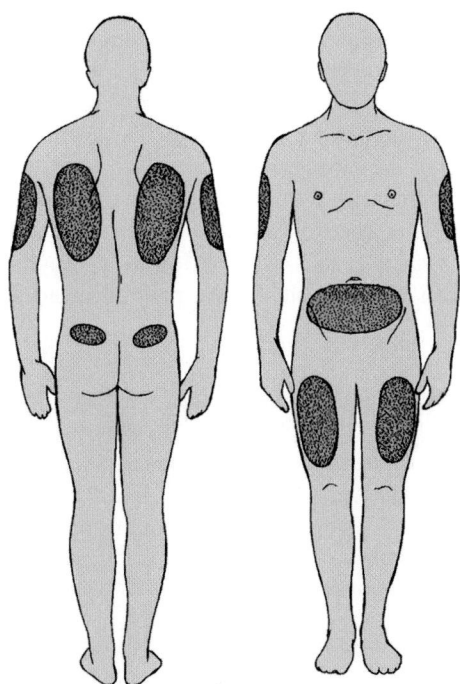

Figure 16-18 ■ Sites recommended for subcutaneous injections.

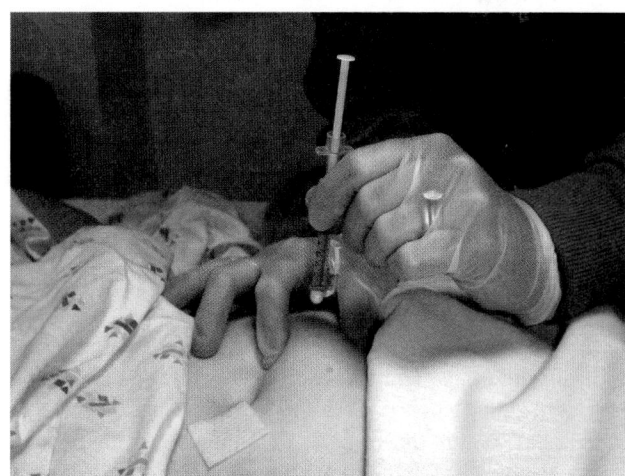

Figure 16-19 ■ Giving subcutaneous heparin in the abdomen.

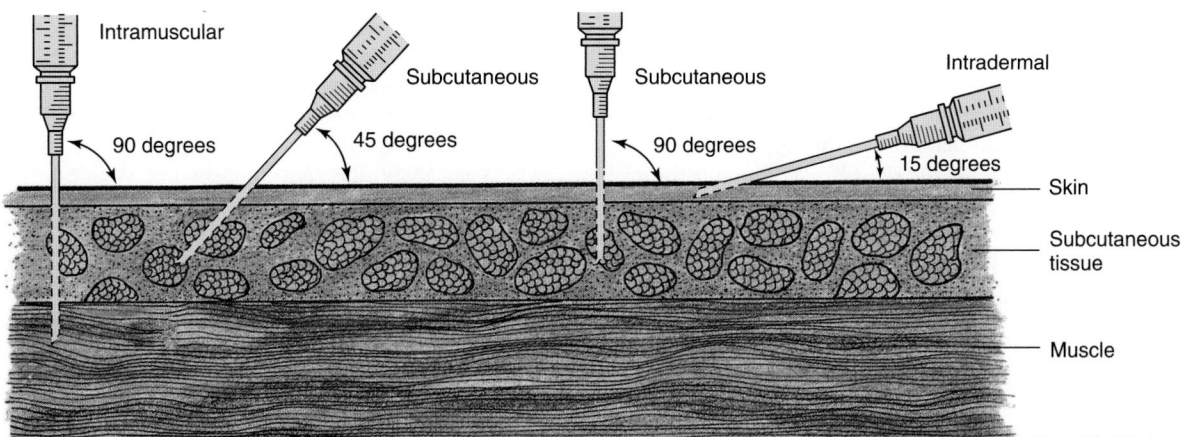

Figure 16-20 ■ Comparison of angles of insertion for IM (90 degrees), subcutaneous (45 and 90 degrees), and ID (15 degrees) injections.

Use a longer and heavier-gauge needle to pass through subcutaneous tissue and penetrate deep muscle tissue (see Skill 16-5). Weight and the amount of adipose tissue influence needle size selection. An obese patient requires a needle 2 to 3 inches long, whereas a thin patient requires only a ½- to 1-inch needle (Nicoll and Hesby, 2002; Zaybak and others, 2007).

Administer IM injections so that the needle is perpendicular to the patient's body and as close to a 90-degree angle as possible (Nicoll and Hesby, 2002) (see Figure 16-20). Muscle is less sensitive to irritating and viscous drugs. A normal, well-developed adult can safely tolerate as much as 2 to 5 mL of medication in a larger muscle without much pain (Nicoll and Hesby, 2002; Prettyman, 2005). However, the body does not absorb larger medication volumes well. Children, older adults, and thin patients tolerate only 2 mL of an IM injection. Give no more than 1 mL of medication in one injection to small children and older infants, and do not give more than 0.5 mL to smaller infants (Hockenberry and Wilson, 2009).

Assess the muscle before giving an injection. Make sure the muscle is free of tenderness. Repeated injections in the same muscle cause severe discomfort. With the patient relaxed, palpate the muscle to rule out any hardened lesions. Help the patient assume a comfortable position to minimize discomfort during an injection.

Sites   When selecting an IM site, consider the following: Is the area free of infection or necrosis? Are there local areas of bruising or abrasions? What is the location of underlying bones, nerves, and major blood vessels? What volume of medication will you administer? Each site has certain advantages and disadvantages (Box 16-22).

Ventrogluteal.   The ventrogluteal site is the preferred and safe site for all adults, children, and infants (Cook and Murtagh, 2006; Hockenberry and Wilson, 2009; Nicoll and Hesby, 2002). This site involves the gluteus medius muscle, which lies on top of the gluteus minimus muscle. Research shows that injuries such as fibrosis, nerve damage, abscess, tissue necrosis, muscle contraction, gangrene, and pain are associated with all of the common IM sites except the ventrogluteal site.

To locate the ventrogluteal muscle, have your patient lie in a supine or lateral position. Flexing the knee and hip helps the patient relax this muscle. Place the palm of your hand against the greater trochanter of the patient's hip with the wrist perpendicular to the femur. Use the right hand for the left hip and the left hand for the right hip. Point your thumb toward the patient's groin with your index finger placed on the anterosuperior iliac spine. Point your middle finger back along the iliac crest toward the buttock. Your index finger, the middle finger, and the iliac crest form a V-shaped triangle (Nicoll and Hesby, 2002). The injection site is the center of the triangle (Figure 16-21).

Vastus Lateralis.   The vastus lateralis muscle is another injection site used in adults and children. The muscle is thick and well developed and is located on the anterior lateral aspect of the thigh. It extends in an adult from a handbreadth

above the knee to a handbreadth below the greater trochanter of the femur (Figure 16-22). Use the middle third of the muscle for injection. The width of the muscle usually extends from the midline of the thigh to the midline of the thigh's outer side. With young children or cachectic patients, grasp the body of the muscle during injection to be sure that you deposit the medication in muscle tissue. To help relax the muscle, have the patient lie flat with the knee slightly flexed or assume a sitting position. The vastus lateralis site is preferable for infants, toddlers, and children receiving biologicals (e.g., immune globulins, vaccines, or toxoids) (Nicoll and Hesby, 2002).

Deltoid.   Because the radial and ulnar nerves and brachial artery lie within the upper arm along the humerus (Figure 16-23), use this site only for small medication volumes or when other sites are inaccessible because of dressings or casts. Locate the deltoid muscle by fully exposing the patient's upper arm and shoulder and having the patient relax the arm at the side and flex the elbow. Do not roll up a tight-fitting sleeve. Have the patient sit, stand, or lie down. Palpate the lower edge of the acromion process, which forms the base of a triangle in line with the midpoint of the lateral aspect of the upper arm. The injection site is in the center of the triangle, about 2.5 to 5 cm (1 to 2 inches) below the acromion process. You also can locate the site by placing four fingers across the

BOX 16-22   Characteristics of Intramuscular Sites

VENTROGLUTEAL
- A deep site, situated away from major nerves and blood vessels
- Less chance of contamination in incontinent patients or infants
- Easily identified by prominent bony landmarks
- Preferred site for medications (e.g., antibiotics) that are larger in volume, more viscous, and irritating for adults, children, and infants over 7 months of age

VASTUS LATERALIS
- Lacks major nerves and blood vessels
- Rapid drug absorption
- Often used for biologicals (e.g., immunizations) in infants, toddlers, and children

DELTOID
- Easily accessible but muscle not well developed in most patients
- Used for small amounts of drugs
- Not used in infants or children with underdeveloped muscles
- Potential for injury to radial and ulnar nerves or brachial artery
- Used for immunizations for toddlers, older children, and adults (Nicoll and Hesby, 2002)
- Recommended site for hepatitis B vaccine and rabies injections

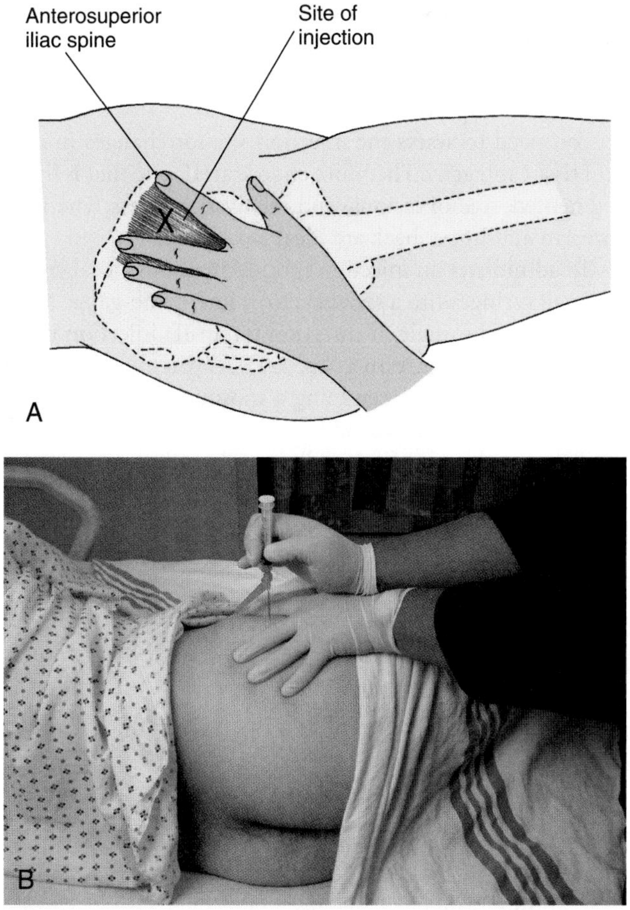

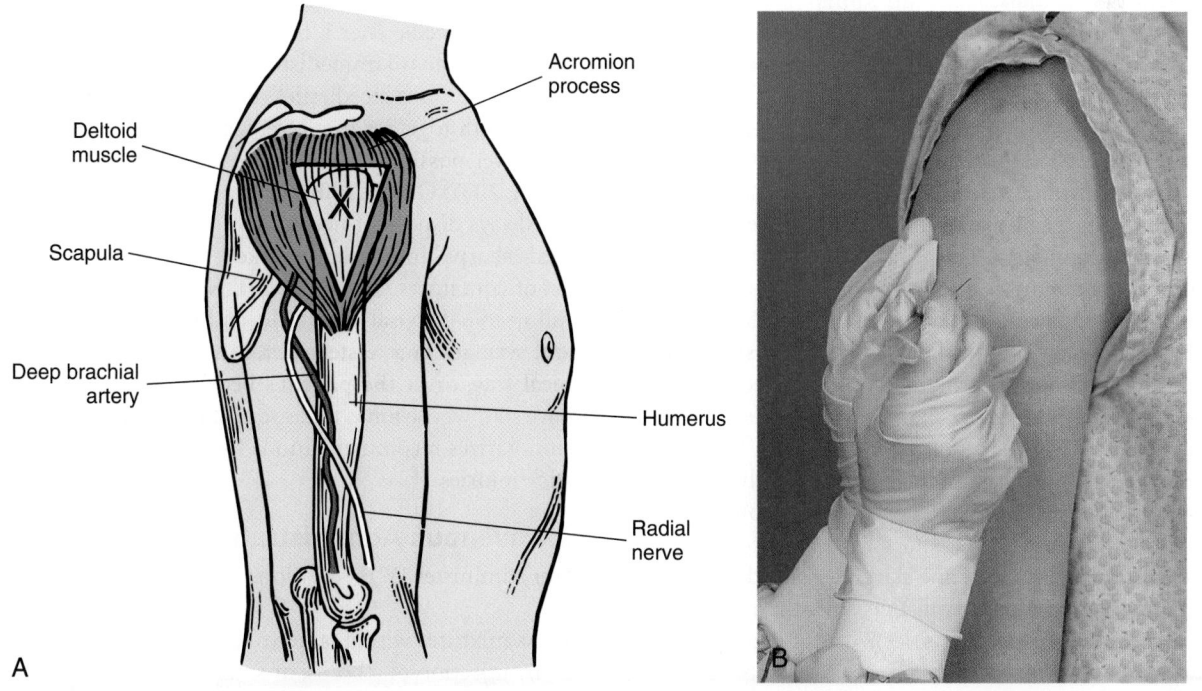

Anterosuperior
iliac spine

Site of
injection

A

Figure 16-21 ■ A, Landmarks for ventrogluteal site.
B, Giving IM injection in ventrogluteal muscle.

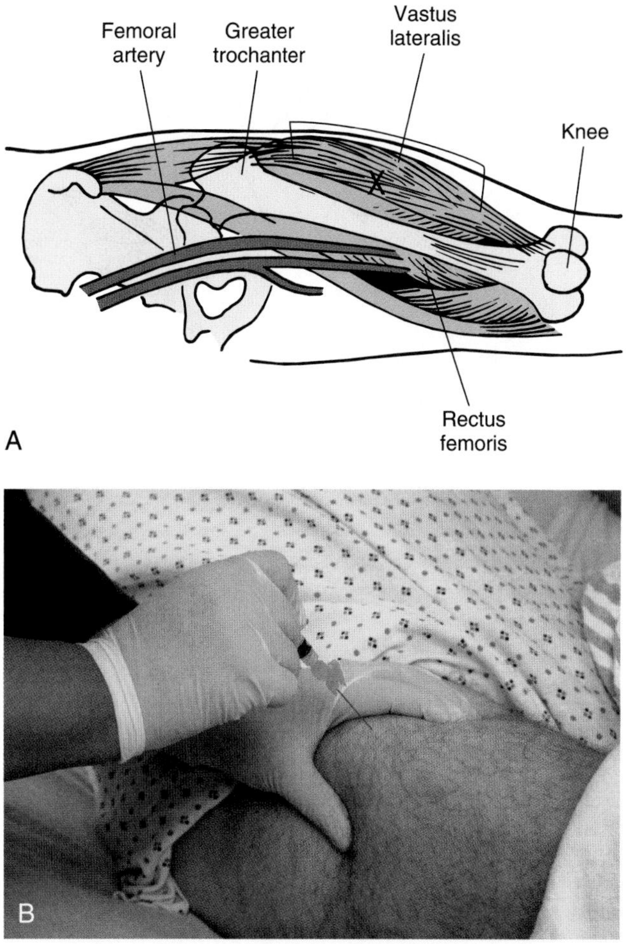

Femoral
artery   Greater
trochanter   Vastus
lateralis

Knee

Rectus
femoris

A

Figure 16-22 ■ A, Landmarks for vastus lateralis site.
B, Giving IM injection in vastus lateralis muscle.

Acromion
process

Deltoid
muscle

Scapula

Deep brachial
artery

Humerus

Radial
nerve

A

Figure 16-23 ■ A, Landmarks for deltoid site. B, Giving IM injection in deltoid
muscle.

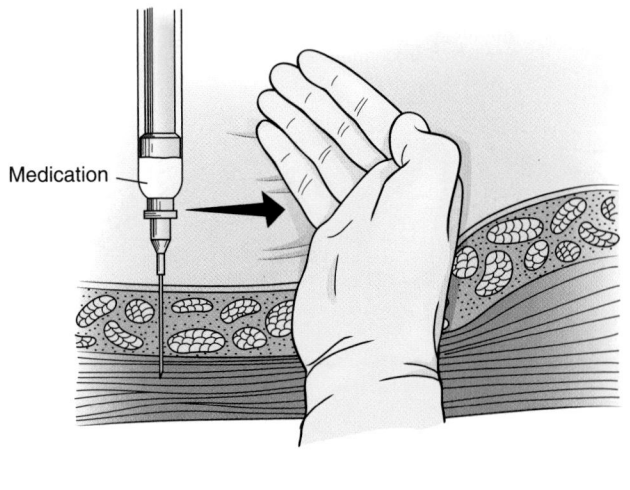

During injection

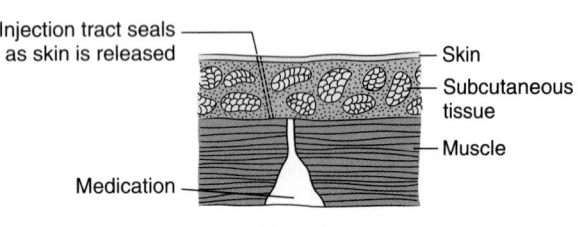

After release

Figure 16-24 ■ Z-Track method of injection prevents deposit of medication into sensitive tissues.

deltoid muscle, with the top finger along the acromion process. The injection site is then three fingerwidths below the acromion process.

Technique in Intramuscular Injections

Z-Track Method. It is recommended that you use the **Z-track injection** method when giving IM injections to minimize irritation by sealing the medication in muscle tissue (Nicoll and Hesby, 2002). To use the Z-track method, apply a new needle to the syringe after preparing the medication so that no solution remains on the outside needle shaft. Then choose an IM site, preferably in a larger, deeper muscle such as the ventrogluteal muscle. Place the ulnar side of the nondominant hand just below the site, and pull the overlying skin and subcutaneous tissues approximately 2.5 to 3.5 cm (1 to 1½ inches) laterally to the side. Hold the skin in this position until you administer the injection. After preparing the site with an antiseptic swab, inject the needle deep into the muscle. Grasp the barrel of the syringe with the thumb and index finger of the nondominant hand. Slowly inject the medication if there is no blood return on aspiration. Keep the needle inserted for 10 seconds to allow the medication to disperse evenly. Then release the skin after withdrawing the needle. This leaves a zigzag path that seals the needle tract where tissue planes slide across each other (Figure 16-24). The medication cannot escape from the muscle tissue.

INTRADERMAL INJECTIONS ID injections are usually used for skin testing (e.g., tuberculin screening or allergy

tests). Because these medications are potent, you inject them into the dermis, where blood supply is reduced and medication absorption occurs slowly. Some patients experience a severe anaphylactic reaction if the medications enter the circulation too rapidly.

You need to assess the injection site for changes in color and tissue integrity. Therefore choose an ID site that is lightly pigmented, free of lesions, and relatively hairless. The inner forearm and upper back are ideal locations.

To administer an injection intradermally, use a tuberculin or small syringe with a short (¼ to ½ inch), fine-gauge (26 or 27) needle. The angle of insertion for an ID injection is 5 to 15 degrees (see Figure 16-20, p. 423). As you inject the medication, a small bleb resembling a mosquito bite will appear on the skin's surface (see Skill 16-5). If a bleb does not appear or if the site bleeds after needle withdrawal, there is a good chance the medication entered subcutaneous tissues. In this case, test results will not be valid.

SAFETY IN ADMINISTERING MEDICATIONS BY INJECTION

Needleless Devices The most frequent route of exposure to blood-borne disease is from needlestick injuries (ANA, 2007; Occupational Safety and Health Administration [OSHA], 2007). These injuries commonly occur when health care workers recap needles, mishandle IV lines and needles, or leave stray needles at a patient's bedside. Exposure to blood-borne pathogens is one of the deadliest hazards nurses are exposed to on a daily basis. However, over 80% of needlestick injuries are preventable with the implementation of safe needle devices (ANA, 2007). The Needlestick Safety and Prevention Act requires health care facilities to use safe needle devices to reduce the frequency of needlestick injury.

Special syringes are designed with a sheath or guard that covers the needle after it is withdrawn from the skin (Figure 16-25). The guard immediately covers the needle, eliminating the chance for a needlestick injury. Dispose of the syringe and sheath together in a receptacle. Use "needleless" devices whenever possible to reduce the risk for needlestick injuries (ANA, 2007; OSHA, 2007).

Always dispose of needles and other instruments considered "sharps" into clearly marked, puncture-proof and leak-proof containers (Figure 16-26). Never force a needle into a full needle disposal receptacle, and never place used needles and syringes in a wastebasket, in your pocket, on a patient's meal tray, or at the patient's bedside. Health care agencies have staff whose job is to dispose of full containers. Box 16-23 summarizes recommendations for the prevention of needlestick injuries.

Intravenous Administration

You administer IV medications by the following methods:

1. As mixtures within large volumes of IV fluids
2. By injection of a bolus, or small volume, of medication through an existing IV infusion line or intermittent venous access (heparin or saline lock)

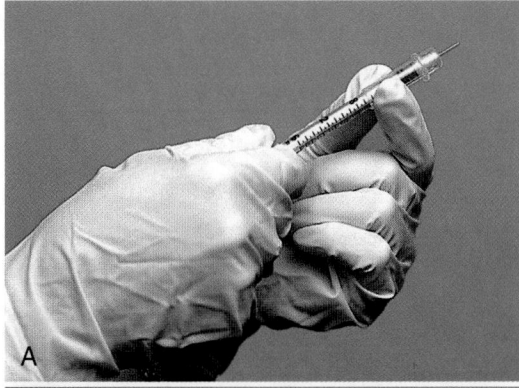

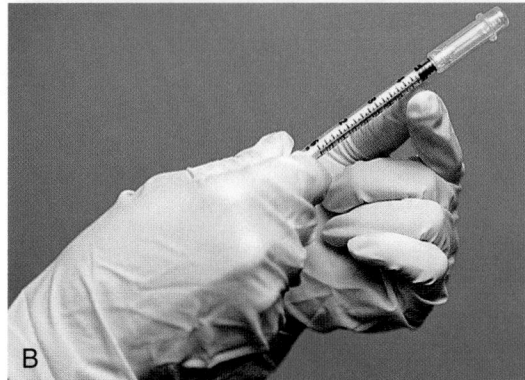

Figure 16-25 ■ Needle with plastic guard to prevent needle sticks. **A,** Position of guard before injection. **B,** After injection, the nurse locks the guard in place, covering the needle.

3. By piggyback, intermittent infusion sets, and mini-infusion pumps, which infuse a solution containing the prescribed medication and a small volume of IV fluid through an existing IV line

In all three methods the patient has either an existing IV infusion line or an IV site that is accessed intermittently for infusions (sometimes called a heparin or saline lock). In most institutions, policies and procedures identify the medications that nurses are allowed to administer intravenously. These policies are based on the medication, capability and availability of staff, and type of monitoring equipment available.

Chapter 17 describes the technique for performing venipuncture and establishing continuous IV fluid infusions. Medication administration is only one reason for supplying IV fluids. You use IV fluid therapy primarily for fluid replacement in patients unable to take oral fluids and as a means of supplying electrolytes and nutrients.

When using any method of IV medication administration, observe patients closely for symptoms of adverse reactions. After a medication enters the bloodstream, it begins to act immediately and there is no way to stop its action. Therefore avoid errors in dose calculation and preparation. Follow the six rights of safe medication administration, and understand the desired action and side effects of the medication. If the medication has an antidote, have it available during adminis-

BOX 16-23   Recommendations for the Prevention of Needlestick Injuries

- Avoid using needles when effective needleless systems or Sharps with Engineered Sharps Injury Protections (SESIP) safety devices are available.
- Do not recap needles of any kind.
- Plan safe handling and disposal of needles before beginning the procedure.
- Immediately dispose of needles, needleless systems, and SESIP into puncture-proof and leak-proof sharps disposal containers.
- Agencies maintain sharps injury logs as part of employee health programs.

From Occupational Safety and Health Administration: *Bloodborne pathogens and needlestick prevention: OSHA standards,* 2007, http://www.osha.gov/SLTC/bloodbornepathogens/standards.html.

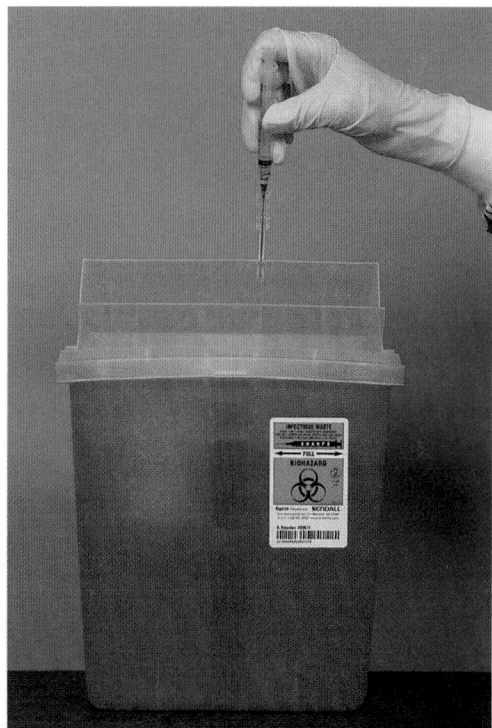

Figure 16-26 ■ Sharps disposal using only one hand.

tration. When administering potent medications, assess vital signs before, during, and after the infusion.

Administering medications by the IV route has advantages. Often you use the IV route in emergencies when you need to deliver a fast-acting medication quickly. The IV route is also best when it is necessary to establish constant therapeutic blood levels. Some medications are highly alkaline and irritating to muscle and subcutaneous tissue. These medications cause less discomfort when given intravenously.

LARGE-VOLUME INFUSIONS Medications can be mixed in large volumes (500 mL or 1000 mL) of compatible

IV fluids, such as normal saline or lactated Ringer's solution. Because the medication is not in a concentrated form, the risk for side effects or fatal reactions is lessened when infused over the prescribed time frame. Vitamins and potassium chloride are two types of medications commonly added to IV fluids. However, there is a danger with continuous infusion. If the IV fluid infuses too rapidly, the patient will suffer circulatory fluid overload.

Although nurses mixed medications in IV fluids in the past, this practice is no longer supported on a routine basis (TJC, 2008b; U.S. Pharmacotherapy Associates, 2006). Many safety risks, such as inaccurate calculations, nonaseptic preparation, and incorrect labeling occur when nurses have to prepare these medications on clinical units. Therefore the preparation of IV medications in IV fluids is usually completed by the manufacturer or occurs in the pharmacy whenever possible (TJC, 2008b). Nurses should mix medications into IV fluids only in emergency situations. However, **never** prepare high-alert medications (e.g., heparin, dopamine, dobutamine, nitroglycerin, potassium, antibiotics, or magnesium). If you have to mix a medication in a bag of IV fluids, first verify that you have to do this with the pharmacist. If the pharmacist confirms that you need to mix the medication, you prepare the medication in a syringe (see Skill 16-4) using strict aseptic technique. Make sure that the medication is compatible with the IV fluids. Verify medication calculations with another nurse, and have the nurse watch you during every step to ensure that you prepare the medication correctly and safely. After the medication is prepared, clean the injection port of the IV container with an alcohol swab, take the sheath off the syringe, and stick the needle through the injection port. Then you push the medication into the IV fluid and mix the solution by turning the IV container gently end to end. Finally, attach a label following the ISMP's safe IV label guidelines (2008d), and administer the medication to the patient at the ordered rate (see Chapter 17). **Do not** add medications to IV bags that are already hanging because there is no way to determine the exact concentration of the medication. Only add medications to new IV fluid containers.

To administer medications in large IV infusions, regulate the IV rate according to the prescriber's order. Monitor patients closely for adverse reactions to the medications and fluid volume overload. Also check the IV site frequently for signs of infiltration and phlebitis (see Chapter 17).

INTRAVENOUS BOLUS An IV bolus involves introducing a concentrated dose of a medication directly into the systemic circulation (see Skill 16-6). Because a bolus requires only a small amount of fluid to deliver the medication, it is an advantage when the amount of fluid the patient takes is restricted. The IV bolus is the most dangerous method for administering medications because the body absorbs the medications as soon as you administer them, so there is no time to correct errors. In addition, a bolus sometimes causes direct irritation to the lining of blood vessels. Before administering a bolus, confirm placement of the IV line. Never give an IV medication if the insertion site appears puffy or red or

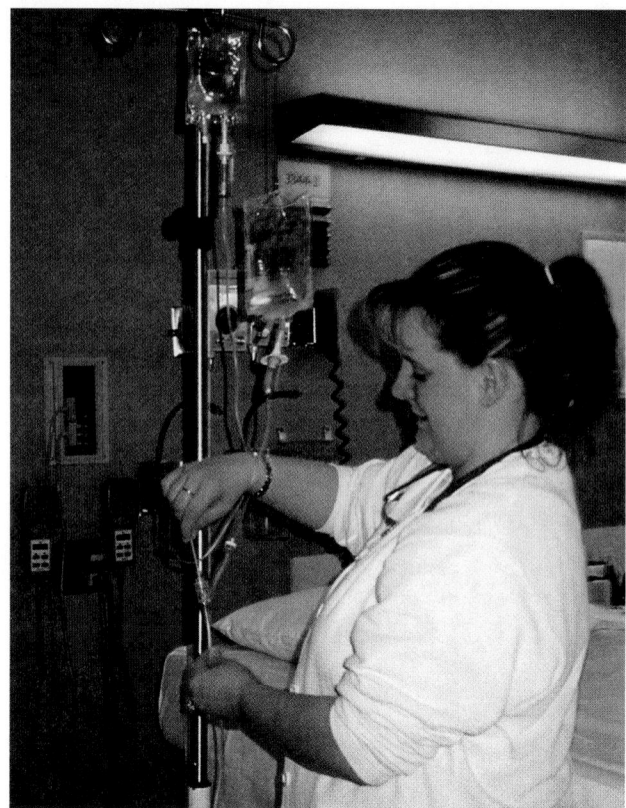

Figure 16-27 ■ Piggyback setup.

the IV fluid does not flow at the proper rate. Accidental injection of a medication into the tissues around a vein often causes pain, sloughing of tissues, and abscesses.

Determine the rate of administration of an IV bolus medication by the amount of medication that can be given each minute. For example, if a patient is to receive 4 mL of a medication over 2 minutes, give 2 mL of the IV bolus medication every minute or give 1 mL every 30 seconds. Look up each medication to determine the recommended concentration and rate of administration. Consider the purpose for which a medication is prescribed and any potential adverse effects related to the rate or route of administration when giving a medication by IV push.

VOLUME-CONTROLLED INFUSIONS Another way of administering IV medications is through small amounts (25 to 100 mL) of compatible IV fluids (see Skill 16-7). The fluid is in a secondary fluid container separate from the primary fluid bag. The container connects directly to the primary IV line or to separate tubing that inserts into the primary line. Different types of containers used include volume-control administration sets (e.g., Volutrol or Pediatrol), piggyback sets (Figure 16-27), and mini-infusers. Using volume-controlled infusions has the following advantages:

1. Volume-controlled infusions dilute and infuse medications over longer time intervals (e.g., 30 to 60 minutes), reducing risks to the patient associated with IV push.

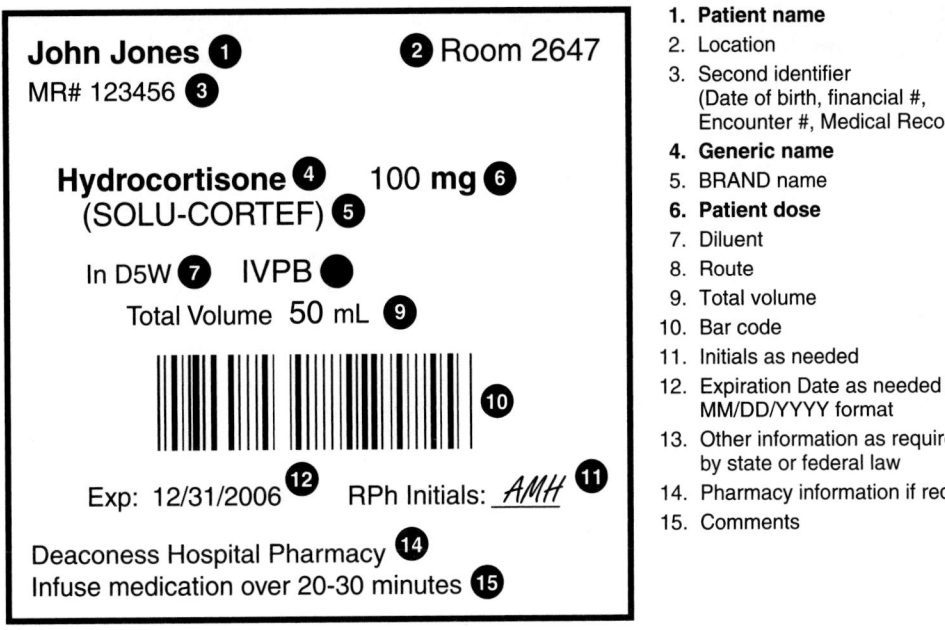

Figure 16-28 ■ IV piggyback medication with label following ISMP safe labeling.

1. **Patient name**
2. Location
3. Second identifier
   (Date of birth, financial #,
   Encounter #, Medical Record #)
4. **Generic name**
5. BRAND name
6. **Patient dose**
7. Diluent
8. Route
9. Total volume
10. Bar code
11. Initials as needed
12. Expiration Date as needed in a
    MM/DD/YYYY format
13. Other information as required
    by state or federal law
14. Pharmacy information if required
15. Comments

2. You can administer medications (e.g., antibiotics) that are stable for a limited time in solution.
3. It controls IV fluid intake.

Piggyback A piggyback is a small (25 to 250 mL) IV bag or bottle connected to a short tubing line that connects to the *upper* Y-port of a primary infusion line or to an intermittent venous access. The IV container that holds the medication is labeled following the ISMP's IV piggyback medication format (2008d) (Figure 16-28). The piggyback's tubing is a microdrip or macrodrip system (see Chapter 17). The set is called a piggyback because the small bag or bottle is set higher than the primary infusion bag or bottle. In the piggyback setup, the main line does not infuse when the piggybacked medication is infusing. The port of the primary IV line contains a back-check valve that automatically stops flow of the primary infusion once the piggyback infusion flows. After the piggyback solution infuses and the solution within the tubing falls below the level of the primary infusion drip chamber, the back-check valve opens and the primary infusion begins to flow again.

Volume-Control Administration Volume-control administration sets (e.g., Volutrol, Buretrol, or Pediatrol) are small (50 to 150 mL) containers that attach just below the primary infusion bag or bottle. The set is attached and filled in a manner similar to that used with a regular IV infusion.

However, the priming of the set is different, depending on the type of filter (floating valve or membrane) within the set. Follow package directions for priming sets.

Mini-infusion Pump The mini-infusion pump is battery operated and delivers medications in very small amounts of fluid (5 to 60 mL) within controlled infusion times. It uses standard syringes.

INTERMITTENT VENOUS ACCESS An intermittent venous access device (commonly called a heparin lock or saline lock) is an IV catheter with a small "well" or chamber covered by a rubber cap. You insert special rubber-seal injection caps into most IV catheters (see Chapter 17). Advantages to intermittent venous access include the following:

1. Cost savings resulting from the omission of continuous IV therapy
2. Saving nurses' time by eliminating constant monitoring of IV flow rates
3. Increased mobility, safety, and comfort for patient by eliminating the need for a continuous IV line

After you administer an IV bolus or piggyback medication through an intermittent venous access device, flush with a solution to keep it patent. Generally, saline is effective as a flush solution. Some institutions require the use of heparin. Be sure to check and follow institutional policies regarding the care and maintenance of the IV site.

SAFETY CONSIDERATIONS

Ensuring patient safety is an essential role of the professional nurse. To ensure patient safety, communicate clearly with members of the health care team, assess and incorporate the patient's priorities of care and preferences, and use the best evidence when making decisions about your patient's care. When performing skills in this chapter, remember the following points to ensure safe, individualized patient care.

- Be vigilant during the entire process of medication administration, and make sure that your patients receive the appropriate medications. Know why your patient is receiving each medication; know what you need to do before, during, and after medication administration; and evaluate the effectiveness and assess for adverse effects after your patients take medications.
- Take care of yourself. Ensure that you are as healthy as possible to allow yourself the ability to think as clearly and critically as possible. Healthy behaviors such as getting adequate sleep, making healthy food choices, and coping with stress in positive ways will help you better process information and make safe decisions during the process of medication administration.
- Prepare medications in areas that are free from distractions, and verify that medications have not expired while preparing them.
- Use at least two identifiers before administering medications to your patients.
- Clarify unclear orders, and ask for help whenever you are uncertain about a medication order or calculation. Consult with your peers, pharmacists, and other health care providers, and be sure you have resolved all concerns related to medication administration before preparing and giving medications.
- Use technology (e.g., bar scanning, electronic MARs) that is available in your agency when preparing and giving medications. Follow all policies related to use of the technology, and do not use "work arounds." Nurses who use "work arounds" fail to follow agency protocols, policies, or procedures during medication administration in an attempt to get medications administered to patients in a more timely fashion. Failing to follow the standard of care greatly increases the risk for making a medication error and impairs patient safety.
- Educate your patients about each medication they take while you are administering medications. Patients often are able to identify inappropriate medications. Make sure you answer all their questions before administering medications. Include family members and significant others in medication education if appropriate.
- Most of the time, you cannot delegate medication administration. Ensure that you follow standards set by your state's Nurse Practice Act and guidelines established by your health care agency. Licensed practical nurses (LPNs) or licensed vocational nurses (LVNs) usually can administer medications via the oral (PO), subcutaneous, IM, and ID routes. Sometimes they can give medications intravenously if they have had special training and if the medications are not high-alert medications. Some states also allow certified medical assistants (CMAs) to administer some types of medications (e.g., oral medications) in some health care settings (e.g., long-term care facilities). The skills in this chapter assume that you are not in a setting where you can delegate medication administration to NAP. If you are in a state and a health care setting that allow you to delegate medication administration, make sure you follow guidelines for safe delegation (see Chapter 12), your agency's policies, and the standards outlined in your state Nurse Practice Act.

| **SKILL 16-1** | ADMINISTERING ORAL MEDICATIONS | View Video! |

DELEGATION CONSIDERATIONS
The skill of administering oral medications cannot be delegated to nursing assistive personnel (NAP). The nurse informs NAP about:
- Potential side effects of medications and to report their occurrence

EQUIPMENT
- Disposable medication cups
- Glass of water, juice, or preferred liquid
- Drinking straw
- Pill-crushing device (optional)
- MAR (electronic or printed)

| **STEP** | **RATIONALE** |

ASSESSMENT

1 Check accuracy and completeness of each MAR with prescriber's original medication order. Check patient's name, drug name and dosage, route of administration, and time for administration. Recopy or re-print any portion of printed MAR that is difficult to read.

2 Assess for contraindications to patient receiving oral medication: Is patient able to swallow? Is patient able to have food and drink by mouth? Is patient suffering from nausea and vomiting? Was patient diagnosed as having bowel inflammation or reduced peristalsis? Has patient had recent GI surgery? Does patient have gastric suction?

The prescriber's order is the most reliable source and only legal record of drugs patient is to receive. Ensures patient receives the right medications. Handwritten MARs are a source of medication errors (Eisenhauer, Hurley, and Dolan, 2007; Furukawa and others, 2008).

Alterations in GI function interfere with drug absorption, distribution, and excretion. Patients with GI suction will not receive benefit from the medication because it may be suctioned from the GI tract before it can be absorbed. Giving medications to patients who cannot swallow increases the risk for aspiration.

STEP	RATIONALE
3 Assess risk for aspiration (see Chapter 32). Is patient able to swallow? Assess patient's swallow, cough, and gag reflexes.	Aspiration occurs when fluid or medication inadvertently enters the respiratory tract. Patients with impaired swallowing are at higher risk for aspiration.
4 Assess patient's medical history, history of allergies, medication history, and diet history. Make sure patient's food and drug allergies are listed on each page of the MAR and prominently displayed on the patient's medical record per agency policy.	Identifies potential food and drug interaction. Reflects patient's need for medications. Effective communication of allergies is essential for all health care providers to provide safe, effective care.
5 Gather and review assessment and laboratory data that influence drug administration, such as vital signs and renal and liver function laboratory findings.	Physical examination or laboratory data sometimes contraindicate drug administration. Alterations in liver and kidney function affect metabolism and excretion of medications (McKenry and others, 2006).

- **Critical Decision Point:** If patient has any contraindications to receiving oral medications or if in doubt about patient's ability to swallow oral medications, withhold medication and notify prescriber.

6 Assess patient's knowledge regarding health and medication usage.	Determines patient's need for medication education and assists in identifying patient's adherence to drug therapy at home. Assessments can reveal drug use problems, such as nonadherence, abuse, or addiction.
7 Assess patient's preferences for fluids. Maintain ordered fluid restriction (when applicable). Can medication be given with preferred fluid?	Fluids ease swallowing and facilitate absorption from the GI tract. It is necessary to maintain fluid restrictions. Some fluids (e.g., grapefruit juice) may interfere with drug absorption.

PLANNING

1 Expected outcomes following completion of procedure:	
• Medication administered safely with desired therapeutic effect achieved.	Medication has exerted its therapeutic action.
• Patient denies adverse effects of medications.	Absence of adverse effects improves adherence to drug therapy (Ebersole and others, 2008).
• Patient explains purpose of medications and dosage schedule.	Demonstrates understanding of medication therapy.

IMPLEMENTATION

1 Prepare medications:	
a Perform hand hygiene.	Reduces transfer of microorganisms.
b If using a medication cart, move it outside patient's room.	Organization of equipment saves time and reduces error.
c Unlock medicine drawer or cart, or log onto computerized medication dispensing system.	Medications are safeguarded when locked in cabinet, cart, or computerized medication dispensing system.
d Prepare medications for one patient at a time. Keep all pages of MARs or computer printouts for one patient together, or look at only one patient's electronic MAR at a time.	Preventing distractions reduces medication preparation errors (Beyea, 2007a).
e Select correct drug from stock supply or unit-dose drawer. Compare label of medication with MAR computer printout (see illustration) or computer screen.	Reading label and comparing it with transcribed order reduce errors. *This is the first check for accuracy.*
f Check expiration date on each medication, one at a time.	Medications used past their expiration date are sometimes inactive, less effective, or harmful to patient.
g Calculate drug dose as necessary. Double-check calculation. Ask another nurse to check calculations if needed.	Double-checking reduces risk for error.
h If preparing controlled substance, check record for previous drug count and compare with supply available.	Controlled substance laws require careful monitoring of dispensed opiates.

SKILL 16-1	ADMINISTERING ORAL MEDICATIONS—cont'd

STEP	RATIONALE

i Prepare solid forms of oral medications:

(1) To prepare tablets or capsules from a floor stock bottle, pour required number into bottle cap and transfer medication to medication cup. Do not touch medication with fingers. Return extra tablets or capsules to bottle.

Maintains clean technique required of medication administration.

• **Critical Decision Point:** Splitting tablets in half, even if they are prescored with a line down the middle, leads to medication errors. Medications need to be provided in the correct dose whenever possible. In inpatient settings if a pill *must* be split, the pharmacist splits the pill, repackages and labels it, and sends it to the nurse for administration. Nurses **should not** split pills (ISMP, 2006).

---

(2) To prepare unit-dose tablets or capsules, place packaged tablet or capsule directly into medicine cup. (Do not remove wrapper; see illustration.)

Wrapper maintains cleanliness of medications and identifies drug name and dosage.

(3) Place all tablets or capsules to be given to patient at same time in one medicine cup. Place medications requiring preadministration assessments (e.g., pulse rate, blood pressure) in separate cups.

Keeping medications that require preadministration assessments separate from others makes it easier for you to remember to make special assessments and withhold drugs as necessary.

(4) If patient has difficulty swallowing and liquid medications are not an option, use a pill-crushing device, such as a mortar and pestle, to grind pills. Clean device before and after use. If a pill-crushing device is not available, place tablet between two medication cups and grind with a blunt instrument. Mix ground tablet in small amount of soft food (e.g., custard, applesauce).

Large tablets are difficult to swallow. Ground tablet mixed with palatable soft food is usually easier to swallow. Cleaning pill-crushing device decreases risk for contaminating medications.

• **Critical Decision Point:** Not all drugs can be crushed (e.g., capsules, enteric-coated drugs). Consult pharmacist and/or "Do Not Crush List" when in doubt (ISMP, 2008b).

---

j Prepare liquids:

(1) Gently shake container. Remove bottle cap from container and place cap upside down, or open the unit-dose container. If unit-dose container has correct amount to administer, no further preparation is necessary.

Shaking container ensures medication is mixed before administration. Placing cap of bottle upside down prevents contamination of inside of cap.

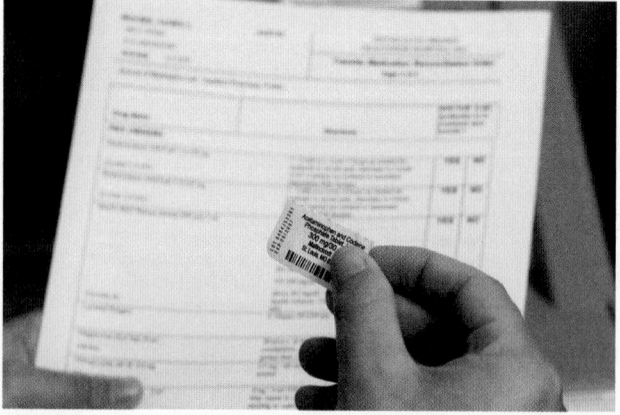

Step 1e ■ Check the label of the medication with the patient's MAR.

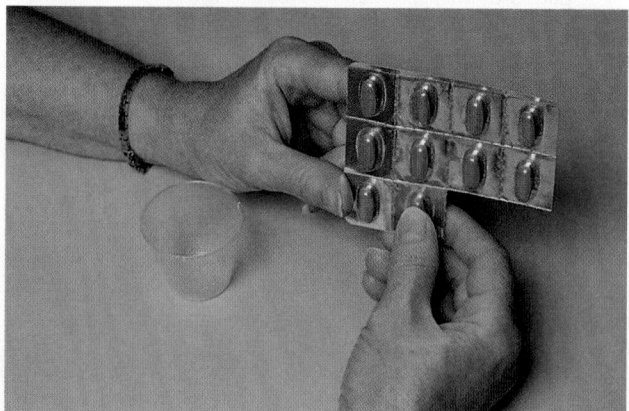

Step 1i(2) ■ Place tablet into medicine cup without removing wrapper.

STEP	RATIONALE
(2) Hold bottle with label against palm of hand while pouring.	Spilled liquid will not soil or fade label.
(3) Place medication cup on hard surface (e.g., countertop), bend over if needed so that you are at eye level with the medication cup, and fill to desired level (see illustration *A*). Make sure scale is even with fluid level at its surface or base of meniscus, not edges. For small doses of liquid medications, draw liquid into a calibrated 10-mL syringe designed for enteral administration (see illustration *B*).	Ensures accuracy of measurement. Use of syringe is more accurate for measuring small doses of liquid medications.
(4) Discard any excess liquid into sink. Wipe lip and neck of bottle with paper towel.	Prevents contamination of bottle's contents and prevents bottle cap from sticking.
(5) Administer liquid medications packaged in single-dose cups directly from the single-dose cup. Do not pour them into medicine cups.	Avoids unnecessary manipulation of dose.
k Compare MAR with prepared drug and container.	*This is the second check for accuracy to reduce medication error.*
l Return unused multiple-dose medications to shelf, drawer, or refrigerator, and read label again.	Checking label of medications in multiple-dose containers reduces administration errors.
m Do not leave drugs unattended.	Nurse is responsible for safekeeping of drugs.
2 Administer medications:	
a Take medications to patient at correct time, within 30 minutes before or after prescribed time, and perform hand hygiene.	Ensures intended therapeutic effect. Give STAT medications immediately or single-order medications at the time ordered. Hand hygiene decreases transfer of microorganisms.
b Identify patient using two identifiers (e.g., name and birthday or name and account number, according to facility policy). Compare identifiers with information on patient's MAR or medical record.	Complies with TJC (2008b) requirements and improves medication safety. In most acute care settings, patient's name and identification number on armband and MAR are used to identify patients. Identification bracelets are made at time of patient's admission and are most reliable source of identification. Patient's room number is **not** an acceptable identifier.

• ***Critical Decision Point:*** Replace patient identification bracelets that are missing, illegible, or faded.

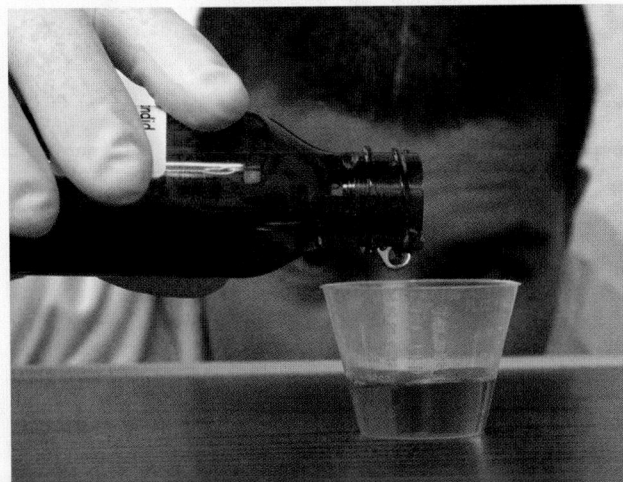

Step 1j(3)A ■ Pour the desired volume of liquid so that base of meniscus is level with line on scale.

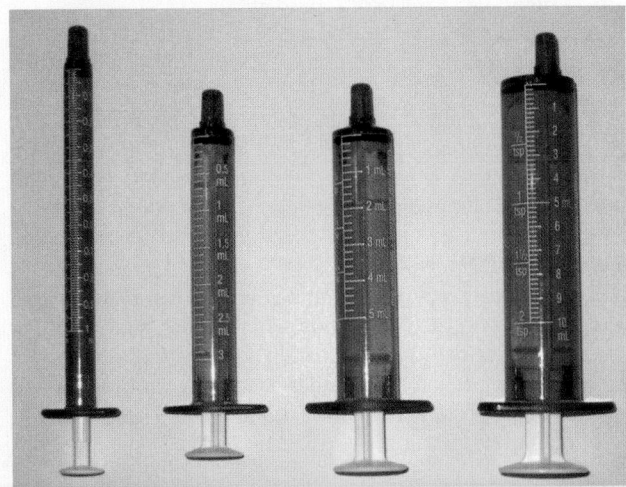

Step 1j(3)B ■ Use special enteric syringe to draw up liquid medications.

SKILL 16-1	ADMINISTERING ORAL MEDICATIONS—cont'd

STEP	RATIONALE
c Compare label of medications with MAR at patient's bedside (see Figure 16-9, p. 405).	Final check of medication label against MAR at patient's bedside reduces medication administration errors. *This is the third check for accuracy.*
d Explain purpose of each medication and its action to patient. Allow patient to ask any questions about drugs.	Patient has right to be informed about medication therapy. Questions often indicate need for teaching, nonadherence to therapy, or potential medication error.
e Assist patient to sitting or Fowler's position. Use side-lying position if sitting is contraindicated. Have patient stay in this position for 30 minutes.	Sitting position prevents aspiration during swallowing (Metheny, 2006). Remaining seated for 30 minutes helps medications move through the stomach.
f Administer medication:	
(1) **For tablets:** Patients sometimes wish to hold solid medications in hand or cup before placing in mouth.	Patient will become familiar with medications by seeing each drug.
(2) Offer water or juice to help patient swallow medications. Give a full glass of water if not contraindicated.	Choice of fluid promotes patient's comfort and will improve fluid intake. Taking tablets and capsules with a full glass of water or other liquid helps medications enter stomach.
(3) **For sublingual medications:** Have patient place medication under tongue and allow it to dissolve completely. Caution patient against swallowing tablet whole (see Figure 16-3, p. 384).	Drug is absorbed through blood vessels of undersurface of tongue. If it is swallowed, gastric juices will destroy the drug or the liver will rapidly detoxify it so that the patient will not attain therapeutic blood levels.
(4) **For buccal medications:** Have patient place medication in mouth against mucous membranes of the cheek until it dissolves (see Figure 16-4, p. 384). Avoid administering liquids until buccal medication has dissolved.	Buccal medications act locally on mucosa or systemically as the patient swallows them in saliva.
(5) Caution patient against chewing or swallowing lozenges.	Drug acts through slow absorption through oral mucosa, not gastric mucosa.
(6) **For powdered medications:** Mix with liquids at bedside, and give to patient to drink.	When prepared in advance, powdered drugs thicken and even harden, making swallowing difficult.
(7) Give effervescent powders and tablets immediately after dissolving.	Effervescence improves unpleasant taste of drug and often relieves GI problems.
g If patient is unable to hold medications, place medication cup to the lips, and gently introduce each drug into the mouth, one at a time. Do not rush.	Administering single tablet or capsule eases swallowing and decreases risk for aspiration.
h If tablet or capsule falls to the floor, discard it and repeat preparation.	Drug is contaminated when it touches floor.
i Stay until patient has completely swallowed each medication. Ask patient to open mouth if uncertain whether patient has swallowed medication.	You are responsible for ensuring that patient receives ordered dosage. If left unattended, patient may not take dose or may save drugs, causing risk to health.
j For highly acidic medications (e.g., aspirin), offer patient nonfat snack (e.g., crackers) if not contraindicated by patient's condition.	Reduces gastric irritation.
k Assist patient in returning to comfortable position.	Maintains patient's comfort.
l Dispose of soiled supplies, and perform hand hygiene.	Reduces transmission of microorganisms.
m Replenish stock, such as cups and straws, return cart to medicine room if used, and clean work area.	Clean working space assists other staff in completing duties efficiently.

EVALUATION

1 Evaluate patient's response to medications at times that correlate with the medication's onset, peak, and duration. Evaluate patient for both desired and adverse effects.	Evaluates drug's therapeutic benefit and detects onset of side effects or allergic reactions.
2 Ask patient or family member to identify drug name and explain purpose, action, dose schedule, and potential side effects of medication.	Determines how well patient or family member understands medication.

RECORDING AND REPORTING

- Record administration of oral medications on MAR immediately after administering medication. If using paper copy of MAR, include your initials or signature.
- If you withheld any medication, record the reason and follow agency policy to record withheld medication on MAR.

- Report adverse effects to prescriber.
- Report evaluation of medication effect to prescriber if required.

UNEXPECTED OUTCOMES AND RELATED INTERVENTIONS

- Patient exhibits adverse effects (e.g., side effect, toxic effect, allergic reaction).
  - Assess for symptoms such as urticaria, rash, pruritus, rhinitis, and wheezing that indicate allergic reaction.
  - Always notify prescriber and pharmacy when the patient exhibits adverse effects.
  - Withhold further doses.
  - Add allergy information to patient's chart.

- Patient refuses medication.
  - Explore reasons why patient does not want medication.
  - Educate if misunderstandings of medication therapy are apparent.
  - Do not force patient to take medication; patients have the right to refuse treatment.
  - If patient continues to refuse medication despite education, record why the drug was withheld on patient's chart and notify prescriber.

| SKILL 16-2 | ADMINISTERING EYE MEDICATIONS | |

DELEGATION CONSIDERATIONS

The skill of administering eye medications cannot be delegated to nursing assistive personnel (NAP). The nurse informs NAP about:

- Potential side effects of medications and to report their occurrence
- Potential for patient's vision to become blurred after administration of eye medications

EQUIPMENT

- Medication bottle with sterile eye dropper or ointment tube or medicated intraocular disk
- Cotton ball or tissue
- Washbasin filled with warm water and washcloth if eyes have crust or drainage
- Eye patch and tape (optional)
- Clean gloves
- MAR (electronic or printed)

STEP	RATIONALE

ASSESSMENT

1 Check accuracy and completeness of each MAR with prescriber's original medication order. Check patient's name, drug name and dosage (e.g., number of drops [if a liquid] and which eye), route of administration, and time for administration. Recopy or re-print any portion of the MAR that is difficult to read.

The prescriber's order is the most reliable source and only legal record of drugs patient is to receive. Ensures patient receives the right medications. Handwritten MARs are a source of medication errors (Eisenhauer and others, 2007; Furukawa and others, 2008).

2 Assess condition of external eye structures (see Chapter 15). (You may do this just before drug instillation.)

Provides baseline to later determine if local response to medications occurs. Also indicates need to clean eye before drug application.

3 Determine whether patient has any known allergies to eye medications. Also ask if patient has allergy to latex.

Protects patient from risk for allergic drug response. If patient has a latex allergy, use latex-free gloves.

4 Determine whether patient has any symptoms of visual alterations.

Certain eye medications act to either lessen or increase these symptoms. Provides baseline data to allow you to recognize change in patient's condition.

5 Assess patient's level of consciousness and ability to follow directions.

If patient becomes restless or combative during procedure, a greater risk for accidental eye injury exists.

6 Assess patient's knowledge regarding drug therapy and desire to self-administer medication.

Patient's level of understanding indicates need for health teaching. Motivation influences teaching approach.

STEP	RATIONALE
7 Assess patient's ability to manipulate and hold equipment necessary for eye medication (e.g., dropper, tube of ointment, intraocular disk).	Reflects patient's ability to self-administer drug.

PLANNING

1 Expected outcomes following completion of procedure:	
• Medication administered safely with desired therapeutic effect achieved.	Medication is administered correctly and has exerted its therapeutic action.
• Patient denies discomfort or other adverse effects of medication.	Absence of adverse effects improves adherence to drug therapy (Ebersole and others, 2008).
• Patient is able to discuss information about medication.	Demonstrates understanding of medication therapy.
• Patient is able to self-administer medication correctly.	Demonstrates learning.

IMPLEMENTATION

1 Perform hand hygiene and prepare medication: See Skill 16-1, Implementation steps 1a-h, k-m. Be sure to check the label two times while preparing medication.	Following the same routine when preparing medications, eliminating distractions, and checking the label of the medication with MAR reduce error. *First and second check ensures right medication is administered.*
2 Take medications to patient at correct time, within 30 minutes before or after prescribed time, and perform hand hygiene.	Ensures intended therapeutic effect. Give STAT medications immediately or single-order medications at the time ordered.
3 Identify patient using two identifiers (e.g., name and birthday or name and account number, according to facility policy). Compare identifiers with information on patient's MAR or medical record.	Complies with TJC (2008b) requirements and improves medication safety. In most acute care settings, you will use the patient's name and identification number on armband and MAR to identify patients. Identification bracelets are made at time of patient's admission and are most reliable source of identification. Patient's room number is **not** an acceptable identifier.
4 Compare label of medication against MAR for third time.	*Third check for accuracy ensures right medication is administered.*
5 Explain procedure to patient regarding positioning and sensations to expect, such as burning or stinging of eye.	Relieves anxiety about medication being instilled into eye.
6 Arrange supplies at bedside; apply clean gloves. If eye drops are stored in refrigerator, allow eye drops to come to room temperature before administering.	Reduces transmission of microorganisms. Warming eye drops reduces irritation to eye.
7 Gently roll container.	Ensures medication is mixed before administration. Shaking container creates bubbles, which affects size of drops.
8 Ask patient to lie supine or sit back in chair with head slightly hyperextended.	Position provides easy access to eye for medication instillation and minimizes drainage of medication through tear duct.

• ***Critical Decision Point:*** If the patient has a cervical spine injury, do not hyperextend the neck.

---

9 If crusts or drainage are present along eyelid margins or inner canthus, gently wash away. Apply damp washcloth or cotton ball over eyelid for a few minutes to soak crusts that are dried and difficult to remove. Always wipe clean from inner to outer canthus.	Crusts or drainage harbors microorganisms. Soaking allows easy removal and prevents pressure from being applied directly over eye. Cleansing from inner to outer canthus avoids entrance of microorganisms into lacrimal duct.
10 Hold cotton ball or clean tissue in nondominant hand on patient's cheekbone just below lower eyelid.	Cotton or tissue absorbs medication that escapes eye.
11 With tissue or cotton resting below lower lid, gently press downward with thumb or forefinger against bony orbit.	Technique exposes lower conjunctival sac. Retraction against bony orbit prevents pressure and trauma to eyeball and prevents fingers from touching eye.

STEP	RATIONALE
12 Ask patient to look at ceiling.	Action retracts sensitive cornea up and away from conjunctival sac and reduces stimulation of blink reflex.
13 Administer ophthalmic medication.	
a To instill eye drops:	
(1) With dominant hand resting on patient's forehead, hold filled medication eye dropper or ophthalmic solution approximately 1 to 2 cm (½ to ¾ inch) above conjunctival sac (see illustration).	Helps prevent accidental contact of eye dropper with eye structures, thus reducing risk for injury to eye and transfer of infection to dropper. Ophthalmic medications are sterile.
(2) Drop prescribed number of medication drops into conjunctival sac.	Conjunctival sac normally holds 1 or 2 drops. Provides even distribution of medication across eye.
(3) If patient blinks or closes eye or if drops land on outer lid margins, repeat procedure.	Therapeutic effect of drug is obtained only when drops enter conjunctival sac.
(4) After instilling drops, ask patient to close eye gently.	Helps to distribute medication. Squinting or squeezing of the eyelids forces medication out of conjunctival sac (VisionRx, 2005).
(5) When administering drugs that cause systemic effects, apply gentle pressure with your finger and clean tissue on the patient's nasolacrimal duct for 30 to 60 seconds.	Prevents overflow of medication into nasal and pharyngeal passages. Prevents absorption into systemic circulation.
b To instill eye ointment:	
(1) Ask patient to look at ceiling.	Action retracts sensitive cornea up and away from conjunctival sac and reduces stimulation of blink reflex.
(2) Holding ointment applicator above lower lid margin, apply thin stream of ointment evenly along inner edge of lower eyelid on conjunctiva (see illustration) from the inner canthus to outer canthus.	Distributes medication evenly across eye and lid margin.
(3) Have patient close eye and roll eye behind closed eyelid.	Further distributes medication without traumatizing eye.
c To administer intraocular disk:	
(1) Application:	
(a) Open package containing the disk. Apply gloves. Gently press finger of dominant hand against the disk so that it adheres to your finger. Position the convex side of the disk on your fingertip (see illustration).	Allows you to inspect disk for damage or deformity.
(b) With your other hand, gently pull the patient's lower eyelid away from the eye. Ask patient to look up.	Prepares conjunctival sac for receiving medicated disk.
(c) Place the disk in the conjunctival sac so that it floats on the sclera between the iris and lower eyelid (see illustration).	Ensures delivery of medication (Alvarez-Lorenzo and others, 2006).
(d) Pull the patient's lower eyelid out and over the disk (see illustration).	Ensures accurate medication delivery.

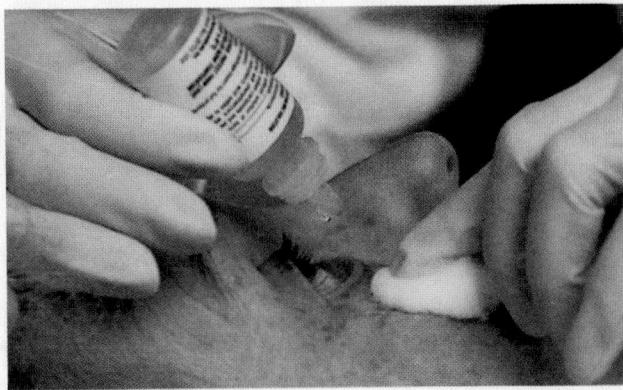

Step 13a(1) ■ Hold eye dropper above conjunctival sac.

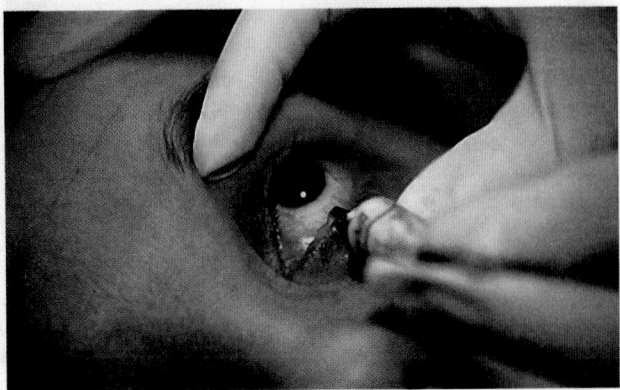

Step 13b(2) ■ Apply ointment along lower eyelid.

SKILL 16-2   ADMINISTERING EYE MEDICATIONS—cont'd

STEP	RATIONALE

- ***Critical Decision Point:*** You should not be able to see the disk at this time. Repeat step 13c(1)(d) if you can see the disk.

---

(2) Removal:
  (a) Perform hand hygiene, and put on gloves.   Reduces transmission of microorganisms.
  (b) Explain procedure to patient.   Relieves anxiety about manipulation of disk in eye.
  (c) Gently pull down on the patient's lower eyelid.   Exposes intraocular disk.
  (d) Using your forefinger and thumb of your opposite hand, pinch the disk and lift it out of the patient's eye (see illustration).

14 If excess medication is on eyelid, gently wipe it from inner to outer canthus.   Promotes comfort and prevents trauma to eye (VisionRx, 2005).

15 If patient had eye patch, apply clean one by placing it over affected eye so entire eye is covered. Tape securely without applying pressure to eye.   Clean eye patch reduces chance of infection.

16 If patient receives more than one eye medication to the same eye at the same time, wait at least 5 minutes before administering the next medication.   Allows medication to absorb and avoids interaction between medications (VisionRx, 2005).

17 If patient receives eye medication to both eyes at the same time, use a different tissue or cotton ball with each eye.   Prevents cross contamination between eyes.

18 Remove gloves, dispose of soiled supplies in proper receptacle, and perform hand hygiene.   Maintains neat environment at bedside and reduces transmission of microorganisms.

EVALUATION

1 Note patient's response to instillation; ask if he or she felt any discomfort.   Determines if you performed procedure correctly and safely and if patient is experiencing adverse effects of medication.

2 Observe response to medication by assessing visual changes and noting any side effects.   Evaluates effects of medication.

3 Ask patient to discuss drug's purpose, action, side effects, and technique of administration.   Determines patient's level of understanding.

4 Have patient or caregiver demonstrate self-administration during next dose.   Provides feedback regarding competency with skill.

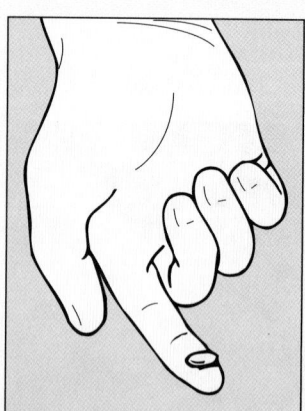

Step 13c(1)(a) ■ Gently position the convex side of the disk against your fingertip.

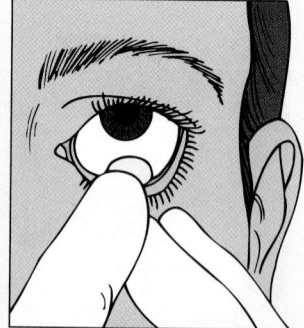

Step 13c(1)(c) ■ Place disk in the conjunctival sac between the iris and lower eyelid.

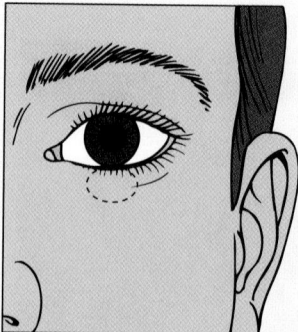

Step 13c(1)(d) ■ Gently pull lower eyelid over the disk.

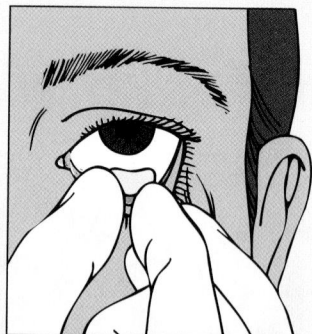

Step 13c(2)(d) ■ Carefully pinch the disk to remove it from patient's eye.

RECORDING AND REPORTING

- Record drug, concentration, number of drops, time of administration, and eye (left, right, or both) that received medication on electronic or printed MAR.

- Record appearance of eye in nurses' notes.

UNEXPECTED OUTCOMES AND RELATED INTERVENTIONS

- Patient cannot instill drops without supervision.
  - Reinforce teaching, and allow patient to self-administer drops as much as possible to enhance confidence.
  - If patient cannot self-administer drops, teach others, such as family members, to instill drops into the patient's eye.

- Patient displays signs of allergic reaction (e.g., tearing, reddened sclera) or systemic response (e.g., bradycardia) to medication.
  - Hold medication, and speak with prescriber.
  - Follow institutional policy or guidelines for reporting of adverse or allergic reaction to medications.
  - Add information about allergy to medical record per agency policy.

| SKILL 16-3 | USING METERED-DOSE OR DRY POWDER INHALERS |

DELEGATION CONSIDERATIONS

The skill of administering inhaled medications cannot be delegated to nursing assistive personnel (NAP). The nurse informs NAP about:

- Potential side effects of medications and to report their occurrence
- The need to report to the nurse any change in respiratory status, increased coughing, or breathing difficulties

EQUIPMENT

- MDI or DPI
- Spacer (optional with MDI)
- Facial tissues *(optional)*
- Washbasin or sink with warm water
- Paper towel
- MAR (electronic or printed)

| STEP | RATIONALE |

ASSESSMENT

1 Check accuracy and completeness of each MAR with prescriber's original medication order. Check patient's name, drug name and dosage, route of administration, and time for administration. Recopy or re-print any portion of printed MAR that is difficult to read.

2 Assess respiratory pattern, and auscultate breath sounds.

3 If patient was previously instructed in self-administration of inhaled medicine, assess technique in using an inhaler.

4 Assess patient's ability to hold, manipulate, and depress canister and inhaler.

5 Assess patient's readiness to learn: patient asks questions about medication, disease, or complications; requests education in use of inhaler; is mentally alert; participates in own care.

6 Assess patient's ability to learn: make sure patient is not fatigued, in pain, or in respiratory distress; assess level of understanding of technical vocabulary terms.

The prescriber's order is the most reliable source and only legal record of drugs patient is to receive. Ensures patient receives the right medications. Handwritten MARs are a source of medication errors (Eisenhauer and others, 2007; Furukawa and others, 2008).

Establishes baseline for airway status for comparison during and after treatment.

Nurse's instruction sometimes requires only simple reinforcement, depending on patient's level of dexterity.

Any impairment of grasp or coordination impairs patient's ability to use MDI or DPI correctly.

Influences patient's motivation to understand explanations and actively participate in teaching process (Bastable, 2008).

Mental or physical limitations affect patient's ability to learn and methods nurse uses for instruction (Bastable, 2008).

SKILL 16-3	USING METERED-DOSE OR DRY POWDER INHALERS— cont'd

STEP	RATIONALE
7 Assess patient's knowledge and understanding of disease and purpose and action of prescribed medications.	Knowledge of disease and medications is essential for patient to realistically understand use of inhaler.
8 Determine drug schedule and number of inhalations prescribed for each dose.	Influences explanations nurse provides for use of inhaler.

PLANNING

1 Expected outcomes following completion of procedure:	
• Medication administered safely with desired therapeutic effect achieved. Patient's breathing pattern improves, and airways become clear.	Desired effect of medication achieved.
• Patient has adequate gas exchange.	Medication administered properly and therapeutic effect achieved.
• Patient describes need for medication, dose, frequency, and how to use inhaler.	Demonstrates learning.
• Patient correctly self-administers inhaler.	Patient is able to administer medication correctly.
2 Provide adequate time for teaching session.	Prevents interruptions and enhances learning (Bastable, 2008).

IMPLEMENTATION

1 Perform hand hygiene and prepare medication: See Skill 16-1, Implementation steps 1a-h, k-m. Be sure to check the label two times while preparing medication.	Following the same routine when preparing medication, eliminating distractions, and checking the medication label with the MAR reduces errors. *First and second checks ensures right medication is administered.*
2 Identify patient using two identifiers (e.g., name and birthday or name and account number, according to facility policy). Compare identifiers with information on patient's MAR or medical record.	Complies with TJC (2008b) requirements and improves medication safety. In most acute care settings, you use the patient's name and identification number on armband and MAR to identify patients. Identification bracelets are made at time of patient's admission and are most reliable source of identification. Patient's room number is **not** an acceptable identifier.
3 Compare the label of the medication with the MAR one more time at the patient's bedside.	*Third check for accuracy ensures right medication is administered.*
4 Help patient get into a comfortable position, such as sitting in chair in hospital room or sitting at kitchen table in home.	Patient will be more likely to remain receptive to nurse's explanations in comfortable environment (Bastable, 2008).
5 Have patient manipulate inhaler, canister, and spacer device. Explain and demonstrate how canister fits into inhaler.	Patient needs to be familiar with how to use equipment.

• **Critical Decision Point:** If patient is using an MDI and the inhaler is new or has not been used for several days, push a "test spray" into the air. You do not need to do this for a DPI.

---

6 Explain what metered dose is, and warn patient about overuse of inhaler and medication side effects.	Makes sure patient does not administer excessive inhalations because of risk for serious side effects. Side effects are minimized if patients take medication as ordered.
7 Explain steps for administering squeeze-and-breathe MDI (demonstrate steps when possible):	Use of simple, step-by-step explanations allows patient to ask questions during procedure (Bastable, 2008).
a Insert MDI canister into the holder.	
b Remove mouthpiece cover from inhaler.	

• **Critical Decision Point:** If dirt or foreign objects are in mouthpiece, clean before using inhaler to avoid inhalation of unwanted material.

STEP	RATIONALE

c Shake inhaler strongly five or six times.

Aerosolizes fine particles.

d Tell patient to sit up straight or stand and take a deep breath and exhale.

Empties lungs and prepares the patient's airway to receive the medication.

e Have patient position the inhaler in one of two ways:

Proper positioning of inhaler is essential to administering medication correctly.

  (1) Close mouth around MDI with opening toward back of throat (see illustration).

  (2) Position MDI 2 to 4 cm (1 to 2 inches) in front of the mouth (see illustration).

f With the inhaler positioned correctly, have patient hold inhaler with thumb at the mouthpiece and the index finger and middle finger at the top. This is called a three-point or lateral hand position.

MDIs work best when patients use a three-point or lateral hand position to activate canisters.

g Instruct patient to tilt head back slightly and inhale slowly and deeply through mouth for 3 to 5 seconds while fully pressing down on canister.

Medication is distributed to airways during inhalation. Inhalation through mouth rather than nose draws medication into airways better.

h Have patient hold breath for as long as comfortable, up to 10 seconds.

Allows the medication to settle into the patient's airway (MayoClinic.com, 2008).

i Remove MDI from mouth and exhale slowly through pursed lips.

Keeps small airways open during exhalation.

8 Explain steps to administer MDI using a spacer, such as an Aerochamber (demonstrate steps when possible):

Use of simple, step-by-step explanations allows patient to ask questions at any point during procedure.

a Remove mouthpiece cover from inhaler and spacer. Inspect spacer for foreign objects, and if the spacer has a valve, make sure it is intact.

Inhaler fits into end of spacer.

b Insert MDI into end of spacer.

Spacer breaks up and slows down the medication particles, increasing the absorption of medication into the airway (MayoClinic.com, 2008).

c Shake inhaler strongly five or six times.

Ensures fine particles are aerosolized.

d Have patient take a deep breath and exhale completely before closing mouth around spacer's mouthpiece. Tell patient to avoid covering small exhalation slots with the lips (see illustration).

Empties the lungs and prepares the patient's airway to receive the medication.

e Have patient press medication canister one time, spraying one puff into spacer.

MDI releases spray that allows finer particles to be inhaled. Large droplets are kept in spacer.

f Instruct patient to inhale slowly and deeply through mouth for 3 to 5 seconds.

Maximizes amount of medication that enters the lungs.

g Instruct patient to hold breath for approximately 10 seconds.

Allows distribution of all medication.

h Remove MDI and spacer before exhaling.

Allows patient to exhale normally.

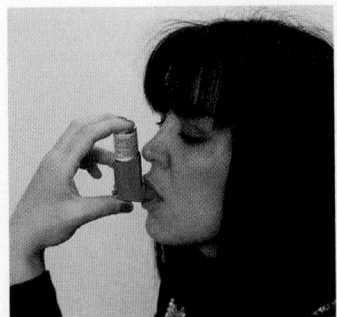

Step 7e(1) ■ One technique for use of the inhaler. The patient opens lips and places inhaler in mouth with opening toward back of throat.

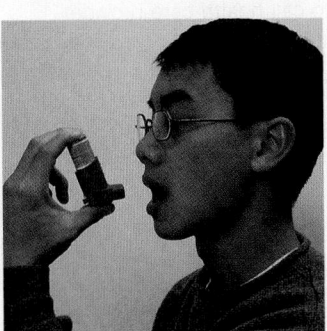

Step 7e(2) ■ One technique for use of the inhaler. The patient positions the mouthpiece 1 to 2 inches from the mouth. This is considered the best way to deliver the medication.

STEP	RATIONALE
9 Explain steps to administer DPI or breath-activated MDI (demonstrate when possible):	Use of simple step-by-step explanations allows patient to ask questions at any point during the procedure (Bastable, 2008).
a Remove mouthpiece cover. Do not shake inhaler.	
b Prepare medication as directed by manufacturer (e.g., hold inhaler upright and turn wheel to the right and then to the left until a click is heard, load medication pellet).	Primes inhaler, ensuring medication will be delivered to patient (Capriotti, 2005).
c Exhale away from the inhaler.	Prevents loss of powder.
d Position mouthpiece between lips (see illustration).	Keeps medication from escaping through mouth.
e Inhale deeply and forcefully through the mouth.	Creates aerosol.
f Hold full breath for 5 to 10 seconds.	Allows distribution of medication.
10 Instruct patient to wait at least 20 to 30 seconds between inhalations of the same medication and 2 to 5 minutes between inhalations of different medications or as ordered by prescriber.	Patients need to inhale medications slowly. First inhalation opens airways and reduces inflammation. Second or third inhalation penetrates deeper airways.

- *Critical Decision Point:* If patient uses a corticosteroid, have patient rinse mouth with water or salt water or brush teeth after inhalation to reduce risk for fungal infection. Also teach patient to inspect oral cavity daily for redness, sores, or white patches. Report abnormal assessment findings to the patient's health care provider (MayoClinic.com, 2008).

STEP	RATIONALE
11 Tell patient not to repeat inhaler doses until next scheduled dose.	Health care providers prescribe medications at intervals during the day to provide constant drug levels and minimize side effects.
12 Explain that patient may feel gagging sensation in throat caused by droplets of medication on pharynx or tongue.	Results when inhalant is sprayed and inhaled incorrectly.
13 Instruct patient in how to clean inhaler:	
a Once a day, rinse inhaler and cap in warm running water. Make sure inhaler is completely dry before using.	Accumulation of spray around mouthpiece interferes with proper distribution during use (MayoClinic.com, 2008).
b Twice a week, wash the L-shaped plastic mouthpiece with antibacterial soap and warm water. Rinse and air dry well before putting canister back into mouthpiece.	Removes residual medication and decreases transfer of microorganisms. Do not place inhalers holding cromolyn, nedocromil, or hydrofluoroalkane (HFA) in water.

EVALUATION

1 Ask if patient has any questions.	Clarifies information.
2 Have patient explain and demonstrate steps in use of inhaler.	Return demonstration provides feedback for measuring patient's learning.
3 Ask patient to explain medication schedule, side effects, and when to call health care provider.	Understanding improves likelihood of compliance with therapy.
4 Ask patient to calculate how many days the inhaler will last.	Helps patient determine when to reorder prescription.

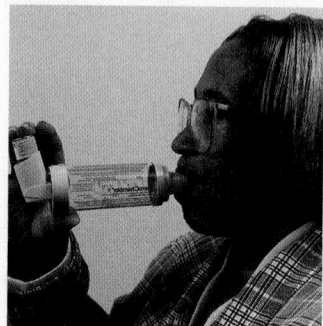

Step 8d ■ Have patient place mouthpiece in mouth and close lips, being careful to keep exhalation slots exposed.

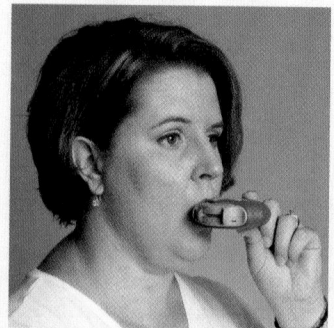

Step 9d ■ Have patient place mouthpiece of DPI between lips.

STEP	RATIONALE
5 After medication has been taken, assess patient's respiratory status, including ease of respirations, auscultation of lungs, and use of pulse oximetry to assess patient's oxygenation status (see Chapter 15).	Determines status of breathing pattern and adequacy of ventilation and confirms desired effect of medication.

RECORDING AND REPORTING

- Document skills you taught and patient's ability to perform skills.
- Record medication, time of administration, and the amount of puffs on the MAR.

- Record patient's response to medication in nurses' notes.
- Report any undesirable effects from medication.

UNEXPECTED OUTCOMES AND RELATED INTERVENTIONS

- Patient needs a bronchodilator more than every 4 hours.
  - Indicates respiratory problems; reassess type of medication and delivery methods needed.
  - Consult with health care provider.
- Patient experiences cardiac dysrhythmias, light-headedness, and/or syncope especially if receiving beta-adrenergics.
  - Withhold all further doses of medication.
  - Discuss with prescriber.

- Patient is not able to self-administer medication properly.
  - Explore alternative delivery routes or methods.
- Patient experiences paroxysms of coughing.
  - Aerosolized particles irritate posterior pharynx. Notify prescriber; need to reassess type of medication or delivery method.

SKILL 16-4   PREPARING INJECTIONS FROM VIALS AND AMPULES

DELEGATION CONSIDERATIONS
The skill of preparing injections cannot be delegated to nursing assistive personnel (NAP).

EQUIPMENT
Medication in an Ampule
- Safety syringe, needle, and filter needle
- Small gauze pad or unopened alcohol swab

Medication in a Vial
- Safety syringe
- Needles:
  - Blunt tip vial access cannula (if needleless system used)
  - Filter needle if indicated
  - Needle for drawing up medication (if needed)
  - Needle for injection
- Small gauze pad or alcohol swab
- Diluent (e.g., normal saline or sterile water) (if indicated)

Both
- Medication in vial or ampule
- MAR (electronic or printed)

STEP	RATIONALE
ASSESSMENT	
1 Check accuracy and completeness of each MAR or computer printout with prescriber's written medication order. Check patient's name, drug name and dosage, route of administration, and time for administration. Recopy or reprint any portion of the MAR that is difficult to read.	The prescriber's order is the most reliable source and only legal record of drugs patient is to receive. Ensures patient receives the right medications. Handwritten MARs are a source of medication errors (Eisenhauer and others, 2007; Furukawa and others, 2008).
2 Review pertinent information related to medication, including action, purpose, side effects, and nursing implications.	Allows you to administer drug properly and to monitor patient's response.
3 Assess patient's body build, muscle size, and weight if giving subcutaneous or IM medication.	Determines type and size of syringe and needles for injection.
PLANNING	
1 Expected outcomes following completion of procedure: • Proper dose is prepared. No air bubbles are in syringe barrel.	Ensures right dose. Air bubbles take up space in syringe. Elimination of air ensures that you give accurate medication dose.

SKILL 16-4	PREPARING INJECTIONS FROM VIALS AND AMPULES—cont'd

STEP	RATIONALE

IMPLEMENTATION

1 Perform hand hygiene, and assemble supplies.

Reduces transmission of microorganisms and saves nursing time.

2 Prepare medication: See Skill 16-1, p. 430, Implementation steps 1a-h, k-m. Be sure to check the label two times while preparing medication.

Following the same routine when preparing medications, eliminating distractions, and checking the label of the medication with the MAR reduce error. *First and second checks ensure right medication is administered.*

A Ampule Preparation:

(1) Tap top of ampule lightly and quickly with finger until fluid moves from neck of ampule (see illustration).

Dislodges any fluid that collects above neck of ampule. All solution moves into lower chamber.

(2) Place small gauze pad or unopened alcohol pad around neck of ampule (see illustration).

Placing pad around neck of ampule protects fingers from trauma as glass tip is broken off.

(3) Snap neck of ampule quickly and firmly away from hands (see illustration).

Protects nurse's fingers and face from shattering glass.

(4) Draw up medication quickly, using a filter needle long enough to reach bottom of ampule.

System is open to airborne contaminants. Makes sure needle is long enough to access medication for preparation. Filter needles filter out any fragments of glass (Nicoll and Hesby, 2002; Preston and Hegadoren, 2004).

(5) Hold ampule upside down, or set it on a flat surface. Insert filter needle into center of ampule opening. Do not allow needle tip or shaft to touch rim of ampule.

Broken rim of ampule is considered contaminated. When ampule is inverted, solution dribbles out if needle tip or shaft touches rim of ampule.

(6) Aspirate medication into syringe by gently pulling back on plunger (see illustrations).

Withdrawal of plunger creates negative pressure within syringe barrel, which pulls fluid into syringe.

(7) Keep needle tip under surface of liquid. Tip ampule to bring all fluid within reach of the needle.

Prevents aspiration of air bubbles.

(8) If you aspirate air bubbles, do not expel air into ampule.

Air pressure forces fluid out of ampule, and medication will be lost.

(9) To expel excess air bubbles, remove needle from ampule. Hold syringe with needle pointing up. Tap side of syringe to cause bubbles to rise toward needle. Draw back slightly on plunger, and then push plunger upward to eject air. Do not eject fluid.

Withdrawing plunger too far will remove it from barrel. Holding syringe vertically allows fluid to settle in bottom of barrel. Pulling back on plunger allows fluid within needle to enter barrel so you do not expel fluid. You then expel air at top of barrel and within needle.

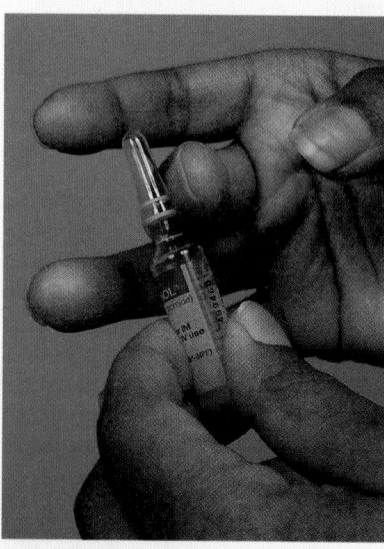

Step 2A(1) ■ Tapping ampule moves fluid down neck.

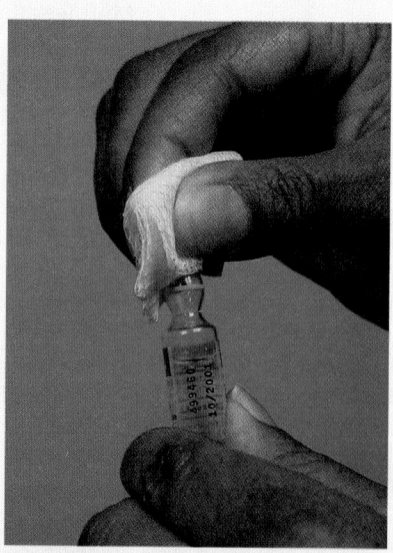

Step 2A(2) ■ Gauze pad placed around neck of ampule.

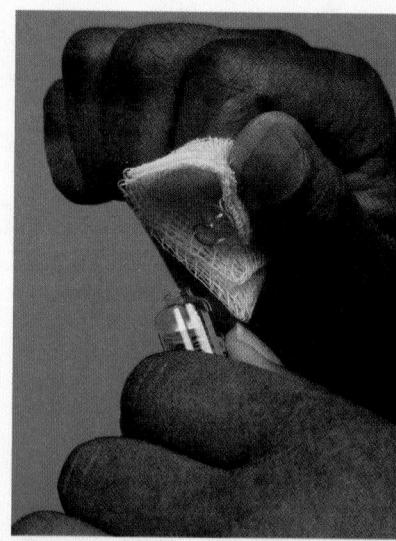

Step 2A(3) ■ Snapping neck away from hands.

STEP	RATIONALE
(10) If syringe contains excess fluid, use sink for disposal. Hold syringe vertically with needle tip up and slanted slightly toward sink. Slowly eject excess fluid into sink. Recheck fluid level in syringe by holding it vertically.	Safely disperses medication into sink. Position of needle allows you to expel medication without it flowing down needle shaft. Rechecking fluid level ensures proper dose.
(11) Cover needle with its safety sheath or cap. Replace filter needle with regular needle.	Do not use filter needles for injection.
B Vial Containing a Solution:	
(1) Remove cap covering top of unused vial to expose sterile rubber seal. If a multidose vial has been used before, cap is already removed. Firmly and briskly wipe surface of rubber seal with alcohol swab, and allow it to dry.	Vial comes packaged with cap that cannot be replaced after seal removal. Not all drug manufacturers guarantee that caps of unused vials are sterile. Swabbing reduces transmission of microorganisms. Allowing alcohol to dry prevents it from coating needle and mixing with medication.
(2) Pick up syringe, and remove needle cap or cap covering needleless vial access device (see illustration). Pull back on plunger to draw amount of air into syringe equivalent to volume of medication to be aspirated from vial.	Injecting air into vial prevents buildup of negative pressure in vial when aspirating medication.

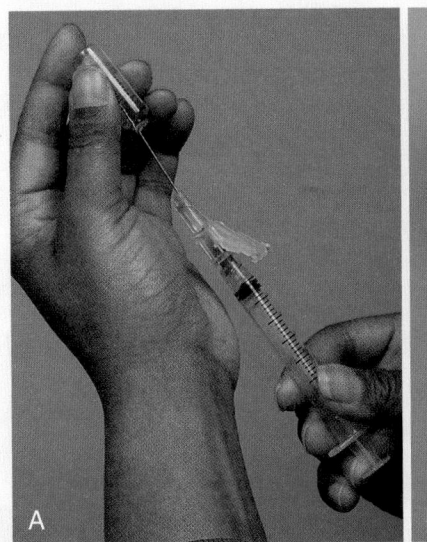 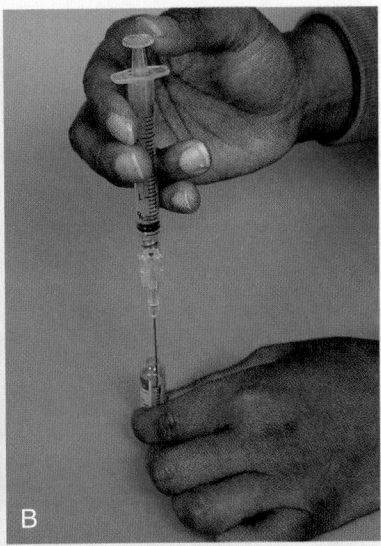

Step 2A(6) ■ **A,** Medication aspirated with ampule inverted.
B, Medication aspirated with ampule on flat surface.

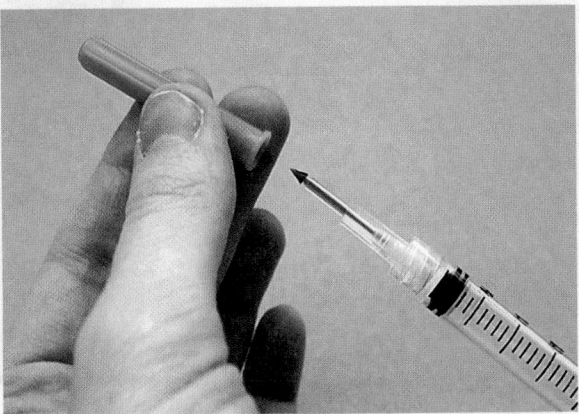

Step 2B(2) ■ Syringe with needleless adapter.

SKILL 16-4	PREPARING INJECTIONS FROM VIALS AND AMPULES— cont'd

STEP	RATIONALE

• *Critical Decision Point:* Some medications and some agencies require use of filter needle when preparing medications from vials. Check agency policy or medication reference to determine if filter needle is required. If you use a filter needle to aspirate medication, then you need to change it to a regular needle of the appropriate size to administer the medication (Nicoll and Hesby, 2002).

STEP	RATIONALE
(3) With vial on flat surface, insert tip of needle or needleless vial access device through center of rubber seal (see illustration). Apply pressure to tip of needle during insertion.	Center of seal is thinner and easier to penetrate. Using firm pressure prevents coring of rubber seal, which could enter vial or needle.
(4) Inject air into the vial's air space, holding on to plunger. Hold plunger with firm pressure; plunger sometimes is forced backward by air pressure within the vial.	You need to inject air before aspirating fluid to create vacuum needed to get medication to flow into syringe. Injecting into vial's air space prevents formation of bubbles and inaccuracy in dosage.
(5) Invert vial while keeping firm hold on syringe and plunger (see illustration). Hold vial between thumb and middle fingers of nondominant hand. Grasp end of syringe barrel and plunger with thumb and forefinger of dominant hand to counteract pressure in vial.	Inverting vial allows fluid to settle in lower half of container. Position of hands prevents forceful movement of plunger and permits easy manipulation of syringe.
(6) Keep tip of needle below fluid level.	Prevents aspiration of air.
(7) Allow air pressure from the vial to fill syringe gradually with medication. If necessary, pull back slightly on plunger to obtain correct amount of solution.	Positive pressure within vial forces fluid into syringe.
(8) When you obtain desired volume, position needle into vial's air space; tap side of syringe barrel carefully to dislodge any air bubbles. Eject any air remaining at top of syringe into vial.	Forcefully striking barrel while needle is inserted in vial may bend needle. Accumulation of air displaces medication and causes dosage errors.
(9) Remove needle or needleless vial access device from vial by pulling back on barrel of syringe.	Pulling plunger rather than barrel causes plunger to separate from barrel, resulting in loss of medication.

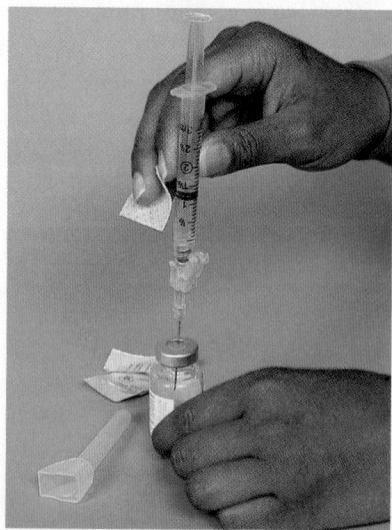

Step 2B(3) ■ Insert safety needle through center of vial diaphragm (with vial flat on table).

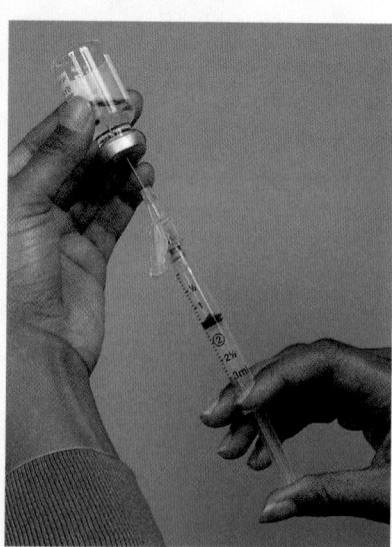

Step 2B(5) ■ Withdraw fluid with vial inverted.

STEP	RATIONALE
(10) Hold syringe at eye level, at 90-degree angle, to ensure correct volume and absence of air bubbles. Remove any remaining air by tapping barrel to dislodge any air bubbles (see illustration). Draw back slightly on plunger; then push plunger upward to eject air. Do not eject fluid.	Holding syringe vertically allows fluid to settle in bottom of barrel. Pulling back on plunger allows fluid within needle to enter barrel so you do not expel fluid. You then expel air at top of barrel and within needle.
(11) If you need to inject medication into patient's tissue, change needle to appropriate gauge and length according to route of medication administration.	Inserting needle through a rubber stopper dulls beveled tip. New needle is sharper. Because no fluid is along shaft, needle will not track medication through tissues. You cannot inject needleless access device into the body.
(12) For multidose vial, make label that includes date of opening vial and your initials.	Ensures that nurses will prepare future doses correctly. You discard some drugs after certain number of days after opening a vial.
C Vial Containing a Powder (Reconstituting Medications):	
(1) Remove cap covering vial of powdered medication and cap covering vial of proper diluents. Firmly swab both caps with alcohol swab, and allow to dry.	Not all drug manufacturers guarantee that caps of unused vials are sterile. Allowing alcohol to dry prevents it from coating needle and mixing with medication.
(2) Draw up diluents into syringe following steps 2B(2) through 2B(10).	Prepares diluents for injection into vial containing powdered medication.
(3) Insert tip of needle or needleless access device through center of rubber seal of vial of powdered medication. Inject diluents into vial. Remove needle.	Diluent begins to dissolve and reconstitute medication.
(4) Mix medication thoroughly. Roll in palms. Do not shake.	Ensures proper dispersal of medication throughout solution.
(5) Reconstituted medication in vial is ready for you to draw into new syringe. Read label. Carefully determine dose after reconstitution.	Once you add diluent, concentration of medication (mg/mL) determines dose you give. Reading medication label carefully decreases administration errors.
(6) Draw up reconstituted medication in syringe following steps 2B(2) through 2B(12).	Prepares medication for administration.

- *Critical Decision Point:* Some agencies require that you verify medications prepared for parenteral administration for accuracy by another nurse. Check guidelines before administering medication.

---

3 Compare label of medication with MAR for the final time at the patient's bedside before administering medication.	*Third check for accuracy ensures right medication is administered.*

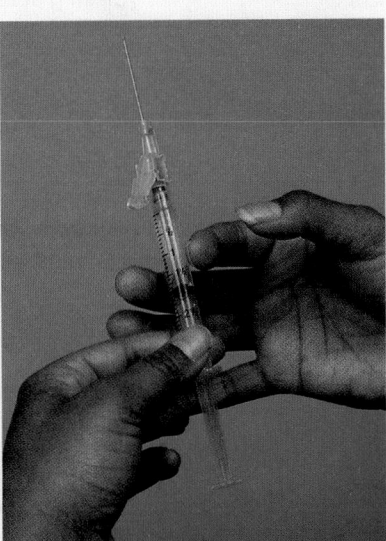

Step 2B(10) ■ Hold syringe upright, tap barrel to dislodge air bubbles.

SKILL 16-4	PREPARING INJECTIONS FROM VIALS AND AMPULES—cont'd

STEP	RATIONALE
4 Dispose of soiled supplies. Place broken ampule and/or used vials and used needle or needleless access device in puncture-proof and leakproof container. Clean work area, and perform hand hygiene.	Proper disposal of glass and needle prevents accidental injury to staff. Controls transmission of infection.

EVALUATION

1 Compare dose in syringe with desired dose.	Determines dose is accurate.

UNEXPECTED OUTCOMES AND RELATED INTERVENTIONS

- Air bubbles remain in syringe.
  - Expel air from syringe, and add medication to syringe until you prepare the correct dose.

- You prepared incorrect dose.
  - Discard prepared dose, and prepare corrected new dose.

SKILL 16-5	ADMINISTERING INJECTIONS

DELEGATION CONSIDERATIONS

The skill of administering injectionable medications cannot be delegated to nursing assistive personnel (NAP). The nurse informs NAP about:

- Potential side effects of medications and to report their occurrence to the nurse
- Reporting change in the patient's vital signs or level of consciousness

EQUIPMENT

- Proper-size syringe and needle:
  - *Subcutaneous:* syringe (1 to 3 mL) and needle (25 to 27 gauge, ¼ to ⅝ inch)
  - *Subcutaneous U-100 insulin:* insulin syringe (0.3, 0.5, or 1 mL) with preattached needle (31 to 28 gauge, ¼ to ½ inch)
  - *Subcutaneous U-500 insulin:* 1-mL tuberculin syringe with needle (25 to 27 gauge, ½ to ⅝ inch)
  - *IM:* Syringe (2 to 3 mL for adult, 0.5 to 1 mL for infants and small children)
    - Needle length corresponds to site of injection and age and size of patient. Refer to following guidelines; length needed may vary outside these guidelines in patients who are smaller or larger than average.

Site	Child (Hockenberry and Wilson, 2009)	Adult (Nicoll and Hesby, 2002)
Ventrogluteal	½ to 1 inch	1½ inch
Vastus lateralis	⅝ to 1 inch	⅝ to 1 inch
Deltoid	½ to 1 inch	1 to 1½ inch

- Needle gauge often depends on length of needle. Administer most biologicals and medications in aqueous solutions with 20- to 25-gauge needle. Use 18- to 25-gauge needles for medications in oil-based solutions (Nicoll and Hesby, 2002).
- *ID:* 1-mL tuberculin syringe with needle (25 to 27 gauge, ½ to ⅝ inch)
- Small gauze pad
- Alcohol swab
- Vial or ampule of medication or skin test solution
- Clean gloves
- MAR (electronic or printed)

STEP	RATIONALE

ASSESSMENT

1 Check accuracy and completeness of each MAR with prescriber's original medication order. Check patient's name, drug name and dosage, route of administration, and time for administration. Recopy or re-print any portion of printed MAR that is difficult to read.	The prescriber's order is the most reliable source and only legal record of drugs patient is to receive. Ensures patient receives the right medications. Handwritten MARs are a source of medication errors (Eisenhauer and others, 2007; Furukawa and others, 2008).
2 Assess patient's medical and medication history.	Identifies need for medication.
3 Assess patient's history of allergies, including latex allergy, and know patient's normal allergic reaction.	Certain substances have similar compositions; it is harmful to give patients a medication if they have a known allergy to it.

STEP	RATIONALE
4 Observe verbal and nonverbal responses toward receiving injection.	Injections are sometimes painful. Patients often have anxiety, which increases pain.
5 Assess for contraindications:	
a **For subcutaneous injections:** Assess for factors such as circulatory shock or reduced local tissue perfusion. Assess adequacy of patient's adipose tissue.	Reduced tissue perfusion interferes with drug absorption and distribution. Physiological changes of aging or patient illness influences the amount of subcutaneous tissue a patient has. This influences methods for administering injections.
b **For intramuscular injections:** Assess for factors such as muscle atrophy, reduced blood flow, or circulatory shock.	Atrophied muscle absorbs medication poorly. Factors interfering with blood flow to muscles impair drug absorption.
c **For intradermal injections:** Assess for history of severe adverse reactions or necrosis that happened after a previous ID injection.	Medications are potent and can cause severe anaphylaxis.
6 Assess patient's knowledge regarding medication to be received.	Determines need for patient education.

- ***Critical Decision Point:*** Because of documented adverse effects of IM injections, other routes of medication injection are safer. Consider calling prescriber for alternate route of medication administration (Nicoll and Hesby, 2002; Pandian and others, 2006; World Health Organization, 2006).

PLANNING

1 Expected outcomes following completion of procedure:	
• Patient experiences no pain or mild burning at injection site.	Medications cause minor irritation to tissues.
• Medication administered safely. Desired effect of medication achieved with no signs of adverse effects.	Medication administered without injury to patient.
• Patient explains purpose of medication, dosage, and effects of medication.	Demonstrates learning.

IMPLEMENTATION

1 Perform hand hygiene and prepare medication using aseptic technique (see Skill 16-4). Check label of medication carefully with the MAR two times while preparing medication.	Ensures medication is sterile; preparation techniques differ for ampule and vial. *First and second checks ensure right medication is administered.*
2 Take medications to patient at correct time, within 30 minutes before or after prescribed time, and perform hand hygiene.	Ensures intended therapeutic effect. Give STAT medications immediately or single-order medications at the time ordered. Decreases transfer of microorganisms.
3 Close room curtain or door.	Provides privacy.
4 Identify patient using two identifiers (e.g., name and birthday or name and account number, according to facility policy). Compare identifiers with information on patient's MAR or medical record.	Complies with TJC (2008b) requirements and improves medication safety. In most acute care settings, patient's name and identification number on armband and MAR are used to identify patients. Identification bracelets are made at time of patient's admission and are most reliable source of identification. Patient's room number is **not** an acceptable identifier.
5 Compare the label of the medication with the MAR one more time at the patient's bedside.	*Third check for accuracy ensures right medication is administered.*
6 Explain steps of procedure, and tell patient injection will cause a slight burning or sting.	Helps minimize patient's anxiety.
7 Apply clean gloves. NOTE: If patient has a latex allergy, use latex-free gloves.	Reduces transmission of microorganisms.
8 Keep sheet or gown draped over body parts not requiring exposure.	Respects dignity of patient while exposing injection area.
9 Select appropriate injection site. Inspect skin surface over sites for bruises, inflammation, or edema.	Injection sites are free of abnormalities that interfere with drug absorption. Sites used repeatedly become hardened from lipohypertrophy (increased growth in fatty tissue). Do not use an area that is bruised or has signs associated with infection.

SKILL 16-5   ADMINISTERING INJECTIONS—cont'd

STEP	RATIONALE
a *Subcutaneous:* Palpate sites, and avoid those with masses or tenderness. Rotate insulin sites within an anatomic area. Be sure needle is correct size by grasping skinfold at site with thumb and forefinger. Measure fold from top to bottom. Make sure needle is one-half length of fold.	You can mistakenly give subcutaneous injections in the muscle, especially in the abdomen and thigh sites. Appropriate size of needle ensures that you inject the medication in the subcutaneous tissue (Cocoman and Baron, 2008; Shin and Kim, 2006).
b *IM:* Note integrity and size of muscle, and palpate for tenderness or hardness. Avoid these areas. If you give injections frequently, rotate sites. Use ventrogluteal site if possible.	The ventrogluteal site is the preferred injection site for adults. This site is also preferred for children who are receiving irritating or viscous solutions (Cook and Murtagh, 2006; Hockenberry and Wilson, 2009; Nicoll and Hesby, 2002).
c *ID:* Note lesions or discolorations of skin. If possible, select site three to four finger widths below antecubital space and one hand width above wrist. If you cannot use the forearm, inspect the upper back. If necessary, use sites appropriate for subcutaneous injections.	An ID injection site is free of discolorations or hair so that you can see the results of skin test and interpret them correctly (Centers for Disease Control and Prevention [CDC], 2008).
10 Assist patient to comfortable position:	
a *Subcutaneous:* Have patient relax arm, leg, or abdomen, depending on site chosen for injection.	Relaxation of site minimizes discomfort.
b *IM:* Position patient depending on site chosen (e.g., sitting, supine, on side).	Reduces strain on muscle and minimizes discomfort of injections.
c *ID:* Have patient extend elbow and support it and forearm on flat surface.	Stabilizes injection site for easiest accessibility.
d Talk with patient about subject of interest.	Distraction reduces anxiety.

> • ***Critical Decision Point:*** Ensure that patient's position is not contraindicated by medical condition.

STEP	RATIONALE
11 Relocate site using anatomical landmarks.	Injection into correct anatomical site prevents injury to nerves, bones, and blood vessels.
12 Cleanse site with an antiseptic swab. Apply swab at center of the site, and rotate outward in a circular direction for about 5 cm (2 inches) (see illustration).	Mechanical action of swab removes secretions containing microorganisms.
13 Hold swab or gauze between third and fourth fingers of nondominant hand.	Gauze or swab remains readily accessible when withdrawing needle.
14 Remove needle cap from needle by pulling it straight off.	Preventing needle from touching sides of cap prevents contamination.
15 Hold syringe between thumb and forefinger of dominant hand:	
a *Subcutaneous:* Hold as dart, palm down (see illustration).	Quick, smooth injection requires proper manipulation of syringe parts.
b *IM:* Hold as dart, palm down.	
c *ID:* Hold bevel of needle pointing up.	With bevel up, you are less likely to deposit medication into tissues below dermis.
16 Administer injection:	
A Subcutaneous:	
(1) For average-size patient, pinch skin with nondominant hand.	Pinching skin elevates subcutaneous tissue and desensitizes area.
(2) Inject needle quickly and firmly at 45- to 90-degree angle. Then release skin, if pinched. *Option:* Continue to pinch skin and release after injecting medications.	Quick, firm insertion minimizes discomfort. (Injecting medication into compressed tissue irritates nerve fibers.) Correct angle prevents accidental injection into muscle.
(3) For obese patient, pinch skin at site and inject needle at 90-degree angle below tissue fold.	Obese patients have fatty layer of tissue above subcutaneous layer.

> • ***Critical Decision Point:*** Aspiration after injecting a subcutaneous medication is not necessary. Piercing a blood vessel in a subcutaneous injection is very rare.

STEP	RATIONALE

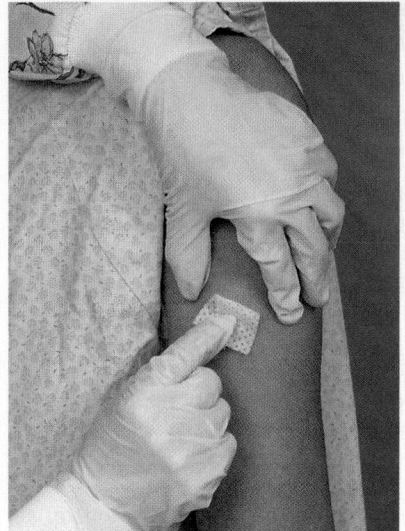 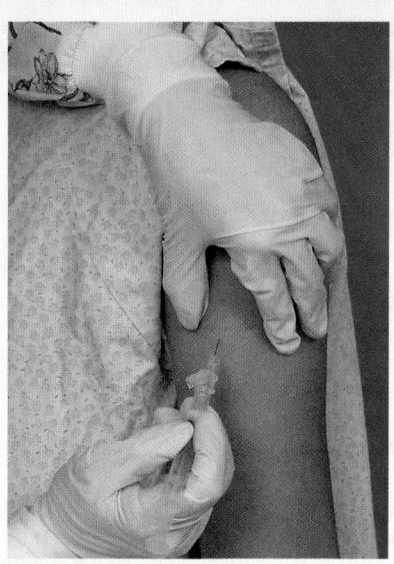 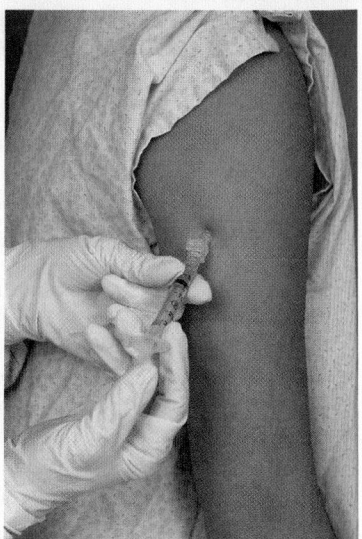

Step 12 ■ Cleanse site with circular motion.

Step 15a ■ Hold syringe as if grasping a dart.

Step 16A(4) ■ Inject medication slowly.

(4) Inject medication slowly (see illustration).

Minimizes discomfort.

B Intramuscular:

(1) Position ulnar aspect of nondominant hand just below site, and pull skin approximately 2.5 to 3.5 cm down or laterally to administer in a Z-track. Hold position until medication is injected. With dominant hand, inject needle quickly at 90-degree angle into muscle.

Z-track creates zigzag path through tissues that seals needle track to avoid tracking of medication (Nicoll and Hesby, 2002). A quick, dartlike injection reduces discomfort.

(2) *Option:* If patient's muscle mass is small, grasp body of muscle between thumb and fingers.

Ensures that medication reaches muscle mass (Hockenberry and Wilson, 2009).

(3) After needle pierces skin, grasp syringe barrel with thumb and forefinger of nondominant hand to stabilize syringe. Continue to pull skin tightly with nondominant hand. Move dominant hand to end of plunger. Do not move syringe.

Smooth manipulation of syringe reduces discomfort from needle movement. Skin remains pulled until after you inject drug to ensure Z-track administration.

(4) Pull back on plunger 5 to 10 seconds. If no blood appears, inject medication slowly at a rate of 1 mL/10 sec.

Aspiration of blood into syringe indicates IV placement of needle. Slow injection reduces pain and tissue trauma (Hockenberry and Wilson, 2009; Nicoll and Hesby, 2002).

• **Critical Decision Point:** If blood appears in syringe, remove needle, dispose of medication and syringe properly, and prepare another dose of medication for injection.

(5) Wait 10 seconds, then smoothly and steadily withdraw needle and release skin.

Allows time for medication to absorb into muscle before removing syringe (Nicoll and Hesby, 2002).

C Intradermal:

(1) With nondominant hand, stretch skin over site with forefinger or thumb.

Needle pierces tight skin more easily.

(2) With needle almost against patient's skin, insert it slowly at a 5- to 15-degree angle until resistance is felt. Then advance needle through epidermis to approximately 3 mm (⅛ inch) below skin surface. You will see needle tip through skin.

Ensures that needle tip is in dermis. You will obtain inaccurate results if you do not inject needle at correct angle and depth (CDC, 2008).

(3) Inject medication slowly. Normally you feel resistance. If not, needle is too deep; remove and begin again.

Slow injection minimizes discomfort at site. Dermal layer is tight and does not expand easily when you inject solution.

SKILL 16-5	ADMINISTERING INJECTIONS—cont'd

STEP	RATIONALE
(4) While injecting medication, note that small bleb (approximately 6 mm [¼ inch]) resembling mosquito bite appears on skin surface (see illustration).	Bleb indicates you deposited medication in dermis.
17 After withdrawing needle, apply alcohol swab or gauze gently over site.	Support of tissue around injection site minimizes discomfort during needle withdrawal. Dry gauze minimizes discomfort associated with alcohol on nonintact skin.
18 Apply gentle pressure. **Do not massage site.** Apply bandage if needed.	Massage damages underlying tissue. Massage of ID site disperses medication into underlying tissue layers and alters test results.
19 Assist patient to comfortable position.	Gives patient sense of well-being.
20 Discard uncapped needle or needle enclosed in safety shield and attached syringe into puncture-proof and leak-proof receptacle.	Prevents injury to patient and health care personnel. Recapping needles increases risk for needlestick injury (OSHA, 2007).
21 Remove gloves, and perform hand hygiene.	Reduces transmission of microorganisms.
22 Stay with patient, and observe for any allergic reactions.	Dyspnea, wheezing, and circulatory collapse are signs of severe anaphylactic reaction.

EVALUATION

1 Return to room within 30 minutes, and ask if patient feels any acute pain, burning, numbness, or tingling at injection site.	Continued discomfort indicates injury to underlying bones or nerves.
2 Inspect site, noting any bruising or induration. Document findings, and notify health care provider. Provide warm compress to site.	Bruising or induration indicates complication associated with injection.
3 Observe patient's response to medication at times that correlate with the medication's onset, peak, and duration.	The body rapidly absorbs IM medications. Adverse effects of parenteral medications develop rapidly. Evaluation determines effectiveness of medication.
4 Ask patient to explain purpose and effects of medication.	Evaluates patient's understanding of medication.
5 *For ID injections:* Use skin pencil to draw circle around perimeter of injection site. Read site within appropriate amount of time, designated by type of medication or skin test you give.	Pencil mark makes site easy to find. You determine the results of skin testing at various times, based on the type of medication used or the type of skin testing completed. Refer to the manufacturer's directions to determine when to read the test's results.

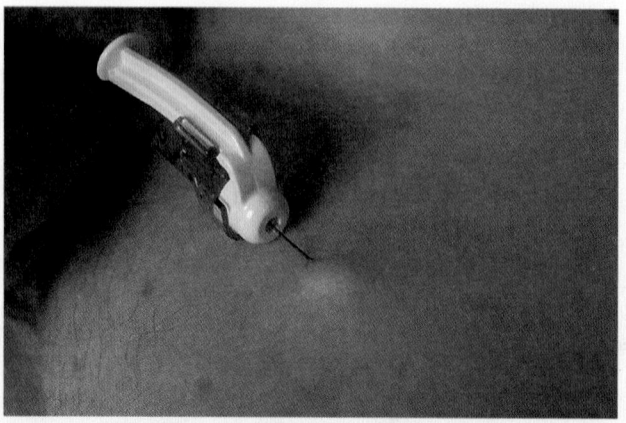

Step 16C(4) ■ Injection creates a small bleb.

STEP	RATIONALE

- *Critical Decision Point:* Read tuberculin test at 48 to 72 hours. Induration (hard, dense, raised area) of skin around injection site indicates positive tuberculin reaction of:
  - 15 mm or more in patients with no known risk factors for tuberculosis (TB)
  - 10 mm or more in patients who are recent immigrants; injection drug users; residents and employees of high-risk settings; patients with certain chronic illnesses; children less than 4 years of age; and infants, children, and adolescents exposed to high-risk adults
  - 5 mm or more in patients who are human immunodeficiency virus (HIV) positive, immunocompromised patients, or patients recently exposed to TB (CDC, 2008)

RECORDING AND REPORTING

- Document medication, dose, route, site, time, and date given on MAR.
- Record patient's response to medications in nurses' notes.
- Report any undesirable effects from medication to prescriber.
- Document if medication is withheld or refused per agency policy.

UNEXPECTED OUTCOMES AND RELATED INTERVENTIONS

- Raised, reddened, or hard zone (induration) forms around ID test site.
  - Notify patient's health care provider.
  - Document sensitivity to injected allergen or positive test if tuberculin skin testing was completed.
- Hypertrophy of skin develops from repeated subcutaneous injections.
  - Do not use this site for future injections.
  - Instruct patient not to use site for 6 months.
- Patient develops signs and symptoms of allergy or side effects.
  - Follow agency policy or guidelines for appropriate response to adverse drug reactions.
  - Notify patient's health care provider immediately.
  - Document allergy information in patient's medical record.
- Patient states has localized pain, numbness, tingling, or burning at injection site.
  - Assess injection site.
  - Notify patient's health care provider.

SKILL 16-6 ADMINISTERING MEDICATIONS BY INTRAVENOUS BOLUS

DELEGATION CONSIDERATIONS

The skill of administering medications by intravenous bolus cannot be delegated to nursing assistive personnel (NAP). The nurse informs NAP about:

- Potential side effects of medications and the need to report their occurrence
- The need to report discomfort at infusion site as soon as possible
- Obtaining any required vital signs and reporting these findings

EQUIPMENT

- Watch with second hand
- MAR (electronic or printed)
- Clean gloves
- Antiseptic swab
- Medication in vial or ampule
- Safety syringe for medication preparation
- Needleless device or sterile needle (21 to 25 gauge)
- Intravenous lock: vial of appropriate flush solution (saline most common, but heparin flush may also be used; if heparin flush is used, most common concentration is 10 to 100 units per mL; check agency policy)

SKILL 16-6	ADMINISTERING MEDICATIONS BY INTRAVENOUS BOLUS—cont'd

STEP	RATIONALE

ASSESSMENT

1 Check accuracy and completeness of each MAR with prescriber's original medication order. Check patient's name, drug name and dosage, route of administration, and time for administration. Recopy or re-print any portion of printed MAR that is difficult to read.

The prescriber's order is the most reliable source and only legal record of drugs patient is to receive. Ensures patient receives the right medications. Handwritten MARs are a source of medication errors (Eisenhauer and others, 2007; Furukawa and others, 2008).

- *Critical Decision Point:* Some IV medications can be pushed safely only when the patient is continuously monitored for dysrhythmias, blood pressure changes, or other adverse effects. Therefore you can push some medications only in specific areas within a health care agency. Confirm agency guidelines regarding requirements for special monitoring and the recommended rate of injection before giving these medications (ISMP, 2003).

2 Collect drug reference information necessary to administer drug safely, including action, purpose, side effects, normal dose, time of peak onset, how slowly to give the medication, and nursing implications, such as the need to dilute the medication or administer it through a filter.

Allows you to give drug safely and to monitor patient's response to therapy (ISMP, 2003).

3 If you will give drug through existing IV line, determine compatibility of medication with IV fluids and any additives within IV solution.

IV medication is sometimes not compatible with IV solution and/or additives.

4 Perform hand hygiene. Assess condition of IV needle insertion site for signs of infiltration or phlebitis.

Do not administer medication if site is edematous or inflamed.

5 Check patient's medical history and drug or latex allergies.

IV bolus delivers drug rapidly. Allergic reaction could prove fatal.

6 Assess patient's understanding of the purpose of drug therapy.

Reveals need for education.

PLANNING

1 Expected outcomes following completion of procedure:
- Desired effect of medication achieved with no signs of adverse reactions.

Medication administered safely with desired therapeutic effect achieved.

- Intravenous site remains clear, without swelling.

Medication administered without complications to IV site.

- Patient explains the purpose and side effects of medication.

Demonstrates learning.

- *Critical Decision Point:* Some IV medications require dilution before administration. Verify with agency policy. If a small amount of medication is given (e.g., less than 1 mL), dilute medication in small amount (e.g., 5 mL) of normal saline or sterile water so that the medication does not collect in the "dead spaces" (e.g., Y-site injection port, IV cap) of the IV delivery system. Verify medication can be diluted by consulting medication reference or checking with pharmacist first.

IMPLEMENTATION

1 Perform hand hygiene and prepare medication from ampule or vial using aseptic technique (see Skill 16-4). Check label of medication carefully with MAR two times.

Ensures that medication is sterile. Preparation techniques differ for ampule and vial. *First and second checks ensure right medication is administered.*

2 Take medication to patient at correct time, within 30 minutes before or after prescribed time, and perform hand hygiene.

Ensures intended therapeutic effect. Give STAT medications immediately or single-order medications at the time ordered. Hand hygiene decreases transfer of microorganisms.

3 Identify patient using two identifiers (e.g., name and birthday or name and account number, according to facility policy). Compare identifiers with information on patient's MAR or medical record.

Complies with TJC (2008b) requirements and improves medication safety. In most acute care settings, patient's name and identification number on armband and MAR are used to identify patients. Identification bracelets are made at time of patient's admission and are most reliable source of identification. Patient's room number is **not** an acceptable identifier.

STEP	RATIONALE
4 Compare the label of the medication with the MAR one more time at the patient's bedside.	*Third check for accuracy ensures right medication is administered.*
5 Explain procedure to patient. Encourage patient to report symptoms of discomfort at IV site.	Keeps patient informed and involved in care; helps identify possible infiltration early.
6 Put on clean gloves. NOTE: If patient has a latex allergy, use latex-free gloves.	Reduces transmission of microorganisms.
7 **Intravenous push (existing line):**	
a Select injection port of IV tubing closest to patient. Whenever possible, use needleless injection port. Use IV filter if required by medication reference or agency policy.	Follows provisions of The Needle Safety and Prevention Act of 2001 (OSHA, 2007).

 • *Critical Decision Point:* Never administer IV medications through tubing that is infusing blood, blood products, or parenteral nutrition solutions.

---

b Clean port with antiseptic swab.	Prevents transfer of microorganisms during needle insertion.
c Connect syringe to IV line: Insert needleless tip of syringe or small-gauge needle containing drug through center of port (see illustration).	Prevents damage to port diaphragm.
d Occlude IV line by pinching tubing just above injection port (see illustration). Pull back gently on syringe's plunger to aspirate for blood return.	*Final check ensures that medication is delivered into bloodstream.*

 • *Critical Decision Point:* In some cases, especially with a smaller-gauge IV needle, blood return sometimes is not aspirated, even if IV line is patent. If IV site does not show signs of infiltration and IV fluid is infusing without difficulty, proceed with IV push.

---

e Release tubing, and inject medication within amount of time recommended by institutional policy, pharmacist, or medication reference manual. Use a watch to time administrations (see illustration). You can pinch the IV line while pushing medication and release it when not pushing medication. Allow IV fluids to infuse when not pushing medication.	Ensures safe drug infusion. Rapid injection of IV drug can be fatal. Allowing IV fluids to infuse while pushing IV drug enables medication to be delivered to patient at prescribed rate.

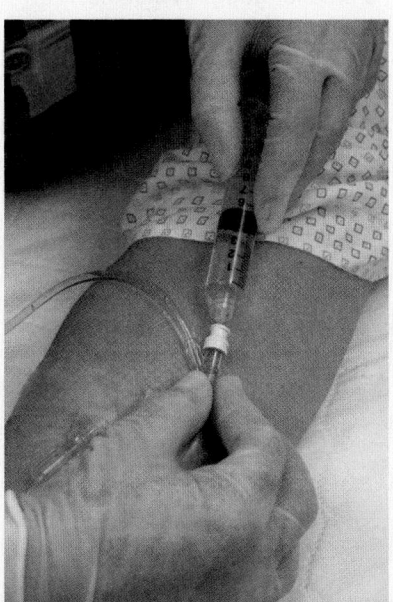

Step 7c ■ Connecting syringe to IV line with blunt needleless cannula tip.

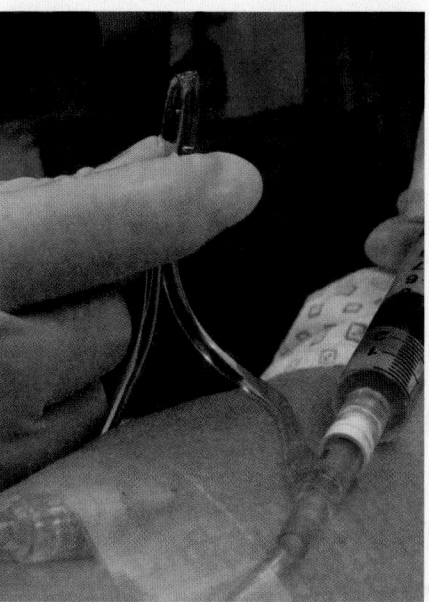

Step 7d ■ IV line pinched above injection port to aspirate for blood return.

SKILL 16-6   ADMINISTERING MEDICATIONS
BY INTRAVENOUS BOLUS—cont'd

STEP	RATIONALE

- *Critical Decision Point:* If IV medication is incompatible with IV fluids, stop the IV fluids, clamp the IV line, flush with 10 mL of normal saline or sterile water, give the IV bolus over the appropriate amount of time, flush with another 10 mL of normal saline or sterile water at the same rate as the medication was administered, and then restart the IV fluids at the prescribed rate. This allows you to give IV push medication through the existing line without creating potential risks associated with IV incompatibilities. If IV infusion that is currently hanging is a medication (e.g., ranitidine), disconnect IV line and administer IV push medication as outlined in step 8 to avoid giving a sudden bolus of the medication in the existing IV line to the patient. Verify institutional policy regarding the stopping of IV fluids or continuous IV medications. If unable to stop IV infusion, start a new IV site (see Chapter 17) and administer medication using the IV push (IV lock) method.

f After injecting medication, withdraw syringe, and recheck fluid infusion rate.	Injection of bolus often alters rate of fluid infusion. Rapid fluid infusion causes circulatory fluid overload.
8 Intravenous push (intravenous lock):	
a Prepare flush solutions according to hospital policy.	
(1) Saline flush method (preferred method): Prepare two syringes filled with 2 to 3 mL of normal saline (0.9%).	Normal saline is effective in keeping IV locks patent and is compatible with a wide range of medications.
(2) Heparin flush method (traditional method):	
(a) Prepare one syringe with ordered amount of heparin flush solution.	
(b) Prepare two syringes with 2 to 3 mL of normal saline (0.9%).	
b Administer medication:	
(1) Clean lock's injection port with antiseptic swab.	Prevents transfer of microorganisms during needle insertion.
(2) Insert syringe with normal saline (0.9%) through injection port of IV lock (see illustrations).	
(3) Pull back gently on syringe plunger, and check for blood return.	Indicates if needle or catheter is in vein.

- *Critical Decision Point:* In some cases, especially with a smaller-gauge IV needle, blood return is usually not aspirated, even if IV line is patent. If IV site does not show signs of infiltration, and IV flushes without difficulty, proceed with IV push.

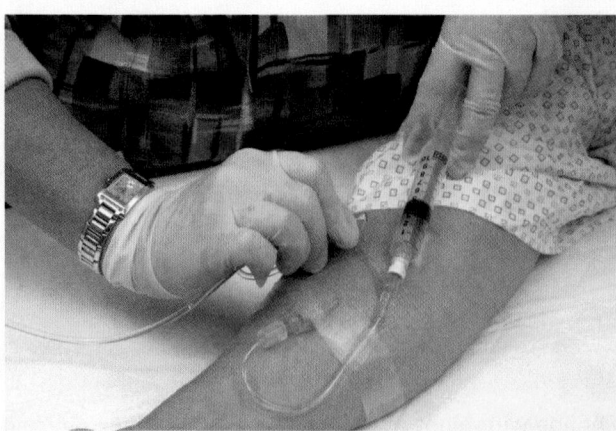

Step 7e ■ Using a watch to time an IV push medication.

STEP	RATIONALE
(4) Flush IV site with normal saline by pushing slowly on plunger.	Cleans needle and reservoir of blood. Flushing without difficulty indicates patent IV line.

• **Critical Decision Point:** Carefully observe the area of skin above the IV catheter. Note any puffiness or swelling as you flush the IV line. Swelling indicates infiltration into the vein and requires removal of catheter.

STEP	RATIONALE
(5) Remove saline-filled syringe.	
(6) Clean lock's injection port with antiseptic swab.	Prevents transmission of infection.
(7) Insert syringe containing prepared medication through injection port of IV lock.	Allows administration of medication.
(8) Inject medication within amount of time recommended by agency policy, pharmacist, or medication reference manual. Use a watch to time administration.	Many medication errors are associated with IV pushes being administered too quickly. Following guidelines for IV push rates promotes patient safety (ISMP, 2003; Karch and Karch, 2003).
(9) After administering bolus, withdraw syringe.	
(10) Clean lock's injection site with antiseptic swab.	Prevents transmission of infection.
(11) Flush injection port.	
(a) Attach syringe with normal saline, and inject normal saline flush at the same rate the medication was delivered.	Flushing IV line with saline prevents occlusion of IV access device and ensures all medication delivered. Flushing IV site at same rate as medication ensures that any medication remaining within IV needle is delivered at the correct rate.
(b) *Heparin flush option:* After instilling saline, attach syringe containing heparin flush. Inject heparin slowly, and then remove syringe.	Maintains patency of IV needle by inhibiting clot formation. SASH method: *S*aline, *A*dministration of medication, *S*aline, *H*eparin.
9 Dispose of uncapped needles and syringes in puncture-proof and leakproof container.	Prevents accidental needlestick injuries and follows CDC guidelines for disposal of sharps (OSHA, 2007).
10 Remove gloves, and perform hand hygiene.	Reduces transfer of microorganisms.

EVALUATION

1 Observe patient closely for adverse reactions during administration and for several minutes thereafter.	Intravenous medications act rapidly.
2 Observe IV site during injection for sudden swelling.	Swelling indicates infiltration into tissues surrounding vein.
3 Assess patient's status after giving medication to evaluate the effectiveness of the medication.	Some IV bolus medications cause rapid changes in the patient's physiological status. Some drugs require careful monitoring and assessment and possibly future laboratory testing (e.g., vasopressors and antiarrhythmics require blood pressure and heart rate monitoring, whereas heparin requires laboratory studies after administration to determine if it is in a therapeutic level).

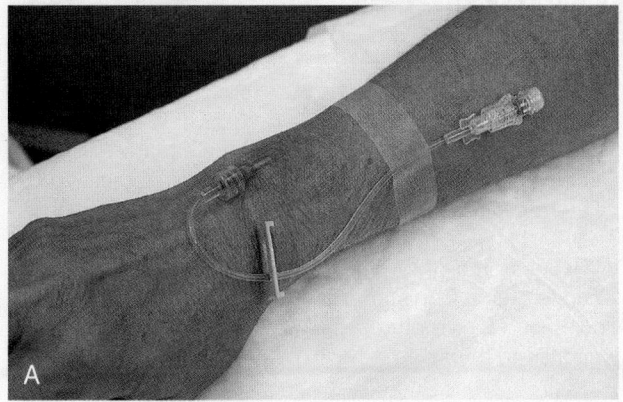
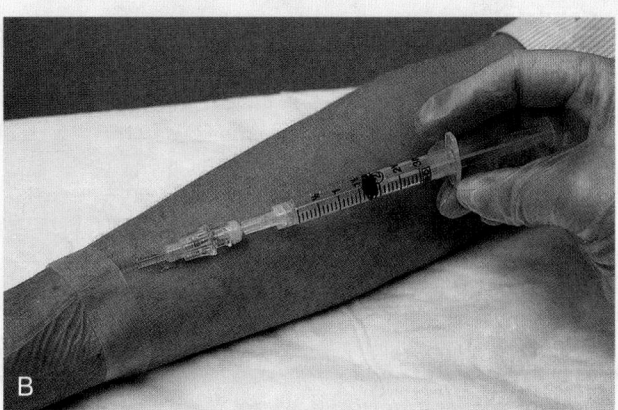

Step 8b(2) ■ **A,** IV catheter with saline lock adapter. **B,** Syringe inserted into injection port.

SKILL 16-6   ADMINISTERING MEDICATIONS BY INTRAVENOUS BOLUS—cont'd

STEP	RATIONALE
4 Ask patient to explain drug's purpose and side effects.	Evaluates learning.

RECORDING AND REPORTING

- Record medication administration, including drug name, dose, route, and time of administration.
- Record patient's response to medication in nurses' notes.

- Report any adverse reactions to patient's health care provider. Patient's response may indicate need for additional medical therapy.

UNEXPECTED OUTCOMES AND RELATED INTERVENTIONS

- Patient develops adverse reaction to medication.
  - Stop delivering medication immediately, and follow agency policy or guidelines for appropriate response and reporting of adverse drug reactions.
  - Add allergy information to patient's medical record per agency policy.

- IV site shows symptoms of infiltration or phlebitis (see Chapter 17).
  - Stop infusing medication.
  - Treat IV site as indicated by agency policy.
  - Insert new IV site if continuing IV therapy.
- Patient is unable to explain medication information.
  - Patient requires reinstruction or is unable to learn at this time.

SKILL 16-7   ADMINISTERING INTRAVENOUS MEDICATIONS BY PIGGYBACK, INTERMITTENT INTRAVENOUS INFUSION SETS, AND MINI-INFUSION PUMPS

DELEGATION CONSIDERATIONS
The skill of administering IV medications cannot be delegated to nursing assistive personnel (NAP). The nurse informs NAP about:
- Potential side effects of medications and to report their occurrence
- Reporting patient's report of any discomfort at infusion site to nurse
- Reporting any change in the patient's condition or vital signs to nurse

EQUIPMENT
- Adhesive tape (optional)
- Antiseptic swab
- IV pole
- MAR (electronic or printed)

Piggyback or Mini-infusion Pump
- Medication prepared in 5- to 250-mL labeled infusion bag or syringe
- Short microdrip, macrodrip, or mini-infusion IV tubing set, preferably with needleless system attachment
- Needleless device or stopcocks preferred if available
- Needles (21 or 23 gauge, **only** if stopcocks or other needleless methods are not available)
- Mini-infusion pump if indicated

Volume-Control Administration Set
- Volutrol or Buretrol
- Infusion tubing (may have needleless system attachment)
- Syringe (1 to 20 mL)
- Vial or ampule of ordered medication

STEP	RATIONALE

ASSESSMENT

1 Check accuracy and completeness of each MAR with prescriber's written medication order to determine type of IV solution you will use, type of medication, dose, route, and time of administration. Recopy or re-print any portion of MAR that is difficult to read. Also check patient's name.

The prescriber's order is the most reliable source and only legal record of drugs patient is to receive. Ensures patient receives the right medications. Handwritten MARs are a source of medication errors (Eisenhauer and others, 2007; Furukawa and others, 2008).

2 Determine patient's medical history.

Determines type of IV solution used. Ensures safe and accurate drug administration.

3 Collect information necessary to administer drug safely, including action, purpose, side effects, normal dose, time of peak onset, and nursing implications.

Allows you to give drug safely and to monitor patient's response to therapy.

STEP	RATIONALE
4 Assess compatibility of drug with existing IV solution.	Drugs that are incompatible with IV solutions result in clouding or crystallization of solution in IV tubing, which will harm the patient.

> • *Critical Decision Point:* Never administer IV medications through tubing that is infusing blood, blood products, or parenteral nutrition solutions.

STEP	RATIONALE
5 Assess patency of patient's existing IV infusion line (see Chapter 17).	In order for medication to reach venous circulation effectively, IV line needs to be patent and fluids should infuse easily.

> • *Critical Decision Point:* If the patient's IV site is saline locked, cleanse the port with alcohol and assess the patency of the IV line by flushing the IV line with 2 to 3 mL of sterile normal saline. Attach appropriate IV tubing to the saline lock, and administer the medication via piggyback, mini-infusion, or volume-control administration set. When the infusion is completed, disconnect the tubing, cleanse the port with alcohol, and flush the IV line with 2 to 3 mL sterile normal saline. Maintain sterility of IV tubing between intermittent infusions.

STEP	RATIONALE
6 Perform hand hygiene. Assess IV insertion site for signs of infiltration or phlebitis: redness, pallor, swelling, or tenderness on palpation.	Confirmation of placement of IV needle or catheter and integrity of surrounding tissues ensures you administer medication safely.
7 Assess patient's history of drug allergies.	Effects of medications develop rapidly after IV infusion. Be aware of patients at risk.
8 Assess patient's understanding of purpose of drug therapy.	Reveals need for education.

PLANNING

1 Expected outcomes following completion of procedure:
* Medication administered safely with desired therapeutic effect achieved.
* Medication infuses within desired time frame.
* IV site remains intact without signs of swelling or inflammation or symptoms of tenderness at site.
* Patient is able to explain drug purposes, action, side effects, and dosage.

Patient tolerates medication.

IV line remains patent.
Fluid infuses into vein, not tissues.

Demonstrates learning.

IMPLEMENTATION

STEP	RATIONALE
1 Perform hand hygiene and prepare medication: See Skill 16-1, Implementation steps 1a-h, k-m. Be sure to check the label two times while preparing medication.	Following the same routine when preparing medications, eliminating distractions, and checking the label of the medication with transcribed order reduce error. *First and second checks ensure right medication is administered.*
2 Take medications to patient at correct time, within 30 minutes before or after prescribed time, and perform hand hygiene.	Ensures intended therapeutic effect. Give STAT medications immediately or single-order medications at time ordered. Hand hygiene decreases transfer of microorganisms.
3 Identify patient using two identifiers (e.g., name and birthday or name and account number, according to facility policy). Compare identifiers with information on patient's MAR or medical record.	Complies with TJC (2008b) requirements and improves medication safety. In most acute care settings, patient's name and identification number on armband and MAR are used to identify patients. Identification bracelets are made at time of patient's admission and are most reliable source of identification. Patient's room number is **not** an acceptable identifier.
4 Explain purpose of medication and side effects to patient, and explain that you will give medication through existing IV line. Encourage patient to report symptoms of discomfort at site.	Keeps patient informed of planned therapies, minimizing anxiety. Patients who verbalize pain at the IV site help detect IV infiltrations early, lessening damage to surrounding tissues.
5 Compare the label of the medication with the MAR one more time at patient's bedside.	*Third check for accuracy ensures right medication is administered.*
6 Administer infusion:	
A Piggyback Infusion:	
(1) Connect infusion tubing to medication bag (see Chapter 17). Allow solution to fill tubing by opening regulator flow clamp. Once tubing is full, close clamp and cap end of tubing.	Filling of infusion tubing with solution and freeing of air bubbles prevent air embolus.

SKILL 16-7	ADMINISTERING INTRAVENOUS MEDICATIONS BY PIGGYBACK, INTERMITTENT INTRAVENOUS INFUSION SETS, AND MINI-INFUSION PUMPS—cont'd

STEP	RATIONALE
(2) Hang piggyback medication bag above level of primary fluid bag (see Figure 16-27, p. 428). (Use hook to lower main bag.)	Height of fluid bag affects rate of flow to patient.
(3) Connect tubing of piggyback infusion to appropriate connector on upper Y-port of primary infusion line:	Connection allows IV medication to enter main IV line.
(a) *Needleless system:* Wipe off needleless port of main IV line, and insert tip of piggyback infusion tubing (see illustration).	Use needleless connections to prevent accidental needle-stick injuries (OSHA, 2007).
(b) *Stopcock:* Wipe off stopcock port with alcohol swab, and connect tubing. Turn stopcock to open position.	Stopcock eliminates need for needle.
(c) *Tubing port:* Connect sterile needle to end of piggyback infusion tubing, remove cap, cleanse injection port on main IV line, and insert needle through center of port. Secure by taping connection.	**Only** use this method if needleless system is unavailable.
(4) Regulate flow rate of medication solution by adjusting regulator clamp or IV pump infusion rate (see Chapter 17). Infusion times vary. Refer to medication reference or agency policy for safe flow rate.	Provides slow, safe infusion of medication and maintains therapeutic blood levels.
(5) After medication has infused, check flow rate on primary infusion. The primary infusion automatically begins to flow after the piggyback solution is empty. If stopcock is used, turn stopcock to off position.	Back-check valve on piggyback stops flow of the primary infusion until medication infuses. Checking flow rate ensures proper administration of IV fluids.
(6) Regulate main infusion line to ordered rate if necessary.	Infusion of piggyback sometimes interferes with the main line infusion rate.

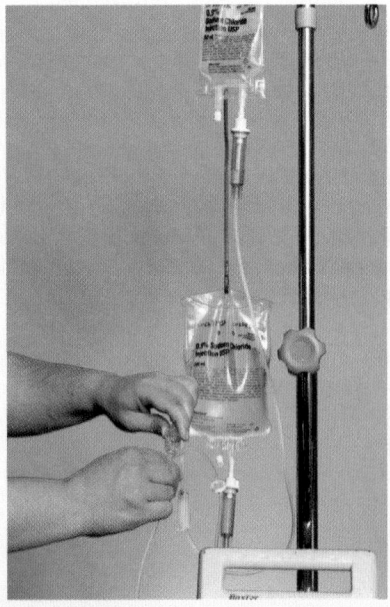

Step 6A(3)(a) ■ For the needleless system, insert tip of piggyback infusion tubing into port.

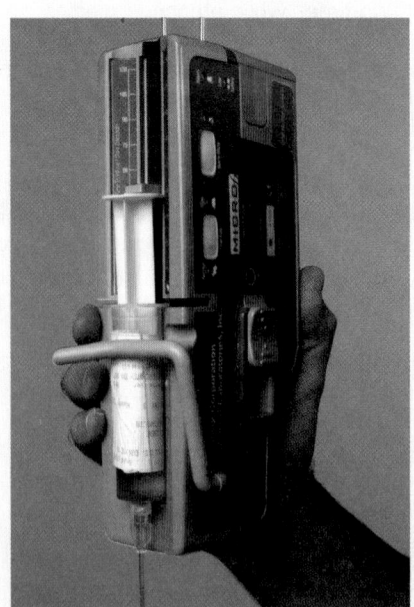

Step 6B(3) ■ Ensure syringe is secure after placing it into mini-infusion pump.

STEP	RATIONALE
(7) Leave IV piggyback bag and tubing in place for future drug administration, or discard in appropriate containers.	Establishment of secondary line produces route for microorganisms to enter main line. Repeated changes in tubing increase risk for infection transmission (check agency policy).
B Mini-infusion Administration:	
(1) Connect prefilled syringe to mini-infusion tubing.	Special tubing designed to fit syringe delivers medication to main IV line.
(2) Carefully apply pressure to syringe plunger, allowing tubing to fill with medication.	Ensures tubing is free of air bubbles to prevent air embolus.
(3) Place syringe into mini-infusion pump (follow product directions). Be sure syringe is secured (see illustration).	Correct placement is necessary for proper infusion.
(4) Connect mini-infusion tubing to main IV line.	
(a) *Needleless system:* Wipe off needleless port of IV tubing, and insert tip of the mini-infusion tubing.	OSHA (2007) recommends needleless system to reduce risk for needle-stick injuries.
(b) *Stopcock:* Wipe off stopcock port with alcohol swab, and connect tubing. Turn stopcock to open position.	Stopcock reduces risk for needle-stick injuries.
(c) *Needle system:* Connect sterile needle to mini-infusion tubing, remove cap, cleanse injection port on main IV line or saline lock, and insert needle through center of port. Consider placing tape where IV tubing enters port to keep connection secured.	Use this method **only** if needleless system is not available.
(5) Hang infusion pump with syringe on IV pole alongside main IV bag. Set pump to deliver medication within time recommended by agency policy, a pharmacist, or a medication reference manual. Press button on pump to begin infusion.	Pump automatically delivers medication at safe, constant rate based on volume in syringe.
(6) After medication has infused, check flow rate on primary infusion. The infusion automatically begins to flow once the pump stops. Regulate main infusion line to desired rate as needed. (NOTE: If using a stopcock, turn off mini-infusion line.)	Maintains patency of primary IV line.
C Volume-Control Administration Set (e.g., Volutrol):	
(1) Fill Volutrol with desired amount of fluid (50 to 100 mL) by opening clamp between Volutrol and main IV bag.	Small volume of fluid dilutes IV medication and reduces risk for fluid infusing too rapidly.
(2) Close clamp, and check to be sure clamp on air vent of Volutrol chamber is open.	Prevents additional leakage of fluid into Volutrol. Air vent allows fluid in Volutrol to exit at regulated rate.
(3) Clean injection port on top of Volutrol with antiseptic swab.	Prevents introduction of microorganisms during needle insertion.
(4) Remove needle cap or sheath, and insert syringe needle through port, then inject medication (see illustrations). Gently rotate Volutrol between hands.	Rotating mixes medication with solution in Volutrol to ensure equal distribution.
(5) Regulate IV infusion rate to allow medication to infuse in time recommended by agency policy, a pharmacist, or a medication reference manual.	For optimal therapeutic effect, drug needs to infuse in prescribed time interval.
(6) Label Volutrol with name of drug, dosage, total volume including diluent, and time of administration following ISMP (2008d) safe IV medication label format (see Figure 16-28, p. 429).	Alerts nurses to drug being infused. Prevents other medications from being added to Volutrol.
(7) If patient is receiving a continuous IV infusion, check continuous infusion after Volutrol infusion is complete to ensure the appropriate rate of IV fluid administration.	Ensures appropriate fluid balance.
(8) Dispose of uncapped needle or needle enclosed in safety shield and syringe in proper container.	Prevents accidental needle sticks.

SKILL 16-7	ADMINISTERING INTRAVENOUS MEDICATIONS BY PIGGYBACK, INTERMITTENT INTRAVENOUS INFUSION SETS, AND MINI-INFUSION PUMPS—cont'd

STEP	RATIONALE
(9) Discard supplies in appropriate container. Perform hand hygiene.	Reduces transmission of microorganisms.

EVALUATION

1 Assess patient's status after giving medication.	Evaluates effect of medication.
2 Observe patient for signs of adverse reactions.	IV medications act rapidly.
3 During infusion, periodically check infusion rate and condition of IV site.	IV system needs to remain patent for proper drug administration. Development of infiltration requires discontinuing infusion.
4 Ask patient to explain purpose and side effects of the medication.	Evaluates patient's understanding of instruction.

RECORDING AND REPORTING

- Record drug, dose, route, and time administered on MAR.
- Record volume of fluid in medication bag or Volutrol as fluid intake.

- Report any adverse reactions to patient's health care provider.

UNEXPECTED OUTCOMES AND RELATED INTERVENTIONS

- Patient develops adverse drug reaction.
  - Stop medication infusion immediately.
  - Follow agency policy or guidelines for appropriate response and reporting of adverse drug reactions.
  - Add allergy information to patient's medical record.

- Medication does not infuse over desired period.
  - Determine reason (e.g., improper calculation of flow rate, poor positioning of IV needle at insertion site, infiltration)
  - Take corrective action as indicated.
- IV site shows symptoms of infiltration or phlebitis (see Chapter 17).
  - See related interventions in Skill 16-6.

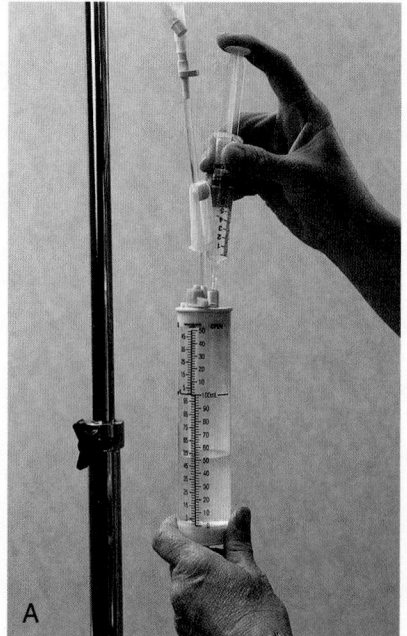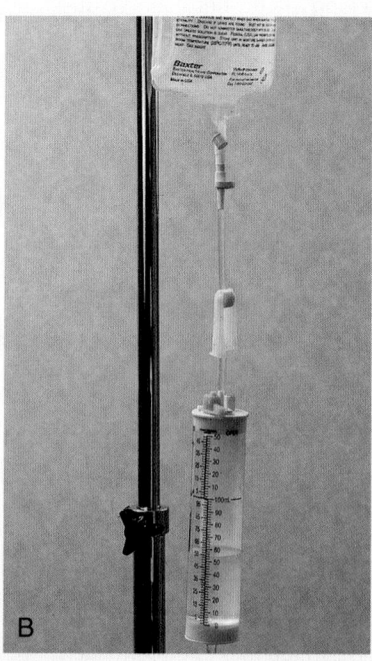

Step 6C(4) ■ **A,** Inject medication into device. **B,** Prepared dose.

KEY POINTS

- Learning medication classifications helps you better understand nursing implications for administering medications with similar characteristics.
- Handle all controlled substances according to strict procedures that account for each medication.
- Apply understanding of the physiology of medication action when timing administration, selecting routes, initiating interventions to promote the potency of the medication, and observing responses to medications.
- The older adult's body undergoes structural and functional changes that alter medication actions and influence the manner in which nurses provide medication therapy.
- Always prepare and calculate medication doses in a location without distractions, and use the calculation method that works best for you.
- The body absorbs medications given parenterally more quickly than medications administered by other routes.
- Each medication order includes the patient's name; the time and date the order was written; the medication name; dosage, route, and time and frequency of administration; and the prescriber's signature.
- Always clarify medication orders that are not clear to you (e.g., written illegibly, contain dangerous abbreviations).

- When you take a patient's medication history, include allergies, medications—including prescription medications, over-the-counter medications, vitamins, and herbal supplements—and the patient's adherence to therapy.
- The six rights of medication administration enhance safe medication preparation and administration.
- Only administer medications you prepare, and never leave medications unattended.
- Document medications immediately after administration.
- Use clinical nursing judgment when determining the best time to administer prn medications.
- Report any actual and potential medication errors immediately.
- When preparing medications, check the medication container label against the MAR or computer printout three times before administration.
- When administering medication to patients, verify your patients' identity by using at least two patient identifiers. Ask your patients to state their name if possible for a third identifier.
- The Z-track method for IM injections protects subcutaneous tissues from irritating parenteral fluids.
- Failure to select injection sites by anatomical landmarks leads to tissue, bone, or nerve damage.

CRITICAL THINKING EXERCISES

While Emilio is caring for Esther, her nurse practitioner (NP) comes to assess Esther and evaluate her progress. Emilio tells the NP that Esther's blood pressure has been a little higher than usual the past few days and that she has 2+ edema in her ankles bilaterally. The NP orders 60 mg furosemide IVP now and q8h.

1. What information does Emilio need to know before he gives the furosemide?
2. Three 8-mL vials of furosemide arrive from the pharmacy. The label on each vial says, "80 mg furosemide in 8 mL." Using dimensional analysis, calculate how much medication Emilio will prepare in the syringe.
3. Esther has a saline lock in her right wrist. After Emilio verifies that the medication is correct, performs hand hygiene, prepares the medication, and verifies Esther's identity, what will he do next in administering the IV push medication?
   a. Push the medication in slowly.
   b. Flush the IV site with heparin.
   c. Observe for adverse reactions.

   d. Assess the IV insertion site for signs of infiltration or phlebitis.
   e. Check the medication one more time at the beside with the MAR.
4. While Emilio flushes Esther's saline lock with saline before administering the IV furosemide, he assesses swelling, warmth, redness, and tenderness at the IV site. Which of the following interventions does Emilio implement at this time? Select all that apply.
   a. Stop flushing the IV line with normal saline.
   b. Infuse the medication slowly.
   c. Reposition the IV cannula.
   d. Discontinue the saline lock.
   e. Insert a new saline lock at a different site.

⊜volve   *Answers to Critical Thinking Questions can be found on the Evolve website.*

REVIEW QUESTIONS

1. A patient receiving an antihypertensive medication states he is having trouble maintaining an erection when he has sex with his wife. This is an example of:
   1. A side effect
   2. A toxic effect
   3. An allergic reaction
   4. An idiosyncratic reaction

2. A patient takes a diuretic, an ACE inhibitor, and a beta-blocker to effectively manage his hypertension. This is an example of:
   1. Alternative medicine
   2. Medication tolerance
   3. Nontherapeutic polypharmacy
   4. A desirable medication interaction

3. You receive a telephone order to mix 20 mEq of potassium in an IV bag of 250 mg normal saline and administer it to your patient STAT. What do you need to do first?
   1. Make sure that the patient wants to take the medication.
   2. Prepare 20 mEq of potassium in a syringe using aseptic technique.
   3. Contact the pharmacist to see if the medication can be prepared in the pharmacy.
   4. Gather all the supplies you will need to mix the medication in the medication room.

4. A patient is to receive a subcutaneous injection of heparin. The patient is 5 feet, 2 inches tall and weighs 135 pounds. The nurse plans to administer the injection in the abdomen. The most appropriate needle size to use for this injection is:
   1. 18 gauge, 1¼ inch
   2. 20 gauge, 1 inch
   3. 22 gauge, 1½ inch
   4. 25 gauge, ½ inch

5. The patient has an order for 1 tablespoon of Robitussin for a cough. The nurse, converting this to the metric system, would give the patient:
   1. 5 mL
   2. 10 mL
   3. 15 mL
   4. 30 mL

6. A physician's order for a medication states: "Insulin 5u reg and 10 u L BID." The physician is very busy, does not like to be bothered, and is known for being difficult to work with. The nurse should:
   1. Consult a pharmacist to interpret the order
   2. Call the physician and have the order verified
   3. Administer 5 units of regular insulin and 10 units of Lente insulin subcutaneously 2 times a day
   4. Talk to the unit secretary on the floor who is good at reading the physician's handwriting

7. A patient is to receive cephalexin (Keflex), 500 mg PO. The drawer of the automated medication dispensing system opens. There are five tablets, each labeled 250 mg cephalexin, in the drawer. The nurse should give:
   1. ½ tablet
   2. 1 tablet
   3. 1½ tablets
   4. 2 tablets

8. You have to give the following medications to the patients listed below. Which patient should you give medications to first?
   1. A patient who is to receive 325 mg aspirin who has a history of coronary artery disease
   2. A patient who needs 2 tablets of Vicodin (acetaminophen and hydrocodone) who is rating his incisional pain at a 10 on a 0 to 10 pain scale
   3. A patient who is to get Capoten (Captopril) 25 mg for a history of hypertension whose current blood pressure is 125/72 mm Hg
   4. A patient who is receiving Bactrim DS (trimethoprim-sulfamethoxazole) for a urinary tract infection

9. A patient is taking a medication via the buccal route and states that she is experiencing some burning in her right cheek. Which of the following statements made by the nurse is the most appropriate after the patient makes this comment?
   1. "I won't give you this medication until the burning and irritation goes away."
   2. "Put your medication under your tongue to prevent further burning to your cheek."
   3. "This is a serious adverse effect; I will ask your health care provider to change the route of your medication."
   4. "Are you alternating the medication between your right and left cheeks when you take your medication?"

10. You give 1000 mg of a medication to a patient at 1200. The biologic half-life of the medication is 3 hours. How much of the total medication will the patient excrete at 1800?
    1. 250 mg
    2. 500 mg
    3. 750 mg
    4. 1000 mg

Answers to Review Questions can be found on pages 1197-1198.

REFERENCES

Alertness Solutions: *New survey uncovers how insomnia affects job performance and safety: first study uncovers how insomnia affects job performance and safety*, 2007, http://www.prnewswire.com/cgi-bin/stories.pl?ACCT=104&STORY=/www/story/06-12-2007/0004606266&EDATE.

Alvarez-Lorenzo C, Hiratani H, Concheiro A: Contact lenses for drug delivery: achieving sustained release with novel systems, *Am J Drug Deliv* 4(3):131, 2006.

American Diabetes Association: Insulin administration: position statement, *Diabetes Care* 27(1S): S106, 2004.

American Diabetes Association: Standards of medical care in diabetes—2009: position statement, *Diabetes Care* 32(1):S13, 2009.

American Hospital Association: *The patient care partnership*, 2003, http://www.aha.org/aha/issues/Communicating-With-Patients/pt-care-partnership.html.

American Nurses Association: *Facts about needlestick injury*, 2007, http://nursingworld.org/MainMenuCategories/OccupationalandEnvironmental/occupationalhealth/SafeNeedles/NeedlestickInjuryFacts.aspx.

Association of periOperative Registered Nurses: *Perioperative standards and recommended practices*, Denver, 2008, The Association.

Bastable SB: *Nurse as educator: principles of teaching and learning for nursing practice*, ed 3, Sudbury, Mass, 2008, Jones & Bartlett.

Beyea SC: Distractions, interruptions, and patient safety, *AORN J* 86(1):109, 2007a.

Beyea SC: Medication reconciliation: what every nurse needs to know, *AORN J* 85(1):193, 2007b.

Bridge L: Reducing the risk of wrong route errors, *Paediatr Nurs* 19(6):33, 2007.

Capriotti T: Changes in inhaler devices for asthma and COPD, *Medsurg Nurs* 14(3):185, 2005.

Carpi V: When consistency counts, *Health Manag Technol* 29(2):60, 2008.

Centers for Disease Control and Prevention: *Division of Tuberculosis Elimination*, 2008, http://www.cdc.gov/tb/.

Cocoman A, Barron C: Administering subcutaneous injections to children: what does the evidence say? *Journal of Children's and Young People's Nursing* 2(2):84, 2008.

Cook IF, Murtagh J: Ventrogluteal area—a suitable site for intramuscular vaccination of infants and toddlers, *Vaccine* 24(13):2403, 2006.

Dennison RD: A medication safety education program to reduce the risk of harm caused by medication errors, *J Contin Educ Nurs* 38(4):176, 2007.

deWit S: *Fundamental concepts and skills for nursing*, ed 2, Philadelphia, 2005, WB Saunders.

Dopson A: Confidence and competence in paediatric drug calculations, *Nurse Prescribing* 6(5):208, 2008.

Ebersole P and others: *Toward healthy aging: human needs and nursing response*, ed 7, St. Louis, 2008, Mosby.

Eisenhauer LA, Hurley AC, Dolan N: Nurses' reported thinking during medication administration, *J Nurs Scholarsh* 39(1):82, 2007.

Foote SO, Coleman JR: Medication administration: the implementation process of barcoding for medication administration to enhance medication safety, *Nurs Econ* 26(3):207, 2008.

Furukawa MF and others: Adoption of health information technology for medication safety in U.S. hospitals, 2006, *Health Affairs* 27(3):865, 2008.

Gray Morris D: *Calculate with confidence*, ed 4, St. Louis, 2006, Mosby.

Greenfield S, Whelan B, Cohn E: Use of dimensional analysis to reduce medication errors, *J Nurs Educ* 45(2):91, 2006.

Haynes RB and others: Interventions for enhancing medication adherence, *Cochrane Database Syst Rev* 2:2008.

Hess DR: Aerosol delivery devices in the treatment of asthma, *Respir Care* 53(6):699, 2008.

Hockenberry MJ, Wilson D: *Wong's essentials of pediatric nursing*, ed 8, St. Louis, 2009, Mosby.

Howland RH: Medication adherence, *J Psychosoc Nurs Ment Health Serv* 45(9):15, 2007.

Institute of Medicine: *Report brief: to err is human: building a safer health system*, 2003, http://www.iom.edu/CMS/8089/5575/4117.aspx.

Institute of Safe Medication Practices: *How fast is too fast for IV push medications?* 2003, http://www.ismp.org/Newsletters/acutecare/articles/20030515.asp.

Institute of Safe Medication Practices: *Tablet splitting: do it only if you "half" to, and then do it safely*, 2006, http://www.ismp.org/Newsletters/acutecare/articles/20060518.asp.

Institute of Safe Medication Practices: *Humulin R concentrate U-500*, 2007a, http://www.ismp.org/Newsletters/ambulatory/archives/200708_2.asp.

Institute of Safe Medication Practices: *ISMP's list of error-prone abbreviations, symbols, and dose designations*, 2007b, http://www.ismp.org/Tools/errorproneabbreviations.pdf.

Institute of Safe Medication Practices: *Confused drug name list*, 2008a, http://www.ismp.org/Tools/confuseddrugnames.pdf.

Institute of Safe Medication Practices: *Oral dosage forms that should not be crushed*, 2008b, http://www.ismp.org/Tools/DoNotCrush.pdf.

Institute of Safe Medication Practices: *Patches: what you can't see can harm patients*, reprinted from ISMP Medication Safety Alert! Nurse Advise-ERR (April 2007, Volume 5, Issue 4), with permission by the Institute for Safe Medication Practices, *KBN Connect* 14:8, Winter 2008c.

Institute of Safe Medication Practices: *Principles of designing a medication label for intravenous piggyback medication for patient specific, inpatient use*, 2008d, http://www.ismp.org/tools/guidelines/labelFormats/IVPB.asp.

Kairuz T and others: Identifying compliance issues with prescription medications among older people: a pilot study, *Drugs Aging* 25(2):153, 2008.

Karch AM, Karch FE: Not so fast! *Am J Nurs* 103(8):71, 2003.

Katz MG, Kripalani S, Weiss BD: Use of pictorial aids in medication instructions: a review of the literature, *Am J Health Syst Pharm* 63(1):2391, 2006.

Kripalani S and others: Medication use among inner-city patients after hospital discharge: patient-reported barriers and solutions, *Mayo Clin Proc* 83(5):529, 2008.

Lewis SL and others: *Medical-surgical nursing*, ed 7, St. Louis, 2007, Mosby.

Maneesakorn S and others: An RCT of adherence therapy for people with schizophrenia in Chiang Mai, Thailand, *J Clin Nurs* 16(7):1302, 2007.

Manno MS: Preventing adverse drug events, *Nursing* 36(3):56, 2006.

MayoClinic.com: *Asthma inhalers*, 2008, http://www.mayoclinic.com/health/asthma-inhalers/AS00019.

McIntyre LJ, Courey TJ: Safe medication administration, *J Nurs Care Qual* 22(1):40, 2007.

McKenry L, Tessier E, Hogan M: *Mosby's pharmacology in nursing*, ed 22, St. Louis, 2006, Mosby.

Metheny NA: Preventing aspiration in older adults with dysphagia, *Medsurg Nurs* 15(2):110, 2006.

Mills PD and others: Improving the bar-coded administration system at the Department of Veterans Affairs, *Am J Health Syst Pharm* 63:1442, 2006.

National Coordinating Council for Medication Error Reporting and Prevention: *Recommendations to reduce medication errors associated with verbal medication orders and prescriptions*, 2006, http://www.nccmerp.org/council/council2001-02-20.html.

Nicoll LH, Hesby A: Intramuscular injection: an integrative research review and guideline for evidence-based practice, *Appl Nurs Res* 16(2):149, 2002.

Novo Nordisk: *Levemir*, 2008, http://www.levemir-us.com/.

Occupational Safety and Health Administration: *Bloodborne pathogens and needlestick prevention: OSHA standards*, 2007, http://www.osha.gov/SLTC/bloodbornepathogens/standards.html.

Pandian JD and others: Nerve injuries following intramuscular injections: a clinical and neurophysiological study from northwest India, *J Peripher Nerv Syst* 11:165, 2006.

Paoletti RD and others: Using bar-code technology and medication observation methodology for safer medication administration, *Am J Health Syst Pharm* 64:536, 2007.

Phillips DP, Barker GEC, Eguchi MM: A steep increase in domestic fatal medication errors with use of alcohol and/or street drugs, *Arch Intern Med* 168(14):1561, 2008.

Preston ST, Hegadoren K: Glass contamination in parenterally administered medicine, *J Adv Nurs* 48(3):266, 2004.

Prettyman J: Subcutaneous or intramuscular? Confronting a parenteral administration dilemma, *Medsurg Nurs* 14(2):93, 2005.

Ptasinski C: Develop a medication reconciliation process, *Nurs Manage* 38(3):18, 2007.

Ross J: Collaboration—integrating nursing, pharmacy and information technology into a barcode medication administration system implementation, *Caring: Connecting, Sharing, & Advancing Healthcare Informatics* 23(1):1, 2008.

Rushing J: How to administer a subcutaneous injection, *Nursing* 34(6):32, 2004.

Sanofi-Aventis: *Dosing and administration of Lovenox*, 2007, http://www.lovenox.com/hcp/dosingAdministration/default.aspx.

Shin H, Kim MJ: Subcutaneous tissue thickness in children with type 1 diabetes, *J Adv Nurs* 54(1):29, 2006.

Sidhu AK: Polypharmacy and the elderly: a review of the literature, *Singapore Nurs J* 34(4):11, 2007.

Skibinski KA and others: Effects of technologic interventions on the safety of a medication-use system, *Am J Health Syst Pharm* 64:90, 2007.

Sunil TS, McGehee MA: Social and religious support on treatment adherence among HIV/AIDS patients by race/ethnicity, *HIV/AIDS Soc Serv* 6(1-2):83, 2007.

Sweet E and others: Relationships between skin color, income, and blood pressure among African Americans in the CARDIA study, *Am J Public Health* 97(12):2253, 2007.

Tang TS and others: Social support, quality of life, and self-care behaviors among African Americans with type 2 diabetes, *Diabetes Educ* 34(2):266, 2008.

The Joint Commission: *Joint Commission alert: prevent pediatric medication errors: children are three times more at risk than adults*, 2008a, http://www.jointcommission.org/NewsRoom/NewsReleases/nr_04_11_08.htm.

The Joint Commission: *2009 national patient safety goals: hospital program*, 2008b, http://www.jointcommission.org/PatientSafety/NationalPatientSafetyGoals/09_hap_npsgs.htm

Tseng C and others: Race/ethnicity and economic differences in cost-related medication underuse among insured adults with diabetes, *Diabetes Care* 31(2):261, 2007.

U.S. Department of Health and Human Services Substance Abuse and Mental Health Services Administration: *The NSDUH report: nonmedical use of pain relievers in substate regions, 2004-2006*, 2008, http://www.oas.samhsa.gov/2k8/pain/substate.cfm.

U.S. Food and Drug Administration: *MedWatch*, 2009, http://www.fda.gov/medwatch/index.html.

U.S. Pharmacopeia: *Similar drug names continue to be reported*, 2003, http://www.usp.org/patientSafety/newsletters/practitionerReportingNews/prn1082003-10-23.html.

U.S. Pharmacotherapy Associates, LLC: *USP chapter 797: compounding sterile preparations Q & A*, 2006, http://www.upa-llc.com/pdf/USP%20Chapter%20797newsletter%20FINAL%201-2006.pdf.

VisionRx: *Encyclopedia: eye drops*, 2005, http://www.visionrx.com/library/enc/enc_eye-drops.asp#top.

Weisner AM and others: Implication of food allergies and intolerances on medication administration, *Orthopedics* 31(2):149, 2008.

World Health Organization: *Injection safety: misuse and overuse of injection worldwide*, 2006, http://www.who.int/mediacentre/factsheets/fs231/en/.

Yin HS and others: Association of low caregiver health literacy with reported use of nonstandardized dosing instruments and lack of knowledge of weight-based dosage, *Ambul Pediatr* 7(4):292, 2007.

Zaybak A and others: Does obesity prevent the needle from reaching muscle in intramuscular injections? *J Adv Nurs* 58(6):552, 2007.

17 Fluid, Electrolyte, and Acid-Base Balances

MEDIA RESOURCES

 CD COMPANION 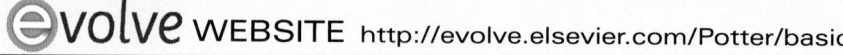 WEBSITE http://evolve.elsevier.com/Potter/basic

- Video Clips
- Crossword Puzzle
- Butterfield's Fluids and Electrolytes Tutorial
- English/Spanish Audio Glossary

OBJECTIVES

- Describe the basic physiological mechanism responsible for maintaining fluid and electrolyte balance.
- Describe the processes involved in acid-base balance.
- Discuss common disturbances in fluid, electrolyte, and acid-base balances.
- Discuss and identify factors that affect normal fluid, electrolyte, and acid-base balances.
- Discuss clinical assessments for determining fluid, electrolyte, and acid-base imbalances.

- List and discuss appropriate nursing interventions for patients with fluid, electrolyte, and acid-base imbalances.
- Describe purpose and procedures for initiation and maintenance of intravenous therapy.
- Calculate an intravenous flow rate.
- Discuss complications of intravenous therapy.
- Demonstrate how to change intravenous solutions, tubing, and dressings.
- Describe the procedure for initiating a blood transfusion and the complications of blood therapy.

KEY TERMS

acidosis, p. 474
active transport, p. 469
allogeneic (homologous)
 transfusion, p. 493
aldosterone, p. 470
alkalosis, p. 474
angiotensin, p. 470
anion gap, p. 476
anions, p. 468

antidiuretic hormone
 (ADH), p. 469
arterial blood gas (ABG),
 p. 473
atrial natriuretic peptide
 (ANP), p. 470
autologous transfusion,
 p. 492
buffer, p. 471

cations, p. 468
colloid osmotic
 pressure, p. 469
colloids, p. 486
concentration gradient,
 p. 468
crystalloids, p. 486
dehydration, p. 469
diffusion, p. 468

electrolyte, p. 468
electronic infusion
 device (EID), p. 488
filtration, p. 468
fluid volume deficit
 (FVD), p. 477
fluid volume excess
 (FVE), p. 486

KEY TERMS, CONT'D

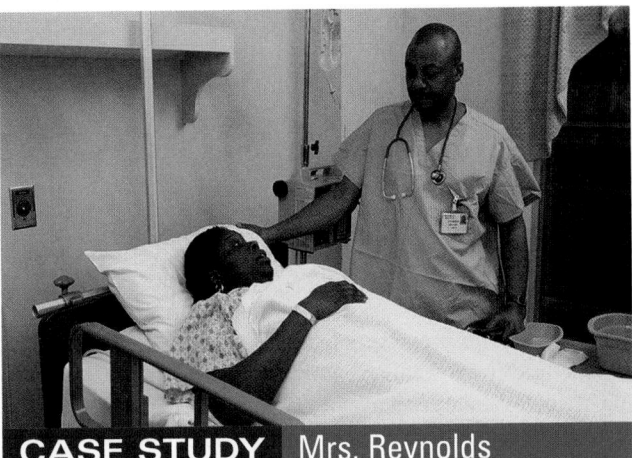

CASE STUDY Mrs. Reynolds

Susan Reynolds, a 42-year-old married accountant, has just been admitted to the acute care unit with a history of nausea, loss of appetite, and vomiting and diarrhea for 7 days. She feels her symptoms are related to "bad food" she had on her recent business trip. Past medical history includes hypertension controlled by furosemide (Lasix) 40 mg by mouth once a day and a no-salt-added diet.

Robert is a junior nursing student assigned to Mrs. Reynolds. He has cared for other patients with gastrointestinal problems but never one with fluid and electrolyte problems. Robert plans his care by reviewing Mrs. Reynolds' chart and health care provider's orders.

longed episodes of vomiting or diarrhea. Acid-base balance is necessary for many physiological processes. Imbalances alter respiration, metabolism, and cardiovascular, renal, muscular, hematological, immunological, and nervous system function (Monahan and others, 2007). Your knowledge and understanding of the mechanisms that contribute to fluid, electrolyte, and acid-base imbalances are essential.

SCIENTIFIC KNOWLEDGE BASE

Water is the largest single component of the body; 60% of the average adult male's weight is fluid. The proportion of water is lower in women and older adults, but higher in infants (Brownie, 2006; Weinstein, 2006). A healthy, mobile, well-oriented adult usually maintains normal fluid, electrolyte, and acid-base balances because of the body's adaptive physiological mechanisms.

Distribution of Body Fluids

Body fluids are distributed in two distinct compartments, one containing intracellular fluid (ICF) and the other extracellular fluid (ECF). ICF comprises all fluid within body cells. This fluid contains dissolved solutes essential for cell fluid and electrolyte balance and metabolism. In adults approximately 42% of body weight is ICF (Edwards, 2006).

ECF is all fluid outside a cell, which is divided into three smaller compartments: interstitial, intravascular fluids, and transcellular fluid. ECF makes up about 17% of total body weight, or one third of the total body water. Interstitial fluid is the fluid between cells and outside the blood vessels. Intravascular fluid is blood plasma found in the vascular system. A cellular barrier separates transcellular fluid, which consists of cerebrospinal, pleural, gastrointestinal (GI), intraocular, peritoneal, and synovial fluids. A loss of or significant increase in transcellular fluid produces fluid and electrolyte disturbance (e.g., ascites) (Lewis and others, 2007).

Fluid, electrolyte, and acid-base balance within the body maintains health and function in all body systems. The body maintains a balance through the intake and output (I&O) of water and electrolytes, their distribution in the body, and regulation by the renal and pulmonary systems. Imbalances result from illness, altered fluid intake, or pro-

Composition of Body Fluids

Body fluid contains substances that are sometimes called minerals or salts but are technically electrolytes. An **electrolyte** is an element or compound that, when dissolved in water or another **solvent,** separates into ions that are electrically charged. Positively charged electrolytes are **cations** (e.g., sodium [Na^+]). Negatively charged electrolytes are **anions** (e.g., chloride [Cl^-]). Although the level of individual electrolytes differs in ECF and ICF, the total number of anions and cations in each fluid compartment is usually the same. Electrolytes are measured in **milliequivalents per liter (mEq/L).**

Movement of Body Fluids

A cell wall and capillary membrane separate each body compartment. Fluids and electrolytes constantly shift from compartment to compartment to meet a variety of metabolic needs, such as urine formation. The movement of fluids between the ICF and ECF spaces depends on cell membrane permeability. Fluids and solutes move across cell membranes by four processes: diffusion, osmosis, filtration, and active transport.

Diffusion is a process in which a **solute** (gas or solid) in a **solution** moves from an area of higher concentration to an area of lower concentration (Figure 17-1). The initial difference in the two concentrations is known as a **concentration gradient.** The outcome is an even distribution of the solute within the solution. For example, when a small amount of cream is poured into a cup of black coffee, the cream mixes or diffuses through the whole cup (Chernecky and others, 2006). For fluids and electrolytes to diffuse across the cellular membrane, the membrane must be permeable.

Osmosis is the movement of a solvent such as water across a semipermeable membrane from an area of lower concentration to one that has a higher concentration (Figure 17-2). Osmosis equalizes the concentration of molecules (ions) on each side of the membrane. Boiling a hot dog is an example

of osmosis. The concentration of molecules inside the hot dog is greater than in water. The water passes through the hot dog skin, which is a semipermeable membrane, to equalize the number of molecules on both sides of the membrane. Finally, when the hot dog is unable to hold more water, the skin, or semipermeable membrane, ruptures.

When a solution is more concentrated on one side of a selectively permeable membrane and a less concentrated on the other side, there is a pull called **osmotic pressure.** Water is drawn through the membrane to the more concentrated side. When the solutions on both sides of the semipermeable membrane have reached an equilibrium, or are equal in concentration, they are isotonic. The osmotic pressure of a solution, or the ability to affect the movement of water, is **osmolality.** It is measured in milliosmoles per kilogram (mOsm/kg). Changes in extracellular osmolality result in changes in both ECF and ICF volume. Another term that describes the concentration of solutions is **osmolarity,** which reflects the number of molecules in a liter of solution. It is measured in milliosmoles per liter (mOsm/L). Water loss increases osmolality, whereas overhydration (water gain) decreases it (Goertz, 2006).

Solutions are **hypertonic, isotonic,** or **hypotonic.** Infusion of hypertonic intravenous (IV) solutions (a solution of higher-than-normal osmotic pressure), such as 3% sodium chloride, pulls fluid from cells, causing them to shrink. Isotonic solutions such as 0.9% sodium chloride (a solution of equal osmotic pressure) expand the body's intravascular fluid volume without causing a fluid shift from one compartment to another. Hypotonic solutions (a solution of lower-than-normal osmotic pressure), such as 0.45% sodium chloride, moves fluid from the intravascular space into the cells, causing them to enlarge. Each of these actions occurs through osmosis. Diffusion and osmosis are passive processes that do not require energy from the body's cells.

Filtration is a process in which water and diffusible substances move across a membrane, in response to fluid pres-

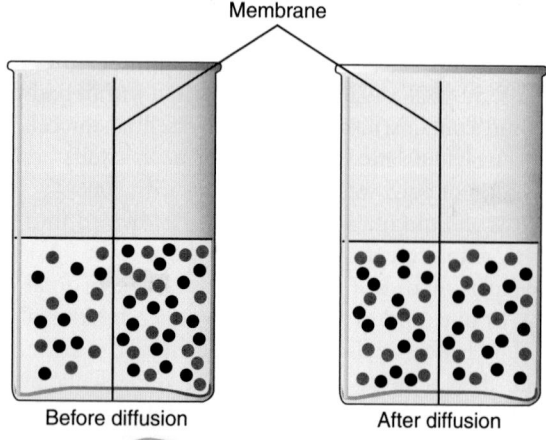

Figure 17-1 ■ Diffusion across a semipermeable membrane. (From Lewis SM and others: *Medical-surgical nursing: assessment and management of clinical problems,* ed 7, St. Louis, 2007, Mosby.)

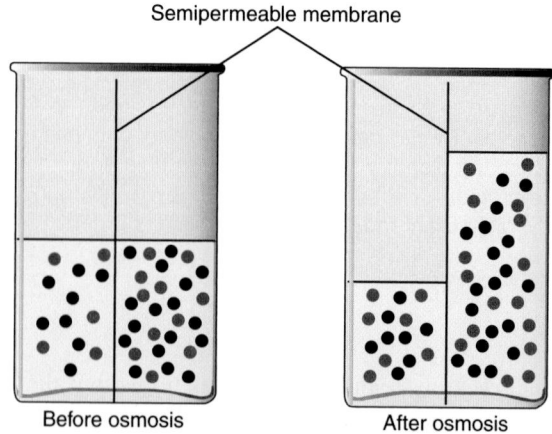

Figure 17-2 ■ Osmosis through a semipermeable membrane. (From Lewis SM and others: *Medical-surgical nursing: assessment and management of clinical problems,* ed 7, St. Louis, 2007, Mosby.)

sure, from an area of higher pressure to lower pressure. **Hydrostatic pressure** is the force of the fluid pressing outward against a surface. At the arterial end of a capillary, the hydrostatic pressure is greater than the **colloid osmotic pressure (oncotic pressure)**, causing fluid and diffusible solutes to move out of the capillary into the interstitial space. At the venous end, the colloid osmotic pressure, or pull, is greater than the hydrostatic pressure, and fluids and some solutes move into the capillary from the interstitial space. The lymph channels return excess fluid and solutes in the interstitial space to the intravascular compartment. The pressure at the capillary bed is the colloid osmotic pressure. The body does not allow blood plasma proteins, especially albumin, to pass freely out of the vasculature because the capillary membrane is impermeable to proteins (colloids). Maintaining blood proteins within the capillary enhances the osmotic pressure.

Active transport is the movement of molecules or ions "uphill" against osmotic pressures to an area of higher concentration. Metabolic activity and energy consumption move substances across cell membranes. An example of active transport is the sodium-potassium-ATPase pump, which moves sodium out of the cell and returns potassium to the inside of the cell (Figure 17-3).

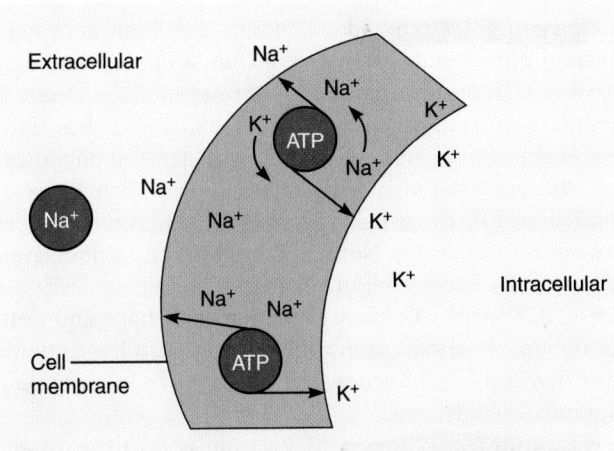

Figure 17-3 ■ The sodium-potassium pump. (From Lewis SM and others: *Medical-surgical nursing: assessment and management of clinical problems,* ed 7, St. Louis, 2007, Mosby.)

Regulation of Body Fluids

Homeostasis is body fluid balance throughout the internal environment of the body. Fluid intake, hormonal controls, and fluid output regulate body fluids. In health, the body readily responds to fluid and electrolyte disturbances to prevent or repair damage so as to maintain homeostasis.

FLUID INTAKE A major factor that influences fluid intake is the thirst mechanism (Chernecky and others, 2006). The thirst-control center is in the hypothalamus of the brain. The **osmoreceptors** continually monitor serum osmotic pressure and when osmolality increases, the hypothalamus stimulates thirst. Eating salty foods increases the osmotic pressure of the body fluids and stimulates the thirst mechanism (Monahan and others, 2007). Increased plasma osmolality occurs as a result of any condition that restricts the oral ingestion of fluids or increases the intake of hypertonic fluids. The hypothalamus is stimulated when excess fluid is lost and **hypovolemia** occurs, as in excessive vomiting and hemorrhage.

The average adult's daily fluid intake (Table 17-1) ranges between 2200 and 2700 mL and consists of oral intake of fluids and solid foods as well as oxidative metabolism (Heitz and Horne, 2005). Water oxidation (oxidative metabolism) is the by-product of cellular metabolism of ingested foods. Oral fluid intake requires an alert state. Infants, patients with neurological or psychological problems, and some older adults who are unable to perceive or respond to the thirst mechanism are at risk for **dehydration** (Brownie, 2006; Goertz, 2006).

HORMONAL REGULATION Hormones regulate fluid intake through different mechanisms. **Antidiuretic hormone (ADH)** is stored in the posterior pituitary gland and is released in response to changes in blood osmolarity. ADH prevents diuresis, thus causing the body to reabsorb water. An increase in serum osmolarity stimulates the osmoreceptors in the hypothalamus to release ADH. ADH works directly on the renal tubules and collecting ducts to make them more permeable to water. This in turn causes water to return to the systemic circulation, which dilutes the blood and decreases its osmolarity. The patient will experience a temporary decrease in urinary output as the body tries to compensate. When the blood becomes diluted, the osmoreceptors stop the release of ADH to restore urine output.

TABLE 17-1	Adult Average Daily Intake and Output			
FLUID INTAKE	(mL)		**FLUID OUTPUT**	(mL)
Oral fluids	1100-1400		Kidneys	1200-1500
Solid foods	800-1000		Skin	500-600
Oxidative metabolism	300		Lungs	400
			Gastrointestinal	100-200
Total gains	**2200-2700**		**Total losses**	**2200-2700**

From Heitz UE, Horne MM: *Mosby's pocket guide series: fluid, electrolyte, and acid-base balance,* ed 5, St. Louis, 2005, Mosby.

Alterations in renal perfusion stimulate the renin-angiotensin-aldosterone mechanism. The body releases **renin,** a proteolytic enzyme, in response to decreased renal perfusion caused by a decrease in extracellular volume. Renin acts to produce **angiotensin** I, which causes some vasoconstriction. However, angiotensin I almost immediately becomes reduced by an enzyme that converts angiotension I into angiotensin II. Angiotensin II then causes massive selective vasoconstriction of many blood vessels to relocate and increase blood flow to the kidneys, improving renal perfusion. In addition, angiotensin II also stimulates the release of aldosterone.

The adrenal cortex releases **aldosterone** to counteract hypovolemia in response to increased plasma potassium levels or as a part of the renin-angiotensin-aldosterone mechanism. Aldosterone acts on the distal portion of the renal tubule to increase the reabsorption (saving) of sodium and the secretion and excretion of potassium and hydrogen. Because sodium retention leads to water retention, the release of aldosterone acts as a volume regulator (Heitz and Horne, 2005). The outcome of the renin-angiotensin-aldosterone mechanism is retention of sodium and water, leading to increased blood volume (Chernecky and others, 2006).

Atrial natriuretic peptide (ANP) is a hormone that promotes vasodilation. ANP is secreted from cells of the atria of the heart in response to atrial stretching and an increase in circulating blood volume. ANP acts as a diuretic that causes sodium loss and diminishes the thirst mechanism. There is value in monitoring ANP when evaluating fluid and electrolyte balance (Martinez-Rumayor and others, 2008).

FLUID OUTPUT REGULATION Fluid output (see Table 17-1) occurs through four organs of water loss: the kidneys, skin, lungs, and GI tract. The kidneys are the major regulatory organs of fluid balance. They receive approximately 180 L of plasma to filter each day and produce 1200 to 1500 mL of urine (Heitz and Horne, 2005). Urine volume changes based on intake.

Insensible water loss is continuous and occurs through the skin and lungs. This type of fluid loss increases with fever (Madara and Pomarico-Denino, 2008). **Sensible water loss** occurs through visible perspiration. The amount of sensible perspiration is directly related to the stimulation of the sweat glands. The sympathetic nervous system regulates water loss from the skin by activating sweat glands. Water loss from the skin occurs both sensibly and insensibly through diffusion or perspiration. An average of 500 to 600 mL of sensible and insensible fluid is lost via the skin each day (Heitz and Horne, 2005).

The lungs expire about 400 mL of water daily (Heitz and Horne, 2005). This insensible water loss changes in response to respiratory rate and depth. In addition, the administration of nonhumidified supplemental oxygen increases insensible water loss from the lungs.

Under normal conditions, the GI tract accounts for only 100 to 200 mL of fluid loss through the feces each day, but plays a vital role in fluid regulation. Approximately 3 to 6 L of isotonic fluid moves in and out of the GI tract daily. When diseased, the GI tract can become a site of major fluid loss.

Regulation of Electrolytes

CATIONS Major cations within the body fluids include sodium (Na^+), potassium (K^+), calcium (Ca^{2+}), and magnesium (Mg^{2+}). Cations interchange when one cation leaves the cell and is replaced by another. This occurs because cells tend to maintain electrical neutrality.

Sodium Regulation Sodium is the most abundant cation (90%) in ECF. Sodium ions are the major contributors to maintaining water balance through their effect on serum osmolality, nerve impulse transmission, regulation of acid-base balance, and participation in cellular chemical reactions (Huether and McCance, 2008). Dietary intake and aldosterone secretion regulate sodium intake. The normal extracellular sodium concentration is 135 to 145 mEq/L.

Potassium Regulation Potassium is the predominant intracellular electrolyte (Monahan and others, 2007). Only 2% of the body's potassium is located within the ECF. It regulates many metabolic activities and is necessary for glycogen deposits in the liver and skeletal muscle, transmission and conduction of nerve impulses, normal cardiac conduction, and skeletal and smooth muscle contraction (Huether and McCance, 2008). The normal range for serum potassium concentrations is 3.5 to 5 mEq/L. Dietary intake and renal excretion regulate potassium. The body conserves potassium poorly, so any condition that increases urine output decreases serum potassium.

Calcium Regulation Bone, plasma, and body cells store calcium. Ninety-nine percent of calcium is in bone, and only 1% is in ECF. Approximately 50% of calcium in the plasma is bound to protein, primarily albumin, and 40% is free (ionized) calcium. The ionized calcium participates in physiological changes associated with hypocalcemia. High levels of ionized calcium in the ECF cause lethargy and coma, whereas low levels cause tetany. Normal serum ionized calcium levels range from 4.5 to 5.5 mg/dL. Normal total calcium levels are 8.5 to 10.5 mg/dL. Calcium is necessary for bone and teeth formation, blood clotting, hormone secretion, cell membrane integrity, cardiac conduction, transmission of nerve impulses, and muscle contraction.

Magnesium Regulation Magnesium is essential for enzyme and neurochemical activities and cardiac and skeletal muscle excitability. Normal plasma concentrations of magnesium range from 1.5 to 2.5 mEq/L. Dietary intake, renal mechanisms, and parathyroid hormone (PTH) regulate serum magnesium levels.

ANIONS The three major body fluid anions are chloride (Cl^-), bicarbonate (HCO_3^-), and phosphate (PO_4^{3-}).

Chloride Regulation Chloride is the major anion in ECF. The transport of chloride follows sodium. Normal serum concentrations of chloride range from 95 to 105 mEq/L. Dietary intake and the kidneys regulate serum chloride level. A person with normal renal function who has a high chloride intake will excrete a higher amount of urine chloride.

Bicarbonate Regulation Bicarbonate is the major chemical base buffer within the body. Bicarbonate ions are found in both ECF and ICF and are a key component of the carbonic acid–bicarbonate buffering system essential to acid-base balance. The kidneys regulate bicarbonate levels. Normal arterial bicarbonate levels range between 22 and 26 mEq/L; normal venous bicarbonate (carbon dioxide content) is 24 to 30 mEq/L.

Phosphorus-Phosphate Regulation. Nearly all the phosphorus in the body exists in the form of phosphate (PO_4^{3-}), which assists in the regulation of acid-base balance. The terms *phosphate* and *phosphorus* are often used interchangeably. Phosphate and calcium are required to develop and maintain bones and teeth. Phosphate also promotes normal neuromuscular action and participates in carbohydrate metabolism. Calcium and phosphate are inversely proportional; if one rises, the other falls. The body normally absorbs phosphate through the GI tract. Dietary intake, renal excretion, intestinal absorption, and PTH regulate phosphate. The normal serum level is 2.8 to 4.5 mg/dL.

Regulation of Acid-Base Balance

Metabolic processes require a steady balance between acids and bases for optimal cell functioning. Acids are a product of cellular metabolism and are continuously buffered by body systems. The lungs and kidneys are the buffering systems that neutralize acids and bases. A **buffer** is a substance or a group of substances that absorb or release hydrogen ion (H^+) to correct an acid-base imbalance. Arterial pH is an indirect measurement of H^+ concentration. For example, the greater the concentration of H^+, the more acidic the solution and the lower the pH; the lower the concentration of H^+ ions, the more alkaline the solution and the higher the pH. The pH is also a reflection of the balance between carbon dioxide (CO_2), an acid, which the lungs regulate, and bicarbonate (HCO_3^-), a base, which the kidneys regulate (Arnett, 2008). Acid-base balance exists when the rate at which the body produces acids or bases equals the rate of excretion. This balance results in a stable concentration of H^+ in body fluids, expressed as the pH value. Normal hydrogen ion levels are necessary to maintain cell membrane integrity and regulate cellular enzymatic reactions. The pH is a scale for measuring fluid acidity or alkalinity. A pH value of 7 is neutral; below 7 is acid, and above 7 is alkaline. Normal values in arterial blood range from 7.35 to 7.45. The three general types of acid-base regulators within the body are chemical (the carbonic acid–bicarbonate buffer system), biological (the absorption and release of hydrogen ions by cells), and physiological buffering systems (the lungs and the kidneys).

Disturbances in Electrolyte, Fluid, and Acid-Base Balances

Disturbances in electrolyte, fluid, or acid-base balances seldom occur alone, and they disrupt normal body processes (Table 17-2). It is important for you as a nurse to be familiar

TABLE 17-2   Electrolyte Imbalances

IMBALANCE AND RELATED CAUSES	SIGNS AND SYMPTOMS
HYPONATREMIA GI loss: Vomiting, diarrhea, NG suction Renal loss: Kidney disease resulting in salt wasting; diuretics; adrenal insufficiency Skin loss: Excessive perspiration; burns Psychogenic polydipsia Syndrome of inappropriate ADH (SIADH)	*Physical examination:* Apprehension, postural hypotension, postural dizziness, abdominal cramping, nausea and vomiting, diarrhea, tachycardia, dry mucous membranes, confusion, seizures, and coma *Laboratory findings:* Serum sodium level **below** 135 mEq/L, serum osmolality **below** 280 mOsm/kg, and urine specific gravity **below** 1.010 (if not caused by SIADH)
HYPERNATREMIA Excess salt intake: Ingestion of large amounts of concentrated salt solutions; iatrogenic administration of hypertonic saline solution parenterally Excess aldosterone secretion Diabetes insipidus Increased sensible and insensible water loss Water deprivation	*Physical examination:* Extreme thirst, dry and flushed skin, dry and sticky tongue and mucous membranes, postural hypotension, fever, agitation, seizures, restlessness, and irritability *Laboratory findings:* Serum sodium levels **above** 145 mEq/L, serum osmolality **above** 300 mOsm/kg, and urine specific gravity **above** 1.030 (if not caused by diabetes insipidus)
HYPOKALEMIA Use of potassium-wasting diuretics Diarrhea, vomiting, or other GI losses Alkalosis Excess aldosterone secretion Polyuria Excessive perspiration Excessive use of potassium-free IV solutions Treatment of diabetic ketoacidosis with insulin	*Physical examination:* Weakness and fatigue, muscle weakness, abdominal distention, decreased bowel sounds, ventricular dysrhythmias, paresthesias, and weak, irregular pulse *Laboratory findings:* Serum potassium level **below** 3.5 mEq/L and electrocardiogram (ECG) abnormalities: flattened T wave; ST segment depression; U wave; ventricular dysrhythmias*

*Data from Heitz U, Horne MM: *Mosby's pocket guide series: fluid, electrolyte, and acid-base balance,* ed 5, St. Louis, 2005, Mosby.

Continued

TABLE 17-2   Electrolyte Imbalances—cont'd

IMBALANCE AND RELATED CAUSES	SIGNS AND SYMPTOMS
HYPERKALEMIA Renal failure Fluid volume deficit Massive cellular damage (e.g., burns and trauma) Iatrogenic administration of large amounts of potassium intravenously Adrenal insufficiency Acidosis, especially diabetic ketoacidosis Rapid infusion of stored blood Use of potassium-sparing diuretics Ingestion of K^+ salt substitutes	*Physical examination:* Anxiety, dysrhythmias, paresthesia, weakness, abdominal cramps, and diarrhea *Laboratory findings:* Serum potassium level 5.3 mEq/L and ECG abnormalities: peaked T wave and widened QRS complex (bradycardia, heart block, dysrhythmias); eventually QRS pattern widens and cardiac arrest occurs*
HYPOCALCEMIA Rapid administration of blood transfusions containing citrate Hypoalbuminemia Hypoparathyroidism Vitamin D deficiency Pancreatitis Alkalosis Chronic renal failure Chronic alcoholism	*Physical examination:* Numbness and tingling of fingers and circumoral (around mouth) region, hyperactive reflexes, positive Chvostek's sign (contraction of facial muscles when facial nerve is tapped), tetany, muscle cramps, and pathological fractures (chronic hypocalcemia) *Laboratory findings:* Serum ionized calcium level **below** 4.5 mEq/L or total serum calcium **below** 8.5 mg/100 dL; ECG abnormalities: ventricular tachycardia
HYPERCALCEMIA Hyperparathyroidism Osteometastasis Paget's disease Osteoporosis Prolonged immobilization Acidosis Thiazide diuretics	*Physical examination:* Anorexia, nausea and vomiting, hypoactive reflexes, lethargy, flank pain (from kidney stones), decreased level of consciousness, personality changes, and cardiac arrest *Laboratory findings:* Serum ionized calcium level **above** 5.5 mEq/L or total serum calcium level **above** 10.5 mg/dL; x-ray examination showing generalized osteoporosis, urinary stones; elevated BUN level **above** 25 mg/100 mL and elevated creatinine level **above** 1.5 mg/100 mL caused by FVD or renal damage caused by urolithiasis (renal stones); ECG abnormalities: heart block
HYPOMAGNESEMIA Inadequate intake: Malnutrition and alcoholism Inadequate absorption or loss: Diarrhea, vomiting, nasogastric drainage, fistulas; diseases of small intestine Excessive loss from thiazide diuretics Aldosterone excess Polyuria	*Physical examination:* Muscular tremors, hyperactive deep tendon reflexes, confusion and disorientation, tachycardia, hypertension, dysrhythmias, and positive Chvostek's sign *Laboratory findings:* Serum magnesium level **below** 1.5 mEq/L
HYPERMAGNESEMIA Renal failure Excess oral or parenteral intake of magnesium	*Physical examination:* Acute elevations in magnesium levels: hypoactive deep tendon reflexes, decreased depth and rate of respirations, hypotension, and flushing *Laboratory findings:* Serum magnesium level **above** 2.5 mEq/L; ECG abnormalities: prolonged QT interval, AV block

ADH, Antidiuretic hormone; *AV,* atrioventricular; *BUN,* blood urea nitrogen; *FVD,* fluid volume deficit; *GI,* gastrointestinal; *NG,* nasogastric.

with the types of imbalances and their effects on body functioning.

ELECTROLYTE IMBALANCES

Sodium Imbalances **Hyponatremia** is a lower-than-normal concentration of sodium in the blood (serum), which occurs when there is a net sodium loss or a net water excess (see Table 17-2). Clinical indicators and treatment of hyponatremia depend on the cause and whether ECF volume is normal, decreased, or increased (Verbalis and others, 2007). The common causes are sodium deficit or free water excess. Both of these cause intracellular overhydration. When there is a sodium deficit, the osmotic pressure of the ECF decreases and water moves into the cells. Plasma volume decreases, leading to signs of hypovolemia. With free water excess, both the ICF and ECF volume increase, causing symptoms of hypervolemia (McCance & Huether, 2006).

Hypernatremia is a greater-than-normal concentration of sodium in ECF caused by excess water loss or an overall sodium excess (see Table 17-2). When increased aldosterone secretion causes hypernatremia, sodium is retained and potassium is excreted. When hypernatremia occurs, the body conserves as much water as possible through renal reabsorption.

Potassium Imbalances **Hypokalemia** is one of the most common electrolyte imbalances, produced by an inadequate amount of potassium in the ECF (see Table 17-2). When severe, hypokalemia affects cardiac conduction and function. Because the normal amount of serum potassium is so small, the body cannot tolerate fluctuations. The most common causes of hypokalemia are vomiting and the use of potassium-wasting diuretics.

Hyperkalemia is a greater-than-normal amount of potassium in the blood. Severe hyperkalemia produces marked cardiac conduction abnormalities (see Table 17-2). The primary cause of hyperkalemia is renal failure, because any decrease in renal function diminishes the amount of potassium a kidney can excrete.

Calcium Imbalances **Hypocalcemia** represents a drop in total serum and/or ionized calcium. It results from several illnesses that affect the thyroid or parathyroid glands (see Table 17-2). Another cause of hypocalcemia is renal insufficiency. When the kidneys cannot excrete sufficient phosphorus, the phosphorus level rises and the calcium level declines. Signs and symptoms are related to the physiological role of serum calcium in neuromuscular and cardiac function.

Hypercalcemia is an increase in the total serum concentration of calcium and/or ionized calcium. Hypercalcemia is frequently a symptom of an underlying disease such as a neoplasm, resulting in excess bone resorption with release of calcium. Prolonged immobilization also causes bone loss of calcium.

Magnesium Imbalances **Hypomagnesemia,** a drop in serum magnesium levels, occurs with malnutrition and malabsorption disorders. **Hypermagnesemia,** an increase in serum magnesium levels, is often the result of excess magnesium intake. Table 17-2 summarizes magnesium level disturbances. Symptoms are the result of changes in neuromuscular excitability.

Chloride Imbalances **Hypochloremia** occurs when the serum chloride level falls below normal. It is frequently associated with sodium imbalance. Vomiting or excessive nasogastric or fistula drainage results in hypochloremia because of the hydrochloric acid loss. The use of loop and thiazide diuretics also increases chloride excretion in conjunction with sodium excretion. When serum chloride levels fall, metabolic alkalosis results. The body adapts by increasing reabsorption of bicarbonate ions to maintain electrical neutrality.

Hyperchloremia occurs when the serum chloride level rises above normal, which usually occurs when the serum bicarbonate value falls or sodium level rises. Hypochloremia and hyperchloremia rarely occur as single disease processes but are commonly associated with acid-base imbalance. There are no unique signs and symptoms associated with these two ion alterations.

FLUID DISTURBANCES The two basic types of fluid imbalances are isotonic and osmolar (Table 17-3). An isotonic deficit or excess exists when water and electrolytes are gained or lost in equal proportions. In contrast, osmolar imbalances are losses or excesses of only water, which in turn affect the concentration (osmolality) of the serum.

ACID-BASE BALANCE Acid or alkaline levels in the blood regulate the body's chemical balance. **Arterial blood gas (ABG)** analysis is an effective method of evaluating acid-base balance and oxygenation. Measurement of ABG levels involves understanding six components: pH, $PaCO_2$, PaO_2, oxygen saturation, base excess, and HCO_3^-. Deviation from a normal value indicates that the patient is experiencing an acid-base imbalance.

pH The pH measures H^+ concentration in body fluids. Even a slight change is potentially life threatening. An increase in concentration of H^+ makes a solution more acidic; a decrease makes the solution more alkaline. Normal arterial blood pH value is 7.35 to 7.45 (acidic is less than 7.35, and alkalotic is greater than 7.45).

$PaCO_2$ $PaCO_2$ is the partial pressure of carbon dioxide in arterial blood and is a reflection of pulmonary ventilation. The normal range is 35 to 45 mm Hg. Hyperventilation produces a $PaCO_2$ of less than 35 mm Hg. As rate and depth of respiration increase, more carbon dioxide is exhaled and the carbon dioxide concentration decreases. Hypoventilation produces a $PaCO_2$ of more than 45 mm Hg. As rate and depth of respiration decrease, less carbon dioxide is exhaled and more is retained, which increases the concentration of carbon dioxide dissolved in the blood.

PaO_2 PaO_2 is the partial pressure of oxygen in arterial blood. Normal range is 80 to 100 mm Hg. When PaO_2 is within normal range, it has no primary role in acid-base regulation. A PaO_2 less than 60 mm Hg leads to anaerobic metabolism, resulting in lactic acid production and metabolic acidosis. There is a normal decline in PaO_2 in older adults (Reuben and others, 2008). Hypoxemia can result in hyperventilation leading to respiratory alkalosis.

Oxygen Saturation Oxygen saturation is the percentage of hemoglobin molecules saturated by oxygen (O_2). Changes

TABLE 17-3 Fluid Disturbances

IMBALANCE AND RELATED CAUSES	SIGNS AND SYMPTOMS
ISOTONIC IMBALANCES	
Fluid Volume Deficit (FVD)—Water and Electrolytes Lost in Equal or Isotonic Proportions	
GI loss: Diarrhea, vomiting, or drainage from fistulas or tubes Loss of plasma or whole blood, such as with burns or hemorrhage Excessive perspiration Fever Decreased oral intake of fluids Use of diuretics Confusion or depression	*Physical examination:* Postural hypotension, tachycardia, dry mucous membranes, poor skin turgor, thirst, confusion, rapid weight loss, slow vein filling, flat neck veins, lethargy, oliguria (urine output **below** 30 mL/hr), weak pulse *Laboratory findings:* Urine specific gravity **above** 1.030, increased hematocrit level **above** 50%, and increased BUN level **above** 25 mg/100 mL (hemoconcentration)
Fluid Volume Excess (FVE)—Water and Sodium Retained in Isotonic Proportions	
Heart failure Renal failure Cirrhosis of the liver Increased serum aldosterone and steroid levels Excessive sodium intake or administration	*Physical examination:* Rapid weight gain, edema (especially in dependent areas), hypertension, polyuria (if renal mechanisms are normal), neck vein distention, increased blood and venous pressure, crackles in lungs, confusion *Laboratory findings:* Decreased hematocrit level **below** 38% and decreased BUN level **below** 10 mg/100 mL (hemodilution)
OSMOLAR IMBALANCES	
Hyperosmolar Imbalance—Dehydration	
Diabetes insipidus Interruption of neurologically driven thirst drive Diabetic ketoacidosis Osmotic diuresis Administration of hypertonic parenteral fluids or tube feedings	*Physical examination:* Dry and sticky mucous membranes, flushed and dry skin, thirst, elevated body temperature, irritability, seizures, coma *Laboratory findings:* Increased serum sodium level **above** 145 mEq/L and increased serum osmolality **above** 295 mOsm/kg
Hypoosmolar Imbalance—Water Excess	
Syndrome of inappropriate antidiuretic hormone (SIADH) Excess water intake	*Physical examination:* Decreased level of consciousness, seizures, coma *Laboratory findings:* Decreased serum sodium level **below** 135 mEq/L and decreased serum osmolality **below** 280 mOsm/kg

BUN, Blood urea nitrogen; *GI,* gastrointestinal.

in temperature, pH, and $PaCO_2$ affect oxygen saturation levels. Normal range is greater than 90%.

Base Excess Base excess (or deficit) is the amount of blood buffer (hemoglobin and bicarbonate) present in the blood. A positive value indicates **alkalosis,** and a negative value indicates **acidosis.** The normal range is ±2 mEq/L.

Bicarbonate Serum bicarbonate (HCO_3^-) is the major renal determinant of acid-base balance and the principal buffer of the extracellular fluid. The kidneys excrete or retain HCO_3^- to maintain a normal acid-base environment. The normal range is 22 to 26 mEq/L. Levels less than 22 mEq/L usually indicate metabolic acidosis; a level greater than 26 mEq/L indicates metabolic alkalosis.

Types of Acid-Base Imbalances Acid-base imbalances are either respiratory or metabolic. The four primary types of acid-base imbalance are respiratory acidosis, respiratory al-

kalosis, metabolic acidosis, and metabolic alkalosis (Table 17-4). However, mixed conditions also exist.

Respiratory acidosis is an increased arterial carbon dioxide concentration ($PaCO_2$), excess carbonic acid (H_2CO_3), and an increased hydrogen ion concentration (pH less than 7.35). Hypoventilation causes respiratory acidosis, which causes the cerebrospinal fluid and brain cells to become acidic, producing neurological changes. Respiratory depression can also cause hypoxemia, resulting in further neurological impairment. Electrolyte changes such as hyperkalemia and hypercalcemia accompany acidosis.

Respiratory alkalosis is a decreased $PaCO_2$ and increased pH (greater than 7.45). Respiratory alkalosis begins outside the respiratory system (e.g., toxins or anxiety-producing hyperventilation) or within the respiratory system (e.g., initial phase of an asthma attack).

TABLE 17-4   Acid-Base Imbalances

IMBALANCE AND RELATED CAUSES	SIGNS AND SYMPTOMS
RESPIRATORY ACIDOSIS	
Hypoventilation Resulting From Primary Respiratory Problems	
Atelectasis (obstruction of small airways often caused by retained mucus) Pneumonia Cystic fibrosis Respiratory failure Airway obstruction Chest wall injury	*Physical examination:* Confusion, dizziness, lethargy, headache, dysrhythmias, warm and flushed skin, muscular twitching, seizures, and coma *Laboratory findings:* Arterial blood gas alterations pH **below** 7.35, PaCO$_2$ **above** 45 mm Hg, PaO$_2$ **below** 80 mm Hg, and bicarbonate level normal (if uncompensated) or **above** 26 mEq/L (if compensated)
Hypoventilation Resulting From Factors Outside of the Respiratory System	
Drug overdose with a respiratory depressant Paralysis of respiratory muscles caused by various neurological alterations Head injury Obesity	
RESPIRATORY ALKALOSIS	
Hyperventilation Resulting From Primary Respiratory Problems	
Asthma Pneumonia Inappropriate mechanical ventilator settings	*Physical examination:* Dizziness, confusion, dysrhythmias, tachypnea, numbness and tingling of extremities, seizures, and coma *Laboratory findings:* Arterial blood gas alterations: pH **above** 7.45, PaCO$_2$ **below** 35 mm Hg, PaO$_2$ normal, and bicarbonate level normal (if short lived or uncompensated) or **below** 22 mEq/L (if compensated)
Hyperventilation Resulting From Factors Outside of the Respiratory System	
Anxiety Hypermetabolic states (fever, exercise) Disorders of the central nervous system (head injuries, infections) Salicylate overdose	
METABOLIC ACIDOSIS	
High Anion Gap	
Starvation Diabetic ketoacidosis Renal failure Lactic acidosis from heavy exercise Use of drugs (e.g., methanol, ethanol, formic acid, paraldehyde, aspirin)	*Physical examination:* Headache, lethargy, confusion, dysrhythmias, tachypnea with deep respirations, abdominal cramps, and flushed skin *Laboratory findings:* Arterial blood gas alterations: pH **below** 7.35, PaCO$_2$ normal (if uncompensated) or **below** 35 mm Hg (if compensated), PaO$_2$ normal or increased (with rapid, deep respirations), bicarbonate level **below** 22 mEq/L, and oxygen saturation normal
Normal Anion Gap	
Renal tubular acidosis Diarrhea	
METABOLIC ALKALOSIS	
Excessive vomiting Prolonged gastric suctioning Hypokalemia or hypercalcemia Excess aldosterone Use of drugs (steroids, sodium bicarbonate, diuretics)	*Physical examination:* Dizziness; dysrhythmias; numbness and tingling of fingers, toes, and circumoral region; muscle cramps; tetany *Laboratory findings:* Arterial blood gas alterations: pH **above** 7.45, PaCO$_2$ normal (if uncompensated) or **above** 45 mm Hg (if compensated), PaO$_2$ normal, and bicarbonate level **above** 26 mEq/L

Metabolic acidosis results from a high acid content in the blood, which decreases sodium bicarbonate levels. A common cause of metabolic acidosis is diabetic ketoacidosis. An analysis of serum electrolytes to detect an anion gap is useful for identifying the cause of metabolic acidosis. An **anion gap** reflects unmeasurable anions present in plasma. You calculate an anion gap by summing the chloride and bicarbonate levels and subtracting this number from the plasma sodium concentration.

Metabolic alkalosis results from heavy acid loss from the body or an increase in levels of bicarbonate. The most common causes are vomiting and gastric suction.

NURSING KNOWLEDGE BASE

Fluid and electrolyte imbalances occur in all patients regardless of age, gender, race, or culture. Your nursing knowledge base with regard to these variables helps you in understanding how fluid and electrolyte alterations affect patients. For example, you can apply knowledge of growth and development when managing patients with fluid and electrolyte alterations. Infants and older adults are at significant risk because of their limited ability to respond independently to early warnings of a problem (Lecko, 2008; Owen and others, 2008). Your knowledge of normal growth and development can be helpful in recognizing behavioral changes from fluid and electrolyte alterations. Similarly, severely ill adults, disoriented patients, and immobile patients also have difficulty expressing symptoms when fluid and electrolyte imbalances develop. A nursing knowledge base with regard to communication and health assessment techniques will prove invaluable in detecting problems early.

CRITICAL THINKING

Synthesis

You will apply elements of critical thinking whenever you perform the nursing process with a patient. Consider the scientific knowledge you have learned, your experience, critical thinking attitudes, and standards to ensure an individualized approach to patient care (Box 17-1). Patients' conditions can change quickly in the presence of a fluid and electrolyte imbalance. Clinical decision making and judgment are necessary to analyze clinical data and make decisions regarding patient care. Use professional standards as guidelines for comprehensive assessment.

KNOWLEDGE   To provide care for patients with alterations in fluid and electrolyte or acid-base imbalance, use previously learned nursing knowledge and related knowledge acquired in anatomy, physiology, pharmacology, and/or chemistry courses. Be sure to consider all factors contributing to a patient's health problem. *For example, Mrs. Reynolds is at risk for dehydration from her vomiting, diarrhea, and decreased fluid intake. Her nurse, Robert, knows she is at risk for becoming dizzy getting out of bed because of orthostatic hypotension from fluid loss. In this case study, synthesizing previously learned knowledge about fluid volume loss and hypotension will help Robert plan and provide appropriate patient care.*

EXPERIENCE   Professional experience assists you when caring for patients with fluid and electrolyte or acid-base imbalances. Understanding the relationship between patients' clinical signs and symptoms helps you identify and make appropriate clinical decisions when presented with a similar assessment. Prior patient care experiences make you more adept at future problem solving and decision making.

BOX 17-1   SYNTHESIS IN PRACTICE

Robert reviews Mrs. Reynolds' clinical condition. The patient's history reveals that Mrs. Reynolds has loss of appetite, episodes of diarrhea, and continued use of furosemide (Lasix, a potassium-wasting diuretic) for hypertension. She is at risk for a fluid and electrolyte imbalance from a gastrointestinal (GI) disturbance and continued use of a diuretic. The cause of her GI symptoms is unclear; therefore her health care provider plans further diagnostic tests. Robert reviews the physiology of potassium as an electrolyte and studies the pathological findings of potassium excess and deficiency. He also reads recommendations in a pharmacology text on how to minimize the risk for hypokalemia when taking diuretics. Robert anticipates the need to perform a focused physical assessment and to manage and monitor Mrs. Reynolds' intravenous (IV) therapy. He knows that patient education will eventually be important for this patient because her therapy for hypertension will continue after discharge.

Just a few weeks ago, Robert cared for a patient with ulcerative colitis. Although Mrs. Reynolds' condition is different, both patients had diarrhea. Robert knows that Mrs. Reynolds will require careful monitoring of intake and output, as well as stabilization of GI function. The lessons learned from his previous patient will help Robert to be more alert if Mrs. Reynolds' clinical condition changes under his care.

Robert applies the critical thinking attitude of discipline by completing a thorough examination and assessment. The attitude of curiosity is important when a clinical sign or symptom may be unclear and further information is needed.

When Robert checks the policy and procedure manual at his institution for an IV therapy protocol, he applies professional standards in practice. He reviews the standards for IV site dressing changes to be familiar with the procedure.

ATTITUDES Accountability and discipline are two of the critical thinking attitudes to use when caring for patients with fluid and electrolyte and acid-base imbalances. Be accountable by reporting changes in patient behavior or physical assessment findings immediately, and follow standards of practice. Patients with fluid and electrolyte alterations often present with complicated physical signs and symptoms, so use discipline in conducting a thorough and comprehensive assessment.

STANDARDS Apply intellectual standards of accuracy, relevancy, and significance in obtaining a health history for a patient with fluid and electrolyte alterations. Apply Infusion Nurses Society (INS) standards of care for establishing, maintaining, monitoring, and discontinuing IV therapy (INS, 2006). In addition, it is necessary to apply the standards of infection control for invasive procedures, such as IV therapy (The Joint Commission [TJC], 2008). Also review laboratory standards for normal electrolyte values.

NURSING PROCESS

■■■ASSESSMENT

It is necessary to understand the importance of fluid, electrolyte, and acid-base balance in relationship to body homeostasis. By gathering assessment data and using critical thinking skills, nurses identify patients at risk and those with alterations. Thorough assessment leads to the development of appropriate nursing diagnoses.

NURSING HISTORY Assessment begins with a patient history, which reveals any risk factors or preexisting conditions that will cause or contribute to a disturbance of fluid and electrolytes and acid-base balance. Explore with the patient any factors that may contribute to a disturbance, and integrate the information with knowledge of fluid volume regulation, electrolyte concentration, and acid-base regulation.

Age is an important assessment consideration. Infants and young children have relatively more body water than older children and adults, making them more vulnerable to fluid volume alterations. The very young also have a greater fluid I&O relative to their size (Hockenberry and Wilson, 2007). Infants are at greater risk for **fluid volume deficit** (FVD), a condition involving water and electrolytes lost in equal or isotonic proportions. With FVD, an infant is at risk because of body water loss being proportionately greater per kilogram of weight. Children ages 2 through 12 have less stable regulatory responses to imbalances, so they have a narrow range of tolerance for severe fluid or electrolyte alterations. Adolescents have an increased metabolism and increased water production. Adolescent girls have greater fluid volume changes because of hormonal changes.

Older adults experience a number of age-related changes that affect fluid, electrolyte, and acid-base balances. These changes include a reduction in body water, diminished thirst sensation, decreased glomerular filtration, and a change in normal concentration of electrolytes (Ignatavicius and Workman, 2008; Mentes, 2006). In addition, older adults are at risk for decreased excretion of medication because of decreased glomerular filtration of the kidneys. These changes often cause sodium depletion or overload in the older adult who may be unable to maintain homeostasis. The changes in lung function that accompany aging lead to a reduced ability to compensate for metabolic acidosis.

A patient's prior medical history provides valuable data about fluid, electrolyte, and acid-base imbalances. When patients have chronic diseases (e.g., cancer, heart failure [HF], and renal disease), review the findings associated with these conditions to understand how they affect fluid and electrolyte and acid-base status. It is important to assess the duration of the disease and treatment regimens. In addition to chronic health problems, determine if the patient has a history of recent GI alterations (e.g., diarrhea or vomiting), nasogastric suctioning, or intestinal drainage. Loss of fluids and potassium and chloride ions predisposes patients to dehydration and a variety of electrolyte disturbances.

Recent surgery, head injury, respiratory disorders, and burns are conditions that place patients at high risk for fluid and electrolyte alterations. The stress response of surgery causes fluid balance changes in the second to fifth postoperative day if excess fluids have not been mobilized. The body increasingly secretes aldosterone, glucocorticoids, and ADH, causing sodium and chloride retention, potassium excretion, and decreased urinary output.

Assess for environmental factors in the patient history. Patients who have vigorously exercised or who have been exposed to temperature extremes may have clinical signs of fluid and electrolyte alterations. Exposure to environmental temperatures exceeding 28° to 30° C (82.4° to 86° F) can result in excessive sweating with weight loss.

Another important component of assessment is the patient's current dietary history. Recent changes in appetite or the ability to chew and swallow affect nutritional status and fluid hydration. Severe weight loss regimens lead to acidosis from rapid water loss, which will lead to hyperosmolar fluid imbalance.

Patient history should also include lifestyle factors. A patient with lifestyle risks, such as a history of smoking or alcohol consumption, will have an impaired ability to adapt to fluid, electrolyte, and acid-base alterations. For example, chronic tobacco use can cause respiratory depression, which can result in respiratory acidosis and an alteration in fluid and electrolyte balance.

Another important area to include in the assessment is a history of medication use (Box 17-2). If the assessment reveals a medication that may cause an electrolyte or acid-base disorder, closely assess pertinent laboratory values.

PHYSICAL EXAMINATION A thorough physical examination (see Chapter 15) is necessary because fluid and electrolyte imbalances or acid-base disturbances affect all body systems. While examining each system, carefully consider the signs and symptoms to expect as a result of any imbalance

BOX 17-2 Medications That Cause Fluid, Electrolyte, and Acid-Base Disturbances

- **Diuretics:** Metabolic alkalosis, hyperkalemia, and hypokalemia
- **Steroids:** Metabolic alkalosis
- **Potassium supplements:** Gastrointestinal disturbances, including intestinal and gastric ulcers and diarrhea
- **Respiratory center depressants** (e.g., opioid analgesic): Decreased rate and depth of respirations, resulting in respiratory acidosis
- **Antibiotics:** Nephrotoxicity (e.g., vancomycin, methicillin, aminoglycosides); hyperkalemia and/or hypernatremia (e.g., azlocillin, carbenicillin, piperacillin, ticarcillin)*
- **Calcium carbonate** (Tums): Mild metabolic alkalosis with nausea and vomiting*
- **Magnesium hydroxide** (Milk of Magnesia): Hypokalemia*
- **Nonsteroidal antiinflammatory drugs:** Nephrotoxicity

*Data from McKenry LM and others: *Mosby's pharmacology in nursing,* ed 22, St. Louis, 2006, Mosby.

(Table 17-5). For example, an examination of the oral cavity reveals signs of dehydration (e.g., dry mouth) when the patient is experiencing a fluid deficit. Table 17-6 provides an example for evaluation of fluid and electrolyte status.

DAILY WEIGHTS AND FLUID INTAKE AND OUTPUT MEASUREMENT Measuring and recording all liquid I&O during a 24-hour period is an important part of the patient's assessment database. Recognizing trends in the I&O is important (e.g., a gradually decreasing urine output indicates that the body is trying to adapt to an FVD). Accurate assessment of fluid status, including I&O, identifies both patients at risk and patients who are experiencing actual fluid, electrolyte, and acid-base disturbances. Patients with alterations need to also have their weight monitored daily. Daily weights are the single most important indicator of fluid status (Browne and others, 2007; Heitz and Horne, 2005). Each kilogram (2.2 lb) of weight gained or lost is equal to 1 L of fluid gained or lost. Obtain the weight at the same time each day on the same scale after a patient voids. Calibrate the scale on a routine basis. Have patients wear clothes that weigh the same each time they weigh. If you are using a bed scale, always use the same number of linens.

TABLE 17-5 Physical and Behavioral Nursing Assessment for Fluid, Electrolyte, and Acid-Base Imbalances

ASSESSMENT	IMBALANCE
WEIGHT CHANGES	
2%-5% loss	Mild fluid volume deficit (FVD)
5%-8% loss	Moderate to severe FVD
8-15% loss	Severe FVD
>15% loss	Death
2% gain	Mild fluid volume excess (FVE)
5%-8% gain	Moderate to severe FVE
HEAD	
History	
Headache	FVD, metabolic or respiratory acidosis, metabolic alkalosis
Dizziness	FVD, respiratory acidosis or alkalosis, hyponatremia
Observation	
Irritability	Metabolic or respiratory alkalosis, hyperosmolar imbalance, hypernatremia, hypokalemia
Lethargy	FVD, metabolic acidosis or alkalosis, respiratory acidosis, hypercalcemia
Confusion, disorientation	FVD, hypomagnesemia, metabolic acidosis, hypokalemia
EYES	
History	
Blurred vision	FVE
Inspection	
Sunken, dry conjunctivae, decreased or absent tearing	FVD
Periorbital edema, papilledema (swelling of ocular disc)	FVE

TABLE 17-5 Physical and Behavioral Nursing Assessment for Fluid, Electrolyte, and Acid-Base Imbalances—cont'd

ASSESSMENT	IMBALANCE
THROAT AND MOUTH	
Inspection	
Sticky, dry mucosa, dry cracked lips, decreased salivation, longitudinal tongue furrows	FVD, hypernatremia
CARDIOVASCULAR SYSTEM	
Inspection	
Flat neck veins	FVD
Distended neck veins	FVE
Dependent body parts: legs, sacrum, back	FVD
Slow venous filling	
Palpation	
Edema: dependent body parts (back, sacrum, legs)	FVE
Dysrhythmias (also noted as ECG changes)	Metabolic acidosis, respiratory alkalosis and acidosis, potassium imbalance, hypomagnesemia
Increased pulse rate	Metabolic alkalosis, respiratory acidosis, hyponatremia, FVD, FVE, hypomagnesemia
Decreased pulse rate	Metabolic alkalosis, hypokalemia
Weak pulse	FVD, hypokalemia
Decreased capillary filling	FVD
Bounding pulse	FVE
Auscultation	
Blood pressure low or without orthostatic changes	FVD, hyponatremia, hyperkalemia, hypermagnesemia
Third heart sound (except in young children)	FVE
Hypertension	FVE
RESPIRATORY SYSTEM	
Inspection	
Increased rate	FVE, respiratory alkalosis, metabolic acidosis
Dyspnea	FVE
Auscultation	
Crackles	FVE
GASTROINTESTINAL SYSTEM	
History	
Anorexia	Metabolic acidosis
Abdominal cramps	Metabolic acidosis
Inspection	
Sunken abdomen	FVD
Distended abdomen	Third-space syndrome
Vomiting	FVD, hypercalcemia, hyponatremia, hypochloremia, metabolic alkalosis
Diarrhea	Hyponatremia, metabolic acidosis
Auscultation	
Loud "growling" sounds from hyperperistalsis with diarrhea, or no sounds from hypoperistalsis	FVD, hypokalemia
RENAL SYSTEM	
Inspection	
Oliguria or anuria	FVD, FVE
Diuresis (if kidneys are normal)	FVE
Increased urine specific gravity	FVD

ECG, Electrocardiogram.

Continued

TABLE 17-5 Physical and Behavioral Nursing Assessment for Fluid, Electrolyte, and Acid-Base Imbalances—cont'd

ASSESSMENT	IMBALANCE
NEUROMUSCULAR SYSTEM	
Inspection	
Numbness, tingling	Metabolic alkalosis, hypocalcemia, potassium imbalances
Muscle cramps, tetany	Hypocalcemia, metabolic or respiratory alkalosis
Coma	Hyperosmolar or hypoosmolar imbalances, hyponatremia
Tremors	Respiratory acidosis, hypomagnesemia
Palpation	
Hypotonicity	Hypokalemia, hypercalcemia
Hypertonicity	Hypocalcemia, hypomagnesemia, metabolic alkalosis
SKIN	
Body temperature	
Increased	Hypernatremia, hyperosmolar imbalance, metabolic acidosis
Decreased	FVD
Inspection	
Dry, flushed	FVD, hypernatremia, metabolic acidosis
Palpation	
Inelastic skin turgor, cold, clammy skin	FVD

Data from Heitz U, Horne MM: *Mosby's pocket guide series: fluid, electrolyte, and acid-base balance,* ed 5, St. Louis, 2005, Mosby.

TABLE 17-6 FOCUSED PATIENT ASSESSMENT

FACTORS TO ASSESS	QUESTIONS	PHYSICAL ASSESSMENT
Vital signs	Are you experiencing dizziness when changing positions?	Monitor patient's blood pressure when moving from a lying or sitting to standing position for changes in blood pressure.
		Observe patient behaviors for dizziness (unsteady gait).
Intake and output	Do you feel your heart "racing"?	Palpate patient's pulse, and auscultate heart rate.
	What are your usual I&O patterns?	Monitor patient's 24- and/or 36-hour I&O amount.
	Has there been a significant increase or decrease in your I&O?	Inspect patient's urine and vomitus or diarrhea, if applicable.
		Obtain a baseline weight, and monitor daily.
Skin turgor	Has your skin been dry?	Inspect patient's skin; palpate for turgor and edema.
	Have you noticed any swelling anywhere on your body?	Inspect for any skin changes.
	Have you had any itching or changes in your skin?	

I&O, Intake and output.

For patients in health care settings, I&O measurement is a routine nursing assessment for patients at risk for a fluid imbalance. You will routinely measure I&O for patients after surgery; those with unstable or declining conditions, a temperature elevation, or fluid restriction; and those who receive diuretic or IV therapy. You will also measure I&O for any patient with chronic cardiopulmonary or renal illness. You are able to delegate measurement of I&O to nursing assistive personnel (NAP). Stress the importance of measurement accuracy and timely reporting of findings.

Parenteral intake includes IV fluids (including continuous infusions and intermittent IV piggybacks) and blood or its components. GI intake includes all liquids taken by mouth (e.g., gelatin, ice cream, broth, juice, and water) and through nasogastric or jejunostomy feeding tubes (see Chapter 32). Occasionally patients receive a specific amount of a liquid medication every 1 to 2 hours. A patient receiving tube feedings may receive numerous liquid medications, and you may use water to flush the tube before and/or after the medications. Over a 24-hour period, these liquids amount to a significant intake. Always record them on the I&O record. Liquid output includes urine, diarrhea, vomitus, gastric suction, and blood and drainage from postsurgical wounds, burns, or other tubes (see Chapter 38).

Instruct ambulatory patients to save their urine in a calibrated (graduated) insert that attaches to the rim of the toilet bowl (Figure 17-4). Record urinary output, or instruct patients to measure and record their own output after each trip to the bathroom. When a patient has an indwelling urinary catheter, or any drainage tube, you record that output as well (e.g., at the end of each nursing shift or every hour) as the patient's condition requires.

Patient and family cooperation is essential for maintaining accurate I&O measurements. Teach the patient and family the purpose of the measurements, and instruct the patient and family either to notify the nurse that there is voided fluid to measure or how to measure and empty the container themselves. It is important for the patient to have good vision and motor skills to perform these assessments.

In the hospital, forms for recording I&O are available on a patient's chart or in an electronic medical record. Recording I&O is essential for accurate patient assessment. This information maintains an ongoing evaluation of the patient's hydration status to prevent severe imbalances.

LABORATORY STUDIES Review the patient's laboratory test results to obtain further objective data about fluid, electrolyte, and acid-base balances (Box 17-3 and Table 17-7). These tests include serum and urinary electrolyte levels, hematocrit, blood creatinine level, blood urea nitrogen (BUN) levels, urine specific gravity, and ABG readings. You measure serum electrolyte levels to determine hydration status, plasma electrolyte concentrations, and acid-base balance. The frequency of electrolyte level measurement depends on the severity of the patient's illness. You routinely perform serum electrolyte tests on any patient entering a hospital to screen for alterations and to serve as a baseline for future comparisons. For example, a patient with the flu may have decreased fluid intake from nausea and needs to be screened for dehydration through serum electrolyte measurement.

PATIENT EXPECTATIONS Fluid and electrolyte or acid-base disturbances may cause serious illness, which prevents a review of patient expectations. If a patient is alert enough to discuss care, a review of expectations may reveal short-term needs (e.g., provision of comfort from nausea) or long-term needs (e.g., understanding how to prevent alterations from occurring in the future). The patient must be able to understand the implications of fluid and electrolyte or acid-base changes to express expectations of care. Strengthen the patient's trust through a competent response to sudden changes in condition and through communication with patients and/or family members. Keep patients informed of any changes so that they become active participants in their care.

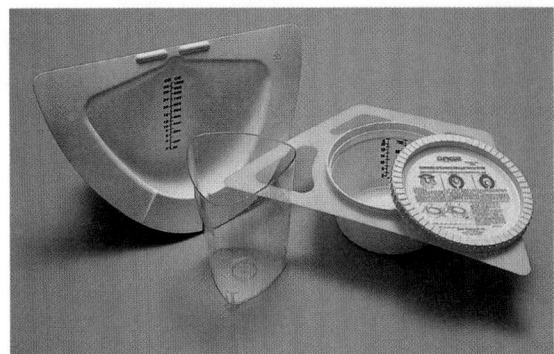

Figure 17-4 ■ Graduated measuring containers. *Clockwise from top left:* "hat" receptacle, specimen, and measurement container.

■■■NURSING DIAGNOSIS

When caring for patients with suspected fluid, electrolyte, or acid-base imbalances, it is important to use critical thinking to formulate nursing diagnoses. The assessment data that establish the risk for or the actual presence of a nursing diagnosis are sometimes subtle, but patterns and trends emerge after a complete assessment. Because multiple body systems may be involved, analyze the defining characteristics carefully. For example, relevant assessment data for the nursing diagnosis *deficient fluid volume* will include defining characteristics such as insufficient oral intake, weight loss, dry skin and mucous membranes, decreased skin turgor, decreased blood pressure, and increased heart rate.

In addition to the accurate clustering of assessment data, another part of developing nursing diagnoses is identifying the relevant causes or related factor. For example, *deficient fluid volume related to loss of gastrointestinal fluids from vomiting* will require interventions to manage the patient's vomiting and restore fluid volume (e.g., administer antiemetics, remove sights and odors that induce nausea, and provide IV fluid replacement). The same nursing diagnosis that has different defining characteristics such as *deficient fluid volume related to elevated body temperature* will require interventions to lower the patient's body temperature and replace lost body fluids (e.g., administer antipyretics and provide oral fluids).

Possible nursing diagnoses for patients with fluid, electrolyte, and acid-base alterations include the following:

- *Decreased cardiac output*
- *Acute confusion*
- *Diarrhea*
- *Deficient fluid volume*
- *Excess fluid volume*
- *Risk for imbalanced fluid volume*
- *Impaired gas exchange*
- *Risk for injury*
- *Ineffective peripheral tissue perfusion*
- *Risk for decreased cardiac tissue perfusion*
- *Risk for ineffective cerebral tissue perfusion*
- *Risk for ineffective gastrointestinal perfusion*
- *Risk for ineffective renal perfusion*
- *Risk for shock*

BOX 17-3   Laboratory Data Reflecting Fluid, Electrolyte, and Acid-Base Imbalances

FLUID AND ELECTROLYTES

- Alterations in sodium, potassium, magnesium, calcium, phosphates, chloride, and bicarbonate (venous CO_2 concentrations)
- Increase in hematocrit, BUN, sodium, and osmolality in serum (related to loss of ECF fluid or gain of solutes)
- Decrease in hematocrit, BUN, sodium, and osmolality in serum (related to gain of ECF fluid or loss of solutes)
- Concentrated urine demonstrated by urine specific gravity >1.030
- Dilute urine demonstrated by a specific gravity <1.010

METABOLIC ALKALOSIS

- pH >7.45
- $PaCO_2$ normal or >45 mm Hg if lungs are compensating
- PaO_2 normal
- O_2 saturation (SaO_2) normal
- HCO_3^- >26 mEq/L
- Ionized calcium <4.5 mg/dL
- K^+ <3.5 mEq/L

METABOLIC ACIDOSIS

- pH <7.35
- $PaCO_2$ normal or <35 mm Hg if lungs are compensating
- PaO_2 normal

- O_2 saturation (SaO_2) normal
- HCO_3^- <22 mEq/L
- K^+ >5.0 mEq/L

RESPIRATORY ALKALOSIS

- pH >7.45
- $PaCO_2$ <35 mm Hg
- PaO_2 normal
- O_2 saturation (SaO_2) normal
- HCO_3^- <22 mEq/L if kidneys are compensating
- Ionized calcium <4.5 mg/dL
- K^+ <3.5 mEq/L

RESPIRATORY ACIDOSIS

- pH <7.35
- $PaCO_2$ >45 mm Hg
- PaO_2 normal or <80 mm Hg, depending on cause of acidosis
- O_2 saturation (SaO_2) normal or <95%, depending on cause of acidosis
- HCO_3^- normal if early respiratory acidosis or >26 mEq/L if kidneys are compensating
- K^+ >5.0 mEq/L

BUN, Blood urea nitrogen; *ECF*, extracellular fluid.

TABLE 17-7   Laboratory Data for Acid-Base Assessment

TEST	NORMAL RANGE FOR ADULTS		SIGNIFICANCE OF ABNORMAL FINDINGS
	ARTERIAL	VENOUS	
pH >90 years of age	7.35-7.45 7.25-7.45	7.32-7.43	Increased: Metabolic alkalosis, loss of gastric fluids, decreased potassium intake, diuretic therapy, fever, salicylate toxicity
			Decreased: Metabolic or respiratory acidosis, ketosis, renal failure, starvation, diarrhea, hyperthyroidism
PaO_2 (mm Hg) >90 years of age	83-108 >50		Increased: Increased ventilation, oxygen therapy, exercise
			Decreased: Respiratory depression, high altitude, carbon monoxide poisoning, decreased cardiac output
$PaCO_2$ (mm Hg)	35-48	41-55	Increased: Respiratory acidosis, emphysema, pneumonia, cardiac failure, respiratory depression
			Decreased: Respiratory alkalosis, excessive ventilation, diarrhea
Bicarbonate (mEq/L or mmol/L)	22-26	24-29	Increased: Bicarbonate therapy, metabolic alkalosis
			Decreased: Metabolic acidosis, diarrhea, pancreatitis
Lactate (mg/100 mL)	<11.3	8.1-15.3	Increased: Hypoxia, exercise, insulin infusion, alcoholism, pregnancy
			Decreased: Fluid overload

From Ignatavicius DD, Workman, ML: *Medical-surgical nursing: critical thinking for collaborative care*, ed 5, Philadelphia, 2008, Saunders.

■■■PLANNING

GOALS AND OUTCOMES During the planning phase collaborate with the patient to establish goals and expected outcomes for each nursing diagnosis (see Care Plan). Make sure goals are individualized and realistic with measurable outcomes. *In the nursing care plan, Robert will set goals for improving Mrs. Reynolds' dehydration status. Robert will later determine if Mrs. Reynolds' goals are met, for example by monitoring the outcome of serum electrolyte balance and I&O. Each goal and outcome needs a time frame for achievement. For Mrs. Reynolds, this time frame was for her goals to be met before discharge from therapy.*

CARE PLAN Deficient Fluid Volume

ASSESSMENT

Mrs. Susan Reynolds, a 42-year-old married accountant, has just been admitted to the acute care unit with a history of nausea, loss of appetite, and vomiting and diarrhea for 7 days. After obtaining a blood sample for electrolyte levels, complete blood count, and an electrocardiogram (ECG), her health care provider has admitted her for observation. Orders include nothing by mouth (NPO), an intravenous (IV) infusion of 0.9% saline at 125 mL/hr, intake and output (I&O) recordings, and vital signs every 4 hours, in addition to daily weights.

ASSESSMENT ACTIVITIES	FINDINGS/DEFINING CHARACTERISTICS*
Ask Mrs. Reynolds to describe when her nausea began and what accompanying signs and symptoms she is experiencing.	Mrs. Reynolds states that she became nauseous after a business trip. She has no appetite, is nauseous, and has been vomiting and has had diarrhea for 7 days. She is still taking her furosemide (Lasix).
Conduct an examination of gastrointestinal (GI) and urinary function.	Bowel sounds are present in all four quadrants but hyperactive. Abdomen is soft to palpation. The patient has had less nausea and vomiting since yesterday and only two loose stools since midnight. Twenty-four–hour intake equaled 1850 mL, with output of 2200 mL **(urine output accounted for only 1000 mL)**. Mrs. Reynolds voids without difficulty, with **dark yellow urine.**
Assess her vital signs.	Vital signs are temperature 99.6° F (37.6° C); **pulse, 100 beats per minute** and regular; and **blood pressure, 110/60 mm Hg** with no changes when standing.
Assess Mrs. Reynolds' skin and mucous membranes for indicators of dehydration.	Her skin is **dry,** without discoloration, but **turgor is decreased.** Inspection of **mucous membranes** shows they **are dry** with thick, clear mucus. Respirations are 18 breaths per minute and nonlabored with bilateral breath sounds clear to auscultation. Her admission **weight** of 143 lb (65 kg) was **down 1 lb** (0.45 kg) since admission.
Evaluate her laboratory values and ECG results.	Mrs. Reynolds' laboratory results are as follows: hematocrit 44% (suggesting hypovolemia); potassium 3.6 mEq/L; and sodium 138 mEq/L (both low normal because of prolonged vomiting and diarrhea). Mrs. Reynolds' ECG showed normal sinus rhythm.

NURSING DIAGNOSIS: Deficient fluid volume related to excessive diarrhea, vomiting, and use of potassium-wasting diuretic.

PLANNING

GOAL	EXPECTED OUTCOMES (NOC)†
	Fluid Balance
• Mrs. Reynolds' fluid volume will return to normal by time of discharge.	• Urine output will equal intake of approximately 1500 mL in 2 days.
	• Mucous membranes will be moist in 24 hours.
	• Skin turgor will return to normal within 24 hours.
	• Daily weights will not vary ± 2 lb over next 2 days.
	Electrolyte and Acid-Base Balance
• Mrs. Reynolds will achieve normal electrolyte balance by discharge.	• Serum electrolyte and blood counts will be within normal limits within 48 hours.
	• Mrs. Reynolds will not have any nausea or vomiting in 24 hours.
	• Mrs. Reynolds will not have more than 1 stool a day in 3 days.

*Defining characteristics are shown in **bold** type.
†Outcomes classification labels from Moorhead S and others, editors: *Nursing outcomes classification (NOC),* ed 4, St. Louis, 2008, Mosby.

CARE PLAN   Deficient Fluid Volume—cont'd

INTERVENTIONS (NIC)‡

Fluid and Electrolyte Management

- Administer IV fluids (0.9% normal saline) at 125 mL/hr.
- Provide patient with an additional 480 mL of noncaffeinated oral fluids every 8 hours.
- Administer as ordered bismuth subsalicylate (Pepto-Bismol) for diarrhea.

- Maintain accurate I&O measurements.
- Weigh Mrs. Reynolds daily, and monitor trends.

- Teach Mrs. Reynolds and family about specific dietary modification (potassium-rich foods). Begin patient teaching regarding types of foods that offer source of potassium.

RATIONALE

Replacement of body fluid restores blood volume and normal serum electrolyte levels; an isotonic solution expands the body's intravascular fluid volume without causing a fluid shift from one compartment to another

Pepto-Bismol is an antidiarrheal to inhibit GI secretions, stimulate absorption of fluid and electrolytes, inhibit intestinal inflammation, and suppress the growth of *Helicobacter pylori* (McKenry and others, 2006).

Documents hydration and fluid balance for directing therapy.

Daily weights provide reliable data of fluid balance (Flanagan and others, 2007).

Furosemide (Lasix) is a potassium-wasting diuretic (McKenry and others, 2006). The body does not store potassium, thus requiring dietary supplements rich in potassium.

EVALUATION

NURSING ACTIONS	PATIENT RESPONSE/FINDING	ACHIEVEMENT OF OUTCOME
Monitor electrolyte levels and daily weights.	Serum electrolyte levels: potassium 4.0 mEq/L and sodium 140 mEq/L; weight, 143 lb (65 kg).	Electrolyte levels within normal range. Daily weight stable.
Inspect oral mucous membranes.	Mucous membranes remain dry.	Fluid balance has not returned to normal.
Assess skin turgor.	Skin turgor normal.	Fluid balance has begun to return to normal.
Evaluate I&O trends during next 48 hours.	Mrs. Reynolds' 24-hour intake is 2800 mL, and output is 2200 mL with 1800 mL urine. Urine specific gravity is 1.025, and weight has now returned to 143 lb (65 kg).	Mrs. Reynolds' fluid balance is improving with urine output exceeding stool output.

‡Interventions classification label from Bulechek GM and others, editors: *Nursing interventions classification (NIC),* ed 5, St. Louis, 2008, Mosby.

In the acute care setting, a long-term goal will be to anticipate the needs of a patient and family to ease the transition to home or long-term care. *For example, Mrs. Reynolds will likely be discharged home with new medications or recommendations for a diet that causes less gastrointestinal upset.* It is important to determine the knowledge and skills of the patient and any family caregiver. When creating a patient care plan, remember to take into consideration the patient's personal preferences and available resources.

SETTING PRIORITIES The patient's clinical condition determines which of the diagnoses takes the greatest priority. Many nursing diagnoses in the area of fluid, electrolyte, and acid-base balance are of highest priority, because the consequences for the patient can be serious or even life threatening. *For example, in the Concept Map (Figure 17-5) Mrs. Reynolds has diarrhea and vomiting, which has created the problem of deficient fluid volume. The nursing diagnosis defi-*cient fluid volume *ranks highest priority, requiring intervention to stabilize her status and prevent further complications.* As the patient's status changes, the priority nursing diagnoses also change. For example, the priority nursing diagnosis may change to *deficient knowledge* once a patient is well enough to be discharged home. The priority at this time is to ensure that the patient and family can return safely to the home which often requires extensive patient education (see Chapter 11).

COLLABORATIVE CARE Consultation with the patient's health care provider will identify realistic time frames for the goals of care, particularly when the patient's physiological status is unstable. Planning care for a patient requires collaboration with other members of the health care team, such as the dietitian or pharmacist. You cannot delegate administration of IV medications and/or oxygen therapy and hemodynamic assessments to the NAP. When the patient

CONCEPT MAP

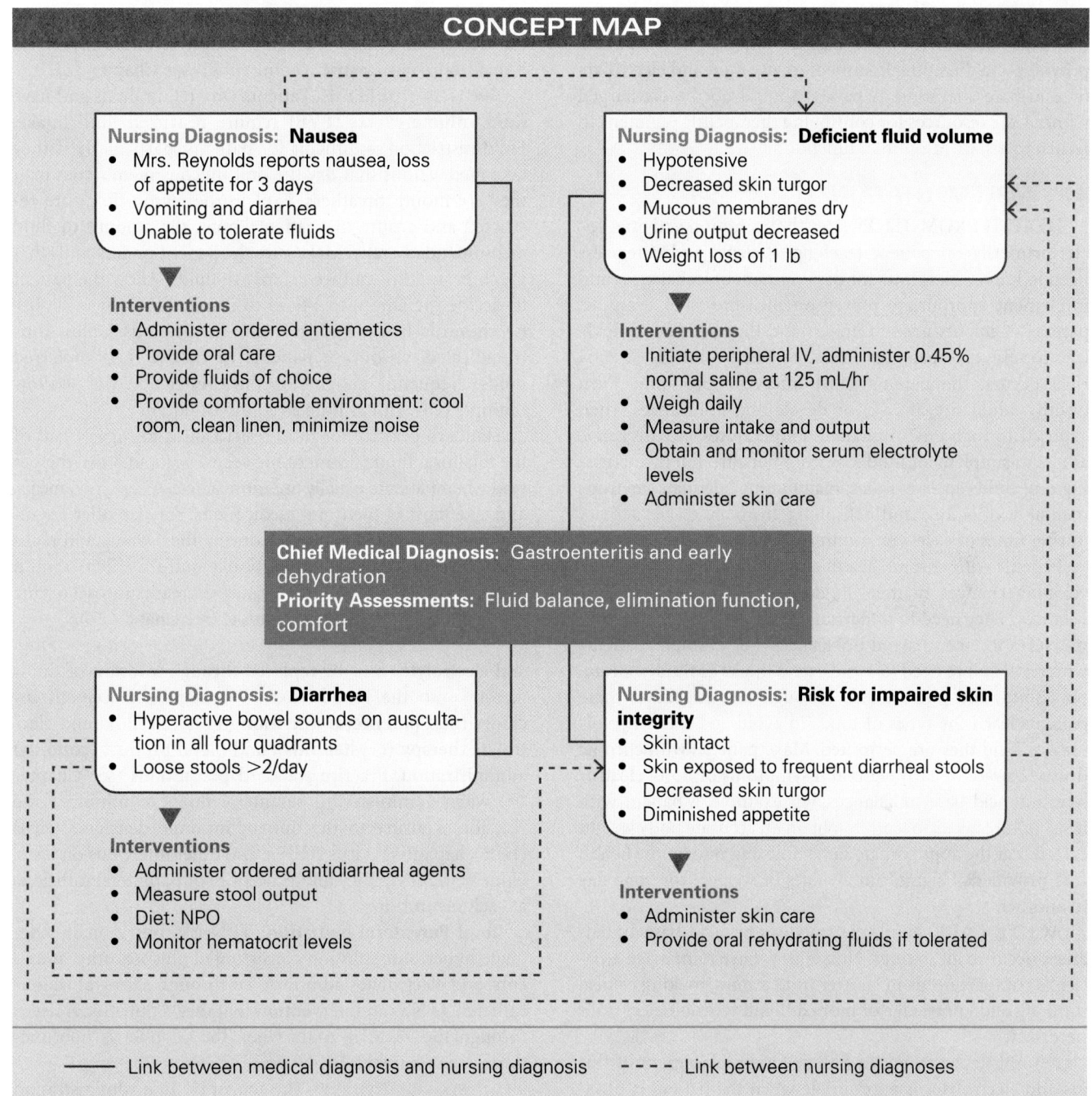

Nursing Diagnosis: Nausea
- Mrs. Reynolds reports nausea, loss of appetite for 3 days
- Vomiting and diarrhea
- Unable to tolerate fluids

▼

Interventions
- Administer ordered antiemetics
- Provide oral care
- Provide fluids of choice
- Provide comfortable environment: cool room, clean linen, minimize noise

Nursing Diagnosis: Deficient fluid volume
- Hypotensive
- Decreased skin turgor
- Mucous membranes dry
- Urine output decreased
- Weight loss of 1 lb

▼

Interventions
- Initiate peripheral IV, administer 0.45% normal saline at 125 mL/hr
- Weigh daily
- Measure intake and output
- Obtain and monitor serum electrolyte levels
- Administer skin care

Chief Medical Diagnosis: Gastroenteritis and early dehydration
Priority Assessments: Fluid balance, elimination function, comfort

Nursing Diagnosis: Diarrhea
- Hyperactive bowel sounds on auscultation in all four quadrants
- Loose stools >2/day

▼

Interventions
- Administer ordered antidiarrheal agents
- Measure stool output
- Diet: NPO
- Monitor hematocrit levels

Nursing Diagnosis: Risk for impaired skin integrity
- Skin intact
- Skin exposed to frequent diarrheal stools
- Decreased skin turgor
- Diminished appetite

▼

Interventions
- Administer skin care
- Provide oral rehydrating fluids if tolerated

——— Link between medical diagnosis and nursing diagnosis   - - - - Link between nursing diagnoses

Figure 17-5 ■ Concept Map.

becomes stable, you can delegate daily weights, I&O measurement, and direct physical patient care. Establishing a rapport of open communication and teamwork with NAP is important, as with any member of the interdisciplinary team, to ensure timely and effective administration of care.

Continuity of care is essential as the patient moves from one health care setting to another or to the home. Therapeutic regimens established in one setting continue until completed in the next setting. For example, a patient who will

continue to monitor I&O at home needs to know how to measure and document fluid I&O. When the patient's discharge has been ordered, it is important to identify what resources are available for the patient to promote positive patient outcomes. Dietitians are a valuable resource for recommending food sources to either increase or reduce intake of certain electrolytes. Chapter 32 describes various therapeutic diets (e.g., low sodium). Pharmacists can provide information about a patient's prescription medications, potential side effects, and over-the-counter medications that may cause electrolyte or acid-base alterations. The health care provider will direct the treatment of any fluid and electrolyte or acid-base alteration. A patient should not be discharged without the resources for continuing therapeutic regimens to return to a state of optimal functioning.

■■■ IMPLEMENTATION

HEALTH PROMOTION Health promotion activities focus primarily on patient teaching. Patients and caregivers need to know risk factors for development of imbalances and implement appropriate preventive measures. For example, parents of infants need to understand that GI losses quickly lead to serious imbalances; therefore when vomiting or diarrhea occurs, the parents must intervene promptly. Even healthy adults are at risk for developing imbalances when exposed to high environmental temperatures. Advise active adults to supplement fluid loss from perspiration by increasing oral fluids such as water, maintaining adequate environmental ventilation, and refraining from excessive activity during times of excess environmental heat.

Patients with chronic health alterations are at risk for developing changes in their fluid, electrolyte, and acid-base balances. They need to understand their own risk factors and measures to take to avoid imbalances. For example, patients with renal failure need to avoid excess intake of fluid, sodium, potassium, and phosphorus. Through diet education these patients learn the types of foods to avoid and the daily volume of fluid they are permitted. Make patients with chronic diseases aware of early signs and symptoms of fluid, electrolyte, and acid-base imbalances. For example, a patient with heart failure needs to learn to obtain an accurate body weight each day at the approximate same time and inform the health care provider of significant changes of weight from one day to another.

ACUTE CARE Fluid, electrolyte, and acid-base imbalances occur in all settings. Nurses now have to manage a patient's complex needs in shorter time frames, making critical thinking and knowledge of more difficult technological skills necessary.

Enteral Replacement of Fluids Oral replacement of fluids and electrolytes is appropriate when the patient is physiologically stable enough for oral fluids to be replaced rapidly. Oral replacement of fluids is contraindicated when the patient is vomiting, has a mechanical obstruction of the GI tract, is at risk for aspiration, has an altered level of consciousness, or has impaired swallowing. Some patients unable to tolerate solid foods are still able to ingest fluids.

When replacing fluids by mouth in a patient with a fluid deficit, choose fluids with adequate calories and electrolyte content (e.g., fruit juices, gelatin, and replacements such as Pedialyte and Gastrolyte). However, it is important to remember that liquids containing lactose, caffeine, or low-sodium content are not appropriate when the patient has diarrhea. Caffeine, for example, causes diuresis, furthering fluid loss.

A feeding tube is appropriate when the patient's GI tract is healthy but the patient cannot ingest fluids (e.g., after oral surgery or with impaired swallowing). You replace fluids through feeding tubes (e.g., gastrostomy, jejunostomy, or via a small-bore nasogastric feeding tube) (see Chapter 32).

Restriction of Fluids Patients who retain fluids and have fluid volume excess (FVE) require restricted fluid intake. Fluid restriction is difficult for patients, particularly if they take medications that dry the oral mucous membranes or if they are mouth breathers. Explain the reason fluids are restricted and ensure the patient knows the amount of fluid recommended orally. Make sure the patient understands that ice chips, gelatin, and ice cream are fluids. Allow the patient to decide the amount of fluid to drink with each meal, between meals, before bed, and with medications. Unless contraindicated, encourage patients to choose their preferred fluids. Frequently patients on fluid restriction will swallow multiple pills with as little as 30 mL of liquid.

Standard practice for fluid restriction is to suggest half of the total oral fluid allotment between 7 AM and 3 PM, the period when patients usually are more active, receive two meals, and take most of their oral medications. You can offer the remainder of the fluid allowance during the evening and night shifts. Patients on fluid restriction require frequent mouth care to moisten mucous membranes, decrease mucosal drying and cracking, and maintain comfort (see Chapter 28).

Parenteral Replacement of Fluids and Electrolytes Fluid and electrolytes may be replaced through infusion of fluids directly into the bloodstream. Parenteral replacement includes total parenteral nutrition (TPN), IV fluid and electrolyte therapy (crystalloids), and blood product (colloids) administration. Practice standard precautions (see Chapter 13) when administering parenteral fluids to minimize the risk for exposure to the human immune deficiency virus (HIV), hepatitis B virus (HBV), and other infectious diseases. Understand the policy and procedure of parenteral infusions at each institution.

Total Parenteral Nutrition. TPN is a nutritionally adequate hypertonic solution consisting of glucose, other nutrients, and electrolytes administered through a central venous catheter. TPN is an intervention that meets nutritional needs through the vascular route when the GI tract is nonfunctional (see Chapter 32).

Intravenous Therapy. The goal of IV fluid administration is to correct or prevent fluid and electrolyte disturbances. It allows for direct access to the vascular system, permitting the continuous or intermittent infusion of fluids and medications over a period of time. Intravenous fluid therapy requires frequent monitoring because of potential changes in the patient's fluid and electrolyte balance. When patients require IV fluid administration, you need to have knowledge of the correct solution ordered and the equipment needed, as well as evidence-based procedures required to initiate an infusion, regulate the infusion rate, and maintain the system. You also need to know how to identify and correct problems and how to discontinue the infusion to maintain patient safety.

Vascular Access Devices. Vascular access devices (VADs) are catheters, cannulas, or infusion ports inserted into large veins of the body and designed for repeated access to the vascular system (Skill 17-1). Peripherally placed cannulas are inserted into veins of the hand and arm for short-term use (e.g., to restore fluid volume). Centrally placed catheters, peripherally inserted central catheters (PICCs), tunneled catheters, and implanted ports are VADs designed for long-term use. These devices are more effective than peripherally placed catheters for administering medications and solutions that are irritating to the veins. Education in the care of these devices is needed to provide safe and appropriate therapy.

Administration of Intravenous Therapy

Types of Solutions. Many prepared IV solutions are available for use (Table 17-8). IV solutions fall into the following general categories: isotonic, hypotonic, and hypertonic. Isotonic solution is the solution used for extracellular volume replacement (e.g., FVD after prolonged vomiting). A health care provider bases the decision to use a hypotonic or hypertonic solution on the patient's specific fluid and electrolyte imbalance. For example, the patient with a hypertonic fluid imbalance will generally receive a hypotonic solution to dilute the ECF and rehydrate the cells. Administer all IV fluids carefully, especially hypertonic solutions, because they can cause circulatory changes quickly. Hypertonic solutions pull fluid into the vascular space by osmosis, resulting in an increased vascular volume, which can lead to pulmonary edema, particularly in patients with heart or renal failure.

It is common to place additives such as vitamins and potassium chloride (KCl) into IV solutions. An IV therapy order will include the IV solution and additives plus the volume and prescribed infusion time or rate. A pharmacist will always prepare the solution, except in emergency situations. An example of an order follows:

Infusion #1: 1000 mL $D_5\frac{1}{2}NS$ with 20 mEq KCl and 1 ampule of multivitamins at 125 mL/hr

Patients with normal renal function who are receiving nothing by mouth need to have potassium added to IV solutions. The body does not store potassium, and even when serum levels fall, the kidneys will continue to excrete potassium. If there is no potassium intake orally or parenterally, hypokalemia develops quickly. Conversely, failure to verify that the patient has adequate kidney function and urine output before administering an IV solution containing potassium could result in hyperkalemia. ***Under no circumstances should you give KCl in an IV push. A direct IV infusion of KCl may be fatal. IV administration of KCl requires dilution in solution and infusion over a period of time.***

TABLE 17-8 Intravenous Solutions

SOLUTION	CONCENTRATION	OTHER NAMES
DEXTROSE IN WATER SOLUTIONS		
Dextrose 5% in water*	Hypotonic	D_5W
Dextrose 10% in water	Hypertonic	$D_{10}W$
SALINE SOLUTIONS		
0.45% sodium chloride (half normal saline)	Hypotonic	½NS 0.45% NS
0.33% sodium chloride (one-third normal saline)	Hypotonic	⅓NS
0.9% sodium chloride† (normal saline)	Isotonic	NS 0.9% NS 0.9% NaCl
3%-5% sodium chloride	Hypertonic	3%-5% NS 3%-5% NaCl
DEXTROSE IN SALINE SOLUTIONS		
Dextrose 5% in 0.9% sodium chloride	Hypertonic	$D_5$0.9% NaCl $D_5$0.9% NS D_5NS
Dextrose 5% in 0.45% sodium chloride	Hypertonic	$D_5$0.45% NaCl $D_5$0.45% NS D_5½NS
MULTIPLE ELECTROLYTE SOLUTIONS		
Lactated Ringer's‡	Isotonic	LR
Dextrose 5% in lactated Ringer's	Hypertonic	D_5LR

*Dextrose is quickly metabolized, leaving free water to be distributed evenly in all fluid compartments (Heitz and Horne, 2005).
†Although it is isotonic because the total concentration of electrolytes equals plasma concentration, it contains 154 mEq of both sodium and chloride, which is a higher concentration of these electrolytes than is found in the plasma, which can cause fluid volume excess, hyperchloremia, and acidosis (Heitz and Horne, 2005).
‡Contains sodium, potassium, calcium, chloride, and lactate.

Equipment. Correct selection and preparation of IV equipment assists in safe and quick placement of an IV line. Sterile technique is necessary because fluids are instilled directly into the bloodstream. For efficient insertion of peripheral IV catheters, organize all equipment at the bedside. IV equipment includes needles or cannulas, tourniquet, clean gloves, dressings, solution containers, various types of tubing, and IV pumps or volume-control devices. IV cannulas and needles are available in a variety of gauges (e.g., 20 gauge, 22 gauge). The larger the gauge, the smaller the diameter of the IV cannula or needle.

You will use different types of infusion tubing to administer medications or IV fluids. A solution given rapidly needs to be infused with macrodrip tubing, which delivers large drops (standard drop size is 10 or 15 gtt/mL depending on the manufacturer) to maintain the prescribed rate. Macrodrip tubing is typically connected to an **electronic infusion device (EID),** to ensure a constant, regulated rate. In contrast, microdrip tubing provides a standard drop size of 60 gtt/mL. Microdrip tubing facilitates precise regulation of IV fluids at slow rates. Some patients require IV extension tubing to increase mobility, decrease manipulation and contamination of the insertion site, increase the number of infusion ports, facilitate tubing changes, or to facilitate changes in position. You will use EIDs or volume-control devices for children, patients with renal or cardiac failure, medications that require precise rates, or for critically ill patients to ensure a prescribed infusion rate and to prevent uncontrolled fluid administration.

Initiating Peripheral Intravenous Access. After organizing collected equipment at the bedside, prepare to insert the IV catheter by assessing the patient for a venipuncture site. Common peripheral IV access sites include veins in the hand and the arm (Figure 17-6). The use of the foot for an IV site is common with children but is not recommended in the adult because of the danger of thrombophlebitis (INS, 2006). When assessing patients for potential venipuncture sites, consider conditions and contraindications that exclude certain sites. For example, because very young children, older adults, and patients receiving steroids have fragile veins, avoid sites that are easily bumped or moved, such as the dorsal surface of the hand (Rosenthal, 2007) (Box 17-4).

Venipuncture is contraindicated in a site that is swollen, reddened, or tender to the touch resulting from inflammation, infiltration, or thrombosis. An infected site is red, tender, swollen, and possibly warm to the touch. Avoid using an extremity with a vascular (dialysis) graft or fistula or on the same side as a mastectomy (breast surgery). Initially place IV catheters at the most distal point when possible, which allows for the use of proximal sites later if the patient needs subsequent venipuncture sites.

Venipuncture is the technique for accessing a vein by puncture through the skin. To start an IV infusion, you will use either a stylet partially covered with a plastic cannula (over-the-needle cannula [ONC]) or a sharp rigid stylet (e.g., butterfly needle or straight metal needle). You will use aseptic technique to prepare the skin. Peripherally and centrally inserted cannulas placed into a central vein, such as the subclavian vein, deliver large volumes of fluids and TPN or allow administration of irritating medications. Large-gauge cannulas, such as 14 or 16 gauge, also allow for the administration of large volumes of fluids. Although specially trained staff members are usually responsible for inserting central cannulas, both types of cannulas require close monitoring and maintenance. Only experienced practitioners should perform venipuncture on patients with fragile veins (e.g., infants or older persons).

The general purposes of venipuncture are to collect a blood specimen, to instill a medication, to start an IV fluid infusion, or to inject a radiopaque or radioactive tracer for special examinations. Intermittent infusion is used when a patient requires medications only at certain times, in an emergency situation, and to avoid the discomfort of repeated injections. An intermittent infusion involves the same techniques as an intravenous drip (pump or gravity drip), but after the complete dose of medication has been given, the

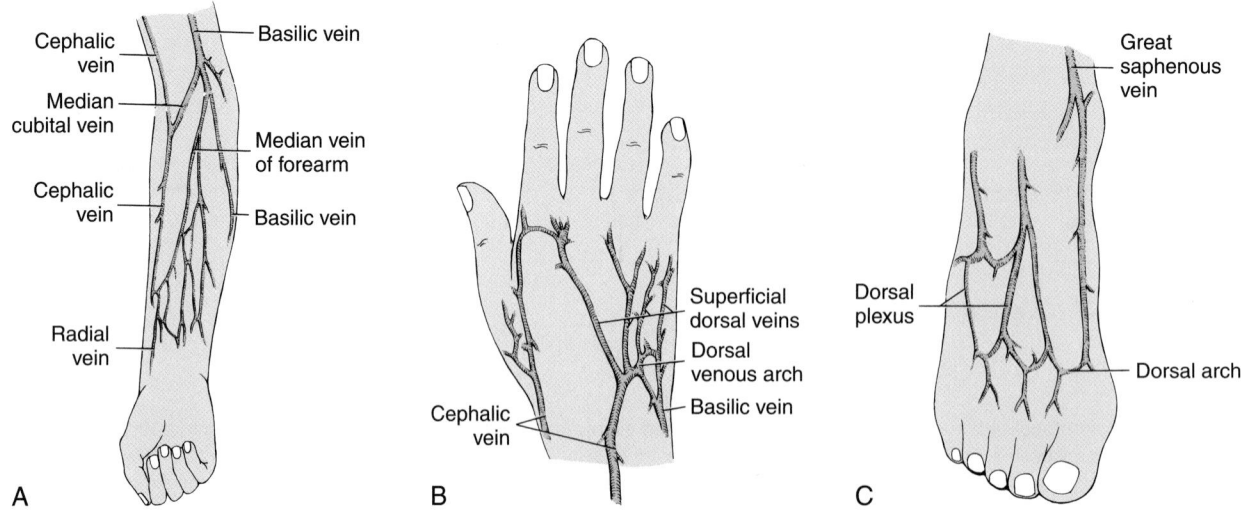

Figure 17-6 ■ Common IV sites. **A,** Inner arm. **B,** Dorsal surface of hand. **C,** Dorsal surface of foot (children only).

tubing is disconnected from the IV access device. A continuous infusion of fluids, with or without medications, is achieved over a 24-hour period through use of a VAD. Skill 17-1 describes the technique for initiating an IV fluid infusion and incorporates INS (2006) standards of practice.

Regulating the Infusion Flow Rate. After initiating an IV infusion and checking the infusion line for patency, regulate the rate of infusion according to the health care provider's orders (Skill 17-2). An infusion rate that is too slow fails to reverse cardiovascular and circulatory collapse in a critically ill patient who is in shock or dehydrated. An IV infusion that is running too slowly is at risk for becoming clotted. An infusion rate that is too rapid can cause fluid and electrolyte overload.

Calculate IV infusion rates to maintain a consistent flow at the ordered rate. There are different methods to ensure an accurate hourly infusion rate for IV therapy. Nonelectronic infusion devices, such as a flow control/regulator (e.g., Dial-a-Flow), deliver small amounts of fluid with the aid of gravity. The rate of infusion with an IV gravity controller depends on the height of the IV fluid container, IV tubing size, and fluid viscosity. An EID or IV volume controller are electronic pumps that deliver a measured amount of fluid over a prescribed period of time (e.g., 125 mL/hr). These devices maintain flow rates and cannula patency, but all patients receiving IV fluids require monitoring to detect and prevent complications.

Patency of the IV cannula means that there are no clots at the tip of the cannula, no kinks or compression of the cannula, and the cannula tip is not against the vein wall. A blocked cannula affects the infusion rate of IV fluids. Infiltration (fluid leaking into tissues), a knot or kink in the tubing, the height of the solution, a restrictive IV dressing, and position can all affect IV flow rates. Whenever an infusion problem occurs with the IV line, perform an assessment of the system until you locate the problem. Start the assessment at the cannula insertion site for signs and symptoms of infiltration (Table 17-9) and phlebitis (Table 17-10). Systematically continue the assessment by inspecting the tubing and area around the insertion site for anything blocking the flow of IV fluids (e.g., a knot or kink in the tubing will decrease the flow rate). Occasionally the cannula is kinked under the dressing, which requires removal of the dressing for inspection. Frequently the flow rate resumes after removing the tubing obstruction. The patient may lie or sit on the tubing, or the roller clamp is closed, which would cause an occlusion. The height of an IV container affects flow rates. Just raising the bag increases the rate because of increased hydrostatic pressure.

If the IV cannula is in an extremity, particularly at the wrist or elbow, the position of the extremity may decrease flow rates by pushing the tip of the catheter against the vein wall. Occasionally the use of an arm board helps to keep the joint extended and provides some protection to the site (Tripathi and others, 2008). However, use armboards with caution because they restrict patient movement. An IV protection device is a better option for protecting an IV site. Sometimes it is more comfortable for the patient to have an infusion started in a new location rather than relying on a site that causes problems. Before discontinuing the infusion, choose another site and start the infusion to verify that the patient has other accessible veins.

Children, older adults, patients with severe head trauma, and patients susceptible to volume overload need protection from sudden increases in infusion volumes through use of an infusion device to regulate IV fluid flow. When an IV controller device is open, it allows a free flow of the IV fluid. An excessive amount of solution infuses until the tubing clamp is regulated. For example, a restless patient loosens the roller clamp with a sudden movement and increases the flow rate, or the flow rate

---

BOX 17-4   CARE OF THE OLDER ADULT

Venipuncture Guidelines

- A tourniquet is not always required. Position the arm in a dependent position to fill the veins sufficiently for a venipuncture, or use a blood pressure cuff, which better protects the older adult's skin.
- Avoid access in the hands if it limits the older adult patient's ability to perform activities of daily living.
- Use the smallest-gauge IV cannula possible, such as 22 or 24 gauge.
- Take time to find the most suitable vein.
- Use strict aseptic technique, because the older adult patient is typically immunocompromised.
- Do not slap or vigorously scrub the arm to visualize the patient's veins.
- Use a decreased angle for insertion—usually between 5 and 15 degrees.

- Set the flow rate for IV medications, especially antibiotics, to no more than 100 mL/hr; for patients with heart failure or renal failure set the rate at 50 mL/hr.
- Use a protective skin preparation before applying a transparent dressing over the venous access device (VAD) insertion site; dry gauze pads are best for patients with tissue-thin skin.
- Cover the VAD dressing with flexible netting. If netting is unavailable, use minimal tape or an elastic bandage to secure the dressing and protect the site; keep the insertion site visible at all times.
- Do not use circumferential restraints on the extremity with the VAD.
- Assess the patient's mental status at least every 4 hours.
- Use electronic infusion devices or controllers to titrate infusion volume and rate.

Modified from Ignatavicius DD, Workman, ML: *Medical-surgical nursing: critical thinking for collaborative care,* ed 5, Philadelphia, 2008, Saunders.

TABLE 17-9 Infiltration Scale

GRADE	CLINICAL CRITERIA
0	No symptoms
1	Skin blanched Edema, <1 inch in any direction Cool to touch With or without pain
2	Skin blanched Edema 1-6 inches in any direction Cool to touch With or without pain
3	Skin blanched, translucent Gross edema >6 inches in any direction Cool to touch Mild to moderate pain Possible numbness
4	Skin blanched, translucent Skin tight, leaking Skin discolored, bruised, swollen Gross edema >6 inches in any direction Deep pitting tissue edema Circulatory impairment Moderate to severe pain Infiltration of any amount of blood product, irritant, or vesicant

From Infusion Nurses Society: Infusion nursing standards of practice, *J Infus Nurs* 29(Suppl 1):S1, 2006.

TABLE 17-10 Phlebitis Scale

GRADE	CLINICAL CRITERIA
0	No clinical symptoms
1	Erythema at access site with or without pain
2	Pain at access site with erythema and/or edema
3	Pain at access site with erythema and/or edema Streak formation Palpable venous cord
4	Pain at access site with erythema and/or edema Streak formation Palpable venous cord >1 inch in length Purulent drainage

From Infusion Nurses Society: Infusion nursing standards of practice, *J Infus Nurs* 29(Suppl 1):S1, 2006.

is accidentally increased when the patient ambulates. A sudden increase in IV infusion rate causes a rapid increase in vascular volume, which can make the patient critically ill or even cause death. Volume control devices, such as the Volutrol burette, limit the amount of sudden excessive increases in the volume of IV solution infused by limiting the volume of fluid in the device. Safeguards are in place for EIDs to prevent free flow of infusion and sudden volume infusion when regulators are removed from the tubing housing.

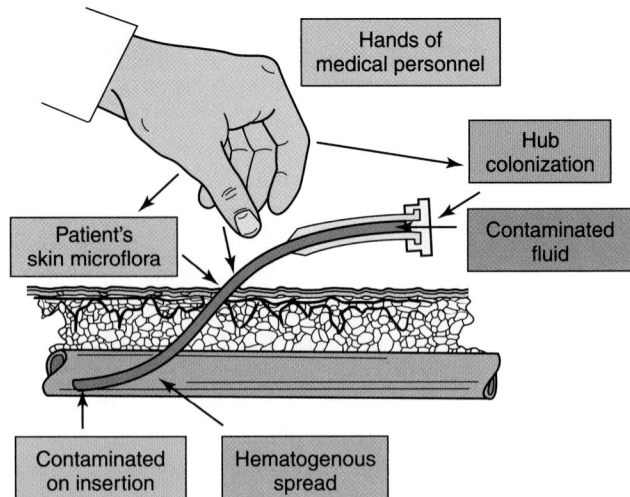

Figure 17-7 ■ Potential sites for contamination of an intravascular device.

Maintaining the System. You must maintain an IV system once the cannula is in place and the flow rate is regulated. Agency policies regulate the maintenance of IV lines. IV line maintenance includes (1) keeping the system sterile; (2) changing solutions, tubing, and site dressings; and (3) assisting the patient with self-care activities (e.g., bathing and gown changes), so the IV system is not disrupted.

An important part of maintaining the integrity of an IV is to prevent infection (Box 17-5). Figure 17-7 demonstrates the potential sites for contamination of an intravascular device. The procedure for IV insertion is designed to minimize contamination during cannula insertion. Other factors are controlled through conscientious ongoing use of infection control principles. This begins with the use of thorough hand hygiene before and after you handle any part of the IV system.

Always maintain the integrity of the IV system. Never disconnect tubing because it becomes tangled or because it is more convenient in positioning or moving a patient. If a patient needs more room to maneuver, add extension tubing to an IV line. Avoid stopcocks for connecting more than one solution to a single IV because they are sources of contamination (INS, 2006). When disconnecting an IV line from a stopcock, plug each port with a sterile cap. Do not allow a port to remain exposed to air, which will cause contamination. Intravenous tubing contains injection ports through which you can insert adapters for medication administration. Clean an injection port thoroughly with 70% alcohol, chlorhexidine, or povidone-iodine before accessing the system (INS, 2006).

Patients receiving IV therapy over several days will require intermittent changing of solution bags. It is important to organize tasks so that you can change solutions before the cannula becomes occluded. The Centers for Disease Control and Prevention (CDC) (2002) has no recommendations for the hang time of IV fluids; therefore refer to agency policies. Intravenous tubing administration sets can remain sterile for 72 hours (CDC, 2002; INS, 2006). The exception is tubing

BOX 17-5   BEST PRACTICES

SUMMARY OF EVIDENCE

You use intravenous (IV) catheters to administer fluids or medications or to withdraw blood samples via open systems, closed systems, or with needleless access devices. Needleless IV access devices were introduced into practice to reduce the rate of IV catheter needlestick injuries and to better meet the standards of practice for safety. Researchers analyzed data from numerous studies and found that the needlestick injury rates from manipulating IV tubing and needle assemblies were associated with the highest rate of needlestick injury.

A review of experimental studies was performed to evaluate the rate of IV contamination from the use of needleless IV access devices. There have been conflicting research reports that suggest there has been an increase and a decrease in catheter-related bloodstream infections since the implementation of needleless devices in practice.

APPLICATION TO NURSING PRACTICE

- Provide training for all health care workers before using needleless devices in practice.
- Develop a defined policy for needleless IV access device care.
- Audit for catheter-related infections.
- Current guidelines suggest changing needleless devices at least every 72 hours or per manufacturer's recommendations.

REFERENCE
Casey A, Elliott T: Infection risks associated with needleless intravenous access devices, *Nurs Stand* 22(11):38, 2007.

---

containing blood products, TPN, and lipids, which need to be changed more often because they are more likely to promote bacterial growth. When possible, schedule tubing changes when it is time to hang a new IV container (Skill 17-3). To prevent entry of microorganisms into the bloodstream, use filters when indicated and maintain sterility during tubing and solution changes.

Dressings over IV sites reduce the entrance of bacteria into the insertion site. The two forms of dressings are transparent and gauze. Transparent dressings reliably secure the IV device and allow continuous visual inspection of the IV site. They also stay cleaner and drier and require less-frequent changes than standard gauze (Winfield and others, 2007). Change gauze dressings every 48 hours (INS, 2006). You must change either form of dressing when the IV device is removed or when the dressing becomes damp, loosened, or soiled (INS, 2006). Agency policy may require routine dressing changes in different time frames (Skill 17-4).

To prevent the accidental disruption of an IV system, the patient may need assistance with hygiene, comfort measures, meals, and ambulation. Because a patient with an infusion in the arm finds it difficult to perform hygiene, you will often need to assist patients with bathing and changing gowns. Use a specially made gown with snaps along the top sleeve seam to change the gown without disturbing the venipuncture site. Traditional tie-back gowns are changed for maximum extremity mobility and speed by following these six steps:

1. Remove the sleeve of the gown from the arm without the IV, keeping the patients draped.
2. Remove the sleeve of the gown from the arm with the IV.
3. Remove the IV solution container from its stand, and pass it and the tubing through the sleeve starting with the end of the sleeve. (If this involves removing the tubing from an EID, use the roller clamp to slow the infusion.)

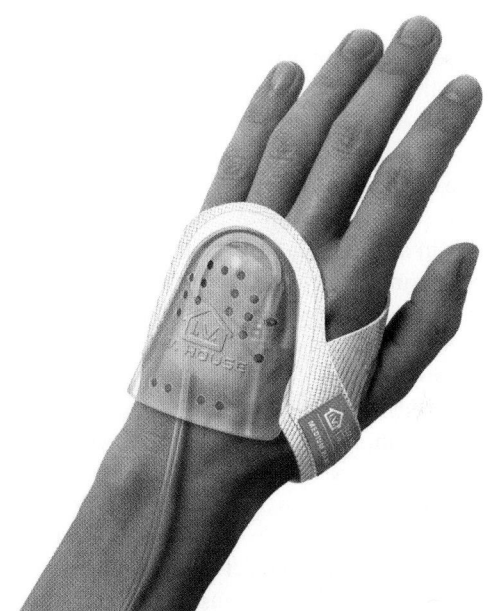

Figure 17-8 ■ I.V. House protective device. (Courtesy I.V. House, St. Louis, Mo.)

4. Place the IV solution container and tubing through the sleeve of the clean gown, and hang it back on the stand. (If the IV is connected to an EID, reassemble into the pump and open the roller clamp. Turn the pump on.)
5. Place the arm with the IV through the new gown sleeve.
6. Place the arm without the IV through the new gown sleeve. (Breaking the integrity of an IV line to change a gown leads to contamination.)

There are commercial protective devices designed to prevent accidental dislodgment of an IV cannula (Figure 17-8). Mechanical catheter-securing devices extend the time a cannula remains in the vein (Smith, 2006).

The patient with an arm, hand, or subclavian infusion is able to walk, unless contraindicated. Offer a rolling IV pole on wheels. Place the pole next to the involved arm and instruct the patient to hold on to the pole with the involved hand and to push it while walking. Check the equipment to ensure that the IV container is at the proper height, that there is no tension on the tubing, and that the flow rate is correct. Instruct the patient to report any blood in the tubing, stoppage in flow, an EID alarm, or increased discomfort.

Complications of Intravenous Therapy   An **infiltration** occurs when IV fluids seep into the subcutaneous tissue around the venipuncture site. Infiltration causes swelling (from increased tissue fluid) and possible pallor and coolness (caused by decreased circulation) around the venipuncture site. Early warning of infiltration is an IV infusing at a decreased rate or one that stops flowing. Pain is also present, usually resulting from tissue edema. Pain increases proportionately as the infiltration progresses.

When infiltration occurs, discontinue the infusion and remove the cannula. If IV therapy is still necessary, insert a new cannula in a vein at a new location. To reduce discomfort, elevate the extremity to promote venous drainage and decrease edema. Apply warm, moist towels to the site for 20 minutes three to four times during the day to promote venous return and reduce pain and edema

Certain IV medications, especially antibiotics and potassium, cause discomfort and burning sensations at the IV site. Evaluate the source of discomfort, and be prepared to start a new IV line in a larger vein if needed.

Phlebitis is inflammation of the vein. Selected risk factors include the size and type of cannula material, chemical irritation of additives and drugs given intravenously, and the anatomical position of the cannula. Signs and symptoms may include pain, edema, erythema, and increased skin temperature over the vein, and in some instances redness traveling along the path of the vein (INS, 2006).

When phlebitis develops, discontinue the IV line and insert a new line in another vein. Warm, moist heat on the site of phlebitis will offer some relief to the patient (see Chapter 36). Phlebitis is dangerous because blood clots (thrombophlebitis) can form, increasing the risk for an emboli. An embolus is a clot that becomes dislodged and travels to the heart, brain, or lungs, causing serious patient injury or death. The routine removal and rotation of IV sites reduces the risk for phlebitis. You should replace peripheral venous cannulas and rotate sites every 72 hours (INS, 2006; Powell and others, 2008).

Another complication of IV therapy is FVE that occurs when IV fluids have infused too rapidly. Assessment findings include shortness of breath, crackles in the lungs, and tachycardia. If these clinical signs are present, slow the rate of IV infusion, notify the health care provider, raise the head of the bed, provide supplemental oxygen as ordered, and monitor the patient's vital signs.

Discontinuing Intravenous Cannulas and Infusions
Discontinuing a cannula or infusion is necessary after the prescribed amount of fluid has been infused, when an infil-

tration occurs, if phlebitis is present, or if a clot develops in the cannula. Review the health care provider's order before discontinuing an infusion or cannula. Explain to patients that they might feel a burning sensation when the catheter is removed. Perform hand hygiene, and apply clean gloves. Move the IV tubing roller clamp to the "off" position, or turn the EID off and then set the clamp to "off" position. This prevents spillage of IV fluid. Remove the IV site dressing, stabilize the IV device, and then remove any tape securing the cannula. Apply clean sterile gauze over the venipuncture site, apply light pressure, and then remove the cannula by pulling straight away from the insertion site in a slow, steady motion (Figure 17-9). Keep the cannula parallel to the skin during withdrawal. Inspect the catheter for intactness after removal. Keep gauze in place and apply continuous pressure to the site for 2 to 3 minutes to control bleeding and minimize hematoma formation (INS, 2006). If a patient has a bleeding tendency, it might be necessary to apply pressure for a longer period of time. Apply a clean, folded gauze dressing over the removal site, and secure it with tape. Record the amount of fluid infused and the time the IV was discontinued. Routinely inspect the site for redness, edema, and tenderness for 48 hours. In some settings NAP are allowed to discontinue peripheral IVs (consult agency policy or Nurse Practice Act).

Blood Replacement   Blood replacement or transfusion is the IV administration of whole blood or a blood component such as plasma, packed red blood cells (RBCs), or platelets. The objectives for blood transfusions include (1) increasing circulating blood volume after surgery, trauma, or hemorrhage; (2) increasing the number of RBCs to maintain hemoglobin levels in patients with severe anemia; and (3) providing selected cellular components as replacement therapy (e.g., clotting factors, platelets, or albumin).

Autologous Transfusion.   The collection and reinfusion of a patient's own blood is referred to as **autologous transfusion** (autotransfusion). The blood for an autologous transfusion can be obtained by preoperative donation up to 5 weeks before the scheduled procedure, depending on the type of surgery and the ability of the patient to maintain an acceptable hematocrit. An autologous transfusion can also be obtained during perioperative blood salvage (e.g., during vascu-

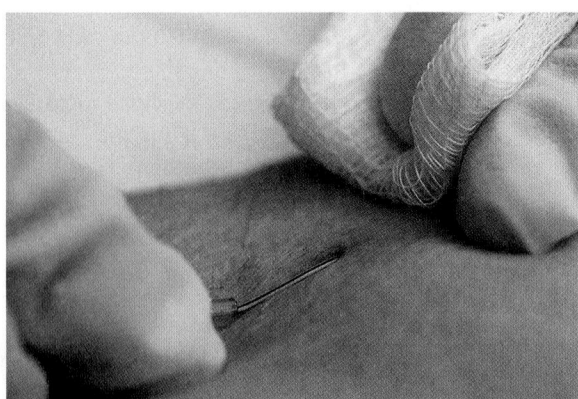

Figure 17-9 ■ IV catheter is withdrawn slowly, keeping catheter parallel to vein.

lar and orthopedic surgery, organ transplant surgery, and traumatic injuries) and reinfused during the surgery. Blood can also be salvaged postoperatively from mediastinal and chest tube drains and after joint and spinal surgery. Autologous transfusions are safer for the patient because they decrease the risk for complications such as mismatched blood and exposure to blood-borne infections.

Allogeneic Transfusion. The collection and reinfusion of a donor's blood into a patient is **allogeneic (or homologous) transfusion.** In the United States, the blood is collected in a donation center and goes through nine different tests to ensure the blood is free from infectious diseases before it is infused. The tests include: hepatitis B (HbsAg and Anti-Hbc), hepatitis C (Anti-HcV), syphilis, human immunodeficiency virus (HIV-1 and HIV-2), human T-lymphotropic virus (TLV-I and -II), and nucleic acid amplification testing (NAT). If the blood tests positive for any of these diseases, the blood is discarded and the donor is notified and placed on a list that prohibits the donor from donating blood again (AAB, 2006).

ABO System. There are three blood typing systems, ABO, Rh, and HLA typing, used to ensure a close match between transfused products and a patient's blood. The presence or absence of specific antigens on the surface of red blood cells determines blood type in the ABO system. When the type A antigen is present, the blood group is called type A. When the type B antigen is present, the blood group is type B. When both A and B antigens are present, the blood group is type AB, and when neither A nor B antigens are present, the blood group is type O.

Antibodies that react against the A and B antigens are naturally present in the plasma of people whose red blood cells do not carry the antigen. These antibodies react against the foreign antigens. For example, if a person who is type A accidentally receives type B blood, the antibodies in the person's blood will attack the type B antigens. Incompatible red blood cells agglutinate (clump together) and result in a life-threatening hemolytic transfusion reaction. People with type A blood have anti-B antibodies; people with type B blood have anti-A antibodies. People with type AB blood have neither antibody and can receive all blood types. People with type O blood have both A and B antibodies and can receive only type O blood.

Rh System. Another system for matching blood transfusions is the presence of the Rh factor, an antigenic substance on the erythrocytes of most people. A person with the Rh factor is Rh positive, whereas a person without it is Rh negative. Unlike the ABO antigens, there are not naturally occurring antibodies to the Rh antigen. A person with Rh-negative blood must first be exposed to Rh-positive blood before developing antibodies. The same applies to a person with Rh-positive blood. However, antibodies can develop after repeated transfusions.

Blood Transfusions. Transfusing blood components is a nursing procedure. Nurses complete thorough patient assessments before, during, and after the transfusion and for regulation of the transfusion. If the patient has IV access already in place, assess the site for signs of infection, infiltration, and patency. Determine the gauge of the IV cannula. A large cannula such as 18 or 19 gauge is preferred because blood is viscous. You can use smaller gauges, but a catheter no smaller than a 20 or 22 gauge is appropriate for a blood transfusion (Gray and others, 2007; Hadaway, 2007). The tubing for blood administration has a 20-μm in-line filter (Figure 17-10). Prime the tubing with 0.9% normal saline to reduce **hemolysis** (breakdown of RBCs).

Before the transfusion, assess the patient to determine if he or she knows the reason for the blood transfusion and whether the patient has ever had a previous transfusion or **transfusion reaction.** A transfusion reaction is an antigen-antibody reaction that ranges from a mild response to a severe anaphylactic reaction and is potentially fatal (Davis and others, 2006; Paris and Grant-Casey, 2007). A patient who has had a transfusion reaction may be at greater risk for a reaction with a subsequent transfusion. Some patients are anxious about the transfusion, requiring nursing intervention such as education. Before starting a transfusion, explain the procedure and instruct the patient to report any side effects (e.g., chills, dizziness, or fever) once the transfusion begins. Ensure the patient or representative has signed the informed consent. Persons from certain cultures may require different assessment techniques, may abstain from blood transfusions, or may seek alternatives to the transfusion (Gray and others, 2007; Tolich, 2008; Whyte, 2008). Be sensitive to these differences (Box 17-6).

ABO incompatibility is one of the most serious errors with transfusions. It commonly involves misidentification of the patient, unit of blood, or label on the pretransfusion blood sample. Use precautions in administering blood or blood products. To ensure that the right patient receives the

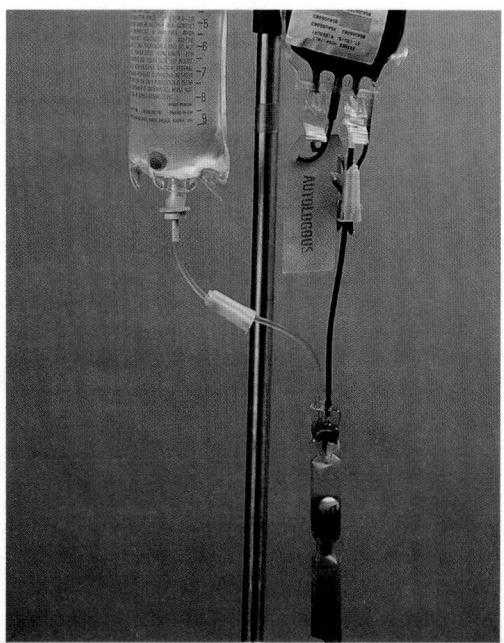

Figure 17-10 ■ Tubing for blood administration has an in-line filter.

BOX 17-6 CULTURAL FOCUS

Robert understands that the current standards of nursing and evidence-based practice dictate the need for culturally competent practices in health care settings. These standards promote an environment and plan of care that is inclusive of cultural and other forms of diversity. He knows that communication and education are essential components of positive therapeutic outcomes with diverse populations. To educate Mrs. Reynolds regarding intravenous (IV) therapy he must be sensitive to cultural and linguistic differences. Mrs. Reynold's education should include clear and concise terms for all aspects of IV therapy and individualized training to include self-care practices (INS, 2006; Pearson and others, 2007). In addition, certain cultures may require different assessment techniques, may abstain from blood transfusions, or may seek alternatives to the transfusion. Robert uses his understanding of culture to develop a plan of care for Mrs. Reynolds.

IMPLICATIONS FOR PRACTICE

- Robert encourages Mrs. Reynolds to identify any aspects of her intravenous care that she did not understand.
- He explains things in simple lay terms and tries to ensure that she understood what he was teaching her.
- Robert provides all care regarding Mrs. Reynold's IV with knowledge of her personal self-care practices, including activities of daily living.
- Robert tries to determine if a blood transfusion should become necessary, whether Mrs. Reynold's culture allows for a transfusion.
- Robert assesses Mrs. Reynold's social support network to aid her during her hospitalization.

Data from Gray and others: Safe transfusion of blood and blood components, *Nursing Standard* 21(51): 40, 2007; Tolich D: Alternatives to blood transfusion, *J Infus Nurs* 31(1): 46, 2008; Whyte A: A serious ethical dilemma, *Nursing Standard* 22(30):18, 2008.

correct crossmatched blood product, follow the health care facility's procedure to check the blood products and the patient, and verify the compatibility of the blood and the patient. Some hospitals use bar code technology to identify patients and verify compatible blood before beginning transfusions. Although not involved in the blood-labeling process, nurses are responsible for determining that the blood delivered to the patient corresponds to the patient's blood type documented in the medical record. Together, two registered nurses or one registered nurse (RN) and a licensed practical nurse (LPN) (check agency policy) must simultaneously check the label on the blood product against the patient's identification number, blood group, and complete name. *If even a minor discrepancy exists, do not give the blood. Notify the blood bank immediately.* Evidence-based transfusion processes prevent infusion errors (Gray and others, 2007).

Obtain the patient's baseline vital signs before a transfusion begins. These data will allow you to determine when changes in vital signs occur, which can indicate the development of a transfusion reaction. Initiation of a transfusion begins slowly to allow for the early detection of a transfusion reaction. Maintain the infusion rate, monitor for side effects, assess vital signs, and promptly record all findings. It is important to stay with the patient during the first 15 minutes, the time when a reaction is most likely to occur. After that time period, continue to monitor the patient and obtain vital signs periodically during the transfusion as directed by agency policy. If a transfusion reaction is suspected, STOP the transfusion immediately. Disconnect the blood tubing, and connect the normal saline infusion to maintain an open IV line. Once the normal saline line is established, obtain vital signs, and notify the health care provider. The unused blood product is returned to the blood bank.

The rate of transfusion is usually specified in the health care provider's orders. A unit of packed RBCs will transfuse in 2 hours. This time can be lengthened to 4 hours if the patient is at risk for FVE. Beyond 4 hours there is an increased risk for bacterial contamination of the blood (Davis and others, 2006). If the patient cannot tolerate the volume of fluid within this time frame, the blood bank can divide the unit into smaller volumes.

When patients have a severe blood loss such as with hemorrhage, they receive rapid transfusions through a central venous catheter or a large-gauge peripheral cannula. A blood-warming device is often necessary, because most blood products are stored at 40° F. Rapid administration of substances can irritate the heart and produce cardiac dysrhythmias (Gray and others, 2007), hypothermia, and coagulopathies.

Transfusion Reactions. A transfusion reaction is a systemic response by the body to incompatible blood. Causes include red cell incompatibility or allergic sensitivity to the components of the transfused blood or to the potassium or citrate preservative in the blood.

A second category of reactions includes diseases transmitted by infected blood donors who are asymptomatic or symptomatic. Diseases transmitted through transfusions include malaria, hepatitis B and C, and HIV. Because all units of blood collected in developed countries undergo serological testing and screening for HIV and HBV, the risk for acquiring these blood-borne infections from blood transfusions is minimal. Blood transfusion reactions are life threatening, but prompt nursing intervention can maintain the patient's physiological stability (Box 17-7).

Circulatory overload is a risk when a patient receives massive transfusions for hemorrhagic shock or when a patient with normal intravascular volume receives blood. Older adults and those with cardiopulmonary diseases are at risk for circulatory overload.

Interventions for Acid-Base Imbalances Nursing interventions to promote acid-base balance aim to reverse the underlying disorder causing the acid-base imbalance. Such imbalances may be life threatening and require rapid correction. It is important to maintain vascular access and frequently check for changes in existing therapies. Give prescribed drugs, such as insulin or sodium bicarbonate, fluid and electrolyte replacement, and oxygen therapy promptly. In addition, monitor patients closely for changes in acid-base

BOX 17-7   Nursing Interventions for Blood Transfusion Reaction

1 If you suspect a blood reaction, *STOP the transfusion immediately.*
2 Keep the intravenous line open, disconnect the blood tubing at the hub of the cannula, and directly connect the primed tubing of 0.9% normal saline. Place a sterile cap on the end of the blood tubing to maintain a sterile system.
3 Do not turn off the blood and simply turn on the 0.9% normal saline that is connected to the Y-tubing infusion set. This causes blood remaining in the Y-tubing to infuse into the patient. Even a small amount of mismatched blood can cause a major reaction.
4 Immediately notify the health care provider.
5 Remain with the patient, observing signs and symptoms and monitoring vital signs as often as every 5 minutes.
6 Prepare to administer emergency drugs such as antihistamines, vasopressors, fluids, and steroids per health care provider's order or agency protocol.
7 Activate the rapid response team.
8 Prepare to perform cardiopulmonary resuscitation.
9 Obtain a urine specimen, and send it to the laboratory to determine the presence of hemoglobin as a result of red blood cell hemolysis.
10 Save the blood container, tubing, attached labels, and transfusion record, and return them to the laboratory.
11 Document the transfusion reaction, description, treatment, and outcome.

balance. Often these patients require repeated ABG analysis, a procedure that involves obtaining arterial blood samples for analysis of hydrogen ion concentration.

Arterial Blood Gas Collection. ABG levels require removal of a sample of blood from an artery to assess the patient's acid-base status and the adequacy of ventilation and oxygenation. A qualified registered nurse (RN) or other health care provider draws arterial blood from a peripheral artery (usually the radial) or from an arterial line (check agency policy). Before obtaining the specimen, perform an Allen's test to ensure that the patient has an ulnar pulse. This protects the hand from loss of blood flow in the event of radial artery damage. After obtaining the specimen, take care to prevent air from entering the syringe because this will affect blood gas results. To reduce red cell metabolism, submerge the syringe in crushed ice and transport it immediately to the laboratory for analysis. After the arterial puncture, apply pressure to the puncture site for at least 5 minutes to reduce hematoma formation. A hematoma could occlude an artery or reduce blood flow. Apply pressure for a longer period if the patient is on anticoagulant medications or has a coagulopathy. Reassess the radial pulse after removing pressure.

RESTORATIVE AND CONTINUING CARE   After experiencing acute alterations in fluid, electrolyte, or acid-base balance, patients often require ongoing maintenance therapy to prevent a recurrence of health alterations. Older adults and the chronically ill require special considerations to prevent complications from developing.

Home Intravenous Therapy   Intravenous therapy often continues in the home setting for patients requiring long-term hydration, parenteral nutrition, or extended medication administration. A home IV therapy nurse will work closely with the patient or caregiver to ensure that a sterile IV system is maintained and that complications are avoided or promptly recognized. Box 17-8 summarizes patient education guidelines for home IV therapy.

Nutritional Support   Most patients who have had electrolyte disorders or acid-base disturbances require ongoing nutritional support. Depending on the type of disorder, certain fluids or food may be encouraged or restricted. If patients are still responsible for meal preparation, they need to learn to understand the nutritional content of foods and learn to read the labels of commercially prepared foods.

Medication Safety   Numerous medications, over-the-counter (OTC) drugs, and herbal supplements contain components or create potential side effects that can alter fluid and electrolyte balance. Patients with chronic disease who are receiving multiple medications and patients with renal or liver disorders are at significant risk for alterations in fluid and electrolyte status. Patient and family education are essential to provide information regarding potential side effects, drug and herbal interactions, or over-the-counter medications to avoid. Review all medications with patients and family caregivers, and encourage them to consult with their local pharmacist before trying a new over-the-counter medication.

■■■EVALUATION

PATIENT CARE   Evaluation of a patient's clinical status is important if an acute alteration in fluid and electrolyte or acid-base disturbance exists. It is important to recognize the signs and symptoms of impending problems by considering the patient's presenting risk factors, clinical status, the effects of the present treatment regimen, and the potential causative agent. Perform an evaluation to determine if changes have occurred from the previous patient assessment. For example, if the patient's hypokalemia is improving, the signs and symptoms of hypokalemia should begin to diminish. The patient's heart rate and rhythm becomes more regular, muscle tone improves, and bowel function returns. The serum potassium level will return to normal levels.

For patients with less acute alterations, evaluation occurs over a longer period of time. In this situation, evaluation may focus more on behavioral changes (e.g., the patient's ability to follow dietary restrictions and medication schedules). The family's ability to anticipate alterations and prevent problems from recurring is also an important component of evaluation.

The patient's rate of progress determines whether the current plan of care needs to be continued or revised. If goals remain unmet, communicate with other members of the health care team to discuss alternative interventions. Additional methods to improve outcomes may include increasing the frequency of an intervention (e.g., provide more fluids to

BOX 17-8 PATIENT TEACHING

Home Intravenous Therapy

Often patients require home intravenous (IV) therapy. It is essential that the patient and family caregiver are prepared to manage a continuous infusion and that the home environment offer the necessary resources. The following is an example of a teaching plan.

OUTCOME

• At the end of the teaching sessions the patient/or family caregiver will be able to demonstrate understanding and competence with IV therapy for safe delivery in the home setting.

TEACHING STRATEGIES

• Explain the importance of IV therapy in maintaining hydration and access for delivery of medications.
• Emphasize the risks involved when the IV system is not kept sterile.
• Show the patient and/or family caregiver how to manipulate the required equipment, and provide opportunity to handle the equipment.
• Instruct in aseptic technique and hand hygiene in the handling of all IV equipment.
• Instruct in how to change IV solutions, tubing, and dressing when they become soiled or dislodged. (NOTE: The home care nurse may be able to visit frequently enough to perform scheduled tubing and dressing changes.)
• Instruct in procedures for safe disposal, in appropriate containers, of all sharps and IV materials exposed to blood.
• Instruct in signs and symptoms of infiltration, phlebitis, and infection and reporting symptoms immediately.
• Instruct patient and/or primary caregiver to report if the infusion slows or stops or if blood is seen in the tubing.
• Teach patient with caregiver's assistance how to ambulate, perform hygiene, and participate in other activities of daily living without dislodging or disconnecting cannula and tubing.

EVALUATION STRATEGIES

• Ask patient and caregiver reasons why it is necessary to maintain hydration and IV access for the delivery of medications.
• Ask what to do if the IV stops.
• Ask patient and/or family caregiver to describe signs and symptoms of complications and what action they should take.
• Observe the patient and caregiver changing the IV container, tubing, and dressing.
• Observe the patient ambulating and participating in activities of daily living.

BOX 17-9 EVALUATION

Robert continues to be assigned to Mrs. Reynolds, 2 days after her admission. He asks Mrs. Reynolds how she feels and prepares to conduct a brief physical examination. Mrs. Reynolds remarks, "I feel much better. I have had no nausea since early yesterday and no diarrhea since late yesterday afternoon." The IV of 0.9% normal saline is still in place, infusing now at 100 mL/hr. However, the patient's physician has just visited and has ordered you to reduce the rate to 40 mL/hr. She has been tolerating oral fluids. During examination, Robert notices the oral mucosa is still slightly dry; skin turgor has returned to normal. Mrs. Reynolds' vital signs are blood pressure, 126/78 mm Hg; pulse, 88 beats per minute; and respirations, 18 breaths per minute. She is afebrile. The serum potassium level drawn at 7 AM was 4.0 mEq/L.

Robert is encouraged by Mrs. Reynolds' progress. He prepares her breakfast meal tray, which includes the first soft food Mrs. Reynolds has had since being hospitalized. Robert sits down and discusses with Mrs. Reynolds the information she has learned from their discussion about food sources for potassium. Robert asks, "After discussing the importance of potassium in your diet, tell me what foods to select that include potassium." Mrs. Reynolds is able to identify five different sources of potassium among foods that she enjoys and can routinely include in her diet.

DOCUMENTATION NOTE

"Denies nausea and reports feeling better. No diarrheal stool since yesterday afternoon around 3 PM. On inspection, oral mucosa remains dry, without lesions or inflammation. Skin turgor is normal. Bowel sounds are normal in all four quadrants, abdomen soft to palpation. IV of 0.9% normal saline is infusing in left cephalic vein in forearm at 40 mL/hr per MD order. No tenderness or inflammation at IV site. Is able to identify five food sources for potassium to include in diet. Is resting comfortably, out of bed in a chair, ate all of breakfast. Will continue to monitor."

a dehydrated patient), introducing a new therapy (e.g., initiate insertion of an IV), or discontinuing a therapy. Once outcomes have been met, the nursing diagnosis is resolved and you can focus on other priorities.

PATIENT EXPECTATIONS Review with the patient his or her perceptions about success at meeting the expectations of care. "Do you feel less nauseous?" is a question to ask if the patient's expectations revolve around symptom management (Box 17-9). If the patient's concerns involve having a better understanding of a newly diagnosed problem, evaluate the patient's satisfaction with the education provided. Often the patient's level of satisfaction with care also depends on success in involving family and friends. If the patient has concerns about returning home or to a different care setting, it is important to evaluate if the patient feels prepared for the transition from acute care. Care plan modification occurs if any planned outcomes are not achieved, so new outcomes can be developed.

SAFETY GUIDELINES FOR NURSING SKILLS

Ensuring patient safety is essential before parenteral infusion therapy. Communicate clearly the goals of therapy with members of the health care team. Assess and incorporate the patient's priorities of care and preferences into your approaches. Use the best evidence when making patient care decisions. When performing skills in this chapter, remember the following points for safe, individualized patient care:

- Conduct a preprocedure verification process to ensure all documents, information, and/or equipment are available before the start of any procedure.
- Before initiation of therapy, check patient identification using two patient identifiers, and assess appropriate route

and rate of infusion and potential incompatibilities between infusing fluids and medications (INS, 2006).

- Use aseptic and sterile techniques, follow standard precautions, and maintain equipment sterility in all IV skills to prevent development of bloodstream infections (INS, 2006).
- Dispose of all disposable blood-contaminated and sharp items in puncture-resistant biohazard containers.
- Ensure that patient does not have latex allergy, and use nonlatex supplies when allergy is present.
- Specific infusion tubing is required for most EIDs and some infusions. Refer to manufacturer's specifications.

SKILL 17-1   INITIATING INTRAVENOUS THERAPY

View Video!

DELEGATION CONSIDERATIONS

The skill of initiating peripheral IV therapy cannot be delegated to nursing assistive personnel (NAP). Delegation to licensed practical nurses (LPNs) varies by state Nurse Practice Act. The nurse directs the NAP to:

- Inform the nurse if the patient complains of burning, bleeding, swelling, or coolness at the catheter insertion site
- Inform the nurse if the patient's IV dressing becomes wet
- Inform the nurse if the solution of fluid in the IV bag is low or the EID alarm is sounding

EQUIPMENT

- Facility-approved, proper IV safety access device for venipuncture (Figure 17-11) (will vary with patient's body size and reason for IV fluid administration). In an adult a peripheral 22-gauge cannula is appropriate for fluid maintenance (Rosenthal, 2007). Use a steel-winged infusion set for short-term therapy (INS, 2006).
- IV start kit (available in some agencies): may contain a sterile drape, tourniquet, cleansing and antiseptic preparations, dressings, and a small roll of sterile tape
- Local anesthetic (e.g., intradermal lidocaine, topical transdermal anesthetic) *(optional)*.

For IV Fluid Infusion

- Correct IV solution
- Administration set (choice depends on type of solution and rate of administration; infants and children, patients with cardiac and renal disease, and certain medications require microdrip tubing, which administers 60 gtt/mL)
- 0.22-μm filter (if required by agency policy or if particulate matter is likely; size appropriate to type of solution)

- Extension tubing
- Antiseptic swabs or sticks (e.g., chlorhexidine gluconate, povidone-iodine, alcohol) (INS, 2006)
- Clean gloves
- Protective equipment: Goggles, mask *(optional,* check agency policy)
- Tourniquet (Determine type of tourniquet based on patient assessment; e.g., blood pressure cuff [older adult], rubber band [infants]. Tourniquets are a source of contamination; use a single-use product)
- Nonallergenic tape and sterile tape
- Manufactured catheter stabilization device (e.g., StatLock), if available
- Transparent dressing or gauze sponge and sterile tape
- Towel (to place under patient's hand or arm)
- IV pole, rolling or ceiling mounted
- Special patient gown with snaps at shoulder seams, if available
- Needle-disposal container (sharps container)
- IV site protection device *(optional)*

For Heparin or Normal Saline Lock

- Injection cap (also called IV plug, prn adapter)
- IV loop or short piece of extension tubing, if necessary
- Syringe filled with 1 to 3 mL of 0.9% sodium chloride or heparin flush (10 units/mL as ordered)

Transparent Dressing Only

- Transparent dressing

Gauze Dressing Only

- 2 × 2 or 4 × 4 gauze sponge
- Sterile tape

SKILL 17-1   INITIATING INTRAVENOUS THERAPY—cont'd

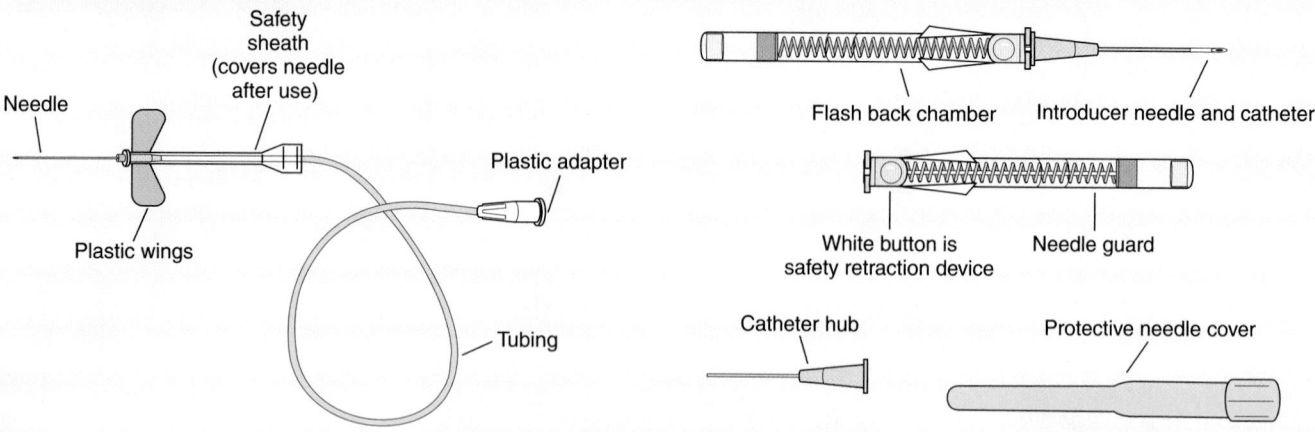

Figure 17-11 ■ IV access device options.

STEP	RATIONALE

ASSESSMENT

1 Review accuracy and completeness of health care provider's order for type and amount of IV fluid, medication additives, infusion rate, and length of therapy. Follow the six rights of medication administration (see Chapter 16).

Before implementing this procedure, you need an order from a health care provider to initiate a peripheral VAD and administration of an IV solution. Ensures safe and correct administration of IV therapy.

• *Critical Decision Point:* In most medical facilities, health care providers do not write an order to "initiate peripheral access" or "perform venipuncture." The statement "start IV" is written followed by the exact IV therapy order. The order to perform the venipuncture is implied. If the order is confusing or in question, clarify with the health care provider before proceeding.

2 Assess for clinical factors/conditions that will be affected by IV fluid administration:

Provides baseline to determine effect IV fluids have on patient's fluid and electrolyte balance.

a Peripheral edema—rate severity by assessing pitting over bony prominences; +1 indicates barely detectable edema to +4 for deep persistent pitting (see Chapter 15)

Indicates expanded interstitial volume. This is usually most evident in dependent areas (i.e., feet and ankles). Fluid overload will worsen edema.

b Body weight

Daily weights document fluid retention or loss. Change in body weight of 1 kg corresponds to 1 L of fluid retention or loss (Heitz and Horne, 2005).

c Dry skin and mucous membranes

Suggests fluid volume deficit (FVD).

d Distended neck veins

Suggests fluid volume excess (FVE).

e Blood pressure changes

Elevated blood pressure indicates volume excess or vasoconstriction resulting from an increase in stroke volume. Decreased blood pressure indicates fluid volume deficit caused by a decrease in stroke volume.

f Irregular pulse rhythm; increased pulse rate

Rhythm changes occur with potassium, calcium, and/or magnesium abnormalities; rate change occurs with fluid volume deficit or overload (e.g., atrial fibrillation).

g Auscultation of crackles or rhonchi in lungs

May signal fluid buildup in the lungs resulting from fluid volume excess.

h Poor skin turgor (after pinching skin over forearm or sternum, fails to return to normal position within 3 seconds)

With a fluid volume deficit, the pinched skin stays elevated for several seconds. This is called "tenting."

• *Critical Decision Point:* Tenting is a less-reliable indicator for older adults because their skin has lost elasticity naturally due to aging (Meiner and Lueckenotte, 2006).

STEP	RATIONALE
i Anorexia, nausea, and vomiting	May occur with acute FVD or FVE.
j Thirst	Symptomatic of FVD.
k Decreased urine output	During dehydration, kidney tries to restore fluid balance by reducing urine production. Average daily adult urine output is 1500 mL; urine output of less than 400 mL/24 hr (oliguria) signals the retention of metabolic wastes (Heitz and Horne, 2005).
l Behavioral changes (e.g., restlessness, confusion)	May occur with FVD or acid-base imbalance.
m Decreased capillary refill	May suggest poor tissue perfusion caused by fluid deficit.
3 Assess patient's previous or perceived experience with IV therapy and arm placement preference.	Determines level of emotional support and instruction needed. If hypersensitive to venipunctures, a local anesthetic may be indicated.
4 Obtain information from drug reference books or pharmacist about composition of IV fluids, purposes of administration, potential incompatibilities, and possible side effects. Include information about the most appropriate type of catheter to use for administration.	Allows detection of an inadvisable IV fluid order and helps to determine priority assessments.
5 Determine if patient is to undergo any planned surgeries or procedures.	Allows anticipation and placement of appropriate VAD and size for fluid infusion and avoids placement in area that will interfere with medical procedures.
6 Assess for the following risk factors: child or older adult; presence of heart failure or renal failure, skin lesions, infection, low platelet count; or receiving anticoagulants.	Persons at extremes in age develop fluid imbalances more rapidly because they have a proportionately larger extracellular fluid volume; persons with heart failure cannot adapt to sudden increases in vascular volume, and persons with renal failure cannot eliminate excess extracellular fluid. Skin lesions or infection influence choice of access site. Low platelet count or use of anticoagulants increases patient's risk for bleeding from VAD site and affects venous integrity, increasing the risk for seepage of blood from puncture site during venipuncture attempt.
7 Assess laboratory data.	Establishes baseline for determining if therapy is effective.
8 Assess patient's history of allergies, especially to iodine, adhesive, or latex.	Equipment used during insertion may contain substances to which patient is allergic.
9 Assess patient's understanding of purpose of IV therapy.	Poses implications for patient education.

PLANNING

1 Collect and organize equipment.	
2 Identify patient using two identifiers (e.g., name and birthday or name and account number, according to facility policy).	Complies with The Joint Commission requirements and improves medication safety. In most acute care settings you will use the patient's name and identification number on armband and MAR to identify patients.
3 Instruct patient about the rationale for IV, fluids, and medications, procedure for initiating an IV, and signs and symptoms of complications.	Provides patient with information about procedure and promotes compliance
4 Assist patient to comfortable sitting or supine position. Position yourself level with patient. Provide adequate lighting.	Promotes comfort and relaxation to patient. Provides proper body mechanics for nurse. Aids in successful vein location.

IMPLEMENTATION

1 Perform hand hygiene. Organize equipment on clean, clutter-free bedside stand or over-bed table.	Reduces transmission of infection and risk for accidents.
2 Change patient's gown to the more easily removed gown with snaps at the shoulder, if available.	Use of special IV gown makes it easier to safely remove the gown once the IV is inserted.
3 Open sterile packages using sterile aseptic technique (see Chapter 13).	Maintains sterility of equipment and reduces spread of microorganisms.

SKILL 17-1 INITIATING INTRAVENOUS THERAPY—cont'd

STEP	RATIONALE

4 Prepare IV infusion tubing and solution.

a Check IV solution, using the six rights of medication administration (see Chapter 16). Be sure prescribed additives, such as potassium and vitamins, have been added. Check solution for color, clarity, and expiration date. Check bag for leaks. This is easier to do before you reach the bedside.

IV solutions are medications and need to be carefully checked to reduce risk for error. Do not use solutions that are discolored, contain particles, or are expired. Do not use leaky bags because they present an opportunity for infection.

b Open infusion set, maintaining sterility of both tubing ends. Many sets allow for priming of tubing without removal of end cap. EID pumps sometimes have a special dedicated administration set.

Prevents touch contamination, which allows microorganisms to enter infusion equipment and bloodstream.

c Place roller clamp about 2 to 5 cm (1 to 2 inches) below drip chamber, and move roller clamp to "off" position (see illustrations).

Close proximity of roller clamp to drip chamber allows more accurate regulation of flow rate. Moving clamp to "off" prevents accidental spillage of IV fluid on patient, nurse, bed, or floor.

d Remove protective sheath from IV tubing port on plastic IV solution bag (see illustration) or top of bottle.

Provides access for insertion of infusion tubing into the solution.

e Insert infusion set into fluid bag or bottle. Remove protector cap from tubing insertion spike, not touching spike, and insert spike into opening of IV container (see illustration). Cleanse rubber stopper on glass bottled solution with single-use antiseptic, and insert spike into black rubber stopper of IV bottle. NOTE: Glass bottles need vented tubing.

Flat surface on the top of bottled solution may contain contaminants, whereas opening to plastic bag is recessed. Prevents contamination of bottled solution during insertion of spike.

• **Critical Decision Point:** Do not touch spike because it is sterile. If contamination occurs (e.g., spike is accidentally dropped on the floor), then discard that IV tubing and obtain a new one).

---

f Prime infusion tubing by filling with IV solution: Compress drip chamber and release, allowing it to fill one-third to one-half full (see illustration).

Ensures tubing is cleared of air before connection with VAD. Creates suction effect; fluid enters drip chamber to prevent air from entering tubing.

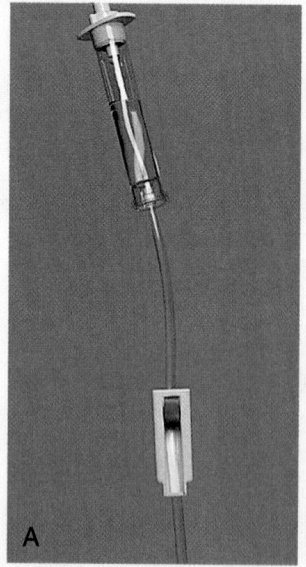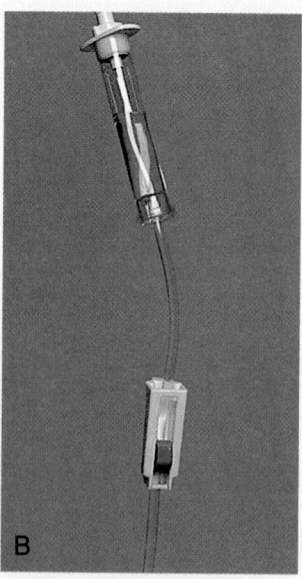

Step 4c ■ **A,** Roller clamp in open position. **B,** Roller clamp in closed or off position.

STEP	RATIONALE

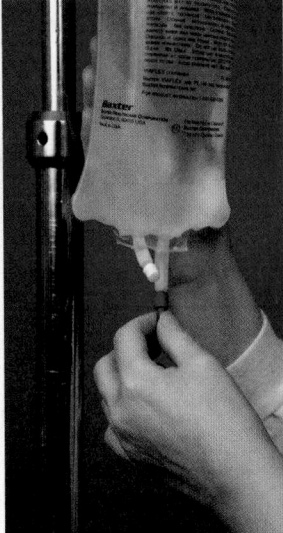 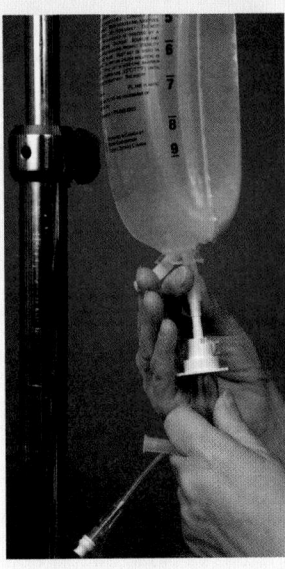 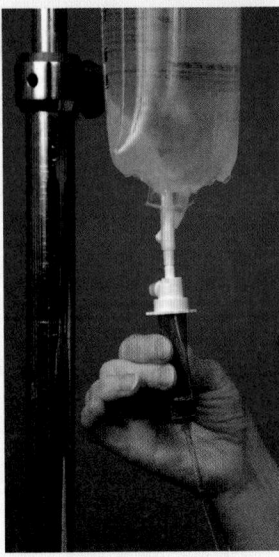 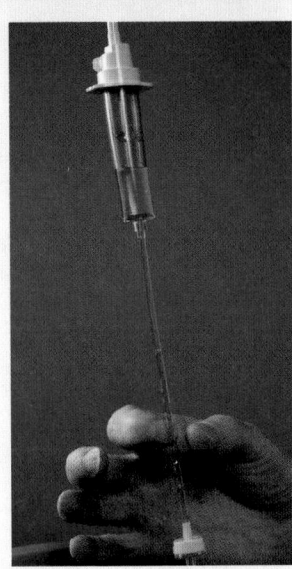

Step 4d ■ Remove protective covering from IV solution.

Step 4e ■ Insert tubing spike into IV container.

Step 4f ■ Squeeze drip chamber to fill with fluid.

Step 4h ■ Remove air bubbles from tubing.

g Remove protector cap on end of tubing (you can prime some tubing without removal), and slowly open roller clamp to allow fluid to travel from drip chamber through tubing to needle adapter. Return roller clamp to "off" position after priming tubing (filled with IV fluid).

Slow fill of tubing decreases turbulence and chance of bubble formation. Removes air from tubing and permits tubing to fill with solution. Closing the clamp prevents accidental loss of fluid.

h Be certain tubing is clear of air and air bubbles. To remove small air bubbles, firmly tap IV tubing where air bubbles are located. Check entire length of tubing to ensure that all air bubbles are removed (see illustration). If using multiple port tubing, turn ports upside down and tap to fill and remove air.

Large air bubbles act as emboli.

i Replace cap protector on end of infusion tubing.

Maintains system sterility.

• **Critical Decision Point:** You can add extension tubing to IV tubing to allow for more length, which will enable patient to move more freely while still keeping IV line stable.

---

5 *Option:* Saline lock (capped catheter)

a If you need a loop or short extension tubing because of awkward VAD placement, use sterile technique to connect extension to the IV tubing.

Used when continuous infusions are not needed.

b Swab injection cap with antiseptic swab. Insert syringe with 1 to 3 mL saline or heparin flush solution, and inject through the injection cap into the loop or short extension tubing.

Removes air from tubing and prevents air from being introduced into the vein.

• **Critical Decision Point:** Gloves are not required to assess veins, but you need to apply them before cannula insertion.

---

6 Apply clean gloves. Wear eye protection and mask (check agency policy) if splash or spray of blood is possible.

Reduces transmission of microorganisms. Decreases exposure to HIV, hepatitis, and other blood-borne organisms (INS, 2006; Occupational Safety and Health Administration [OSHA], 2006). Prevents spraying blood from contacting nurse's mucous membranes.

SKILL 17-1   INITIATING INTRAVENOUS THERAPY—cont'd

STEP	RATIONALE
7 Identify accessible vein for placement of VAD. Apply tourniquet around arm above antecubital fossa (see illustration) or 4 to 6 inches (10 to 15 cm) above proposed insertion site. Do not apply tourniquet too tightly to avoid injury or bruising to skin. One option is to apply tourniquet over top of a thin layer of clothing such as a gown sleeve. Sometimes it is necessary to remove tourniquet and move it along arm. *Option:* Use a blood pressure cuff instead of a tourniquet. Inflate it to a level just below the patient's normal diastolic pressure (less than 50 mm Hg.) Maintain inflation until venipuncture is completed.	Tourniquet slows down venous return but should not occlude arterial flow. If you cannot find a vein in the hand or lower arm, move up to the antecubital fossa. Use of blood pressure cuff reduces trauma to the underlying skin and tissues.

8 Vein distention
  a Select well-dilated vein. Methods to foster venous distention include:
    (1) Stroking the extremity from distal to proximal below the proposed venipuncture site.
    (2) Applying warmth to the extremity for several minutes, for example, with a warm washcloth.
	Increases the volume of blood in the vein at the venipuncture site.
	Promotes venous filling.
	
	Increases blood supply and fosters venous dilation.

• *Critical Decision Point:* Vigorous friction and multiple tapping of the veins, especially in older adults, will cause hematoma and/or venous constriction.

9 *Vein selection:* Select the vein for VAD insertion. Veins found on the dorsal and ventral surfaces of upper extremities (e.g., cephalic, basilic, and median veins) are preferred in adults.	Ensures adequate vein that is easier to puncture with needle and less likely to rupture.
a Use the most distal site in the nondominant arm, if possible. Clip arm hair with scissors if necessary.	You perform venipuncture distal to proximal, which increases the availability of other sites for future IV therapy. Hair impedes venipuncture or adherence of dressing.

• *Critical Decision Point:* Do not shave area with a razor. Shaving may cause microabrasions and increase patient's risk for infection (INS, 2006).

b If possible, place extremity in dependent position.	Permits venous dilation and visibility.
c Select a vein large enough for a VAD.	Prevents interruption of venous flow while allowing adequate blood flow around the catheter.
d With the index finger, palpate the vein by pressing downward. Note the resilient, soft, bouncy feeling when releasing the pressure (see illustration).	Fingertip is more sensitive and is better to assess vein location and condition.

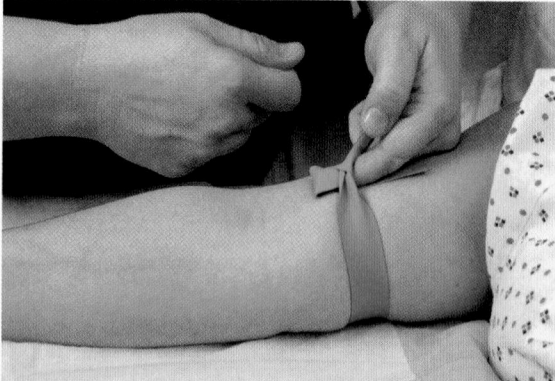

Step 7 ■ Tourniquet placed on arm for initial vein selection.

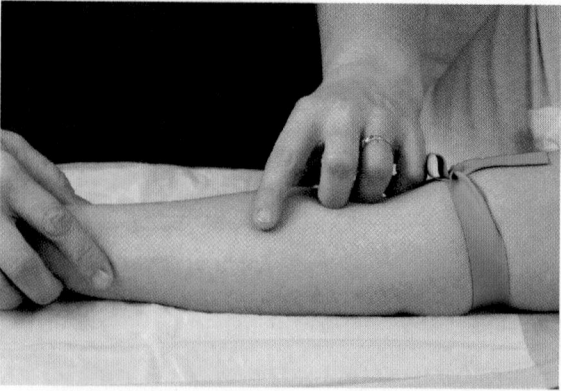

Step 9d ■ Palpate vein for resilience.

STEP	RATIONALE

e Avoid areas for vein selection affected by:

(1) Pain, infection, or wound

Indicates inflammation.

(2) Previous cerebrovascular accident (CVA), paralysis, or mastectomy

Increases risk for complications such as infection, lymphedema, or vessel damage.

(3) Site distal to previous venipuncture site, veins in antecubital fossa or inner wrist, sclerosed or hardened veins, infiltrate site or phlebotic vessels, bruised areas, and areas of venous valves

Such sites cause infiltration of newly placed VAD and excessive vessel damage. Antecubital fossa area is for blood draws; limits mobility (Otto, 2005).

(4) Fragile dorsal veins in older adult patients and vessels in an extremity with compromised circulation (e.g., in cases of mastectomy, dialysis graft, or paralysis)

Venous alterations increase risk for complications (e.g., infiltration and decreased catheter dwell time).

f Choose a site that will not interfere with patient's activities of daily living (ADLs) or planned procedures.

Keeps patient as mobile as possible.

10 Release tourniquet temporarily and carefully. *Option:* At this point in the procedure there is the option of applying a local anesthetic to site. Monitor patient for allergic reaction.

Restores blood flow and prevents venospasm when preparing for venipuncture. Most patients prefer a local anesthetic (Earhart and others, 2007).

11 Apply clean gloves if not done in Step 6.

Reduces transmission of microorganisms.

12 Place adapter end of infusion tubing or extension/injection cap nearby on sterile gauze or sterile towel.

Permits smooth, quick connection of infusion to VAD once vein is accessed.

13 If area of insertion appears to need cleansing, use soap and water first. Then use antiseptic swab, cleanse insertion site working in a horizontal plane with first swab, vertical plane with second swab, and a circular motion, moving outward with third swab (see illustration). Allow to dry completely. Refrain from touching the cleansed site unless using sterile technique.

Mechanical friction in this pattern allows penetration of the antiseptic solution into the cracks and fissures of the epidermal layer of the skin (INS, 2006). INS, 2006Hadaway, 2006INS, 2006TJC, 2008Allowing antiseptic solutions to air-dry completely effectively reduces microbial counts (). Drying allows time for maximum microbiocidal activity of agents (). Chlorhexidine 2% preparation is preferred (;). Touching cleansed area introduces microorganisms from finger to site. If this happens, prep the site again.

14 Reapply tourniquet 10 to 12.5 cm (4 to 5 inches) above anticipated insertion site. Check presence of distal pulse.

Diminished arterial flow prevents venous filling. The pressure of the tourniquet causes the vein to dilate.

15 Perform venipuncture. After the antiseptic dries, anchor vein below site by placing thumb over vein and by stretching the skin against the direction of insertion 1½ to 2 inches (4 to 5 cm) distal to the site (see illustration). Warn patient of a sharp, quick stick.

Stabilizes vein for needle insertion. Places VAD parallel to vein.

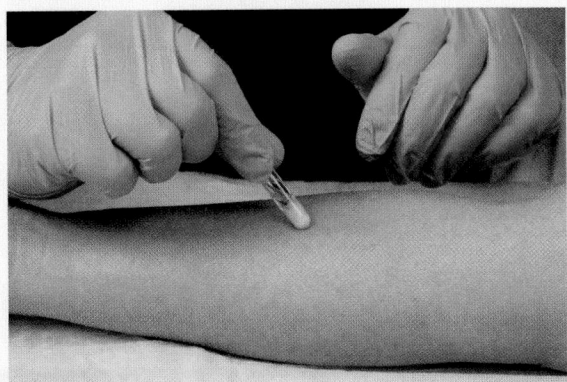

Step 13 ■ Cleanse site with chlorhexidine.

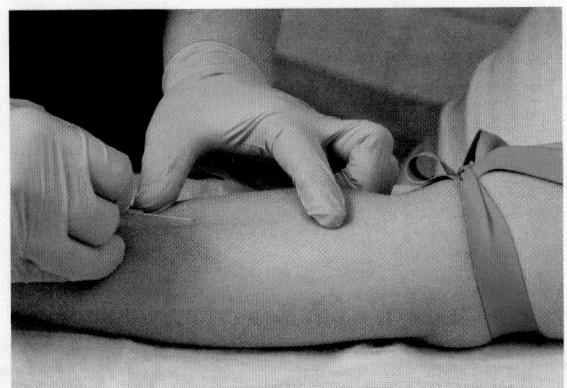

Step 15 ■ Stabilize vein below insertion site.

SKILL 17-1	INITIATING INTRAVENOUS THERAPY—cont'd

STEP	RATIONALE
a *Over-the-needle catheter (ONC) with safety device:* Insert with the bevel up at 5- to 15-degree angle slightly distal to actual site of venipuncture in the direction of the vein (see illustration). **b** *Winged needle:* Hold needle at 5- to 15-degree angle with bevel up, slightly distal to actual site of venipuncture.	Places needle at a 10- to 30- degree angle to the vein. When vein is punctured, risk for puncturing posterior vein wall is reduced. Superficial veins require a smaller angle. Deeper veins require a greater angle.

• *Critical Decision Point:* Use each VAD only once for each insertion attempt.

16 Observe for blood return through flashback chamber of catheter or tubing of winged catheter, indicating that bevel of needle stylet/needle has entered vein (see illustration A). Lower catheter until almost flush with skin. Advance catheter approximately ¼ inch into vein, and then loosen stylet if using ONC. Continue to hold skin taut while stabilizing the catheter, and advance it off the stylet to thread just the catheter into vein until hub is almost at insertion site. *Do not reinsert the stylet once it is loosened.* Advance the catheter while the safety device automatically retracts the stylet (see illustration B). (NOTE: Techniques for retracting stylet will vary with each IV device.) Advance a winged needle until hub rests at venipuncture site. Place needle/stylet directly into sharps container. Follow manufacturer's guidelines for specific safety catheter use.	Increased venous pressure from tourniquet increases backflow of blood into catheter or tubing. Allows for full penetration of the vein wall, placement of the catheter in the vein's inner lumen, and advancement of the catheter off the stylet. Reduces risk for introduction of microorganisms along catheter. Advancing the entire stylet into the vein may penetrate the wall of the vein, resulting in a hematoma. Reinsertion of stylet causes catheter shearing in the vein and potential catheter embolization.

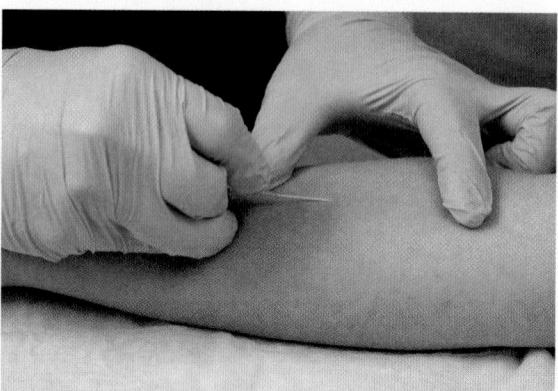

Step 15a ■ Puncture skin with VAD at 5 to 15 degrees above vein.

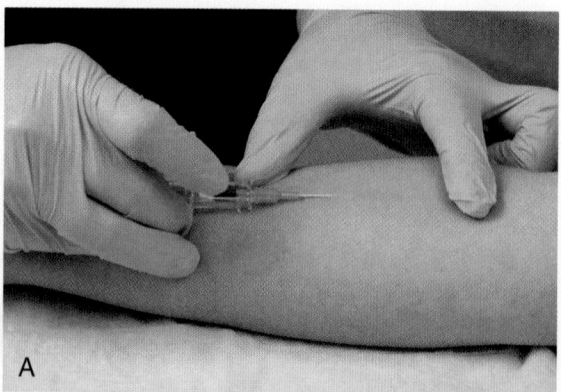

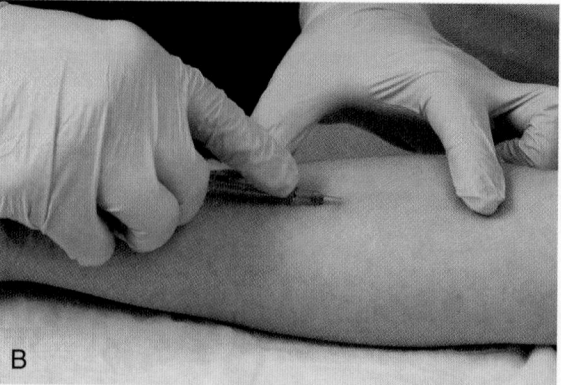

Step 16 ■ **A,** Blood return in flashback chamber. **B,** Advance device into vein.

STEP	RATIONALE

• *Critical Decision Point:* An individual nurse makes no more than two attempts at initiating the IV access (INS, 2006).

17 Stabilize catheter with one hand, and release tourniquet or blood pressure cuff with other. Apply gentle but firm pressure with middle finger of nondominant hand 1¼ inches (3 cm) above the insertion site. Keep catheter stable with index finger.

Permits venous flow, reduces backflow of blood, and allows connection with the administration set with minimal blood loss.

18 Quickly connect end of the infusion tubing set (see illustration) or the prepared saline lock to end of cannula. Do not touch point of entry of connection. Secure connection.

Prompt connection of infusion set maintains patency of vein and prevents risk for exposure to blood. Maintains sterility.

19 Begin infusion by slowly opening the slide clamp or adjusting the roller clamp of the IV tubing or flush injection cap of lock (see illustration).

Initiates flow of fluid through IV catheter, preventing clotting of device.

20 Observe site for swelling.

Swelling indicates infiltration, and you would need to remove the catheter and start over.

• *Critical Decision Point:* Be sure to calculate rate to regulate IV solution at prescribed rate.

21 Secure catheter (procedures differ; check agency policy):

a *Manufactured catheter stabilization device:* Wipe selected area with single-use skin protectant, and allow to dry. Slide device under catheter hub, and center hub over device. Holding catheter in place, peel off half of liner, press to adhere to skin. Repeat on other side. Holding catheter in place, pull tab out from center of device to create opening; insert catheter into slit. This frames the IV site (see illustration). Cover insertion site with a transparent or sterile gauze dressing.

The manufactured catheter stabilization device is a sterile, adhesive pad that holds the catheter in place and reduces the risk for infection and needlestick injuries and improves patient outcomes (INS, 2006; Rosenthal, 2007).

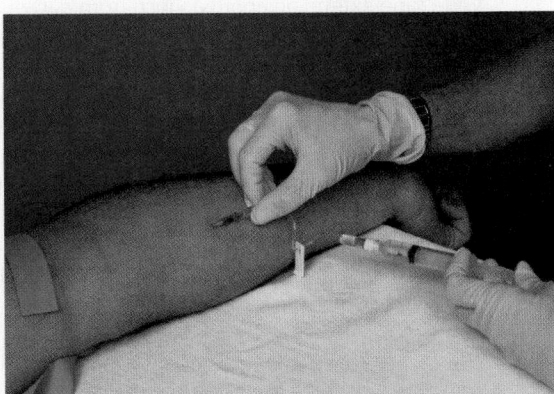

Step 19 ■ Flush injection cap.

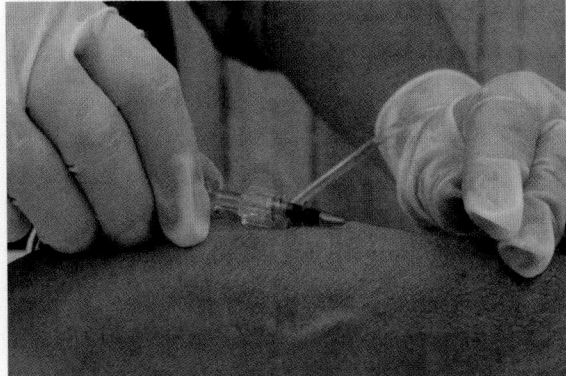

Step 18 ■ Connect end of infusion tubing.

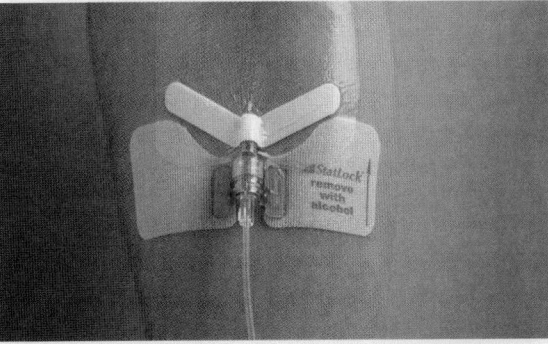

Step 21a ■ Manufactured catheter stabilization device. (Courtesy C. R. Bard, Inc., Murry Hill, NJ.)

| **SKILL 17-1** | INITIATING INTRAVENOUS THERAPY—cont'd |

STEP	**RATIONALE**

b *Transparent dressing:* Secure catheter with nondominant hand while preparing to apply dressing.

Prevents accidental dislodgment of catheter.

c *Sterile gauze dressing:* Place narrow piece (½ inch) of sterile tape over catheter hub. If sterile tape is not available, apply nonsterile tape around catheter hub or stabilization device. Place tape only on the catheter, *never* over the insertion site. Secure site to allow easy visual inspection. Avoid applying tape or gauze around arm.

Use only sterile tape under a sterile dressing to prevent site contamination. Prevents back-and-forth motion, which will irritate the vein and introduce microorganisms on the skin into the vein.

Wrapping anything around the arm prevents visualization of the insertion site.

22 Apply sterile dressing over site.

a Transparent Dressing:

(1) Carefully remove adherent backing. Apply one edge of dressing, and then gently smooth remaining dressing over IV site, leaving connection between IV tubing and catheter hub uncovered. Remove outer covering, and smooth dressing gently over site (see illustration).

Occlusive dressing protects site from bacterial contamination. Connection between administration set and hub needs to be uncovered to facilitate changing the tubing if necessary.

(2) Take a 1-inch piece of tape, and place it over extension tubing or administration set (see illustration). Do not apply tape on top of transparent dressing.

Removal of tape from a transparent dressing will possibly cause accidental removal of the catheter.

Tape on top of a transparent dressing prevents moisture from being carried away from the skin.

b Sterile Gauze Dressing:

(1) Place 2 × 2 gauze pad over insertion site and catheter hub. Secure all edges with tape. Do not cover connection between IV tubing and catheter hub (see illustration).

(2) Fold a 2 × 2 gauze in half, and cover with a 1-inch-wide tape extending about an inch from each side. Place under the tubing/catheter hub junction (see illustration).

Tape on top of gauze makes it easier to access hub/tubing junction. Gauze pad elevates hub off skin to prevent pressure area.

23 Curl a loop of tubing alongside the arm, and place a second piece of tape directly over the tubing and secure (see illustration).

Securing loop of tubing reduces risk for dislodging catheter if the IV tubing is pulled (i.e., the loop comes apart before the catheter dislodges).

24 For IV fluid administration, recheck flow rate to correct drops per minute (see Skill 17-2), and connect to EID as per agency policy.

Manipulation of catheter during dressing application alters flow rate. Maintains correct rate of flow for IV solution. Flow fluctuates, so you must check it at intervals for accuracy.

25 Label dressing per agency policy. Include date and time of IV insertion, VAD gauge size and length, and your initials (see illustration).

Provides immediate access to data as to when IV was inserted and when to change dressing and rotate site.

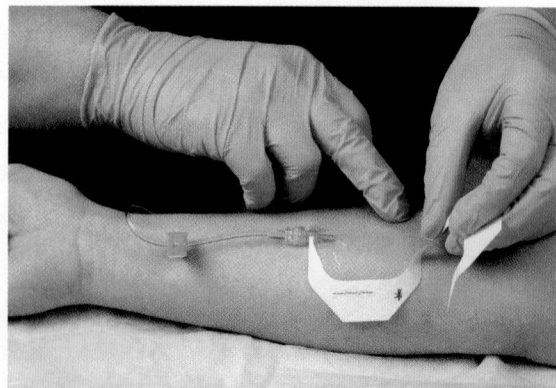

Step 22a(1) ■ Applying transparent dressing.

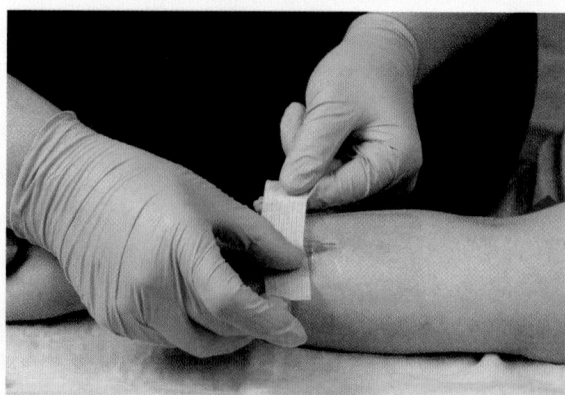

Step 22a(2) ■ Place tape over extension tubing.

STEP	RATIONALE
26 Dispose of used stylet or other sharps in appropriate sharps container. Discard supplies. Remove gloves, and perform hand hygiene.	Reduces transmission of microorganisms and prevents accidental needlestick injuries and follows CDC guidelines for disposal of sharps (OSHA, 2006).
27 Instruct patient in how to move or turn without dislodging VAD.	Prevents accidental dislodgment of catheter.

EVALUATION

1 Observe peripheral IV access. Change peripheral IV access every 72 hours (INS, 2006) or per health care provider's orders or more frequently if complications occur.

Incidence of complications is higher when peripheral IV remains in a vein over 72 hours (INS, 2006; Rosenthal, 2007).

2 Observe patient every 1 to 2 hours:

  a Check if correct amount of IV solution has infused by comparing time tape on IV container or by checking EID record.

Correct administration of fluid volume will prevent fluid imbalance.

  b Count drip rate (if gravity drip), or check rate on infusion pump.

Accurate monitoring of drip rate further ensures correct volume administration.

  c Check patency of VAD.

Flow rate will slow or stop if there is a patency problem.

  d Observe patient during palpation of vessel for signs of discomfort.

Tenderness is an early sign of phlebitis.

  e Inspect insertion site, noting color (e.g., redness or pallor). Inspect for presence of swelling, infiltration (see Table 17-9), and phlebitis (see Table 17-10, p. 490). Palpate temperature of skin above dressing.

Redness, inflammation, tenderness, and warmth indicate vein inflammation or phlebitis. Swelling above insertion site and cool temperature indicate infiltration of fluid into tissues.

3 Observe patient to determine response to therapy (e.g., I&O, weights, vital signs, postprocedure assessments).

IV fluids and additives help maintain or restore fluid and electrolyte balance. Early recognition of complications leads to prompt treatment.

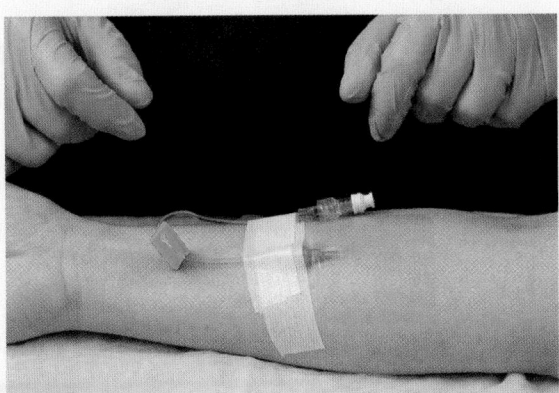

Step 22b(1) ■ Place 2 × 2 gauze over insertion site.

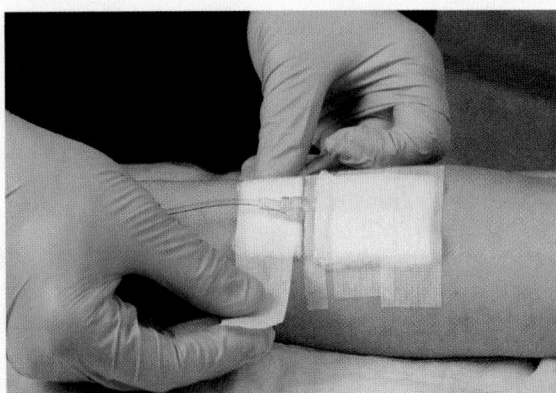

Step 22b(2) ■ Apply 2 × 2 gauze under tubing junction.

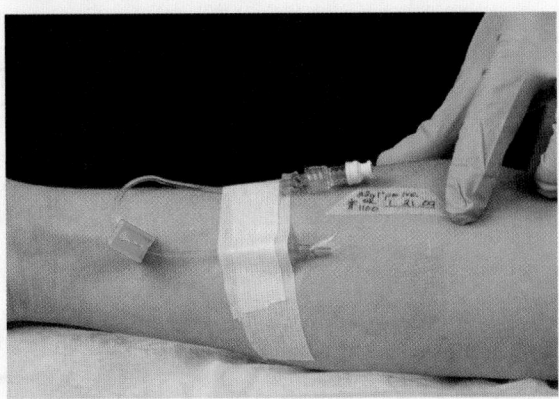

Step 23 ■ Loop and secure tubing.

Step 25 ■ Label IV dressing.

SKILL 17-1   INITIATING INTRAVENOUS THERAPY—cont'd

RECORDING AND REPORTING

- Record in nurses' notes number of attempts and site of insertion; precise description of insertion site (e.g., cephalic vein on dorsal surface of right lower arm, 2.5 cm above wrist); flow rate; size and type, length, and brand of catheter; and time infusion started. Use an infusion therapy flow sheet when available.
- If using an EID, document type and rate of infusion and device identification number.

- Record patient's status, IV fluid, amount infused, and integrity and patency of system according to agency policy.
- Report to oncoming nursing staff: type of fluid, flow rate, status of VAD, amount of fluid remaining in present solution, expected time to hang subsequent IV container, and patient condition.
- Report to health care provider adverse reactions such as pulmonary congestion, shock, or thrombophlebitis.

UNEXPECTED OUTCOMES AND RELATED INTERVENTIONS

- FVD as manifested by decreased urine output, dry mucous membranes, decreased capillary refills, a disparity in central and peripheral pulses, hypotension, tachycardia, shock.
  - Notify health care provider; infusion rate requires readjustment.
  - Adjust infusion rate per order.
- FVE as manifested by crackles in the lungs, shortness of breath, edema, and increased urinary output.
  - Reduce IV flow rate if symptoms appear.
  - Notify health care provider.
- Electrolyte imbalances indicated by abnormal serum electrolyte levels, changes in mental status, alterations in neuromuscular function, cardiac dysrhythmias, changes in vital signs.
  - Notify health care provider.
  - Adjust additives in IV or type of IV fluid per order.
- Infiltration as indicated by swelling and possible pitting edema, pallor, coolness, pain at insertion site, possible decrease in flow rate (see Table 17-9, p. 490).
  - Stop infusion, and discontinue IV.
  - Elevate affected extremity.
  - Restart new IV if continued therapy is necessary.
  - Document degree of infiltration (see Table 17-9, p. 490) and nursing intervention.

- Phlebitis as indicated by pain, increased skin temperature, erythema along path of vein.
  - Stop infusion, and discontinue IV.
  - Restart new IV if continued therapy is necessary.
  - Place moist warm compress over area of phlebitis.
  - Document degree of phlebitis (see Table 17-10, p. 490) and nursing intervention.
- Bleeding occurs at venipuncture site.
  - Verify that the system is intact, and place a dressing over site or change dressing. NOTE: If using gauze dressing, remove it and accurately assess insertion site.
  - Restart new IV if bleeding from site does not stop or if IV is dislodged.

SKILL 17-2   REGULATING INTRAVENOUS FLOW RATE   View Video!

DELEGATION CONSIDERATIONS

The skill of regulating intravenous flow rate cannot be delegated to nursing assistive personnel (NAP). Delegation to LPNs varies by State Nurse Practice Act. The nurse directs the NAP to:

- Inform the nurse when the electronic infusion device alarm signals
- Inform the nurse when the fluid container is almost empty
- Report any patient complaints of any discomfort at the IV site

EQUIPMENT

- Watch with second hand
- Calculator, paper, and pencil
- Tape
- Label
- IV flow-control device: EID (optional), volume-control device (optional)

STEP	RATIONALE

ASSESSMENT

1 Review accuracy and completeness of health care provider's order for type and amount of IV fluid, medication additives, infusion rate, and length of therapy. Follow the six rights of medication administration (see Chapter 16).

Ensures safe and correct administration of IV therapy.

2 Perform hand hygiene.

Reduces transmission of microorganisms.

3 Assess patient's knowledge of how positioning of IV site affects flow rate.

Fosters patient participation in maintaining most effective position of arm with IV equipment. Nurse is responsible for positioning or setting control clamp or infusion device drip rate.

4 Inspect IV site, and verify with patient how venipuncture site feels (e.g., determine if there is pain, burning, or tenderness at site).

Pain or burning is an early indication of phlebitis. Includes patient in decision making.

5 Observe for patency of VAD and IV tubing.

For fluid to infuse at proper rate, IV tubing and VAD must be free of kinks, knots, and clots.

6 Identify patient risk for fluid imbalance (e.g., neonate, history of cardiac or renal disease, electrolyte imbalance).

Volume control needs to be strict. Guides choice of infusion device.

PLANNING

1 Collect and organize equipment.

2 Identify patient using two identifiers (e.g., name and birthday or name and account number, according to facility policy). Compare identifiers with information on patient's MAR or medical record.

Complies with The Joint Commission requirements and improves medication safety. In most acute care settings, you will use the patient's name and identification number on armband and MAR to identify patients (TJC, 2010).

3 Have paper and pencil or calculator to calculate flow rate.

Use mathematical calculations to determine correct IV flow rate.

4 Know calibration (drop factor) in drops per milliliter (gtt/mL) of infusion set used by agency:
Microdrip: 60 gtt/mL

Microdrip tubing universally delivers 60 gtt/mL. Used when small or very precise volumes are to be infused.

Macrodrip: 10 to 15 gtt/mL is clearly noted on administration set packaging.

There are different commercial parenteral administration sets for macrodrip tubing. Used when large volumes or fast rates are necessary. Know the drip factor for the tubing being used.

5 Determine how long each liter of fluid should run. Calculate milliliters per hour (hourly rate) by dividing volume by hours:
mL/hr = total infusion (mL)/hours of infusion
Example: to determine hourly rate when you need to infuse 1 L (1000 mL) over 8 hours:
  1000 mL/8 hr = 125 mL/hr
or if 3 L is ordered for 24 hours:
  3000 mL/24 hr = 125 mL/hr

Provides even infusion of fluid over prescribed hourly rate.

6 Select one of the following formulas to calculate minute flow rate (drops per minute) based on drop factor of infusion set:
  mL/hr/60 min = mL/min
  Drop factor × mL/min = drops/min
  or
  mL/hr × drop factor/60 min = drops/min

Once you determine the hourly rate, these formulas compute correct flow rate.

• *Critical Decision Point:* It is common for health care providers to write an abbreviated IV order such as: "D$_5$W with 20 mEq KCl 125 mL/hr continuous." This order implies that the IV is maintained at this rate until order has been written for IV to be discontinued.

SKILL 17-2 REGULATING INTRAVENOUS FLOW RATE—cont'd

STEP	RATIONALE

IMPLEMENTATION

1 Obtain IV fluid/medication and appropriate tubing if new solution needs to be hung.

Use of correct tubing ensures accurate calculation for infusion delivery. Determines volume of fluid that infuses hourly.

2 Confirm hourly infusion rate, and place marked adhesive tape or commercial fluid indicator tape on existing IV container next to volume markings (see illustration). Document each IV fluid bag sequentially, and note type of fluid, patient's name, infusion span, and expected start and end time of infusion.

Provides a visual scale to assess progress of hourly infusion. Use time tapes for all IV infusions, including those on EIDs.

NOTE: Some patients receive secondary infusions that affect the visual time tape scale.

- **Critical Decision Point:** On IV bags made of polyvinylchloride (PVC), avoid drawing directly with felt-tip pens or permanent markers because the ink could contaminate the solution (Hadaway and Millam, 2005).

3 *For gravity infusions:* Confirm hourly rate and minute rate based on drop factor of infusion set. Microdrip infusion set has a drop factor of 60 gtt/mL. Regular drip or macrodrip infusion set, used in this example, has a drop factor of 15 gtt/mL. Using formula (see Planning Step 6), calculate minute flow rate.

For example, to infuse 1000 mL with 20 mEq KCl at the rate of 125 mL/hr:

Microdrip:

   125 mL/hr × 60 gtt/mL = 7500 gtt/hr
   7500 gtt ÷ 60 minutes = 125 gtt/min

Macrodrip:

   125 mL/hr × 15 gtt/mL = 1875 gtt/hr
   1875 gtt ÷ 60 minutes = 31-32 gtt/min

4 Regulate flow rate by counting drops in drip chamber for 1 minute by watch, then adjust roller clamp to increase or decrease rate of infusion (see illustration).

Calculates minute flow rate for regulation of infusion.

When using microdrip, milliliters per hour (mL/hr) always equals drops per minute (gtt/min).

Multiply volume by drop factor, and divide the product by time (in minutes).

Regulates flow to prescribed rate.

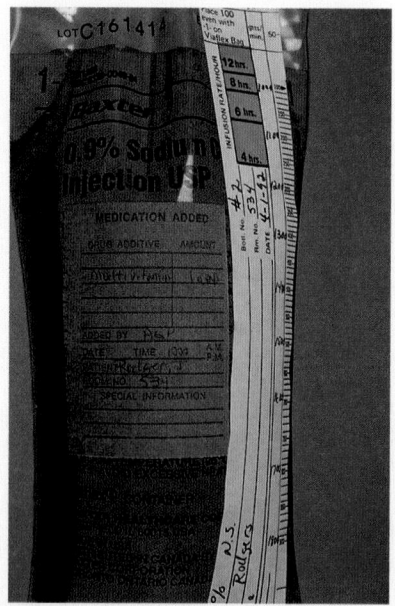

Step 2 ■ IV fluid bag with time tape.

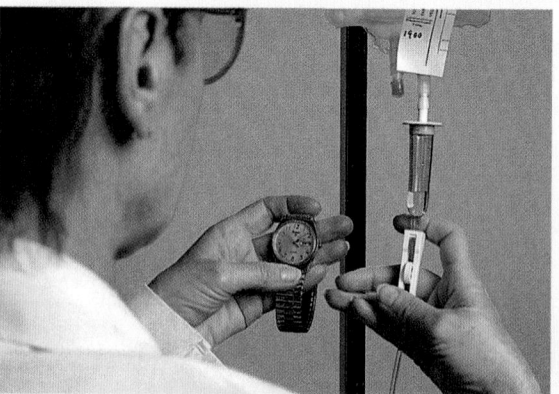

Step 4 ■ Nurse counts drops infusing.

STEP	RATIONALE
5 *For use of EID for infusion:* Follow manufacturer's guidelines for setup of EID.	EID sometimes regulates by positive pressure (pump) or gravity (controller).
a Consult manufacturer's directions for setup of the infusion. If using a gravity controller, ensure that IV container is 36 inches above IV site.	IV controller works by gravity. Heights of 36 to 48 inches will overcome venous pressure and other resistance from tubing and catheter (INS, 2006).
b Insert IV tubing into chamber of control mechanism (see manufacturer's directions) (see illustration).	Most electronic **infusion pumps** use positive pressure to infuse. Infusion pumps propel fluid through tubing by compressing and milking the IV tubing.
c Turn on power button, select required drops per minute or volume per hour, close door to control chamber, and press start button (see illustration).	

- *Critical Decision Point:* An anti–free flow safeguard (preventing bolus infusion in the event of machine malfunction or when tubing removed from machine) is an important element of an electronic infusion device and is required. Always check manufacturer's recommendations for specific device features.

---

d Open drip regulator completely while EID is in use.	Ensures that pump freely regulates infusion rate.
e Monitor infusion rate and IV site for complications according to agency policy. Use watch to verify rate of infusion, even when using EID.	Infusion controllers or pumps are not perfect and do not replace frequent, accurate nursing evaluation. EIDs continue to infuse IV fluids after a complication has begun.
f Assess patency of system when alarm signals.	Alarm indicates some blockage in the system. Empty solution container, tubing kinks, closed clamp, infiltration, clotted catheter, air in the tubing, and/or low battery will all trigger the EID alarm.
6 *For smart pump* (see illustration):	
a Place pump module into the computer.	
b Insert the IV tubing into the pump module, and close the door.	
c Computer screen will need for the patient unit to be identified.	Manufacturer's guidelines and health care facility programming automatically configure the computer to the specific unit (e.g., critical care, pediatrics).
d From the list on screen, choose the medication and concentration.	
e Program the dose and infusion rate ordered. If the entered order matches the database, the pump will begin the infusion.	The pump checks the programming against the medication database.
f If the programming does not match the database, a visual and audible alarm sounds.	Prevents medication and infusion errors.
g If an alarm sounds, the pump will automatically turn off. You must reprogram it within the facility's database.	Prevents medication and infusion errors.

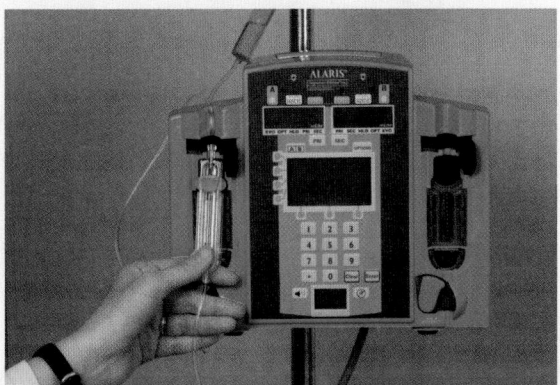

Step 5b ■ Place tubing into control mechanism.

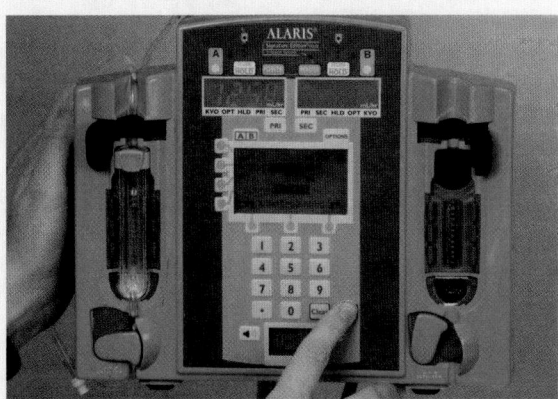

Step 5c ■ Press start button.

SKILL 17-2	REGULATING INTRAVENOUS FLOW RATE—cont'd

STEP	RATIONALE
h Reconfirm that the medication is infusing at the ordered rate.	The pump maintains a log of all alarms, including alarms for time, date, medication, medication concentration, rate, and any actions.
7 *For a volume-control device:*	
a Place volume-control device between IV container and insertion spike of infusion set using aseptic technique (see illustration).	Delivers small fluid volumes, but needs refilling as volume becomes low. Reduces risk for sudden fluid infusion.
b Place no more than 2 hours' worth of fluid into device by opening clamp between IV bag and device.	Allows for a continuous infusion of fluid if you do not return in exactly 60 minutes to refill volume. If infusion rate accidentally increases, patient receives only a 2-hour portion of fluid.
c Assess system at least hourly; add fluid to volume control device. Regulate flow rate.	Maintains patency of system and patient monitoring.
8 Instruct patient about the purpose of the alarms, to avoid raising hand or arm that affects flow rate, and to avoid touching the control clamp.	Information allows patient to protect IV site and informs patient about rationale for not altering control rate.

EVALUATION

1 Monitor IV infusion at least every hour, noting volume of IV fluid infused and rate.	Ensures correct volume infuses over prescribed time period.
2 Observe patient for signs of overhydration or dehydration to determine response to therapy and restoration of fluid and electrolyte balance.	Signs and symptoms of dehydration or overhydration necessitate changing rate of fluid infused.
3 Evaluate for signs of complications with IV flow rate: infiltration, inflammation at site, occluded VAD, or kink or obstruction in infusion tubing.	Prevents complications that can decrease or stop flow rate.

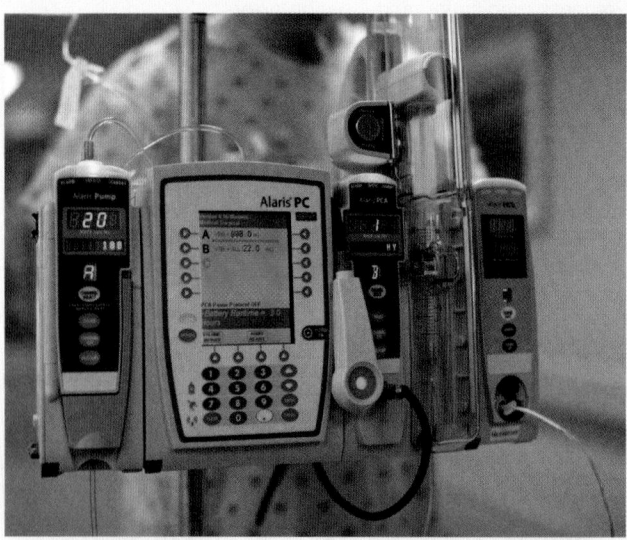

Step 6 ■ Smart pump. (Courtesy CareFusion, San Diego, Calif.)

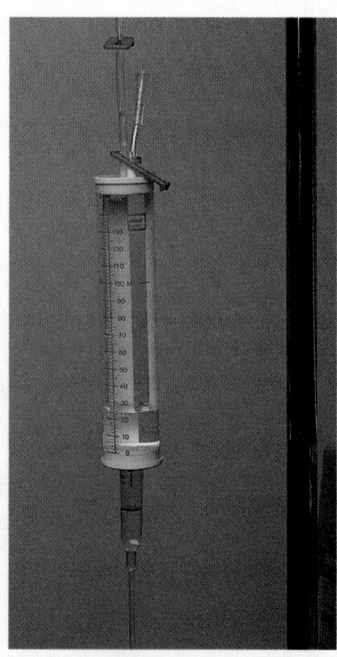

Step 7a ■ Volume-metric device.

RECORDING AND REPORTING

- Record rate of infusion, drops per minute or milliliters per hour in nurses' notes or parenteral fluid form according to agency policy.
- Immediately record in nurses' notes any new IV fluid rates.

- Document use of any electronic infusion device or controlling device and identification number on that device.
- At change of shift or when leaving on break, report rate of and volume left in infusion to nurse in charge or next nurse assigned to care for patient.

UNEXPECTED OUTCOMES AND RELATED INTERVENTIONS

- Sudden infusion of large volume of solution occurs with patient having symptoms of dyspnea, crackles in the lung, and increased urine output, indicating fluid overload.
  - Notify health care provider immediately.
  - Slow infusion to keep vein open (KVO) rate.
  - Place patient in high-Fowler's position.
  - Anticipate new IV orders.
  - Administer diuretics if ordered.

- IV fluid container is completed with subsequent loss of IV line patency.
  - Discontinue present IV, and restart new VAD.
- The IV infusion is slower than ordered rate.
  - Check patient for positional change that affects rate, height of IV container, kinking of tubing or obstruction.
  - Check VAD site for complications.
  - Consult health care providers for new order to provide necessary fluid volume.

SKILL 17-3   CHANGING INTRAVENOUS SOLUTION AND TUBING

DELEGATION CONSIDERATIONS

The skill of changing IV solutions and tubing cannot be delegated to nursing assistive personnel (NAP). Delegation to LPNs varies in State Nurse Practice Acts. The nurse directs the NAP to:

- Report any leakage from or around the IV tubing to the nurse
- Report any cloudiness or precipitate in IV solution
- Inform the nurse when an IV container is near completion

EQUIPMENT

- Clean gloves
- 0.22-μm filter and extension (for TPN and certain medications)
- IV solution as ordered by the health care provider
- Time tape

Continuous IV Infusion

- Microdrip or macrodrip infusion tubing, as appropriate
- 0.22-μm filter and extension tubing (if necessary)
- Tubing label
- Antiseptic swab (2% chlorhexidine)

Intermittent Saline Lock

- 5-mL syringe filled with preservative-free normal saline
- Loop or short extension tubing (if necessary), injection cap or prn adapter
- Antiseptic swab

STEP	RATIONALE

ASSESSMENT

1 Review accuracy and completeness of health care provider's order for type and amount of IV fluid, medication additives, infusion rate, and length of therapy. Follow the six rights of medication administration (see Chapter 16).

Ensures safe and correct administration of IV therapy.

2 Note date and time when IV tubing and solution were last changed.

INS recommends a hang time no longer than 24 hours after addition of an administration set, to ensure sterility of solutions in bag or bottle (INS, 2006). Administration sets need to be changed every 72 hours (INS, 2006).

3 Determine the compatibility of all IV fluids and additives by consulting appropriate literature or the pharmacy.

Incompatibilities cause physical, chemical, and therapeutic patient changes.

4 Determine patient's understanding of need for continued IV therapy.

Reveals need for patient instruction.

5 Assess patency of current VAD site. *Lowering IV container below level of IV site for presence of blood return (retrograde) is an unreliable indicator of patency.*

New IV access site needed if IV is not patent.

SKILL 17-3	CHANGING INTRAVENOUS SOLUTION AND TUBING— cont'd

STEP	RATIONALE
6 Assess IV insertion site for swelling, coolness to touch, or tenderness around site.	Indicates infiltration.
7 Assess IV tubing for puncture, contamination, or occlusions.	Indicates need for tubing change.

PLANNING

1 Collect appropriate equipment. Have next solution prepared at least 1 hour before needed. If solution is prepared in pharmacy, ensure it has been delivered to the patient care unit. Allow solution to warm to room temperature if it has been refrigerated. Check that solution is correct and properly labeled. Check solution expiration date.	Adequate planning reduces risk for clot formation in vein caused by empty IV container. Checking that solution is correct prevents medication error.
2 Identify patient using two identifiers (e.g., name and birthday or name and account number, according to facility policy). Compare identifiers with information on patient's MAR or medical record.	Complies with The Joint Commission requirements and improves medication safety. In most acute care settings, you will use the patient's name and identification number on armband and MAR to identify patients (TJC, 2010).
3 Prepare to change solution when about 50 mL of fluid remains in container.	Prevents air from entering tubing and vein from clotting from lack of flow.
4 Change administration set tubing with new fluid container whenever possible.	Decreases number of times system is open and maintains sterility.
5 Prepare patient and family by explaining the procedure, its purpose, and what is expected of patient.	Decreases anxiety and promotes cooperation.

IMPLEMENTATION

1 Perform hand hygiene.	Reduces transmission of microorganisms.
2 Open new infusion set, and connect add-on pieces (e.g., filters, extension tubing). Keep protective coverings over infusion spike and distal adapter. Secure all connections.	Securing connections reduces the risk later of air emboli, hemorrhage, and infection. Protective covers reduce entrance of microorganisms.
3 *Change new solution with existing tubing of continuous IV infusion:*	Permits quick, smooth, and organized change from old to new solution.
a If using plastic bag, remove protective cover from IV tubing port. If using glass bottle, remove metal cap and metal and rubber disks.	
b Position roller clamp on existing solution to stop flow rate. Remove tubing from EID (if used. Then remove old IV fluid container from IV pole). Hold container with tubing port pointing upward.	Prevents solution remaining in drip chamber from emptying while changing solutions. Prevents solution from spilling.
c Quickly remove spike from old solution container, and without touching tip, insert spike into new container.	Reduces risk for drip chamber becoming empty and maintains sterility.

• *Critical Decision Point:* If spike is contaminated, you will need a new IV tubing set. You can use sterile IV tubing for 72 hours unless compromised.	

d Hang new solution container on IV pole.	Gravity assists with delivery of fluid into drip chamber.
e Check for air in tubing. If bubbles form, remove them by closing the roller camp, stretching the tubing downward, and tapping the tubing with fingers (bubbles rise in fluid to drip chamber). For a larger amount of air, swab port below the air, allow to dry, and insert needleless syringe into the port. Aspirate air into the syringe.	Reduces risk for air entering the tubing. Use of an air-eliminating filter also reduces this risk.
f Make sure drip chamber is one-third to one-half full. If the drip chamber is too full, pinch off tubing below the drip chamber, invert the container, squeeze the drip chamber, release, turn the solution container upright, and unpinch the tubing.	Reduces risk for air entering tubing. If chamber is completely filled, you cannot observe or regulate drip rate.

STEP	RATIONALE
4 *Change new solution and tubing on existing continuous IV infusion:*	
a Move roller clamp on new IV tubing to "off" position.	Prevents fluid spillage.
b Slow rate of infusion to existing IV by regulating roller clamp on old tubing to KVO rate.	
c Compress and fill drip chamber of old tubing.	Ensures fluid chamber remains full until new tubing is changed.
d Remove old tubing from IV container. *Optional:* Tape old drip chamber to IV pole without contaminating spike.	Fluid in drip chamber will continue to run and maintain catheter patency.
e Place insertion spike of new tubing into new solution container. Hang solution bag on IV pole, compress and release drip chamber on new tubing, and fill drip chamber one-third to one-half full.	Permits flow of fluid from solution into new infusion tubing.
f Slowly open roller clamp, remove protective cap from adapter (if necessary), and flush new tubing with solution. Stop infusion, and replace cap. Place end of adapter near patient's IV site.	Removes air from tubing, and replaces it with IV solution. Equipment is positioned for a quick connection of new tubing.
g Turn roller clamp on old tubing to "off" position.	Prevents fluid spillage.
h Apply gloves. Gently disconnect old tubing from IV catheter, and quickly insert adapter of new tubing into IV catheter hub.	Allows smooth transition from old to new tubing, minimizing time system is open.
5 *Change of intermittent saline lock:*	
a If a loop or short extension tubing is needed, use sterile technique to connect the new injection cap to the loop or tubing.	Removes air from tubing and prevents air from being introduced into the vein. Maintains sterility of IV site.
b Swab injection cap with antiseptic swab. Insert syringe with 1 to 3 mL of saline solution, and inject through the injection cap into the loop of the extension tubing.	Maintains patency of catheter. Volume of saline solution should not exceed 30 mL in a 24-hour period (INS, 2006).
c Apply gloves. Gently disconnect old tubing from extension tubing, and quickly insert adapter of saline lock into tubing connection (see illustrations).	Allows smooth transition from old to new tubing, minimizing time system is open.
6 For continuous infusion, open roller clamp and allow to run for 30 seconds. Then regulate drip rate to ordered rate using roller clamp or reprogram EID.	Ensures proper infusion rate and IV catheter patency.
7 Attach a time label with date and time of solution change on side of bag. Attach a time label with date and time of tubing change onto tubing below the drip chamber.	Provides reference to determine next time for solution or tubing change.
8 When adding new tubing, form a loop of tubing, and secure it to patient's arm with a strip of tape.	Avoids accidental pulling against site and stabilizes the catheter.
9 Remove and discard used supplies. If necessary, apply new IV site dressing (see Skill 17-4). Remove and dispose of gloves. Perform hand hygiene.	Reduces transmission of microorganisms.

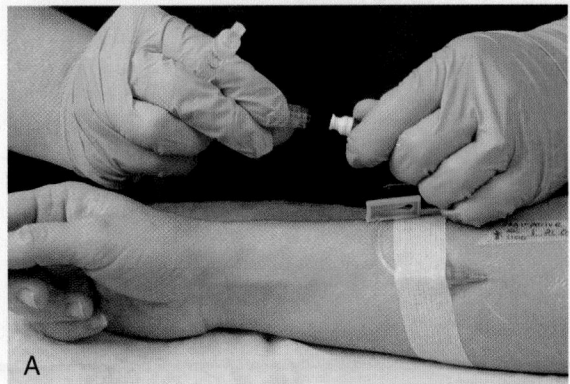 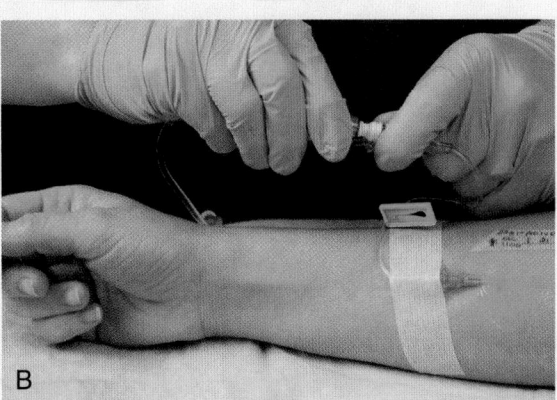

Step 5c ■ **A,** Disconnect old tubing. **B,** Insert adapter of new tubing.

SKILL 17-3	CHANGING INTRAVENOUS SOLUTION AND TUBING—cont'd

STEP	RATIONALE

EVALUATION

1 Evaluate flow rate hourly, and observe connection site for leakage.

2 Observe patient for signs of overhydration or dehydration to determine response to IV therapy.

3 Check IV system for patency and development (e.g., infiltration, phlebitis).

Maintains prescribed rate of flow of IV fluid and determines if fit is secure.
Determines response to IV fluid therapy.

Provides ongoing evaluation of patient's fluid and electrolyte status.

RECORDING AND REPORTING

• Record tubing change, type of solution, volume, and rate of infusion on patient's record. Use a special IV therapy flow sheet for parenteral fluids.

• Mark a piece of tape or preprinted label with date and time of tubing change, and attach to tubing below the level of drip chamber.

UNEXPECTED OUTCOMES AND RELATED INTERVENTIONS

• Obstructed flow with decreased or absent flow of IV fluid.
  • Assess infusion system for patency by opening roller clamp, slide clamps, and check for kinks in tubing.
  • Recalibrate drip rate.
  • Assess patient for complaints of pain or discomfort at IV site.

• Flow rate is incorrect; patient receives too little or too much fluid.
  • Readjust infusion rate to ordered rate.
  • Evaluate patient for adverse effects of infusion.
  • Determine and correct the cause of incorrect flow rate (e.g., change in position, tubing kink).
  • Use EID when accurate flow rate is critical.
  • Notify health care provider.

SKILL 17-4	CHANGING A PERIPHERAL INTRAVENOUS DRESSING

DELEGATION CONSIDERATIONS

The skill of changing a peripheral intravenous dressing cannot be delegated to nursing assistive personnel (NAP). The nurse directs the NAP to:
• Report to the nurse if a patient complains of moistness or loosening of IV dressing
• Protect intravenous dressing during hygiene and ADLs

EQUIPMENT
• Antiseptic swabs (2% chlorhexidine)
• Skin protectant swab

• Adhesive remover *(optional)*
• Clean gloves
• Strips of nonallergenic tape
• Commercially available IV site protection device *(optional)*

For Transparent Dressing
• Sterile transparent semipermeable dressing

For Gauze Dressing
• Sterile 2 × 2 gauze pad or
• Sterile 4 × 4 gauze pad

STEP	RATIONALE

ASSESSMENT

1 Determine when dressing was last changed. Many institutions require dressing label to include date and time dressing applied, size and type of VAD, and date the VAD was inserted.

2 Observe present dressing for moisture and intactness. Determine if moisture is from site leakage or external source.

3 Observe IV system for proper functioning or complications (e.g., current flow rate, tubing or catheter kinks). Palpate the catheter site through the intact dressing for complaints of tenderness, pain, or burning. (NOTE: Apply clean gloves if dressing is moist.)

Provides information regarding length of time that present dressing has been in place. In addition, you are able to plan for dressing change.

Moisture is medium for microorganism growth and renders dressing contaminated. Nonadhering dressing increases risk for bacterial contamination to venipuncture site or displacement of IV catheter.
Unexplained decrease in flow rate indicates problems with VAD placement and patency. Pain is associated with phlebitis and infiltration.

STEP	RATIONALE
4 Monitor body temperature.	Elevated temperature is possibly related to infection at VAD site.
5 Assess patient's understanding of the need for continued IV infusion.	Reveals need for patient instruction.

PLANNING

1 Explain procedure and purpose to patient and family. Explain that patient will need to hold the affected extremity still. Explain how long the procedure will take.

Decreases anxiety, promotes cooperation, and gives patient time frame around which to plan personal activities.

2 Collect equipment.

IMPLEMENTATION

1 Perform hand hygiene. Apply clean gloves.	Reduces transmission of microorganisms. Infections related to IV therapy are most often caused by catheter hub contamination, so you need to use careful technique throughout the dressing change (INS, 2006).
2 Identify patient using two identifiers (e.g., name and birthday or name and account number, according to facility policy).	Complies with The Joint Commission requirements and improves patient safety. In most acute care settings, you will use the patient's name and identification number on armband and MAR to identify patients (TJC, 2010).
3 Remove tape from old dressing one layer at a time by pulling toward the insertion site, leaving tape that secures VAD to skin intact. Be cautious if IV tubing becomes tangled between two layers of dressing. Remove transparent semipermeable dressing by pulling up one corner and pulling the side laterally while holding the catheter hub (see illustration). Repeat on other side. When removing transparent dressing, hold catheter hub and tubing with nondominant hand.	Prevents accidental displacement of VAD.
4 Observe insertion site for signs and/or symptoms of infection: Redness, swelling, and exudate. If complication exists or if ordered by health care provider, discontinue the infusion.	Presence of infection or complication indicates need to remove VAD at current site.
5 Prepare new tape strips for use. If IV is infusing properly, gently remove tape securing VAD. Stabilize VAD with one hand. Use adhesive remover to cleanse skin and remove adhesive residue, if needed.	Exposes venipuncture site. Stabilization prevents accidental displacement of VAD. Adhesive residue decreases ability of new tape to adhere tightly to skin.

• **Critical Decision Point:** Keep one finger over catheter at all times until tape or dressing secures placement. If patient is restless or uncooperative, it is helpful to have another staff member assist with procedure.

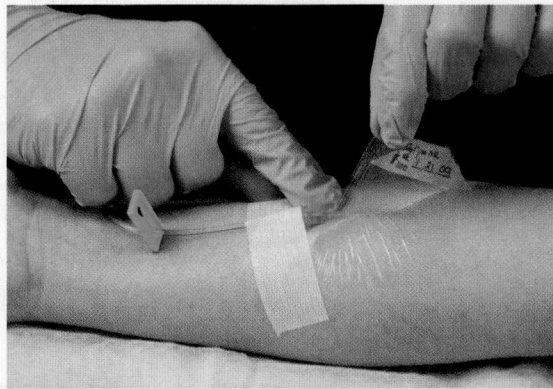

Step 3 ■ Remove transparent dressing by pulling side laterally.

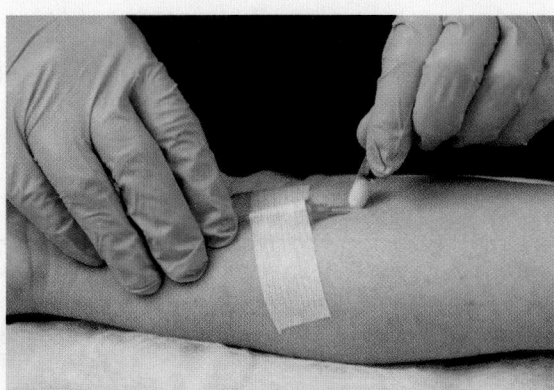

Step 6 ■ Cleanse peripheral insertion site with antiseptic swab.

SKILL 17-4	CHANGING A PERIPHERAL INTRAVENOUS DRESSING— cont'd

STEP	RATIONALE
6 While stabilizing IV, cleanse insertion site with antiseptic swab using friction in a horizontal plane, then a vertical plane, followed by a circular pattern moving from the insertion site outward (see illustration). Allow antiseptic to dry completely.	Mechanical friction in this pattern allows penetration of the antiseptic solution into the epidermal layer of the skin (Hadaway and Milam, 2005).
	Allowing antiseptic solutions to dry completely reduces microbial counts (INS, 2006).
7 *Option:* Apply skin protectant solution (e.g., Skin-Prep, No Sting Barrier Film) to the area where you will apply the tape or transparent dressing. Allow to dry.	Coats the skin with protective solution to maintain skin integrity, prevents irritation from the adhesive, and promotes adhesion of the dressing.
8 While securing catheter, apply sterile dressing over site (procedures differ; follow agency policy).	
a *Manufactured catheter stabilization device:* Apply catheter stabilization as directed in Skill 17-1, Implementation Step 21a.	The manufactured catheter stabilization device is a sterile, adhesive pad that holds the catheter in place and reduces the risk for infection and needlestick injuries. It improves patient outcomes (INS, 2006; Rosenthal, 2007).
	Prevents accidental dislodgment of catheter.
b *Transparent dressing:* As directed in Skill 17-1, Implementation Step 21b, apply transparent dressing.	Occlusive dressing protects site from bacterial contamination. Connection between administration set and hub needs to be uncovered to facilitate changing the tubing if necessary.
c *Sterile gauze dressing:* As directed in Skill 17-1, Implementation Step 21c, apply sterile gauze dressing.	Use only sterile tape under a sterile dressing to prevent site contamination. Prevents back-and-forth motion, which will irritate the vein and introduce microorganisms on the skin into the vein.
	Tape on top of gauze makes it easier to access hub/tubing junction. Gauze pad elevates hub off skin to prevent pressure area. Securing loop of tubing reduces risk for dislodging catheter if the IV tubing is pulled (i.e., the loop will come apart before the catheter dislodges).
9 Remove and discard gloves.	Prevents transmission of microorganisms.
10 *Option:* Apply site protection device (e.g., I.V. House protective device).	Reduces the risk for phlebitis and infiltration from mechanical motion.
11 Anchor IV tubing with additional pieces of tape if necessary. When using transparent dressing, avoid placing tape over dressing.	Prevents accidental displacement of VAD.
12 Label dressing per agency policy. Information on label includes date and time of IV insertion, VAD gauze size and length, and your initials.	Communicates type of device and time interval for dressing change and site rotation.
13 Discard equipment, and perform hand hygiene.	Reduces transmission of microorganisms.

EVALUATION

1 Observe function, patency of IV system, and flow rate after changing dressing.	Validates that IV is patent and functioning correctly. Manipulation of catheter and tubing will affect rate of infusion.
2 Inspect condition of VAD site, noting color. Palpate for skin temperature, edema, and tenderness.	Complications such as phlebitis and infiltration require removal of VAD and insertion of new VAD at another site.
3 Monitor patient's body temperature.	Elevated temperature indicates an infection that is possibly associated with contamination of the venipuncture site.

RECORDING AND REPORTING

- Record time peripheral IV dressing was changed, reason for change, type of dressing material used, patency of system, and description of venipuncture site.
- Report to nurse in charge or oncoming nursing shift the dressing was changed and any significant information about integrity of system.

- Report to health care provider, and document any complications.

UNEXPECTED OUTCOMES AND RELATED INTERVENTIONS

- VAD is infiltrated, as evidenced by decreased flow rate or edema, pallor, or decreased temperature around insertion site.
  - Stop infusion, and remove VAD.
  - Restart new VAD in other extremity or above previous insertion site if continued therapy is necessary.
  - Elevate affected extremity.
- Phlebitis is present, as evidenced by erythema and tenderness along vein pathway.
  - Stop infusion, and remove VAD.
  - Restart new VAD in other extremity if continued therapy is necessary.
  - Apply warm moist compress to affected site until resolved (see Chapter 36).

- VAD is accidentally removed.
  - Restart VAD if continued therapy is needed.
- Patient has an elevated temperature.
  - Notify health care provider.
  - Prepare to obtain blood culture or culture of IV site to evaluate source of infection.
- Insertion site is red and/or edematous and/or painful and/or has presence of exudate, indicating infection at venipuncture site.
  - Notify health care provider. Culture of catheter tip and/or exudate will probably be ordered. (Confirm before removal of IV.)
  - Remove VAD.
  - Antibiotic therapy may be ordered. Do not begin until blood cultures obtained, if ordered.

KEY POINTS

- Body fluids, consisting of electrolytes, cellular components, proteins, and water, are distributed in ECF and ICF compartments.
- Volume disturbances include both isotonic and osmolar deficits or excesses.
- Dietary intake, medications, hormonal controls, environmental factors, and disease states regulate electrolyte levels.
- Chronic and serious illnesses or injuries increase the risk for fluid, electrolyte, and acid-base imbalances.
- Patients who are very young or very old are at greatest risk for fluid, electrolyte, and acid-base imbalances.
- Treatment for electrolyte disturbances includes dietary and pharmacological interventions.
- Acid-base status is determined by the concentration of hydrogen ions in the blood.
- The body's chemical buffering systems are the first to respond to acid-base imbalances.
- Enteral or parenteral fluid administration corrects osmolar imbalances and fluid volume deficit.

- Common complications of IV therapy include infiltration, phlebitis, infection, fluid volume excess, and bleeding at the insertion site.
- Blood transfusions are given to replace fluid volume lost from hemorrhage, to treat anemia, or to replace coagulation factors.
- Transfused blood can be obtained from volunteer donors, autologous donation, or through perioperative salvage.
- Administration of blood products entails a specific procedure for identification of the patient and the blood product.
- In addition to transfusion reactions, the risks of transfusion include hyperkalemia, hypocalcemia, hypothermia, fluid volume excess, coagulopathies, and infection.
- The goals of therapy for acid-base imbalances are to treat the underlying disorders and to restore the arterial pH to normal.

CRITICAL THINKING EXERCISES

During Robert's assessment he finds that Susan Reynolds has decreased skin turgor and dry mucous membranes. The health care provider has ordered assessing vital signs every 4 hours, nothing by mouth, intake and output measurement, blood chemistry analysis, an IV of 0.9% NS at 125 mL/hr, and an abdominal radiograph.

1. What additional information should the nurse obtain from Mrs. Reynolds?
2. What considerations does Robert include before he proceeds with starting the IV?
3. Robert determines that a priority nursing diagnosis for Mrs. Reynolds is *deficient fluid volume*. What nursing in-

terventions are appropriate for Robert to implement at this time?

4. Upon further assessment, Mrs. Reynolds presents with a temperature of 38.2° C (100.9° F). How does this affect her condition?
5. What other indicators does Robert expect to find with Mrs. Reynolds' dehydration?
6. What is the primary cause of Mrs. Reynolds' fluid imbalance?

evolve *Answers to Critical Thinking Questions can be found on the Evolve website.*

REVIEW QUESTIONS

1. The following four patients are all at risk for fluid volume deficit. Which of the patients do you see **first**?
   1. An 80-year-old with a fractured hip scheduled for surgery
   2. A 60-year-old with a recent history of severe vomiting and hypotension
   3. A 40-year-old with pneumonia
   4. An alert 10-year-old with acute otitis media

2. You assess four patients. Which patient is at greatest risk for the development of hyperkalemia?
   1. A 65-year-old with acute renal failure and cardiac dysrhythmias
   2. A 25-year-old with rheumatoid arthritis, with swollen, hot joints
   3. An 80-year-old with heart failure, on digoxin orally once per day by mouth
   4. A 60-year-old taking furosemide (Lasix), with a potassium level of 4.2 mEq/L

3. Your patient presents with arterial blood gas levels as follows: pH, 7.56; PaO_2, 90 mm Hg; $PaCO_2$, 28 mm Hg; HCO_3^-, 18 mEq/L. You would expect the health care provider to order:
   1. Oxygen at 4 L/min via mask
   2. Sodium bicarbonate 1 amp every 12 hours
   3. Deep breathing exercises and use of incentive spirometer
   4. Potassium chloride 20 mEq in ½NS (normal saline)

4. Place the following steps for discontinuing peripheral IV access in the correct order:
   1. Clamp the IV tubing.
   2. Apply continuous pressure to site for 2 to 3 minutes.
   3. Review the discontinuation order.
   4. Place clean sterile gauze over the puncture site, and remove the cannula by pulling it straight away from insertion site.
   5. Perform hand hygiene, and apply clean gloves.
   6. Explain to the patient what removing the catheter will feel like.
   7. Remove the IV site dressing, and then remove any tape securing cannula.
   8. Apply a clean dressing over the site, and secure with tape.

5. You just started a blood transfusion on your patient, and within 5 minutes he states, "My throat feels like it is closing up." Which of the following nursing interventions should you do first?
   1. Give the patient some ice chips.
   2. Notify the health care provider.
   3. Stop the blood transfusion.
   4. Check the patient's vital signs.

6. Your patient presents with arterial blood gas levels as follows: pH, 7.59; PaO_2, 90 mm Hg; $PaCO_2$, 42 mm Hg; HCO_3^-, 39 mEq/L; base excess, positive. You understand that the patient's acid-base imbalance is:
   1. Metabolic acidosis
   2. Metabolic alkalosis
   3. Respiratory acidosis
   4. Respiratory alkalosis

7. A patient who is admitted with acute renal failure and has a 24-hour urine output of 75 mL is at risk for developing:
   1. Hypercalcemia
   2. Hyperkalemia
   3. Hypokalemia
   4. Metabolic alkalosis

8. The health care provider orders potassium chloride (KCl) 20 mEq/L in normal saline to be given intravenously at 125 mL/hour. Which of the following methods is the most appropriate?
   1. Direct IV push
   2. IV piggyback
   3. Hang a new intravenous fluid bag that has 1 L of normal saline and 20 mEq of KCl in it as soon as possible.
   4. Wait until the next primary fluid is due to be infused and then change the IV fluids to match the new order.

Answers to Review Questions can be found on pages 1197-1198.

REFERENCES

AABB: Testing of donor blood for infectious diseases, 2006, accessed 7/29/09 at: http://www.aabb.org/Content/About_Blood/Facts_About_Blood_and_Blood_Banking/fabloodtesting.htm.

Arnett T: Extracellular pH regulates bone cell function, *J Nutr* 138:S415, 2008.

Browne N and others: *Nursing care of the pediatric surgical patient*, ed 2, Boston, 2007, Jones & Bartlett.

Brownie S: Why are elderly individuals at risk of nutritional deficiency? *Int J Nurs Pract* 12:110, 2006.

Bulechek GM and others, editors: *Nursing interventions classification (NIC)*, ed 5, St. Louis, 2008, Mosby.

Casey A, Elliott T: Infection risks associated with needleless intravenous access devices, *Nurs Stand* 22(11):38, 2007.

Centers for Disease Control and Prevention: Guidelines for the prevention of intravascular catheter-related infections, *MMWR Morb Mortal Wkly Rep* 51(RR-10):1, 2002.

Chernecky C and others: *Saunders' nursing survival guide: fluid and electrolytes*, ed 2, Philadelphia, 2006, Saunders.

Davis K and others: Transfusing safely: a 2006 guide for nurses, *Am J Nurs* 13(6):4, 2006.

Earhart A and others: Assessing pediatric patients for vascular access and sedation, *J Infus Nurs* 30(4):226, 2007.

Edwards S: Tissue viability: understanding the mechanisms of injury and repair, *Nurs Stand* 21(13):48, 2006.

Flanagan J and others: Interpreting laboratory values in the rehabilitation setting, *Rehabil Nurs* 32(2):77, 2007.

Goertz S: Gauging fluid balance with osmolality, *Nursing* 36(10):70, 2006.

Gray A and others: Safe transfusion of blood and blood components, *Nurs Stand* 21(51):40, 2007.

Hadaway LC: Practical considerations in administering intravenous medications, *J Neurosci Nurs* 38(2):119, 2006.

Hadaway LC: Intermittent intravenous administration sets: survey of current practices, *J Assoc Vasc Access* 12(3):143, 2007.

Hadaway LC, Millam, DA: On the road to successful IV starts, *Nursing* 35(Suppl):1, 2005.

Heitz U, Horne MM: *Mosby's pocket guide series: fluid, electrolyte, and acid-base balance*, ed 5, St. Louis, 2005, Mosby.

Hockenberry MJ, Wilson D: *Wong's nursing care of infants and children*, ed 8, St. Louis, 2007, Mosby.

Huether SE, McCance KL: *Understanding pathophysiology*, ed 4, St. Louis, 2008, Mosby.

Ignatavicius DD, Workman ML: *Medical-surgical nursing: critical thinking for collaborative care*, ed 5, Philadelphia, 2008, Saunders.

Infusion Nurses Society: Infusion nursing standards of practice, *J Infus Nurs* 29(Suppl 1):S1, 2006.

Lecko C: Improving hydration: an issue of safety, *Nurs Residential Care* 10(3):150, 2008.

Lewis SM and others: *Medical-surgical nursing: assessment and management of clinical problems*, ed 7, St. Louis, 2007, Mosby.

Madara B, Pomarico-Denino V: *Quick look nursing: pathophysiology*, ed 2, Boston, 2008, Jones & Bartlett.

Martinez-Rumayor A and others: Biology of the natriuretic peptides, *Am J Cardiol* 101(3):S3, 2008.

McKenry LM and others: *Mosby's pharmacology in nursing*, ed 22 rev, St. Louis, 2006, Mosby.

Meiner S, Lueckenotte A: *Gerontologic nursing*, ed 3, St. Louis, 2006, Mosby.

Mentes J: Oral hydration in older adults: greater awareness is needed in preventing, recognizing, and treating dehydration, *Am J Nurs* 106(6):40, 2006.

Monahan F and others: *Phipp's medical-surgical nursing: health and illness perspectives*, ed 8, St. Louis, 2007, Mosby.

Moorhead S and others, editors: *Nursing outcomes classification (NOC)*, ed 4, St. Louis, 2008, Mosby.

Occupational Safety and Health Administration: Occupational exposure to blood borne pathogens, needlestick, and other sharps injuries: final rule, *Federal Register*, CFR 29, part 1910 (*Fed Regist* 66:5317, Jan 18, 2001), updated April, 2006, http://www.osha.gov/SLTC/bloodbornepathogens/index.html.

Otto S: *Pocket guide to infusion therapy*, ed 5, St. Louis, 2005, Mosby.

Owen P and others: Implementing and assessing an evidence-based electrolyte dosing order form in the medical ICU, *Intensive Crit Care Nurs* 24(1):8, 2008.

Paris E, Grant-Casey J: Promoting safer blood transfusion practice in hospital, *Nurs Stand* 21(41):35, 2007.

Pearson A and others: Systematic review on embracing cultural diversity for developing and sustaining a health work environment in healthcare, *Int J Evid Based Healthc* 5:54, 2007.

Powell J and others: The relationship between peripheral intravenous catheters indwell time and the incidence of phlebitis, *J Infus Nurs* 31(1):39, 2008.

Reuben DB and others: *2007-2008 Geriatrics at your fingertips*, ed 10, Malden, Mass, 2008, Blackwell.

Rosenthal K: Reducing the risk of infiltration and extravasation, *Nursing* 37(4):8, 2007.

Smith B: Peripheral intravenous catheter dwell times: a comparison of three securement methods for implementation of a 96-hours scheduled change protocol, *J Infus Nurs* 29(1):17, 2006.

The Joint Commission: *2009 National Patient Safety Goals Hospital Program*, Oakbrook Terrace, Ill, 2008, The Joint Commission, http://www.jointcommission.org, accessed July 2008.

The Joint Commission: *National Patient Safety Goals: 2010*, Chicago, 2009, The Joint Commission, http://www.jointcommission.org/PatientSafety/NationalPatientSafetyGoals, accessed September, 2009.

Tolich D: Alternatives to blood transfusion, *J Infus Nurs* 31(1):46, 2008.

Tripathi S and others: Peripheral IVs: factors affecting complications and patency—a randomized controlled trial, *J Infus Nurs* 31(3):182, 2008.

Verbalis J and others: Hyponatremia treatment guidelines 2007: expert panel recommendations, *Am J Med* 120(11):S1, 2007.

Weinstein S: *Plumer's principles and practice of intravenous therapy*, ed 8, Philadelphia, 2006, Lippincott Williams & Wilkins.

Whyte A: A serious ethical dilemma, *Nurs Stand* 22(30:18, 2008.

Winfield C and others: Evidence: the first work in safe I.V. practice, *Am Nurse Today* 2(5):31, 2007.

18 Caring in Nursing Practice

MEDIA RESOURCES

 CD COMPANION   evolve WEBSITE   http://evolve.elsevier.com/Potter/basic

- Crossword Puzzle
- English/Spanish Audio Glossary

OBJECTIVES

- Discuss the role that caring plays in building nurse-patient relationships.
- Describe the commonalities among theories of caring.
- Discuss the evidence that exists about patients' perceptions of caring.

- Describe ways to express caring in practice.
- Describe the therapeutic benefit of listening to patients.
- Discuss qualities of spiritual caring.
- Explain the relationship between knowing a patient and clinical decision making.

KEY TERMS

caring p. 523   nurturant, p. 524   presence, p. 529   transcultural, p. 524

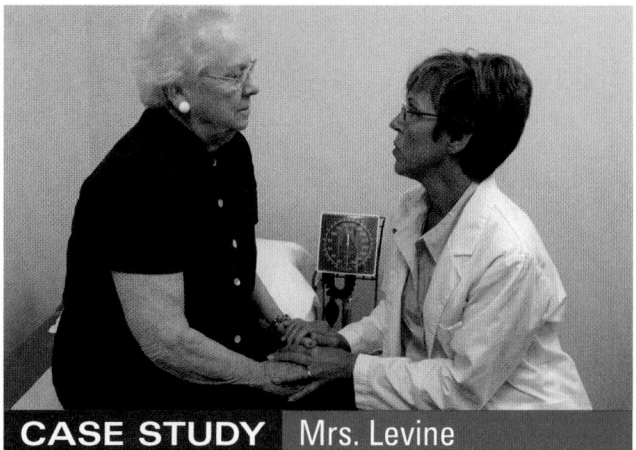

CASE STUDY   Mrs. Levine

Mrs. Levine is an 82-year-old patient diagnosed 2 months ago with lymphoma, a cancer of the lymph tissue. She has been experiencing weakness and fatigue. Over the last 4 weeks she has lost 8 pounds. Mrs. Levine has been relatively independent before her diagnosis, playing bridge each week with friends and going to lunch with fellow church members. But now she has much less energy to do the things she enjoys. Her son, Jim, lives only a few miles away and is a consistent resource when she needs transportation to the physician or trips to the grocery. She will begin a research protocol for chemotherapy treatments this week at the oncology clinic.

Sue is a nurse who has worked in the oncology clinic for over 10 years. She enters the examination room where Mrs. Levine is waiting, introduces herself, and sits down next to her patient. Sue states, "Mrs. Levine, I am here to understand your story. I want to listen and learn how I can best help you." Sue uses eye contact while talking and leans toward Mrs. Levine to establish a physical presence. Mrs. Levine, nods, smiles, and begins her story. "I have had a good life. I just don't know what is going to happen." Sue replies, "Go on." Mrs. Levine explains, "The doctor tells me the cancer is serious. I worry about what is going to happen to me and how it will affect my son, Jim. I do not want to become a burden to him." Sue responds in a calm, soothing tone, "Mrs. Levine, your concerns are very normal. It is important for you to remain as independent as possible; let's talk about how we can do that."

In this case study Sue displays caring through her words and actions. Her calm presence, eye contact, and attention to the patient's concerns all convey a relationship-centered, comforting approach to care. Caring is central to nursing practice, but perhaps it has never been more important because of today's fast-paced health care environment. Financial pressures and fewer resources place demands on nurses that make it difficult to establish interpersonal connections that are an important part of caring practice. Despite these

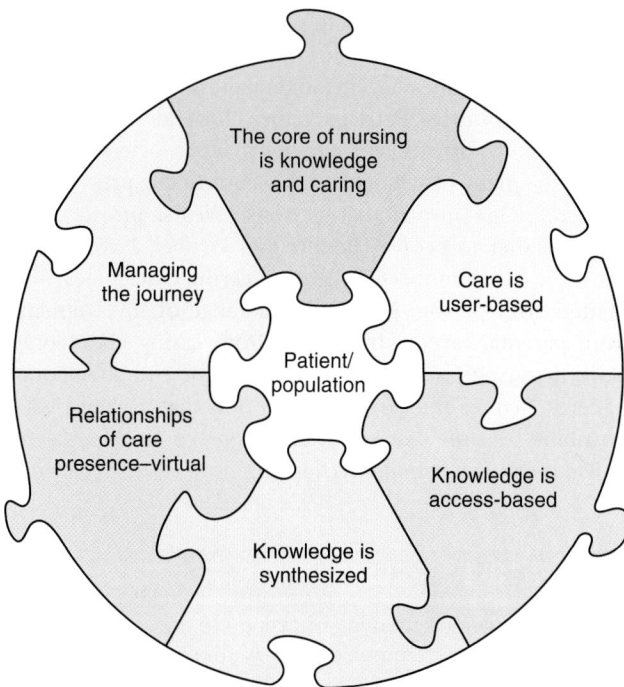

Figure 18-1 ■ AONE guiding principles for future care delivery. (From American Organization of Nurse Executives: *Guiding principles for patient care delivery toolkit,* 2005, http://www.aone.org/aone/resource/toolkit.html, accessed May 9, 2006.)

challenges, more professional organizations are stressing the importance of nurse caring in health care. The American Nurses Association (ANA) states in *Nursing's Agenda for the Future,* "Nursing is *the* pivotal health care profession highly valued for its specialized knowledge, skill, and *caring* in improving the health status of the public . . ." (ANA, 2002). In addition, the American Organization of Nurse Executives (AONE) (2005) describes caring and knowledge as the core of nursing, with caring being a key component of what a nurse brings to a patient experience (Figure 18-1). Now more than ever, it is time to value and embrace caring practices that are the heart of competent nursing practice (Lesnaik, 2005). When you engage patients in a caring and compassionate way, you learn that the therapeutic gain in caring contributes to the health and well-being of your patients.

THEORETICAL VIEWS ON CARING

Caring is universal. It affects the way we think, feel, and behave in relation to one another. Since Florence Nightingale, nurses have studied caring from a variety of philosophical and ethical perspectives. A number of nursing scholars developed theories on caring because of its importance to the practice of nursing. This chapter does not detail all of the theories of caring, but it helps you understand how caring is at the heart of a nurse's ability to work with all patients in a respectful and therapeutic way.

Caring Is Primary

After spending time studying and analyzing the clinical stories of expert nurses, Patricia Benner (1984) describes caring as the essence of excellent nursing practice. The stories revealed the many behaviors and decisions that express nurses' caring. Caring means that persons, events, projects, and things matter to people (Benner and Wrubel, 1989). It is a word for being connected. Because caring determines what matters to a person, it describes a range of involvements, from parental love to friendship, from caring about one's work to caring for one's pet, to caring for and about one's patients. Benner and Wrubel (1989) note that "caring creates possibility." *In the case study, Sue's concern for Mrs. Levine provides motivation and direction for Sue to better understand*

the meaning cancer has for Mrs. Levine and to provide the best approach in helping the patient cope with her cancer.

Patients are not all the same. Each person brings a unique background of experiences, values, and cultural perspectives to a health care encounter. Caring is always specific and relational for each nurse-patient encounter. As nurses acquire more experience, they learn that caring helps them to focus on the patients for whom they care. Caring facilitates a nurse's ability to know a patient, allowing the nurse to recognize a patient's problems and to find and implement individualized solutions.

In addition to their work in understanding caring, Benner and Wrubel (1989) describe the relationship between health, illness, and disease. Health is not the absence of illness, nor is illness identical with disease (see Chapter 1). Health is a state of being that people define in relation to their own values, personality, and lifestyle. Health exists along a continuum. Illness is the experience of loss or dysfunction. Disease is the manifestation of an abnormality at the cellular, tissue, or organ level. Some persons have a disease (e.g., arthritis or diabetes) but do not experience the sense of being ill. An individual usually does not seek health care until there is a disruption, loss, or concern. For example, when Mrs. Levine first began to feel fatigued, she thought it was just a part of being older. However, once the fatigue became serious enough to threaten her ability to manage her home and care for herself, she sought medical care. Illness has meaning only within the context of a person's life.

Because illness is the human experience of loss or dysfunction, any treatment or intervention given without consideration of its meaning to an individual is likely to be much less effective. Expert nurses understand the difference between health, illness, and disease. Through caring relationships, nurses listen to patients' stories to understand the meaning of their illness. With this understanding, they provide therapeutic, patient-centered care.

Transcultural Caring

Madeleine Leininger (1978) offers a **transcultural** view of caring. She describes the concept of care as the essence and unifying domain that sets nursing apart from other health care disciplines. Care is an essential human need, necessary for the health and survival of all individuals. Care, unlike cure, assists an individual or group in improving a human condition. Acts of caring refer to the direct or indirect **nurturant** and skillful activities, processes, and decisions that assist people in ways that are empathetic, compassionate, and supportive. Caring acts depend on the needs, problems, and values of the patient. Leininger's studies of numerous cultures around the world found that care helps protect, develop, nurture, and provide survival to people. Care is vital to recovery from illness and to the maintenance of healthy life practices in all cultures.

Leininger (1988) stresses the importance of nurses' understanding cultural caring behaviors. Even though human caring is universal, the expressions, processes, and patterns of caring vary among cultures. Caring is also very personal. One

---

BOX 18-1	**CULTURAL FOCUS**

When the various theories of caring are analyzed, a common theme is communication. A nurse shows caring through listening, showing patients respect, talking to and being honest with patients, and maintaining confidentiality. Caring communication is in many ways culturally universal. When a nurse cares for patients from different cultural backgrounds it is not possible to become familiar with all the patients' cultural beliefs that may conflict with his or her own cultural beliefs. Often clinicians believe that "knowing" a culture involves familiarizing oneself with a list of beliefs, but this tendency is the clinician's way to systematize or "tidy up" culture. In fact, people often have overlapping membership in several cultural communities. A barrier to effective communication is the languages a patient and nurse speak, both verbally and nonverbally. When communicating with patients of different cultures, it helps to acknowledge one another's difficulty in talking to put all involved at ease.

IMPLICATIONS FOR PRACTICE

- Explore with patients your difficulty in understanding their cultural frame for communication. For example, say, "In my culture we believe that . . ." or "As a nurse, I tend to value . . . ."
- By admitting your own ideas are not the only way of thinking, you allow your patients to share their perspective.
- In some cultures, discussion of a patient's common customs and popular culture can create a common ground for communication.
- Understand how patients choose to communicate their feelings. For example, the Chinese people who embrace Confucian ethics believe it is dangerous to express opinion.

Data from Chambers T: Cross-cultural issues in caring for patients with cancer, *Cancer Treat Res* 140:45, 2008; Heikkila K, Sarvimaki A, Ekman SL: Culturally congruent care for older people: Finnish care in Sweden, *Scand J Caring Sci* 21(3):354, 2007; Lai A: Eye on religion: cultural signs and caring for Chinese patients, *South Med J* 99(6):688, 2006; Simpson RL: Caring communications: how technology enhances interpersonal relations, part I, *Nurs Adm Q* 32(1):70, 2008.

challenge is to find ways to communicate with patients so as to learn the culturally specific behaviors and words that reflect human caring (Box 18-1) (see Chapter 19).

Watson's Transpersonal Theory of Caring

Most patients and their families expect a high quality of human interaction from nurses. Unfortunately, many of the conversations occurring today between patients and their nurses are very brief and disconnected. Workload demands create situations in which the development of a "close" relationship with a patient is limited (Henderson and others, 2007). Watson's transpersonal theory of caring (1979, 1985) is a holistic model that describes a conscious recognition that caring for a person involves sensitivity, respect, and a high moral and ethical commitment (Hoover, 2002). The theory integrates human caring processes with healing environments, incorporating the life-generating and life-receiving processes of caring and healing for nurses and their patients (Watson, 2006b). The theory describes a consciousness that allows nurses to raise new questions about nursing, illness, and caring. Transpersonal caring theory rejects the disease orientation of health care and places care before cure (Watson, 1988). A nurse looks beyond a patient's disease and its treatment. Instead, transpersonal caring looks for deeper sources of inner healing to protect, enhance, and preserve a person's dignity, wholeness, and inner harmony.

In Watson's view (2006b), caring becomes almost spiritual, because it preserves human dignity in a cure-dominated health care system. The nurse connects with the patient at a deep spiritual level, sometimes only for a moment, and that "connectedness" allows both the nurse and patient to heal. The emphasis of the theory and its method of caring is focused on the care of the whole patient rather than the pathologic condition and treatment of the patient's disease (Childs, 2006).

The theory supports a holistic approach that allows a caring nurse to gain a level of understanding that is unique. Consider the example of performing a nursing assessment. A nurse who applies Watson's theory during an assessment will be able to plan care in a way that goes beyond the physical aspect of a disease. *For example, Sue wants to assess Mrs. Levine's nutritional status to ensure a holistic approach to her patient's nutritional needs. Her assessment would go beyond what Mrs. Levine eats, her weight, and her sense of an appetite. Sue would also consider Mrs. Levine's desire for food, food preferences, hunger, availability of food, social environment, and emotional attachment to food.* When applying a transpersonal theory of caring, the nurse accurately assesses the patient's physical needs and combines those needs with the patient's preferences, social environment, and emotional needs (Childs, 2006).

The emphasis in Watson's theory is on the nurse-patient relationship. How a nurse chooses to be with a patient and family in any given moment influences the caring-healing relationship. Watson (2003) has identified 10 carative factors that offer a framework for nursing care (Table 18-1). The carative factors are tools for providing caring and humane nursing therapies.

TABLE 18-1 Watson's 10 Carative Factors

CARATIVE FACTOR	EXAMPLE IN PRACTICE
Forming a human-altruistic value system	Use loving-kindness to extend yourself. Use self-disclosure appropriately to promote a therapeutic alliance with your patient.
Instilling faith and hope	Provide a connectedness with the patient that offers purpose and direction when trying to find the meaning of an illness.
Cultivating a sensitivity to one's self and to others	Learn to accept yourself and others for their full potential. A caring nurse matures into becoming a self-actualized nurse.
Developing a helping-trusting, human caring relationship between the care-receiver and the caregiver	Learn to develop and sustain a helping-trusting, authentic caring relationship through effective communication with your patients.
Promoting and accepting the expression of positive and negative feelings	Support and accept your patients' feelings. When connecting with your patients, show a willingness to take risks in what you share with one another.
Using the scientific-problem-solving method for decision-making	Apply the nursing process in a systematic way to provide patient-centered care.
Promoting transpersonal teaching-learning	Learn together while educating the patient to acquire self-care skills. The patient assumes responsibility for learning.
Providing for a supportive, protective, and/or corrective mental, physical, societal, and spiritual environment	Create a healing environment at all levels, physical and nonphysical. This promotes wholeness, beauty, comfort, dignity, and peace.
Meeting human needs	Assist patients with basic needs with an intentional care and caring consciousness.
Allowing for existential-phenomenological-spiritual forces	Allow spiritual forces to provide a better understanding of oneself and your patient.

Modified from Watson J: Love and caring: ethics of face and hand—an invitation to return to the heart and soul of nursing and our deep humanity, *Nurs Adm Q* 27(3):197, 2003.

Swanson's Theory of Caring

Kristen Swanson (1991) studied patients and professional caregivers develop a theory of caring for nursing practice. She interviewed three different groups: women who miscarried, parents and health care professionals in a newborn intensive care unit, and socially at-risk mothers who received long-term, public health care. All groups were in a perinatal (before, during, or after the birth of a child) setting and experienced caring by their nurses. Researchers asked each group questions about how they experienced or expressed caring in their situation. After analyzing the stories and descriptions of the three groups, Swanson developed a theory of caring that consists of five categories or processes (Table 18-2). Swanson (1991) defines caring as a nurturing way of relating to a valued other, toward whom one feels a personal sense of commitment and responsibility. The theory supports the claim that caring is a central nursing phenomenon but not necessarily unique to nursing practice.

Swanson's theory (1991) is valuable in providing direction for how to develop useful and effective caring strategies. Each of the caring processes has definitions and subdimensions that serve as the basis for nursing interventions. For example, if a nurse provides an intervention by "doing for" patients, he or she will anticipate the risks associated with the procedure, administer the intervention skillfully, and explain aspects of the procedure to minimize the patient's anxiety.

An example would be in the way Sue would administer chemotherapy. Knowing that chemotherapy is toxic and can cause adverse reactions, Sue will begin the administration slowly as ordered, have the necessary equipment available should a reaction develop, and explain the reasons for each step of the administration. Nursing care and caring are crucial in making positive differences in patients' health and well-being outcomes. The theory is useful in guiding clinical nursing practice.

Summary of Theoretical Views

There are commonalities among all of the theoretical views on caring. Duffy, Hoskins, and Siefert (2007) identify these commonalities as human interaction or communication, mutuality, appreciating the uniqueness of individuals, and improving the welfare of patients and families. Caring is highly relational. The nurse and the patient enter into a relationship that is much more than one person simply "doing tasks for" another. There is a mutual give-and-take that develops as nurse and patient begin to know and care for one another.

Caring seems invisible at times, when a nurse and patient enter a relationship of respect, concern, and support. The nurse's empathy and compassion become a natural part of each patient encounter. However, when caring is absent, it becomes very obvious. For example, if a nurse shows disinterest or chooses to avoid a patient's request for help, the nurse's inaction quickly conveys an uncaring attitude. Henderson and others (2007) observed nurse-patient interactions on medical-surgical nursing units in Australia and then interviewed patients' perceptions of those interactions. The nurse researchers found that negative nurse-patient interactions were best described as "forgetfulness," incidences in which

TABLE 18-2 Swanson's Theory of Caring		
CARING PROCESS	**DEFINITIONS**	**SUBDIMENSIONS**
Knowing	Striving to understand an event as it has meaning in the life of the other	Avoiding assumptions Centering on the one cared for Assessing thoroughly Seeking cues Engaging the self or both
Being with	Being emotionally present to the other	Being there Conveying ability Sharing feelings Not burdening
Doing for	Doing for the other as he or she would do for the self if it were at all possible	Comforting Anticipating Performing skillfully Protecting Preserving dignity
Enabling	Facilitating the other's passage through life transitions (e.g., birth, death) and unfamiliar events	Informing/explaining Supporting/allowing Focusing Generating alternatives Validating/giving feedback
Maintaining belief	Sustaining faith in the other's capacity to get through an event or transition and face a future with meaning	Believing in/holding in esteem Maintaining a hope-filled attitude Offering realistic optimism "Going the distance"

From Swanson K: Empirical development of a middle-range theory of caring, *Nurs Res* 40(3):161, 1991.

nurses did not remember or follow-up with patient requests. Patients are perceptive of nurses' behaviors and capable of recognizing when nurses show an uncaring approach. Benner and Wrubel (1989) relate the story of a clinical nurse specialist who learned from a patient what caring is all about:

> I felt that I was teaching him a lot, but actually he taught me. One day he said to me (probably after I had delivered some well-meaning technical information about his disease), "You are doing an OK job, but I can tell that every time you walk in that door you are walking out."

In this nurse's story, the patient perceived that the nurse was simply going through the motions of teaching and showed little caring toward the patient. Patients quickly know when nurses fail to relate to them.

When you practice caring, patients sense your commitment and are willing to enter into a relationship, allowing you to gain an understanding of their experience of illness. Patients particularly sense caring when nurses are accessible and optimistically able to look forward to the future, whatever it holds (Duffy and others, 2007). As the nurse-patient relationship forms, the nurse becomes a coach and partner rather than a detached provider of care.

In the case study, Sue works with Mrs. Levine to find ways that will help her remain independent. By considering Mrs. Levine's relationship with her son, the effects of her cancer, and upcoming treatment, Sue's caring behavior becomes enabling. When a nurse practices enabling, the patient and nurse work together to identify alternatives and resources. For example, are there ways for Mrs. Levine to organize her day so that she can take frequent rest periods and still complete her daily tasks? As Sue enables Mrs. Levine, she explains the effects of cancer and chemotherapy and supports the patient in identifying ways to complete self-care activities. By understanding Mrs. Levine's unique needs, Sue is able to improve her patient's sense of well-being.

PATIENTS' PERCEPTIONS OF CARING

Research has shown a connection between patient satisfaction and nurse caring (Box 18-2). Put simply, when the nurses within an organization successfully demonstrate caring, more patients are satisfied and more likely to return to the health care setting. In addition, when patients sense that health care providers are sensitive, sympathetic, compassionate, and interested in them as people, they usually become active partners in the plan of care (Attree, 2001). Thus more health care settings are adapting models of care that focus on relationship-centered caring approaches. It therefore becomes important for organizations to be able to measure caring from a patient's point of view and to thus determine the value of nursing. Duffy and others (2007) have developed the Caring Assessment Tool (CAT) for that purpose. The tool has been tested among hospitalized patients, representing diverse ethnic groups. The tool is useful to you as a beginning nurse to appreciate the type of behaviors hospitalized patients identify as caring.

The CAT was initially designed on the basis of Watson's carative factors. The tool includes eight major factors, with three to six items that describe nursing behaviors for each (Box 18-3). The researchers have shown that each of the major factors is very consistent with the caring theories in nursing (Duffy and others, 2007).

Mutual Problem Solving

A caring nurse helps hospitalized patients understand how to think about their health and illness and to figure out questions to ask of their health care providers (Duffy and others, 2007). In addition, a caring nurse will help patients explore

---

BOX 18-2 **BEST PRACTICES**

The Effects of Nurse Caring on Patient Satisfaction

SUMMARY OF EVIDENCE

Patient satisfaction is an indicator for the quality of health care. Researchers have shown a strong, positive relationship between nurse caring behavior and patient satisfaction. The higher the patient satisfaction with nursing care, the higher their overall satisfaction with their health care experience. One aspect of caring behavior is nurses' willingness to respond to patients' specific requests. Patients value nurses' responding within a suitable time frame to meet their needs. There is evidence to show that patient satisfaction is more likely to be improved if nurses adapt their work to accommodate patients' requests or communicate why these requests cannot be immediately addressed.

APPLICATION TO NURSING PRACTICE

- Respond promptly to a patient request, either personally or by directing nursing assistive personnel to respond.
- Prioritize specific requests from patients to show your response to their needs.
- When a patient makes a request, explore with the patient the degree to which you can adapt the request and provide care.
- Discuss any limitations that may lead to a delay in responding to requests (e.g., having to assist another patient first or choosing to wait until a pain medication takes effect).

REFERENCES

Al-Mailam FF: The effect of nursing care on overall patient satisfaction and its predictive value on return-to-provider behavior: a survey study, *Qual Manag Health Care* 14(2):116, 2005.

Henderson A and others: "Caring for" behaviours that indicate to patients that nurses "care about" them, *J Adv Nurs* 60(2):146, 2007.

Wolf Z, Miller PA, Devine M: Relationship between nurse caring and patient satisfaction in patients undergoing invasive cardiac procedures, *Medsurg Nurs* 12(6):391, 2003.

BOX 18-3 Factors and Items Constituting the Caring Assessment Tool (CAT)

Each item begins with the stem: Since I have been a patient here the nurse(s)

MUTUAL PROBLEM SOLVING
- Help me understand how I am thinking
- Ask me how I think treatment is going
- Help me explore alternative ways of dealing
- Ask me what I know
- Help me figure out questions to ask

ATTENTIVE REASSURANCE
- Are available
- Seem interested
- Support sense of hope
- Help me believe in self
- Anticipate my needs

HUMAN RESPECT
- Listen to me
- Accept me
- Treat me kindly
- Respect me
- Pay attention to me

ENCOURAGING MANNER
- Support my beliefs
- Encourage to ask questions
- Help me to see some good
- Encourage me to go on
- Help me deal with bad feelings

APPRECIATION OF UNIQUE MEANINGS
- Are concerned how I view things
- Know what is important to me
- Acknowledge my inner feelings
- Show respect for things having meaning

HEALING ENVIRONMENT
- Check up on me
- Pay attention to me when I am talking
- Make me feel comfortable
- Respect my privacy
- Treat my body carefully

AFFILIATION NEEDS
- Are responsive to my family
- Talk openly with my family
- Allow my family to be involved

BASIC HUMAN NEEDS
- Make sure I get food
- Help me with routine needs for sleep
- Help me feel less worried

Modified from Duffy JR, Hoskins L, Seifert RF: Dimensions of caring: psychometric evaluation of the Caring Assessment Tool, *Adv Nurs Sci* 30(3):235, 2007.

options for resolving health problems and provide information and instruction. Using evidence in practice is an aspect of mutual problem solving, with a nurse continuously learning and engaging patients and families in discussions about their health issues.

Attentive Reassurance

Patients perceive nurses to be caring when they are accessible and show interest in the patient's well-being. Being able to foresee the future (whatever it holds) and confidently express possibilities often gives patients hope (Duffy and others, 2007). Attentive reassurance is consistent with Watson's faith-hope, sensitivity, and helping-trust relationship factors. It is also consistent with Swanson's maintaining belief.

Human Respect

Respect for patients is integral to the provision of care. In the CAT, human respect refers to nurses being able to appreciate the value of human beings and displaying behaviors that demonstrate value, such as accepting or paying attention to a patient (Duffy and others, 2007). By showing respect, a nurse honors the worth of individuals.

Encouraging Manner

Hospitalized patients face very difficult situations: numerous diagnostic tests, anxiety and fear of not knowing what the future holds, family role changes, and multiple physical ailments. When a nurse remains poised and cheerful and points out the good in a difficult situation, patients perceive these behaviors as caring (Duffy and others, 2007). Having an encouraging manner also involves helping a patient deal with bad feelings. Patients perceive how both nurses' attitudes and mannerisms reflect an encouraging manner.

Appreciation of Unique Meanings

In Swanson's theory of caring (1991), knowing involves nurses' attempts at understanding the lived experiences of patients. Duffy and others (2007) have identified that hospitalized patients recognize when nurses know what is important to them and their families. This is especially important because nurses care for patients from different ethnic groups, with different levels of illness, and with unique life experiences. This aspect of caring is challenging because it takes time for a nurse to develop a relationship with patients that allows for an appreciation of a patient's inner feelings.

Healing Environment

Florence Nightingale was the first nurse to understand how manipulating patients' environments (e.g., providing nutrition, hygiene, and comfort) promoted healing. The CAT includes several items that measure patients' perceptions of nurses providing a healing environment. A healing environment, for example, is one in which nurses check patients frequently, respect patient privacy, and treat the body carefully. Such an environment leads patients to a sense of security and protection from harm (Duffy and others, 2007).

Affiliation Needs

Basic to nursing practice is the inclusion of family members in a patient's care. It is a key element in discharge planning (see Chapter 2). With respect to caring, hospitalized patients perceive nurses as caring when they are responsive to patients' families and allow them to be involved in the patient's health care situation (Duffy and others, 2007). This means that nurses are not reluctant to engage families in conversation and to explain (when appropriate) the care a patient is receiving. Family members influence decisions regarding how a patient will manage health care needs in the home. A caring nurse involves the family in such decisions.

Basic Human Needs

All humans require the basic needs of fluids, nutrition, oxygen, elimination, body temperature, shelter, and sex (Maslow, 1987) (see Chapter 1). Unfortunately, these basic needs are not readily met when nurses instead become focused on managing technological demands and complex therapies. Typically nurses are now delegating basic human needs to nursing assistive personnel (see Chapter 12). However, patients tested using the CAT clearly viewed nurses as caring when they took the patients' basic needs into account (Duffy and others, (2007).

As you begin clinical practice, consider how patients perceive caring and what are the best approaches to providing care. Behaviors associated with caring offer an excellent starting point. It is important to determine each patient's perceptions and unique expectations. Always focus on building a relationship that allows you to learn what is important to your patients.

CARING IN NURSING PRACTICE

It is impossible to prescribe ways that will ensure you will become a caring professional. For those who find caring a normal part of their life, caring is a product of their culture, values, experiences, and relationships with others. Persons who do not experience care in their lives often find it difficult to act in caring ways. As nurses deal with health and illness in their practice, most grow in the ability to care. Caring nurses use a caring approach in each patient encounter.

Providing Presence

The concept of **presence** is an interpersonal process that is characterized by sensitivity, holism, intimacy, vulnerability, and adaptation to unique circumstances (Finfgeld-Connett, 2006). Put more simply, providing presence is a person-to-person encounter conveying closeness and a sense of caring. Presence occurs within an atmosphere of intimacy and sensitivity and is characterized by open and honest interactions (Finfgeld-Connett, 2008). The process of presence is mutual. Patients demonstrate a need for and openness to presence. Then in turn a nurse is willing to display presence and practice in an environment that is conducive to it (Finfgeld-Connett, 2006).

Presence involves "being there" and "being with." "Being there" is more than a physical presence; it also includes communication and understanding. The interpersonal relationship of "being there" depends on a nurse being attentive and receptive to a patient. *For example, in the case study Sue decides it is important to be with Mrs. Devine during her first chemotherapy treatment. Sue tells her patient, "You know, I want to be the one who gives you the first chemotherapy treatment. I know this has been an anxious moment for you." Sue sits down next to Mrs. Devine and prepares the infusion supplies carefully while continuing their conversation. When Sue sees Mrs. Devine's son at the doorway, she invites him in to sit with his mother.*

Receptivity is intuitively sensed by patients, and it is read in nurses' faces, body language, and expressions (Carr, 2008). This type of presence is something the nurse offers to the patient with the purpose of achieving some goal, such as support, comfort, or encouragement; to diminish the intensity of unwanted feelings; or for reassurance (Fareed, 1996).

"Being with" is interpersonal. The nurse and patient share personal insights in verbal and nonverbal ways (Finfgeld-Connett, 2008). The nurse gives himself or herself, which means being available and at a patient's disposal. If patients accept the nurse, they will invite him or her to see, share, and touch their vulnerability and suffering. One's human presence never leaves one unaffected (Watson, 2003). Through presence a nurse enters the patient's world. A patient is able to put words to feelings and to understand himself or herself in a way that leads to identifying solutions, seeing new directions, and making choices.

When a nurse establishes presence, eye contact, body language, voice tone, listening, and having a positive and encouraging attitude act together to create an openness and understanding (Figure 18-2). The message conveyed is that the other's experience matters to the one caring (Swanson, 1991). Establishing presence with a patient enhances the nurse's ability to appreciate the unique meanings in a patient's life and to learn from the patient. This strengthens the nurse's ability to provide adequate and appropriate nursing care.

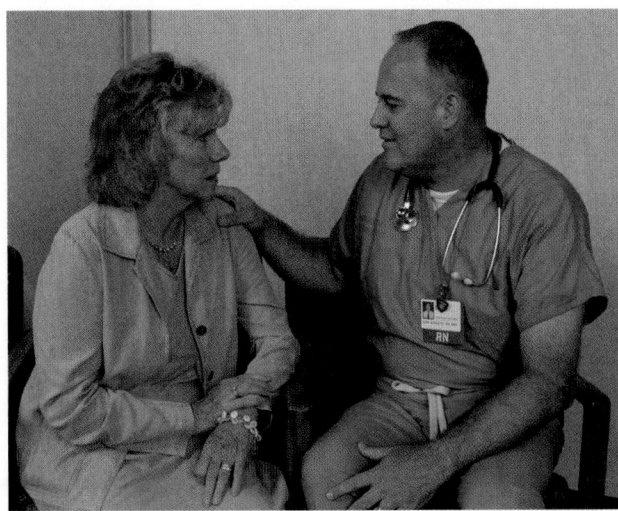

Figure 18-2 ■ Nurse conveying presence to a patient.

It is important to establish presence when patients are experiencing stressful events or situations. Awaiting a doctor's report of test results, preparing for an unfamiliar procedure, and planning for a return home after serious illness are just a few examples of events in the course of a person's illness that can create unpredictability and dependency on nurses. The nurse's presence calms anxiety and fear related to stressful situations. Giving reassurance and thorough explanations about a procedure, remaining at the patient's side, and coaching the patient through the experience all convey a presence that is invaluable to the patient's well-being.

Touch

Patients face situations that are embarrassing, frightening, and painful. Whatever the feeling or symptom, patients look to nurses for comfort. Many patients associate touch with fear and pain, because nurses touch patients while performing painful procedures (Brill and Kashurba, 2001). However, a simple touch offered in a compassionate way by a health care professional can be comforting, allowing a nurse to reach out to patients to communicate concern and support. Nonetheless, a simple gesture of touching a patient on the arm can, according to different cultures, be either consoling and sympathetic or invasive and offensive (Chambers, 2008).

Touch is relational and leads to a connection between nurse and patient. Fredriksson (1999) describes three categories of touch: task-oriented, caring, and protective. Nurses use task-oriented touch when performing a task or procedure. The skillful and gentle performance of a nursing procedure conveys security and competence. Expert nurses learn that any procedure is more effective when they administer it carefully and in consideration of any patient concern. For example, if a patient is anxious about the insertion of a nasogastric tube, offer comfort through a full explanation of the procedure and what the patient will feel. Then you convey that you will perform the procedure safely, skillfully, and successfully in the way you prepare supplies, position the patient, and gently manipulate and insert the nasogastric tube. Throughout any procedure talk quietly with a patient to provide reassurance and support. Patients report their worries are alleviated when they know that they are in caring, competent hands (Carr, 2008).

Caring touch is a form of nonverbal communication that successfully influences a patient's comfort and security, enhances self-esteem, and improves reality orientation (Boyek and Watson, 1994). You express this in the way you hold a patient's hand, give a back massage, gently position a patient, or participate in a conversation. When using caring touch, you are making a connection with the patient and showing acceptance of the individual.

Protective touch is a form of touch that protects the nurse and/or patient (Fredriksson, 1999). The patient views it either positively or negatively. The most obvious form of protective touch is preventing an accident, for example, holding and bracing the patient to avoid a fall. Protective touch is also a kind of touch that protects the nurse emotionally. A nurse withdraws from a patient when he or she is unable to tolerate suffering or needs to escape from a situation that is causing tension. When used in this way, protective touch elicits negative feelings in a patient (Fredriksson, 1999).

Because touch conveys many messages, use it with discretion. Touch itself is a concern when crossing cultural boundaries of either the patient or the nurse (Benner, 2004). However, do not assume that touch is only a cultural issue. In a recent study involving trauma patients, researchers found that patients did not like to be touched a lot and that it would not be a caring thing for them (Hayes and Tyler-Ball, 2007). Most patients allow task-oriented touch, as most individuals give nurses and doctors a license to enter their personal space to provide care. Know and understand if patients are accepting of touch and how they interpret your intentions.

Listening

Caring is an interpersonal interaction that is much more than two persons simply talking back and forth. In a caring relationship the nurse establishes trust, opens lines of communication, and listens to what the patient has to say. Listening is key, because it conveys the nurse's full attention and interest. Listening includes "taking in" what a patient says, as well as an interpretation and understanding of what the patient is saying, and giving back that understanding to the person talking. Listening to the meaning of what a patient says creates a mutual relationship. True listening leads to knowing and responding to what really matters to the patient and family (Boykin and others, 2003).

When an individual becomes ill, he or she usually has a story to tell about the meaning of their illness. Any critical or chronic illness affects all of a patient's life choices and decisions, sometimes affecting the individual's identity. Being able to tell that story helps the patient break the distress of illness. Thus a story needs a listener. Through listening, a nurse is receptive and able to hear not only what is said but what is not being said by the patient (Carr, 2008).

Frank (1998) described his own feelings during his experience with cancer: "I needed a [health care professional's] gift of listening in order to make my suffering a relationship between *us,* instead of an iron cage around *me.*" He needed to be able to express what he needed when he was ill. The personal concerns that are part of a patient's illness story determine what is at stake for the patient. Caring through listening enables you to participate in a patient's life.

You can also listen by recognizing that big things can come out of small talk (Carr, 2008). Often patients may seem to be talking about trivial topics, such as the weather, a favorite pastime, what a relative did yesterday. But patients explain that these topics are important. Having their stories heard, no matter how trivial, is affirming and shows patients that they are important people (Carr, 2008). Patients want to know that their life and experiences matter to nurses.

Through active listening, you begin to know your patients and what is important to them (Bernick, 2004). Learning to listen to a patient is sometimes difficult. It is easy to become distracted by tasks at hand, colleagues shouting instructions, or other patients waiting to have their needs met. However, the time you take to listen effectively is worthwhile both in the information gained and in the strengthening of the nurse-patient relationship. Listening allows nurses to help patients find meaning, release fears, and answer their own questions (Carr, 2008).

Knowing the Patient

One of the five caring processes described by Swanson (1991) is knowing the patient. The concept comprises both the nurse's understanding of a specific patient and the nurse's subsequent selection of interventions (Radwin, 1995). Knowing develops over time as a nurse learns the clinical conditions within a specialty and the behaviors and physiological responses of patients. Knowing helps a nurse respond to what really matters to a patient (Bulfin, 2005). To know a patient means that you avoid assumptions, focus on the patient, and engage in a caring relationship that reveals information and cues that facilitate critical thinking and clinical judgments (see Chapter 7). Knowing the patient is at the core of clinical decision making. Through caring you develop an understanding that helps you to better know the patient as a unique individual and choose the most appropriate and efficacious nursing therapies.

The caring relationships that a nurse develops over time, coupled with the nurse's growing knowledge and experience, provide a rich source of meaning that allows a nurse to recognize changes in a patient's clinical status. Expert nurses develop the ability to detect changes in patients' conditions almost effortlessly. Clinical decision making involves various aspects of knowing the patient, including responses to therapies, routines and habits, coping resources, physical capacities and endurance, and body typology and characteristics (Tanner and others, 1993). The experienced nurse knows additional facts about his or her patients such as their experiences, behaviors, feelings, and perceptions (Radwin, 1995). When you make clinical decisions accurately in the context of knowing a patient well, improved patient outcomes will result. Swanson (1999) notes that when nurses base care on knowing the patient, the patients perceive care as personalized, comforting, supportive, and healing.

Success in knowing a patient lies in the relationship you form together. To know a patient is to enter into a caring, social process. You and the patient form a bond that sets the stage for a positive "working" relationship so that you can help the patient become involved in his or her care and accept help when needed (Bulfin, 2005).

Spiritual Caring

Spiritual caring is about developing caring relationships with patients through fostering connections to promote spiritual comfort and well-being (Carr, 2008). A growing body of research in nursing and other fields shows that spirituality influences health. In a study involving the perspectives of nurses, patients, and families, Carr (2008) discovered that most patients and families seek spiritual care from nurses. This is not a conscious or planned process, but simply a way of being human. All human beings desire to be cared for; they desire connectedness, and they desire to be recognized as individuals with a past, present, and future.

Establishing a caring relationship with a patient involves an interconnectedness between the nurse and the patient. This interconnectedness is why Watson (1979, 2006a, 2006b) describes the caring relationship in a spiritual sense. Spirituality offers a sense of connectedness, intrapersonally (connected with oneself), interpersonally (connected with others and the environment), and transpersonally (connected with the unseen, God, or a higher power). In a caring relationship the patient and the nurse come to know one another so that both move toward a healing relationship by doing the following (Watson, 2003):

- Mobilizing hope for the patient and for the nurse
- Finding an understanding of illness, symptoms, or emotions that is acceptable to the patient
- Assisting the patient in using social, emotional, or spiritual resources
- Recognizing that caring relationships connect us human to human

Family Care

Each individual experiences life through relationships with others. Thus caring for a patient cannot occur in isolation from that person's family. As a nurse, it is important for you to know the family almost as thoroughly as you know a patient. The family is an important resource. Success with nursing interventions often depends on the family's willingness to share information about the patient, their acceptance and understanding of therapies, whether the interventions fit with the family's daily practices, and whether the family supports and delivers the therapies recommended.

There are many nurse caring behaviors that families of patients with cancer perceive as important to patients' well-being. Ensuring the patient's well-being and being able to be active participants in care are critical for family members. *In the case study, Sue spends time discussing with Mrs. Levine's son how he can help his mother manage her side effects from the chemotherapy. Sue prepares him to deal with any nausea or loss of appetite his mother might experience.* Although specific to families of patients with cancer, the behaviors listed in Box 18-4 offer useful guidelines for developing a caring relationship with all families. Begin a relationship by learning who makes up the patient's family and what their roles are in the patient's life. Showing the family care and concern for the patient creates an openness that then enables you to form a relationship with the family. Caring for the family considers the context of the patient's illness and the stress it imposes on all members (see Chapter 23).

BOX 18-4 Nurse Caring Behaviors as Perceived by Families

- Being honest
- Advocating for patient's care preferences
- Giving clear explanations
- Keeping family members informed
- Asking permission before doing something to a patient
- Providing comfort: Offering a warm blanket, finding food a patient can swallow, rubbing a patient's back
- Reading patients passages from religious texts, a favorite book, cards or mail
- Providing for and maintaining patient privacy
- Assuring the patient that nursing services will be available
- Helping patients to do as much for themselves as possible
- Teaching the family how to keep the patient physically comfortable

Data from Brown CL and others: Caring in action: the patient care facilitator role, *Int J Hum Caring* 9(3):51, 2005; Radwin L: Oncology patients' perceptions of quality nursing care, *Res Nurs Health* 23(3):179, 2000; Carr T: Mapping the processes and qualities of spiritual nursing care, *Qual Health Res* 18(5):686, 2008.

THE CHALLENGE OF CARING

Assisting individuals during a time of need is the reason many enter nursing. When nurses are able to affirm themselves as caring individuals, they achieve a meaning and purpose to their lives (Benner, 2004; Hoover, 2002). Caring is a motivating force for people to become nurses, and it is a source of satisfaction when nurses know they have made a difference in their patients' lives. It is a challenge to care in today's health care system. Being a part of the helping professions is difficult and demanding. Nurses are torn between the human caring model and the task-oriented biomedical model and institutional demands that consume their practice (Watson and Foster, 2003). Nurses have increasingly less time to spend with patients, making it much harder to know who they are. A reliance on technology and cost-effective health care strategies and efforts to standardize and refine work processes all undermine the nature of caring. Too often patients become just a number, with their real needs either overlooked or ignored.

The ANA, National League for Nursing, AONE, and American Association of Colleges of Nursing recommend strategies to reverse the current nursing shortage. A number of the strategies have potential for creating work environments that enable nurses to demonstrate more caring behaviors. Finfgeld-Connett (2008) argues that environmental factors promote artful nursing, presence, and caring. A conducive work setting is one that consists of aesthetic surroundings, adequate resources, and time. To create environments conducive to nursing, health care organizations must introduce greater flexibility into the work environment structure, reward experienced nurse mentors, improve nurse staffing, and provide nurses with autonomy over their practice (Brown and others 2005; Watson and Foster, 2003).

If health care is to make a positive difference in their lives, human beings cannot be treated like machines or robots. Instead, health care has to become more humanizing. Nurses play an important role in making care an integral part of health care delivery. This begins by nurses' making caring a part of the philosophy and environment in the workplace. Incorporating care concepts into standards of nursing care establishes the guidelines for professional conduct. Finally, during day-to-day practice with patients and families, nurses need to be committed to caring and be willing to establish the relationships necessary for personal, competent, compassionate, and meaningful nursing care.

KEY POINTS

- Caring is the essence of clinical nursing practice.
- Human caring is universal; the expressions, processes, and patterns of caring vary among cultures.
- When the nurses within an organization successfully demonstrate caring, more patients are satisfied and more likely to return to the health care setting
- Watson's 10 carative factors offer tools for providing caring and humane nursing therapies.
- An understanding of the behaviors that patients associate with caring offers you an excellent starting point to establish a caring practice.
- When a nurse establishes presence, eye contact, body language, voice tone, listening, and having a positive attitude act together to create an openness and understanding.
- Because touch conveys many messages, use it with discretion.
- Listening includes "taking in" what a patient says, as well as an interpretation and understanding of what the patient is saying, and giving back that understanding to the person talking.
- Through caring you develop an understanding that helps you to better know the patient as a unique individual and choose the most appropriate and efficacious nursing therapies.
- Most patients and families seek spiritual care from nurses, not as a conscious or planned process, but simply as a way of being human.
- Showing the family care and concern for the patient creates an openness that then enables you to form a relationship with the family.

CRITICAL THINKING EXERCISES

Mrs. Levine has consistently relied on her son, Jim, to provide caregiving support through transportation and being a day-to-day resource. Jim brings his mother to the outpatient oncology clinic for her first chemotherapy infusion. The total treatment will last for approximately 5 hours. Sue invites Jim to sit in the treatment area with his mother.

1. As Sue prepares to administer the chemotherapy, identify three ways that she can demonstrate to Jim her caring for Mrs. Levine.

2. Jim asks Sue outside of the treatment room, "How will my mother respond to this chemotherapy? What should we be expecting?" Based on Swanson's theory of caring, what might be an appropriate response on Sue's part in "maintaining belief"?

3. Three hours into the infusion, Mrs. Levine asks Sue for a glass of water and begins talking about her pet cat and her desire to return home and be able to visit with one of her bridge partners tomorrow. Sue has another patient down the hall who has an infusion that has been under way for about an hour. What should Sue do to show her caring for Mrs. Levine?

evolve Answers to Critical Thinking Questions can be found on the Evolve website.

REVIEW QUESTIONS

1. A nurse hears a colleague tell a nursing student she never touches patients unless she is performing a procedure or doing an assessment. The nurse tells the colleague that:
   1. When performing procedures, touch is a form of protection
   2. Touch is a type of verbal communication
   3. Touch forms a connection between nurse and patient
   4. There is never a problem with using touch

2. A young Mexican American woman has come to the clinic for the first time to undergo a gynecological examination. Which nursing behavior applies Swanson's caring process of "knowing" the patient?
   1. Sharing feelings about the importance of having regular gynecological examinations
   2. Explaining risk factors for cervical cancer
   3. Recognizing the patient is modest, keeping the patient covered as much as possible during the examination
   4. Gaining an understanding of what a vaginal examination means to the patient

3. Helping a surgical patient adapt his learning style to discharge teaching demonstrates which of the following caring behaviors?
   1. Being with
   2. Doing for
   3. Enabling
   4. Knowing

4. When a nurse helps a patient find the meaning of cancer by supporting his beliefs about life, this is an example of:
   1. Instilling faith and hope
   2. Forming a human-altruistic value system
   3. Cultural caring
   4. Being with

5. A number of strategies have potential for creating work environments that enable nurses to demonstrate more caring behaviors. Some of these include:
   1. Increased technological support
   2. Increasing working hours
   3. Flexibility, autonomy, and improved staffing
   4. Increased input concerning nursing functions from health care providers

6. An example of a nurse caring behavior that families of cancer patients perceive as important to a patient's well-being is:
   1. Making health care decisions for the patient
   2. Having family members provide a patient's total personal hygiene
   3. Injecting the nurse's personal views about death into a patient's story
   4. Asking permission before performing a procedure on a patient

7. A nurse is caring for an older adult male who will have to go to an assisted living facility following discharge. Which of the descriptions below is an example of listening that displays caring?
   1. The nurse encourages the patient to talk about his concerns while reviewing a computer screen at the patient's bedside.
   2. The nurse sits at the patient's bedside, listens as he relays his fear of never seeing his home again, and then asks if he needs anything for pain.
   3. The nurse listens to the patient's story while sitting on the side of the bed, then summarizes an interpretation of the patient's story.
   4. The nurse enters the patient's room, listens as he talks about his fears of not returning home, and tells the patient to think positively.

8. Jean is a nursing student assigned to care for a young Vietnamese patient diagnosed with a serious heart ailment. Jean's instructor discusses the importance of finding ways to support and reinforce the young patient's healthy life practices in order to help him adjust to limitations of his disease. This is an example of applying which theory of caring?
   1. Swanson's ten carative factors
   2. Leininger's transcultural view of caring
   3. Watson's transpersonal theory of caring
   4. Benner's theory of caring as the essence of excellent nursing practice

9. In the health clinic in a large metropolitan urban area, Frank meets patients from a wide variety of cultural backgrounds. In his attempt to show caring communication, he knows it is not possible to know all patients' cultural beliefs that may conflict with his own. Which of the following statements displays an effort to show caring communication with a Latino patient?
    1. "I have seen many patients with your illness, and it helps if you tell your children about what is wrong."
    2. "It seems to me that there is really only one way to tell your children about your illness. What do you think?"
    3. "I know my ideas for what to tell my children when I become ill are not the same as everyone else's. What are your thoughts?"
    4. "Now, when your children come back into the waiting room, I will walk out so you can tell them about your illness."

10. A nursing student enters a patient's room, arranges the supplies for an enema administration, and tells the patient what she plans to do, step by step. Just before giving the enema, she tells the patient, "Try to relax, this will just take a few minutes, and once you have this enema, you will feel much less uncomfortable." The nursing student then administers the enema gently and skillfully. This is an example of:
    1. Caring touch
    2. Protective touch
    3. Task-oriented touch
    4. Interpersonal touch

Answers to Review Questions can be found on pages 1197-1198.

REFERENCES

Al-Mailam FF: The effect of nursing care on overall patient satisfaction and its predictive value on return-to-provider behavior: a survey study, *Qual Manag Health Care* 14(2):116, 2005.

American Nurses Association: *Nursing's agenda for the future: a call to the nation,* 2002, http://www.nursingworld.org/naf, accessed May 9, 2008.

American Organization of Nurse Executives: *Guiding principles for patient care delivery toolkit,* 2005, http://www.aone.org/aone/resource/toolkit.html, accessed May 9, 2006.

Attree M: Patients' and relatives' experiences and perspectives of "good" and "not so good" quality care, *J Adv Nurs* 33(4):456, 2001.

Benner P: *From novice to expert,* Menlo Park, Calif, 1984, Addison-Wesley.

Benner P: Relational ethics of comfort, touch, solace-endangered arts, *Am J Crit Care* 13(4):346, 2004.

Benner P, Wrubel J: *The primacy of caring: stress and coping in health and illness,* Menlo Park, Calif, 1989, Addison Wesley.

Bernick L: Caring for older adults: practice guided by Watson's care-healing model, *Nurs Sci Q* 17(2):128, 2004.

Boyek K, Watson R: A touching story, *Elderly Care* 3:20, 1994.

Boykin and others: Transforming practice using a caring-based nursing model, *Nurs Admin Q* 27(3):223, 2003.

Brill C, Kashurba M: Each moment of touch, *Nurs Adm Q* 25(3):8, 2001.

Brown CL and others: Caring in action: the patient care facilitator role, *Int J Hum Caring* 9(3):51, 2005.

Bulfin S: Nursing as caring theory: living caring in nursing practice, *Nurs Sci Q* 18(4):313, 2005.

Carr T: Mapping the processes and qualities of spiritual nursing care, *Qual Health Res* 18(5):686, 2008.

Chambers T: Cross-cultural issues in caring for patients with cancer, *Cancer Treat Res* 140:45, 2008.

Childs A: The complex gastrointestinal patient and Jean Watson's Theory of Caring in Nutrition Support, *Gastroenterol Nurs* 29(4):483-488, 2006.

Duffy JR, Hoskins L, Seifert RF: Dimensions of caring: psychometric evaluation of the caring assessment tool, *Adv Nurs Sci* 30(3):235, 2007.

Fareed A: The experience of reassurance: patients' perspectives, *J Adv Nurs* 23:272, 1996.

Finfgeld-Connett D: Meta-synthesis of presence in nursing, *J Adv Nurs* 55:708, 2006.

Finfgeld-Connett D: Qualitative convergence of three nursing concepts: art of nursing, presence, and caring, *J Adv Nurs* 63(5):527, 2008.

Frank AW: Just listening: narrative and deep illness, *Fam Syst Health* 16(3):197, 1998.

Fredriksson L: Modes of relating in a caring conversation: a research synthesis on presence, touch, and listening, *J Adv Nurs* 30(5):1167, 1999.

Hayes JS, Tyler-Ball S: Perceptions of nurses' caring behaviors by trauma patients, *J Trauma Nurs* 14(4):187, 2007.

Heikkila K, Sarvimaki A, Ekman SL: Culturally congruent care for older people: Finnish care in Sweden, *Scand J Caring Sci* 21(3):354, 2007.

Henderson A and others: "Caring for" behaviours that indicate to patients that nurses "care about" them, *J Adv Nurs* 60(2):146, 2007.

Hoover J: The personal and professional impact of undertaking an educational module on human caring, *J Adv Nurs* 37(1):79, 2002.

Lai A: Eye on religion: cultural signs and caring for Chinese patients, *South Med J* 99(6):688, 2006.

Leininger M: *Transcultural nursing: concepts, theories and practices,* New York, 1978, John Wiley & Sons.

Leininger M: *Care: the essence of nursing and health,* Detroit, 1988, Wayne State University Press.

Lesnaik R: Caring through technological competence, *J School Nurs* 21(4):199, 2005.

Maslow AH: *Motivation and personality,* ed 3, Upper Saddle River, NJ, 1987, Prentice Hall.

Radwin L: Knowing the patient: a process model for individualized interventions, *Nurs Res* 44:364, 1995.

Radwin L: Oncology patients' perceptions of quality nursing care, *Res Nurs Health* 23(3):179, 2000.

Simpson RL: Caring communications: how technology enhances interpersonal relations, part I, *Nurs Adm Q* 32(1):70, 2008.

Swanson KM: Empirical development of a middle-range theory of caring, *Nurs Res* 40(3):161, 1991.

Swanson KM: Effects of caring, measurement, and time on miscarriage impact and women's well-being, *Nurs Res* 48(6):288, 1999.

Tanner C and others: The phenomenology of knowing the patient, *Image J Nurs Sch* 25:273, 1993.

Watson MJ: *Nursing: the philosophy and science of caring,* Boston, 1979, Little, Brown.

Watson MJ: *Nursing: human science and human care: a theory of nursing.* Norwalk, Conn, 1985, Appleton-Century-Crofts.

Watson MJ: New dimensions of human caring theory, *Nurs Sci Q* 1:175, 1988.

Watson J: Love and caring: ethics of face and hand—an invitation to return to the heart and soul of nursing and our deep humanity, *Nurs Adm Q* 27(3):197, 2003.

Watson J: Can an ethic of caring be maintained? *J Adv Nurs* 15:125, 2006a.

Watson J: Caring theory as an ethical guide to administrative and clinical practices, *Nurs Adm Q* 30(1): 8, 2006b.

Watson J, Foster R: The Attending Nurse Caring Model®: integrating theory, evidence and advanced caring-healing therapeutics for transforming professional practice, *J Clin Nurs* 12:360, 2003.

Wolf Z, Miller PA, Devine M: Relationship between nurse caring and patient satisfaction in patients undergoing invasive cardiac procedures, *Medsurg Nurs* 12(6):391, 2003.

Cultural Diversity

MEDIA RESOURCES

 CD COMPANION 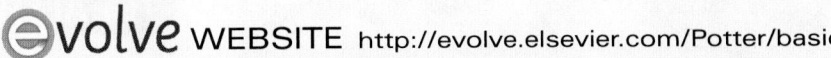 **WEBSITE** http://evolve.elsevier.com/Potter/basic

- Crossword Puzzle
- English/Spanish Audio Glossary

OBJECTIVES

- Identify the impact of ethnic demographic trends on health and nursing.
- Describe health disparities linked with racial and ethnic differences.
- Compare dominant and variant cultural contexts of health and illness.
- Analyze the impact of culture on health, illness, and caring patterns.

- Describe steps toward developing cultural competence.
- Use cultural assessment to plan culturally competent care.
- Apply research findings in culturally competent care.

KEY TERMS

acculturation, p. 542
assimilation, p. 542
biases and prejudices, p. 537

cultural assessment, p. 540
cultural competence, p. 538

culturally congruent care, p. 539
Culture Care Theory, p. 539
emic worldview, p. 537

ethnicity, p. 536
etic worldview, p. 537
subcultures, p. 536
transcultural nursing, p. 539

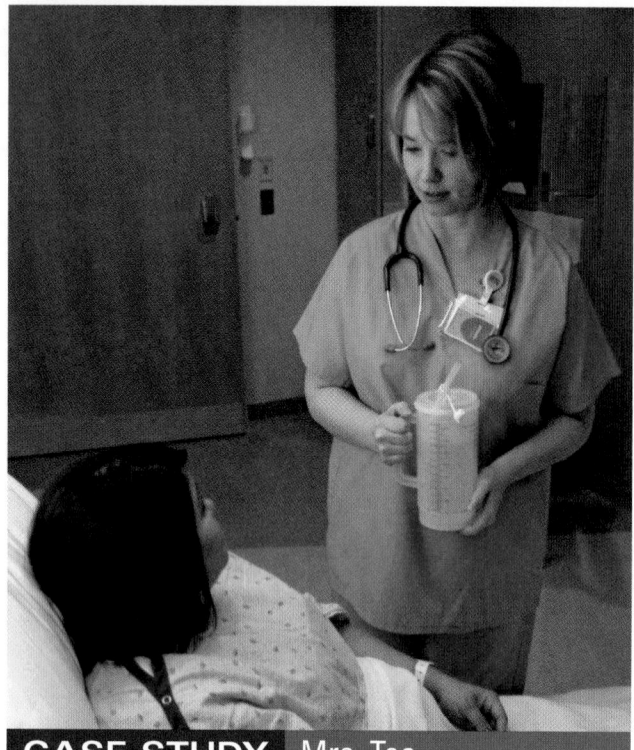

CASE STUDY   Mrs. Tao

Mrs. Tao is 27 years old and immigrated to the United States from China 3 years ago. She is in the hospital because she gave birth to a baby girl yesterday. She is breast-feeding her baby and plans to go home tomorrow. Jenny is a 23-year-old nursing student assigned to care for Mrs. Tao. Jenny knows that it is important to provide education to Mrs. Tao so she will be able to take care of her daughter at home. Jenny teaches Mrs. Tao that it is important to drink fluids to replace fluids lost during birth and to facilitate production of breast milk. Jenny then gives Mrs. Tao a fresh pitcher of ice water and suggests that Mrs. Tao drink at least 8 ounces of water every hour.

Several hours later, Jenny checks Mrs. Tao's water pitcher and notices that Mrs. Tao did not drink any of it. Jenny adds new ice to the pitcher and explains again to Mrs. Tao the importance of drinking fluids. Mrs. Tao nods that she understands. Jenny leaves Mrs. Tao, expecting that she will drink the ice water.

The U.S. population is increasing in diversity. According to the U.S. Bureau of the Census (2009), ethnic or racial minority groups constitute approximately 33% of the U.S. population. By the year 2050 the percentage of minority groups in the United States is expected to climb to 50%. In most countries, there is a dominant culture that exists along with a variety of subcultures. The Anglo American culture, which has its origins in Western Europe, is dominant in the United States. **Subcultures** have similarities with the dominant culture but also have unique life patterns, values, and norms that represent various ethnic, religious, and other groups with distinct characteristics from the dominant culture. Appalachian, Amish, and Cajun cultures are examples of subcultures in the United States. **Ethnicity** refers to a shared identity related to social and cultural heritage such as values, language, geographical space, and racial characteristics. Members of an ethnic group feel a common sense of identity. For example, individuals declare their ethnic identity as Peruvian, Bosnian, or Korean. The term *race*, which is often wrongly interchanged with *ethnicity*, refers to the common biological characteristics shared by a group of people such as skin color (Leininger and McFarland, 2002; Spector, 2004). Some examples of racial classifications are Asian and Caucasian.

HEALTH DISPARITIES

Health disparities are unequal burdens of disease morbidity and mortality rates experienced by racial and ethnic groups (Baldwin, 2003). Although the overall health of Americans has improved over the past few decades, the health of some minority groups has actually declined (Centers for Disease Control and Prevention [CDC], 2009). Infant mortality is more than twice as high in African American infants compared with white infants. African American women are more than twice more likely to die of cervical cancer than are white women. In addition, African American women are more likely to die of breast cancer than are women of any other racial or ethnic group. In 2000, rates of death from diseases of the heart were 29% higher among African American adults than among white adults and death rates from stroke were 40% higher. American Indians and Alaska Natives were 2.6 times more likely to be diagnosed with diabetes in 2000 than non-Hispanic whites. In 2006, 66% of newly diagnosed acquired immunodeficiency syndrome (AIDS)/human immune deficiency virus (HIV) cases were racial minorities. In addition, 81% of babies born with HIV were from minority mothers (Office of Minority Health and Health Disparities, 2009).

Visiting a regular primary health care provider increases the chances that an individual will receive adequate preventive care and appropriate health care services. Research has shown that 30% of adult Hispanics and 20% of adult African Americans lack a regular primary health care provider, as opposed to 16% of adult white Americans. More alarming is that Hispanic American children are three times as likely as white American children to lack regular access to a health care provider (Agency for Healthcare Research and Quality [AHRQ], 2000). In addition, Hispanics who have diabetes are at a much higher risk for needing an amputation of a foot or leg compared with white Americans (AHRQ, 2008). According to the Office of Minority Health and Health Disparities (2009), minority populations are more likely to have poor health and to die at an earlier age because of a complex interaction between genetic differences, environmental and socioeconomic factors, and specific health behaviors.

TABLE 19-1	Comparative Cultural Worldviews About Health and Illness	
	DOMINANT UNITED STATES	**VARIANT CULTURES**
Illness causation	Biomedical Scientific	Cosmological Supernatural Magicoreligious
Treatment	Organ-specific Specialty-driven	Holistic Mixed (magicoreligious, supernatural, herbal, biomedical, etc.)
Providers/healers	Universal standards of practice Uniform qualifications for practice	May be learned through apprenticeship Criteria for practice not uniform Reputation established in community
Caring pattern	Self-care Self-determination	Caring provided by others Group reliance and interdependence

CULTURAL CONFLICTS

Culture significantly influences patients and health care providers. Because culture influences the way that we think about things, members of a cultural group tend to hold their own way of life as superior to that of others. Culture is also the source of **biases and prejudices** composed of beliefs and attitudes associating negative characteristics with people who are perceived to be different from oneself. When a person acts with prejudice, discrimination occurs. Health care providers who are culturally ignorant about differences often resort to cultural imposition. This happens when health care providers use their own values and customs as their guide in interacting with patients and interpreting their behaviors. Although knowledge about particular cultures is important, it is also important to avoid stereotypes, which result in a tendency to fit every person into a particular pattern without further assessment (Leininger and McFarland, 2002).

CULTURE IN HEALTH AND ILLNESS

Culture is a concept that applies to a group of people whose members share values and ways of thinking and acting that are different from those of people who are outside the group (Srivastava, 2007). Culture provides the framework in which the meaning of illness is defined. Illness is the way that people react to disease, whereas disease is a malfunctioning of biological or psychological processes. People tend to react differently to disease based on their unique cultural perspective (Kleinman, 1980). Understanding the effect culture has on health is evident in the priorities for research funded by the National Institutes of Health and the initiative taken by the U.S. Department of Health and Human Services in eliminating health disparities.

Culture-bound syndromes are illnesses restricted to a particular culture or group of people (Andrews, 2003). They explain the behaviors and reactions of members of the culture. For example, among the Bena people of Tanzania, where communal values are the norm, the condition of *baridi* is attributed to disrespectful behavior within the family or transgression of cultural taboos. The person experiences physical symptoms (feeling cold, fatigue, restlessness, and loss of appetite and weight), psychological symptoms (mental disturbances, sexual disability), and social and economic losses (loss of job, property, partner). Traditional healers detect the illness and treat it by having the ill person make a public admission and an apology, having the person make amends toward the family, or by using herbal remedies (Juntunen, 2005). In the United States, these symptoms might be diagnosed as a depressive disorder (National Institute of Mental Health [NIMH], 2004).

Comparative Worldviews About Health and Illness

A worldview is the framework of beliefs through which a cultural group perceives the world. Note that professional worldviews about health and illness are often different from those of patients. Table 19-1 presents a comparison between distinct worldviews held by the dominant U.S. culture and those of variant groups. Health care providers are educated in the dominant cultural norms of the society in which they practice. Consequently, they have a particular worldview that can be different from that of other subcultures. In any encounter of two cultures, there are two simultaneous perspectives about the situation. There is an insider or native perspective (**emic worldview**) and an outsider's perspective (**etic worldview**).

For example, the Asian Indian belief in karma attributes mental illness to past deeds in one's previous life, which leads them to believe that the individual deserves suffering. This would be considered an emic worldview (from the insider's perspective). Unfortunately, with the cultural stigma attached to the illness, patients generally express their symptoms in physical symptoms and seek help only when the family is no longer able to manage the condition (Conrad and Pacquiao, 2005).

The dominant Anglo American culture in the United States encourages self-care. The focus of care is the individual patient, who is responsible for changing his or her behavior to achieve health and well-being. In contrast, members of some subcultures rely on their family to care for the sick member. Family members will make decisions about care and perform the tasks of caring in these cases.

Folk healers share a group's naturalistic, holistic, and supernatural worldview about causes of illness (Table 19-2). Treatments are more holistic and not focused on one specific organ. The healers use different methods, combining the spiritual, religious, and supernatural with natural means. Heat, massage, acupuncture, and herbs are commonly used. Some folk healers learn their trade through apprenticeship, and some guard their trade with great secrecy such as in Santeria and voodoo.

CULTURALLY COMPETENT CARE

Cultural competence is a process in which the health care provider continually strives to work effectively with individuals, families, and communities (Campinha-Bacote, 2003). Cultural desire is the motivation to develop the following:

- *Cultural awareness:* Gaining in-depth awareness of one's own background, stereotypes, biases, prejudices, and assumptions about other people
- *Cultural knowledge:* Obtaining knowledge of other cultures; gaining sensitivity to, respect for, and appreciation of differences
- *Cultural skills:* Developing cultural skills such as communication, cultural assessment, and culturally competent care
- *Cultural encounters:* Engaging in cross-cultural interactions, refining intercultural communication skills, gaining in-depth understanding of others and avoiding stereotypes, and cultural conflict management

To provide culturally competent health care, it is important to acknowledge and value diversity. Characteristics of cultural competence include the ability to give care to diverse populations, an openness to cultural differences, and flexibility or adaptability to different situations. Outcomes of cultural competence are evident in patients (they are satisfied with their care and they adhere to treatment), health care

TABLE 19-2 Folk Healers

CULTURAL GROUP	HEALER	NATURE OF PRACTICE
Chinese and Southeast Asian	Herbalist	Combination of plant, animal, and mineral products in restoring balance based on yin-yang concepts
	Acupuncturist	Yin treatment using needles to restore balance and flow of *qi;* yang treatment using moxibustion or heat with acupuncture; may be indicated to restore yin-yang balance
	Fortune teller	Consultation to foretell outcomes of plans and seek spiritual advice to enhance good fortune and deal with misfortune
	Shaman	Combination of prayers, chanting, and herbs to treat illnesses caused by supernatural, psychological, and physical factors
Asian Indians	Ayurvedic provider	Combination of dietary, herbal, and other naturalistic therapies to prevent and treat illness
	Homeopath	Use of natural remedies in titrated doses
Native American	Shaman	Combination of prayers, chanting, and herbs to treat illnesses caused by supernatural, psychological, and physical factors
African American	Old lady "granny midwife"	Consultation in diagnosing and treating common illnesses and care of women in childbirth and children
	Spiritualist	Spiritual advisement, counseling, and prayers to treat illness or cope with personal and psychosocial problems
	Voodoo provider *Hougan* (male) *Mambo* (female)	Combination of herbs, drumming, and symbolic offerings to cure illness, remove curses, and protect a person
Hispanic	*Curandero/a*	Combination of prayers, herbs, and other rituals to treat traditional illnesses, especially in children
	Partera Lay midwife	Assistance for women in childbirth and newborn care
	Yerbero Herbalist	Consultation for herbal treatment of traditional illnesses
	Sabador Bonesetter	Massage and manipulation of bones and joints used to treat a variety of ailments, including musculoskeletal conditions
	Espiritista Spiritualist	Foretelling of future and interpretation of dreams; combination of prayers, herbs, potions, amulets, and prayers for curing illnesses, including witchcraft
	Santeria provider	Combination of prayers, symbolic offerings, herbs, potions, and amulets against witchcraft and curses

providers (they feel personal growth and development), and cost-effective quality health care outcomes (Suh, 2004).

Leininger's **Culture Care Theory** emphasizes that the central purpose of nursing is to provide **culturally congruent care.** This is care that fits an individual's personally valued life patterns and meanings, which are sometimes different from the health care provider's perspectives of the person's care. Leininger developed **transcultural nursing** as a distinct discipline to understand cultural similarities (culture universal) and differences (culture-specific) among groups of people. Because of rapid globalization in health care, providing trans-

cultural nursing care has become important. The Transcultural Nursing Society (http://www.tcen.org) is an international nursing organization with a mission to advance culturally congruent care (Webber, 2008). Leininger's Sunrise Model (Figure 19-1) demonstrates how culturally congruent care comes from the cultural and social structure of a particular group of people. This helps health care providers to make decisions and act in ways that are appropriate for a specific group of people. Leininger also describes folk care as a form of caring that is defined by the people. Folk care is different from medical care (Leininger and McFarland, 2002).

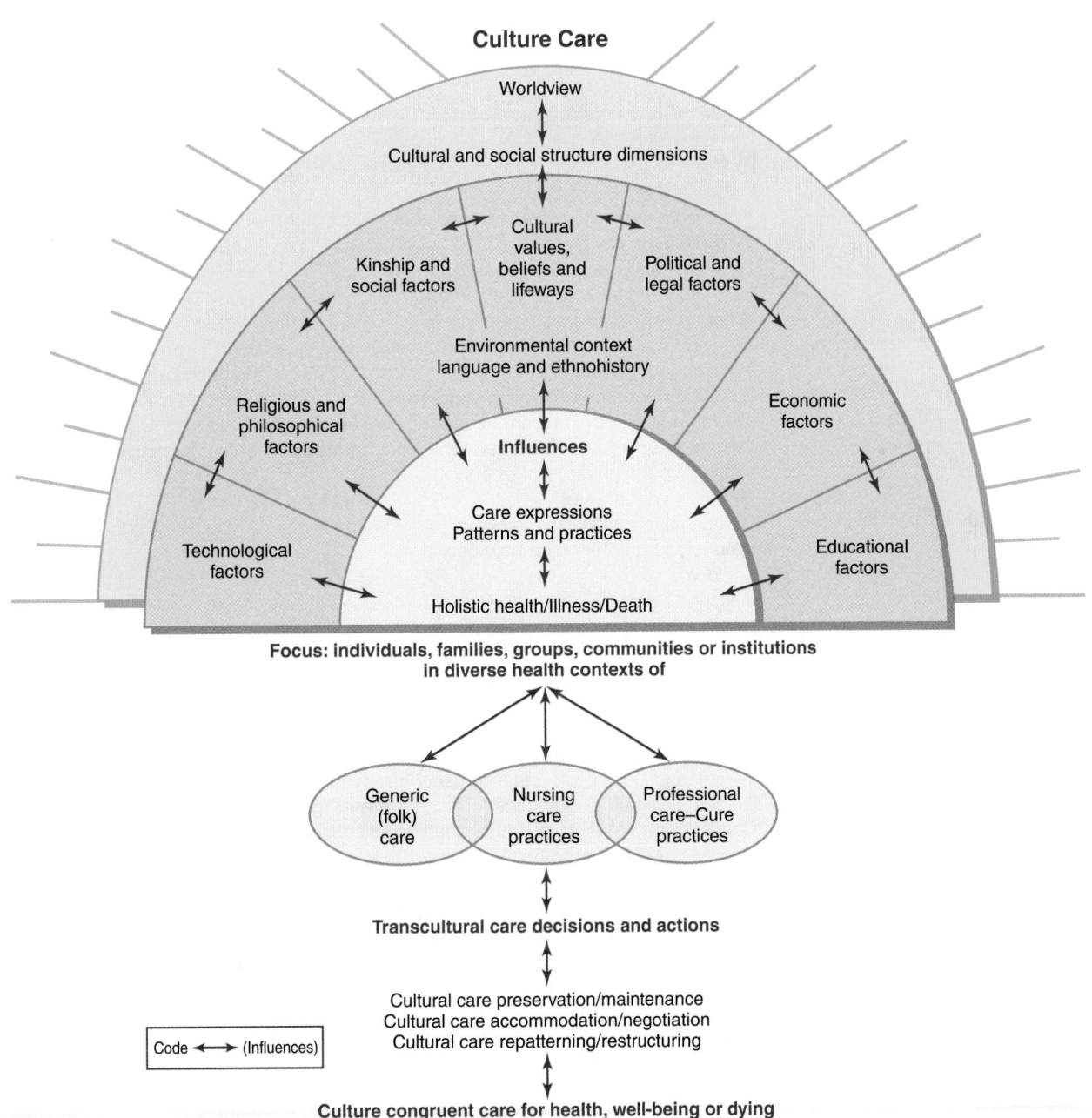

Figure 19-1 ■ Leininger's Culture Care Theory and Sunrise Model. (Reprinted with permission of the McGraw-Hill Companies.)

CULTURAL ASSESSMENT

Cultural assessment (Andrews, 2003) is a systematic and comprehensive examination of the cultural care values, beliefs, and practices of individuals, families, and communities. The goal of cultural assessment is to gather information and understanding from patients that will help the nurse implement culturally congruent care (Leininger and McFarland, 2002). There are several models for cultural assessment, such as Purnell's Model for Cultural Competence (Purnell and Paulanka, 2008), Giger and Davidhizar's Transcultural Assessment Model (2008), Spector's HEALTH Traditions Model (2004), Andrews and Boyle's Assessment Guide (Andrews, 2003), and Leininger's Culture Care Theory and Sunrise Model (see Figure 19-1, p. 539). Using a model helps nurses perform comprehensive cultural assessments by focusing on categories of information that are most relevant to the problems at hand. The models also provide nurses with a guide to understanding how factors influence a culture and making decisions about nursing care. Background knowledge of the culture assists with conducting a focused assessment when time is limited (Table 19-3).

INTERCULTURAL COMMUNICATION

One challenge nurses sometimes face is assessing the insider or emic perspective of patients and using the patient's own context for interpreting the information. Three types of questions can be used: open-ended, structured or focused, and contrast questions (Box 19-1). Encourage patients to

TABLE 19-3   Cultural Assessment Guide

CATEGORIES	QUESTIONS
Cultural identity/ancestry/heritage	What is your (or your parents'/ancestors') place of birth?
	Why did you immigrate?
Ethnohistory	How long have you been in the United States?
	How old were you when you came to the United States?
Social organization	What are your living arrangements?
	Describe your family. How much contact do you have with them?
	What is your position in the family hierarchy? Who makes decisions in your family?
	Describe the different roles in your family. Which role do you play?
	To what extent do you want your family involved in your care?
Socioeconomic status	What was your occupation before you immigrated? What is your occupation now?
	What is your highest level of education?
	Describe your home.
	Do you have medical insurance?
	Who is your primary care provider? What other health care providers and specialists do you see?
Biocultural ecology and health risks	Describe why you are here.
	What do you think caused the problem?
	Do other people in your family or community have similar problems?
	What folk treatments or home remedies have you used?
	What effect has this problem had on you and your family?
	What do you expect me/us to do for you today?
Language and communication	What language do you normally speak at home?
	What language do you prefer to use when writing and reading?
	Do you have any preferences for an interpreter (gender, age, etc.)?
	Do you sometimes have trouble reading or understanding English?
Religion/spirituality	Whom can I contact to help meet your religious/spiritual needs?
	Do you have any religious/spiritual needs?
	What religious rituals do you observe or follow?
	What special dietary practices do you follow?
Caring beliefs and practices	Describe what you do to promote your health.
	How do you take care of yourself/your family during illnesses?
	Describe your normal routines.
	How do age and gender influence your beliefs and practices?
	What are your beliefs and practices in regard to life transitions (e.g., birth, death, marriage)?
Experience with professional health care	Describe your previous experiences with health care providers.
	What characteristics do you value in your caregivers?

describe values, beliefs, and practices that are significant to their care and would be taken for granted unless otherwise uncovered. Culturally oriented questions are broad and require a lot of descriptions. Prepare a set of questions to elicit the patients' descriptions.

Rather than asking a global question such as, "Do you have any cultural practices that we should know about?" ask patients more specific questions about their cultural practices, such as routines regarding mealtimes, praying, bathing, etc. Global questions require a higher level of understanding and expression in English and are especially difficult for patients who are not proficient in English or have a low level of literacy.

Building Relationships

Cultural assessment is essential. To be effective, establish a trusting relationship with the patient and the family. Miscommunication occurs when there are differences in language and communication styles between you and your patients or when you and your patients interpret behaviors differently. Use impression management skills to avoid miscommunication. Impression management is the ability to interpret another person's behavior within the context of that person's culture and behave in a culturally congruent way. In a sense it is managing the impression that you make on the other person to achieve desired outcomes of communication (Pacquiao, 2000). Impression management requires linguistic skills, culturally congruent interpretation of behaviors of others, and listening and observation skills (Box 19-2). If your behavior is offensive, your patients will not be likely to share important information with you. Communicate respect by not rushing your patients, being attentive, demonstrating genuine interest in your patients, and using appropriate group-centered approaches. Avoid making judgmental comments about patients' beliefs and statements.

It is a federal mandate that patients have access to interpreters at no cost. Therefore you need to determine a patient's spoken and written language(s) and need for an interpreter on admission to any health care facility. Working with interpreters, as well as patients who speak little or no English, requires skill development. Participate in educational pro-

---

BOX 19-2 Rules of Impression Management

1 Address the group or individuals who are present with the patient.
2 Introduce your name and identify your role.
3 Ask people who are with the patient to introduce themselves and explain how they are related to the patient.
4 Welcome the group, and thank them for coming to visit.
5 Request to privately talk with the patient, and offer to accompany the group to the waiting room.
6 Inform the group that you will get them when you are done.
7 Tell the patient your purpose.
8 Ask the patient if he or she wants a family member to be present.
9 Avoid asking the patient questions in front of family/spouse.
10 Ask the patient if there is a person who needs to be consulted for major decisions and how to contact this person.
11 Observe nonverbal behavior, and match degree of distance exhibited by the patient.
12 If the patient needs an interpreter:
   • Introduce yourself to the interpreter.
   • Determine qualifications of interpreter.
   • Make sure that the interpreter can speak the dialect of the patient.
   • Make sure that the interpreter is appropriate for the topic that is to be discussed (assess gender, age, and ethnicity).
   • Watch for differences in educational and socioeconomic status between the patient and the interpreter.
   • Orient the interpreter to your purpose and expectation.
   • Make sure that both the patient and interpreter are compatible and that both understand the expectations of the interpreter role.
   • Introduce the interpreter to the patient.
   • Remember the distinct difference between interpretation and translation. Do not expect the interpreter to translate your statements word for word.
   • Pace your speech slowly, and allow time for the patient's response to be interpreted.
   • Direct your questions to the patient.
   • Request the interpreter to ask the patient for feedback and clarification at regular intervals.
   • Observe the patient's nonverbal and verbal behaviors.
   • Thank both patient and interpreter.

BOX 19-1 Examples of Questions Used in Cultural Care Assessment

Mrs. Tao's husband comes in to visit his wife at noon. Jenny decides to ask Mrs. Tao an *open-ended question.* "Please help me understand why you aren't drinking your water." Mr. Tao replies, "My wife needs to avoid cold during the next 30 days to return the balance between yin and yang to her body. She needs the warm energy force of yang right now, so she cannot drink cold water." Jenny then asks a *focused question.* "According to your beliefs, what beverages can you drink?" Mrs. Tao replies that she prefers to drink hot tea right now. Jenny then asks a *contrast question.* "Would you prefer hot herbal tea or is hot decaffeinated tea better for you?" Mrs. Tao replies, "I would like some hot herbal tea, please." Jenny gives Mrs. Tao a cup of herbal tea and conveys Mrs. Tao's preferences to the cafeteria to make sure she continues to receive the appropriate fluids on her meal trays. Mrs. Tao drinks three cups of hot tea in the next hour.

grams, and practice applications of principles of impression management before an intercultural encounter. It is not appropriate for family members to translate health care information, but they can help with ongoing interaction during the patient's care.

Ethnic Heritage and Ethnohistory

Ethnohistory refers to significant historical experiences of a particular group. Knowledge of a patient's country of origin and the country's history is significant to health care. For example, African cultures in the Caribbean colonized by Great Britain speak English, whereas those colonized by France speak French. Colonial influence is also apparent in the family names of those populations.

People immigrate to another country for various reasons and have different motivations for adapting to the new country. **Acculturation** is the process of adapting to and adopting a new culture and results in varying degrees of affiliation with the dominant culture. For instance, refugees sometimes enter another country in desperation or because they have no choice. This group of individuals may not experience acculturation to the degree of other immigrants who enter a country with the option of returning to their homeland. Age of immigrants may also determine the level of acculturation. Younger immigrants usually acculturate faster than older immigrants. Similarities shared by an immigrant group with the dominant culture in the new country are strong predictors that the group will successfully acculturate.

Assimilation results when an individual gives up his or her ethnic identity in favor of the dominant culture (Spector, 2004). Historically, white European immigrants have experienced less difficulty in America and had greater motivation to assimilate than nonwhite immigrants. Although acculturation and length of residence in the new culture are related, other factors such as education, racial characteristics, and familiarity with the language and religion are factors in how individuals assimilate into other cultures.

Biocultural History

Identify patients' health risks related to sociocultural and biological history during admission to a health care facility. Some distinct health risks are related to the ecological context of a culture. For example, Hispanics living in the United States are almost twice as likely to die from diabetes as non-Hispanic whites. African American women have a higher death rate from breast cancer than white women, despite having nearly identical mammography screening rates. The rate of diabetes for Native Americans, Alaska Natives, and Pacific Islanders is more than twice that for whites (National Centers for Chronic Disease and Health Promotion, 2008). Japanese Americans have a greater incidence of cancer of the stomach, colon, rectum, and liver than whites (Giger and Davidhizar, 2008).

Social Organization

In the dominant American society, the most common unit of social organization is the nuclear family, with married or adult children expected to establish separate residences from their parents. In collective cultures, such as Hispanics and Filipinos, the family may include distant blood relatives across three generations and nonblood kin. Kinship is extended bilineally to both the father's and mother's side of the family or may be limited to the side of either father (patrilineal) or mother (matrilineal). Some Chinese and Hindu cultures have patrilineally extended families, in which a woman moves into her husband's family after marriage and minimizes her kinship ties with her parents and siblings.

The status of people within their social hierarchy is sometimes based on age, gender, or achieved status such as education, job or position. The dominant culture in the United States emphasizes achievement as the determinant of status, whereas most collectivistic cultures give higher priority to age and gender. The eldest male is next to his father in terms of authority in many Arabic and African cultures.

Cultures based on age and gender define the roles of their members. Certain behaviors are acceptable in children, but not tolerated among adults. For example, in Muslim families, females perform the family caretaking tasks, whereas men make the major decisions about the care of family members. Make sure to determine the family social hierarchy as soon as possible to prevent offending patients and their families.

Religious and Spiritual Beliefs

Religious and spiritual beliefs are major influences in the patient's worldview about health and illness, pain and suffering, and life and death. Unlike the United States, the distinction between religion and spirituality can be blurred in other cultures. It is advisable to understand the emic perspective of the patient. Many cultures do not separate religion and spirituality, whereas other cultures have a totally distinct concept between the two (see Chapter 20).

Many patients expect to continue their religious rituals in the hospital. For example, Mormons who have gone through the sacraments and are deemed worthy wear a white undergarment at all times except when taking a bath or shower. Devout Muslims pray five times daily and must clean some parts of their body before praying. During Sabbath (sundown Friday to sundown Saturday) Orthodox Jewish patients do not use electrical appliances. This calls for creative accommodations by the nursing staff. For instance, articles of care need to be placed near the patient so he or she does not need to use the call light or telephone to get assistance. Battery-operated candles may also need to be provided for use during Sabbath.

Religious beliefs often influence a patient's dietary practices. For example, devout Muslims eat *halal*, or foods prepared in a way that is permissible for Muslims to eat. These foods include meat, fish, fresh fruit, vegetables, eggs, milk, and cheese. *Halal* meat comes from animals that have been slaughtered during a prayer ritual. *Haram*, or prohibited foods, include non-*halal* meat, animals with fangs, pork products, gelatin products, and alcohol (Akhtar, 2002). During the 28 days of Ramadan, observed during the ninth lunar month, Muslims fast during the daylight hours. Although children and sick individuals are exempt from fasting, do not assume that these individuals will eat regular meals during Ramadan. Sometimes treatments and medications will need to be rescheduled to prevent complications such as hypoglycemia. Observant Mormons avoid drugs, alcohol, and beverages containing stimulants such as coffee and cola. Some people of the Jewish faith follow strict kosher dietary guidelines that dictate the manner in which acceptable food is prepared and consumed. In addition, they may experience cultural pain if visitor limitations prohibit them from praying in groups at the bedside of a dying patient. Maintain open communication with families and their religious/spiritual leaders to facilitate culturally congruent care (Pacquiao, 2003).

Communication Patterns

Different cultural groups have distinct linguistic and communication patterns that reflect the core cultural values of the society. The dominant American culture values assertive and direct communication. This communication pattern reflects the ideal of individual autonomy and self-determination. The individual is expected to say what he or she means and mean what he or she says. Promoting group harmony is a priority in collectivistic cultures, so participants interact based on their positions and relationships within the social structure. Differences in status and position, age, gender, and outsider versus insider determine the content and process of communication.

In many cultures, conflict is seen as embarrassing or demeaning. Face-saving communication promotes harmony by indirect communication and avoiding conflict. This communication pattern is associated with East Asian, African, and Hispanic cultures. An example of an indirect communication style that a nurse uses when providing health teaching is, "A person who is experiencing symptoms such as yours should . . . ." Observing a patient's behavior and clarifying messages heard from a trusted insider prevents misinterpretation (Srivastava, 2007).

In cultural groups with distinct linear hierarchy, negotiation of conflict occurs between persons within the same level of position or authority. Identifying and working with established family hierarchy prevents miscommunication. In cultures with highly differentiated gender roles, some patients place more value on the advice of a male than a female. By recognizing and working within this cultural context, the male nurse becomes more effective in achieving positive outcomes.

Culture also shapes nonverbal communication. Examples of nonverbal communication include the amount of personal space that is comfortable, the degree of eye contact, the extent of touching, and how much private information is shared with others. Individuals commonly use less distance when speaking to trusted insiders and persons of the same age, gender, and position in the social hierarchy. Many ethnic groups tend to speak their own dialect with insiders for ease and privacy and as a marker of insider status. To effectively communicate with patients, establish rapport and behave in a culturally congruent manner.

Time Orientation

It is important to be aware of and appreciate cultural differences regarding perceptions of time. Some cultures, such as the dominant Anglo American culture, are future time oriented. For instance, people have schedules for both work and leisure. Time orientation is reflected in communication patterns, which tend to be direct and focused on task achievement. When working with patients who are future oriented, it is important to plan patient teaching in relation to the future and also to adhere to a schedule (Srivastava, 2007).

In contrast, some cultures emphasize present time to preserve social standing and promote group harmony. Time is perceived as flexible, and events begin when they arrive. Within these cultures it is acceptable to be 30 minutes to an hour late. Communication is sometimes indirect to avoid offending and disrespecting others. Patients may perceive rushed, hurried, and businesslike communication as uncaring or disrespectful. Patients from these subcultures tend to trust caregivers who interact with them in a personal, warm, friendly, and respectful manner (Zoucha, 1998).

Present time orientation often causes challenges in health care settings that emphasize punctuality and adherence to appointments. Expect conflicts, and make adjustments when dealing with ethnic groups who value present time orientation. When making appointments and referrals, explore anticipated barriers to time adherence and manage them with the patient. Some of the groups who value present time orientation include African Americans, Puerto Ricans, Mexicans, Chinese, and American Indians (Giger and Davidhizer, 2008).

Caring Beliefs and Practices

Care meanings, values, and beliefs are expressed in practices associated with life transitions. Determine how patients and their families define meaningful and supportive caring. Caring expressions are part of the central values of a culture. In some cultures, caring means active involvement of the group, emphasizing the need for members to care for each other. This caring norm is different from the individualism and self-care values of the dominant Anglo American culture. Determine your patient's definition of caring, and use it when working with patients and their families, especially when providing patient education (Box 19-3).

CULTURAL PRACTICES DURING LIFE TRANSITIONS

Rituals that symbolize cultural values and meanings generally mark life transitions. Religious and spiritual beliefs are often integrated in these rituals. Examining the practices surrounding these life transitions provides a glimpse of the cultural meanings and expressions that are important.

Pregnancy Most cultures associate pregnancy with caring practices symbolic of its significance as a life transition in women. Some Asian, African, and Hispanic cultures believe that a mother's activities also affect the fetus. These cultures often believe that if a pregnant woman's food craving is not met, negative consequences to the baby will occur.

Some cultures believe in the hot and cold theory of illness. For example, many Hindus view pregnancy as a hot state, so

BOX 19-3   PATIENT TEACHING

Nutritional Education Following Pregnancy

 After doing some reading about the Chinese culture, Jenny finds out the yin-yang (hot-cold) theory is important and influences what a patient eats and drinks, especially during pregnancy, following delivery, and in times of illness. Jenny uses cultural care concepts to provide education about breast-feeding to Mrs. Tao.

OUTCOME
- At the end of the teaching session, Mrs. Tao will verbalize dietary measures and fluid needs used to promote lactation.

TEACHING STRATEGIES
- Provide an interpreter or patient education information written in Chinese if needed.
- Assess Mrs. Tao's dietary and fluid preferences.
- Assess the meanings of foods and fluids within Mrs. Tao's cultural context.
- Explain that a breast-feeding mother requires more fluids than normal to produce milk.
- Provide brochures that describe information about breast-feeding, including information regarding sufficient fluid intake.

EVALUATION STRATEGIES
- Monitor fluid intake over the remainder of Mrs. Tao's hospitalization.
- Assess hydration and nutritional status of Mrs. Tao's daughter (e.g., weight, sunken fontanels, moistness of mucous membranes).
- Ask Mrs. Tao to list at least three fluids she will drink to promote lactation.

they encourage a pregnant woman to eat "cold" foods such as milk and milk products, yogurt, sour foods, and vegetables. They believe "hot" foods such as chilies, ginger, and animal products cause miscarriage and fetal abnormality. Although many cultures share the hot and cold theory, there is no agreement on what foods and beverages are classified as hot or cold. These classifications are specific to each culture.

Modesty is a strong value among most Arab women (Kulwicki, 2008). Many Arab women avoid prenatal visits because of embarrassment, and sometimes they demand to be examined by a female provider. Religious beliefs sometimes interfere with prenatal testing, as in the case of a Filipino couple that refuses amniocentesis because they believe that the outcome of pregnancy is God's will. Supernatural beliefs associated with pregnancy are evident among some Hispanics who believe that baby showers early in pregnancy will bring bad luck (Spector, 2004). Orthodox Jews often avoid baby showers and do not announce the baby's name before the naming ceremony for the same reason.

Childbirth Expressing pain and treating suffering vary across different cultures. Some Puerto Rican and Mexican women are verbally expressive of their pain during labor. *Parteras,* or lay midwives, commonly advise a screaming woman in labor to close her mouth because an open mouth will cause the uterus to rise (Juarbe, 2008). Middle Eastern mothers may verbally express their labor pain by crying and screaming aloud. They often refuse pain medication.

Fear of drug addiction and belief that pain is a form of spiritual atonement for one's past deeds motivate many Filipino mothers to tolerate pain without much complaining or requests for medication (Pacquiao, 2001). Southeast Asian women frequently believe that crying and screaming are shameful and expect to endure labor pains.

Some religious beliefs prohibit the presence of males, including husbands, from the delivery room. This is common among devout Muslims, Hindus, and Orthodox Jews. Husbands generally leave the room with the appearance of the bloody show. As soon as the child is born, a Muslim father or mother whispers the Islamic call to prayer in the newborn's ear, welcoming the baby into the life of the world where they feel the responsibility to Allah's call is the greatest (Emerick, 2002).

Health care providers other than physicians attend childbirth in some cultural groups, such as *parteras* among Mexicans, "granny midwives" among Appalachian and southern African Americans, and *hilots* among Filipinos (Pacquiao, 2008). Known in their communities, these providers are affordable and accessible in remote areas. They use a combination of naturalistic, religious, and supernatural methods combining herbs, massage, and prayers.

Newborn The age of the newborn varies in some cultures. Among traditional Vietnamese and Koreans, a newborn is a year old at birth. Once acculturated to Western culture, they often assume a bicultural view and deduct 1 year from the age of the child when speaking to outsiders.

The name of the child often reflects the cultural values of the group. It is typical for a Hispanic baby to have several first names followed by the surnames of the father and mother (e.g., Maria Kristina Lourdes Lopez Vega). Some bilineal tracing of descent from both the mother's and father's side in the Hispanic group is different from the patrilineal system, in which the last name of the father precedes the child's first name. In the Chinese culture, descent is traced only from the paternal side. Hence the name Chen Lu means that Lu is the daughter of Mr. Chen.

In many countries (e.g., in the Middle East, South and Central America), the evil eye is believed to cause illness, injury, or bad luck to a person. These societies often consider newborns and young children vulnerable and use a variety of ways to prevent the evil eye, using amulets, religious medals, herbs, or spices. For example, some Catholic Filipinos keep newborns inside the home until after the baptism to ensure the baby's health and protection. The practice of using a cotton binder or *fajita* on the baby's abdomen to prevent gas and umbilical hernia is also evident among some Filipinos and Hispanic groups (Pacquiao, 2008). Filipinos sometimes rub warm oil on the baby's belly to prevent and relieve gas. Some traditional Iranians believe babies are vulnerable to cold and wind; hence they are not bathed for a number of days. They remain indoors with their mothers for a period of 30 to 40 days following their birth (Hafizi and Lipson, 2008).

Some cultures do not regard the colostrum (initial cloudy breast secretion following delivery) as healthy for the baby. Some Hindus and Muslims believe the colostrum is dirty and not fit for a newborn, so they postpone breast-feeding until regular milk appears. In this case, use alternative measures to promote lactation (Jambunathan, 2008).

Postpartum Period In many non-Western cultures, people associate postpartum with the mother's vulnerability to cold. To restore balance, mothers sometimes refuse to shower and prefer a sponge bath. Cultural groups have preferences in terms of what types of foods are appropriate to restore balance in women after birth. Some Chinese mothers prefer soups, eggs, and tea, whereas rural Iranian women may prefer pistachio nuts and eggs (Hafizi and Lipson, 2008; Wang, 2008). The length of the postpartum period is generally much longer (30 to 40 days) in non-Western cultures to provide attention and support for the mother and her baby. This is one of the reasons given for the rarity of postpartum depression in these cultures compared with the United States. Some Hispanic women go into a 40-day period of *la cuarentena,* when they follow a special diet and restrict physical activity. This cultural belief that the mother needs much rest and relaxation after delivery conflicts with the Western belief in early ambulation.

Some Filipinos, Mexicans, and Pacific Islanders use an abdominal binder to prevent air from entering the woman's uterus and to promote healing (Pacquiao, 2008; Zoucha and Purnell, 2008). Orthodox Jewish, Islamic, and Hindu cultures may associate postpartum bleeding with pollution. In these cultures a woman will often go into a ritual bath after the bleeding stops before she is able to resume sexual relations with her husband (Hafizi and Lipson, 2008; Selekman, 2008). In some African cultures in Ghana and Sierra Leone, women will not resume sexual relations with their husbands until after weaning the baby.

Grief and Loss

Dying and death bring a reappearance of cultural traditions that have been meaningful to groups of people most of their lives (see Chapter 25). Cultures assign different meanings to the death of a child, a young person, or an older adult. In Western cultures with strong future time orientation such as the dominant Anglo American culture, a child is expected to survive his or her parent. The death of a young person is devastating. However, in cultures in which infant mortality is high, such as Haiti and some countries in Africa, the reality that many children do not live to adulthood sometimes lessens the emotional distress over a child's death. These cultures often mourn the untimely death of an adult more deeply.

Societies such as devout Hindus and Buddhists believe in the concept of reincarnation and view death as a step toward rebirth. Care of the dying focuses on supporting the patient's preparation for a good death. The family prays and reads religious scriptures to the patient to improve his or her chances in the next cycle of life.

Advance directives, informed consent, and consent for hospice are examples of mandates that may violate some cultural values. Informed consent and advance directives (see Chapter 4) protect the right of the individual to know and make decisions ensuring continuity of these rights even when the individual is unable to act on his or her own behalf. However, in some cultures such as Korean Americans or Mexican Americans, the group or family assumes decision making and is trusted to make the right decision for the dying individual. These cultures value group interdependence and view individual autonomy as an unnecessary burden for a loved one who is ill (Giger and Davidhizar, 2008).

In the case of cultures that share the religious belief that events in their life are God's will, predicting the outcome of a disease is not an acceptable human practice. Hence devout Muslims sometimes object to a diagnosis of terminal illness or cancer. This belief may hinder their willingness to get into hospice programs unless organizational policies are flexibly applied to accommodate their cultural values and beliefs (Pacquiao, 2002, 2003).

Cultural Rituals Associated With Dying and Death

Many Orthodox Jews tend to rally behind members of their congregation and provide care for the dying, as well as assistance to the family. They generally come in groups of about 10 and pray together with the patient and the family at the bedside. After the patient dies, Orthodox Jews and Muslims call a special group who are knowledgeable in religious rituals to perform postmortem care. They strictly observe same-gender care and provision of privacy as a show of respect for the dead person. Because they generally schedule an immediate burial, it is important to plan preparations with the family before the patient dies. Orthodox Jews generally bury the dead before sundown (Bonura and others, 2001). Some Buddhists refuse to move the dead body after death because of their belief that the spirit of the dead takes some time to leave the body. They define death as the absence of consciousness and loss of body warmth, and they do not agree with using brain death as a criterion of death.

Religious beliefs also affect attitudes toward cremation or organ donation. Devout Muslims sometimes refuse an autopsy for fear of desecrating the dead and because of their belief that one has to be whole to appear in front of the creator. They prefer burial to cremation.

Experience With Professional Health Care

Understanding the patient's emic perspective of professional care is valuable in preventing misconceptions and culturally offensive actions. Previous encounters with health care providers affect patients' decisions to seek health care. For example, southern African Americans generally prefer their family members to make end-of-life decisions for them. Their reluctance to execute advance directives may come from a mistrust of the health care system, past experience with racism, or discrimination by the white majority. There are a large number of African Americans who may even regard an advance directive as a way to legitimize neglect or as a way to commit genocide of their race (Dupree, 2000; Giger and Davidhizar, 2008). To gain information about advance directives, there needs to be a trusting relationship between providers and patients.

CULTURALLY COMPETENT CARE

After completing the cultural care assessment, use evidence-based information to plan culturally competent care (Box 19-4). Also, identify potential conflicts between patients' health care needs and their values and practices. To do this, identify similarities and differences between the way care is normally delivered and the patient's cultural practices. Leininger and McFarland (2002) identified three nursing decision and action modes to achieve culturally congruent care. Use any or all of these action modes simultaneously. These actions require knowledge of the patient's culture and the willingness, commitment, and skills to work with patients and their families in decision making.

- *Cultural care preservation or maintenance:* Retain and/or preserve relevant care values so that patients are able to maintain their well-being, recover from illness, or face handicaps and/or death.
- *Cultural care accommodation or negotiation:* Adapt or negotiate with the patient/family to achieve beneficial or satisfying health outcomes.
- *Cultural care repatterning or restructuring:* Reorder, change, or greatly modify patient's/family's customs for new, different, and beneficial health care pattern.

In the following scenario a nurse uses the action modes with a male Pakistani patient admitted for terminal pancreatic cancer. On admission the patient denies presence of pain. His main complaint is the inability to sleep. He admits to having "discomfort that goes away only when I am sleeping." Knowing that the patient is a South Asian male Muslim who appears to be controlling his emotions, the nurse understands the patient's behavior is consistent with the behavioral norms of his culture. Stoicism is a valued trait and demonstrates a male's inner strength. Because of this cultural knowledge, the nurse interprets the patient's behavior in a culturally congruent manner.

BOX 19-4 BEST PRACTICES

Promoting Culturally Appropriate Nursing Interventions

SUMMARY OF EVIDENCE

Culturally diverse populations often require different approaches from those used for the dominant culture in order to improve patient care outcomes. It is crucial to use evidence-based practice to customize nursing interventions so that they are appropriate for the population for which they are intended. Research studies have shown that when interventions are implemented in a way that is culturally appropriate, patients are more likely to have more positive outcomes. The health status of minority populations improves when culturally competent and culturally sensitive interventions are used. For example, one study found that African American smokers who went to a smoking cessation program that took their culture into consideration were more successful in their plans to stop smoking.

APPLICATION TO NURSING PRACTICE
- Develop nursing interventions that take the cultural norms of the patient into consideration.
- Be flexible in your approach to providing care.
- Have a self-awareness of your own cultural values.
- Use a collaborative approach with patients in order to be aware of cultural issues that may impact care.

REFERENCE
Giger J, Davidhizar R: Promoting culturally appropriate interventions among vulnerable populations, *Annu Rev Nurs Res* 25:293, 2007.

The nurse selects the nursing diagnosis: *disturbed sleep pattern related to discomfort* and decides on the following plan of action: obtain an order for pain medication as an aid to promote sleep, institute environmental controls to minimize disruption. The nurse communicates the plan to the other members of the team. This is an example of repatterning the health care team's thinking regarding the use of pain medication to promote sleep. The nurse accommodates the patient's interpretation of his problem and does not try to convince him that his pain causes his difficulty sleeping. The nurse's decision is culturally congruent with the patient's life patterns and demonstrates the nurse's cultural competence.

KEY POINTS

- Nurses need to provide culturally competent and congruent care.
- Even when there is access to health services, racial and ethnic differences contribute to health care disparities.
- Health care providers often misinterpret the impact of culture on health.
- When providers disregard a patient's valued way of life, the patient experiences cultural pain.
- Collectivistic cultures rely on family to care for sick members.
- Attributes or characteristics of cultural competence are the ability to give care to diverse populations, openness to cultural differences, and flexibility or adaptability to different situations.
- The goal of cultural assessment is to gather significant information from patients that will help the nurse implement culturally congruent care.
- Hospitals are required to provide a trained interpreter to communicate information about medical conditions to patients.
- Life transitions are generally marked by rituals that symbolize cultural values and meanings attached to these transitions.
- Strong cultural traditions typically surround the process of dying and death.

CRITICAL THINKING EXERCISES

Upon Mrs. Tao's discharge from the hospital, Jenny has discovered that the Chinese American population in her community has been growing. Jenny learns that a local church has sponsored many of the new Chinese immigrants who speak very little English. Based on her experience with the Tao family, Jenny understands that there is an opportunity for the health care providers in her community to acquire cultural knowledge so that they can provide culturally congruent care for this population. Jenny knows that by becoming more aware of the beliefs within the Chinese American culture in her community, she will feel more confident in providing nursing care.

1. List strategies for Jenny to use when performing a cultural assessment on a patient from a different culture.
2. Based on a cultural assessment of Mrs. Tao, Jenny discovers that the Chinese believe in the yin-yang theory. Describe how this influences the dietary preferences of a Chinese American patient.

3. In order for Jenny to develop cultural awareness, she first needs to examine which of the following?
   a. The geography of China
   b. Her own cultural background
   c. The percentage of minority populations in her community
   d. Community resources available for indigent patients
4. Before Jenny's realization of her own cultural ignorance, she used her own values and customs to care for Mrs. Tao. This behavior is known as:
   a. Cultural imposition
   b. Cultural repatterning
   c. Cultural competence
   d. Cultural awareness

ⓔvolve   *Answers to Critical Thinking Questions can be found on the Evolve website.*

REVIEW QUESTIONS

1. An older adult Filipino patient asked his wife to ask the nurse manager not to have the same nurse assigned to him. He refused to give any explanation to the nurse manager. His communication pattern demonstrates:
   1. Assertive communication
   2. Face-saving communication
   3. Direct communication
   4. Biased communication
2. An Arab female patient who is pregnant refuses to have an abdominal examination done by a male care provider despite attempts to drape her. After several attempts, explaining the reason for the procedure, the care provider finally stepped out of the room. The behavior of the care provider is an example of:
   1. Cultural imposition
   2. Stereotypes
   3. Cultural accommodation
   4. Ethnocentrism
3. The behavior of the patient in the previous situation is congruent with the Arabian cultural value of:
   1. Female modesty
   2. Short distance between unrelated males and females
   3. Female subservience to males
   4. Supernatural beliefs associated with pregnancy
4. The nurse enters the room to find her postpartum patient, a Filipino woman, rubbing warm oil on her baby's belly. The mother explains the purpose is to prevent and relieve gas. The mother believes that this practice will:
   1. Prevent the evil eye from affecting the newborn
   2. Prevent the baby from getting an infection
   3. Ensure the baby's protection from disease
   4. Reinforce her religious beliefs

5. A Mexican woman's refusal to walk frequently during her postpartum stay in the hospital is a manifestation of:
   1. Poor health habits
   2. Belief in hot and cold theory of illness
   3. Fear of bleeding
   4. a 40-day period *la cuarantena*
6. One potential challenge when working with patients from present time–oriented cultures is:
   1. Ensuring patients do not miss scheduled appointments
   2. Providing discharge teaching
   3. Performing hospital admission process
   4. Complying with a therapy regimen
7. Mrs. de la Cruz, an older adult Cuban matriarch, is hospitalized with heart failure. The nurses are concerned that the numerous visitors who stay at her bedside from early morning until late evening are exhausting her. She denies being exhausted by her visitors. The constant presence of extended family members at the bedside of Mrs. de la Cruz is a manifestation of the Cuban cultural value of:
   1. Having close ties among extended kin
   2. Caring by others through presence and attention to the ill member
   3. Extending of kinship ties to both the father's and mother's side of the family
   4. Maintaining present time orientation

8. Cultural accommodation of the de la Cruz family is best done by:
    1. Collaborating with the family decision maker to schedule turns of limited number of visitors at her bedside
    2. Explaining repeatedly the visiting policy to Mrs. de la Cruz's visitors
    3. Instructing the information desk not to allow all visitors to go up at the same time
    4. Requesting an early discharge for Mrs. de la Cruz
9. In some cultures, such as Asian, Hispanic, and African, food cravings of the pregnant woman are satisfied because:
    1. The mother will be in danger of malnutrition
    2. It strengthens bonds between husband and wife
    3. It will result in twin births
    4. A mother's stressful condition creates stress in her baby
10. The devout Muslim husband of a 46-year-old woman who is in end-stage renal disease becomes angry when the female nurse suggests discussing hospice with the health care provider. This is most likely because many Muslims:
    1. Want their loved ones to die at home
    2. Do not believe in hospice
    3. Do not believe in predicting the outcome of a disease
    4. Do not want to discuss personal family matters with a person of the opposite gender

Answers to Review Questions can be found on pages 1197-1198.

REFERENCES

Agency for Healthcare Research and Quality: *Addressing racial and ethnic disparities in health care fact sheet*, Publication No. 00-PO41, 2000, http://www.ahrq.gov/research/disparit.htm.

Agency for Healthcare Research and Quality News and Numbers: *Diabetes-related amputations increase for Hispanics*, 2008, http://www.ahrq.gov/news/nn/nn032108.htm.

Akhtar S: Nursing with dignity. VIII. Islam, *Nurs Times* 98(16):40, 2002.

Andrews M: Cultural competence in the health history and physical examination. In Andrews M, Boyle J: *Transcultural concepts in nursing care,* ed 4, Philadelphia, 2003, Lippincott Williams & Wilkins.

Baldwin DM: Disparities in health and health care: focusing efforts to eliminate unequal burdens, *Online J Issues Nurs* 8(1):2, 2003.

Bonura D and others: Culturally-congruent end-of-life care for Jewish patients and their families, *J Transcult Nurs* 12(3):211, 2001.

Campinha-Bacote J: *The process of cultural competence in the delivery of healthcare services: a culturally competent model of care*, ed 4, Cincinnati, 2003, Transcultural C.A.R.E. Associates.

Centers for Disease Control and Prevention, Office of Minority Health and Health Disparities: *About minority health*, 2009, http://www.cdc.gov/omhd/AMH/AMH.htm.

Conrad M, Pacquiao DF: Manifestation, attribution and coping with depression among Asian Indians from the perspective of healthcare providers, *J Transcult Nurs* 16(1):23, 2005.

Dupree CY: The attitudes of black Americans toward advance directives, *J Transcult Nurs* 11(1):12, 2000.

Emerick Y: *The complete idiot's guide to understanding Islam*, Indianapolis, 2002, Pearson Education, Inc.

Giger J, Davidhizar R: Promoting culturally appropriate interventions among vulnerable populations, *Annu Rev Nurs Res* 25:293, 2007.

Giger J, Davidhizar R: *Transcultural nursing: assessment and intervention*, ed 5, St. Louis, 2008, Mosby.

Hafizi H, Lipson J: People of Iranian heritage. In Purnell LD, Paulanka BJ: *Transcultural health care: a culturally competent approach*, ed 3, Philadelphia, 2008, FA Davis.

Jambunathan J: People of Hindu heritage. Chapter on CD-ROM. In Purnell LD, Paulanka BJ: *Transcultural health care: a culturally competent approach*, ed 3, Philadelphia, 2008, FA Davis.

Juarbe J: People of Puerto Rican heritage. In Purnell LD, Paulanka BJ: *Transcultural health care: a culturally competent approach*, ed 3, Philadelphia, 2008, FA Davis.

Juntunen A: Baridi: a culture-bound syndrome among the Bena peoples in Tanzania, *J Transcult Nurs* 16(1):15, 2005.

Kleinman A: *Patients and healers in the context of culture*, Berkeley, 1980, University of California Press.

Kulwicki AD: People of Arab heritage. In Purnell LD, Paulanka BJ: *Transcultural health care: a culturally competent approach*, ed 3, Philadelphia, 2008, FA Davis.

Leininger MM, McFarland M: *Transcultural nursing concepts, theories, research and practice*, ed 3, New York, 2002, McGraw-Hill.

National Centers for Chronic Disease and Health Promotion: Racial and Ethnic Approaches to Community Health (REACH U.S.) finding solutions to health disparities, 2008, http://www.cdc.gov/nccdphp/publications/aag/reach.htm.

National Institute of Mental Health: *Depression: a treatable illness (fact sheet)*, NIH Publication No. 03-5299, Bethesda, Md, 2004, National Institute of Mental Health.

Office of Minority Health and Health Disparities: *HIV/AIDS data/statistics*, 2009, http://www.omhrc.gov/templates/browse.aspx?lvl=3&lvlid=70.

Pacquiao DF: Impression management: an alternative to assertiveness in intercultural communication, *J Transcult Nurs* 11(1):5, 2000.

Pacquiao DF: Cultural incongruities of advance directives, *Bioethics Forum* 17(1):27, 2001.

Pacquiao DF: Ethics and cultural diversity: a framework for decision-making, *Bioethics Forum* 17(3-4):12, 2002.

Pacquiao DF: Cultural competence in ethical-decision-making. In Andrews M, Boyle J: *Transcultural concepts in nursing care*, ed 4, Philadelphia, 2003, Lippincott Williams & Wilkins.

Pacquiao DF: People of Filipino heritage. In Purnell LD, Paulanka BJ: *Transcultural health care: a culturally competent approach*, ed 3, Philadelphia, 2008, FA Davis.

Purnell LD, Paulanka BJ: The Purnell model for cultural competence. In Purnell LD, Paulanka BJ: *Transcultural health care: a culturally competent approach*, ed 3, Philadelphia, 2008, FA Davis.

Selekman J: People of Jewish heritage. In Purnell LD, Paulanka BJ: *Transcultural health care: a culturally competent approach*, ed 3, Philadelphia, 2008, FA Davis.

Spector R: *Cultural diversity in health and illness*, ed 6, Upper Saddle River, NJ, 2004, Prentice Hall.

Srivastava, RH: *The healthcare professional's guide to clinical competence*, Toronto, 2007, Elsevier.

Suh EE: The model for cultural competence through an evolutionary concept analysis, *J Transcult Nurs* 15(2):93, 2004.

U.S. Bureau of the Census: *National and state population estimates*, 2009, http://www.census.gov/popest/states/NST-ann-est.html.

Wang Y: People of Chinese heritage. In Purnell LD, Paulanka BJ: *Transcultural health care: a culturally competent approach*, ed 3, Philadelphia, 2008, FA Davis.

Webber PB: Yes, Virginia, nursing does have laws, *Nurs Sci Q* 21(1):68, 2008.

Zoucha R: The experience of Mexican Americans receiving professional nursing care: an ethnonursing study, *J Transcult Nurs* 9(3):34, 1998.

Zoucha R, Purnell LD: People of Mexican heritage. In Purnell LD, Paulanka BJ: *Transcultural health care: a culturally competent approach*, ed 3, Philadelphia, 2008, FA Davis.

Spiritual Health

20

MEDIA RESOURCES

 CD COMPANION   **evolve WEBSITE**   http://evolve.elsevier.com/Potter/basic

- Crossword Puzzle
- English/Spanish Audio Glossary

OBJECTIVES

- Describe the relationship between faith, hope, and spiritual well-being.
- Compare and contrast the concepts of religion and spirituality.
- Discuss the relationship of spirituality to an individual's total being.
- Assess a patient's spirituality and spiritual health.
- Discuss nursing interventions designed to promote spiritual health.
- Establish presence with your patients.
- Evaluate how patients attain spiritual health.

KEY TERMS

agnostic, p. 552
atheist, p. 552
connectedness, p. 558

faith, p. 551
holistic, p. 550
hope, p. 553

self-transcendence, p. 551
spiritual distress, p. 553

spiritual well-being, p. 552
spirituality, p. 550

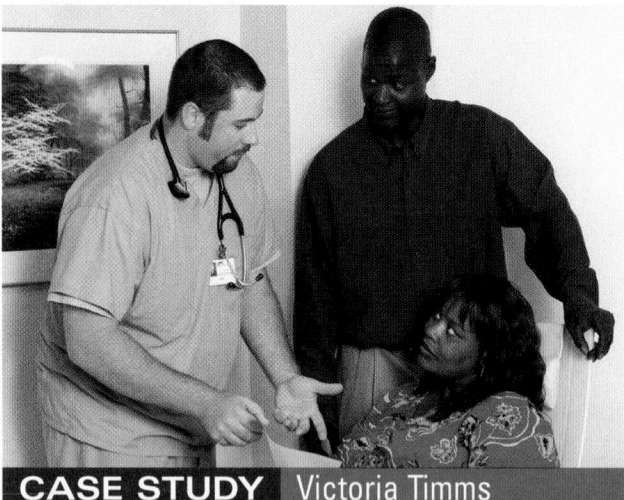

CASE STUDY Victoria Timms

Victoria Timms is a 48-year-old African American college professor, diagnosed 3 months ago with breast cancer. She is married to Joe, an insurance salesman, and is the mother of two children: Valerie, who is 16 years old, and Peter, who is 12. Victoria describes her family as being very close and supportive. Surgeons removed Victoria's cancerous tumor and two involved lymph nodes. Because of the lymphatic involvement, Victoria is at increased risk for the cancer to spread. Victoria has completed a course of radiation and now visits the local cancer clinic with her husband 3 times a week for chemotherapy treatments. Both Victoria and Joe discuss their concern for their children. Valerie and Peter attend Sunday school weekly after going to church with their parents. Their Sunday school teacher informed Victoria and Joe that Valerie and Peter are very angry about their mother's illness.

Jeff is a 36-year-old, married student nurse assigned to the oncology clinic. One of the clinic case managers, who is Jeff's preceptor, assigns Jeff to follow Victoria during her clinic visits. Jeff is in his last semester at school and hopes to get a position in the clinic after graduation. Victoria's experience is significant for Jeff because he has children who are the same age as Victoria's, and he wonders how his children would react if his spouse became ill.

During one of their clinic visits, Victoria and Joe appear very calm and relaxed when discussing cancer therapy. Joe explains, "We both have a lot of faith in God." Victoria responds, "Even though I know I have cancer, I hope to be able to continue to go to church with my family and my children. My family is very supportive, and together I know we will make it through this experience. But I am worried about my children. With God's help, I can help them cope with my illness better."

The word *spirituality* comes from the Latin word *spiritus,* which refers to breath or wind. The spirit gives life to a person. It signifies whatever is at the center of all aspects of a person's life (Nelson-Becker, Nakashima, and Canda, 2007). **Spirituality** is an awareness of one's inner self and a sense of connection to a higher being, nature, or to some purpose greater than oneself (Hermann, 2007). A person's health depends on a balance of physical, psychological, sociological, cultural, emotional, developmental, and spiritual variables. This **holistic** view of health is the focus and heart of nursing practice. Spiritual care is often an overlooked part of nursing; however, the spiritual dimension does not exist in isolation from our physical and psychological being (Hermann, 2007). Spirituality is an important factor that helps people achieve the balance needed to maintain health and well-being and to cope with illness. Research focused on patients with chronic illness and survivors of abuse has shown that spirituality reduces a person's distress and even enhances personal growth and empowerment (Chang, Wallis, and Tiralongo, 2007; Leak, Hu, and King, 2008; MacMaster and others, 2007).

Too often, nurses and other health care providers fail to recognize the spiritual dimension of human nature. In addition, there are health care providers who do not believe in God or an ultimate being. Frequently people use the concepts of spirituality and religion interchangeably, but spirituality is a much broader and more unifying concept than religion (Hollins, 2005). Florence Nightingale believed that spirituality is a force that provides energy needed in a healthy hospital environment. She also believed that caring for a person's spiritual needs is just as important as caring for a person's physical needs (Delgado, 2005). The human spirit is powerful, and spirituality has different meanings for different people. Therefore you need to understand your own spirituality in order to integrate spirituality into your patients' care. Nursing care involves helping patients use their spiritual resources as they identify and explore what is meaningful in their lives and to find ways to cope with illness and life's stressors (Tanyi and Werner, 2007).

SCIENTIFIC KNOWLEDGE BASE

Recently health care research has shown the association between spirituality and health. There are beneficial health outcomes when an individual is able to engage personal beliefs in a higher power and sense a source of strength or support. For example, Drentea and Goldner (2006) found that African American caregivers who cared for patients outside the home experienced less depression when they had strong religious beliefs. Many people use prayer frequently as a method of coping because it is effective in minimizing physical stressors. Attending church often positively influences health and the decision to participate in health promotion practices (Holt and McClure, 2006; Van Dover and Pfeiffer, 2007). The increased interest in studying the effect of spirituality and health has greatly contributed to nursing science (Ross, 2006) (Box 20-1).

Researchers do not fully understand the relationship between spirituality and healing. However, the individual's intrinsic spirit seems to be one factor in healing. Current evidence shows a link among the mind, body, and spirit (Hermann, 2007). An individual's beliefs and expectations have effects on the person's physical well-being (Nelson-

BOX 20-1 BEST PRACTICES

Enhancing Spirituality and Spiritual Health

SUMMARY OF EVIDENCE

Spirituality and spiritual health are essential parts of nursing care. People who are spiritually healthy and who participate in spiritual activities often have better health and will participate in health-promoting activities. In addition, people often use spiritual interventions to help them cope with a variety of crises, including acute and chronic illnesses, domestic violence, and substance abuse. It is important for patients to feel connected to themselves and others. Spiritual connectedness results in hope and a sense of encouragement. Even though nurses are aware of the spiritual needs of their patients, it is sometimes difficult to implement spiritual interventions for a variety of reasons. Many times patient care is complex, and nurses often have limited time to spend in personal conversation with patients and their families. In addition, you can provide effective spiritual care only if you are aware of your own spirituality. Sometimes nurses do not attend to their own spiritual needs, making it difficult to meet the spiritual needs of their patients.

APPLICATION TO NURSING PRACTICE

- It is essential to provide spiritual care as a component of holistic care to your patients.
- Pray with your patients if they want you to; prayer enhances connectedness to God or another higher being and often provides a source of strength, enhancing coping and other positive outcomes such as improving quality of life and decreasing anxiety.
- Establish presence, and connect with your patients by spending time with them, actively listening, and respecting them as individuals.
- Include spouses, children, and significant others in your care; patients need to continue to feel connected to others, especially during times of illness or crisis.

REFERENCES
Gillum TL, Sullivan CM, Bybee DI: The importance of spirituality in the lives of domestic violence survivors, *Violence Against Women* 12(3):240, 2006.
Holt CL, McClure SM: Perceptions of the religion-health connection among African American church members, *Qual Health Res* 16(2):268, 2006.
Lamb M and others: The psychosocial spiritual experience of elderly individuals recovering from stroke: a systematic review, *Int J Evid Based Healthc* 6(2):173, 2008.
Lewis FM and others: Helping her heal: a pilot study of an educational counseling intervention for spouses of women with breast cancer, *Psycho-Oncology* 17:131, 2008.

Becker and others, 2007; Smith, 2006). Many of these effects are tied to hormonal and neurological function. For example, relaxation exercises and guided imagery improve individuals' immune function (Lindberg, 2005) and reduce perceptions of pain and anxiety (Carrico, Peters, and Diokno, 2008). Laughter raises pain thresholds, boosts antibody production, reduces stress hormones, relieves tension, and elevates mood (Bennett and Langacher, 2006; Facente, 2006; Hsieh and others, 2005). In one study, researchers found that older Mexican Americans who attended religious services regularly had lower rates of declining cognitive status (Hill and others, 2006). A person's inner beliefs and convictions are powerful resources for healing. As a nurse you will be more successful in helping patients achieve desirable health outcomes after learning to support patients and families spiritually.

NURSING KNOWLEDGE BASE

Concepts in Spiritual Health

It is important for you to understand the fundamental concepts of spiritual health. The concepts of spirituality, faith, hope, spiritual well-being, and religion give direction in understanding the view each individual has of life and its value.

SPIRITUALITY Spirituality is unique for each of us and exists in everyone, regardless of religious beliefs (Delgado, 2005). Our culture, development, life experiences, beliefs, and values about life influence our definition of spirituality (Delgado, 2005). There are two important common characteristics of spirituality: (1) it is a unifying theme in people's lives, and (2) it is a state of being. Current definitions of spirituality include eight distinct but overlapping constructs or ideas (Figure 20-1). Spirituality gives people the *energy* needed to maintain health and cope with difficult situations. **Self-transcendence** refers to the belief that there is a positive force outside of and greater than oneself. This force allows a person to develop new perspectives that are beyond physical boundaries (Teixeira, 2008). Examples of transcendent moments include the feelings of awe when holding a new baby or watching the sun rise over the mountains (Delgado, 2005; Hollins, 2005). Spirituality also offers a sense of connectedness intrapersonally (connected with oneself), interpersonally (connected with others and the environment), and transpersonally (connected with God, the unseen, or a higher power). Through connectedness, patients are able to move beyond the stressors of everyday life and find comfort, faith, hope, peace, and empowerment (Delgado, 2005; Nelson-Becker and others, 2007; Villagomeza, 2005).

Faith allows you to have firm beliefs about something despite the lack of physical evidence. Although many associate faith with religious beliefs, faith can exist without them (Villagomeza, 2005). *Existential reality* allows people to have unique subjective experiences and find meaning and purpose in life. This search for purpose is often connected to vocation or a calling in life (Delgado, 2005). Existential reality helps you deal with the unknown and to love, comfort, and forgive others (Chiu and others, 2004). *Beliefs and values* help you

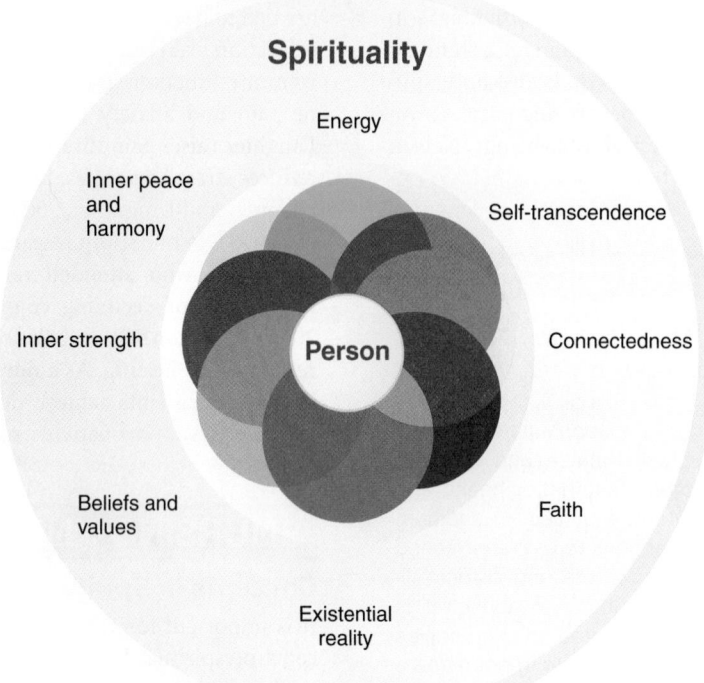

Figure 20-1 ■ The concept of spirituality has eight distinct but overlapping constructs. (Modified from Villagomeza LR: Mending broken hearts: the role of spirituality in cardiac illness: a research synthesis, 1991-2004, *Holistic Nurs Pract* 20(4):169, 2006.)

determine what is important to you and provide the foundation of truth (Hollins, 2005; Villagomeza, 2005). *Inner strength* is an energy source that instills hope, provides motivation, and promotes a positive outlook on life, even during difficult times (Banks-Wallace and Parks, 2004; Chiu and others, 2004; Villagomeza, 2005). *Inner peace and harmony* foster calm and positive feelings despite life experiences of chaos, fear, and uncertainty. These feelings help people feel comforted and find peace even in times of great distress (Banks-Wallace and Parks, 2004; Villagomeza, 2005).

Spirituality is an important concept for individuals who either do not believe in the existence of God (**atheist**) or who believe that any ultimate reality is unknown or unknowable (**agnostic**) (Tanyi, 2006). Atheists search for meaning in life through their work and relationships with others. It is important for agnostics to discover meaning in what they do or how they live because they find no ultimate meaning for the way things are. They believe that we, as people, bring meaning to what we do.

Spirituality is an integrating theme in life. A person's concept of spirituality begins in childhood and continues to grow throughout adulthood (Hendricks-Ferguson, 2008; Lamb and others, 2008; McSherry and Smith, 2007). Spirituality represents the totality of one's being, serving as the overriding perspective that unifies the various aspects of an individual. Spirituality spreads throughout the physiological, psychological, and sociocultural dimensions of a person's life, whether or not the individual acknowledges or develops it.

SPIRITUAL WELL-BEING There are two dimensions to **spiritual well-being.** The vertical dimension supports the transcendent relationship between you and some higher power (e.g., God, Buddha). The horizontal dimension describes positive relationships you have with others (Gray, 2006; Smith, 2006). Spiritual well-being has a positive effect on health and leads to spiritual health. If you are spiritually healthy, you experience joy, forgive yourself and others, accept hardship and mortality, experience enhanced quality of life, and have a positive sense of physical and emotional well-being (Van Dyke and Elias, 2007; Yampolsky and others, 2008).

FAITH In addition to being a part of the definition of spirituality, the concept of faith has two other common definitions. First, faith is defined as a cultural or institutional religion, such as Buddhism, Christianity, or Islam. Second, faith is a relationship with a divinity, higher power, authority, or spirit that incorporates a reasoning faith (belief) and a trusting faith (action). Reasoning faith is a person's belief and confidence in something for which there is no proof. It is an acceptance of what our reasoning cannot reach. Sometimes it involves a belief in a higher power, spirit guide, God, or Allah. However, faith also is the manner in which a person chooses to live life. Faith in this sense enables action. For example, a person believes that having a positive outlook on life is the best way to achieve life's goals. The belief that comes with faith involves self-transcendence (Perry, 2004). It gives purpose and meaning to an individual's life. *For example, Victoria (in the case study) is living with breast cancer. She has* *faith; thus she has a positive outlook on life and continues to pursue daily activities rather than resigning to the symptoms caused by her breast cancer. Her faith becomes stronger because she is able to view her cancer as an opportunity for personal growth.*

RELIGION Religion is associated with the "state of doing," or a specific system of practices associated with a particular denomination, sect, or form of worship. Religion refers to the system of organized beliefs and worship that a person practices to outwardly express spirituality. Many people practice a faith or belief in the doctrines of a specific religion or sect, such as the Lutheran church within Christianity or Orthodox Judaism. People from different religions view spirituality differently (Nelson-Becker and others, 2007). For example, a Buddhist believes in Four Noble Truths: life is suffering, suffering is caused by clinging, suffering can be eliminated by eliminating clinging, and to eliminate clinging and suffering, one follows an eightfold path. The path includes the right understanding, intention, speech, action, livelihood, effort, mindfulness, and concentration. This path promotes wisdom, moral behavior, and meditation (Smith-Stoner, 2005). A Buddhist turns inward, valuing self-control, whereas a Christian looks to the love of God to provide enlightenment and direction in life.

When providing spiritual care to patients, you need to know the differences between religion and spirituality. Although closely related, these terms are not synonymous (Hermann, 2007). Religious care helps patients follow their belief systems and worship practices. Spiritual care helps people maintain personal relationships and a relationship with a higher being or life force in order to identify meaning and purpose in life. Both enhance positive patient outcomes (Choumanova and others, 2006).

HOPE Spirituality and faith bring hope (Chiu and others, 2004). When a person has the attitude of something to live for and look forward to, hope is present. **Hope** is multidimensional and gives comfort while a person endures hardship and personal challenges (Hendricks-Ferguson, 2008). It is closely associated with faith. Hope is energizing, giving individuals a motivation to achieve and the resources to use toward that achievement. People express hope in all aspects of their lives as a force that helps them deal with life stressors. Hope is a valuable personal resource and brings comfort when people face a loss (see Chapter 25) or a challenge that seems difficult to achieve (Mednick and others, 2007).

Spiritual Health

People gain spiritual health by finding a balance between their life values, goals, and belief systems and their relationships within themselves and with others. Throughout life a person sometimes grows more spiritual, becoming increasingly aware of the meaning, purpose, and values of life. In times of stress, illness, loss, or recovery, a person often turns to previous ways of responding or adjusting to a situation. Often these coping styles lie within the person's spiritual beliefs.

Spiritual beliefs change as patients grow and develop (Table 20-1). Spirituality begins as children learn about themselves and their relationships with others. When you understand a child's spiritual beliefs, it is easier to care for and comfort the child (Hufton, 2006; McSherry and Smith, 2007). As children mature into adulthood, they experience spiritual growth by entering into lifelong relationships. An ability to care meaningfully for others and self is evidence of a healthy spirituality. Older adults often turn to important relationships and the giving of themselves to others as spiritual tasks.

Spiritual Problems

When illness, loss, grief, or a major life change affects a person, spiritual resources help the person move to recovery. Without spiritual resources, concerns and doubts develop within an individual. **Spiritual distress** is a nursing diagnosis, defined as "the impaired ability to experience and integrate meaning and purpose in life through connectedness with self, others, art, music, literature, nature, and/or a power greater than oneself" (NANDA International, 2009). For example, a catastrophic illness, like a stroke, can upset a person's spiritual well-being enough to cause doubt and a loss of faith (Lamb and others, 2008). Spiritual distress causes the person to feel alone or even abandoned. Individuals question their spiritual values, raising questions about their way of life and purpose for living. Spiritual distress also occurs when there is conflict between a person's beliefs and prescribed health treatment plan or the inability to practice usual rituals.

ACUTE ILLNESS Sudden, unexpected illness that threatens a patient's life, health, and/or well-being creates significant spiritual distress. For example, a 50-year-old man who has a heart attack and a 20-year-old who is injured in a motor vehicle accident both face crises that threaten their spiritual health. The illness or injury creates an unanticipated scramble to integrate and cope with new realities (e.g., disability). People look for ways to remain faithful to their beliefs and value systems through use of spiritual resources. Often conflicts develop around a person's beliefs and the meaning of life. Anger is common, and patients sometimes express it against God, their families, themselves, and their nurses or other health care providers. The strength of patients' spirituality influences their ability to cope with sudden illness and their ability to begin recovery. You play a key role in helping patients resolve feelings of spiritual distress. You create a healing environment and maximize recovery by enhancing your patients' spiritual well-being (Carpenter and others, 2008).

CHRONIC ILLNESS People with chronic illnesses often suffer debilitating symptoms that change their lifestyles. The uncertain and long-term nature of chronic illness, along with the potential for outcomes such as pain, changes in body image, and the need to confront death, all lead to spiritual distress. Patients struggle with questions about the meaning and purpose of their lives because their independence is threatened, causing fear, anxiety, and an overall dispiritedness. The nursing diagnosis *spiritual distress* is appropriate to use for patients who experience these symptoms. A person's spirituality is a significant factor in how he or she adapts to the changes resulting from chronic illness. Successfully adapting to those changes strengthens a person spiritually, but it sometimes takes a long-term plan to help the patient with a

TABLE 20-1   Relationship Between Developmental Stage and Spiritual Beliefs

ERICKSON'S DEVELOPMENTAL STAGE	SPIRITUAL BELIEFS
Trust versus mistrust Birth to 18 months	Spiritual well-being provided by parents Trust provides a basis for hope Love, affection, security, and a stimulating environment promote spirituality
Autonomy versus shame and doubt 20-36 months	Fascination with magic and mystery Often believes illness is related to bad behavior Begins to learn the difference between right and wrong Imitates parents' spiritual or religious actions, recites prayers and sings simple religious songs but does not understand their meanings Interprets meanings literally
Initiative versus guilt 3-6 years	Feels guilty when not acting responsibly Influenced by spiritual and religious stories, examples, moods, and actions Models moral behaviors of parents Begins to ask about God or supreme beings
Industry versus inferiority 6-12 years	Wants to learn about spirituality Has a clear picture of God or supreme being, morality, and the difference between right and wrong Sorts fantasy from fact Demands proof of reality and believes literal meanings of spiritual stories
Identity versus identity confusion Adolescence	Reflects on inconsistencies in stories Begins to question spiritual practices, forms own opinions, and occasionally discards parents' beliefs Abstract reasoning leads to exploration of moral issues Spirituality comes from connectedness with family, nature, and God or a supreme being
Intimacy versus isolation and loneliness Young adulthood	Establishes self-identity and world view Forms independent beliefs, attitudes, and lifestyles Uses principles to solve problems when individual's and a society's rules conflict
Generativity versus stagnation Middle-age adulthood	Develops appreciation of past spiritual experiences Embraces people from different faiths and religions Reviews value system during crisis Values others
Ego identity versus despair and disgust Older adulthood	Values love and interactions with others Focuses on overcoming oppression and violence Beliefs vary based on many factors, such as gender, past experiences, religion, economic status, and ethnic background

Data from Edelman CL, Mandle CL: *Health promotion throughout the life span,* ed 6, St. Louis, 2006, Mosby; McSherry W, Smith J: How do children express their spiritual needs? *Paediatr Nurs* 19(3):17, 2007.

chronic illness achieve spiritual well-being. As a nurse, you are in a unique position to help patients reevaluate their lives and achieve spiritual health (Burkhart, Solari-Twadell, and Haas, 2008). Patients who have a sense of spiritual well-being are often better able to cope with their illnesses and experience enhanced quality of life (Tanyi and Werner, 2007).

TERMINAL ILLNESS Terminal illness commonly causes fears of physical pain, isolation, the unknown, and dying. When patients feel uncertain about what death means, they are susceptible to spiritual distress. On the other hand, spirituality helps patients and families find resolution and peace at the end of life. Their spiritual sense of peace enables them to face death without fear (Prince-Paul, 2008). Individuals experiencing a terminal illness often find themselves reviewing their life and questioning its meaning. Common ques-

tions asked include, "Why is this happening to me?" or "What have I done?" Terminal illness affects family and friends just as much as the patient. It causes members of the family to ask important questions about life's meaning and how it will affect their relationship with the patient (see Chapter 25).

When caring for dying patients, help them gain a greater sense of control over their illness regardless if they are in a health care setting (e.g., the hospital) or in the home. Dying is a holistic process encompassing the patient's physical, social, psychological, and spiritual health (Lhussier, Carr, and Wilcockson, 2007; Peters and Sellick, 2006).

NEAR-DEATH EXPERIENCE You may care for a patient or have a family member who has had a near-death experience (NDE). NDE is a psychological phenomenon in which people who have either been close to clinical death or have recovered

BOX 20-2   SYNTHESIS IN PRACTICE

Jeff plans for Victoria and Joe's return to the oncology clinic. He spent time learning more about Victoria's disease and treatment plan so he is able to better explain what to expect as chemotherapy progresses. Jeff recognizes that Joe usually comes to the clinic, and Victoria describes him as a strong source of support. However, Jeff does not know enough about the couple's relationship and wants to explore this further. The role of family members in providing support, particularly with regard to decision making, is important for Jeff to understand before he develops a plan of care. In reviewing information about loss and grieving, Jeff recognizes that Victoria shows acceptance of her disease because she is able to discuss cancer and the plan for treatment. Jeff knows that as patients begin to accept the fact of being diagnosed with a life-threatening disease, it is important to offer opportunities to share feelings and to begin to provide time to discuss future plans.

Jeff's previous experiences with patients who have cancer taught him that when patients express hope, they seem to be able to move forward and cope with the challenges of their disease. During the last clinic visit Victoria expressed an intermediate hope, to be able to continue to attend religious services at her church. Jeff reflected on that experience and thinks that Victoria and Joe have a strong sense of spiritual well-being that will help them cope with cancer. However, further assessment is necessary.

Jeff wants to completely assess Victoria and Joe's level of spiritual health. Jeff is Lutheran and does not know very much about the Baptist faith, the couple's religion. However, he knows that the Baptist sense of community is very strong and that it is important to learn more about how members of the Timms' church play a role in offering support to the family. Jeff recognizes that spiritual well-being is more complex than religion. He spends time reflecting on his own value and belief systems so that he will remain open and receptive to understanding Victoria and Joe's spiritual belief systems. By understanding his own beliefs, Jeff will also be better able to help Victoria and Joe cope with Victoria's diagnosis of cancer.

---

after being declared dead. It is not associated with a mental disorder. Instead, experts agree that NDE describes a powerfully close brush with physical, emotional, and spiritual death. Persons who have an NDE after cardiopulmonary arrest, for example, often tell the same story of feeling themselves rising above their bodies and watching caregivers initiate lifesaving measures. Commonly, patients who experience an NDE describe feeling totally at peace, having an out-of-body experience, being pulled into a dark tunnel, being surrounded by bright light, and encountering people who preceded them in death. Instead of moving toward the light, they learn it is not time for them to die, and they return to life (Betty, 2006; Duffy, 2007).

Patients who have an NDE are often reluctant to discuss it, thinking family or caregivers will not understand. Isolation and depression often occur. However, individuals experiencing an NDE who discuss it openly with family or caregivers find acceptance and meaning from this powerful experience. They are often no longer afraid of death, and they have a decreased desire to achieve material wealth. They also report increased sensitivity to different chemicals, such as alcohol and medications. After patients have survived an NDE, promote spiritual well-being by remaining open and give patients a chance to explore what happened, and support patients as they share the experience with significant others (Betty, 2006; Duffy, 2007).

CRITICAL THINKING

Synthesis

You will apply elements of critical thinking whenever you perform the nursing process with a patient. Consider the scientific knowledge you have learned, your experience, critical thinking attitudes, and standards to ensure an individualized approach to patient care (Box 20-2).

KNOWLEDGE The helping role is an important domain of nursing practice (Benner, 1984). Patients look to nurses for help that is different from the help they seek from other health care professionals. To effectively care for your patients' spiritual needs, you first need to be comfortable with your own spirituality (Miner-Williams, 2006). By fostering your own personal, emotional, and spiritual health, you become a resource for your patient (Gray, 2006). Use your awareness of your own spirituality as a tool when caring for yourself and your patients (Carpenter and others, 2008). Differentiate your personal spirituality from that of the patient. This becomes important during the delivery of care, when you need to be able to engage a patient spiritually rather than try to exercise personal spiritual convictions. Your role is not to solve the spiritual problems of patients but to provide an environment for your patients to express their spirituality.

After becoming comfortable with your own spirituality, use your nursing expertise to anticipate your patients' personal issues and the resulting effect on spiritual well-being. Your knowledge about the concept of spirituality and a patient's faith and belief systems helps to provide appropriate spiritual care. Knowledge of a patient's culture will provide additional insight into a person's spiritual practices (Box 20-3). Application of therapeutic communication principles (see Chapter 10) and caring (see Chapter 18) will help you to establish therapeutic trust with patients. An individual's spiritual beliefs are very personal. When you convey caring and openness to individuals, you will be more successful in promoting honest discussion about spiritual beliefs.

When caring for patients who have a terminal illness or are experiencing some other type of loss, knowledge of loss and grief dynamics is important (see Chapter 25). Spirituality influences personal reactions to loss and response to grief. Also consider family dynamics while providing spiritual care (see Chapter 23). For many individuals, their spiritual health is often integrated with the relationships between family members. Therefore consider the family's beliefs when planning spiritual care for your patient.

BOX 20-3   CULTURAL FOCUS

Through studying, Jeff found that breast cancer makes up about 26% of all new cancer diagnoses in American women. African American women have the second-highest breast cancer incidence rate and the highest mortality rate. Jeff also discovered that spiritual needs are often associated with cultural beliefs. Spiritual and cultural beliefs affect how women of different cultures experience health and illness. African American women generally express a deep relationship with God and strong moral and ethical values. Spirituality for African Americans often provides a source of healing, coping, and peace. Jeff uses this understanding of breast cancer and spirituality among African American women to develop a culturally competent plan of care for Victoria and her family.

IMPLICATIONS FOR PRACTICE

- Jeff encourages Victoria and her family to strengthen their spiritual health as they continue to cope with Victoria's breast cancer diagnosis and cancer treatment.
- Victoria's church has a parish nurse. Parish nurses care for the spiritual, emotional, and physical health of the members of a congregation. Because of their holistic approach to health, African American people usually consider parish nurses to be helpful. Jeff talks with Victoria about the services her parish nurse provides. With Victoria's permission, he shares her health problems and concerns with the parish nurse. The parish nurse agrees to contact Victoria and arrange a time for them to meet.
- Many African American women study the Bible and pray regularly. Jeff prays with Victoria and Joe during their visits to the oncology clinic and encourages them to continue to read the Bible together at home.
- African American churches provide a great deal of social support and companionship, which is helpful to people who have cancer and their caregivers. Therefore Jeff encourages Joe to attend church even if Victoria is too ill to attend. He also contacts the Timms' pastor and arranges times for people from the church to come sit with Victoria for a few hours 2 days a week to allow Joe some time to take care of himself.

Data from Boyd AS, Wilmoth MC: An innovative community-based intervention for African American women with breast cancer: the witness project, *Health Soc Work* 31(1):77, 2006; Gibson LM, Smith Hendricks C: Integrative review of spirituality in African American breast cancer survivors, *ABNF J* 17(2):67, 2006; Leak A, Hu J, King CR: Symptom distress, spirituality, and quality of life in African American breast cancer survivors, *Cancer Nurse* 31(1):E15, 2008; Underwood SM and others: Pilot study of the breast cancer experiences of African American women with a family history of breast cancer: implications for nursing practice, *ABNF J* 19(3):107, 2006.

Finally, a sound understanding of ethics and values (see Chapter 5) is essential when providing spiritual care. A person's values or beliefs about the worth of a given idea, attitude, or custom are linked to the individual's spiritual well-being. Application of ethical principles ensures respect for a patient's spiritual and religious convictions.

EXPERIENCE You often will care for patients who are in spiritual distress. Use these experiences when helping others select coping options. Because spirituality is more than religion, you need to consider personal views and philosophies about life and reflect on whether your own spirituality is beneficial in assisting patients (Baldacchino, 2006). If you sense a personal faith and hope regarding life, it is likely that you will be better able to help patients. Previous personal and professional experiences with dying patients, patients with chronic disease, or patients who have experienced significant losses provide lessons in how to help patients face difficult challenges and how to offer support to family and friends (Wright, 2005).

ATTITUDES Do not take a patient's reaction to illness or loss for granted. Humility becomes very important, particularly when caring for patients from diverse cultural and/or religious backgrounds. Recognize any limitations in your own knowledge about a patient's spiritual beliefs and religious practices, and be willing to pursue the knowledge needed to provide appropriate, individualized care. Show genuine concern for patients as you ask them about their beliefs and how spirituality influences their health (Baldacchino, 2006). Also exhibit integrity; realize the importance of refraining from expressing your opinions about religion or spirituality when they conflict with that of the patient. Finally, show confidence in dealing with spiritual issues as you build a caring relationship with the patient. Confidence works to build trust (Skalla and McCoy, 2006).

STANDARDS A good critical thinker is thorough and ensures that information about a patient is significant and relevant when making decisions about patients' spiritual needs. The nature of a person's spirituality is complex and highly individualized. Therefore avoid making assumptions about the patient's religion and beliefs. Significance and relevance are standards of critical thinking that ensure you explore the issues that are most meaningful to patients and most likely to affect their spiritual well-being. Also, apply ethical standards of care when providing spiritual care.

The Joint Commission sets standards for quality health care. The Joint Commission requires health care organizations to acknowledge patients' rights to spiritual care and provide for patients' spiritual needs through pastoral care or others who are certified, ordained, or lay individuals. The standards also require that you assess and provide for your patients' denomination, beliefs, and spiritual practices (The Joint Commission [TJC], 2008).

The American Nurses Association's Code of Ethics for Nurses (Fowler, 2008) sets standards for quality nursing care. The Code requires you to practice nursing with compassion by accepting the dignity and worth of all your patients despite their socioeconomic status, personal characteristics, or type of health problems. You promote an environment that respects your patients' values, customs, and spiritual beliefs.

NURSING PROCESS

Understanding a patient's spirituality and then appropriately identifying the level of support and resources needed requires a broad perspective and an open mind. As a nurse, you make a commitment to care. In order to care for and meet the spiritual needs of your patients, it is essential to respect each patient's personal beliefs. People experience the world and find meaning in life in different ways. Application of the nursing process from the perspective of a patient's spiritual needs is not simple. It goes beyond assessing a patient's religious practices. Caring for your patients' spiritual needs requires you to be compassionate and remove any personal biases or misconceptions. Be willing to share and discover your patients' meaning and purpose in life, illness, and health. Identify common values and respect unique commitments and values with your patients by having quiet conversations, listening effectively, and communicating using presence and touch (Smith and McSherry, 2004; Villagomeza, 2005).

You need to recognize that not all patients have spiritual problems. Patients bring certain spiritual resources that help them assume healthier lives, recover from illness, or face impending death. Supporting and recognizing the positive side of a patient's spirituality goes a long way in delivering effective, individualized nursing care (McSherry, 2006).

■■■ ASSESSMENT

Before you complete a spiritual assessment on your patient, be aware of your own spiritual beliefs, values, and biases. Understanding your own spirit is essential when you provide spiritual care to your patients. Remember that spirituality is very subjective and has different meanings for different people. You are able to gather an accurate assessment of your patients' spirituality when you take time to build therapeutic relationships with them. Once you establish a trusting relationship with a patient, you and the patient will reach a point of learning together, and spiritual caring will occur (O'Brien, 2008). Conduct an ongoing spiritual assessment the entire time you care for a patient (McSherry, 2006). Focus your as-

sessment on aspects of spirituality most likely to be influenced by life experiences, events, and questions in the case of illness and hospitalization (Table 20-2). Conducting an assessment is therapeutic for you and your patient because it conveys a level of caring and support.

Assess a patient's spiritual health in several different ways. One way is to ask the patient direct questions. This approach requires you to feel comfortable asking others about their spirituality. Some health care agencies and researchers have created assessment tools to clarify values and assess spirituality (Elkins and Cavendish, 2004). For example, the Spiritual Well-Being Scale (SWB) has 20 questions that assess a patient's view of life and relationship with a higher power (Gray, 2006). The B-E-L-I-E-F assessment tool (McEvoy, 2003) helps nurses evaluate a child and family's spiritual and religious needs. The acronym stands for the following:

B—Belief system
E—Ethics or values
L—Lifestyle
I—Involvement in a spiritual community
E—Education
F—Future events

Effective assessment tools like the SWB and B-E-L-I-E-F help you remember important areas to assess and create a spiritual plan of care. Responses to the assessment items on the tools indicate areas you need to investigate further. For example, if a patient has difficulty accepting life situations, you need to spend time learning how the patient accepts and manages his or her illness. Remember, when using any spiritual assessment tool, do not impose your personal values on your patient. This is sometimes difficult, especially when the patient's values and beliefs are similar to yours, because it is very easy for you to make false assumptions. When you understand the overall approach to spiritual assessment, you are able to enter into thoughtful discussions with the patient, gain a greater awareness of the personal resources the patient brings to a situation, and incorporate the resources into an effective plan of care.

FAITH/BELIEF Assess the source of authority and guidance that your patients use to lead their lives and guide their actions and beliefs. The authority is sometimes a supreme

TABLE 20-2 FOCUSED PATIENT ASSESSMENT

FACTORS TO ASSESS	QUESTIONS	PHYSICAL ASSESSMENT
Past experiences with loss	How would you describe the ways you cope spiritually when faced with difficult times?	Observe patient's facial expressions and mannerisms during the discussion.
Fear of the unknown resulting from a terminal illness	Describe the people who mean the most to you. In what way do you look to them for support? Do you consider yourself a spiritual person? If so, what gives you comfort? If not, what provides you a sense of peace?	Fear is associated with anxiety. Be alert for changes in vital signs. Observe the patient's mood, willingness to initiate conversation, and interest in surroundings.

being, a code of conduct, a religious leader, family or friends, oneself, or a combination of sources. Faith in an authority provides a sense of confidence that guides a person in exercising beliefs and experiencing growth. Assess a person's faith in an authority by asking, "Who do you look to for guidance in life?" The patient's response will likely open the door for a meaningful discussion. Listen carefully, and explore what is meaningful to the patient (O'Brien, 2008; Skalla and McCoy, 2006).

Determine if the patient has a religious source of guidance that conflicts with medical treatment plans. This seriously affects the treatment options nurses and other health care providers are able to offer patients. For example, if a patient is a Jehovah's Witness, blood products are not an acceptable form of treatment. Christian Scientists often refuse any medical intervention, believing that their faith will heal them.

It is also important to understand a patient's philosophy of life. Asking the patient, "Describe for me what is most important in your life" or "Tell me what gives your life meaning or purpose" helps to assess the basis of the patient's spiritual belief system. This information reveals the patient's spiritual focus and will help to reflect the impact illness, loss, or disability has on the person's life. A patient's religious practices, views about health, and response to illness influence how you will provide support (Table 20-3).

LIFE AND SELF-RESPONSIBILITY Assessing spiritual well-being includes looking at your patient's life and self-responsibility. People who accept change, make decisions about their lives, and are able to forgive themselves and others in times of difficulty have a higher level of spiritual well-being. During illness, patients often are unable to accept limitations or know what to do to regain a functional and meaningful life. Their sense of helplessness reflects spiritual distress. However, if a patient is able to adapt to changes and seek solutions for how to deal with any limitations, spiritual well-being reflects an important coping resource. Assess the extent to which a patient understands any limitations or threats posed by an illness and the manner in which the patient chooses to adjust to them. Ask, "Tell me how you feel about the changes caused by your illness" and "How do these changes affect what you now need to do?"

CONNECTEDNESS Connectedness is a dimension of spirituality. Patients who are connected to themselves, others, nature, and God or another supreme being cope with the stress brought on by crisis and chronic illness (Narayanasamy, 2004). Patients remain connected with God by praying (Figure 20-2). Prayer is personal communication with one's god. It provides a sense of hope, strength, and security and is woven into one's faith (Cavendish and others, 2006; Narayanasamy and Narayanasamy, 2008). You help patients become or remain connected by respecting each patient's unique sense of spirituality. Assess whether the patient loses the ability to express a sense of relatedness to something greater than the self. You assess a patient's connectedness by asking, "What feelings do you have after you pray?" or "Who do you feel is the most important person to you?"

LIFE SATISFACTION Spiritual well-being is tied to a person's satisfaction with life and what he or she has accomplished (Katerndahl, 2008). When people are satisfied with

TABLE 20-3   Religious Beliefs About Health

RELIGIOUS OR CULTURAL GROUP	HEALTH CARE BELIEFS	RESPONSE TO ILLNESS	IMPLICATIONS FOR HEALTH AND NURSING
Hinduism	Accepts modern medical science.	Past sins cause illness. Prolonging life is discouraged.	Allow time for prayer and purity rituals. Allow use of amulets, rituals, and symbols.
Sikhism	Accepts modern medical science.	Females to be examined by females. Removing undergarments causes great distress.	Provide time for devotional prayer. Allow use of religious symbols.
Buddhism	Accepts modern medical science.	Sometimes refuses treatment on holy days. Nonhuman spirits invading the body cause illness. May want a Buddhist priest. May permit withdrawal of life support. Does not practice euthanasia. Often will not take time off from work or family responsibilities when sick.	Health is an important part of life. Good health is maintained by caring for yourself and others. Does not always accept medications because of belief that chemical substances in the body are harmful.

TABLE 20-3 Religious Beliefs About Health—cont'd

RELIGIOUS OR CULTURAL GROUP	HEALTH CARE BELIEFS	RESPONSE TO ILLNESS	IMPLICATIONS FOR HEALTH AND NURSING
Islam	Must be able to practice the Five Pillars of Islam. Sometimes has a fatalistic view of health.	Uses faith healing. Family members are a comfort. Group prayer is strengthening. May permit withdrawal of life support. Does not practice euthanasia. Believes time of death is predetermined and cannot be changed. Maintains a sense of hope and often avoids discussions of death.	Women prefer female health care providers. During month of Ramadan, Muslims do not eat anything from dawn until sunset. Health and spirituality are connected. Family and friends visit during times of illness. Organ transplantation or donation and postmortem examinations are usually not considered.
Judaism	Believes in the sanctity of life. God and medicine have a balance. Observance of the Sabbath is important. Some refuse treatments on the Sabbath.	Visiting the sick is an obligation. Obligation to seek care, exercise, and sleep, eat well, and avoid drug and alcohol abuse. Euthanasia is forbidden. Life support is discouraged.	Believes it is important to keep yourself healthy. Expects nurses to provide competent health care. Allow patients to express their feelings. Allow family to stay with the dying patient.
Protestants and Catholics	Accept modern medical science.	Use prayer, faith healing. Appreciate visits from clergy. Some will use laying on of hands. Commonly take holy communion. Anointing of the sick is given when individual is ill, in acute setting or near death (Catholic). Catholics do not practice euthanasia. Extraordinary measures not required to prolong life.	Are in favor of organ donation. Health is important to maintain. Allow time for patients to pray by themselves, with family or friends.
Navajos	Concepts of health have a fundamental place in their concept of humans and their place in the universe.	Blessingway is a practice that attempts to remove ill health by means of stories, songs, rituals, prayers, symbols, and sand paintings.	Prefer holistic approach to health care. Often are not on time for appointments. Promote physical, mental, spiritual, and social health of persons, families, and communities. Allow family members to visit. Provide teaching about wellness, not disease prevention, when possible.
Appalachians	Nature controls life and health. Accept folk healers. Good Christian members of community are called as servants to minister to disabled.	Dislike hospitals. Tend to not follow medical regimens but expect help when seeking episodic treatment.	Become anxious in unfamiliar settings. Encourage communication with family and friends when ill.

Data from Giger JN, Davidhizar RE: *Transcultural nursing: assessment and intervention,* ed 5, St. Louis, 2008, Mosby; Hockenberry MJ, Wilson D: *Wong's essentials of pediatric nursing,* ed 8, St. Louis, 2009, Mosby.

life and how they are using their abilities, there is more energy available to deal with new difficulties and to resolve problems. You assess a patient's satisfaction with life by asking, "How happy or satisfied are you with your life?" or "Tell me to what extent you feel satisfied with what you have accomplished in life."

FELLOWSHIP AND COMMUNITY Fellowship is one kind of relationship an individual has with other people, including immediate family, close friends, associates at work or school, fellow members of a church, and neighbors. More specifically, this includes the extent of the community of shared faith between patients and their support networks. Many times, social support from faith-based groups helps patients cope with illness (Schneider and Mannell, 2006) and participate in health promotion behaviors (Underwood and Powell, 2006). To assess the patient's supportive community, ask questions such as, "Who do you have a bond with?" "Who do you find is the greatest source of support in times of difficulty?" or "When you have faced difficult times in the past, who has been your greatest resource?"

Explore the extent and nature of a person's support networks and their relationship with the patient. It is unwise to assume that a given network offers the kind of support a patient desires. For example, calling the patient's clergy-person to request a visit is inappropriate if the patient finds little fellowship with that individual or the community that the individual represents. Does the patient have one significant fellowship or several? What is the level of support received from the community? Do they visit, say prayers, or support the patient's immediate family? Learn whether openness exists between the patient and those persons with whom a fellowship has formed.

RITUAL AND PRACTICE The use of rituals and practice is easy to assess and will help you understand a patient's spirituality. Rituals include participation in a religious group or private worship, prayer, sacraments such as baptism or communion, fasting, singing, meditating, scripture reading,

and making offerings or sacrifices. Different religions have different rituals for life events. For example, Buddhists practice baptism later in life and find burial or cremation acceptable at death. Muslims wash the body of a dead family member and wrap it in white cloth with the head turned toward the right shoulder. Orthodox and Conservative Jews have their newborn sons circumcised 8 days after birth. Determine whether illness or hospitalization has interrupted a patient's usual rituals or practices. A ritual provides a patient with structure and support during difficult times. If rituals are important to the patient, use them as part of your nursing intervention (O'Brien, 2008).

VOCATION Individuals express their spirituality daily in their work, play, and relationships. Spirituality is often a part of a person's identity and vocation in life. Determine if illness or hospitalization has altered the ability to express some aspect of spirituality as it relates to the person's work or daily activities. Expression of spirituality is highly individual and includes showing an appreciation for life in the variety of things people do, living in the moment and not worrying about tomorrow, appreciating nature, expressing love toward others, and being productive (McSherry, Cash, and Ross, 2004). Assess how the patient routinely expresses spirituality. Questions to ask include, "Has your illness affected the way you live your life spiritually, at home or where you work?" or "Has your illness affected your ability to express what's important in life for you?"

PATIENT EXPECTATIONS Before completing your spiritual assessment, learn what the patient expects from you and other caregivers. Patients expect you to maintain a compassionate, trusting, and open relationship. They also expect you to understand the psychological, social, and spiritual implications of their care, especially when illness or loss prevents them from exercising their spirituality. Learn to find ways to offer guidance and support. In addition, it is important for you to accept your patients' religious practices or rituals. Ask patients what they expect of you to establish a therapeutic nurse-patient relationship.

■■■ NURSING DIAGNOSIS

When you review your patient's spiritual assessment, you will know a great deal about the patient's spirituality. Exploring a patient's spirituality sometimes reveals responses to health problems that require nursing intervention, or it reveals a strong set of resources for the patient to use in coping. Use your critical thinking skills to analyze data and discover patterns of defining characteristics. Potential nursing diagnoses affected by spiritual health include the following:

- *Anxiety*
- *Ineffective coping*
- *Fear*
- *Impaired religiosity*
- *Readiness for enhanced religiosity*
- *Spiritual distress*
- *Risk for spiritual distress*
- *Readiness for enhanced spiritual well-being*

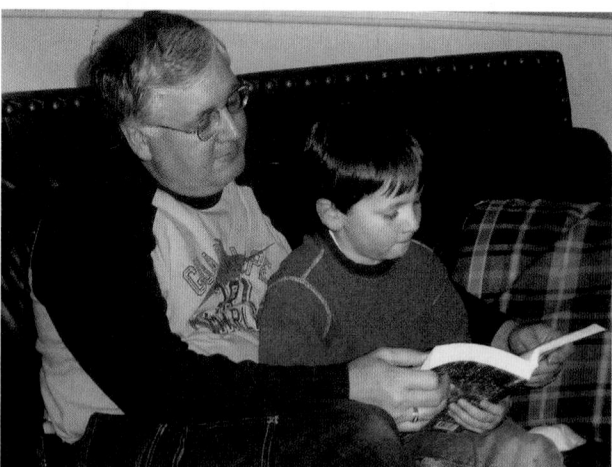

Figure 20-2 ■ Praying together enhances the connectedness between parents and their children.

As you identify nursing diagnoses for a patient, it is important to recognize the significance that spirituality has for all types of health problems. You may need to apply spiritual care principles if your patient has nursing diagnoses such as *acute pain, chronic pain, fear, anxiety,* and *compromised family coping.*

Three nursing diagnoses accepted by NANDA International (2009) pertain specifically to spirituality. *Readiness for enhanced spiritual well-being* is based on defining characteristics that show a pattern of inner strength and interconnectedness that comes from inner faith and hope. Patients with this nursing diagnosis have a strong faith; are in harmony with self, others, and a higher power; and have a good sense of purpose and meaning of life. A patient with enhanced spiritual well-being has resources to draw on when faced with other nursing diagnoses. You will help the patient explore how to use these resources when facing health problems.

The nursing diagnoses of *spiritual distress* and *risk for spiritual distress* create different clinical pictures. Defining characteristics from your assessment will show patterns that reflect a person's actual or potential dispiritedness (e.g., expressing concern with the meaning of life and beliefs, anger toward God, and verbalizing conflicts about personal beliefs). Patients likely to be at risk for spiritual distress include those who have poor relationships, have experienced a recent loss, or are suffering some form of mental or physical illness.

Validate defining characteristics and clarify them with the patient before you make a diagnosis and develop a plan of care. With spiritual care the importance of your own spiritual well-being and perceptions cannot be overemphasized. Do not impose your personal beliefs. Be sure any diagnosis has an accurate related factor (e.g., a situational loss or relationship conflict) so that your interventions are purposeful and goal directed.

■■■PLANNING

During planning, integrate the knowledge gathered from assessment and knowledge relating to resources and therapies available for spiritual care to develop an individualized plan of care (see Care Plan). Match the patient's needs with evidence-based interventions that are supported and recommended in the clinical and research literature. Use a Concept Map (Figure 20-3) to organize your patient's care and to show how the patient's medical diagnosis, assessment data, and nursing diagnoses are interrelated. Focus on building a caring relationship with the patient so that you will enter into a healing relationship together.

GOALS AND OUTCOMES A spiritual plan of care includes realistic and individualized goals along with relevant outcomes. This will require you to work closely with the patient in setting goals and outcomes and ultimately choosing nursing interventions. In cases in which spiritual care re-

---

CARE PLAN Readiness for Enhanced Spiritual Well-Being

ASSESSMENT
Jeff learns that Victoria has been told her prognosis is promising, although she will need treatment to prevent spread of her disease. Joe has been helping Victoria more at home and has been trying to arrange work so that he is able to take her to the clinic. This means that he has less time in the evening to spend with the children. In the past, Joe and Victoria have always had discussions with the children during mealtime, but recently this has been difficult. Jeff knows that current evidence shows many African American women use spirituality to cope with breast cancer, so he decides to assess Victoria's spirituality.

ASSESSMENT ACTIVITIES	FINDINGS/DEFINING CHARACTERISTICS*
Assess Victoria's connections with herself.	Victoria used to feel good about herself. However, since she has received cancer treatments, she has been more tired and feels less positive at times. She states, **"I wish I had more hope about my prognosis."**
Assess Victoria's connections with her family and significant others.	Before Victoria's illness the **children were very close to their parents and shared their faith in God.** However, **now they are not coping well with Victoria's illness.** Victoria and Joe **attend their church regularly and hope to continue** doing so even during the chemotherapy. **Members of their church have offered support** by taking Victoria to the clinic if Joe is unable.
Determine Victoria's connections with a power greater than herself.	Victoria **expresses a connectedness with her God,** "I do not feel alone; God is with me. I have a better appreciation of each day God gives me, and I believe God's strength will help me continue to be active in my church."

NURSING DIAGNOSIS: Readiness for enhanced spiritual well-being related to desire to be more connected with self, family, and God.

*Defining characteristics are shown in bold type.

Continued

PLANNING

GOAL

Spiritual Health
- Victoria will restore connectedness with children within 2 months.

- Victoria will remain connected with herself, her husband, and God within 1 month.

INTERVENTIONS (NIC)‡

Spiritual Support
- Use therapeutic communication (see Chapter 10) to establish presence and trust and to demonstrate empathy with Victoria and Joe.
- Pray with Victoria and her family.

- Encourage Victoria and her family to continue to attend church and to participate in religious practices.

Family Integrity Promotion
- Identify typical family coping mechanisms during a conference scheduled late in afternoon at the cancer clinic when the children are able to attend. Provide discussion of their mother's progress. Establish a presence, and express a realistic hope of mother's prognosis.

- Encourage Joe to communicate frequently and openly with Victoria so he can better understand Victoria's feelings, and encourage him to create special times in which they spend time with each other every day to talk about feelings and fears and connect with each other.

EXPECTED OUTCOMES (NOC)†

- In 2 weeks, Victoria, Joe, and children will discuss patient's beliefs about the future and her hope of having the cancer cured.
- In 4 weeks Victoria will report son and daughter's ability to discuss fears with mother.
- By the end of this week, Victoria will make a formal time in her day to pray with family members.
- In 3 weeks Victoria will report that she and Joe are able to discuss their feelings and fears on a daily basis.

RATIONALE

Establishing rapport, active listening, and trust are necessary when caring for people with spiritual needs (Grange and others, 2008).
When people pray, they recognize the importance of their relationships with others and experience enhanced connectedness (O'Brien, 2008).
African Americans who attend church and actively participate in religious activities experience improved spiritual, mental, and physical health (Holt and McClure, 2006).

Diagnosis of cancer causes entire family to grieve. Discussing coping mechanisms used in the past helps children cope with illness. Discussion of illness ensures children will have accurate perception of mother's clinical condition and treatment. Some children experience spiritual growth when they effectively grieve a loss through personal reflection (Leighton, 2008).
Connection between a couple is enhanced when men whose wives have breast cancer are encouraged to communicate openly, support their wives' experience with breast cancer, and spend time with their wives. In addition, the wife experiences less anxiety and is better able to care for herself (Lewis and others, 2008).

EVALUATION

NURSING ACTIONS	PATIENT RESPONSE/FINDING	ACHIEVEMENT OF OUTCOME
Ask Victoria about her daily routine. Determine if her routine includes time for prayer with the family.	Victoria reports she spends at least 10 minutes every morning in prayer while sitting in her garden. Husband has joined her at times. She meditates for 10 to 15 minutes every day and reports she is going to church regularly.	Victoria is attending to her spiritual health daily and is maintaining connections with herself and with God.
Ask Victoria and Joe about their relationship with themselves and their children.	Victoria and Joe set time aside every day to talk about what is going on that day, but they are having difficulty finding time to spend with their children because of their hectic school schedule.	Victoria is spending time with her husband regularly; she needs some help working out a schedule that will allow her to spend time with her children. Suggest that Victoria plan a family game night or some other fun family activity to allow time for enhanced interaction with children.

†Outcomes classification label from Moorhead S and others, editors: *Nursing outcomes classification (NOC)*, ed 4, St. Louis, 2008, Mosby.
‡Intervention classification labels from Bulechek GM and others, editors: *Nursing interventions classification (NIC)*, ed 5, St. Louis, 2008, Mosby.

CONCEPT MAP

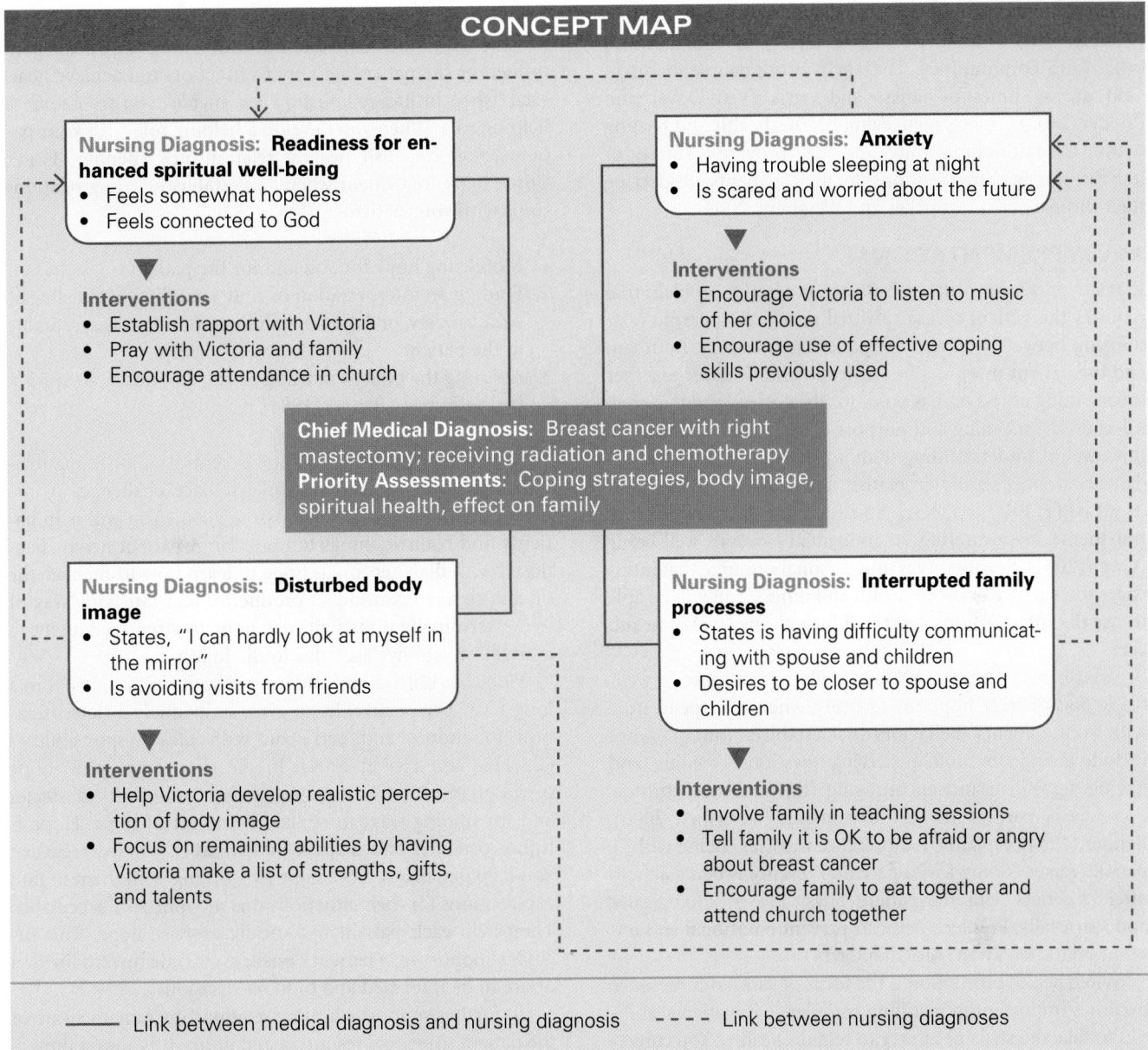

Figure 20-3 ■ Concept Map.

quires helping patients adjust to loss or stressful situations, some goals are long term (e.g., regaining spiritual comfort or affirming a purpose in life). Short-term goals, such as renewing participation in religious practices, are helpful to allow a patient to move toward a more spiritually healthy situation. Outcomes need to relate to what you have learned about the patient. For example, if you know a patient once practiced regular prayer and meditation, you state an outcome for the goal of regaining spiritual comfort as "Patient will pray and meditate daily."

SETTING PRIORITIES Spiritual care is very personalized. Your relationship with the patient allows you to understand your patient's priorities. If you have developed a mutually agreed-on plan with the patient, he or she is able to relate what is most important. Spiritual priorities need not be sacrificed for physical care priorities. For example, if your pa-

tient is in acute distress, focus your care to help the patient gain a sense of control. In the case of a terminally ill patient, spiritual care is possibly the most important intervention you will provide (Prince-Paul, 2008).

COLLABORATIVE CARE To ensure ongoing spiritual care, it sometimes becomes necessary to involve family members, significant others, and clergy to lend support. This means you learned from the assessment which individuals or groups have formed a fellowship with the patient. These individuals become involved in all levels of your care plan. The patient's support network will assist in sharing quiet moments of prayer, reading scripture to the patient, and even giving physical care. In a hospital setting the pastoral care department is a valuable resource. These professionals provide insight about how and when to best support patients and families. When caring for patients with spiritual needs in the community setting, make a referral to a parish nurse if possible. Parish nurses work in a variety of churches and other faith communities. They help bring people closer to God during times of illness and crisis (Van Dover and Pfieffer, 2007). Their practice emphasizes health and healing within the faith community, and they provide a variety of holistic nursing interventions to their patients, respecting their diverse needs (Smucker and Weinberg, 2008).

■■■ IMPLEMENTATION

If a patient is in spiritual distress or has a health problem that requires the patient to use spiritual resources, a caring relationship between you and the patient is necessary. Both you and the patient must feel free to let go and discover together the meaning illness or loss poses for the patient and the effect it has on the meaning and purpose of life. When you achieve this level of understanding with a patient, it enables you to deliver care in a sensitive, creative, and appropriate manner.

HEALTH PROMOTION   Spiritual care needs to be a central theme in promoting an individual's overall well-being (Grant, 2004). Spirituality is one personal resource that influences the balance between health and illness. You will be able to use the interventions described here at any level of health care.

Establishing Presence   You contribute to a sense of well-being and provide hope for recovery when you spend time with your patients. Behaviors that establish your presence include giving attention, answering questions, listening, and having a positive and encouraging (but realistic) attitude. Presence is part of the art of nursing (Tavernier, 2006). Benner (1984) explains that presence involves "being with" a patient versus "doing for" a patient. Presence is being able to offer closeness with the patient physically, psychologically, and spiritually. Presence helps to prevent emotional and environmental isolation (see Chapter 18).

When health promotion is the focus of care, your presence becomes important in instilling confidence in patients' abilities to take the steps necessary to remain healthy. You convey a caring presence by listening to patients' concerns, willingly involving family in discussions about the patient's health, showing self-confidence when providing health instruction, and supporting your patients when they make decisions about their health.

Trust is fundamental to any relationship. The attitude you convey when first interacting with a patient sets the tone for all conversations (see Chapter 10). Actively listening to the meaning of what a patient says is most important. It involves paying attention to the person's words and tone of voice and entering his or her frame of reference. By observing the patient's expressions and body language, you will find cues to help the patient explore ways to achieve inner peace, take action, or manage pain. Your role as a nurse is not to solve the spiritual problems of patients but to provide an environment where your patients can express spirituality (O'Brien, 2008).

Supporting a Healing Relationship   When giving spiritual care, look beyond isolated patient problems and recognize the broader picture of a patient's holistic needs. For ex-

ample, do not look at a patient's back pain as just a problem to solve with quick remedies but rather look at how the pain influences the patient's ability to function and achieve goals established in life. A holistic view enables you to assume a helping role. When you develop a helping role with your patients, you establish healing relationships (Benner, 1984). Three steps are evident when you establish healing relationships with your patients:

1. Mobilizing hope for you and for the patient
2. Finding an interpretation or understanding of the illness, pain, anxiety, or other stressful emotion that is acceptable to the patient
3. Assisting the patient in using social, emotional, or spiritual resources (Benner, 1984)

Mobilizing the patient's hope is central to a healing relationship. Hope motivates people to face challenges in life (Chi, 2007; Lohne and Severinsson, 2006). You will help patients find realistic things to hope for. A patient newly diagnosed with diabetes might hope to learn how to manage the disease so as to continue a productive and satisfying way of life. A terminally ill patient may hope to attend a daughter's graduation and live each day to the fullest.

Hope has both short- and long-term implications. From a long-term perspective, hope gives individuals a determination to endure and carry on with life's responsibilities (Buckley and Herth, 2004). In the short-term view, hope provides an incentive for constructive coping with obstacles and for finding ways to realize the object of hope. Hope is future oriented and helps a patient work toward recovery. You help patients achieve hope by working with them to find explanations for their situations that are mutually acceptable. Then help each patient realistically exercise hope. This includes supporting a patient's positive attitude toward life or a desire to be informed and to make decisions.

To further support a healing relationship, remain aware of the patient's spiritual resources and needs. It is always important for patients to be able to express and exercise their beliefs and to find spiritual comfort. When illness or treatment creates confusion or uncertainty for the patient, recognize the possible effect this can have on a patient's well-being. How can spiritual resources be used and strengthened? Having a clear sense of what illness will be like for an individual helps the person to apply all resources toward recovery.

ACUTE CARE   Within an acute care setting, support and enhancement of a patient's spiritual well-being is a challenge because the focus of health care seems to be one of treatment and cure rather than care. Patients also experience multiple stressors and frequently feel like they are losing control. To overcome these challenges, display a soothing presence and supportive touch as you implement nursing interventions. Some patients are fearful of experiencing an illness that threatens their loss of control, and they look for someone to offer competent direction. Your artful use of hands, encouraging words of support, promotion of connectedness, and calm and decisive approach will establish a presence that builds trust (Tavernier, 2006). Work closely with patients to maximize resources that support their spirituality. For example, you build trust with your patients when you perform procedures competently. You promote connectedness and build trust by listening to the dying patient's concerns, providing reassurance and comfort, and helping the patient complete unfinished business (Narayanasamy and others, 2004).

Support Systems Using support systems is important in any health care setting. Support systems serve as a human link connecting the patient, the nurse, and the patient's lifestyle before an illness. In today's society, support comes from many areas, including the family, friends, and support groups. Nolan and others (2006) found that an Internet-based chat room for family members of patients who had pancreatic cancer helped family members express hope, accept the power of God and eternal life, and find positive meaning in cancer. The members of the chat room formed a special bond with each other and prayed with and for each other, even though many of them had never met in person. Part of the patient's caregiving environment is the regular presence of supportive family and friends. Families often influence how patients perceive their illness. You enhance the patient's support network when you include the patient's family and friends in planning care. The patient's support system is a source of coping, faith, and hope (Black and Lobo, 2008).

When a patient depends on family, friends, spiritual advisors, and members of the clergy for support, encourage them to visit the patient regularly. Make all the patient's visitors welcome on nursing units, and ensure privacy during visits to provide spiritual comfort. If the patient desires, ask the pastoral care department to notify the patient's clergy of the patient's admission. Often illness and the hospital environment produce uncertainty that frightens family members and friends. Help the family to feel welcome, and use their support and presence to promote the patient's healing. For example, including family members in prayer is a thoughtful gesture if it is appropriate to the patient's religion and if family members are comfortable participating. Encouraging the family to bring meaningful religious symbols to the patient's bedside and facilitating the administration of sacraments, rites, and rituals offers significant spiritual support. Do not forget to support the family as well. When you support the family's spirituality and faith practices, you decrease their anxiety and feelings of uncertainty (Kloos and Daly, 2008).

Diet Therapies Food and nutrition are important aspects of nursing care. Food is also an important component of some religious observances. For example, people in some Hindu and Islamic sects are vegetarian. Muslims are not allowed to eat pork, and they fast during the month of Ramadan. Orthodox Jewish patients observe kosher dietary restrictions. Native Americans have food practices influenced by individual tribal beliefs. Like many aspects of a particular culture or religion, food and the rituals surrounding the preparation and serving of food are important to a patient's spirituality. Integrate the patient's dietary preferences into daily care when possible, and consult with the health care institution's dietitian. In the event that a hospital or other health care agency cannot prepare food in the preferred way, ask the family to bring meals that are appropriate for dietary restrictions posed by the patient's condition.

Supporting Rituals You become active in your patients' spiritual care by supporting patients' participation in spiritual rituals and activities. This is especially important for older adults (Box 20-4). Plan care to allow time for religious readings, spiritual visitations, or even attendance at religious services. Some churches and synagogues offer audiotapes of religious services. Allow family members to plan a prayer session or an organized reading when appropriate. Taped meditations, religious music, and televised religious services provide other effective treatment options. Be respectful of icons, medals, prayer rugs, or crosses that patients bring to a health care setting, and make sure they are not accidentally lost or misplaced.

BOX 20-4   CARE OF THE OLDER ADULT
Supporting Older Adults' Spirituality

- Religious activities, attitudes, and spiritual experiences are very common among older adults. Those who experience spiritual well-being have strong social support, better emotional health, and to some extent, improved physical health (Yoon, 2006).
- Respecting privacy and dignity is an essential part of nursing care, especially when meeting spiritual needs of the older adult (Anderberg and others, 2007).
- Older adults use a variety of strategies such as exercise, physical therapy, and complementary medicine to cope with pain and chronic illness. Including religious activities positively enhances coping (Yeun and others, 2007).
- Feelings of connectedness are important for the older adult (Lamb and others, 2008). Enhance connectedness by helping the older patient find meaning and purpose in life, listening actively to concerns, and being present (Narayanasamy and others, 2004).
- Beliefs in the afterlife increase as adults grow older. Make visits from clergy, social workers, lawyers, and even financial advisors available so patients feel as though they have completed all unfinished business. Leaving a legacy to loved ones prepares the older adult to leave the world with a sense of meaning (Ebersole and others, 2008). Legacies include oral histories, works of art, publications, photographs, or other objects of significance.

RESTORATIVE AND CONTINUING CARE

Prayer and Meditation The act of prayer gives an individual the opportunity to renew personal faith and belief in a higher being in a specific, focused way that is either highly ritualized and formal or quite spontaneous and informal. Prayer is an effective coping resource for physical and psychological symptoms (Narayanasamy and Narayanasamy, 2008). Patients pray in private or pursue opportunities for group prayer with family, friends, or clergy. Some patients pray while listening to music. Be supportive of prayer by giving the patient privacy if desired, by learning if the patient wishes to have you participate, and by suggesting prayer when you know it is a coping resource for the patient. If prayer is not suitable for a patient, alternatives include listening to calming music or reading a book, poetry, or inspirational texts selected by the patient.

Meditation is effective in creating a relaxation response that reduces daily stress. Patients who meditate often state they have an increased awareness of their spirituality and of the presence of God or a supreme being (Box 20-5). Meditation exercises give patients relief from chronic pain, insomnia, anxiety, and depression and help in coping with the side effects of uncomfortable therapy (Bormann and others, 2008; Wachholtz and Pargament, 2008). Meditation involves sitting quietly in a comfortable position with eyes closed and repeating a sound, phrase, or sacred word in rhythm with breathing, while disregarding intrusive thoughts. Individuals who meditate regularly (twice a day, for 10 or 20 minutes) experience decreased metabolism and heart rate, easier breathing, and slower brain waves. Chapter 31 addresses relaxation approaches.

BOX 20-5   PATIENT TEACHING

Teaching Plan for Meditation Techniques

At one of her clinic visits, Victoria tells Jeff, "My friend told me yesterday that when she had cancer, she used meditation to help her cope with the side effects of her chemotherapy. I was thinking that I might try meditating to see if it would help me, but I don't know how to meditate. Can you help me?" Jeff develops the following teaching plan for Victoria:

OUTCOME
- Victoria will verbalize feelings of relaxation and self-transcendence after meditation.

TEACHING STRATEGIES
- Provide a brief description of what will be taught.
- Give Victoria a patient teaching sheet that describes how to meditate.
- Help Victoria identify at least one quiet place in her home that has minimal interruptions.
- Encourage her to use soft background noise like a fan or soft music during meditation to block out distractions.
- Teach Victoria the steps of meditation—sit in a comfortable position with the back straight; breathe slowly; and focus on a sound, a prayer, or an image.
- Encourage Victoria to meditate for 10 to 20 minutes 2 times a day.
- Answer any questions.
- Reinforce information as needed.

EVALUATION STRATEGIES
- Ask Victoria to identify what she learned about herself and how she feels after meditating.

BOX 20-6   EVALUATION

Victoria returns to the clinic 1 week after making a plan to enhance her spiritual health with Jeff. A member of her church accompanies Victoria because Joe is out of town on a business trip. Jeff wants to evaluate whether Victoria continues to feel connected with herself, Joe, her children, and God. Jeff asks, "Tell me, Mrs. Timms, have you had a chance yet to try any of the approaches we talked about last week to give yourself, Joe, and the kids a chance to talk about their feelings? If so, what were the results?" Victoria reports, "Yes, I spend at least 10 minutes every morning in prayer while I sit in my garden, and I have been meditating for 10 to 15 minutes every day. Joe and I set aside at least 15 minutes a day to talk in private after the kids go to bed. If he is not in town, we talk on the phone. Joe and I planned a family game night last Saturday evening with the kids. We shared lots of funny family stories and began to talk with them about my cancer treatment. The kids really seemed to enjoy being together as a family. They asked many questions, and we talked about chores they could do to help me. They are looking forward to coming to the clinic Thursday. I hope this will help them feel less frightened." Jeff also determines that Victoria has spoken with close friends from her church, and they plan to visit her this week. Victoria states she is going to see the physical therapist today.

In an effort to evaluate whether the clinic has met Victoria's expectations, Jeff asks, "Your faith is strong, and it is my hope you have felt comfortable in talking about your worries. Do you believe we have helped you so far with your concerns about your family?" Victoria replies, "The best thing you have done is listen and recognize how important my family is to me. Your suggestions have helped so far; I am truly blessed to have met all of you nice people at the clinic."

DOCUMENTATION NOTE
"Visited the clinic for the third week of chemotherapy. Denies nausea but is complaining of some soreness in the mouth and a loss of hair. Asks questions readily and made an appointment with the physical therapist as recommended. States has enhanced her connectedness with herself and her family by taking time to pray and meditate, talking and listening with her family, and having fun with her children. Expresses hope that her children will feel less frightened over the diagnosis and states her children will be coming to the next clinic visit."

■■■EVALUATION

PATIENT CARE Attainment of spiritual health is a lifelong goal. Patients will experience the need to clarify values (see Chapter 5), reshape philosophies, and live those experiences that help to shape purpose in life. As you provide spiritual care, always evaluate whether the patient achieved planned outcomes and goals (Box 20-6). Compare the patient's level of spiritual health with the behaviors and perceptions noted in the nursing assessment. For example, if your assessment found the patient losing hope, the follow-up evaluation involves a discussion to determine if the patient has regained an attitude that life is worth living. Family and friends are a useful source of evaluative information. Successful outcomes reveal the patient developing an increased or restored sense of connectedness with family; maintaining, reviewing, or reforming a sense of purpose in life; and, for some, a confidence and trust in a supreme being or higher power.

For patients with a serious or terminal illness, evaluation focuses on the goal of helping the patient retain faith and hope or express openly the uncertainties life poses. Evaluate how well the patient is accepting the illness and whether hope has enabled the patient to recognize individual mortality and focus on living for each day. You cannot assume all patients have faith in a higher power. However, your support helps patients find meaning in life and death, accept their destiny, and be at peace (Wong and others, 2004).

PATIENT EXPECTATIONS Evaluate whether you met your patient's expectations. When you evaluate spiritual care, determine if you respected the patient's spiritual practices and if the quality of the nurse-patient relationship was supportive. Both the patient and family should relate that opportunities were offered for religious rituals. With respect to the nurse-patient relationship, does the patient express trust and confidence in you? Is the patient able to discuss those things that are important spiritually? Taking time to ask the patient to reflect on the quality of the nurse-patient relationship is time well spent. Asking the patient, "Have you felt comfortable in saying what you feel is important to you spiritually?" will determine whether you developed an effective healing relationship.

KEY POINTS

- Attending to a patient's spirituality ensures a holistic focus to nursing practice.
- Frequently the concepts of spirituality and religion are interchanged, but spirituality is a much broader and more unifying concept than religion.
- An individual's beliefs and spiritual well-being influence physical health status.
- Faith and hope are closely linked to a person's spiritual well-being, providing an inner strength for dealing with illness and disability.
- Research suggests there is a link between a patient's spirituality and potential for healing.
- Acute and chronic illness, terminal illness, and near-death experiences pose spiritual problems for individuals.
- The provision of appropriate spiritual care requires you to critically apply knowledge from principles related to caring, cultural care, loss and grief, and therapeutic communication.
- Avoid biases when assessing and planning spiritual care.

- Learning to practice caring and compassion helps you to discover a patient's life values and meaning.
- Connectedness and fellowship with other persons are a source of hope for a patient.
- Patients often have spiritual strengths that you will use as resources to help them assume healthier lives.
- Interruptions or changes to customary religious practices affect the support that religion contributes to a person's well-being.
- Common religious rituals include private worship, prayer, singing, use of a rosary, and scripture reading.
- The personal nature of spirituality requires open communication and the establishment of trust between you and the patient.
- Establishing presence involves giving attention, answering questions, having an encouraging attitude, and conveying a sense of trust.
- Part of a patient's caregiving environment is the regular presence of family, friends, and spiritual advisors.

CRITICAL THINKING EXERCISES

Victoria and Joe return to the oncology clinic with their children for Victoria's first chemotherapy treatment. Jeff continues his spiritual assessment of the family unit and determines how well they are coping with Victoria's diagnosis.

1. During his assessment, Jeff pays close attention to what Victoria and her family say. Jeff answers their questions about breast cancer and Victoria's treatments and remains with the family while the nurse begins Victoria's chemotherapy treatment. These interventions are examples of how Jeff establishes _____ with Victoria and her family.

2. While Victoria is receiving her chemotherapy, Jeff takes her children to the family waiting room to have a snack. While they are sitting in the family room, the children tell Jeff that they are angry about their mother's breast cancer and they are really upset that she is going to lose her hair because of her treatments. They both ask Jeff why God has done this to their family and say they are no longer inviting friends over to their house. What nursing diagnosis should Jeff develop next in his care plan?

3. After the children finish their snack, Jeff walks with them back to Victoria. He begins to speak with Joe. Joe says, "I am having trouble sleeping at night because I am so worried about Victoria. I also am having trouble focusing at work because I can't get her off my mind." Based on this information, Jeff determines that *anxiety related to change in health status of wife* is an appropriate nursing diagnosis for Joe at this time. List two nursing interventions that will enhance Joe's spiritual health and decrease his anxiety.

4. Based on the assessment data Jeff gathers, he decides that he needs to further assess Joe's feelings of connectedness. Which of the following questions will assess Joe's feelings of connectedness? Select all that apply.
   a. How happy or satisfied are you with your life?
   b. How do you feel after you pray?
   c. Who is the most important person in your life?
   d. How satisfied are you with your accomplishments in your life so far?
   e. Describe the relationship you have with your wife.
   f. Who has helped you the most when you have faced difficult times in the past?

ⓔvolve   *Answers to Critical Thinking Questions can be found on the Evolve website.*

REVIEW QUESTIONS

1. You are caring for a patient who has just had a heart attack. When you walk into the waiting room, your patient's spouse is wringing her hands and she is tearful when she speaks. You place your hand on the spouse's shoulder and softly ask, "Can you tell me what is bothering you?" In this example you are demonstrating:
   1. Presence
   2. Connecting
   3. Establishing hope
   4. Offering social resource

2. You are completing a spiritual assessment on a 27-year-old male patient admitted to the hospital following a spinal cord injury. When you ask him if he prays to God, he replies, "I don't pray. I just try to find meaning in what I do and in my relationships with my family and friends." Based on his reply, this man most likely is an:
   1. Agenic
   2. Atheist
   3. Agnostic
   4. Anarchist

3. You are caring for a 21-year-old female patient who recently had her first baby. During your assessment you learn that the patient recently lost her job. After completing the referral, you ask the patient to describe her feelings now that she has lost her job. The patient states that even though she is going through a tough time, her family and the baby's father have been very supportive. She knows that her situation is only temporary, and this situation has helped her "put things into perspective." This patient is likely experiencing the nursing diagnosis of:
   1. *Spiritual distress*
   2. *Ineffective coping*
   3. *Risk for spiritual distress*
   4. *Readiness for enhanced spiritual well-being*

4. You are working in an emergency department when a patient comes in because of severe abdominal pain. The patient's clothes are torn and do not match. You note an odor when you walk into the room, and you know from the patient's admission database that the patient is homeless. You can tell that there is something that is really bothering him. You pull up a chair next to the patient's bed, sit in the chair, and ask the patient, "Tell me what concerns you have." You are demonstrating an intellectual standard for critical thinking called:
   1. Risk taking
   2. Significance
   3. Compassion
   4. Completeness

5. You are caring for a patient who is dealing with terminal cancer. The patient is in pain and is contemplating hospice care. After assessing your patient, you discover that he is very anxious about making this decision. You know that your patient is a farmer and that he likes to fish. Based on this information, which of the following interventions might help reduce the patient's pain and elevate his mood? Select all that apply.
   1. Ask the patient if he would like to pray with you.
   2. Tell the patient a funny joke about a fisherman.
   3. Give the patient an antihypertensive medication.
   4. Lead the patient through a guided imagery exercise of fishing at a peaceful place.

6. A patient who recently was severely injured following a motorcycle accident shows faith when she states:
   1. "My pain medicine helps me feel better."
   2. "I know I will get better if I just keep trying."
   3. "I have had a great life and a good marriage."
   4. "My daughter is a major source of support for me."

7. You are caring for a patient who is very angry and depressed. His brother betrayed his trust several years ago, and he still has not been able to forgive his brother. His son and daughter-in-law recently had a new baby, and you overhear him saying, "Great, just what they need—another mouth to feed. What were they thinking when they decided to have another child?" Based on this information, you determine that this patient is experiencing challenges with his:
   1. Faith
   2. Spirituality
   3. Overall health
   4. Spiritual health

8. Which of the following statements made by a patient who has experienced a miscarriage recently most requires follow-up by the nurse?
   1. "I believe that my child is in heaven."
   2. "My husband sits with me when I cry."
   3. "I have not eaten lunch with my friends since my miscarriage."
   4. "Sometimes it is hard to understand why bad things happen to good people."

9. You are caring for a patient who had a near-death experience 2 months ago. He tells you that he remembers seeing paramedics and physicians giving him cardiopulmonary resuscitation (CPR), and he is asking you questions about the event. Your priority intervention is to:
   1. Inform the patient that it was probably just a dream
   2. Sit with the patient and ask him to describe what he remembers
   3. Encourage him to share this experience with his wife immediately
   4. Ask the patient's health care provider to answer the patient's questions

10. You are caring for a patient who is supposed to go to surgery in about 10 minutes. The patient starts to cry. She tells you that she is very anxious about the surgery and she is in pain. Your priority intervention is to:
    1. Reposition the patient
    2. Help her gain a sense of control
    3. Give her a sedative-hypnotic medication
    4. Call the pastoral care department to ask someone to come pray with the patient

Answers to Review Questions can be found on pages 1197-1198.

REFERENCES

Anderberg P and others: Preserving dignity and caring for older adults: a concept analysis, *J Adv Nurs* 59(6):635, 2007.

Baldacchino DR: Nursing competencies for spiritual care, *J Clin Nurs* 15(7):885, 2006.

Banks-Wallace J, Parks L: It's all sacred: African American women's perspectives on spirituality, *Issues Ment Health Nurs* 25(1):25, 2004.

Benner P: *From novice to expert*, Menlo Park, Calif, 1984, Addison-Wesley.

Bennett MP, Langacher C: Humor and laughter may influence health. II. Complementary therapies and humor in a clinical population, *eCAM* 3(2):187, 2006.

Betty LS: Are they hallucinations or are they real? The spirituality of detached and near-death experiences, *Omega* 53(1-2):37, 2006.

Black K, Lobo M: A conceptual review of family resilience factors, *J Fam Nurs* 14(1):33, 2008.

Bormann JE and others: A spiritually based group intervention for combat veterans with posttraumatic stress disorder: feasibility study, 26(2):109, 2008.

Boyd AS, Wilmoth MC: An innovative community-based intervention for African American women with breast cancer: the witness project, *Health Soc Work* 31(1):77, 2006.

Buckley J, Herth K: Fostering hope in terminally ill patients, *Nurs Stand* 19(10):33, 2004.

Bulechek GM and others, editors: *Nursing interventions classification (NIC)*, ed 5, St. Louis, 2008, Mosby.

Burkhart L, Solari-Twadell PA, Haas S: Addressing spiritual leadership: an organizational model, *J Nurs Admin* 38(1):33, 2008.

Carpenter K and others: Spirituality: a dimension of holistic critical care nursing, *Dimens Crit Care Nurs* 27(1):16, 2008.

Carrico DJ, Peters KM, Diokno AM: Guided imagery for women with internal cystitis: results of a prospective, randomized, controlled pilot study, *J Altern Complement Med* 14(1):53, 2008.

Cavendish R and others: Patients' perceptions of spirituality and the nurse as a spiritual care provider, *Holist Nurs Pract* 20(1):41, 2006.

Chang H, Wallis M, Tiralongo E: Use of complementary and alternative medicine among people living with diabetes: literature review, *J Adv Nurs* 58(4):307, 2007.

Chi GC: The role of hope in patients with cancer, *Oncol Nurs Forum* 34(2):415, 2007.

Chiu L and others: An integrative review of the concept of spirituality in the health sciences, *West J Nurs Res* 26(4):405, 2004.

Choumanova I and others: Religion and spirituality in coping with breast cancer: perspectives of Chilean women, *Breast J* 12(4):349, 2006.

Delgado C: A discussion of the concept of spirituality, *Nurs Sci Q* 18(2):157, 2005.

Drentea P, Goldner MA: Caring outside of the home: the effects of race on depression, *Ethn Health* 11(1):41, 2006.

Duffy N: Supporting a patient after a near-death experience, *Nursing* 37(4):46, 2007.

Ebersole P and others: *Toward healthy aging*, ed 7, St. Louis, 2008, Mosby.

Edelman CL, Mandle CL: *Health promotion throughout the life span*, ed 6, St. Louis, 2006, Mosby.

Elkins M, Cavendish R: Developing a plan for pediatric spiritual care, *Holist Nurs Pract* 18(4):179, 2004.

Facente A: Humor in health care: irreverent or invaluable? *Nursing* 36(4):64hn6, 2006.

Fowler MDM: *Guide to the code of ethics for nurses: interpretation and application*, Silver Spring, Md, 2008, American Nurses Association.

Gibson LM, Smith Hendricks C: Integrative review of spirituality in African American breast cancer survivors, *ABNF J* 17(2):67, 2006.

Gillum TL, Sullivan CM, Bybee DI, The importance of spirituality in the lives of domestic violence survivors, *Violence Against Women* 12(3):240, 2006.

Giger JN, Davidhizar RE: *Transcultural nursing: assessment and intervention*, ed 5, St. Louis, 2008, Mosby.

Grange CM and others: Identifying supportive and unsupportive responses of others: perspectives of African American and Caucasian cancer patients, *J Psychosoc Oncol* 26(1):81, 2008.

Grant D: Spiritual interventions: how, when, and why nurses use them, *Holist Nurs Pract* 18(1):36, 2004.

Gray J: Measuring spirituality: conceptual and methodological considerations, *Journal of Theory Construction and Testing* 10(2):58, 2006.

Hendricks-Ferguson V: Hope and spiritual well-being in adolescents with cancer, *West J Nurs Res* 30:385, 2008.

Hermann CP: The degree to which spiritual needs of patients near the end of life are met, *Oncol Nurs Forum* 34(1), 2007.

Hill TD and others: Religious attendance and cognitive functioning among older Mexican Americans, *J Gerontol B Psychol Sci Soc Sci* 61(B1):3, 2006.

Hockenberry MJ, Wilson D: *Wong's essentials of pediatric nursing*, ed 8, St. Louis, 2009, Mosby.

Hollins S: Spirituality and religion: exploring the relationship, *Nurs Manage* 12(6):22, 2005.

Holt CL, McClure SM: Perceptions of the religion-health connection among African American church members, *Qual Health Res* 16(2):268, 2006.

Hsieh C and others: Positive psychological measure: constructing and evaluating the reliability and validity of a Chinese humor scale applicable to professional nursing, *J Nurs Res* 13(2):206, 2005.

Hufton E: Parting gifts: the spiritual needs of children, *J Child Health Care* 10(3):240, 2006.

Katerndahl DA: Impact of spiritual symptoms and their interactions on health services and life satisfaction, *Ann Fam Med* 6(5):412, 2008.

Kloos JA, Daly BJ: Effect of a family-maintained progress journal on anxiety of families of critically ill patients, *Crit Care Nurse Q* 31(2):96, 2008.

Lamb M and others: The psychosocial spiritual experience of elderly individuals recovering from stroke: a systematic review, *Int J Evid Based Healthc* 6(2):173, 2008.

Leak A, Hu J, King CR: Symptom distress, spirituality, and quality of life in African American breast cancer survivors, *Cancer Nurse* 31(1):E15, 2008.

Leighton S: Bereavement therapy with adolescents: facilitating a process of spiritual growth, *J Child Adolesc Psychiatr Nurs* 21(1):24, 2008.

Lewis FM and others: Helping her heal: a pilot study of an educational counseling intervention for spouses of women with breast cancer, *Psycho-Oncology* 17:131, 2008.

Lhussier M, Carr SM, Wilcockson J: The evaluation of an end-of-life integrated care pathway, *Int J Palliat Nurs* 13(2):74, 2007.

Lindberg DA: Integrative review of research related to mediation, spirituality, and the elderly, *Geriatr Nurs* 26(6):372, 2005.

Lohne V, Severinsson E: The power of hope: patients' experiences of hope a year after acute spinal cord injury, *J Clin Nurs* 15(3):315, 2006.

MacMaster SA and others: Evaluation of a faith-based culturally relevant program for African American substance users at risk for HIV in the Southern United States, *Res Soc Work Pract* 17(2):229, 2007.

McEvoy M: Culture and spirituality as an integrated concept in pediatric care, *MCN Am J Matern Child Nurs* 28(1):39, 2003.

McSherry W: The principal components model: a model for advancing spirituality and spiritual care within nursing and health care practice, *J Clin Nurs* 15(7):905, 2006.

McSherry W, Cash K, Ross L: Meaning of spirituality: implications for nursing practice, *J Clin Nurs* 13(8):934, 2004.

McSherry W, Smith J: How do children express their spiritual needs? *Paediatr Nurs* 19(3):17, 2007.

Mednick L and others: Hope more, worry less: hope as a potential resilience factor in mothers of very young children with type I diabetes, *Child Health Care* 36(4):385, 2007.

Miner-Williams D: Putting a puzzle together: making spirituality meaningful for nursing using an evolving theoretical framework, *J Clin Nurs* 15(7):811, 2006.

Moorhead S and others, editors: *Nursing outcomes classification (NOC)*, ed 4, St. Louis, 2008, Mosby.

NANDA International: *NANDA nursing diagnoses: definitions and classifications 2009-2011*, Philadelphia, 2009, Wiley-Blackwell.

Narayanasamy A: Spiritual coping mechanisms in chronic illness: a qualitative study, *J Clin Nurs* 13(1):116, 2004.

Narayanasamy A, Narayanasamy M: The healing power of prayer and its implications for nursing, *Br J Nurs* 17(6):394, 2008.

Narayanasamy A and others: Responses to the spiritual needs of older people, *J Adv Nurs* 48(1):6, 2004.

Nelson-Becker H, Nakashima M, Canda ER: Spiritual assessment in aging: a framework for clinicians, *J Gerontol Soc Work* 48(3/4):331, 2007.

Nolan MT and others: Spiritual issues of family members in a pancreatic cancer chat room, *Oncol Nurs Forum* 33(2):239, 2006.

O'Brien ME: *Spirituality in nursing: standing on holy ground*, ed 3, Sudbury, Mass, 2008, Jones & Bartlett.

Perry DJ: Self-transcendence: Lonergan's key to integration of nursing theory, research, and practice, *Nurs Philos* 5(1):67, 2004.

Peters L, Sellick K: Quality of life of cancer patients receiving inpatient and home-based palliative care, *J Adv Nurs* 53(5):524, 2006.

Prince-Paul M: Relationships among communicative acts, social well-being, and spiritual well-being on the quality of life at the end of life in patients with cancer enrolled in hospice, *J Palliat Med* 11(1):20, 2008.

Ross L: Spiritual care in nursing: an overview of the research to date, *J Clin Nurs* 15(7):852, 2006.

Schneider MA, Mannell RC: Beacon in the storm: an exploration of the spirituality and faith of parents whose children have cancer, *Issues Compr Pediatr Nurs* 29(1):3, 2006.

Skalla KA, McCoy JP: Spiritual assessment of patients with cancer: the moral authority, vocational, aesthetic, social, and transcendent model, *Oncol Nurs Forum* 33(4):745, 2006.

Smith AR: Using the synergy model to provide spiritual nursing care in critical care settings, *Crit Care Nurse* 26(4):41, 2006.

Smith J, McSherry W: Spirituality and child development: a concept analysis, *J Adv Nurs* 45(3):307, 2004.

Smith-Stoner M: End of life needs of patients who practice Tibetan Buddhism, *J Hospice Palliat Nurs* 7(4):228, 2005.

Smucker CJ, Weinberg L: *Faith community nursing: developing a quality practice*, Silver Spring, Md, 2008, American Nurses Association.

Tanyi RA: Spirituality and family nursing: spiritual assessment and interventions for family, *J Adv Nurs* 53(3):287, 2006.

Tanyi RA, Werner JS: Spirituality in African American and Caucasian women with end-stage renal disease on hemodialysis treatment, *Health Care Women Int* 28:141, 2007.

Tavernier SS: An evidence-based conceptual analysis of presence, *Holist Nurs Pract* 20(3):152, 2006.

Teixeira ME: Self-transcendence: a concept analysis for nursing praxis, *Holist Nurs Pract* 22(1):25, 2008.

The Joint Commission: *Standards*, 2008, http://www.jointcommission.org/Standards/.

Underwood SM, Powell RL: Religion and spirituality: influence on health/risk behavior and cancer screening behavior of African Americans, *ABNF J* 17(1):20, 2006.

Underwood SM and others: Pilot study of the breast cancer experiences of African American women with a family history of breast cancer: implications for nursing practice, *ABNF J* 19(3):107, 2006.

Van Dover L, Pfeiffer JB: Spiritual care in Christian parish nursing, *J Adv Nurs* 57(2):213, 2007.

Van Dyke CJ, Elias MJ: How forgiveness, purpose, and religiosity are related to the mental health and well-being of youth: a review of the literature, *Mental Health, Religion, and Culture* 19(4):395, 2007.

Villagomeza LR: Spiritual distress in adult cancer patients, *Holist Nurs Pract* 19(6):285, 2005.

Villagomeza LR: Mending broken hearts: the role of spirituality in cardiac illness: a research synthesis, 1991-2004, *Holistic Nurs Pract* 20(4):169, 2006.

Wachholtz A, Pargament K: Migraines and meditation: does spirituality matter? *J Behav Med* 31(4):351, 2008.

Wong FKY and others: Health problems encountered by dying patients receiving palliative home care until death, *Cancer Nurs* 27(3):244, 2004.

Wright LM: *Spirituality, suffering, and illness: ideas for healing*, Philadelphia, 2005, FA Davis.

Yampolsky MA and others: The role of spirituality in coping with visual impairment, *J Vis Impair Blind* 102(1):28, 2008.

Yeun HK and others: Actions and personal attributes of community-dwelling older adults to maintain independence, *Phys Occup Ther Geriatr* 25(3):35, 2007.

Yoon DP: Factors affecting subjective well-being for rural elderly individuals: the importance of spirituality, religiousness, and social support, *Journal of Religion and Spirituality in Social Work* 25(2):59, 2006.

Growth and Development

 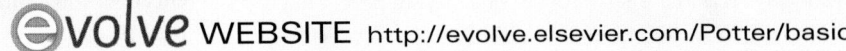
OBJECTIVES

- Compare the frameworks for growth and development as described by major developmental theorists.
- Describe the growth and development changes that occur in individuals from conception through old age.
- Identify factors that promote or interfere with normal growth and development of individuals at each stage of life.

- Specify the physical and psychosocial health concerns of infants, children, adolescents, and adults.
- Use knowledge of growth and development to enhance use of the nursing process for individuals across the life span.
- Identify specific nursing interventions for the health promotion of patients across the life span.
- Use critical judgment to determine appropriate teaching topics for individual patients across the life span.

KEY TERMS

adolescence, p. 579
Alzheimer's disease, p. 587
climacteric, p. 584
delirium, p. 586

dementia, p. 586
depression, p. 587
development, p. 572
geriatrics, p. 585
growth, p. 572

maturation, p. 572
menarche, p. 580
menopause, p. 584
neonate, p. 574
polypharmacy, p. 588

puberty, p. 579
reality orientation, p. 588
reminiscence, p. 587
teratogens, p. 574

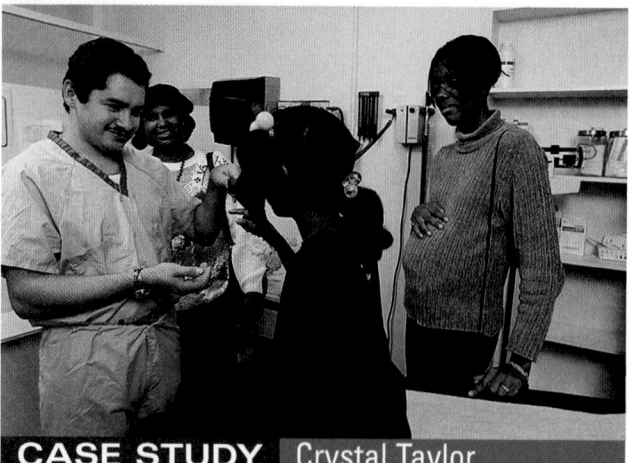

CASE STUDY Crystal Taylor

Crystal Taylor, a 25-year-old African American woman, is a single parent of 2½-year-old Zachary and 6-year-old Monica and is in the sixth month of a current pregnancy. She lives with her 44-year-old mother and 15-year-old brother. Crystal's 68-year-old maternal grandmother and aunt live next door and often help care for Zachary and Monica. Crystal has a strong family history for breast cancer. Her grandmother and aunt are both breast cancer survivors. Crystal mentioned that her mother had a mammogram 6 years ago but has not had routine screenings. Crystal's family has used the health care center for years, and she now brings her children to the neighborhood clinic for their health care. Today she has brought Monica to the clinic for her checkup before beginning school.

Louis Ruiz is a 28-year-old student assigned to the clinic. He has to select a family to follow throughout the semester. Louis, who is married and has a 4-year-old son who attends day care, was a medical technician in the army for 4 years. The clinic is Louis' first clinical experience as a nursing student, and he is eager to become involved in health promotion activities but also anxious about his new role as a professional nurse.

As a nurse, you care for individuals of all ages. Human growth and development are orderly, predictable processes beginning with conception and continuing until death. Knowledge of these patterns helps you help your patients reach their full potential (Behrman and others, 2004).

SCIENTIFIC KNOWLEDGE BASE

Growth and Development Theory

The terms *growth* and *development* used together include all of the many changes that take place throughout an individual's lifetime (Hockenberry and Wilson, 2007). **Growth** is the measurable aspect of a person's increase in physical dimensions. Measurable growth indicators include changes in height, weight, teeth and skeletal structures, and sexual characteristics. **Development** occurs gradually and refers to

changes in skill and capacity to function. These changes are qualitative in nature and difficult to measure in exact units. There are, however, certain predictable characteristics that are measurable, such as development proceeds from simple to complex. An example of this is learning to walk before learning to run.

Maturation is the biological plan for the predictable milestones for growth and development. Physical growth and motor development are a function of maturation. Examples of age-related behaviors that follow a specific sequence are sitting, walking, and reading, which are a result of maturation.

A critical period of development refers to a specific phase or period when the presence of a function or reasoning has its greatest effect on a specific aspect of development. For example, if a child does not walk by 20 months, there is delayed gross motor ability, which slows exploration and manipulation of the environment. The success or failure experienced within a phase affects the child's ability to complete the next phases.

THEORIES OF HUMAN DEVELOPMENT Developmental theories provide a framework for examining, describing, and appreciating human development. They are intended to describe how and why people become what they are (Santrock, 2007). Useful theories explain behavior, as well as predict behavior that is testable and observable (Table 21-1). Some theories view development as a continuous process, moving from the simple to the more complex. Others consider it as discontinuous, with alternating periods of relative equilibrium and disequilibrium.

Sigmund Freud Sigmund Freud (1856-1939) provided the first formal structured theory of personality development. Freud's psychoanalytic model of personality development is grounded in the belief that two internal biological forces drive the psychological change in a child: sexual (libido) and aggressive energies. Each of the five stages is associated with a pleasurable zone, serving as the focus of gratification. In the first stage, oral stage, sucking and oral satisfaction are not only vital to life, but also very pleasurable. During the anal stage, the focus of pleasure changes to the anal zone. In Stage 3, phallic stage, the genital organs become the focus of pleasure. In the latency stage, Freud believed that the sexual urges from the earlier phallic stage are repressed and channeled into productive activities that are socially acceptable. The genital stage occurs during adolescence and is a turbulent time for the child and the family. The child's sexual urges reawaken, and social activities begin to occur outside the family circle.

Erik Erikson's Eight Stages of Development Erik Erikson (1902-1994) expanded Freud's psychoanalytic stages into a psychosocial model that covered the whole life span (Santrock, 2007). In this theory, Erikson divided life into eight stages, known as Erikson's eight stages of development (Erikson, 1963, 1997). According to this theory, individuals need to accomplish a particular task before successfully completing the stage. Each task is framed with opposing conflicts, such as trust versus mistrust. Each stage builds upon the successful attainment of the previous developmental conflict. In addition to the five stages in Table 21-1, three additional

TABLE 21-1   Comparison of Major Development Theories of Childhood

DEVELOPMENTAL STAGE (APPROXIMATE AGE)	FREUD (PSYCHOSEXUAL DEVELOPMENT)	ERIKSON (PSYCHOSOCIAL DEVELOPMENT)	PIAGET (LOGICAL AND COGNITIVE DEVELOPMENT AND MORAL DEVELOPMENT)	KOHLBERG (DEVELOPMENT OF MORAL REASONING)
Infancy (birth to 18 months)	Oral stage	Trust versus mistrust Ability to trust others	Sensorimotor period Progress from reflex activity to simple repetitive actions	
Early childhood/ toddler (18 months to 3 years)	Anal stage	Autonomy versus shame and doubt Self-control and independence	Preoperational period—thinking using symbols; egocentric	Preconventional level Punishment-obedience orientation
Preschool (3-5 years)	Phallic stage	Initiative versus guilt Highly imaginative	Use of symbols; egocentric	Preconventional level Premoral Instrumental orientation
Childhood (6-12 years)	Latent stage	Industry versus inferiority Engaged in tasks and activities	Concrete operations period Logical thinking	Conventional level Good-boy, nice-girl orientation
Adolescence (12-19 years)	Genital stage	Identity versus role confusion Sexual maturity, "Who am I?"	Formal operations period Abstract thinking	Postconventional level Social contract orientation

stages occur from young adulthood to the older adulthood years. Stage 6, intimacy versus isolation, occurs as young adults develop a sense of identity and deepen their capacity to love others and care for them. Generativity versus self-absorption and stagnation (Stage 7) occurs during the middle adult years. The last stage, ego integrity versus despair, occurs through the aging process. As the adult ages, he or she begins to struggle with losses, such as the loss of loved ones, changes in family, or losses in functional status. These changes challenge the person to adjust while continuing to live a full and rich life.

Piaget's Theory of Cognitive Development Jean Piaget (1896-1980) developed the theory of cognitive development, which describes children's intellectual organization and how they think, reason, and perceive the world. The theory includes four periods: sensorimotor, preoperational, concrete operations, and formal operations (see Table 21-1). As the child grows from infancy into adolescence, the intellectual development progresses, starting with reflex and repetitive motion responses, to the use of symbols and objects from the child's point of view, to logical thinking, and finally to abstract thinking (Santrock. 2007).

Kohlberg's Moral Developmental Theory Lawrence Kohlberg (1927-1987) expanded on Piaget's work. According to Kohlberg (1964), moral development is one component of psychosocial development. It involves the reasons an individual makes a decision about right and wrong behaviors within a culture. Moral development depends on the child's ability to accept social responsibility and to integrate personal principles of justice and fairness. In addition, the child's

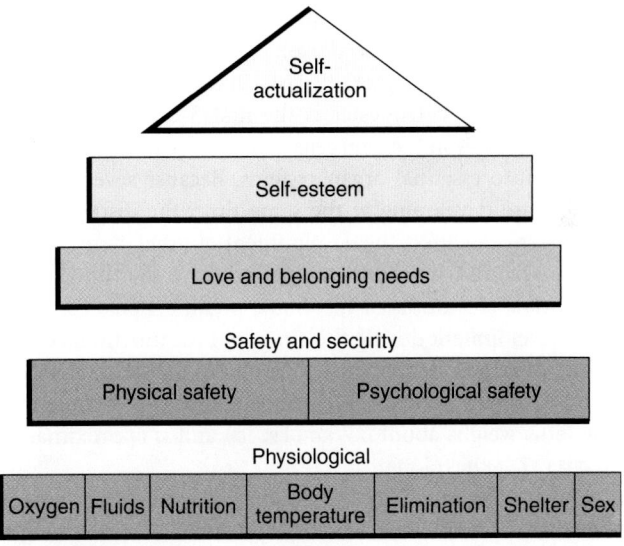

Figure 21-1 ■ Maslow's hierarchy of needs. (Redrawn from Maslow AH: *Motivation and personality,* ed 3, Upper Saddle River, NJ, 1970, Prentice Hall.)

knowledge of right and wrong and behavioral expression of this knowledge must be founded on respect and regard for the integrity and rights of others (Santrock, 2007). Cognitive development aids the progression of a person's morality from level to level.

Maslow's Theory of Human Needs Abraham Maslow (1908-1970) developed a theory of human needs from his study of individuals without physical or mental illness (Figure 21-1). He described an ordering (hierarchy) of needs that motivate human behavior. This ordering is often depicted as a pyramid composed of five levels (Maslow, 1970). When the most basic needs, such as hunger and oxygen, are met, the person strives to satisfy those needs for safety and security on the next highest level. Disturbances at lower levels interfere with the highest level, self-actualization or the realization of one's potential. This theory has made a valuable contribution to understanding human development through its positive viewpoint and recognition of needs that motivate all humans. However, critics have noted that it does not differentiate according to age-groups.

NURSING KNOWLEDGE BASE

A strong body of knowledge about growth and development gives you good insight regarding how individuals perceive an event or behave in response to a given situation at a particular age or stage of life. The following is an overview of the stages of life and related health concerns.

Conception and Fetal Development

From the moment of conception, human development proceeds rapidly. The ovum and sperm each carry half the genetic material that guides biochemical processes essential to the developing organism. Abnormalities in the genes or chromosomes alter health. Other health problems, such as fetal alcohol syndrome, result from environmental factors (e.g., the mother's diet or tobacco use).

Intrauterine life generally lasts 9 calendar or 10 lunar months. The first trimester is the first 3 calendar months. After implantation the fetal cells continue to differentiate and develop into essential organ systems. Because several organ systems are developing at the same time, the disruption of one system can affect the development of other systems.

The second trimester is the period from the third to the sixth prenatal months of life. Some organ systems continue basic development during this time, and the functional capabilities of others are refined. By the end of the second trimester most organ systems are complete and able to function. The fetus weighs about 0.7 kg (1½ lb) and is approximately 30 cm (12 inches) long.

During the last 3 months of intrauterine life the fetus grows to approximately 50 cm (20 inches) in length. Weight increases to approximately 3.2 to 3.4 kg (7 to 7½ lb). The skin thickens, lanugo (soft, downy hair) begins to disappear, and the fetal body becomes rounder and fuller. A tremendous spurt in brain growth begins during this trimester and lasts well into the first few years of life. The central nervous system has established its total number of neurons and connections between neurons, and myelination of nerve fibers progresses rapidly. Damage to the central nervous system during the third trimester can potentially alter higher-level cognitive functions. Exposure to potential teratogens can affect fetal development during any of the trimesters; however, vulnerability is increased during the first trimester when fetal cells are differentiating and organs are forming.

HEALTH PROMOTION Because the placenta is extremely porous, teratogens pass easily from mother to fetus. **Teratogens** are chemical or physiological agents capable of having adverse effects on the fetus. Some examples of teratogens are viruses, drugs (prescribed, over-the-counter, and street drugs), alcohol, and environmental pollutants, such as lead. The fetal effect of these harmful agents depends on the developmental stage in which exposure takes place. Some teratogens produce defects only if the fetus is exposed to the agent at a critical time when the vulnerable organ is developing. For example, the rubella or measles virus is primarily dangerous if a fetus is exposed to it in the first trimester. This virus can cause spontaneous abortion, stillbirth, or defects of the eyes, ears, and heart.

Many drugs are teratogenic during the period of rapid organ growth in the first trimester. Barbiturates, alcohol, anticonvulsants, antibiotics, anticoagulants, and over-the-counter medications can cause fetal abnormalities. Health care providers weigh the benefits of prescribed medications against potentially harmful fetal effects. In addition, there is evidence that mothers who smoke deliver infants with lower birth weights than nonsmoking mothers.

You will explore lifestyle changes that can help women abstain from tobacco, alcohol, and drugs not only during pregnancy but also while planning for pregnancy. Preconception counseling is a growing trend in health care. The goal is to secure the best outcome for mother, fetus, and significant others through good prenatal care.

Neonate

The neonatal period is the first 28 days of life. The newborn's physical functioning is primarily reflexive, and stabilization of major organ systems is the body's primary task. The average full-term **neonate** weighs 3.4 kg (about 7½ lb), is 50 cm (20 inches) in length, and has a head circumference of 35 cm (14 inches). Neonates lose up to 10% of their birth weight in the first few days of life, primarily through fluid losses by respirations, urination, defecation, and low fluid intake. They usually regain the weight by the second week of life.

Physically, the neonate may have lanugo on the skin of the back; cyanosis of the hands and feet (acrocyanosis), especially during activity; and a soft, protuberant abdomen. Behaviorally, the newborn has periods of sucking, crying, sleeping, and activity. The newborn's movements are generally sporadic, but they are symmetrical and involve all extremities. Newborns respond to sensory stimuli, particularly the caregiver's face, voice, and touch.

Early cognitive development begins with innate behaviors, reflexes, and sensory functions. For example, neonates instinctively turn to the nipple. Newborns are able to focus on objects 20 to 25 cm (8 to 10 inches) from their faces and respond to auditory stimuli. Therefore you need to teach parents the importance of talking to their babies and providing appropriate visual stimulation.

HEALTH PROMOTION Parental concerns during the neonatal period most frequently center on the baby's crying, feeding, eliminating, and sleeping behaviors (Box 21-1). New parents are not always aware of the newborn's immature im-

BOX 21-1 Health Promotion Guidelines for Parents of Newborns

- Selection of a crib with slats less than 2⅜ inches (approximately 6 cm) apart (Hockenberry and Wilson, 2007)
- Mattress fitting snugly against the slats
- No pillows or bumper pads in baby's crib
- Positioning infants on their backs in the crib, "face up to wake up" (American Academy of Pediatrics, 2008)
- Expected physiological newborn behaviors
- Variability of behavioral cycles (sleep-awake states)
- Principles and techniques for feeding method chosen; the American Academy of Pediatrics (2005) recommends breast-feeding, and breast-feeding moms need support and interventions for some minor problems such as sore nipples, temporary decline in milk production
- Appropriate stimulation techniques and support for parents' attempts to provide sensory stimulation to the newborn
- Feeding patterns and behaviors
- Schedule of well-baby visits and immunization schedule
- Care measures, including hygiene, dressing, comfort
- Protective measures, including asepsis, safety, cardiopulmonary resuscitation (CPR), thermoregulation
- Cleansing of umbilical cord stump with alcohol until it falls off
- Circumcision care
- Signs and symptoms of the newborn requiring evaluation by a health care professional

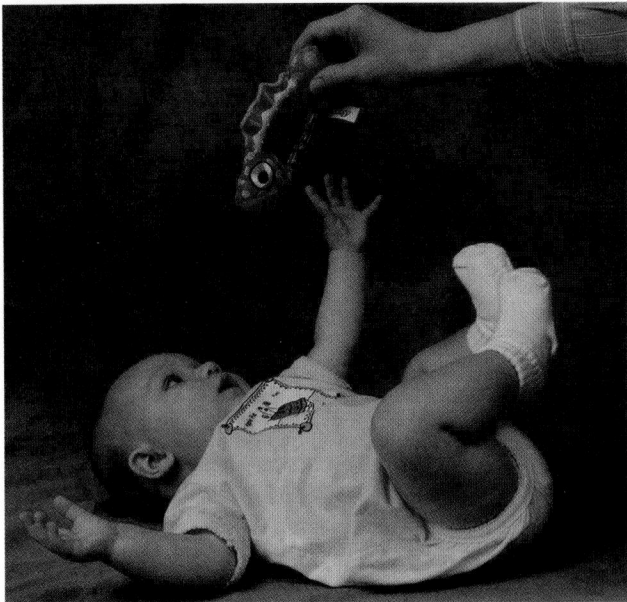

Figure 21-2 ■ Three-month-old infant focuses on visual subject and reaches toward it. (Courtesy Paul Vincent Kuntz, Texas Children's Hospital, Houston, Tex. From Hockenberry ML, Wilson D: *Wong's nursing care of infants and children,* ed 8, St. Louis, 2007, Mosby.)

mune system and need information about how to protect the baby from infection (e.g., avoiding exposure to crowds of people, such as at church or the grocery store).

The American Academy of Pediatrics (AAP) recommends placing healthy infants on their backs while they sleep to decrease the risk for sudden infant death syndrome (SIDS). Side sleeping is not advised because it is not as safe as back sleeping. The AAP also recommends not placing infants on thick bedding, sheepskins, waterbeds, or cushions. Research shows these preventive measures are associated with a decreased incidence of SIDS (AAP, 2008). Nurses assist parents in attaining the knowledge and skills required to foster the newborn's physical, psychosocial, and cognitive well-being and development. You help new parents by teaching the phrase "face up to wake up" as a reminder to always place children on their backs.

Infant

Growth and development are more rapid during the first 12 months of life than they will ever be again. The infant depends completely on caretakers to provide for basic needs of food and sucking, warmth and comfort, love and security, and sensory stimulation.

Typically infants double their birth weight by 5 to 6 months and triple it by 12 months. Their length increases about 1 inch

per month during the first 6 months and then ½ inch per month to the end of their first year. Play provides opportunities for the infant to develop many motor skills. Rattles, plastic stacking rings, and wooden blocks are just a few examples of toys that promote fine motor development of the hands and fingers (Figure 21-2).

HEALTH PROMOTION In addition to health promotion activities regarding feeding, crying, eliminating, and sleeping for the newborn, new health promotion activities for the 1- to 12-month-old infant are often related to dentition, immunizations, and safety.

The first tooth to erupt is usually one of the lower central incisors at the average age of 7 months. Most babies have six teeth by their first birthday (Hockenberry and Wilson, 2007). The use of a frozen teething ring and medication to numb the gums is helpful to comfort the irritable infant during teething episodes. Tooth decay is preventable by providing adequate fluoride through formula or otherwise, cleaning inside the baby's mouth at least once a day with a wet washcloth, and not allowing the baby to take the bottle to bed (Hockenberry and Wilson, 2007).

The quality and quantity of nutrition influence the infant's growth and development. Breast-feeding is recommended for infants. It is associated with a decreased frequency of gastroenteritis, otitis media, and food allergies (Behrman and others, 2004; Hockenberry and Wilson, 2007; U.S. Department of Health and Human Services [USDHHS], 2000). However, when breast-feeding is not possible or desired by the parent, an acceptable alternative is iron-fortified commercially prepared formula. Infants should not have any type of cow's milk (skim, 2%, or whole) or imitation milk (soy products) during the first year because of the infant's decreased ability to digest fat.

The use of immunizations has resulted in a dramatic decline of infectious diseases over the past 50 years. However, recently complacency and fears regarding side effects of vaccines have resulted in inadequate immunization of children less than 2 years (Behrman and others, 2004). Nurses play a major role in assisting community organizations in promoting immunizations and eliminating preventable childhood disease.

Infants' quickly developing motor skills increase their mobility and their ability to place all types of objects in their mouths. Infants need constant supervision when not sleeping. You need to help parents raise their level of awareness regarding potential hazards in their homes. Common accidents during infancy include automobile accidents, aspiration, burns, drowning, falls, poisoning, and suffocation (Box 21-2).

ACUTE CARE   When an infant becomes ill, it is important that you maintain the infant's routine daily care. Whenever this is impossible, limit the number of caregivers who have contact with the infant, and follow the parents' directions for care. If hospitalization is necessary, infants sometimes have difficulty establishing physical boundaries because of repeated bodily intrusions and painful sensations. Limiting these negative experiences and providing pleasurable sensations support early psychosocial development.

Toddler

The toddler period ranges from 12 to 36 months of age. The rapid development of motor skills allows the child to participate in feeding, dressing, and toileting. Toddlers walk in an upright position with a broad-stance gait, bowed legs, protu-

---

BOX 21-2   Health Promotion Guidelines for Parents of Infants

- Keeping crib away from radiators, the blast of air ducts, and cords from drapes or blinds
- Expected growth and developmental norms
- Play activities to stimulate gross and fine motor development
- Techniques to encourage development of language
- Readiness for weaning from breast or bottle to cup
- Addition of solid foods (usually at 6 months) and other fluids by introducing only one new food at a time to assess for food allergies
- Need for immunizations and immunization schedule
- Safety measures related to use of approved car seats, falls, drowning, and use of mouth to explore everything in environment
- Avoiding exposure to secondhand smoke
- Development of attachment, stranger awareness, and separation anxiety
- Use of voice, eyes, and facial gestures as disciplinary measures
- Signs of illness, measures for assessment (temperature taking), and appropriate action
- Criteria to use when choosing day care

---

berant abdomen, and arms flung out to the sides for balance. Soon the child begins to navigate stairs, run, jump, stand on one foot for several seconds, and kick a ball.

Because moral development is closely associated with cognitive ability, the moral development of toddlers is just beginning. Toddlers are also egocentric. Toddlers do not understand concepts of right and wrong. However, they do grasp that some behaviors bring pleasant results and others bring unpleasant results.

Toddlers are generally able to speak in short sentences. Common questions they ask are, "Who's that?" and "What's that?" By 3 years of age, toddlers have a beginning mastery of speech, are possessive of their toys, and are often heard to say, "That's mine!" They begin to learn that sharing is a desirable behavior when they offer parents toys to hold and the parents express pleasure. Play is frequently solitary in nature. However, toddlers often participate in parallel play, playing beside another child with a similar toy or object but not actively interacting through their play. Gradually play begins to include the exchanging or sharing of objects when playing beside another toddler engaged in a similar activity.

HEALTH PROMOTION   Slower growth rates often occur with a decrease in caloric needs and a smaller food intake. Confirming the child's pattern of growth with standard growth charts is reassuring to parents concerned about their toddler's decreased appetite (physiological anorexia). Encourage parents to offer a variety of nutritious foods, in reasonable servings, for mealtime and snacks. Special dietary considerations are necessary for the toddler who is ill, is going to have surgery, or is on a vegetarian diet. Finger foods allow the toddler to be independent.

Toilet training is a major task of toddlerhood. The success of toilet training is based on three primary factors: physical ability to control anal and urethral sphincters (after the child learns to walk), the child's ability to recognize urge and communicate it to the parent, and the desire to please the parent by holding on and letting go at appropriate times. The average age for achieving control is 2 years for daytime and 3 years for nighttime control. Girls usually toilet train earlier than boys (Hockenberry and Wilson, 2007).

The natural curiosity and the mobility of toddlers, without good reasoning abilities, make them an accident waiting to happen. Toddlers want to put everything into their mouths (e.g., bugs, bleach, or electrical cords) or place their hands, feet, or entire bodies into dangerous sites (e.g., electrical outlets, clothes dryers, tubs with very hot water). They need constant supervision unless they are in a totally childproofed area such as their crib or playpen. Toddlers have little awareness of physical safety, and accidents continue to be the leading cause of death and injury. The most common accidents are burns, drowning, falls, motor vehicle accidents, and poisoning (Behrman and others, 2004). You will often help parents anticipate the safety needs of their toddlers and make appropriate suggestions (Box 21-3).

ACUTE CARE   Whenever toddlers are ill, it is important to provide care consistent with the child's developmental needs. Use the responses of children and their parents to determine children's specific care. For a young child, being separated from one's family in an unfamiliar environment during an illness is a stressful experience. Parents are more likely to remain with their young child when the nurse and members of the health care team create a comfortable environment for them. Whenever possible encourage the family to bring in the child's favorite toy, blanket, or familiar object. If a significant caretaker cannot remain with the toddler, it is especially important that one nurse assume responsibility for providing the toddler with consistent and appropriate care. Limiting the number of strange caretakers will help establish trust and reduces separation anxiety for the toddler. During times of stress or illness children often regress to behaviors of an earlier time that provide them comfort and security. This regression of behavior is often disturbing to parents, and they need reassurance that this behavior is normal and that the child will return to more mature behavior patterns when the stressful situation is resolved.

Toddlers cannot clearly identify where they feel pain and often find anything that causes pressure intrusive or extremely painful. Reduce physical discomfort by keeping periods of restraint or immobility to a minimum. A soft voice, physical contact, and a security item will also comfort the child.

Preschool Child

Early childhood is a period between the ages of 3 and 5 years when children refine the mastery of their bodies and eagerly await the beginning of formal education. Many parents find this age-group more enjoyable than toddlerhood because children are more cooperative, share thoughts with greater accuracy, and interact and communicate more effectively. Physical development continues to slow, whereas cognitive and psychosocial development accelerates.

Three-year-olds are able to recognize persons, objects, and events by their outward appearance. For example, they prefer having two nickels over a dime because it appears to be more. The continued egocentricity of early thinking makes it difficult to suggest acceptable alternatives to the preschooler. When they are hungry, they expect others also to be hungry, and they think they must eat now!

In addition, preschoolers are increasingly able to solve problems intuitively on the basis of one aspect of a situation. For example, they can classify objects according to either size or to color, but not both. They also ask questions such as, "Why do they call it the thirty-first day of the month instead of the thirty-last?" They also have a great sense of imagination. Adults often misinterpret preschoolers' "tall tales" as lying; however, they are actually presenting their own reality. Their imagination also contributes to the development of fears, the greatest of which in this age-group is the fear of bodily harm. For example, this manifests as fear of various animals, the dark, or of procedures such as having their blood pressure measured.

If two events are related in time or space, children link them causally. The hospitalized child, for example, reasons, "I cried last night and that's why the nurse gave me the shot." As children near age 5, they begin to use rules to understand cause and effect. They then begin to reason from the general to the particular.

HEALTH PROMOTION Ingestion of large amounts of carbohydrates and fats from junk foods results in overweight and undernourishment. Encourage parents to be role models for good eating habits and to offer their children a varied diet that prevents deficiencies and excesses. Children enjoy helping prepare healthy snacks such as fruit slices, carrot sticks, celery stuffed with peanut butter, and popcorn. Family meals also help improve the quality of food eaten.

Preschoolers require role models and instruction to develop good hygiene measures such as brushing their teeth after meals and sugary snacks, covering their mouths and noses when coughing or sneezing, keeping their fingers out of their noses and eyes, and washing their hands before eating and after using the toilet.

Accidents are the major cause of mortality for this age-group, and motor vehicle accidents (usually as a pedestrian) are the major cause of death. Parents need education to assist in meeting the health promotion needs of their child (Box 21-4). This is a good time for you to teach children what to do in case of fire, safety regulations for crossing the street, the necessity of riding in the back seat of the car, and how to get help when someone is hurt.

ACUTE CARE When preschoolers become ill, their beginning abilities to reason and understand make illness less stressful. Although preschoolers have developed object permanence and recognize their parents still exist when out of sight, most

---

BOX 21-3   Health Promotion Guidelines for Parents of Toddlers

- Play activities to stimulate gross and fine motor development (e.g., push/pull, nesting toys)
- Reading to the child
- Good nutritional habits and feeding of self
- Techniques to encourage development of language
- Readiness and appropriate methods for toilet training
- Need for independence and setting limits on behavior
- Need to set limits and provide firm, gentle discipline to resolve negativism and temper tantrums
- Continued separation anxiety and development of ritualism
- Safety measures, including childproofing the home environment (e.g., storage of cleaning products and medication, use of car seats, selection of appropriate safe toys, pool and water precautions, outdoor play, placing plants out of reach and getting rid of poisonous ones)
  - Keeping electrical cords out of reach and covering unused electrical outlets
  - Blocking stairways and balconies and not leaving infant unsupervised near water
  - Reducing the risk for injuries: not leaving iron on ironing board, turning handles of saucepans and frying pans to the inside of the stove when cooking
- Continued need for immunization and developmental assessments

BOX 21-4   Health Promotion Guidelines for Parents of Preschool Children

- Encouraging parents to support their child's sense of initiative and recognizing that the child will be unable to complete all activities begun
- Nutritional requirements for optimal growth
- Methods to stimulate continued progress in the development of motor skills, language, cognitive skills, and social skills: Reading to the child, using play groups, encouraging the child to do small chores and activities for the family
- Signs of common childhood communicable diseases and measures to reduce their risk and spread
- Beginning instruction for children for personal safety (e.g., do not talk to strangers; tell an adult about inappropriate touching, strangers in the area)
- Criteria to use when evaluating preschool education programs:
  - Teaching methods used to help preschoolers learn about their health, including nutrition, exercise, and rest
  - Safety measures and education related to motor vehicles, tricycles, and fire
- Increased sexual curiosity and need for use of correct anatomical terminology
- Child abuse, including how to protect children, identify signs of abuse, and know community agencies available for assistance

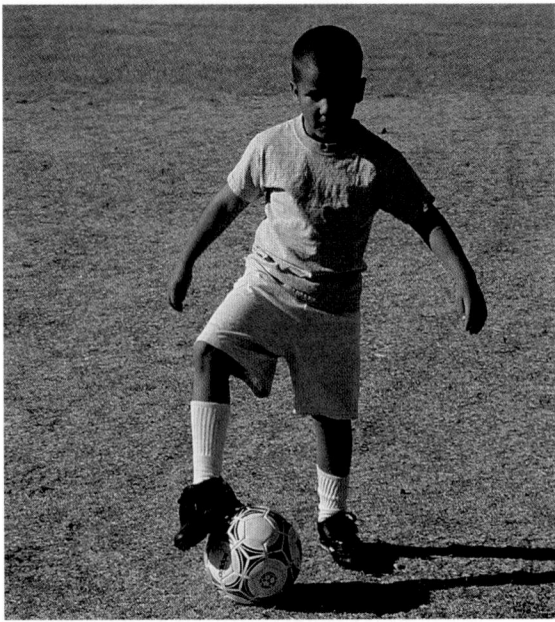

Figure 21-3 ■ Coordination improves in school-age children as they gain control over their bodies.

tolerate only short absences without becoming distressed. Encourage parents to tell the child when they are leaving and when they will return in terms the child can understand (e.g., "I am leaving and will be back after lunch"). Be present when parents leave to provide distraction and support for the child. Reduce children's fear by allowing the child to sit up for assessments and procedures when possible and demonstrating procedures on another person or doll. Also allow the child to see and handle equipment, and allow the child to assist with a procedure as appropriate. Encouraging parents to be present during procedures and leaving the room door open at night if the child requests it reduce fear as well. Simple and factual information is especially important to this age-group because of their great sense of imagination (Hockenberry and Wilson, 2007).

School-Age Child

The foundation for adult roles in work, recreation, and social interaction occurs during the "middle years" of childhood (ages 6 to 12). Great developmental strides are made in physical, cognitive, and psychosocial skills. Children become "better" at things. For example, they run faster and farther as proficiency and endurance develop.

Educational experience in school expands the child's world and transitions the child from a life of relatively free play to a life of structured play, learning, and work. The school and home influence growth and development. For optimal devel-

opment to occur, the child has to learn to cope with the rules and expectations of school and peers.

School-age children become more graceful as they gain increasing control over their bodies (Figure 21-3). Strength doubles, and large muscle coordination improves. Participation in the basic gross motor skills of running, jumping, balancing, throwing, and catching refines neuromuscular function and skills. Holding a pencil and printing letters and words are evidence of fine motor coordination improvement in 6-year-olds. By age 12 the child makes detailed drawings and writes sentences. Assessment of neurological development is often based on fine motor coordination. Teachers often ask school nurses to conduct fine motor assessment of children if they observe a lack of these motor skills.

The middle childhood years are often referred to as the "age of the loose tooth," because children often lose all of their primary teeth during this period. The secondary teeth are much larger in proportion and are often referred to as "tombstone teeth." Regular dental visits confirm that children are brushing their teeth with regularity and good technique.

As children begin to move into the world of school, there are many opportunities for them to gain a sense of competence as they learn reading, writing, and other academic skills. They also have the ability to follow the rules of a new authority person and to compete and cooperate with peers in play and work. The recognition that a child receives at home for achievements also improves the child's developing self-esteem and provides reason to put forth further good efforts. Children's success in work and play leads to an increasing sense of independence and a need to participate in any decisions that involve them. As children move through these middle years of childhood, they confront a number of stressors in the school, in their home, and from peers.

The school-age child prefers same-sex peers to opposite-sex peers. In general, girls and boys view the opposite sex negatively. Peer influence becomes diverse during this stage.

HEALTH PROMOTION Accidents and injuries are major health problems affecting school-age children and are the causative factor in a large number of deaths in this age-group. Motor vehicle accidents, followed by drowning, fires, burns, and firearms are the most frequent fatal accidents. Other major causes of accidents involve recreational activity, most frequently involving bicycles, swings, skateboards, and contact sports. Encourage parents of school-agers to have their children assume some responsibility for their own safety by establishing rules and acting as good role models (Box 21-5).

Blood pressure elevation in childhood is the single best predictor of adult hypertension. This recognition has reinforced the significance of making blood pressure measurement a part of every annual assessment of the child (Behrman and others, 2004; Hockenberry and Wilson, 2007; National High Blood Pressure Education Program [NHBPEP], 2003). Measure on at least three separate occasions with the appropriate-size cuff and in a relaxed situation before concluding that the child's blood pressure is elevated and needs further medical attention.

Childhood obesity is a prominent health problem, which increases the child's risk for hypertension, diabetes, coronary artery disease, and other chronic health problems. In addition, overweight children are frequently the targets of teasing and bullying, and these children are less likely to be chosen for team or peer activities. Daily exercise and maintaining normal body weight are important as both interventions and prevention (Hockenberry and Wilson, 2007).

ACUTE CARE During illness, school-agers usually tolerate the absence of their parents better than the younger child because of their reasoning abilities. Although they understand their parents often need to be elsewhere, they want and expect daily visits and intervening phone calls. The items school-agers often bring from home, such as their own pillows and favorite books, give them a sense of security and independence. Honesty, factual information, and interest in their concerns are helpful in establishing a trusting relationship with this age-group.

School-agers are usually able to pinpoint their pain, describe it with moderate assistance, and sometimes attempt to explain its cause. They often use play to cope with their pain or withdraw in an attempt to deal with their discomfort. They are usually aware that they receive medication for pain but sometimes do not ask for it until the pain is intense. They are quick to learn to use a scale to assess their discomfort. Most school-agers are eager learners who enjoy learning to find their various pulses, read a thermometer, or operate the blood pressure machine during hospitalization. Many school-agers are able to assist in checking their urine for sugar or protein or to learn to do their own fingersticks for blood samples. School-agers who become ill are often threatened by a loss of their recently developed independence by needing to use a bedpan, having help with bathing, bed rest, or having someone else select their menus.

BOX 21-5	Health Promotion Guidelines for School-Agers and Their Parents

- Expected growth parameters and developmental tasks, including the middle childhood growth spurt and puberty
- Measures to enhance adjustment to school and reduce school-related stressors
- Influence and importance of peers as they learn to follow rules and be competitive
- Development and expression of sexuality, including sex play (e.g., masturbation)
- Parental modeling of safety practices
- Instruction for children for personal safety (e.g., do not talk to strangers, tell an adult about inappropriate touching, strangers in the area, bullying)
- Monitoring of and limiting recreational screen time (computer, video games, television) to 1 to 2 hours a day
- Educate parent to read violence and sexual language ratings on video and computer games and media
- Reinforce Internet safety (e.g., placing the computer in an interactive family area rather than in the child's room, blocking inappropriate e-mail messages and pop-up messages, emphasizing the need to tell an adult when there is "something funny" on the screen or in the e-mail)
- Recreational safety, including helmets for sports, bicycling, and skateboarding
- Substance abuse (tobacco, alcohol, drugs), including dangers, signs of use, and available community agency support
- Responsibility for health-promoting activities, including nutrition, exercise, and safety

Preadolescent

At present, children experience more emotional and social pressures than youngsters 30 years ago. As a result, children 10 to 12 years of age are now having experiences that were once unique to 14- and 15-year-old youths. This transitional period between childhood and adolescence is preadolescence. Others refer to this period as late childhood, early adolescence, pubescence, and transescence. Physically it refers to the beginning of the second skeletal growth spurt, when the physical changes such as the development of pubic hair and female breasts begin. Children also become more social, and their behavioral patterns become much less predictable.

Adolescent

Adolescence is the transition from childhood to adulthood, usually between 13 and 18 years of age but sometimes extending until graduation from college. The term *adolescence* refers to the psychological maturation of the individual, whereas **puberty** refers to the point when reproduction is possible. A steady progression of physical, social, cognitive, psychological, and moral changes all characterize this period. The adaptations required by these changes push adolescents to develop individualized coping mechanisms and styles of behaviors, which they will continue to use or adapt throughout life. Most teenagers successfully meet the challenges of this period.

PHYSICAL DEVELOPMENT Although timing varies greatly, physical changes occur rapidly during adolescence. Sexual maturation occurs with the development of primary and secondary sexual characteristics. Primary characteristics are physical and hormonal changes necessary for reproduction. Secondary characteristics externally differentiate males from females.

Girls attain 90% to 95% of their adult height by **menarche,** the onset of menstruation, and reach their full height by 1 to 2 years after menarche. Boys continue to grow taller until 18 to 20 years of age. Adolescents are sensitive about physical changes that make them different from peers. Thus they are generally interested in the normal pattern of growth, as well as in their personal growth curves.

PUBERTY A wide variation exists between the sexes and within the same sex as to when the physical changes of puberty begin. Use the ranges of normal growth to assess the progress of growth for an adolescent patient. As with increases in height and weight, the pattern of sexual changes is more significant than their time of onset. Large deviations from normal time frames require attention. Visible and invisible changes take place during puberty as a result of hormonal changes.

The physical changes of puberty enhance achievement of sexual identity. These changes encourage the development of masculine and feminine behaviors. If these physical changes involve deviations, the person has more difficulty developing a comfortable sexual identity. Adolescents depend on these physical clues because they want assurance of maleness or femaleness and because they do not wish to be different from peers. Cultural attitudes, expectations of sex role behavior, and available role models also influence sexual identity. The masculine and feminine behaviors teenagers see and the expectations they perceive for behaving as a man or woman affect how they express sexuality. Adolescents master age-appropriate sexuality when they feel comfortable with sexual behaviors, choices, and relationships (Figure 21-4).

Language development is fairly complete by adolescence, although vocabulary continues to expand. The primary focus becomes developing diverse communication skills to use effectively in many situations, which the person will refine later in life. Adolescents need to communicate thoughts, feelings, and facts to peers, parents, teachers, and other persons of authority.

Developing moral judgment depends on cognitive and communication skills and peer interaction. Moral development, begun in early childhood, matures. Adolescents learn to understand that rules are cooperative agreements that can be changed to fit the situation, rather than absolutes. Adolescents learn to apply rules by using their own judgment rather than simply to avoid punishment as in the earlier years. They judge themselves by internalized ideals, which often leads to conflict between personal and group values.

Adolescents are more likely to engage in risk-taking behaviors that often jeopardize their safety. The prefrontal area

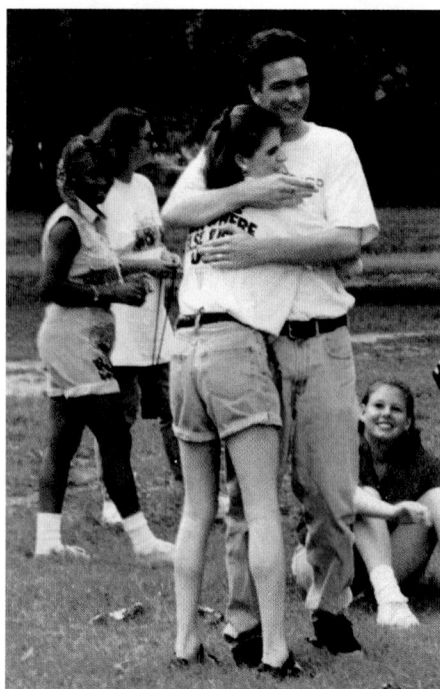

Figure 21-4 ■ Heterosexual relationships are an important part of adolescence. (From Hockenberry ML, Wilson D: *Wong's nursing care of infants and children,* ed 8, St. Louis, 2007, Mosby.)

of the brain, which is responsible for impulse control, is not fully developed until 25 years of age. Adolescents have a sense of invulnerability, which also increases risk-taking behavior. It is during adolescence that the incidence of motor vehicle accidents, sexually transmitted infections, and substance experimentation and addiction increases.

The search for personal identity is the major task of adolescent psychosocial development. Teenagers establish close peer relationships or remain socially isolated. Erikson (1963) sees identity (or role) confusion as the prime danger of this stage. Teenagers have to become emotionally independent from their parents and yet retain family ties. They also need to develop their own ethical systems based on personal values.

HEALTH PROMOTION A component of personal identity is perception of health. Healthy adolescents evaluate their own health according to feelings of well-being, ability to function normally, and absence of symptoms. Health problems causing severe or long-term alteration of these factors permanently alter self-identity. Along with parents, you will assist adolescents in taking responsibility for their own health status and practices (Box 21-6).

The major causes of mortality in the adolescent age period are injuries, homicide, and suicide (Hockenberry and Wilson, 2007). Motor and other vehicular accidents, pregnancy, STIs, and substance abuse are major causes of morbidity. Mental disorders, chronic illness, and eating disorders are other causes.

Females are more likely to have eating disorders and emotional distress, and males are more often involved in vehicular

BOX 21-6   Health Promotion Guidelines for Adolescents and Their Parents

- Clear, reasonable limits for acceptable behavior and consequences for breaking the rules
- Automobile safety, including driver's education course; use of seat belts; risks to self and others associated with drinking, drugs, and driving; use of helmets by bicyclists and motorcyclists
- Developing a mutual plan so that the adolescent never gets into a car when the driver has been drinking or the adolescent never drives if he or she has been drinking; plan to include whom to call to pick up the child
- Awareness of warning signs of depression and suicide, alternatives to suicide, and methods to deal with a suicidal peer
- Potential of social isolation and the excessive use of computer for recreational activities (e.g., searching the Internet, solitary computer games)
- Discuss threats to safety from the Internet (e.g., identity theft, sexual predators)
- Dealing with peer pressure, school-related stressors, anger, and violent feelings through decision-making skills, conflict resolution, and positive coping strategies
- Prevention of unintentional injuries (e.g., classes on use of firearms, danger of swimming alone or under the influence of alcohol or drugs)
- Sexual experimentation and measures to prevent STIs and pregnancy, including abstinence, transmission of infection, symptoms of disease, prophylactic measures, and community organizations that provide assistance
- Support development of sexual identity (i.e., homosexual, heterosexual, and bisexual)
- Importance of routine HIV testing for at-risk adolescents
- Allowing increasing independence within limits of safety and well-being
- Breast self-examination and testicular self-examination

HIV, Human immune deficiency virus; *STIs,* sexually transmitted infections.

accidents (Behrman and others, 2004). Homicide is the most frequent cause of death among older African American adolescents, whereas vehicular accidents are the leading cause of death among white males (Edelman and Mandel, 2006).

Health services for adolescents need to be readily available, affordable, and approachable if parents and communities expect teens to use them. Adolescents also tend to use school-based programs. Health care workers need skills in interviewing adolescents and identifying those more at risk. Successful health promotion activities actively involve teenagers at all times. The involvement of teens in organizations that promote responsible behaviors such as Students Against Destructive Decisions (SADD, formerly Students Against Drunk

Driving) is a key element. Through your efforts in the school and community, you will make a contribution in meeting the *Healthy People 2010* objectives (USDHHS, 2000).

Substance abuse is a major concern to those who work with teenagers. All adolescents are at risk for experimental or recreational substance use. You assess those at risk, educate them to prevent accidents related to substance abuse, and counsel those in rehabilitation.

Suicide is the third leading cause of death in persons between 15 and 24 years of age and the second leading cause of death for white males in this age-group (Edelman and Mandel, 2006). Depression and social isolation commonly precede a suicide attempt, but suicide most likely results from a combination of several factors. Be alert to the following warning signs, which often occur for at least 1 month before a suicide attempt (Behrman and others, 2000; Hockenberry and Wilson, 2007):

1. Decrease in school performance
2. Withdrawal
3. Loss of initiative
4. Loneliness, sadness, or crying
5. Appetite and sleep disturbances
6. Verbalization of suicidal thoughts

Make immediate referrals to mental health professionals when your assessment suggests an adolescent is considering suicide. Guidance helps focus on the positive aspects of life and strengthen coping abilities.

Sexual experimentation is common among adolescents. Peer pressure, physiological and emotional changes, and societal expectations contribute to heterosexual and homosexual relations. About 50% of adolescent students have had sexual intercourse during their lifetime, and two thirds of these sexually active teenagers are inconsistent in their use of safe sex. The risk-taking behaviors of adolescent sexual activity and drug use make adolescents vulnerable to the threat of human immune deficiency virus (HIV) infection and acquired immunodeficiency syndrome (AIDS). AIDS is the sixth leading cause of death among individuals between 15 and 24 years of age (USDHHS, 2000).

The United States has one of the highest rates of teenage pregnancy in the world. Pregnancy rates are higher among older adolescents than they are among younger adolescents (Hockenberry and Wilson, 2007). Adolescent pregnancy occurs across socioeconomic classes, in public and private schools, among all ethnic and religious backgrounds, and all parts of the country.

ACUTE CARE Hospitalization imposes rules and separates adolescents from their usual support system, restricts their independence, and threatens their personal identity. Adolescents who are forced into dependency or have their need for privacy ignored respond with frustration, anger, or self-assertion. Although most hospitals allow peers to visit, some adolescents will isolate themselves until they are able to compete on an equal basis with peers. The telephone is often the lifeline between adolescents and their friends and helps them maintain their place in their social group. Many adolescents welcome peer visitors, and hospitals often allow the patient to go to a lounge or cafeteria with them.

Adolescents who are more independent from their parents usually do well with intermittent visiting but expect some type of daily contact. Some will request that their parent remain with them throughout the hospitalization, and others will not object to it, demonstrating that they also experience regression with the stress of illness. It is important that you address the patient rather than the parents during the assessment process.

Adolescents usually describe their pain with minimal assistance, pinpoint its location, and often explain its cause. They are usually aware of the medication they receive for pain and like to be in control of when you give it to them. Many of them are able to use distraction and relaxation techniques to decrease their discomfort.

Young Adult

Adult developmental changes are based on earlier characteristics that help shape subsequent behaviors. Each person's development is a unique process. Young adulthood is somewhere between the late teens and the mid to late 30s (Edelman and Mandel, 2006). During this phase the individual moves away from the family and marries or remains single. Young adults are active and adapt to new experiences and newly acquired independence.

Young adults have reached physical maturity, have achieved the highest level of cognitive ability according to Piaget, and are expected to exhibit a high degree of psychosocial maturity. Many young adults recognize that they are continuously in the process of becoming more mature in their behavior.

PHYSICAL DEVELOPMENT Young adults usually complete their physical growth by the age of 20. They are usually at their peak of health and less commonly experience severe illnesses compared with other adults. Although physical changes associated with aging have begun, the effects are not great enough to be noticed or require attention.

COGNITIVE DEVELOPMENT Rational thinking habits and flexibility of thought increase steadily through the adult years. Formal and informal educational experiences, general life experiences, and occupational opportunities dramatically increase conceptual, problem-solving, and motor skills. A rich, stimulating environment for the growing and maturing adult encourages the development of full creative potential. An understanding of how adults learn will assist you in developing teaching plans for them (see Chapter 11).

PSYCHOSOCIAL DEVELOPMENT The emotional health of young adults is related to their ability to effectively address personal and social tasks. According to developmental theorists, certain patterns or trends are relatively predictable. Once young adults have begun to work in their chosen area, they have more time and energy to select a mate (if they have not already done so) and develop a greater sense of intimacy. Many will choose to marry, but an increasing number of young adults are choosing to remain single.

Identifying a preferred occupational area is a major task of young adults. When individuals know their skills, talents, and personality characteristics, occupational choices are easier and they are generally more satisfied with their choices. In the young and middle adult years, job satisfaction is a major factor in achievement and responsibility.

The developmental tasks of young adults are potentially filled with stressful situations. Most young adults have the physical and emotional resources and support systems to meet the many challenges, tasks, and responsibilities they face. You will often assist young adults in developing time management skills or in mobilizing their resources and support systems, especially when one of their immediate family members is ill or hospitalized.

HEALTH PROMOTION Health teaching and health counseling are often directed at assisting patients in improving their health habits. Understanding the dynamics of behavior and habits will assist you in designing interventions that will help the patient develop or reinforce health-promoting behaviors. To help patients form positive health habits, you become a teacher and facilitator. You need to remember that you will not always change patients' habits but you are able to raise their level of knowledge regarding the potential impact of behavior on health. Patients have control and are responsible for their own behaviors. When working with the patient, explain psychological principles of changing habits, offer information about health risks, and provide positive reinforcement of health-directed behaviors and decisions. Minimize or eliminate barriers to change, such as lack of knowledge or motivation, to bring about change.

Young adults are generally active and have no major health problems. However, their fast-paced lifestyles put them at risk for illnesses or disabilities during their middle or older adult years. Motor vehicle accidents and violence are the greatest cause of mortality and morbidity among young adults. Poor adherence to routine screening schedules puts the patient at risk for severe illnesses because of failed early detection. Encourage your patients to follow cancer screening guidelines for breast self-examination (BSE), testicular self-examination (TSE), and genital self-examination (see Chapter 15).

Family stressors occur at any time. Family life has peaks, when everyone in the family works together, and valleys, when everyone appears to pull apart. Situational stressors occur during events such as births, deaths, illnesses, marriages, divorces, and job losses. The psychosocial assessment allows you to identify areas of particular stress for the young adult (see Chapter 24). After identifying these stressors, work with the patient to modify the stress response.

ACUTE CARE Many young adults do not experience hospitalization, but when they do, it is often threatening because it interferes with their employment and fulfillment of family responsibilities. Scheduled hospitalizations allow adults to effectively plan to meet the needs of their families and expectations of their employment. Unanticipated hospitalizations often cause chaos for adults and all those directly involved in their lives. If they do not have a strong support system, they usually welcome your help to establish priorities and mobilize their resources. Adults are often impatient with the time and energy requirements that a chronic health problem requires for good management. Support groups often help patients deal with these challenges.

Middle-Age Adult

Middle adulthood usually refers to those years between 40 and 65. For many it is a period when one has both grown children and older adult parents. Most have experienced personal and career achievements, along with socioeconomic stability. Using leisure time in satisfying and creative ways is a challenge that, if met satisfactorily, will enable middle-age adults to prepare for retirement.

PHYSICAL CHANGES Accepting and adjusting to the physiological changes of middle age is one of the major developmental tasks of this age period. Because middle adulthood spans 25 years, many of the physical changes described usually do not occur until later in the developmental period. Middle-age adults use much energy to adapt self-concept and body image to physiological realities and changes in physical appearance. Table 21-2 summarizes these expected physical assessment findings.

TABLE 21-2 Physical Assessment Findings in the Middle-Age Adult

BODY SYSTEM	NORMAL OR EXPECTED FINDINGS
Integument	Intact
	Appropriate distribution of pigmentation
	Slow, progressive decrease in skin turgor
	Graying and loss of hair
Head and neck	Symmetry of scalp, skull, and face
Eyes	Visual acuity by Snellen chart that is less than 20/50
	Loss of accommodation of lens to focus light on near objects
	Pupillary reaction to light and accommodation
	Normal visual fields and extraocular movements
	Normal retinal structures
Ears	Normal auditory structures; acuity of high-pitched sounds declines
Nose, sinuses, and throat	Patent nares and intact sinuses, mouth, and pharynx
	Location of trachea at midline
	Nonpalpable lateral thyroid lobes
Thorax and lungs	Increased anteroposterior diameter
	Respiratory rate 10-20 breaths per minute and regular
	Normal tactile fremitus, resonance, and breath sounds
Heart and vascular system	Normal heart sounds
	Systole: S_1 less than S_2 at base
	Diastole: S_1 less than S_2 at apex
	Point of maximal impulse: at fifth intercostal space in midclavicular line and 2 cm or less in diameter
	Vital signs
	Temperature: 36.0°-37.6° C (96.8°-99.6° F)
	Pulse: 60-100 beats per minute (conditioned athlete, 50 beats per minute)
	Blood pressure: <120 mm Hg systolic
	<80 mm Hg diastolic
	All pulses palpable
Breasts	Decreased size resulting from decreased muscle mass
	Normal nipples and areola
Abdomen	No tenderness or organomegaly
	Decreased strength of abdominal muscles
Female reproductive system	Change in menstrual cycle and in duration and quality of menstrual flow
	"Hot flashes"
	Change in cervical mucosa
Male reproductive system	Normal penis and scrotum
	Prostatic enlargement in some individuals
Musculoskeletal system	Decreased muscle mass
	Decreased range of joint motion
Neurological system	Appropriate affect, appearance, and behavior
	Lucidity and appropriate level of cognitive ability
	Intact cranial nerves
	Adequate motor responses
	Responsive sensory system

Climacteric is a term used to describe the decline of reproductive capacity and accompanying changes brought about by the decrease in sexual hormones. This affects men and women differently. Men begin to experience decreased fertility, but they are able to continue to father children. **Menopause,** when a woman stops ovulating and menstruating, occurs only when 12 months have passed since the last menstrual flow.

COGNITIVE DEVELOPMENT Changes in the cognitive function of middle-age adults are few except during illness or trauma. Performance on intelligence tests indicates increases in some areas, particularly verbal abilities and tasks involving stored knowledge. Although middle-age adults sometimes perform more slowly and are not as adept at solving new or unusual problems, the ability to solve practical problems based on experience peaks at midlife because of the ability for integrative thinking.

PSYCHOSOCIAL DEVELOPMENT According to Erikson (1963), the primary developmental task of the middle-age adult years is to achieve generativity, which is the willingness to establish and guide the next generation and care for others. Many find particular joy in assisting their children and other young people to become productive and responsible adults.

Expected changes in the middle-age adult involve expected events such as children moving away from home or unexpected events such as a marital separation or the death of a spouse or parent. These changes result in stress that affect the middle-age adult's overall level of health.

Career changes occur by choice or as a result of changes in the workplace or society as a whole. In recent decades, middle-age adults more often change occupations because they find themselves less satisfied with their present employment. In some cases, technological advances or changes in the direction of industry force middle-age adults to change work situations. Such changes, especially when unanticipated, result in stress that affects family relationships, self-concept, and financial security for the later years.

Marital changes that occur during middle age include death of a spouse, separation, divorce, and the choice of remarrying or remaining single. A widowed, separated, or divorced patient goes through a period of loss and grief during which it is necessary to adapt to the change in marital status. If the single middle-age adult decides to marry, the stressors of marriage are similar to those for the young adult. In addition, the couple sometimes has to cope with the social expectations and pressures related to middle-age marriage.

The increasing life span in the United States and Canada has led to increased numbers of older adults in the population. Therefore greater numbers of middle-age adults address the personal and social issues confronting their aging parents. Adult children frequently assume partial or total caregiving responsibilities for their older parents. This means adult children assist with personal care, decision-making, housekeeping, financial, transportation, and medical care management tasks. The burden placed on adult caregivers increases if they are also employed and continuing to raise children. The middle-age adult and the older adult parent have conflicting relationship priorities. The older adult often desires to remain independent, whereas the adult child strives to protect the parent. Negotiations and compromises are useful in defining and resolving such problems.

HEALTH PROMOTION Because middle-agers experience physiological changes and face certain health realities, their perceptions of health and health behaviors are often important factors in maintaining health. Middle-age adults are more prone to stress-related illnesses such as heart attacks, hypertension, migraine headaches, backache, arthritis, cancer, and autoimmune diseases.

The leading causes of death in persons between the ages of 45 and 64 years are heart disease, cancer (primarily lung, breast, and colorectal), stroke, accidental injuries, and chronic obstructive pulmonary diseases. Middle-age adults need to continue the same recommended health practices outlined in the discussion on the young adult. It is also important that you understand cultural implications when providing health screening to your patients (Box 21-7). It is also important for middle-age patients to follow cancer screening guidelines (see Chapter 15).

When middle-age adults seek health care, you need to develop goals for positive health behaviors. For example, women need to increase the calcium in their diets to decrease the risk for osteoporosis. Simple things like increasing dietary calcium and calcium supplements are effective. In addition, exercise and fitness clubs, for example, give men and women the opportunity to participate in many physical activities. These activities help improve balance, coordination, and activity tolerance.

ACUTE CARE Middle-agers hold the same family and occupational concerns regarding hospitalization as do young adults. There is sometimes less stress because of the security of employment or because the children who are still at home are usually old enough to care for themselves. However, underinsured middle-agers face serious financial threats. Middle-age adults are at risk for a decline in their physical health. Chronic health problems such as sickle cell anemia, arthritis, asthma, diabetes, and lung disease require ongoing medical care and often require brief hospitalizations. The middle-age adult is usually interested in his or her health and wants to be informed.

Older Adult

Most older adults are physically active, intelligent, and socially engaged (Figure 21-5). Extended life spans allow many older adults to enjoy their retirement by pursuing interests for which they previously had little time. The number of older adults in the United States continues to grow. In addition, statistics project that the diversity of this population will increase. By 2030 it is expected that the older adults from minority groups (e.g., African American, American Indians, Asian/Pacific Islanders, Hispanics, and Islamic) will account for 25.4% of the total over the age of 65 (Administration on Aging, 2008).

Older adulthood traditionally begins after retirement, but the time when people retire varies greatly. Some people retire

BOX 21-7   CULTURAL FOCUS

As Louis prepared to assist in developing health promotion activities for Crystal and her family, he read about the impact of a patient's culture on health care practices. Louis knows that it is important to respect his patient's cultural beliefs and practices, but he also understands the value of routine health screenings. Because there is a strong family history for breast cancer, Louis wants to help Crystal and her mother develop strong breast health practices. He knows that breast cancer survival rates are increasing, but he also recognizes that cultural beliefs and practices influence breast cancer screening practices and for some cultures the breast cancer survival rate did not increase. Although the 5-year survival rate for breast cancer is steadily improving, the survival rate for African American women remains lower. African American women are not as diligent in having routine clinical breast examinations (CBEs) or mammograms as are white women. As a result, more African American women delay breast cancer screening and at time of diagnosis are often diagnosed with late-stage breast cancer. Louis also learns that an African American woman might be more receptive to learning about breast health practices and having CBEs from a female health care provider.

IMPLICATIONS FOR PRACTICE

- Louis assesses Crystal to determine her family's beliefs and practices about breast self-examination, CBE, and mammography.
- Ask Crystal about the role of their family's spirituality and spiritual practices in coping with illness, symptoms, and other life stressors.
- Contact the breast health center at the city clinic, and identify a mechanism for Crystal and her mother to be introduced to culturally specific breast health practices from a female health care provider.

Data from Leak A, Hu J, King CR: Symptom distress, spirituality, and quality of life in African American breast cancer survivors, *Cancer Nurs* 31(1):E15, 2008; Phillips JM and others: African American women's experiences with breast cancer screening, *J Nurs Scholarsh* 33(2):135, 2001.

at 50, and others work into their 80s and 90s. It is not unusual for those who write about older adults to divide them into the "young old," who are vital, vigorous, and active, and the "old old," who are frail and infirm. The fastest growing subset is the nearly 3 million people over the age of 85, whose growth rate is nearly three times that of the overall older adult population (Meiner and Lueckenotte, 2006).

Geriatrics is the branch of health care dealing with the physiology and psychology of aging and with the diagnosis and treatment of diseases affecting older adults. Gerontology is the study of all aspects of the aging process and its consequences.

Nursing care of older adults poses special challenges because of diversity in patients' physical, cognitive, and psychosocial health. Older adults vary in level of function and productivity. Before making a health assessment, be aware of the

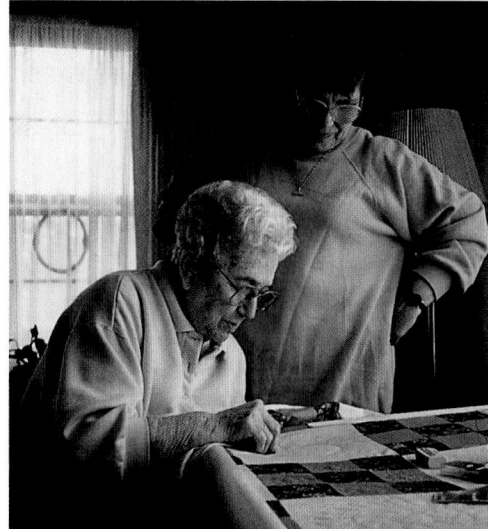

Figure 21-5 ■ Quilting keeps this older adult active.

normal expected findings on physical and psychosocial assessment for an older adult and consider the normal changes of aging.

PHYSICAL DEVELOPMENT The older adult must adjust to the physical changes of aging. These changes are not associated with a disease state but are the normal changes anticipated with aging. The physiological changes that occur with advancing age vary with the patient. Table 21-3 describes the common types of physiological changes. They occur in all persons but take place at different rates and depend on accompanying circumstances in an individual's life.

COGNITIVE DEVELOPMENT Older adults often remain alert and highly perceptive until the time of their death. Nevertheless, the misconception that older adults always have cognitive impairments and suffer from memory loss and confusion persists. Because cognitive impairment occurs in this age-group, be aware of the nature and type of these impairments.

Certain aspects of short-term memory (e.g., numbers) decrease with age, but visual memory, which allows a person to remember how to read, remains strong. Long-term memory for newly learned information decreases significantly with age, but recall for distant experiences and procedural experiences (e.g., driving) do not seem to be affected in the later years of life. Both intelligence and memory vary greatly among individuals. Most older people who want and need to learn new skills and information do so when it is presented more slowly over a long period. Continuing mental activity is essential to keeping older adults alert, and older people benefit from memory training (Ebersole and others, 2008; Edelman and Mandel, 2006).

Three common conditions affect cognition in older adults: delirium, dementia, and depression (Box 21-8). It is important that you learn how to distinguish between these three conditions in order to select appropriate among interventions for your patients (Foreman and others, 1996; Lemiengre and others, 2006). Use a valid assessment tool to accurately assess

TABLE 21-3 Common Physical Changes of Aging

SYSTEM	NORMAL OR EXPECTED FINDINGS
Integument	
Skin color	Brown age spots and spotty pigmentation in areas exposed to sun; pallor even in absence of anemia
Moisture	Dry, scaly
Temperature	Extremities cooler; perspiration decreased
Texture	Decreased elasticity; wrinkles; folding, sagging
Fat distribution	Decreased on extremities; increased on abdomen
Hair	Thinning and graying on scalp; axillary and pubic hair and hair on extremities sometimes decreased; facial hair in men decreased; chin and upper lip hair is present in women
Nails	Decreased growth rate
Head and neck	
Head	Nasal and facial bones sharp and angular; loss of eyebrow hair in women; men's eyebrows become bushier
Eyes	Decreased visual acuity; decreased accommodation; reduced adaptation to darkness; sensitivity to glare; diminished light reflex
Ears	Decreased pitch discrimination; diminished hearing acuity
Nose and sinuses	Increased nasal hair; decreased sense of smell
Mouth and pharynx	Use of bridges or dentures; decreased sense of taste; atrophy of papillae of lateral edges of tongue; occasionally change in voice pitch
Neck	Thyroid gland nodular; slight tracheal deviation resulting from muscle atrophy
Thorax and lungs	Increased anterior-posterior diameter; increased chest rigidity; increased respiratory rate with decreased lung expansion
Heart and vascular system	Blood pressure (BP) remains within normal limits, <120/80 mm Hg (NHBPEP, 2003); BP between 120/80 and 139/89 mm Hg is considered prehypertension; elevations in BP are not a normal aspect of aging, and older adults need minor elevations monitored (NHBPEP, 2003); peripheral pulses easily palpated; pedal pulses weaker and lower extremities colder, especially at night; orthostatic hypertension common
Breasts	Diminished breast tissue; pendulous
Gastrointestinal system	Decreased salivary secretions, which make swallowing more difficult; decreased peristalsis; decreased production of digestive enzymes, hydrochloric acid, pepsin, and pancreatic enzymes, leading to indigestion and constipation
Reproductive system	
Female	Decreased estrogen; decreased uterine size; decreased secretions; atrophy of epithelial lining of the vagina; vaginal dryness
Male	Decreased testosterone; decreased sperm count; erections less firm and slower to develop; decreased testicular size
Urinary system	Decreased renal filtration and renal efficiency; subsequent loss of protein from kidney; nocturia
Female	Urgency and stress incontinence from decrease in perineal muscle tone
Male	Frequent urination resulting from prostatic enlargement
Musculoskeletal system	Decreased muscle mass and strength; bone demineralization (more pronounced in women); shortening of trunk from intervertebral space narrowing; decreased joint mobility; decreased range of joint motion; kyphosis (usually in women); slowed reaction time
Neurological system	Decreased rate of voluntary or automatic reflexes; decreased ability to respond to multiple stimuli; insomnia; shorter sleeping periods

Modified from Ebersole P and others: *Toward healthy aging: human needs and nursing response*, ed 7, St. Louis, 2008, Mosby.
NHBPEP, National High Blood Pressure Education Program.

for patient's cognitive changes. In addition, take time to learn how to correctly use these cognitive assessment tools (Lemiengre and others, 2006).

Delirium is an acute confusional state and requires prompt assessment. It is a potentially reversible cognitive impairment that is often due to physiological causes. Some of these causes include electrolyte imbalance, hypoglycemia, infection, and medications. In addition, very slight body temperature alterations cause delirium in older adults. This condition often accompanies infections, such as pneumonia. The characteristics of delirium usually include fluctuations in cognition that develop over a short time, such as a reduced ability to focus, sustain, or shift attention, and there are acute changes in mood, arousal, and self-awareness. Other signs are hallucinations, transient incoherent speech, disturbed sleep pattern, and disorientation.

Dementia is a broad category of disorders that refers to a generalized impairment of intellectual functioning that in-

BOX 21-8 BEST PRACTICES

Caring for the Patient With Cognitive Impairment

SUMMARY OF EVIDENCE

Understanding the cognitive and neurological function in older adults is important when caring for this population. Altered thought processes occur with cognitive decline or disturbances in cognitive function. Because of the interaction between physical illness and cognitive changes, it is important to accurately assess for the causes of cognitive change, specifically acute confusion. Acute confusion is a common geriatric syndrome in older adults who reside in long-term care facilities. Sensory impairments, specifically vision and hearing impairment, are even more common in this population, and these impairments often contribute to cognitive changes.

APPLICATION TO NURSING PRACTICE

- Older adults living in long-term care facilities are at risk for acute confusion. Nurses in this setting need to be aware of the residents' sensory status and correctly assess for sensory functioning.
- Encourage routine visual acuity examinations, and obtain the best-corrected visual acuity glasses. For some patients magnification devices for reading are helpful.
- Establish routine assessment of ear canals and use of cerumen-softening agents or referrals for cerumen removal as needed.
- Major surgery, infection, drug interactions, and polypharmacy are all risks for cognitive impairment in hospitalized older adults.
- Slight temperature elevations increase confusion and agitation, so frequently assess for and intervene when a fever is present.

REFERENCES

Cacchione PZ and others: Risk for acute confusion in sensory-impaired, rural long-term care elders, *Clin Nurs Res* 12(4):340, 2003.

Naylor MD and others: Cognitively impaired older adults: from hospital to home, *Am J Nurs* 105(2):52, 2005.

terferes with social and occupational functioning. Dementia differs from delirium in that it is a gradual, progressive, irreversible dysfunction. Early recognition is thus important, requiring you to make thorough observations of patient behavior, neurological function (see Chapter 15), and laboratory diagnostic studies. Family and friends are valuable resources in detecting behavioral changes.

Alzheimer's disease is the most common form of dementia. Alzheimer's disease is a progressive loss of memory (amnesia), loss of ability to recognize objects (agnosia), loss of the ability to perform familiar tasks (apraxia), and loss of language skills (aphasia). As the disease progresses, some patients also experience changes in personality and behavior, such as anxiety, suspiciousness, or agitation, as well as delusions or hallucinations (Alzheimer's Association, 2008).

Depression among older adults is increasing. This diagnosis was once overlooked and assumed to be a normal response

to aging, physical losses, or other life events. Like delirium, depression is reversible, and with individualized collaborative care that includes appropriate medication, treatment of underlying conditions, control for polypharmacy, physical rehabilitation when needed, and individualized psychotherapeutic techniques, the patient's depression improves (National Institute of Mental Health, 2007; Raj, 2004).

PSYCHOSOCIAL DEVELOPMENT The older adult has to adapt to many psychosocial changes that occur with aging. Among the more common transitions that occur with aging are retirement, volunteerism, and loss of spousal roles (Ebersole and others, 2008). Despite the changes that occur, the older adult has the potential for developing new and fulfilling life patterns.

Most older adults desire to work as long as they are physically able (Ebersole and others, 2008). The time a person chooses to retire is often based on type of work, status achieved, and length of time employed. When a patient describes retirement, it is important to know whether the individual is fully retired, partially retired, or retired from one position to assume another.

Retirement represents a developmental stage that may occupy 30 years of one's life. It also represents a highly productive and fulfilling period of life. Help patients and their families prepare for retirement by gathering information as to why the patient is considering retirement. Retirement also affects more individuals than the retired person; it affects spouses, adult children, and grandchildren. In addition, the retired person may be spending more time alone for the first time in his or her life.

Death The majority of older adults experience death of spouses, friends, and in some cases children. These losses require individuals to go through a process of grieving (see Chapter 25). Some older adults experience loss when they lose a partner after many years in a satisfying relationship (Ebersole and others, 2008). For many older adults the grief associated with loss of a spouse lasts for many years. Experiencing the grieving process requires support from family, nurses, and other health professionals. You lend support by showing warmth and caring to help patients feel they are not alone.

A common misconception is that the death of an older adult is always a blessing and the culmination of a full and rich life. Many dying older adults still have life goals and are not emotionally prepared to die. **Reminiscence,** or life review, is a technique that facilitates the individual's preparation for the end of life. It is an adaptive function of older adults that allows them to recall the past for the purpose of assigning new meaning to past experiences. Reminiscence is the natural way older adults revive their past in an attempt to establish order and meaning and to reconcile conflicts and disappointments as they prepare for death.

Aloneness and Loneliness With advancing age, more people live alone. This is particularly common for older white women. However, living alone is not equivalent to the feeling of loneliness. A person can be surrounded by others yet still feel lonely. Ebersole and others (2008) define loneliness as an affective state of longing and emptiness, whereas being alone is to be solitary, apart from others, and undisturbed. Many patients choose to be alone or isolated simply because of the desire for privacy or an opportunity for self-reflection and creativity. Loneliness, on the other hand, is sometimes a passive and painful emotion, influenced by psychological, economic, sociological, and physiological factors.

Housing and Environment Changes in social roles, family responsibilities, and health status influence the older patient's choice of living arrangements. An older adult sometimes needs to change living arrangements because of the death of a spouse or a change in health status. A change in an older patient's living arrangements requires an extended period of adjustment during which assistance and support will be needed from family and friends and health care professionals.

HEALTH PROMOTION The possibility of an individual being reasonably healthy and fit in later life often depends on the person's lifestyle. Older adults need to continue the same recommended health practices introduced in the young adult section. Some older adults will need encouragement to maintain a pattern of physical exercise and activity. It is not too late for an older person to begin an exercise program; however, older adults need to have a complete physical examination, which usually includes a stress cardiogram or stress test. Assessment of activity tolerance will help you and the patient plan a program that meets physical needs while allowing for physical impairments (Box 21-9).

BOX 21-9   CARE OF THE OLDER ADULT

Health Promotion and Independence

- Provide information from the American Association of Retired Persons (http://www.aarp.org) regarding supplemental health insurance, group discounts for older adults, and medical and legal information.
- Discuss housing alternatives to help the older adult make a decision regarding the sale of the home, relocation to another area of the country, or retirement communities.
- Instruct patient in health maintenance programs, such as exercise activities, that are designed to increase exercise tolerance, flexibility, and socialization.
- Teach patient that the need for annual influenza and routine pneumonia vaccines increases, especially when chronic illness is present.
- Teach patient about safe and appropriate administration of prescribed drugs: purpose; effect; possible other prescription, over-the-counter, or dietary interactions; and reportable side effects.
- Encourage patient to use one pharmacy for prescription and over-the-counter preparations.
- Instruct patient regarding environmental safety issues (e.g., home lighting, floor coverings, stairs, shoes, electrical cords) to reduce the risk for falling.
- Instruct patient in nutritional aspects related to disease (e.g., a low-fat diet with hypertension, the need for a balanced diet with reduced total calories because of aging changes and lower energy expenditures).

Most older adults are in good health; however, chronic medical conditions increase dramatically with age. The effect of a particular chronic health problem on mobility and independence depends greatly on the individual. Most older adults are capable of taking charge of their lives and assume responsibility for preventing disability.

Sensory impairments are common in the older adult (see Chapter 37). These changes are frequently the result of the normal aging process. Help the older adult identify resources to help correct visual and auditory problems. The sense of touch usually remains strong. Older adults who often become victims of social isolation are often deprived of touching and holding, which convey affection and friendliness. The touch of nurses and all caregivers who work with older adults serves to provide sensory stimulation, reduce anxiety, relieve physiological and emotional pain, orient the person to reality, and provide comfort, particularly during the dying process.

As a group, adults over 65 years of age are the greatest users of prescription drugs. Many drugs interact with one another, potentiating or negating the effect of another drug. Some drugs cause confusion; affect balance; cause dizziness, nausea, or vomiting; or promote constipation or urinary frequency. **Polypharmacy,** the prescription, use, or administration of more medications than are indicated clinically, is a common problem of older adults. The combined use of multiple drugs causes serious problematic effects.

ACUTE CARE Hospitalization of older adults is often disturbing to them because they are not accustomed to the environment and routines. Even those who are able to live independently with some assistance from their families become temporarily disoriented by the strange surroundings of a hospital. Monitor the patient for confusion, and encourage frequent visitation by family members. In addition, use reality orientation techniques to help reorient the older adult who has been disoriented by a change in environment, surgery, illness, or emotional stress.

Reality orientation is a communication modality used for making the patient aware of time, place, and person. The major purposes of reality orientation include the following:

- Restoring patients' sense of reality
- Improving their level of awareness
- Promoting socialization
- Elevating patients to a maximal level of independent functioning
- Minimizing confusion, disorientation, and physical regression

Environmental changes within a hospital, such as the bright lights and lack of windows in intensive care and the noise from nearby roommates, often lead to disorientation and confusion. The patient's environment and the nursing personnel are constantly changing in the hospital, and the immediate environment is unstable, making coping and adaptation difficult. Anticipate disorientation and confusion as a consequence when older adults are hospitalized, and incorporate reality orientation interventions into their care.

When an older adult is hospitalized or has an acute or chronic illness, the related physical dependence makes it difficult for the person to maintain a positive body image. You are able to have an influence on the older adult patient's appearance. Help the patient maintain a pleasant appearance and present a socially acceptable image.

CRITICAL THINKING

Synthesis

You will apply elements of critical thinking whenever you perform the nursing process with a patient. Consider the scientific knowledge you have learned, your experience, critical thinking attitudes, and standards to ensure an individualized approach to patient care. When caring for an individual patient or family, a variety of factors will influence your care. In addition to your knowledge, you and your patients bring unique backgrounds and personal experiences to each care setting. Although you do not always discuss these individual perspectives openly, they do influence your care. Both you and your patients will have preexisting ideas as to how to best meet their developmental needs.

KNOWLEDGE Before assessing your patient, review the developmental theories that relate to the patient. In addition, as you work with your patients in attaining an optimal level of health, it is essential that you know the expected physical developmental milestones, psychosocial developmental crises, cognitive development, and health concerns for each age-group.

Another important area of knowledge to consider when caring for a patient's developmental needs is that of cultural diversity (see Chapter 19). Together with the patient, explore the cultural variations in family roles and relationships as they influence an individual's development, to have a clear understanding of patient needs.

EXPERIENCE If you are a parent or have been involved in the teaching of children, you are aware that the thinking abilities of individuals of different ages differ, and it is necessary to change your approach to gain their cooperation. In addition, your family, social, and educational experiences with individuals of various ages will make it easier for you to determine age-specific appropriate or inappropriate behaviors and health concerns.

ATTITUDES Humility is an important attitude for you to apply when collecting data about a patient's developmental history. It is easy to form opinions about patients' developmental needs on the basis of developmental theory and related psychosocial principles. However, as is the case in any nursing situation, do not assume you know what the patient's needs are without gathering a clear picture of a patient's physical and psychosocial health concerns. Often information about the patient's health practices will reflect the patient's cultural background, which is sometimes very different from yours. Creativity is a valuable critical thinking attitude when you conduct an assessment of an infant or child. Often you will incorporate play or other activities into the assessment to better visualize the child's physical developmental capacities.

STANDARDS Critical thinking standards help to ensure that you are making the right decisions. When developing a plan of care that incorporates growth and development principles and approaches, strive to apply the intellectual standards of relevance and completeness. It is important that you employ a developmental approach that fits with the patient's level of maturation. *Referring to the case study, for example, asking Zachary to attempt a motor skill, such as coloring a detailed picture or successfully using eating utensils, is not within his ability, is irrelevant, and is inappropriate for promoting developmental enrichment.* When selecting a plan of care, you need to be sure the plan uses psychosocial, cognitive, and physical approaches that complement and strengthen the patient's developmental abilities.

Also use professional standards when providing care to patients of various age-groups. For example, when supporting parents' health promotion practices, it is important to refer to the Centers for Disease Control and Prevention or the American Academy of Pediatrics standards for adult and childhood immunizations (Box 21-10). These standards help to determine the required immunizations for certain age-groups. Similarly, the American Cancer Society lists a variety of health screenings for adults. Refer to these standards when providing patient education.

NURSING PROCESS

■ ■ ■ ASSESSMENT

Nursing assessment of individuals across the life span requires you to be familiar with the physiological, cognitive, and psychosocial changes that occur during each stage of development and the health concerns for each age-group. Table 21-4 is an example of a focused assessment for a school-age child, like Crystal's daughter, Monica. A number of assessment tools facilitate concise but comprehensive data collection for individuals of various ages. Observe the interactions between the individual and any family member present during the health history, physical assessment, and developmental assessment. Data gathered will provide information regarding the patient's lifestyle, level of functioning, family relationships, health concerns, and health promotion activities.

Throughout life, illness and hospitalization are stressful experiences. Many factors affect the ability of individuals to cope, such as their level of development, their coping skills, their previous experiences with illness and hospitalization, and the seriousness of the diagnosis. The degree to which the illness interferes with activities of daily living and lifestyle and the availability of a support system also have an impact on how individuals cope. Your assessment needs to demonstrate an awareness of specific patient concerns at various stages of life.

PATIENT EXPECTATIONS During your assessment it is important to determine what patients and/or their families

BOX 21-10   SYNTHESIS IN PRACTICE

 Louis selected Crystal Taylor and her family to follow throughout this semester of his nursing program. As he prepares to begin an assessment, he focuses on 6-year-old Monica, whom Crystal has brought to the clinic for a checkup before beginning school. Louis recalls the physical, psychosocial, and cognitive developmental characteristics that are typical of the older preschool child and prepares to use this information as a basis for his observations. He plans to engage Monica in play activities with dolls to ensure that observations of her physical abilities are relevant and complete. He is also interested in any concerns Crystal has regarding Monica's health. In preparation for doing anticipatory guidance with Monica and her mother, he reviews types of accidents common among her age-group and appropriate health promotion activities. He is also interested in observing the quality of the interaction between Monica and her mother and assessing how Crystal copes with being a single parent.

As the parent of a 4-year-old, Louis knows the importance of immunizations in keeping children free of many contagious diseases with serious consequences, and he is aware that children are not admitted to school without the completion of certain immunizations. His own child has made him very conscious of the great fear young children have for bodily harm and the fact that Monica may have difficulty cooperating with an injection. He recalls the approach he has used to help his own son cooperate with and recover from the discomfort of an injection. Louis refers to the standards for immunizations that the American Academy of Pediatrics, the American Academy of Family Physicians, and the Centers for Disease Control and Prevention update twice yearly to determine Monica's immunization needs. Louis knows that the key to having a positive effect on the practice of health promotion activities by Crystal Taylor's family members is the development of trust through positive interactions.

Louis' nursing instructors have informed him that he is responsible for encouraging health promotion activities among his patients. Louis recognizes that *Healthy People 2010: National Objectives for Improving Health* is a guide for choosing health promotion activities for Crystal's family (see Chapter 1). Louis knows he cannot be judgmental of Ms. Taylor as a single parent. He knows he needs to assess the resources she has to support health promotion in her family. Understanding that Crystal probably has some definite ideas about parenting and health promotion will ensure that Louis is complete in assessing patient needs and in offering appropriate suggestions to support Crystal and her family.

expect from the caregiver. At the beginning of a home visit ask, "What do you think is most important for us to accomplish today?" or when preparing to leave, ask, "Have I met your expectations for this visit?" In the outpatient setting ask what expectation(s) the patient and/or family have for the visit. In the hospital setting it is wise to determine if family members want to participate in the care of the patient and how members of the health team can help. As the patient's primary nurse, you will begin each day with a brief assessment to determine any change in condition and the patient's perceptions of the care received.

■■■NURSING DIAGNOSIS

Your nursing assessment of the patient, and when appropriate the family, reveals clusters of data from the nursing history, physical examination, and developmental assessment. These data include defining characteristics, which you analyze through critical thinking to select the nursing diagnoses that apply. Accuracy is important because the defining characteristics help to differentiate the nursing diagnosis that applies to the clinical situation. For example, *parental role conflict* and *impaired parenting* are two distinctly different nursing diagnoses. Carefully review all information before selecting the nursing diagnosis that applies to the patient's and family's needs. Defining characteristics for the nursing diagnosis of *ineffective sexuality pattern* include factors such as difficulties or limitations in sexual functioning, expressions of concern about sexuality, and inappropriate verbal and nonverbal sexual behavior. The following are more examples of nursing diagnoses for patients with developmental problems throughout the life span:

- *Risk for delayed development*
- *Caregiver role strain*
- *Compromised family coping*
- *Delayed growth and development*
- *Readiness for enhanced self health management*
- *Risk for injury*
- *Impaired social interaction*

The second part of the nursing diagnostic statement states suspected causes or related factors for the patient's response to the health problem. Revealed in the assessment data, the related factors allow you to target specific interventions toward the patient's diagnosis. For example, the nursing diagnosis of *ineffective sexuality pattern* might be related to the stress of an impaired relationship with a significant other, fear of pregnancy, or lack of a significant other. The related factors are different, and each requires different nursing strategies.

■■■PLANNING

GOALS AND OUTCOMES The plan addresses each identified nursing diagnosis by determining goals, patient outcomes, and interventions for the alleviation or resolution of the diagnosis. The goal for each nursing diagnosis identifies a specific and measurable patient outcome that is realistic and reflects the patient's highest level of wellness and independence in function. An example of a goal is "Patient ac-

TABLE 21-4 **FOCUSED PATIENT ASSESSMENT**

FACTORS TO ASSESS	QUESTIONS	PHYSICAL ASSESSMENT
Home safety	Where do you keep household cleaners, medications?	Observe patient's home environment. Observe child's play area.
	Has your child had any accidents playing at home or other home-based accidents during the last year? If so, please tell me about them.	
	Does your family have a home evacuation plan and a meeting place?	Along with parent, play out a situation when the home needs to be evacuated (e.g., fire), and observe the evacuation and congregation of the family at the meeting place.
	Where do you keep your computer? Does your child have unsupervised use of the Internet? Do you have any parental controls that block unsafe sites?	If able, observe the child's use of a home computer if a home visit is made.
Health promotion activities	Does your child have all the immunizations? How current are your immunizations? Where do you keep this information?	Obtain actual immunization history. Obtain serial weight and height measurements, and compare with standards.
	Tell me about your child's usual food intake.	
Sibling interaction	How do your children get along? Do they play together?	Observe child playing and interacting with sibling.
	Are there any changes in your child's behavior, independence?	

quires healthy physical and mental health behaviors within 3 months." An example of an outcome is "Patient participates in scheduled exercise activities within 6 weeks." See the Care Plan for detailed examples of goals and outcomes.

Collaboration with patients and their families is essential when determining goals and outcomes. Patients' degree of participation in planning depends on their developmental status, as well as physiological and psychological condition. For example, because young children are often unable to articulate feelings and needs, their parents need to become involved in establishing goals. The participation of patients and their families in this process will increase their motivation for achievement of identified goals and outcomes (see Care Plan).

SETTING PRIORITIES During the planning phase of the nursing process, formulate a plan of care directed toward the identified nursing diagnoses. Patients and their families often have multiple nursing diagnoses, and these diagnoses often interact with one another (Figure 21-6, p. 594). Then address the nursing diagnoses in order of priority, giving the most pressing problems immediate attention. Base your priorities of nursing diagnoses on such factors as the nature of the problem (e.g., whether it is life threatening, interferes with activities of daily living, or affects level of comfort) and the degree of importance attributed to the problem by the patient or family. Maslow's theory of human needs is helpful as a guide when arranging nursing diagnoses in order of priority. A high-priority nursing diagnosis is not always a physiological problem. *For example, in the case study Louis has*

concerns over Monica's fear of injections, so he views fear as a priority for care in the initial clinic visit, especially when immunizations are necessary.

COLLABORATIVE CARE Collaboration and consultation with other members of the health care team provide valuable resources for care for patients. Such collaboration identifies community resources to help parents of a child with developmental disabilities or help a family find adult day care activities for an older adult. In addition, these resources often assist in providing continuity in discharge planning.

Begin discharge planning at the time of admission to the hospital because the length of stay is usually very brief. Effective planning involves the health care team, the patient, and the patient's support system. Make sure you individualize nursing interventions for the patient and modify them accordingly for home- or hospital-based nursing care. Make needed referrals to community agencies coincide with the patient's arrival home.

■■■**IMPLEMENTATION**

Provide developmental interventions in collaboration with the patient and the family or significant others. It is important that you keep patients and their families as active in this process as possible. Interventions are appropriate for both the patient's developmental level and the patient's unique needs to support and promote normal developmental processes. Collaboration with a variety of health team members facilitates the provision of optimal care for patients.

CARE PLAN   Ineffective Health Maintenance

 ASSESSMENT

Louis knows that this family has multiple health promotion needs. He wants to ensure that the children are on target with their growth and development and developmental tasks, especially Monica, who is entering school. In addition, he wants to determine any of Crystal's concerns as she enters the last trimester of her pregnancy.

ASSESSMENT ACTIVITIES

Complete height and weight examination on Monica.

Using the Denver II (Denver Developmental Screening Test), observe Monica as she completes developmental tasks.

Ask Crystal about how the children interact with each other.

Ask about immunizations and safety concerns.

Ask Crystal about preparation for the new baby.

FINDINGS/DEFINING CHARACTERISTICS*

Monica is in the 60th percentile for weight and the 75th percentile for height of a 6-year-old.
Monica balances on each foot for 6 seconds.
Monica defines words such as *house* and *banana*.
She can copy a square.
Crystal says that she independently brushes her teeth and dresses, prepares her own cereal, and plays board games.
Monica enjoyed showing and telling Louis about the pictures she is coloring and often giggles.
Crystal explains that **Monica is very protective of and bossy with her brother,** and she always **wants to sit on Crystal's lap when she is holding Zachary.**
Crystal is **unsure of the status of the children's immunizations and states, "I'm not sure they help."**
Crystal states that all medications and cleaning agents are locked in a cabinet in the garage, and she has the only key.
Monica tries to **play with a cigarette lighter.**
Crystal states that she has **done nothing in particular.**
Monica asks **how the baby will get out.**
Crystal asks about **suggestions to prepare her children for the arrival of the new baby.**

NURSING DIAGNOSIS: Ineffective health maintenance related to a lack of knowledge regarding age-related health promotion activities.

PLANNING

GOAL

• Crystal will become more knowledgeable about health concerns related to her children's ages within the next 3 months.

EXPECTED OUTCOMES (NOC)†

Knowledge: Health Promotion

• Crystal will begin to discuss the safety needs of her children with all other family members who participate in their care before her next clinic visit.
• Crystal will talk to other family caregivers and Monica about protecting Monica from the danger of playing with fire before the next clinic visit.
• Crystal will begin to prepare Monica and Zachary for the birth of a sibling within the next month.

Health Promotion Behavior

• Crystal will keep her children's appointments for well-baby or well-child checkups and have the children receive appropriate immunizations during the next clinic visit.

***Defining characteristics** are shown in **bold** type.
†Outcomes classification labels from Moorhead S and others, editors: *Nursing outcomes classification (NOC)*, ed 4, St. Louis, 2008, Mosby.

CARE PLAN Ineffective Health Maintenance—cont'd

INTERVENTIONS (NIC)‡

Health Education

- Provide Crystal with literacy-appropriate handouts that describe safety measures according to age of child.
- Discuss with Crystal measures to decrease Monica's risk for playing with fire.

- Provide Crystal with a list of books about preparing children for a new sibling.
- Enroll Crystal in a child health class.

Decision-Making Support

- Provide Crystal with a pocket schedule for required childhood immunizations.
- Provide a copy of her children's actual immunization records.

RATIONALE

Handouts provide initial information and allow for a quick review of information whenever needed (Bass, 2005).

Adults need to keep potentially hazardous items out of reach of children; a lighter, like a match, is an adult tool (Hockenberry and Wilson, 2007).

The list will assist Crystal in finding these books in a bookstore or at the local library.

Class provides alternative learning approach.

Immunization education that includes immunization schedules, appointment reminder methods, and the importance for routine immunizations is essential.

EVALUATION

NURSING ACTIONS	PATIENT RESPONSE/FINDING	ACHIEVEMENT OF OUTCOME
Provide Crystal with handouts describing safety measures.	Crystal continues to lock up medicines and cleaning agents, but also locks up any lighters and matches in her own home.	Crystal's home is improved for safety.
	She was able to get grandmother to move medicines and cleaning agents to a locked cabinet.	Crystal is modifying her grandmother's home for safety risks.
Ensure Crystal receives appointment card for next visit and an up-to-date immunization schedule.	Crystal kept next appointment. Crystal provided child's school with an up-to-date record of immunizations.	This is ongoing, and Crystal needs to maintain appointments for checkups and immunizations.
Ask Crystal if she received list of books and tapes to prepare children for arrival of new sibling.	Children were able to talk about the "almost new baby." "Baby is coming for Halloween."	Preparation for new sibling is progressing, but remains ongoing.

‡Intervention classification labels from Bulechek GM and others, editors: *Nursing interventions classification (NIC)*, ed 5, St. Louis, 2008, Mosby.

Many of the interventions related to your patients' developmental stage include a component of patient education (see Chapter 11). Patient education is an effective tool to teach your patients about health promotion practices, desired behavioral changes, and the need for age-appropriate screening practices. However, patients from different cultures or countries have different languages and beliefs that affect their ability to understand or talk to a health care provider (Edmunds, 2005). Effective patient education considers your patient's health literacy, and it is planned according to the patient's needs (Box 21-11).

Earlier in this chapter, nursing strategies for health promotion and acute care were discussed for each age-group. Restorative care measures for older adults were also outlined. Refer to each of the developmental age-groups for specific interventions regarding age-related health concerns. It is important to remember to incorporate a patient's developmental needs into any plan of care, regardless of the nature of the patient's health problem. Whether the patient has serious physiological alterations or merely is seeking health promotion information, developmental care considerations ensure a more individualized and thorough nursing approach.

■■■EVALUATION

PATIENT CARE During evaluation, measure the patient's progress and the degree to which the planned interventions were effective in meeting the expected outcomes and goals of care (see Case Study). Evaluate the patient's behavioral response to the interventions, and thus determine the success or failure of the nursing action. This includes observing family members interact, having the patient describe health promotion habits, or visiting the home to see if your patient followed suggestions for improving child safety. Both you and the patient and/or family evaluate if the expected out-

CONCEPT MAP

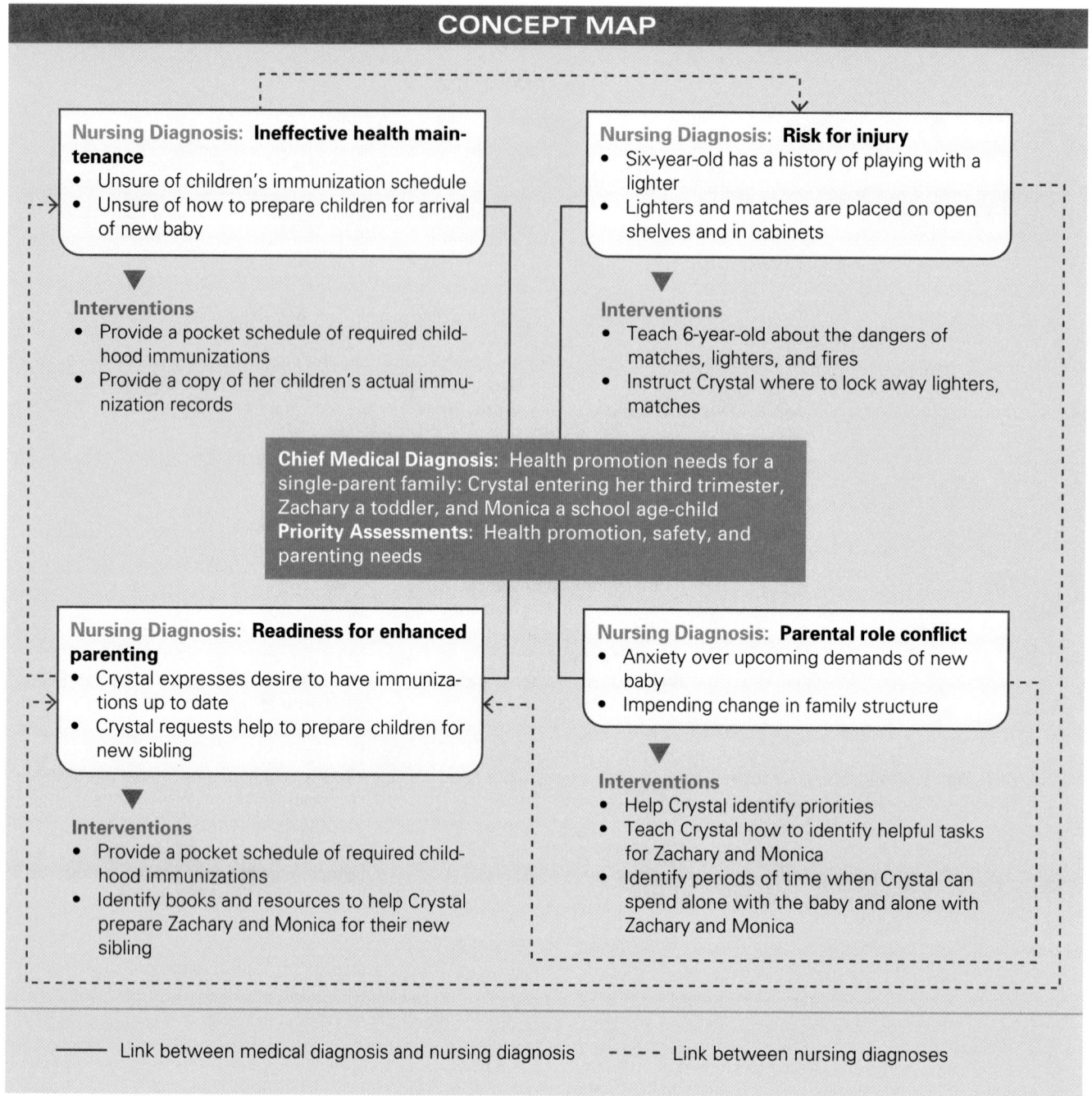

Nursing Diagnosis: Ineffective health maintenance
- Unsure of children's immunization schedule
- Unsure of how to prepare children for arrival of new baby

Interventions
- Provide a pocket schedule of required childhood immunizations
- Provide a copy of her children's actual immunization records

Nursing Diagnosis: Risk for injury
- Six-year-old has a history of playing with a lighter
- Lighters and matches are placed on open shelves and in cabinets

Interventions
- Teach 6-year-old about the dangers of matches, lighters, and fires
- Instruct Crystal where to lock away lighters, matches

Chief Medical Diagnosis: Health promotion needs for a single-parent family: Crystal entering her third trimester, Zachary a toddler, and Monica a school age-child
Priority Assessments: Health promotion, safety, and parenting needs

Nursing Diagnosis: Readiness for enhanced parenting
- Crystal expresses desire to have immunizations up to date
- Crystal requests help to prepare children for new sibling

Interventions
- Provide a pocket schedule of required childhood immunizations
- Identify books and resources to help Crystal prepare Zachary and Monica for their new sibling

Nursing Diagnosis: Parental role conflict
- Anxiety over upcoming demands of new baby
- Impending change in family structure

Interventions
- Help Crystal identify priorities
- Teach Crystal how to identify helpful tasks for Zachary and Monica
- Identify periods of time when Crystal can spend alone with the baby and alone with Zachary and Monica

———— Link between medical diagnosis and nursing diagnosis   - - - - Link between nursing diagnoses

Figure 21-6 ■ Concept Map.

comes were met in the manner anticipated. When outcomes are not met, a review will determine if they were realistic and appropriate, or if there is a need to modify an approach. Ongoing evaluation is necessary to ensure that progress toward defined goals is achieved (Box 21-12).

PATIENT EXPECTATIONS Nurse-patient relationships are often long term when you start a developmental plan of care. Always remember to determine if the patient's expectations of care are continuing to be met. Over time the patient's expectations sometimes change. To add to the complexity of evaluation, expectations sometimes vary when family members are involved. Basic to understanding the patient's and family members' expectations is trust. When you and the patient have established trust, it becomes easier to evaluate on a frequent basis how your relationship with the patient is proceeding and whether the patient senses his or her health care needs are being adequately and professionally addressed.

BOX 21-11 PATIENT TEACHING

Immunizations

Louis knows that he is developing a therapeutic nurse-patient relationship with Crystal. Crystal told Louis that she wants to provide good health care for her children, but she does not understand the suggested immunization schedule for her children.

OUTCOME
- At the end of the teaching session, Crystal will be able to state the routine immunization schedule for her children.

TEACHING STRATEGIES
- Provide Crystal with the American Academy of Pediatrics schedule for routine immunizations.
- Using Crystal's personal calendar, highlight the dates when the immunizations are due.

- Provide Crystal with the phone contact for the appropriate clinic for immunizations.
- Show Crystal how to safely keep a permanent record of the immunizations.
- Tell Crystal to provide only copies of the immunization records to the children's school.

EVALUATION STRATEGIES
- Ask Crystal when the next immunizations are due.
- Review Crystal's personal calendar for a scheduled appointment for immunizations.
- Ask Crystal where she keeps the children's immunization records.

BOX 21-12 EVALUATION

Louis sees Crystal 1 month later when she returns to the clinic for a scheduled prenatal visit. She has left the children at home with their grandmother. While Crystal waits to see her primary caregiver, Louis takes the opportunity to evaluate the progress she has made in meeting expected outcomes. Louis asks Crystal if she has been able to find any of the books on the list he had given her about preparing young children for the birth of a sibling. Crystal reports that the librarian helped her locate two books, one appropriate for her toddler and the other one for Monica. She adds that the children loved the books and want her to read them every night at bedtime. Louis asks her if she thinks the content of the books was the kind of information she wanted to share with her children, and she replies that they explained childbirth so simply it really made it easy for her to talk about the new baby with both children.

During the previous clinic visit, Louis had also given Crystal pamphlets that described important safety measures for infants and young children. He asks her if she has discussed any of this information with any family members. Crystal tells him that her mother and grandmother have looked at the pamphlets and have told her it is a big responsibility to watch those two grandchildren and that they are very hard to keep up with. She also reports that they have all talked to Monica about not playing with candles, matches, or lighters, and Crystal locks up these items as well. She tells Louis about the evening news on TV talking about a child who hid in her bedroom playing with a

lighter and caught herself and the mattress on fire and almost died. The story seemed to scare Monica, and they talked about what young children should do if anything caught fire around them. She says Monica has often brought up the situation and asked what happened to the little girl on TV.

Crystal asks Louis if he will be there for her next prenatal appointment, and he tells her that he plans to be. He asks if there is anything in particular that she would like to talk about next time, and Crystal replies, "Just tell me how I can manage a new baby and my other two at the same time!" Before leaving, Crystal again tells Louis she likes having him be with her at each clinic visit and that he has given her helpful information. Louis is satisfied that they are developing a therapeutic relationship and that he has assisted her in developing her knowledge base for managing health promotion activities for her children.

DOCUMENTATION NOTE

After the primary caregiver has documented Crystal's prenatal visit, Louis adds the following documentation in Crystal's clinic chart:

"While waiting for primary caregiver, reports she has begun to prepare her two children for the birth of a new sibling through reading books and talking about the event. States she has shared safety measures for children, particularly in regard to fire, with family caregivers. Has requested additional information pertaining to child rearing; will assess further during next visit."

KEY POINTS

- Growth and development are orderly, predictable, inter-dependent processes that continue throughout the life span.
- Growth is most rapid during the prenatal and infancy stages and continues to slow until the second skeletal growth spurt announces that puberty is approaching.
- People progress through similar stages of growth and development but at an individual pace and with individual behaviors.
- Theories of growth and development, such as those of Freud, Erikson, and Piaget, provide nurses with a frame-work for understanding individual behaviors.
- Physiological, cognitive, and psychosocial development continue across the life span. You must be familiar with normal expectations to determine potential problems and promote normal development.

- Patients need specific immunizations throughout life, not just in childhood. These immunizations help to protect individuals against illness and infections.
- Young adults have few health problems but need to develop positive health habits to avoid many health problems in middle and late adulthood.
- The health concerns of the middle adult commonly involve hormonal changes, stress-related illnesses, situational stressors, screening for health problems, and adoption of positive health habits.
- The health concerns of older adults are related to chronic illnesses, lifestyle changes, functional ability changes, accidents, and infectious diseases, such as the flu.

CRITICAL THINKING EXERCISES

As indicated in the case study, Monica, 6 years old, is having a checkup in preparation for beginning school. Louis needs to perform a number of procedures, which Monica may perceive as threatening because of their intrusive or invasive nature (e.g., measure her blood pressure, check her throat, and look in her ears).

1. What nursing approaches can Louis use to gain the child's cooperation?
2. During the checkup Monica was able to help with the examination by answering questions and reading the eye chart. She also had the opportunity to play with the equipment and has had her blood pressure and other vital signs taken. During the review of immunizations Louis has noted that up to now Monica's vaccinations have been up-to-date, but she will need two shots at this visit. How should Louis approach this?

3. Crystal is also concerned that her 15-year-old brother may soon become sexually active and wants to be sure that he knows the risks involved and how to protect himself from STIs (including AIDS) and from becoming a father before he is ready for the responsibility. How should Louis advise her?
4. As noted in the case study, Crystal is pregnant with her third child; she is a single parent as well. After Louis does the well-child examination on the children, he is able to turn his attention to Crystal. What information should he obtain from Crystal?

e̶volve   *Answers to Critical Thinking Questions can be found on the Evolve website.*

REVIEW QUESTIONS

1. While assessing for a toddler's growth and developmental status, it is important to remember that:
   1. Each toddler has the same set of communication skills
   2. Each toddler progresses at the same rate of development
   3. The toddler may have sufficient motor skills to assist in self-care activities
   4. The toddler does not have sufficient motor skills to assist in self-care activities
2. When teaching safety tips to the parents of a preschooler, you need to tell the parents that the major cause of mortality is:
   1. Violence
   2. Poisonings
   3. Infectious illness
   4. Motor vehicle accidents

3. During an assessment a patient indicates that the school performance of her 16-year-old daughter has declined and the girl is withdrawn, appears bored, and no longer takes pride in caring for possessions. You feel that these assessment findings indicate:
   1. A dislike of school
   2. An increased risk for suicide
   3. Normal adolescent changes
   4. A breakup with her boyfriend
4. You are working in an adolescent health clinic. A 16-year-old girl enters the clinic and is concerned that she might have a sexually transmitted infection (STI) because she had unprotected sex 6 weeks ago. You perform a pregnancy test, which is negative. At the patient's request you obtain appropriate specimens and requests for STI testing, including HIV infection and hepatitis. What is your next priority of care?

1. Notify the young girl's parents.

2. Initiate education regarding safe sex.

3. Obtain a prescription for birth control pills.

4. Ask the girl's sexual partner to make a clinic appointment.

5. When assessing young adults, you know that this population usually has a high level of wellness. However, it is important to direct health care education toward the priority of:

1. Health promotion

2. Primary prevention

3. Tertiary prevention

4. Secondary prevention

6. When you suspect that your patient is a victim of domestic violence, you need to know that patients' risk for violence increases when:

1. They seek medical treatment

2. They experience their first violent attack

3. They seek law enforcement intervention

4. They initiate a plan to remove themselves from the abusive environment

7. Women need to increase their daily calcium intake to prevent:

1. Arthritis

2. Osteoporosis

3. Hypertension

4. Coronary artery disease

8. Which statement made by the parent of a toddler indicates a need for further teaching?

1. "My son likes the apple slices I give him as a snack."

2. "Now that my son is 3, he won't need a car seat anymore."

3. "I use time-out as a form of discipline."

4. "I have moved all of the plants off of the floor."

9. Karen selects *ineffective coping* as a priority diagnosis. You work with her to develop realistic interventions. Which of the following interventions is (are) appropriate for this diagnosis? Select all that apply.

1. Counseling sessions

2. Stress management techniques

3. 1800-calorie diet

4. Yoga classes

10. Common conditions affecting cognition in the older adult include:

1. Blindness, hearing loss, and stroke

2. Delirium, dementia, and depression

3. Delirium, Alzheimer's disease, and visual impairment

4. Stroke, hearing loss, and depression

Answers to Review Questions can be found on pages 1197-1198.

REFERENCES

Administration on Aging: *Statistics on the aging population*, Washington, DC, 2008, U.S. Department of Health and Human Services, http://www.aoa.gov/AoARoot/Aging_Statistics/index.aspx, accessed July 2009.

Alzheimer's Association: *Alzheimer's disease symptoms*, Chicago, 2008, The Association, http://www.alz.org/alzheimers_disease_symptoms_of_alzheimers.asp, accessed July 2008.

American Academy of Pediatrics: Policy statement: breast feeding and the use of human milk, *Pediatrics* 115(2):496, 2005, http://aappolicy.aappublications.org/cgi/content/full/pediatrics;115/2/496#ABS, accessed January 2009.

American Academy of Pediatrics: *A childcare provider's guide to safe sleep*, revised 2008, http://www.healthychildcare.org/pdf/SIDSchildcaresafesleep.pdf, accessed July 2008.

Bass L: Health literacy: implications for teaching the adult patient, *J Infus Nurs* 28 (1):15, 2005.

Behrman RE and others: *Nelson textbook of pediatrics*, ed 17, Philadelphia, 2004, WB Saunders.

Bulechek GM and others, editors: *Nursing interventions classification (NIC)*, ed 5, St. Louis, 2008, Mosby.

Cacchione PZ and others: Risk for acute confusion in sensory-impaired, rural long-term care elders, *Clin Nurs Res* 12(4):340, 2003.

Ebersole P and others: *Toward healthy aging: human needs and nursing response*, ed 7, St. Louis, 2008, Mosby.

Edelman C, Mandel C: *Health promotion throughout the life span*, ed 6, St. Louis, 2006, Mosby.

Edmunds M: Health literacy: a barrier to patient education, *Nurse Pract* 30(3):54, 2005.

Erikson E: *Childhood and society*, New York, 1963, WW Norton.

Erikson E: *The lifecycle completed*, New York, 1997, WW Norton.

Foreman M and others: Assessing cognitive function, *Geriatr Nurs* 17(5):239, 1996.

Hockenberry M, Wilson D: *Wong's nursing care of infants and children*, ed 8, St. Louis, 2007, Mosby.

Kohlberg L: Development of moral character and moral ideology. In Hoffman ML, Hoffman LNW, editors: *Review of child development research*, vol 1, New York, 1964, Russell Sage Foundation.

Leak A, Hu J, King CR: Symptom distress, spirituality, and quality of life in African American breast cancer survivors, *Cancer Nurs* 31(1):E15, 2008.

Lemiengre J and others: Detection of delirium by bedside nurses using the confusion assessment method, *J Am Geriatr Soc* 54:685, 2006.

Maslow AH: *Motivation and personality*, ed 3, Upper Saddle River, NJ, 1970, Prentice Hall.

Meiner SE, Lueckenotte AG: *Gerontologic nursing*, ed 3, St. Louis, 2006, Mosby.

Moorhead S and others, editors: *Nursing outcomes classification (NOC)*, ed 4, St. Louis, 2008, Mosby.

National High Blood Pressure Education Program; National Heart, Lung, and Blood Institute; National Institutes of Health: The seventh report of the Joint National Commission on Detection, Evaluation, and Treatment of High Blood Pressure, *JAMA* 289(19):2560, 2003. http://www.nhlbi.nih.gov/guidelines/hypertension/jnc8/index.htm

National Institute of Mental Health: *Older adults: depression and suicide facts*, Bethesda, Md, 2007, National Institutes of Health, http://www.nimh.nih.gov/publicat/elderlydepsuicide.cfm, accessed July 2008.

Naylor MD and others: Cognitively impaired older adults: from hospital to home, *Am J Nurs* 105(2):52, 2005.

Phillips JM and others: African American women's experiences with breast cancer screening, *J Nurs Scholarsh* 33(2):135, 2001.

Raj A: Symposium on geriatric psychiatry: depression in the elderly, *Postgrad Med* 115(6):26, 2004, http://www.postgradmed.com/issues/2004/06_04/raj.html.

Santrock J: *Life-span development*, ed 9, New York, 2007, McGraw Hill.

U.S. Department of Health and Human Services, Public Health Service: *Healthy people 2010 objectives*, Washington, DC, 2000, Office of Disease Prevention and Health Promotion.

22 Self-Concept and Sexuality

 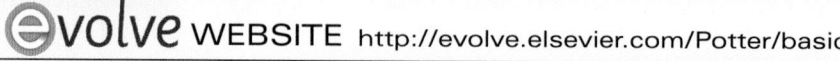
OBJECTIVES

- Discuss factors that influence the following components of self-concept: identity, body image, and role performance.
- Identify stressors that affect self-concept, self-esteem, and sexuality.
- Describe the components of self-concept as each relates to Erikson's developmental stages.

- Discuss ways in which your self-concept and nursing actions affect your patient's self-concept and self-esteem.
- Discuss your role in maintaining or enhancing a patient's sexual health.
- Apply the nursing process to promote a patient's self-concept and sexual health.

KEY TERMS

body image, p. 601
identity, p. 600
role performance, p. 601

self-concept, p. 599
self-esteem, p. 601

sexual dysfunction, p. 604
sexual orientation, p. 601

sexuality, p. 599
sexually transmitted infection, p. 604

Self-concept and sexuality include a complex mixture of unconscious and conscious thoughts, attitudes, and perceptions. As a nurse, you will care for patients who face a variety of health problems that threaten their self-esteem and their sexuality. For example, patients who experience a loss of body function or a change in their physical appearance are at risk for experiencing a change in self-concept and sexuality. Help your patients adjust to alterations in self-concept and sexuality to promote successful coping.

SCIENTIFIC KNOWLEDGE BASE

Self-concept is your view of who you are. It is a combination of unconscious and conscious thoughts, attitudes, and perceptions. Self-concept, or how you think about yourself, directly affects your self-esteem and how you feel about yourself. What you think and how you feel about yourself affect the way in which you care for yourself physically and emotionally. It also influences the way in which you are able to care for others. As a nurse, you need to have knowledge of factors that affect self-concept and self-esteem. Be aware of differences across age and gender, and be sensitive to ethnic and cultural differences in self-concept and self-esteem to individualize your approach to patient care (see Chapter 19).

Sexuality is a broad term that refers to all aspects of being sexual. It is a part of who a person is and is important for overall health. It is possible for people to be sexually healthy in numerous ways. Sex is considered a basic physiological need, and sexual intimacy throughout the life span is equally important for sexual health. Healthy sexuality enables a person to develop and maintain the fullest potential. Sexuality includes a person's thoughts and feelings about the body, a sense of femaleness or maleness, romantic and erotic attachments toward others, and attitudes toward sexual functioning. Our sexual health is based on our ability to form healthy relationships with others (Figure 22-1).

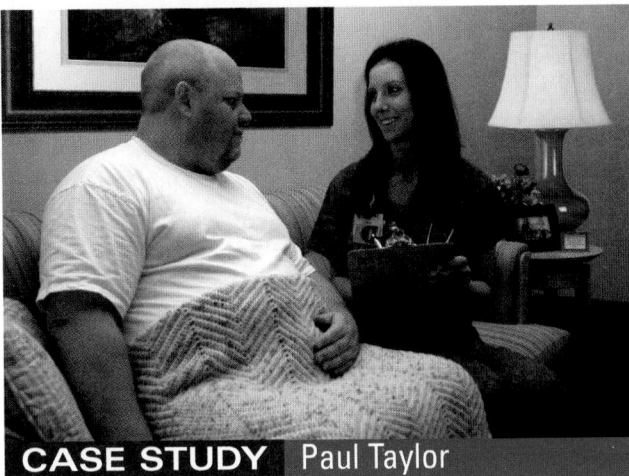

CASE STUDY   Paul Taylor

Paul Taylor, a 58-year-old man, suffered a stroke. The stroke was unexpected and sudden. He did not know that he had hypertension because he had not been getting yearly checkups. Mr. Taylor woke up in the hospital bed to find that he could not move his hand. He was not able to care for himself or to turn himself for days. With his nurses' constant encouragement, he is finally able to transfer from his bed into a chair. Mr. Taylor wonders what lies ahead for him. His body image has dramatically changed from that of a man of strength to that of a helpless individual. Mr. Taylor worries about his family and what will happen. He and his wife, Meredith, are terrified. Although Mrs. Taylor works, they have not saved enough money to meet monthly expenses or to educate their children without both incomes. Mr. Taylor's role as primary breadwinner for the family will be drastically changed if his condition does not improve.

Mr. Taylor's self-esteem lessens as his recovery and rehabilitation move slowly. His self-concept has changed from that of a strong laborer, one who did his own plumbing and car repairs, to a man who must rely on others. Although he is now at home in the rehabilitation process, Mr. Taylor is not able to perform tasks for the family and waits until his wife and son get home to help him with things that require strength. Moreover, because of the sexual side effects of the antihypertensive medication he is taking, his sexual health has been dramatically altered, and the lack of intimacy with his wife is affecting their relationship. Mr. Taylor's adaptation capabilities are stretched to the maximum. Mr. Taylor's identity is not clear to him anymore. He has no clear role within the family, his body image has been drastically altered, his sexual health has suffered, and his self-esteem has never been lower.

Maria Kendal is a 27-year-old nursing student assigned to care for Mr. Taylor. Ms. Kendal is divorced, has two school-age children, and works part-time as a certified nurse assistant (CNA) at a local long-term care facility while in school. She recognizes that changes in health status often result in stressors that affect a person's self-concept and sexuality. Such stressors influence a person's ability to interact with others and to function effectively. Ms. Kendal's knowledge of self-concept and sexuality will aid in identifying stressors that affect Mr. Taylor and promote effective planning to support his growth and adaptation to change.

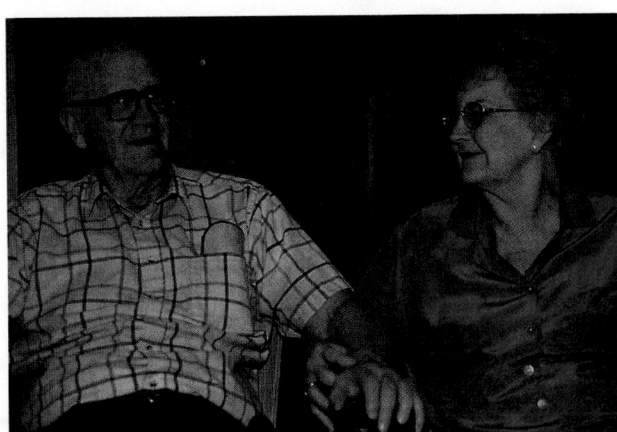

Figure 22-1 ■ Sexuality is important across the life span.

BOX 22-1　Erikson's Developmental Tasks and Impact on Self-Concept and Sexuality

TRUST VERSUS MISTRUST (BIRTH TO 1 YEAR)
- Develops trust following consistency in caregiving and nurturing interactions
- Distinguishes self from environment

AUTONOMY VERSUS SHAME AND DOUBT (1 TO 3 YEARS)
- Begins to communicate likes and dislikes
- Increasingly independent in thoughts and actions
- Appreciates body appearance and function (including dressing, feeding, talking, and walking)

INITIATIVE VERSUS GUILT (3 TO 6 YEARS)
- Takes initiative
- Identifies with a gender
- Enhances self-awareness
- Increases language skills, including identification of feelings

INDUSTRY VERSUS INFERIORITY (6 TO 12 YEARS)
- Incorporates feedback from peers and teachers
- Increases self-esteem with new skill mastery (e.g., reading, math, sports, music)
- Sexual identity strengthens
- Aware of strengths and limitations

IDENTITY VERSUS ROLE CONFUSION (12 TO 20 YEARS)
- Accepts body changes/maturation
- Examines attitudes, values, and beliefs; establishes goals for the future
- Feels positive about expanded sense of self

INTIMACY VERSUS ISOLATION (MID-20s TO MID-40s)
- Has intimate relationships with family and significant others
- Has stable, positive feelings about self
- Experiences successful role transitions and increased responsibilities

GENERATIVITY VERSUS SELF-ABSORPTION (MID-40s TO MID-60s)
- Able to accept changes in appearance and physical endurance
- Reassesses life goals
- Shows contentment with aging

EGO INTEGRITY VERSUS DESPAIR (LATE 60s TO DEATH)
- Feels positive about one's life and its meaning
- Interested in providing a legacy for the next generation

NURSING KNOWLEDGE BASE

To provide evidence-based care to patients, incorporate professional nursing knowledge developed from the humanities and sciences, nursing research, and clinical practice. A broad knowledge base allows you to have a holistic view of patients, thus promoting quality patient care that will best meet the self-concept and sexual health needs of each patient and family.

Development of Self-Concept

The development of self-concept is a complex process that involves many factors. Erikson's psychosocial theory of development (1963) is helpful in understanding key tasks that individuals face at various stages of development. Each stage builds on the tasks of the previous stage. Completing each developmental stage successfully leads to a solid sense of self. The development of self-concept and self-esteem begins at a young age and continues throughout life with a general tendency for males to report higher self-esteem than females (Birndorf and others, 2005).

As a nurse, you will use Erikson's theory to identify the stage of psychosocial development a patient is in based first on his or her biological age and adjusted based on any significant life events. You will also assess where the patient actually is and determine how the patient is handling the tasks of that stage. Awareness of these developmental tasks (Box 22-1) allows you to select appropriate nursing actions.

Components and Interrelated Terms of Self-Concept

A positive self-concept gives a sense of meaning and wholeness to a person. The components of self-concept frequently considered by nurses are identity, body image, and role performance. Sexuality also has an effect on self-concept. Likewise, identity, body image, role performance, and self-esteem affect sexual health. Although overlap exists between concepts, this chapter will present each one separately.

Identity involves the sense of individuality and completeness of a person over time and in various circumstances. Identity implies being distinct and separate from others. Being "oneself" or living a life that is genuine and authentic is the basis of true identity.

The achievement of identity is necessary for intimate relationships because you express your identity in relationships with others. Sexuality is a part of your identity. Gender identity is a person's private view of maleness or femaleness, and gender role is the feminine or masculine behavior exhibited.

Racial or cultural identity develops from identifying and socializing within an established group and through incorporating the responses of individuals who do not belong to that group into one's self-concept. The opinion or approval of others affects self-esteem differently among racial and cultural groups. Demographic, physical, and behavioral characteristics influence body image and self-esteem (Kornblau and others, 2007). One group of researchers found that family income above the federal poverty level, positive family communication, and involvement in a religious community were associated with high self-esteem in boys; for girls, being of African American or Hispanic race/ethnicity, positive family communication, and feeling safe were predictive of higher self-esteem (Birndorf and others, 2005). Sensitivity to factors that affect self-concept and self-esteem in diverse cultures is essential to ensure an individualized approach to health care.

Body image involves attitudes related to the body, including physical appearance, femininity and masculinity, youthfulness, health, and strength. These views are not always the same as the person's actual physical structure or appearance. When a change in health status occurs, as in the case of Mr. Taylor, exaggerated disturbances in body image sometimes occur. The way others view a person's body and the feedback offered is also influential. For example, a controlling, violent husband tells his wife that she is ugly and that no one else would want her. Over the years of marriage, she incorporates this criticism into her self-concept.

Cultural and societal attitudes and values influence body image and sexuality. Culture and society influence the accepted norms of body image and affect one's attitudes. Values such as ideal body weight and shape, as well as attitudes toward body markings, piercing, and tattoos are culturally based. Racial and ethnic background affects body satisfaction in adolescent girls as reflected in the higher incidence of body satisfaction among African American girls compared with white girls (Kelly and others, 2005). American society typically emphasizes youth, beauty, and wholeness. This is apparent in television programs, movies, and advertisements. Western cultures have been socialized to dread the normal aging process. In contrast, Eastern cultures view aging very positively and respect the older adult.

Body image depends only partly on the reality of the body. When physical changes occur, individuals may or may not incorporate these changes into their body image. For example, people who have experienced significant weight loss do not perceive themselves as thin and may still tell you there is still a "fat person" inside. Body image issues are often associated with negative self-concept and self-esteem. The majority of men and women experience some degree of body dissatisfaction, which can affect body image and overall self-concept. As a nurse, you are in an ideal position to influence a patient's body image.

Normal developmental changes such as puberty and aging have a more obvious effect on body image than on other aspects of self-concept. Hormonal changes during puberty and menopause in later adulthood influence body image. The development of secondary sex characteristics and changes in body fat distribution have a tremendous impact on the self-concept of an adolescent. For both male and female adolescents, negative body image is a risk factor for suicidal thoughts (Brausch and Muehlenkamp, 2007). Changes associated with

aging (e.g., wrinkles; graying hair; and decrease in visual acuity, hearing, and mobility) affect body image in older adults.

As a person grows and develops, so does his or her sexuality. Each stage of development brings changes in sexual functioning, sexual focus, and sexual relationships (see Chapter 21). Knowledge of sexual development and changes throughout the life span is essential for a nurse. The adult has achieved physical maturation, but is continuing to explore and define emotional maturation in relationships. Even into adulthood, we continue to struggle with questions of who we are, how we want to present ourselves, and what type of partners we find most attractive. A clear sense of your sexual orientation and the ability to form open relationships also influences sexual health. You will provide care to individuals whose **sexual orientation** is heterosexual (attracted to different-sex partners), homosexual (same-sex partners), or bisexual (both male and female partners). Also, you will care for patients who are involved in intimate relationships with several partners and for patients whose sexual relationships occur outside of marriage.

Role performance is the way in which a person views his or her ability to carry out significant roles. Common roles include mother or father, wife or husband, daughter or son, sister or brother, employee or employer, and nurse or patient. For example, stating, "I am a good mother" or "I am a caring and competent nurse" reflects a positive self-concept and self-esteem. Each role involves meeting certain expectations. Fulfillment of these expectations leads to an enhanced sense of self. Difficulty or failure in meeting role expectations leads to decreased self-esteem or altered self-concept.

Self-esteem is an individual's overall sense of self-worth or the emotional evaluation of self-concept. It represents the overall judgment of personal worth or value. Self-esteem is positive when one feels capable, worthwhile, and competent (Rosenberg, 1965). Once established, basic feelings about the self tend to be constant, even though there is sometimes a little fluctuation. A situational crisis, like a hospitalization, often temporarily affects one's self-esteem.

Self-evaluation is an ongoing mental process. A positive sense of self-worth, or self-esteem, is an important factor in determining how an individual functions in the world. A person's ability to contribute in a meaningful way to society often affects self-concept and self-esteem. Some individuals who are chronically ill feel a sense of worthlessness. Your acceptance of a patient as an individual with worth and dignity will help maintain and improve the patient's self-esteem.

Stressors Affecting Self-Concept and Sexuality

A self-concept stressor is any real or perceived change that threatens identity, body image, or role performance (Figure 22-2). The individual's perception of the stressor is the most important factor in determining his or her response. For example, a man who has had a heart attack believes that he will no longer be able to be the aggressive businessman he has

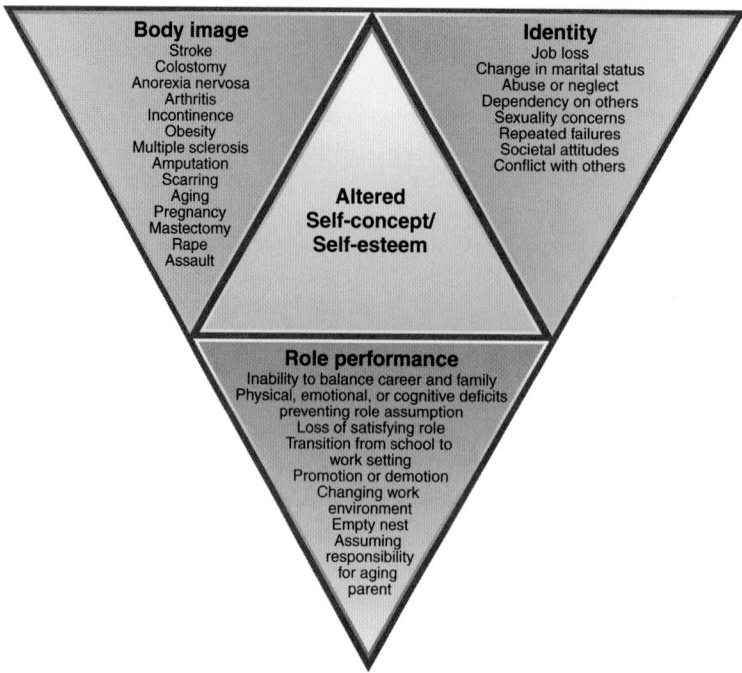

Figure 22-2 ▪ Common stressors that influence self-concept.

prided himself as being. This perception of what the heart attack will mean to his lifestyle leads to depression. However, another man views his heart attack as a message to slow down and enjoy his life.

Any change in health is a stressor that potentially affects self-concept. A physical change in the body leads to an altered body image, affecting identity and self-esteem. Chronic illnesses often alter role performance, which frequently alter a person's identity and self-esteem. Living with a chronic illness requires a person to cope with a lost sense of self while a new self emerges. After adjustment to the loss, the person has to develop a new self-concept. For example, the loss of a partner sometimes leads to a loss of identity and a lower self-esteem.

A crisis occurs when a person cannot cope with stressors with usual methods of problem solving and adaptation. Any crisis potentially threatens self-concept and self-esteem. Some crises, like the one with Paul Taylor in the case study, directly affect all components of self-concept. If people are unable to adapt to such stressors, their health may be at risk and illness may result.

IDENTITY STRESSORS Stressors throughout life affect an individual's identity, but identity is particularly vulnerable during adolescence, which is a time of great change. Adolescents are trying to adjust to the physical, emotional, and mental changes of increasing maturity, which results in insecurity and anxiety. For example, an adolescent who wants to be identified as part of the popular crowd at school develops a poor self-concept if not included in that group. Family and cultural factors sometimes influence negative health practices, such as cigarette smoking (Box 22-2). Promoting a change in self-concept demands an evidence-based practice approach, supported by the entire health care team. This means the team uses the best knowledge available about self-concept to drive patient care decisions.

An adult generally has a stable identity and thus a more firmly developed self-concept. Once a person has established his or her identity, the adult is better able to handle stressors such as marriage, divorce, menopause, aging, and retirement. Retirement for some means the loss of an important means of achievement. Some people at retirement begin to reevaluate their identities and accomplishments. More and more older people are working past the traditional retirement age or change careers following retirement. Some do so because of a financial need, whereas others have a desire to remain involved and productive (Ebersole and others, 2005). Sometimes loss of a significant other also leads a person to reexamine aspects of his or her identity.

BODY IMAGE STRESSORS Changes in the appearance or function of a body part require an adjustment in body image. An individual's perception of the change and the relative importance placed on body image in the individual's self-concept will affect the significance of the loss or change. For example, if a woman considers her breasts key to her femininity, a mastectomy will negatively affect her body image. Changes in the appearance of the body, such as an amputation, facial disfigurement, or burns, are obvious stressors affecting body image. Surgical procedures, potentially undetected by others, have a significant impact on the individual. Elective changes such as breast augmentation or reduction also affect body image. Chronic illnesses such as heart and lung disease involve a change in function, in which the body no longer performs at an optimal level. Physical changes associated with aging or treatment for medical conditions negatively affect body image as well. In addition, the effects of

BOX 22-2   BEST PRACTICES

The Impact of Body Image, Self-Esteem, and Stress on Adolescent Smoking Behaviors

SUMMARY OF EVIDENCE

The prevalence of tobacco use in the United States is highest between ages 18 and 24, with college students representing the highest portion of smokers. Half of all college students have tried tobacco in the past year, and about a third are current tobacco users. Previous studies have shown weight concerns, especially in women, motivate users to continue smoking and predict smoking relapse. Smokers were more likely to perceive higher amounts of stress and lower self-esteem. The majority of smokers, regardless of gender, consider tobacco use an important stress management practice. Enhancing opportunities for physical activity may reduce adolescent risk behaviors, including smoking.

APPLICATION TO NURSING PRACTICE

- Smoking cessation efforts need to include stress management and self-esteem and body image improvement.
- A priority nursing action is the assessment of child and adolescent coping strategies. Appropriate techniques include effective communication, conflict resolution, and stress management.
- Body weight concerns, as well as family, social environment, and behavioral factors, are important issues you need to address during preadolescence and adolescence.
- Implement effective, healthy, and realistic weight management methods for adolescents. Techniques include promoting fun, family-oriented physical activity, monitoring and reducing sedentary activities like TV viewing and gaming, and eliminating dieting.
- Identification of risk factors for early drug and alcohol use, including genetic predisposition, family environment, and sedentary behaviors, need to be a priority for nurses and other health care providers.

REFERENCES

Croghan IT and others: Is smoking related to body image satisfaction, stress, and self esteem in young girls? *Am J Health Behav* 30(3):322, 2006.

Nelson MC, Gordon-Larsen P: Physical activity and sedentary behavior patterns are associated with selected adolescent risk behaviors, *Pediatrics* 117(4):1281, 2006.

pregnancy, significant weight gain or loss, medication management of an illness, or radiation therapy all change body image. Negative body image sometimes leads to adverse health outcomes. Many people associate success with a specific body part or function. For example, some athletes consider their bodies and physical activities to be the focus of personal success. If they are never again able to participate in athletics because of an accident or injury, this can affect their adaptation and rehabilitation. Body image changes require reevaluation of long-accepted self-perceptions, as well as alterations in lifestyle.

ROLE PERFORMANCE STRESSORS Throughout life a person undergoes many role changes. Normal changes associated with maturation result in changes in role performance. For example, when a man has a child, he becomes a father. The new role of father will involve many changes in behavior if the man is going to be successful. Group interventions aimed at improving fathering experiences have led to significant improvements in the father's participation in the family, including role performance, involvement, communication, self-esteem, a sense of increased competence, and decreased stress in parenting (Gearing and others, 2008). Another shift is necessary when a middle-age woman with young children assumes responsibility for the care of her older parents. Acute and chronic illnesses alter a person's ability to carry out various roles, which will affect self-esteem and identity.

All people must adapt to two major changes that occur with aging: changes in the work role and in the role of spouse or partner (Ebersole and others, 2005). Role performance changes associated with retirement differ for men and women. Many women have adjusted to several different roles throughout their lifetime and are more likely than men to have developed friendships that are not work related. Adjusting to changes in role performance has an impact on the marital relationship. Changes in role performance following the loss of a spouse or partner also affect self-concept. A widow who has never paid bills or one who needs to learn to cook will need assistance in changing roles.

SELF-ESTEEM STRESSORS Individuals with high self-esteem are generally better able to cope with demands and stressors than those with low self-esteem. Low self-worth contributes to feeling unfulfilled and misunderstood and results in depression and anxiety. Illness, surgery, or accidents that change life patterns also influence feelings of self-worth. The more that chronic illness such as diabetes, arthritis, and heart disease interfere with the ability to engage in activities contributing to feelings of worth or success, the more they affect self-esteem.

Self-esteem stressors vary with developmental stages. If a child believes that he is unable to meet his parents' expectations or if his parents harshly criticize or inconsistently discipline him, this will reduce his level of self-worth. The self-esteem of an adolescent is also vulnerable because the adolescent directs so much energy to worrying about appearance, searching for identity, and being overly concerned about what others think. Stressors affecting the self-esteem of an adult include failures at work and failures in relationships. Box 22-3 discusses potential self-esteem stressors in older adults.

SEXUALITY STRESSORS As a nurse you will work with patients who are making decisions or dealing with issues related to sexuality on a regular basis. For example, people of all ages face reproductive health issues including contraception, infertility, sexual dysfunction, and sexual satisfaction. Understanding some of the decisions and issues patients face increases your effectiveness in helping patients to reach their maximum level of health in the area of sexuality.

Alterations in sexual health occur from a variety of situations such as illness, infertility, trauma, and abuse. **Sexual**

BOX 22-3 CARE OF THE OLDER ADULT

Promoting Self-Concept and Self-Esteem

Self-concept can be negatively affected in older adulthood because of life changes such as spousal loss or decline in health. Gender differences exist in body image, with many men becoming more negative about appearance and function of their bodies than women. In some individuals, aging promotes improved coping strategies that protect against the declining feelings of self-esteem, despite all the physical and emotional changes associated with aging. Nursing interventions aimed at promoting resiliency and enhancing self-concept and self-esteem in older adults are essential.
- Clarify what the life changes mean and the impact on self-concept for the older adult.

- Be alert to preoccupation with physical complaints. Assess complaints thoroughly, and if no physical explanation exists, encourage the older adult to verbalize needs (fear, insecurity, loneliness) in a nonphysical way.
- Identify positive and negative coping mechanisms. Support and teach effective strategies.
- Encourage the use of storytelling and review of old photographs.
- Communicate that the older adult is worthwhile by actively listening to and accepting the person's feelings, being respectful, and praising healthy behaviors.
- Allow additional time to complete tasks. Reinforce the older adult's efforts at independence.

Data from Collins A, Smyer MA: The resilience of self-esteem in late adulthood, *J Aging Health* 17(4):471, 2005; Ebersole P and others: *Gerontological nursing and healthy aging,* ed 2, St. Louis, 2005, Mosby; Kaminski PL, Hayslip B: Gender differences in body esteem among older adults, *J Women Aging* 18(3):19, 2006.

dysfunction interferes with sexual health and is a problem with desire, arousal, or orgasm. Erectile dysfunction is a common problem among older men. It is generally related to chronic diseases such as diabetes, kidney disease, alcohol dependence, depression, neurological disorders, vascular insufficiency, and diseases of the prostate (Ebersole and others, 2005). In addition, side effects of medications also contribute to sexual dysfunction. Although patients take medications to stay healthy, the side effects sometimes negatively affect sexuality. The causes of sexual dysfunction are physiological or psychological. Sometimes the cause of a dysfunction cannot be identified or is a result of a combination of several factors.

Because sexual dysfunction sometimes results from the use of medications such as antidepressants and antihypertensives, it is important to include sexual side effects in patient teaching. Your patient is more likely to adhere to a treatment plan if you discuss side effects of medications that alter sexual function with both partners and the patient is able to make an informed decision. Our current state of health greatly influences sexual response (from desire to arousal to orgasm). The availability of sexual performance–enhancing medication like Viagra (sildenafil) and Cialis (tadalafil) has changed the lives of many couples. These medications treat erectile dysfunction but are contraindicated in men with coronary artery disease or those taking common cardiac drugs.

Changing physical appearance and concerns about physical attractiveness affect sexual functioning. The loss of sexual activity and the absence of a self-concept that includes being a sexual person is not an inevitable aspect of aging. Some older people face health concerns and societal attitudes that make it difficult for them to continue sexual activity. Although declining physical abilities sometimes make sex as they knew it painful or impossible, with intervention, older adults are able to experiment with and learn alternative ways of sexual expression.

Hormonally stimulated changes brought on by developmental maturation are also stressors that affect sexuality across the life span. Menarche, the onset of menstrual cycle in girls, is occurring at an earlier age in the United States, and some adolescent girls are unaware that it is normal to grow pubic, underarm, and body hair and deposit more fat on their hips and breasts, all of which will also affect body image. Early maturation is often associated with lower psychological well-being and lower enjoyment of physical activity, which in turn, could negatively affect body image (Davison and others, 2007). As boys approach puberty, physical changes include nocturnal emissions and ejaculation, increasing sexual desire, and increased hygiene needs. Older women experiencing menopause, the cessation of menstrual periods, experience changes in vaginal lubrication and sexual interest. The majority of menopausal woman recognize the importance of maintaining an active sex life, but many report reduced sex drive, decreased sexual interest, and mood changes that may require intervention by a health care provider (Nappi and Nijland, 2008). Additional patient teaching needs to include instruction on breast and testicular self-examinations as well as prevention of **sexually transmitted infection,** an infection spread through oral, anal, or vaginal activity. The use of latex condoms to prevent sexually transmitted disease and unintended pregnancy is essential because approximately 50% of new human immune deficiency virus (HIV) infections in the United States occur in teenagers, with a high incidence in African American females (Aronowitz and others, 2007). African Americans also have higher rates of gonorrhea, chlamydial infection, and syphilis than any other group in the United States (Barrow and others, 2008).

Sexual abuse, assault, and rape are also stressors that affect self-concept. Be alert to clues that suggest abuse (Box 22-4). In addition, observe the interaction between the patient and partner for additional clues. Controlling behaviors such as speaking for the person or refusing to leave him or her alone with a caregiver are suggestive of emotional and perhaps physical or sexual abuse. If you suspect abuse, interview the patient privately. A patient will probably not admit to prob-

BOX 22-4	Signs and Symptoms That May Indicate Current Sexual Abuse or a History of Sexual Abuse

- Unexplained bruises, lacerations, or abrasions especially around breasts or genital or anal areas
- Unexplained vaginal or anal soreness or bleeding
- Unexplained venereal disease or genital infection
- Frequent visits to health care providers
- Headaches
- Gastrointestinal problems
- Abdominal pain
- Dysmenorrhea
- Premenstrual syndrome
- Sleep pattern disturbances
- Nightmares
- Repetitive dreams
- Depression
- Social withdrawal
- Anxiety
- Eating disorders
- Substance abuse
- Decreased self-esteem
- Difficulty developing trust
- Difficulties with intimate relationships
- Impaired school or work performance
- Reports of being sexually assaulted or raped

NOTE: No physical symptoms may be present.

Modified from Meiner SE, Lueckenotte A: *Gerontologic nursing*, ed 3, St. Louis, 2006, Mosby; Stuart GW: *Principles and practice of psychiatric nursing*, ed 9, St. Louis, 2009, Mosby.

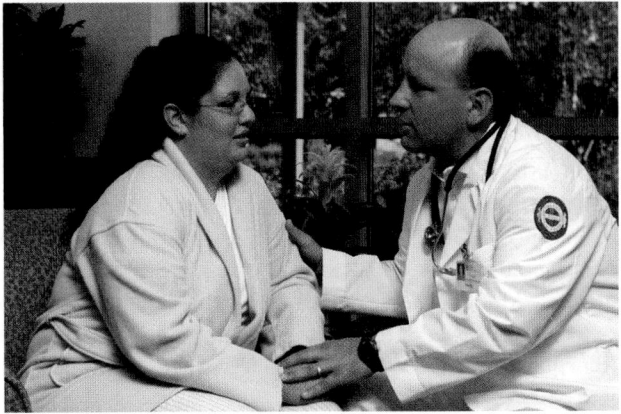

Figure 22-3 ■ Nurses use touch and eye contact to enhance a patient's self-esteem.

lems of abuse with the abuser present. Some of the following questions are useful: "Are you in a relationship in which someone is hurting you?" or "Have you ever been forced to have sex when you didn't want to?" When you recognize or report abuse, mobilize treatment immediately for the victim and the family. The most important factor to consider is the safety of the suspected victim. Often, all family members require therapy to promote healthy interactions and relationships.

The Nurse's Influence on the Patient's Self-Concept and Sexuality

As a nurse, you have the ability to positively influence a patient's self-concept. Your acceptance of a patient with an altered self-concept helps promote positive change. Your words and actions convey sincere interest and acceptance and have a profound effect on the patient. When a patient's physical appearance has changed, both the patient and the family will watch your verbal and nonverbal responses and reactions to the changed appearance. A positive and matter-of-fact approach to care provides a model for the patient and family to follow. It is important that health care providers understand the degree to which self-esteem and sexuality affect patient outcomes (Figueroa-Hass, 2007).

How you respond to patients who have experienced changes in body appearance sets the stage for how they come to see themselves. The patient with a change in body functioning or appearance is often extremely sensitive to your verbal and nonverbal responses (Figure 22-3). General nursing interventions, such as building a trusting nurse-patient relationship and appropriately including the patient in decision making, supports most patients' self-concept. Sometimes individualized approaches, including supporting the use of alternative healing techniques or methods of spiritual expression, will help a patient adapt to changes in self-concept.

As a nurse, you can affect your patient's body image. For example, perceived acceptance has a positive impact on the body image and self-esteem of homosexual males (Levesque and Vichesky, 2006). You will influence the body image of a woman who has had a mastectomy in a positive way by showing acceptance of the mastectomy scar. On the other hand, a shocked or disgusted facial expression will influence the woman to develop a negative body image. It is very important to monitor your responses toward the patient. Matter-of-fact statements such as "This wound is healing nicely" or "This looks healthy" enhance the body image of the patient.

Inadvertently frowning or grimacing when performing procedures has a profound effect on the patient. Your nonverbal behavior conveys the level of caring that exists for your patient and affects your patient's self-esteem. For example, when an incontinent patient perceives that you find the situation unpleasant, this threatens the patient's self-concept. Anticipate your own reactions, acknowledge them, and focus on the patient instead of the unpleasant task or situation. Put yourself in the patient's position, to lessen the patient's embarrassment, frustration, and anger.

When you consider the sexuality of patients, think about your own knowledge regarding sexual development, sexual orientation, sexual response, sexually transmitted diseases, contraception, and alterations in sexual health. Also consider your knowledge base about communication (see Chapter 10). Your own sexuality, sexual experiences, and communication style are valuable when trying to understand your patient's experiences. Attempts at self-exploration teach us about our bodies and the potential for providing pleasure. Your attitude about masturbation may have stemmed from personal experience or from values or beliefs communicated by other people. Games like "doctor" and "nurse" may have provided other early sex play and exploration. In addition, your own sexual experiences add to understanding about what a first sexual encounter may have been like or what it is like to introduce the topic of sexually transmitted diseases or intercourse. In addition to personal experiences related to sexuality, use what you have learned through working with other patients as you assess and develop trust with current patients.

It is important that you understand the reason for changes in the patient's sexual health. The response to changes in sexuality and intimacy following an illness depends on the person's self-concept, support of sexual partner, and attitudes regarding sexuality. Many health professionals fail to address sexual needs of their patients. To promote sexual health, understand the effect of a diagnosis, as well as its treatment and medications, on your patient's perception of sexuality or sexual performance as you develop a treatment plan. For example, when caring for an older man who has had a heart attack, you say, "Following a heart attack, many older men have questions about sexuality, such as when they are able to resume sexual intercourse. Do you have questions like this that I can answer?" A professional specializing in altered sexual health is sometimes necessary to help the patient and partner resume a satisfying sexual relationship. Before making a referral, though, use therapeutic communication techniques to open the discussion about sexual concerns and provide information about sexual health.

CRITICAL THINKING

Synthesis

You will apply elements of critical thinking whenever you perform the nursing process with a patient. Consider the scientific knowledge you have learned, your experience, critical thinking attitudes, and standards to ensure an individualized approach to patient care. Your nursing expertise will allow you to anticipate and respond to stressors that affect your patient's self-concept and sexual health. Consider changes in your patient's identity, body image, role performance, and self-esteem as important aspects of care (Box 22-5).

KNOWLEDGE In addition to considering the various aspects of a patient's self-concept, use knowledge of how various medications and chronic pain influence your patient's ability to perform self-care and function at an optimal level. Many medications have actions and side effects that influence a patient's self-concept and sexuality. When you care for patients who have alterations in self-concept, be particularly alert to the patient who is experiencing chronic pain. Chronic pain predisposes a person to decreased ability to function, irritability, and decreased sleep. These changes negatively af-

BOX 22-5   SYNTHESIS IN PRACTICE

As Maria prepares to care for Mr. Taylor, she thinks about what she knows about self-concept and sexuality. She realizes that Mr. Taylor's stroke and resulting neurological deficits along with the sexual side effects of his antihypertensive medications are significant stressors in regard to his self-concept and sexuality. Mr. Taylor's independence is threatened because he is in the hospital and is dependent upon the nurses for most of his care. He may never be able to go back to work again, and he does not consider himself a strong man anymore. Therefore his family role as provider is threatened. Maria recognizes the significance of these changes and their potential influence on his self-concept and sexuality.

Maria's father experienced a stroke 2 years ago. Although his neurological symptoms finally improved enough to allow him to go back to work, Maria remembers the struggle her father went through as he coped with the physical and emotional changes the stroke created. Maria's experience as a single mother also provides insight into what it is like to assume a new role within a family. Maria uses these two different experiences to guide her assessment of Mr. Taylor's concerns.

Maria needs to learn as much as she can about Mr. Taylor's thoughts and feelings about his self-concept and sexuality. In order to do this, she realizes that she must first establish a trusting relationship with Mr. Taylor and his wife, Meredith. Because Maria feels uncomfortable in discussing sexuality with her patients, she reviews the PLISSIT* assessment of sexuality the night before she cares for Mr. Taylor and writes out some questions that she wants to ask him. Maria also plans to talk with both Mr. and Mrs. Taylor about their relationship before and after the stroke.

*See Box 22-8, p. 608.

fect self-concept. Another area of knowledge to consider is the patient's cultural background. Culture influences the importance people place on such things as appearance, role performance, and acceptance by others (see Chapter 19).

EXPERIENCE Throughout life all individuals, including nurses, have experience with self-concept issues. Personal memories of changes in appearance or times when you were unable to carry out usual roles because of a temporary illness will help you be empathetic with patients who are experiencing stressors to their self-concept or sexuality. Past experiences with patients who have undergone changes in self-concept or experienced self-concept stressors also provide useful insight into how to work effectively with a current patient.

ATTITUDES Attitudes to adopt when caring for patients with threats to self-concept and sexuality are acceptance, respect, and compassion. Some patients will have values, attitudes, or behaviors that differ from your own (Box 22-6). Developing a therapeutic nurse-patient relationship based on

BOX 22-6   CULTURAL FOCUS

Racial and cultural identity are important components of a person's self-concept. Early in growth and development, an individual develops this identity within the context of family. As the individual grows, the cultural aspects of his or her self-concept are reinforced through social, family, or cultural experiences. In addition, a person's self-concept is strengthened or questioned through political, social, or cultural influences experienced in the school and workplace environments. Positive or negative role cultural modeling or past experiences influence self-concept.

IMPLICATIONS FOR PRACTICE
- Develop an open, nonrestrictive attitude for assessing and encouraging cultural practices to improve patients' self-concept.
- Ask patients what they think is important to help them feel better or gain a stronger sense of self.
- Encourage cultural identity by individualizing self-care practices and offering treatment choices to meet patients' self-concept needs.
- Facilitate culturally sensitive health promotion activities that address at-risk behaviors identified through evidence-based practice (e.g., sexual risk behaviors, weight and shape issues).

Data from Birndorf S and others: High self-esteem among adolescents: longitudinal trends, sex differences , and protective factors, *J Adolesc Health* 37:194, 2005; Sterk CE and others: Self-esteem and at risk women; determinants and relevance to sexual and HIV-related risk behaviors, *Women Health* 40(4):75, 2004.

BOX 22-7   Behaviors Suggestive of Altered Self-Concept and Sexuality

- Avoidance of eye contact
- Slumped posture
- Unkempt appearance
- Overly apologetic
- Hesitant speech
- Overly critical or angry
- Frequent or inappropriate crying
- Negative self-evaluation
- Excessively dependent
- Hesitant to express views or opinions
- Lack of interest in what is happening
- Passive attitude
- Difficulty in making decisions

---

mutual respect, professional compassion, and unconditional acceptance promotes positive patient outcomes.

STANDARDS There are several codes of professional conduct for nurses; each reflects a commitment to the principle of respect for patient autonomy. Autonomy means that individuals have the freedom to choose their own life plan. Supporting your patients' autonomy to make choices and live in an authentic way consistent with personal values and beliefs supports the development and maintenance of a strong and positive self-concept.

NURSING PROCESS

■■■ASSESSMENT

When assessing self-concept and self-esteem, focus on each component of self-concept (identity, body image, and role performance); behaviors suggestive of altered self-concept, self-esteem, or sexuality (Box 22-7); and actual and potential self-concept stressors (see Figure 22-2, p. 602). Determining the patient's current and past coping patterns is also important. In addition to direct questioning, you will effectively gather much of the data regarding self-concept through ob-

servation of the patient's nonverbal behavior and by paying attention to what a patient says. Take note of the manner in which patients talk about the people in their lives, because this provides clues to both stressful and supportive relationships. It also suggests key roles the patient assumes.

Use knowledge of developmental stages (see Box 22-1, p. 600) to determine what areas are likely to be important to the patient, and inquire about these aspects of the person's life. For example, ask a 65-year-old male patient about his life and what has been important to him. This is the stage of development in life in which individuals are examining their lives and considering the impact they have had in the world. The individual's conversation will likely provide data relating to role performance, identity, self-esteem, stressors, and coping patterns. At appropriate times, specific questions are useful (Table 22-1).

You also need to assess all relevant factors to determine a patient's sexual well-being. Assessment of sexuality involves physical, psychological, social, and cultural variables. In approaching patients about their sexuality and sexual functioning, it is sometimes unnerving to inquire about another person's sexual functioning. You may worry that the patient will not appreciate being asked about sexuality and sexual practices. However, patients want to know how medications, treatments, and surgical procedures influence their sexual relationships. With experience you will come to recognize that many patients welcome the opportunity to talk about their sexuality, especially when they are experiencing difficulty in sexual functioning. Once you approach the topic, the patient is able to talk about concerns and explore possible ways to resolve the problem. When you address sexuality in a sensitive, relaxed, matter-of-fact manner, patients feel safe to bring up areas of concern. The intimacy of the nurse-patient relationship, whether it is involved in providing physical care or discussing the impact of a recent diagnosis, provides a unique opportunity for discussing a person's sexual concerns. The acronym PLISSIT is a helpful format for discussing sexuality with patients (Box 22-8).

TABLE 22-1 FOCUSED PATIENT ASSESSMENT

FACTORS TO ASSESS	QUESTIONS	PHYSICAL ASSESSMENT
Identity	How would you describe yourself?	Assess for verbal and nonverbal responses. Watch for hesitant speech, poor eye contact, and slumped posture. Derogatory answers (e.g., "I don't know; there's not too much worth mentioning") raise concern.
Body image	What aspects of your appearance do you like? Are there any aspects of your appearance that you would like to change? If yes, describe the changes you would make.	Assess for ability to identify something about their appearance or the way their body functions that they like (e.g., "People have always told me I have nice eyes" or "I am strong"). People who do not identify positive characteristics often have negative body image and poor self-esteem.
Self-esteem	Tell me about the things you do that make you feel good about yourself. How do you feel about yourself?	Assess verbal and nonverbal responses. With prompting, most patients can identify something favorable. Statements about not having any strengths or being able to do anything well raise concern and require additional assessment.
Role performance	Tell me about your primary roles (e.g., partner, parent, friend, sister, professional role, and volunteer). How effective are you at carrying out each of these roles?	Listen for the number of primary roles identified. A large number of primary roles will put the patient at risk for role conflicts and role overload. Patients who do not feel that these roles are adequately met may be experiencing alterations in self-concept.
Sexuality	How has your illness, medication, or surgery affected your sex life? Are your needs for intimacy being met? Do you have any concerns about your sexual functioning?	Assess for concerns about sexual functioning (e.g., erectile dysfunction in men, changes in vaginal lubrication in women) or overall change in sex drive. Determine if patient is hesitant to bring up issues of sexuality.

BOX 22-8 PLISSIT Assessment of Sexuality

- **P**ermission to discuss sexuality issues
- **L**imited **I**nformation related to sexual health problems being experienced
- **S**pecific **S**uggestions—Only when the nurse is clear about the problem
- **I**ntensive **T**herapy—Referral to professional with advanced training if necessary

Modified from Annon J: The PLISSIT model: a proposed conceptual scheme for the behavioral treatment of sexual problems, *J Sex Educ Ther* 2(2):1, 1976.

Every complete nursing history needs to include a few questions related to sexual functioning. Start with a general statement such as "Sex is an important part of life and can be affected by health status" or "To better understand your health, it is useful to know if you have concerns about your sexual functioning." Explore sexual decision making, including the patient's use of contraception and safe sex practices. Adolescents best respond to a question such as "Many teenagers have questions about sexually transmitted infections or whether their bodies are developing at the right rate. What questions about sex can I answer?"

In gathering a sexual history, consider physical, functional, relationship, lifestyle, and self-esteem factors that influence sexual functioning. A variety of physical factors positively or negatively influence sexual desire and function. For example, sexual intercourse sometimes results in pain or discomfort from arthritis, angina, endometriosis, or lack of vaginal lubrication. Even anticipation that sex may hurt, such as during the postpartum period or postoperatively, will lessen sexual desire. Learn to what extent these physical factors affect a patient's sexual performance. Also, perceptions of body image are related to adherence to medical and treatment regimens. Therefore you need to assess a patient's sexual concerns and ask questions about body image changes and effects on sex life. For example, begin a discussion with, "It's common for women to be self-conscious and concerned they are not sexually attractive after losing a breast. Have you and your partner talked about how this change will affect your sexual intimacy?"

Some medications affect sexual desire or cause physical changes that affect performance. Drinking alcohol or using drugs clouds judgment and results in sexual intercourse or other activities that lead to sexually transmitted infections or pregnancy. Gather a complete history of any medications or illicit drugs the patient is taking or has taken in the past. You will also need to obtain the same information for the patient's partner.

Reviewing sexuality changes associated with aging is also important. Women experience a reduction in vaginal secretions, and the vagina becomes shorter and does not expand as well to accommodate the penis (Meiner and Lueckenotte, 2006). Orgasmic contractions are fewer and are sometimes accompanied by painful uterine contractions. In men, the penis does not become firm as quickly and is not as firm as it is at a younger age. Ejaculation takes longer to achieve and is shorter in duration, and the erection often diminishes more quickly. When assessing sexual changes, you need to ask about the patient's past sexual experiences, perceptions, and difficulties.

Your nursing assessment includes consideration of previous coping behaviors; the nature, number, and intensity of stressors; and the patient's internal and external resources. Knowing how a patient has dealt with self-concept stressors in the past provides insight into the patient's style of coping. Not all patients address issues in the same way, but often a person uses a familiar coping pattern for newly encountered stressors. As you identify previous coping patterns, it is useful to determine whether these patterns have contributed to healthy functioning or created more problems. For example, the use of drugs or alcohol during times of stress often creates additional stressors.

Exploring resources and strengths, such as availability of significant others or prior use of community resources, is important when formulating a realistic and effective plan. You also need to determine how the patient views the situation. For example, some women grow accustomed to changes in their health status as they get older. For these women, experiencing heart disease is one more aspect of growing older. For others, a cardiac event is less expected and more problematic, especially for middle-age women who still have family and career responsibilities. As a nurse, be aware of women's changing roles in society such as increased caregiving responsibilities. You are in a unique position to reinforce the need for women to make lifestyle changes after a myocardial infarction and to identify and remove barriers to attending cardiac rehabilitation classes (McSweeney and Coon, 2004).

Valuable assessment data often evolve out of conversations with family and significant others. Sometimes significant others have insights into the person's way of dealing with stressors and have knowledge about what is important to the person's self-concept. The way in which the loved one talks about the patient, including his or her nonverbal behaviors, provides information about what kind of support is available for the patient. Ask patients if they feel comfortable when they are relating to their partner and whether there is openness in the interaction.

PATIENT EXPECTATIONS The patient's expectations are also important to assess. Asking the patient how he or she believes medical and nursing interventions will make a difference provides useful information regarding the patient's expectations. This provides an opportunity to discuss the patient's goals. For example, when working with a patient who

is experiencing anxiety related to an upcoming diagnostic study, ask the patient about his expectations of the relaxation exercise that you have been practicing together. The patient's response provides valuable information about his beliefs and attitudes regarding the effectiveness of the interventions, as well as the potential need to modify the nursing approach. When nursing care involves consideration of the patient's sexuality, you need to be sensitive and understanding and always maintain the patient's confidentiality.

■■■NURSING DIAGNOSIS

Carefully consider assessment data to identify a patient's actual or potential problem areas. You rely on knowledge and experience, apply appropriate critical thinking attitudes and professional standards, and look for clusters of defining characteristics that indicate a nursing diagnosis. Possible nursing diagnoses (NANDA International, 2009) related to self-concept and sexual functioning include the following:

- *Disturbed body image*
- *Disturbed personal identity*
- *Ineffective role performance*
- *Readiness for enhanced self-concept*
- *Chronic low self-esteem*
- *Situational low self-esteem*
- *Sexual dysfunction*
- *Ineffective sexuality pattern*

Forming nursing diagnoses about self-concept or sexuality is complex. Often, isolated data are defining characteristics for more than one nursing diagnosis. If a person who has recently been laid off from work expresses a predominantly negative self-appraisal, including inability to handle situations or events and difficulty making decisions, these characteristics suggest a nursing diagnosis of *situational low self-esteem related to inability to fulfill previous roles*. Assessing information regarding recent events in the patient's life and how the patient has viewed himself or herself in the past is important. Likewise, identifying a nursing diagnosis regarding sexuality often requires you to clarify that defining characteristics exist and that the patient perceives difficulty with regard to sexuality. Clues to help you identify defining characteristics of a possible nursing diagnosis include surgery of reproductive organs or changes in appearance, chronic fatigue or pain, past or current physical abuse, chronic illness, and developmental milestones such as puberty or menopause. Determining the contributing factors is important. Interventions depend on selecting the correct related factors. When you include all relevant contributing factors, you plan effectively. For example, the nursing diagnosis *ineffective sexuality pattern related to difficulty with acceptance of recent loss and fear of pain* is appropriate for a woman who has recently undergone a mastectomy. Further expanding the "related to" section to include more about how the mastectomy is affecting sexuality is helpful. For example, altered sexuality is possibly related to postoperative pain or fear of pain, fear of diminished attractiveness, and/or difficulty in moving.

■ ■ ■ **PLANNING**

GOALS AND OUTCOMES Develop an individualized plan of care for each nursing diagnosis, and help the patient set realistic expectations for care. Individualize goals, and set realistic and measurable outcomes. While establishing goals, consult with the patient about whether the goals are perceived as realistic (see Care Plan). Consult with significant others to develop a more comprehensive and workable plan. Once you have formulated a goal, consider how the data that illustrated the problem would change if the problem were diminished. Reflect these changes in the outcome criteria. For example, Mr. Taylor was diagnosed with *situational low self-esteem related to negative view of self and uncertainty about future roles.* He described feeling like "less than a man" and

---

CARE PLAN Situational Low Self-Esteem

ASSESSMENT

After Maria completes Mr. Taylor's physical assessment and helps him with his self-care activities, she sits down with Mr. and Mrs. Taylor to discuss how the stroke has affected Mr. Taylor's self-concept and sexual health.

ASSESSMENT ACTIVITIES

Assess identity concerns (e.g., sexual role, masculinity, breadwinner). Ask how the stroke has affected Mr. Taylor's sense of self.

Observe Mr. Taylor's mood and affect and his nonverbal communication and interactions with others; interview family as appropriate.

Determine Mr. Taylor's interest and involvement in self-care activities.

Offer opportunities to participate in treatment and provide supportive-educative nursing care.

FINDINGS/DEFINING CHARACTERISTICS*

Mr. Taylor **looks away, shakes his head,** and states, "**I feel like less of a man.** My wife says she's just thankful I'm alive, but that's not enough for me."

Mrs. Taylor reports that Mr. Taylor demonstrates **intermittent eye contact, frequent crying when alone, blank staring** at his flaccid hand, and **superficial conversations** with family members.

Mr. Taylor **refuses to bathe or comb his hair.** He **eats less** than 50% of meals and **demonstrates avoidance** of the prescribed rehabilitation activities.

Mr. Taylor does not ask questions about his condition and answers, "I don't know" to most questions about the future.

NURSING DIAGNOSIS: Situational low self-esteem related to negative view of self as less than whole following stroke and uncertainty of future personal, family, and professional roles.

PLANNING

GOAL

- Mr. Taylor will experience fewer alterations in self-concept, including low self-esteem, disturbed body image, altered role performance, and impaired sexuality, and will discuss concerns with staff members and significant others before discharge.

EXPECTED OUTCOMES (NOC)†

Self-Esteem

- Mr. Taylor will verbalize feelings of self-acceptance and self-worth within 4 days.
- Mr. Taylor will demonstrate maintenance of basic grooming and hygiene needs within 2 days.

Role Performance

- Mr. Taylor will describe role changes associated with his stroke and will verbalize commitment to participating in rehabilitation and community resources to fulfill role performance by day of discharge.

Body Image

- Mr. Taylor will demonstrate adjustment to changes in body function and appearance within 1 week.

Sexual Identity

- Mr. Taylor will challenge negative images of sexual self within 1 week.

---

*Defining characteristics are shown in **bold** type.

†Outcomes classification labels from Moorhead S and others, editors: *Nursing Outcomes Classification (NOC)*, ed 4, St. Louis, 2008, Mosby.

CARE PLAN   Situational Low Self-Esteem—cont'd

INTERVENTIONS (NIC)‡	RATIONALE
Self-Esteem Enhancement • Facilitate an environment and activities (e.g., writing in a journal, reflection, praying, talking with a nurse) that will increase self-esteem. • Monitor Mr. Taylor's statements of self-worth. • Encourage increased responsibility for self, and assist patient with accepting dependence on others, as appropriate.	A therapeutic nurse-patient relationship promotes positive patient outcome, including the patient's assuming responsibility for his own care (Stuart, 2009). Assessing thoughts and feelings, including depression and suicide risk, ensure the patient's safety (Folse and others, 2006). Self-esteem and body image are strong predictors of depression (MacPhee and Andrews, 2006). Promoting self-care enhances self-concept, including improving role performance (Stuart, 2009).
Role Enhancement • Help Mr. Taylor identify specific role changes brought on by the stroke.	Alternative choices can be proposed only after the problem is accurately defined. Assessment of role performance is necessary to modify maladaptive behavior and promote optimal functioning. Injuries, such as a stroke, often disrupt role performance (Stuart, 2009).
Body Image Enhancement • Discuss changes in function and physical appearance caused by change in medical condition.	A threat to body image and overall self-concept often influences adherence to recommended health regimens, including diet and taking medications as prescribed (Thomas, 2007).
Sexual Counseling • Include Mrs. Taylor while teaching that sexuality is an important part of life and that illness, medications, and stress often alter sexual functioning and self-concept.	Family involvement is essential for comprehensive care. Sexuality is a basic need and concern for both men and women, yet is one of the most difficult discussions for patients to initiate. Many nurses believe that patients do not expect the nurse to address sexuality concerns and lack comfort and confidence in addressing concerns (Magnan and Reynolds, 2006).

EVALUATION

NURSING ACTIONS	PATIENT RESPONSE/FINDING	ACHIEVEMENT OF OUTCOME
Ask Mr. Taylor how effective he feels in his ability to identify and express feelings verbally and nonverbally.	Mr. Taylor reports, "I've been able to talk with my wife, even about my concerns that she won't find me attractive anymore."	Improved verbal and nonverbal communication noted.
Monitor changes in Mr. Taylor's statements about himself.	Mr. Taylor is making fewer negative comments and is evaluating body image more realistically but remains dissatisfied with appearance and strength of hand.	Small improvement in self-esteem; body image more realistic but remains negative. Discusses body image with wife and primary nurse.

‡Intervention classification labels from Bulechek GM and others, editors: *Nursing interventions classification (NIC)*, ed 5, St. Louis, 2008, Mosby.

Continued

CARE PLAN Situational Low Self-Esteem—cont'd

NURSING ACTIONS	PATIENT RESPONSE/FINDING	ACHIEVEMENT OF OUTCOME
Ask Mr. Taylor to describe how his roles have changed since his stroke.	Mr. Taylor states, "Although I can't work right now, Meredith is going to pick up some extra hours at her job to help make ends meet. I may not be able to bring home any money right now, but I can do other things around the house to help out."	Relationship with wife is strengthened. Beginning to accept change in family role.
Observe Mr. Taylor's participation in self-care related to stroke.	Mr. Taylor assumed responsibility for basic hygiene; able to do most of his bath independently, and although his gait remains unsteady, he is able to walk short distances with a walker.	Meeting self-care needs. Seeks assistance as needed.
Encourage Mr. Taylor to identify resources outside the hospital.	Mr. Taylor expresses interest in attending local stroke recovery support group and connecting with friends.	Scheduled to attend stroke recovery support group 2 days after discharge and plans to invite a close friend over within 1 week of discharge, which indicate adjustment to changes in body function and appearance.

lost interest in self-care activities. These are the defining characteristics. Formulate the goals that Mr. Taylor will experience fewer alterations in self-concept and will discuss his concerns before discharge. Expected outcomes include that Mr. Taylor will perform self-care within 2 days and verbalize feelings of self-acceptance in 4 days. As you develop your patient's plan of care, remember that patients have more than one interrelated problem (Figure 22-4).

With the nursing diagnosis *ineffective sexuality pattern related to recent mastectomy and fear of pain*, you explore with the patient what she sees as a satisfactory recovery after her mastectomy. This gives the patient the opportunity to share that she wants to return to her presurgical sexual relationship with her partner. She specifies that she wants to feel comfortable having her remaining breast caressed and to engage in intercourse within 2 weeks, without experiencing pain.

SETTING PRIORITIES The care plan presents the goals, expected outcomes, and interventions for a patient with an alteration in self-concept. Your interventions focus on helping the patient adapt to the stressors that led to the self-concept disturbance and on supporting and reinforcing the development of coping methods. The patient often needs time to adapt to physical changes. Self-concept priorities include maximizing the patient's ability to address physical and psychological needs. Priorities for sexual health typically include resuming sexual activities. Look for strengths in both the individual and the family, and provide resources and education to turn limitations into strengths. Patient teaching communicates the normalcy of certain situations (e.g., nature of a chronic disease, change in relationships, effect of a

loss). It is important to determine if this is your patient's need and plan accordingly. For example, when caring for a patient whose sexual health is altered, include private time for your patient and partner to quietly sit in the room and have dinner and watch a movie without any interruptions.

COLLABORATIVE CARE The perceptions of significant others are important to incorporate into the plan of care. Sometimes individuals who have experienced deficits in self-concept before the current episode of treatment have established a system of support, including mental health clinicians, clergy, and other community resources. Before involving the family, consider the patient's desires for significant others to be involved and cultural norms regarding who most frequently makes decisions in the family. Sexual conflict in marriage, intimacy issues stemming from past sexual assault, or incest often require intensive treatment with mental health professionals. Resolving self-concept issues is a long-term goal and includes referrals to a clinical psychologist, advanced practice psychiatric nurse, social worker, or professional counselor.

■ ■ ■ IMPLEMENTATION

As with all of the steps of the nursing process, a therapeutic nurse-patient relationship is central to the implementation phase. Once you have developed goals and outcomes, consider nursing interventions that will help move your patient toward the goals. To develop effective nursing interventions, consider the nursing diagnosis and related interventions that address the diagnosis. Individualize standard interventions to your patient. You develop additional nursing interventions based on the "related to" component of the nursing diagnosis.

CONCEPT MAP

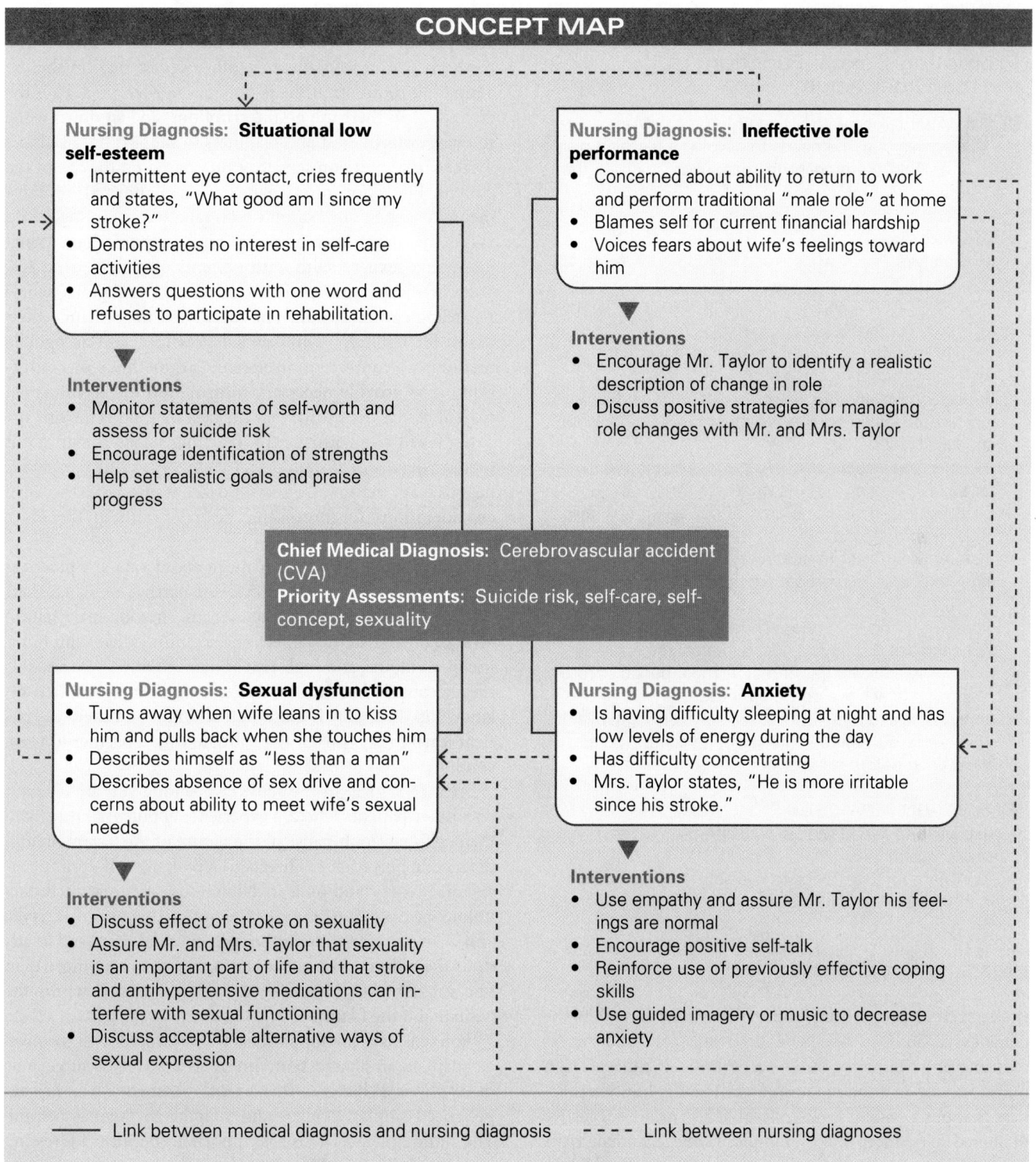

Nursing Diagnosis: Situational low self-esteem
- Intermittent eye contact, cries frequently and states, "What good am I since my stroke?"
- Demonstrates no interest in self-care activities
- Answers questions with one word and refuses to participate in rehabilitation.

▼

Interventions
- Monitor statements of self-worth and assess for suicide risk
- Encourage identification of strengths
- Help set realistic goals and praise progress

Nursing Diagnosis: Ineffective role performance
- Concerned about ability to return to work and perform traditional "male role" at home
- Blames self for current financial hardship
- Voices fears about wife's feelings toward him

▼

Interventions
- Encourage Mr. Taylor to identify a realistic description of change in role
- Discuss positive strategies for managing role changes with Mr. and Mrs. Taylor

Chief Medical Diagnosis: Cerebrovascular accident (CVA)
Priority Assessments: Suicide risk, self-care, self-concept, sexuality

Nursing Diagnosis: Sexual dysfunction
- Turns away when wife leans in to kiss him and pulls back when she touches him
- Describes himself as "less than a man"
- Describes absence of sex drive and concerns about ability to meet wife's sexual needs

▼

Interventions
- Discuss effect of stroke on sexuality
- Assure Mr. and Mrs. Taylor that sexuality is an important part of life and that stroke and antihypertensive medications can interfere with sexual functioning
- Discuss acceptable alternative ways of sexual expression

Nursing Diagnosis: Anxiety
- Is having difficulty sleeping at night and has low levels of energy during the day
- Has difficulty concentrating
- Mrs. Taylor states, "He is more irritable since his stroke."

▼

Interventions
- Use empathy and assure Mr. Taylor his feelings are normal
- Encourage positive self-talk
- Reinforce use of previously effective coping skills
- Use guided imagery or music to decrease anxiety

—— Link between medical diagnosis and nursing diagnosis   - - - - Link between nursing diagnoses

Figure 22-4 ■ Concept Map.

Developing interventions that affect the "related to" factors will often decrease the problem reflected in the nursing diagnosis. In the case of Mr. Taylor (see Care Plan), the "related to" component of the nursing diagnosis focuses on the areas to explore when talking with the patient.

Nursing interventions are designed to promote a patient's healthy self-concept and sexuality. Strategies help patients regain or restore the elements that contribute to a strong and

secure sense of self. The approaches that you choose will vary according to the level of care required. Effective nursing care includes promoting sexual health in acute and restorative settings by helping patients understand their problems and by exploring methods to deal with them effectively.

HEALTH PROMOTION Work with patients to help them develop healthy lifestyle behaviors that contribute to a positive self-concept. Measures that support adaptation to

BOX 22-9 PATIENT TEACHING

Promoting Sexual Function for the Older Adult

 After talking with Mr. and Mrs. Taylor, Maria determines that she needs to develop a teaching plan to help them adapt to changes in sexuality that resulted from Mr. Taylor's stroke.

OUTCOME
- Mr. and Mrs. Taylor will state at least three ways to attain satisfactory level of sexual activity.

TEACHING STRATEGIES
- Provide teaching on normal sexual changes that occur with aging and following a stroke.
- Encourage Mr. and Mrs. Taylor to discuss what types of intimate behavior provide the most sexual stimulation and satisfaction.
- Discuss side effects of medications that commonly alter sexual function and response.
- Encourage selection of a time of day when Mr. Taylor feels most rested.
- Instruct Mrs. Taylor to use a water-based lubricant during intercourse to promote comfort.
- Encourage alternative positions for intercourse (e.g., side-lying, lying on a bed with legs over the side) that will decrease discomfort during intercourse.
- Inform Mr. and Mrs. Taylor that a longer period of foreplay helps to achieve penile firmness.
- Instruct Mr. and Mrs. Taylor to conserve strength by not working hard at the beginning of intercourse, so as to avoid tiring before climax.

EVALUATION STRATEGIES
- Ask Mr. and Mrs. Taylor to verbalize plan for improved sexual health.
- Ask Mr. and Mrs. Taylor to evaluate their satisfaction with their sexual relationship.

Modified from Meiner SE, Lueckenotte A: *Gerontologic nursing,* ed 3, St. Louis, 2006, Mosby.

stress, such as proper nutrition, regular exercise within the patient's capabilities, adequate sleep and rest, and stress-reducing practices contribute to a healthy self-concept. As a nurse, you are in a unique position to identify lifestyle practices that put a patient's self-concept at risk or are suggestive of altered self-concepts. For example, a college student visits an outpatient clinic with complaints of being unable to sleep and anxiety attacks. In gathering the patient history, you learn of lifestyle practices such as too little rest, a large number of life changes occurring simultaneously, and excessive use of alcohol. These data suggest actual or potential self-concept disturbances. You then talk with the patient to determine how she views the various lifestyle elements, to facilitate the patient's insight into behaviors, and to make appropriate referrals or provide needed health teaching.

Exploring a person's sexuality and providing useful sex education require good communication skills. Make sure the environment and timing provide privacy, uninterrupted time, and patient comfort. For example, discuss contraception methods with a woman in an office rather than in the examination room when she is only partially clothed. Plan the discussion so there are no interruptions, and sit down while showing your interest and readiness to support her needs.

Teaching topics on sexuality vary based on the age of the patient. Education offers explanation of normal developmental changes. For example, you talk to a school-age child about the appearance of breast buds or pubic hair. When discussing sexual health with patients of childbearing age, always consider your patient's cultural and religious beliefs regarding contraception. The discussion may include their desire for children, usual sexual practices, and acceptable methods of contraception. Review all methods of contraception to provide necessary information for an informed patient choice. Reinforce that the best method is the one the patient will use consistently. Teaching needs for an adult include details of physiological changes resulting from illness or from treatment effects. Box 22-9 summarizes special considerations for promoting sexual health in the older adult.

Individuals need to learn more about safe sex practices when they have more than one sex partner or when their partner had other sexual experiences. Provide information on sexually transmitted infections, including their symptoms, use of condoms, and high-risk sexual activities. Safe sex also means considering the patient's emotional risks within a relationship. Role play is a useful teaching tool to help the patient learn to say "no" or to negotiate with a partner to use a condom.

ACUTE CARE In the acute care setting you are likely to encounter patients who are experiencing potential threats to their self-concept because of the nature of the treatment and diagnostic procedures. Threats to a patient's self-concept result in anxiety and/or fear. Numerous stressors, including unknown diagnoses, the need to make changes in lifestyle, and change in functioning, are present, and you need to address them. In the acute care setting there is often more than one stressor, thus increasing the overall stress level for the patient and the family.

You will also care for patients who are faced with the need to adapt to an altered body image as a result of surgery or other physical change. Often a visit by someone who has experienced similar changes and adapted to them is helpful. The timing of such a visit is important. Because addressing these needs is often difficult to do while in an acute care setting, appropriate follow-up and referrals, including home care, are essential. Be sensitive to the patient's level of acceptance of the change. Forcing confrontation with the change before the patient is ready delays the patient's acceptance. Signs that a person is receptive to such a visit include the patient's asking questions related to how to manage a particular aspect of what has happened or looking at the changed area. As the patient expresses readiness to integrate the body change into his or her self-concept, you either let the patient know about groups that are available or ask the patient if he or she wants you to make the initial contact. In addition, you facilitate adjustment to a change in physical appearance through your own response to the wound or change. As you respond with acceptance, you model acceptance for both the patient and the family.

Both physical and psychological aspects of illness have the potential to affect sexuality. Never assume that sexual functioning is not a concern merely because of an individual's age or severity of prognosis. After identifying concerns, address them in the context of the patient's value system. When a patient experiences physical limitations to sexual performance, provide the following suggestions: planning sexual activity when the patient is rested, experimenting with positions that are more comfortable, encouraging partners to give one another more time, and encouraging the use of foreplay to achieve arousal.

RESTORATIVE AND CONTINUING CARE If you work in a home care or restorative care environment, you will have the opportunity to work with a patient to attain a more positive self-concept. Interventions designed to help a patient reach the goal of adapting to changes in self-concept or attaining a positive self-concept are based on the premise that the patient first develops insight and self-awareness concerning problems and stressors and then acts to solve the problems and cope with the stressors. You can incorporate this approach into patient teaching for alterations in self-concept, including situational low-self esteem, which is sometimes present in the home care setting (Box 22-10).

Increase the patient's self-awareness by establishing a trusting relationship that allows the patient to openly explore thoughts and feelings. A priority nursing intervention continues to be the expert use of communication skills to clarify the expectations of the patient and family. Open exploration will make the situation less threatening for the patient and encourages behaviors that expand self-awareness. Encourage the patient's self-exploration by accepting the patient's thoughts and feelings, by helping the patient to clarify interactions with others, and by being empathetic. Also encourage self-expression and stress the patient's self-responsibility.

Promoting the patient's self-evaluation involves helping the patient define problems clearly and identify positive and negative coping mechanisms. Work closely with the patient to help analyze adaptive and maladaptive responses, consider alternatives, and discuss outcomes. Collaborating with the patient in establishing realistic goals involves helping the patient identify alternative solutions and develop realistic goals based on them. This facilitates real change and encourages further goal-setting behaviors. You design opportunities that result in success, reinforce the patient's skills and strengths, and help the patient get needed assistance.

Teach the patient to move away from ineffective coping mechanisms and develop successful coping strategies. Supporting attempts that are health promoting is essential because with each success, the patient is more motivated to make another attempt at promoting health. Supporting adaptive, flexible coping is critical to intervening in self-concept alterations. Patients who are experiencing threats to or altera-

---

BOX 22-10 PATIENT TEACHING

Promoting Self-Concept and Self-Esteem

 Maria Kendal sees Mr. Taylor following discharge to his home. His physical condition has stabilized, but his self-concept and self-esteem remain a concern for both Mr. Taylor and his wife. After meeting with Mr. and Mrs. Taylor, Maria develops the following teaching plan:

OUTCOME
- Mr. Taylor will reduce his risk for low self-esteem in the home care setting.

TEACHING STRATEGIES
- Reinforce Mr. Taylor's expression of thoughts and feelings; clarify meaning of verbal and nonverbal communication.
- Encourage opportunities for Mr. Taylor to care for himself.
- Elicit Mr. Taylor's perceptions of strengths and weaknesses.
- Convey verbally and behaviorally that Mr. Taylor is responsible for his behavior.
- Identify relevant stressors, and discuss Mr. Taylor's perception of each stressor.
- Explore with Mr. Taylor his adaptive and maladaptive coping responses to problems.
- Collaboratively identify alternative solutions; encourage alternatives not previously tried.
- Continue to reinforce strengths and successes.

EVALUATION STRATEGIES
- Ask Mr. Taylor how involved he is in making decisions that affect his care.
- Determine if increase in activities and tasks has been a positive experience.
- Ask Mr. and Mrs. Taylor how they will apply new coping resources during this time of change.

Modified from Stuart GW: *Principles and practice of psychiatric nursing*, ed 9, St. Louis, 2009, Mosby.

tions in self-concept often benefit from collaboration with mental health and community resources to promote increased awareness. Knowledge of available community resources allows you to make appropriate referrals.

You will frequently be in a position to establish relationships with couples that encourage honest and open discussions about sexual health. Address sexuality issues by taking a sexual health history and implementing a basic model such as PLISSIT to provide options for patients (see Box 22-8, p. 608). Assessment and management of sexuality concerns is important as you promote sexual intimacy and provide closeness and closure between partners at the end of life (Stausmire, 2004). Give priority to patients in middle and older adulthood when you address sexuality concerns due to illness, medications, or physical changes. Provide information on how the specific illness will limit sexual activity and ideas for adapting or facilitating sexual activity. Interventions range from giving permission for a partner to lie in bed and hold a patient to coordinating nursing care and medications in a way that provides opportunity for privacy and intimacy. In the home environment it is important to help patients create an environment comfortable for sexual activity. This sometimes involves making recommendations for ways to rearrange the patient's bedroom to accommodate any limitations. Patients and partners need to know how to accommodate barriers such as Foley catheters or drainage tubes that make sexual positioning difficult.

In the long-term care setting, facilities need to make proper arrangements for privacy during an older patient's sexual experience (Meiner and Lueckenotte, 2006). The ideal situation is to set up a pleasant room that is used for a variety of activities that the older adult is able to reserve for private visits with a spouse or partner. This is not always possible. Another option is to use the patient's room and make other arrangements for the patient's roommate. Although privacy of patients is important, do not leave patients alone in a situation in which they will injure themselves (Meiner and Lueckenotte, 2006).

Establishing a therapeutic relationship is critical to successfully intervening with patients who have alterations in self-concept, whether care is focused on health promotion, dealing with an acute process, or addressing restorative care. To support the development of a positive self-concept in a patient, convey genuine caring for the patient (see Chapter 18). Then, and only then, will you establish a partnership with the patient to address underlying problems.

■■■EVALUATION

PATIENT CARE Expected outcomes for a patient with a self-concept disturbance include nonverbal behaviors indicating a positive self-concept, statements of self-acceptance, and acceptance of change in appearance or function (see Care Plan, p. 610, and Box 22-11). For example, a patient who has had difficulty making eye contact will demonstrate a more positive self-concept by making more frequent eye contact and smiling during conversation. Adequate self-care and acceptance of the use of prosthetic devices indicate progress. A positive attitude toward rehabilitation and increased movement toward independence facilitate a return to preexisting roles at work or at home. Patterns of interacting will often reflect changes in self-concept. For example, a patient who has been hesitant to express his or her views will more readily offer opinions and ideas as self-esteem increases.

Sometimes initial goals are unrealistic or require modification as the patient's condition changes. You and the patient will need to revise the plan in these cases. Patient adaptation to major changes sometimes takes a year or longer, but the fact that this period is long does not suggest problems with adaptation. Look for signs that the patient has reduced some

---

BOX 22-11   EVALUATION

Because Mr. Taylor was in the hospital for 2 weeks, Maria was able to care for Mr. Taylor and watch him adapt to the changes he experienced as a result of his stroke. On the last day Maria cared for Mr. Taylor, he reported that he was going to a rehabilitation center that specializes in helping people who have had strokes. Mr. Taylor is able to complete most of his bath independently. Although his gait is a little unsteady, he is able to walk short distances with a walker. During his bath he jokes, "I think my new haircut makes me look a lot younger!" This improvement in function and acceptance of self has helped Mr. Taylor become more satisfied with himself and his progress in therapy. He is hopeful that he will be able to return to work after he leaves the rehabilitation center. Both Mr. and Mrs. Taylor have worked with a therapist who specializes in helping couples who have sexual problems. Mr. Taylor states that the therapy sessions have helped him grow closer to his wife and have strengthened their relationship. Several of his bowling friends visited him last night. Mr. Taylor states, "I can't wait to get better. I have a lot of things to do, and I have a lot to live for."

DOCUMENTATION NOTE
"Ability to perform ADLs improving. Only needs help to wash back during bath. Improvements in function have led to reports of enhanced self-esteem and acceptance of body image. Actively participates in sexual therapy with spouse and is maintaining relationships with friends. States is highly motivated to get better and return to work soon. Plans to continue to work on improving neurological deficits at the stroke rehabilitation center."

ADLs, Activities of daily living.

---

stressors and that some behaviors have become more adaptive. This will require a follow-up discussion with the patient to determine if the level of satisfaction with sexual performance or sexual function has improved. Sometimes the patient has achieved the goal and outcome criteria, but sexual functioning is still not ideal. Consider what other steps will be appropriate. Changes in self-concept and sexuality take time. Although change is slow, care of the patient with a self-concept disturbance is rewarding.

PATIENT EXPECTATIONS In evaluating care provided to patients with alterations in self-concept and sexual health, determine if the patient's expectations are met. After determining the achievement of targeted outcomes, ask if the patient thinks that nursing care was effective and supportive. Remain aware of any personal limitations in being able to counsel the patient. In some cases, referrals to other health care providers will still be necessary.

KEY POINTS

- Self-concept is an integrated set of conscious and unconscious attitudes and perceptions about the self.
- Components of self-concept are identity, body image, and role performance. Self-esteem and sexuality are closely related terms.
- Each developmental stage involves factors that are important to the development of a healthy, positive self-concept.
- Identity is particularly vulnerable during adolescence.
- Body image is the mental picture of one's body and is not necessarily consistent with a person's actual body structure or appearance.
- Body image stressors include changes in physical appearance, structure, or functioning caused by normal developmental changes or illness.
- Self-esteem is the emotional appraisal of self-concept and reflects the overall sense of being capable, worthwhile, and competent.
- Self-esteem stressors include developmental and relationship changes, illness (particularly chronic illness involving changes in what were normal activities), surgery, accidents, and the responses of other individuals to changes resulting from these events.
- The nurse's self-concept and nursing actions often have an effect on a patient's self-concept.
- Planning and implementing nursing interventions for self-concept disturbance involve expanding the patient's self-awareness, encouraging self-exploration, aiding in self-evaluation, helping formulate goals in regard to adaptation, and assisting the patient in achieving those goals.
- Sexuality is related to all dimensions of health. Therefore address sexual concerns or problems as part of nursing care.
- Sexual health involves physical and psychosocial aspects and contributes to an individual's sense of self-worth and positive interpersonal relationships.
- Development and life changes, ethical decisional issues, fertility, personal and emotional conflicts, illness, and hospitalization all affect a patient's sexuality.

CRITICAL THINKING EXERCISES

Mr. Taylor has become more depressed and less interested in his rehabilitation. During the morning he has shared with you some of his concerns about when he will be able to return to work. He says to you, "I just want to get back to my normal self."

1. Describe how you would respond to Mr. Taylor's comment regarding "getting back to normal."
2. Mrs. Taylor reports that Mr. Taylor has no interest in being intimate and he rejects her when she attempts to initiate sexual contact. How will you approach issues of sexuality with the Taylors?

3. You suspect that Mr. Taylor's depressed mood and loss of interest in usual activities is now a higher priority than your previous diagnosis of *situational low self-esteem*. Describe what assessment data are needed to modify your plan of care. Identify your priority actions.

⊜volve   *Answers to Critical Thinking Questions can be found on the Evolve website.*

REVIEW QUESTIONS

1. When a nurse is caring for a patient after mastectomy, interventions to promote physiological stability and pain control are necessary. Once this occurs, the nurse also needs to design nursing interventions directed toward improving the patient's:
   1. Mobility
   2. Self-concept
   3. Activity tolerance
   4. Self-care activities
2. Developing an individualized treatment plan for a 15-year-old girl considers that a primary developmental task of adolescence is to:
   1. Become aware of strengths and weaknesses
   2. Separate from parents and live independently
   3. Achieve positive self-esteem through experimentation
   4. Feel positive about the changes that are happening in her body

3. After completing an assessment, you determine that a 36-year-old woman has an internal sense of individuality and wholeness that has been consistent over time and in various circumstances. You document this assessment as a part of the patient's:
   1. Identity
   2. Body image
   3. Self-concept
   4. Role performance
4. You are providing health education to a very thin female adolescent who is at risk for body image disturbance. Additional teaching and intervention are needed if the adolescent verbalizes which of the following statements?
   1. "I look like I need to lose 10 pounds today."
   2. "My friends think I dress nicely, and they really like my hair."
   3. "My body image includes what I actually look like and how I think I look."

4. "I am okay with the physical changes that have happened to me since I started going through puberty."

5. A depressed patient is crying and verbalizes feelings of low self-esteem and self-worth such as "I'm such a failure . . . I can't do anything right." The best nursing response would be to:
   1. Remain with the patient until the patient stops crying
   2. Tell the patient that is not true and that every person has a purpose in life
   3. Review recent behaviors or accomplishments that demonstrate skill ability
   4. Reassure the patient you know how he is feeling and that things will get better

6. A patient who has just been diagnosed with breast cancer and had a mastectomy states, "I am no longer a complete woman." She verbalizes fear that she will no longer be able to maintain her relationship with her husband and has become very dependent upon the nursing staff for her care. This patient is having problems with which of the following? Select all that apply.
   1. Her identity
   2. Her body image
   3. Low self-esteem
   4. Low self-concept
   5. Fear of the unknown

7. The nurse asks a patient who recently experienced severe burns over the majority of his body, "How do you feel about yourself?" and "What can we do today to help you feel better about yourself?" The nurse is assessing the patient's:

1. Identity
2. Self-esteem
3. Body image
4. Role performance

8. A nurse who wants to increase a patient's self-awareness needs to:
   1. Accept the patient's thoughts and feelings
   2. Help the patient define her problems clearly
   3. Have the patient identify positive and negative coping mechanisms
   4. Establish a trusting relationship that allows the patient to explore thoughts and feelings

9. Your teaching plan for a 70-year-old man includes discussing which normal change in male sexual response associated with aging?
   1. Loss of sex drive
   2. Loss of firm erection
   3. Loss of ability to ejaculate
   4. Increase in semen production

10. You know an older female patient understands your teaching about normal changes in female sexual responses associated with aging when she states she will probably experience which of the following as she continues to age?
    1. Loss of orgasm
    2. Loss of sex drive
    3. Less clitoral response
    4. Less vaginal lubrication

Answers to Review Questions can be found on pages 1197-1198.

REFERENCES

Annon J: The PLISSIT model: a proposed conceptual scheme for the behavioral treatment of sexual problems, *J Sex Educ Ther* 2(2):1, 1976.

Aronowitz T and others: Attitudes that affect the ability of African American preadolescent girls and their mothers to talk openly about sex, *Issues Ment Health Nurs* 28(1):7, 2007.

Barrow RY and others: Taking positive steps to address STD disparities for African-American communities, *Sex Transm Dis* 35(Supp 12):S1, 2008.

Birndorf S and others: High self-esteem among adolescents: longitudinal trends, sex differences, and protective factors, *J Adolesc Health* 37:194, 2005.

Brausch AM, Muehlenkamp JJ: Body image and suicidal ideation in adolescents, *Body Image* 4(2):207, 2007.

Bulechek GM and others, editors: *Nursing interventions classification (NIC)*, ed 5, St. Louis, 2008, Mosby.

Collins A, Smyer MA: The resilience of self-esteem in late adulthood, *J Aging Health* 17(4):471, 2005.

Croghan IT and others: Is smoking related to body image satisfaction, stress, and self esteem in young girls? *Am J Health Behav* 30(3):322, 2006.

Davison KK and others: Why are early maturing girls less active: links between pubertal development, psychological well-being, and physical activity among girls ages 11 and 13, *Soc Sci Med* 64(12):2391, 2007.

Ebersole P and others: *Gerontological nursing and healthy aging*, ed 2, St. Louis, 2005, Mosby.

Erikson E: *Childhood and society*, ed 2, New York, 1963, WW Norton.

Figueroa-Hass CL: Effect of breast augmentation mammoplasty on self-esteem and sexuality: a quantitative analysis, *Plast Surg Nurs* 27(1):16, 2007.

Folse VN and others: Detecting suicide risk in adolescents and adults in an emergency department: a pilot study, *J Psychosoc Nurs Ment Health Serv* 44(3):1, 2006.

Gearing RE and others: Remembering fatherhood: evaluating the impact of a group intervention on fathering, *J Spec Group Work* 33(1):22, 2008.

Kaminski PL, Hayslip B: Gender differences in body esteem among older adults, *J Women Aging* 18(3):19, 2006.

Kelly AM and others: Adolescent girls with high body satisfaction: who are they and what can they teach us? *J Adolesc Health* 37:391, 2005.

Kornblau IS and others: Demographic, behavioral, and physical correlates of body esteem among low- income female adolescents, *J Adolesc Health* 41(6):566, 2007.

Levesque MJ, Vichesky DR: Raising the bar on the body beautiful: an analysis of the body image concerns of homosexual men, *Body Image* 3(1):45, 2006.

MacPhee AR, Andrews J: Risk factors for depression in early adolescence, *Adolescence* 41(163):435, 2006.

Magnan MA, Reynolds K: Barriers to addressing patient sexuality concerns across five areas of specialization, *Clin Nurse Spec* 20(6):285, 2006.

McSweeney JC, Coon S: Women's inhibitors and facilitators associated with making behavioral changes after myocardial infarction, *Medsurg Nurs* 13(1):49, 2004.

Meiner SE, Lueckenotte A: *Gerontologic nursing*, ed 3, St. Louis, 2006, Mosby.

Moorhead S and others, editors: *Nursing outcomes classification (NOC)*, ed 4, St. Louis, 2008, Mosby.

NANDA International: *NANDA International nursing diagnoses: definitions and classifications 2009-2011*, Oxford, UK, 2009, Wiley-Blackwell.

Nappi RE, Nijland EA: Women's perception of sexuality around the menopause: outcomes of a European telephone survey, *Eur J Obstet Gynecol Reprod Biol* 137(1):10, 2008.

Nelson MC, Gordon-Larsen P: Physical activity and sedentary behavior patterns are associated with selected adolescent risk behaviors, *Pediatrics* 117(4):1281, 2006.

Rosenberg M: *Society and the adolescent self-image*, Princeton, NJ, 1965, Princeton University Press.

Stausmire J: Sexuality at the end of life, *Am J Hosp Palliat Care* 21(1):33, 2004.

Sterk CE and others: Self-esteem and at risk women: determinants and relevance to sexual and HIV-related risk behaviors, *Women Health* 40(4):75, 2004.

Stuart GW: *Principles and practice of psychiatric nursing*, ed 9, St. Louis, 2009, Elsevier.

Thomas CM: The influence of self-concept on adherence to recommended health regimens in adults with heart failure, *J Cardiovasc Nurs* 22(5):405, 2007.

Family Context in Nursing

CHAPTER 23

MEDIA RESOURCES

 CD COMPANION 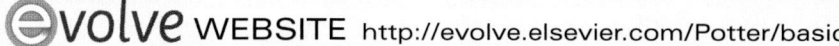 **evolve WEBSITE** http://evolve.elsevier.com/Potter/basic

- Crossword puzzle
- English/Spanish Audio Glossary

OBJECTIVES

- Examine current trends in the American family.
- Discuss how the term *family* is defined to reflect family diversity.
- Discuss common family forms and their health implications.
- Explain how the relationship between family structure and patterns of functioning affects the health of individuals within the family and the family as a whole.
- Discuss the role of families and family members as caregivers.
- Compare family as context to family as patient and family as system and explain the way that these perspectives influence nursing practice.
- Use the nursing process to provide for the health care needs of the family.

KEY TERMS

family, p. 621
family as context, p. 624
family as patient, p. 624
family as system, p. 624
family forms, p. 621
hardiness, p. 624
resiliency, p. 624

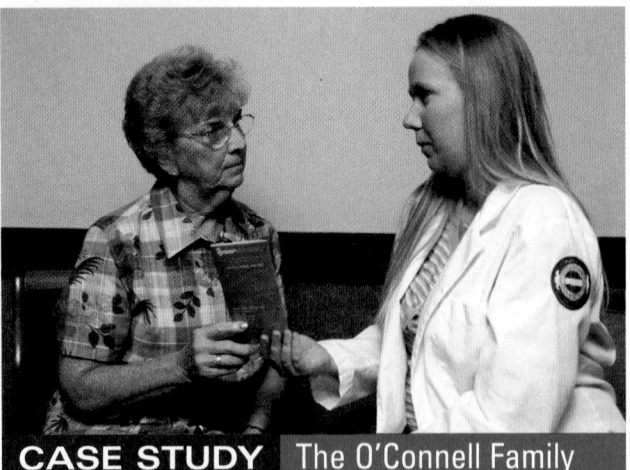

CASE STUDY   The O'Connell Family

Patrick and Michelle O'Connell have been married for 10 years. Patrick is 38 years old and works in the Department of Public Safety. Recently he learned that he is in danger of being laid off in the next round of cuts. Patrick has borderline hypertension and admits his stress level is an 8 on a scale of 0 to 10. He enjoys watching TV, playing war games on the computer, and playing with the family's pet dogs and cats. The family has health insurance through Patrick's job. Michelle is 32 years old, is employed part-time as a receptionist at a building supply company, and attends nursing school. They are a childfree couple by choice. Michelle was diagnosed with cervical cancer 3 months after their wedding and had a hysterectomy. Michelle is very worried about their financial problems and the health problems of her grandmother, Lois. She describes herself as spiritual and attends church occasionally.

Michelle is the oldest daughter in her family and is the only one of the siblings to maintain routine contact with her 80-year-old grandmother. Her two sisters live about 4 to 6 hours away by car. Michelle has learned that Lois has become more forgetful and less tolerant of physical activity related to severe heart disease. Michelle worries about what she will do about this because she lives 2 hours away. Lois needs support, and it is probable that this needed support will increase over time. Michelle worries that the only alternative is for Lois to move in with the O'Connells. If so, Michelle would have to rid the house of pets, which Lois is allergic to, and her home would require major renovations.

Bethany, age 28, is the nursing student assigned to care for Lois in her community health rotation. She sees Lois living alone in a clean mobile home in a nice park. Although Lois receives Social Security and has Medicare, she cannot afford supplemental insurance.

The family remains a central institution in American society. However, the concept, structure, and functioning of the family unit continue to change over time. Although the family is in transition and looks very different from the families of the 1950s, the family unit is here to stay. Families face many challenges, including the effects of health and illness, childbearing and child rearing, changes in family structure and dynamics, and caring for an older parent. However, family characteristics or attributes, such as durability, resiliency, and diversity, assist in adapting to these challenges.

Family durability is the intrafamilial system of support and structure that sometimes extends beyond the walls of the household. Through divorce, remarriages, or cohabitation new members are added to a family. In addition, an extended family also includes contact with former spouses or partners. For example, in the case study Patrick and Michelle are part of an extended family because of their relationship with Lois. Michelle keeps her husband connected with her grandmother. The players may change, the parents may remarry, the children may or may not leave home as adults, but the "family" transcends long periods and inevitable lifestyle changes.

Family resiliency is the ability to cope with expected and unexpected stressors. One stressor on the O'Connell family is Patrick's potential job loss. Not only does Patrick's job provide income and insurance benefits, it defines part of Patrick's role in the family. Both Patrick's and Michelle's resiliency will show how they adjust to this stressor. For example, if Michelle needs to resume full-time work with benefits, will Patrick be able and willing to take over household tasks and care for Lois? The family's ability to adapt to role changes, developmental milestones, and crises shows resilience (see Chapter 24). The goal of the family is not only to survive "the challenge" but also to thrive and grow as a result of the newly gained knowledge.

Family diversity is the attention to the uniqueness of each family. You will work with many different kinds of families. Some families will be experiencing marriage for the first time and having children in later life, whereas other families of the same age will be grandparents. Every person within a familial unit has specific needs, strengths, and important developmental considerations.

As nurses, we are responsible for first understanding the makeup (configuration), structure, function, and coping capacity of the family and then building on the family's relative strengths and resources (Feeley and Gottlieb, 2000). The goal of family-centered nursing care is to promote, support, and provide for the well-being and health of the family and individual family members (Astedt-Kurki and others, 2002; Joronen and Astedt-Kurki, 2005).

SCIENTIFIC KNOWLEDGE BASE

Concept of Family

For some, the term family evokes a visual image of adults and children living together in a satisfying, harmonious manner. For others this term has the exact opposite image. Families represent more than a set of individuals, and a family is more than a sum of its individual members (Astedt-Kurki and others, 2001). Families are, however, as diverse as the individuals that compose them, and patients have deeply ingrained values about their families that deserve respect. Each individual de-

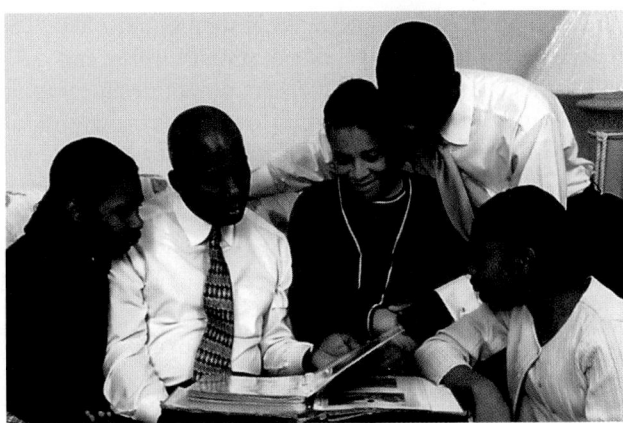

Figure 23-1 ■ Family celebrations and traditions strengthen the family.

fines the family. In other words, think of the family as a set of relationships that the patient identifies as family or as a network of individuals who influence each other's lives whether there are actual biological or legal ties (Figure 23-1).

Definition: What Is Family?

Defining family may at first seem simple. However, different definitions cause debates among social scientists and legislators. The definition of family has a significant impact on who is included on health insurance policies, who has access to children's school records, who files joint tax returns, and who has eligibility for sick-leave benefits or public assistance programs. A **family** is a set of interacting individuals related by blood, marriage, or adoption who are interdependent in carrying out the relative roles and responsibilities of the family unit (Astedt-Kurki and others, 2004). Your personal beliefs do not have to coincide with those of the patient. To provide individualized family care, understand that families take many forms and have diverse cultural and ethnic orientations. In addition, no two families are alike. Each has its own strengths, weaknesses, resources, and challenges.

Family Forms

Family forms are patterns of people who are considered to be family members. Although all families have some things in common, each family form has unique problems and strengths. As a nurse, keep an open mind about what makes up a family so that you do not overlook potential resources and concerns. Box 23-1 describes several family forms.

CURRENT TRENDS AND NEW FAMILY FORMS Families are smaller today. People are marrying later, women are delaying childbirth, and couples are choosing to have fewer children or none at all. The number of people living alone is expanding and accounts for approximately 26% of households. Divorce rates have tripled since the 1950s, and although the rate appears to have stabilized, it is estimated that 55% of all marriages will end in divorce (U.S. Census Bureau, 2007).

The number of single-parent families doubled from the 1970s to the 1990s but now appears to be stabilizing at about

BOX 23-1 Family Forms

NUCLEAR FAMILY
Nuclear family consists of husband and wife (and perhaps one or more children).

EXTENDED FAMILY
The extended family includes relatives (aunts, uncles, grandparents, and cousins) in addition to the nuclear family. The case study with Michelle and Patrick is an example of an extended family.

SINGLE-PARENT FAMILY
The single-parent family is formed when one parent leaves the nuclear family because of death, divorce, or desertion or when a single person decides to have or adopt a child.

BLENDED FAMILY
The blended family is formed when parents bring unrelated children from prior or foster parenting relationships into a new, joint living situation.

ALTERNATIVE PATTERNS OF RELATIONSHIPS
These relationships include multiadult households, "skip-generation" families (grandparents caring for grandchildren), and communal groups with children, "nonfamilies" (adults living alone), and cohabitating partners.

26% of all families with children. Although mothers head 83% of single-parent families, father-only families are on the rise. Forty-one percent of children are living with mothers who have never married; many of these children result from an adolescent pregnancy (U.S. Census Bureau, 2007).

Adolescent pregnancy is an ever-increasing concern. The majority of these adolescents continue to live with their families. A teenage pregnancy tends to have long-term consequences for the mother and often severely stresses family relationships and resources. In addition, there is an increased risk for continued poverty for the family (Raneri and Wiemann, 2007; SmithBattle, 2000). Teenage fathers also have stressors placed on them when their partner becomes pregnant. These young men have poorer support systems and fewer resources to teach them how to parent (James-Childs, 2000). As a result, both of these adolescents often struggle with the normal tasks of development and identity, but are also forced to accept a responsibility that they are not ready for physically, emotionally, socially, and/or financially (Sangalang and Rounds, 2005).

Although unable to marry by law in many states, homosexual couples define their relationship in family terms. Approximately half of all gay male couples live together, compared with three fourths of lesbian couples. Individuals in same-sex relationships have become more open about their sexual preference and more vocal about their legal rights.

FACTORS INFLUENCING FAMILY FORMS Families face many challenges, including changing structures and roles related to the changing economic status of society. There are family challenges related to divorce and the aging of its older members. There are three additional trends that social scientists identify as threats or concerns facing the family: (1) changing economic status (e.g., declining family income, need for dual incomes), decreased health insurance, or lack of access to health care; (2) homelessness; and (3) domestic violence.

Economic Factors Making ends meet is a daily concern for many people because of the declining economic status of families. Economics have particularly affected families at the lower end of the income scale, and single-parent families are especially vulnerable. As a result, many families have inadequate or no health insurance and they have difficulty accessing health care. There are 13.3 million children living below the poverty level, and 9 million children are uninsured (Children's Defense Fund [CDF], 2008). As you read in the case study, the O'Connell family is faced with a potential decline in economic resources. Not only will this loss affect the family finances, but there is a potential loss of health insurance benefit if Patrick loses his job.

Homelessness Another factor influencing family forms is homelessness. The fastest growing segment of the homeless population is families with children. This includes complete nuclear families and single-parent families. Families with children account for 36% of the homeless population (National Coalition for the Homeless, 2008). Poverty, lack of affordable housing, chronic mental illness, and substance abuse are primary causes. Homelessness severely affects the functioning, health, and well-being of the family and its members. Children of homeless families are often in fair or poor health and have higher rates of asthma, ear infections, stomach problems, and mental illness. As a result, usually the only access to health care for these children is through the emergency department (Haldenby, Berman, and Forchuk, 2007).

Homeless adults face health risks as well. They are more likely to suffer from mental health issues, as well as chronic health problems. They are exposed to the elements and have poor nutrition and limited access to health care. When a shelter is present, it is usually an evening/night shelter only. Because of the homelessness and the fact that these adults are "on the street," they are vulnerable to physical and emotional violence, injury, and trauma.

Homeless children face barriers, such as meeting residency requirements for public schools and inability to obtain previous enrollment records, when enrolling and attending school. As a result, these children are more likely to drop out of school and become unemployable. Homeless families and their children are at serious risk for developing long-term health, psychological, and socioeconomic problems, thus posing a major challenge for our entire society (Schanzer and others, 2007).

Domestic Violence Domestic violence includes not only the intimate partner relationships of spousal, live-in partners, and dating relationships, but also familial, elder, and child abuse. Abuse generally falls into one or more of the following categories: physical battering, sexual assault, and emotional or psychological abuse; and it generally escalates over a period of time (Family Violence Prevention Fund, 2008). The statistics regarding family violence are disturbing and difficult to calculate because researchers do not use a common definition of abuse. Some count only victims of physical abuse, whereas others include data for both physical and sexual abuse. Still other investigators also include emotional abuse (Lewis-O'Connor, 2004). The cause of family violence is complex and multidimensional. Stress, poverty, social isolation, psychopathology, and learned family behavior are all factors associated with violence.

In addition, other factors such as alcohol and drug abuse, pregnancy, sexual orientation, and mental illness increase the incidence of abuse within a family. Although abuse sometimes ends when a person leaves a specific family environment, there are often negative long-term physical and emotional consequences. One of these consequences includes moving from one abusive situation to another. For example, a child sees marriage as a way to leave an abusive home and in turn marries a person who continues the abuse within the marriage (Wathen and MacMillan, 2003).

STRUCTURE AND FUNCTION Each family has a unique structure and way of functioning. Family structure is based on organization (i.e., the ongoing membership of the family and the pattern of relationships). Relationships are often numerous and complex. For example, in the case study you see that Michelle has relationships with her husband, mother, employer, and colleagues in school. Each of these relationships has different demands, roles, and expectations. The multiple relationships and their expectations are often sources for personal and family stress (see Chapter 24).

Although the definitions of structure vary, you can assess family structure by asking the following questions: "Who is included in the family?" "Who performs which tasks?" and "Who makes which decisions?" Structure either enhances or detracts from the family's ability to respond to the expected and unexpected stressors of daily life. Structures that are too rigid or flexible can threaten family functioning. Rigid structures specifically dictate who accomplishes different tasks and also limits the number of persons outside the immediate family allowed to assume these tasks. For example, in a rigid family the mother is the only acceptable person to provide emotional support for the children and/or to perform all of the household chores. The husband is the only acceptable person to provide financial support, maintain the vehicles, do the yard work, and/or do all of the home repairs. A change in the health status of the person responsible for a task places a burden on a rigid family because no other person is available, willing, or considered acceptable to assume that task. An extremely flexible structure also presents problems for the family. There is sometimes an absence of stability that would otherwise lead to automatic action during a crisis or rapid change.

Family functioning is how the family performs every day. Specific functional aspects include how a family reproduces, interacts to socialize its young, cooperates to meet economic needs, and relates to the community or larger society. Family functioning also focuses on the processes used by the family to achieve its goals. These processes include communication among family members, goal setting, conflict resolution, nurturing, and use of internal and external resources. Although many families pursue these goals at various times during their development, the provision of psychological support remains an important goal throughout the life span.

DEVELOPMENTAL STAGES Families, like individuals, change and grow over time. Although families are far from identical to one another, they have a basic pattern and similarity in experiences resulting in predictable stages. Each of these developmental stages has its own challenges, needs, and resources and includes tasks that need to be completed before the family is able to successfully move on to the next stage (Table 23-1).

FAMILY AND HEALTH Family health influences family functioning. The family is one primary social context in which health promotion and disease prevention take place. The family's beliefs, values, and practices strongly influence health-promoting behaviors of its members. When the family satisfactorily meets its goals through adequate functioning, its members tend to feel positive about themselves and their family. Conversely, when they do not meet goals, families view themselves as ineffective. Constant stress resulting from inadequate functioning adversely affects an individual family member's health. Constant stress affects cardiovascular function, blood pressure, and blood glucose levels, which can affect a person's level of health (see Chapter 24).

TABLE 23-1 Stages of the Family Life Cycle

FAMILY LIFE CYCLE STAGE	EMOTIONAL PROCESS OF TRANSITION: KEY PRINCIPLES	CHANGES IN FAMILY STATUS REQUIRED TO PROCEED DEVELOPMENTALLY
Unattached young adults	Accepting parent-offspring separation	Differentiation of self in relation to family of origin Development of intimate peer relationships Establishment of self in work
Joining of families through marriage: newly married couple	Commitment to new family system	Formation of marital system Realignment of relationships with extended families and friends to include spouse
Family with young children	Accepting new generation of members into system	Adjusting marital system to make space for children Taking on parenting roles Realignment of relationships with extended family to include parenting and grandparenting roles
Family with adolescents	Increasing flexibility of family boundaries to include children's independence	Shifting of parent-child relationships to permit adolescents to move into and out of system Refocus on midlife marital and career issues Beginning shift toward concerns for older generation
Family with young adults	Accepting multitude of exits from and entries into family system	Renegotiation of marital system as couple or unit of only two Development of adult-to-adult relationships between grown children and their parents Realignment of relationships to include in-laws and grandchildren Dealing with disabilities and death of parents (grandparents)
Family without children		Refocus on new career opportunities Refocus on marital and career issues Renegotiation of recreational activities
Family in later life	Accepting shifting of generational roles	Maintaining own or couple functioning and interests in the face of physiological decline; exploration of new familial and social role options Support for more central role for middle generation Making room in system for wisdom and experience of older adults; supporting older generation without overfunctioning for them Retirement; change in role Dealing with loss of spouse, siblings, and other peers, and preparation for own death; life review and integration

Data from Duvall EM, Miller BC: *Marriage and family development,* ed 6, Boston, 2005, Allyn and Bacon.

Good health is not always highly valued; in fact, harmful practices are acceptable in some families. A long-term illness in one of the family members affects the well-being and health of the entire family (Tarkka and others, 2003). Although illness strains relationships, research indicates that family members have the potential to be a primary force for coping.

Hardiness and **resiliency** are factors that moderate a family's stress. Family hardiness is the internal strengths and durability of the family unit. A sense of control over the outcome of life, a view of change as beneficial and growth producing, and an active rather than passive orientation in adapting to stressful events characterize family hardiness (McCubbin, McCubbin, and Thompson, 1996). Resiliency helps to evaluate healthy responses when individuals and families are experiencing stressful events. Resources and techniques a family or individuals within the family use to maintain a balance or level of health assist in understanding a family's level of resiliency. Hardiness and resiliency are important for the O'Connell family. The strong marital bond between Patrick and Michelle will assist in balancing the new demands as Lois' health declines.

NURSING KNOWLEDGE BASE

To begin work with families, you need a scientific knowledge base in family theory and knowledge base in family nursing. The two concepts interact to affect the care that you deliver to the family. All practice settings and all health care environments emphasize family nursing.

Family Nursing: Family as Context, as Patient, and as System

In caring for a family, your goal is to help the family and its individual members reach and maintain maximum health in any given situation. Family nursing is based on the assumption that all people regardless of age are a member of some type of family form (see Box 23-1). The goal of family nursing is to help the family and its individual members reach and maintain maximum health throughout and beyond the illness experience (Tapp, 2004). *In the case study, Bethany strives to offer Michelle strategies that allow her to help Lois adapt to the physical limits of her heart disease. In addition, Bethany also offers Patrick and Michelle preparation strategies to adjust to the impending changes in their family life resulting from Lois' illness and the change in the family's finances.*

There are different approaches for family nursing practice. For this chapter, family nursing practice has three levels of approaches: (1) **family as context,** (2) **family as patient,** and (3) **family as system.** Family as system is a newer model and includes both relational and transactional concepts. All approaches recognize that a nursing intervention for one member influences all members and affects family functioning. Families are continually changing. As a result, the need for family support changes over time, and it is important for you to understand that the family is more complex than simply a combination of individual members (Tapp, 2004).

FAMILY AS CONTEXT When you view the family as context, your primary focus is on the health and development of an individual member existing within a specific environment (i.e., the patient). Although you focus the nursing process on the individual's health status, you will also assess the extent to which the family provides the individual's basic needs. These needs vary, depending on the individual's developmental level and situation. Because families provide more than just material essentials, you need to consider their ability to help the patient meet psychological needs.

FAMILY AS PATIENT When you view the family as patient, the family processes and relationships (e.g., parenting or family caregiving) are your primary focus of care. In the case study, Bethany focuses on the O'Connell family as the patient. The nursing assessment focuses on family patterns versus individual characteristics. The nursing process concentrates on the extent to which these patterns and processes are consistent with reaching and maintaining family and individual health.

FAMILY AS SYSTEM It is important to understand that although you make theoretical and practical distinctions between the family as context and the family as patient, they are not necessarily mutually exclusive. You will use both simultaneously, such as with the perspective of the family as system. When you view the family as a system, you will see that the effect one member has creates a "trickle-down" effect. This affects all members of the family, including the extended family members (Duhamel and Talbot, 2004).

CRITICAL THINKING

You will apply elements of critical thinking whenever you perform the nursing process with a patient. Consider the scientific knowledge you have learned, your experience, critical thinking attitudes, and standards to ensure an individualized approach to patient care. Critical thinking is crucial in the care of patients and their families. As a nurse, you must synthesize all aspects of critical thinking to give individualized, compassionate family care. The care of a family is an ongoing mutually acceptable relationship. As you begin to provide family-centered care, you continually assess, analyze, and reflect on the changing needs and health care goals of your patients and their families.

Synthesis

Scientific and family nursing knowledge, experience, critical thinking attitudes, and standards enable you to identify the needs of both patients and their families. Synthesis of these elements enables you to assess the family as context, as patient, or as a system and to gain information about the family life cycle perspective, family structure and functioning, and family health (Box 23-2).

KNOWLEDGE The health and functioning of each member in the family to some degree depends on the health of the family system as a whole. Family care draws on knowledge from growth and development, psychology, communication,

BOX 23-2   SYNTHESIS IN PRACTICE

Bethany assesses Lois' health care demands and basic physiological needs. She analyzes the role strain on Michelle and how this affects her relationship with Patrick. She also is aware of the impact of stress on Patrick's hypertension. She understands that Lois wants to stay in her home and Michelle wants Lois to do what will make her happiest. Bethany asks about any extended family members, and Michelle says that she has two sisters, who live 4 and 6 hours away. They are willing to come and help care for Lois. Michelle's two sisters plan on alternating visits every month to assist Patrick and Michelle.

If Bethany views the family as the context, she focuses on each member of the family. Lois' changes in health affect the family greatly, and care is directed toward improving Lois' ability to tolerate exercise as much as possible and maximizing her independence. In addition, Bethany helps Michelle to reduce stress by teaching her relaxation and meditation techniques, helping her to plan "down

time," and giving her some time management techniques. Bethany assesses Patrick's knowledge of ways to manage his blood pressure (e.g., reducing the number of high-sodium foods and using stress reduction techniques).

If she views the family as a patient, Bethany assesses the family's goals for Lois' care and independence. She will assess the family's caregiving strengths and needs, weaknesses, and the resources available to the family as they assume the role of caregiver. Bethany observes the impact that caregiving has on Michelle and Patrick and also inquires about Michelle's siblings who are assisting in the care.

If Bethany views the family as a system, she needs to work with the entire family to help Lois transition from her own home. One solution to this problem may be to help the family select an assisted living community located halfway between the O'Connell home and the homes of Michelle's two sisters.

family theories, sociology, and the family life cycle. When a family is in a transitional phase of the life cycle perspective (e.g., birth of a first child) or there is an additional stressor to the family unit (e.g., chronic illness), it creates considerable anxiety and stress within the family system. Your knowledge of stress and coping will assist in family care.

EXPERIENCE Your past experiences in related situations help you to problem solve. We all draw on life experience even if we are not able to draw on nursing knowledge. Experiences in your own family assist in designing family-centered care. Carefully appraise past experiences and your use of experience-related information, because no two families are alike.

It is possible for illness to bring family members closer together because they all share duties, roles, and responsibilities. Conversely, illnesses, especially critical or life-threatening illnesses, have the potential to pull families apart. *In the case study, as Lois' health declines, Patrick and Michelle look for ways to assist her. As the case study progresses, you will see that Michelle begins to reach out to her siblings to help.*

ATTITUDES Keep an open mind to identify the patient's needs and begin to solve problems and apply critical thinking attitudes such as creativity, perseverance, and risk taking. Partner with the patient and family to use the strengths from your patient's family structure and function, beliefs, values, and expectations to develop a comprehensive, multidisciplinary plan of care.

STANDARDS As a nurse, you will apply nursing standards (e.g., critical care, obstetrical, or gerontological) that apply to the family. In the case study, Bethany applies gerontological standards when offering guidelines for Lois' care. In addition, it is important to apply ethical principles when supporting family decisions, such as assisting family members with accepting the advance directives of their loved ones. Because you can provide a portion of family-centered care in community-based, clinic, or restorative care settings, as well as in the acute care setting, any information about the family

must be kept confidential. In family-centered care, there may be many health care providers, so be sure to document the pertinent information accurately and consistently.

NURSING PROCESS

The nursing process is the same whether the focus is family as patient, context, or a system. It is also the same as that used with individuals and incorporates the needs of the family and those of the patient.

■■■ ASSESSMENT

It is essential to assess the patient and family thoroughly (Table 23-2). The family as a whole differs from individual members. The measure of family health is more than a summation of the health of all members. Areas included in family assessment are the form, structure, and function of the family; its developmental stage; and its progress toward or accomplishment of developmental tasks. Begin assessment by considering the views of the patient toward the family. To determine the family form and membership, ask the patient to tell you about the family: "Who do you consider your family?" or "Who do you share your concerns with?" If the patient is unable to express a concept of family, ask with whom the patient lives, spends time, and shares confidences. Then ask the patient to confirm that people mentioned are his or her family: "Do you consider this person to be family or like family to you?"

STRUCTURE AND FUNCTION It is important to assess family structure and function and determine the effects of illness and the support the family requires (Hanson and others, 2005). Family structure provides information about composition of the family, for example, whether it is a nuclear or extended family. To assess family structure it is helpful to determine the following: who is the head of the household, who is the wage earner, how are decisions made, and who maintains

TABLE 23-2   FOCUSED PATIENT ASSESSMENT

FACTORS TO ASSESS	QUESTIONS	PHYSICAL ASSESSMENT
Family resources	Are there significant relatives and friends not occupying immediate residence? How does your family cope? What do you see as your family's coping strengths/coping challenges, or needs? How does your family obtain health services?	When possible, observe family member interaction. Review past medical experiences of the family. Observe for physical signs of stress or coping difficulties, such as rapid speech, difficulty focusing, weight gain/loss, increased blood pressure, heart rate, etc. (see Chapter 24).
Family patterns	Who works outside the home, type of work, and hours worked? How does your family divide the work of the family, such as household chores (e.g., housekeeping, shopping, repairs), child-rearing responsibilities, and care of older parents? How are decisions made (e.g., day-to-day decisions, financial decisions, health care decisions)?	Observe communication patterns with individual family members. Observe family members as they make decisions (e.g., regarding health care, discharge planning) to help obtain this information.
Family function	Does your family have any short- and long-term goals regarding a variety of subjects (e.g., child rearing, retirement, health care)? Do these goals change because of an illness of a family member?	Observe communication and interaction patterns within the family.

the household. To assess family functioning, ask questions to determine the power structure and patterning of roles and tasks. For example, "How are financial decisions made?" "Who makes decisions for the family?" "How are the tasks divided in your family (e.g., who does the laundry and who mows the lawn)?" and "Who decides where to go on vacation?"

CULTURAL ASPECTS A comprehensive, culturally sensitive family assessment is critical to forming an understanding of family life, current changes in family life, and overall goals and expectations. A family's cultural background (see Chapter 19) is an important variable when assessing the family because race and ethnicity affect structure, function, health beliefs, values, and the way a family perceives events (Box 23-3). The United States is increasingly more diverse. A large number of immigrants enter the country daily, adding to both the number and the variety of ethnic groups that make up the population. American health care institutions tend to operate from a white, middle-class perspective, and immigrant populations often have particular difficulty understanding and "fitting into" the system.

Forming conclusions about families' needs based on cultural backgrounds requires critical thinking. It is imperative to remember that categorical generalizations are often misleading (e.g., Asian Americans consume low-fat diets). Overgeneralizations in terms of racial and ethnic group characteristics do not lead to greater understanding of the culturally diverse family. Culturally different families vary in meaningful and significant ways; however, neglecting to examine similarities will lead to inaccurate assumptions and stereotyping (see Chapter 19).

To determine the influence of culture on a family, you might want to ask the patient about his or her cultural background. Then ask questions concerning cultural practices. For example, "What type of foods do you eat?" "Who cares for sick family members?" "Have you or anyone in your family been hospitalized?" "Did family members remain at the hospital?" "Do you use some of your culture's health practices, such as acupuncture or meditation?" "What role do grandparents play in raising your children?"

PSYCHOSOCIAL NEEDS Assessment of family functions includes determining the family's ability to cope with their current health problem or situation, the need for social and emotional support for members, the appropriateness of their goal setting, and progress toward achievement of developmental tasks (see Table 23-1, p. 623). Because families' goals vary, make sure measures of family health are flexible. During assessment, assess whether the family is able to provide and distribute sufficient economic resources and if the family's social network is extensive enough to provide support.

COMMUNITY ASSESSMENT Assess the family's home environment and community. When assessing the patient's home, determine the size of the home, provision for privacy, and safety factors, such as presence of smoke detectors and safe bathrooms and stairwells (see Chapter 27). When assessing the community, determine the presence of health care resources, proximity of emergency services, and municipal services (see Chapter 3). If there is a strong extended family, how far away does the extended family live from the patient? Do they live together, in the same neighborhood, or the same city? If the family lives together, how large is the space?

PATIENT EXPECTATIONS Families, like individual patients, have certain expectations for care. Some families expect to be consulted as a whole unit when discussing care of

BOX 23-3   CULTURAL FOCUS

 Bethany knows that families have their unique perspectives and characteristics. Families have differences in values, beliefs, and philosophies. The cultural heritage of the family often affects religious, child-rearing, and nutritional practices; recreational activities; and health promotion behaviors. As she studies and reviews the literature, Bethany learns that nurses need to have cultural competence and sensitivity when caring for culturally diverse patients. Incorporating cultural preferences into the plan of care increases the patient's adherence to therapy, assists in transition from hospital to home, and provides a unique aspect to the patient's care.

IMPLICATIONS FOR PRACTICE

- Perception of certain events varies across cultural groups and has particular impact on families. For example, the care of the grandmother has a great significance to the extended family.
- Caregiving values and practices vary across cultures. Bethany knows that in some cultures it is a sign of disrespect to your elders to place them in nursing homes, even those older adults with severe dementia. Bethany knows that Lois' family wants to assist her in living as independently as possible.
- Intergenerational support and patterns of living arrangements are related to cultural background. For example, traditional Chinese, African American, Japanese, and Hispanic persons are more likely to live in extended family households than their white counterparts.
- Health beliefs differ among various cultures, which affects the decision of a family and its members about when and where to seek help. For example, some Asian families rarely consider symptoms as psychological and are not likely to go to mental health providers.

Data from Cox C, Monk A: Strain among caregivers: comparing the experiences of African-American and Hispanic caregivers of Alzheimer's relatives, *Int J Aging Hum Dev* 43(2):93, 1996; Wang Y: People of Chinese heritage. In Purnell LD, Paulanka BJ: *Transcultural health care: a culturally competent approach*, ed 2, Philadelphia, 2003, FA Davis; Bonura D and others: Culturally-congruent end-of-life care for Jewish patients and their families, *J Transcult Nurs* 12(3):211, 2001; Galanti GA: *Caring for patients from different cultures*, ed 3, Philadelphia, 2004, University of Pennsylvania Press.

their loved one. Others wish to have a designated decision maker. The family sometimes expects the health care system to meet all of their needs, not only those related to health issues. When assessing the family's expectations, be clear whether the family is the patient and receiver of care or whether the family member is the patient and receiver of care. Determining these expectations early in the assessment will help to avoid problems resulting from misunderstandings in the future.

■■■ NURSING DIAGNOSIS

Nursing assessment results in clustering relevant data and seeing patterns that support nursing diagnoses. The nursing diagnoses selected often include the family's health needs,

current and potential health problems, level of wellness, or a combination of these areas. Examples of nursing diagnoses for family-focused care include the following:

- *Risk for caregiver role strain*
- *Compromised family coping*
- *Disabled family coping*
- *Interrupted family processes*
- *Impaired parenting*
- *Ineffective role performance*
- *Risk for other-directed violence*

The nursing diagnosis often focuses on the family's ability to cope with its current situation, whether it is an acute illness, an anticipated developmental transition, or negative behaviors that threaten short-term or long-term health. Appropriate use of internal and external resources allows the family to cope with day-to-day challenges and with unexpected occurrences that threaten health and equilibrium. A nursing diagnosis might also focus on changes in family processes or roles of members. During times of acute illness the family becomes extremely distressed and focuses solely on the ill member, neglecting the needs of the other family members. For example, consider the diagnosis of *risk for caregiver role strain* a possibility when extended care of a family member is necessary.

The diagnostic statement indicates related factors contributing to the health problem. For example, unrealistic expectations is a possible related factor. *In the case study, Michelle initially wanted to assume responsibility for Lois. However, after making repeated trips to Lois' home and trying to support Patrick, Michelle becomes more stressed when trying to handle all the demands of care. In this case the nursing diagnosis* risk for caregiver role strain related to unrealistic expectations *is appropriate. Another potential nursing diagnosis,* interrupted family processes related to caregiving demands, *is due to a change in the relationship between Michelle and Patrick. Because of the caregiving demands, Michelle and Patrick are not able to relax and spend time together as a couple.*

■■■ PLANNING

GOALS AND OUTCOMES After you develop nursing diagnoses, the next step is to plan care with the family. Goal setting is mutual. The goals need to be concrete, realistic, compatible with the family's developmental stage and expectations, and acceptable to the family. The plan of care of the O'Connell family is represented in a Concept Map (Figure 23-2) and nursing Care Plan.

A family-focused approach enhances nursing practice. Goals for a plan of care incorporating a family approach include those that view the family as context, the family as patient, the family as system, or a combination. The patient situation and availability of family members define the types of goals that are feasible. For example, a goal might read, "The family functions at its optimal level," with the expected outcome being "Communication between family members is clear." Family members are able to confront and resolve conflict in a healthy way. *The broader the goals, however, the less*

CONCEPT MAP

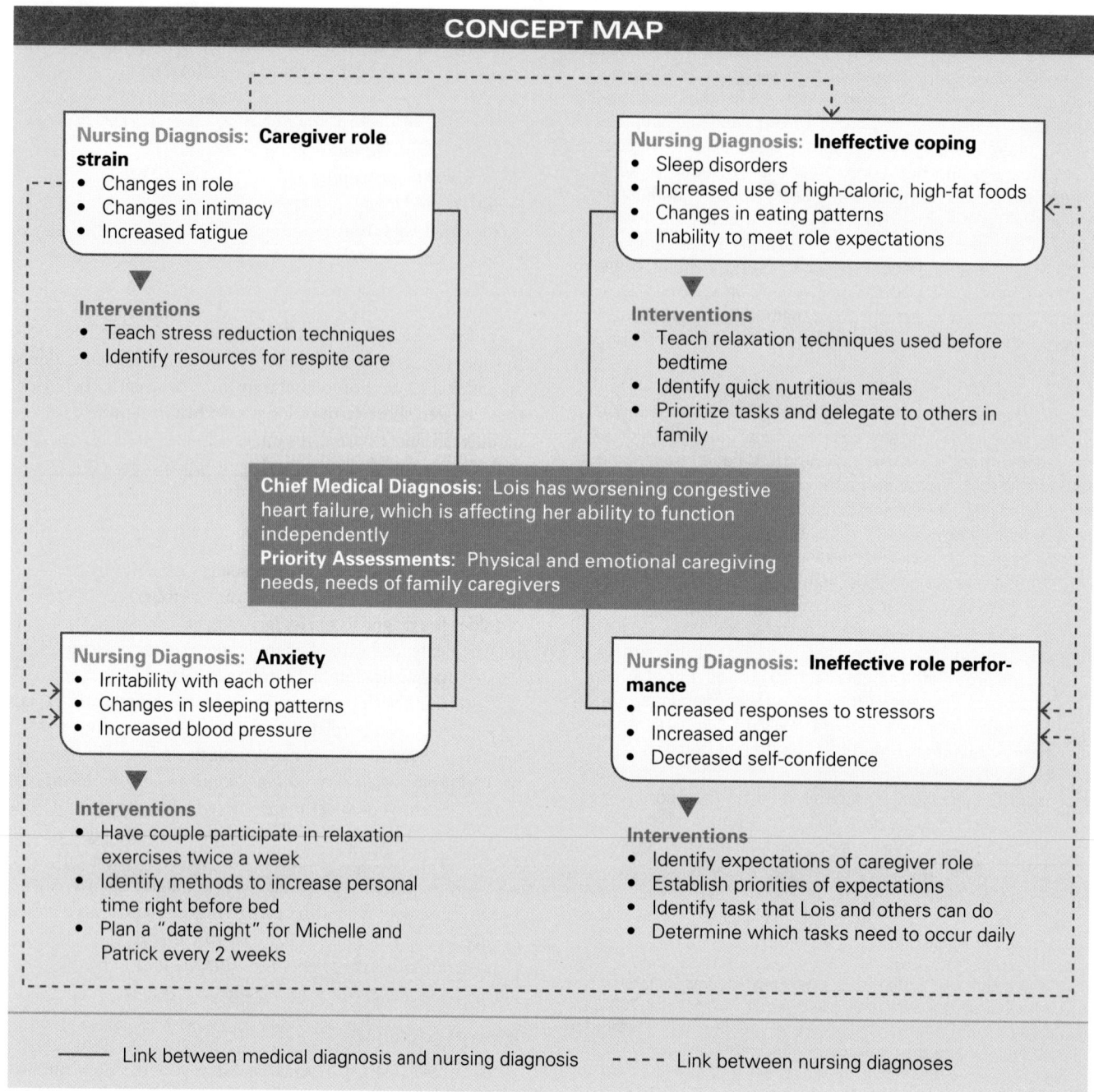

Nursing Diagnosis: Caregiver role strain
- Changes in role
- Changes in intimacy
- Increased fatigue

Interventions
- Teach stress reduction techniques
- Identify resources for respite care

Nursing Diagnosis: Ineffective coping
- Sleep disorders
- Increased use of high-caloric, high-fat foods
- Changes in eating patterns
- Inability to meet role expectations

Interventions
- Teach relaxation techniques used before bedtime
- Identify quick nutritious meals
- Prioritize tasks and delegate to others in family

Chief Medical Diagnosis: Lois has worsening congestive heart failure, which is affecting her ability to function independently
Priority Assessments: Physical and emotional caregiving needs, needs of family caregivers

Nursing Diagnosis: Anxiety
- Irritability with each other
- Changes in sleeping patterns
- Increased blood pressure

Interventions
- Have couple participate in relaxation exercises twice a week
- Identify methods to increase personal time right before bed
- Plan a "date night" for Michelle and Patrick every 2 weeks

Nursing Diagnosis: Ineffective role performance
- Increased responses to stressors
- Increased anger
- Decreased self-confidence

Interventions
- Identify expectations of caregiver role
- Establish priorities of expectations
- Identify task that Lois and others can do
- Determine which tasks need to occur daily

—— Link between medical diagnosis and nursing diagnosis   - - - - Link between nursing diagnoses

Figure 23-2 ■ Concept Map.

measurable and practical they become. For specific examples, see the Care Plan.

SETTING PRIORITIES Setting priorities focuses on the patient, the patient/family unit, or the family alone. It is imperative that the family and the patient clearly understand and agree on the plan of care and priorities. The priorities for the patient and family are sometimes different. For example, the priority for your patient is to obtain physiological or emotional stability, self-care, or progress to a rehabilitation facility. However, the family priorities include obtaining temporary housing so they are near their ill family member,

spiritual support, assistance with decision making, or understanding the complexities of the health care delivery system. In some instances the priorities of the family and patient are different but require simultaneous interventions.

COLLABORATIVE CARE Collaboration with family members is essential. Collaborate with all appropriate family members when planning care. You base a positive collaborative relationship on mutual respect and trust. The family needs to feel "in control" as much as possible. By offering alternative actions and asking family members for their own ideas and suggestions, you will help to reduce the family's feelings of powerlessness.

CARE PLAN Caregiver Role Strain

ASSESSMENT

Patrick and Michelle are caregivers to Michelle's grandmother, Lois, who has heart disease, and who is still living in her own home. Lois suffers fatigue and forgetfulness and poses numerous caregiving demands. She frequently complains about how Michelle offers assistance with household chores. Michelle and Patrick have frequent arguments over how to best help Lois, because they live 2 hours away. They both share concerns as to what will happen to Lois.

ASSESSMENT ACTIVITIES

Ask Michelle if she notices any changes in her sleeping or eating.

Ask Patrick to describe changes in lifestyle since Michelle increased her caregiving activities.

Ask Patrick about any changes in his health status.
Use a scale of 0 to 10 to ask Patrick and Michelle to rate their stress level.
Ask Michelle to describe how she feels about taking care of her grandmother.

FINDINGS/DEFINING CHARACTERISTICS*

Difficulty sleeping—includes both **falling asleep** and **remaining asleep**
Poor eating habits—Michelle notes that she does not eat regularly, and when she eats, it is frequently a high-fat, high-carbohydrate fast-food meal.
There is decreased time spent together.
They have **increased arguments** with one another.
He **complains about the time Michelle spends with her grandmother and the amount of time she spends worrying about her grandmother.**
He admits to doing less around the home to help Michelle.
Patrick notes that his **blood pressure is higher.**
Patrick rates his stress as a 8.
Michelle rates her stress as a 7.
She describes being fearful of "not doing things well for her grandmother."
She **feels anxious** when actually helping with tasks and when at home with Patrick.

NURSING DIAGNOSIS: Caregiver role strain related to Lois' increasing health care needs and unrealistic expectations.

PLANNING

GOAL

- Michelle and Patrick will gain improved understanding of stress and adaptive management techniques within 1 month.

- Patrick and Michelle will use community-based resources within 1 month.

EXPECTED OUTCOMES (NOC)†

Caregiver Well-Being
- Michelle and Patrick will be able to identify and share four caregiving activities within 1 week.
- Michelle and Patrick will demonstrate correct meditation techniques within 1 month.
- Michelle and Patrick will meditate together 4 nights a week within 6 weeks.
- Michelle and Patrick will contact the local council on aging within 3 weeks.

INTERVENTIONS (NIC)‡

Caregiver Support
- Discuss with Patrick and Michelle the effects of stress on themselves and the family.
- Listen to their individual concerns.
- Teach them techniques, relaxation exercises, and meditation to reduce their response to stress.

RATIONALE

Identification of specific stressors and their effects needs to occur before techniques to reduce the stress will be effective (Stajduhar and others, 2008). Caring and support through listening and accepting the needs and expectations of the members of the family enhance coping (Maijala and others, 2004).

*Defining characteristics are shown in bold type.
†Outcomes classification label from Moorhead S and others, edtiros: *Nursing outcomes classification (NOC)*, ed 4, St. Louis, 2008, Mosby.
‡Intervention classification labels from Bulechek GM and others, editors: *Nursing interventions classification (NIC)*, ed 5, St. Louis, 2008, Mosby.

CARE PLAN Caregiver Role Strain—cont'd

INTERVENTIONS (NIC)‡

Caregiver Support

- Provide a list of support services, such as volunteers from faith-based group or the local council on aging, who provide respite care, for Patrick and Michelle.

- Contact community support groups, such as American Heart Association, to obtain a list of reputable house-cleaning services.
- Consult with Patrick and Michelle to establish a list of community resources, assisted living facilities, and family support to assist with caregiver tasks.

RATIONALE

Intergenerational assistance is complex and at times requires some support. Identification of community-based groups that provide support to families helps reduce strain on the caregiver and provides assistance with some health care issues (Tarkka and others, 2003).

Community service groups frequently maintain lists of reputable household service providers. Such a listing assists the family in identifying the service in a timely manner.

A potential list of resources provides the family with an organized system of providing supportive, safe care for an older adult who is living in the community (Abbott, Shaw, and Bryar, 2004).

EVALUATION

NURSING ACTIONS	PATIENT RESPONSE/FINDING	ACHIEVEMENT OF OUTCOME
Ask Patrick and Michelle to describe how they will divide caregiving activities.	Patrick and Michelle describe the new activities they assumed responsibility for and those activities that remained shared.	Patrick is sharing more caregiving activities.
Ask Patrick and Michelle how often they meditate each week and how they feel after they meditate.	Patrick and Michelle state they meditate three times per week. Michelle states, "It is difficult to find the time to meditate, but we are much more relaxed after we do it."	Meditation is effective. Need to work with couple to work out a schedule that will allow meditation four times per week.
Ask Patrick and Michelle to identify resources found through the local agency on aging.	Patrick and Michelle state they were able to locate resources through their church. Patrick states, "The ladies from church come once a week to stay with Lois so Michelle and I can run errands and spend some time together."	Michelle and Patrick have located community resources to help meet caregiving demands.

For example, offering options for how to prepare a low-fat diet or how to rearrange the furnishings of a room to accommodate a family member's disability gives the family an opportunity to express their preferences, make choices, and ultimately feel as though they have contributed. Collaborating with other disciplines, such as physical therapy and social service, increases the likelihood of a comprehensive approach to the family's health care needs, and it ensures better continuity of care. Using other disciplines is particularly important when discharge planning from a health care facility to home or an extended care facility is necessary (Bluvol and Ford-Gilboe, 2004).

■■■IMPLEMENTATION

Family nursing is used in a variety of health care settings whether the nurse is providing health promotion, acute care, or restorative and continuing care. Regardless of the setting, some general facts about family nursing are applied across all health care settings. Knowing about challenges for family

nursing and principles for implementing family-centered nursing is important to assist you in developing individualized care for your patients and their families.

CHALLENGES FOR FAMILY NURSING Delegation in the management of nursing care activities is a challenge in family nursing. Often nurses are trying to affect family health by delegating duties to family members or to other members of the health care team. For example, you help family members learn how to provide certain types of procedures to care for an ill family member. With earlier discharge and more complex family needs at the time of discharge, planning for discharge begins with the initiation of care.

Using family caregivers is an important resource and challenge for family nursing. Family caregivers need to learn aspects of physical and emotional care for the patient. For example, many family caregivers are now faced with having to perform complex nursing procedures at home, such as wound care, enteral nutrition, and intravenous therapy. However, family care-

BOX 23-4   PATIENT TEACHING

Medication Administration

 chelle tells Bethany that Lois' medications were changed. Some of these medications may need to be "held" if Lois' pulse changes. Michelle is fearful of giving her grandmother the wrong medication or giving the medication incorrectly.

OUTCOMES

At the end of the teaching sessions, Michelle and Patrick will be able to do the following:

- Correctly place all Lois' medications in the weekly medication dispenser
- Correctly obtain an apical pulse
- State that if Lois' pulse rate is 60 beats per minute or less or 100 beats per minute or greater, she should not be given the digoxin 0.25 mg, and they should notify the home care nurse

TEACHING STRATEGIES

- Provide Michelle and Patrick with a laminated card that lists all medications: include action, side effects, precautions, and premedication assessments (e.g., need for pulse measurement).
- Demonstrate to both Michelle and Patrick how to fill the weekly medication dispenser.
- Demonstrate how to take an apical pulse.
- Discuss with Michelle and Patrick situations in which digoxin is not given.

EVALUATION STRATEGIES

- Ask Michelle and Patrick to identify which medication requires a preadministration apical pulse.
- Observe weekly medication dispenser to determine accurate medication administration.
- Observe and validate Michelle and Patrick obtaining an apical pulse.
- Ask Michelle and Patrick about situation in which digoxin should not be given.

givers have physical and emotional health care needs as well. Teach caregivers how to meet their needs as well. Family caregivers are often used in restorative and continuing care areas, and this is discussed in a later section of this chapter.

IMPLEMENTING FAMILY-CENTERED CARE It is important to (1) guide the family in problem solving, (2) provide practical services, and (3) convey a sense of acceptance and caring by listening carefully to family members' concerns and suggestions. Whether you provide care for the family as context, patient, or system, nursing interventions aim to increase family members' abilities in certain areas, to remove barriers to health care, and to do things that the family is not able to do for itself.

For example, as a health educator, you provide accurate health information about diagnosis and prognosis that helps the family caregiver to understand and anticipate needs and concerns of a care recipient. Caregivers are not born with the knowledge of how to be caregivers, and older adults are not born with the knowledge of how to accept dependency (Box

23-4). A moderately flexible structure is generally most beneficial to the family. Nursing interventions will therefore involve changing the family patterns away from extremely rigid or flexible structures if either extreme causes problems related to the health of an individual or the family as a whole. Work within the family structure when providing care, and do not attempt to change the structure.

HEALTH PROMOTION It is important to include health promotion activities as part of your family-centered nursing care. When implementing family nursing, design health promotion interventions, such as low-fat, low-carbohydrate meals or a family exercise program, to improve or maintain the physical, social, emotional, and spiritual well-being of the family unit and its members (Ford-Gilboe, 2002). Often health promotion behaviors are also linked to the developmental stage of the family. For example, the childbearing family needs effective prenatal care, and the child-rearing family needs encouragement to follow immunization schedules. Encourage patients and families to reach their optimum level of wellness. "Strong" families that adapt to transitions, crises, and change tend to have clear communication, problem-solving skills, a commitment to each other and to the family unit, and a sense of cohesiveness and spirituality (Schumacher, Beck, and Marren, 2006).

One approach for meeting goals and promoting health is the use of family strengths. Families do not look at their own system as one that has inherent, positive components. Help the family recognize and use their own unique strengths. For example, in the case study Michelle and Patrick clearly communicated with each other regarding dividing household tasks. Family strengths can include clear communication, adaptability, healthy child-rearing practices, support and nurturing among family members, and the use of crisis for growth.

Help family members focus on their strengths instead of their problems and weaknesses. For example, Bethany points out to Patrick and Michelle that their 10-year marriage probably endured a variety of crises and transitions. As a result, they are likely to have the capabilities to adapt to this latest challenge. Prevention programs aimed at enhancing or developing these attributes are available for families and children in many communities. You need to be aware of family-oriented offerings so that you are able to refer patients as needed.

ACUTE CARE The family is becoming more of the focus within the context of health care delivery in a managed care environment. Acute care settings discharge patients very quickly. Thus you need to take more of a role in understanding and supporting family and patient needs. Family members often have to maintain their jobs while also providing assistance during the patient's recovery. It is a challenge to prepare family members to assist with health care or to locate appropriate community resources.

Discharge Planning Discharge planning with a family is important during the acute care phase of an illness. This planning involves an accurate assessment of what is needed at time of discharge, including resources in the community and the patient's home as well. For example, when a postoperative patient is discharged with an open healing wound, a member of the family needs to know how to take care of the wound, to recognize complications, and when to contact the health care professional. In some cases the family may also have home care services, which can include some short-term assistance with wound care.

Communication Communication is an important aspect of family health, and it is important in all family activities and all health care settings. In the acute care setting clear communication is essential. Help the family identify methods to maintain open lines of communication. For example, when a family member is ill, how will the family inform the nuclear and extended family about any progress or setbacks? In this electronic age, some families are using blogs on the Internet as a way of providing consistent information. Identify who makes decisions for the family, and consistently go to the decision maker. In some situations the decision maker also needs assistance in developing a method to clearly communicate any decisions.

Likewise it is important that the health care team uses communication techniques that are supportive and clear to understand the family's expectation. In addition, clear communication from the health care team enables the family to understand the health care issues, types of decisions, and health care outcomes (see Chapter 10).

RESTORATIVE AND CONTINUING CARE Family nursing emphasizes maintenance of a patient's functional abilities. This means working closely with the family in making sure the home environment is adaptive to the patient's strengths and limitations. Referral to home care nursing is essential. The home care nurse will assist in educating family members about providing ongoing care and making changes in the home so that the patient becomes self-sufficient.

Family Caregiving Family caregiving involves the routine provision of services and personal care activities for a family member by spouses, siblings, or parents. Caregiving activities include personal care (bathing, feeding, and grooming), monitoring for complications or side effects of medications, performing instrumental activities of daily living (shopping or housekeeping), and providing ongoing emotional support and decision making that is necessary.

The fastest-growing age-group is 65 years and older. For the first time in history the average American has more living parents than children, and children are more likely to have living grandparents and even great-grandparents. This "graying" of America affects the family life cycle; it is perhaps most

significant for the middle generation. These caregivers are part of the "sandwich generation" (Box 23-5). These individuals find that they need to balance their own needs with those of their offspring and the needs of their aging parents. This balance often occurs at the expense of their well-being and resources. In addition, many of these caregivers report that support received from professional health professionals is often lacking (Isaksen, Thuen, and Hanestad, 2003).

The majority of these caregivers frequently provide an average of 20 hours of care per week (Schumaker and others, 2006). Caring for a frail or chronically ill relative is a primary concern for a growing number of families. It is not uncommon for people in their 60s and 70s to be the major caregivers for one another, and as a result there are major caregiver concerns for this age-group (Box 23-6).

When family members assume the role of caregiver, they sometimes lose support from significant others. One way you best provide family care is through support of family caregivers. In some cases the family caregiver must provide nursing skills and needs assistance in learning how to perform and evaluate the skill. Whenever an individual becomes dependent on another family member for care and assistance, there is significant stress affecting both the caregiver and the care recipient. In addition, the caregiver needs to continue to meet the demands of his or her usual lifestyle (e.g., raising children, working full time, or dealing with personal problems or illness). In many instances adult children are trying to take care of their parents while meeting the needs of their own family. You can support the caregiver in many ways; for ex-

---

BOX 23-6   CARE OF THE OLDER ADULT

Caregiver Concerns

- Assess the family for additional caregivers to provide respite care for older adult family members. For example, determine additional roles for members of the family (e.g., providing additional financial support; designating someone to obtain groceries and medications or providing someone to assist with household tasks).
- Assess for caregiver stress, such as tension in relationships with family and care recipient, changes in level of health, changes in mood, and anxiety and depression.
- Caregivers are either spouses, who are sometimes an older adult with declining physical stamina, or middle-age children, who often have other responsibilities.
- Later-life families have a different social network than younger families because friends and same-generation family members often have died or been ill themselves. Look for social support within the community and church affiliation.
- Identify family members, friends, and neighbors who will take the time to socialize with caregiver to avoid caregiver's feeling isolated.
- Abuse of older adults in families occurs across all social classes. Spouses are the most frequent abusers. Nurses need to report unexplained bruises and skin trauma to state protective agencies.

BOX 23-5   Sandwich Generation

- Usually a daughter or daughter-in-law is the caregiver
- Conflicting responsibilities for aging parents, children, spouse, and job
- Frequently tries to "do it all"
- May not recognize need for or request help
- Potential interventions
  - Help families set realistic priorities
  - Assess for application of "flex time" with caregiver's employer
  - Identify available resources (e.g., respite care, meal delivery, housekeepers)

ample, simply listening to the caregiver's stories and offering suggestions on how to deliver care or how to find community resources are often beneficial. Also connect the caregiver with other caregivers in the community and when appropriate online resources. Last, help the caregiver develop ways to effectively communicate with the extended family.

Caregiving is more than simply a series of tasks and often occurs within the context of a family. Whether it is a wife caring for a husband or a daughter caring for a mother, caregiving is an interactional process. The interpersonal dynamics between family members influence the ultimate quality of caregiving. Thus you have a key role in helping family members develop better communication and problem-solving skills to build the relationships needed for caregiving to be successful. Caregiving occurs in all aspect of care. As health care costs continue to increase, families are important caregivers. One expanding area for family caregivers is end-of-life care (Box 23-7). You can assist family members in their role as caregiver by showing them how to do specific aspects of physical care (e.g., dressing changes), assisting them with finding home care equipment (e.g., oxygen therapy), and helping them identify community resources. Preparing members of the family for care activities and responsibilities helps caregiving become a meaningful experience for the caregiver as well as for the patient.

■■■ EVALUATION

PATIENT CARE When the patient's family functions as context, evaluation focuses on attainment of patient needs. Thus evaluation is patient centered, although nursing measures have involved assisting the patient in adapting to the family environment. You compare the response of the patient with predetermined outcomes (see Care Plan).

When the family is the patient, the measure of family health is more than an evaluation of the health of all family members. For example, the family's attainment of family developmental tasks is a useful criterion. You evaluate the family's change in functioning and its satisfaction with the new level of functioning.

BOX 23-7   BEST PRACTICES

Family and End-of-Life Care

SUMMARY OF EVIDENCE

Meeting the needs of the family and family caregivers is essential when assisting with end-of-life care. It does not matter if the patient is at home, in a critical care setting, a hospital, or other facility. Some families desire to help their loved one die at home in familiar surroundings. These families may have a combination of a variety of family members and end-of-life care professionals assisting with overall care. Other families may choose to have their loved one at home but have home-based nursing care services, as well as assistance of end-of-life care professionals. Last, other families may choose to have their loved one in a health care facility. Although these settings are different and each family makes the decision based on their own needs and resources, the families usually participate as caregivers. Family caregivers are concerned about their abilities to manage end-of-life symptoms, such as pain control, comfort measures, and hygiene and nutrition needs. Families appreciate information on symptom management, communication strategies, information that detangles medical language, and compassion and caring from the professional caregiver. For the most part families do not fear having their loved one die in their home or in the family caregivers' presence. What they do fear is an inability to meet the end-of-life needs of the patient, such as not knowing how to provide physical and emotional comfort to the patient, or how to manage breathlessness, anorexia, and fatigue.

APPLICATION TO NURSING PRACTICE

- Assess what the family understands and what they expect for end-of-life care. This helps in developing patient-centered care for the dying family member.
- Avoid needless medical jargon and terminology. Use the words "dying" or "death."
- Identify the patient's priority symptoms, and provide specific tips for managing patient-specific symptoms. Avoid the temptation to give too much information about pharmacology or pathophysiology.
- Provide opportunities for caregiver to express the burdens of caregiving, such as emotional, physical, and economic burdens.
- Help caregivers understand that their silent presence next to their loved one's bedside is beneficial; they do not need to be "doing something" all the time.
- Assist the family caregivers with developing an action plan when death is imminent or has occurred.
- Family caregivers need and want to know the signs and symptoms of impending death.
- Be sure that family members have bereavement resources.

REFERENCES

Ferrell BR and others: End-of-life nursing education consortium (ELNEC) training program: improving palliative care in critical care, *Crit Care Nurs Q* 30(3):206, 2007.

Heyland DK and others: What matters most in end-of-life care: perceptions of seriously ill patients and their family members, *CMAJ* 174(5):627, 2007.

Lautreet A and others: End-of-life conferences: rooted in the evidence, *Crit Care Med* 34(11):S364, 2006.

London MR, Lundstedt J: Families speak about inpatient end-of-life care, *J Nurs Care Qual* 22(2):152, 2006.

Ruder S: The challenges of family member care giving: how the home health and hospice clinician can help at the end of life, *Home Healthc Nurse* 26(2):131, 2008.

BOX 23-8   EVALUATION

 Recently Lois' health status declined, and she needed more supervision with medication administration and her activities. As a result, she needed to move in with Michelle and Patrick. Michelle's two sisters alternate monthly visits to give Patrick and Michelle a 3-day weekend.

Bethany visits Lois periodically throughout the semester and checks to see how the family's short-term goals are coming along for caregiving and maintaining their own family life. She checks to see how Lois' goals are being fulfilled regarding her care in her granddaughter's home, activity tolerance, and forgetfulness. Bethany assesses Michelle's and Patrick's stress levels with school, home, and meeting Lois' health care needs. To assess Michelle and Patrick, she requests that the family arrange a meeting once a month. This ongoing evaluation requires a multidisciplinary effort from the home care nurse who knows the family best, the family members themselves, their physician, the chaplain, the social worker, and the nutritionist. The nurse is the true coordinator and evaluator of care provided, and Bethany knows this.

Michelle has more free time to concentrate on her studies every other night so she is able to "hurry through school to get a better job to help their financial future plans," as she and Patrick have wanted. One evening a week another family member comes to Michelle and Patrick's home to stay with Lois so the couple can have an evening out.

Bethany discussed the long-term goals of including the community in Lois' care. A registered nurse visits for 1 hour per week, a volunteer from their church takes Lois to the Senior Enrichment Program on Mondays, and a clergyman visits once per week. Lois sees the nurse practitioner one month and the physician every 4 months. Michelle's sisters are great resources, and the plan is working well. However, they are also in the process of investigating assisted living/nursing home facilities for Lois as her health declines.

DOCUMENTATION NOTE

"Patrick and Michelle both report that sitting down together helps them deal with the stress of their jobs, school, and the care of Lois. Michelle feels that she and Patrick are partners in the work of the family. Both Patrick and Michelle know that Lois will eventually need an assisted living setting or nursing home care and have begun looking at placements together along with other family members."

When you care for the family as a system, evaluation focuses on the effects interventions have on the entire family, including extended family. For example, if you are caring for an older adult who has begun chemotherapy for a new cancer diagnosis, you evaluate how the frequent trips to the oncology clinic and the cancer diagnosis affect the patient, the spouse, the children, and the grandchildren.

Evaluation is an ongoing process. Use critical thinking skills and clinical decision making to evaluate your patient's responses to interventions (Box 23-8). Often the patient and/or family does not know the best way to deliver care. For example, the family thinks a pain medication does not work at all. However, you make an adjustment in scheduling and the medication is more effective. Each patient and family is unique. Family nursing requires the use of therapeutic communication skills, scientific and family nursing knowledge, critical thinking skills, knowledge of oneself, and extensive learning about the patients and their families.

PATIENT EXPECTATIONS It is important to obtain the family's perspective of nursing care: how you planned and delivered the care with them, whether it was satisfactory, whether it met the family's goals, and if not, what they think was needed instead. This evaluation is continuous to modify or adjust care delivery techniques (e.g., how soon the home care nurse was able to make a visit, adequacy of comfort measures, or timeliness of care) or even to adjust care delivery personnel.

KEY POINTS

- The family has a significant effect on the lives of its members.
- Because the concept of family is highly individualized, base care on the patient's attitude toward family.
- Families are as diverse as the individuals who compose them, and patients have deeply ingrained values about their families that deserve respect.
- Family functioning involves the processes used by the family to achieve its goals.
- The goal of family nursing is to help the family and its individual members reach and maintain maximum health throughout and beyond the illness experience.
- The nurse views the family as an important context for the individual family member or views the family unit as the patient, or as a system. The approach for any family depends in part on the situation.

- Families face many challenges, including changing structures and roles, especially as the economic status of society changes.
- The family is the primary social context in which health promotion and disease prevention take place.
- As you begin to provide family-centered care, you continually assess, analyze, and reflect on the changing needs and health care goals of patients and their families.
- Goals for a care plan that incorporate a family approach include those that view the family as patient, as context, as system, or as a combination of the three.
- Whether you are caring for a patient with the family as context, family as patient, or family as system, you direct your nursing interventions to increasing family members' abilities in certain areas, to removing barriers to health care, and to doing things that the family cannot do for itself.

CRITICAL THINKING EXERCISES

Patrick and Michelle are caring for Michelle's grandmother, Lois, who is in the last stages of heart failure. They are married without children. At present they have health insurance and are facing potential reduction in income because Patrick may lose his job. As mentioned earlier in the case study, Lois lives 2 hours away, she is easily fatigued, and she needs more assistance in her activities of daily living. The following are the nursing diagnoses for this family:

- *Risk for caregiver role strain*
- *Compromised family coping*
- *Ineffective coping*
- *Interrupted family processes*

- *Impaired parenting*
- *Ineffective role performance*

1. What are the stressors placed on this family?
2. As Lois' health status changes, what additional stressors do you anticipate?
3. Identify priority nursing interventions for ineffective coping and interrupted family processes, and state why they are priority.
4. What family experiences do you bring to this situation?

⊖volve   *Answers to Critical Thinking Questions can be found on the Evolve website.*

REVIEW QUESTIONS

1. The Collins family includes a mother, Jean; stepfather, Adam; two teenage biological daughters of the mother, Lisa and Laura; and a biological daughter of the father, 25-year-old Stacy. Stacy just moved home following the loss of her job in another city. This is an example of a(n):
   1. Alternative family
   2. Blended family
   3. Extended family
   4. Nuclear family

2. The Collins family (question 1) is converting a study into Stacy's bedroom and is in the process of distributing household chores. When you talk to the family, they all feel that their family can adjust to these lifestyle changes. This is an example of:
   1. Configuration
   2. Diversity
   3. Durability
   4. Resiliency

3. Kathy Lind and Sharon Johnson are both single parents and have four daughters between them. All the girls go to the same school. Both Kathy and Sharon have good jobs and have active social lives. Three years ago they decided to form a household and share living expenses, housing costs, and child care responsibilities. This is an example of what family form?
   1. Alternate pattern
   2. Blended family
   3. Diverse family
   4. Extended family

4. The Carson family is composed of John, 52 years old; his wife, Sandy, 54 years old; and Sandy's two daughters, Kera, who is 21 years old, and Kathy, who is 23 years old. John's mother, Agnes, who is 78 years old, lives with them. Everyone is healthy. The two girls are teachers, Sandy is a head nurse, John is an aerospace engineer, and Agnes occasionally cooks for the family. Each New Year's Day the family has a brunch, and the five of them sit down and discuss their personal and family goals for the year, vacations, and activities. This family brunch is an example of:
   1. Family functioning
   2. Family forms

   3. Family structure
   4. Family support

5. The Carson family structure (in Question 4) includes blended family members as well as intergenerational family members. Which of the following best describes family structure?
   1. The process used by the family to achieve its goals
   2. The patterns of people who are considered to be family members
   3. The ongoing membership of the family and the pattern of relationships
   4. The intrafamilial system of support and structure extending beyond the walls of the household

6. The most common reason grandparents are called on to raise their grandchildren is due to:
   1. Dual-income families
   2. Increased divorce rate
   3. Legal intervention
   4. Single parenthood

7. Family assessment includes:
   1. Assessing individual family members separately
   2. Assessing only those members living in the household
   3. Assessing only the patient's perception of family interaction
   4. Assessing individual family members and their interactions with one another and the patient

8. When planning care for the family as a patient, you need to: Select all that apply.
   1. Consider the developmental stage of the family
   2. Include only the ill family member and the significant other
   3. Understand that the family will always help to achieve the health goals of an ill member of the family
   4. Understand that cultural background is an important variable to consider when developing nursing interventions

9. You are caring for an intergenerational family. The family consists of a single parent with two school-age children (5 and 8 years old) and a grandfather who is 65 years old with end-stage kidney disease. The family enters the

clinic for a follow-up visit to evaluate the grandfather's renal failure. During the course of the history, you notice that the mother has a black eye, which she attributes to a fall. However, the oldest child states that the mother's boyfriend did it. What is your priority?

1. Continue with the evaluation of the grandfather's kidney disease.
2. Assume that the 8-year-old does not have all the facts.
3. Tell the mother to terminate the relationship with the boyfriend.
4. Refer the mother to a battered victims resource center.

10. When working with a family with a rigid family structure, you design interventions to:
1. Attempt to change the family structure
2. Include only the most flexible family member
3. Create interventions that require minimal change
4. Provide solutions for problems only when they arise

Answers to Review Questions can be found on pages 1197-1198.

REFERENCES

Abbott S, Shaw S, Bryar R: Family-centered public health practice: is health visiting ready? *Community Pract* 77(9):338, 2004.

Astedt-Kurki P and others: Methodological issues in interviewing families in family nursing research, *J Adv Nurs* 35(2):288, 2001.

Astedt-Kurki P and others: Development and testing of a family nursing scale, *West J Nurs Res* 24(5):567, 2002.

Astedt-Kurki P and others: Determinants of perceived health in families of patients with heart disease, *J Adv Nurs* 48(2):115, 2004.

Bluvol A, Ford-Gilboe M: Hope, health work and quality of life in families of stroke survivors, *J Adv Nurs* 48(4):322, 2004.

Bonura D and others: Culturally-congruent end-of-life care for Jewish patients and their families, *J Transcult Nurs* 12(3):211, 2001.

Bulechek GM and others, editors: *Nursing interventions classification (NIC)*, ed 5, St. Louis, 2008, Mosby.

Children's Defense Fund: *CDF statement on new data show nearly 9 million uninsured children and 13.3 million in poverty in 2007*, August 26, 2008, http://www.childrensdefense.org/site/news, accessed September 5, 2008.

Cox C, Monk A: Strain among caregivers: comparing the experiences of African-American and Hispanic caregivers of Alzheimer's relatives, *Int J Aging Hum Dev* 43(2):93, 1996.

Dewit SC: *Fundamental concepts and skills for nursing*, ed 2, St. Louis, 2004, Saunders.

Duhamel F, Talbot LR: A constructivist evaluation of family systems nursing interventions with families experiencing cardiovascular and cerebrovascular illness, *J Fam Nurs* 10(1):12, 2004.

Duvall EM, Miller BC: *Marriage and family development*, ed 6, Boston, 2005, Allyn and Bacon.

Family Violence Prevention Fund: *Domestic violence is a serious widespread social problem in America: the facts*, 2008, http://www.endabuse.org/programs/printable/display, accessed September 5, 2008.

Feeley N, Gottlieb LN: Nursing approaches for working with family strengths and resources, *J Fam Nurs* 6(1):9, 2000.

Ferrell BR and others: End-of-life nursing education consortium (ELNEC) training program: improving palliative care in critical care, *Crit Care Nurs Q* 30(3):206, 2007.

Ford-Gilboe M: Developing knowledge about family health promotion by testing the developmental model of health and nursing, *J Fam Nurs* 8:140, 2002.

Galanti GA: *Caring for patients from different cultures*, ed 3, Philadelphia, 2004, University of Pennsylvania Press.

Haldenby AM, Berman H, Forchuk: Homelessness and health in adolescents, *Qual Health Res* 17(9):1232, 2007.

Hanson SM and others: *Family health care nursing, theory, practice and research*, ed 3, Philadelphia, 2005, FA Davis.

Heyland DK and others: What matters most in end-of-life care: perceptions of seriously ill patients and their family members, *CMAJ* 174(5):627, 2007.

Isaksen AS, Thuen F, Hanestad B: Patients with cancer and their close relatives: experiences with treatment, care, and support, *Cancer Nurs* 26(1):68, 2003.

James-Childs EY: *Adolescent and young adult male parenting: the forgotten half*, doctoral dissertation, Denver, 2000, University of Colorado Health Sciences Center.

Joronen K, Astedt-Kurki P: Familial contribution to adolescent subjective well being, *Int J Nurs Pract* 11:125, 2005.

Lautreet A and others: End-of-life conferences: rooted in the evidence, *Crit Care Med* 34(11):S364, 2006.

Lewis-O'Connor A: "Dying to tell?": Do mandatory reporting laws benefit victims of domestic violence? *Am J Nurs* 104(10):75, 2004.

London MR, Lundstedt J: Families speak about inpatient end-of-life care, *J Nurs Care Qual* 22(2):152, 2006.

Maijala H and others: Caregiver's experiences of interaction with families expecting a fetally impaired child, *J Clin Nurs* 13(3):376, 2004.

McCubbin MA, McCubbin HI, Thompson AI: Family Hardiness Index (FHI). In McCubbin HI, Thompson AI, McCubbin MS, editors: *Family assessment: resiliency, coping, and adaptation, inventories for research and practice*, Madison, 1996, University of Wisconsin Press.

Moorhead S and others, editors: *Nursing outcomes classification (NOC)*, ed 4, St. Louis, 2008, Mosby.

National Coalition for the Homeless: *Who is homeless?* NCH fact sheet No. 3, Washington, DC, June 2008, The Coalition, http://www.nationalhomeless.org/publications/who.html, accessed September 5, 2008.

Raneri LG, Wiemann CM: Social ecological predictors of repeat adolescent pregnancy, *Perspect Sex Reprod Health* 39(1):39, 2007.

Ruder S: The challenges of family member caregiving: how the home health and hospice clinician can help at the end of life, *Home Healthc Nurse* 26(2):131, 2008.

Sangalang BB, Rounds K: Differences in health behaviors and parenting knowledge between adolescents and parenting adolescents, *Soc Work Health Care* 42(2):1, 2005.

Schumacher K, Beck C, Marren JM: Family caregivers, *Am J Nurs* 106(8):40, 2006.

Schanzer B and others: Homelessness, health status, and health care use, *Am J Public Health* 97:464, 2007.

SmithBattle L: The vulnerabilities of teenage mothers: challenging prevailing assumptions, *Adv Nurs Sci* 23(1):29, 2000.

Stajduhar KI and others: Factors influencing family caregivers' ability to cope with providing end-of-life cancer care at home, *Cancer Nurs* 31(1):77, 2008.

Tapp DM: Dilemmas of family support during cardiac recovery: nagging as a gesture of support, *West J Nurs Res* 26(5):561, 2004.

Tarkka MT and others: In-hospital social support for families of heart patients, *J Clin Nurs* 12(5):736, 2003.

U.S. Bureau of the Census: *Population profile of the United States: 2000 (Internet release, 2007 update)*, Washington, DC, 2001, The Bureau, http://www.census.gov, accessed August 15, 2008.

Wang Y: People of Chinese heritage. In Purnell LD, Paulanka BJ: *Transcultural health care: a culturally competent approach*, ed 2, Philadelphia, 2003, FA Davis.

Wathen CN, MacMillan HL: Interventions for violence against women: scientific review, *JAMA* 289:589, 2003.

Stress and Coping

MEDIA RESOURCES

 CD COMPANION 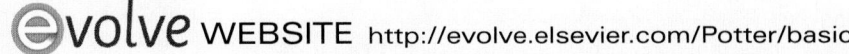 WEBSITE http://evolve.elsevier.com/Potter/basic

- Crossword Puzzle
- English/Spanish Audio Glossary

OBJECTIVES

- Describe the three stages of the general adaptation syndrome.
- Discuss the integration of stress theory with nursing theories.
- Formulate nursing diagnoses based on assessment data.
- Describe stress management techniques beneficial for coping with stress.

- Discuss the process of crisis intervention.
- Develop a care plan for a patient experiencing stress.
- Discuss how stress in the workplace affects nurses.

KEY TERMS

coping, p. 640
crisis, p. 641
crisis intervention, p. 650

endorphins, p. 639
flashback, p. 643
general adaptation syndrome (GAS), p. 639

primary appraisal, p. 640
secondary appraisal, p. 640

stress, p. 638
stress management, p. 640
stressor, p. 638

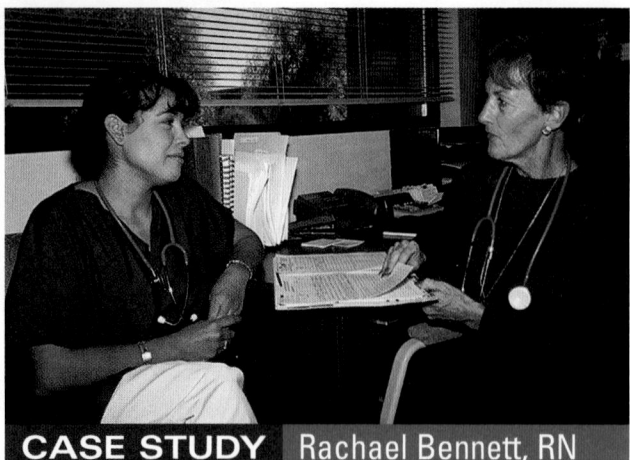

CASE STUDY   Rachael Bennett, RN

Rachael Bennett, a 32-year-old married mother of three children, works as the nurse manager in a medical intensive care unit. Until recently she has felt very happy with her job. However, patient and staff satisfaction have been declining, and Rachael feels pressured to improve the satisfaction scores. In addition, within the past year Rachael's husband has had several hospitalizations related to heart disease, and he is unable to work. For the past 6 weeks, she has been feeling defeated and hopeless, she has no energy, and she has difficulty organizing her thoughts. When her supervisor noticed Rachael's frequent severe headaches, reported lack of sleep, and use of wine at night to relax, her supervisor referred her to the hospital's employee health office. One of this department's duties is to help employees cope with their stress.

Becky Howard, a nurse practitioner in the employee health office, does preliminary screening and crisis intervention with staff members experiencing stress and potential substance abuse problems. The behavioral health care resources are included in Rachael's employee health benefit package.

Stress affects all of us. **Stressors** are disruptive forces operating within or on any system (Neuman and Fawcett, 2002). You need to know about **stress,** not only so you recognize stress in patients and families and intervene effectively, but also because stressful events that occur in the course of clinical practice will affect you as a nurse. How you react to stress depends on how you view and evaluate the impact of the stressor, its effect on your situation, your support at the time of the stress, and your usual coping mechanisms (Box 24-1).

Stress, emotion, and coping occur together. Our appraisal of stressors activates our emotions, which in turn affects the neuroendocrine and immune systems. Anger, envy, jealousy, anxiety, fright, shame, and sadness are stress emotions. Stress also relates to positive emotions such as happiness, pride, gratitude, and even love (Lazarus, 2007). You need to understand the role of emotions in stress and be aware of your own feelings.

BOX 24-1   Factors Influencing the Response to Stressors

ASPECTS OF A STRESSOR THAT INFLUENCE THE STRESS RESPONSE

As Becky interviews Rachael, she learns more about Rachael's stressors and how she perceives them.

Intensity
Rachael experiences pressures at work, as well as at home. This combination of stressors creates continuous intensity.

Scope
Rachael's stress pervades her life, both at work and at home, day and night.

Duration
Rachael has been feeling the effects of stress for about 6 weeks, having problems sleeping and feelings of hopelessness.

Number and Nature of Other Stressors Present
Rachael has multiple stressors. Rachael has stress at home from her husband's hospitalizations and at work with low staff and patient satisfaction scores.

Predictability
Rachael is unable to anticipate or control the stressor of her husband's illness and is unable to control the poor satisfaction scores.

CHARACTERISTICS OF THE INDIVIDUAL THAT INFLUENCE THE STRESS RESPONSE

Level of Personal Control
Rachael feels no control over patient and staff satisfaction at work and no control over her husband's disability.

Feelings of Competence
Rachael questions her competence at work with the lower satisfaction scores.

Cognitive Appraisal
Rachael is telling herself that she is a failure, and she is afraid of losing her job. Her identity as a nurse and her image of nursing conflict with the events in her life.

Availability of Social Supports
Rachael does not report having the support of other people who could help reduce her stress.

SCIENTIFIC KNOWLEDGE BASE

Nearly 80 years ago Walter Cannon proposed the fight-or-flight response to stress, an arousal of the sympathetic nervous system. This reaction prepares a person for action by increasing heart rate; diverting blood from the intestines to the brain and striated muscles; and increasing blood pressure,

TABLE 24-1 Indicators of Stress

SYSTEM	ASSESSMENT FINDINGS	SYSTEM	ASSESSMENT FINDINGS
PHYSICAL		**PSYCHOLOGICAL**	
Cardiovascular	Tightness of chest Increased heart rate Elevated blood pressure	Cognitive	Forgetfulness/preoccupation Denial Poor concentration
Respiratory	Breathing difficulty Tachypnea		Inattention to detail Orientation to past instead of present
Neuroendocrine	Headaches, migraines Fatigue, exhaustion Insomnia, sleep disturbances Feeling uncoordinated Restlessness, hyperactivity Tremors (lips, hands) Profuse sweating (palms) Dry mouth Cold hands and feet		Decreased creativity Slower thinking, reactions Learning difficulties Apathy Confusion Decreased attention span Calculation difficulties Memory problems

Gastrointestinal/
    genitourinary
	Urinary frequency
	Nausea, diarrhea, vomiting
	Weight gain or loss of more than
	    10 pounds
	Change in appetite
	Gastrointestinal bleeding
		Emotional	Disruption of logical thinking
			Blaming others
			Lack of motivation to get up in the
			    morning
			Crying tendencies
			Lack of interest

Diagnostic	Blood in stools/vomitus Elevated blood glucose level Elevated cortisol levels		Irritability Isolation Diminished initiative
Musculoskeletal	Backaches, muscle aches Bruxism (clenched jaw) Slumped posture	Behavior/lifestyle	Worrying Decreased involvement with others Withdrawal
Reproductive	Amenorrhea Failure to ovulate Impotency in men Loss of libido		Change in interactions with others Increased or decreased food intake Increased smoking or alcohol intake Overvigilance to environment
Immunological	Frequent or prolonged colds/flu		Excessive humor or silence No exercise

heart rate, respiratory rate, and blood glucose levels. In the 1930s, 1940s, and 1950s, Hans Selye expanded Cannon's fight-or-flight hypothesis to describe the **general adaptation syndrome (GAS),** a three-stage reaction to stress. The GAS reflects how the body responds to stressors through the alarm reaction, the resistance stage, and the exhaustion stage. The GAS is triggered either directly by a physical event or indirectly by a psychological event. The mind, the neuroendocrine system, and the immune system respond to stress in a coordinated way (Lazarus, 2007).

General Adaptation Syndrome

The GAS is an immediate physiological response of the body to stress. It involves several body systems, especially the autonomic nervous system and the endocrine system (Table 24-1). When an injury or some physical demand occurs, the pituitary gland secretes adrenocorticotropic hormone (ACTH). In response to ACTH, the adrenal glands release hormones, including corticosteroids and the catecholamines, adrenaline and noradrenaline, into the bloodstream. In addition, the hypothalamus, another part of the brain, secretes endor-

phins. **Endorphins** are hormones that act on the mind such as morphine and opiates, and they produce a sense of well-being and reduce pain. In this way the GAS defends us against stress both by activating the neuroendocrine system and by providing endorphins that decrease our awareness of the pain (Lazarus, 2007).

While the hormonal system activates the body, the autonomic, or involuntary, nervous system also influences the action of hormones and affects all the tissues of the body. The sympathetic nerves arouse us during stress and use body resources for energy and emergencies. The parasympathetic nerves dampen this arousal and facilitate relaxation and restore energy (Lazarus, 2007).

During the alarm reaction rising hormone levels result in increased blood volume, blood glucose levels, epinephrine and norepinephrine amounts, heart rate, blood flow to muscles, oxygen intake, and mental alertness. In addition, the pupils of the eyes dilate to produce a greater visual field. This change in body systems prepares an individual for fight or flight and lasts from 1 minute to many hours. If the stressor poses an extreme threat to life or remains for a long time, the person progresses to the second stage, resistance (Lazarus, 2007).

During the resistance stage the body stabilizes and responds in an opposite manner to the alarm reaction. The injured tissues become inflamed to isolate them from the rest of the body. Antiinflammatory adrenocortical hormones are released, and healing occurs. Hormone levels, heart rate, blood pressure, and cardiac output return to normal, and the body repairs any damage that occurred. However, if the stressor remains and adaptation does not happen, the person enters the third stage, exhaustion. The exhaustion stage occurs when the body is no longer able to resist the effects of the stressor and the struggle to maintain adaptation drains all available energy. The physiological response intensifies, but the person has so little energy left that adaptation to the stressor diminishes (Lazarus, 2007). The body can no longer defend itself against the impact of the event, and if the stress continues, it damages the heart and lowers resistance to illness (McEwen and Lasley, 2007). Unhealthy coping choices, such as the use of alcohol or tobacco, negatively affect a person's health as well as increasing the perception of stress (Jones and Bright, 2007).

Mind-Body Connection

The limbic system in the brain mediates emotions and includes the hypothalamus, the pituitary gland, and the amygdala. The limbic system possesses receptors for neuropeptides, such as endorphins, insulin, and angiotension, and makes the connection with the rest of the body to provide the physiological basis for the emotions (Pert, 2007).

Physiological responses to stress also include immunological responses. In the immune system the cells move, in contrast to brain cells, which stay in one place. One type of immune system cells, monocytes, travel throughout the body to recognize and digest foreign bodies, as well as to heal wounds and repair tissue. The brain, the glands, and the immune system communicate in a network with each other by using the neuropeptides as messengers (Pert, 2007).

The immune system differentiates between self and nonself. This means that under normal conditions your immune system does not treat your own cells as threats but treats bacteria, viruses, parasites, or toxins as threats. Problems occur when the immune system makes a too-vigorous response and an autoimmune illness develops.

REACTION TO PSYCHOLOGICAL STRESS Lazarus (2007) maintained that a person experiences stress only if the person evaluates the event or circumstance as personally significant. Evaluating an event for its personal meaning, or **primary appraisal,** happens very quickly and automatically in the person's mind. If primary appraisal results in the person identifying the event or circumstance as a harm, loss, threat, or challenge, the person has stress. Therefore you need to determine how the patient perceives the event or circumstance. Following the recognition of stress, **secondary appraisal** focuses on possible coping strategies.

Coping means trying to manage a situation a person appraised as potentially harmful or stressful (Kleinke 2007). No single coping strategy works for everyone or for every stressor. The same person copes differently from one time to another. In stressful situations we use both problem-focused coping and emotion-focused coping. In other words, when we are under stress and we believe we can do something about the problem, we use problem-focused coping. We obtain information and take action to change the situation. On the other hand, if a problem or challenge seems to be beyond our control, we are more likely to rely on emotion-focused coping and regulate our emotions tied to the stress. In some cases we avoid thinking about the situation or change the way we think about it, without changing the actual situation itself (Lazarus, 2007).

Psychological adaptive behaviors, or ego-defense mechanisms, regulate emotional distress and thus protect a person from anxiety and stress (Box 24-2). When you recognize that a patient is using an ego-defense mechanism such as denial or displacement, do not point this out to the patient or suggest that the defense mechanism is unhealthy. Denial often helps the patient reduce stress to a manageable level until he or she can cope with it. Displacement means transferring emotions from a stressful situation to a less-anxiety-producing substitute. This can happen, for example, if a patient acts angrily toward the nurse when he or she is worried about his or her own illness, pain, or trauma.

Stress management techniques, used to cope with generalized stress and arousal, aim to relax and soothe the body and mind. For example, physical exercise, relaxation strategies, and letting go of excess anger reduce a person's level of

---

BOX 24-2 | Examples of Ego-Defense Mechanisms

- **Compensation:** Making up for a deficiency in one aspect of self-image by strongly emphasizing a feature considered an asset. (*Example:* A person who is a poor communicator relies on organizational skills.)
- **Conversion:** Unconsciously repressing an anxiety-producing emotional conflict and transforming it into nonorganic symptoms (e.g., difficulty sleeping, loss of appetite).
- **Denial:** Avoiding emotional conflicts by refusing to consciously acknowledge anything that causes intolerable emotional pain. (*Example:* A person refuses to discuss or acknowledge a personal loss.)
- **Displacement:** Transferring emotions, ideas, or wishes from a stressful situation to a less-anxiety-producing substitute. (*Example:* A person transfers anger over a job conflict to a malfunctioning computer.)
- **Identification:** Patterning behavior after that of another person and assuming that person's qualities, characteristics, and actions.
- **Dissociation:** Experiencing a subjective sense of numbing and a reduced awareness of one's surroundings.
- **Regression:** Coping with a stressor through actions and behaviors associated with an earlier developmental period.

physical and psychological tension. Exercise improves circulation and triggers the release of endorphins. The relaxation response, elicited by meditation or progressive muscle relaxation, lowers blood pressure, pulse rate, and respiratory rate. Forgiveness, or letting go of excess anger, reduces stress-provoking hormone levels. Other well-known stress management techniques include massage, mindfulness-based stress reduction, yoga, cognitive therapy, and nutrition (Monat, Lazarus, and Reevy, 2007).

Crisis

A **crisis** occurs in response to a perception, event, or situation that exceeds the person's current resources and coping mechanisms. Developmental crises often arise during the normal flow of human growth, such as with the birth of a child, graduation from college, or a midlife career change. Situational crises emerge from the occurrence of extraordinary events such as terrorist attacks, car crashes, rapes, or job loss. Existential crises refer to inner conflicts and anxieties arising from concerns about life's purpose, responsibilities, independence, or commitment. Finally, ecosystemic crises occur following a natural or human-caused disaster, such as a hurricane, flood, war, or severe economic depression (James, 2008).

Crisis differs from stress in the degree of severity, although stress and crisis share many characteristics. A patient with stress so severe that the patient is unable to cope using previous stress reduction strategies often experiences a crisis. A crisis devastates a person and requires use of all resources available. Unlike stress, which ends when the stressor disappears, the effects of a crisis sometimes last for years (James, 2008).

NURSING KNOWLEDGE BASE

Nursing Theory and the Role of Stress

Many nursing theories explain and describe stress. For example, explanation of the concepts of stress and reaction to stress constitute Betty Neuman's Neuman Systems Model. Because the Neuman Systems Model uses a systems approach, it helps you understand your patients' individual responses to stressors and also families' and communities' responses. A systems approach explains that a stressor at one place in a system affects other parts of the system; a system is a person, a family, or a community. Events are multidimensional and not caused or affected by only one thing. Every person develops a set of responses to stress that constitute the "normal line of defense" (Neuman and Fawcett, 2002). This line of defense helps to maintain health and wellness. Physiological, psychological, sociocultural, developmental, or spiritual influences buffer stress. When the patient cannot buffer stress, the normal line of defense breaks, resulting in disease. Neuman Systems Model of nursing views the patient, family, or community as constantly changing in response to the environment and stressors.

Pender's Health Promotion Theory, on the other hand, focuses on promoting health and managing stress. She contends that people want to live in ways that enable them to be as healthy as possible and to be capable of assessing their own abilities and assets. Pender and co-workers (2006) advocate increasing physical activity, improving diet and nutrition, and using stress management strategies to become healthy and remain healthy.

Situational, Maturational, and Sociocultural Factors

Potential stressors and coping mechanisms vary across the life span. For example, adolescence, adulthood, and old age bring different stressors related to separating from family, establishing oneself as an adult, and making a contribution to society. Likewise, coping strategies fluctuate from an emphasis on primarily emotional coping to problem solving as our minds grow and thinking develops.

SITUATIONAL FACTORS Work stress for nurses happens with work overload, heavy physical work, shift work, patient concerns (dealing with death and medical treatment), and interpersonal problems with other health care professionals and staff (Sulsky and Smith, 2007). Coping strategies vary with the individual and the situation. People often ease their coping with shift work by knowing their own circadian rhythms. People who function best in the morning have the greatest difficulty with night work and changing shifts. As people age, they tend to become more morning oriented. Morning people need to be counseled about the potentially negative effects of night work for them. In general, people doing shift work need to maintain as consistent a sleep and mealtime schedule as possible.

Research shows an association between chronic interpersonal stress and vulnerability to a cold following exposure to a rhinovirus, as well as delayed wound healing among students under stress. However, studies about the relationship of stress and illness are correlational and not experimental. Consequently, causation of stress and illness is not completely established (Aldwin, 2007).

Adjusting to chronic illness can also result in situational stress. Common diseases, such as obesity, hypertension, diabetes, depression, asthma, and coronary artery disease, provoke stress. Furthermore, being a family caregiver for someone with a chronic illness such as Alzheimer's disease causes stress.

MATURATIONAL FACTORS Stressors and coping strategies vary with life stage. Babies use the emotion-focused coping mechanisms of thumb sucking, rocking, and crying. Children learn to manage the reactions of their caregivers using problem-focused coping strategies. In general, problem-focused coping strategies aim to alter the situation, to alter the behavior of others, to change the person's own attitudes, and to develop new skills and responses. Emotion-focused coping strategies aim to manage emotional distress. Examples of emotion-focused coping among adults include physical exercise, meditation, expressing feelings, and seeking support (Kleinke, 2007). Older adults may use dyadic coping, which occurs when older adults work with partners, friends, or family members to adapt to stress (Box 24-3) (Aldwin, 2007).

BOX 24-3   CARE OF THE OLDER ADULT

Coping Strategies Used by Older Adults

Some older adults report better mental health than younger adults because older adults appraise and cope with stress differently. For example, for older adults healthy coping includes the following:

- Organizing objects in their environment such as using canes, walkers, hand railings, hearing aids, amplifiers on telephones, and magnifying glasses to enhance their daily functioning.
- Making their daily activities routine and predictable.
- De-emphasizing their health problems by using positive comparisons with their peers, finding others who are more disabled to compare themselves with.
- Dissociating their body from an illness by attributing the illness episode to external factors such as food poisoning or a hazardous environment.
- Making a fatalistic appraisal by attributing control of their health to inevitability, fate, or luck.
- Using dyadic coping, or joint coping, to compensate for memory problems and other physical deficits. This happens when one spouse or partner anticipates the other's needs and helps as needed, often without being asked.
- Arranging one's schedule or actions to help the spouse or partner to facilitate the other person's coping.

Data from Aldwin C: *Stress, coping, and development: an integrative perspective*, ed 2, New York, 2007, Guilford.

BOX 24-4   CULTURAL FOCUS

Stress and anxiety may lead to insomnia, as it did for Rachael. There are also cultural factors that are related to poor sleeping. There are significant differences in rates of insomnia among the ethnic groups. Seventy-one percent of the African American women in one study experienced trouble getting to sleep, waking up during the night, or awakening too early in the morning. European American, Eastern European, and Dominican women had similar high rates. On the other hand, only about a third of Caribbean and Haitian women reported insomnia-related symptoms.

IMPLICATIONS FOR PRACTICE

- Ethnic differences in sleep and insomnia influence interventions for insomnia. Interventions for anxiety-related sleep problems need to be culturally appropriate.
- Suggesting daytime naps may be more culturally acceptable for some cultures, such as African American and Spanish women.
- Ask patients what their family members, especially their parents, do when they cannot sleep in order to learn about their cultural values associated with insomnia.
- Help patients connect their insomnia with the stress they are experiencing by asking them what they think about while they are lying in bed awake.
- Ask women with insomnia what coping strategies they have tried.
- When assessing women with insomnia, determine if their coping measures include sleep medication.

Data from Jean-Louis G and others: Insomnia symptoms in a multi-ethnic sample of American women, *J Womens Health* 17(1):15, 2008.

People who cope successfully take responsibility for finding a solution to their problems. They assess the situation, get advice and support, and make a plan. They view challenges as growth-producing opportunities, and they use hope, patience, and a sense of humor. On the other hand, people who do not cope successfully meet challenges with denial and avoidance. They may become angry and aggressive or depressed and passive; they blame themselves or others for their problems (Kleinke, 2007).

SOCIOCULTURAL FACTORS Potential stressors affect any age-group, but they are especially stressful for young people. These include prolonged poverty, physical handicap, and chronic illness. The vulnerability of children escalates when they lose relationships with parents and caregivers through divorce, imprisonment, death, or when parents have mental illness or substance abuse disorders. Furthermore, living under conditions of continuing violence, disintegrated neighborhoods, or homelessness affects people of any age, but these factors are especially stressful to young people (Pender and others, 2006).

Cultural variations produce stress, particularly if the person's values differ from the dominant culture in aspects of gender roles, family relationships, and religious beliefs (Box 24-4). Other aspects of cultural variations begin with language difference, geographical location, family relationships, time orientation, access to health care programs, and dispari-

ties in health care (Pender and others, 2006). Uncertainty about immigration status and citizenship increases stress.

The culture of being a nurse carries many expectations for people who are nurses. For example, nurses expect themselves to be altruistic and to be a role model of adaptive and growth-producing behavior. Nurses expect themselves to approach life with a sense of growing, hopefulness, and adapting (Stuart, 2009). When a nurse's home and /or professional life becomes chaotic or overwhelming, the nurse might feel unsuccessful and subsequently stressed.

Cultural differences exist in both problem-focused and emotion-focused coping. Because problem-focused coping attempts to control or manage a situation, culture heavily influences these coping strategies. For example, Americans or Israelis might confront a problem directly. On the other hand, people from Asian cultures might use indirect methods that nevertheless confront a problem situation, such as asking an older relative to address a difficult interpersonal situation. Indirect action does not necessarily indicate passive behavior, however (Aldwin, 2007).

In the realm of emotion-focused coping strategies, various ethnic groups use social support differently. European Americans might go outside the family to social support groups, whereas Africans and Hispanics might rely more heavily on family members rather than on friends. Culture strongly influences expression of feelings or control of feelings. Generally, people from northern European cultures prefer emotional control, yet Italian and Jewish ethnic groups are more expressive. Many cultures view mental illness as temporary reactions to stress, not necessarily pathological as long as they are time limited (Aldwin, 2007).

Posttraumatic Stress Disorder

Posttraumatic stress disorder (PTSD) affects people who have experienced accidents, violent events such as rape or domestic abuse, war, and natural disasters. PTSD symptoms appear to be a normal response to a traumatic event; however, if the symptoms persist beyond 3 months, health care providers often make a diagnosis of PTSD. Nevertheless, symptoms may first appear months or years after the traumatic event. Because intense stress can cause permanent physical changes in the brain, people with PTSD sometimes experience a **flashback**. Sights, sounds, and smells associated with the original trauma stimulate the neuroendocrine system and cause a stress reaction (James, 2008).

CRITICAL THINKING

Synthesis

You will apply elements of critical thinking whenever you perform the nursing process with a patient. Consider the scientific knowledge you have learned, your experience, critical thinking attitudes, and standards to ensure an individualized approach to patient care. This approach helps you identify specific health care needs and design individualized interventions (Box 24-5).

KNOWLEDGE Physiological changes occur in the patient experiencing the alarm reaction, resistance stage, and exhaustion stage of the GAS. Apply knowledge of those physiological changes. Your knowledge of communication principles helps you to assess the patient's behaviors. Consider your patient's perception of the stress. Determine the ability of the patient to cope with the stress. If the patient does not succeed with his or her usual coping skills, you need to refer the patient to crisis intervention counseling.

EXPERIENCE Your experience teaches you to understand the patient's unique perception of stressors and responses to stress. View every person as an individual, recognizing that no two people are exactly alike. Experience with patients also helps you to recognize responses to stress. In addition, your own personal experiences with stress and coping increase your ability to empathize with a patient temporarily immobilized by stress. Understanding the patient's position enables you to intervene more effectively.

ATTITUDES Use confidence, and believe that you and the patient are able to manage stress effectively. Patients respect your advice and counsel and gain confidence from your belief in their ability to move past the stressful event or illness. Patients experiencing a crisis often lack the ability, at least initially, to act on their own behalf. They require either

BOX 24-5	SYNTHESIS IN PRACTICE

When Becky talks with Rachael, she learns that Rachael worries about losing her job because of the declining quality of patient care. Rachael provides sole support for her family at this time. She also learns about Mr. Bennett's recent illness and the effect it has on Rachael's overall well-being. Becky has also talked with Rachael's supervisor and knows that Rachael has been having headaches and difficulty concentrating when making decisions.

Becky takes time to reflect on other employees she sees in Employee Health. Many of the registered nurses have had physical complaints of stress, including headaches, sleep problems, changes in eating habits, and flare-ups of existing medical problems. Becky knows she wants to be thorough in assessing the responses and symptoms Rachael has been experiencing. Previous experience with other employees taught Becky the importance of learning about the employee's family and the type of support they offer and the person's appraisal of the situation.

direct intervention or guidance. You need to have an attitude of integrity through which you respect the patient's perception of or perspective about the stressor. Make the effort to have patients explain their unique viewpoint and situation.

STANDARDS Make accurate assessment of a patient's stress, coping mechanisms, and support system before intervening. Clearly and precisely understand a patient's perception of the stress, and focus on factors significant to the patient's well-being. In addition, select interventions that respect the individuality of the patient. Be especially aware of your ethical responsibility in caring for someone who has less independence because of being in a crisis state.

NURSING PROCESS

■ ■ ■ ASSESSMENT

Assessment of a patient's stress level and coping resources requires that you first establish a trusting nurse-patient relationship. You will ask the patient and family to share personal and sensitive information (see Chapter 8). Learn from the patient both by asking questions and by making observations of nonverbal behavior, interactions with the family, and the patient's environment. Synthesize the information you obtain, and adopt a critical thinking attitude while observing and analyzing patient behaviors. Often the patient has difficulty describing the most bothersome aspects of the situation until someone else has time to listen and encourage the patient to explore it.

SUBJECTIVE FINDINGS When you assess a patient's stress level and coping resources, sit with the patient in comfortable chairs in a private setting facing one another. Assume a listening posture, establish eye contact, and allow time for the patient to talk. Gather information about the health status of the patient from the patient's perspective, and begin the process of developing a trusting relationship with the patient.

Use the interview to determine the patient's view of the situation that provoked stress, assess safety issues, coping resources, any possible maladaptive coping, and adherence to prescribed medical recommendations, such as medication or diet (Table 24-2) (James, 2008). If the patient uses denial as a coping mechanism, be alert to whether the person overlooks necessary information. Listen for any recurrent themes in the patient's conversation. As in all interactions with the patient, respect the confidentiality and sensitivity of the information shared.

If your patient is experiencing a crisis, assess safety concerns such as potential for suicide or homicide and ability to care for one's own activities of daily living. Assessment includes determining the patient's emotions, behaviors, cognitive state, and precrisis level of functioning. In addition, as-

sess for prior trauma, symptoms of mental illness, and use of legal and illegal drugs. Assess whether this crisis is a one-time situation or part of a pattern of a crisis-oriented life history. Finally, assess alternatives, coping mechanisms, and support systems (James, 2008).

OBJECTIVE FINDINGS Obtain objective findings related to stress and coping through your observation of the appearance and nonverbal behavior of the patient. Observe grooming and hygiene, gait, characteristics of the patient's handshake, actions of the patient while sitting, quality of speech, eye contact, and the attitude of the patient toward you during the interview (see Chapter 15). Before the interview begins or at the end of the interview, depending upon the anxiety level of the patient, take basic vital signs to assess for physiological signs of stress such as elevated blood pressure, heart rate, or respiratory rate.

PATIENT EXPECTATIONS Recognize the importance of the meaning of the precipitating event to the patient and the ways in which stress affects the patient's life. Allow time for the patient to express priorities for coping with stress. For example, you are caring for a woman who has just found out

TABLE 24-2 FOCUSED PATIENT ASSESSMENT

FACTORS TO ASSESS	QUESTIONS	PHYSICAL ASSESSMENT
Patient safety	Do you have thoughts of harming yourself? How are you sleeping? Do you have problems going to sleep or awakening during the night? How has your appetite changed? How does your stress affect your work? Are you having problems concentrating? Have you had accidents at home, in the car, or on the job?	Observe for indicators of anxiety, anger, or tension. For example, you may observe such nonverbal behaviors as irritability, crying, and inappropriate laughing.
Perception of stressor	What do you believe is stressing you? What do you think about when you can't sleep? What does this situation or stressor mean, in your opinion?	Observe for nonverbal indicators of stress, such as rapid talking, crying, changes in posture (e.g., folding arms over chest). Listen for recurrent themes.
Available coping resources	Are you keeping in touch with your friends? How often do you see your family members? What have you done before to cope with similar problems or stress? What do you do for fun? How do you spend your leisure time?	Observe whether the person is alone or with others. Observe the person's communication skills. Observe if the person is able to ask for help. Observe developmental level and sociocultural circumstances.
Maladaptive coping used	How much do you smoke? How much do you drink? Do you use any over-the-counter or herbal medications for your stress? How much coffee or soda do you drink in a day?	Observe for effects of smoking, alcohol, drugs, and caffeine, for example, difficulty sleeping, nervousness, or difficulty concentrating.
Adherence to healthy practices	How long has it been since you saw a health care provider? Do you get regular check-ups? What kind of a diet do you follow? Do you eat regular meals at home? What kind of exercise do you get?	Obtain vital signs, and palpate for any tender areas. Obtain weight.

about a breast mass identified on a routine mammogram. It is important for you to know what the patient wants and needs most from you. Ask the patient what she wants to know about the next steps (e.g., surgical or diagnostic procedure). Although some persons in this situation identify their need for information about biopsy or mastectomy as their personal priority, other women need guidance and support in discussing how to share the news with family members. Remember that there are some cases when nothing will change or improve the situation. Allowing the patient to use denial as a coping mechanism is helpful. Gaining an understanding of patient expectations does not mean that you will exclude certain types of care that are important simply because a patient does not identify them as needs. However, by inquiring about patient expectations and priorities, you are better able to ensure that the patient's needs are addressed in some way.

■■■ NURSING DIAGNOSIS

Nursing diagnoses for people experiencing stress generally focus on problems with coping. Examples of stress-related nursing diagnoses include the following:

* *Anxiety*
* *Caregiver role strain*
* *Compromised family coping*
* *Ineffective coping*
* *Fear*
* *Chronic pain*
* *Post-trauma syndrome*

Specifically, when selecting a diagnosis be sure the defining characteristics confirm the diagnosis. For example, major defining characteristics of *ineffective coping* include verbalization of an inability to cope and an inability to ask for help. Identify defining characteristics by asking the patient what concerns him or her most at the time of the interview, and, importantly, allow the patient sufficient time to answer (see Table 24-1, p. 639). Observe for psychological indicators of stress and nonverbal signs of anxiety, fear, anger, and irritability.

■■■ PLANNING

GOALS AND OUTCOMES Desirable goals for persons experiencing stress are (1) coping, (2) family coping, and (3) psychosocial adjustment: life change (Moorhead and others, 2008). Expected outcomes are behavioral markers that show progress toward goal achievement. For example, if a patient is to cope with stress, outcomes may include increasing interaction with others and improved sleep. After setting goals and outcomes, select interventions for managing the specific stressor and improving coping.

Plan care using nursing interventions designed within the framework of primary, secondary, and tertiary prevention. At the primary level of prevention, nursing interventions

include preparing patients for life's turning points, such as the birth of a baby or the death of a parent. Nursing interventions at the secondary level include actions directed at symptoms, such as protecting the patient from self-harm. Tertiary-level interventions assist your patient in readapting and often include relaxation training and time management training.

Patients' perceptions of stress and coping depend on recognition of the problem and use of coping resources. Similarly, selecting appropriate interventions requires a partnership with the patient and support system, usually the family. In the case of a family or community stressor and impaired family or community coping, your view of the situation and resources would be broader (see Care Plan).

SETTING PRIORITIES People experiencing stress have multiple nursing diagnoses that interact with one another. Prioritizing their diagnoses is important in planning care (see Figure 24-1, p. 648). One way to prioritize is to first ask, "What has happened that caused you to come for help today?" or "What happened in your life that is *different?*" This requires some focusing by the patient. Next, learn about the patient's perception of the event, available situational supports, and what the patient usually does about a problem the patient is not able to solve (James, 2008). As in all areas of nursing, make the safety of the patient and others in the patient's environment the highest priority. For example, if a patient is suicidal, determine if the patient is at risk for harming himself or herself. Ask, "Are you thinking of hurting yourself?" If the answer is yes, ask for more information such as whether or not the person has attempted suicide previously, has a plan for committing suicide, and has the means to carry out the specific plan. These questions are sometimes difficult to ask, but a patient who is highly stressed has thought about suicide at some point and is usually relieved when someone else brings up the subject.

Prioritize diagnoses by determining the degree of disruption in the person's life with work, school, home, and family. If your assessment was thorough, you will be able to prioritize problems, ensure the patient's safety, and begin the problem-solving process (James, 2008).

COLLABORATIVE CARE An effective plan requires you to collaborate with occupational therapists, dietitians, or pastoral care professionals. There will be times when nursing practice alone does not meet all of the patient's needs. Patients experiencing stress from medical conditions or psychiatric disorders will present needs that will make it necessary for you to consult with advanced practice mental health nurses, psychiatrists, psychologists, or psychiatric social workers. Such a multidisciplinary approach to care addresses the holistic needs of the patient. Recognize the need for collaboration and consultation, inform the patient about potential resources, and make arrangements for consultations, group sessions, or therapy as needed.

CARE PLAN Stress and Individual Coping

 ASSESSMENT

During her initial contact with Rachael, Becky detects a great deal of anxiety but also some anger. Becky knows it is important to build trust with Rachael as quickly as possible. She knows that Rachael's anger is not directed at her, but reflects Rachael's frustration. As a single parent herself, Becky identifies with Rachael's crisis of being the sole financial support for the family. Yet Becky decides not to tell her life history to Rachael because she recognizes that no two persons have exactly the same experience or use the same coping strategies to get through difficult times. Becky wants to be able to work closely with Rachael and establish priorities that are realistic for her to achieve.

ASSESSMENT ACTIVITIES	FINDINGS/DEFINING CHARACTERISTICS*
Observe for signs of stress.	She observes Rachael **frequently licking her lips, picking at her fingernails, and being easily startled.** Rachael **uses poor eye contact** and then **bursts into tears and expresses feelings of being overwhelmed.**
Measure vital signs.	Rachael's **vital signs show changes in response to stress:** pulse, 120 beats per minute; respirations, 24 breaths per minute; blood pressure, 168/84 mm Hg.
Ask Rachael about recent weight loss.	Rachael appears thin and pale and reports that she has **lost 20 pounds in the last 3 months.**
Ask Rachael about changes in sleep.	She also reports **difficulty in falling and remaining asleep at night.**
Assess Rachael's perception of the stress.	Rachael expresses fear of both losing her job and being unable to support her family. Rachael also expresses **feelings of shame and embarrassment.** She **thinks of herself as a failure for not coping better.**
Ask Rachael about current coping methods.	Rachael admits to having started **drinking at night to help herself "unwind."**

NURSING DIAGNOSIS: Ineffective coping related to increased pressure at work and multiple family stresses and responsibilities.

PLANNING

GOAL

Coping
- Rachael will manage stressors that have been taxing her individual resources.

EXPECTED OUTCOMES (NOC)†

- Rachael will differentiate effective and ineffective coping patterns.
- Rachael will verbalize a decrease in stress.
- Rachael will modify her lifestyle to reduce stress.
- Rachael will use her personal support system.
- Rachael will verbalize need for assistance.

INTERVENTIONS (NIC)‡

Coping
- Encourage Rachael to identify a realistic description of her changing roles.

- Use a calm, reassuring approach.

- Assist Rachael with developing an objective appraisal of her situation.

RATIONALE

A cognitive reappraisal will help Rachael to reframe the satisfaction scores so she does not take all the responsibility upon herself. How she defines the reality and the personal meaning it has for her directly affects her stress level (Stuart, 2009).

In order for treatment goals to be accomplished in a short time, Rachael will see the nurse as being nonthreatening, reliable, and understanding (Varcarolis and Halter, 2009).

Rachael's primary appraisal of the stressor and her secondary appraisal of her coping strategies define the stressful situation (Kleinke, 2007).

---

*__Defining characteristics__ are shown in **bold** type.
†Outcomes classification label from Moorhead S and others, editors: *Nursing outcomes classification (NOC),* ed 4, St. Louis, 2008, Mosby.
‡Intervention classification labels from Bulechek GM and others, editors: *Nursing interventions classification (NIC),* ed 5, St. Louis, 2008, Mosby.

CARE PLAN Stress and Individual Coping—cont'd

INTERVENTIONS (NIC)‡

Coping

- Explore with Rachael previous methods of dealing with life problems.
- Explore Rachael's previous achievements.

- Encourage Rachael to identify own strengths and abilities.

- Assist Rachael in breaking down complex goals into small, manageable steps.

- Help Rachael identify available support systems, such as family members and support groups.

- Teach Rachael strategies to increase her resistance to stress.

RATIONALE

A problem-solving approach will empower Rachael and improve her self-confidence (Kleinke, 2007).

Emphasizing the positive helps a person feel more optimistic, which leads to positive actions and results (Stuart, 2009).

To manage stress and cope with change, people need to know their strengths and abilities and what is important to them (Stuart, 2009).

Changing her cognitive view of her situation will reduce her stress. Small successes will accumulate for her and reduce the magnitude of her stress (Stuart, 2009).

Talking with others relieves tension for a person, and helping others, as in a support group, reduces self-absorption and stress (Stuart, 2009).

Increasing resistance to stress is one of the primary modes for intervention for stress management (Pender and others, 2006).

EVALUATION

NURSING ACTIONS	PATIENT RESPONSE/FINDING	ACHIEVEMENT OF OUTCOME
Ask Rachael about her perception of stress on her life and changes she has made.	Rachael appears less anxious. She exercises by walking with her husband 3 times a week. Her blood pressure is 140/82 mm Hg, and pulse is 88 beats per minute. She has a 3-lb weight gain and is eating healthy foods. She is not drinking wine to reduce her stress. During the past week she began sleeping through the night.	Rachael is decreasing the effect of stress by using healthy lifestyle habits.
Ask Rachael about the use of new and former support systems.	Rachael resumed a friendship with a neighbor. She now asks her husband for assistance at home and her co-workers for assistance at work.	Rachael is increasing her use of personal support systems at home and at work. Consider helping Rachael locate a support group to provide further support.

■■■IMPLEMENTATION

HEALTH PROMOTION Intervention for stress has a three-pronged approach: (1) decrease stress-producing situations, (2) increase resistance to stress, and (3) learn skills that reduce physiological response to stress (Pender and others, 2006). First, help patients reduce the frequency of stress-inducing situations by such strategies as instituting positive workplace habits, avoiding excessive change, and effectively managing one's personal time. Next, increase the patient's resistance to stress by recommending physical and psychological conditioning, which includes enhancing self-esteem, increasing assertiveness, setting realistic goals, and building

coping resources. Finally, use relaxation strategies to reduce physiological arousal (Pender and others, 2006). As a nurse, you educate patients and families about the importance of health promotion (Box 24-6).

Regular Exercise A regular exercise program improves muscle tone and posture, controls weight, reduces tension, improves circulation, triggers release of endorphins, and promotes relaxation. In addition, exercise reduces the risk for cardiovascular disease and improves cardiopulmonary functioning.

Support Systems A support system of family and friends who will listen, offer advice, share recreation time, and provide emotional support benefits a patient experiencing stress

CONCEPT MAP

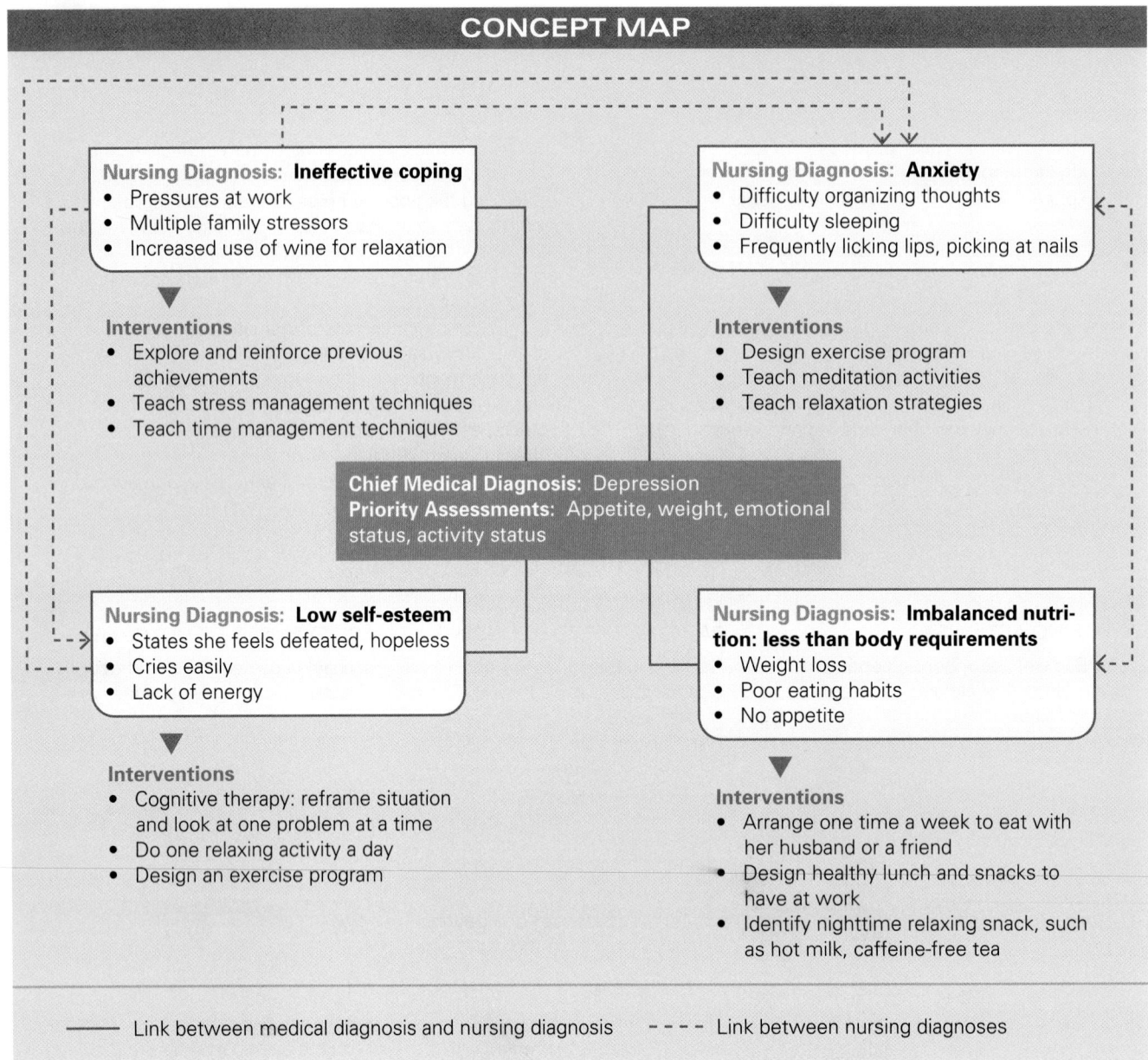

Nursing Diagnosis: Ineffective coping
- Pressures at work
- Multiple family stressors
- Increased use of wine for relaxation

Interventions
- Explore and reinforce previous achievements
- Teach stress management techniques
- Teach time management techniques

Nursing Diagnosis: Anxiety
- Difficulty organizing thoughts
- Difficulty sleeping
- Frequently licking lips, picking at nails

Interventions
- Design exercise program
- Teach meditation activities
- Teach relaxation strategies

Chief Medical Diagnosis: Depression
Priority Assessments: Appetite, weight, emotional status, activity status

Nursing Diagnosis: Low self-esteem
- States she feels defeated, hopeless
- Cries easily
- Lack of energy

Interventions
- Cognitive therapy: reframe situation and look at one problem at a time
- Do one relaxing activity a day
- Design an exercise program

Nursing Diagnosis: Imbalanced nutrition: less than body requirements
- Weight loss
- Poor eating habits
- No appetite

Interventions
- Arrange one time a week to eat with her husband or a friend
- Design healthy lunch and snacks to have at work
- Identify nighttime relaxing snack, such as hot milk, caffeine-free tea

—— Link between medical diagnosis and nursing diagnosis   - - - - Link between nursing diagnoses

Figure 24-1 ■ Concept Map.

(Figure 24-2). People with strong networks of friends, neighbors, and family tend to be healthier than those without support systems (Box 24-7). Many organizations, such as the American Heart Association, the American Cancer Society, local hospitals and churches, and mental health organizations offer support group services to individuals. Acceptable support systems vary by cultural group. For example, one cultural group relies heavily upon church members for support. Another cultural group values individual privacy and prefers to avoid a self-help group with "strangers."

Progressive Muscle Relaxation In the presence of anxiety-provoking thoughts and events, muscles tense. Physiological tension diminishes through a systematic approach to releasing tension in major muscle groups. Typically the patient achieves a relaxed state through deep chest breathing,

and then the facilitator directs the patient to alternately tighten and relax muscles in specific groupings.

Cognitive Therapy Cognitive therapy teaches patients how certain thinking patterns cause symptoms of stress or depression. For example, all-or-none thinking leads people to believe that consequences of a situation are catastrophic. Cognitive therapy focuses on changing ways of thinking so that the patient feels empowered and in control of his or her own life. People using cognitive therapy examine whether or not they are overestimating the catastrophic nature of a situation by asking, "What is the worst thing that can happen?" or "Would it be so terrible if that really took place?" (Stuart, 2009).

Cognitive therapy uses reframing of perceptions, a strategy that involves focusing on other aspects of a problem and

BOX 24-6   PATIENT TEACHING

Stress Reduction

 Becky recognizes that Rachael wants to learn how to increase her resistance to stress. Becky develops the following teaching plan for Rachael:

OUTCOME
- At the end of the teaching session, Rachael will use two methods to reduce her stress.

TEACHING STRATEGIES
- Meet with Rachael in a quiet and private setting at a time when Rachael has about 1 hour to talk without interruptions.
- Schedule a follow-up hour about a week after the first session.
- Based on Rachael's identified needs in the areas of physical exercise, assertiveness skills, coping resources, meditation, self-esteem, and insight about personal and professional responsibilities, encourage Rachael to focus on two stress management strategies.
- For a goal of increasing physical exercise, ask Rachael to discuss and explore her reasonable alternatives for exercise. Ask her to maintain a daily record of her physical exercise.
- For increasing assertiveness skills, explain assertive behavior and suggest Rachael keep a log of her assertive, aggressive, or passive responses for the next week.

- For coping resources, explore with Rachael her support system, possibilities for continuing education, financial status, and her personal appearance, depending upon her identified needs (Pender and others, 2006). Ask her to explore these resources and prepare a summary of her findings.
- For self-esteem describe cognitive skills such as positive self-talk and becoming successful in a particular skill (Pender and others, 2006). Ask her to keep a daily log of her experiences with positive self-talk and her thoughts about a skill at which she excels.
- For developing insight about maintaining appropriate boundaries between work and personal space, explore with Rachael ways she will increase awareness of her feelings of anger, pain, hurt, sadness, and joy. Discuss with her how she will recognize the limits of her responsibilities. Ask her to keep a personal journal of her feelings for the next week.

EVALUATION STRATEGIES
- During the follow-up meeting ask Rachael to report her progress on the two strategies she chose, exercise and meditation.
- Review with Rachael her record of the week's exercise and meditation activities.
- Ask Rachael to evaluate her progress toward her goal of increased resistance to stress.

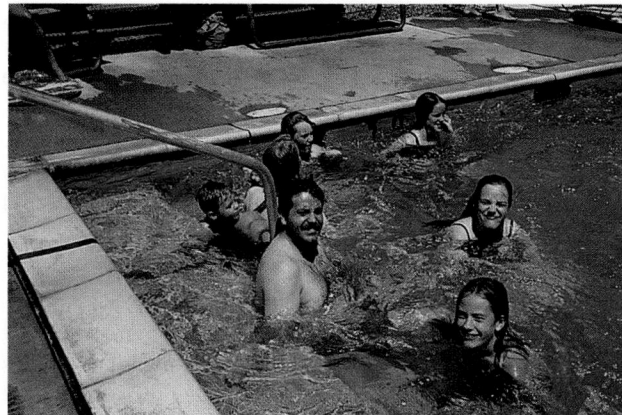

Figure 24-2 ■ Sharing recreation with family and friends promotes relaxation. (Courtesy Michael S. Clement, MD, Mesa, Ariz.)

encouraging a person to see the issue from a different perspective. Reframing helps a person see an adversity as a potentially positive event. For example, a job loss may be perceived as a stressor, but by reframing the situation, a person could see the job loss as an opportunity to pursue a new job or career (Stuart, 2009). In the process, however, be cautious about minimizing the patient's view of the stressor. Suggest that the patient reframe the perception rather than offering your own reframing.

Assertiveness Training Assertiveness training teaches individuals to communicate effectively regarding their needs and desires. The ability to resolve conflict with others through assertiveness training reduces stress. When a group leader teaches assertiveness, the effects of interacting with other people increase the benefits of the experience.

Stress Management in the Workplace The interventions described above address activities and responses that you can make in your personal life or teach your patients to use. Dealing with stress in the workplace requires a different approach. Rapid changes in health care technology, diversity in the workforce, organizational restructuring, and changing work systems place stress on nurses. Additional causes of job stress include particular job assignments, difficult schedules, shift work, fear of failure, and inadequate support services. Burnout occurs as a result of chronic stress and is often associated with the human service professions (Sulsky and Smith, 2007).

If you recognize feelings of burnout, make changes in your behavior to cope with workplace stress. Identify the limits and scope of your responsibilities at work (James, 2008). Recognize the areas over which you have control and the ability to change and those for which you do not have responsibility. Make a clear separation between work and home life as well. Strengthening friendships outside of the workplace, socially isolating oneself for personal "recharging" of emotional energy, and spending off-duty hours in interesting activities all help reduce burnout.

BOX 24-7   BEST PRACTICES

Impact of Social Support on Stress Reduction

SUMMARY OF EVIDENCE

Among a sample of 159 women, 55 to 84 years of age, those who were lonely but had a cat or dog had better general health than those who were lonely but did not have a pet. Having a pet reduced the negative effects of loneliness on the women's general health. The women in this study either lived in an independent living housing community or lived at home and participated in a senior citizen community center. Most of the women lived alone, and some wanted a cat or dog but were not permitted to have a pet in their living facility. In some situations in which pets were allowed, the security deposits for pets were prohibitive.

This research also supports a theory that states that women respond to stress by caring for others and joining social networks. The fight-or-flight theory may be only part of the natural response to stress for women. More research is needed about women's response to stress.

APPLICATION TO NURSING PRACTICE

- Assess your patients for loneliness.
- Teach older adults about the health benefits of social relationships and of pets as companions.
- Advocate for changes in public policy that would allow pets in senior citizen housing complexes, nursing homes, rehabilitation centers, and retirement communities.
- Explore the current pet ownership policy where your patients live and assist them to address concerns when appropriate.
- Consider developing a pet ownership contract outlining the patient's responsibilities to keep the pet healthy, licensed, and trained if issues about pet ownership arise.

REFERENCE

Krause-Parello CA: The mediating effect of pet attachment support between loneliness and general health in older females living in the community, *J Community Health Nurs* 25:1, 2008.

ACUTE CARE

Crisis Intervention When stress overwhelms a person's usual coping mechanisms and demands mobilization of all available resources, the stress becomes a crisis. **Crisis intervention** is different from counseling and focuses on how intensely the patient views the problems as intolerable or how emotionally unstable the patient is. Crisis intervention provides more direction than brief psychotherapy or counseling. Any member of the interdisciplinary health care team who has been trained in its techniques is able to initiate crisis intervention (James, 2008). Crisis intervention requires excellent nurse-patient communication skills (see Chapter 10).

Crisis intervention begins with defining the problem, ensuring patient safety, and providing support. First, determine that the patient is safe and is not at risk for injury to self or others, then use crisis intervention to examine alternatives, make plans, and obtain a commitment to positive action from the patient. Ideally, these last three steps are completed collaboratively with the patient, but a patient in crisis may be unable to participate actively and may need a very directive approach by the nurse or crisis interventionist (James, 2008).

When using crisis intervention, help the person become aware of present feelings, such as anger, grief, guilt, or tension. Using open-ended questions elicits feelings and responses with deeper meaning. Close-ended questions provide important information early in the crisis intervention process. Emphasize focusing on the specific problem, and help the patient to avoid all-encompassing, catastrophic interpretations. You may need to provide guidance and direction for obtaining resources and assistance. Provide an atmosphere of calm acceptance, yet be aware of situations that require a direct approach to ensure the safety of the patient. Capitalize on the patient's strengths when identifying coping strategies with the patient; these might include previous hobbies, an interest in music or sports, or religious faith (James, 2008).

RESTORATIVE AND CONTINUING CARE A person under stress recovers when the stress disappears or coping strategies succeed. However, a person who experienced a crisis has changed, and the effects sometimes last for years or for the rest of the person's life. In the final stage of adapting to a crisis, the patient acknowledges the long-term implications of the crisis. If a person successfully coped with a crisis and its consequences, he or she becomes a more mature and healthy person. When a person has recovered from a stressful situation, teach the patient stress management skills to reduce the number and intensity of the stress response in future situations.

■■■EVALUATION

PATIENT CARE By evaluating the goals and expected outcomes of care, you know if your nursing interventions were effective and if the patient copes with the identified stress. Assess the patient's perception of the effectiveness of the plan. Review the behaviorally stated, measurable goals, and evaluate whether or not the patient has met the criteria for success as stated in the outcomes. If the nursing interventions have not been effective in helping the patient achieve targeted goals, reevaluate the strategies implemented and revise the plan of care in consideration of the patient's current health status.

To evaluate the patient experiencing stress, observe patient behaviors and talk with the patient and family, if appropriate (Box 24-8). Remember that coping with stress takes time. If you are in a setting in which contact with a patient ends before achieving goals or resolution, refer your patient to appropriate resources so as not to delay or interrupt progress.

PATIENT EXPECTATIONS Maintain ongoing communication with patients regarding the plan of care. Patients under severe stress often experience feelings of powerlessness, vulnerability, and loss of control. Actively involve patients and families in problem identification (assessment), prioritizing, and goal setting and evaluation. Involving patients in these processes gives them an opportunity to direct their energy in a positive way and moves them toward taking greater responsibility for health maintenance and promotion.

Engaging the patient as a partner in health care sets the stage for open communication. This gives the patient a sense of control and begins to promote independence, which are both crucial to the patient's successful resolution of the situation. In such an environment the patient feels more freedom to give important feedback to you about interventions that are successful. This helps you better understand why some interventions fail to meet the established goals.

BOX 24-8   EVALUATION

 Three weeks after their initial discussion, Rachael makes her routine appointment at the employee health office to see Becky. Becky is relieved to see that Rachael is less anxious and looking better. The nervous behaviors previously assessed are no longer present. Feeling less drained, Rachael is making progress on developing professional and personal boundaries. Her neighbors and friends know about her situation and provide casseroles for the family to eat. Rachael accepts this help by reminding herself that it will only be temporary. She is encouraged by the insight she gets from individual and group counseling sessions. Although the Bennett family has not yet found full resolution for their stress, they are making progress toward achievable, short-term goals.

DOCUMENTATION NOTE
"Reports that she feels 'more hopeful.' Blood pressure is 140/82 mm Hg, and pulse is 88 beats per minute. Weight increased by 3 lb since her last visit, and this week began sleeping through the night. States is going with husband to a family support group meeting held every week at the rehabilitation facility."

KEY POINTS

- The general adaptation syndrome (GAS), an immediate physiological response to stress, involves several body systems, especially the autonomic nervous system and the endocrine system.
- Physiological responses to stress also include immunological changes.
- Stress makes people ill as a result of both increased levels of powerful hormones that change bodily processes and coping choices that are unhealthy, such as not getting enough rest or a proper diet or use of tobacco, alcohol, or caffeine.
- A person experiences psychological stress only if the person evaluates the event or circumstance as personally significant; this is called primary appraisal.

- Stress includes work stress, family stress, chronic stress, acute stress, daily hassles, trauma, and crisis.
- Potential stressors and coping mechanisms vary across the life span, from childhood through adolescence, adulthood, and old age, and from one culture to another.
- Coping, a process that constantly changes to manage demands on a person's resources, means making an effort to manage psychological stress.
- Posttraumatic stress disorder affects people who have experienced accidents, violent events, war, and natural disasters.
- A patient who has such severe stress that he or she is unable to cope in ways that worked before is experiencing a crisis.

CRITICAL THINKING EXERCISES

Rachael Bennett, a 32-year-old married mother of three children, works as the nurse manager in a medical intensive care unit. Until recently she has felt very happy with her job. The stress in both her personal life and professional life is increasing. She feels defeated and hopeless, she has no energy, and she has difficulty organizing her thoughts. She has severe headaches, reports a lack of sleep, and use of wine at night to relax. Her supervisor referred her to the hospital's employee health office. One of this department's duties is to help employees cope with the stress. Use this information and the information from the case study in the chapter to answer the following questions.

1. At this point in Rachael's care there are three relevant nursing diagnostic labels: *caregiver role strain, compromised family coping,* and *ineffective coping.* Prioritize these potential nursing diagnoses for Rachael Bennett. Provide the rationale for your priority selection.

2. Which of the following is an appropriate goal for crisis intervention for Rachael?
    a. Rachael will leave her job and return to school to prepare for a less stressful career.
    b. Rachael will mobilize community resources for meeting her family's basic needs on a temporary basis.
    c. Rachael will arrange for her children to stay with a relative for the rest of the school year.

3. List three cultural factors to assess when meeting with Rachael.

4. The type of crisis that Rachael is experiencing is called:
    a. Developmental
    b. Situational
    c. Existential
    d. Ecosystemic

ⓔvolve   *Answers to Critical Thinking Questions can be found on the Evolve website.*

REVIEW QUESTIONS

1. While assessing a person for the effects of the general adaptation syndrome, be aware that:
    1. Heart rate increases in the resistance stage
    2. Blood volume increases in the exhaustion stage
    3. Vital signs return to normal in the exhaustion stage
    4. Blood glucose level increases during the alarm reaction stage

2. Your 52-year-old female patient has hypertension and is in the middle of a bitter divorce. You see her in the clinic, and you want to help her understand the potential impact of increased stress level on her existing hypertension. You explain:
    1. Hypertension causes stress by suppressing immunity
    2. Stress causes forgetfulness and it is important to remember to take hypertensive medication
    3. Some antihypertensive medications cause stress and illness
    4. A person who takes antihypertensive medication has an immunity to stress

3. A colleague is describing the stress she feels on the job. Stress in the health care workplace results from:
    1. Nurses who feel stress pass the stress along to their patients
    2. Nurses who are ineffective and should not be working
    3. Unprofessional discussion about the stress
    4. The rapid changes in health care technology and organizational restructuring

4. A family has three children. Over the last year, the husband lost his job and the wife had a serious illness. The parents are worried about the impact of stress on their children. When assessing the children, it is important to remember:
    1. Children are resilient and cope with stress better than adults

2. Children provoke more stress in others than they experience themselves
3. Stressors and coping methods are different for children than older people
4. Ways of coping that will be effective for a child are similar to those of the child's parents

5. You are evaluating the coping success of a patient experiencing stress from a new diagnosis of multiple sclerosis, a progressive neurological disease. Which of the following responses lets you know that the patient is beginning to successfully cope with this situation? Select all that apply.
    1. "I am attending a support group to learn more about multiple sclerosis."
    2. "I am going to learn to drive a car so I can be more independent."
    3. "My sister says she feels better when she goes shopping, so I will go shopping."
    4. "I have always felt better when I go for a long walk. I will do that when I get home."

6. When assessing a young woman who was in an automobile accident 6 months before, you learn that the woman has vivid images of the crash whenever she hears a loud, sudden noise. You recognize this as:
    1. Social phobia
    2. Acute anxiety
    3. Posttraumatic stress disorder
    4. Borderline personality disorder

7. A family tells the community mental health nurse that their adult mentally disabled son is experiencing hallucinations. This has begun very recently and had not happened before. They are frightened for him and do not know what to do. In addition, they are living below the poverty level on their pensions and have only enough money to last from one month to the next. The nurse helps them set the following goal:

1. After a psychiatric evaluation, investigate a group home for the son
2. With help from the nurse, obtain suitable housing and additional financial resources
3. Develop a plan to take in a renter so that they can have a better income
4. Obtain a psychiatric assessment and stabilize the son on Medicaid-covered medications

8. The mother of a 4-year-old child who sustained burns on his hands when he was helping his mother bake cookies is experiencing stress. She cries easily and tells you she is having trouble sleeping. Which of the following are important assessment questions? Select all that apply.
   1. What stresses you the most when you think of your son's burns?
   2. Tell me more about your problem sleeping.
   3. Do you have friends or family members to help you and your son?
   4. Are you able to do your routine activities, such as caring for your family, working?

9. A patient newly diagnosed with type 2 diabetes exhibits denial when she says, "My blood sugar was just a little high. I don't have diabetes." The nurse responds:
   1. "Let's talk about something cheerful."
   2. "Do other members of your family have diabetes?"
   3. "I can tell that you feel stressed to learn that you have diabetes."
   4. With silence; the nurse understands the denial is a defense mechanism that assists in coping with a shock.

10. A nurse experiencing work-related stress should take which of the following actions first?
    1. Determine the particular cause of the workplace stress for him or her.
    2. Begin an aerobic exercise program.
    3. Use relaxation strategies.
    4. Increase assertiveness and set realistic goals.

Answers to Review Questions can be found on pages 1197-1198.

REFERENCES

Aldwin C: *Stress, coping, and development: an integrative perspective,* ed 2, New York, 2007, Guilford.

Bulechek GM and others, editors: *Nursing interventions classification (NIC),* ed 5, St. Louis, 2008, Mosby.

James RK: *Crisis intervention strategies,* ed 6, Belmont, Calif, 2008, Thomson Brooks/Cole.

Jean-Louis G and others: Insomnia symptoms in a multiethnic sample of American women, *J Womens Health* 17(1):15, 2008.

Jones F, Bright J: Stress: health and illness. In Monat A, Lazarus RS, Reevy G, editors: *The Praeger handbook on stress and coping,* Westport, Conn, 2007, Praeger.

Kleinke CL: What does it mean to cope? In Monat A, Lazarus RS, Reevy G, editors: *The Praeger handbook on stress and coping,* Westport, Conn, 2007, Praeger.

Krause-Parello CA: The mediating effect of pet attachment support between loneliness and general health in older females living in the community, *J Community Health Nurs* 25:1, 2008.

Lazarus RS: Stress and emotion: a new synthesis. In Monat A, Lazarus RS, Reevy G, editors: *The Praeger handbook on stress and coping,* Westport, Conn, 2007, Praeger.

McEwen B, Lasley EN: Allostatic load: when protection gives way to damage. In Monat A, Lazarus RS, Reevy G, editors: *The Praeger handbook on stress and coping,* Westport, Conn, 2007, Praeger.

Monat A, Lazarus RS, Reevy G, editors: *The Praeger handbook on stress and coping,* Westport, Conn, 2007, Praeger.

Moorhead S and others, editors: *Nursing outcomes classification (NOC),* ed 4, St. Louis, 2008, Mosby.

Neuman B, Fawcett J: *The Neuman systems model,* ed 4, Upper Saddle River, NJ, 2002, Prentice Hall.

Pender NJ, Murdaugh CL, Parsons MA: *Health promotion in nursing practice,* ed 5, Upper Saddle River, NJ, 2006, Prentice Hall.

Pert CB: The wisdom of the receptors: neuropeptides, the emotions, and bodymind. In Monat A, Lazarus RS, Reevy G, editors: *The Praeger handbook on stress and coping,* Westport, Conn, 2007, Praeger.

Stuart GW: *Principles and practice of psychiatric nursing,* ed 9, St. Louis, 2009, Mosby.

Sulsky L, Smith C: Work stress: macro-level work stressors. In Monat A, Lazarus RS, Reevy G, editors: *The Praeger handbook on stress and coping,* Westport, Conn, 2007, Praeger.

Varcarolis EM, Halter MJ: *Essentials of psychiatric mental health nursing: a communication approach to evidence-based care,* St. Louis, 2009, Saunders.

25 Loss and Grief

MEDIA RESOURCES

 CD COMPANION 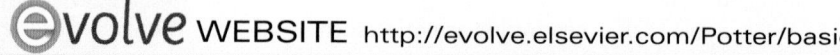 **WEBSITE** http://evolve.elsevier.com/Potter/basic

- Crossword Puzzle
- English/Spanish Audio Glossary

OBJECTIVES

- Discuss five basic categories of loss.
- Compare theories on grief and loss.
- Describe types of grief.
- Discuss variables that influence a person's response to grief.
- Identify elements in an assessment of a patient experiencing loss and grief.
- Identify nursing interventions for helping patients cope with loss, death, and grief.
- Develop a care plan for a patient and family members experiencing loss and grief.

- Discuss the principles of palliative and hospice care.
- Identify ways to educate and involve family members in providing palliative care.
- List the steps in the procedure for care of the body after death.
- Discuss the nurse's experiences of loss when caring for dying patients.

KEY TERMS

acceptance, p. 656
actual loss, p. 655
advance directive, p. 661
anger, p. 656
anticipatory grief, p. 657
autopsy, p. 671
bargaining, p. 656
bereavement, p. 656

complicated grief, p. 658
denial, p. 656
depression, p. 656
disenfranchised grief, p. 658
disorganization and despair, p. 657
grief, p. 656

hope, p. 658
hospice, p. 668
maturational loss, p. 655
mourning, p. 656
necessary losses, p. 655
normal or uncomplicated grief, p. 657
numbing, p. 656

palliative care, p. 667
perceived loss, p. 655
postmortem care, p. 671
reminiscence, p. 657
reorganization, p. 655
situational loss, p. 655
yearning and searching, p. 656

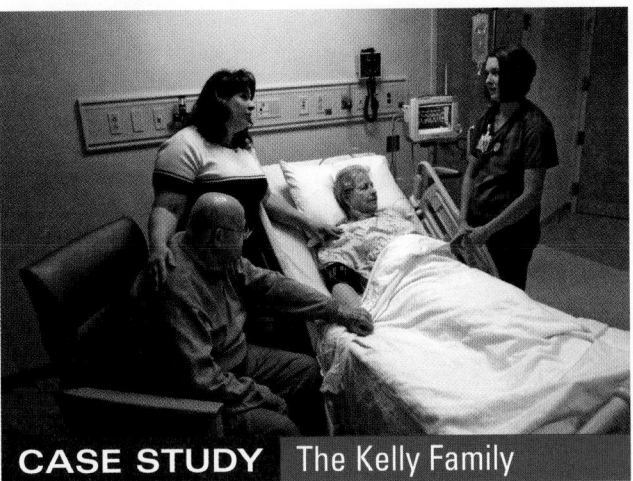

CASE STUDY | The Kelly Family

Mrs. Kelly is 79 years old and is in end-stage heart disease secondary to diabetes mellitus. Her mobility has declined greatly because of shortness of breath, poor food intake, decreased strength, and lack of oxygen. She takes pain medication for severe back and joint pain and has trouble with constipation. She was admitted to the hospital four times in the past year for heart failure or for care of her stasis ulcers. She is now in the intensive care unit for chest pain and congestive heart failure. Tests indicate that her heart function is worsening. Mrs. Kelly no longer wants to be hospitalized for her medical conditions, and she wants to go home to die. Mrs. Kelly is being evaluated for home hospice care and will temporarily receive home care.

Mrs. Kelly lives with her husband of 54 years. Her daughter, Lilly, lives near her parents and visits them every day. Lilly does not agree with the plan to begin hospice care. She cannot accept her mother's plan to "give up." Mr. Kelly does not understand hospice and is not sure if he will be a good caregiver.

Nursing student Jennifer Brown will be caring for the Kelly family as she learns how to give care in the home. She has never given end-of-life care and feels anxious about her abilities to care for Mrs. Kelly. Not only will she be taking care of Mrs. Kelly's physical needs, Jennifer will also have to address the family's grief and coping issues.

People need nursing care for many reasons. They want to learn how to stay healthy or prevent illness, they need help to recover from an acute illness or injury, or need to learn how to live with chronic illness. At some point, all patients and families need end-of-life care. Nurses have a long and proud history of caring for patients who face loss, grief, and death (Blum, 2006). Care situations that involve loss and grief elicit fear and uncertainty in many caregivers (Weigel and others, 2007). Fortunately, nursing knowledge regarding the care of the dying and bereaved has expanded greatly in the last decade (American Association of Colleges of Nursing [AACN], 2008; Ferrell and Coyle, 2006; Matzo and Sherman, 2006). Grief and loss affect a person's health physically, psy-

chologically, socially, and spiritually. Nurses therefore need to offer holistic care. Patients at the end of life need our knowledge and compassion, expressed in expert nursing care, as they live with illnesses that cannot be cured and come to the end of their lives.

SCIENTIFIC KNOWLEDGE BASE

Loss

Throughout our lives, from birth to death, we form attachments and suffer losses. We become independent from our parents, leave home to attend school, begin careers, and form relationships. Growing up is natural and positive, yet throughout life we experience **necessary losses.** We learn that many losses are replaced by something different or better. A person, for example, leaves behind family members to begin college but makes new friends and learns to live independently. Other necessary losses, such as death of a loved one, challenge a person's sense of security and coping skills.

How we perceive loss depends on what we value. Our family, friends, society, culture, and faith traditions shape our priorities and help us determine what matters most in life. A person experiences loss when a meaningful object, person, body part or function, emotion, or idea is no longer present. There are several types of loss (Table 25-1). People experience an **actual loss** when they can no longer touch, hear, see, or have near them valued people or objects. Examples include the loss of a body part, pet, friend, life partner, or role at work. People feel grief when a valued object becomes worn out, lost, stolen, or ruined by disaster. A child often grieves after losing a favorite toy. **Perceived losses** are uniquely experienced by a grieving person and are often less obvious to others. A perceived loss is "real" to the person who feels the loss. A person may perceive that she is less loved by her parents, for example, and experiences a loss of self-esteem. Others often overlook or misunderstand perceived losses.

People experience **maturational losses** as they go through a lifetime of normal developmental processes. When a child goes to school for the first time, for example, she will spend less time with her parent and the parent-child relationship changes. Acknowledging and grieving maturational losses help a person cope with the change. **Situational loss** occurs as a result of a sudden, unpredictable life event. A situational loss often involves multiple losses. A divorce, for example, begins with the loss of a life companion, but often leads to financial strain, changes in living arrangements, less contact with one's children, and loss of friends who were part of the couple's married life.

How an individual interprets the meaning of any loss and the type of the loss determines, in part, how that person will grieve. People respond to loss differently. Do not assume, for example, that the loss of a possession or social status could not generate the same level of grief as loss of a person. The value an individual places on the absent object or changed social status (e.g., loss of job and income) influences his or her emotional response to the loss.

TABLE 25-1 Types of Loss

DEFINITION	IMPLICATIONS OF LOSS
Loss of external objects (e.g., loss, misplacement, theft, destruction by nature)	Extent of grieving depends on object's value, sentiment attached to it, and its usefulness.
Loss of a known environment (e.g., moving from a neighborhood, hospitalization, a new job, moving to a long-term care facility)	Loss occurs through maturational or situational events and with injury or illness. Loneliness in unfamiliar setting threatens self-esteem and makes grieving difficult.
Loss of a significant other (e.g., being promoted, moving, loss of a family member, friend, trusted nurse, or pet)	Significant others meet a person's need for psychological safety, love and belonging, and self-esteem.
Loss of an aspect of self (e.g., body part, psychological or physiological function)	Illness, injury, or developmental changes result in a loss that causes changes in body image, self-concept, and level of independence.
Loss of life (e.g., death of family member, friend, or acquaintance; own death)	Loss of a life creates grief for those left behind. Persons facing death often fear pain and loss of control or independence.

People usually experience multiple losses when they become ill or need to be hospitalized. When patients enter a hospital, they often lose their privacy, modesty, and control over body functions and daily routines. They often lose a sense of safety and their perception of themselves as a once-healthy person. Chronic, debilitating illness or hospitalization often adds financial concerns, necessitates job changes, threatens independence, forces changes in lifestyle, and challenges family relationships.

Death is the ultimate loss. Although death is a part of life and is universally experienced by all living things, death's mysterious, uncertain character often produces anxiety and fear (Matzo and Sherman, 2006). Death ends relationships with family and friends and separates people from the physical presence of people important to them. Persons at the end of life and their caregivers often experience sorrow, uncertainty, fear, or physical, emotional, and spiritual challenges throughout the dying process. Close friends and caregivers of a dying person are reminded of their own mortality. Most people do not want to become completely dependent on others at the end of life, yet they do not want to die alone.

Facing death often brings out emotions such as guilt, anger, sadness, and fear. Some family members and caregivers, fearful of the intensity of the experience, withdraw at a time when the dying person most needs their love and support. A person's basic beliefs and values, culture, spirituality, and the quality of the emotional support available influence the way a person and his or her family members approach dying. They need understanding and individually designed, compassionate end-of-life care.

Grief

Grief is the emotional response to a loss, manifested in ways unique to an individual, based on personal experiences, cultural expectations, and spiritual beliefs (Hooyman and Kramer, 2006); (see Chapters 19 and 20). Grief involves **mourning,** the conscious and unconscious behaviors associated with loss. **Bereavement** includes grief and mourning, the inner feelings and outward behaviors of a survivor. Many

theorists have described the grief process. Note the similarities among the theories to identify the key elements involved in a grief or loss experience (Table 25-2). Theories of grief apply to all forms of loss, including death, chronic illness, or sudden loss of body function. Each describes commonly experienced psychological and behavioral characteristics that follow phases or stages of response (Corless, 2006).

KÜBLER-ROSS' FIVE STAGES OF GRIEF Kübler-Ross' classic behavior-oriented theory (1969) includes five stages. The theory applies to any person undergoing a significant loss. At the end of life, dying persons and people close to them experience these stages of loss. Individuals in the **denial** stage act as though nothing has changed. They cannot believe or understand that a loss has occurred. In the **anger** stage, a person resists the loss and feels and expresses anger about his or her situation or sometimes feels angry with God. During **bargaining,** the individual postpones awareness of the loss and tries to prevent the loss from happening by making deals or promises, in subtle or overt ways. A person realizes the full impact and significance of the loss during the **depression** stage. When depressed, the person feels overwhelmingly lonely or sad and withdraws from interactions with others. Finally, during the stage of **acceptance,** the individual begins to accept the reality and inevitability of loss and begins to look to the future.

BOWLBY'S FOUR PHASES OF MOURNING Attachment theory serves as the foundation for Bowlby's phases of mourning (1980). Attachment, an instinctive behavior, leads to the development of bonds of affection between children and their primary caregivers that remain present throughout life. Later in life, people generalize attachment bonds to other individuals with whom they form close relationships. Attachment behavior ensures survival by keeping people in close contact with others who offer them protection and support.

Bowlby describes four phases of mourning. In the **numbing** phase, a person has periods of extremely intense emotion and reports feeling "stunned" or "unreal." The numbing phase can last from several hours to 1 week. The **yearning and searching** phase evokes emotional outbursts, tearful sobbing, and acute distress. Theorists explain that in order to

TABLE 25-2   Theories of Grief, Loss and Mourning

KÜBLER-ROSS' FIVE STAGES OF GRIEF	BOWLBY'S FOUR PHASES OF MOURNING	WORDEN'S FOUR TASKS OF MOURNING	RANDO'S R PROCESS MODEL
Denial Anger Bargaining Depression Acceptance	Numbing Yearning and searching Disorganization and despair Reorganization	Accepting the reality of loss Working through the pain of grief Adjusting to the environment without the deceased Emotionally relocating the deceased and moving on with life	Recognize and accept the reality of the loss React to, experience, and express the pain of separation Reminiscence Relinquish old attachments Readjust and Reinvest

move forward, bereaved persons must experience this painful phase of grief. Common physical symptoms include tightness in the chest and throat, shortness of breath, a feeling of weakness and lethargy, insomnia, and loss of appetite. This phase lasts for months or, intermittently, for years. During the phase of **disorganization and despair** an individual spends much time thinking about how and why the loss occurred. It is common for the person to express anger at anyone he or she believes to be responsible. Gradually this phase gives way to an acceptance that the loss is permanent. During the final phase of **reorganization,** which usually requires a year or more, the person begins to accept unaccustomed roles, acquire new skills, and build new relationships.

WORDEN'S FOUR TASKS OF MOURNING Worden's four tasks of mourning theory (1982) describes individuals as able to actively help themselves through mourning and as able to ask others for help. Although the time needed varies from person to person, moving through Worden's tasks typically takes a minimum of 1 year.

- Task I: *To accept the reality of the loss.* People experience a period of disbelief and surprise that a loss has really happened, even when a death is expected. This task involves moving toward the realization that the person or object is gone and will not return.
- Task II: *To work through the pain of grief.* It is impossible to experience a loss without some degree of emotional pain. Individuals who deny or suppress the pain often prolong their grief.
- Task III: *To adjust to the environment in which the deceased is missing.* A person does not realize the full impact of a loss for at least 3 months. After the first few weeks after a death, visitors and friends become less attentive and the person must experience the full impact of the loss alone. People show signs of adjustment by taking on roles formerly filled by the deceased and participating in new activities.
- Task IV: *To emotionally relocate the deceased and move on with life.* People who move on with life do not forget the deceased or devalue the relationship but begin the difficult task of giving the deceased a less central place in their emotional life. Eventually a person realizes that it is

possible to love other people without loving the deceased person less.

RANDO'S R PROCESS MODEL Rando (1993) developed her model of mourning specifically in relation to Western society. She describes mourning as an action-oriented process involving recognizing the loss, reacting to the pain of separation, reminiscence, relinquishing old attachments, and readjusting to life after loss. Rando's model includes reminiscence as an important activity in grief and mourning. In **reminiscence** a person recollects and reexperiences the deceased and the relationship by mentally or verbally reliving and remembering the person and past experiences.

Theories of loss, death, grief, or mourning help us understand common, shared pathways through complex human experiences. You need to remember, however, that people do not go through stages or phases or complete tasks in a linear fashion. Rather, they move back and forth between stages, experience phases in an overlapping manner, or even skip some of the steps. People rarely "get over" a significant loss, but instead heal and learn to live with loss. Knowledge of grief theories and the types of grief will assist you in the selection of appropriate, individualized nursing interventions.

TYPES OF GRIEF

Normal Grief **Normal** or **uncomplicated grief** consists of commonly expected emotional and behavioral reactions to a loss (e.g., resentment, sorrow, anger, crying, loneliness, and temporary withdrawal from activities). When patients feel supported and valued as they grieve, they often come to view the experience later as growth-producing and positive (Egan and Arnold, 2003).

Anticipatory Grief The process of "letting go" that occurs before an actual loss or death has occurred is called **anticipatory grief.** For example, after a person and family members accept the reality of a terminal diagnosis, they begin saying good-bye and completing life affairs. After a prolonged dying process, a patient's family members often do not respond with the shock and disbelief at the time of death, and feelings of sadness might mingle with some relief that the suffering is finally over. There are risks associated with anticipatory grieving. Some family members begin withdrawing emotionally from the patient as a self-protective mechanism, leaving the patient with less support as death approaches. On the other hand, if a person thought to be near death survives longer than anticipated, others can have difficulty reconnecting or feel resentful that the stressors associated with anticipating a death continue.

Complicated Grief When a person has difficulty progressing through his or her loss experience, he or she experiences **complicated grief.** The person does not accept the reality of the loss, and the intense feelings associated with acute grief do not go away. A person experiencing complicated grief feels strain in his or her relationships and finds it hard to go forward in life. The following are four types of complicated grief:

- *Chronic grief:* When the active acute mourning experienced in normal grief reactions does not decrease and continues over long periods of time, a person experiences chronic grief. The person verbalizes an inability to "get past" the grief.
- *Delayed grief:* When a person consciously or unconsciously avoids the pain of loss and does not experience common grief reactions at the time of the loss, he or she may experience a delayed grief reaction. The grief arises later, often in response to a different, seemingly lesser loss. For example, a wife suppresses the pain of loss after the death of her husband and quickly resumes her busy career life. A year later she becomes severely depressed and withdraws from her children when one of them moves out of town. The extreme reaction to the relocation is, in part, a delayed response to the death of her husband.
- *Exaggerated grief:* Persons overwhelmed by their loss cannot function or display significant behavioral dysfunction in an exaggerated grief response. Evidence of exaggerated grief includes severe phobias, deep depression, or self-destructive behaviors such as alcoholism, substance abuse, or suicide.
- *Masked grief:* After a significant loss some people are unable to recognize that the behaviors making normal functioning difficult are a result of their loss. For example, a person who has lost a pet develops changes in sleeping patterns but does not see the connection between the two events. "Unmasking" the connections between grief and unwanted behaviors helps the healing process.

Disenfranchised Grief Individuals experience disenfranchised grief when they cannot openly acknowledge a loss and experience full social support from others. **Disenfranchised grief** happens most often in situations in which others regard the person's loss as less significant or "legitimate." It is often difficult to feel support when a person loses a loved one in a relationship of devalued social standing (e.g., same-sex partnership, ex-spouse, or unmarried cohabitants) or when the loss is deeply private or secretly experienced (e.g., early miscarriage or death of a family member due to acquired immune deficiency syndrome or alcoholism).

NURSING KNOWLEDGE BASE

Nurses interact with people who have experienced all types of losses and who express their grief in different ways. You will give care using interventions validated through research and evidence-based practice to support patients through difficult life transitions. Many factors influence the way an individual experiences loss and responds to it.

Factors Influencing Loss and Grief

HUMAN DEVELOPMENT A person's age and stage of development partly determine his or her ability to understand loss and what it means for his or her future and well-being (see Chapter 21). Expressions of grief evolve as individuals mature. Toddlers, for example, cannot understand the permanence of death but feel anxiety over loss of objects and separation from parents. School-age children, although able to understand the significance of loss more completely, regard their loss as a challenge to their emerging identity or self-concept. Middle-age adults often use grief experiences to reexamine or reprioritize their lives. Older adults begin to anticipate grief as they encounter declining physical function or life opportunities, give up employment or social status, or lose loved ones to death.

PSYCHOLOGICAL PERSPECTIVES OF GRIEF AND LOSS Individuals first respond to loss by using coping mechanisms that worked for them in the past. Sometimes when a person has multiple losses or loses something of great significance, usual coping strategies are inadequate for the challenge. The person must then use new coping mechanisms (see Chapter 24).

SOCIOECONOMIC STATUS Socioeconomic status influences a person's access to resources and support for coping with loss. Generally people feel greater burden from a loss when they lack financial, educational, or occupational resources. For example, a person with limited financial resources is unable to replace a home lost in a fire or purchase necessary medications to manage a newly diagnosed disease. Community agencies often provide needed material and educational resources.

NATURE OF PERSONAL RELATIONSHIPS In situations of loss from a death, gaining information about the quality and meaning of the relationship a grieving person had with the deceased helps you better understand that person's grief. When a relationship between two people has been very close and well connected, the surviving person often finds it very difficult to cope with the loss. If there was conflict or abuse in the relationship, the survivor may feel guilt, remorse, regret, or relief.

NATURE OF THE LOSS The visibility of a loss often influences the amount of support a person receives. For example, the loss of one's home from a tornado will bring support from the community, whereas the loss of an early-term pregnancy may bring less support. Many people empathize with the first, very public loss. In the second case of a private loss, fewer people may know about it or appreciate its significance to the woman and family. People respond differently to sudden, unexpected, or stigmatized deaths (e.g., suicide) than to anticipated or seemingly inevitable losses.

CULTURE AND ETHNICITY A person's cultural practices influence one's responses to grief and loss (Box 25-1). One's cultural belief systems provide a person with the structures and interpretations he or she needs to cope with change, loss, illness, or death (Hattori, McCubbin, and Ishida, 2006). For example, in Western societies many people grieve privately and with restrained emotional expressions. In other cultures, survivors wail loudly and publically display their sorrow to communicate the significance of their loss to others. Some Chinese communities consider death to be a taboo subject and believe that discussion of the topic brings bad luck. Most people practicing the Hindu religion believe in reincarnation and use those beliefs to interpret events surrounding the death of a loved one (Clements and others, 2003). Although members of a cultural or religious group often share similar beliefs, members of any group still respond in their own unique way. Gain knowledge and appreciation of values and beliefs as they apply generally to a cultural group, but assess each person for his or her individualized responses as well (Doorenbos, Wilson, and Coenen, 2006; Kikuchi, 2005). Research supports that ethnicity is strongly related to attitudes toward life-sustaining treatments during terminal illness and the use of hospice services (Campbell, 2007; Rosenfeld and others, 2007).

SPIRITUAL BELIEFS People use their faith in a higher power, a community of friends, their sources of hope and meaning in life, and religious rituals and practices to cope with life challenges and grief (Chochinov and Cann, 2005); (see Chapters 20 and 24). Murray and others (2004) found that whether or not patients and their family caregivers held religious beliefs, they expressed needs for love, meaning, and purpose. Loss causes conflicts about spiritual values and the meaning of life. Spirituality helps patients buffer the stress of chronic illness and other life challenges (Delgado, 2007).

HOPE People facing life-changing experiences need to maintain hope. **Hope** is the anticipation of a continued good or an improvement or lessening of something unpleasant. Hope energizes and comforts people as they face personal challenges and enhances their coping skills (Buckley and Herth, 2004; Nowotny, 1991). Some people view hope as encouragement to work toward recovery. People often reveal their sense of hope when they talk about their expectations for the present and the future. A terminally ill patient often places his or her hope on getting to a milestone (e.g., living to experience a child's wedding), significant event (e.g., an upcoming birthday), or on believing that pain or other disabling symptoms can be managed. Spiritual distress is often tied to lack of hope. People who feel hopeless cannot imagine any favorable outcomes. Hope and help are related. When a person has strong relationships and a sense of emotional connectedness to others, he or she knows that help is available for moving into the future. Nurses provide patients with a personal connection essential to fostering hope.

BOX 25-1 CULTURAL FOCUS

Loss, Death, and Grieving

People across the world rely on culturally specific rituals and mourning practices to achieve a sense of acceptance and inner peace and participate in socially accepted expressions of grief. One's culture greatly influences what behaviors and rituals are expected at the time of death. Institutional guidelines and end-of-life care procedures for patients from all cultures provide standards based on compassion, maintaining privacy and dignity, and respect for patients' and family members' cultural beliefs and practices. Expert end-of-life care allows time for patients and their families to make private and public preparations and complete unfinished communication. Understanding the uniqueness of cultural expectations at the end of life helps you know what questions to ask. You need to understand patients' culture-specific practices surrounding end-of-life care. The cultural or religious practices described below are not necessarily exclusive to the culture named, but are offered to give you ideas of some culturally specific concerns you may encounter in end-of-life care.

- European Americans affirm the life of the whole person and seek closure and a sense of completion at the end of life.
- Orthodox Jews stay with a person who is dying throughout the entire process and have community members (minyan) praying at the bedside.
- Members of religious faiths that believe in reincarnation (e.g., Hindu religion) support refusal of nourishment and pain medications because of the implications for the dying person's next life.
- Religious leaders in devout Muslim and Jewish communities play a key role in resolving conflicts between medical practices and religious beliefs.
- Some religious groups or cultures object to a person being told that he or she has a terminal condition.
- Members of Christian religious traditions often receive an anointing by a priest and receive Holy Communion. Christian traditions usually have a belief in heaven or an afterlife for believers.

IMPLICATIONS FOR PRACTICE

- Provide end-of-life care with cultural sensitivity to postmortem care practices and the timing, form, and type of support provided to grieving patients and families.
- Cultural care includes knowing who makes decisions in a family.
- Care provided at the end of life within the patient and family's cultural context draws on the resources of their whole lives.

Data from Jenko M, Moffitt S: Transcultural nursing principles, *J Hosp Palliat Nurs* 8(3):173, 2006; Kemp C: Cultural issues in palliative care, *Semin Oncol Nurs* 21(1):44, 2005.

CRITICAL THINKING

Synthesis

You will apply elements of critical thinking whenever you perform the nursing process with a patient. Consider the scientific knowledge you have learned, your experience, critical thinking attitudes, and standards to ensure an individualized approach to patient care. Each patient you care for has different developmental, spiritual, and cultural backgrounds. Consider all of these factors when developing a comprehensive, holistic plan of care (Box 25-2). You will use all of your critical thinking skills to review data, recognize patterns, interpret the meaning of the data, make nursing diagnoses, and plan, implement, and evaluate a plan of care.

KNOWLEDGE Knowledge of loss and grief theories helps you understand a patient's unique responses to grief, loss, and death. Applying knowledge of therapeutic communication principles (see Chapter 10) allows you to have helpful discussions with patients and family members to better understand their experience and perspectives. When loss is related to a particular disease or illness, knowledge about the disease process helps you design educational interventions and offer patients a realistic description of what to expect. Understanding cultural and religious diversity allows you to individualize your approach. Finally, principles of caring (see Chapter 18) and family dynamics (see Chapter 23) enable you to provide inclusive, compassionate care.

EXPERIENCE Most of us have experienced some type of loss. Personal experience with loss prepares you to understand and empathize with others going through difficult times. Each time you care for a patient or family member who is coping with grief, loss, or death, you gain valuable nursing wisdom and experience. Reflect upon those experiences, and consider how to apply what you have learned when caring for other patients.

ATTITUDES Critical thinking attitudes of risk taking, self-confidence, and humility help you make accurate assessments and decisions about your patients (see Chapter 7). Many nurses become anxious when caring for dying patients or people coping with grief and loss (Weigel and others, 2007). When you care for an actively mourning person, you take a personal risk. Self-confidence goes hand in hand with risk taking. Confidence helps you to understand that even if there is nothing you can do or say to change the situation, the patient needs your compassionate presence and a personal connection with someone who cares. Confidence helps you accept the responsibility to remain present even in difficult situations. By silently sharing a moment of sadness with a patient or family member, you communicate caring and send the message that you respect and accept their feelings in the moment. You cannot know everything there is to know about a patient's loss. Humility helps you put aside personal assumptions about how the patient interprets loss and keeps you open to hearing and understanding his or her beliefs and concerns.

STANDARDS The use of appropriate intellectual standards (e.g., determining significance and relevance) guides you during the assessment phase of the nursing process so that you gather the data most pertinent to the patient's situation. Professional standards, including bioethical principles (see Chapter 5), the *Dying Person's Bill of Rights* (Box 25-3), the End-of-Life Nursing Consortium's basic and advanced curricula for end-of-life care (AACN, 2008), and clinical standards such as the guidelines for assessing pain in the nonverbal patient (Herr, Bjoro, and Decker, 2006) provide dependable information for expert symptom management and end-of-life care.

BOX 25-2   SYNTHESIS IN PRACTICE

 Before Jennifer meets the Kelly family for the first time, she reviews the information essential for making a thorough assessment. She identifies the key symptoms to look for in a person with end-stage heart disease with chronic pain and will be sensitive to any embarrassment Mrs. Kelly feels about her constipation and decreased functional abilities. Jennifer understands that people experience grief differently, and she anticipates that the members of the Kelly family may not agree on the plan of care.

Jennifer worries that she will be asked questions for which she has no answer. She feels more comfortable talking about heart disease than about end-of-life decisions and care. She knows that attitudes of humility and willingness to take risks will help her form helping, trusting relationships. If they ask her difficult questions about death or ask her to predict what will happen, Jennifer plans to use open-ended questions to explore the family members' concerns. She knows that she cannot "fix things" for the Kelly family, but she can assure them that they will have help. If family members share intense emotions, Jennifer will listen carefully and validate their feelings.

Jennifer will ensure that Mrs. Kelly's pain is well managed before asking about her other priorities for care. Jennifer knows that many families have never given end-of-life care, so she plans to provide teaching for their priority concerns. She anticipates that they may want to learn how to help Mrs. Kelly conserve her energy, give medications, assist with ambulation, and position her for comfort. Jennifer knows that above all, she will honor patient and family preferences, culture, and religious traditions during this meaningful event in the Kelly's family history.

NURSING PROCESS

■■■ ASSESSMENT

Begin with an open mind and accepting, humble attitude as you assess a patient or family experiencing a loss. The assessment process continues throughout the entire scope of your interactions. Be aware that your assumptions can interfere with making an accurate assessment of a patient or family unit. Do not assume that other people react to loss or grief as you do or that a particular behavior necessarily indicates grief. Crying, for example, expresses different feelings—grief, relief, sorrow, happiness, or gratitude. Encouraging patients to tell stories about their loved one or about what is happening gives them an opportunity to provide information in a natural, unstructured but meaningful way. Remain attuned to verbal and nonverbal communication as you ask questions and gather information about the way patients and family members seem to be handling their situation (Table 25-3).

Provide opportunities and safe places for patients and family members to talk about their feelings with others (Figure 25-1). To maintain confidentiality and encourage conver-

BOX 25-3 The Dying Person's Bill of Rights

- I have the right to be treated as a living human being until I die.
- I have the right to be in control.
- I have the right to maintain a sense of hopefulness, however changing its focus may be.
- I have the right to be cared for by those who can maintain a sense of hopefulness, however changing this might be.
- I have a right to have a sense of purpose.
- I have the right to express my feelings and emotions about my approaching death in my own way.
- I have the right to participate in decisions concerning my care.
- I have the right to expect continuing medical and nursing attention even though "cure" goals must be changed to "comfort" goals.
- I have the right not to die alone.
- I have the right to be free from pain.
- I have the right to have a respected spirituality.
- I have the right to have my questions answered honestly.
- I have the right not to be deceived.
- I have the right to have help from and for my family in accepting my death.
- I have the right to die in peace and dignity.
- I have the right to retain my individuality and not be judged for my decisions that may be contrary to beliefs of others.
- I have the right to discuss and enlarge my religious and/or spiritual experiences, whatever these may mean to others.
- I have the right to expect that the sanctity of the human body will be respected after death.
- I have the right to be cared for by caring, sensitive, knowledgeable people who will attempt to understand my needs and will be able to gain some satisfaction in helping me face my death.

Modified from Barbus AJ: The dying person's bill of rights, *Am J Nurs* 75:99, 1975; *Dying person's bill of rights*, 2004.

sation, talk to patients and family members separately unless they want to speak in each other's presence. Listen carefully, and observe the patient's responses and behaviors. Assume a neutral but interested perspective, and remain alert for nonverbal cues such as facial expressions, voice tones, and avoidance of certain topics. Collaborate with other members of the health care team to complete your assessment.

TYPE AND STAGES OF GRIEF Most people will exhibit some signs and symptoms of grief (Box 25-4). As you identify the type and/or stage of grief, your assessment becomes more specific. Application of a theorist's phase of grief will help you to assess a situation accurately. For example, a patient who complains of loneliness and difficulty falling asleep may be in a yearning or searching phase. To gather more data, ask questions such as, "When did the loss occur?" or "How long have you been feeling this way?" Ask patients to describe their losses and how their lives have changed. You will understand the patient's grief better by assessing in detail those factors that influence grieving (Table 25-4). Use information from appropriate specialty areas (e.g., spiritual health and family assessment) to better assess a patient's situation (see Chapters 20 and 23).

COPING RESOURCES Determine what coping patterns and resources a patient typically uses to get through difficult challenges. Use open-ended questions when you try to learn more about coping patterns: "Tell me how you usually adjust to change or loss." Use direct questioning to find out if certain activities (e.g., relaxation exercises, massage, meditation, reading, or exercise) help a patient cope with stress (see Chapter 24). Include some of those interventions in your care plan. Assess family members' coping patterns and methods too. If they are coping well, their care for the patient is enriched. A change in roles can become very stressful for a family member. For example, if the mother of a young child dies, the father must take on more parenting and household responsibilities. The child's relationship with the father changes when he becomes the primary source for love, discipline, and guidance. Refer the family to a nurse case manager, counselor, or social worker in a complicated situation such as this.

END-OF-LIFE DECISIONS Patients who have the capacity to make their own decisions determine their wishes for end-of-life care. Sometimes when a patient can no longer speak for himself or herself, family members must make stress-producing decisions on the patient's behalf. Their ability to make difficult decisions is helped when they have some understanding of the patient's wishes for end-of-life care and the use of life-sustaining medical interventions (Davis and others, 2005). **Advance directives** provide people with a means to communicate their health care wishes, including end-of-life care, when they can no longer participate in decision making (Dobbins, 2005). As part of your assessment, ask the patient if he or she has an advance directive or look for a copy in the patient's medical record. Some patients designate a durable power of attorney, a person who will make decisions for them if they cannot communicate. Find out who that person is. Most people, however, do not have an advance directive. Ask patients or family members about their prefer-

TABLE 25-3 FOCUSED PATIENT ASSESSMENT

FACTORS TO ASSESS	QUESTIONS	PHYSICAL ASSESSMENT
Phase of grief	Tell me how you are feeling now. Validate patient's feelings: You seem (angry/sad); tell me more about that . . . This can be a confusing time . . .	Observe patient's behaviors: 　Frequent sighing or crying 　Withdrawn behaviors (e.g., decreased communication, silence, does not want visits) 　Poor eye contact 　Unwilling to talk about feelings and disagreements
Family member's response to loss	It is so difficult to deal with these kinds of decisions. What do you think your wife is going through right now? What are *you* feeling right now? You feel guilt/sad/regret because . . . ? So you believe you could have changed what is happening?	Observe nonverbal behaviors as members of family interact: Tone of conversation Frequency of interaction Detachment behaviors (e.g., changing topic, walking away) Seeks physical closeness

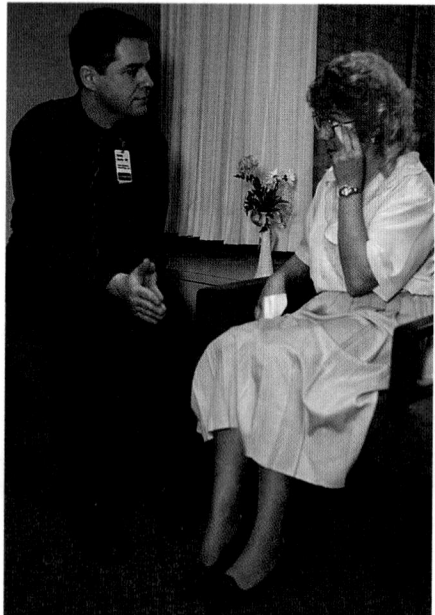

Figure 25-1 ■ Nurses use the resources of the interdisciplinary team for family member support.

ence for place for death, their wishes for the use of life-sustaining measures, and their expectations about pain control and symptom management (McSteen and Peden-McAlpine, 2006). If you feel uncomfortable in assessing a patient's wishes, find a health care team member (e.g., social worker or spiritual care provider) who has experience with discussing sensitive, complex issues. Remember that patients' cultural or religious beliefs often influence their wishes for end-of-life care.

PATIENT EXPECTATIONS A patient's perceptions and expectations for care will influence how you prioritize nursing diagnoses (Box 25-5). Carefully assess patients' and family members' expectations for nursing care. Attend to acute, distressing symptoms before attempting to have a discussion with a patient about his or her care expectations. For example, if a patient has severe pain, he or she will be less able to

identify other needs. Assess patient or family member expectations within the context of the loss by asking questions such as "What is the most important thing I could do to help you through this?" Ask family members if they understand the roles of other health care team members and offer clarification if necessary. Teno and others (2004) note that family members want their loved ones to get relief from pain and dyspnea and want health care providers to communicate with them in a way that helps them make good decisions. Early communication about expectations and goals provides clarity and helps prevent misunderstandings.

■■■ NURSING DIAGNOSIS

After reviewing and interpreting the data you have collected, identify the relevant nursing diagnoses, and cluster defining characteristics to identify the most applicable nursing diagnoses. Clustering data concerning patient or family behaviors, actual or potential losses, observed coping mechanisms, and information about the nature and meaning of the loss will lead to individualized nursing diagnoses. You need three or four defining characteristics to make an accurate diagnosis. Examples of nursing diagnoses frequently identified in situations of grief, loss, and end of life include the following:

- *Death anxiety*
- *Readiness for enhanced comfort*
- *Compromised family coping*
- *Ineffective denial*
- *Fear*
- *Grieving*
- *Hopelessness*
- *Risk for loneliness*
- *Social isolation*
- *Spiritual distress*
- *Readiness for enhanced spiritual well-being*

Next determine if competing diagnoses exist. For example, you may identify more than one nursing diagnosis for a patient who cries often, displays anger, and reports nightmares.

BOX 25-4   Symptoms of Normal Grief

FEELINGS
- Sadness
- Anger
- Guilt or self-reproach
- Anxiety
- Loneliness
- Fatigue
- Helplessness
- Shock/numbness (lack of feeling)
- Yearning
- Relief

COGNITIONS (THOUGHT PATTERNS)
- Disbelief
- Confusion
- Preoccupation about the deceased
- Sense of the presence of the deceased
- Hallucinations
- Hopelessness ("I'll never be OK again")

PHYSICAL SENSATIONS
- Hollowness in the stomach
- Tightness in the chest
- Tightness in the throat
- Oversensitivity to noise
- Sense of depersonalization ("Nothing seems real")
- Feeling short of breath
- Muscle weakness
- Lack of energy
- Dry mouth

BEHAVIORS
- Sleep disturbances
- Appetite disturbances
- Dreams of the deceased
- Sighing
- Crying
- Carrying objects that belonged to the deceased

TABLE 25-4   Assessment of Factors Influencing Grieving

FACTORS	AREAS/SUGGESTED QUESTIONS TO EXPLORE
Hope	Goals, worth, adaptations to future changes *Examples:* Tell me what you think about your treatment plan. What do you expect will happen to you? What do you most want to accomplish?
Nature of relationships	Functions of family, community, society *Examples:* How have you and your husband coped during other hospitalizations? Tell me about your relationship with _____. Will it change? I see you have lots of cards from church friends. Tell me about your church activities.
Social support system	Explore availability of health care workers, timing, family needs *Examples:* How do other people best give you help? Tell me about the family/friends who are available to help you. Tell me about the people you talk to about your _____.
Nature of loss	Actual versus perceived; death issues; impact on roles *Examples:* How is the loss affecting your daily life? What past experiences have you had with loss? Tell me how you usually cope with disappointment or loss.
Cultural and spiritual beliefs	Values, practices, beliefs, and attitudes are shaped by culture/religion *Examples:* What do you believe about death? Who makes health care decisions in your family/culture? Tell me about your family's/culture's funeral practices.
Personal life goals	Actual or perceived losses affect future decisions and options *Examples:* How will your life change as a result of your diagnosis/loss? How does this loss change your personal goals? Tell me what you know about advance directives.

These defining characteristics are common with *acute or chronic pain, ineffective coping,* and *spiritual distress.* Look for other behaviors and symptoms to validate your selection of an accurate nursing diagnosis.

Identify the appropriate related factor for each diagnosis. For example, *complicated grieving related to loss of the ability to walk due to lower limb paralysis* will require different interventions than *complicated grieving related to the loss of a*

BOX 25-5   BEST PRACTICES
Patients' and Family Members' Perceptions of Care at the End of Life

SUMMARY OF EVIDENCE

In palliative care, nurses base their planning and interventions on patient and family needs, perceptions, and priorities. Researchers have studied how patients in hospice perceive their care, what patients identify as their priority concerns when receiving palliative care, and family members' perspectives regarding their deceased loved ones' end-of-life care. Pevey (2005) asked patients if and how their hospice experience was comforting for them. All but 2 of the 38 patients interviewed had very positive experiences with hospice. One participant wanted a schedule to better predict the time when the hospice nurse would visit, and another patient needed help with a home maintenance problem. Participants identified good communication skills, opportunities for human contact, physical attention, competence, and practical assistance as comforting. Shah and others (2008) asked a group of palliative care patients, "What bothers you most?" Although 44% identified a physical problem, a majority of patients also mentioned one or more emotional, spiritual, relational, or existential concerns. Patients were distressed about loss of function and normalcy, had questions about the dying process, or were distressed by medical providers or treatments. Palliative care philosophy includes care for family members. After a patient dies, family members continue to remember their loved one's end-of-life care. Marco, Buderer, and Thum (2005) studied the responses of 969 family members whose loved ones had died. Overall, the respondents were satisfied with nursing, physician, and pastoral care. Most responded that caregivers honored patient and family wishes and their advance directives. Effective communication was identified as a major component of good palliative care.

APPLICATION TO NURSING PRACTICE
- Patients report high levels of satisfaction with hospice care. Nurses often explain the purposes of hospice to patients and family members. They may benefit from hearing that most people receive excellent care from hospice teams.
- Participants in the studies identify good communication skills as essential to providing comfort in end-of-life care. Human contact also brought comfort. Nurses must recognize the power of their presence with patients who are dying and their families.
- Patients experience a range of physical, emotional, social, spiritual, and existential symptoms. Their responses underscore the importance of providing holistic hospice and palliative care with interdisciplinary teams.
- Family members in one study believed it was important for caregivers to honor a patient's advance directives. Ask patients about their preferences for the use of life-sustaining interventions, and find out if they have any form of advance directive.

REFERENCES

Marco C, Buderer N, Thum D: End of life care: perspectives of family members of deceased patients, *Am J Hosp Palliat Med* 22(1):26, 2005.
Pevey C: Patient speaking: hospice patients discuss their care, *Am J Hosp Palliat Med* 22(2):129, 2005.
Shah M and others: "What bothers you most?" Initial responses from patients receiving palliative care consultation, *Am J Hosp Palliat Med* 25(2):88, 2008.

pregnancy. Clarification of the related factor will help you select appropriate interventions. Several related nursing diagnoses apply to patients who experience loss, grief, or death (Figure 25-2). In addition to diagnoses specific to grieving, you will likely diagnose problems related to the patient's physical or mental states.

■■■PLANNING

Plan your nursing care to meet the patient's and family members' physical, emotional, developmental, and spiritual needs, and select interventions to alleviate symptoms as much as possible (see Care Plan). Support the patient's self-esteem and autonomy by including him or her in care plan decisions. Patient preferences and priorities are of primary importance in planning end-of-life care.

GOALS AND OUTCOMES Establish realistic goals and expected outcomes based on the patient's nursing diagnoses. Consider the patient's available resources, such as supportive family members, methods for coping, spiritual beliefs, and physical energy when establishing goals of care. For example, if a terminally ill patient has the diagnosis of *powerlessness related to cancer diagnosis and treatment,* a goal of "Patient will discuss expected course of disease" will be realistic if the patient has accepted his diagnosis enough that he can talk about the disease without excessive anxiety. An expected outcome of "Patient will participate in series of short planned teaching discussions about disease" takes into account a patient's need for short, nonthreatening sessions to reduce uncertainty and anxiety.

Goals of care for a patient dealing with loss can be long- or short-term, depending on the nature of the loss and the nature of the patient's grief and how long the patient has to live. Because a patient sometimes moves back and forth between phases of grief, revise goals and outcomes with patient input to ensure they are still relevant. Some nursing care goals include accommodating grief, accepting the reality of a loss, and renewing relationships.

SETTING PRIORITIES When a patient has multiple nursing diagnoses, it is not possible to address all of them at the same time. Address the patient's most urgent physical or psychological needs first, and then gather information about the patient's expectations and preferences for prioritizing care. If the patient meets a high-priority goal, address other unmet needs. *For example, Mrs. Kelly (see Care Plan) now feels*

CONCEPT MAP

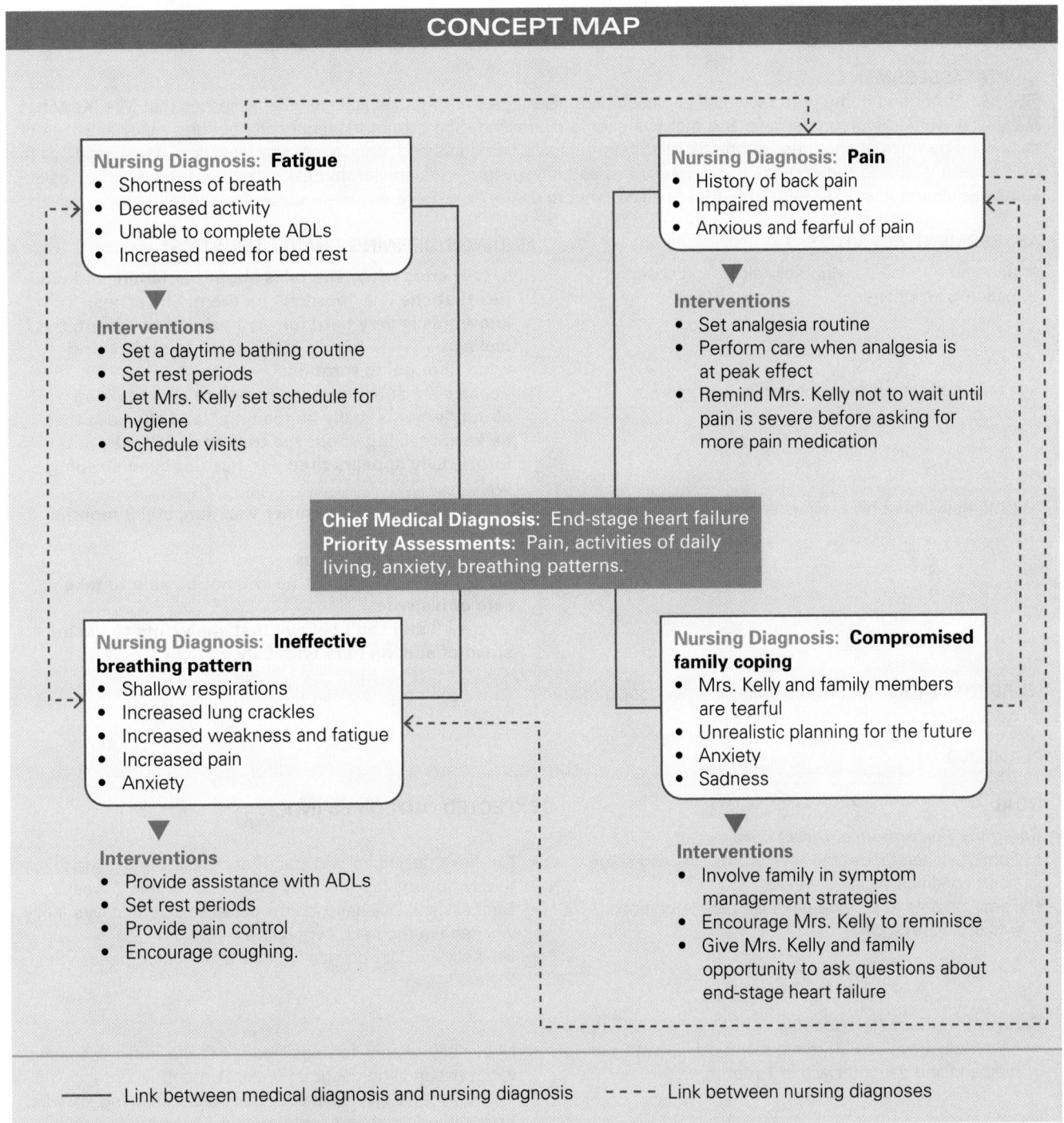

Nursing Diagnosis: Fatigue
- Shortness of breath
- Decreased activity
- Unable to complete ADLs
- Increased need for bed rest

Interventions
- Set a daytime bathing routine
- Set rest periods
- Let Mrs. Kelly set schedule for hygiene
- Schedule visits

Nursing Diagnosis: Pain
- History of back pain
- Impaired movement
- Anxious and fearful of pain

Interventions
- Set analgesia routine
- Perform care when analgesia is at peak effect
- Remind Mrs. Kelly not to wait until pain is severe before asking for more pain medication

Chief Medical Diagnosis: End-stage heart failure
Priority Assessments: Pain, activities of daily living, anxiety, breathing patterns.

Nursing Diagnosis: Ineffective breathing pattern
- Shallow respirations
- Increased lung crackles
- Increased weakness and fatigue
- Increased pain
- Anxiety

Interventions
- Provide assistance with ADLs
- Set rest periods
- Provide pain control
- Encourage coughing.

Nursing Diagnosis: Compromised family coping
- Mrs. Kelly and family members are tearful
- Unrealistic planning for the future
- Anxiety
- Sadness

Interventions
- Involve family in symptom management strategies
- Encourage Mrs. Kelly to reminisce
- Give Mrs. Kelly and family opportunity to ask questions about end-stage heart failure

—— Link between medical diagnosis and nursing diagnosis   - - - - Link between nursing diagnoses

Figure 25-2 ■ Concept Map. *ADLs,* Activities of daily living.

more secure using a walker, but she continues to have problems with constipation. Reassess her bowel pattern and frequency, and recommend dietary or medication changes. Base your goal setting and prioritization on the patient's expectations and preferences. If Mrs. Kelly wants comfort interventions and spiritual support rather than maintaining mobility, address her priority needs first.

COLLABORATIVE CARE End-of-life care draws on the resources of an interdisciplinary team. Social workers, spiri-

tual care providers, and psychologists have skills to help patients and family members deal with grief, anger, or depression. A pain management specialist can offer an individualized plan to address chronic pain. A coordinated team approach ensures that the patient's plan of care will be managed well and thoroughly addressed. When patients choose to go home for end-of-life care, home care and hospice nurses collaborate closely with family members and other health care providers to ensure continuity of care.

CARE PLAN   Loss and Grief

ASSESSMENT
At her first home visit 1 week after Mrs. Kelly's discharge from the hospital, Jennifer assesses that Mrs. Kelly has a worried look on her face and that she seems distressed. She cannot independently perform many activities of daily living because of shortness of breath. Mrs. Kelly eats small amounts and reports that she feels dizzy, weak, and "wobbly" when walking to the commode. Mrs. Kelly shares her feelings with Jennifer and asks many questions. When asked about her daughter, she replies, "She doesn't know what to do."

ASSESSMENT ACTIVITIES

Arrange time to talk to Mrs. Kelly alone and observe patient's emotions.

Ask Mrs. Kelly about how she thinks her family is doing.

Ask Mr. Kelly about his feelings and needs.

FINDINGS/DEFINING CHARACTERISTICS*

Mrs. Kelly **cries when she talks about her family and worries that she is a "burden" on them.** She states, **"I know this is very hard for my husband to accept, but I feel alone when people don't seem to understand what I am going through."**

She confides that her husband **seems to avoid talking about "what is really happening," and she says that he keeps talking about the trips they will take in the future. Lilly appears tired and has not been sleeping well.**

Talks about **plans for a summer vacation, still 9 months away.**

He appears **sad** and **anxious.**

He talks about **his fear that he will not be able to take care of his wife.**

He states, **"I still can't believe that she wants to die instead of staying here with Lilly and me."**

NURSING DIAGNOSIS: Compromised family coping related to stress of impending death of wife/mother.

PLANNING

GOAL

Caregiver Performance: Direct Care
- Family understands the symptoms of end-stage heart condition within 2 weeks.
- Family is able to provide palliative care interventions within 2 weeks.

Caregiver-Patient Relationship
- Mrs. Kelly develops affirming relationships with her husband and daughter within 1 month.

EXPECTED OUTCOMES (NOC)†

- Mr. Kelly describes end-stage heart disease and identifies the symptoms his wife may experience within 2 weeks.
- Mr. Kelly and Lilly describe the palliative care that Mrs. Kelly will need in the next 2 weeks.
- Mr. Kelly and Lilly provide hygiene and comfort needs within 2 weeks.

- Mrs. Kelly shares feelings about her life and relationship with husband and daughter within 1 month.
- Mr. Kelly and Lilly verbalize their understanding of Mrs. Kelly's need for their support within 1 month.

INTERVENTIONS (NIC)‡

Reminiscence Therapy
- Ask Mrs. Kelly to reminisce by sharing stories with her family.

- Discuss with Mr. Kelly and Lilly the value of reminiscence as part of looking back and evaluating life and its meaning.

RATIONALE

Encouraging patients to tell anecdotes and stories about events and people allows patients to sense life was meaningful and worth living (Meiner and Lueckenotte, 2006).

Engaging in this process will help move the family along the process of anticipatory grieving (Jenko and others, 2007).

***Defining characteristics** are shown in **bold** type.

†Outcomes classification label from Moorhead S and others, editors: *Nursing outcomes classification (NOC)*, ed 4, St. Louis, 2008, Mosby.

‡Intervention classification labels from Bulechek GM and others, editors: *Nursing interventions classification (NIC)* ed 5, St. Louis, 2008, Mosby.

CARE PLAN Loss and Grief—cont'd

INTERVENTIONS (NIC)‡	RATIONALE
Reminiscence Therapy **Caregiver Support** • Involve the Kelly family in a discussion about symptom recognition and management. • Offer the Kelly family a chance to ask questions about end-stage heart disease, the projected course of the condition, and Mrs. Kelly's wishes regarding the use of medications. • Explain that setting easily achievable goals helps give hope. Enlist family help to establish goals for the next week.	Even with a poor prognosis, social support and prompt symptom relief help maintain a higher quality of life (Green, 2006). Clarifying expectations better prepares individuals to face changes that will happen as the disease progresses (Hemani and Letizia, 2008; Mellar and others, 2005). Restructuring goals to be more short-term and achievable is a means of supporting and sustaining hope in terminally ill patients (Buckley and Herth, 2004).

EVALUATION

NURSING ACTIONS	PATIENT RESPONSE/FINDING	ACHIEVEMENT OF OUTCOME
Ask Mr. Kelly and Lilly about any changes they see in Mrs. Kelly.	Both note that Mrs. Kelly has less activity tolerance. She is able to rest with oxygen in place. They ask Mrs. Kelly about any pain more frequently instead of waiting until Mrs. Kelly states she is in pain.	Mr. Kelly and Lilly are more skillful in recognizing subtle symptoms in Mrs. Kelly's status, and they are more proactive in controlling her symptoms.
Observe family members' caregiving activities and their level of comfort and involvement in care. Ask Mrs. Kelly to describe her feelings after sharing stories and life review with family.	After 1 week, Mr. Kelly and Lilly note that they were more at ease with their care activities. After 2 weeks the Kelly family notices that they look forward to sharing these stories and are becoming at ease with Mrs. Kelly's decision and their role in palliative care.	Family continues to increase their knowledge of and ability to provide palliative care. Developing and strengthening the relationship between her husband and daughter remains ongoing.

■■■ IMPLEMENTATION

HEALTH PROMOTION A person experiencing grief needs support as he or she learns how to live with loss and move toward grief resolution. Persons facing significant disability, loss of body function, or even death want to achieve optimal physical and emotional well-being. Patients and family members will feel sadness or emotional turmoil along the way, but still want to cope with their life stressors. Nurses help patients learn how to deal with their loss, make effective decisions about their health care, and adjust to the disappointment, frustration, and anxiety created by their loss. Remember that with good care and support, patients at the end of life often experience high levels of wellness (Wayman and Gaydos, 2005).

PALLIATIVE CARE IN ALL SETTINGS

Palliative Care Interventions for patients with serious chronic illness or those near the end of life are based on a philosophy of total care called palliative care. **Palliative care** focuses on the prevention, reduction, or relief of physical, emotional, social, and spiritual symptoms of disease or treatment at the end of life when cure is no longer possible. People of any age or diagnosis can receive palliative care at any time and in any setting. Expert palliative care involves an interdisciplinary team composed of health care professionals—nurses, social workers, spiritual care professionals, nutritionists, physicians, psychologists, and pharmacists. Therapists who use complementary healing interventions (e.g., massage, music, healing touch, or aromatherapy) also work with palliative care teams (Mariano, 2006). The World Health Organization (2006) summarizes palliative care philosophy and practice as follows:

- Affirms life and regards dying as a normal process
- Neither hastens nor postpones death
- Provides relief from pain and other distressing symptoms
- Integrates psychological and spiritual aspects of patient care
- Offers a support system to help patients live as actively as possible until death
- Offers a support system to help families cope during the patient's illness and their own bereavement

- Enhances the quality of life
- Uses a team approach to meet the needs of patients and families

Above all, palliative care ensures that patients with advanced chronic illness or those near death receive care that is as free of avoidable pain and suffering as possible, in accord with the patient's and family's wishes, and reasonably consistent with clinical, cultural, and ethical standards (Kehl, 2006).

Hospice Care **Hospice** care provides services for patients who are at the end of life. Many people do not know about this option for care and will depend on you to explain hospice services and care philosophy to them (Mee, 2007). Patients who meet the criteria for hospice care generally have less than 6 months to live. Hospice teams provide care in many settings—home, hospital, or extended care facilities—and provide physical, emotional, and spiritual care for patients and family members. Hospice care focuses exclusively on palliative care interventions to relieve the symptoms and burdens of illness or treatment and help patients live as fully as possible until death. Nurses base hospice care on the patient's goals and support patient and family preferences for maintaining comfort and a high quality of life. Hospice programs are built on the following core beliefs and services:

- Patient and family as the unit of care
- Coordinated home care with access to inpatient and nursing home beds when needed
- Symptom management
- Physician-directed services
- Provision of an interdisciplinary care team
- Medical and nursing services available at all times
- Bereavement follow-up after a patient's death
- Use of trained volunteers for visitation and respite support

For a patient to receive home hospice care, a primary caregiver must be living in the home. The primary caregiver receives support from professional and volunteer hospice team members who are available 24 hours a day. At times, patients receiving home hospice care must go to the hospital for the management of acute symptoms. In this case, the hospice nurse coordinates care between the home and hospital settings. Figure 25-3 shows the relationship between palliative care and hospice.

Communicate Therapeutically Nurses giving palliative care must first develop a relationship of trust. Trust develops as you relate to patient and family members with an open, non-assuming communication style (Lowey, 2008). Open-ended questions invite patients to expand on their thoughts and tell their stories. Closed-ended questions usually lead patients to give short answers (yes or no) to your limited inquiry. Use active listening, learn to be comfortable with silence, and use prompts (e.g., "go on" or "tell me more") to encourage continued conversation. Verbally empathize with the patient's grief, and build a trusting relationship by offering your caring presence and using intentional, meaningful touch (Newman, 2008).

Some people resist invitations to talk about their feelings of loss or grief with others. Do not take personally a person's inability or lack of desire to communicate with you. Some people cope with stress and loss by talking things out, whereas others need to process their loss privately before they can talk to others. Cultural or gender expectations also influence the degree to which people talk about their loss. If a patient does not want to share his or her feelings or concerns, convey a willingness to be available if they want to talk later. If you are respectful of patients' personal or cultural values and their need for dignity, respect, and privacy, a therapeutic relationship will likely develop.

Grief brings out intense feelings such as anger, denial, depression, or guilt. People often take out their anger on family or caregivers or become demanding and accusing. Recall that denial, anger, and depression are normal reactions to loss. Reflect on how you react to people who exhibit intense feelings or negative behaviors. If you show fear or disappointment when people express intense emotions, they may not find it easy to confide in you at a later time. Offer support by saying, "I can see this is very upsetting to you. I just want you to know I am available to talk if you want." Avoid creating barriers to communication (see Chapter 10) such as denying the patient's grief, offering false reassurance, or offering unsolicited advice.

Do not avoid a topic that a dying patient wishes to discuss. When you sense that patients want to talk, find the time to listen. In a busy, acute care setting, you may have to reprioritize your responsibilities so you can talk to the patient when he or she is ready. Respond to questions openly and honestly. Provide information to help patients understand their condition, consider the benefits and burdens of treatment choices, and clarify their personal values and goals (Green, 2006; Griffie, Melson-Marten, and Muchka, 2004).

Promote Hope Hope is an energizing resource for patients experiencing loss. To help patients feel more hopeful remind them of their strengths and reinforce their expressions of courage, positive thinking, and realistic goal setting. Patients feel more hopeful when they have a sense of control. Offer information to patients about their illness, correct misinformation, and clarify patient's perceptions. Patients can behave in hopeful ways also. Help them practice healthy behaviors (e.g., enjoying meals, talking with friends, and getting

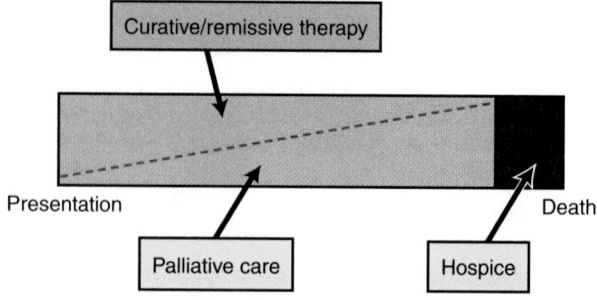

Figure 25-3 ■ Continuum of palliative and hospice care. (From Emanuel L, VonGunten C, Ferris F: *Education in Palliative and End of Life Care (EPEC) curriculum: The EPEC Project*, Chicago, 2003, Northwestern University Press.)

rest), and suggest that they develop a workable schedule for each day. People give hope to one another. Encourage patients to nurture important relationships. For patients near the end of life, set short-term, achievable goals and ask them to tell you about positive moments and achievements in their lives.

Facilitate Mourning Nursing interventions and communication strategies often help patients move through uncomplicated grief. The following care suggestions, based on Worden's theory of mourning (1982), relate to each task in the process of coping with a loss.

- *Help the patient accept that the loss is real.* Discuss how the loss or illness occurred or was discovered, when, under what circumstances, who told them about it, and other similar topics to help make the event more real and place it in perspective.
- *Support efforts to live without the deceased person or in the face of disability.* Ask patients or family members to list their concerns and prioritize them, and then facilitate a step-by-step discussion of how they will address each concern. Encourage them to rely on their support network of family members, friends, professionals, and community resources.
- *Encourage establishment of new relationships.* Some people fear that seeking new relationships devalues or disrespects their deceased loved one. Reassure them that this is not the case, and suggest that they begin by reaching out to others in welcoming groups (e.g., religious communities or volunteer activities).
- *Allow time to grieve.* Some people have "anniversary reactions" (heightened or renewed feelings of loss or grief) months or years after a loss. They worry that they are losing ground when signs of grief reappear after a period of relative calm. Offer reassurance that anniversary reactions are common, and encourage pleasant reminiscence.
- *Interpret "normal" behavior.* Common, "normal" grief responses, although often intense, do not mean a person has a mental or emotional disorder. Reinforce the understanding that people grieve differently and that those feelings resolve over time.
- *Provide continuing support.* Patients and their families will need to talk and may look to you for support for some time after a loss. If you have occasion to see the patient or family after an extended time, it is appropriate to ask them how they are doing after the loss. This gives them the opportunity to talk if they wish to and lets them know that their loved one is remembered.
- *Be alert for signs of ineffective coping.* Be on the alert for evidence of potentially harmful coping behaviors (e.g., alcohol or other substance abuse, excessive use of sleep aids or prescribed medications for anxiety or pain).

Manage Symptoms Expert palliative care focuses primarily on managing the distress caused by the unwanted symptoms of disease or treatments. Worry or fear concerning symptoms heightens a patient's perception of distress. Assess the character of the patient's symptoms carefully, and individualize therapies. For a detailed discussion of pain management, so vital for achieving high-level palliative care, see Chapter 31. Patients at the end of life commonly experience physical symptoms (e.g., pain, dyspnea, fatigue, urinary incontinence, or nausea), psychological symptoms (e.g., anxiety, fear, or depression), social symptoms (e.g., loneliness, isolation, or loss of community), and spiritual symptoms (e.g., hopelessness, despair, or loss of meaning). Pain medications, especially opioids, cause constipation, which can be very distressing for patients. A comprehensive care plan addresses those symptoms identified by the patient as most distressing. Extended discussions of evidence-based care interventions for managing symptoms in palliative care are available (Ferrell and Coyle, 2006; Matzo and Sherman, 2006). See Table 25-5 for a summary of the implications of commonly experienced symptoms.

Maintain Dignity and Self-Esteem Help patients maintain dignity and self-esteem by providing spiritual care (Chochinov, 2007) (see Chapter 20). You can also enhance patients' self-esteem by helping them maintain a pleasing physical appearance. Cleanliness, absence of body odors, attractive clothing, and personal grooming often elevate a patient's mood. Demonstrate respect, patience, and willingness when helping patients with toileting and bathing, especially as they become increasingly dependent on caregivers. Patients experience added grief and embarrassment when they can no longer tend to their basic needs. Include patients in making care decisions (e.g., how to perform personal hygiene, diet preferences, and timing of activities). Inform patients in advance about planned activities and their anticipated effects on the patient. Provide privacy while giving care, and give patients and family members quiet, uninterrupted time together.

Prevent Feelings of Abandonment and Isolation Many people fear dying alone. In hospitals or extended care facilities, answer patients' call lights promptly and assure them that caregivers are available throughout the day and night. Be readily available to answer questions or interpret changes in the patient's condition. Offer your calm, comforting presence, and use gentle touch when providing care (Coyle, 2006; Shubha, 2007). Unless family members need privacy or are remaining with the patient around the clock, avoid placing patients in a private room. Patients who are dying often feel a sense of involvement and companionship when sharing a room and have more opportunities to interact with staff and visitors.

Family members who are having difficulty accepting the patient's impending death sometimes avoid visits. When family members do come, reassure them that their presence is important and offer information about what the patient was talking about or has recently experienced. Encourage family members to discuss normal family activities, reminisce about enjoyable times, and ask about the patient's concerns. Suggest simple and appropriate tasks for family members to perform (e.g., offering help with meals, simple hygiene or comfort activities, or filling out a menu).

TABLE 25-5   Managing Symptoms in the Terminally Ill Patient

SYMPTOMS	CHARACTERISTICS OR CAUSES	NURSING IMPLICATIONS
Discomfort	Any source of physical irritation (e.g., dehydration, immobility) that causes pressure injuries and pain.	Provide thorough skin care, including daily baths, lubrication of skin, and dry, clean bed linens to reduce irritants (Pitorak, 2005).
	As patient approaches death, he or she breathes through the mouth, tongue becomes dry, and lips become dry and cracked.	Provide oral care at least every 2 to 4 hours.
		Use soft toothbrushes or foam swabs dipped in water for frequent mouth care. Apply a light film of petroleum jelly to lips and tongue (Stricker and Sullivan, 2003) (see Chapter 28).
	Blinking reflexes diminish near death; eyes often remain open, causing drying of cornea.	Gently remove crusts from eyelid margins.
		Artificial tears reduce corneal drying (Pitorak, 2005).
Fatigue	Increased metabolic demands, disease progression, pain, or declining heart function cause weakness and fatigue.	Help patient to identify valued or desired tasks; conserve energy for only those tasks. Assist with activities of daily living (Whitecar and others, 2004).
	Exhaustion phase of the general adaptation syndrome causes energy depletion.	Plan frequent rest periods in a quiet environment, and pace nursing care activities.
Nausea	Occurs as a side effect of medications, disease progression, or as a result of severe pain.	Give antiemetics: provide oral care at least every 2 to 4 hours; offer clear liquids and ice chips; avoid liquids that cause stomach acidity such as coffee, milk, and citrus juice.
Constipation	Opioid medications and immobility slow peristalsis.	Increase fluid intake or fiber intake if possible. Give prophylactic stool softeners (Economou, 2006).
	Lack of bulk in diet or reduced fluid intake occurs as appetite decreases.	
Diarrhea	Diarrhea results from some disease processes and side effects of medications.	Assess for fecal impaction.
		Confer with health care provider to change medication if possible.
		Provide low-residue diet.
Urinary incontinence	Incontinence results from disease progression, decreased level of consciousness.	Protect skin from irritation or breakdown. Change linens frequently.
		Use indwelling urinary catheter or condom catheters if indicated (Pitorak, 2005).
Decreased appetite	Decreased blood flow to the intestines at the end of life causes anorexia.	Give patient whatever food or fluids patient prefers. Do not force people to eat. Offer small portions of desired foods or home-cooked meals if patient prefers.
	Nausea and vomiting decrease appetite.	
Dyspnea or shortness of breath	Disease progression involves lung tissue (e.g., pneumonia, pulmonary edema).	Treat or control underlying cause.
	Anemia reduces oxygen-carrying capacity.	Maximize lung expansion and ease of breathing (e.g., position patient upright, provide supplemental oxygen if patient prefers; decrease anxiety or fever).
	Anxiety increases oxygen demands.	Give medications (e.g., bronchodilators, anxiolytics, inhaled steroids, opioids) to suppress cough and ease breathing (Wheeler, 2004; Whitecar and others, 2004).
	Fever increases oxygen demands.	Provide antipyretics as ordered.

Many people feel particularly lonely or fearful at night and may want a family member to stay with them. In acute care settings or extended care facilities, allow visitors to remain at all times with patients who are dying, and relax other visiting restrictions (e.g., visits from children and number of visitors) to accommodate the patient's circumstances. Know how to contact family members so they can be notified at any time if a patient wants to see them or if the patient's condition changes.

Provide a Comfortable and Peaceful Environment Promote patient comfort by repositioning, keeping bed linens dry, and controlling environmental noise. Keep the patient's immediate surroundings pleasant and clean. Open curtains so patients can experience the natural changes from day to night. Remove sources of unpleasant odors (e.g., stale food and used bedpans or emesis basins) promptly. Pictures, cherished objects, cards from friends and family, or plants create a comforting and familiar environment. Offer the patient frequent body massage, if desired, and provide opportunities for patients to hear their favorite music. Aromatherapy combined with massage can improve a patient's ability to sleep (Soden and others, 2004). A comfortable environment often

BOX 25-6   PATIENT TEACHING

Preparing the Dying Patient's Family

 Jennifer establishes a teaching plan for Mr. Kelly and Lilly to help them learn how to perform palliative care interventions.

OUTCOME

- At the end of the teaching session Mr. Kelly and Lilly will demonstrate ways to help Mrs. Kelly with activities of daily living, pain management, and mobility safety.

TEACHING STRATEGIES

- Describe and demonstrate techniques for helping a person experiencing fatigue to eat safely and select easily chewed and swallowed foods.
- Demonstrate bathing, mouth care, and other hygiene interventions, and allow family to perform a return demonstration.
- Show video on simple transfer techniques and use of walker to prevent injury to themselves and the patient. Observe family members practice the techniques.
- Describe ways the family can promote patient's comfort (e.g., frequent rest periods, giving massage, repositioning).
- Discuss medication purposes and side effects.
- Discuss ways to assess fatigue, bowel and bladder symptoms, and shortness of breath.
- Demonstrate how to assess pain, record pain intensity, and give medications.
- Teach family to recognize signs and symptoms of impending death and whom to call in an emergency and when death occurs.
- Invite questions from family, and provide information as needed.

EVALUATION STRATEGIES

- Observe Mr. Kelly and Lilly as they provide supportive care to Mrs. Kelly.
- Ask Mr. Kelly and Lilly to describe the purpose and dosage of pain medications and how frequently they administer them to Mrs. Kelly.
- Ask Mr. Kelly and Lilly to describe hospice services and who they will call when Mrs. Kelly dies.

BOX 25-7   Signs of Impending Death

- Minimal intake of food or water
- Increased sleeping and decreased consciousness
- Disorientation and restlessness
- Decreased urinary output and/or incontinence
- Cool hands and feet
- Noisy breathing
- Irregular breathing patterns with long pauses
- At the time of death, you will note:
  - Absence of breathing and heartbeat
  - Bowel and bladder release`
  - Unresponsiveness
  - Eyes fixed on a certain spot
  - Dilated pupils

helps patients relax, promotes sleep, and minimizes severity of symptoms.

Support Family Members   When a patient chooses to be at home at the end of life, family members become primary caregivers. Caring for a person dying at home, while rewarding, can also be emotionally and spiritually stressful and physically exhausting (Buck and McMillan, 2008). Family members benefit from education regarding the physical, emotional, and spiritual issues that often arise through each phase of the dying process (Box 25-6). They also need information about home care services, hospice, and community service resources. Hospice programs offer respite care for family caregivers to temporarily relieve them of their duties

so they can get needed rest and rejuvenation. In some cases, families will need assistance and support in making the difficult decision about nursing home placement.

Provide family members with a description of common symptoms the patient will likely experience, the signs and symptoms of impending death, and the implications for care (Box 25-7). Encourage family members to talk openly with their loved one to give everyone a chance to discuss lingering concerns or requests. Family members often appreciate the opportunity to share their concerns with you in private. As death approaches, encourage the use of silent vigil at the patient's bedside, touch, and verbal reassurances that the person is loved and not alone. After death, help family members notify the funeral home, family members, and friends who were not present at the bedside; arrange for safe transportation; and gather the patient's belongings.

Provide Care After Death   The nurse assumes responsibility for **postmortem care,** care of the body after death. Give postmortem care with dignity and sensitivity and in a manner consistent with the patient's religious or cultural beliefs. Because the body undergoes many physical changes after death, provide postmortem care as soon as possible to prevent tissue damage or disfigurement of body parts. For example, immediately after death, elevate the head of the bed to 30 degrees or place the head on pillows to prevent pooling of blood, which can discolor the face (Marthaler, 2005).

Be aware that federal and state legislation require that health care agencies formulate policies and procedures based on current laws to validate death, identify potential organ or tissue donors, request autopsy, and provide postmortem care. Following some deaths, family members will be asked to consent to an **autopsy,** the surgical dissection of a body after death to determine cause of death, how the person died, or to contribute to knowledge of the disease. State legislation determines when an autopsy must be obtained, usually in circumstances when death may have resulted from accident, homicide, or suicide. You will make some alterations in your care of the body after death if an autopsy is planned.

Provide a private area for the family to discuss organ donation. Professionals educated in organ procurement and transplant procedures (e.g., transplant coordinators, social workers, or spiritual care providers) make the first contact with family members regarding requests for donation of organs or tissues. They consider the family's personal, religious, and cultural needs and discuss what tissues or organs are suitable for transplant; offer a description of the process, costs, and impact of donation on funeral plans; and answer family members' questions. For example, many people do not understand "brain death." For their loved one to donate major organs (e.g., heart, lungs, and liver), the body must be kept in good functional condition so the organs will not become damaged before donation. The patient remains on a ventilator until his or her organs are removed. Family members often believe that the person is still alive because his or her heart is still beating. Be available to reinforce explanations of the organ retrieval process during this most stressful, tragic time. Nonvital tissues such as corneas, skin, long bones, and middle ear bones can be removed at the time of death without maintaining vital functions. If the patient left no communication regarding his or her preferences for organ donation, family members make that decision with support and conversation. Review your state's laws regarding organ retrieval and the formal consent process.

Nurses coordinate all aspects of care surrounding a patient's death. Box 25-8 summarizes the steps in providing postmortem care. If a hospitalized patient dies while in a semiprivate room, transfer the other patient temporarily to another room to provide privacy for the deceased patient and family and avoid exposing the roommate to the stressors related to postmortem care. Use postmortem care guidelines to make the body appear as natural and comfortable as possible.

After a patient's death, shift your care to surviving family members. Make all appropriate resources available to them. They may want their family priest, minister, or rabbi to be with them, or they may appreciate the presence of the spiritual care staff at the health care agency. Social workers and counselors also offer valuable support. Remember that this is a very stressful but important event in this family's history. Do all you can to help things proceed calmly and smoothing, facilitate family members' requests, attend to their needs, and always ask them about their preferences. Some family members prefer to be left alone and are unable to talk about the event until they have processed it privately.

Nurses must carefully document all of the activities surrounding a death to provide an accurate record of the final events of the patient's life. Your complete and accurate summary of activities may be used for risk management or legal investigations. Include in your documentation the time and date of death, the name of the health care provider who pronounces the death, organ or tissue donation status (e.g., request made and donation decision), preparation of the body, medical devices left in or on the body, valuables or belongings left with the patient (e.g., dentures, glasses, or wedding ring) or given to the family (e.g., clothing, mail, or photographs), the time of discharge, and destination of the body (e.g., morgue at the agency or funeral home). Become familiar with the policies and procedures for postmortem care

used in your agency, and be sure your care and documentation reflect those guidelines.

▪▪▪EVALUATION

PATIENT CARE Nurses care for patients and families throughout a grief experience. You learn to recognize the behaviors and symptoms of a grief response. Use your observations of behaviors and symptoms as criteria for evaluating how the patient or family member is coping with loss and progressing through the grief process. Critical thinking ensures that the evaluation process is thorough and relevant to the patient's situation.

Refer to the goals and expected outcomes in your care plan, and use evaluative indicators to identify actual patient behaviors. Compare the actual behaviors with expected outcomes to determine the patient's progress and to make care plan revisions, as needed. For example, if the goal is to have a patient share her feelings about death through reminiscing, you evaluate her verbal and nonverbal communication for cues that reflect normal grieving and healthy coping. Your patient's responses will determine if the problem is resolving, if the patient needs new interventions, or if you need to revise existing strategies. Include patients and family members as active participants in the evaluation process (Box 25-9).

PATIENT EXPECTATIONS Maintain open lines of communication with patients so they will feel free to evaluate their nursing care honestly. Patients who have developed a good relationship with a nurse will comfortably discuss their perceptions of care and ask for what they need to improve care. Consider it a sign of a trusting relationship when a patient or family member offers feedback or suggestions for improving care. When providing end-of-life care, ask often about patient and family satisfaction. Revise the care plan to include changing patient needs or requests for a different approach. Similarly, be encouraged when patients or family members tell you that the care plan is helping them achieving their established goals.

NURSES' SELF-EVALUATION Nurses who care for patients at the end of life and their family members often find their work to be very fulfilling and rewarding. Experiencing repeated deaths of patients with whom you develop a close connection, however, can feel overwhelming at times. Nurses grieve, too. Frequently evaluate your own emotional well-being. We all carry with us feelings and memories about previous illnesses and death. Use self-reflection, a critical thinking activity, or journaling to consider if your personal sadness is related to a patient or to an unresolved personal experience from your past. Knowing more about your own grief and past experiences will help you care for others more insightfully.

If you work in an area in which you experience multiple losses and fail to acknowledge your own feelings of loss, you may begin to feel overwhelmed by intense emotions (e.g., frustration, anger, guilt, sadness, or dissatisfaction with life). Being a professional caregiver involves knowing when to get away from a situation and how best to take care of one's self. Many nurses, especially those who routinely provide hospice

BOX 25-8 Care of the Body After Death

HEALTH CARE PROVIDER RESPONSIBILITIES

1 Certify the time of death and the actions taken.
2 Request an autopsy, especially under unusual circumstances.
3 A staff member educated in making requests for organ and tissue donation discusses with family the donation options.

NURSE RESPONSIBILITIES

1 Provide care with dignity and sensitivity to the patient and family members. Place the patient in a supine position and elevate the head 30 degrees or elevate with pillows to prevent discoloration of the face as you prepare for and complete postmortem care.
2 Check orders for any specimens to be collected or special postmortem instructions, such as autopsy or retrieval of donated tissues.
3 Ask family members if and how they would like to help care for the body. Make arrangements for a member of the professional staff (e.g., spiritual care provider) to stay with family members if they do not wish to participate in body care. Ask family members if they have any special requests for body preparation (e.g., shaving, a special gown, Bible or rosary with the body).
4 Ask family about shaving male facial hair. Some cultures or religions prohibit shaving facial hair or cutting hair.
5 Remove all catheters, tubes, or indwelling devises from the patient's body, except in the case of autopsy. In that case, leave medical devices in place. Remove medical equipment, supplies, and dirty linens from the room to create a clean, natural environment.
6 Cleanse the body thoroughly, keeping the head of the bed elevated; apply clean sheets.
7 Brush and comb patient's hair. Apply patients' hairpieces, if possible, for natural appearance.
8 Position according to protocol. Close eyes gently by holding eyelids down briefly. Some cultural groups prefer that the eyes remain open. Dentures remain in the mouth to maintain facial alignment.
9 Cover the body with a clean sheet up to the chin with arms outside covers if possible.
10 Lower the lighting and reduce unpleasant odors as able.
11 Give family members an opportunity to view the body, and accompany them to the bedside. Some will not want to view their dead loved one, so make it clear that either choice is acceptable.
12 Encourage the family to say goodbye with words and touch.
13 Do not rush the process of family visitation and body viewing. Once the family is more comfortable, *ask* if they would like to be left alone. Tell them how to find you easily.
14 Ask which personal belongings remain with or on the body. Give remaining personal items to a family member, and document a description of the item and the date and time you transferred the belongings to the family's possession.
15 Do not throw away any personal belongings accidentally left behind by the family. Call a family member to describe the item(s) and arrange for someone to retrieve the items they want to keep.
16 Apply name tags to the body according to agency protocol, usually on the right big toe, and/or outside a shroud before transporting the body. Clearly mark the outside of the shroud if the body presents an isolation or contamination risk.
17 Document all care in the nursing notes.
18 Remain sensitive to other hospitalized patients or visitors when transporting the body. Cover the body with a clean sheet and avoid moving the body past groups of visitors when transporting the body to the morgue or funeral home.
19 Follow all agency protocols and policies, and comply with national or state laws regarding end-of-life issues.

BOX 25-9 EVALUATION

 Two weeks after discussing her plan of care with the Kelly family, Jennifer observes Mr. Kelly helping his wife with her bath. He explains that Lilly is "taking a break to catch up on her schoolwork." Mr. Kelly has obtained a walker, and Mrs. Kelly states that she feels less afraid of walking now. Walking relieves the back pain that has become worse with bed rest. Mrs. Kelly explains that she and Lilly have enjoyed looking through old photo albums together, and yesterday Mr. Kelly "wanted to join in the fun, too." Mr. Kelly tells Jennifer that his wife's constipation is not worse, but she still reports problems with it. He carefully records her pain medication schedule and frequency of bowel movements. He also tells Jennifer that he and his daughter have received information about a support group for family caregivers sponsored by the hospital's palliative care service.

DOCUMENTATION NOTE

"Uses walker to ambulate in the home. States she feels more secure. Husband involved in bathing and interaction with patient. Husband and daughter working together in care activities. Bath in progress at time of visit. Skin has no redness, tenderness, or evidence of tissue breakdown. Continues to have problems with constipation. Assessed current bowel medication regimen and bowel movement frequency. States has some constant back pain, but current pain medication keeps in control. Sleeps well at night, waking once a night for pain meds. Family contacted palliative care team regarding support group."

care, attend a viewing at the mortuary or the funeral to show support for the family, honor the deceased's memory, and cope with their own grief. As a caregiver, you were an important part of the patient's story at a very meaningful time of life. Develop your own support systems, take restful time away from your work, and find a person with whom you can safely share your feelings and concerns. Stress management techniques (e.g., meditation, yoga, deep breathing, or healing touch) will help to restore your energy and enjoyment in your work.

KEY POINTS

- The type of loss and the meaning of the loss influence how a person experiences and expresses grief.
- Theorists describe grief as a series of stages, phases, processes, or tasks experienced by people as they adapt to loss and move on with life.
- Individuals move back and forth through the theoretical stages, phases, or tasks of grieving or experience them simultaneously over a period of time, often several years.
- Knowing specific types of grief helps develop an effective plan of care.
- A person's age, developmental stage, beliefs, roles, culture, relationships, and socioeconomic status influence reactions to loss and expressions of grief.
- When assessing patients experiencing grief or loss, do not make assumptions about how you think they behave or feel. Ask patients to share their experience in their own words and tell their stories.
- Therapeutic communication fosters the development of trust and provides an opportunity for patients and family members talk about their concerns.
- Nursing care of a grieving or dying patient focuses on enhancing the patient's sense of identity, dignity, and self-esteem and maintaining the highest possible quality of life.
- Patients of any age or diagnosis benefit from palliative care at any time in the course of their illness.
- Palliative and hospice care principles include involving patients and family members in determining the plan of care; helping patients make informed choices; providing relief for physical, emotional, or spiritual symptoms; and offering support from an interdisciplinary team.
- Provide education and opportunities for family members who want to be involved in end-of-life care.
- Care of a body after death and care for surviving family members are provided with respect and sensitivity for their preferences, culture, and/or religion and based on evidence-based protocols and standards.
- Base your ongoing evaluation of nursing care on identifiable behaviors and communication.
- Nurses benefit from acknowledging and attending to their own grief when caring for dying patients and their family members.

CRITICAL THINKING EXERCISES

Two months have passed, and Mrs. Kelly is approaching death. She is having increased pain, weakness, confusion, and eats very little. She requires increased doses of pain medication. She becomes fatigued easily and speaks only in short sentences. Mrs. Kelly is receiving home hospice care, and Mr. Kelly and Lilly are the primary care providers. Mr. Kelly says to Jennifer, "This is happening so fast. I don't know what to expect next. Do you think she will get better again for a while?"

1. Mr. Kelly indicates that he does not know what to expect in the final phase of his care for his wife. What assessments should Jennifer make to help her design a teaching intervention to help Mr. Kelly?

2. Identify the four tasks of mourning, according to Worden, that might best explain Mr. Kelly's experience at this time. Discuss how a grieving patient might act in this phase and how the nurse provides support.

3. What is the best response to Mr. Kelly's question: "Do you think she will get better again for a while?"
   a. "In reality, she has had heart disease for a very long time. This has been a slow process for her."
   b. "It's hard to find meaning in an illness like this. This must be very difficult for you."
   c. "Are the hospice nurses helping her get out of bed every day?"
   d. "Have you been able to record your wife's pain medications accurately? Maybe she is sleeping because she has had too much medication."

4. Identify a goal of care and expected outcome for Mr. Kelly and Lilly as primary caregivers.

ⓔvolve *Answers to Critical Thinking Questions can be found on the Evolve website.*

REVIEW QUESTIONS

1. How should the nurse best determine end-of-life care activities and priorities?
   1. Learn about preferences by listening to the patient and by asking questions.
   2. Guide the selection of priorities by offering advice based on your experiences.
   3. Rely primarily on close family members to make decisions for the patient.
   4. 1, 2, and 3

2. Which of the following statements best illustrates the bargaining stage of loss?
   1. "I have always taken such good care of my health. This isn't fair!"
   2. "If I get over this cancer, I'll never smoke again."
   3. "It doesn't really matter what happens anymore."
   4. "I don't think my disease is really as serious as they say."

3. Place the following postmortem care activities in the correct order.
   1. Bathe the body.
   2. Ask family members if they wish to participate in care.
   3. Elevate the head of the bed, or place patient's head on pillows.
   4. Ask if an autopsy will be done on the body.
   5. Place identification tags on the body.

4. Which of the following nursing diagnoses is most appropriate for a patient recently diagnosed with a serious, life-limiting disease who withdraws from others, stops taking his medications, and repeatedly states that he sees no reason to go on living?
   1. *Complicated grieving*
   2. *Anxiety*
   3. *Risk for loneliness*
   4. *Spiritual distress*

5. A patient's wife asks you to explain hospice services to her. What points would you include in your teaching? Select all that apply.
   1. Hospice care must be given in the home.
   2. People who are likely to have less than 6 months to live may be eligible for hospice care.
   3. Hospice care is designed to meet the needs of cancer patients exclusively.
   4. You may continue to receive treatments to cure your disease while receiving hospice care.
   5. Hospice interventions focus on providing symptom relief and maintaining a high quality of life.
   6. A person may not be admitted to the hospital while on hospice care.
   7. A person eligible for hospice receives care from an interdisciplinary team and volunteers.

6. A patient who is near the end of life tells you that she no longer feels hungry but does not want to disappoint her daughter by not eating the home-cooked foods her daughter prepares. How should you respond?
   1. "Could you eat just a little, tell your daughter that you love the food but you will eat it later?"
   2. "Tell me about your decreased appetite. Do you have nausea or stomach pain, too?"
   3. "It sounds like your relationship with your daughter is very important to you. Tell me more about it."
   4. "Your daughter is trying to show you she cares about you. She probably feels pretty helpless."

7. How can the nurse best apply knowledge of grief theories to the care of patients?
   1. Use theoretical knowledge to better understand the grief and loss experience.
   2. Select a theory that best applies to a particular patient, and teach the patient about it.
   3. Use theories to predict how long a person will stay in each phase of grief.
   4. If you can identify the stages of loss, you can determine where that person is in his or her grief experience.

8. Mr. R is a 49-year-old hospitalized patient who has recently been diagnosed with advanced pancreatic cancer. You enter the room and notice he is staring out the window. He does not acknowledge your presence, nor does he respond to you when you greet him. What should you do?
   1. Encourage him until he talks to you, knowing that people are helped when they share their feelings with others.
   2. Go about your activities, and quickly leave the room without saying anything.
   3. Try to cheer him up by reminding him that his family is coming soon to visit.
   4. Briefly acknowledge that this must be a difficult time for him, and assure him that you are available to help in any way you can.

9. Mr. R was raised in a culture in which males should be touched or bathed only by female caregivers. Now that his strength is declining, Mr. R needs help with all activities of daily living. There are more male caregivers scheduled for a shift than female caregivers. How would you proceed when making patient care assignments?
   1. Inform Mr. R that a male nurse will be caring for him to keep the assignments fair, but assure him that that this nurse will provide excellent care.
   2. Honor the patient's cultural values, and be sure that a female nurse performs activities that involve bodily contact.
   3. Discuss with Mr. R the importance of not making distinctions based on gender, and explain that both males and females work as nurses and should be treated equally.

4. Tell him that he should get a family member to take care of him if he does not want to comply with routine practices in this hospital and culture.

10. Mr. R reports abdominal pain. You also note that he is taking an opioid pain medication and that he has had decreased fluid intake for 2 days. What action would you take first based on this information?

1. Call the doctor to see if abdominal pain could be related to his cancer.

2. Encourage Mr. R to drink more fluids and increase his activity.

3. Further assess Mr. R's pain and bowel movement patterns.

4. Administer an as-needed (prn) medication for constipation.

Answers to Review Questions can be found on pages 1197-1198.

REFERENCES

American Association of Colleges of Nursing, City of Hope: *ELNEC-Core: End-of-life Nursing Education Consortium (Core)*, Duarte, Calif, 2008, The Authors.

Barbus AJ: The dying person's bill of rights, *Am J Nurs* 75:99, 1975.

Blum C: "Till death do us part?" The nurse's role in the care of the dead: a historical perspective—1850-2004, *Geriatr Nurs* 27(1):58, 2006.

Bowlby J: *Attachment and loss*,vol 3, *Loss, sadness, and depression*, New York, 1980, Basic Books.

Buck H, McMillan S: The unmet spiritual needs of caregivers of patients with advanced cancer, *J Hosp Palliat Nurs* 10(2):91, 2008.

Buckley J, Herth K: Fostering hope in terminally ill patients, *Nurs Stand* 19(10):33, 2004.

Bulechek GM and others, editors: *Nursing interventions classification (NIC)*, ed 5, St. Louis, 2008, Mosby.

Campbell C: Respect for persons: engaging African Americans in end-of-life research, *J Hosp Palliat Nurs* 9(2):74, 2007.

Chochinov H: Dying, dignity and new horizons in palliative end of life care, *CA Cancer J Clin* 56(2):84, 2007.

Chochinov H, Cann B: Interventions to enhance the spiritual aspects of dying, *J Palliat Med* 8(1):S103, 2005.

Clements P and others: Cultural perspectives on death, grief, and bereavement, *J Pychosoc Nurse Ment Health Serv* 41(7):18, 2003.

Corless I: Bereavement. In Ferrell B, Coyle N, editors, *Textbook of palliative nursing*, New York, 2006, Oxford University Press.

Coyle N: The hard work of living in the face of death, *J Pain Symptom Manage* 32(3):266, 2006.

Davis B and others: Family stress and advance directives, *J Hosp Palliat Nurs* 7(4):219, 2005.

Delgado C: Coherence, spirituality, stress, and quality of life in chronic illness, *J Nurs Scholarsh* 39(3):229, 2007.

Dobbins E: Helping your patient to a "good death, *Nurs J Clin Excel* 35(2):43, 2005.

Doorenbos A, Wilson S, Coenen A: A cross-cultural analysis of dignified dying, *J Nurs Scholarsh* 38(4):352, 2006.

Dying person's bill of rights, 2004, http://learningplaceonline.com/stages/together/dying-rights.htm.

Economou D: Bowel management: constipation, diarrhea, obstruction and ascites. In Ferrell B, Coyle N, editors: *Textbook of palliative nursing*, ed 2, New York, 2006, Oxford University Press.

Egan K, Arnold R: Grief and bereavement care, *Am J Nurs* 103(9):42, 2003.

Emanuel L, VonGunten C, Ferris F: *Education in palliative and end of life care (EPEC) curriculum: the EPEC Project*, Chicago, 2003, Northwestern University.

Ferrell B, Coyle N, editors: *Textbook of palliative nursing*, ed 2, New York, 2006, Oxford University Press.

Green A: A person-centered approach to palliative care nursing, *J Hosp Palliat Nurs* 8(5):293, 2006.

Griffie J, Melson-Marten P, Muchka S: Acknowledging the elephant in the room: communication in palliative care, *Am J Nurs* 104(1):48, 2004.

Hattori K, McCubbin M, Ishida D: Concept analysis of good death in the Japanese community, *J Nurs Scholarsh* 38(2):141, 2006.

Hemani S, Letizia M: Providing palliative care in end-stage heart failure, *J Hosp Palliat Nurs* 10(2):100, 2008.

Herr K, Bjoro K, Decker S: Pain assessment in the nonverbal patient: position statement with clinical practice recommendations, *J Pain Symptom Manage* 31(2):170, 2006.

Hooyman N, Kramer B: *Living through loss: interventions across the lifespan*, New York, 2006, Columbia University Press.

Jenko M, Moffitt S: Transcultural nursing principles, *J Hosp Palliat Nurs* 8(3):173, 2006.

Jenko M and others: Life review with the terminally ill, *J Hosp Palliat Nurs* 9(3):159, 2007.

Kehl K: Moving toward peace: an analysis of the concept of a good death, *Am J Hosp Palliat Med* 23(4):277, 2006.

Kemp C: Cultural issues in palliative care, *Semin Oncol Nurs* 21(1):44, 2005.

Kikuchi J: Cultural theories of nursing responsive to human needs and values, *J Nurs Scholarsh* 37(4):302, 2005.

Kübler Ross E: *On death and dying*, New York, 1969, Macmillan.

Lowey S: Communication between the nurse and family caregiver in end of life care: a review of the literature, *J Hosp Palliat Nurs* 10(1):35, 2008.

Marco C, Buderer N, Thum D: End of life care: perspectives of family members of deceased patients, *Am J Hosp Palliat Med* 22(1):26, 2005.

Mariano C: Holistic integrative therapies in palliative care. In Matzo J, Sherman D, editors: *Palliative care nursing: quality care to the end of life*, New York, 2006, Springer.

Marthaler M: End of life care: practical tips, *Dimens Crit Care Nurs* 24(5):215, 2005.

Matzo M, Sherman D: *Palliative care nursing: quality care to the end of life*, New York, 2006, Springer.

McSteen K, Peden-McAlpine C: The role of the nurse as advocate in ethically difficult care situations with dying patients, *J Hosp Palliat Nurs* 8(5):259, 2006.

Mee C: Hospice care, *Nursing* 37(11):43, 2007.

Meiner SE, Lueckenotte AG: *Gerontologic nursing*, ed 3, St. Louis, 2006, Mosby.

Mellar P and others: Palliation of heart failure, *Am J Hosp Palliat Med* 22(3):211, 2005.

Moorhead S and others, editors: *Nursing outcomes classification (NOC)*, ed 4, St. Louis, 2008, Mosby.

Murray SA and others: Exploring the spiritual needs of people dying of lung cancer or heart failure: a prospective qualitative interview study of patients and their carers, *Palliat Med* 18(1):39, 2004.

Newman M: *Transforming presence*, Philadelphia, 2008, FA Davis.

Nowotny M: Every tomorrow a vision of hope, *J Psychosoc Oncol* 9(3):117, 1991.

Pevey C: Patient speaking: hospice patients discuss their care, *Am J Hosp Palliat Med* 22(2):129, 2005.

Pitorak E: Care at the time of death, *Home Healthc Nurs* 23(5):318, 2005.

Rando T: *Treatment of complicated mourning*, Champaign, Ill, 1993, Research Press.

Rosenfeld and others: Are there racial differences in attitudes toward hospice care? A study of hospice-eligible patients at the Visiting Nurse Service of New York, *Am J Hosp Palliat Med* 24(5):408, 2007.

Shah M and others: "What bothers you most?" Initial responses from patients receiving palliative care consultation, *Am J Hosp Palliat Med* 25(2):88, 2008.

Shubha CT: Psychological issues in end of life care, *J Psychosoc Nurs* 45(8):25, 2007.

Soden K and others: A randomized controlled trial of aromatherapy massage in hospice setting, *Palliat Med* 18(2):87, 2004.

Stricker CT, Sullivan J: Evidence-based oncology oral care practice guidelines: development implementation and evaluation, *Clinic J Oncol Nurs* 7(2):222, 2003.

Teno J and others: Family perspectives on end-of-life care at the last place of care, *JAMA* 291(1):88, 2004.

Wayman L, Gados H: Self-transcending through suffering, *J Hosp Palliat Nurs* 7(5):52, 2005.

Weigel C and others: Apprehension among hospital nurses providing end of life care, *J Hosp Palliat Nurs* 9(2):86, 2007.

Wheeler M: Palliative care is more than pain management, *Home Healthc Nurs* 22(4):251, 2004.

Whitecar P and others: Principles of palliative care medicine. II. Pain and symptom management, *Johns Hopkins Adv Studies Med* 4(2):8, 2004.

Worden JW: *Grief counseling and grief therapy*, New York, 1982, Springer.

World Health Organization: *Palliative care*, 2006, http://www.who.int/hiv/topics/palliative/care/en.

Exercise and Activity

26

MEDIA RESOURCES

 CD COMPANION 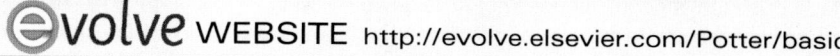 **evolve WEBSITE** http://evolve.elsevier.com/Potter/basic

- Video Clips
- Crossword Puzzle
- English/Spanish Audio Glossary

OBJECTIVES

- Describe the role of the skeleton, skeletal muscles, and nervous system in the regulation of movement.
- Discuss physiological and pathological influences on body alignment and joint mobility.
- Assess patients for impaired body alignment, exercise, and activity.
- Formulate nursing diagnoses for patients experiencing problems with exercise and activity.

- Write a nursing care plan for a patient with impaired body alignment and activity.
- Describe the interventions for maintaining proper alignment, assisting a patient in moving up in bed, repositioning a patient needing assistance, and transferring a patient from a bed to a chair.
- Evaluate the nursing care plan for maintaining body alignment and activity.

KEY TERMS

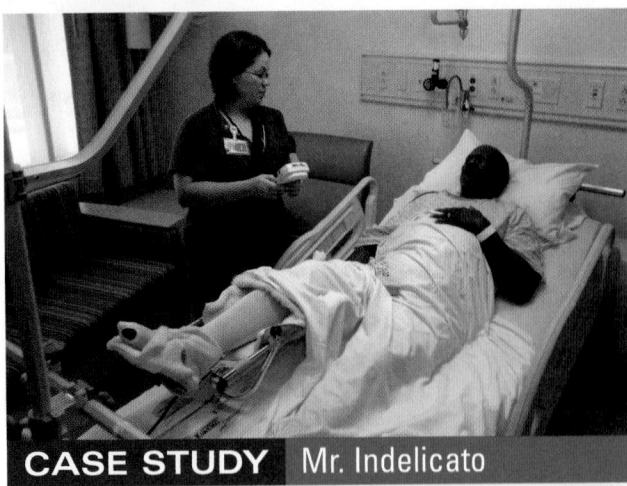

CASE STUDY   Mr. Indelicato

Mr. Indelicato is a 72-year-old African American who is hospitalized for surgery on his right knee. His general level of health is good. He does not have any underlying chronic illnesses. He relates the problem with his knee to previous sports injuries. He repeatedly "twisted the knee" while playing racquetball and knows that he hurt his knee at least six times over the last 30 years while playing the sport. He first sought medical advice and treatment about 6 years ago. His last injury to his knee was approximately "5 or 6 years ago, and it hasn't worked the same since." He has tried various treatments, including physical therapy, rest, and pain medication. His only preoperative medication is ibuprofen 600 mg every 6 to 8 hours. He has not taken his ibuprofen for the past few days because of the impending surgery. He wants the surgery so he can get back to being active. He and his wife are very active and enjoy golf, tennis, and bike riding. Mr. Indelicato's wife is in good health as well.

Marilyn Sweeney is a 40-year-old nursing student. She has just finished rotating through a general surgical unit and is spending the remaining 6 weeks in the orthopedic/rehabilitation division of the agency. Her assignment is to follow this patient through his surgery and rehabilitation.

The actions of walking, turning, lifting, or carrying are all common in the provision of nursing care. Such activities require muscle exertion. Know and practice proper body mechanics, and remain knowledgeable of current research, standards, and guidelines concerning safe transfer and positioning techniques to reduce the risk for injury (Box 26-1). This includes knowledge of the actions of various muscle groups, understanding of the factors involved in the coordination of body movement, and familiarity with the integrated functioning of the skeletal, muscular, and nervous systems.

SCIENTIFIC KNOWLEDGE BASE

The coordinated efforts of the musculoskeletal and nervous systems to maintain balance, posture, and body alignment during lifting, bending, moving, and performing activities of daily living provide the foundation for body mechanics. Proper implementation of these activities decreases the risk for musculoskeletal system injury and allows physical mobility without muscle strain and excessive use of muscle energy.

Body Alignment

Body alignment refers to the relationship of one body part to another body part along a horizontal or vertical line. Correct alignment reduces strain on musculoskeletal structures, maintains adequate **muscle tone,** and contributes to balance.

Body Balance

You achieve body balance when you balance a relatively low **center of gravity** over a wide, stable base of support. A vertical line falls from the center of gravity through the base of support. The base of support is the foundation. When the vertical line from the center of gravity does not fall through the base of support, the body loses balance.

Posture also enhances body balance. The term **posture** means maintaining optimal body position. It means a position that most favors function, requires the least muscular work to maintain, and places the least strain on muscles, ligaments, and bones (Thibodeau and Patton, 2007).

Maintain proper body alignment and posture by using two simple techniques. First, widen your base of support by separating your feet to a comfortable distance. Second, bring the center of gravity closer to your base of support to increase balance. You achieve this by bending the knees and flexing the hips until squatting and maintaining proper back alignment by keeping the trunk erect.

Coordinated Body Movement

Weight is the force exerted on a body by gravity. When you lift an object, you must overcome the object's weight and be aware of its center of gravity. In symmetrical objects, the center of gravity is located at the exact center of the object. The force of weight is always directed downward. An object that is unbalanced has its center of gravity away from the midline and falls without support. Like unbalanced objects, patients who fail to maintain a balance with their center of gravity are unsteady, placing them at risk for falling. Be able to identify such patients and intervene in a way to maintain safety.

Friction

Friction is the effect of rubbing or the resistance that a moving body meets from the surface on which it moves. As you turn, transfer, or move a patient up in bed, you need to overcome friction. Remember, the greater the surface area of the object you are moving, the greater the friction.

A passive or immobilized patient produces greater friction to movement. Thus when possible, use some of the patient's strength and mobility when lifting, transferring, or moving the patient up in bed. You do this by explaining the procedure and telling the patient when to move. For instance, you de-

BOX 26-1　BEST PRACTICES

Safe Patient Transfer

SUMMARY OF EVIDENCE

Musculoskeletal disorders are the most prevalent and debilitating occupational health hazards among nurses. Little improvement in the incidence of musculoskeletal injuries in health care workers has taken place. For example, 4.2 lost-workday injury cases per 100 were reported in 1989; while in the year 2000, there were 4.1 cases per 100 (Baptiste and others, 2006; Bureau of Labor Statistics, 2003). The American Nurses Association (ANA) (2003, 2007) put forth a position statement calling for the use of assistive equipment and devices to promote a safe health care environment for nurses and their patients. The use of assistive equipment and continued use of proper body mechanics significantly reduces the risk for musculoskeletal injuries and promotes safe patient transfer (ANA, 2003, 2007). In addition, the Occupational Safety and Health Administration (OSHA) (2005) recommends that nurses minimize or eliminate manually lifting patients in all cases when possible. Many facilities are moving toward limited lift policies (LLP) that minimize patient handling by nurses (de Castro and others, 2006; Miami Valley Hospital, 2007; UC Davis Health System, 2005). Instead, lift devices are used to reduce on-the-job injuries (Pelczarski, 2007). For example, a compre-hensive program initiated by the Veterans Health Administration was designed to reduce job-related musculoskeletal injuries in nurses. The program included an algorithm for each major patient transfer and repositioning task and the purchase of lift devices. One year after the inception of the program, preliminary data projected a cost savings of approximately $5 million over the next 9 years due to reduction in job-related musculoskeletal injuries (Nelson and others, 2003a, 2003b).

APPLICATION TO NURSING PRACTICE

- Partner with health care facilities to provide employees with safety information and training concerning the transfer, positioning, and lifting of patients.
- Inform your health care facility about needed safe patient handling resources. OSHA (2005) has identified recommendations on back safety and guidelines on the prevention of musculoskeletal injuries.
- Remain current about the research, standards, and guidelines regarding safe positioning and transfer of patients, so you will safely transfer patients without causing injury to the patient or yourself.

REFERENCES

American Nurses Association: Position statement on elimination of manual patient handling to prevent work-related musculoskeletal disorders, 2003, http://www.nursingworld.org/readroom/position/workplac/pathand.htm.

American Nurses Association: Nursing's legislative and regulatory initiatives for the 110th Congress: workplace health and safety, 2007, Department of Government Affairs, http//www.anapoliticalpower.org.

Baptiste A and others: Friction-reducing devices for lateral patient transfers: a clinical evaluation, *AAOHN J* 54(4):173, 2006.

Bureau of Labor Statistics: Occupational industries and illnesses: industry data, 2003, http://stats.bls.gov/bls/occupation.html.

de Castro A and others: Prioritizing safe patient handling, *J Nurs Adm* 36(7/8):363, 2006.

Miami Valley Hospital: *Lift team case study,* June 2007, http://www.miamivalleyhospital.com/.

Nelson A and others: Myths and facts about back injuries in nursing, *Am J Nurse* 103(2):32, 2003a.

Nelson A and others: Safe patient handling and movement: preventing back injury among nurses requires careful selection of the safest equipment and techniques, *Am J Nurs* 103(3):32, 2003b.

Occupational Safety and Health Administration: Ergonomics standard proposal, *Fed Reg* 29 CFR part 1910, 2005, http://www.osha-slc.gov/SLTC/ergonomics/index.html

Pelczarski K: Take a proactive approach to bariatric patient needs, *Materials Management,* June 2007.

UC Davis Health System: New team gives nurses a lift in handling patients, http:ucdavis.edu/, March 2005.

Wound Ostomy and Continence Nurses Society: *Guidelines for prevention and management of pressure ulcers,* WOCN Clinical Practice Guidelines Series, Glenview, Ill, 2003, The Society.

crease friction if the patient is able to bend his or her knees and lift the hips while being moved up in bed. You also reduce friction by lifting rather than pushing a patient. Lifting has an upward component and decreases the pressure between the patient and the bed or the chair. The use of a drawsheet reduces friction because you are able to move the patient more easily along the bed's surface. However, there are several commercially available products to assist in the task of positioning and moving patients in bed such as transfer boards and Maxi Slides (Hughes, 2006).

Regulation of Movement

Coordinated body movement involves the integrated functioning of the skeletal, muscular, and nervous systems. Because these three systems cooperate so closely in mechanical support of the body, they are often considered as a single functional unit.

SKELETAL SYSTEM Bones perform five functions in the body: support, protection, movement, mineral storage, and hematopoiesis (blood cell formation). Two of these functions, support and movement, are most important during activity and exercise. In support, bones serve as the framework and contribute to the shape, alignment, and positioning of the body parts. In movement, bones with their joints constitute levers for muscle attachment. When muscles contract and shorten, they pull on bones, producing joint movement (Thibodeau and Patton, 2007).

Joints An articulation, or **joint,** is the connection between bones. Each joint is classified according to its structure and degree of mobility. On the basis of connective structures, joints are classified as fibrous, cartilaginous, and synovial (Huether and McCance, 2008). Fibrous joints consist of a ligament or membrane that unites two bony surfaces such as the paired bones of the tibia and fibula. The joint is flexible but permits limited movement. The cartilaginous joint has little movement but is elastic. This type of joint allows for bone growth while providing stability, such as the joint between the sternum and second rib. The synovial, or true joint, is a freely movable joint. Bony surfaces are covered by cartilage and connected by ligaments lined with a synovial membrane. An example is the hip joint.

Ligaments Ligaments are white, shiny, flexible bands of fibrous tissue that bind joints and connect bones and cartilages. Ligaments are elastic and aid joint flexibility and support. In some areas of the body, ligaments also have a protective function.

Tendons Tendons are white, glistening, fibrous bands of tissue that connect muscle to bone. Tendons are strong, flexible, and inelastic and occur in various lengths and thicknesses.

Cartilage Cartilage is nonvascular, supporting connective tissue with the flexibility of a firm, plastic material. The gristlelike nature of cartilage permits it to sustain weight and serve as a shock-absorber pad between articulating bones (Thibodeau and Patton, 2007).

SKELETAL MUSCLE In addition to facilitating movement, muscles determine body form and contour. Muscles span at least one joint and attach to both articulating bones. When contraction occurs, one bone is fixed while the other moves. The origin is the point of attachment that remains still; the insertion is the point that moves when the muscle contracts (Thibodeau and Patton, 2007).

Muscles Concerned With Movement The muscles of movement are near the skeletal region, where a lever system causes movement (Thibodeau and Patton, 2007). The lever system makes the work of moving a weight or load easier. It occurs when specific bones, such as the humerus, ulna, and radius, and the associated joints, such as the elbow, act as a lever. Thus the force applied to one end of the bone to lift a weight at another point tends to rotate the bone in the opposite direction of the applied force. Muscles that attach to bones of leverage provide the necessary strength to move the object.

Muscles Concerned With Posture Gravity pulls on parts of the body all the time; the only way the body stays in position is for muscles to exert pull on bones in the opposite direction. Muscles accomplish this counterforce by maintaining a low level of sustained contraction. Poor posture places more work on muscles to counteract the force of gravity. This leads to fatigue and will eventually interfere with bodily functions and cause deformities.

Muscle Groups The nervous system coordinates the antagonistic, synergistic, and antigravity muscle groups that maintain posture and initiate movement. Antagonistic muscles bring about movement at the joint. During movement the active mover muscle contracts while its antagonist relaxes. For example, during **extension** of the arm, the active mover,

the triceps brachii, contracts, and the antagonist, the biceps brachii, relaxes.

Synergistic muscles contract to accomplish the same movement. When you flex your arm, you increase the strength of the contraction of the biceps brachii by contraction of the synergistic muscle, the brachialis.

Antigravity muscles are involved with joint stabilization. These muscles continuously oppose the effect of gravity on the body and permit a person to maintain an upright or sitting posture. In an adult the antigravity muscles are the extensors of the leg, the gluteus maximus, the quadriceps femoris, the soleus muscles, and the muscles of the back.

Skeletal muscles support posture and carry out voluntary movement. The muscles are attached to the skeleton by tendons, which provide strength and permit motion.

NERVOUS SYSTEM The nervous system regulates movement and posture. The major voluntary motor area, located in the cerebral cortex, is the motor strip (precentral gyrus). A majority of motor fibers descend from the motor strip and cross at the level of the medulla. The motor fibers from the right motor strip initiate voluntary movement for the left side of the body, and motor fibers from the left motor strip initiate voluntary movement for the right side of the body. Transmission of the impulse from the nervous system to the musculoskeletal system is an electrochemical event that requires a neurotransmitter, a chemical that transfers the electric impulse from the nerve to the muscle.

Proprioception The nervous system also regulates posture. Posture requires coordination of proprioception and balance. **Proprioception** is the awareness of the position of the body and its parts and is dependent on impulses from the inner ear and from receptors in joints and ligaments (Huether and McCance, 2008). Proprioceptors located on nerve endings in muscles, tendons, and joints monitor proprioception. While a person carries out activities of daily living, proprioceptors monitor muscle activity and body position. When a person walks, the proprioceptors on the bottom of the feet monitor pressure changes. Thus when the bottom of the moving foot comes in contact with the walking surface, the individual automatically moves the stationary foot forward.

Balance The cerebellum and the inner ear control **balance** through the nervous system. The major function of the cerebellum is to coordinate all voluntary movement. Within the inner ear are the fluid-filled semicircular canals. When you rotate your head suddenly in one direction, the fluid remains stationary for a moment, whereas the canal turns with the head. This allows a person to change position suddenly without losing balance.

Principles of Body Mechanics

Using principles of **body mechanics** during routine activities helps to prevent injury. Teach colleagues and patients' families to lift, transfer, or position patients properly. For example, teaching a patient's family how to transfer the patient from bed to chair increases and reinforces the family's knowledge and provides opportunity to consistently demonstrate proper body mechanics (Box 26-2).

BOX 26-2 Principles of Body Mechanics

- A wide base of support increases stability.
- A lower center of gravity increases stability.
- You maintain the equilibrium of an object as long as the line of gravity passes through its base of support.
- Facing the direction of movement prevents abnormal twisting of the spine.
- Dividing balanced activity between arms and legs reduces the risk for back injury.
- Leverage, rolling, turning, or pivoting requires less work than lifting.
- When you reduce friction between the object and the surface, it requires less force to move it.
- Reducing the force of work reduces the risk for injury.
- Maintaining good body mechanics reduces fatigue of the muscle groups.
- Alternating periods of rest and activity helps to reduce fatigue.

Pathological Influences on Body Alignment, Exercise, and Activity

Many pathological conditions affect body alignment, exercise, and activity. A few of these conditions include congenital defects; disorders of bones, joints, and muscles; central nervous system damage; and musculoskeletal trauma.

CONGENITAL DEFECTS Congenital abnormalities affect the musculoskeletal system in regard to alignment, balance, and appearance. Osteogenesis imperfecta is an inherited disorder that affects bone. Some characteristics of this are fractures and bone deformity (Hockenberry and Wilson, 2007). Bones are porous, short, bowed, and deformed; as a result, children experience curvature of the spine and shortness of stature. Scoliosis is a structural curvature of the spine associated with vertebral rotation. Muscles, ligaments, and other soft tissues become shortened. This affects balance and mobility in proportion to the severity of abnormal spinal curvatures (Huether and McCance, 2008).

DISORDERS OF BONES, JOINTS, AND MUSCLES Osteoporosis is a well-known and well-publicized disorder of aging in which the density or mass of bone is reduced. The bone remains biochemically normal but has difficulty maintaining integrity and support. There are many factors that cause this, varying from hormonal imbalances to insufficient intake of nutrients (Huether and McCance, 2008).

Inflammatory and noninflammatory joint diseases and articular disruption all alter joint mobility. Some characteristics of inflammatory joint disease (e.g., arthritis) are inflammation or destruction of the synovial membrane and articular cartilage and systemic signs of inflammation. Noninflammatory diseases have none of these characteristics, and the synovial fluid is normal (Huether and McCance, 2008).

CENTRAL NERVOUS SYSTEM DAMAGE Damage to any component of the central nervous system that regulates voluntary movement results in impaired body alignment and mobility. For example, your patient has experienced head trauma with damage to the motor strip in the cerebrum. The amount of voluntary motor impairment is directly related to the amount of destruction of the motor strip. A patient with a right-sided cerebral hemorrhage and damage to the right motor strip sometimes has left-sided hemiplegia.

MUSCULOSKELETAL TRAUMA Trauma to the musculoskeletal system sometimes results in bruises, contusions, sprains, and fractures. A fracture is a disruption of bone tissue continuity. Fractures most commonly result from direct external trauma. They also occur because of some deformity of the bone, as with pathological fractures of osteoporosis.

NURSING KNOWLEDGE BASE

Knowledge from areas of nursing practice enables you to meet the activity and exercise needs of the patient. Growth and development changes, behavioral aspects, and cultural and ethnic origin are a few areas of knowledge that you will incorporate into the plan of care.

Growth and Development

Throughout the life span the body's appearance and functioning undergo change. Knowledge of growth and development (see Chapter 21) enables you to anticipate types of activities patients are able to perform. The newborn infant's spine is flexed and lacks the anteroposterior curves of the adult. As growth and stability increase, the thoracic spine straightens, and the lumbar spinal curve appears, which allows sitting and standing. As the baby grows, musculoskeletal development permits support of weight for standing and walking. The toddler's posture is awkward because of the slight swayback and protruding abdomen (Hockenberry and Wilson, 2007). From the third year through the beginning of adolescence, the musculoskeletal system continues to grow and develop. Greater coordination enables the child to perform tasks that require fine motor skills. With aging, changes in musculoskeletal function limit patient activity.

Behavioral Aspects

It is important to take into consideration the patient's knowledge of exercise and activity, barriers to a program of exercise and physical activity, and current exercise behavior or habits. Patients are more open to developing an exercise program if they are at the stage of readiness to change their behavior (Prochaska and others, 1994). Patients' decisions to change behavior and include a daily exercise routine in their lives often occur gradually with repeated information individualized to their needs and lifestyle (Box 26-3).

Cultural and Ethnic Origin

Exercise and physical fitness is beneficial to all people. When developing a physical fitness program for culturally diverse populations, consider what motivates individuals to exercise and what activities will be appropriate and enjoyable (Box 26-4).

BOX 26-3   General Guidelines for Initiating an Exercise Program

STEP 1: ASSESS FITNESS LEVEL
- Seek approval from a health care provider to begin.
- Record baseline fitness scores such as pulse rate, how long it takes to walk 1 mile, waist circumference, and body mass index.

STEP 2: DESIGN THE FITNESS PROGRAM
- Consider fitness goals. Make goals attainable.
- Plan a logical progression of activities (e.g., walk a mile and gradually increase the pace).
- Build the program into a daily routine.
- Plan the fitness program with creativity and different activities.

STEP 3: ASSEMBLE EQUIPMENT
- Choose athletic shoes designed for the chosen exercise.
- Try equipment at a fitness center before purchasing to make sure it fits into the fitness program.
- Buy used equipment.
- Try homemade equipment (e.g., half-gallon milk jugs filled with sand for weights).

STEP 4: GET STARTED
- Start slowly, including a warm-up and cool-down period.
- Divide exercise time throughout day if time or fatigue is a barrier. Ten minutes of exercise 3 times a day instead of a single 30-minute workout may be better for some patients' schedules and medical conditions.

STEP 5: MONITOR PROGRESS
- Retake fitness assessment at 6 weeks and then every 3 to 6 months.
- If losing motivation: set new goals, exercise with a friend, or incorporate new activities.

Data from Mayo Clinic Tools for Healthier Lives: *Fitness programs: ready to get started?* 2005, http://www.mayoclinic.com/health/fitness/HQ00171.

CRITICAL THINKING

Synthesis

You will apply elements of critical thinking whenever you perform the nursing process with a patient. Consider the scientific knowledge you have learned, your experience, critical thinking attitudes, and standards to ensure an individualized approach to patient care. Doing so helps prevent complications, promotes rehabilitation, and promotes a timely return of patients to their homes (Box 26-5).

KNOWLEDGE When you begin the process of problem solving for patient care, you need to consider a variety of concepts and weave them together to provide the best outcome for your patient. Knowledge of the musculoskeletal

BOX 26-4   CULTURAL FOCUS

 As Marilyn studies about activity and exercise, she learns that physical inactivity is one of the risk factors associated with type 2 diabetes. In the United States, type 2 diabetes is more common in African Americans. Physical activity plays an important role in the prevention and treatment of type 2 diabetes (Morrato and others, 2006). However, African Americans have a disproportionate number of poor, unemployed, and disadvantaged individuals who lack access to health care systems and recreational facilities. Marilyn determines that Mr. Indelicato has three major risk factors for the development of type 2 diabetes: African American culture, age, and inactivity. She uses this information in her plan of care to increase his activity and prevent type 2 diabetes in the future.

IMPLICATIONS FOR PRACTICE
- Support promotion of physical activity through formal programs in schools, churches, and government agencies within African American communities (Boltri and others, 2008).
- Incorporate motivational factors into the exercise program, such as providing a healthy snack or meal for the participants and furnishing each with a log to monitor weight loss and blood glucose levels.
- Develop an exercise and prevention program that removes barriers such as transportation and cost to facilitate commitment to the program.

Data from Boltri J and others: Diabetes prevention in a faith-based setting: results of translational research, *J Public Health Manag Pract* 14(1):29, 2008; Morrato E and others: Are health care professionals advising patients with diabetes or at risk for developing diabetes to exercise more? *Diabetes Care* 29(3):543, 2006; O'Brien-Gillespie H: Exercise. In Edelman CL, Mandle CL, editors: *Health promotion throughout the life span*, ed 6, St. Louis, 2006, Mosby.

system, exercise physiology, and health alterations that create problems for the patient in the area of exercise and activity provide the foundation for decision making and planning care.

EXPERIENCE Past experiences with exercise or caring for patients with problems related to activity and exercise help you anticipate patients' needs such as pain control, positioning, transferring, and support of activities of daily living. Visits to a physical or occupational therapy unit in a hospital or community setting will increase your experiential base.

ATTITUDES You need to possess creativity because problems with activity and exercise are often prolonged. The more creative your approach for improving activity tolerance and mobility skills, the greater the chance for success. This is especially important with children. For example, creating a game that incorporates the goal of improving activity tolerance will elicit better cooperation and participation from the child. Also, providing colorful stickers to symbolize success is a creative approach to enhance cooperation (Hockenberry and Wilson, 2007).

BOX 26-5   SYNTHESIS IN PRACTICE

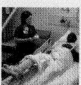

As Marilyn prepares to assess Mr. Indelicato, she reviews anatomy and physiology related to the musculoskeletal system and exercise physiology. She gathers information about the expected surgery, anticipated recovery, and physical therapy. During her previous rotation she cared for postoperative patients and knows relevant postoperative care measures to promote patient comfort and the implications of inactivity on postoperative recovery.

Marilyn knows that it is important to assist Mr. Indelicato in a prompt immediate postoperative recovery and to engage him in a steady, progressive physical therapy program. Although she has cared for patients who have required physical therapy, Marilyn has never cared for a patient requiring continuous passive motion equipment. She has acquired and read literature about this equipment, and she consulted with the physical therapist who will be assigned to Mr. Indelicato.

Marilyn approaches this clinical experience with energy and creativity. She plans to collaborate and implement individualized care to promote Mr. Indelicato's comfort, to increase activity, and to improve range of motion.

STANDARDS Professional standards and guidelines, such as those from the American Nurses Association (ANA) (2003, 2007) and Occupational Safety and Health Administration (OSHA) (2003, 2005) concerning the use of assistive equipment and devices to safely transfer and position patients, provide valuable guidelines for the safety of you and your patient. In addition, these standards help you promote the patient's independence while safely adhering to the prescribed rehabilitation plan.

NURSING PROCESS

■■■ASSESSMENT

An assessment includes the patient's present activity tolerance and information about preillness functioning. Assess body alignment and posture with the patient standing, sitting, or lying down. Table 26-1 offers examples of factors to assess, related questions, and physical assessment related to activity intolerance.

Through assessment you are able to determine normal physiological changes in growth and development; deviations related to poor posture, trauma, muscle damage, or nerve dysfunction; and any learning needs of patients. In addition, assessment provides opportunities for you to observe patients' posture and obtain important information about other factors that contribute to poor alignment, such as fatigue, malnutrition, and psychological problems.

BODY ALIGNMENT The first step in assessing body alignment is to put the patient at ease, so he or she does not assume unnatural or rigid positions. Remove pillows and positioning supports from the bed (if not contraindicated), and place the patient in the **supine** position.

Standing Assessment of the patient includes the following:

- The head is erect and midline.
- Body parts are symmetrical.
- The spine is straight with normal curvatures (cervical concave, thoracic convex, and lumbar concave).
- The abdomen is comfortably tucked.
- The knees are in a straight line between the hips and ankles and slightly flexed.
- The feet are flat on the floor and pointed directly forward and slightly apart to maintain a wide base of support.
- The arms hang comfortably at the sides (Figure 26-1).

The patient's center of gravity is in the midline, and the line of gravity is from the middle of the forehead to a midpoint between the feet. Laterally the line of gravity runs vertically from the middle of the skull to the posterior third of the foot (Wilson and Giddens, 2005).

Sitting Assess your patient for the following: the head is erect, and the neck and vertebral column are in straight alignment; the body weight is distributed on the buttocks and thighs; the thighs are parallel and in a horizontal plane (be careful to avoid pressure on the popliteal nerve and blood supply); the feet are supported on the floor; and the forearms are supported on the armrest, in the lap, or on a table in front of the chair.

Assessment of alignment in the sitting position is particularly important for the patient with neuromuscular disorders, muscle weakness, muscle paralysis, or nerve damage. A patient with these alterations has diminished sensation in affected areas and is unable to perceive pressure or decreased circulation. Proper sitting alignment reduces the risk for musculoskeletal system damage in such a patient.

Recumbent Position your patient in the lateral position with all but one pillow and all positioning supports removed from the bed. Make sure the vertebrae are in straight alignment without observable curves. This assessment provides baseline data concerning the patient's body alignment.

Conditions that create a risk for damage to the musculoskeletal system when lying down include impaired mobility (e.g., spinal curvature), use of immobilization devices (e.g., traction), decreased sensation (e.g., hemiparesis from a stroke), impaired circulation (e.g., diabetes), and lack of voluntary muscle control (e.g., spinal cord injuries).

When a patient is unable to change position voluntarily, assess the position of body parts while the patient is lying down. Make sure the vertebrae are in straight alignment without any observable curves. Normally the extremities are in alignment and do not cross over one another. The head and neck are aligned without excessive flexion or extension.

MOBILITY The adequacy of your patient's mobility affects his or her coordination and balance while walking, the ability to carry out activities of daily living, and the ability to participate in an exercise program. The assessment of mobility has three components: range of motion, gait, and exercise.

TABLE 26-1   FOCUSED PATIENT ASSESSMENT

FACTORS TO ASSESS	QUESTIONS	PHYSICAL ASSESSMENT
Range of motion (ROM)	Do you have limited movement in your joints? Do you have a history of connective tissue disorders, fractures, and/or damage to ligaments or tendons?	Observe patient's gait and ability to carry out activities of daily living (ADLs). Inspect joints for deformity. Measure range of motion of affected joints.
Pain	Do you experience pain or discomfort upon movement? Do you need pain medication before ambulating (with assistance), particularly after your surgical procedure? Please rate your pain on a scale of 0 to 10 with 10 representing the worst pain.	Inspect joints for redness or swelling indicating potential inflammatory process. Observe for objective signs of pain such as grimacing, moaning, increasing respiratory rate, pulse, and blood pressure. (NOTE: These objective signs are not always present, and it is best to ask patient if pain is present.)
Activity tolerance	Do you feel fatigued? Do you have any difficulty with your daily activities because of muscle weakness? Do you feel short of breath, palpitations, light-headed, or dizzy?	Observe for signs of fatigue. Observe patient's performance of ADLs. Observe patient for paleness, obtain vital signs, and compare to baseline measures.

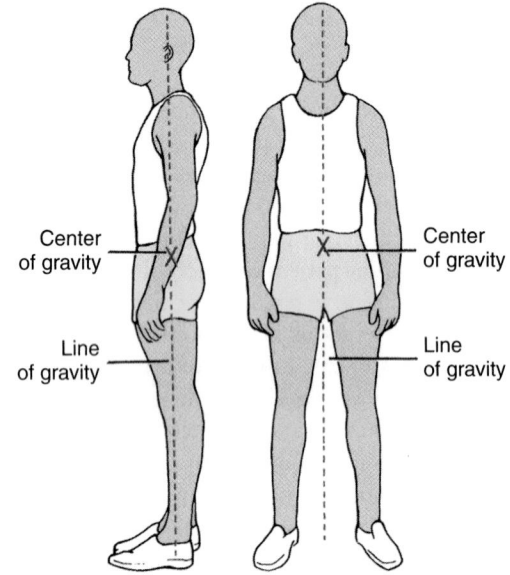

Figure 26-1 ■ Correct body alignment with standing.

Range of Motion Observing **range of motion (ROM)** is one of the first assessment techniques used to determine the degree of limitation or injury to a joint. Assess ROM to further clarify the extent of joint stiffness, swelling, pain, limited movement, and unequal movement. Chapter 35 covers a thorough ROM assessment. Limited ROM indicates inflammation such as arthritis, fluid in the joint, altered nerve supply, or contractures. Increased mobility (beyond normal) of a joint indicates connective tissue disorders, ligament tears, and possible joint fractures.

Gait **Gait** is the manner or style of walking, including rhythm, cadence, and speed. Assessing gait allows for conclusions about balance, posture, and the ability to walk without assistance (see Chapter 15). While the patient walks in a room, look for conformity, a regular smooth rhythm, symmetry in the length of leg swing, smooth swaying related to the gait phase, and a smooth, symmetrical arm swing (Wilson and Giddens, 2005).

Exercise Exercise is physical activity for conditioning the body, improving health, maintaining fitness, or providing therapy for correcting a deformity or restoring the body to a maximal state of health. When a person exercises, physiological changes occur in body systems (Box 26-6).

During exercise you improve muscle tone, size, and strength and cardiopulmonary conditioning. As a result, you are able to exercise longer with each strengthening of the muscles. Exercise also enhances joint mobility because the exercise itself requires movement of body parts.

Activity Tolerance **Activity tolerance** is the kind and amount of exercise or work a person is able to perform without undue exertion or injury (Box 26-7). Observe patients after ambulation, self-bathing, or sitting in a chair for several hours, and assess their verbal report of fatigue and weakness. Assess heart rate and blood pressure response to activity.

PATIENT EXPECTATIONS In assessing the patient's expectations concerning body alignment and joint mobility, determine your patient's perception of what is normal or acceptable in regard to mobility. For example, if exercising is painful or tiresome to patients, they may lack adherence and commitment to desired interventions. Some patients are content with their present range of motion or mobility and do not perceive a need for improvement. Unless there is a real threat to health maintenance, forcing patients to accept perspectives not in accordance with their own beliefs is a breach of standards of care.

■■■NURSING DIAGNOSIS

The patient's assessment provides related clusters of data or defining characteristics that lead to the identification of nursing diagnoses, including these examples:

BOX 26-6   Effects of Exercise

CARDIOVASCULAR SYSTEM
- Increased cardiac output
- Improved myocardial contraction, thereby strengthening cardiac muscle
- Decreased resting heart rate
- Improved venous return

PULMONARY SYSTEM
- Increased respiratory rate and depth followed by a quicker return to resting state
- Improved alveolar ventilation
- Decreased work of breathing
- Improved diaphragmatic excursion

METABOLIC SYSTEM
- Increased basal metabolic rate
- Increased use of glucose and fatty acids
- Increased triglyceride breakdown
- Increased gastric motility
- Increased production of body heat

MUSCULOSKELETAL SYSTEM
- Improved muscle tone
- Increased joint mobility
- Improved muscle tolerance to physical exercise
- Possible increase in muscle mass
- Reduced bone loss

ACTIVITY TOLERANCE
- Improved tolerance
- Decreased fatigue

PSYCHOSOCIAL FACTORS
- Improved tolerance to stress
- Reports of "feeling better"
- Reports of decrease in illness (e.g., colds, influenza)

Data from Huether SE, McCance KL: *Understanding pathophysiology,* ed 4, St. Louis, 2008, Mosby; Hoeman SP: *Rehabilitation nursing: process, application, and outcomes,* ed 4, St. Louis, 2008, Mosby.

BOX 26-7   Factors Influencing Activity Tolerance

PHYSIOLOGICAL FACTORS
- Skeletal abnormalities
- Muscular impairments
- Endocrine or metabolic illnesses (e.g., diabetes mellitus, thyroid disease)
- Hypoxemia
- Decreased cardiac function
- Decreased endurance
- Impaired physical stability
- Pain
- Sleep pattern disturbance
- Prior exercise patterns
- Infectious processes and fever

EMOTIONAL FACTORS
- Anxiety
- Depression
- Chemical addictions
- Motivation

DEVELOPMENTAL FACTORS
- Age
- Sex
- Pregnancy
- Physical growth and development of muscle and skeletal support

Modified from Monahan F and others: *Phipps' medical surgical nursing,* ed 8, St. Louis, 2007, Mosby.

nursing diagnosis and not the actual nursing diagnosis. Nursing diagnoses often focus on the individual's ability to move. Make sure the diagnostic label directs nursing interventions. For example, the diagnostic label *impaired physical mobility related to pain and muscle weakness* will direct you to initiate pain relief and exercise measures.

- *Activity intolerance*
- *Risk for activity intolerance*
- *Disturbed body image*
- *Fatigue*
- *Risk for injury*
- *Impaired physical mobility*
- *Acute pain*
- *Chronic pain*
- *Impaired skin integrity*
- *Risk for impaired skin integrity*

Alterations in body alignment and joint mobility result from developmental changes, postural and bone formation abnormalities, impaired muscle development, damage to the central nervous system, or direct trauma to the musculoskeletal system. In some cases alterations in joint mobility or alignment are one of the defining characteristics of a separate

■■■PLANNING

During planning for your patient, use data gathered during assessment and critical thinking to develop an individualized plan of care. You will identify patient needs and, in collaboration with the patient and family, integrate these needs with the goals and outcomes of care, care priorities, and restorative and continuing care needs. This will enable you to develop a plan of care to optimize the patient's exercise and activity levels (Figure 26-2).

GOALS AND OUTCOMES Once you define the nursing diagnoses, work with the patient to set goals and expected outcomes, which then direct nursing interventions. For example, the goal of achieving optimum ROM in the right knee will have the outcome of achieving 90-degree flexion in the right knee by discharge. Nursing therapies will include ROM and muscle strengthening. The plan considers risks for injury to the patient and preexisting health concerns. It is especially important to have knowledge of your patient's previous functional status and home environment.

CONCEPT MAP

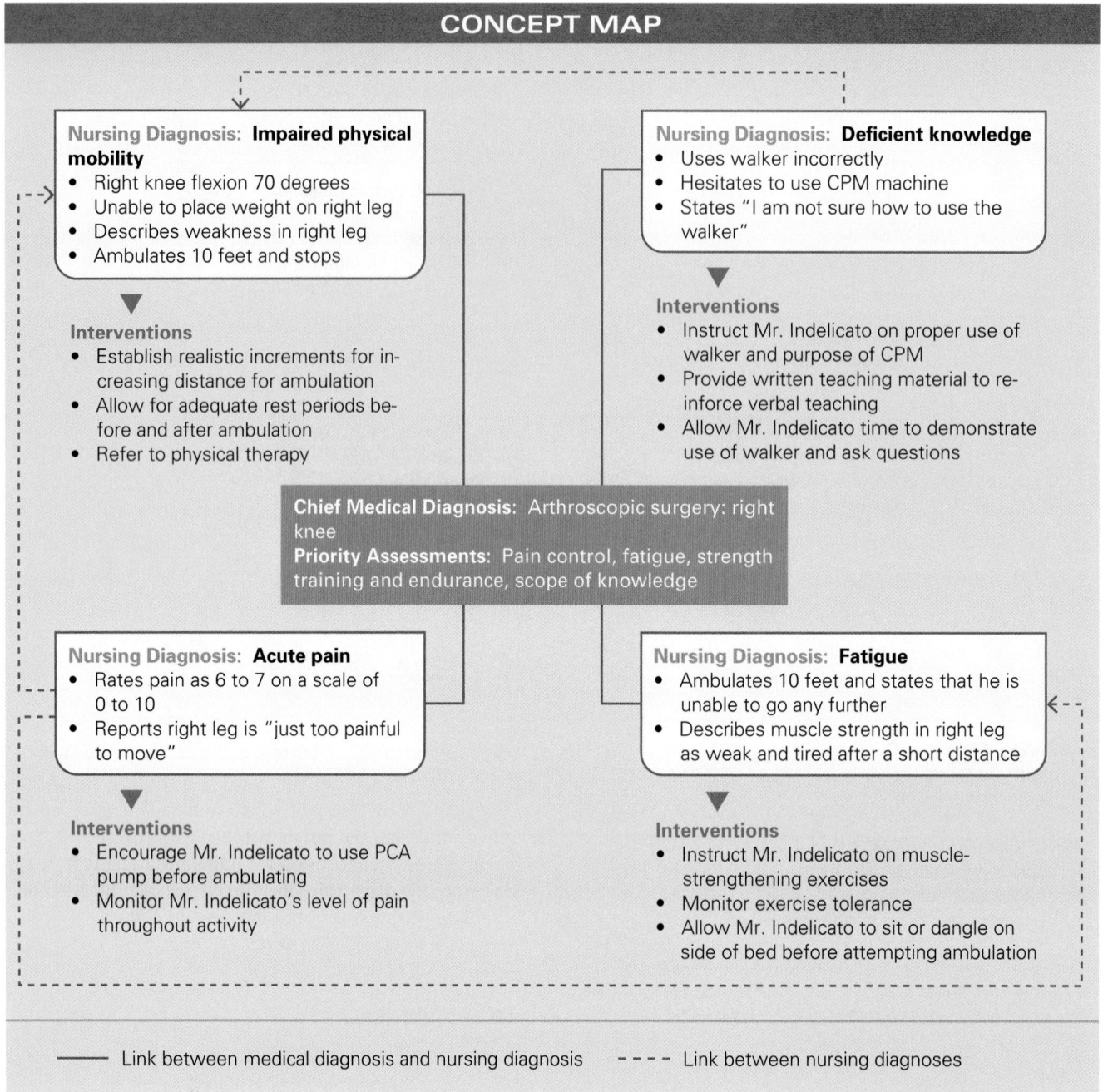

Nursing Diagnosis: Impaired physical mobility
- Right knee flexion 70 degrees
- Unable to place weight on right leg
- Describes weakness in right leg
- Ambulates 10 feet and stops

Interventions
- Establish realistic increments for increasing distance for ambulation
- Allow for adequate rest periods before and after ambulation
- Refer to physical therapy

Nursing Diagnosis: Deficient knowledge
- Uses walker incorrectly
- Hesitates to use CPM machine
- States "I am not sure how to use the walker"

Interventions
- Instruct Mr. Indelicato on proper use of walker and purpose of CPM
- Provide written teaching material to reinforce verbal teaching
- Allow Mr. Indelicato time to demonstrate use of walker and ask questions

Chief Medical Diagnosis: Arthroscopic surgery: right knee
Priority Assessments: Pain control, fatigue, strength training and endurance, scope of knowledge

Nursing Diagnosis: Acute pain
- Rates pain as 6 to 7 on a scale of 0 to 10
- Reports right leg is "just too painful to move"

Interventions
- Encourage Mr. Indelicato to use PCA pump before ambulating
- Monitor Mr. Indelicato's level of pain throughout activity

Nursing Diagnosis: Fatigue
- Ambulates 10 feet and states that he is unable to go any further
- Describes muscle strength in right leg as weak and tired after a short distance

Interventions
- Instruct Mr. Indelicato on muscle-strengthening exercises
- Monitor exercise tolerance
- Allow Mr. Indelicato to sit or dangle on side of bed before attempting ambulation

—— Link between medical diagnosis and nursing diagnosis   - - - - Link between nursing diagnoses

Figure 26-2 ■ Concept Map. *CPM,* Continuous passive motion; *PCA,* patient-controlled analgesia.

SETTING PRIORITIES Consider your patient's most immediate needs when individualizing a plan of care. Determine the immediacy of any problem by the effect the problem has on the patient's mental and physical health. For example, if a patient is in acute pain, relieving pain is a priority before you begin exercise therapy. Safety becomes a priority whenever you are assisting with the many skills associated with the care of patients with activity intolerance, improper body mechanics, and/or impaired mobility. For example, you must use caution to avoid a patient fall during transferring. Your priorities will change from short term to long term when you plan for patients' return to their homes. For those who remain disabled or limited in mobility, be sure family members are prepared to assist with positioning and transfer techniques. When you perform skills that promote a patient's activity, always be vigilant in monitoring your patients and supervising nursing assistive personnel in carrying out activities to prevent complications and potential injury.

COLLABORATIVE CARE Planning also involves an understanding of the patient's need to maintain motor function and independence. Collaborate with other members of the health care team, such as physical or occupational therapists. Long-term rehabilitation is sometimes necessary, and you begin discharge planning when a patient enters the health care system. In addition, always individualize a plan of care directed at meeting the actual or potential needs of the patient (see Care Plan).

CARE PLAN Impaired Physical Mobility

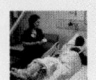 **ASSESSMENT**

Joseph Indelicato is a 72-year-old African American hospitalized for surgery on his right knee. Over the past 5 years, he has continued to experience pain and decreased mobility. He is now 2 days *postoperative* following right total knee replacement. His incision is healing, and there is no edema or redness.

ASSESSMENT ACTIVITIES	FINDINGS/DEFINING CHARACTERISTICS*
Assess Mr. Indelicato's pain level.	Mr. Indelicato is hesitant to ambulate or use his continuous passive motion (CPM) machine. He rates his **pain as 6 to 7 on a scale of 0 to 10** and is using a patient-controlled analgesia (PCA) pump. He states, **"I can't put all my weight on my right leg, it is just too painful."**
Assess Mr. Indelicato's baseline mobility and endurance.	His degree of **knee flexion is now 70 degrees.** He is able to **ambulate 10 feet with a walker but states, "I can't go any further."** In addition, he further describes his muscle strength in his right leg as **feeling weak and tired after walking a short distance.**
Assess Mr. Indelicato's knowledge about proper use of his walker.	The nurse observes Mr. Indelicato using the walker incorrectly.

NURSING DIAGNOSIS: Impaired physical mobility related to pain, muscle weakness, and limited joint motion.

PLANNING

GOAL

- Mr. Indelicato will obtain a tolerable level of pain during ambulation.

- Mr. Indelicato will gain optimal functioning of the right knee with independent, purposeful movement.

- Mr. Indelicato will demonstrate proper use of walker while ambulating.

EXPECTED OUTCOMES (NOC)†

Pain Control
- Mr. Indelicato's pain will be 2 to 3 on a scale of 0 to 10 during ambulation.

Endurance
- Mr. Indelicato will ambulate 50 to 75 feet with aid of walker without reports of increasing fatigue.
- Mr. Indelicato will gain a minimum of 90-degree flexion in right knee by discharge.

Knowledge: Prescribed Activity
- Mr. Indelicato will perform a return demonstration of proper use of walker.

INTERVENTIONS (NIC)‡

Exercise Therapy: Ambulation
- Encourage Mr. Indelicato to use patient-controlled analgesia (PCA) pump before ambulation.
- Encourage Mr. Indelicato to sit in bed or on side of bed (dangle) before standing to ambulate.

- Establish realistic increments for Mr. Indelicato to increase walking distance during ambulation.

Exercise Promotion: Strength Training
- Monitor exercise tolerance.

RATIONALE

Peak actions of analgesic will occur as patient begins activity (Berry and others, 2006; Gahart and Nazareno, 2008).

Allowing the patient to dangle before changing positions prevents orthostatic hypotension; maintains safety and prevents injury to the patient (Dingle, 2003).

Gradually increasing physical activity and setting realistic goals for ambulation encourage activity in older adults (Yen, 2005).

Presence of such symptoms as breathlessness, rapid pulse, pallor, or light-headedness indicates need for patient to stop activity.

*****Defining characteristics** are shown in **bold** type.
†Outcomes classification labels from Moorhead S and others, editors: *Nursing outcomes classification (NOC)*, ed 4, St. Louis, 2008, Mosby.
‡Intervention classification labels from Bulechek GM and others, editors: *Nursing interventions classification (NIC)*, ed 5, St. Louis, 2008, Mosby.

CARE PLAN Impaired Physical Mobility—cont'd

INTERVENTIONS (NIC)‡

Teaching: Prescribed Activity/Exercise
- Consult with physical therapist on proper use of walker.
- Instruct Mr. Indelicato and family caregivers on the proper use of walker. Provide written material that reinforces verbal instructions.

RATIONALE

Ensures safe use of assistive device.

Providing instructions in a quiet environment and giving written instructions in large, easy-to-read print enhances learning for the older adult (Mamaril, 2006).

EVALUATION

NURSING ACTIONS	PATIENT RESPONSE/FINDING	ACHIEVEMENT OF OUTCOME
Ask Mr. Indelicato to rate the level of pain on a scale of 0 to 10.	Mr. Indelicato rates his pain at a 3 and states, "I am able to walk now that my knee doesn't hurt so bad anymore."	Mr. Indelicato's pain is under control and is able to ambulate with minimal discomfort.
Observe Mr. Indelicato's range of motion (ROM) or use of CPM machine.	Able to perform ROM and use CPM machine.	Outcome met. Mr. Indelicato expresses understanding of need for ROM and CPM machine.
Observe Mr. Indelicato's ambulation.	Steady gait with aid of walker.	Outcome met. Demonstrates correct use of walker.

■■■ IMPLEMENTATION

HEALTH PROMOTION In recent years the rate of injuries in occupational settings has increased dramatically (Baptiste and others, 2006). The most common back injury is strain on the lumbar muscle group, which includes the muscles around the lumbar vertebrae. Injury to these areas affects the ability to bend forward, backward, and side-to-side. This also decreases the ability to rotate the hips and lower back. You and your patients need to learn and master proper body mechanics to prevent injury to your patients and yourself.

Lifting Techniques Before lifting, assess the weight you will lift and what assistance, if any, you will need. If you need help, assess if a second person is adequate or if you will need mechanical assistance. Once you determine the amount of assistance you need, follow these steps:

1. Keep the weight you are lifting as close to the body as possible; this action places the object in the same plane as the lifter and close to the center of gravity for balance.
2. Bend at the knees; this maintains the center of gravity and uses the stronger leg muscles to do the lifting (Figure 26-3). Avoid twisting. Twisting overloads the spine and leads to serious injury.
3. Tighten abdominal muscles and tuck the pelvis; this provides balance and helps protect the back.
4. Maintain the trunk erect and knees bent so that multiple groups work together in a coordinated manner.

However, note that injuries are not only related to lifting. You spend time in many activities involving bending and

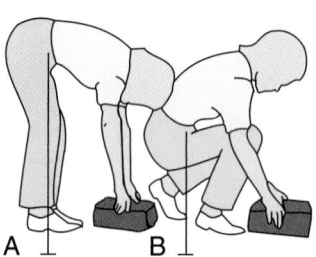

Figure 26-3 ■ Incorrect **(A)** and correct **(B)** body position for lifting.

twisting that also cause injury. Examples of such activities include bathing, feeding, dressing, and undressing patients (Nelson and others, 2003a).

ACUTE CARE

Positioning Techniques Patients with impaired nervous or musculoskeletal system functioning, patients with increased weakness, or those restricted to bed rest benefit from therapeutic positioning (Hoeman, 2008). During patient positioning determine areas of bony prominences where pressure, friction, and shear cause the most wear and tear. Through the use of proper positioning and pressure-relief methods, you are able to protect these areas (see Chapter 36).

In general, you reposition patients as needed and at least every 2 hours if they are in bed and every 20 to 30 minutes if they are sitting in a chair. Those patients with contractures or who are at greater risk for skin breakdown over bony prominences need repositioning more frequently. The following

TABLE 26-2   Devices Used for Proper Positioning

DEVICES	USES AND DESCRIPTIONS
Pillows	Make sure pillows are appropriate size for the body part you will position. They provide support, elevate body parts, and splint incisional areas.
Foot boots	**Foot boots** maintain feet in **dorsiflexion.** Remove boots at least 2 to 3 times per day to assess skin integrity and joint mobility.
Trochanter rolls	**Trochanter rolls** prevent external rotation of legs when immobile patients are in the supine position. To form a trochanter roll, fold a cotton bath blanket or a sheet lengthwise to a width extending from the greater trochanter of the femur to the lower border of the popliteal space (Figure 26-4). Place the roll under the buttocks, and then roll it away from the patient until the thigh is in a neutral position or an inward position with the patella facing upward.
Sandbags	**Sandbags** provide support and shape to body contours; they immobilize extremities and maintain specific body alignment. You use them in place of or in addition to the trochanter roll.
Hand rolls	**Hand rolls** maintain the thumb slightly adducted and in opposition to the fingers; they maintain fingers in a slightly flexed position (Figure 26-5). You make hand rolls by folding a washcloth in half, rolling it lengthwise, and securing the roll with tape. Place the roll against the palmar surface of the hand. Evaluate the position of the hand to make certain the hand is in a functional position.
Hand-wrist splints	**Hand-wrist splints** are individually molded for the patient to maintain proper alignment of the thumb in slight **adduction** and the wrist in slight dorsiflexion. Use these splints only for the patient for whom they were made.
Trapeze bar	The **trapeze bar** descends from a securely fastened overhead bar attached to the bed frame (Figure 26-6). The trapeze allows the patient to use upper extremities to raise the trunk off the bed, to assist in transfer from bed to wheelchair, or to perform upper arm–strengthening exercises.
Side rails	**Side rails** are bars positioned along the sides of the length of a hospital bed. They are designed to increase patient's ability to move and turn in bed, for example, rolling from side to side or sitting up in bed.
Bed boards	**Bed boards** are plywood boards placed under the entire surface of the mattress. They are useful for increasing back support and alignment, especially with a soft mattress.
Wedge pillow	A wedge or abductor pillow is a triangular-shaped pillow made of heavy foam. You use it to maintain the legs in **abduction** following total hip replacement surgery.

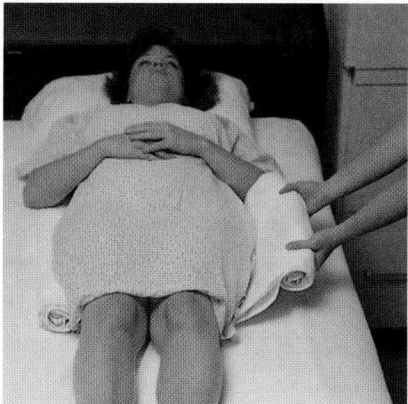

Figure 26-4 ■ Trochanter roll.

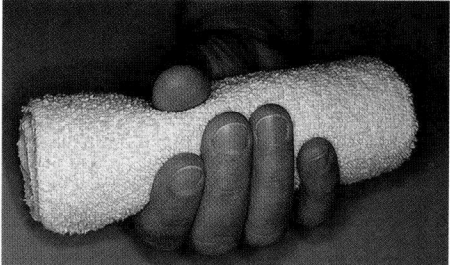

Figure 26-5 ■ Hand roll.

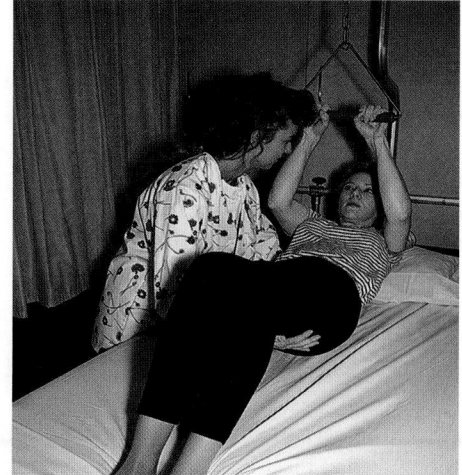

Figure 26-6 ■ Patient using a trapeze bar.

also influence the frequency of position changes: level of comfort, amount of spontaneous movement, presence of edema, loss of sensation, and overall physical and mental status (Hoeman, 2008). Several devices are available for you to use in maintaining a patient's body alignment after positioning (Table 26-2). Select the therapeutic position that maximizes your patient's comfort, safety, and ability to still use remaining function. Skill 26-1 describes the methods of positioning patients.

Fowler's and Semi-Fowler's Positions. Elevate the head of the patient's bed 45 to 60 degrees, and slightly elevate the patient's knees, avoiding pressure on the popliteal vessels. The head rests against the mattress or a small pillow for support. Use pillows to maintain natural alignment of the hands, wrists, and forearms. In semi-Fowler's position the head of the bed is at a 30-degree angle; you will use this position for patients who will not tolerate a supine position, such as those with cardiac and respiratory problems. In high-Fowler's position, the head of the bed is 90 degrees. Patients with severe respiratory distress breathe more easily in high-Fowler's position. The following are common trouble areas for the patient in the Fowler's position:

- Increased cervical flexion because the pillow at the head is too thick and head thrusts forward
- Extension of the knees, allowing the patient to slide to the foot of the bed
- Pressure on the posterior aspect of the knees, decreasing circulation to the feet
- External rotation of the hips
- Arms hanging unsupported at the patient's sides
- Unsupported feet or pressure on the heels
- Unprotected pressure points at the sacrum and heels
- Increased shearing force on the back and heels when you raise the head of the bed greater than 60 degrees

Supine Position. In the **supine** position the patient rests on the back. A small, flat pillow supports the head, neck, and upper shoulders (Hoeman, 2008). When a patient is immobile, use pillows, trochanter rolls (see Table 26-2), and hand rolls or arm splints to increase comfort and reduce injury to the skin or musculoskeletal system. The risk for aspiration is greater with this position; thus avoid the supine position when the patient is confused, agitated, experiencing a decreased level of consciousness, or at risk for aspiration.

Make sure the mattress is firm enough to support the cervical, thoracic, and lumbar vertebrae. Avoid pressure on the back of the legs. Use a foot boot to prevent **footdrop,** maintain proper alignment, and provide freedom of movement for the feet. The following are some common trouble areas for patients in the supine position:

- Pillow at the head that is too thick, increasing cervical flexion
- Head flat on the mattress
- Shoulders unsupported and internally rotated
- Elbows extended
- Thumb not in opposition to the fingers
- Hips externally rotated
- Unsupported feet
- Unprotected pressure points at the vertebrae, coccyx, elbows, heels, and the occipital region of the head

Prone Position. When prone, the patient is in the face-down position. Before placing a patient in the prone position, assess the patient's medical record for any possible complica-

tions such as increasing intracranial pressure or cardiopulmonary disease.

Assist the patient in lying on the abdomen. Have the patient turn the head to the side. This facilitates respiration and drainage of oral secretions. Place a pillow under the head for comfort and relief from pressure. As an alternative, place a wedge under the patient's chest, or arms flexed over the head, if it is more comfortable. Place a pillow under the lower leg; this promotes relaxation. If a pillow is unavailable, make sure the patient's ankles are in **dorsiflexion** over the end of the mattress. Body alignment is poor when the ankles are continuously in **plantar flexion** and the lumbar spine remains in **hyperextension.** Sometimes lung expansion is compromised in this position, especially in persons who are obese. Monitor your patient for signs of respiratory distress. You assess for and correct any of the following potential trouble points:

- Neck hyperextension
- Hyperextension of the lumbar spine
- Plantar flexion of the ankles
- Unprotected pressure points at the chin, elbows, hips, knees, and toes

Lateral Position. In the lateral (or side-lying) position, the patient is supported on the right or left side with the opposite arm, thigh, and knee flexed and resting on the bed. Place a pillow under the patient's head to keep the head, neck, and spine in alignment. The upper arm is flexed and supported with a pillow. The upper leg is flexed at the hip and knee and positioned on a small pillow (Hoeman, 2008). Patients who are obese or older are often not able to tolerate this position for any length of time. The 30-degree lateral position is recommended as a position to avoid development of pressure ulcers (WOCN, 2003). The position differs from the side-lying in that the dependent hip is brought forward so that less pressure is directly on the bony prominence (Figure 26-7) The following trouble points are common in the side-lying position:

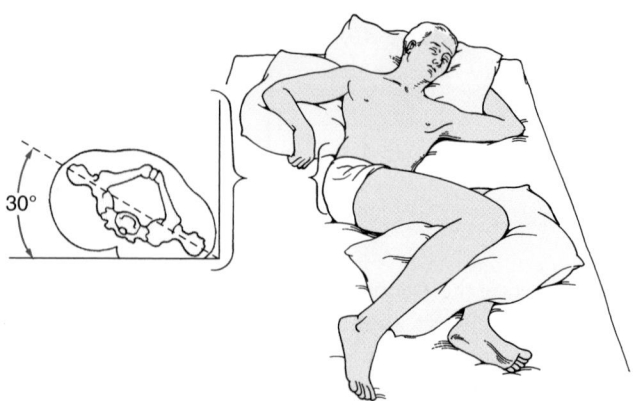

Figure 26-7 ■ Thirty-degree lateral position at which pressure points are avoided. (From Pieper B: Mechanical forces, pressure, shear, and friction. In Bryant RA, Nix DP eds: *Acute and chronic wounds: current management concepts,* ed 3, St. Louis, 2007, Mosby.

- Lateral flexion of the neck
- Spinal curves out of normal alignment
- Shoulder and hip joints internally rotated, adducted, or unsupported
- Lack of support for the feet
- Lack of protection for pressure points at the ear, shoulder, anterior iliac spine, trochanter, and ankles
- Excessive lateral flexion of the spine if the patient has large hips and a pillow is not placed superior to the hips at the waist

Sims' Position. In the Sims' position the patient is semi-prone on the right or left side with the opposite arm, thigh, and knee flexed and resting on the bed (Figure 26-8). The Sims' position differs from the side-lying position in the distribution of the patient's weight. In this position you place the patient's weight on the anterior ilium, humerus, and clavicle.

Improper positioning causes unnecessary harm to patients, such as pressure ulcers and joint contractures, especially if they have certain preexisting conditions (e.g., peripheral vascular disease or diabetes). Positions that compromise peripheral blood flow damage nerves as well. Every time you reposition the patient, make certain to check total body alignment, placement of extremities, skin breakdown, and joint contractures. Trouble points common in Sims' position include the following:

- Lateral flexion of the neck
- Internal rotation, adduction, or lack of support to the shoulders and hips
- Lack of support for the feet
- Lack of protection for pressure points at the ilium, humerus, clavicle, knees, and ankles

Transfer Techniques You will often care for immobilized patients who need a position change, who need to be moved up in bed, or who need to be transferred from a bed to a chair or a bed to a stretcher. Proper use of body mechanics enables you to move, lift, or transfer patients safely and also protects you from injury to your musculoskeletal system (Skill 26-2). Transferring is a skill that helps the dependent patient regain optimal independence as quickly as possible. Physical activity maintains and improves joint motion, increases strength, promotes circulation, relieves pressure on skin, and improves urinary and respiratory functions. It also benefits the patient psychologically by increasing social activity and mental stimulation and providing a change in environment. Thus mobilization plays a crucial role in the patient's rehabilitation.

One of the major concerns during transfer is the safety of you and your patient. You prevent self-injury by using correct posture, minimal muscle strength, and effective body mechanics and lifting techniques. Always be aware of the patient's motor deficits, ability to aid in transfer, and body weight. As a rule of thumb, GET HELP to transfer a patient. If you or any other caregiver needs to lift more than 35 lb (Nelson, 2006), use assistive devices for the transfer (Figure 26-9). Explain the assistive device and procedure to the patient before the transfer.

When preparing to transfer patients, consider the type of problems that can develop. A patient who has been immobile for several days or longer is often weak or dizzy or sometimes develops **orthostatic hypotension** (a drop in blood pressure of 20 mm Hg or more systolic or 10 mm Hg or more diastolic when rising from a sitting position) when transferred (Jarvis, 2008; Monahan and others, 2007; Schrezenmaier and others, 2005). A patient with neurological deficits sometimes has paresis (muscle weakness) or paralysis unilaterally or bilaterally, which complicates safe transfer. A flaccid arm sustains injury during transfer if unsupported. As a general rule, use a transfer belt and obtain assistance for mobilization of such patients.

Joint Mobility and Ambulation

Range-of-Motion Exercises. The easiest intervention to maintain or improve joint mobility for patients and one that you are able to coordinate with other activities is the use of range-of-motion exercises. In **active range-of-motion exercises,** the patient is able to move his or her joints. In contrast, the nurse moves the patient's joints in **passive range-of-motion exercises.** The use of these exercises enables you to systematically assess and improve the patient's joint mobility (see Chapter 35).

Joints that are not moved periodically develop contractures, a permanent shortening of a muscle followed by the eventual shortening of associated ligaments and tendons. Over time the joint becomes fixed in one position, and the patient loses normal use of the joint. For the patient who does not have voluntary motor control, passive range-of-motion exercises are the exercises of choice.

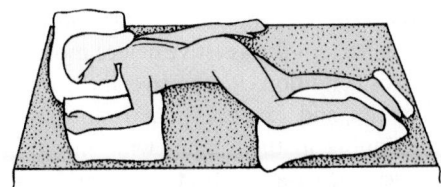

Figure 26-8 ■ Patient in Sims' position.

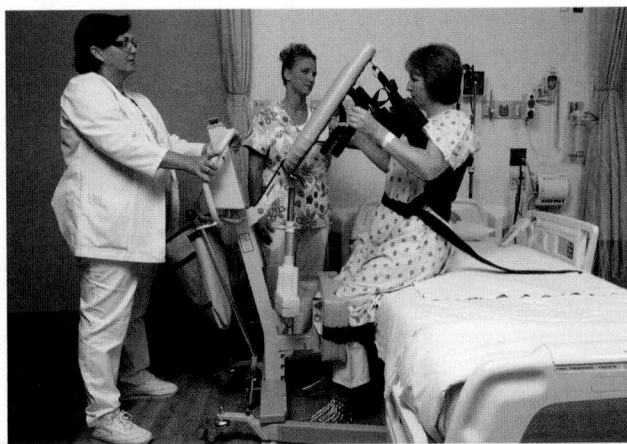

Figure 26-9 ■ Patient grasps handles as nurse enables motorized lift.

BOX 26-8   CARE OF THE OLDER ADULT

General Guidelines for Initiating an Exercise Program With the Older Adult

- Encourage the older adult patient to avoid prolonged sitting and to get up and stretch. Frequent stretching decreases joint contractures. Tai Chi exercise may be a suitable exercise alternative for the older adult (Choi, Moon, and Song, 2005).
- Be sure patient maintains proper body alignment when sitting. Proper alignment minimizes joint and muscle stress.
- Teach patients how to use stronger joints or larger muscle groups to manipulate spray cans, container lids, etc. Efficient distribution of workload decreases joint stress and pain.
- Provide resources for planned exercise programs. Proper exercise activities slow further bone loss and prevent fractures in the older adult with osteoporosis (Monahan and others, 2007).
- It is never too late to begin an exercise program (O'Brien-Gillespie, 2006). Consult a health care provider before beginning an exercise program, particularly in the presence of heart or lung disease and other chronic illnesses.

Mechanical devices are available for specific joints, which place these joints through continuous passive motion (CPM). Use these CPM machines postoperatively to place joints through a selective repetitive range of motion (see Chapter 35). Set the machine to certain degrees of joint mobility with increasing joint mobility or flexion as the goal. The most common patients who use the CPM machine are those who have undergone some form of total joint replacement surgery.

Unless contraindicated, the nursing care plan includes exercising each joint through as nearly a full range of motion as possible. Initiate passive range-of-motion exercises as soon as the patient loses the ability to move the extremity or joint (see Chapter 35).

The older adult often experiences a decline in physical activity and changes in joints that predispose to problems with mobility and limit joint flexibility. You will recommend approaches that help older adults to use proper body mechanics and prevent injury (Box 26-8).

Walking. Walking also increases joint mobility. In the normal walking posture the head is erect; the cervical, thoracic, and lumbar vertebrae are aligned; the hips and knees have appropriate flexion; and the arms swing freely in alternation with the legs. Illness or trauma reduces activity tolerance, necessitating a need for assistance with walking or the use of mechanical devices such as crutches, canes, or walkers.

Assisting a Patient in Walking. Assisting a patient in walking requires preparation. Assess the patient's activity tolerance, strength, coordination, and balance to determine the type of assistance needed. Also assess the patient's orientation, and determine if there are any signs of distress. This precludes attempts at ambulation.

Evaluate the environment for safety before ambulation. Remove obstacles, be sure the floor is clean and dry, and establish rest points in case the patient's activity tolerance decreases or if the patient becomes dizzy. Also, make sure the patient wears supportive, nonslip shoes.

When preparing a patient for ambulation, dangling is an important technique. You assist the patient to a sitting position with the legs dangling off the side of the bed and have

the patient rest for 1 to 2 minutes before standing. The longer the period of immobility, the greater the physiological changes. This is especially true with changes in circulation. When the patient has been flat for extended periods, blood pressure drops when the patient stands. Dangling helps to prevent this. After standing, have the patient remain stationary for a minute or two before moving. If the patient becomes dizzy, the bed is still nearby and you are able to quickly ease him or her back to bed.

You can use several methods for assisting a patient with ambulation. Use a gait belt to support the patient and maintain a midline center of gravity. Make sure patients do not lean to one side because their center of gravity is no longer midline, which distorts their balance and increases their risk for falling.

Return the patient who appears unsteady or complains of dizziness to the closest bed or a chair. If the patient has a syncopal episode or begins to fall, assume a wide base of support with one foot in front of the other, thus supporting the patient's body weight. Gently lower the patient to the floor, protecting the patient's head. Although lowering a patient to the floor is not difficult, practice this technique with a friend or classmate before attempting it in a clinical setting (Figure 26-10). Assess the patient for injuries at this time and notify the patient's health care provider. Even if the patient is stable, get the assistance of a lift team to help you get the patient off the floor and back in bed or a chair.

RESTORATIVE AND CONTINUING CARE Restorative and continuing care involving activity and exercise involves implementing strategies to assist the patient in activities of daily living (ADLs) after the patient's need for acute care is no longer warranted. In collaboration with other health care professionals such as physical therapists, you promote activity and exercise by teaching the use of canes, walkers, or crutches, depending on the assistive device most appropriate for the patient's condition. Restorative and continuing care includes activities and exercises that restore and improve optimal functioning in the patient with chronic musculoskeletal illnesses, such as arthritis, trauma, and other chronic illnesses, such as coronary artery disease (CAD).

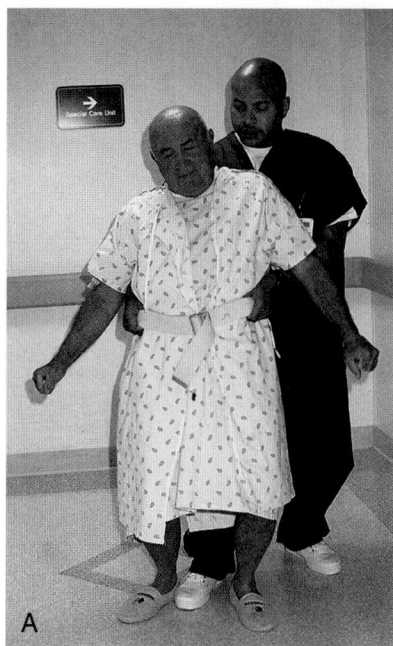
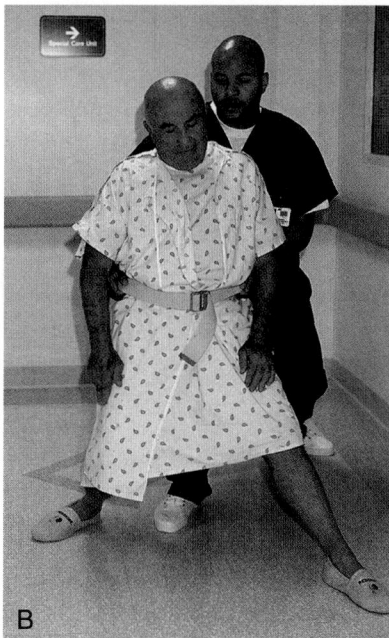
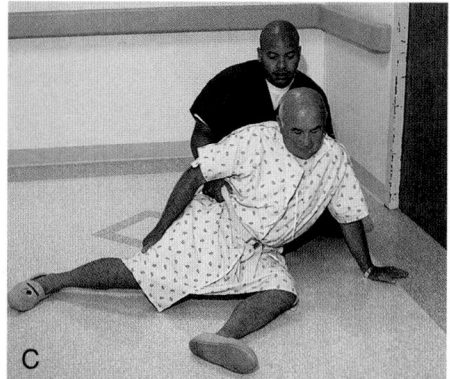

Figure 26-10 ■ **A,** Stand with feet apart to provide a broad base of support. **B,** Extend one leg, and let patient slide against it to the floor. **C,** Bend knees to lower body as patient slides to the floor.

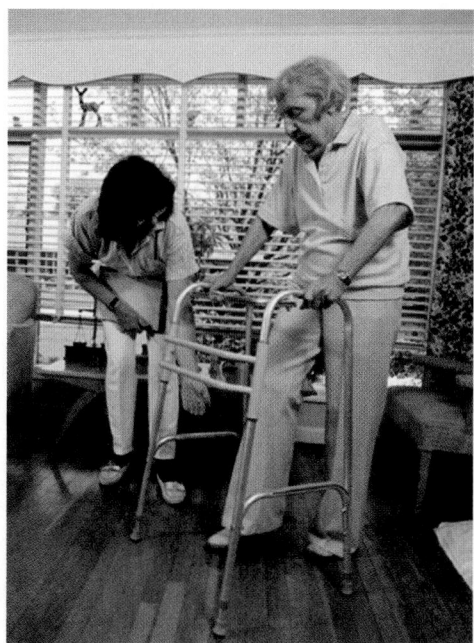

Figure 26-11 ■ Patient using a walker.

Assistive Devices for Walking

Walkers. Walkers are extremely light, movable devices, about waist high and made of metal tubing (Figure 26-11). They have four widely placed, sturdy legs. A walker is fitted correctly by having the patient step inside the walker. The person's elbow should bend comfortably, about 30 degrees, while holding onto the grips. When the person relaxes the arms at the side of the body, the top of the walker should line up with the crease on the inside of the wrist. When walking,

the patient holds the handgrips on the upper bars, takes a step, moves the walker forward, and takes another step. The patient should not lean over the walker or walk behind it; otherwise he or she might lose balance and fall.

Canes. Canes are lightweight, easily movable devices about waist high, made of wood or metal. Two common types of canes are the single straight-legged cane and the quad cane. The single straight-legged cane is used to support and balance a patient with decreased leg strength. Make sure the patient keeps the cane on the stronger side of the body (Pierson and Fairchild, 2008). The nurse stands on the patient's weak side for support (Pierson and Fairchild, 2008). For maximum support when walking, the patient places the cane forward 15 to 25 cm (6 to 10 inches), keeping body weight on both legs. The patient moves the weaker leg to the cane, which divides body weight between the cane and the stronger leg. The patient then advances the stronger leg past the cane so the weaker leg and the body weight is supported by the cane and weaker leg. During walking, the patient continually repeats these three steps. Teach the patient that two points of support, such as both feet or one foot and the cane, are present at all times.

The quad cane provides the most support and is used when there is partial or complete leg paralysis or some hemiplegia (Figure 26-12). You teach the same three steps used with the straight-legged cane to the patient.

Crutches. The use of crutches is usually temporary, such as after ligament damage to the knee. However, some patients, such as those with paralysis of the lower extremities, need crutches permanently. A crutch is a wooden or metal staff. The two types of crutches are the double adjustable Lofstrand or forearm crutch (Figure 26-13) and the axillary wooden or metal crutch. The forearm crutch has a handgrip and a metal band that fits around the patient's forearm. The metal band and the handgrip are adjustable to fit the patient's height. The axillary crutch has a padded curved surface at the top, which fits under the axilla. The patient holds a handgrip in the form of a crossbar at the level of the palms to support the body. It is important to measure crutches for the appropriate length and to teach patients to use their crutches safely. This includes teaching the patient to achieve a stable gait, to ascend and descend stairs, and to rise from a sitting position. You or a physical therapist will teach the patient safety measures and guidelines associated with the use of crutches (Box 26-9).

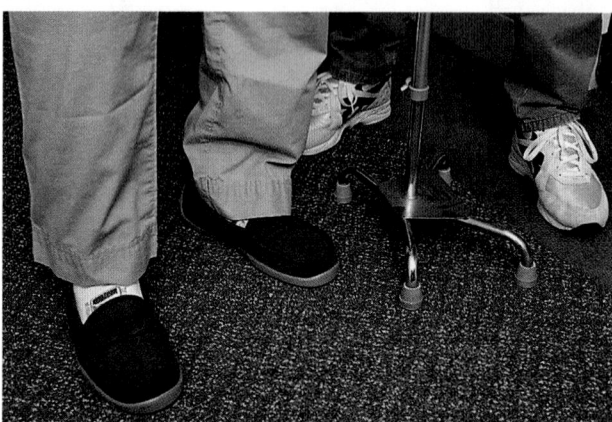

Figure 26-12 ■ Base of quad cane.

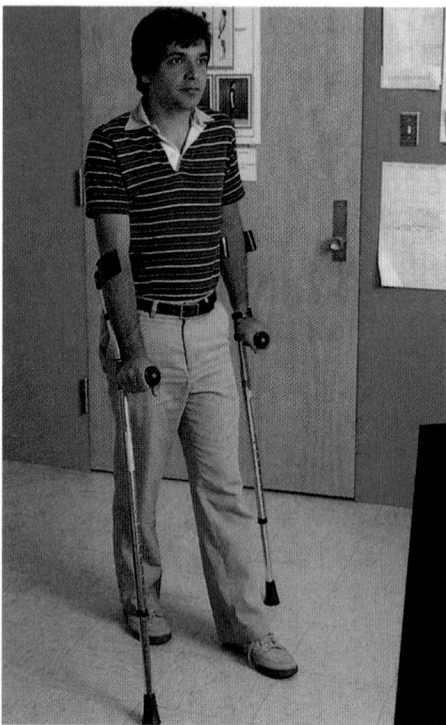

Figure 26-13 ■ Double adjustable Lofstrand or forearm crutch.

Measuring for Crutches. The axillary crutch is the crutch more commonly used. Measurements include the patient's height, the angle of elbow flexion, and the distance between the crutch pad and the axilla. When fitting crutches, the appropriate length of the crutch is from three to four finger widths from the axilla to a point 15 cm (6 inches) lateral to the patient's heel (Hoeman, 2008) (Figure 26-14).

BOX 26-9   PATIENT TEACHING

Crutch Safety

 The physical therapist (PT) told Marilyn that Mr. Indelicato will need crutches for a short period of time because of limited weight bearing on the affected knee. It is important that Mr. Indelicato begin to use the crutches before discharge. Marilyn and the PT work together to develop the following teaching plan:

OUTCOMES
- Patient will state the steps needed for safe crutch walking.
- Patient will describe how to identify axillary pressure points.
- Patient will demonstrate safe crutch walking.

TEACHING STRATEGIES
- Tell patient about the dangers of pressure on the axilla and how to identify pressure in the axillary region.
- Instruct patient not to lean on his crutches to support body weight.
- Demonstrate to patient how to inspect the crutch tips routinely. Make sure the rubber tips are securely attached to the crutches. When the tips are worn, they need replacing immediately. Rubber crutch tips increase surface friction and prevent the crutches from slipping.
- Inform patient about the importance of keeping the crutch tips dry. If the tips become wet, the patient needs to dry them. Water decreases surface friction and increases the risk that the crutches will slip.
- Show patient how to inspect the structure of the crutches routinely. Cracks in a wooden crutch decrease the crutch's ability to support weight. Bends in aluminum crutches alter body alignment, increasing the risk for further damage to the musculoskeletal system.
- Give patients a list of medical suppliers in their community. This allows the patients to obtain repairs and new rubber tips, handgrips, and crutch pads.
- Suggest that patient investigate the possibility of having a set of spare crutches and tips.

EVALUATION STRATEGIES
- Ask patient to describe how he will maintain crutch safety.
- Observe patient inspect his crutch tips and structure.
- Observe patient using the crutches.
- Observe axillae for signs of pressure or skin breakdown.
- Ask patient what he will do if his crutch breaks or he needs additional crutch tips.

Make sure you position the handgrips so the axillae do not support all of the patient's body weight. Pressure on the axillae increases risk to underlying nerves, which sometimes results in partial paralysis of the arm. You determine the correct position of the handgrips with the patient upright, supporting weight by the handgrips with the elbows slightly flexed (20 to 25 degrees). You verify elbow flexion with a goniometer (Figure 26-15). When you have determined the height and placement of the handgrips, you again verify that the distance between the crutch pad and the patient's axilla is three to four finger widths (Figure 26-16).

Crutch Gait. The patient assumes the **crutch gait** by alternately bearing weight on one or both legs and on the crutches. The health care provider determines the gait by assessing the patient's functional abilities, strength and weight bearing ability, and the disease or injury that resulted in the need for crutches. This section summarizes the basic crutch stance and the four standard gaits: four-point alternating gait, three-point alternating gait, two-point gait, and swing-through gait.

The basic crutch stance is the tripod position, formed when the crutches are placed 15 cm (6 inches) in front of and 15 cm to the side of each foot (Figure 26-17). This position improves the patient's balance by providing a wider base of support. The body alignment of the patient in the tripod position includes erect head and neck, straight vertebrae, and extended hips and knees. No weight should be borne by the axillae. The tripod position is used before crutch walking.

Four-point alternating or four-point gait gives stability to the patient but requires weight bearing on both legs. Each leg is moved alternately with each opposing crutch so that three points of support are on the floor at all times (Figure 26-18, *A*).

Three-point alternating or three-point gait requires the patient to bear all of the weight on one foot. In a three-point gait, the patient puts weight on both crutches and then on the uninvolved leg, and then repeats the sequence (Figure 26-18, *B*). The affected leg does not touch the ground during the early phase of the three-point gait. Gradually the patient progresses to touchdown and full weight bearing on the affected leg.

The two-point gait requires at least partial weight bearing on each foot (Figure 26-18, *C*). The patient moves a crutch at

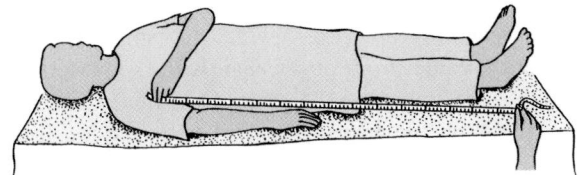

Figure 26-14 ■ Measuring for crutch length.

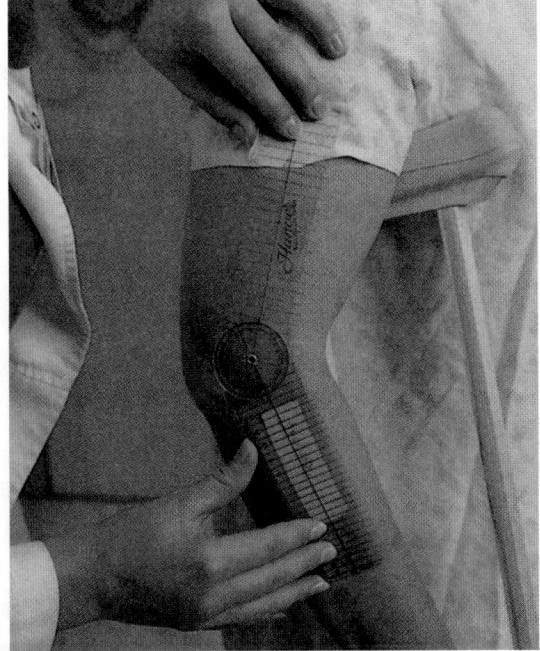

Figure 26-15 ■ Using the goniometer to verify correct degree of elbow flexion for crutch use.

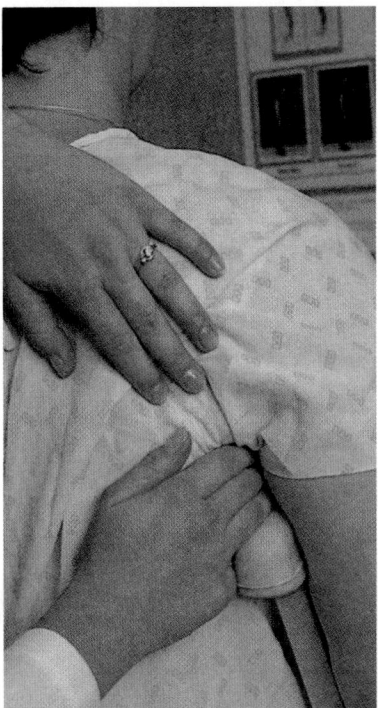

Figure 26-16 ■ Verifying correct distance between crutch pad and axilla.

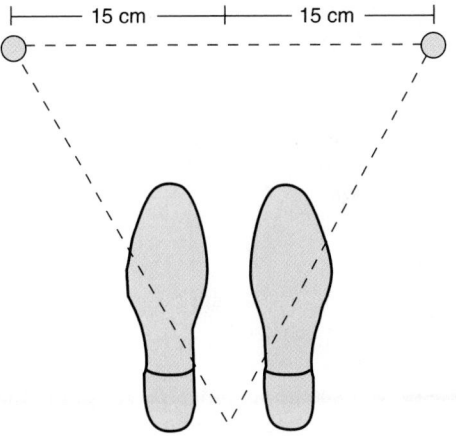

Figure 26-17 ■ Tripod position, basic crutch stance.

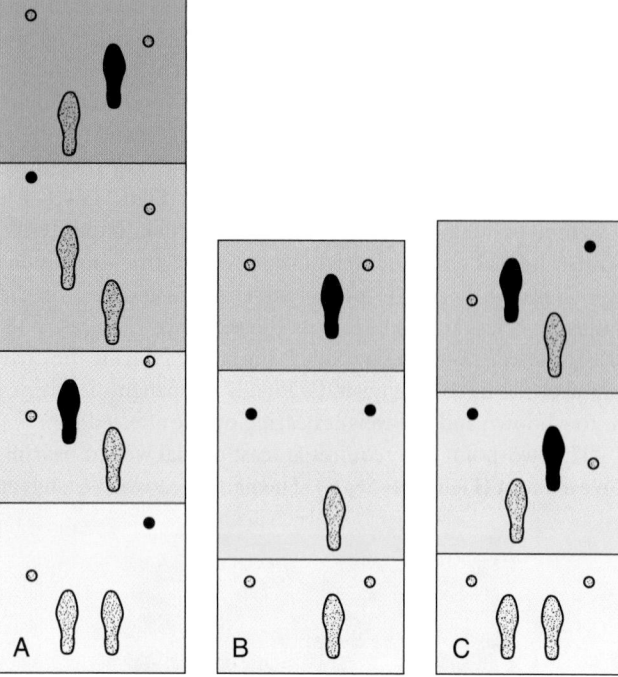

Figure 26-18 ■ **A,** Four-point alternating gait. Solid feet and crutch tips show foot and crutch tip moved in each of the four phases. (Read from bottom to top.) **B,** Three-point gait with weight borne on unaffected leg. Solid foot and crutch tips show weight bearing in each phase. **C,** Two-point gait with weight borne partially on each foot and each crutch advancing with opposing leg. Solid areas indicate leg and crutch tips bearing weight.

the same time as the opposite leg, so the crutch movements are similar to arm motion during normal walking.

Paraplegics who wear weight-supporting braces on their legs frequently use the swing-through gait. With weight placed on the supported legs, the patient places the crutches one stride in front and then swings to or through the crutches while they support the patient's weight.

Crutch Walking on Stairs. When ascending stairs on crutches, the patient usually uses a modified three-point gait (Figure 26-19). The patient stands at the bottom of the stairs and transfers body weight to the crutches. The patient advances the unaffected leg between the crutches to the stairs. The patient then shifts weight from the crutches to the unaffected leg. Finally, the patient aligns both crutches on the stairs. The patient repeats this sequence until the patient reaches the top of the stairs.

To descend the stairs (Figure 26-20), the patient also uses a three-phase sequence. The patient transfers body weight to the unaffected leg. The patient places crutches on the stair, and then begins to transfer body weight to the crutches, moving the affected leg forward. Finally, the patient moves the unaffected leg to the stairs with the crutches. Again, the patient repeats the sequence until reaching the bottom of the stairs.

Sitting in a Chair With Crutches. As with crutch walking and crutch walking up and down stairs, the procedure for sitting in a chair involves phases and requires the patient to transfer weight (Figure 26-21). First, the patient gets positioned at the center front of the chair with the posterior aspect of the legs touching the chair. Then the patient holds both crutches in the hand opposite the affected leg. If both

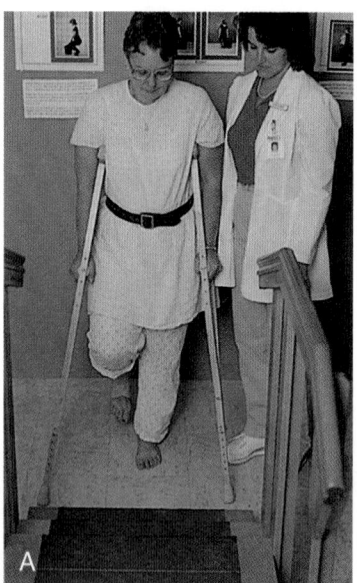
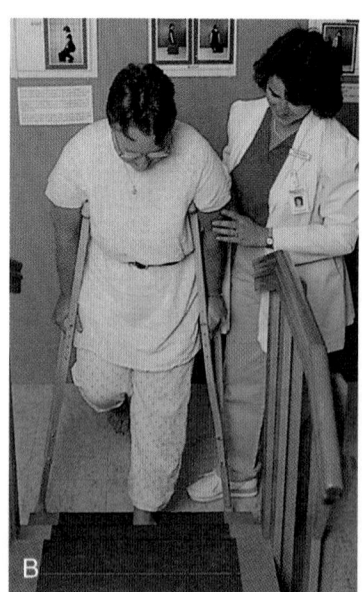
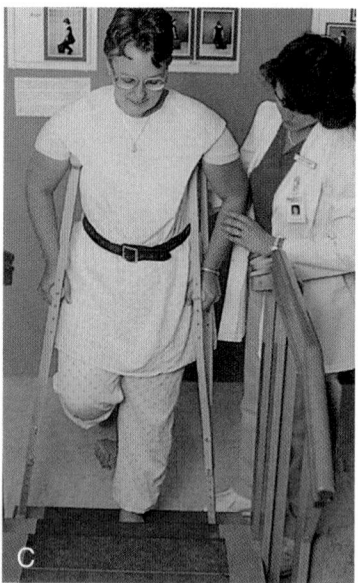

Figure 26-19 ■ Ascending stairs. **A,** Weight is placed on crutches. **B,** Weight is transferred from crutches to unaffected leg on stairs. **C,** Crutches are aligned with unaffected leg on stairs.

legs are affected, as with a paraplegic who wears weight-supporting braces, the patient holds the crutches in the hand on the patient's stronger side. With both crutches in one hand, the patient supports body weight on the unaffected leg and crutches. While still holding the crutches, the patient grasps the arm of the chair with the remaining hand and lowers the body into the chair. To stand, the patient reverses the procedure and, when fully erect, assumes the tripod position before beginning to walk.

■■■EVALUATION

PATIENT CARE You evaluate all nursing interventions by comparing the patient's actual response to the expected outcomes for each goal. You evaluate specific outcomes designed to demonstrate improved activity and exercise. If the patient does not achieve the expected outcomes, you need to revise the care plan. The success in meeting each outcome is based on the use of evaluative measures such as ROM, ability

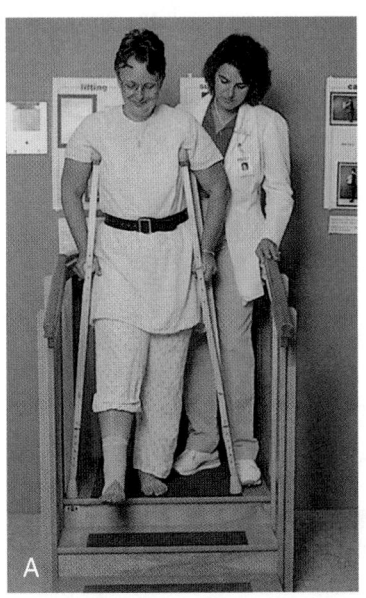
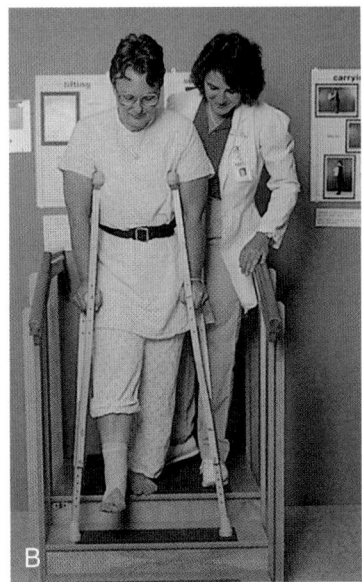
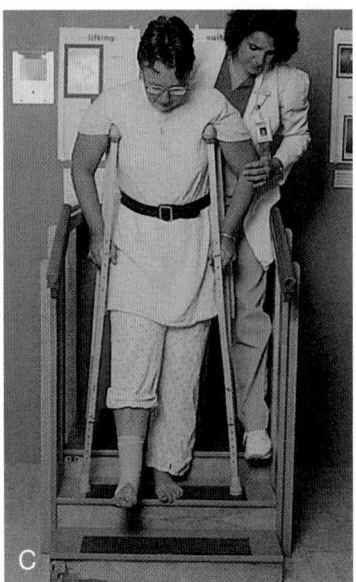

Figure 26-20 ■ Descending stairs. **A,** Body weight on unaffected leg. **B,** Body weight transferred to crutches. **C,** Unaffected leg aligned on stairs with crutches.

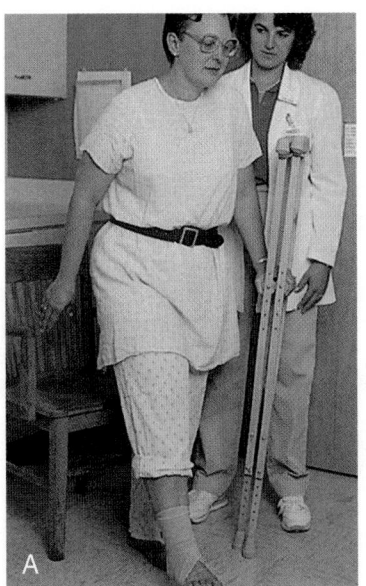
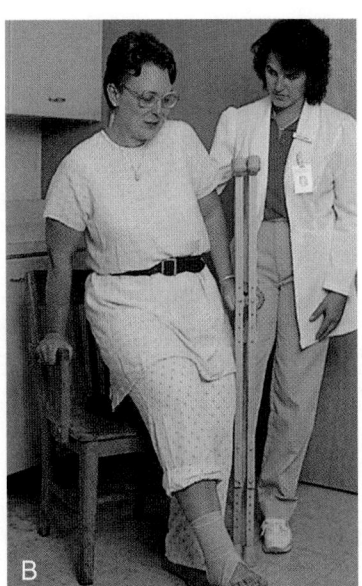
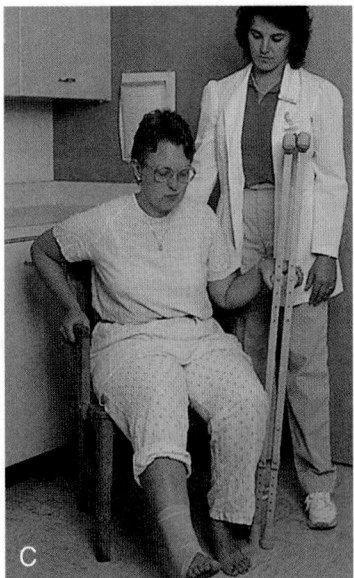

Figure 26-21 ■ Sitting on chair. **A,** Both crutches are held by one hand. Patient transfers weight to crutches and unaffected leg. **B,** Patient grasps arm of chair with free hand and begins to lower herself into chair. **C,** Patient completely lowers herself into chair.

of patient to ambulate, distance of ambulation, and activity/exercise tolerance (Box 26-10).

PATIENT EXPECTATIONS For the patient with alterations in body mechanics or joint mobility, you measure the effectiveness of nursing interventions by the success of meeting the patient's expected outcomes and goals of care. For some patients with altered body mechanics or joint mobility, maintenance of joint mobility will be easily accomplished and will not be a priority goal. For others, return of joint mobility and maintenance of body alignment will be the most important outcome, and you will direct all interventions toward its accomplishment.

For you to evaluate the patient's perception of the interventions, first you need to know the patient's expectations concerning joint mobility, posture, or body alignment. What is acceptable or anticipated on your part is sometimes vastly different from what the patient and family members anticipate or accept.

BOX 26-10   EVALUATION

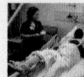 It has been 5 weeks since Marilyn began to care for Mr. Indelicato. For the last 4 weeks she has followed him in the outpatient rehabilitation setting. Mr. Indelicato has progressed steadily to increase both weight bearing and range of joint motion on the affected knee. His pain was more difficult to manage. Mr. Indelicato expected pain to be completely resolved on hospital discharge and did not expect pain to follow his physical therapy. Marilyn and the physical therapist worked with Mr. Indelicato and his orthopedic surgeon to identify pain-control measures following physical therapy. Currently Mr. Indelicato takes 600 mg of ibuprofen 45 minutes before physical therapy and every 8 to 12 hours thereafter. Mr. Indelicato reports that his pain is now almost totally gone. He is now working on increasing strength so he is able to return to golf and bike riding. He says he will probably give up racquetball and tennis.

DOCUMENTATION NOTE

"Weight bearing and range of motion continue to improve. States takes 600 mg ibuprofen 45 minutes before coming to therapy and every 8 to 12 hours as needed for pain. Rates pain a 1 when exercising. States would like to begin riding bike and playing golf again in next 1 to 2 months."

SAFETY GUIDELINES FOR NURSING SKILLS

Ensuring patient safety is an essential role of the professional nurse. To ensure patient safety, communicate clearly with members of the health care team, assess and incorporate the patient's priorities of care and preferences, and use the best evidence when making decisions about your patient's care. When performing the skills in this chapter, remember the following points to ensure safe, individualized patient care.

- Mentally review the transfer steps before beginning to ensure both the patient's and your safety.
- Assess the patient's mobility and strength to determine the assistance he or she is able to offer during transfer. Stand on the patient's weak side when assisting (Pierson and Fairchild, 2008).
- Determine the amount and type of assistance you require. This includes determining the type of transfer equipment

and the number of personnel it will take to safely transfer and prevent harm to the patient and yourself.

- Explain the procedure, and describe what you expect of the patient.
- Raise the side rail on the side of the bed opposite of where you are standing to prevent the patient from falling out of bed on that side.
- Position the level of the bed to a comfortable and safe height.
- Arrange equipment (e.g., intravenous [IV] lines, feeding tube, Foley catheter) so it will not interfere with the transfer.
- Evaluate patient for correct body alignment and pressure areas after the transfer.

SKILL 26-1   MOVING AND POSITIONING PATIENTS IN BED

DELEGATION CONSIDERATIONS

The skill of moving and positioning patients in bed can be delegated to nursing assistive personnel (NAP). The nurse informs the NAP about:

- Any limitations affecting movement and positioning of patient in bed
- Scheduled times to reposition patient throughout the shift
- When to request assistance, such as when the patient is unable to assist the nurse or has a lot of equipment or is confused, etc.

EQUIPMENT

- Pillows
- Therapeutic boots, splints, ankle support device, if needed
- Trochanter roll
- Sandbag
- Hand rolls
- Side rails
- Appropriate safe-patient-handling assistive device

STEP	RATIONALE

ASSESSMENT

1 Assess patient's body alignment and comfort level while patient is lying down.

Provides baseline data for later comparisons. Determines ways to improve position and alignment.

2 Assess for risk factors that will contribute to complications of immobility:

Increased risk factors require you to reposition the patient more frequently (see Chapter 35).

  a Paralysis: Hemiparesis resulting from cerebrovascular accident (CVA); decreased sensation

Paralysis impairs movement; muscle tone changes; affects sensation. Because of difficulty in moving and poor awareness of involved body part, patient is unable to protect and position body part for self.

  b Impaired mobility: Traction or arthritis or other contributing disease processes

Traction or arthritic changes of affected extremity result in decreased ROM.

  c Impaired circulation

Decreased circulation predisposes patient to pressure ulcers.

  d Age: Very young, older adult

Premature and young infants require frequent turning because their skin is fragile. Normal physiological changes associated with aging predispose older adults to greater risks for developing complications of immobility.

  e Level of consciousness and mental status

Comatose or semicomatose patients are unable to verbalize areas of skin pressure, increasing the risk for skin breakdown.

3 Assess patient's physical ability to help with moving and positioning:

Enables nurse to use patient's mobility, coordination and strength. Determines need for additional help. Ensures the patient's and the nurse's safety.

  a Age

Some older adult patients move more slowly with less strength.

  b Level of consciousness and mental status

Determines need for special aids or devices.

Patients with altered levels of consciousness do not always understand instructions and are often unable to help.

  c Disease process

Cardiopulmonary disease requires patient to have head of bed elevated.

  d Strength, coordination

Determines amount of assistance provided by patient during position change.

  e ROM

Limited ROM contraindicates certain positions.

4 Assess patient's height, weight, and body shape.

Devices for safe patient handling have different weight restrictions; bariatric patients require special beds, lifts, wheelchairs, and toileting and bathing equipment (Nelson and others, 2003b).

5 Assess health care provider's orders. Clarify whether patient's condition contraindicates any positions (e.g., spinal cord injury; respiratory difficulties; certain neurological conditions; presence of incisions, drain, or tubing).

Placing patient in an inappropriate position causes injury.

6 Assess for presence of tubes, incisions, and equipment (e.g., traction).

Will alter positioning procedure and affect patient's ability to independently change positions.

7 Assess condition of patient's skin.

Provides baseline to determine effects of positioning.

8 Assess ability and motivation of patient, family members, and primary caregiver to participate in moving and positioning patient in bed in anticipation of discharge to home.

Determines ability of patient and caregivers to assist with positioning.

PLANNING

1 Collect appropriate equipment. Get extra help as needed. Close door to room or close bedside curtains.

Having appropriate number of people to position patient prevents patient and nurse injury. Provides for patient privacy.

2 Perform hand hygiene.

Reduces transfer of microorganisms.

3 Verify patient's identity by using at least two patient identifiers. Compare patient's name and one other identifier, such as hospital identification number, with medical record. Ask patient to state name as a third id entifier. Explain procedure.

Complies with The Joint Commission requirements and improves patient safety. In most acute care settings you will use the patient's name and identification number on armband and medical record to identify patients (The Joint Commission, 2010). Decreases anxiety and increases patient cooperation.

4 Raise level of bed to comfortable working height. Remove all pillows and devices used for positioning.

Raises work toward nurse's center of gravity. Reduces any interference during positioning.

SKILL 26-1   MOVING AND POSITIONING PATIENTS IN BED—cont'd

STEP	RATIONALE

IMPLEMENTATION

1 Position patient flat in bed on back if tolerated. Keep patient aligned.

Repositioning from a flat position decreases friction and possible shear on patient's skin.

• **Critical Decision Point:** Before flattening bed, account for all tubing, drains, and equipment to prevent dislodgment or tipping if caught in mattress or bed frame as bed is lowered.

A Assist Patient in Moving Up in Bed (Two Nurses)

This is not a one-person task. Assisting a patient in moving up in bed without help from other co-workers or without the aid of an assistive device (i.e., friction-reducing pad) is no longer recommended or considered safe for the patient or nurse (ANA, 2003, 2007). If a patient is unable to fully assist, then refer to Step 1B.

(1) Remove pillow from under head and shoulders, and place pillow at head of bed.

Prevents striking patient's head against head of bed.

(2) Face head of bed.

Facing direction of movement prevents twisting of your body while moving patient.

(3) Each nurse places one arm under patient's head and shoulders and one arm under patient's thighs.

Provides support across length of patient's body.

(4) Alternative position if patient can assist: Position one nurse at patient's upper body. Nurse's arm nearest head of bed is under patient's head and opposite shoulder; other arm is under patient's closest arm and shoulder. Position other nurse at patient's lower torso. The nurse's arms are under patient's lower back and torso.

Prevents trauma to patient's musculoskeletal system by supporting shoulder and hip joints and evenly distributing weight.

(5) Place feet apart, with foot nearest head of bed in front of other foot (forward-backward stance).

Wide base of support increases balance. Stance enables you to shift body weight as you move patient up in bed, thereby reducing force needed to move load.

(6) Before moving patient, instruct patient to flex knees with feet flat on bed.

Decreases friction and enables patient to use leg muscles during movement.

(7) Also instruct patient to flex neck, tilting chin toward chest.

Prevents hyperextension of neck when moving patient up in bed.

(8) Have patient assist moving by pushing with feet on bed surface.

Reduces friction. Increases patient mobility. Decreases workload.

(9) Flex your knees and hips, bringing forearms closer to level of bed.

Increases balance and strength by bringing your center of gravity closer to patient. Uses thighs instead of back muscles.

(10) Instruct patient on a count of 3 to push with heels and elevate trunk while breathing out, thus moving toward head of bed.

Prepares patient for move. Reinforces assistance in moving up in bed. Increases patient cooperation. Breathing out avoids Valsalva maneuver.

(11) On count of 3, rock and shift weight from front to back leg. At the same time patient pushes with heels and elevates trunk.

Rocking enables you to improve balance and overcome inertia. Shifting weight counteracts patient's weight and reduces force needed to move load. Patient's assistance reduces friction and workload.

B Move Immobile Patient Up in Bed With Drawsheet (Two Nurses)

• **Critical Decision Point:** Use safe nursing judgment by increasing number of nurses or NAP when moving a larger patient up in bed. If in doubt, acquire more help.

(1) Place drawsheet under patient by turning side to side. Extend sheet from shoulders to thighs. Return patient to supine position.

Supports patient's body weight and reduces friction during movement.

STEP	RATIONALE
(2) Position one nurse at each side of the patient's hips.	Distributes weight equally between nurses.
(3) Grasp drawsheet firmly near the patient.	
(4) Place feet apart with forward-backward stance. Flex knees and hips. On count of three shift weight from front to back leg, and move patient and drawsheet to desired position in bed (see illustration).	Facing direction of movement ensures proper balance. Shifting weight reduces force needed to move load. Flexing knees lowers center of gravity and thighs instead of back muscles.
(5) Realign patient in correct body alignment.	Prevents injury to musculoskeletal system.
C Position Patient in Supported Fowler's Position (see illustration)	
(1) Elevate head of bed 45 to 60 degrees, if not contraindicated.	Increases comfort, improves ventilation, and increases patient's opportunity to socialize or relax.
(2) Rest head against mattress or on small pillow.	Prevents flexion contractures of cervical vertebrae.
(3) Use pillows to support arms and hands if patient does not have voluntary control or use of hands and arms.	Prevents shoulder dislocation from effect of downward pull of unsupported arms, promotes circulation by preventing venous pooling, and prevents flexion contractures of arms and wrists.
(4) Position pillow at lower back.	Supports lumbar vertebrae and decreases flexion of vertebrae.
(5) Place small pillow under thigh.	Prevents hyperextension of knee and occlusion of popliteal artery caused by pressure from body weight.
(6) Position patient's heels in heel boots or other heel pressure-relief device.	Heel pressure-relief devices are more effective than pillows for consistently reducing pressure from the mattress on the heels.

- ***Critical Decision Point:*** To keep feet in proper alignment and prevent footdrop, use foot support devices, such as ankle or foot boots. In addition, a foot cradle is often used for patients with poor peripheral circulation as a means of reducing pressure on the tips of a patient's toes (check agency policy).

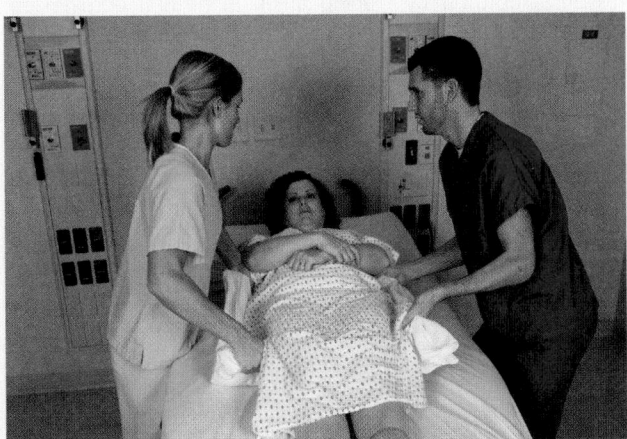

Step 1B(4)

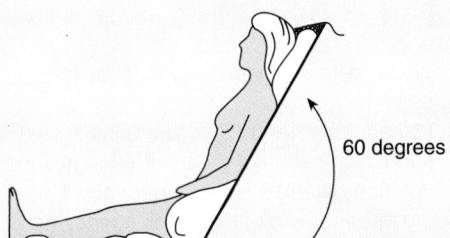

60 degrees

Step 1C ■ Supported Fowler's position.

STEP	RATIONALE
D Position Hemiplegic Patient in Supported Fowler's Position	
(1) Elevate head of bed 45 to 60 degrees.	Increases comfort, improves ventilation, and increases patient's opportunity to relax.
(2) Position patient in sitting position as straight as possible.	Counteracts tendency to slump toward affected side. Improves ventilation, cardiac output, and decreases intracranial pressure. Improves patient's ability to swallow and helps to prevent aspiration of food, liquids, and gastric secretions (Glenn-Molali, 2008).
(3) Position head on small pillow with chin slightly forward. If patient is totally unable to control head movement, avoid hyperextension of the neck.	Prevents hyperextension of neck. Too many pillows under head cause neck flexion contracture.

- *Critical Decision Point:* If the patient has a paralyzed extremity, provide support for involved arm and hand on over-bed table in front of patient. Place arm away from patient's side, and support elbow with pillow.
- Position flaccid hand in normal resting position with wrist slightly extended, arches of hand maintained, and fingers partially flexed; use section of rubber ball cut in half; clasp patient's hands together.
- Position spastic hand with wrist in neutral position or slightly extended; extend fingers with palm down or leave fingers in relaxed position with palm up. At times it is difficult to position spastic hands without the use of specially made splints for the patient.

STEP	RATIONALE
(4) Flex knees and hips by using pillow or folded blanket under knees.	Ensures proper alignment. Flexion prevents prolonged hyperextension, which impairs joint mobility.
(5) Place trochanter rolls along side patient's legs.	Prevents external rotation of hips that often contributes to contractures.
(6) Support feet in dorsiflexion with foot support such as ankle or foot boots (check agency policy).	Prevents footdrop by placing ankle in neutral dorsiflexion. Stimulation of ball of foot by hard surface has tendency to increase muscle tone in patient with extensor spasticity of lower extremity.
E Position Patient in Supine Position	
(1) Be sure patient is comfortable on back with head of bed flat.	Some patients' physical conditions will not tolerate supine position.
(2) Place small rolled towel under lumbar area of back.	Provides support for lumbar spine.
(3) Place pillow under upper shoulders, neck, or head.	Maintains correct alignment and prevents flexion contractures of cervical vertebrae.
(4) Place trochanter rolls or sandbags parallel to lateral surface of patient's thighs, if patient is immobile.	Reduces external rotation of hip.
(5) Position patient's heels in heel boots or other heel pressure-relief device (check agency policy).	Heel pressure-relief devices are more effective than pillows for consistently reducing pressure from the mattress on the heels.
(6) If needed support feet in dorsiflexion with foot support such as ankle or foot boots (check agency policy).	Prevents footdrop by placing ankle in neutral dorsiflexion. Stimulation of ball of foot by hard surface has tendency to increase muscle tone in patient with extensor spasticity of lower extremity.
(7) Place pillows under pronated forearms, keeping upper arms parallel to patient's body (see illustrations).	Reduces internal rotation of shoulder and prevents extension of elbows. Maintains correct body alignment.
(8) Place hand rolls in patient's hands. Consider physical therapy referral for use of hand splints.	Reduces extension of fingers and abduction of thumb. Maintains thumb slightly adducted and in opposition to fingers.

STEP	RATIONALE

F Position Hemiplegic Patient in Supine Position

(1) Be sure patient is comfortable on back with head of bed flat.

Some patients' physical conditions will not tolerate supine position.

(2) Place folded towel or small pillow under shoulder of affected side.

Decreases possibility of pain, joint contracture, and subluxation. Maintains mobility in muscles around shoulder to permit normal movement patterns.

(3) Keep affected arm away from body with elbow extended and palm up. (*Alternative* is to place arm out to side, with elbow bent and hand toward head of bed.)

Maintains mobility in arm, joints, and shoulder to permit normal movement patterns. (*Alternative* position counteracts limitation of ability of arm to rotate outward at shoulder [external rotation]. Need external rotation to raise arm overhead without pain.)

• *Critical Decision Point:* Position affected hand in one of the recommended positions for flaccid or spastic hand. (See Critical Decision Point on p. 702.)

---

(4) Place folded towel under hip of involved side.

Diminishes effect of spasticity in entire leg by controlling hip position.

(5) Flex affected knee 30 degrees by supporting it on pillow or folded blanket.

Slight flexion breaks up abnormal extension pattern of leg. Extensor spasticity is most severe when patient is supine.

(6) Position patient's heel in heel sboots or other heel pressure-relief device (check agency policy).

Heel pressure-relief devices are more effective than pillows for consistently reducing pressure from the mattress on the heels. In addition, a heel boot also maintains the feet in dorsiflexion, which prevents footdrop.

(7) If needed support feet in dorsiflexion with foot support such as ankle or foot boots (check agency policy).

Prevents footdrop by placing ankle in neutral dorsiflexion. Stimulation of ball of foot by hard surface has tendency to increase muscle tone in patient with extensor spasticity of lower extremity.

G Position Patient in Prone Position (see illustration)

(1) With patient supine, place arm on side to be turned, alongside the body. Roll patient over arm positioned close to body, with elbow straight and hand under hip. Position on abdomen in center of bed.

Positions patient correctly to maintain alignment.

(2) Turn patient's head to one side, and support head with small pillow.

Reduces flexion or hyperextension of cervical vertebrae.

(3) Place small pillow under patient's abdomen below level of diaphragm.

Reduces pressure on breasts of some female patients and decreases hyperextension of lumbar vertebrae and strain on lower back.

(4) Support arms in flexed position level at shoulders.

Maintains proper body alignment. Support reduces risk for joint dislocation.

(5) Support lower legs with pillow to elevate toes.

Prevents footdrop. Reduces external rotation of hips. Reduces mattress pressure on toes.

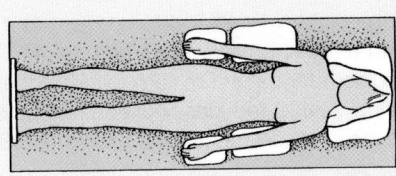
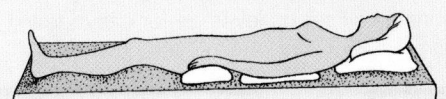
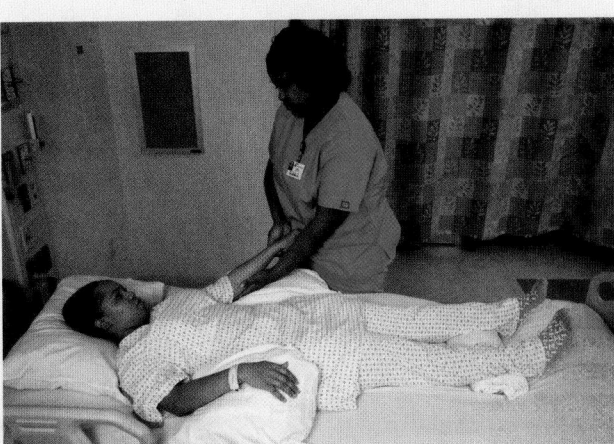

Step 1E(7) ■ Supine position with pillows in place.

SKILL 26-1	MOVING AND POSITIONING PATIENTS IN BED—cont'd

STEP	RATIONALE

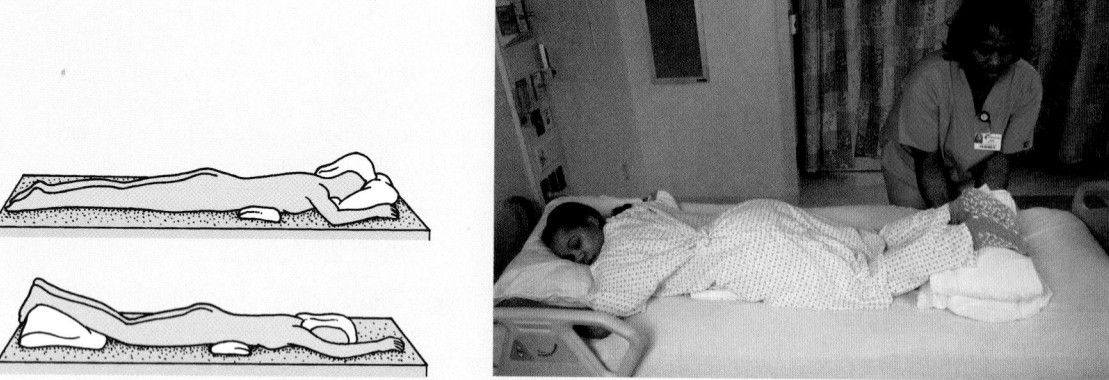

Step 1G ■ Prone position with supporting pillows.

H Position Hemiplegic Patient in Prone Position

- *Critical Decision Point:* Increase frequency of positioning if pressure areas begin to appear, joint mobility becomes impaired or worsened, or patient demonstrates signs of discomfort. Consult with physical and occupational therapists as needed.

STEP	RATIONALE
(1) Move patient toward unaffected side, with patient remaining supine.	Creates room for proper patient alignment in center of bed when patient is rolled onto abdomen.
(2) Place pillow on patient's abdomen.	Prevents sagging of abdomen when patient is rolled over; decreases hyperextension of lumbar vertebrae and strain on lower back.
(3) Roll patient onto affected side.	
(4) Roll patient onto abdomen by positioning involved arm close to patient's body, with elbow straight and hand under hip. Roll patient carefully over arm.	Prevents injury to affected side.
(5) Turn head toward involved side.	Promotes development of neck and trunk extension, which is necessary for standing and walking.
(6) Position involved arm out to side, with elbow bent, hand toward head of bed, and fingers extended (if possible).	Counteracts limitation of arm's ability to rotate outward at shoulder (external rotation). Need external rotation to raise arm over head without pain.
(7) Flex knees slightly by placing pillow under legs from knees to ankles.	Flexion prevents prolonged hyperextension, which impairs joint mobility.
(8) Support feet with foot support devices, such as ankle or foot boots (check agency policy).	Maintains feet in dorsiflexion.

I Position Patient in 30-Degree Lateral (Side-Lying) Position

STEP	RATIONALE
(1) Patient lies supine with head of bed as low as patient tolerates.	Provides position of comfort for patient and removes pressure from bony prominences on back and buttocks.
(2) Position patient to one side of bed. Then move to opposite side of bed toward which patient is to be turned. Use friction-reducing device or mechanical lift per manufacturer's guidelines if patient cannot assist with moving.	Provides room for patient to turn to side. Use of safe patient-handling device reduces workload of caregivers and enhances safety (de Castro and others, 2006).
(3) Prepare to turn patient onto side. Flex patient's knee that will not be next to mattress. Place one hand on patient's hip and one hand on patient's shoulder.	Positioning will set up leverage for easy turning.

STEP	RATIONALE
(4) Roll patient onto side toward you.	Rolling patient toward you decreases trauma to tissues. In addition, positioning patient so leverage is on hip makes turning easy.
(5) Place pillow under patient's head and neck.	Maintains alignment. Reduces lateral neck flexion. Decreases strain on sternocleidomastoid muscle.
(6) Place hands under patient's dependent shoulder, and bring shoulder blade forward.	Prevents patient's weight from resting directly on shoulder joint.
(7) Position both arms in slightly flexed position. Support upper arm with pillow level with shoulder, other arm by mattress.	Decreases internal rotation and adduction of shoulder. Supporting both arms in slightly flexed position protects joints. Improves ventilation because chest is able to expand more easily.
(8) Place hands under dependent hip and bring hip slightly forward so that angle from hip to mattress is approximately 30 degrees (see Figure 26-7, p. 690).	The 30-degree lateral position reduces pressure on trochanter.
(9) Place tuck-back pillow behind patient's back. (Make by folding pillow lengthwise. Smooth area is slightly tucked under patient's back.)	Provides support to maintain patient on side.
(10) Place pillow under semiflexed upper leg level at hip from groin to foot.	Maintains leg in correct alignment. Prevents pressure on bony prominence.
(11) Support feet with foot support devices, such as ankle or foot boots (check agency policy).	Maintains dorsiflexion of foot. Prevents footdrop.

J Position Patient in Sims' (Semiprone) Position

STEP	RATIONALE
(1) Be sure patient is comfortable in supine position.	Provides for proper body alignment while patient is lying down.
(2) Position patient in side-lying position, lying partially on abdomen, with dependent arm straight along patient's body.	Facilitates turning onto side. Avoids injury to arm; semiprone position places less pressure on abdomen.
(3) Carefully lift patient's dependent shoulder, and bring arm back behind patient.	Patient is rolled only partially on abdomen.
(4) Place small pillow under patient's head.	Maintains proper alignment and prevents lateral neck flexion.
(5) Place pillow under flexed upper arm, supporting arm level with shoulder.	Prevents internal rotation of shoulder. Maintains alignment.
(6) Place pillow under flexed upper leg, supporting leg level with hip (see Figure 26-8, p. 691).	Prevents internal rotation of hip and adduction of leg. Flexion prevents hyperextension of leg. Reduces mattress pressure on knees and ankles.
(7) Support feet with foot support devices, such as ankle or foot boots (check agency policy).	Maintains foot in dorsiflexion. Prevents footdrop.

K Logrolling the Patient (Three Nurses)

• **Critical Decision Point:** Supervise and assist NAP when there is a health care provider's order to **logroll** a patient. Patients who have suffered from a spinal cord injury or are recovering from neck, back, or spinal surgery often need to keep the spinal column in straight alignment to prevent further injury.

STEP	RATIONALE
(1) Place small pillow between patient's knees.	Prevents tension on the spinal column and adduction of the hip.
(2) Cross patient's arms on chest.	Prevents injury to arms.
(3) Position two nurses on side of bed to which the patient will be turned. Position third nurse on the other side of bed (see illustration). If needed, use a fourth caregiver who stands on the same side as the third person.	Distributes weight equally between nurses.
(4) Fanfold or roll the drawsheet along side of patient.	Provides strong handles in order to grip the drawsheet without slipping.

SKILL 26-1	MOVING AND POSITIONING PATIENTS IN BED—cont'd

STEP	RATIONALE
(5) Move the patient as one unit in a smooth, continuous motion on the count of three (see illustration).	This maintains proper alignment by moving all body parts at the same time, preventing tension or twisting of the spinal column.
(6) Nurse on the opposite side of the bed places pillows along the length of the patient (see illustration).	Pillows keep patient aligned.
(7) Gently lean the patient as a unit back toward the pillows for support (see illustration).	Ensures continued straight alignment of spinal column, preventing injury.
2 Perform hand hygiene.	Reduces transmission of microorganisms.

EVALUATION

1 Evaluate patient's body alignment, position, and level of comfort.	Determines effectiveness of positioning. Add or remove additional supports (e.g., pillows, bath blankets) to promote comfort and correct body alignment.
2 Measure ROM (see Chapter 35).	Determines if joint contracture is developing.
3 Observe for areas of erythema or breakdown involving skin.	Indicates complications of immobility or improper positioning of body part. Determines if need for increasing frequency of repositioning patient.

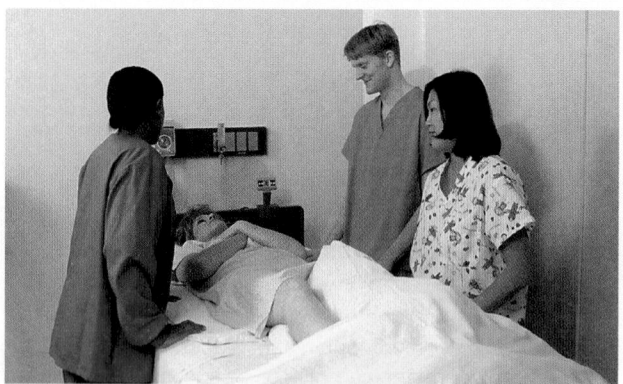

Step 1K(3) ■ Position nurses on each side of patient.

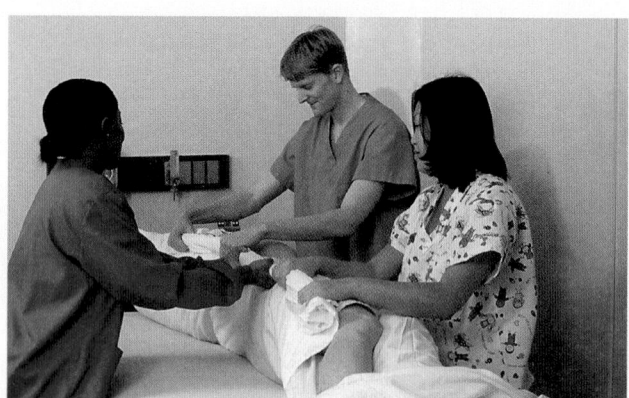

Step 1K(5) ■ Move patient as a unit, maintaining proper alignment.

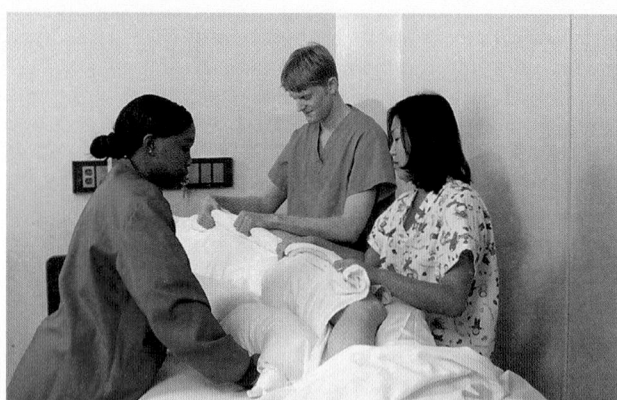

Step 1K(6) ■ Place pillows along patient's back for support.

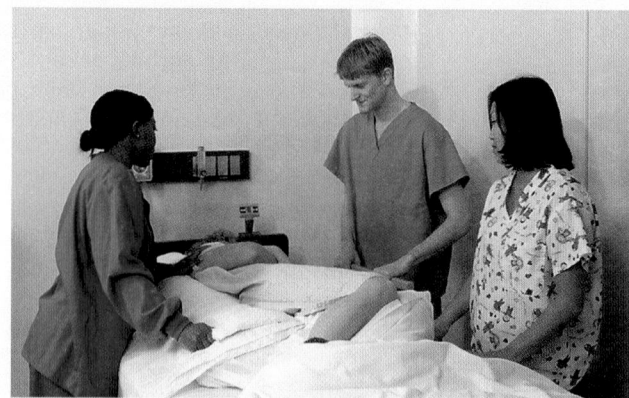

Step 1K(7) ■ Gently lean patient as a unit against pillows.

RECORDING AND REPORTING

- Record procedure and observations (e.g., condition of skin, joint movement, patient's ability to assist with positioning and patient's tolerance of position).

- Report observations at change of shift and document in nurses' notes.
- Report turning schedule and frequency of repositioning patient at change of shift.

UNEXPECTED OUTCOMES AND RELATED INTERVENTIONS

- Joint contractures develop or worsen.
  - Ensure patient is positioned properly.
  - Consider referral to physical or occupational therapy.
- Skin shows areas of erythema and breakdown.
  - Increase frequency of repositioning.
  - Place turning schedule above patient's bed.
  - Initiate skin care protocol (check agency policy) (Chapter 36).

- Patient avoids moving.
  - Medicate for pain as ordered by a health care provider to ensure patient's comfort before moving.
  - Allow pain medication to take effect before proceeding.

| SKILL 26-2 | USING SAFE AND EFFECTIVE TRANSFER TECHNIQUES |

 View Video!

DELEGATION CONSIDERATIONS

The skill of transfer techniques can be delegated to NAP. Patients whom you are transferring for the first time after prolonged bed rest, extensive surgery, critical illness, or spinal cord trauma require supervision by professional nurses. Before delegation, inform NAP about:

- Seeking assistance when moving or lifting a patient, for example, when the patient is overweight or confused
- Patient limitations (e.g. changes in blood pressure, mobility restrictions) that affect safe transfer techniques

EQUIPMENT

- Transfer belt, sling, or lapboard (as needed),
- Nonskid shoes, bath blankets, pillows
- Wheelchair: Position chair at 45-degree angle to bed, lock brakes, remove footrests, lock bed brakes
- Stretcher: Position next to bed, lock brakes on stretcher, lock brakes on bed
- Mechanical lift: Use frame, canvas strips or chains, and hammock or canvas strips

---

| STEP | RATIONALE |

ASSESSMENT

1 Assess physiological capacity to transfer:

Provides information relative to the patient's abilities, physical status, ability to comprehend, and the number of individuals needed to provide safe transferring.

  a Muscle strength (legs and upper arms)

Immobile patients have decreased muscle strength, tone, and mass. Affects ability to bear weight or raise body.

  b Joint mobility (ROM) and contracture formation

Immobility or inflammatory processes (e.g., arthritis) lead to contracture formation and impaired joint mobility.

  c Paralysis or paresis (spastic or flaccid)

Patient with central nervous system damage sometimes has bilateral paralysis (requiring transfer by swivel bar, sliding bar, or **mechanical lift**) or unilateral paralysis, which requires belt transfer to "best" side. Weakness (paresis) requires stabilization of knee while transferring. Flaccid arm needs support with sling during transfer.

  d Risk for orthostatic (postural) hypotension (e.g., previously on bed rest, first time arising from supine position following surgical procedure, history of dizziness when arising)

Determines risk for fainting or falling during transfer. Immobile patients have decreased ability for autonomic nervous system to equalize blood supply, resulting in drop of 20 mm Hg or more in blood pressure when rising from sitting position (Jarvis, 2008; Monahan and others, 2007).

  e Activity tolerance

Determines ability of patient to assist with transfer.

  f Level of comfort

Pain reduces patient's motivation and ability to be mobile. Pain relief before transfer enhances patient participation.

SKILL 26-2   USING SAFE AND EFFECTIVE TRANSFER TECHNIQUES—cont'd

STEP	RATIONALE
g Vital signs	Vital sign changes such as increased pulse and respiration and change in blood pressure indicate activity intolerance (see Chapter 14).
2 Assess patient's sensory status: a Adequacy of central and peripheral vision b Adequacy of hearing c Loss of peripheral sensation	Determines influence of sensory loss on ability to make transfer. Visual field loss decreases patient's ability to see in direction of transfer. Peripheral sensation loss decreases proprioception. Patients with visual and hearing losses need transfer techniques adapted to deficits. Patients with CVA sometimes lose area of visual field, which profoundly affects vision and perception.

• *Critical Decision Point:* Patients with hemiplegia also often "neglect" one side of the body (inattention to or unawareness of one side of body or environment), which distorts perception of the visual field. If patient experiences neglect of one side, instruct patient to scan all visual fields when transferring.

STEP	RATIONALE
3 Assess patient's cognitive status.	Determines patient's ability to follow directions and learn transfer techniques.

• *Critical Decision Point:* Patients with head trauma or CVA have perceptual cognitive deficits that create safety risks. If patient has difficulty in comprehension, simplify instructions and maintain consistency.

STEP	RATIONALE
4 Assess patient's level of motivation: a Patient's eagerness versus unwillingness to be mobile b Whether patient avoids activity and offers excuses	Altered psychological states reduce patient's desire to engage in activity.
5 Assess previous mode of transfer (if applicable).	Determines mode of transfer and assistance required to provide continuity. Use of transfer belts is necessary with all patients being transferred.
6 Assess patient's specific risk for falling or being injured when transferred (e.g., neuromuscular deficits, motor weakness, calcium loss from long bones, cognitive and visual dysfunction, altered balance).	Certain conditions increase patient's risk for falling or potential for injury.
7 Assess special transfer equipment needed for home setting. Assess home environment for hazards.	Prior teaching of family and support persons, assessment of home for safety risks and functionality, and provision of applicable aids greatly enhances transfer ability at home.

PLANNING

STEP	RATIONALE
1 Gather appropriate equipment.	
2 Determine number of people needed to assist with transfer. Do not start procedure until all caregivers are available.	Ensures safe patient transfer.
3 Perform hand hygiene. Verify that bed's brakes are locked.	Reduces transmission of microorganisms. Promotes patient and caregiver safety.
4 Explain procedure to patient.	Increases patient participation.

IMPLEMENTATION

1 Transfer patient.

   A **Assist Cooperative Patient to Sitting Position in Bed**

• *Critical Decision Point:* Careful assessment of your patient's ability to assist in the following positioning technique is extremely important. Consider the use of a mechanical lift. Your role in assisting your patient to a sitting position is to guide and instruct. If your patient can bear weight and move to a sitting position independently, allow the patient to do so and offer assistance.

STEP	RATIONALE
(1) Raise bed to waist level. Place patient in supine position.	Enables you to assess your patient's body alignment continually.
(2) Face head of bed at a 45-degree angle, and remove pillows.	Proper positioning reduces twisting of your body when moving the patient. Pillows cause interference when the patient is sitting up in bed.
(3) Place feet in a wide base of support, with foot closest to bed in front of other foot.	Improves balance and allows transfer of body weight as you move patient to sitting position.
(4) Place hand nearer head of bed under patient's shoulders, supporting patient's head and cervical vertebrae.	Maintains alignment of head and cervical vertebrae and allows for even lifting of patient's upper trunk.
(5) Place other hand on bed surface.	Provides support and balance.
(6) Raise patient to sitting position by shifting weight from front to back leg.	Improves balance, overcomes inertia, and transfers weight in direction in which you move patient.
(7) Push against bed using arm that is placed on bed surface.	Divides activity between arms and legs and protects back from strain. By bracing one hand against mattress and pushing against it as you lift the patient, you transfer weight away from your back muscles through your arm onto the mattress.
B Assist Cooperative Patient Who Can Partially Bear Weight to Sitting Position on Side of Bed	
(1) With bed flat and at waist level, turn patient to side, using assistance of another caregiver, if necessary. Patient needs to face nurse on side of bed that patient will be sitting (see illustration).	Decreases amount of work needed by you and your patient.
(2) Raise head of bed 30 degrees.	Facilitates raising patient to sitting position and protects patient from falling.
(3) Stand opposite patient's hips. Turn diagonally so that you face the patient and far corner of the foot of bed.	Places your center of gravity nearer the patient. Reduces twisting of your body because you are facing direction of movement.
(4) Place feet apart with foot closest to bed in front of other foot (see illustration).	Improves balance and allows transfer of body weight as you move patient to sitting position.
(5) Place arm nearer head of bed under patient's shoulders, supporting patient's head and cervical vertebrae.	Maintains alignment of head and cervical vertebrae and allows for even lifting of patient's upper trunk.
(6) Place other arm over patient's thighs (see illustration).	Supports hip and prevents patient from falling backward during procedure.
(7) Move patient's legs and feet over side of bed. Pivot toward rear leg, allowing patient's upper legs to swing downward. At same time shift weight to back leg and elevate patient (see illustration).	Decreases friction and resistance. Weight of patient's legs when off the bed allows gravity to lower legs, and weight of legs assists in pulling upper body to a sitting position.

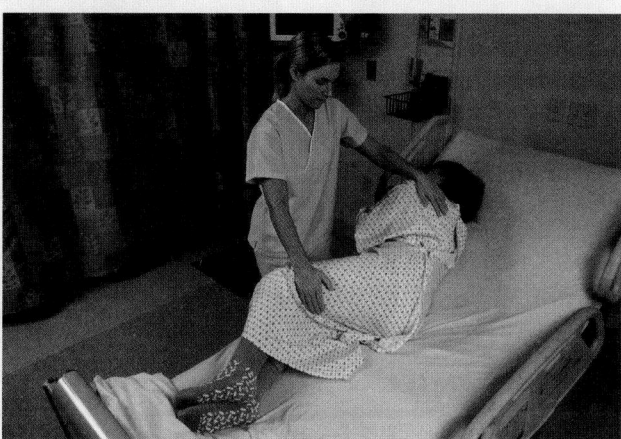

Step 1B(1) ■ Side-lying position.

| SKILL 26-2 | USING SAFE AND EFFECTIVE TRANSFER TECHNIQUES— cont'd |

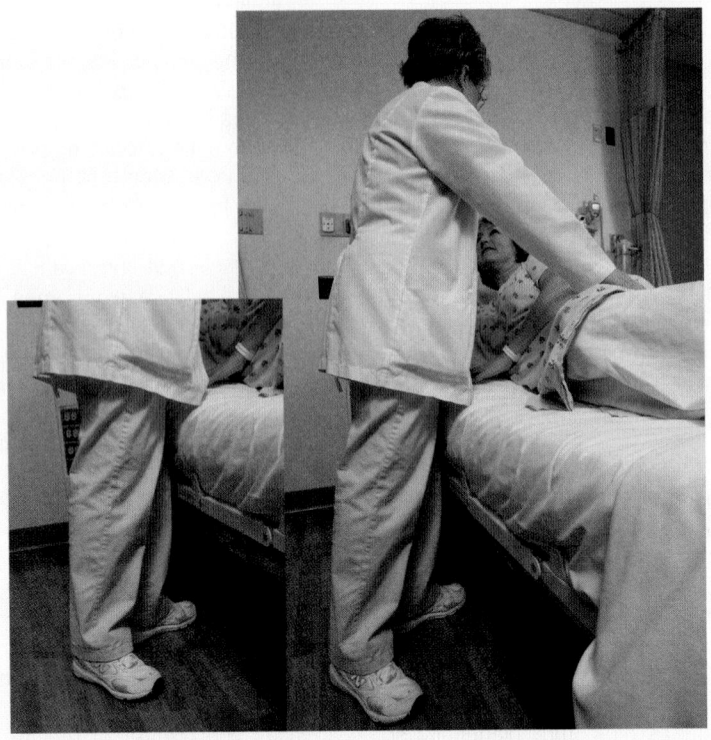

Step 1B(4) ■ Proper foot placement.

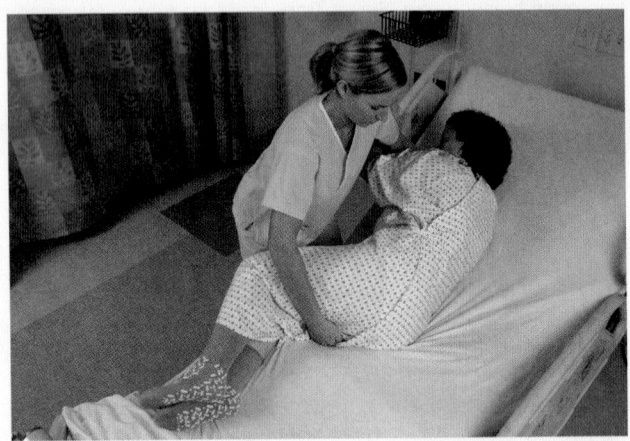

Step 1B(6) ■ Nurse places arm over patient's thighs.

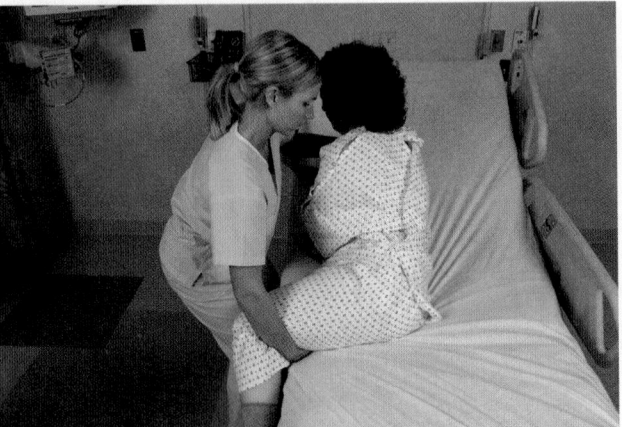

Step 1B(7) ■ Nurse shifts weight to rear leg and elevates patient.

STEP	RATIONALE

C Transferring Cooperative Patient Who Is Partially Weight Bearing From Bed to Chair

- *Critical Decision Point:* Allow patient to transfer independently if able to fully bear weigh. Stand by as needed to promote safe transfer (Nelson and others, 2003b).

(1) Assist patient to sitting position on side of bed (see Step 1B). Have chair in position at 45-degree angle to bed on the patient's strong side. Allow patient to sit on side of the bed (dangling) for a few minutes before transferring. Ask if patient feels dizzy. Do not leave unattended while dangling.

Positions chair within easy access for transfer. Placing the chair on the patient's stronger side will allow the patient to assist when transferring. Dangling helps equilibrate blood pressure, reducing risk for dizziness or fainting when standing (Koval, 2004).

(2) Apply transfer belt or other transfer aids.

Transfer belt maintains stability of patient during transfer and reduces risk for falling (Nelson and others, 2003a, 2003b). Put patient's arm in sling if flaccid paralysis is present.

(3) Ensure that patient is wearing stable nonskid shoes. Place weight-bearing or strong leg forward, with weak foot back.

Nonskid soles decrease risk for slipping during transfer. Always have patient wear shoes during transfer; bare feet increases risk for falls. Patient will stand on stronger, or weight-bearing, leg.

(4) Spread your feet apart.

Ensures balance with wide base of support.

(5) Flex your hips and knees, aligning knees with patient's knees (see illustration).

Flexion of knees and hips lowers the center of gravity to object to be raised; aligning knees with patient's allows for stabilization of knees when patient stands.

(6) Grasp transfer belt from underneath along patient's sides.

Grasping transfer belt at patient's side provides movement of patient at center of gravity. Never lift patients by arms or under arms (Nelson and others, 2003b).

- *Critical Decision Point:* Use a transfer belt or walking belt with handles in place of the under-axilla technique. The under-axilla technique is physically stressful for nurses and uncomfortable for patients (Owens and others, 1999).

(7) Rock patient up to standing position on count of 3 while straightening hips and legs and keeping knees slightly flexed (see illustration). Unless contraindicated, instruct patient to use hands to push up, if applicable.

Rocking motion gives patient's body momentum and requires less muscular effort to lift patient.

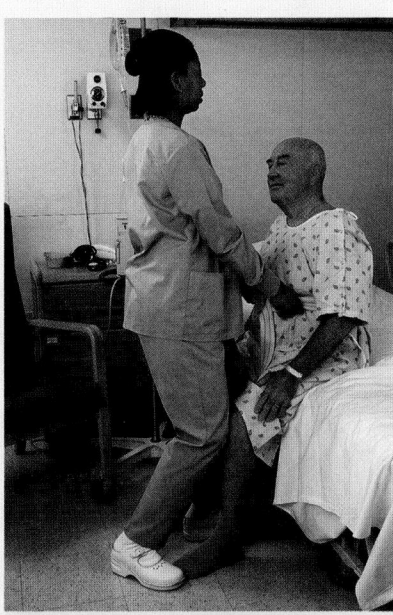

Step 1C(5) ■ Nurse flexes hips and knees, aligning knees with patient's knees.

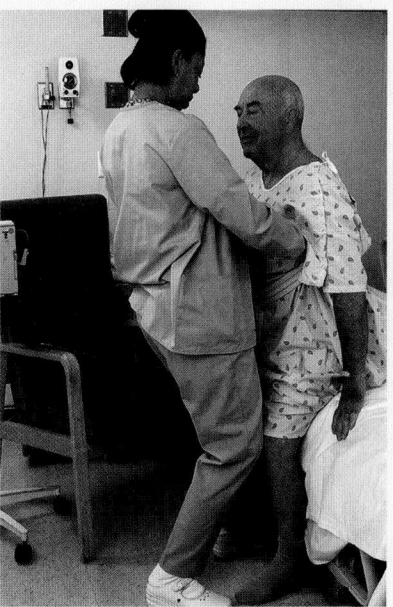

Step 1C(7) ■ Nurse rocks patient to standing position.

SKILL 26-2 USING SAFE AND EFFECTIVE TRANSFER TECHNIQUES— cont'd

STEP	RATIONALE
(8) Maintain stability of patient's weak or paralyzed leg with knee.	Often patient maintains ability to stand on paralyzed or weak limb with support of knee to stabilize (Pierson and Fairchild, 2008).
(9) Pivot on foot farther from chair.	Maintains support of patient while allowing adequate space for patient to move.
(10) Instruct patient to use armrests on chair for support, and ease into chair (see illustration).	Increases patient stability.
(11) Flex hips and knees while lowering patient into chair (see illustration).	Prevents injury from poor body mechanics.
(12) Assess patient for proper alignment for sitting position. Provide support for paralyzed extremities. Lapboard or sling will support flaccid arm. Stabilize leg with bath blanket or pillow.	Prevents injury to patient from poor body alignment.
(13) Praise patient's progress, effort, or performance.	Continued support and encouragement provide incentive for patient perseverance.
D Use Mechanical Lift and Full Body Sling to Transfer Uncooperative Patient Who Can Bear Partial Weight or Patient Who Cannot Bear Weight and Is Either Uncooperative or Does Not Have Upper Body Strength to Move From Bed to Chair	
(1) Position lift properly at bedside.	Ensures safe elevation of patient off bed. (Before using lift, be thoroughly familiar with its operation.)
(2) Position chair near bed, and allow adequate space to maneuver lift.	Prepares environment for safe use of lift and subsequent transfer.
(3) Raise bed to high position with mattress flat. Lower side rail.	Maintains nurses' alignment during transfer.
(4) Keep bed side rail up on the side opposite to you.	Maintains patient safety.
(5) Roll patient away from you.	Positions patient for use of lift sling.
(6) Place sling under patient. Place lower edge under patient's knees (wide edge) and upper edge under patient's shoulders (narrow piece).	Allows positioning of patient on mechanical/hydraulic lift. Places sling under patient's center of gravity and greatest portion of body weight.

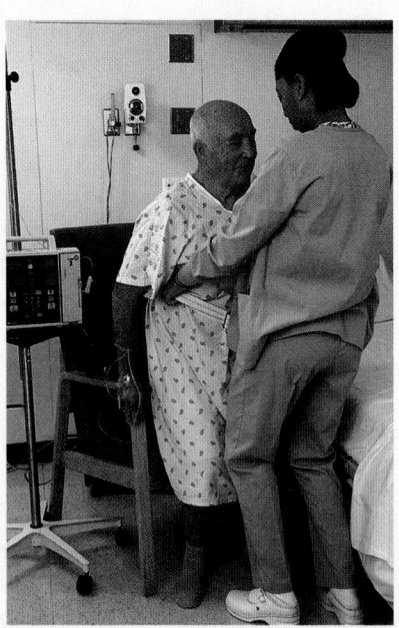

Step 1C(10) ■ Patient uses armrests for support.

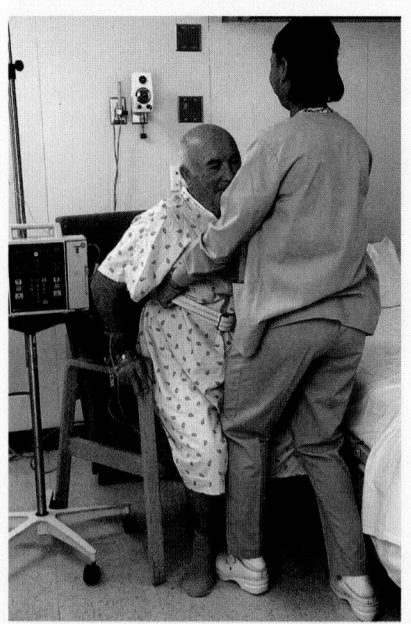

Step 1C(11) ■ Nurse eases patient into chair.

STEP	RATIONALE
(7) Roll patient to opposite side toward you, and pull body sling through.	Completes positioning of patient on mechanical/hydraulic sling.
(8) Roll patient supine onto canvas seat.	Sling extends from shoulders to knees (hammock) to support patient's body weight equally.
(9) Remove patient's glasses, if appropriate.	Swivel bar is close to patient's head and could break eyeglasses.
(10) If using a transportable Hoyer life, place lift's horseshoe-shaped base under side of bed (on side with chair).	Positions lift efficiently and promotes smooth transfer.
(11) Lower horizontal bar to sling level following manufacturer's directions. Some lifts require valve to be locked.	Positions hydraulic lift close to patient. Locking valve prevents injury to patient.
(12) Attach hooks on strap to holes in sling. Short straps hook to top holes of sling; longer straps hook to bottom of sling.	Secures hydraulic lift to sling.
(13) Elevate head of bed.	Positions patient in sitting position.
(14) Fold patient's arms over chest.	Prevents injury to paralyzed arms.
(15) Use lift to raise patient off bed (see illustration).	Moves patient off bed.
(16) Use steering handle to pull lift from bed and maneuver to chair.	Moves patient from bed to chair.
(17) Move lift to chair.	Positions lift in front of the chair.
(18) Position patient, and lower slowly into chair following manufacturer's guidelines (see illustration).	Safely guides patient into back of chair as seat descends.
(19) Remove straps and mechanical/hydraulic lift.	Prevents damage to skin and underlying tissues from canvas or hooks.
(20) Check patient's sitting alignment, and correct if necessary.	Prevents injury from poor posture.
E Transfer Patient From Bed to Stretcher (Bed at Stretcher Level).	
(1) Raise the bed to the height of the stretcher.	Bed and stretcher need to be at same level to allow patient to slide from bed to stretcher.
(2) Lower head of bed as much as patient can tolerate. Cross patient's arms on chest. Ensure bed brakes are locked.	Prevents injury to arms during transfer.
(3) Lower side rails. Two caregivers stand on the side where the stretcher will be while third caregiver stands on the other side.	Minimizes caregivers' stretching. Prevents patient from falling out of bed and promotes safety.
(4) Two caregivers help patient roll onto side toward them (use of drawsheet is *optional*) with a smooth, continuous motion.	Positions patient for placing friction-reducing lateral transfer device.

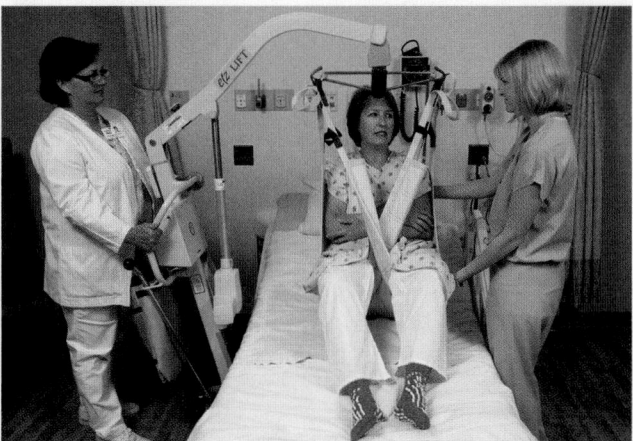

Step 1D(15) ■ Use mechanical lift to raise patient off the bed.

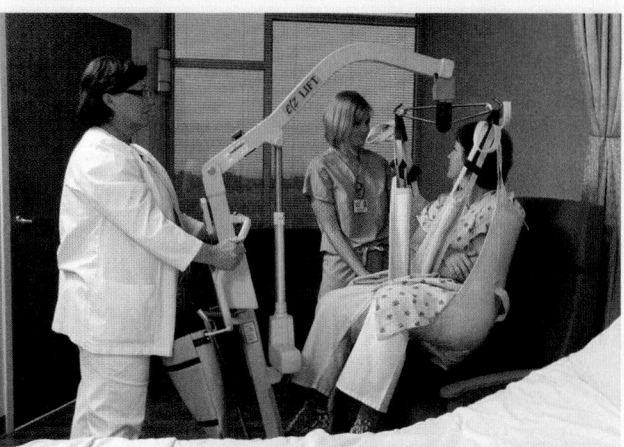

Step 1D(18) ■ Use mechanical lift to lower patient into chair.

SKILL 26-2   USING SAFE AND EFFECTIVE TRANSFER TECHNIQUES—
cont'd

STEP	RATIONALE
(5) Place slide board under drawsheet or follow manufacturer's guidelines (see illustrations). Gently roll patient back onto the slide board.	Patient needs to be placed on transfer device properly to allow safe transfer.
(6) Align stretcher alongside the bed. Lock wheels of stretcher once it is in place. Instruct the patient not to move.	Positions stretcher in correct position for transfer and prevents patient falling out of bed.
(7) All three caregivers place feet widely apart with one slightly in front of the other, and grasp the fiction-reducing device.	Prepares for transfer. Wide base of support allows nurse to shift weight and minimizes back strain.
(8) On the count of three, the two caregivers pull the drawsheet or patient from the bed onto the stretcher while the third person holds the slide board in place. Using the friction-reducing device, shift weight from front foot to back foot (see illustrations). Position patient in center of stretcher.	Transfers patient smoothly and efficiently to the stretcher.

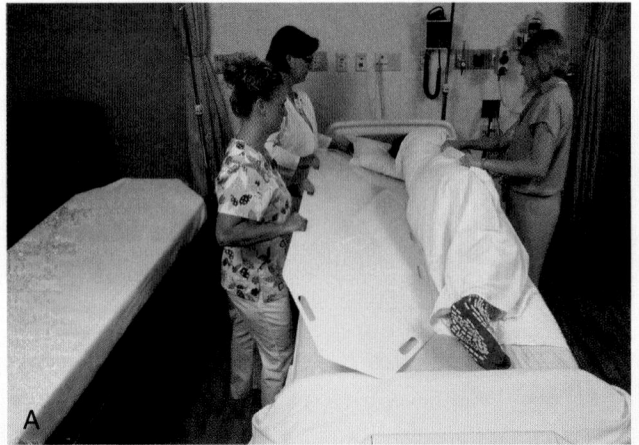

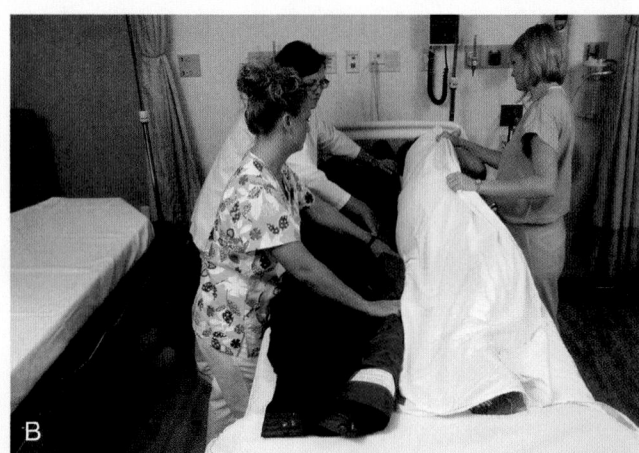

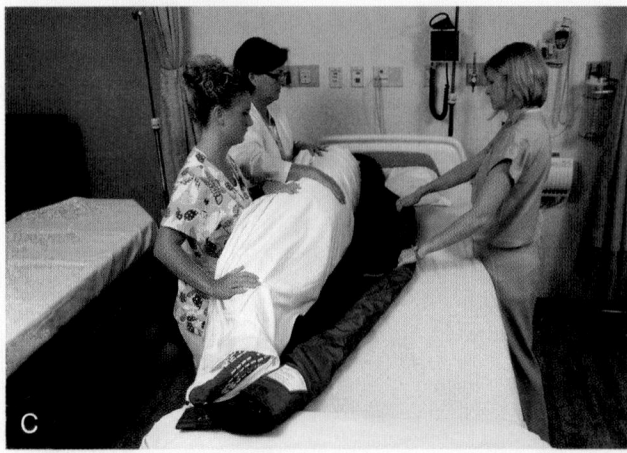

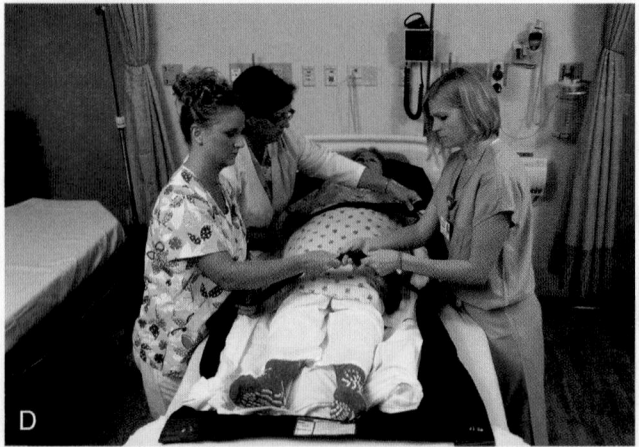

Step 1E(5) ■ **A,** Two caregivers position sliding board under patient. **B,** Two caregivers place air-assisted device under patient. **C,** Patient rolls to opposite side while other caregiver unrolls air-assisted device. **D,** Secure safety straps.

STEP	RATIONALE
(9) Put up side rail of stretcher on side where caregivers are then roll stretcher away from bed and put side rail up on that side.	Side rails prevent patient from falling off stretcher.
(10) Cover patient with a sheet or blanket.	Promotes comfort and provides patient dignity.
(11) Perform hand hygiene.	Reduces transmission of microorganisms.
(12) Following transfer, evaluate patient's body alignment.	Prompt identification of poor alignment reduces risks to the patient's skin and musculoskeletal systems.
2 Perform hand hygiene.	Reduces transmission of microorganisms.

EVALUATION

1 Evaluate vital signs. Ask if patient feels fatigued.	Evaluates patient's response to postural changes and activity.
2 Observe for correct body alignment and presence of pressure points on skin.	Minimizes risk for immobility complications.
3 Ask if patient experienced pain during transfer.	Determines need for additional pain control or alteration of technique of transferring.

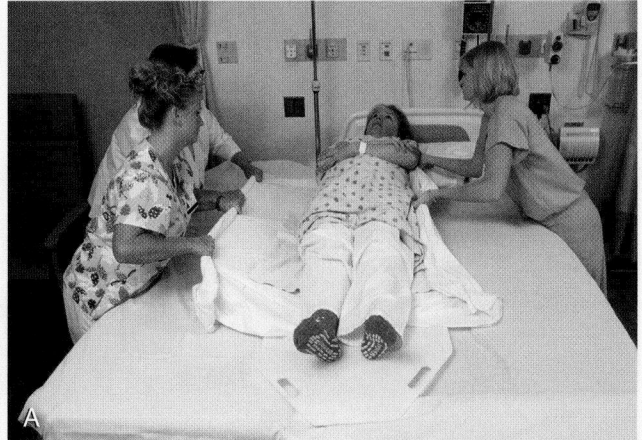

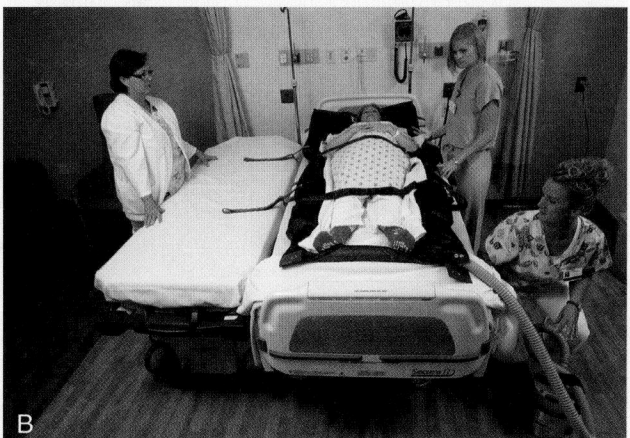

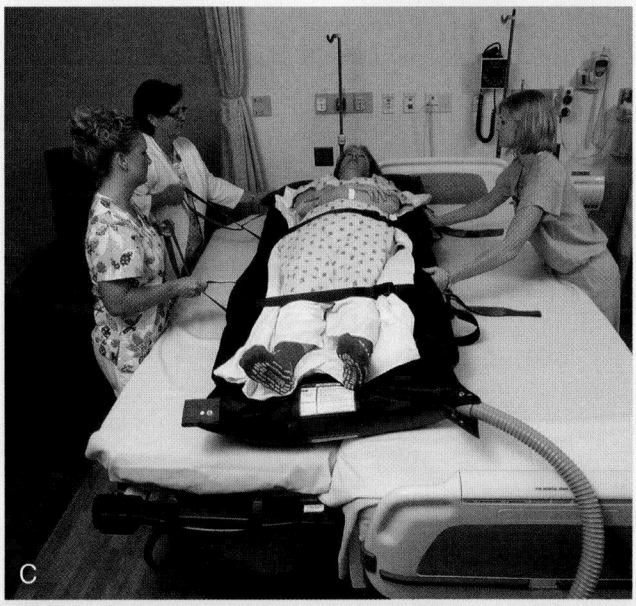

Step 1E(8) ■ **A,** Transfer of patient from bed to stretcher using sliding board. **B,** Inflating air-assisted transfer device. **C,** Transfer of patient using air-assisted device.

SKILL 26-2   USING SAFE AND EFFECTIVE TRANSFER TECHNIQUES— cont'd

RECORDING AND REPORTING

- Record procedure, including pertinent observations: weakness, ability to follow directions, weight-bearing ability, balance, ability to pivot, number of personnel needed to assist, and amount of assistance (muscle strength) required.

- Report any unusual occurrence to nurse in charge. Report transfer ability and assistance needed to next shift or other caregivers. Report progress or transfer difficulties to rehabilitation staff (physical therapist or occupational therapist).

UNEXPECTED OUTCOMES AND RELATED INTERVENTIONS

- Patient unable to comprehend and follow directions for transfer.
  - Reassess continuity and simplicity of instructions.
- Patient sustains injury on transfer.
  - Evaluate incident that caused injury (e.g., assessment inadequate, change in patient status, improper use of equipment).
  - Complete occurrence report according to institution policy.
- Patient's level of weakness does not permit active transfer.
  - Obtain assistance from additional nursing personnel.
  - Increase bed activity and exercise to heighten tolerance.

- Patient continues to bear weight on non–weight-bearing limb.
  - Reinforce information about weight-bearing status.
- Patient transfers well on some occasions, poorly on others.
  - Assess patient for factors that affect ability to transfer (e.g., pain, fatigue, confusion) before transfer.
  - Allow for a rest period before transferring, medicate for pain if indicated, or reorient patient.
  - Periodic confusion also alters performance.
- Patient is unable to stand for time required in transfer to chair.
  - Provide for adequate assistance during transfer.
  - Assess for orthostatic changes in blood pressure when transferring patient.
- Localized areas of erythema develop that do not disappear quickly (see Chapter 36).
  - Establish individualized skin care regimen.
  - Position patient in 30-degree lateral position.

KEY POINTS

- Muscles primarily associated with movement are located near the skeletal region, where movement results from leverage.
- Muscles primarily associated with posture are located in the lower extremities, trunk, neck, and back.
- Body alignment is the positioning of joints, tendons, ligaments, and muscles in various body positions.
- You achieve body balance when there is a wide base of support, the center of gravity falls within the base of support, and a vertical line falls from the center of gravity through the base of support.
- Conditions that affect body alignment and mobility include postural abnormalities, altered bone formation or joint mobility, impaired muscle development, central nervous system damage, and musculoskeletal system trauma.

- Assessment of a patient's mobility enables you to determine the patient's coordination, balance, and ability to complete activities of daily living and makes it possible to evaluate or plan an exercise program.
- Assessing gait allows you to draw some conclusions about the patient's balance, posture, and ability to walk without assistance.
- Patients with impaired body alignment require nursing interventions to maintain them in the supported Fowler's, supine, prone, side-lying, and Sims' positions.
- Transfer techniques require the use of correct body mechanics.
- Mechanical devices, such as canes and walkers, require specific nursing interventions to promote walking.

CRITICAL THINKING EXERCISES

Mr. Timber is 65 years old and had a knee replacement 2 days ago. He has type 2 diabetes mellitus. The nurse tells you that he is "uncooperative" and refuses to use his crutches or get up in the chair. He is allowed partial weight bearing on his right leg.

1. During your assessment of Mr. Timber, what potential barriers is he experiencing that are preventing him from participating in his treatment?
2. Which of the following statements from Mr. Timber do you address first?
   a. "My pain level is 8 out of 10. I just can't take it."
   b. "I don't understand how to use those crutches."
   c. "I've been in this bed for 2 days, and I feel weak."
3. Mr. Timber has agreed to begin crutch training. However, this is his first time out of bed since his surgery. What risk factors does he possess that contribute to orthostatic hypotension, and what interventions do you initiate before attempting to transfer Mr. Timber?

4. Mr. Timber is agreeing to use his crutches. However, as you talk with him, you find out that he is anxious about pain associated with crutch waking and about using the crutches. During an earlier crutch walking experience, his pain increased and he is afraid of his pain getting out of control. In addition, he states that he is afraid of falling when using the crutches and damaging his repaired knee. Describe what measures you will take to control his pain before crutch walking and to assess safety of Mr. Timber's crutch walking.
5. Which is the most appropriate crutch gait for Mr. Timber? Explain your choice.
   a. Two-point
   b. Three-point
   c. Four-point
   d. Swing-through

ℰvolve   *Answers to Critical Thinking Questions can be found on the Evolve website.*

REVIEW QUESTIONS

1. A patient begins to fall during ambulation. To prevent injury to the patient, you:
   1. Call for assistance
   2. Slide the patient down your body to the floor
   3. Instruct the patient to sit in the nearest chair
   4. Contact the health care provider, and document the fall
2. A principle of good body mechanics includes:
   1. Keeping knees in locked position
   2. Maintaining a wide base of support
   3. Bending at the waist to maintain center of gravity
   4. Holding objects away from the body for better leverage
3. Passive range-of-motion exercises prevent:
   1. Contractures
   2. Osteoporosis
   3. Muscle atrophy
   4. Renal calculi formation
4. A necessary safety precaution when ambulating a patient is to:
   1. Have family members present
   2. Have patient wear well-fitting rubber-soled shoes or slippers
   3. Have at least two people present to assist the patient
   4. Be sure no pain medication was given for at least 3 hours before ambulation
5. The piece of equipment that works best to help ambulate an unsteady patient is:
   1. A walker
   2. Crutches
   3. A wheelchair
   4. A mechanical lift device
6. A device that helps prevent footdrop is the:
   1. Foot roll
   2. Foot boot

3. Trochanter roll
4. Ankle-foot splint

7. Two nurses are standing on opposite sides of the bed to move a patient up in bed with a drawsheet. In relation to the patient, they stand even with the patient's:
   1. Hips
   2. Chest
   3. Knees
   4. Shoulders
8. A health care provider orders partial weight bearing on the left foot of a patient with a broken ankle and full weight bearing on the right foot. The crutch gait that the patient uses is the:
   1. Two-point
   2. Four-point
   3. Three-point
   4. Swing-through
9. When a patient has left-sided cerebral hemorrhage, what may also be present?
   1. Bilateral hemiplegia
   2. Left-sided hemiplegia
   3. Right-sided hemiplegia
   4. Degenerative hemiplegia
10. Which of the following methods of transfer from the bed to a chair is most appropriate for a patient who weighs 250 lb and is able to minimally assist?
    1. Mechanical lift
    2. Sliding board
    3. Drawsheet with two caregivers
    4. Walker

Answers to Review Questions can be found on pages 1197-1198.

REFERENCES

American Nurses Association: *Position statement on elimination of manual patient handling to prevent work-related musculoskeletal disorders*, 2003, http://www.nursingworld.org/readroom/position/ workplac/pathand.htm.

American Nurses Association: *Nursing's legislative and regulatory initiatives for the 110th Congress: workplace health and safety*, 2007, Department of Government Affairs, http//www.anapoliticalpower.org.

Baptiste A and others: Friction-reducing devices for lateral patient transfers: a clinical evaluation, *AAOHN J* 54(4):173, 2006.

Berry PH and others: *Pain: current understanding of assessment, management, and treatment*, Reston, Va, 2006, National Pharmaceutical Council.

Boltri J and others: Diabetes prevention in a faith-based setting: results of translational research, *J Public Health Manag Pract* 14(1):29, 2008.

Bulechek GM and others, editors: *Nursing interventions classification (NIC)*, ed 5, St. Louis, 2008, Mosby.

Bureau of Labor Statistics: Occupational industries and illnesses: industry data, http://stats.bls.gov/bls/occupation.htlm, 2003.

Choi JH, Moon JS, Song R: Effects of sun-style tai chi exercise on physical fitness and fall prevention in fall-prone older adults, *J Adv Nurs* 51(2):150, 2005.

de Castro AB, Hagan P, Nelson A: Prioritizing safe patient handling, *J Nurs Adm* 36(7/8):363, 2006.

Dingle M: Role of dangling when moving from supine to standing position, *Br J Nurs* 12(6):346, 2003.

Gahart BL, Nazareno AR: *2008 intravenous medications: a handbook for nurses and allied health professionals*, St. Louis, 2008, Mosby.

Glenn-Molali NH: Nourishment and swallowing. In Hoeman SP, editor, *Rehabilitation nursing: process, application, and outcomes*, ed 4, St. Louis, 2008, Mosby.

Hockenberry DL, Wilson D: *Wong's nursing care of infants and children*, ed 8, St. Louis, 2007, Mosby.

Hoeman SP: *Rehabilitation nursing: process, application and outcomes*, ed 4, St. Louis, 2008, Mosby.

Huether SE, McCance KL: *Understanding pathophysiology*, ed 4, St. Louis, 2008, Mosby.

Hughes K: Who's got your back? Reducing the incidence of on-the-job injuries among nurses, *Am J Nurs* 106(7):72A, 2006.

Jarvis C: *Physical examination and health assessment*, ed 5, St. Louis, 2008, Saunders.

Koval K: A clinical pathway for hip fractures in the elderly. *Tech Orthop*, 19(3):181, 2004.

Mamaril ME: Nursing considerations in the geriatric surgical patient: the perioperative continuum of care, *Nurs Clin North Am* 41(2):313, 2006.

Mayo Clinic Tools for Healthier Lives: *Fitness programs: ready to get started?* 2005, http://www.mayoclinic.com/health/fitness/HQ00171.

Miami Valley Hospital: *Lift team case study*, June 2007, http://www.miamivalleyhospital.com/.

Monahan F and others: *Phipps' medical surgical nursing*, ed 8, St. Louis, 2007, Mosby.

Moorhead S and others, editors: *Nursing outcomes classification (NOC)*, ed 4, St. Louis, 2008, Mosby.

Morrato E and others: Are health care professionals advising patients with diabetes or at risk for developing diabetes to exercise more? *Diabetes Care* 29(3):543, 2006.

Nelson A, Baptiste A: Evidence-based practices for safe patient handling and movement, *Online J Issues Nurs* 9(3):4, 2004.

Nelson A and others: Myths and facts about back injuries in nursing, *Am J Nurs* 103(2):32, 2003a.

Nelson A and others: Safe patient handling and movement: preventing back injury among nurses requires careful selection of the safest equipment and techniques, *Am J Nurs* 103(3):32, 2003b.

Nelson A and others: Myths and facts about back injuries in nursing, *Am J Nurse* 103(2):32, 2003a.

Nelson A: Safe patient handling and movement algorithms, 2006, VISN Patient Safety Center, http:visn8med.va.gov/patientsafetycenter/. Last accessed August 3 2009.

O'Brien-Gillespie H: Exercise. In Edelman CL, Mandle CL, editors: *Health promotion throughout the life span*, ed 6, St. Louis, 2006, Mosby.

Occupational Safety and Health Administration: *Ergonomics: guidelines for nursing homes*, 2003, http://www.osha.gov/ergonomics/guidelines/nursinghome/final_nh_guidelines.html.

Occupational Safety and Health Administration: Ergonomics standard proposal, *Fed Regist* 29 CFR part 1910, 2005, http://www.osha-slc.gov/SLTC/ergonomics/index.html.

Occupational Safety and Health Administration: Ergonomics standard proposal, Fed Reg 29 CFR part 1910, 2005, http://www.osha-slc.gov/SLTC/ergonomics/index.html

Owens B and others: What are we teaching about lifting and transferring patients? *Res Nurs Health* 22:3, 1999.

Pelczarski K: Take a proactive approach to bariatric patient needs, *Material Management,* June 2007.

Pierson F, Fairchild S: *Principles and techniques of patient care*, ed 4, St. Louis, 2008, Saunders.

Prochaska J and others: *Changing for good*, New York, 1994, William Morrow.

Schrezenmaier C and others: Evaluation of orthostatic hypotension: relationship of a new self-report instrument to laboratory-based measures, *Mayo Clin Proc* 80(3):330, 2005.

The Joint Commission: *2009 National Patient Safety Goals Hospital Program*, Oakbrook Terrace, Ill, 2008, The Joint Commission, http://www.jointcommission.org, accessed July 2008.

Thibodeau GA, Patton KT: *Anatomy and physiology*, ed 6, St. Louis, 2007, Mosby.

UC Davis Health System: *New team gives nurses a lift in handling patients*, March 2005, http:ucdavis.edu/.

Wilson SF, Giddens JF: *Health assessment for nursing practice*, ed 3, St. Louis, 2005, Mosby.

Wound Ostomy and Continence Nurses Society: *Guidelines for prevention and management of pressure ulcers*, WOCN Clinical Practice Guidelines Series, Glenview, Ill, 2003, The Society.

Yen PK: Physical activity: the "new" nutrition guideline, *Geriatr Nurs* 26(6):341, 2005.

Safety

MEDIA RESOURCES

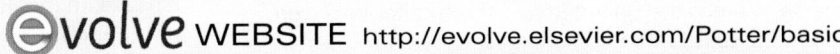

CD COMPANION **evolve WEBSITE** http://evolve.elsevier.com/Potter/basic

- Video Clip
- Crossword Puzzle
- English/Spanish Audio Glossary

OBJECTIVES

- Describe how unmet basic physiological needs of oxygen, nutrition, temperature, and humidity threaten safety.
- Discuss methods to reduce physical hazards and the transmission of pathogens.
- Discuss the specific risks to safety for each developmental age.
- Identify factors to assess when it becomes necessary to physically restrain a patient.
- Describe four categories of safety risks in a health care agency.
- Describe assessment activities designed to identify a patient's physical, psychological, and cognitive status as it relates to safety.

- Identify relevant nursing diagnoses associated with risks to safety.
- Develop a nursing care plan for patients whose safety is threatened.
- Describe nursing interventions specific to the patient's age for reducing risk for falls, fires, poisonings, and electrical hazards.
- Describe methods to evaluate interventions designed to maintain or promote safety.

KEY TERMS

Ambularm, p. 734
carbon monoxide, p. 720
heat exhaustion, p. 720
hypothermia, p. 721
immunization, p. 721
pathogen, p. 721
restraint, p. 733

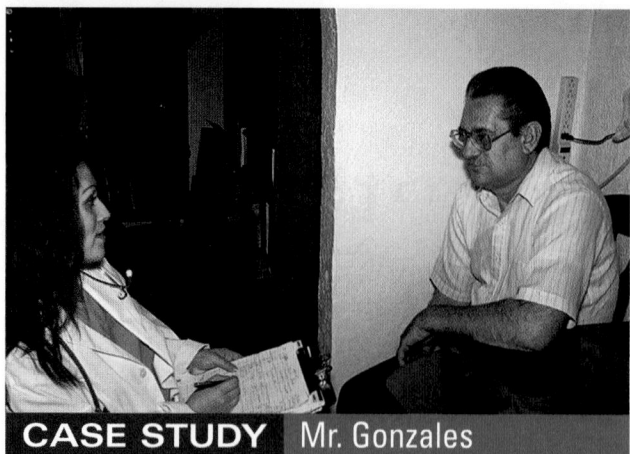

CASE STUDY   Mr. Gonzales

Mr. Gonzales is a 68-year-old man who has lived alone in a senior apartment building since his wife died 6 months ago. He and his wife were born in Mexico but came to live in the United States shortly after they were married. He is retired from a produce warehouse where he worked for 37 years. He and his wife raised three sons. The closest son, Carlos, is 30 minutes away by car. Carlos visits Mr. Gonzales every week to socialize and take him shopping. Mr. Gonzales is generally healthy but has decreased visual acuity, hearing loss from the noisy warehouse job, and some "arthritis." He expects to live at least as long as his father, who lived to be 92 years old. Since his wife's death, Mr. Gonzales has attended Catholic mass every day at his parish church, where his wife had attended daily.

Joani Green, a 25-year-old married mother of two, is currently a nursing student at the local college. As part of the clinical requirements, she and her study partner are conducting health screenings and providing health promotion education for the residents of the apartment building where Mr. Gonzales lives. Part of her screening will include Mr. Gonzales' home environment.

SCIENTIFIC KNOWLEDGE BASE

Safety, the freedom from psychological and physical injury, is a basic human need. Health care provided in a safe manner and a safe community environment is essential for a patient's well-being. A safe environment reduces the risk for accidents and helps to contain the cost of health care. One of your primary responsibilities as a nurse is to protect patients from harm.

Vulnerable groups who often require help in achieving a safe environment include infants, children, older adults, the ill, the physically and mentally disabled, the illiterate, and the poor. To be effective, you need to understand factors that contribute to a safe environment in the home or health care agency and thoroughly assess the environment for threats to safety. You also need to understand how alterations in mobility, sensory function, and cognitive function affect a patient's safety (see Chapters 35 and 37). A safe environment includes meeting basic human needs, reducing physical hazards, and reducing transmission of pathogens.

Basic Human Needs

The physiological needs of adequate oxygen, nutrition, and favorable temperature and humidity are basic human needs often at risk from a variety of environmental hazards.

OXYGEN A common environmental hazard in the home is an improperly functioning heating system. A furnace, stove, or fireplace that is not properly vented introduces carbon monoxide into the environment. **Carbon monoxide** is a colorless, odorless, poisonous gas produced by the combustion of carbon or organic fuels. This gas binds strongly with hemoglobin; preventing the formation of oxyhemoglobin and thus reducing the supply of oxygen delivered to the tissues (see Chapter 29). Low concentrations cause nausea, dizziness, headache, and fatigue. Higher concentrations are often fatal. In the United States, unintentional carbon monoxide poisoning is responsible for about 500 deaths and over 15,000 poisonings every year (Centers for Disease Control and Prevention [CDC], 2007).

NUTRITION In the home, patients need to properly refrigerate, store, and prepare food. The patient needs a refrigerator with a freezer compartment to keep perishable foods fresh. An adequate, clean water supply is necessary for drinking and to wash fresh produce and dishes. Provisions for garbage collection are necessary to maintain sanitary conditions. Foods need to be adequately cooked to kill any residing organisms. If the patient does not adequately prepare or store foods, this will increase the patient's risk for infections and food poisoning. Groups at the highest risk are children, pregnant women, older adults, and people with compromised immune systems (Nix, 2005). Eating food contaminated by bacteria such as *Escherichia coli*, *Salmonella*, *Shigella*, or *Listeria* causes food poisoning. Although most food-borne diseases are bacterial, hepatitis A virus is spread by fecal contamination of food, water, or milk.

TEMPERATURE A person's comfort zone is usually between 18.3° and 23.8° C (65° and 75° F). Temperature extremes, which often occur during the winter and summer, affect comfort, productivity, and safety. Exposure to severe cold for prolonged periods causes frostbite and accidental **hypothermia** (see Chapter 14). Older adults, the very young, patients with cardiovascular conditions, patients who have ingested drugs or excess alcohol, and the homeless are at high risk for hypothermia. Exposure to extreme heat changes the body's electrolyte balance and raises the core body temperature, resulting in heatstroke or **heat exhaustion.** People at risk from high environmental temperatures need to avoid extremely hot, humid environments; otherwise, heat exhaustion will result.

HUMIDITY The relative humidity of the air affects a patient's health and safety. Relative humidity is the amount of water vapor in the air compared with the maximum amount of water vapor that the air could contain at the same temperature. Increasing the environmental humidity with the use of a home humidifier has therapeutic benefits for patients with upper respiratory infections. The increase in humidity helps to liquefy pulmonary secretions and improves breathing.

Physical Hazards

Physical hazards in the environment threaten a person's safety and result in physical or psychological injury or death. Nearly 44% of self-reported episodes of injury occurred in or around the home (CDC, 2006). As a nurse, you play an important role by anticipating potential hazards in the health care setting and the patient's home and then implementing appropriate nursing interventions.

Common physical hazards in the home include inadequate lighting, barriers along normal walking paths and stairways, and a lack of safety devices. Inadequate lighting causes eyestrain while the patient carries out daily activities. Poorly illuminated stairs or walkways increase the risk for injury from falls. Injuries frequently result from accidental contact with objects on stairs, floors, bedside tables, closet shelves, refrigerator tops, and bookshelves. Older adults, patients with impaired vision, and patients with impaired mobility are at greater risk for injury due to falls.

A poison is any substance that impairs health or destroys life when ingested, inhaled, or absorbed by the body. Sources include drugs, medicines, other solid and liquid substances, and gases and vapors. Poisons impair the function of every major organ system. In the home, accidental poisoning is a greater risk for the toddler, preschooler, and young school-age child, who often ingest household cleaning solutions, medications, or personal hygiene products. However, the 2005 poisoning death rate peaked at ages 45 to 54 years with 91% of all poisoning deaths being drug related (CDC, 2008c). Poisoning is also a risk for health care providers who work around chemicals such as mercury and toxic cleaning agents. Mercury is found in glass thermometers and sphygmomanometers. When there is equipment breakage, health care workers and patients are at risk for exposure to mercury. When a person has ingested a poisonous substance or comes in contact with a chemical that is absorbed through the skin, emergency treatment is a necessity. Specific antidotes or treatments are available for only some types of poisons. A poison control center is the best resource for patients and parents needing information about the treatment of an accidental poisoning.

Home fires are a major cause of death and injury. Smoking materials such as cigarettes, cigars, and pipes are the primary source. About 25% of the 3000 home fire deaths in the United States are due to smoking (CDC, 2008b). Many fatal fires are the result of individuals smoking in bed and accidentally falling asleep. Another problem related to fatal fires is a failure to keep fresh batteries in home smoke detectors.

When they strike, natural disasters such as floods, tsunamis, hurricanes, tornadoes, and wildfires are a major cause of death and injury. These types of disasters kill 1 million people around the world each decade and leave millions more homeless (Federal Emergency Management Agency [FEMA], 2004a). It is important for individuals and communities to focus on preparation and mitigation to avoid losses and to reduce the risk for injury associated with these types of disasters.

A new potential environmental health threat is the possibility of a bioterrorist attack. Threats of this type come in the form of biological, chemical, and radiological attacks. A biological attack involves release of a biological agent, such as anthrax, plague, botulism, smallpox, and typhoid, into the environment. A chemical attack includes spreading a toxic agent such as cyanide, mustard gas, chlorine, or nerve agents (e.g., tabun or sarin). Radiological events threaten the community by dispersal of radioactive materials into the food and water supply, over terrain, or as a "dirty bomb." Although the likelihood is low, disaster can strike quickly and without warning. It forces members of a community to evacuate neighborhoods or be confined to their homes. The Federal Emergency Management Agency's (FEMA's) Family Protection Program and the American Red Cross Disaster Education Program provide nationwide efforts to help community members prepare for disasters of all types (FEMA, 2004b).

Pathogen Transmission

Pathogens and parasites pose a threat to patient safety. A **pathogen** is any microorganism capable of producing an illness (see Chapter 13). The most common means of transmission of pathogens is by the hands. For example, if an individual infected with hepatitis A does not wash his or her hands thoroughly after having a bowel movement, the risk for transmitting the disease during food preparation is great. One of the most effective ways to limit the transmission of pathogens is the medical aseptic practice of hand washing.

Human immune deficiency virus (HIV), the pathogen that causes acquired immunodeficiency syndrome (AIDS), and hepatitis B virus are transmitted through blood and other body fluids. Drug abusers frequently share syringes and needles, which increases their risk for acquiring these viruses. Some states and many nonprofit organizations fund syringe exchange programs as a means to slow down the spread of infectious diseases obtained through needle sharing (Coalition for Safe Community Needle Disposal, 2005a). Unsafe sexual practices, such as unprotected sexual intercourse or oral sex, also increase the likelihood of contracting HIV infection or AIDS, as well as other sexually transmitted diseases.

Insects and rodents are carriers of pathogens. For example, some mosquitoes are carriers of malaria and West Nile virus. Rats and mice carry rat-bite fever. Uncontrolled mosquito and rodent populations increase the risk for these diseases. Persons living at the poverty level sometimes live in homes that landlords do not maintain. Rat and roach infestations are common problems. Mosquito repellant and rodent traps help eliminate this risk.

Proper disposal of human waste also controls the transmission of pathogens and parasites. Without a satisfactory sewer and waste system, the population is at risk for illnesses such as typhoid fever and hepatitis.

Immunization is the process by which resistance to an infectious disease is produced or increased. The body acquires active immunity after a small amount of weakened or dead organisms and modified toxins from the organism (toxoids) is injected into the body. Passive immunity occurs when antibodies produced by other persons or animals are introduced into a person's bloodstream for protection against a pathogen. Nurses must inform the public about the importance of immunization in maintaining the health of their children.

Health care agencies are concerned with the processing of biohazardous wastes. It is important to properly dispose of needles, surgical dressings, and syringes to prevent the risk for exposure to the general population and employees. You also need to clean or dispose of bed linens and patient gowns contaminated by body fluids to reduce threats to safety.

NURSING KNOWLEDGE BASE

A person's developmental stage, lifestyle habits, mobility status, sensory and cognitive impairments, and safety awareness all influence threats to safety. In the United States accidents resulting from unintentional injuries are the leading cause of death in people between 1 and 44 years of age and the fifth leading cause overall (Kung and others, 2007). It is important to be aware of the threats to safety and to teach patients, parents, and other caregivers how to lessen the dangers.

Developmental Level

INFANT, TODDLER, AND PRESCHOOLER Injuries in children over age 1 cause more death and disability than do all diseases combined (Hockenberry, 2009). The nature of an injury is closely related to normal growth and development. For example, the incidence of lead poisoning is highest in late infancy and toddlers. Children at this stage explore the environment, and because of an increase in oral activity, put objects in their mouths. Accidents involving children are largely preventable. Parents need to be aware of specific dangers at each stage of growth and development. Accident prevention requires health education for parents and the removal of dangers whenever possible.

SCHOOL-AGE CHILD When children enter school, their environment expands to include the school, the means of transportation to and from school, and after-school activities. School-age children are learning how to perform more complicated motor activities and oftentimes are uncoordinated. Instruct parents and teachers about safe practices to follow at school and during play. Teach school-age children involved in team and contact sports rules for playing safely and how to use protective safety equipment such as helmets. Head injuries are a major cause of death, with bicycle accidents being one of the major causes of such injuries (Hockenberry, 2009). Playground safety is especially important during the summer months. Teach children about safe distances for jumping and climbing, to avoid unsafe and isolated areas, and to keep away from strange dogs.

ADOLESCENT As children enter adolescence, they develop greater independence and a sense of identity. The adolescent begins to separate emotionally from the family, and the peer group begins to have a stronger influence. Wide variations that swing from childlike to mature behavior are characteristic of adolescent behavior (Hockenberry, 2009). To relieve the tensions associated with the physical and psychosocial changes, as well as peer pressure, adolescents often engage in risk-taking behaviors such as smoking, drinking alcohol, and using drugs. This increases the risk for accidents such as drowning and motor vehicle accidents. According to the Insurance Institute for Highway Safety (2006), 33% of deaths among 13- to 19-year-olds in the United States occurred in motor vehicle crashes. To assess for possible substance abuse, have parents look for environmental and psychosocial clues. Environmental clues include the presence of drug-oriented magazines, beer and liquor bottles, drug paraphernalia, blood spots on clothing, and the continual wearing of long-sleeved shirts in hot weather and dark glasses indoors. Psychosocial clues include failing grades, change in dress, increased absenteeism from school, isolation, increased aggressiveness, and changes in interpersonal relationships.

ADULT Threats to an adult's safety are often related to lifestyle habits. The patient who excessively uses alcohol or drugs, for example, is at greater risk for motor vehicle accidents. The adult experiencing a high level of stress is also at a greater risk for accidents and certain stress-related illnesses such as headaches, depression, gastrointestinal disorders, and infections.

OLDER ADULT The physiological changes associated with aging, effects of multiple medications, psychological factors, and acute or chronic disease increase the older adult's risk for falls and other types of accidents. In 2005 almost 16,000 people age 65 and older died from unintentional fall-related injuries (CDC, 2008a, 2008d). Most falls occur within the home, specifically in the bedroom, bathroom, and kitchen. Environmental factors such as broken stairs, icy sidewalks, inadequate lighting, throw rugs, and exposed electrical cords cause many of the accidents. Older adults typically fall while transferring from beds, chairs, and toilets; getting into or out of bathtubs; tripping over carpet edges or doorway thresholds; and slipping on wet surfaces or descending stairs.

Other Risk Factors

LIFESTYLE Lifestyle choices increase safety risks. People who drive or operate machinery while under the influence of chemical substances or work at jobs that are more dangerous are at greater risk for injury. People who are preoccupied by stress or anxiety are more accident-prone because they fail to recognize the source of potential accidents, such as a cluttered stair or a stop sign.

IMPAIRED MOBILITY A patient with impaired mobility has many kinds of safety risks. Immobilization predisposes a patient to physiological and emotional hazards, which in turn further restrict mobility and independence (see Chapter 35). Physically challenged patients are at greater risk for injury when entering motor vehicles and buildings not equipped for the handicapped.

SENSORY IMPAIRMENTS Patients with visual, hearing, tactile, or communication impairments such as aphasia or language barrier are at greater risk for injury. Such patients are not always able to perceive a potential danger or express need for assistance (see Chapter 37).

COGNITIVE IMPAIRMENTS Cognitive impairments associated with delirium, dementia, and depression place patients at greater risk for injury. These conditions contribute to altered concentration and attention span, impaired memory, and orientation changes. Patients with these alterations become easily confused about their surroundings and are more likely to have falls and burns.

SAFETY AWARENESS Some patients are unaware of safety precautions, such as keeping medicine, poisonous plants, or other poisons away from children or reading the expiration date on food products. Your nursing assessment will identify the patient's level of knowledge regarding home safety so that you are able to correct safety problems with an individualized care plan.

Risks in the Health Care Agency

Environmental safety pertains to the health care agency, as well as to the patient's home and community. However, there are specific risks in health care agencies that you also need to address. Various forms of chemicals used are a source of an environmental risk. Chemicals such as mercury and those found in some medications, anesthetic gases, cleaning solutions, and disinfectants are potentially toxic if ingested or inhaled. Material Safety Data Sheets (MSDS) are a necessary resource available in any health care agency (Occupational Safety and Health Administration [OSHA], 1996).

A study by Health Grades Inc reported that nearly 195,000 people in the United States died each year in 2000, 2001, and 2002 as a result of potentially avoidable medical errors (Warner, 2004). In 2005 the Department of Health and Human Services enacted the Deficit Reduction Act, titled by the Centers for Medicare and Medicaid Services (CMS) as the "Hospital-Acquired Conditions and Present on Admission Indicator Reporting" (CMS, 2007a). This act identified eight conditions that are preventable through the application of evidence-based guidelines: object left in surgery, air embolism, blood incompatibility, catheter-associated urinary tract infection, pressure ulcers, vascular catheter–associated infection, surgical site infection following coronary artery bypass graft surgery, and falls and trauma. The government will not financially reimburse acute care hospitals if a patient acquires one of the eight conditions during hospitalization. In addition, The Joint Commission (2008) has identified National Patient Safety Goals in an effort to reduce the risk for medical mistakes. These evidence-based recommendations require health care agencies to focus their attention on a series of specific actions (Box 27-1).

Patients in health care settings are at risk for falls, patient-inherent accidents, procedure-related accidents, and equipment-related accidents. Learn to recognize factors associated with these risks, and take steps to prevent or minimize accidents.

FALLS In 2005 about 1.8 million older adults were treated in emergency departments for nonfatal fall-related injuries, and more than 433,000 of these were hospitalized (CDC,

---

BOX 27-1 The Joint Commission 2009 National Patient Safety Goals

- Improve the accuracy of patient identification.
- Improve the effectiveness of communication among caregivers.
- Improve safety of using medications.
- Reduce the risk for health care–associated infections.
- Accurately and completely reconcile medications across the continuum of care.
- Reduce the risk for patient harm resulting from falls.
- Reduce the risk for influenza and pneumococcal disease in institutionalized older adults.
- Reduce the risk for surgical fires.
- Encourage patients' active involvement in their own care as a patient safety strategy.
- Prevent health care–associated pressure ulcers (decubitus ulcers).
- The organization identifies safety risks inherent in its patient population.
- Improve recognition and response to changes in a patient's condition.
- The organization meets the expectations of the Universal Protocol.

2008a). Gait or lower extremity problems, urinary/stool frequency or incontinence, and use of certain medications increased the likelihood of patient falls in an acute care hospital (Krauss and others, 2005). Of those who fall, many suffer moderate to severe injuries such as hip fractures or head trauma that result in reduced mobility and independence and increase the risk for premature death. Patients who have underlying disease states are more susceptible to fall-related injuries (Hughes, 2008). For example, a patient with a bleeding disorder is more likely to undergo an intracranial bleed; a patient with osteoporosis has a greater chance for fracture. A risk assessment tool helps you assess potential risks before accidents and injuries result (Box 27-2). Based upon the results of this risk assessment, multiple evidence-based interventions should be implemented (Box 27-3).

PATIENT-INHERENT ACCIDENTS Patient-inherent accidents are accidents other than falls in which the patient is the primary factor causing the accident. Examples are self-inflicted cuts, injuries, and burns; ingestion or injection of foreign substances; self-mutilation or setting fires; and pinching fingers in drawers or doors. One of the more common precipitating factors for a patient-inherent accident is a seizure. A seizure leads to sudden, violent, and involuntary muscle contractions that are sometimes paroxysmal and episodic, causing loss of consciousness, falling, tonicity (rigidity of muscles), and clonicity (jerking of muscles). Place patients with a seizure disorder on seizure precautions, which are designed to protect patients when seizures occur.

PROCEDURE-RELATED ACCIDENTS Accidents that are procedure-related accidents are caused by health care

BOX 27-2   Morse Fall Scale

VARIABLES			SCORE
History of falling	No	0	
	Yes	25	_____
Secondary diagnosis	No	0	
	Yes	15	_____
Ambulatory aid	None/bed rest/nurse assist	0	
	Crutches/cane/walker	15	
	Furniture	30	_____
Intravenous therapy/ saline lock	No	0	
	Yes	20	_____
Gait	Normal/bed rest/wheelchair	0	
	Weak	10	
	Impaired	20	_____
Mental status	Oriented to own ability	0	
	Overestimates/forgets limitations	15	_____
		Total	_____

To determine risk, the Morse Fall Scale should be calibrated to each unit. High risk score should not be greater than 55. The patient's actual score should be charted as well as ranking of risk (high, medium, and low).

From Morse JM: *Preventing patient falls: establishing a fall intervention program,* ed 2, New York, 2009, Springer Publishing.

BOX 27-3   BEST PRACTICES

SUMMARY OF EVIDENCE

Most research on falls is conducted in samples from the community and in nursing homes, concentrating on the older adult population (Halfon and others, 2001). Less is known about falls among hospital inpatients, and only a few of the studies use strong methodological design.

Research shows that regardless of clinical setting, fall prevention consists of identifying a patient's risk factors and implementing targeted strategies or interventions aimed at reducing risk. Nurses need to link fall prevention strategies to the patient characteristics that lead to a fall and implement a comprehensive program that targets interventions that are appropriate and effective (Morse, 2002). Assessment of fall risk includes fall history; medication review; acute or chronic medical problems; mobility level; examination of vision, gait, and balance; and basic neurological and cardiovascular function (American Geriatrics Society, 2001). Successful interventions, based upon the patient's assessment, include such things as balance and gait training, exercise programs, medication modification, postural hypotension treatment, environmental hazard modification, and behavioral and educational programs (Tinetti, 2003). Although some interventions, such as assistive devices (bed alarms, canes, and walkers) and behavioral and educational programs, do not prevent falls when used in isolation, they do demonstrate benefit as a part of a multifaceted intervention program (American Geriatrics Society, 2001). Nurses need to select fall prevention equipment carefully and base their selection on empirical outcomes rather than on untested consensus (Brush and Capezuti, 2001). It is clear that the combined effect of multiple interventions produces the best outcomes.

APPLICATION TO NURSING PRACTICE

- Nurses are key to preventing patient falls in any health care setting.
- Assessment of fall risk helps you identify risk factor–specific fall prevention strategies.
- Promote a safe environment for patients, especially those at high risk for falls or a fall-related injury.
- Educate patients about why falls and fall-related injuries occur and how to prevent them.
- Multiple interventions aimed at the patient's specific risk factors produce the best outcomes.

REFERENCES

Data from American Geriatrics Society, British Geriatrics Society, American Academy of Orthopedic Surgeons Panel on Falls Prevention: Guideline for the prevention of falls in older persons, *J Am Geriatr Soc* 49:664, 2001.

Brush BL, Capezuti E: Historical analysis of siderail use in American hospitals, *J Nurs Scholarsh* 33(4):381, 2001.

Halfon P and others: Risk of falls for hospitalized patients: a predictive model based on routinely available data, *J Clin Epidemiol* 54(12):1258, 2001.

Morse JM: Enhancing the safety of hospitalization by reducing patient falls, *Am J Infect Control* 30:376, 2002.

Tinetti ME: Preventing falls in elderly persons, *N Engl J Med* 348:42, 2003.

providers and include medication and fluid administration errors, improper application of external devices, and improper performance of procedures such as dressing changes. Following an organization's policies and procedures and standards of nursing practice helps prevent procedure-related accidents. For example, correct use of body mechanics and transfer techniques reduces the risk for injuries when moving and lifting patients (see Chapter 35).

EQUIPMENT-RELATED ACCIDENTS Accidents that are equipment related result from the malfunction, disrepair, or misuse of equipment or from an electrical hazard. For example, too-rapid infusion of intravenous (IV) fluids can have serious consequences. The Joint Commission (2007) requires that hospitals use programmable infusion pumps when heparin, an anticoagulant medication, is a continuous IV infusion. To avoid injury, understand how to operate all monitoring or therapy equipment. If you discover faulty equipment, place a tag on it to prevent it from being used on another patient, and promptly report any malfunctions.

CRITICAL THINKING

Synthesis

You will apply elements of critical thinking whenever you perform the nursing process with a patient. Consider the scientific knowledge you have learned, your experience, critical thinking attitudes, and standards to ensure an individualized approach to patient care (Box 27-4).

KNOWLEDGE You will need a complete picture of a patient's situation, including physical, cultural, physiological, psychosocial, and environmental information to protect the patient from injury. Consider a wide variety of factors (e.g., the patient's risk for injury, medications being taken, and the

environment where most activities of daily living occur) before you develop a plan of care. Because every patient is different, with various strengths and weaknesses, prioritize factors that are threats to safety, and concentrate on probable threats. After considering a patient's specific strengths and weaknesses, environment, and developmental stage, work with the patient and family to determine creative interventions.

EXPERIENCE Use clinical and personal experience to recall incidents that occurred with another patient or family member and the specific circumstances that led to the situation. For example, your grandmother fell because her slipper became entangled in a throw rug at the top of the stairs. Use the experience of your grandmother's fall, and apply the knowledge gained when you assess a patient's home for safety hazards during a home visit.

ATTITUDES Use of critical thinking attitudes ensures your plan of care for a patient's safety is comprehensive. For example, show perseverance in identifying all potential safety risks and threats. Be responsible for collecting unbiased, accurate data that are relevant to the patient's safety. It is important to show discipline in conducting a thorough review of a patient's home environment. View all situations as opportunities to protect the patient. Once they occur, injuries cause pain, immobility, loss of income, or even death.

STANDARDS The American Nurses Association's (ANA's) Nursing: Scope and Standards of Practice (2004) includes the concept of safety, stating that nurses will implement nursing interventions competently in a safe and appropriate manner. The ANA Code of Ethics (see Chapter 5) includes safety issues in the statement of the nurse's responsibility to promote, advocate for, and strive to protect the health, safety, and rights of the patient. Regulatory agencies such as The Joint Commission and the Occupational Safety and Health Administration (OSHA) define standards and guidelines related to safety in health care settings.

NURSING PROCESS

■■■ASSESSMENT

To conduct a thorough patient assessment, consider possible threats to the patient's safety, including the patient's immediate environment and any individual risk factors (Table 27-1). When caring for a patient in the home, a home hazard assessment is necessary (Box 27-5). A thorough hazard assessment covers topics such as adequacy of lighting, presence of safety devices, placement of furniture or other items that will possibly create barriers, condition of flooring, and safety of the kitchen and bathrooms. To assess the home, walk through the rooms with the patient and discuss how the patient normally conducts daily activities and whether the environment poses problems. For example, when assessing adequacy of lighting, inspect areas where the patient moves and works, particularly outside walkways, steps, interior halls, and doorways. Getting a sense of the patient's routines helps you recognize safety hazards.

BOX 27-4 SYNTHESIS IN PRACTICE

Joani completed the health screening on Mr. Gonzales. She knows she needs to incorporate knowledge about environmental risks as they relate to Mr. Gonzales' age, level of independence, health status, and expectations. In addition, Mr. Gonzales is the third patient Joani has cared for in the home, so she also has an experiential basis for practice. As Joani integrates knowledge with previous experience, she remembers that Mr. Gonzales values his independence. As a result, Joani is able to develop a plan of care to meet Mr. Gonzales' safety needs while assisting him in maintaining his independence. She discovers that the lighting is poor and that several throw rugs are near the chairs and the bedside. The health screening has revealed that Mr. Gonzales has decreased visual acuity and has not had a new pair of glasses for 3 years. He fell in his apartment about a month ago but did not have any injuries.

TABLE 27-1 FOCUSED PATIENT ASSESSMENT

FACTORS TO ASSESS	QUESTIONS	PHYSICAL ASSESSMENT
Environment	Have you ever fallen down? Where did the fall happen? Were you injured? Have you ever burned yourself?	Inspect the home environment both inside and outside for potential hazards: focus on the kitchen and bathroom.
Sensory	When do you wear your glasses? When was the last time you had your eyes checked? Can you tell me what the label on this medication bottle says?	Observe patient's ability to read printed material accurately.
Physical mobility	Do you exercise? What kind of exercise do you do? Are you able to move around safely at home?	Observe patient's posture, gait, and balance during activities of daily living.

BOX 27-5   Home Hazard Assessment

- Proper lighting inside and outside
- Storage areas within easy reach
- Appliances in good working order
- Extension cords placed along walls
- Presence of smoke detectors and a fire extinguisher
- Presence of carbon monoxide detector
- Flammable objects away from stove or heaters
- Gas pilot lights lit
- Hot water thermostat set to 120° F or less
- Handrails or grip bars installed
- Nonskid surfaces in the bathroom and tub or shower
- Floor coverings secured and floors free of clutter
- Furniture and assistive devices promote ease of mobility
- Medications stored properly and not outdated
- Telephone accessible with readily available emergency phone numbers

In a health care facility, determine if any hazards exist in the immediate care environment. Does the placement of equipment pose barriers when the patient attempts to ambulate? Does positioning of the patient's bed allow the patient to safely reach items on a bedside table? Are self-care items in a bathroom arranged for accessibility? Be sure to collaborate with the hospital's clinical engineering staff to ensure equipment functions properly.

Your nursing history will include data about the patient's level of wellness to determine if any underlying conditions pose a threat to safety. For example, assess the patient's activity tolerance, gait, muscle strength and coordination, balance, and vision. Consider the patient's developmental level when you analyze your data. Review whether the patient is taking any medications or undergoing any procedures that pose risks. For example, using a diuretic increases the frequency of voiding and results in more frequent trips to the bathroom. Falls often occur when patients get out of bed quickly to urinate. When you assess an older adult, recognize the types of physical changes that increase the risk for injury (Box 27-6).

PATIENT EXPECTATIONS When you care for patients with safety needs, ask what they expect from your care. For example, "How can I provide care that will make you feel safe?" or "After we walk through your home, tell me what is important that we do to help you feel safe." In some cases a patient's and family's expectations of what is safe are not always appropriate. When this happens, intervene and educate both the patient and family regarding safe practices concerning everyday decisions, use of medications and medical equipment, and the environment. When patients are uninformed or inexperienced, this threatens their safety.

■■■ NURSING DIAGNOSIS

Gather data from your nursing assessment, and analyze clusters of defining characteristics to identify relevant nursing diagnoses (Figure 27-1). Include specific related or contributing factors to individualize your nursing care. Nursing diagnoses for patients with safety risks include the following:

- *Risk for imbalanced body temperature*
- *Risk for falls*
- *Impaired home maintenance*
- *Risk for injury*
- *Deficient knowledge*
- *Risk for poisoning*
- *Disturbed sensory perception*
- *Risk for suffocation*
- *Risk for trauma*

For example, the nursing diagnosis *risk for injury* could be related to altered mobility, or it could be related to sensory alteration (e.g., visual). Altered mobility leads you to select such nursing interventions as range-of-motion (ROM) exercises or teaching the proper use of safety devices such as side rails, canes, or crutches. Visual impairment as the related factor leads you to select different interventions such as keeping the area well lit; orienting the patient to the surroundings; or keeping eyeglasses clean, handy, and well protected. When

BOX 27-6 CARE OF THE OLDER ADULT

Physical Assessment Findings in the Older Adult That Increase the Risk for Accidents

MUSCULOSKELETAL CHANGES
- Muscle strength decreases
- Joints become less mobile
- Brittle bones due to osteoporosis
- Posture changes; some kyphosis is common
- Range of motion (ROM) is limited

NERVOUS SYSTEM CHANGES
- Voluntary or autonomic reflexes are slower
- Decreased ability to respond to multiple stimuli
- Decreased sensitivity of touch

SENSORY CHANGES
- Peripheral vision and lens accommodation decrease
- Decrease in night vision and ability to adjust to changes in light
- Lens develops opacity (cataracts)
- Stimuli threshold for light touch and pain increases
- Hearing is impaired because high-frequency tones are less perceptible

GENITOURINARY CHANGES
- Increased nocturia
- Increased occurrence of incontinence

Modified from Ebersole P, Hess P: *Toward healthy aging*, ed 7, St. Louis, 2008, Mosby.

you do not identify the correct related factor, the use of inappropriate interventions increases a patient's risk for injury. For example, not evaluating the home environment for hazards will possibly result in sending a hospitalized patient back home only to return with an additional injury.

■■■PLANNING

Patients with actual or potential risks to safety require a nursing care plan with interventions that prevent and minimize threats to safety. You need to design your interventions to help a patient feel safe to interact freely within the environment. The total plan of care will address all aspects of patient needs and use resources of the health care team and the community when appropriate.

GOALS AND OUTCOMES Planning and goal setting need to be done in collaboration with the patient, family, and other members of the health care team. Remember to keep goals realistic, within the resources available to the patient. When you involve the patient and family in planning, they become more alert to safety risks and potential hazards. For example, you develop a goal "Reduce the number of falls" in a patient with Parkinson's disease who falls frequently at home. An expected outcome is "Patient reduces barriers to reaching the bathroom." You then suggest the intervention that the patient sleep in a bedroom closest to the bathroom. After collaborating with the family, however, you select the alternative of a bedside commode.

SETTING PRIORITIES Prioritize patient nursing diagnoses and interventions that are most important in terms of risk to safety and health promotion. In some situations you need to select more than one nursing diagnosis that best represents a patient's particular needs. For example, the nursing diagnoses *risk for poisoning* and *deficient knowledge* are important for an older patient who takes several medications and has an impaired memory. Priority nursing interventions include ways to reduce accidental poisoning (e.g., large labels on medication containers, use of dose dispensers, and having a family member prepare medications) and teaching safe

methods of taking medications, within a patient's learning capabilities (see Care Plan).

COLLABORATIVE CARE It is important to help patients with safety needs develop a link within their community that helps to maintain a safe environment. Hospitalized patients need to learn how to identify and select resources within their community that will enhance safety once they return home. For example, an older adult may need to go to an adult day care center during weekdays when family members are working and unable to provide regular assistance.

■■■IMPLEMENTATION

Direct your nursing interventions toward maintaining the patient's safety in all types of settings. Providing a safe environment includes health promotion, developmental interventions, and environmental protection. Each of these areas of implementation is appropriate in acute and restorative care settings.

HEALTH PROMOTION The emphasis in health care today is on health promotion. Edelman and Mandle (2010) describe passive and active strategies aimed at health promotion. Passive strategies are put into practice through government legislation (e.g., sanitation and clean water laws). Active strategies involve the individual and include changes in lifestyle and participation in wellness programs.

Participate in health promotion activities by supporting legislation, by acting as a positive role model, and by recommending safety measures in the home, school, neighborhood, and workplace.

DEVELOPMENTAL INTERVENTIONS

Infant, Toddler, and Preschooler Growing, curious children need adults to protect them from injury. Educate young parents or guardians about reducing risks of injuries to children, and teach ways to promote safety in the home. Some examples are preventing access to poisonous substances; correct use of car seats; use of safe, age-appropriate toys; and placement of safety covers on electrical outlets (see Chapter 21). Encourage parents to position infants on the back ("back to

CONCEPT MAP

Nursing Diagnosis: Risk for injury
- History of decreased visual acuity
- Throw rugs on the floor
- Low lighting in the bathroom and bedroom
- Walks without picking his feet up very far from the floor

Interventions
- Remove the throw rugs from Mr. Gonzales' home
- Increase lighting in Mr. Gonzales' home to a minimum of 75 watts
- Discuss with the health care team a referral to physical therapy for walking exercises

Nursing Diagnosis: Disturbed sensory perceptual: Visual
- Mr. Gonzales is unable to read medication labels
- Last visual examination was 3 years ago
- Mr. Gonzales expressed concern for his safety

Interventions
- Assist Mr. Gonzales to schedule an appointment with an ophthalmologist for a vision check
- Increase lighting in home to a minimum of 75 watts
- Label medication bottles clearly in large print
- Encourage Mr. Gonzales to use a medication organizer

Chief Medical Diagnosis: Decreased visual acuity, decreased hearing, osteoarthritis
Priority Assessments: Ability to see and hear, home environment, pain levels, ability to provide self-care

Nursing Diagnosis: Impaired comfort
- History of osteoarthritis
- Report of discomfort
- Report of stiffness

Interventions
- Encourage Mr. Gonzales to talk to his physician about medication for the arthritis
- Instruct Mr. Gonzales on the use of warm compresses to relieve pain
- Demonstrate range–of–motion exercises to help relieve stiffness
- Evaluate Mr. Gonzales' ability to perform activities of daily living

Nursing Diagnosis: Disturbed sensory perceptual: Auditory
- Hearing loss previous employment
- Expressed concern about safety

Interventions
- Face Mr. Gonzales and speak clearly
- Encourage Mr. Gonzales to have his hearing evaluated by an audiologist

——— Link between medical diagnosis and nursing diagnosis   - - - - Link between nursing diagnoses

Figure 27-1 ■ Concept Map.

CARE PLAN Risk for Injury

ASSESSMENT

Joani knows that people with impaired vision and a history of falls are at increased risk for injury. When Joani met with Mr. Gonzales, he expressed concern about his safety. He wants to remain independent and live to a "ripe old age," but knows that he is not as young as he used to be. His son Carlos recently purchased a medication organizer that Mr. Gonzales has not started using because he is concerned he will make a mistake.

ASSESSMENT ACTIVITIES	FINDINGS/DEFINING CHARACTERISTICS*
Inspect Mr. Gonzales' environment for safety hazards.	Joani discovers **throw rugs on the floors** near the chairs and at the bedside and **poor lighting** in the bedroom and bathroom.
Conduct a physical assessment to determine Mr. Gonzales' risk factors for falling.	Mr. Gonzales is unable to **read the labels on his medication bottles. His last visual examination was 3 years ago.** Gait assessment reveals that Mr. Gonzales **does not pick his feet very high up off the floor** and **his movements are stiff.**

NURSING DIAGNOSIS: Risk for injury related to altered mobility and decreased visual acuity.

PLANNING

GOAL

- Mr. Gonzales will adapt his environment to motor, sensory, and cognitive developmental needs (within 2 months).

EXPECTED OUTCOMES (NOC)†

Safe Home Environment
- Mr. Gonzales will list hazards within 1 week.
- Mr. Gonzales will reduce modifiable hazards by 100% within 1 month.

INTERVENTIONS (NIC)‡

Environmental Management: Safety
- Review with Mr. Gonzales the potential risks for accidents observed in the home.

    a. Remove throw rugs.

    b. Increase lighting to a minimum of 75 watts per light.
    c. Label medication bottles clearly in bold, large print. Use medication organizer for daily medications.
- Stress the importance of making safety modifications in the home, and give specific instructions for prevention of burns, falls, and poisoning.
- Arrange for Mr. Gonzales to visit an ophthalmologist and have a new prescription written for eyeglasses.

Exercise Promotion
Encourage Mr. Gonzales to take 20-minute walks in the neighborhood at least 3 times per week.

RATIONALE

An accurate home assessment identifies threats to a patient's safety (Emergency Care Research Institute, 2006).

Throw rugs often roll up or bunch to create an uneven walking surface.

Adequate lighting reduces the likelihood of falling over objects or bumping into them.

Clearly labeled medication bottles and use of a medication organizer reduce the risk for a medication error.

Advance guidance is important in preventing potential injuries.

Reduced visual acuity is correctable. Routine eye examinations are recommended annually for all persons after the age of 50 (Ebersole and Hess, 2008).

Maintenance of a physically active lifestyle delays age changes associated with cardiovascular, respiratory, and musculoskeletal function (Ebersole and Hess, 2008).

*Defining characteristics are shown in **bold** type.
†Outcomes classification label from Moorhead S and others, editors: *Nursing outcomes classification (NOC)*, ed 4, St. Louis, 2008, Mosby.
‡Intervention classification labels from Bulechek GM and others, editors: *Nursing interventions classification (NIC)*, ed 5, St. Louis, 2008, Mosby.

CARE PLAN   Risk for Injury—cont'd

EVALUATION

NURSING ACTIONS	PATIENT RESPONSE/FINDING	ACHIEVEMENT OF OUTCOME
Observe Mr. Gonzales' environment for elimination of threats to safety.	Throw rugs have been removed or replaced with rubber-backed rugs. Lighting has been increased to 75 watts except in bathroom and bedroom. Mr. Gonzales is able to identify potential hazards.	Mr. Gonzales has reduced hazards. Mr. Gonzales verbalizes adaptation to environmental modifications.
Reassess motor, sensory, and cognitive status for appropriate environmental modifications.	Mr. Gonzales has obtained new glasses. Mr. Gonzales is able to read medication bottle labels and is using the medication organizer. Mr. Gonzales takes 20-minute walks in the neighborhood at least 3 times per week. Mr. Gonzales reports difficulty getting into bathtub due to stiffness. Bathtub floor is without nonskid strips.	Outcome of reducing hazards 100% has not been fully achieved. Mr. Gonzales will purchase nonskid strips for tub floor and bathtub transfer assist device.

sleep") to prevent sudden infant death syndrome (SIDS). As a pediatric nurse, teach new parents about removing poisonous substances from easy-to-reach storage areas and the importance of supervised play. Educate parents about the importance of immunizations and how they protect a child from life-threatening diseases.

School-Age Child School-age children increasingly explore their environment. They have friends outside their immediate neighborhood, and they become more active in school, church, and the community. Teach children to wear seat belts whenever riding in a car; to wear a helmet when riding a bicycle, skateboard, or scooter; and to keep adults informed of where they are. Teach children how to cross the street safely and to refrain from talking to or accepting rides or gifts from strangers. Teach them what to do if a stranger approaches and how to get help.

Adolescent Risks to the adolescent's safety involve many factors outside the home because they spend much of their time away from home and with their peer group. However, adults serve as role models for adolescents. Help adolescents minimize safety risks by setting expectations and providing examples and education. Because adolescence is a time when sexual physical characteristics develop, adolescents often begin to have physical relationships with others. They need prompt accurate instructions about abstinence and safe sexual practices. When adolescents learn to drive, they need education on complying with rules and regulations regarding the use of a car. Most schools have driver's education programs. Make sure you strongly recommend the regular use of a seat belt. Box 27-7 offers an example of patient teaching for preventing automobile accidents during adolescence.

Adult Risks to young and middle-age adults frequently result from lifestyle factors such as child rearing, high-stress states, inadequate nutrition, use of firearms, and abuse of drugs or alcohol. In this fast-paced society there also appears to be more expression of anger. This anger can quickly precipitate motor vehicle collisions resulting from "road rage." Help adults understand their safety risks, and guide them in making lifestyle modifications by referring them to resources such as classes to help quit smoking and for stress management and employee assistance programs. Also encourage adults to exercise regularly, maintain a healthy diet, practice relaxation techniques, and acquire adequate sleep (see Chapters 24, 26, 30, and 32).

Older Adult Elimination of threats to the safety of the older adult focuses primarily on accidents. Advancing age and concurrent physiological changes predispose older adults to falls (Box 27-8) (see Chapter 21). Certain disease states common to older adults, such as arthritis or strokes, increase the chance of injury. The effects of many medications, such as sedatives, diuretics, and anticoagulants, also increase the chance of injury. Table 27-2 lists nursing interventions designed to prevent falls and compensate for the physiological changes of aging.

Provide information about neighborhood resources to help the older adult maintain an independent lifestyle. Older adults frequently relocate to new neighborhoods and must get acquainted with new resources such as modes of transportation, church schedules, and food resources (e.g., Meals on Wheels). Although retired from their jobs, older adults have a wealth of past experience to aid volunteer organizations. Some retirees even enjoy reentering the work force in a new capacity. Information about assistance resources, such as daily "hello" programs, emergency services, and elder abuse hot lines, is also helpful.

ENVIRONMENTAL INTERVENTIONS To eliminate environmental threats, make sure your nursing interventions

BOX 27-7   PATIENT TEACHING

Safe Driving Habits

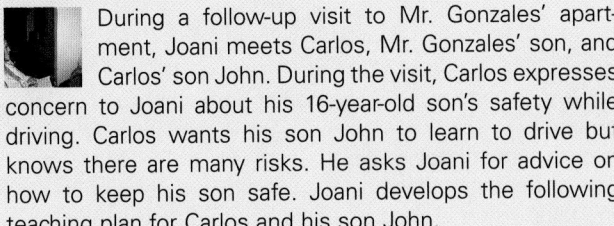 During a follow-up visit to Mr. Gonzales' apartment, Joani meets Carlos, Mr. Gonzales' son, and Carlos' son John. During the visit, Carlos expresses concern to Joani about his 16-year-old son's safety while driving. Carlos wants his son John to learn to drive but knows there are many risks. He asks Joani for advice on how to keep his son safe. Joani develops the following teaching plan for Carlos and his son John.

OUTCOME

- At the end of the teaching session, Carlos and John will verbalize understanding of ways to promote safe driving habits.

TEACHING STRATEGIES

- Establish rapport with Carlos and John, and maintain eye contact.
- Provide a brief description of what will be taught.
- Suggest to Carlos that he enroll John in a driver's education course.
- Explain the importance of using seat belts while driving and as a passenger.
- Stress to Carlos the importance of being a role model by practicing safe driving habits.

- Explain to Carlos the importance of providing John frequent opportunities to practice driving in good and bad weather.
- Explain to John the safety risks associated with driving under the influence of drugs and alcohol.
- Explain the costs associated with traffic violations such as higher insurance premiums and possible loss of driver's license.
- Ask Carlos and John to form a contract regarding not driving and drinking. Instruct John never to enter an automobile when the driver has been using drugs or alcohol.

EVALUATION STRATEGIES

- Ask Carlos to identify when he will provide opportunities for John to practice driving.
- Ask John what he would do if he were drinking at a party and needed to get home.
- Ask John what will happen if he receives a traffic violation.
- Ask Carlos how he will demonstrate safe driving habits to John.
- Ask John to identify the risks of driving without a seat belt.

BOX 27-8   CARE OF THE OLDER ADULT

Educating About Safety

- Because of visual impairments in older adults, teach patients to keep living areas well lighted and free of clutter, to keep eyeglasses in good condition, and to avoid night driving.
- Older adults have musculoskeletal changes that make movement difficult and increase the risk for falling. Teach patients to keep assistive devices in proper working order (canes, rails in tub and bathroom, and elevated seats) and to use nonskid strips in bathtubs.
- Advise older adults to avoid smoking in bed, to lower thermostats on water heaters, to avoid overloading electrical outlets, and to install and maintain smoke and carbon monoxide detectors in the house.
- Older adults are more likely to have automobile accidents as a result of decreased hearing and visual acuity, altered depth perception, slowed reaction time, and poor peripheral vision. Advise older adults to drive only short distances and in the daylight; avoid driving in inclement

weather, such as fog, heavy rain and snow; use side and rear view mirrors carefully; look behind them toward their blind spot before changing lanes; and keep a window rolled down in order to hear sirens and horns.
- Older adults can have some impairment of memory, especially when scheduling medications. Teach patients about the proper handling and storage of medications and safe methods of scheduling and taking medications.
- Older adults have physiological changes that result in slower metabolism of drugs. Teach patients about drug interactions and signs and symptoms of drug toxicity to report to their health care provider.
- Some older adults suffer from irreversible dementia. Assist family caregivers in understanding the nature of dementia. Teach them ways to match expectations with the patient's capabilities, how to incorporate earlier life skills and interests, and to provide a calm, caring, and structured environment.

include general preventive measures and specific measures to reduce the risk for accidental injuries.

General Preventive Measures Your nursing interventions contribute to a safer environment by helping patients meet their basic physiological needs. To ensure that there are no threats to oxygen availability, encourage patients to have their fuel-burning appliances inspected each season for proper

functioning and to install a battery-operated carbon monoxide detector in the home. To achieve a comfortable level of humidity in the home, attach a humidifier to the furnace or, in the case of patients who have upper respiratory tract infections, use a room humidifier while sleeping. Teach patients to follow the manufacturer's directions regarding the cleaning and maintenance of home humidifiers to reduce contamina-

TABLE 27-2   Measures to Prevent Falls in Older Adults

MEASURE	RATIONALE
HOME OR HEALTH CARE FACILITY	
Stairs	
Install treads with uniform depth of 9 inches (22.9 cm) and 9-inch risers (vertical face of steps).	If stairs are of uniform size, older adult does not have to continually adjust vision.
Install uniform-textured or plain-colored surfaces on each tread, and mark edge of tread with contrasting color.	Uniform textures or color help to decrease vertigo. Marking edge of tread provides obvious visual clue to end of stair.
Ensure proper lighting of each tread. Block sun or light bulb glare with translucent shades or screen, or use lower-wattage bulbs.	Older adults' vision is unable to adjust quickly to changes in lighting.
Ensure adequate head room so that users do not have to duck to negotiate stairs.	Sudden changes in head position often result in dizziness, which increase the risk for falling.
Remove protruding objects from staircase walls.	Decreased peripheral vision prevents patient from seeing object. Moving to avoid protruding objects will disrupt balance.
Maintain outdoor walkways and stairs in good condition and free of holes, cracks, and splinters.	Decreased visual acuity prevents patient from seeing any structural defect.
Handrails	
Install smooth but slip-resistant handrail at least 2 inches (5 cm) from wall.	Two-inch distance allows patient to grasp handrail firmly for support.
Secure handrail firmly to support user's weight, especially at bottom and top of stairway.	Older adults have greatest risk for falling at top and bottom of stairs because they shift their center of gravity, making balance unstable.
Install grab rails in bathroom near toilet and tub.	Enables patient to have support while rising from sitting to standing position.
Floors	
Ensure patients wear properly fitting shoes or slippers with nonskid surface.	Reduces chances of slipping.
Secure all carpeting, mats, and tile; place nonskid backing under small rugs.	Sudden slip causes dizziness and inability to regain balance.
Place bath mats or nonskid strips on bathtub or shower stall floors.	Wet surfaces increase the risk for falling.
Secure electrical cords against baseboards.	Prevents tripping.
Maintain proper illumination in areas both inside and outside where the patient moves and walks.	Reduces the risk for falling due to eyestrain.
HEALTH CARE FACILITY	
Orientation	
Admit disoriented patients to a room near nurses' station.	Provides for more frequent observation by nursing staff.
Maintain close supervision of confused patients.	Confused patient often attempts to wander out of bed or room.
Show the patient how to use the call light at the bedside and in bathroom, and place within easy reach. Instruct patient to call for assistance with movement as needed.	Location and use of the call light is essential to patient safety.
Place bedside tables and over-bed tables close to the patient. Place articles within easy reach.	Prevents patient from searching or overreaching for items such as eyeglasses, dentures, hearing aid, or telephone.
Remove clutter from bedside tables, hallways, bathrooms, and grooming areas.	Eliminates potential hazards and promotes patient independence.
Keep the bed in low position. Have the patient rise from the bed or chair slowly.	Prevents dizziness resulting from postural hypotension.
Leave one side rail up and one down on the side where the oriented and ambulatory patient gets out of bed.	Patient is able to use the side rail for support when getting in and out of bed and to position self once in bed.
Transport	
Lock bed and wheelchair when transferring a patient from a bed to a wheelchair or back to bed.	Provides stability and support during transfer.
Place side rails in the up position, and secure safety straps around the patient on a stretcher.	Prevents the patient from rolling off the stretcher.

tion of the water. Teach basic techniques for food handling and preparation so that patients meet all their nutritional needs safely (e.g., wash hands before and after food preparation, clean cutting surfaces thoroughly with soap and water, cook food thoroughly, refrigerate food after preparation, and label and date when leftovers are saved). To prevent injury from exposure to temperature extremes, educate older adults or patients who enjoy outdoor activities about signs and symptoms of frostbite, hypothermia, heatstroke, and heat exhaustion and how to avoid these conditions.

Adequate lighting and security measures in and around the home, including the use of night-lights, exterior lighting, and locks on doors and windows, enable patients to reduce the risk for injury from falls or crime. The local police department and community organizations often have safety classes available on how not to become a victim of crime. If patients have a history of falling and live alone, recommend that they obtain an electronic safety alert device to wear. This device, when activated by the wearer, alerts a monitoring site to call emergency services for assistance.

In the health care setting, color-coded wristbands are often used to help communicate a patient's safety risk. In 2008 the American Hospital Association (AHA) issued an advisory recommending that hospitals standardize wristband colors: red for patient allergies, yellow for fall risk, and purple for do-not-resuscitate preferences. This recommendation came after a near-miss incident in which a nurse, working in two different hospitals, placed a wrong-colored band on a patient. Many state hospital associations and communities are now standardizing colors to reduce confusion both within and across health care organizations (AHA, 2008).

To control pathogen transmission, teach patients how and when to wash hands (e.g., following toileting, before and after food preparation and wound care). Patients also need to know how to dispose of infected material such as wound dressings and used needles in the home. For example, heavy plastic containers such as hard, colored plastic liquid detergent bottles are excellent for needle disposal. The Environmental Protection Agency (EPA) encourages disposal of used needles by way of community drop-off programs, household hazardous waste facilities or sharps mail-back programs or using home needle destruction devices (Coalition for Safe Community Needle Disposal, 2005b). Encourage patients to contact neighborhood community governments for guidelines on waste disposal methods. Teach patients "safe sex" practices, including correct use of condoms and engaging in monogamous relationships to reduce the risk for sexually transmitted diseases. Nurses use standard precautions for all patients to protect themselves from contact with blood and body fluids (see Chapter 13).

Specific Safety Concerns There are specific interventions that you as a nurse implement to ensure patient safety.

Falls. Modifying a patient's environment reduces the risk for falls. For example, a patient who is morbidly obese needs a bed, wheelchair, or commode specifically designed to support the additional weight. A patient with impaired mobility benefits from organizing the home so it becomes unnecessary to walk up or down stairs. In a health care facility, explain to patients how to use the call light or intercom system, and make sure you always place the call device close to the patient. For patients needing assistance to ambulate, a gait belt can provide a secure way to steady or guide patients when transferring or walking. Respond quickly when call lights are on so that the patient does not attempt to get out of bed without help. Removing clutter such as excess furniture and equipment and providing patients with rubber-soled shoes or slippers for walking or during transfer helps keep the immediate environment safe. Provide a clear path to the bathroom, and keep rooms well lit to promote safe ambulation. Inspect canes, walkers, and crutches to be sure rubber tips are intact and connections are tight and that the assistive devices are at the appropriate height for the patient. Additional devices to use at a patient's bedside include a bedside commode, non-skid floor mat, overhead trapeze, and hemi-walker (Figure 27-2).

Implementing certain safeguards and teaching the family ways to reduce the risk for falls further minimizes the risk for falls (see Table 27-2). Confused and disoriented patients or patients who repeatedly fall or try to remove medical devices (e.g., oxygen equipment, IV lines, or dressings) often require the temporary use of restraints to keep them safe. Restraints are not a solution to a patient problem, but rather a temporary means to maintain patient safety.

Restraints. Restraints are either chemical or physical. Chemical restraints are medications, such as anxiolytics and sedatives, used to control the patient's behavior. A physical **restraint** is any manual method, physical or mechanical device, material. or equipment that immobilizes or reduces the ability of a patient to move arms, legs, body, or head freely (Centers for Medicare and Medicaid Services [CMS], 2007b). The use of restraints is associated with serious complications resulting from immobilization, such as pressure ulcers, pneumonia, constipation, and incontinence. In some cases death has resulted because of restricted breathing and circulation. There have been cases in which patients have been strangled while trying to get out of bed while restrained in a jacket or vest restraint. As a result, many health care facilities have eliminated the use of the jacket (vest) restraint because of this risk (Capezuti and others, 2008). For this reason, this text will not describe the use of the vest restraint. Loss of self-esteem, humiliation, and agitation are also serious concerns. Because of these risks, legislation emphasizes reducing the use of restraints. Regulatory agencies such as The Joint Commission and CMS enforce standards for the safe use of restraint devices. A restraint-free environment, either physical or chemical, is your first goal for all patients. Always try alternatives such as more frequent observation, involvement of family during visitation, frequent reorientation, and the introduction of familiar stimuli (e.g., knitting or crocheting or looking at family photos) within the environment to reduce behaviors that often lead to restraint use.

In keeping with current trends toward health promotion, your assessment techniques and modifications of the envi-

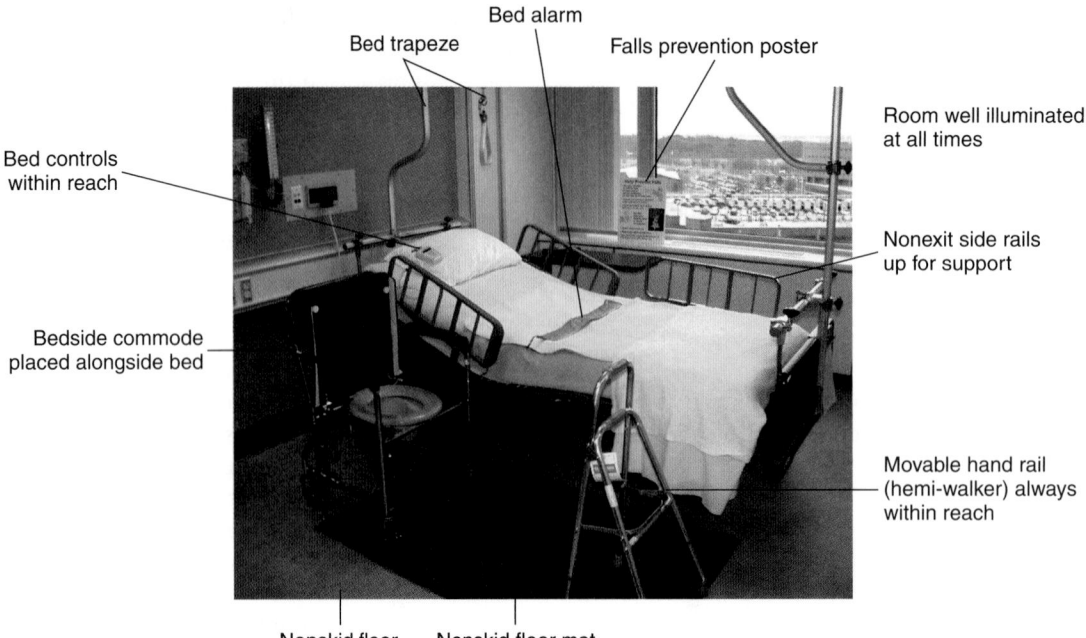

Bed alarm

Bed trapeze

Falls prevention poster

Room well illuminated
at all times

Bed controls
within reach

Nonexit side rails
up for support

Bedside commode
placed alongside bed

Movable hand rail
(hemi-walker) always
within reach

Nonskid floor   Nonskid floor mat

Figure 27-2 ■ Making the hospital patient's environment safe. (From U.S. Department of Veterans Affairs, National Center for Patient Safety: *2004 Falls toolkit, falls notebook interventions,* 2004, http://www.patientsafety.gov/Safetytopics/fallstoolkit/index.html, accessed June 25, 2007.)

BOX 27-9   Alternatives to Restraints

- Involve patients and families in planning care; explain all procedures and treatments to them.
- Encourage family and friends to stay, or use sitters for patients who need continuous supervision.
- Use calm, simple statements and physical cues as needed.
- Use a knee band such as the Ambularm or an alarming seat belt to alert caregivers when the patient reaches a near-vertical position.
- Eliminate full side rails. To reduce injury resulting from falls, use low beds with a floor mat at bedside.
- Assign confused or disoriented patients to rooms near the nurses' station. Observe these patients frequently, and institute regular patient checks.
- Provide appropriate visual and auditory stimuli (e.g., family pictures, clock, radio).
- Eliminate bothersome treatments as soon as possible. For example, discontinue tube feedings and begin oral feedings as quickly as the patient's condition allows.
- Camouflage IV lines with clothing, skin sleeves, or Kling dressing. Camouflage a gastrostomy tube (G-tube) with

an abdominal binder. Use freedom splints and endotracheal tube (ET) holders to maintain ET tubes.
- Provide ongoing pain assessment. Try nonpharmacological interventions first, such as positioning and relaxation techniques (e.g., music, massage).
- Use diversional activities appropriate for the patient (e.g., activity aprons).
- Institute exercise and ambulation schedules as the patient's condition allows.
- Provide scheduled toileting, especially during peak fall times, such as 6 to 8 AM and 4 to 6 PM.
- Consult with physical and occupational therapists to enhance strength, mobility, and exercise.
- Use protective devices such as hip pads, helmet, skid-proof slippers, and nonskid strips near bed.
- Provide prompt treatment and ongoing evaluation of medical problems (e.g., orthostatic hypotension, constipation, fluid overload, dehydration, infection, drug toxicity, medication side effects).

Modified from GeronurseOnline.org: *Want to know: physical restraints,* 2005, http://www.geronurseonline.org/index.dfm?section_id530&geriatric_topic_id510&sub_section_id574&page_id5156&tab52.

---

ronment are effective alternatives to restraints (Box 27-9). For patients who continue to attempt to ambulate without assistance, use electronic bed and chair alarm devices. These devices warn nursing staff that a patient is attempting to leave the bed or chair unassisted. Many devices are available, including a knee band, such as the **Ambularm** (Figure 27-3),

that sounds an alarm when the patient reaches a near-vertical position. Other devices include pressure-sensitive strips placed beneath the patient under the buttocks or a tether alarm that is clipped to the patient's gown. These devices help avoid physical restraints and when responded to immediately, prevent a patient fall.

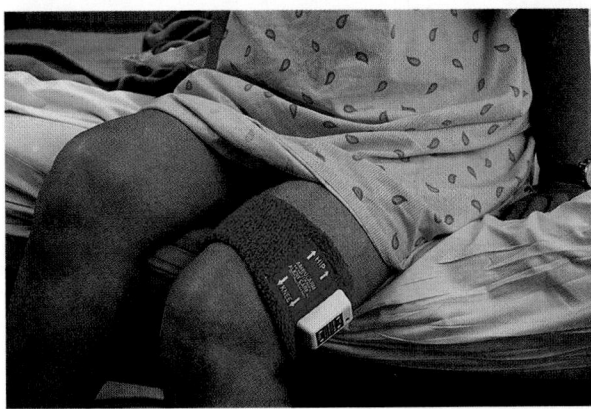

Figure 27-3 ■ Audio alarm will sound when patient approaches a near-vertical position when getting out of bed. (Courtesy Alert Care, Tiburon, Calif.)

When restraints are required to protect the patient or others, involve the patient and family in the decision to use restraints. Assist them in adapting to this change by explaining the purpose of the restraint, expected care while the patient is in restraints, and that the restraint is temporary and protective. It is a requirement for nursing homes to obtain informed consent from family members before using restraints. As with other procedures, follow specific guidelines when using physical restraints (Skill 27-1). The overall objectives for restraint use include the following:

1. Reduce the risk for patient injury from falls
2. Prevent interruption of therapy such as traction, IV infusions, nasogastric tube feeding, or Foley catheter
3. Prevent the confused or combative patient from removing life support equipment
4. Reduce the risk for injury to self or others

For legal purposes, know agency-specific policies for appropriate use and monitoring of a restrained patient. Some medications, such as sedatives or hypnotics given to calm an agitated patient, are a chemical restraint when they are not a standard part of that patient's treatment plan. You must have clinical justification for the use of a restraint, and it must be a part of the patient's prescribed medical treatment and plan of care. A physician's order is required and must be based on a face-to-face assessment of the patient. The order must be current and specify the duration and circumstances under which you will use the restraints. Focus your nursing interventions on preventing complications of restraints, such as hazards of immobility, a decreased sense of self-esteem, and increased agitation. Collaborate with other members of the health care team to design fall prevention programs and a restraint-free environment for the patient. The goal is to discontinue the use of restraints as soon as possible.

Side Rails. Traditionally, side rails were used for patient protection. Recent research shows that raised side rails increase the occurrence of falls (Krauss and others, 2005). When used properly, side rails can increase a patient's mobility and stability in bed when moving from a bed to a chair.

Raising only the top two side rails gives the patient room to exit a bed safely and maneuver within the bed. Side rails also help to prevent the unconscious or sedated patient from rolling out of bed. Always check agency policy about the use of side rails; they are a restraint if they immobilize or reduce the ability of a patient to move freely such as getting out of bed. Side rails also have the potential to trap the head and body in gaps and openings between the bed frame and mattress (Powell-Cope and others, 2005). Use side rail netting or protective padding to prevent the mattress from sliding to one side. Be sure the bed is in the lowest position possible whenever side rails are raised.

The use of side rails alone for a disoriented patient often causes more confusion and further injury. Frequently a confused patient or one determined to get out of bed because of pain, toileting needs, or anxiety attempts to climb over the side rail or out at the foot of the bed. Either attempt often results in a fall. To reduce a patient's confusion, focus your interventions first on the cause. Confusion is frequently mistaken for a patient's attempt to explore the environment or to self-toilet. Additional measures include the use of a low bed with a nonskid mat placed alongside the bed on the floor. A low bed reduces the distance between the bed and floor, facilitating a roll rather than a fall from the bed. If all efforts to reduce confusion or restlessness fail and the patient is at risk for serious injury to self or others, a restraint is sometimes necessary. A less-restrictive restraint for the cognitively impaired is the Posey Bed Canopy. The canopy is a bed enclosure that allows a patient freedom of movement within a protected environment. However, remember the goal is to remove the restraint at the earliest possible time.

Fires. A fire is always possible in the home or health care setting. Accidental home fires typically result from smoking in bed, careless extinguishing of cigarette butts in trash cans, grease fires, or improper use of candles or space heaters; electrical fires resulting from faulty wiring or appliances. Institutional fires typically result from an electrical or anesthetic-related fire. Smoking is generally not permitted in the health care setting; however, because of unauthorized smoking in the bed or bathroom, smoking-related fires continue to pose a risk. Regardless of where the fire occurs, it is important to have an evacuation plan in place. Know where fire extinguishers and gas shut-off valves are located, and know how to activate a fire alarm.

To reduce the risk for fires in the home, instruct patients to quit smoking or smoke outside the home (CDC, 2008b). Have patients inspect the condition of cooking equipment and appliances, particularly irons and stoves. For patients with visual deficits, it helps to have dials installed with large numbers or symbols on temperature controls. Make sure smoke detectors are in strategic positions throughout the home (e.g., in a kitchen and near a bedroom) so that the alarms will alert the occupants in a home when a fire breaks out. Make sure all patients, even young children, are familiar with the phrase "stop, drop, and roll," which describes what to do when a person's clothing or skin is burning.

If a fire occurs in a health care agency, first protect any patients in immediate danger. All personnel help to evacuate patients from the area, especially those patients who are closest to the fire. If a patient requires oxygen but not life support, discontinue the oxygen, which is combustible and will fuel an existing fire. If the patient is on life support, maintain the patient's respiratory status manually with a bag-valve mask (e.g., Ambu-bag) (see Chapter 29) until you move the patient away from the fire. Direct ambulatory patients to walk by themselves to a safe area, or have them assist in moving patients in wheelchairs. Move bedridden patients from the scene by a stretcher, their bed, or a wheelchair, or have one or two rescuers carry them. Use the blanket drag when two or more people are necessary to move a patient. Place the victim on a blanket, and drag the victim head-first along the floor to safety. A variant of the blanket drag is the clothes drag, in which the rescuer drags the victim head first by upper body clothing. Another two-rescuer technique is the chair carry, where the victim is seated in a chair and both rescuers carry the chair (Integrated Publishing, 2004). If you must carry a patient, be careful not to overextend your physical limits for lifting because an injury to you will result in further injury to the patient. If fire department personnel are on the scene, they will also help to evacuate patients.

After a fire has been reported and patients are out of danger, you and other personnel need to take measures to contain or put out the fire, such as closing doors and windows, turning off oxygen and electrical equipment, and using a fire extinguisher. Extinguishers are used for three basic types of fires: paper and rubbish (type A), grease and anesthetic gas (type B), and electrical (type C). Use the appropriate extinguisher for each type.

Your best intervention to prevent fires is to comply with the agency's smoking policies and keep combustible materials away from heat sources. Some agencies have fire doors that are held open by magnets and close automatically when a fire alarm sounds. Make sure that you keep equipment away from these doors.

Poisoning. You help parents reduce the risk for accidental poisoning by teaching them to keep hazardous substances such as medications, cleaning fluids, and batteries out of the reach of children. Drug and other substance poisonings in adolescents and adults are commonly related to suicide attempts or drug experimentation. Teach parents that calling a poison control center for information before attempting home remedies will save their child's life. There are guidelines for accepted interventions for accidental poisonings that you teach a parent or guardian (Box 27-10). Older adults are also at risk for poisoning because diminished eyesight may cause an accidental ingestion of a toxic substance. In addition, the impaired memory of some older adults results in an accidental overdose of prescribed medications. Be sure medications are kept in their original containers and labeled in large print. Recommend the use of medication organizers that are filled once a week by the patient and/or family. Have patients keep poisonous substances out of the bathroom and discard old or unused medications.

In the health care setting it is important for you to know how to respond when exposure to a poisonous substance occurs. OSHA considers mercury a hazardous chemical. Common exposures in a hospital include broken thermometers or sphygmomanometers. Mercury enters the body through inhalation and absorption through the skin. Exposures that occur in a hospital setting are usually short term, some of which affect the brain or kidney. However, full recovery is likely to occur once the body cleans itself of the contamination. Box 27-11 summarizes steps to take in the event of a mercury spill. Many

---

BOX 27-10 PROCEDURAL GUIDELINES

Intervening in Accidental Poisoning

1 Assess for signs or symptoms of ingestion of harmful substances, such as nausea, vomiting, foaming at the mouth, drooling, difficulty breathing, sweating, and lethargy.
2 Terminate the exposure by emptying the mouth of pills, plant parts, or other material.
3 If poisoning is due to skin contact or eye contact, irrigate the skin or eye with copious amounts of tap water for 15 to 20 minutes. In the case of an inhalation exposure, safely remove the victim from the potentially dangerous environment.
4 Identify the type and amount of substance ingested to help determine the correct type and amount of antidote needed.
5 If the victim is conscious and alert, call the local poison control center or the national toll-free poison control center number (1-800-222-1222) before attempting any intervention. Poison control centers have information needed

to treat poisoned patients or to offer referral to treatment centers. The administration of ipecac syrup is no longer recommended for routine home treatment of poisoning (American Academy of Pediatrics, 2003).
6 If the victim has collapsed or stopped breathing, call 911 for emergency transportation to the hospital. Initiate CPR, if indicated, until emergency personnel arrive. Ambulance personnel will be able to provide emergency measures if needed. In addition, parent or guardian is sometimes too upset to drive safely.
7 Position victim with head turned to side to reduce risk for aspiration.
8 Never induce vomiting if the victim has ingested the following poisonous substances: lye, household cleaners, hair care products, grease or petroleum products, and furniture polish, paint thinner, or kerosene.
9 Never induce vomiting in an unconscious or convulsing victim because vomiting increases risk for aspiration.

Modified from Hockenberry MJ: *Wong's essentials of pediatric nursing*, ed 8, St. Louis, 2009, Mosby; American Academy of Pediatrics, Committee on Injury, Violence and Poison Prevention: Poison treatment in the home, *Pediatrics* 112(5):1182, 2003.
CPR, Cardiopulmonary resuscitation.

hospitals are replacing mercury thermometers and sphygmomanometers with electronic and/or aneroid equipment to improve safety.

Bioterrorism. Government agencies such as the Department of Homeland Security and the Centers for Disease Control and Prevention have developed plans to protect the health and safety of people at home and abroad in the event of a biological, chemical, or radiological attack (Perry and Potter, 2010). Preparedness is the first focus of these plans and is the key to responding to any disaster. Health care facilities need to be prepared to treat mass casualties by having an emergency management plan. This plan details how to respond to a terrorist attack. Health care providers play a very important role in preparing for and responding to all types of disasters. Nurses, as the largest sector of the health care workforce, need to have a basic understanding of types of disasters and key components of a plan to deal with any mass casualty event. When disaster strikes, the first priority is to ensure your own personal safety and that of other team members. Rapid response is crucial; therefore be familiar with agency policies for disaster response and specific roles to follow. In addition, know types of transmission, types of isolation and radiation precautions used, treatment options such as fluid and nutrition therapy, and crisis intervention techniques to manage public alarm and fear of the unknown. Participate in disaster planning efforts, education and training, and disaster drills to help prepare for a mass casualty event. The best protection in the event of any disaster is a strong and prepared public health system; well-trained medical personnel; coordinated planning between medical, public health, emergency management, and law enforcement personnel; and an informed public. Instruct patients to inquire about emergency plans at schools, day care centers, and places of work (American Medical Association, 2004).

Electrical Hazards. Much of the equipment used in health care settings is electrical and needs to be well maintained. Biomedical equipment, such as a hospital bed, infusion pump, or ventilator, needs a safety inspection sticker with an expiration date. Decrease the risk for electrical injury and fire by using properly grounded and functional electrical equipment. The ground prong carries any stray electrical current back to the ground. Teach patients and families how to reduce the risk for electrical injury in the home. For example, discuss prevention of electrical shock by avoiding use of electrical appliances near a water source, the importance of grounding appliances, and avoiding operation of unfamiliar equipment.

■■■■ EVALUATION

PATIENT CARE Evaluate your nursing interventions for reducing threats to safety by comparing the patient's response to the expected outcomes for each goal of care. When the expected outcomes are not achieved, revise your interventions. It is also possible that new nursing diagnoses have developed. Apply evaluative measures to determine a patient's progress toward outcomes and goals. An example of a goal, outcome, and evaluative measure includes the goal "Patient's environment is adapted to motor, sensory, and cognitive developmental needs." A possible outcome for this goal is "Modifiable hazards in the home are reduced by 100% within 2 weeks." Your evaluative measures would include "Observe environment for elimination of threats to safety" and "Reassess motor, sensory, and cognitive status for appropriate environmental modifications."

Evaluate the patient's outcome by comparing what you planned with what resulted, and evaluate how well you implemented the plan (Box 27-12). Examine the planned inter-

---

BOX 27-11	Mercury Spill Cleanup Procedure

In the event of a mercury spill, follow these steps:

1 Evacuate the room except for a housekeeping crew (if available).
2 Cleanup personnel need to wear rubber (latex or vinyl) gloves while handling the mercury.
3 Spray the spill area with a mist of water. This diminishes vaporization of mercury.
4 Ventilate the area. Close interior doors, and open any outside windows.
5 Use a suction device, such as a syringe without a needle, to extract as much of the mercury as possible from the spill site. Put recovered mercury in a leakproof glass or plastic container with a nonmetallic cap or lid. **DO NOT VACUUM THE SPILL.**
6 Mop the floor with a mercury cleaner (see agency policy).
7 Dispose of collected mercury according to local environmental safety regulations.

BOX 27-12	EVALUATION

It has been 2 weeks since Joani implemented the plan of care for Mr. Gonzales. She has identified the hazards and made modifications. With regular exercise Mr. Gonzales has found that his walking has improved, and now he feels safer about leaving the apartment. The new medication labels and medication organizer have made it easier for Mr. Gonzales to tell his several medications apart. He reports that his vision is much better with his new glasses. The patient is currently injury free and now feels better about living to a "ripe old age" like his father. He understands that he is able to make changes in his environment that will keep him safe. In the last 2 weeks he has not suffered a fall.

DOCUMENTATION NOTE

"Mr. Gonzales' home has improved lighting, and he has removed the throw rugs. During good weather and during daylight hours he takes walks in his neighborhood. He is able to list all medications by name, dose, when taken, and significant side effects. No reports of injury."

ventions for appropriateness and effectiveness in each situation. By accomplishing goals and outcomes you validate effective care.

PATIENT EXPECTATIONS Patients expect the highest quality care from you and the health care system. Expectations as a result of care include restoration of health, re-duction in risks for falling, a safer home environment, and improved recognition of safety risks. Patients are often un-aware of the dangers in their homes and workplaces, and many will make the necessary adjustments to keep them-selves and loved ones safe and injury free once you identify the dangers.

SAFETY GUIDELINES FOR NURSING SKILLS

Ensuring patient safety is an essential role of the professional nurse. To ensure patient safety, communicate clearly with members of the health care team, assess and incorporate the patient's priorities of care and preferences, and use the best evidence when making decisions about your patient's care. When performing the skill in this chapter, remember the following points to ensure safe, individualized patient care.

- Always attempt restraint alternatives (see Box 27-9, p. 734) before using a restraint.
- If a restraint is needed, always use the least restrictive device.
- Because restraints limit the patient's ability to move freely, make clinical judgments appropriate to patient's condition and agency policy.

SKILL 27-1 APPLYING PHYSICAL RESTRAINTS

DELEGATION CONSIDERATIONS

The skill of applying a restraint can be delegated to trained nursing assistive personnel (NAP). However, the nurse is re-sponsible for assessment of patient's behavior, need for re-straint, type of restraint to use, and patient assessments while restraint is in place. The nurse directs the NAP by:

- Informing NAP of patient's need for restraint
- Reviewing frequency of position changes, range of mo-tion, skin care, toileting, food/fluid, and opportunities for socialization

- Reviewing correct placement of the restraint and how to check patient's circulation, skin integrity, and breathing
- Instructing NAP to report signs and symptoms when pa-tient is not tolerating the restraint (e.g., increased agita-tion, constriction of circulation, impaired skin integrity, change in breathing pattern)

EQUIPMENT

- Proper restraint: belt, extremity, or mitten
- Padding (if needed)

STEP	RATIONALE

ASSESSMENT

1 Assess if a patient needs a restraint. Does the patient continually try to interrupt needed therapy? Is the patient repeatedly trying to ambulate independently, creating a serious risk for injury?

Use restraints only when other less-restrictive measures fail to prevent interruption of therapies. Such instances in-clude traction, endotracheal intubation, IV infusions, or nasogastric tube feedings; preventing a confused or com-bative patient from self-injury by getting out of bed or falling out of bed; preventing a patient from removing uri-nary catheters, surgical drains, or life support equipment; and reducing risk for injury to others by patient.

2 Assess patient's behavior, such as confusion, disorienta-tion, agitation, restlessness, combativeness, or inability to follow directions.

If patient's behavior continues despite attempts to eliminate cause of behavior, use of physical restraint is sometimes necessary.

3 Review agency policies regarding restraints. Check health care provider's order for purpose and type of restraint, lo-cation, and duration of restraint; prn orders for restraint should never be written. Determine if you need a signed consent for use of a restraint.

An order from the health care provider, usually the patient's attending physician, who is responsible for the care of the patient is necessary to apply restraints. The physician must be authorized to order restraints by hospital policy. The patient's attending physician must be consulted as soon as possible if the attending physician did not write the original order. Each original restraint order and renewal is limited to 4 hours for adults, 2 hours for ages 9 through 17, and 1 hour for under age 9. Original orders may be re-newed up to a maximum of 24 hours (CMS, 2007b).

- *Critical Decision Point:* If a nurse or qualified health care provider (check agency policy) restrains a patient in an emergency situation because of violent or self-destructive behavior that presents an immediate danger, a face-to-face physician assessment within 1 hour is required (TJC, 2007).

STEP	RATIONALE

PLANNING

1 Review manufacturer's instructions for restraint application before entering patient's room. Determine the most appropriate size restraint.

Be familiar with all devices used for patient care and protection. Incorrect application of restraint device could result in patient injury or death.

2 Perform hand hygiene, and collect appropriate equipment.

Reduces transmission of microorganisms and promotes organization.

3 Approach patient in a calm, confident manner, and explain what you plan to do.

Reduces patient anxiety and promotes cooperation.

4. Identify patient using two identifiers (e.g., name and birthday or name and account number, according to facility policy).

Ensures correct patient. Complies with Joint Commission requirements (2008) and improves patient safety.

5 Introduce self to patient and family, and assess their feelings about restraint use. Explain that restraint is temporary and designed to protect patient from injury.

Informs patient and family about the use of restraint. In nursing homes, informed consent is mandatory.

6 Inspect area where restraint will be placed. Assess condition of skin, sensation, and circulation.

Sometimes restraints compress and interfere with functioning of devices or tubes. Assessment provides baseline to monitor patient's skin integrity.

- *Critical Decision Point:* Make sure restraints do not interfere with equipment such as IV tubes. Do not place them over access devices, such as an arteriovenous (AV) dialysis shunt.

IMPLEMENTATION

1 Provide privacy. Position and drape patient as needed.

Respects patient's dignity.

2 Adjust bed to proper height, and lower side rail on side of patient contact.

Allows use of proper body mechanics and prevention of injury.

3 Be sure patient is comfortable and in correct anatomical position.

Prevents contractures and neurovascular impairment.

4 Pad skin and bony prominences (if necessary) that will be under the restraint.

Reduces friction and pressure from restraint to skin and underlying tissue.

5 Apply proper-size restraint: Always refer to manufacturer's directions.

   a Belt restraint: Have patient in a sitting position. Apply over clothes, gown, or pajamas. Make sure you place restraint at the waist, not the chest or abdomen. Remove wrinkles or creases in clothing. Bring ties through slots in belt. Help patient lie down if in bed. Avoid applying belt too tightly (see illustrations).

Restrains center of gravity and prevents patient from rolling off stretcher or sitting up while on stretcher or from falling out of bed. Tight application interferes with breathing.

   b Extremity (ankle or wrist) restraint: Restraint designed to immobilize one or all extremities. Commercially available limb restraints are made of sheepskin with foam padding (see illustration). Wrap limb restraint around wrist or ankle with soft part toward skin, and secure snugly in place by Velcro straps.

Maintains immobilization of extremity to protect patient from injury from fall or accidental removal of therapeutic device (e.g., IV tube, urinary catheter). Tight application interferes with circulation.

- *Critical Decision Point:* Patient with wrist and ankle restraints is at risk for aspiration if placed in supine position. Place patient in lateral position rather than supine.

---

   c Mitten restraint: Thumbless mitten device that restrains patient's hands (see illustration). Place hand in mitten, being sure Velcro strap is around the wrist and not the forearm.

Prevents patients from dislodging invasive equipment, removing dressings, or scratching, yet allows greater movement than a wrist restraint.

- *Critical Decision Point:* This text does not address application of vest restraints. Many health care agencies have eliminated the use of the jacket (vest) restraint because of its association with fatal injuries (Capezuti and others, 2008).

SKILL 27-1   APPLYING PHYSICAL RESTRAINTS—cont'd

STEP	RATIONALE

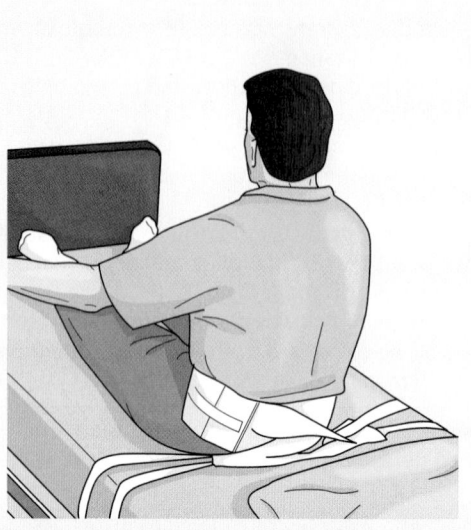
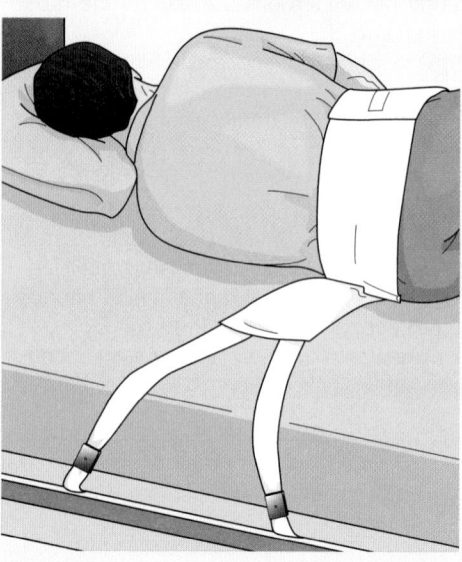

Step 5a ■ Roll belt restraint tied to the bed frame and to an area that does not cause the restraint to tighten when the side rail is raised or lowered. (From Sorrentino SA: *Mosby's textbook for nursing assistants,* ed 6, St. Louis, 2004, Mosby.)

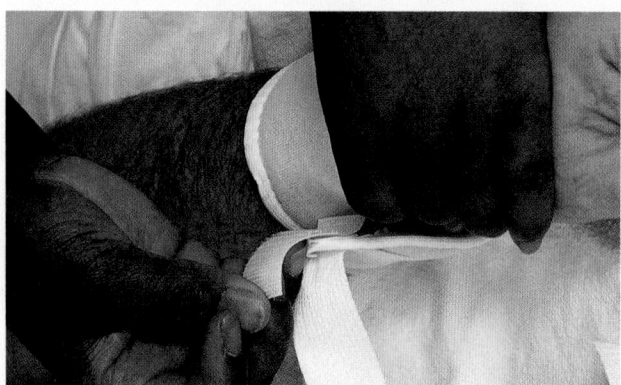

Step 5b ■ Placement of wrist restraint.

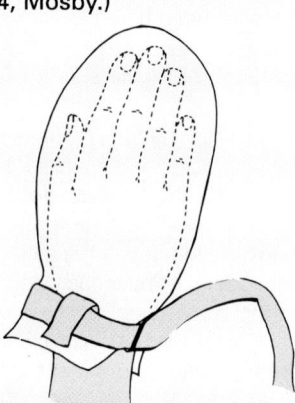

Step 5c ■ Mitten restraint.

6 Attach restraint straps to portion of bed frame that moves when raising or lowering head of bed (see illustration). **Do not attach to side rails.** Check bed frame for a label indicating where restraint should be attached.	Patient will be injured if you secure restraint to a side rail and it is lowered.
7 Secure restraints with a quick-release tie (see illustrations). **Do not tie in a knot. Be sure tie is out of patient reach.**	Quick-release tie allows for easy release in an emergency.
8 Insert two fingers under secured restraint (see illustration).	Checking for constriction prevents neurovascular injury.

• ***Critical Decision Point:*** A tight restraint causes constriction and impedes circulation.

9 Assess proper placement of restraint, skin integrity, pulses, temperature, color, and sensation of the restrained body part. Remove restraints **at least every 2 hours** (TJC, 2007) or more frequently as determined by agency policy. If patient is violent or noncompliant, remove one restraint at a time and/or have staff assistance while removing restraints.	Removal provides opportunity to change patient's position, to offer nutrients, to perform full ROM, and to toilet and exercise patient.

STEP	RATIONALE

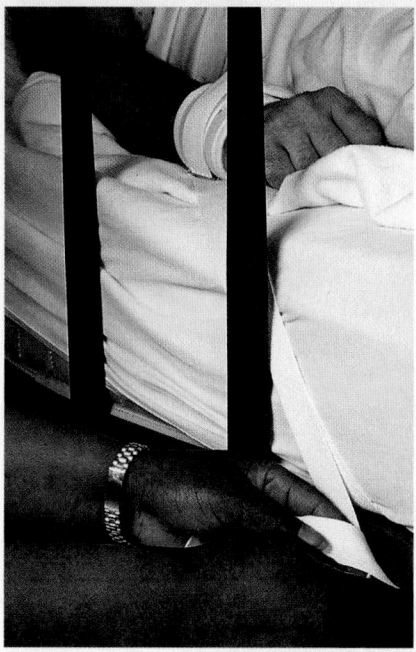

Step 6 ■ Tie restraint strap to bed frame.

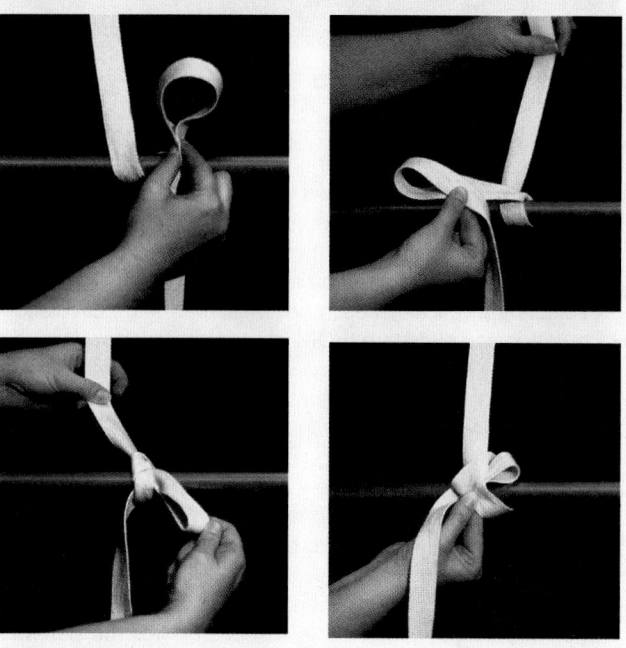

Step 7 ■ The Posey quick-release tie. (Courtesy JT Posey Co, Arcadia, Calif.)

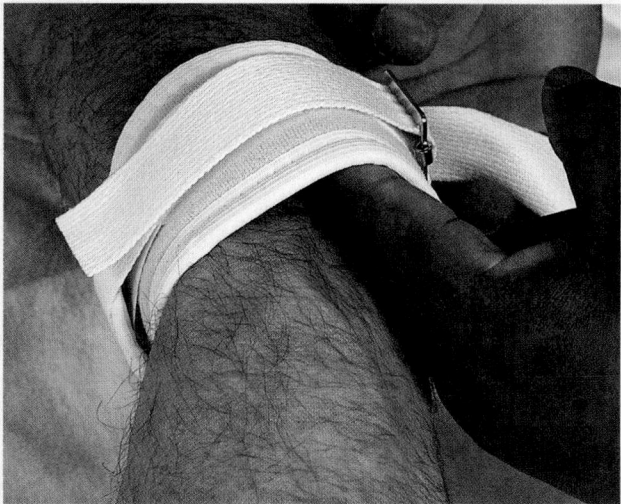

Step 8 ■ Place two fingers under restraint to check tightness.

• **Critical Decision Point:** Do not leave violent or aggressive patients unattended while restraints are off.

---

10 Secure call light or intercom system within reach.

Allows patient, family, or caregiver to obtain assistance quickly.

• **Critical Decision Point:** Restraints restrict movement, making patients unable to perform their activities of daily living without assistance. Providing food and/or fluids and assisting with toileting and other activities are essential.

---

11 Leave bed with wheels locked. Make sure bed is in the lowest position.

Locked wheels prevent bed from moving if patient attempts to get out. If patient falls when bed is in lowest position, this will reduce chances of injury.

12 Perform hand hygiene.

Reduces transmission of microorganisms.

SKILL 27-1	APPLYING PHYSICAL RESTRAINTS—cont'd

STEP	RATIONALE

EVALUATION

1 If patient is restrained for violent or destructive behaviors, evaluate patient's condition for signs of injury every 15 minutes (TJC, 2007). If patient is restrained for nonviolent and non–self-destructive reasons (previously referred to as med-surg restraints), frequent monitoring, such as every 2 hours, is required (check agency policy). Use judgment and consider the patient's condition and the type of restraint when selecting physical assessment measures (e.g., circulation, nutrition and hydration, ROM in extremities, vital signs, hygiene and elimination, physical and psychological status, readiness for discontinuation). Perform visual checks if the patient is too agitated to approach (TJC, 2007).

Frequent assessments prevent injury to the patient and promote removal of restraint at the earliest possible time.

2 The physician, health care provider, or registered nurse (RN) trained according to CMS requirements needs to evaluate the patient within either 1 or 4 hours after initiation of restraint, depending on hospital's Medicare status (see agency policy).

Determines patient's immediate situation, reaction to restraints, medical and behavioral condition, and need to continue or terminate restraints (CMS, 2007b).

3 After 24 hours, before writing a new order, a physician or health care provider who is responsible for the patient's care must see and assess the patient.

Ensures restraint application continues to be medically appropriate.

4 Observe IV catheters, urinary catheters, and drainage tubes to determine that you positioned them correctly.

Reinsertion is uncomfortable and increases risk for infection or interruption of therapy.

5 Provide appropriate sensory stimulation, and reorient patient as needed.

Use of restraints further increases disorientation.

RECORDING AND REPORTING

- Record patient behaviors before you applied restraints.
- Record restraint alternatives you attempted and the patient's response.
- Record patient and/or family's understanding of and consent to restraint application.
- Record type and location of the restraint and time applied.
- Record times that you performed assessments and releases while patient in restraints.

- Record findings from your assessments related to orientation, oxygenation, skin integrity, circulation, and positioning.
- Record patient's behavior and expected or unexpected outcomes after you applied the restraint.
- Record patient's response when you removed restraints (e.g., calm, cooperative).
- Also see behavioral restraint flow sheet (Figure 27-4).

UNEXPECTED OUTCOMES AND RELATED INTERVENTIONS

- Skin integrity becomes impaired.
  - Reassess need for continued use of restraint and if alternatives can be used.
  - If restraint is necessary, make sure you apply restraint correctly and provide adequate padding.
  - Assess skin, provide appropriate therapy, or remove restraints more frequently.
  - Change wet or soiled restraints.
- Patient becomes more confused and agitated after you apply restraints.
  - Determine the cause of the behavior, and eliminate the cause, if possible.
  - Determine the need for more or less sensory stimulation.
  - Reorient as needed, and/or attempt other restraint alternatives.

- Neurovascular status of an extremity is altered, manifested by cyanosis, pallor, edema, or coldness of skin, or patient complains of tingling, pain, numbness, or loss of ROM.
  - Remove the restraint immediately, stay with the patient, and notify the physician.
  - Protect extremity from further injury.
- Patient releases the restraint and suffers a fall or other injury.
  - Attend to patient's immediate physical needs.
  - Notify the physician, and reassess type of restraint and correct application.

Holy Family Hospital and Medical Center
70 East Street, Methuen, MA 01844

BEHAVIORAL RESTRAINT FLOW SHEET

Behavior Requiring Restraint: (Check all that apply)
☐ Confusion/disorientation/combative
☐ Self Harm
☐ Harm to others/surroundings
☐ Removing medical devices
☐ Other: _____

Physician order obtained: ☐ Yes; ☐ No

Type of Restraint: (Check all that apply)
☐ Soft wrist/ankle
☐ Halter type vest
☐ Seat Belt
☐ Mitts
☐ Leather
☐ Other: _____

Less Restrictive Measures Attempted: (Check all that apply)
☐ Pain/comfort measures
☐ Schedule position changes
☐ Schedule toileting
☐ Place closer to Nursing Station
☐ Reorient
☐ Encourage family/friends to visit
☐ Other: _____

Patient/Family Informed: ☐ Yes; ☐ No
If no, Comment: _____
_____

Date Restraint Applied: _____ **Time:** _____
Date Restraint ☐ Ended / ☐ Renewed: _____ **Time:** _____

Date: Time:am/pm	12	2	4	6	8	10	12	2	4	6	8	10
1. Hydration/Nutrition/Elimination												
2. Skin condition												
3. Range of motion/turn & position												
4. Communication (call light in reach)												
5. Circulation/Neurovascular Changes												
6. Assess chg. in clinical condition/behavior												
7. Assess for early release												
8. Restraint reduced/removed*												
9. Behavioral/Safety Check done q15"												
10. Vital Signs (if applicable)**												
Initials of assessor:												

Initials/Signature: _____ Initials/Signature: _____ Initials/Signature: _____

Comments: _____

* New order required when restraint removed or reduced.   ** Temperature not required unless indicated.

KEY: ✓ = Observation / Intervention; NN = Nurses' Notes; O = Patient Off Unit; R = Restraint Removed

Note: It is not necessary to document the Behavioral/Safety Check every 15 minutes but nurse must note every 2 hours in the assessment documentation #7 that the observation was performed. *Any changes in behavior require an assessment.*

Caritas Christi · A Catholic Health Care System · Member

Written: 7/95; Revised: 29 January 1999

Figure 27-4 ■ Behavioral restraint flow sheet. (Courtesy Holy Family Hospital and Medical Center, Methuen, Mass.)

- A safe environment in a health care agency is comfortable; maintains the patient's privacy; and reduces the risks for injury, infection, and negative effects of treatment or medications.
- In the community a safe environment means basic needs are achievable, physical hazards are reduced, transmission of pathogens and parasites is reduced, pollution is controlled, and sanitation is maintained.
- The transmission of pathogens and parasites is reduced through medical and surgical asepsis, food sanitation, insect and rodent control, and disposal of human wastes.
- Every developmental stage involves assessment of specific safety risks.
- The school-age child is at risk for injury at home, at school, and traveling to and from school.

- Adolescents are at risk for injury from motor vehicle accidents and the effects of drug and alcohol abuse.
- Threats to an adult's safety are frequently associated with lifestyle habits.
- Risks of injury for older adults are directly related to the physiological changes of the aging process.
- Risks to patient safety within a health care agency include falls and patient-inherent, procedure-related, and equipment-related accidents.
- Individualize nursing interventions for promoting safety for developmental stage, lifestyle, and the environment.
- Continually evaluate the nursing care plan to promote safety in order to identify new or continued risks to the patient.
- Use physical restraints only as a last resort, when patients' behavior places them or others at risk for injury.

CRITICAL THINKING EXERCISES

Mr. Gonzales is visiting his widowed sister, Mrs. Pruitt, a 73-year-old who recently had a colectomy to remove a mass in her colon. Mrs. Pruitt did very well after her surgery. Although morphine has been effective in relieving her pain, during your assessment she appears agitated and restless and is picking at her tubes. Mr. Gonzales tells you that he is worried because this is unusual behavior for his sister. You are also concerned that Mrs. Pruitt is at risk for removing her nasogastric tube and IV catheter.

1. What are possible sources for Mrs. Pruitt's unusual behavior?
2. How will you prioritize your interventions when addressing these potential sources?
3. What factors about restraints and their safety implications affect your decision to use a restraint on Mrs. Pruitt?

4. If a restraint is necessary to avoid disruption of therapy, what interventions are necessary to ensure Mrs. Pruitt's safety while in restraints?
5. After application of upper extremity restraints, nursing assistive personnel report that Mrs. Pruitt repeatedly tries to remove the restraints. What actions do you take after hearing this report? Select all that apply. Explain your answers.
   a. Notify the physician or health care provider.
   b. Instruct the nursing assistive personnel to continue hourly checks.
   c. Immediately assess Mrs. Pruitt's behavior.
   d. Instruct the nursing assistive personnel to remove the restraints.

evolve   *Answers to Critical Thinking Questions can be found on the Evolve website.*

REVIEW QUESTIONS

1. The nurse discovers an electrical fire in a patient's room. Which action should the nurse take first?
   1. Turn off the oxygen to the unit.
   2. Evacuate any patients/visitors in immediate danger.
   3. Close all doors and windows.
   4. Use the nearest fire extinguisher to put the fire out.
2. A parent calls the pediatrician's office frantic about the bottle of cleaner that her 2-year-old child drank. Which of the following is the most important instruction the nurse gives to this parent?
   1. Contact the local poison control center.
   2. Take the child to the nearest emergency department.
   3. Give the child milk.
   4. Give the child syrup of ipecac.
3. During the nursing assessment of a 52-year-old man, he reports increased alcohol consumption secondary to stress at work. One of the expected outcomes for this patient is to:
   1. Contact the local health department for stress management classes
   2. Decrease his alcohol intake during stress
   3. Decrease stress in his life
   4. Adopt sleep hygiene measures to promote sleep

4. The nurse has just completed a gait assessment on a 78-year-old woman. The assessment reveals shuffling gait, decreased balance, and instability. Based on these data, which one of the following nursing diagnoses indicates an understanding of the assessment findings?
   1. *Activity intolerance*
   2. *Impaired bed mobility*
   3. *Disturbed sensory perception*
   4. *Risk for falls*
5. The nurse has just found a 68-year-old woman wandering in the hallway and exhibiting confused behavior. The patient says she is looking for the bathroom. Which interventions are appropriate to ensure the safety of the patient? Select all that apply.
   1. Ask the physician or health care provider to order a vest restraint.
   2. Insert a urinary catheter.
   3. Provide scheduled toileting rounds every 2 to 3 hours.
   4. Assign a nurse to stay with the patient.
   5. Keep the bed in low position with the upper side rails up.
   6. Keep the pathway from the bed to the bathroom clear.

6. A 62-year-old woman is being discharged to home with her husband after surgery for a hip fracture from a fall at home. When providing discharge teaching about home safety to this patient and her husband, the nurse knows that:
   1. A safe environment promotes patient independence
   2. Assessment focuses on environmental factors only
   3. Teaching the patient and her husband about home safety is difficult to do in the hospital setting
   4. Most accidents in the older adult are due to lifestyle factors

7. A fragile, 87-year-old nursing home resident has just been admitted to the hospital with increased confusion. The patient has upper limb restraints to prevent her from pulling the nasogastric tube. In delegating care of this patient to the nursing assistive personnel (NAP), the nurse tells the NAP to:
   1. Call the physician or health care provider if the patient becomes more agitated
   2. Check the patient's circulation, skin integrity, and breathing every hour
   3. Move the patient to a room down the hall
   4. Check to see if the patient can have a medication for agitation

8. The nursing assistive personnel (NAP) tells the nurse that the portable sphygmomanometer broke during transfer of a bed into a patient's room. There is now mercury on the floor of the room. The NAP asks what to do. The nurse's best answer is:
   1. Spray the mercury with a fire extinguisher
   2. Pick the mercury up carefully with a towel
   3. Evacuate the room
   4. Tell the patient to remain in bed

9. An 80-year-old patient who demonstrates some confusion but without anxiety was recently admitted to the medical unit. The nursing assessment reveals that she is at risk for injury due to falls because she continues to get out of bed without help despite frequent reminders. The initial nursing intervention is to:
   1. Place a bed alarm device on the bed
   2. Place the patient in a belt restraint
   3. Provide one-to-one observation of the patient
   4. Apply wrist restraints

10. The family of a confused, ambulatory patient insists that all four side rails be up when the patient is alone. The best way to handle this situation is to:
    1. Thank them for being conscientious
    2. Restrict their visiting privileges
    3. Report them to the charge nurse
    4. Inform them of the risks associated with side rail use

Answers to Review Questions can be found on pages 1197-1198.

REFERENCES

American Academy of Pediatrics, Committee on Injury, Violence and Poison Prevention: Poison treatment in the home, *Pediatrics* 112(5):1182, 2003.

American Geriatrics Society, British Geriatrics Society, American Academy of Orthopedic Surgeons Panel on Falls Prevention: Guideline for the prevention of falls in older persons, *J Am Geriatr Soc* 49:664, 2001.

American Hospital Association: *Quality advisory: implementing standardized colors for patient alert wristbands,* September 4, 2008, http://www.agaqualitycenter.org.

American Medical Association: *Bioterrorism: frequently asked questions,* 2004, http://www.ama-assn.org/ama/pub/category/6667.html.

American Nurses Association: *Nursing: scope and standards of practice,* Washington, DC, 2004, The Association.

Brush BL, Capezuti E: Historical analysis of siderail use in American hospitals, *J Nurs Scholarsh* 33(4):381, 2001.

Bulechek GM and others, editors: *Nursing interventions classification (NIC),* ed 5, St. Louis, 2008, Mosby.

Capezuti E and others: Least restrictive or least understood? Waist restraints, provider practices, and risk of harm, *J Aging Soc Policy* 20(3):305, 2008.

Centers for Disease Control and Prevention, National Center for Health Statistics: *NCHS data on injuries,* 2006, http://www.cdc.gov/nchs.injury.htm.

Centers for Disease Control and Prevention: *State injury indicators report third edition—2004 data,* Atlanta, 2007, U.S. Department of Health and Human Services.

Centers for Disease Control and Prevention: *Falls among older adults: an overview,* 2008a, http://www.cdc.gov.ncipc/factsheets/adultfalls.htm.

Centers for Disease Control and Prevention: *Reductions in smoking show promise for reducing home fire deaths,* 2008b, http://www.cdc.gov/media/pressrel/2008/r080808.htm.

Centers for Disease Control and Prevention, National Center for Health Statistics: *The three leading causes of injury mortality in the United States, 1999-2005,* 2008c, http://www.cdc.gov/nchs.injury.htm.

Centers for Disease Control and Prevention: *Traumatic brain injuries can result from senior falls,* 2008d, http://www.cdc.gov/media/pressrel/2008/r080623.htm.

Centers for Medicare and Medicaid Services: *Present on admission (POA) indicator reporting and hospital-acquired conditions (HAC),* 2007a, http://www.cms.hhs.gov/HospitalAcqCond.

Centers for Medicare and Medicaid Services: *Revisions to Medicare conditions of participation, 482.13,* Bethesda, Md, 2007b, U.S. Department of Health and Human Services.

Coalition for Safe Community Needle Disposal: *EPA revises needle disposal options,* 2005a, http://www.safeneedledisposal.org/news/ 041216.html.

Coalition for Safe Community Needle Disposal: *Types of sharps disposal programs,* 2005b, http://www.safeneedledisposal.org/gentypes.html.

Ebersole P, Hess P: *Toward healthy aging: human needs and nursing process,* ed 7, St. Louis, 2008, Mosby.

Edelman CL, Mandle CL: *Health promotion throughout the life span,* ed 7, St. Louis, 2010, Mosby.

Emergency Care Research Institute: *Falls prevention strategies in healthcare settings,* Plymouth Meeting, Pa, 2006, The Institute.

Federal Emergency Management Agency: *Disaster facts,* 2004a, http://www.fema.gov/library/df_1.shtm, accessed June 8, 2005.

Federal Emergency Management Agency: *Your family disaster plan,* 2004b, http://www.fema.gov/rrr/famplan/shtm, accessed January 4, 2005.

GeronurseOnline.org: *Want to know: physical restraints,* 2005, http://www.geronurseonline.org/index.dfm?section_id=30& geriatric_topic_id=10&sub_section_id=74&page_id=156& tab=2.

Halfon P and others: Risk of falls for hospitalized patients: a predictive model based on routinely available data, *J Clin Epidemiol* 54(12):1258, 2001.

Hockenberry MJ: *Wong's essentials of pediatric nursing,* ed 8, St. Louis, 2009, Mosby.

Hughes RG, editor: *Patient safety and quality: an evidence-based handbook for nurses,* AHRQ Publication No. 08-0043, Rockville, Md, 2008, Agency for Healthcare Research and Quality.

Insurance Institute for Highway Safety: *Fatality facts 2006: teenagers,* Arlington, Va, 2006, The Institute, http://www.iihs.org/research/fatality/_facts_2006/teenagers.html, accessed September 20, 2008.

Integrated Publishing Inc: *Rescue drag and carry techniques,* 2004, http://www.tpub.com/corpsman/115.htm.

Krauss MJ and others: A case-control study of patient, medication and care related risk factors for falls, *J Gen Intern Med* 20:116, 2005.

Kung H and others: *Deaths: preliminary data for 2005,* Bethesda, Md 2007, Division of Vital Statistics, Centers for Disease Control and Prevention, National Center for Health Statistics.

Moorhead S and others, editors: *Nursing outcomes classification (NOC),* ed 4, St. Louis, 2008, Mosby.

Morse JM: Enhancing the safety of hospitalization by reducing patient falls, *Am J Infect Control* 30:376, 2002.

Morse JM: *Preventing patient falls: establishing a fall intervention program,* ed 2, New York, 2009, Springer Publishing.

Nix S: *Basic nutrition and diet therapy,* St. Louis, 2005, Mosby.

Occupational Safety and Health Administration, U.S. Department of Labor, *Hazard communication,* Standards 29 CFR, 1910.1200, www.osha.gov/pls/oshaweb/owadisp.show_document?p_table5STANDARDS&p_id510099, accessed January 29, 2009.

Perry A, Potter P: *Clinical nursing skills and techniques,* ed 7, St. Louis, 1996, Mosby.

Powell-Cope G and others: Modification of bed systems and use of accessories to reduce the risk of hospital-bed entrapment, *Rehabil Nurs* 30(1):9, 2005.

Sorrentino SA: *Mosby's textbook for nursing assistants,* ed 6, St. Louis, 2004, Mosby.

The Joint Commission: *Comprehensive accreditation manual for hospitals,* Chicago, 2007, The Joint Commission.

The Joint Commission: *2009 National Patient Safety Goals,* Chicago, 2008, The Joint Commission.

Tinetti ME: Preventing falls in elderly persons, *N Engl J Med* 348:42, 2003.

U.S. Department of Veterans Affairs, National Center for Patient Safety: *2004 Falls toolkit, falls notebook interventions,* 2004, http://www.patientsafety.gov/Safetytopics/fallstoolkit/index.html, accessed June 25, 2007.

Warner J: *Medical errors still plague U.S. hospitals,* 2004, http://my.webmd.com/content/Article/91/101128.htm, accessed June 8, 2005.

MEDIA RESOURCES

 CD COMPANION　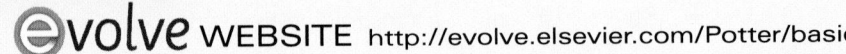 **WEBSITE** http://evolve.elsevier.com/Potter/basic

- Video Clip
- Crossword Puzzle
- English/Spanish Audio Glossary

OBJECTIVES

- Describe factors that influence personal hygiene practices.
- Perform a comprehensive assessment of a patient's hygiene needs.
- Discuss factors that influence the condition of the nails and feet.
- Identify common problems involving the skin, feet, nails, hair, and scalp and their related interventions.
- Describe the types of bathing techniques used for various physical conditions and for patients of various age-groups.

- Correctly perform hygiene procedures for the care of the patient's skin, perineum, feet and nails, mouth, eyes, ears, and nose.
- Explain the importance of foot care for the patient with diabetes.
- Discuss conditions that place patients at risk for impaired oral mucous membranes.
- Describe effect of oral hygiene on periodontal disease.
- Describe how hygiene for the older adult differs from that for the younger patient.
- Make an occupied and unoccupied hospital bed.

KEY TERMS

acne, p. 749
cerumen, p. 756
dental caries, p. 748

effleurage, p. 764
gingivitis, p. 748

halitosis, p. 754
macerated, p. 771

perineal care, p. 763
stomatitis, p. 767

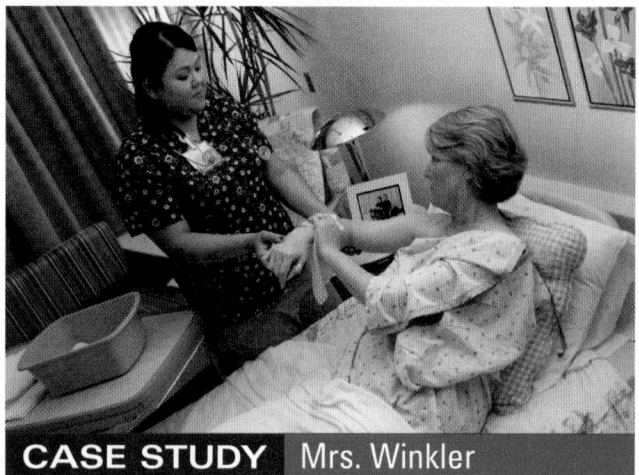

CASE STUDY Mrs. Winkler

Mrs. Winkler is a 58-year-old white woman admitted recently to an assisted living nursing facility. She has a medical history of multiple sclerosis and diabetes mellitus plus a family history of coronary artery disease. Mrs. Winkler uses a wheelchair for mobility. She has recently become weaker, is unable to push the chair herself, and requires assistance in transferring to and from the chair. She has both upper and lower extremity weakness. Mrs. Winkler was married for 37 years; her husband died suddenly 3 months ago of a heart attack. She has three daughters who live about an hour from the facility. Mrs. Winkler states, "I will miss my daughters and grandchildren. I rely on them and am used to seeing them every day. But, I don't want to be a burden to them." Mrs. Winkler wears full dentures. She complains that her mouth is sore when she wears her dentures.

Jamie Johnson is a 20-year-old nursing student assigned to the nursing facility. She is single and works part-time in a skilled nursing facility near her home. Jamie knows how important it is for patients to feel comfortable and have their basic needs met.

To provide basic hygiene, Jamie needs to learn about what is important to Mrs. Winkler's comfort. When hygiene needs are not fulfilled, patients experience complications such as oral lesions and infections. Jamie needs to review the effect of dependency on the patient's self-esteem and review ways to give patients opportunities to maintain self-care needs. At an optimal level of functioning with assistance, Mrs. Winkler is at risk for potential self-care deficits, impaired skin integrity, impaired oral mucosa, and altered health maintenance. During hygiene care Jamie interacts with Mrs. Winkler to assess her readiness to learn and to teach health promotion practices. Jamie wants to preserve as much of Mrs. Winkler's independence as possible, ensure privacy, and foster physical well-being.

Personal hygiene affects your patient's comfort, safety, and well-being. Healthy people are able to meet their own hygiene needs. Ill or physically challenged people often need various levels of assistance. A variety of personal, social, and cultural factors influence hygiene practices. Because hygienic care requires close contact with your patient, use communi-

cation skills to promote a caring therapeutic relationship (see Chapter 10). You can integrate other nursing activities during hygiene care, including patient assessment and interventions such as range-of-motion (ROM) exercises, application of dressings, or inspection and care of intravenous (IV) sites. During hygiene care, try to preserve as much of the patient's independence as possible, assess the patient's ability to perform hygiene care, ensure privacy, convey respect, and foster the patient's physical comfort.

SCIENTIFIC KNOWLEDGE BASE

Providing hygiene to patients requires an understanding of the anatomy and physiology of the skin, nails, oral cavity, eyes, ears, and nose. Hygiene includes cleansing and grooming activities that maintain personal body cleanliness and appearance. Personal hygiene activities such as taking a bath or shower, brushing and flossing the teeth, washing the hair, and performing nail care promote comfort, foster a positive self-image, and help prevent infection and disease. Healthy people usually perform their own hygiene self-care. When ill or injured, patients require varying amounts of help to perform hygiene care. Whether patients perform their own hygiene needs or you help provide their needs, effective hygiene techniques promote the normal structure and function of body tissues.

Skin

The skin is the largest organ in the body with the functions of protection, secretion, excretion, temperature regulation, and sensation (Table 28-1). Three primary layers compose the skin: epidermis, dermis, and subcutaneous. The epidermis (outer layer) shields underlying tissues against water loss and injury, prevents entry of disease-producing microorganisms, and generates new cells to replace the dead cells that are continuously shed from the skin's outer surface. Bacteria (normal flora) commonly reside on the outer epidermis; these bacteria inhibit disease-producing microorganisms. The dermis provides support for the epidermis and contains nerve fibers, blood vessels, sebaceous and sweat glands, and hair follicles. Subcutaneous tissue insulates and cushions the skin.

The skin often reflects a change in a person's physical condition by alterations in color, thickness, texture, turgor, temperature, and hydration (see Chapter 15). Hygiene practices frequently influence skin status, having both beneficial and negative effects on the skin and its functions. For example, too frequent bathing can lead to dry, flaky skin and loss of protective oils.

Feet, Hands, and Nails

The feet, hands, and nails often require special attention to prevent infection, odor, and injury. Problems may result from abuse or improper care. The condition of the patient's hands and feet influences the ability to perform hygiene care. Without ability to bear weight, ambulate, or manipulate the hands the patient is at risk for losing self-care ability. Foot pain often changes the patient's gait, causing strain on different

TABLE 28-1   Functions of the Skin and Implications for Care

FUNCTION/DESCRIPTION	IMPLICATIONS FOR CARE
PROTECTION The epidermis is the relatively impermeable skin layer that prevents entrance of microorganisms. Although microorganisms reside on skin surface and in hair follicles, relative dryness of surface inhibits bacterial growth. Sebum removes bacteria from hair follicles. Acidic pH of skin further slows bacterial growth.	Weakening of epidermis occurs by scraping or stripping its surface as by use of dry razors, tape removal, or improper turning or positioning techniques. Excessive dryness causes cracks and breaks in skin and mucosa that allow bacteria to enter. Emollients soften and prevent moisture loss; soaking improves moisture retention; and hydration of mucosa prevents dryness. Constant exposure to moisture causes maceration or softening, which interrupts dermal integrity and promotes ulcers and bacterial growth. Keep bed linen and clothing dry. Misuse of soap, detergents, cosmetics, deodorant, and depilatories causes chemical irritation. Alkaline soaps neutralize protective acid condition of skin. Cleansing removes excess oil, sweat, dead skin cells, and dirt that promote bacterial growth.
SENSATION The skin contains sensory organs for touch, pain, heat, cold, and pressure.	Minimize friction to avoid loss of stratum corneum, which increases risk for pressure ulcers. Smoothing linen removes sources of mechanical irritation. Remove rings during bathing to prevent injuring patient's skin. Make sure bathwater is not too hot or cold.
TEMPERATURE REGULATION Radiation, evaporation, conduction, and convection control body temperature.	Factors that interfere with heat loss can alter temperature control. Wet bed linen or gowns increase heat loss. Excess blankets or bed coverings interfere with heat loss through radiation and conduction. Coverings conserve heat.
EXCRETION AND SECRETION Sweat promotes heat loss by evaporation. Sebum lubricates skin and hair.	Perspiration and oil sometimes harbor microorganism growth. Bathing removes excess body secretions, although excessive bathing causes dry skin.

muscle groups. Discomfort while standing or walking frequently leads to physical and emotional stress.

The nails are epithelial tissues that grow from the root of the nail bed, located in the skin at the nail groove. A normal healthy nail is transparent, smooth, and convex, with a pink nail bed and translucent white tip. The appearance of the nails reflects level of self-care. Inadequate nutrition and disease can cause changes in the shape, thickness, and curvature of the nail (see Chapter 15).

Oral Cavity and Teeth

Mucous membranes continuous with the skin line the oral cavity. Normal oral mucosa glistens and is pink, soft, moist, smooth, and without lesions. Healthy gums fit tightly around each tooth and appear pink, moist, and smooth. Healthy teeth are white, smooth, shiny, and aligned. The condition of the oral cavity reflects overall health and also indicates oral hygiene needs (see Chapter 15).

The teeth are the organs of chewing designed to cut, tear, and grind ingested food so it can be mixed with saliva and swallowed for digestion. Difficulty in chewing develops when the gums surrounding the teeth become inflamed or infected or when teeth are lost or become loosened. Regular oral hygiene helps to prevent **gingivitis,** inflammation of the gums, and **dental caries,** tooth decay produced by interaction of food with bacteria that form plaque.

Hair

Hair growth, distribution, and pattern indicate general health status (see Chapter 15). Hormonal changes, emotional and physical stress, aging, infection, and certain illnesses can affect hair characteristics. Because the hair shaft is a lifeless structure, it is not affected by physiological factors. A lack of hormones and nutrients to the hair follicle causes changes in hair color or condition.

The Eyes, Ears, and Nose

Chapter 37 describes the structure and function of the eyes, ears, and nose. When you provide hygiene care, the patient's eyes, ears, and nose also require careful attention. These tissues are very sensitive to soap and other chemicals, especially in younger and older patients. Patients with alterations in one or more of these senses often need help to meet their hygiene needs.

NURSING KNOWLEDGE BASE

A number of factors influence personal preferences for hygiene. No two individuals perform hygiene in the same way. You will provide individualized care only after learning about patients' unique hygiene practices and preferences.

Hygiene care is never routine. This care often involves intimate contact with the patient and requires use of communication skills to promote a therapeutic relationship. The time spent with the patient during hygiene care offers the opportunity to convey caring and learn more about the patient's emotional needs.

Body Image

Body image often affects the way in which an individual maintains personal hygiene. A patient's general appearance frequently reflects the importance hygiene holds for that person. The patient's body image may change as the result or surgery, illness, or a change in functional status (see Chapter 22). When a patient experiences discomfort, emotional stress, or fatigue, the ability to perform hygiene self-care diminishes, requiring extra efforts to promote the patient's hygienic comfort and appearance.

Social Practices

Social groups influence hygiene preferences and practices, including the type of hygienic products used and the nature and frequency of personal care. Parents and caregivers perform hygiene care for infants and young children. Family customs play a major role during childhood in determining hygiene practices such as the frequency of bathing, the time of day bathing is performed, and even whether certain hygiene practices such as brushing of the teeth are performed. As children enter adolescence, peer groups and media influence hygiene practices. Young girls, for example, become more interested in their personal appearance and begin to wear makeup. Later in life, friends and work groups shape the expectations people have about personal appearance. The older adult may experience a decrease in social interaction and be less likely to focus on personal care as a result of social isolation.

Developmental Variations in the Skin

Age influences the normal condition of the skin and the type of hygiene required. The neonate's skin is relatively immature and thin. The epidermis and dermis are loosely bound together. A break in the skin easily becomes infected.

The toddler's skin layers become more tightly bound together, resulting in greater resistance to skin irritation and infection. However, because the toddler is more active and does not have regular hygiene habits, caregivers need to take care of the toddler's hygiene needs.

During adolescence, growth and maturation of the skin increase. Sebaceous glands become more active, which may result in **acne** (inflammatory, papulopustular skin eruption, usually on the face, neck, shoulders, and upper back). Sweat glands become fully functional during puberty. More frequent bathing and use of antiperspirants become necessary to reduce body odors.

The condition of the adult's skin depends on hygiene practices and exposure to environmental irritants. Normally the skin is elastic, well hydrated, firm, and smooth. With age the skin loses its resiliency and moisture, and sebaceous and sweat glands become less active. These changes often lead to

dry, cracked skin. Daily bathing, inadequate fluid and nutrition, and the use of some soap products can cause the skin of an older adult to become too dry. As the epithelium thins and elastic collagen fibers shrink, the skin becomes fragile and subject to bruising and breaking. Activities such as turning and repositioning and washing the skin and perineal tissues can cause impaired skin integrity.

Personal Preferences

Patients have individual desires and preferences about when to bathe, shave, and perform hair and oral care. Some patients prefer to shower, whereas others prefer to bathe in the bed. Patients select different hygiene products according to personal preference and needs. Knowing these desires and preferences helps to individualize care for the patient. Safe, effective nursing care respects individual preferences, allows patients to make personal choices whenever possible, and promotes patient involvement and independence.

Socioeconomic Status

A patient's economic resources influence the type and extent of hygiene practices used. A patient's economic status sometimes influences the ability to regularly maintain hygiene. For example, patients who are not able to afford supplies such as deodorant, shampoo, and toothpaste will experience difficulties meeting their hygiene needs. Some patients need to modify the home environment by adding safety devices such as nonskid surfaces in the bath or using a tub chair to perform hygienic self-care safely. When patients have the added problem of limited socioeconomic resources, it is difficult for them to afford these modifications, making it difficult for them to participate and take responsibility in health promotion activities.

Cultural Variables

A patient's cultural beliefs, practices, and personal values influence hygiene care (Box 28-1). People from diverse cultural backgrounds follow different self-care practices (see Chapter 19). Maintaining cleanliness may not hold the same importance for some ethnic groups as it does for others (Galanti, 2004). In North America it is common to bathe or shower daily and to use deodorant to prevent body odors. People from some cultures, however, may not be sensitive to body odor and may prefer to bathe less frequently and to not use deodorant. Religious beliefs associated with culture sometimes influence hygiene practices. Facilitate a patient's religious practices whenever possible.

HEALTH BELIEFS AND MOTIVATION

Knowledge about the importance of hygiene and its implications for a person's well-being influences hygiene practices. Knowledge alone, however, is not enough. Motivation plays a key part in a patient's hygiene practices, too. Patient teaching is often needed to foster hygiene self-care. Our society values

Patients need a culturally competent plan for hygiene care. For some, culture influences hygiene practices, and hygiene care becomes a potential source of conflict and stress in the caregiving environment. Hygiene is a personal matter; patients from different cultures will vary in their care practices and caregiver requirements.

IMPLICATIONS FOR PRACTICE

- Maintain privacy, especially for women from cultures that value female modesty.
- Avoid uncovering the lower torso and exposing the arms of Middle Eastern and East Asian women.
- Allow family members to participate in the care of patients if desired by adapting the schedule of hygiene activities when they are present.
- Provide gender-congruent caregiver as needed or requested.
- If gender-congruent caregivers are not available, ask the family for assistance.
- In some cultures (e.g., Hindu, Orthodox Jewish, Muslim, Amish) touching between unrelated males and females is forbidden.
- Respect cultural and religious practices relevant to hygienic practices.
- Some cultures (e.g., Chinese, Filipino) avoid bathing for 7 to 10 days following childbirth (Galanti, 2004).
- Many Asians (Chinese, Japanese, Koreans, and Hindus) consider the top parts of the body cleaner than the lower parts.
- Hindus and Muslims often use the left hand for cleaning, whereas the right hand is reserved for eating and praying.
- Do not cut or shave hair without discussion with the patient or family (Galanti, 2004).

self-care as a part of health care. Patients and their caregivers make personal decisions daily that influence lifestyle and health care choices (Pender, Murdaugh, and Parsons, 2002). When patients recognize a risk exists and understand that they can take action without risk, they will be more receptive to nursing care and teaching.

Physical Condition

Patients with physical limitations or disabilities associated with disease and injury often lack the physical energy and dexterity to perform hygiene self-care. A patient whose arm is in a cast or who has an intravenous line or other device connected to the body needs help with hygiene care. Inability to use the hands because of disease or injury can make using a toothbrush, washcloth, or hairbrush difficult or ineffective. Sensory deficits not only alter the patient's ability to perform care but also place the patient at risk for injury. Safety is a priority for the patient with a sensory deficit. For example, the inability to feel that the water is too hot can lead to burn injury.

Chronic illnesses (e.g., cardiac disease, chronic lung disease, cancer, or neurological disorders) often exhaust or incapacitate the patient. Patients who become fatigued need complete hygiene care in some instances. Including periods of rest during care often allows patients to participate in their care.

Pain often accompanies illness and injury, limiting a patient's ability to tolerate hygiene and grooming activities or to perform self-care. Pain frequently limits range of motion, resulting in impaired use of the arms or hands or in limited ability to move about in the environment; any of these limitations impairs hygiene self-care ability. Sedation and drowsiness associated with analgesics used for pain management also limit a patient's ability to participate in care.

Limited mobility caused by a variety of factors (e.g., physical injury, weakness, surgery, pain, prolonged inactivity, medication effect, and presence of indwelling catheter or intravenous line) decreases a patient's ability to perform hygiene self-care activities safely. Individualized care considers the patient's ability to perform care, the amount of assistance needed, and the need for assistive and safety devices to facilitate safe hygiene care.

Acute and chronic cognitive impairments, such as stroke, brain injury, psychoses, and dementia, often result in the inability to perform self-care independently. In addition, patients with cognitive impairments are frequently not aware of their hygiene and grooming needs. Because of impaired ability to interpret stimuli, some patients with dementia become fearful and agitated during hygiene care, resulting in aggressive behavior (Hoeffer and others, 2006). Safe, effective patient care takes the impact of cognitive impairment on hygiene care into consideration and allows for appropriate modifications.

CRITICAL THINKING

Synthesis

You will apply elements of critical thinking whenever you perform the nursing process with a patient. Consider the scientific knowledge you have learned, your experience, critical thinking attitudes, and standards to ensure an individualized approach to patient care (Box 28-2).

KNOWLEDGE Knowledge of the anatomy and physiology of the skin, oral cavity, nails, and sense organs helps you understand the implications of proper hygiene for the patient's total health status. As you develop a knowledge base about various pathologic conditions, you will more fully understand risk factors that increase the risk for hygiene problems. You will apply this knowledge to guide the questions you ask patients about their hygiene care as you assess their care needs and their hygiene self-care status. Also use your knowledge to plan and implement patient care. For example, the patient with diabetes has specialized needs for nail and foot care. Knowledge about the pathophysiology of diabetes and its potential effect on the patient's circulation provides you with the scientific knowledge base needed to implement proper foot care practices.

Knowledge about developmental and cultural factors influencing hygiene practices provides a basis for identifying

BOX 28-2   SYNTHESIS IN PRACTICE

Before entering Mrs. Winkler's room, Jamie reviews and synthesizes knowledge about the effect of chronic illness on body image and independence, reviews principles of communication, and reviews the pathophysiology for multiple sclerosis, diabetes, and oral lesions.

Previous clinical experience has taught Jamie that patients need to have an opportunity to determine how nurses implement nursing care. By applying the ethical standard of autonomy, Jamie encourages Mrs. Winkler to make decisions about how to proceed with her hygiene care by engaging Mrs. Winkler in a therapeutic conversation. Jamie learns that Mrs. Winkler likes to have her face and hands washed first and then her teeth brushed before breakfast. But then she tells Jamie that it really is not important. Mrs. Winkler says, "I am not going to have breakfast today because my mouth is sore. I took my dentures out yesterday. They hurt my mouth too much. I guess I just can't wear them anymore." At this time Jamie determines that assisting Mrs. Winkler with oral care is a priority.

Jamie continues to synthesize knowledge and uses previous clinical experiences to appropriately analyze assessment data and make nursing diagnoses. She maintains accurate information and incorporates therapeutic communication skills, which will ensure meeting standards for quality care.

and meeting your patients' hygiene needs in an individualized manner. To effectively identify the hygiene needs of your patient, use your knowledge of communication techniques and cultural influences with regard to hygiene. These principles assist you in establishing a trusting relationship and acquiring a basic understanding of the patient. Knowing your patient as an individual will aid in identifying and meeting your patient's hygiene needs.

Apply knowledge of physical assessment skills (see Chapter 15) when providing hygiene. Doing a thorough examination of the skin, oral and nasal cavities, eyes and ears, peripheral circulation, motor function, and degree of range of motion while providing hygiene needs uses time efficiently and will provide a database to identify hygiene problems and monitor a patient's progress over time.

EXPERIENCE Draw on your own experiences in meeting your personal hygiene needs as you assist with your patients' hygiene care. You may have helped family members with their hygiene. Usually an early clinical experience involves providing hygiene to a patient. As your experience increases, your comfort and expertise in meeting the individualized hygiene needs of your patients increase as well.

ATTITUDES There are multiple critical thinking attitudes applicable to hygiene care. For example, use creativity to collaborate with your patient and determine the best way to meet your patient's individual hygiene needs. You will need to be creative and supportive to help your patient develop new

hygiene practices or adapt existing ones when illness or loss of function impairs self-care abilities. Be nonjudgmental and confident when providing care. Because of variations in individual patient's physical strength and hygiene practices, it is important that you approach care with an attitude of flexibility. Encourage patient involvement while determining how and when care is provided. For example, you may need to include periods of rest to prevent exhaustion during hygiene care. Demonstrate responsibility and accountability when making a plan of care that will promote your patient's well-being.

STANDARDS The use of critical thinking standards ensures that assessment of hygiene needs is relevant and accurate. Apply professional standards of care in your practice. For example, when caring for patients with diabetes, apply standards from the American Diabetes Association to ensure that you give proper foot care. Recommendations from the American Dental Association provide the basis for teaching oral care. Also apply standards of professional responsibility to advocate for the patient. For example, apply the ethical standard of autonomy by letting your patient choose the time and type of bath when possible. You adhere to the principle of beneficence when you use evidence-based, patient-centered bathing measures with a patient who is cognitively impaired and becomes agitated or aggressive when bathed (Hoeffer and others, 2006). Promote your patients' independence as much as possible while still maintaining their safety.

NURSING PROCESS

■■■ ASSESSMENT

Assessment of a patient's hygiene status and self-care abilities requires you to complete a nursing history and perform physical assessment. You will not routinely assess all body regions before providing hygiene. However, you will need to conduct a brief history to determine priority areas and to help you plan individualized hygiene care. While assisting the patient with personal hygiene, carefully assess the skin, nails, oral cavity, hair and scalp, and the sensory organs (see Chapter 15). Visually inspect and palpate tissue, noting alterations in integrity. Pay particular attention to characteristics most influenced by hygiene measures. For example, too frequent bathing with hot water and harsh soaps can cause the skin of the older adult to become dry and easily damaged (Box 28-3). Assessment data will help you determine any hygiene-related issues and identify the type and extent of hygiene care required.

Observe the patient as you are giving care to detect problems associated with inadequate hygiene practices. It is important to assess the patient's ability to tolerate hygiene procedures that are sometimes exhausting. Hygiene care allows you to assess for a variety of health care problems and thus helps to set health care priorities (Table 28-2).

SELF-CARE ABILITY Assessment of a patient's ability to provide self-care will help you make decisions about the kind and amount of hygiene care to provide, as well as the patient's

BOX 28-3 CARE OF THE OLDER ADULT

Skin Changes With Aging

- The turnover rate for the stratum corneum declines by 50% as patients age, resulting in slower healing, reduced barrier protection, and delayed absorption of medications or chemicals placed on the skin (Meiner and Lueckenotte, 2006).
- Older patients produce less sebum and perspire less. Thus they generally need to bathe less frequently. However, always consider their personal preferences.
- Older patients' skin is often more fragile; avoid hot water, and use only a mild cleansing agent. Use bath oils with caution because they increase the danger of falling in a slippery tub.
- The majority of older patients have some degree of itching and skin sensitivity; hydrocortisone cream, superfatted soaps, and petrolatum offer relief.
- Dryness and redness are a common problem as skin ages. Minimize environmental factors that lead to skin drying such as low humidity and exposure to cold.
- According to best available estimates, between 1 and 2 million Americans age 65 or older have been injured, exploited, or mistreated. Because of the risk for elder abuse, do not ignore unexplained bruises and skin trauma (National Center on Elder Abuse, 2005).

ability to participate in care. When a patient is unable to bathe or perform personal skin care, you need to provide assistance. To determine whether a patient requires a bed bath instead of a tub bath or shower, assess your patient's balance, activity tolerance, and muscle strength and coordination as well as presence of treatment-related tubes or equipment. Be alert for activity intolerance during hygiene care. Rapid respirations or difficulty breathing and changes in skin color indicate activity intolerance. Palpate the pulse to detect changes in rate and regularity, and question the patient about dizziness or weakness.

The degree of assistance needed by a patient during bathing also depends on the patient's vision, the ability to sit without support, hand grasps, and ROM of extremities. Assess your patient's physical ability to perform eye, ear, and nose care and to care for any sensory aids. Patients who have limited upper extremity mobility, have reduced vision, are seriously fatigued, or are unable to grasp small objects, such as a hearing aid battery or contact lenses, will require assistance. Current evidence shows that the degree of hand function plays a key role in the adequate removal of dental and denture plaque in institutionalized older people performing their own oral care (Padilha and others, 2007).

Assess your patient's cognitive status using the Mini-Mental State Examination (see Chapter 15). The patient with impaired cognitive function may be unaware of hygiene care needs or may be less able to follow instructions and assist with care. For the patient with cognitive impairments you often need to consult with therapists and specialists from other disciplines, which usually requires an order from the patient's health care provider.

ASSESSMENT OF THE SKIN Use the opportunity when assisting the patient with personal hygiene care to perform an assessment of the skin (see Chapter 15). Examine the skin, noting color, texture, thickness, turgor, temperature, and hydration. Pay special attention to presence and characteristics of any lesions. Note dryness of the skin indicated by flaking, redness, scaling, and cracking. Observing for manifestations of common skin problems will affect how you administer hygiene (Table 28-3). Observe less obvious or difficult-to-reach areas (e.g., under the breasts or scrotum, around the female patient's perineum, and in the groin) for redness, excessive moisture, and soiling or debris.

When caring for patients with dark skin pigmentation, be aware of assessment techniques and skin characteristics unique to highly pigmented skin (see Chapter 15). It is especially important to carefully assess dark skin in patients who are at risk for pressure ulcers (see Chapter 36).

Determine the degree of cleanliness by observing the appearance of the skin and detecting body odors that indicate previous inadequate cleansing or excessive perspiration due to fever or pain. Inspect all surfaces of body structures, and separate skin folds for observation. Carefully assess the skin under orthopedic devices (braces, splints) and beneath items such as support stockings and tape. Assess the condition and cleanliness of the perineal and anal areas during hygiene and with each toileting when patients require hygiene assistance. Most people consider these areas to be private. Your reluctance to expose the patient or your patient's reluctance results in problems because of inadequate hygiene care. Use sensitivity in your approach.

Pay attention to characteristics most influenced by hygiene measures. Is the skin dry from too much bathing or from use of hot water or irritating soap? Are there calluses on the feet that may benefit from soaking? Certain conditions place patients at risk for impaired skin integrity (see Chapter 36). Be particularly alert when assessing patients with reduced sensation, vascular insufficiency, impaired cognition, incontinence, and decreased mobility. Patients are often unaware of skin disorders because they are unable to feel pressure or see their skin in some places (e.g., the back). The development of pressure ulcers is a common complication that extends hospital stays. For the patient who experiences frequent diarrhea or is incontinent of stool or urine, inspect the perineal and anal areas for irritation and cleanliness with each soiling.

ASSESSMENT OF THE FEET AND NAILS Often people are unaware of foot or nail problems until pain or discomfort occurs. A variety of common foot and nail problems can be caused by inadequate hygiene and are detected during hygiene care (Table 28-4). Problems sometimes result from abuse or poor care of the feet and hands, such as nail biting or trimming nails improperly, exposure to harsh chemicals, and wearing poorly fitting shoes. Determine the patient's type of footwear and usual foot and nail care practices.

Thoroughly examine all skin surfaces of the feet, including areas between the toes and over the soles of the feet. Poorly

TABLE 28-2　FOCUSED PATIENT ASSESSMENT

FACTORS TO ASSESS	QUESTIONS	PHYSICAL ASSESSMENT
Skin care	What type of bath do you prefer? How often do you usually bathe? What kind of soap and lotion do you use? Do you need help with your bath and skin care? Have you noticed any skin changes or irritation? Do you have any open sores or rashes?	Observe patient during hygiene activities. Inspect condition of skin and bony prominences. Observe skin surfaces and skin folds for presence of dirt or debris.
Mouth care	Do you have any trouble chewing? Have you had a change in food or fluid intake because of trouble chewing or mouth discomfort? Are you having any mouth pain, or have you noticed any sores in your mouth? Do you wear dentures or a partial plate?	Inspect condition of teeth, gums, and mouth. Observe patient during mouth care or eating to determine presence of oral pain or discomfort that impairs hygiene practices. Observe fit of dentures. Inspect gums for sores or pressure areas.
Foot care	Do you experience pain or discomfort in your legs or feet when walking? Do you have cramping in your legs? Have you noticed any changes in color of the skin on your lower legs or feet? Do you have a history of diabetes? Do you have any sore spots or any hardened areas on your feet or toes? Do you frequently feel tingling or pain in your feet? Have you noticed any loss of feeling in your feet? How do you usually care for your feet and nails? Do you soak your feet?	Watch patient walk; observe for limping, uneven gait. Inspect feet and between toes for pressure or open area. Inspect patient's shoes for unequal wear. Inspect nail beds for open sores, trauma, and proper nail care. Test feet for presence of touch sensation. Palpate pedal pulses. Observe skin and nail bed color.
Assistance with hygiene	Do you use any aids to help you with your bath such as grab bars in your tub or shower? Do you need someone of the same gender or your family to assist in your hygiene care? What parts of personal hygiene can you do for yourself? What parts of hygiene care do you need help with? How can I make assisting you with your hygiene easier and more pleasant?	Observe patient's use of assistive devices, noting proper, safe use. Complete an environmental assessment to detect presence of safety devices or hazards related to hygiene care.
Tolerance of hygiene	Do hygiene activities cause any symptoms such as shortness of breath, pain, or fatigue? What do you do to minimize these symptoms? What can I do to help you complete hygiene care most comfortably?	Observe patient before, during, and after hygiene. Palpate pulse, noting rate and rhythm changes. Observe breathing pattern, noting rate and ease of breathing. Observe patient for pallor and diaphoresis. Notice facial expressions that indicate pain.

fitting shoes often irritate the heels, soles, and sides of the feet. Chronic foot problems are common in older adults, who often have dry feet because of a decrease in sebaceous gland secretion, dehydration, or poor condition of footwear. Fissures result in severe itching. One of the more common problems in the older adult population is foot pain (Meiner and Lueckenotte, 2006).

Observe the patient's gait. A variety of common foot problems contribute to pain and cause alterations in gait. Assess the adequacy of the patient's peripheral circulation and sensation particularly in patients with diabetes or known peripheral vascular disease. Foot ulceration is the most com-

mon single risk factor for lower extremity amputations among persons with diabetes (Frykberg and others, 2006). Palpate the dorsalis pedis and posterior tibial pulses, and assess for intact sensation to light touch, pinprick, and temperature (see Chapter 15).

Inspect the condition of the fingernails and toenails, looking for lesions, dryness, inflammation, or cracking, which are often associated with a variety of common nail problems (see Table 28-4) or with nail care practices. The cuticle that surrounds the nail can grow over the nail and become inflamed if nail care is not performed periodically. Chemicals in nail polish remover cause excessive nail dryness. Disease changes

TABLE 28-3 Common Skin Problems

PROBLEM	CHARACTERISTICS	IMPLICATIONS	INTERVENTIONS
Dry skin	Flaky, rough texture on exposed areas such as hands, arms, legs, or face	Skin may become infected if epidermal layer cracks.	Bathe less frequently. Use superfatted soap (e.g., Dove) for cleansing. Rinse body of all soap well because residue left will cause irritation and breakdown. Use a humidifier to add moisture to air. Increase fluid intake when skin is dry. Use moisturizing lotion to aid healing process; lotion forms protective barrier and helps maintain fluid within skin. Use creams to clean skin that is dry or irritated by soaps and detergents.
Acne	Inflammatory, papulopustular skin eruption, usually involving bacterial breakdown of sebum; appears on face, neck, shoulders, and back	Infected material within pustule will spread if area is squeezed or picked. Permanent scarring can result.	Wash hair and skin each day with soap and warm water to remove oil. Use oil-free cosmetics because oily cosmetics or creams accumulate in pores and make acne worse. Use prescribed topical antibiotics for severe acne.
Skin rashes	Skin eruption that may result from overexposure to sun or moisture or from allergic reaction; appears flat or raised, localized or systemic, pruritic or nonpruritic	If patient scratches skin, inflammation and infection will occur. Rashes also cause discomfort.	Wash area thoroughly, and apply antiseptic spray or lotion to prevent further itching and aid healing process. Warm soaks sometimes relieve inflammation.
Contact dermatitis	Inflammation of skin characterized by abrupt onset with erythema, pruritus, pain, and appearance of scaly oozing lesions; seen on face, neck, hands, forearms, trunk, and genitalia	Dermatitis is often difficult to eliminate because person is usually in continual contact with substance causing skin reaction. Substance is sometimes hard to identify.	Condition usually disappears when patients avoid exposure to causative agents (e.g., cleansers, soaps).
Abrasion	Scraping or rubbing away of epidermis; results in localized bleeding and later weeping of serous fluid	Infection occurs easily as result of loss of protective skin layer.	Be careful not to scratch patients with your jewelry or fingernails. Wash abrasions with mild soap and water. Dressing or bandage sometimes increases risk for infection because of retained moisture.

the condition, shape, and curvature of the nails (see Chapter 15). Inflammatory lesions and fungus of the nail bed cause thickened, horny nails that can separate from the nail bed.

ASSESSMENT OF THE ORAL CAVITY The condition of the oral cavity reflects overall health and also indicates oral hygiene needs. Inspect all areas of the mouth carefully for color, hydration, texture, and lesions (see Chapter 15). Patients who do not perform oral hygiene regularly or correctly frequently develop associated problems. Localized pain and infection are common symptoms of gum disease and some tooth disorders. Apply clean gloves to palpate any tender areas or lesions. Observe for cleanliness, and use olfaction to detect **halitosis** (foul-smelling breath). If during assessment you identify any oral problems (Box 28-4), notify the patient's health care provider. Early identification of poor oral hygiene practices and common oral problems reduces the risk for gum disease and dental caries or cavities. Research also links

poor oral hygiene in older adult patients to a greater prevalence of nosocomial bacterial pathogens and risk for lower respiratory infections (El-Solh and others, 2004).

Include specific questions and observations for the patient with dentures or a dental appliance. Observe under dentures and appliances for evidence of pressure areas or irritation. Note size and location of any lesions. Note how well the dentures or appliance fit. Question patients about any problems associated with dental devices, including tender areas and poor fit. Observe the patient's care of the dentures or appliance.

ASSESSMENT OF THE HAIR AND HAIR CARE Before performing hygiene care, assess the condition of the patient's hair and scalp (Box 28-5). Findings will help you determine the frequency and extent of care needed (Table 28-5). During care observe your patient's ability to perform hair care. A person's appearance and feeling of well-being often are

TABLE 28-4 Common Foot and Nail Problems

PROBLEM	CHARACTERISTICS	IMPLICATIONS	INTERVENTIONS
Callus	Thickened portion of epidermis, consisting of mass of horny, keratotic cells; usually flat, painless, and found on undersurface of foot or on palm of hand; caused by local friction or pressure	Foot calluses often cause discomfort when wearing tight-fitting shoes.	Wear gloves when using tools or objects that create friction on palms. Wear comfortable shoes that fit. Soak callus in warm water and Epsom salts to soften cell layers (soaking of feet is contraindicated in patients with diabetes). Use pumice stone to remove callus after it softens. Be careful not to use stone on noncallused skin. Applications of creams or lotions reduce reoccurrence. Use of orthotic devices (e.g., foam insoles, metatarsal pads, and various cushioning devices) redistributes weight and pressure away from callused area.
Corns	Keratosis caused by friction and pressure from shoes; mainly on toes, over bony prominence; usually cone shaped, round, and raised; calluses with painful core	Conical shape compresses underlying dermis, making it thin and tender. Tight shoes aggravate pain. Tissue will attach to bone if allowed to grow. Patient may suffer alteration in gait because of pain.	Surgical removal is sometimes necessary depending on location and severity of pain and size of corn. Use oval corn pads carefully, because they increase pressure on toes and reduce circulation. Do not use corn pads for patients with diabetes or impaired circulation.
Plantar warts	Fungating lesion that appears on sole of foot; caused by papillomavirus	Warts are sometimes contagious, are painful, and make walking difficult.	Treatment ordered by health care provider may include topical applications of acids, electrodesiccation (burning with electric spark), cryotherapy (freezing with carbon dioxide or liquid nitrogen), or laser therapy.
Athlete's foot (tinea pedis)	Fungal infection of foot; scaliness and cracking of skin between toes and on soles of feet; small blisters containing fluid appear, apparently induced by constricting footwear (e.g., sneakers)	Athlete's foot can spread to other body parts, especially hands. It is contagious and frequently recurs.	Make sure feet are well ventilated. Drying feet well after bathing and applying powder help prevent infection. Wearing clean socks or stockings reduces incidence. Health care provider often orders application of griseofulvin, miconazole nitrate, or tolnaftate.
Ingrown nails	Toenail or fingernail growing inward into soft tissue around nail; results from improper nail trimming, poor shoe fit, or heredity	Ingrown nails cause localized pain in presence of pressure; some become infected.	Treatment is frequent warm soaks in antiseptic solution and removal of portion of nail that has grown into skin. Instruct patient in proper nail trimming techniques and to report purulent drainage. Recommend professional podiatry if needed.
Ram's horn nails	Unusually long, curved nails	Attempt to cut nails sometimes damages nail bed and/or causes infection.	Refer patient to podiatrist.
Paronychia	Inflammation of tissue surrounding nail after hangnail or other injury; occurs in people who frequently have their hands in water; common in patients with diabetes	Area sometimes becomes infected.	Treatment is warm compresses or soaks and local application of antibiotic ointments. Careful manicuring prevents paronychia.
Foot odors	Result of excess perspiration promoting microorganism growth; faulty foot hygiene or improper footwear cause foot odor	Odor frequently embarrasses patient.	Frequent washing, use of foot deodorants and powders, and clean footwear will prevent or reduce this problem.
Nail fungal infection	Results from excess moisture, use of artificial nails	Infection requires treatment with a fungicide.	Wear clean, dry footwear (see entry on athlete's foot).

BOX 28-4   Common Oral Problems

DENTAL CARIES (CAVITIES)
- Most common among young people
- Buildup of plaque causes acid destruction of tooth enamel; initially appears as chalky, white discoloration of the tooth

PERIODONTAL DISEASE (PYORRHEA)
- Most common after age 35
- Involves destruction of gingiva (gums) and other supporting structures with bleeding gums, inflammation, and receding gum lines

OTHER PROBLEMS
- Oral mucositis (oral erythema, ulceration, and pain)
- Glossitis (inflammation of the tongue)
- Gingivitis (inflammation of the gums)
- Halitosis (bad breath)
- Cheilitis (cracked lips)
- Oral malignancy (mouth lumps or ulcers)

BOX 28-5   Assessment of Hair Care

PHYSICAL CHANGES
- Assess condition of hair and scalp (see Chapter 15). Consider age-appropriate changes.
- Consider racial or ethnic differences.
- Determine reasons for change in distribution or loss of hair.
- Check oiliness and texture of hair.
- Inspect scalp for lesions, inflammation, infection, or parasites.

SELF-CARE ABILITY
- Assess patient's ability to grasp comb or brush and to raise arm for brushing or combing.
- Determine patient's ability to physically care for hair.
- Does patient become easily fatigued?

HAIR-CARE PRACTICES
- Assess patient's preferences in hair styling.
- Identify patient's preferences for hair care and shaving products.
- Assess adequacy of patient's hygiene practices.
- Determine patient's perceptions of own appearance.
- Assess patient's socioeconomic background.

person's appearance and feeling of well-being often are related to the way the hair looks and feels. Illness, disability, and conditions such as arthritis, fatigue, and the presence of physical barriers (e.g., cast or IV access) alter a patient's self-care ability and prevent a patient from maintaining daily hair care. Assess the immobilized patient's hair for tangles, and check hair around and beneath dressings for sticky blood residue or antiseptic solutions.

ASSESSMENT OF THE EYES, EARS, AND NOSE Carefully inspect all external eye structures. Normally the conjunctivae are clear and not inflamed. The eyelid margins are in close approximation with the eyeball, and the lashes turn outward. The lid margins are normally without inflammation, drainage, or lesions. Flaking skin around the eyebrows sometimes indicates dandruff.

Assessment of the external ear structures includes inspecting the auricle and external ear canal. Particularly note the presence of accumulated wax called **cerumen** or drainage in the ear canal, local inflammation, or pain.

Inspect the nares for signs of inflammation, discharge, lesions, edema, and deformity. The nasal mucosa is normally pink, clear, and without discharge. For patients with any type of tubing exiting the nose, observe for tissue damage, localized tenderness, inflammation, drainage, and bleeding.

For patients who wear eyeglasses, contact lenses, artificial eyes, or hearing aids, assess the patient's knowledge regarding methods used to care for the aids, as well as any problems caused by them. Have patients describe how they typically care for the aids, and watch patients as they care for their aids when possible. Compare your patients' actions with what you know is the proper care technique. Any inconsistencies in findings indicate a need for patient education.

PATIENTS AT RISK FOR HYGIENE PROBLEMS Some patients present risks that require more attentive and rigorous hygiene care (Table 28-6). These risks result from side effects of medications, lack of knowledge, an inability to perform hygiene, or a physical condition that potentially injures the skin, feet and nails, hair, or oral cavity structures. Anticipate whether a patient is predisposed to any risks, and follow through with a complete assessment. Timely identification of risks and preventive care reduces injury to the patient's skin, feet, nails, or oral mucosa. For example, patients who receive broad-spectrum antibiotics are at risk for the medication destroying normal flora in their mouths, allowing the overgrowth of opportunistic microbes. You will need to more thoroughly and more frequently observe their oral cavity for inflammation and lesions. Also question patients about sores or tenderness in the mouth.

PATIENT EXPECTATIONS With all nursing care it is important to know your patient's expectations. Hygiene is a very personal aspect of care, and patients have varying expectations. Personal preferences reflect both individual and cultural or religious customs and beliefs. Assess your patient's usual practices, and ask questions about cultural, personal, or religious practices affecting hygiene care.

When giving or assisting with hygiene care, ask patients about preferred personal care items such as soap, lotion, toothpaste, and deodorant. Also ask the type of bath patients desire and when they prefer to bathe. Ask about special grooming preferences such as hair styling, makeup, and shaving.

Each culture exhibits unique personal hygiene practices (see Box 28-1, p. 750). When caring for patients from different cultures, learn as much as possible about and be sensitive to the patients' customs, beliefs, and practices. Ask about preferred hygiene methods or any cultural restrictions. Rec-

TABLE 28-5 Hair and Scalp Problems

PROBLEM	CHARACTERISTICS	IMPLICATIONS	INTERVENTIONS
Dandruff	Scaling of the scalp accompanied by itching; in severe cases, dandruff on eyebrows	Dandruff causes embarrassment; if dandruff enters eyes, conjunctivitis may develop.	Shampoo regularly with medicated shampoo; in severe cases seek health care provider's advice.
Ticks	Small gray-brown parasites that burrow into skin and suck blood	Ticks sometimes transmit Rocky Mountain spotted fever, Lyme disease, and tularemia.	To remove ticks, use tweezers to grasp tick firmly at its head or mouth next to the skin. Do not use petroleum jelly or a hot match to kill and remove a tick. Sometimes you need to save the tick to determine what kind it is. In these cases, place the tick into a jar with isopropyl alcohol and screw the lid on tight.
Pediculosis capitis (head lice)	Tiny grayish white parasitic insects that attach to hair strands; eggs look like oval particles, resemble dandruff; bites or pustules often found behind ears and at hairline	Head lice are difficult to remove and if not treated will spread to furniture and other people.	Check entire scalp. Use a special lice comb to remove lice and nits. The National Pediculosis Association (2005) encourages a nonchemical approach with manual removal whenever possible. **Caution against use of products containing lindane because the ingredient is a neurotoxin known to cause adverse reactions** ranging from dermatitis to seizures and death (National Pediculosis Association, 2005). Check the hair for nits, and comb with a nit comb for 2 to 3 days until all lice and nits have been removed. Vacuum infested areas of home and car upholstery.
Pediculosis corporis (body lice)	Tend to cling to clothing, making them difficult to see; body lice suck blood and lay eggs on clothing and furniture	Patient itches constantly; scratches on skin become infected; hemorrhagic spots appear on skin where lice are sucking blood.	Have patient bathe or shower thoroughly; after drying skin, apply lotion for eliminating lice; after 12 to 24 hours have patient take another bath or shower; bag infested clothing or linen until laundered.
Pediculosis pubis (crab lice)	Found in pubic hair; crab lice are grayish white with red legs	Lice spread through bed linen, clothing, furniture, or sexual contact.	Shave hair off affected areas; cleanse as for body lice; if lice were sexually transmitted, patient needs to notify partner.
Alopecia	Balding patches in periphery of hair line; hair becomes brittle and broken; caused by improper use of hair curlers and picks, tight braiding, hot styling tools, certain diseases	Patches of uneven hair growth and loss alter patient's appearance. Alopecia is very distressing for all patients, especially women. Hair care practices do not cause or accelerate male pattern baldness.	Stop hair care practices that damage hair (e.g., teasing hair, hair dyes, excessive heat when blow-drying).

ognize that patients from some cultures may express sensitivity to invasion of personal space and to gender of caregivers. When assessing patients ask, "How would you prefer I do your bath?" "Are you comfortable with someone helping you? Would you feel more comfortable having a nurse of the same gender bathe you?"

■■■NURSING DIAGNOSIS

Thorough assessment of the patient's hygiene status and self-care abilities identifies clusters of data or defining characteristics that support actual or at-risk hygiene-related diagnoses. Identification of the defining characteristics leads you to se-

lect the appropriate NANDA International diagnostic label. For example, when caring for an older adult with degenerative arthritis you observe swollen joints, weakness, and limited range of motion in the patient's dominant hand and a generally unkempt appearance. Closer review of data reveals defining characteristics of an inability to wash body parts and difficulty turning on and regulating the water faucet. You add the nursing diagnosis of *bathing self-care deficit* to the patient's plan of care. Accurate selection of nursing diagnoses requires thorough assessment and critical thinking as you analyze defining characteristics and make an accurate diagnosis.

TABLE 28-6 Risk Factors for Hygiene Problems

RISKS	HYGIENE IMPLICATIONS
ORAL PROBLEMS	
Patients who are unable to use upper extremities because of paralysis, weakness, or restriction (e.g., cast or dressing)	Patient lacks upper extremity strength or dexterity needed to brush teeth, perform hair care, and many aspects of hygiene.
Dehydration, inability to take fluids or food by mouth (NPO)	Causes excess drying and fragility of mucosa; increases accumulation of secretions on tongue and gums.
Presence of nasogastric or oxygen tubes; mouth breathers	Causes drying of mucosa, which increases risk for breakdown and infection.
Chemotherapeutic drugs	Drugs kill rapidly multiplying cells, including normal cells lining oral cavity. Ulcers and inflammation develop with resulting discomfort.
Broad-spectrum antibiotics	Destroy normal oral flora, allowing overgrowth of opportunistic microbes.
Over-the-counter lozenges, cough drops, antacids, and chewable vitamins	Medications contain large amounts of sugar. Repeated use increases sugar or acid content in mouth, increasing risk for tooth and gum problems.
Radiation therapy to head and neck	Causes oral mucositis, which affects all the mucosal folds within the oral cavity, resulting in erythema, ulceration, and pain (Scully and others, 2004).
Oral surgery, trauma to mouth, placement of oral airway	Cause trauma to oral cavity with swelling, ulcerations, inflammation, and bleeding.
Immunosuppression; altered blood clotting	Predisposes to inflammation, infection, and bleeding gums.
Diabetes mellitus	Prone to dryness of mouth, gingivitis, periodontal disease, and loss of teeth.
Poorly fitting dentures	Food trapped under dentures causes mouth odor; increased risk for oral mucosa breakdown.
Inadequate brushing and flossing of teeth	Predisposes patients to periodontal disease.
Cardiovascular disease	Linked to periodontal disease.
SKIN PROBLEMS	
Immobilization	Dependent body parts are exposed to pressure from underlying surfaces. The inability to turn or change position increases risk for pressure ulcers.
Reduced sensation due to stroke, spinal cord injury, diabetes, local nerve damage	Patient does not receive normal transmission of nerve impulses when excessive heat or cold, pressure, friction, or chemical irritants are applied to skin.
Limited protein or caloric intake and reduced hydration (e.g., fever, burns, gastrointestinal alterations, poorly fitting dentures)	Limited caloric and protein intake predispose to impaired tissue synthesis. Skin becomes thinner, less elastic, and smoother with a loss of subcutaneous tissue. Poor wound healing results. Reduced hydration impairs skin turgor.
Excessive secretions or excretions on the skin from perspiration, urine, watery fecal material, and wound drainage	Moisture is a medium for bacterial growth and causes local skin irritation, softening of epidermal cells, and skin maceration.
Presence of external devices (e.g., cast, restraint, bandage, dressing)	Device exerts pressure or friction against skin's surface.
Vascular insufficiency	Arterial blood supply to tissues is inadequate, or venous return is impaired, causing decreased circulation to extremities. Tissue ischemia and breakdown occur. Risk for infection is high.
FOOT PROBLEMS	
Patient unable to bend over or has reduced visual acuity	Patient is unable to fully visualize entire surface of each foot, making it difficult to adequately assess condition of skin and nails.
Decreased sensation	Patient is unable to sense pressure. Patient requires education on importance of regular foot inspection and the potential for referral to podiatrist.
EYE CARE PROBLEMS	
Reduced dexterity and hand coordination	Physical limitations create inability to safely insert or remove contact lenses.

Determine whether the patient has an actual alteration (e.g., impaired oral mucous membrane) or is at risk (e.g., risk for impaired skin integrity) to appropriately focus nursing care. For example, a patient with open oral lesions requires more extensive hygienic oral care than usual, including cleansing and comfort measures, as well as care to promote healing of the lesions. If the patient is at risk for a problem, take preventive measures. In the case of the patient at risk for impaired oral mucous membranes, keep the mucosa well hydrated, minimize foods irritating to oral tissues, and provide adequate cleansing.

The identification of related factors (contributing factors) guides you when selecting interventions. The diagnoses of *impaired oral mucous membrane related to malnutrition* and *impaired oral mucous membrane related to chemical trauma* require different interventions. When poor nutrition is a causal factor, you need to consult with a dietitian for appropriate dietary supplements and incorporate patient education about diet into the plan. When chemotherapy injures the oral mucosa, you will follow cancer nursing guidelines regarding oral care for mucositis, including frequent assessment, gentle brushing with soft toothbrushes, flossing, rinsing with bland rinse, and application of water-based moisturizer to lips (Oncology Nursing Society, 2007). Although many possible nursing diagnoses apply to patients in need of supported hygienic care, the following list represents examples of commonly associated nursing diagnoses:

- *Activity intolerance*
- *Ineffective health maintenance*
- *Risk for infection*
- *Impaired physical mobility*
- *Impaired oral mucous membrane*
- *Bathing self-care deficit*
- *Dressing self-care deficit*

■■■PLANNING

During planning use collected data and critical thinking to develop an individualized plan of care. When planning care it is important to identify patient goals and outcomes, set priorities for care, and plan for continuity of care. In many situations patients have multiple nursing diagnoses. Use a Concept Map (Figure 28-1) to show how numerous nursing diagnoses interrelate. Rely on knowledge, experience, and established standards of care when developing the plan of care. Involvement of the patient and other health care providers (e.g., occupational or physical therapists) in developing the plan whenever possible will promote a successful outcome.

GOALS AND OUTCOMES Work closely with the patient and family to identify goals and outcomes and develop an individualized plan of care for the patient's nursing diagnoses (see Care Plan). Establish goals with the patient's self-care abilities, risks, preferences, and resources in mind. Focus goals on improving self-care abilities and the condition of the skin and mucosa, oral mucosa, or dental hygiene. Make outcomes measurable and achievable within patient limitations. In addition, work with the patient to select individualized hygiene measures.

You will care for a variety of patients with varying self-care abilities and hygienic needs. For example, you and the patient who has right-sided paralysis following a stroke establish the following goal: "Patient's skin remains free of breakdown." Then you create a series of realistic individualized expected outcomes. These outcomes include the following:

- Patient's skin is clean, dry, and intact without signs of inflammation.
- Patient's skin remains elastic and well hydrated.
- Patient's skin is free from pressure areas.
- Patient tolerates bathing without excessive fatigue.

SETTING PRIORITIES The patient's condition influences your priorities for hygiene care. Set priorities based on the necessary assistance required by patients, the extent of hygiene problems, and the nature of the patient's nursing diagnoses. For example, a patient who is seriously ill usually needs a daily bath because body secretions accumulate, and the patient is unable to independently maintain cleanliness. Some older patients at home require a visit from a home care aide to assist with a tub bath or shower. Patients who are normally inactive during the day and have skin that tends to be dry may need to bathe only twice a week, whereas a patient with urinary and bowel incontinence will need perineal cleansing with each episode of soiling. A patient who has acute pain requires a bath, but it is necessary to administer pain medications before giving the bath. Plan to use assistive devices to ensure optimum level of independence and safety. For example, a patient with partial paralysis who has difficulty getting out of the tub needs to have a tub chair, handrails, or extra personnel available for help.

Timing is also important in planning hygiene care. Being interrupted in the middle of the bath for an x-ray examination frustrates and embarrasses the patient. If a patient is tired after extensive diagnostic tests, rest will be an important patient priority. In this situation it is best to delay hygiene and allow the patient to rest.

COLLABORATIVE CARE It is important to plan for care throughout the patient's hospital stay. Also ensure continuity of care when patients are discharged to a rehabilitation facility or home. When your patient needs help because of a self-care deficit, family members often become caregivers and need to be included in the plan of care. Be mindful of the equipment and procedures needed, so that the patient and family are knowledgeable about the care, have the skill needed to provide the care, and have access to necessary equipment on discharge.

Collaborate with other health care providers such as physical or occupational therapists and social workers. For example, physical therapists assist patients with strengthening exercises needed for bathing, and occupational therapists fit patients with useful assistive devices that allow patients to pick up toileting items. Use community resources, such as having home care agencies provide staff to assist with bathing if the patient and/or family are unable to perform hygiene activities.

CONCEPT MAP

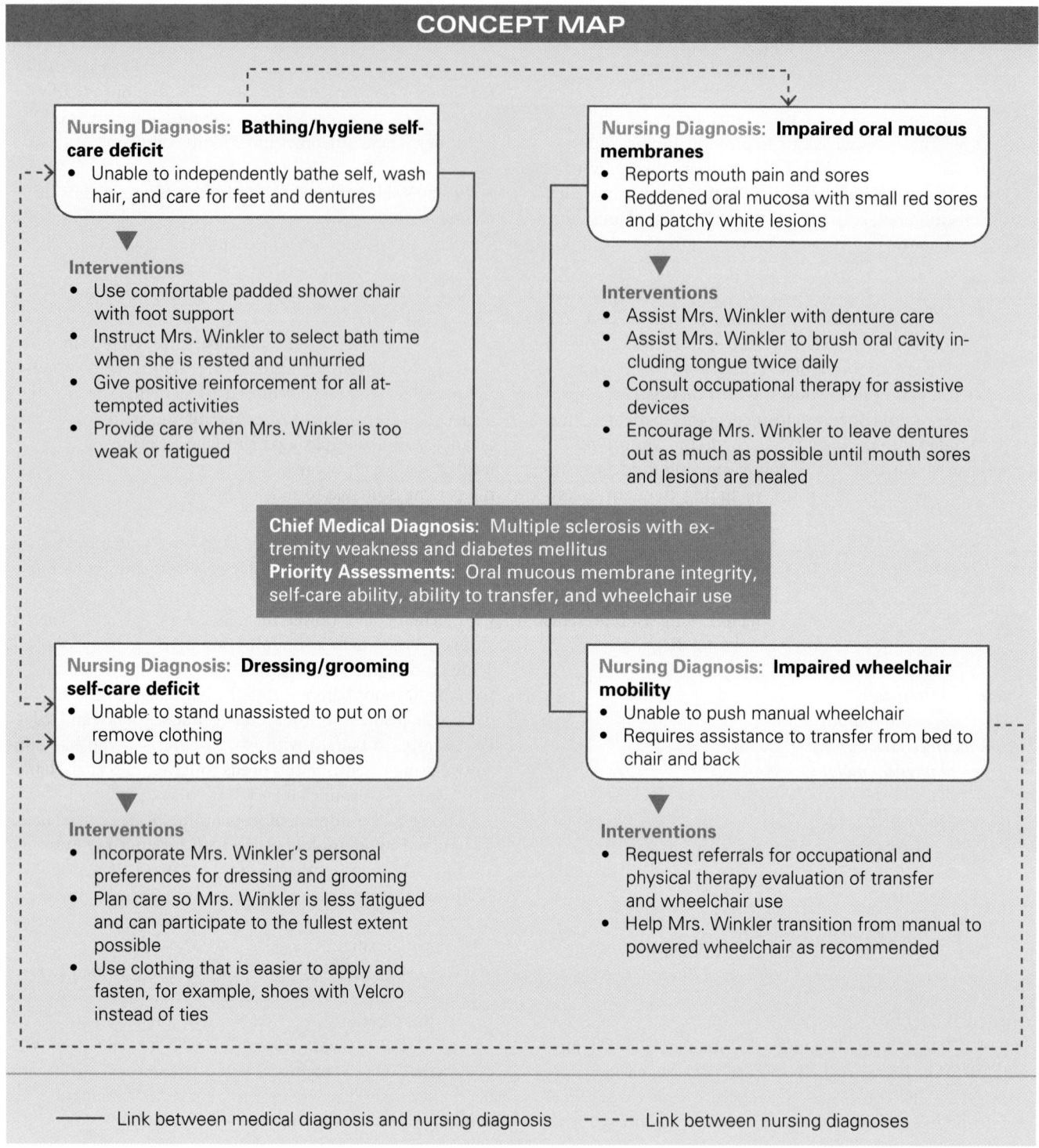

Nursing Diagnosis: Bathing/hygiene self-care deficit
- Unable to independently bathe self, wash hair, and care for feet and dentures

Interventions
- Use comfortable padded shower chair with foot support
- Instruct Mrs. Winkler to select bath time when she is rested and unhurried
- Give positive reinforcement for all attempted activities
- Provide care when Mrs. Winkler is too weak or fatigued

Nursing Diagnosis: Impaired oral mucous membranes
- Reports mouth pain and sores
- Reddened oral mucosa with small red sores and patchy white lesions

Interventions
- Assist Mrs. Winkler with denture care
- Assist Mrs. Winkler to brush oral cavity including tongue twice daily
- Consult occupational therapy for assistive devices
- Encourage Mrs. Winkler to leave dentures out as much as possible until mouth sores and lesions are healed

Chief Medical Diagnosis: Multiple sclerosis with extremity weakness and diabetes mellitus
Priority Assessments: Oral mucous membrane integrity, self-care ability, ability to transfer, and wheelchair use

Nursing Diagnosis: Dressing/grooming self-care deficit
- Unable to stand unassisted to put on or remove clothing
- Unable to put on socks and shoes

Interventions
- Incorporate Mrs. Winkler's personal preferences for dressing and grooming
- Plan care so Mrs. Winkler is less fatigued and can participate to the fullest extent possible
- Use clothing that is easier to apply and fasten, for example, shoes with Velcro instead of ties

Nursing Diagnosis: Impaired wheelchair mobility
- Unable to push manual wheelchair
- Requires assistance to transfer from bed to chair and back

Interventions
- Request referrals for occupational and physical therapy evaluation of transfer and wheelchair use
- Help Mrs. Winkler transition from manual to powered wheelchair as recommended

——— Link between medical diagnosis and nursing diagnosis   - - - - Link between nursing diagnoses

Figure 28-1 ■ Concept Map.

■■■ IMPLEMENTATION

Providing hygiene is a very basic part of patient care. Caring practices reduce patient anxiety and promote comfort and relaxation while performing hygiene interventions. Throughout hygiene care use a gentle approach and speak in a soft, caring manner. Provide for relief of symptoms such as pain or nausea before performing hygiene care.

An important element of implementation is preparing patients to provide their own hygiene care as they become able. This includes teaching patients not only the proper hygiene techniques but also the symptoms of hygiene problems

CARE PLAN Impaired Oral Mucous Membranes

ASSESSMENT

As Jamie is talking with Mrs. Winkler before breakfast is served, she learns that Mrs. Winkler likes to wash her face and hands and then put in her dentures. Mrs. Winkler states, "I just want to stay in bed because I'm tired and I don't feel well. I just get so tired when I do anything. Also, I think I have sores in the roof of my mouth."

ASSESSMENT ACTIVITIES

Ask Mrs. Winkler what care is important this morning.

Assess the condition of Mrs. Winkler's oral cavity.

Assess Mrs. Winkler's ability to bathe and perform oral hygiene care, including an assessment of her range of motion and upper extremity strength.

FINDINGS/DEFINING CHARACTERISTICS*

Mrs. Winkler says, "I want to be able to wear my teeth and to feel clean and look nice."

Mrs. Winkler **reports mouth pain and sores.** Upon visual inspection Jamie observes generalized **reddened oral mucosa** with small **red sores and patchy white lesions** most notable on the roof of the mouth; thick secretions **coating** the gums, cheeks, and tongue; and some **bleeding** from the **inflamed, swollen tissues.** Jamie detects **halitosis.**

Mrs. Winkler admits, **"I have trouble holding my arms up above my waist and I have trouble holding my brush or small things. My muscles are just so weak. I just get so tired doing anything."**

Observed **inability to raise arms over head; inability to grasp** small-handled toothbrush and hair brush.

NURSING DIAGNOSIS: Impaired oral mucous membrane related to difficulty performing oral and denture care due to upper extremity weakness.

PLANNING

GOAL

- Mrs. Winkler will verbalize preventive and routine oral and denture care by discharge.

- Mrs. Winkler will have return of intact oral mucosa within 1 week.

EXPECTED OUTCOMES (NOC)†

Knowledge: Illness Care
- Mrs. Winkler will state importance of reporting symptoms, including mouth tenderness and discomfort, sores, dry mouth, presence of coating within 2 weeks.
- Mrs. Winkler will describe correct preventive oral hygiene care practices within 2 weeks.

Oral Hygiene
- Mrs. Winkler's oral mucosa will be moist and free of thick coating.
- Mrs. Winkler's oral cavity will be odor free.
- Mrs. Winkler will report mouth feels clean.

INTERVENTIONS (NIC)‡

Oral Health Restoration
- Provide oral care at least twice a day, cleansing for a minimum of 90 seconds using a soft-bristled toothbrush or toothette
- Assist patient with rinsing mouth four times a day using a bland rinse (normal saline, sodium bicarbonate, or mixture of saline and sodium bicarbonate).

- Remove, clean, and do not replace dentures except for meals (if desired).

RATIONALE

- Stimulates gums and cleans oral cavity. Recommended oral care protocol for mucositis (Oncology Nursing Society, 2007).
- Rinses remove loose debris and aid in oral hydration. Sodium bicarbonate reduces the acidity of oral fluids, dilutes accumulating mucus, and discourages yeast colonization (Oncology Nursing Society, 2007).
- Promotes healing during cases of mild to moderate stomatitis (Sciubba, 2009).

Defining characteristics are shown in **bold type.*
†Outcome classification labels from Moorhead S and others, editors: *Nursing outcomes classification (NOC)*, ed 4, St. Louis, 2008, Mosby.
‡Intervention classification labels from Bulechek GM and others, editors: *Nursing interventions classification (NIC)*, ed 5, St. Louis, 2008, Mosby.

CARE PLAN   Impaired Oral Mucous Membranes—cont'd

INTERVENTIONS (NIC)‡

Oral Health Restoration
- Refer for dental appointment to check fit of dentures; follow up with routine examinations.

- Carefully observe oral mucosa at least twice daily, noting worsening of manifestations.

RATIONALE

- Denture-induced stomatitis is related in part to dentures that fit poorly, especially if worn while sleeping (Sciubba, 2009).
- Monitor effectiveness of treatment and patient progress toward goal.

EVALUATION

NURSING ACTIONS	PATIENT RESPONSE/FINDING	ACHIEVEMENT OF OUTCOME
Ask patient about reporting of symptoms.	Mrs. Winkler states she now knows that her oral discomfort and sores are related to how she cares for her dentures and that she will report these symptoms if they recur.	Mrs. Winkler is able to participate in prevention of oral problems by reporting symptoms indicating a problem.
Ask patient about preventive oral care.	Mrs. Winkler lists the steps that she needs to take to prevent the recurrence of oral problems. She states, "I now always take my teeth out at night so they can soak."	Although Mrs. Winkler does not have the ability to perform her own care, she is involved in care by requesting oral and denture care.
Assess patient's oral cavity.	Mrs. Winkler's oral cavity mucosa is pink, moist, and not swollen; no lesions are present. No odor is noted. No coating on oral surfaces.	Inflammation and infection in the mouth are resolved.

and available resources in the community for dealing with these problems if they arise.

HEALTH PROMOTION In primary health care situations, educate and counsel patients and caregivers on proper hygiene techniques. For example, a new mother needs help learning how to bathe her newborn, whereas an older adult needs information on the importance of regular ear care to avoid accumulated cerumen and hearing impairment. The skills illustrated throughout this chapter provide standards for excellent physical care. When working with patients in primary health care settings, maintain these standards and incorporate adaptations for the patient's lifestyle, functional status, living arrangements, and preferences. Key points when teaching patients about hygiene include the following:

- Make instructions relevant based on an assessment of the patient's knowledge, motivation, preferences, and situation. For example, when teaching the patient with diabetes, include how circulation to the feet is impaired and how this causes poor healing and infection, especially when the skin is injured or broken.
- Adapt instructions to the patient's bathing facilities and resources. Not all patients have ideal home situations

(e.g., easily accessible shower or tub). Adapt available resources so the patient can comfortably and safely reach and utilize needed items.
- Teach the patient ways to avoid injury. Almost any hygienic procedure poses risks (e.g., cutting a nail too close or failing to adjust the water temperature of the bath). Include safety risks with all instructions.
- Reinforce infection control practices. Damage to the skin, mucosa, eyes, or other tissues creates an immediate risk for infection. Determine that the patient understands the relation between healthy and intact skin and tissues, hand hygiene practices, and the prevention of infection.

ACUTE, RESTORATIVE, AND CONTINUING CARE Nursing knowledge and skills needed for performing hygiene care apply across all health care settings where acute and restorative or continuing care are provided. In addition, some of the skills in this section apply in areas of health promotion.

The variety and timing of hygiene measures varies across health care settings. In the acute care setting, factors such as more frequent diagnostic and treatment plans and the need for more extensive hygiene care due to acute illness or injury affect the scheduling of hygiene care. In extended care facilities and nursing homes, hygiene care is sometimes scheduled less frequently.

Bathing and Skin Care   In hospital settings, you will usually bathe patients in the morning when more staff are available, unless the patient's condition contraindicates or the patient strongly prefers a different option. Follow these guidelines when bathing patients:

- Clean the skin at the time of soiling and at routine intervals. Individualize frequency of cleansing according to patient need and preference. Problems such as incontinence, wound drainage, or excessive diaphoresis require bathing several times a day.
- Avoid hot water, and use a mild cleansing agent to minimize irritation.
- During cleansing of the skin avoid use of force and friction.
- Minimize environmental factors that lead to skin drying such as low humidity and exposure to cold.
- Protect patients from injury by assessing and controlling the bathwater temperature. This is especially important for older adults and others with reduced sensation, such as patients with diabetes, peripheral neuropathy, or spinal cord injuries.
- Use assistive devices such as bath chairs or trolleys when indicated.
- Use bathing as a time to interact with and assess a patient. When giving a complete bath, examine a variety of body systems and discuss issues of concern for the patient.
- During bathing assist patients through joint range-of-motion exercises to promote circulation and joint integrity.
- For patients who fatigue easily, consider administering a partial instead of a complete bed bath.

Teach patients to follow a few general rules for skin health. Have patients routinely inspect their skin for any changes in skin color and texture and report abnormalities to their health care provider. Instruct patients to handle the skin gently, avoiding excessive rubbing. Also encourage patients to eat nutritious foods from all food groups, including those rich in vitamins and minerals and to consume adequate fluids. Stress safety concerns such as failing to adjust the water temperature, cutting nails too close to the skin, and slipping on wet surfaces. Ensure that patients understand that healthy and intact skin and tissues protect them from infection. Reinforce infection control practices, including proper hand hygiene.

There are two categories of baths: cleansing and therapeutic. Cleansing baths include the complete bed bath and partial bed bath, tub bath, shower, sponge bath at the sink, and the bag bath (Box 28-6). The type of cleansing bath you provide depends on the patient's physical capabilities and the degree of hygiene required. You are responsible for deciding what type of bath is most appropriate. Stay informed of new

BOX 28-6   Types of Baths

- **Complete bed bath:** Bath administered to totally dependent patient in bed (see Skill 28-1).
- **Partial bed bath:** Bed bath that consists of bathing only body parts that would cause discomfort if left unbathed, such as the hands, face, axillae, and perineal area. Partial bath also includes washing back and providing a back rub. Give a partial bath to dependent patients in need of partial hygiene or self-sufficient bedridden patients who are unable to reach all body parts.
- **Sponge bath at the sink:** Involves bathing from a bath basin or sink with patient sitting in a chair. Patient is able to perform a portion of the bath independently. You will assist patient with hard-to-reach areas.
- **Tub bath:** Involves immersion in a tub of water that allows more thorough washing and rinsing than a bed bath. Patient may still require assistance. Some institutions have tubs equipped with lifting devices that facilitate positioning dependent patients in the tub.
- **Shower:** Patient sits or stands under a continuous stream of water. The shower provides more thorough cleansing than a bed bath but can be fatiguing.
- **Bag bath/travel bath:** Contains several soft, nonwoven cotton cloths that are premoistened in a solution of no-rinse surfactant cleanser and emollient. The bag bath offers an alternative because of the ease of use, reduced time bathing, and patient comfort.

evidence regarding bathing techniques (Box 28-7). Therapeutic baths include sitz baths or medicated baths (e.g., oatmeal, cornstarch, or Aveeno). A sitz bath cleanses and reduces pain and inflammation of perineal and anal areas. Medicated baths relieve skin irritation and create an antibacterial and drying effect.

Perineal Care. Perineal care is the procedure used to cleanse the genital and anal areas and is part of the daily bath (Skill 28-1). Perineal care is also associated with certain procedures such as catheterization and is performed more frequently for patients with perineal secretions (e.g., patients who have indwelling urinary catheters [see Chapter 33] or who are recovering from rectal or genital surgery or childbirth). Excretions that accumulate along the urinary meatus or a suture line sometimes lead to infection. Allow the patient to perform self-care if possible. Many nurses are embarrassed about providing perineal care, particularly to patients of the opposite sex. This should not cause you to overlook the patient's hygiene needs. A professional, dignified attitude will reduce embarrassment and put the patient and you at ease. When possible have a caregiver of the patient's gender perform this care.

If a patient performs self-care, various problems such as vaginal or urethral discharge, skin irritation, and unpleasant odors may go unnoticed. Stress the importance of perineal care in preventing skin breakdown and infection. Be alert for

BOX 28-7   BEST PRACTICES

Using Person-Centered Care Techniques When Bathing Patients With Cognitive Impairments

SUMMARY OF EVIDENCE

For patients with Alzheimer's disease and related dementia, bathing frequently creates high levels of discomfort. Confusion causes these patients to feel vulnerable or as if they are being attacked during bathing, resulting in screaming, crying, and even aggressively lashing out at caregivers. These bathing scenes leave both the patient and caregiver feeling unsatisfied. Research has focused on techniques to ease the conflict and reduce the aggressive, negative behaviors associated with bathing activities. These efforts include specialized training in a person-centered approach for bathing and use of nontraditional bathing techniques. Use of a patient-centered showering technique and the in-bed towel bath with no-rinse soap results in a reduction of discomfort and aggressive incidents compared with traditional bathing methods.

APPLICATION TO NURSING PRACTICE

- Use person-centered care techniques when bathing patients with cognitive impairments. Develop a therapeutic relationship with the patient. Include the patient in planning care, especially in regard to comfort and personal preferences. For example, let the patient select whether to shower or take a towel bath. Show respect in all interactions and communication. Use a gentle approach, and avoid rushing.
- Recognize triggers for agitation and aggression such as spraying water or touching body parts without a verbal warning, confrontational or disrespectful communication, washing the face first, and hair washing that result in water dripping in the face.
- Develop creative, individualized solutions for bathing conflict. For example, assist the patient with bathing in a recliner using no-rinse soap and towel bathing, or sing favorite songs along with the patient during the bath.
- Provide privacy, and promote comfort. Close the door, or pull room curtains around the bathing area. Control drafts, and keep the patient covered, exposing only the body part being washed. For showering, consider leaving a light gown on during the shower.

REFERENCES

Hoeffer B and others: Assisting cognitively impaired nursing home residents with bathing: effects of two bathing interventions on caregiving, *Gerontologist* 46(4):524, 2006
Perlmutter JS, Camberg L: Better bathing for residents with Alzheimer's, *Nurs Homes Long Term Care Manage* 53(4):40, 2004.
Rader J and others: The bathing of older adults with dementia, *Am J Nurs* 106(4):40, 2006.
Sloane PD and others: Effect of person-centered showering and the towel bath on bathing-associated aggression, agitation, and discomfort in nursing home residents with dementia: a randomized, controlled trial, *J Am Geriatr Soc* 52(11):1795, 2004.
Somboontanont W and others: Assaultive behavior in Alzheimer's disease: identifying immediate antecedents during bathing, *J Gerontol Nurs* 30(9):22, 2004.

complaints of burning during urination, localized soreness or excoriation, or perineal pain. Also inspect vaginal and perineal areas and bed linen for signs of discharge, and use your sense of smell to detect abnormal odors.

Back Rub. A back rub usually follows the bath (see Chapter 31). The back rub promotes relaxation, relieves muscular tension, and decreases perception of pain (Piotrowski and others, 2003). Current evidence supports that **effleurage,** the long, light, gliding strokes used in a massage, is associated with reduced anxiety, heart rate, and respiratory rate (Zullino and others, 2005). A back rub of 3 minutes' duration enhances patient comfort and relaxation (Zullino and others, 2005). Enhance the relaxing effect of the back rub by reducing noise and making sure the patient is comfortable. Always ask if the patient wants a back rub because some patients dislike physical contact. Also, consult the patient's record for contraindications, such as spinal cord injury, rib fractures, or other painful conditions. Because effleurage causes an immediate rise in blood pressure and heart rate in patients who have had coronary artery bypass surgery, this therapy is not recommended for those patients during the first 48 hours after surgery (Zullino and others, 2005).

Nail and Foot Care The feet and nails require special care to prevent infection, odors, pain, and injury to soft tissues. Often people are unaware of foot or nail problems until discomfort or pain develops. For proper foot and nail care, teach your patients to protect their feet from injury, keep their feet clean and dry, and wear footwear that fits properly. Help patients learn the proper way to inspect feet for lesions, dryness, or signs of infection. The patient, family, or delegated nursing assistive personnel need to report any of these conditions to you. This is especially important for patients with peripheral vascular diseases or diabetes mellitus, older adults, and patients with suppressed immune systems. Finally, to maintain and promote foot and nail health, have patients visit a podiatrist when necessary.

Foot and nail care involves soaking to soften cuticles and layers of horny cells, thorough cleansing, drying, and proper nail trimming. Always check agency policy to determine if you can trim nails independently or if a health care provider's order is required. You provide foot and nail care in bed for an immobilized patient or have the patient sit in a chair (Box 28-8). During the procedure is an excellent time to teach the patient proper techniques for cleaning and trim-

BOX 28-8 PROCEDURAL GUIDELINES

Performing Nail and Foot Care

DELEGATION CONSIDERATIONS: You can delegate nail and foot care of patients without diabetes or circulatory compromise to nursing assistive personnel (NAP). Instruct NAP about:
- Proper use of nail clippers
- Use of warm, not hot, water for soaking
- Reporting any changes that may indicate inflammation or injury to tissue

EQUIPMENT: Washbasin, emesis basin, washcloth, towels, nail clippers, orangewood stick *(optional)*, emery board or nail file, lotion, disposable bath mat *(optional)*, paper towels, linen bag or hamper

1. Obtain health care provider's order for cutting nails if agency policy requires.
2. Explain procedure to patient, including fact that proper soaking requires several minutes.
3. Perform hand hygiene. Arrange equipment on over-bed table.
4. Pull curtain around bed, or close room door (if desired).
5. Assist ambulatory patient with sitting in bedside chair. Help bed-bound patient to supine position with head of bed elevated. Place disposable bath mat on floor under patient's feet, or place towel on mattress.
6. Fill washbasin with warm water. Test water temperature.
7. Place basin on bath mat or towel, and help patient place feet in basin. Place call light within patient's reach.
8. With patient sitting in chair or lying in bed, adjust over-bed table to low position, and place table over patient's lap.
9. Fill emesis basin with warm water, and place basin on paper towels on over-bed table.
10. Instruct patient to place fingers in emesis basin and place arms in comfortable position.
11. Have patient soak feet and fingernails for 10 to 20 minutes. Rewarm water after 10 minutes. Exception: Patients with diabetes and peripheral vascular disease should not soak nails in advance.
12. Clean gently under fingernails with orangewood stick while immersing fingers (see illustration). Remove emesis basin, and dry fingers thoroughly.
13. With nail clippers, clip fingernails straight across and even with tops of fingers (see illustration). Shape nails with emery board or file. If patient has circulatory problems, do not cut nails. Only file them.
14. Push cuticle back gently with orangewood stick.
15. Move over-bed table away from patient.
16. Put on clean gloves; scrub callused areas of feet with washcloth.
17. Clean gently under nails with orangewood stick. Remove feet from basin, and dry thoroughly.
18. Clean and trim toenails as in Steps 12 to 14 for fingernails. Do not file corners of toenails.
19. Apply lotion to feet and hands; assist patient back to bed and into comfortable position.
20. Remove gloves, discarding in trash. Perform hand hygiene.
21. Return supplies to appropriate location; place soiled linen in bag or hamper.
22. Perform hand hygiene.
23. Record care given.
24. Report any breaks in skin, any reddened or tender areas, and any discomfort.

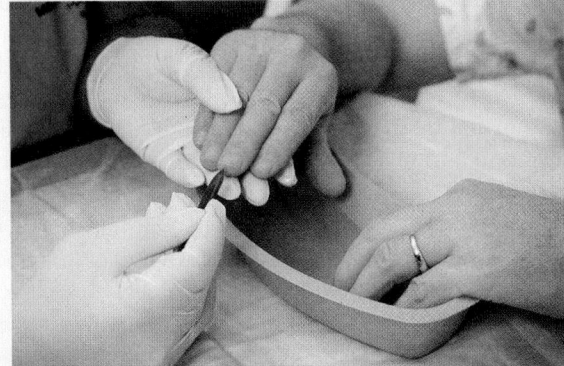

Step 12 ■ Clean under fingernails with orange stick.

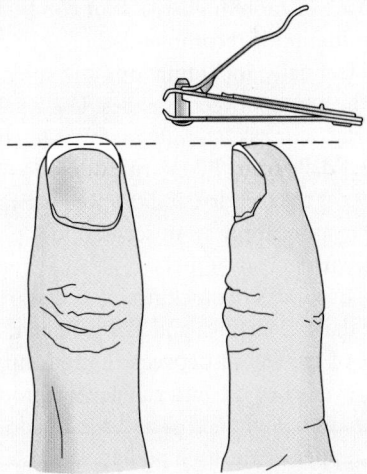

Step 13 ■ Clip fingernails straight across. Use a nail clipper.

ming nails. Stress ways to prevent infection and promote good circulation.

Patients with impaired sensation in the extremities, such as those with diabetes mellitus, require daily foot care and inspection to prevent the development of foot ulcers and subsequent complications that may lead to amputation. The American Diabetes Association (2007) identifies conditions that place patients at increased risk for amputation such as peripheral neuropathy, limited joint mobility, bony deformity, peripheral vascular disease, and a history of skin ulcers or amputation. Assess for signs of peripheral neuropathy or vascular insufficiency (Box 28-9). Advise patients to use the

BOX 28-9   Signs of Peripheral Neuropathy or Vascular Insufficiency

PERIPHERAL NEUROPATHY
- Muscle wasting of lower extremities
- Foot deformities
- Infections
- Abnormal gait
- Decreased or absent vibratory sensation

VASCULAR INSUFFICIENCY
- Decreased hair growth on legs and feet
- Absent or decreased pulses
- Infection of the foot
- Poor wound healing
- Thickened nails
- Shiny appearance of the skin
- Blanching of the skin on elevation

Data from American Diabetes Association: Position statement on standards of medical care in diabetes—2007, *Diabetes Care* 30:S4, 2007; Pinzur MS and others: Guidelines for diabetic foot care, The Diabetes Committee of the American Orthopaedic Foot and Ankle Society, *Foot Ankle Int* 26(1):113, 2005.

following guidelines for routine foot and nail care (American Diabetes Association, 2007; Pinzur and others, 2005):

- Receive a thorough foot examination at least yearly; for those with one or more high-risk foot conditions more frequent evaluation is recommended.
- Inspect the feet daily, including tops and soles of the feet, heels, and the areas between the toes. Use a mirror to inspect all surfaces or ask a family member to check daily.
- Wash the feet daily using lukewarm water; **do not soak.** Thoroughly pat the feet dry, and dry well between the toes.
- If the feet perspire, apply an unscented foot powder. Wear shoes with porous uppers.
- Wear clean, dry socks or stockings. If necessary, change socks twice daily (Martinez and Tripp-Reiner, 2005).
- For dryness of the feet or between the toes, apply lanolin, baby oil, or even corn oil, and rub gently into the skin.
- File the toenails straight across and square; do not use scissors or clippers. Consult a podiatrist as needed.
- Do not use over-the-counter preparations to treat athlete's foot or ingrown toenails or to remove corns or calluses. Consult a health care provider or podiatrist.
- Avoid wearing elastic stockings, knee-high hose, or constricting garters. Do not cross the legs. These activities impair circulation to the lower extremities.
- Wear properly fitted shoes. The soles of the shoes must be flexible and nonskid. Use small amounts of lamb's wool between toes that rub or overlap. Shoes must be sturdy, closed in, and not restrictive to the feet. If you have increased plantar pressure (e.g., erythema or callus), use footwear that cushions and redistributes pressure,

and if you have bony deformity (e.g., bunion or Charcot's joint), wear extrawide or extradeep shoes with cushioned insoles.
- Do not wear new shoes for an extended time. Wear them for short periods over several days to break them in.
- Exercise regularly to improve circulation to the lower extremities.
- Wash minor cuts immediately, and dry thoroughly. Apply only mild antiseptics (e.g., Neosporin ointment). Avoid iodine or Mercurochrome. Contact a health care provider to treat cuts or lacerations.
- Avoid going barefoot.
- Avoid applying hot-water bottles or heating pads to the feet; use extra covers instead.

Oral Hygiene Regular oral hygiene, including brushing, flossing, and rinsing, is necessary for the prevention and control of plaque-associated oral diseases. Proper care prevents inflammation and infection and promotes comfort, nutrition, and verbal communication. Brushing cleanses the teeth of food particles, plaque, and bacteria. It also massages the gums and relieves discomfort from unpleasant odors and taste. Flossing removes tartar that collects at the gum line. Rinsing removes dislodged food particles and excess toothpaste.

When patients become ill, many factors influence their need for oral hygiene. Patients in hospitals or long-term care facilities do not always receive the aggressive oral care they need. Base the frequency of care on the condition of the oral cavity and the patient's level of comfort (Skills 28-2 and 28-3). Some patients will require oral hygiene as often as every 1 to 2 hours.

Acidic fruits in the patient's diet will reduce plaque formation. A well-balanced diet contributes to the integrity of oral tissues. To prevent tooth decay, patients sometimes need to change eating habits (e.g., reducing intake of carbohydrates, especially sweet snacks between meals). All patients need to visit a dentist regularly for checkups. Teaching about common gum and tooth disorders and methods to prevent these problems may motivate patients to follow recommended oral hygiene practices.

Brushing. The American Dental Association (2008) guidelines for effective oral hygiene include brushing your teeth at least twice a day with American Dental Association–approved fluoride toothpaste. A toothbrush with a straight handle and a brush small enough to reach all areas of the mouth is best. Older adult patients with reduced dexterity and grip require an enlarged handle with an easier grip. The American Dental Association (2008) also encourages the use of antimicrobial mouth rinses to inhibit bacterial activity associated with dental plaque, which causes gingivitis.

Brush all tooth surfaces thoroughly. Commercially made foam rubber toothbrushes are useful for patients with sensitive gums. Patients can use electric toothbrushes, but check for electrical hazards. Avoid lemon-glycerin sponges because they dry mucous membranes and erode tooth enamel.

When teaching patients about mouth care, recommend that they not share toothbrushes with family members or drink directly from a bottle of mouthwash. Cross-contamination occurs easily. Instruct patients to obtain a new toothbrush every 3 months or following a cold or strep throat to minimize growth of microorganisms on the brush surfaces (American Dental Association, 2008).

Flossing. Dental flossing removes plaque and tartar between teeth. Flossing involves inserting waxed or unwaxed dental floss between all tooth surfaces, one at a time. The seesaw motion used to pull floss between teeth removes plaque and tartar from tooth enamel. If you apply toothpaste to the teeth before flossing, fluoride comes in direct contact with tooth surfaces, aiding in cavity prevention. According to American Dental Association (2008) recommendations, flossing once a day is sufficient using dental floss or an interdental cleaner. Because it is important to clean all tooth surfaces thoroughly, do not rush to complete flossing. Placing a mirror in front of the patient will help you to demonstrate the proper methods for holding the floss and cleaning between the teeth. Flossing the patient's teeth is not appropriate in all care situations or settings. Research shows that twice-daily rinsing with an essential oil–containing mouth rinse (e.g., Cool Mint Listerine Antiseptic) is at least as effective as daily flossing in reducing plaque and gingivitis (Barouth and others, 2003).

Oral Hygiene for Patients With Special Needs. You will encounter patients who require special oral hygiene care because of dependence on others for care or the presence of oral mucosa problems. Patients who are unconscious or have artificial airways (e.g., endotracheal or tracheal tubes) are susceptible to excessive drying of salivary secretions because they are unable to eat or drink, frequently breathe through the mouth or have their mouths open, and often receive oxygen therapy, which has a drying effect on the mucosal surfaces. In addition, the unconscious patient does not swallow salivary secretions, resulting in accumulation of secretions in the mouth. These secretions often contain gram-negative bacteria that cause pneumonia if aspirated into the lungs. Topical chlorhexidine is accepted for use in oral care, especially in patients on ventilators in the acute setting. Current evidence shows a one-time use of chlorhexidine with oral hygiene reduces the risk for ventilator-associated pneumonia (Berry and others, 2007; Grap and others, 2004; Munro and others, 2006).

Unconscious patients need special attention because they often do not have a gag reflex. Proper oral hygiene requires keeping the mucosa moist and removing secretions that lead to infection. While providing hygiene to an unconscious patient, you need to protect the patient from choking and aspiration. The safest practice is to have two nurses provide the care. You can delegate nursing assistive personnel to participate. One nurse does the actual cleaning, and the other removes secretions with suction equipment. Some agencies use equipment that combines a mouth swab with suction. You can use this equipment safely by yourself. While cleansing the oral cavity, use a small oral airway or a padded tongue blade to hold the mouth open. Never use your fingers. A human bite is highly contaminated. Explain the steps of mouth care and the sensations the patient will feel. Also tell the patient when the procedure is completed (see Skill 28-3).

Researchers have found that foam stick applicators, a popular substitute for the toothbrush, stimulate the mucosal tissues but are ineffective in removing debris from the teeth (Grap and others, 2003). A pediatric-size toothbrush is more effective in removing plaque and tartar and fits better around an endotracheal tube.

Patients receiving cancer chemotherapy, immunosuppressive agents, head and neck radiation therapy, or having nasogastric intubation or an infection of the mouth are susceptible to experiencing **stomatitis** or inflammation of the oral mucosa. Stomatitis causes burning, pain, and a change in food and fluid tolerance. For these patients, perform brushing with a soft toothbrush and floss gently to prevent bleeding of the gums. In some cases, flossing will need to be temporarily omitted from oral care. Rinsing with approximately 30 mL of normal saline on awaking in the morning, after each meal, and at bedtime will help clean the oral cavity. Instruct patients with stomatitis to avoid alcohol and commercial mouthwash and to stop smoking. Health care providers sometimes prescribe oral analgesics for pain control.

Denture Care. Encourage patients to clean their dentures on a regular basis to avoid gingival infection and irritation. When patients become disabled, someone must assume responsibility for denture care (Box 28-10). Dentures are the patient's personal property and need to be handled with care because they break easily. Remove dentures at night to give the gums a rest and prevent bacterial buildup. To prevent warping, keep dentures covered in water when they are not being worn, and always store them in an enclosed, labeled cup with the cup placed in the patient's bedside stand. Discourage patients from removing their dentures and placing them on a napkin or tissue or in the bed or chair because they could be easily thrown away.

Implement measures to prevent denture-induced stomatitis when caring for patients who wear dentures. Also called denture sore mouth, denture-induced stomatitis is a disease of the mouth and gums caused by ill-fitting dentures and poor dental hygiene habits (Columbia University, 2008). Measures to prevent denture-induced stomatitis include rinsing the dentures after meals, cleaning dentures carefully, soaking dentures overnight, brushing and flossing remaining teeth, and teaching the patient how to prevent this complication (Box 28-11).

Hair Care

Brushing and Combing. Frequent brushing helps to keep hair clean and distributes oil evenly along hair shafts. Combing prevents hair from tangling. Encourage patients to maintain routine hair care. However, patients with limited mobility and poor coordination and those who are confused or seriously weakened by illness require help. Patients in a hospital or extended care facility appreciate the opportunity to have their hair brushed and combed before others visit them.

Long hair easily becomes matted when a patient is confined to bed, even for a short period. Blood and topical

BOX 28-10   PROCEDURAL GUIDELINES

Cleaning Dentures

DELEGATION CONSIDERATIONS: You can delegate cleaning dentures to nursing assistive personnel (NAP). Instruct NAP to report:

- Cracked dentures or rough surfaces on the dentures
- Patient complaints of oral discomfort, mouth sore, or poorly fitting appliances

EQUIPMENT: Soft-bristle toothbrush, denture toothbrush *(optional)*, emesis basin or sink, denture cleaning agent or toothpaste, denture adhesive *(optional)*, water glass, 4 × 4 inch gauze, washcloth, denture cup, clean gloves

1 Ask patient if dentures fit and if there is any gum or oral tenderness or irritation.
2 Ask patient about preferences for denture care and products used. You will provide denture care for patients unable to care for their own dentures. Clean dentures for patient during routine mouth care; dentures need to be cleansed as often as natural teeth.
3 Fill emesis basin with tepid water. If using sink, place washcloth in bottom of sink, and fill sink with approximately 1 inch of water.
4 Remove dentures. If patient is unable to do this independently, perform hand hygiene and apply clean gloves, grasp upper plate at front with thumb and index finger wrapped in gauze, and pull downward. Gently lift lower denture from jaw, and rotate one side downward to remove from patient's mouth. Place dentures in emesis basin or sink.
5 Apply cleaning agent or toothpaste and brush surfaces of dentures (see illustration). Hold dentures close to water. Hold brush horizontally, and use back-and-forth motion to cleanse biting surfaces. Use short strokes from top of denture to biting surfaces of teeth to clean teeth surfaces. Hold brush vertically, and use short strokes to clean inner tooth surfaces. Hold brush hori-

zontally, and use back-and-forth motion to clean undersurface of dentures.

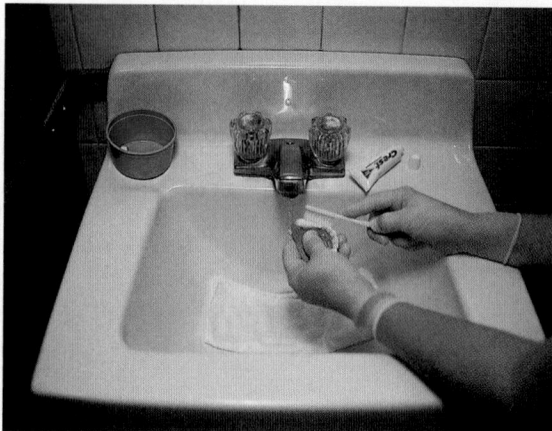

Step 5 ■ Brush surface of dentures.

6 Rinse dentures thoroughly in tepid water.
7 For the patient who uses an adhesive to seal dentures in place, apply a thin layer of adhesive to undersurface before inserting the dentures.
8 If the patient needs help with insertion of dentures, moisten upper denture and press firmly to seal in place. Then moisten and insert lower denture. Ask if dentures feel comfortable.
9 If the patient does not desire dentures to be inserted, place them in a denture cup covered by tepid water. Keeping the dentures moist prevents warping. Store cup in a safe location to prevent loss or breakage.
10 Remove and discard gloves, and perform hand hygiene.

medications also cause tangling when lacerations or incisions involve the scalp. Frequent brushing and combing keep long hair neatly groomed. Braiding helps to avoid repeated tangles. Ask permission before braiding a patient's hair.

To brush hair, part the hair into two sections and separate each into two more sections. It is easier to brush smaller sections of hair. Brushing from the scalp toward the hair ends minimizes pulling. Moistening the hair with water or an alcohol-free detangle product makes the hair easier to comb. Never cut a patient's hair without consent.

Shampooing. Frequency of shampooing depends on a patient's preferences and the condition of the hair. Remind hospitalized patients that staying in bed, excess perspiration, or treatments that leave blood or solutions in the hair may require more frequent shampooing. For patients at home the greatest challenge is to find ways for the patient to shampoo the hair without injury.

The patient who is able to take a shower or bath will usually be able to shampoo the hair without difficulty. Use a shower chair for the ambulatory patient who becomes tired

or faint. Handheld shower nozzles allow patients to wash the hair during a tub bath or shower. If the patient is allowed to sit in a chair, you will usually shampoo the hair in front of a sink. If the patient sits at the bedside, shampoo the hair as the patient leans forward over a washbasin. Bending is limited or contraindicated, however, in certain conditions (e.g., after eye surgery or neck injury). In these situations teach the patient and caregivers the degree of bending allowed.

Transfer patients who cannot sit but can be moved to a stretcher for transportation to a sink or shower equipped with a handheld nozzle. Place a towel or small pillow under the patient's head and neck, allowing the head to hang slightly over the stretcher's edge. Use caution when shampooing patients with neck injuries because hyperextension of the neck will possibly cause further injury. You will need a health care provider's order to shampoo the hair of patients with neck injuries. Another option is to wash the patient's hair in the bed (Box 28-12).

When patients are unable to move, sit in a chair, be transferred to a stretcher, or tolerate a wet hair-washing procedure, there are various "dry" shampoo products available. Read manufacturer's guidelines carefully. In general, you will massage these products into the patient's hair and scalp. Some products require you to apply a towel to remove excess oil and dirt, whereas other products require you to brush the product through the patient's hair.

Shaving. Shave facial hair after the bath or shampoo. Some women will prefer to shave their legs or axillae while bathing. You need to use caution when assisting a patient with shaving to avoid cutting the patient with the razor blade. Patients prone to bleeding (e.g., those receiving anticoagulants or high doses of aspirin) need to use an electric razor. Before using an electric razor, check it for electrical hazards. Use electric razors on only one patient because of the risk for infection transmission.

When using a razor blade for shaving, the skin must be softened to prevent pulling, scraping, or cuts. Placing a warm washcloth over the male patient's face for a few seconds, followed by application of shaving cream or a lathering of mild soap, softens the skin. You will need to shave patients when they are unable to shave themselves independently. To avoid causing discomfort or razor cuts, gently pull the skin taut and use short, firm razor strokes in the direction the hair grows. Short downward strokes work best to remove hair over the upper lip. A patient will usually explain to you the best way to move the razor across the skin. Facial hair of African Americans tends to be curly and becomes ingrown unless shaved close to the skin.

Mustache and Beard Care. Mustaches or beards require daily grooming. Grooming keeps food particles and mucus from collecting in the hair. You will need to groom the patient's mustache and beard if the patient is unable to carry out self-care. Comb out beards gently, and obtain the patient's permission before trimming or shaving off a mustache or beard.

Hair and Scalp Care. To best promote and restore hair and scalp health, instruct patients to keep hair clean, combed, and brushed regularly. Patients may also need to know how to check for and remove parasites (see Table 28-5, p. 757). Tell patients to notify their primary health care provider of changes in the texture and distribution of hair, which may indicate a systemic problem.

Care of Eyes, Ears, and Nose Give special attention to cleansing the eyes, ears, and nose during the patient's bath. Focus care on preventing infection and maintaining normal organ function.

To maintain optimal health, instruct patients in the proper methods of caring for the eyes, ears, and nose. Patients with specific health concerns involving these sensory organs need to see the appropriate specialist regularly for checkups and ongoing care. When active, patients need to know the best ways of protecting these sensitive organs (e.g., eye protective devices). Older adults experience a variety of changes in sensory function (see Chapter 37).

Basic Eye Care. Cleansing the eyes simply involves washing with a clean washcloth moistened in water. Do not use soap because it causes burning and irritation. Always cleanse from

---

BOX 28-11 PATIENT TEACHING
Preventing Denture-Induced Stomatitis

 To help Mrs. Winkler prevent further denture stomatitis, Jamie develops the following teaching plan for Mrs. Winkler:

OUTCOME
- At the end of the teaching session, Mrs. Winkler will verbalize warning signs of denture-induced stomatitis and will assist with performing preventive oral and denture care correctly.

TEACHING STRATEGIES
- Teach Mrs. Winkler the signs and symptoms of denture-induced stomatitis such as redness and swelling under dentures, especially on upper palate, and small red sores on roof of mouth. Although mouth pain may not occur, the patient may experience mouth discomfort with dentures in place or upon inserting or removing dentures.
- Encourage Mrs. Winkler's involvement by encouraging her to report any symptoms to staff.
- Teach Mrs. Winkler that denture-induced stomatitis commonly is caused by the following:
  - Poorly fitting dentures
  - Wearing dentures while you sleep
  - Inadequate cleansing and buildup of the yeast *Candida albicans*
- Teach Mrs. Winkler prevention strategies, and encourage her involvement to prevent recurrence of stomatitis.
- Ask Mrs. Winkler to visit her dentist twice a year.
- Make sure Mrs. Winkler's dentures fit properly. Encourage her to report any problems.
- Instruct Mrs. Winkler what to do if her dentures become damaged (e.g., do not wear them, do not try to fix them, go to the dentist for needed repairs).
- Rinse mouth and dentures after eating. Ask for staff help as needed.
- Encourage Mrs. Winkler to ask for help every night to take her dentures out and cleanse them with dental brush and paste. Leave teeth out overnight, soaking them in clean water. Mark calendar to cleanse once a week with an effervescent cleanser.
- Provide Mrs. Winkler with printed material about denture stomatitis so she can review the material after one-on-one instruction.

EVALUATION STRATEGIES
- Ask Mrs. Winkler to state the signs and symptoms of denture stomatitis and what to do if they occur.
- Ask Mrs. Winkler to state ways she can help to prevent recurrence of denture stomatitis.

Data from Sciubba JJ: *Denture stomatitis*, 2009, http://www.emedicine.com/derm/topic642.htm; Columbia University College of Dental Medicine faculty: *Denture-induced stomatitis*, 2008, http://www.simplestepsdental.com/SS/ihtSS/r.WSIHW000/st.32219/t.25048/pr.3.html.

BOX 28-12 PROCEDURAL GUIDELINES

Shampooing Hair of Bed-Bound Patient

DELEGATION CONSIDERATIONS: You can delegate shampooing hair of bed-bound patients to nursing assistive personnel (NAP). Instruct NAP:

- About any precautions needed in positioning the patient
- To inform the nurse if the patient reports neck pain
- To inform the nurse of any skin or scalp lesions

EQUIPMENT: Bath towels (two or more), washcloths, shampoo, hair conditioner *(optional)*, hydrogen peroxide *(optional)*, water pitcher and warm water supply, shampoo trough, washbasin, bath blanket, waterproof pad, clean gloves if open lesions on scalp, clean comb and brush, hair dryer *(optional)*

1 Before washing patient's hair, determine that there are no contraindications to this procedure. Certain medical conditions, such as head and neck injuries, spinal cord injuries, and arthritis, place the patient at risk for injury during shampooing because of positioning and manipulation of patient's head and neck.

2 Perform hand hygiene. Apply clean gloves if open lesions present.

3 Inspect the hair and scalp before initiating the procedure to determine the presence of any conditions that require the use of special shampoos or treatments (e.g., for the removal of dried blood, dandruff).

4 Place waterproof pad under patient's shoulders, neck, and head. Position patient supine with head and shoulders at top edge of bed. Place trough under patient's head and washbasin at end of trough spout (see illustration). Be sure trough spout or tubing extends beyond edge of mattress.

5 Place rolled towel under patient's neck and bath towel over patient's shoulders.

6 Brush and comb patient's hair.

7 Obtain warm water.

8 Ask patient to close eyes, or hold face towel or washcloth over eyes.

9 Slowly pour water from water pitcher over hair until it is completely wet (see illustration). If hair contains matted blood, put on gloves, apply peroxide to dissolve clots, and then rinse hair with saline. Apply small amount of shampoo.

10 Work up lather with both hands. Start at hairline, and work toward back of neck. Lift head slightly with one hand to wash back of head. Shampoo sides of head. Massage scalp by applying pressure with fingertips.

11 Rinse hair with water. Make sure water drains into basin. Repeat rinsing until hair is free of soap.

12 Apply conditioner or cream rinse if requested, and rinse hair thoroughly.

13 Wrap patient's head in bath towel. Dry patient's face with cloth used to protect eyes. Dry off any moisture along neck or shoulders.

14 Dry patient's hair and scalp. Use second towel if first becomes saturated.

15 Comb hair to remove tangles, and dry with dryer if desired.

16 Apply oil preparation or conditioning product to hair, if desired by patient.

17 Assist patient to comfortable position, and complete styling of hair.

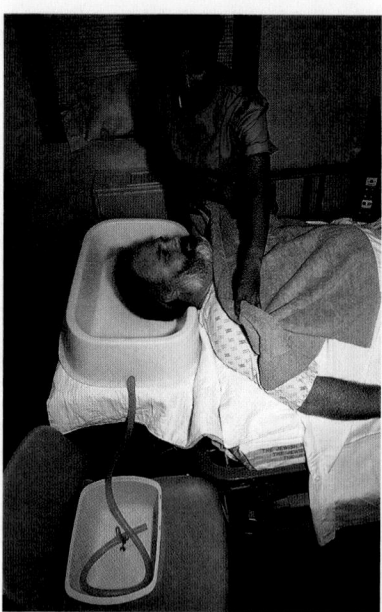

Step 4 ■ Patient positioned for shampoo.

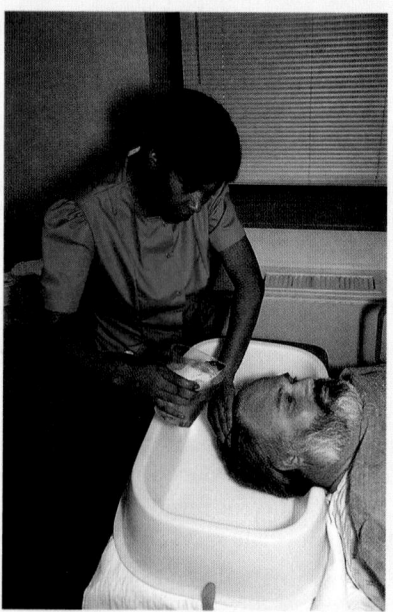

Step 9 ■ Rinsing of hair.

inner canthus to outer canthus, and use a different section of the washcloth for each eye. Never apply direct pressure over the eyeball because it is painful and may cause injury.

The unconscious patient requires more frequent eye care. Secretions collect along the lid margins and inner canthus when the blink reflex is absent or when the eye does not totally close. When an eye remains open, it is sometimes necessary to place an eye patch over the involved eye to prevent corneal drying and irritation. Administer lubricating eye drops according to the health care provider's orders.

Eyeglasses. Eyeglasses are made of hardened glass or plastic that is impact resistant to prevent shattering. Nevertheless, be careful when cleaning glasses and protect them from damage when they are not worn. Put glasses in a case in a drawer of the bedside table when not in use.

Cool water is sufficient for cleaning glass lenses. A soft cloth is best for drying to prevent scratching the lens. Avoid use of paper towels for cleansing or drying glasses. Plastic lenses in particular scratch easily; special cleansing solutions and drying tissues are available.

Contact Lenses. A contact lens is a thin, transparent, circular disk that fits directly over the cornea of the eye. Contact lenses are designed specifically to correct refractive errors of the eye or abnormalities in the shape of the cornea. They are relatively easy to apply and remove. Daily wear lenses are removed nightly for cleansing and disinfection, whereas extended wear lenses may be worn overnight and removed at least weekly for cleansing and disinfection.

Care of contact lenses includes proper cleansing, insertion and removal, and storage. When patients require help to clean their contact lenses, first perform hand hygiene and then clean and disinfect the lenses with the appropriate contact lens solution. Before reinsertion rinse the lenses with the appropriate solution, such as sterile saline. Instruct the patient to never use saliva or homemade solutions when cleansing contacts to avoid potential eye infections. Also instruct the patient to clean the contact lens case frequently with warm water and allow to air dry.

When patients are admitted to hospitals or agencies in unresponsive or confused states, it is important to determine if the patient wears contact lenses and if the lenses are in place. If a seriously ill patient is wearing contact lenses and no one detects this, severe corneal injury results. If you determine that your patient has contact lenses in place and the patient cannot remove them, seek assistance in removing the lenses from the patient's eyes. Once you remove the lenses, be sure to document their removal, the condition of the patient's eyes following removal, and if you gave the lenses to a relative or placed them with the patient's valuables.

Ear Care. Routine ear care involves cleansing the ear with the end of a moistened washcloth, rotated gently into the ear canal. Gentle, downward retraction at the entrance of the ear canal usually causes visible cerumen to loosen and slip out. Instruct your patient never to use objects such as bobby pins, toothpicks, paper clips, or cotton-tipped applicators to remove ear wax. These objects can injure the ear canal and rupture the tympanic membrane. In addition, they may cause ear wax or cerumen to become impacted within the ear canal.

When ear wax is impacted, you can usually remove it by irrigation, which requires a health care provider's order. Review the order for type of solution and ear(s) to receive the irrigation. Before irrigation question the patient for history of perforated eardrum, and inspect the patient's tympanic membrane to be sure it is intact; a perforated tympanic membrane is a contraindication to irrigation. Visually inspect the pinna and external meatus for redness, swelling, drainage, and presence of foreign objects. If vegetable matter (e.g., dried bean) is in the ear canal, do not perform irrigation. Use an otoscope to inspect deeper portions of the auditory canal and the tympanic membrane (see Chapter 15). Determine the patient's ability to hear in the affected ear before irrigation.

To irrigate the ear, have patients sit or lie on their side with the affected ear up. Place a curved emesis basin under the affected ear. For adults and children over 3 years of age, gently pull the pinna up and back. In children 3 years of age or younger, the pinna should be pulled down and back. Using a bulb irrigating syringe, gently wash the ear canal with warm solution (37° C or 98.6° F), being careful to not occlude the canal, which results in pressure on the tympanic membrane. Direct the fluid slowly and gently toward the superior aspect of the ear canal, maintaining the flow in a steady stream. Periodically during the irrigation ask if the patient is experiencing pain, nausea, or vertigo. These symptoms indicate the solution is too hot or too cold or is being instilled with too much pressure. After the canal is clear, wipe off any moisture from the ear with cotton balls and inspect the canal for remaining ear wax.

Hearing Aid Care. Hearing aids amplify sound in a controlled manner; the aid receives normal low-intensity sound inputs and delivers them to the patient's ear as louder outputs. Hearing aids come in a variety of types. Box 28-13 outlines patient teaching for care of a hearing aid.

Nasal Care. The patient usually removes secretions from the nose by gently blowing into a soft tissue. Caution the patient against harsh blowing, which creates pressure capable of injuring the eardrum, nasal mucosa, and even sensitive eye structures. Bleeding from the nares is a key sign of harsh blowing.

If the patient is unable to remove nasal secretions, assist by using a wet washcloth or a cotton-tipped applicator moistened in water or saline. Never insert the applicator beyond the length of the cotton tip. You can also remove excessive nasal secretions by gentle suctioning.

When patients have nasogastric, feeding, or endotracheal tubes inserted through the nose, change the tape anchoring the tube at least once a day. When the tape becomes moist from nasal secretions, the skin and mucosa can easily become **macerated** (softened by soaking). Friction from a tube causes tissue injury. Anchor tubing correctly with tape or fixative devices to minimize tension or friction on the nares (Figure 28-2).

BOX 28-13　Teaching Care and Use of Hearing Aids

- Perform hand hygiene before handling the aid.
- Check battery by holding the hearing aid in your hand and turning up the volume. If the battery is working, you will hear a "whistle." This is feedback noise.
- After inserting or applying the hearing aid, slowly turn up the volume to one-third to one-half volume to obtain a comfortable hearing level for talking at a distance of 1 yard.
- A whistling sound while the patient is wearing the hearing aid indicates incorrect ear mold insertion, improper fit of the aid, or buildup of ear wax or fluid.
- Initially wear a hearing aid 15 to 20 minutes; then gradually increase time to 10 to 12 hours.
- Do not wear aid under heat lamps or a hair dryer or in very wet, cold weather.
- Do not store the aid in a warm place like a windowsill or in a car. The heat can change the shape of the ear mold, causing the aid to not fit properly.
- Remove the battery from the hearing aid when it is not being used for a day or longer.
- Avoid dropping the aid or twisting the cord.
- Remove the aid before radiological examination or radiation therapy to avoid damage.
- Protect the aid from water, alcohol, aerosol sprays, perspiration, and cologne.
- Use the manufacturer-recommended cleaning solution and a soft, lint-free cotton cloth to clean the ear mold. Regularly remove cerumen from the aid using a wax loop or device supplied with the aid.

Data from Ebersole P, Hess P: *Toward healthy aging: human needs and nursing response*, ed 7, St. Louis, 2008, Mosby; Meiner SE, Lueckenotte AG: *Gerontologic nursing*, ed 3, St. Louis, 2006, Mosby; National Institute on Deafness and Other Communication Disorders: *Hearing aids*, Pub No. 99-4340, Bethesda, Md, 2001, National Institutes of Health, http://www.nidcd.nih.gov/health/hearing/hearingaid.asp.

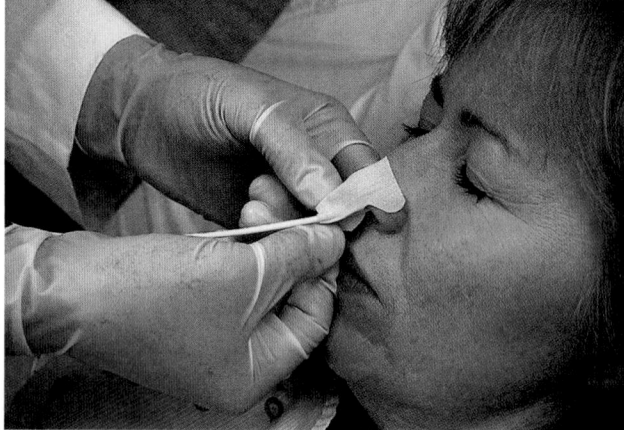

Figure 28-2 ■ Apply new fixative device over feeding tube.

PATIENT'S ROOM ENVIRONMENT

Attempting to make a patient's room as comfortable as the home is one of your priorities. The room needs to be comfortable, safe, and large enough to allow the patient and visitors to move about freely. Control room temperature, ventilation, noise, and odors to create a more comfortable environment. Keeping the room neat and orderly also contributes to the patient's sense of well-being.

Maintaining Comfort

What makes a comfortable environment depends on the patient's age, severity of illness, and level of normal daily activity. Depending on the patient's age and physical condition, maintain the room temperature between 20° and 23° C (68° and 74° F). Infants, older adults, and the acutely ill often need a warmer room. However, certain ill patients benefit from cooler room temperatures to lower the body's metabolic demands.

An effective ventilation system keeps stale air and odors from lingering in the room. Protect acutely ill and older adults from drafts by ensuring they are adequately dressed and covered with a lightweight blanket.

Good ventilation also reduces lingering odors caused by draining wounds, vomitus, bowel movements, and unemptied bedpans and urinals. Always empty and rinse bedpans or urinals promptly. Room deodorizers help remove many unpleasant odors. Before using room deodorizers, determine that your patient is not allergic to or sensitive to the deodorizer itself. Thorough hygiene measures are the best way to control body or breath odors.

Ill patients seem to be more sensitive to noises and lighting commonly found in health care facilities. Try to control the noise level, especially when patients are trying to sleep, and explain the source of unfamiliar noises. Proper lighting is necessary for everyone's safety and comfort. A brightly lit room is usually stimulating, but a darkened room is best for rest and sleep. Adjust room lighting by closing or opening drapes, regulating over-bed and floor lights, and closing or opening room doors. When entering a patient's room at night, avoid abruptly turning on the overhead light unless necessary.

Room Equipment

A typical room contains certain basic pieces of furniture. The over-bed table rolls on wheels and adjusts to various heights over the bed or a chair. Usually two storage areas are under the tabletop. The table provides ideal working space for performing procedures. It also provides a surface on which to place meal trays, toiletry items, and objects the patient frequently uses. Make sure to clean the top of the over-bed table with an antiseptic cleaner before using the table for meals. Do not place bedpans and urinals on over-bed tables. Use the bedside stand to store the patient's personal possessions and hygiene equipment. Patients often use bedside stands for their telephone, water pitcher, and drinking cup.

Hospital rooms often contain different types of chairs. Armless straight-backed chairs are convenient when temporarily transferring your patient from the bed, such as during bed making. Upholstered lounge chairs or recliners tend to be more comfortable when patients are able to sit for an extended period.

Each room usually has an over-bed light and floor level night lighting. Position movable lights that extend over the bed from the wall into the patient's reach, but move them aside when not in use. Gooseneck or portable special examination lights are used to provide extra light during bedside procedures; these lights need to be removed after use. Some facilities have permanent examination lights mounted in the ceiling or wall.

Other equipment usually found in a patient's room includes a call light, a television set or radio, a wall-mounted blood pressure gauge, oxygen and vacuum wall outlets, and personal care items. Special equipment designed for promoting comfort or positioning patients includes footboards and foot boots (Figure 28-3), special mattresses, and bed boards.

BEDS Seriously ill patients often remain in bed for a long time. Because a bed is the piece of equipment patients use most, it is designed for comfort, safety, and adaptability for changing positions.

The typical hospital bed has a firm mattress on a metal frame that you and the patient can raise and lower horizontally. More and more hospitals are converting the standard hospital bed to one in which the mattress surface can be electronically adjusted for patient comfort. You will use different bed positions to promote patient comfort, minimize symptoms, promote lung expansion, and improve access during procedures (Table 28-7).

You change the position of a bed by using electrical controls usually incorporated into the call light or in a panel on the side or foot of the bed. It is important for you to be familiar with use of the bed controls. Instruct patients in the proper use of controls, and caution them against raising the bed to a position that causes harm. Maintain the bed height at the lowest horizontal position when the patient is unattended to promote safety.

Beds contain safety features such as locks on the wheels or casters. Lock wheels when the bed is stationary to prevent accidental movement. Side rails allow patients to move more efficiently in bed and prevent accidents. Do not use side rails to restrict a patient from moving in bed. When using side rails as a restraint, you need a health care provider's order (see Chapter 27). You can remove the headboard from most beds. This is important when the medical team needs to have easy access to the head, such as during cardiopulmonary resuscitation.

Bed Making Keep a patient's bed as clean and comfortable as possible. This requires frequent inspections to be sure linen is clean, dry, and free of wrinkles. When patients are diaphoretic, have draining wounds, or experience incontinence, check frequently for wet or soiled linen.

Usually you make a bed in the morning after the patient's bath or while the patient is bathing, in a shower, sitting in a chair eating, or out of the room for procedures or tests. Throughout the day straighten linen that becomes loose or wrinkled. Also, check the bed linen for food particles after meals and for wetness or soiling. Change linen that becomes soiled or wet.

When changing bed linen, follow basic principles of medical asepsis by keeping soiled linen away from your uniform. Place soiled linen in special linen bags before discarding in the linen hamper. To avoid air currents, which spread microorganisms, never shake linen. To avoid transmitting infection, do not place soiled linen on the floor. Immediately dis-

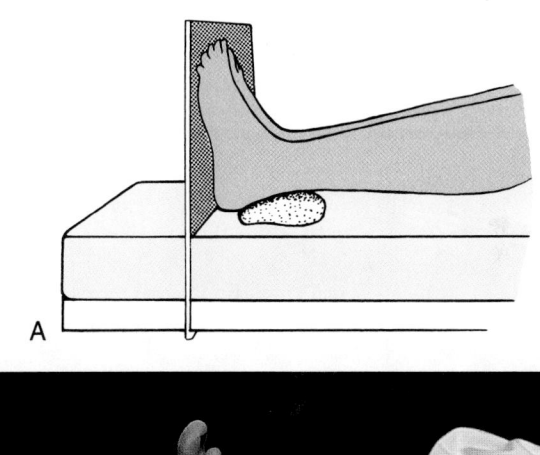

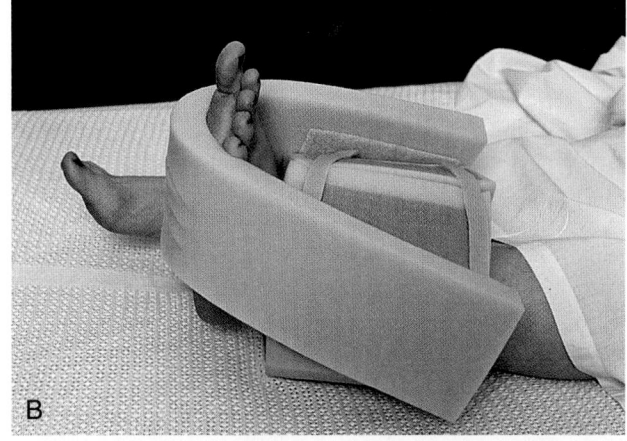

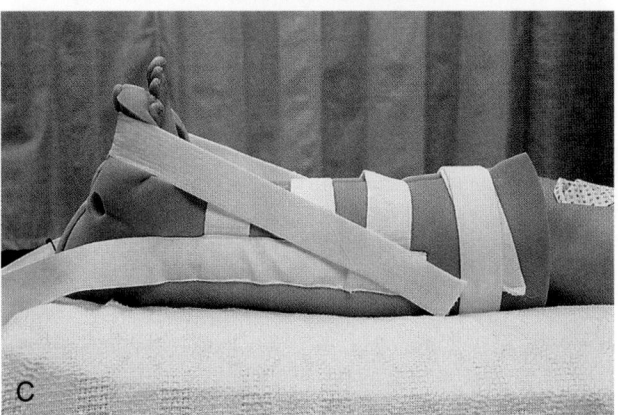

Figure 28-3 ■ **A,** Footboard. **B,** Foot boot. **C,** Foot boot with lower leg extension.

TABLE 28-7 Common Bed Positions

POSITION	DESCRIPTION	USES
Fowler's	Head of bed raised to angle of 45 degrees or more; semisitting position; foot of bed may also be raised at knee	Used during meals, nasogastric tube insertion, and nasotracheal suction Promotes lung expansion
Semi-Fowler's	Head of bed raised approximately 30 degrees; incline is less than Fowler's position; foot of bed may also be raised at knee	Promotes lung expansion Used when patients receive gastric feedings to reduce regurgitation and risk for aspiration
Trendelenburg's	Entire bed tilted with head of bed down	Used for postural drainage Facilitates venous return in patients with poor peripheral venous perfusion
Reverse Trendelenburg's	Entire bed frame tilted with foot of bed down	Used infrequently Promotes gastric emptying Prevents esophageal reflux
Flat	Entire bed frame horizontally parallel with floor	Used for patients with vertebral injuries and in cervical traction Used for patients who are hypotensive Generally preferred by patients for sleeping

card any clean linen that touches the floor or any unclean surface.

During bed making, use safe patient handling procedures and proper body mechanics (see Chapter 26). Make sure you raise the bed to the appropriate height before changing linen so you do not have to bend or stretch over the mattress.

The patient's privacy, comfort, and safety are important when making a bed. If the patient is confined to bed, organize bed-making activities to conserve time and energy (Skill 28-4). Using side rails, keeping call lights within the patient's reach, and maintaining the proper bed position help promote comfort and safety. After making a bed you always return it to the lowest horizontal position and verify that the wheels are locked to prevent accidental falls.

When possible, make the bed while it is unoccupied (Box 28-14). When making an unoccupied bed, follow the same basic principles used for making an occupied bed. The surgical, recovery, or postoperative bed is a modified version of the unoccupied bed. Fold the top covers of the surgical bed to one side or fanfold them to the bottom third of the bed to allow for easy transfer of the patient into the bed. After a patient is discharged, send all bed linen to the laundry. Housekeeping personnel usually clean the mattress and bed and apply new bed linen following discharge.

Linens Before bed making, it is important to collect not only bed linens but also the patient's personal items. Linens come folded to prevent the spread of microorganisms and to make bed making easier. Bed linens have a center crease that you place in the center of the bed from the head to the foot. The linens unfold easily to the sides, with creases often fitting over the mattress edge. Apply new linens whenever there is soiling. Because of the importance of cost control in health care, avoid bringing excess linen into a patient's room. Once you bring the linen into the patient's room, if unused, you need to return it to the laundry for laundering.

▪▪▪EVALUATION

Evaluation of hygiene measures occurs both while giving care and upon completion of care giving activities (Box 28-15). For example, while bathing a patient, inspect the skin carefully to see if soiling or drainage is effectively removed. Once the bath is finished, evaluate the effectiveness of hygiene care by asking patients if they feel more comfortable and relaxed. Observe the patient's behavior during and after hygiene care to detect discomfort that might be associated with movement and hygiene care. Is the patient restless or relaxed? Does the patient's facial expression suggest a feeling of comfort? Is the patient free of body odor?

Include continuing assessment in the plan of care because it often takes time for hygiene care to result in an improvement in the patient's condition. For example, oral lesions and skin excoriation will usually need repeated hygiene interventions.

BOX 28-14 PROCEDURAL GUIDELINES

Making an Unoccupied Bed

DELEGATION CONSIDERATIONS: You can delegate making an unoccupied bed to nursing assistive personnel.

EQUIPMENT: Linen bag, mattress pad (*optional, depending on facility's practice; changed only when soiled*), bottom sheet (flat or fitted), drawsheet (*optional*), top sheet, blanket, bedspread, waterproof pads (*optional*), pillowcases, bedside chair or table, clean gloves (if linen is soiled), washcloth, and antiseptic cleanser

1 Perform hand hygiene.
2 Determine if patient has been incontinent or if excess drainage is on linen. Gloves will be necessary in these cases.
3 Assess activity orders or restrictions in mobility. Assist to bedside chair or recliner if patient can get out of bed.
4 Lower side rails on both sides of bed, and raise bed to comfortable working position.
5 Remove soiled linen, and place in laundry bag. Avoid shaking or fanning linen.
6 Reposition mattress, and wipe off any moisture using a washcloth moistened in antiseptic solution. Dry thoroughly.
7 Apply all bottom linen on one side of bed before moving to opposite side. Apply bottom sheet, flat or fitted.
8 Be sure to place fitted sheet smoothly over mattress. To apply a flat unfitted sheet, allow about 25 cm (10 inches) to hang over mattress edge. Lower hem of sheet lies seam down, even with bottom edge of mattress. Pull remaining top portion of sheet over top edge of mattress.
9 While standing at head of bed, miter top corner of bottom flat sheet (see Skill 28-4, Step 14).
10 Tuck remaining portion of unfitted sheet under mattress.
11 *Optional:* Apply drawsheet, laying center fold along middle of bed lengthwise. Smooth drawsheet over mattress and tuck excess edge under mattress, keeping palms down.
12 Move to opposite side of bed, and spread bottom sheet smoothly over edge of mattress from head to foot of bed.
13 Apply fitted sheet smoothly over each mattress corner. For an unfitted sheet, miter top corner of bottom sheet (see Step 9), making sure corner is stretched tight.
14 Grasp remaining edge of unfitted bottom sheet, and tuck tightly under mattress while moving from head to

foot of bed. Smooth folded drawsheet over bottom sheet, and tuck under mattress, first at middle, then at top, and then at bottom.
15 If needed, apply waterproof pad over bottom sheet or drawsheet.
16 Place top sheet over bed with vertical center fold lengthwise down middle of bed. Open sheet out from head to foot, being sure top edge of sheet is even with top edge of mattress.
17 Make horizontal toe pleat: Stand at foot of bed and fanfold top sheet 5 to 10 cm (2 to 4 inches) across bed. Pull sheet up from bottom to make fold approximately 15 cm (6 inches) from bottom edge of mattress.
18 Tuck in remaining portion of sheet under foot of mattress. Then place blanket over bed with top edge parallel to top edge of sheet and 15 to 20 cm (6 to 8 inches) down from edge of sheet. (*Optional:* Apply additional spread over bed.)
19 Make cuff by turning edge of top sheet down over top edge of blanket and spread.
20 Standing on one side at foot of bed, lift mattress corner slightly with one hand, and with other hand tuck top sheet, blanket, and spread under mattress. Be sure toe pleats are not pulled out.
21 Make modified mitered corner with top sheet, blanket, and spread. After making triangular fold, do not tuck tip of triangle (see illustration).

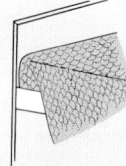

Step 21 ■ Modified mitered corner.

22 Go to other side of bed. Spread sheet, blanket, and spread out evenly. Make cuff with top sheet and blanket. Make modified corner at foot of bed.
23 Apply clean pillowcase(s).
24 Place call light within patient's reach on bed rail or pillow, and return bed to height allowing for patient transfer. Assist patient to bed when desired.
25 Arrange patient's room. Remove and discard supplies. Perform hand hygiene.

Ongoing assessment will be needed to determine if the patient's condition and level of comfort improve over time. Throughout evaluation consider the goals of care and evaluate whether expected outcomes have been achieved. Use the established expected outcomes as the standards for evaluation.

During assessment you collect data about the patient's expectations of care. Both during and after care determine from the patient that care is being provided in an acceptable manner. While giving care encourage the patient to verbalize any discomfort such as cool water temperature or discomfort with movement. To determine the patient's satisfaction with your care ask questions like the following: "Do you feel your bath helped you feel more comfortable?" "Are there ways we can do a better job with your hygiene care?" Being aware of and addressing the patient's expectations and any concerns fosters a caring therapeutic relationship.

BOX 28-15   EVALUATION

Jamie provides Mrs. Winkler with oral and denture care. After several days of careful mouth care, Mrs. Winkler's mouth is now free from infection and inflammation. Jamie includes a teaching plan on oral hygiene to prevent recurrence of dental stomatitis. Mrs. Winkler was able to describe proper oral hygiene but continues to need assistance with her denture care. Mrs. Winkler knows that Jamie provides the extra effort to her care. Mrs. Winkler is satisfied with her care and states, "It is nice to be involved in my oral care. I would like to participate more in the rest of my hygiene needs. Do you think I can help more with my bath tomorrow?" Based on as-

sessment data, Jamie anticipates that Mrs. Winkler will probably need help during her bath to prevent fatigue. Jamie uses this information to plan her care for the next day.

DOCUMENTATION NOTE
"Oral mucous membranes pink, moist, and intact. Unable to perform denture care independently but verbalized understanding of daily denture care and requests to have dentures removed and cleaned nightly. Also verbalized three signs and symptoms of mucositis and when to contact physician about problems with oral cavity. Verbalized desire to be more involved in personal care."

SAFETY GUIDELINES FOR NURSING SKILLS

SAFETY CONSIDERATIONS
Ensuring patient safety is an essential role of the professional nurse. To ensure patient safety, communicate clearly with members of the health care team, assess and incorporate the patient's priorities of care and preferences, and use the best evidence when making decisions about your patient's care. When performing the skills in this chapter, remember the following points to ensure safe, individualized patient care:

- Always perform hygiene measures moving from cleanest to less clean or dirty areas. This often requires you to change gloves and perform hand hygiene during care activities.
- Use clean gloves when you anticipate contact with nonintact skin or mucous membranes or when there is or may likely be contact with drainage, secretions, excretions, or blood during hygiene care.

- When using water or solutions for hygiene care, be sure to test the temperature to prevent burn injury.
- To avoid injury when performing hygiene care, use principles of body mechanics and safe patient handling.
- When giving or assisting with hygiene care, be sensitive to the invasion of privacy and possible loss of self-esteem associated with these procedures. Foster acceptance and comfort by using therapeutic communication techniques, draping and providing privacy, and informing the patient when touching sensitive or private body parts.
- Remember that you are responsible and accountable for assessing the patient both before and after care to detect unexpected outcomes and to give proper direction to nursing assistive personnel when delegating hygiene care.

SKILL 28-1   BATHING AND PERINEAL CARE

DELEGATION CONSIDERATIONS
The skill of bathing and perineal care can be delegated to nursing assistive personnel (NAP). The nurse directs NAP about:
- Not massaging reddened skin areas
- Reporting early signs of impaired skin integrity, including redness or pallor
- Proper ways to position male and female patients with musculoskeletal limitations and indwelling catheters
- Reporting patient fatigue or report of pain during hygiene care

EQUIPMENT
- Washcloths and bath towels
- Bath blanket
- Soap and soap dish
- Toiletry items (deodorant, powder, lotion, cologne)
- Toilet tissue or wipes
- Warm water
- Clean hospital gown or patient's own pajamas or gown
- Laundry bag
- Clean gloves (when risk for contacting body fluids)
- Washbasin

STEP	RATIONALE

ASSESSMENT

1. Assess patient's tolerance for bathing: activity tolerance, comfort level during movement, cognitive ability, musculoskeletal function, and the presence of shortness of breath.

Determines patient's ability to perform or tolerate bathing and level of assistance required (e.g., tub bath, partial bed bath).

- **Critical Decision Point:** Patients with dementia may become agitated and aggressive during bathing activities. Consider using alternative bathing procedures with these patients (see Box 28-7, p. 764).

2. Assess patient's visual status, ability to sit without support, hand grasp, range of motion (ROM) of extremities.

Determines degree of assistance patient will need for bathing.

3. Assess for presence of equipment (e.g., IV line, oxygen tubing, Foley catheter)

Affects how you will plan bathing activities and positioning. Helps determine how to set up supplies.

4. Assess patient's bathing preferences: frequency and time of day preferred for bathing, type of hygiene products used, and other factors related to patient preferences.

Patient participates in plan of care. Promotes patient's comfort and willingness to cooperate. Includes cultural or personal hygiene preferences in care.

5. Ask if patient has noticed any problems related to condition of skin and genitalia: excess moisture, inflammation, drainage or excretions from lesions or body cavities, rashes or other skin lesions.

Provides you with information to direct physical assessment of skin and genitalia during bathing. Also influences selection of skin care products.

6. Before or during bath, assess condition of patient's skin. Note the presence of dryness, indicated by flaking, redness, scaling, and cracking.

Provides a baseline for comparison over time in determining if bathing improves condition of skin.

7. Assess patient's knowledge of skin hygiene in terms of its importance, preventive measures to take, and common problems.

Determines patient's learning needs.

PLANNING

1. Review orders for specific precautions concerning patient's movement or positioning.

Prevents injury to patient during bathing activities. Determines level of assistance required by patient.

2. Check for a health care provider's therapeutic bath order; if there is an order, note type of solution, length of time for bath, and body part to be treated.

Therapeutic baths are ordered for specific physical effect, which usually includes promotion of healing or soothing effects.

3. Explain procedure, and ask patient for suggestions on how to prepare supplies. If partial bath, ask how much of bath patient wishes to complete.

Promotes patient's cooperation and participation.

4. Adjust room temperature and ventilation, close room doors and windows, and draw room divider curtain.

Warm room that is free of drafts prevents rapid loss of body heat during bathing. Privacy ensures patient's mental and physical comfort.

5. Prepare equipment and supplies. If it is necessary to leave room, be sure call light is within patient's reach.

Avoids interrupting procedure or leaving patient unattended to retrieve missing equipment.

IMPLEMENTATION

1. **Complete or Partial Bed Bath**

   a. Offer patient bedpan or urinal. Provide toilet tissue.

   Patient will feel more comfortable after voiding. Prevents interruption of bath.

   b. Perform hand hygiene. If patient has nonintact skin or the skin is soiled with drainage, excretions, or body secretions, apply clean gloves. Ensure patient is not allergic to latex.

   Reduces transmission of microorganisms.
   Prevents allergic reaction if latex gloves used.

   c. Verify that the bed is in locked position, and raise bed to a comfortable working height. Lower side rail closest to you, and assist patient in assuming comfortable supine position, maintaining body alignment. Bring patient toward side closest to you.

   Prevents bed from moving. Helps you reach the patient without stretching and reaching across bed, thus minimizing strain on back muscles.

   d. Place bath blanket over patient, and then loosen and remove top covers without exposing patient. If possible, have patient hold top of bath blanket. Place soiled linen in laundry bag. Take care to not allow linen to touch your uniform. *Optional:* Use top sheet when bath blanket is not available or patient prefers.

   Removal of top linens prevents them from becoming soiled or moist during bath. Blanket provides warmth and privacy.

SKILL 28-1   BATHING AND PERINEAL CARE—cont'd

STEP	RATIONALE

e Remove patient's gown or pajamas.

   (1) If available, use gown with ties or snaps on sleeves for patient with IV or upper extremity injury or limited ROM.

   (2) If a gown with snaps or ties on the arms is not available and patient has limited upper extremity ROM or has an IV access, remove gown from *unaffected side first*.

Provides full exposure of body parts during bathing. Undressing unaffected side first allows easier manipulation of gown over body part with reduced ROM.

   (3) Remove gown from arm without IV line first. Then remove gown from arm with IV. Remove IV bag from pole, and slide IV container and tubing through arm of patient's gown. Rehang IV container, and check flow rate. Regulate if necessary (see illustrations).

Manipulation of IV tubing and container may disrupt flow rate.

   (4) If IV pump is in use, turn pump off, clamp tubing, remove tubing from pump, and proceed as in Step (3). Reinsert tubing into pump, unclamp tubing, and turn pump on at correct rate. Observe flow rate and regulate if necessary. *Do not disconnect tubing.*

Regulation is necessary to prevent improper infusion of fluids. Disconnecting IV tubing places patient at risk for introduction of microorganisms into the IV line.

f Pull side rail up. Lower bed temporarily to lowest position, then raise upon return. Fill washbasin two-thirds full with warm water. Place basin and supplies on overbed table over bed. Check water temperature, and also have patient place fingers in water to test temperature tolerance. Place plastic container of bath lotion in bathwater to warm if desired.

Raising side rail and lowering bed position maintains patient's safety while you leave bedside. Warm water promotes comfort, relaxes muscles, and prevents unnecessary chilling. Testing temperature prevents accidental burns. Bathwater warms lotion for application to patient's skin.

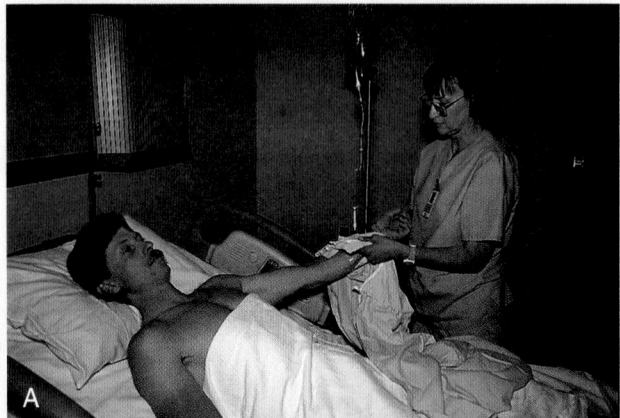
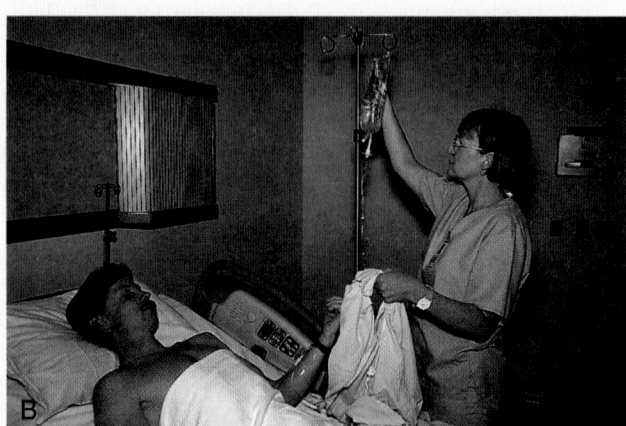
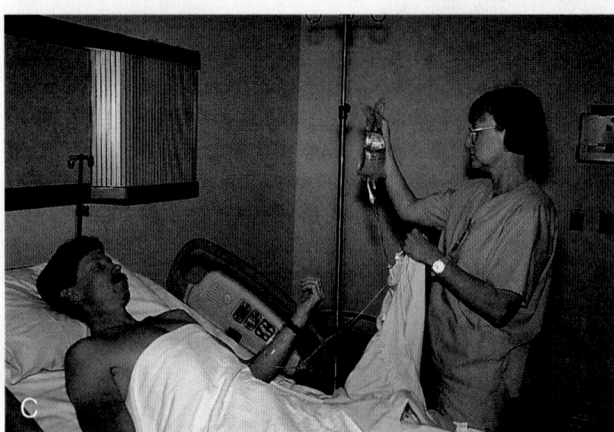
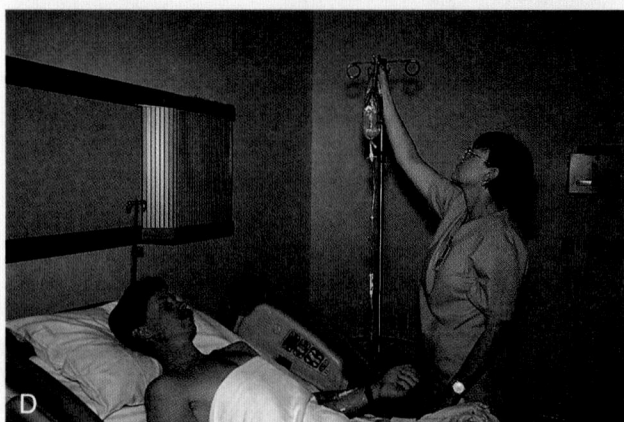

Step 1e(3) ■ **A,** Remove patient's gown. **B,** Remove IV from pole. **C,** Slide IV tubing and bag through arm of patient's gown. **D,** Rehang IV bag.

STEP	RATIONALE

g Lower side rail, remove pillow if tolerated, and raise head of bed 30 to 45 degrees if allowed. Place bath towel under patient's head. Place second bath towel over patient's chest.

Aids your access to patient. You do not have to reach across bed, thus minimizing strain on back muscles. Removal of pillow makes it easier to wash patient's ears and neck. Placement of towels prevents soiling of bed linen and bath blanket.

h Wash face.

  (1) Ask if patient is wearing contact lenses.

Prevents accidental injury to eyes.

  (2) Fold washcloth around fingers of your hand to form a mitt (see illustration). Immerse mitt in water, and wring thoroughly.

Mitt retains water and heat better than loosely held washcloth; keeps cold edges from brushing against patient, and prevents splashing.

  (3) Wash patient's eyes with plain warm water. Use different section of mitt for each eye. Move mitt from inner to outer canthus (see illustration). Soak any crusts on eyelid for 2 to 3 minutes with damp cloth before attempting removal. Dry eyes thoroughly but gently.

Soap irritates eyes. Use of separate sections of mitt reduces infection transmission. Bathing eye from inner to outer canthus prevents secretions from entering nasolacrimal duct. Pressure can cause internal injury.

  (4) Ask if patient prefers to use soap on face. Otherwise, wash, rinse, and dry forehead, cheeks, nose, neck, and ears without using soap. (Men sometimes wish to shave at this point or after bath.)

Soap tends to dry face, which is exposed to air more than other body parts.

i Wash trunk and upper extremities.

  (1) Remove bath blanket from patient's arm that is closest to you. Place bath towel lengthwise under arm. Bathe arm with soap and water using long, firm strokes from distal to proximal areas (fingers to axilla).

Towel prevents soiling of bed. Soap lowers surface tension and facilitates removal of debris and bacteria when friction is applied during washing. Long, firm strokes stimulate circulation; moving distal to proximal promotes venous return.

  (2) Raise and support arm above head (if possible) to wash, rinse, and dry axilla thoroughly (see illustration). Apply deodorant or powder to underarms if desired or needed.

Movement of arm exposes axilla and exercises joint's normal ROM. Alkaline residue from soap discourages growth of normal skin bacteria. Drying prevents excess moisture that can cause skin maceration or softening. Respect patient's preference in use of hygiene products.

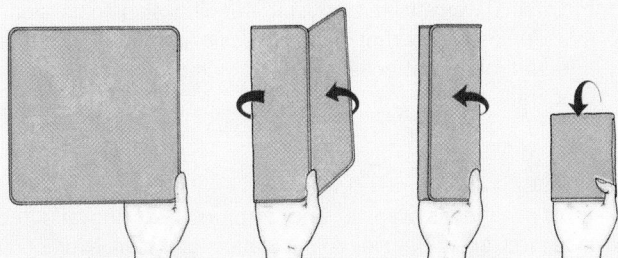

Step 1h(2) ▪ Steps for folding washcloth to form a mitt.

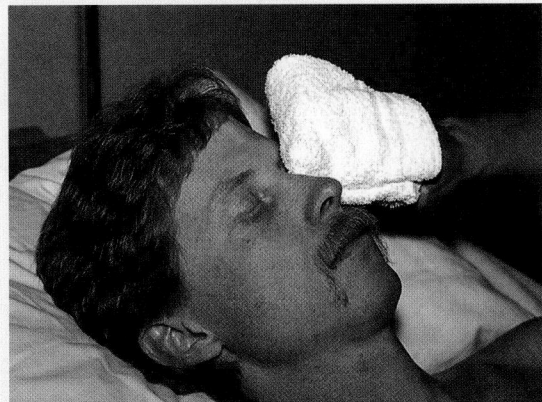

Step 1h(3) ▪ Wash eye from inner to outer canthus.

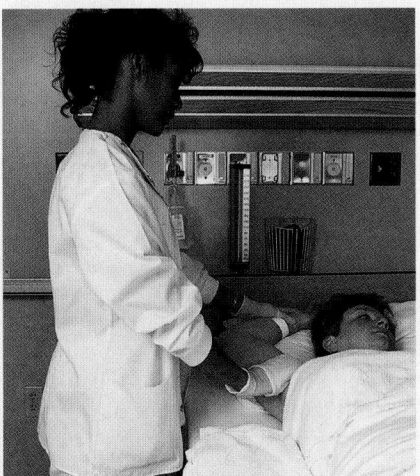

Step 1i(2) ▪ Positioning the patient's arm to wash the axilla.

SKILL 28-1   BATHING AND PERINEAL CARE—cont'd

STEP	RATIONALE
(3) Move to other side of bed, and repeat Steps (1) and (2) with other arm.	Provides for better access to patient and helps prevents back strain.
(4) Cover patient's chest with bath towel, and fold bath blanket down to umbilicus. While lifting edge of towel away from chest with one hand, bathe chest with mitted washcloth on other hand using long, firm strokes. Take special care to wash skin folds under female's breasts. It is often necessary to lift breast upward while bathing underneath the breast. Keep patient's chest covered between wash and rinse periods. Rinse and dry well.	Draping prevents unnecessary exposure of body parts. Towel maintains warmth and privacy. Secretions and dirt collect easily in areas of tight skin folds. Skin under breasts is vulnerable to excoriation if not kept clean and dry.
j Wash hands and nails.	
(1) Fold bath towel in half, and lay it on bed beside patient. Place basin on towel. Immerse patient's hand in water. Allow hand to soak for 2 to 3 minutes before washing hand and fingernails (see Box 28-8, p. 765). Remove basin, and dry hand well. Repeat for other hand.	Soaking softens cuticles and calluses of hand, loosens debris beneath nails, and enhances feeling of cleanliness. Thorough drying removes moisture from between fingers.
k Check temperature of bathwater, and change water when cool or soapy.	Warm water maintains patient's comfort. Alkaline soap residue is irritating to skin, and can decrease the normal protectiveness of acid pH.

- **Critical Decision Point:** If patient is at risk for falling, be sure two side rails are up before obtaining fresh water. Also lower bed when it is necessary to leave bedside. NOTE: Having all side rails raised is often considered a restraint.

STEP	RATIONALE
l Wash the abdomen.	
(1) Place bath towel lengthwise over chest and abdomen. (Two towels may be needed.) Fold bath blanket down to just above pubic region. With one hand, lift bath towel. With mitted hand, bathe and rinse abdomen, giving special attention to umbilicus and skin folds of abdomen and groin. Stroke from side to side. Keep abdomen covered between washing and rinsing. Rinse and dry well.	Draping prevents unnecessary exposure of body parts. Towel maintains warmth and privacy. Keeping skin folds clean and dry helps prevent odor and skin irritation. Moisture and sediment that collect in skin folds predispose skin to maceration.
(2) Apply clean gown or pajama top. If an extremity is injured or immobilized, dress affected side first. *Optional:* You may omit this step until completion of bath; make sure gown does not become damp or soiled during remainder of bath.	Maintains patient's warmth and comfort. Dressing affected side first allows easier manipulation of gown over body part with reduced ROM.
m Wash the lower extremities.	
(1) Cover chest and abdomen with top of bath blanket. Cover legs with bottom of blanket. Expose near leg by folding blanket toward midline. Be sure to drape other leg and perineum.	Prevents unnecessary exposure.
(2) Place bath towel under leg, supporting leg at knee and ankle. If appropriate, place patient's foot in the bath basin to soak while washing and rinsing. (Bend patient's leg at knee, and while grasping patient's heel, elevate leg from mattress slightly and place bath basin on towel). If patient is unable to support leg, cleansing can be done by washing feet thoroughly with washcloth.	Towel prevents soiling of bed linen. Support of joint and extremity during lifting prevents strain on musculoskeletal structures. Sudden movement by patient could spill bathwater. Soaking softens calluses and rough skin.

- **Critical Decision Point:** If patient has diabetes or peripheral vascular disease, do not soak feet.

STEP	RATIONALE
(3) Wash leg using long, firm strokes from ankle to knee and then from knee to thigh (see illustration). Do not rub or massage the back of the calf. Rinse and dry well. Cleanse foot, making sure to bathe between toes. Rinse and dry toes and feet completely. Clean and clip nails as needed (see Box 28-8, p. 765). Remove and discard towel.	Promotes circulation and venous return. Excess massage of calf could loosen deep vein thrombus. Secretions and moisture may be present between toes, predisposing patient to maceration and breakdown.
(4) Raise side rail, move to opposite side of bed, lower side rail, and repeat Steps (2) and (3) for other leg and foot. If skin is dry, apply moisturizer. When finished, cover patient with bath blanket.	When applied within 3 minutes of bathing, moisturizers help prevent dryness and itching by trapping existing water in the skin (American Academy of Dermatology, 2008).

> • ***Critical Decision Point:*** Do not use long, firm strokes to wash the lower extremities of patients with history of deep vein thrombosis or blood-clotting disorder. Use short, light strokes instead.

STEP	RATIONALE
n Cover patient with bath blanket, raise side rail for patient's safety, remove soiled gloves and/or perform hand hygiene. Change bathwater.	Decreased bathwater temperature causes chilling. Clean water reduces microorganism transmission to perineal structures.
o Provide perineal hygiene.	
(1) If patient is able to maneuver and handle washcloth, allow cleansing the perineum on own.	Maintains patient's dignity and self-care ability.
(2) Female Patient	
(a) Apply new pair of clean gloves. Lower side rail. Assist patient in assuming dorsal recumbent position. Note restrictions or limitations in patient's positioning. If patient is totally dependent, provide assistance to support patient in side-lying position and to raise leg as perineum is bathed. Be sure waterproof pad is positioned under patient's buttocks. If position causes patient discomfort, reduce degree of abduction in female's hips. Drape patient with bath blanket placed in the shape of a diamond. Lift lower edge of bath blanket to expose perineum (see illustration).	Provides full exposure of female genitalia. Draping limits exposure and shows respect for patient's dignity.
(b) Fold lower corner of bath blanket up between patient's legs onto abdomen. Wash and dry patient's upper thighs.	Keeping patient draped until procedure begins minimizes anxiety. Buildup of perineal secretions soils surrounding skin surfaces.

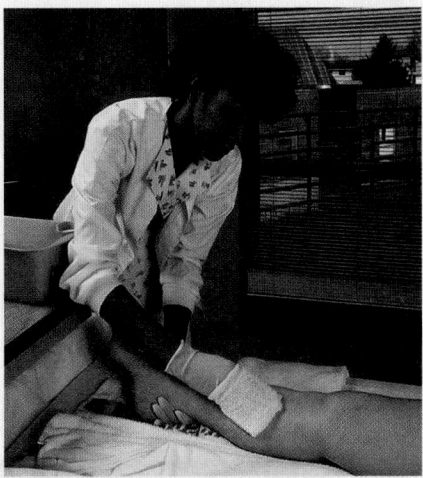

Step 1m(3) ■ Wash patient's leg.

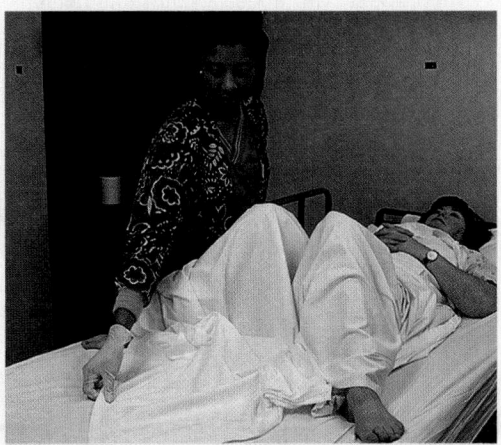

Step 1o(2)(a) ■ Drape the patient for perineal care.

| SKILL 28-1 | BATHING AND PERINEAL CARE—cont'd |

STEP	RATIONALE
(c) Wash labia majora. Use nondominant hand to gently retract labia from thigh: with dominant hand, wash carefully in skin folds. Wipe in direction from perineum to rectum. Repeat on opposite side using separate section of washcloth. Rinse and dry area thoroughly.	Perineal care involves thorough cleansing of the patient's external genitalia and surrounding skin. Skin folds may contain body secretions that harbor microorganisms. Wiping front to back reduces chance of transmitting fecal organisms to urinary meatus.
(d) Gently separate labia with nondominant hand to expose urethral meatus and vaginal orifice. With dominant hand, wash downward from pubic area toward rectum in one smooth stroke (see illustration). Wash the middle and both sides of the perineum. Use separate section of cloth for each stroke. Cleanse thoroughly around labia minora, clitoris, and vaginal orifice. Avoid placing tension on indwelling catheter if present, and clean area around it thoroughly.	Cleansing method reduces transfer of microorganisms to urinary meatus. (For menstruating women or patients with indwelling catheters, may cleanse with cotton balls.)
(e) Provide catheter care as needed (see Chapter 33).	Cleansing along catheter from exit site reduces incidence of nosocomial urinary infection.
(f) Rinse area thoroughly. May use bedpan and pour warm water over perineal area. Dry thoroughly from front to back.	Rinsing removes soap and microorganisms more effectively than wiping. Retained moisture harbors microorganisms.
(g) Fold lower corner of bath blanket back between patient's legs and over perineum. Ask patient to lower legs and assume comfortable position.	
(3) Male Patient	
(a) Apply new pair of clean gloves. Lower side rail. Assist patient to supine position. Note any restriction in mobility.	Provides full exposure of male genitalia. Position patients who are unable to lie supine on their side.
(b) Fold lower half of bath blanket up to expose upper thighs. Wash and dry thighs.	Buildup of perineal secretions soils surrounding skin surfaces.
(c) Cover thighs with bath towels. Raise bath blanket up to expose genitalia. Gently raise penis and place bath towel underneath. Gently grasp shaft of penis. If patient is uncircumcised, retract foreskin. If patient has an erection, defer procedure until later.	Draping minimizes patient anxiety. Towel prevents moisture from collecting in inguinal area. Gentle but firm handling of penis reduces chance of an erection. Secretions capable of harboring microorganisms collect underneath foreskin.
(d) Wash tip of penis at urethral meatus first. Using circular motion, cleanse from meatus outward (see illustration). Discard washcloth, and repeat with a clean cloth until penis is clean. Rinse and dry gently.	Direction of cleansing moves from area of least contamination to area of most contamination, preventing microorganisms from entering urethra.

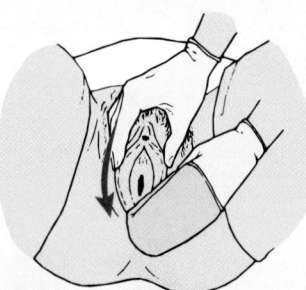

Step 1o(2)(d) ■ Cleanse from perineum to rectum (front to back).

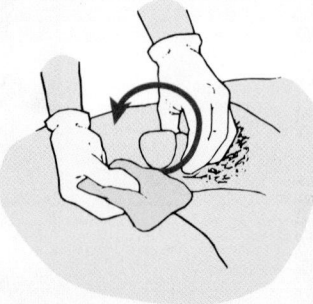

Step 1o(3)(d) ■ Use circular motion to cleanse tip of penis.

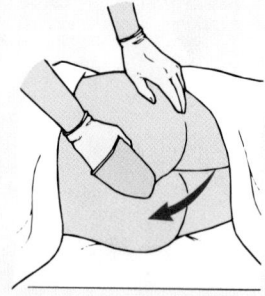

Step 1q(4) ■ Cleanse buttocks from front to back.

STEP	RATIONALE

(e) Return foreskin to its natural position. This is extremely important in patients with decreased sensation in their lower extremities.

Tightening of foreskin around shaft of penis causes local edema and discomfort. Patients with reduced sensation will not feel tightening of foreskin.

(f) Gently cleanse shaft of penis and scrotum by having patient abduct legs. Pay special attention to underlying surface of penis. Lift scrotum carefully, and wash underlying skin folds. Rinse and dry thoroughly.

Vigorous massage of penis may cause an erection. Underlying surface of penis is an area where secretions accumulate. Abduction of legs provides easier access to scrotal tissues. Secretions easily collect between skin folds.

(g) Avoid placing tension on indwelling catheter if present, and clean area around it thoroughly. Provide catheter care (see Chapter 33).

Cleansing along catheter from exit site reduces incidence of nosocomial urinary infection.

p Remove soiled gloves, and throw in trash; raise side rail before leaving bedside to dispose of water and obtain fresh water.

Prevents transmission of infection. Protects patient from injury.

q Wash back. (This follows both female and male perineal care.)

(1) Perform hand hygiene, and apply clean pair of gloves. Lower side rail. Assist patient in assuming prone or side-lying position (as applicable). Place towel lengthwise along patient's side, and keep patient covered with bath blanket.

Exposes back and buttocks for bathing while limiting exposure.

(2) Keep patient draped by sliding bath blanket over shoulders and thighs during bathing. Wash, rinse, and dry back from neck to buttocks using long, firm strokes. Move from back to buttocks and anus. Pay special attention to folds of buttocks and anus.

Cleansing buttocks and anus after back prevents contamination of water.

(3) If fecal material is present, enclose in a fold of underpad or toilet tissue, and remove with disposable wipes.

Skin folds near buttocks and anus may contain fecal secretions that harbor microorganisms.

(4) Cleanse buttocks and anus, washing front to back (see illustration). Cleanse, rinse, and dry area thoroughly. If needed, place a clean absorbent pad under patient's buttocks. Remove contaminated gloves. Raise side rail, and perform hand hygiene.

Cleansing motion prevents contaminating perineal area with fecal material or microorganisms.

(5) Return to bed, and lower side rail; give a back rub.

Promotes patient relaxation. Make sure that a back rub is appropriate for your patient. Back rubs are contraindicated in some patients with cardiac problems.

r Apply additional body lotion or oil to patient's skin as needed.

Moisturizing lotion prevents dry, chapped skin.

s Remove soiled linen, and place in dirty-linen bag. Clean and replace bathing equipment. Perform hand hygiene.

Reduces transmission of microorganisms.

t Assist patient in dressing. Comb patient's hair. Women may want to apply makeup. Assist as needed.

Promotes patient's body image.

u Make patient's bed (see Skill 28-4 and Box 28-14, p. 775).

Provides clean, comfortable environment.

v Check the function and position of external devices (e.g., indwelling urethral catheters, nasogastric tubes, IV lines).

Ensures that systems remain functional after bathing activities.

w Place bed in lowest position.

Maintains patient's safety by deceasing height of bed frame from floor.

x Replace call light and personal possessions. Leave room as clean and comfortable as possible.

Prevents transmission of infection. Clean environment promotes patient's comfort. Keeping call light and articles of care within reach promotes patient's safety.

y Perform hand hygiene.

Reduces transmission of microorganisms.

SKILL 28-1   BATHING AND PERINEAL CARE—cont'd

STEP	RATIONALE

2 Commercial Bag Bath or Cleansing Pack

  a The cleansing pack contains 8 to 10 premoistened towels for cleansing (see illustrations). Warm the package contents in a microwave following package directions.

Provides warm soothing heat.

  b Use a single towel for each general body part cleansed. Follow the same order of cleansing as the total or partial bed bath.

Reduces transmission of microorganisms.

  c Allow the skin to air dry for 30 seconds. It is permissible to lightly cover patient with a bath towel to prevent chilling.

Drying the skin with a towel removes the emollient that is left behind after the water/cleanser solution evaporates.

  d NOTE: If there is excessive soiling (e.g., in the perineal region), use an extra bag bath or conventional washcloths, soap, water, and towels.

3 Tub Bath or Shower

  a Consider patient's condition, and review orders for precautions concerning patient's movement or positioning.

Prevents accidental injury to patient during bathing.

  b Schedule use of shower or tub.

Prevents unnecessary waiting that causes fatigue.

  c Check tub or shower for cleanliness. Use cleaning techniques outlined in agency policy. Place rubber mat on tub or shower bottom. Place disposable bath mat or towel on floor in front of tub or shower.

Cleaning prevents transmission of microorganisms. Mats prevent slipping and falling.

  d Collect all hygienic aids, toiletry items, and linens requested by patient. Place within easy reach of tub or shower.

Placing items close at hand prevents possible falls when patient reaches for them.

  e Help patient to bathroom if necessary. Have patient wear robe and slippers to bathroom.

Assistance prevents accidental falls. Wearing robe and slippers prevents chilling.

  f Demonstrate how to use call signal for assistance.

Bathrooms are equipped with signaling devices in case patient feels faint or weak or needs immediate assistance. Patients prefer privacy during bath if safety is not jeopardized.

  g Place "occupied" sign on bathroom door.

Maintains patient's privacy.

  h Fill bath tub halfway with warm water. Check temperature of bathwater, then have patient test water, and adjust temperature if water is too warm. Explain which faucet controls hot water. If patient is taking shower, turn shower on and adjust water temperature before patient enters shower stall. Use shower seat or tub chair if needed (see illustration).

Adjusting water temperature prevents accidental burns. Older adults and patients with neurological alterations (e.g., diabetes, spinal cord injury) are at high risk for burn as a result of reduced sensation. Use of assistive devices facilitates bathing and minimizes physical exertion.

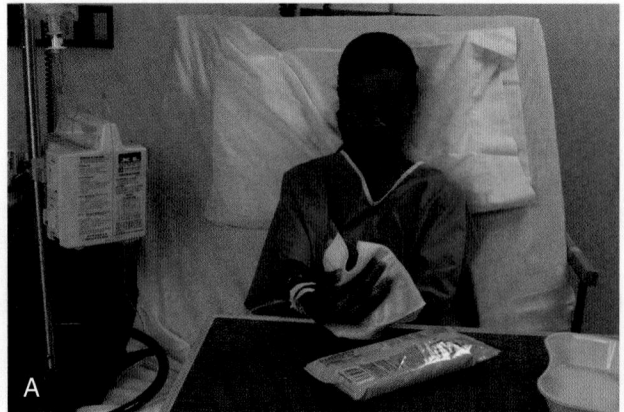

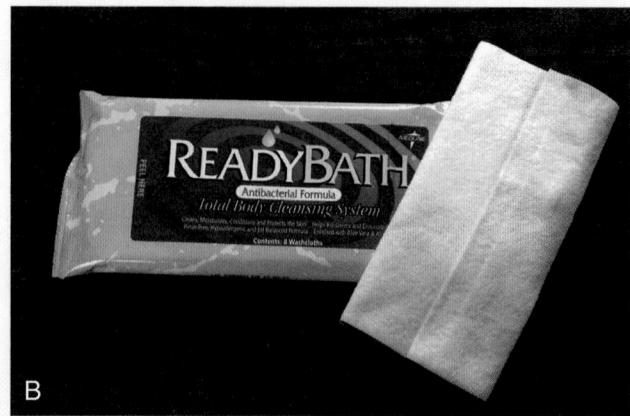

Step 2a ■ Bag bath. **A,** Patient uses individual wipes to bathe. **B,** Bag bath package.

STEP	RATIONALE

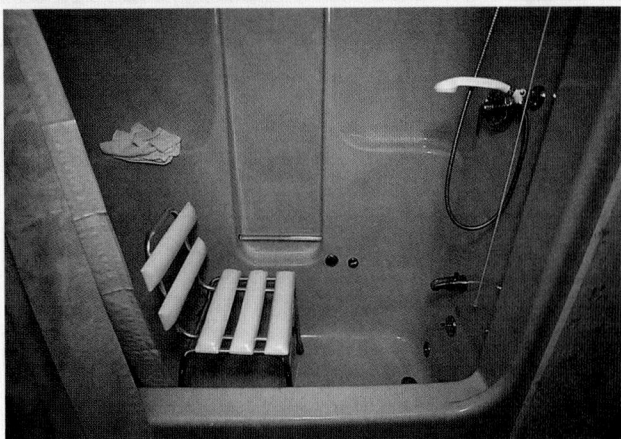

Step 3h ■ Shower seat for patient safety.

i Instruct patient to use safety bars when getting in and out of tub or shower. Also instruct to pull cord to summon assistance (if available). Caution patient against use of bath oil in tub water.

Prevents slipping and falling. Oil causes tub surfaces to become slippery.

j Instruct patient not to remain in tub longer than 10 to 15 minutes. Check on patient every 5 minutes.

Prolonged exposure to warm water causes vasodilation and pooling of blood in some patients, leading to light-headedness or dizziness.

k Return to bathroom when patient signals, and knock before entering.

Provides privacy.

l For patient who is unsteady, drain tub of water before patient attempts to get out of it. Place bath towel over patient's shoulders. Help patient get out of tub as needed, and assist with drying.

Prevents accidental falls. Patient may become chilled as water drains.

• **Critical Decision Point:** Weak or unstable patients need extra assistance getting out of a tub. Planning for additional personnel is essential before attempting to assist the patient from the tub.

---

m Assist patient as needed with getting dressed in a clean gown or pajamas, slippers, and robe. (In home setting, patient may put on regular clothing.)

Maintains warmth to prevent chilling.

n Assist patient to room and comfortable position in bed or chair.

Maintains relaxation gained from bathing.

o Clean tub or shower according to agency policy. Remove soiled linen, and place in dirty-linen bag. Discard disposable equipment in proper receptacle. Place "unoccupied" sign on bathroom door. Return supplies to storage area.

Prevents transmission of infection through soiled linen and moisture.

p Perform hand hygiene.

Reduces transfer of microorganisms.

EVALUATION

1 Observe skin, paying particular attention to areas previously soiled, reddened, dry, or showing early signs of breakdown.

Techniques used during bathing leave skin clean and clear. Over time dry skin will diminish. If patient shows areas of redness, use the Braden Scale to measure risk for pressure ulcers (see Chapter 36).

2 Observe ROM during bath.

Measures joint mobility.

3 Ask patient to rate level of comfort.

Determines patient's tolerance of bathing activities.

4 Ask patient to rate level of fatigue.

Determines patient's tolerance of bathing activities.

SKILL 28-1   BATHING AND PERINEAL CARE—cont'd

RECORDING AND REPORTING

- Record procedure and observations (e.g., breaks in skin, inflammation, ulcerations).

- Report any breaks in skin or ulcerations to nurse in charge or health care provider. These are serious in patients with altered circulation to the lower extremities. Patient may need special foot care treatments.

UNEXPECTED OUTCOMES AND RELATED INTERVENTIONS

- Areas of excessive dryness, rashes, or pressure ulcers appear on skin.
  - Complete pressure ulcer assessment (see Chapter 36).
  - Apply moisturizing lotions or topical skin applications per agency policy.
  - Limit frequency of complete baths.
  - Obtain special bed surface if patient is at risk for skin breakdown.
- Joint ROM decreases.
  - Increase frequency of ROM exercises unless contraindicated.
  - Encourage more self-care by patient.
- Patient becomes excessively fatigued and unable to cooperate or participate in bathing.
  - Reschedule bathing to a time when patient is more rested.
  - Leave pillow or elevate head of bed during bath for patient with breathing difficulties.
  - Notify health care provider if this is a change in patient's fatigue level.

- Patient seems unusually restless or complains of discomfort.
  - Schedule patient rest periods.
  - Consider analgesia if patient complains of pain or discomfort before the bath.
  - Consider use of patient-centered bathing techniques for patients with Alzheimer's or related dementia.
- The rectum, perineum, or genital area is inflamed or swollen or has foul-smelling odor.
  - Bathe perineal area frequently enough to keep clean and dry.
  - Obtain an order for a sitz bath.
  - Apply protective barrier ointment or antiinflammatory cream.
  - Report findings to health care provider.

SKILL 28-2   PROVIDING ORAL HYGIENE

DELEGATION

The skill of performing oral hygiene can be delegated to nursing assistive personnel (NAP). However, the nurse is responsible for the assessment of risk for aspiration. The nurse directs NAP to:
- Position the patient to avoid aspiration
- Immediately report to the nurse excessive patient coughing or choking during or after oral hygiene
- Report any bleeding of oral mucosa or gums, any patient report of pain, or any lesions

EQUIPMENT

- Tongue depressor
- Soft-bristle toothbrush
- Nonabrasive fluoride toothpaste or dentifrice
- Dental floss
- Water glass with cool water
- Normal saline or an essential oil–antiseptic mouth rinse (optional; follow patient preference)
- Emesis basin
- Face towel
- Paper towels
- Clean gloves

STEP	RATIONALE
ASSESSMENT	
1 Perform hand hygiene, and apply clean gloves.	Reduces transmission of microorganisms. Gloves prevent contact with microorganisms in blood or saliva.
2 Instruct patient to not bite down. Then, using a tongue depressor, inspect integrity of lips, teeth, buccal mucosa, gums, palate, and tongue (see Chapter 15).	Determines status of patient's oral cavity and extent of need for oral hygiene.

STEP	RATIONALE
3 Identify presence of common oral problems:	Helps determine type of hygiene patient requires and information patient requires for self-care.
a Dental caries—chalky white discoloration of tooth or presence of brown or black discoloration	
b Gingivitis—inflammation of gums	
c Periodontitis—receding gum lines, inflammation, gaps between teeth	
d Halitosis—bad breath	
e Cheilosis—cracking of lips	
f Stomatitis—inflammation of the mouth	Patients receiving immunosuppressive chemotherapy (e.g., cancer chemotherapy, antirejection medication after organ transplant) or those with suppressed immune function are at risk for stomatitis.
4 Remove gloves, and perform hand hygiene.	Prevents spread of microorganisms.
5 Assess patient's risk for aspiration: impaired swallowing, reduced gag reflex.	Accumulation of secretions and cleansing agent increase patient's risk for aspiration because of reduced ability to control oral secretions.
6 Assess risk for oral hygiene problems (see Table 28-6, p. 758).	Certain conditions increase likelihood of impaired oral cavity integrity and need for preventive care.
7 Remove gloves, and perform hand hygiene.	Prevents transmission of microorganisms.
8 Determine patient's oral hygiene practices and willingness to attend to hygiene needs:	
a Frequency of toothbrushing and flossing	Identifies errors in patient's technique, deficiencies in preventive oral hygiene, and patient's level of knowledge regarding dental care.
b Type of toothpaste or dentifrice used	Toothpaste needs to contain fluoride.
c Last dental visit	Provides reference for subsequent visits.
d Frequency of dental visits	American Dental Association recommends regular visits to the dentist for professional cleanings and oral examinations at least twice a year (American Dental Association, 2008).
e Type of mouth rinse or moistening preparation	Lemon-glycerin preparations are harmful. Glycerin is an astringent that dries and shrinks mucous membranes and gums. Lemon exhausts salivary reflex and erodes tooth enamel. Mouthwash provides pleasant aftertaste but dries mucosa after extended use if it has an alcohol base. An essential oil–antiseptic mouthwash such as Cool Mint Listerine is effective in reducing plaque and gingivitis (Bauroth and others, 2003). However, mouthwashes are not a replacement for flossing (American Dental Association, 2008).
9 Assess patient's ability to grasp and manipulate toothbrush. Assessment determines level of assistance required from you.	Older adult patients or persons with musculoskeletal or nervous system alterations are sometimes unable to hold toothbrush with firm grip or manipulate brush.
PLANNING	
1 Explain procedure to patient, discussing preferences regarding use of hygiene aids.	Some patients feel uncomfortable about having you care for their basic needs. Patient involvement with procedure minimizes anxiety.
2 Place paper towels on over-bed table, and arrange other equipment within easy reach.	Creates organized work space.
IMPLEMENTATION	
1 Raise bed to comfortable working position. Raise head of bed (if allowed), and lower side rail. Move patient or help patient move closer. Use side-lying position if needed.	Raising bed and positioning patient prevent you from straining muscles. Semi-Fowler's position helps prevent patient from choking or aspirating.
2 Place towel over patient's chest.	Prevents soiling of patient's gown.
3 Apply clean gloves.	Prevents contact with microorganisms or blood in saliva.
4 Apply enough toothpaste to brush to cover length of bristles. Hold brush over emesis basin. Pour small amount of water over toothpaste.	Moisture aids in distribution of toothpaste over tooth surfaces.

SKILL 28-2   PROVIDING ORAL HYGIENE—cont'd

STEP	RATIONALE
5 Patient may assist with brushing. Hold toothbrush bristles at 45-degree angle to gum line. Be sure tips of bristles rest against and penetrate under gum line. Brush inner and outer surfaces of upper and lower teeth by brushing from gum to crown of each tooth. Clean biting surfaces of teeth by holding top of bristles parallel with teeth and brushing gently back and forth (see illustration). Brush sides of teeth by moving bristles back and forth (see illustrations).	Angle allows brush to reach all tooth surfaces and to clean under gum line, where plaque and tartar accumulate. Back-and-forth motion dislodges food particles caught between teeth and along chewing surfaces.
6 Have patient hold brush at 45-degree angle and lightly brush over surface and sides of tongue. Avoid initiating gag reflex.	Microorganisms collect and grow on tongue's surface and contribute to bad breath. Gagging will sometimes cause aspiration of toothpaste.
7 Allow patient to rinse mouth thoroughly by taking several sips of water (may use straw), swishing water across all tooth surfaces, and spitting into emesis basin.	Irrigation removes food particles.
8 Have patient rinse teeth with antiseptic mouth rinse for 30 seconds. Then have patient spit rinse into emesis basin.	Mouth rinse leaves a pleasant taste but dries mucosa after extended use if it has an alcohol base. Using an essential oil–antiseptic mouth rinse a minimum of twice daily is at least as effective as flossing daily in reducing plaque and gingivitis (Bauroth and others, 2003).
9 Assist in wiping patient's mouth.	Promotes sense of comfort.
10 Allow patient to floss. Floss between all teeth. Hold floss against tooth while moving floss up and down sides of teeth and under gum line.	Reduces tartar on tooth surfaces and prevents gum disease. The American Dental Association (2008) recommends flossing once daily.
11 Allow patient to rinse mouth thoroughly with cool water and spit into emesis basin. Assist in wiping patient's mouth.	Irrigation removes plaque and tartar from oral cavity.
12 Wipe off over-bed table, discard soiled linen and paper towels in appropriate containers, remove and discard soiled gloves, raise side rail, and return bed to low position.	Proper disposal of soiled equipment prevents spread of infection.
13 Perform hand hygiene.	Prevents spread of microorganisms.
14 Assist patient to comfortable position, and lower bed to original position. Return supplies to appropriate location.	Provides for patient comfort and safety.

EVALUATION

1 Ask patient if any area of oral cavity feels uncomfortable or irritated.	Pain indicates more chronic problem.
2 Apply gloves, and inspect condition of oral cavity.	Determines effectiveness of hygiene and rinsing.
3 Ask patient to describe proper hygiene techniques.	Evaluates patient's learning.
4 Observe patient brushing and flossing.	Evaluates patient's ability to use correct technique.

RECORDING AND REPORTING

- Record procedure on flow sheet. Note condition of oral cavity in nurses' notes.

- Report bleeding or presence of lesions to nurse in charge or health care provider.

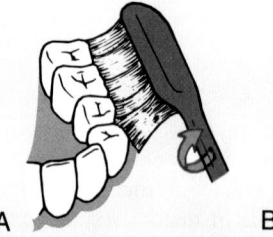 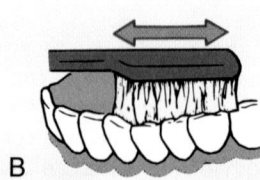 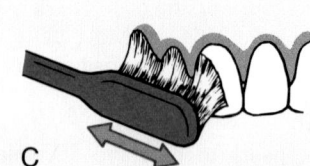

Step 5 ■ Direction for toothbrush placement. **A,** Forty-five degree angle brushes gum line. **B,** Parallel position brushes biting surfaces. **C,** Lateral position brushes side of teeth.

UNEXPECTED OUTCOMES AND RELATED INTERVENTIONS

- Mucosa is dry and inflamed. Tongue has thick coating.
  - Increase patient's hydration.
  - Apply protectant to patient's lips.
  - Increase frequency of oral hygiene, including tongue brushing.
- Gum margins are retracted from teeth, with localized areas of inflammation. Bleeding occurs around gum margins.
  - Report findings because patient may have an underlying bleeding tendency.
  - Use a soft-bristle toothbrush.
  - Avoid too vigorous brushing and flossing.
  - Increase frequency of oral hygiene.

- Teeth show signs of dental caries.
  - Review patient's hygiene routines at home.
  - Refer patient to dentist upon order from health care provider.
  - Teach patient proper oral hygiene.

SKILL 28-3   PERFORMING MOUTH CARE FOR AN UNCONSCIOUS OR DEBILITATED PATIENT

DELEGATION CONSIDERATIONS

The skill of performing mouth care of an unconscious or debilitated patient can be delegated to nursing assistive personnel (NAP). However, the nurse is responsible for assessment of the patient's risk for aspiration before care, including determining presence of gag reflex. The nurse instructs NAP about:

- Proper positioning of patient to lessen chance of aspiration
- Using oral suction catheter for clearing oral secretions (see Chapter 29, Skill 29-1)
- Signs of impaired integrity of oral mucosa and report to nurse.
- Reporting any bleeding of mucosa or gums, painful reaction by patient, or excessive coughing or choking to the nurse

EQUIPMENT

- Small pediatric soft-bristled toothbrush
- Antiinfective solution (e.g., commercial diluted hydrogen peroxide and sodium bicarbonate solution) that loosens crusts; check agency policy
- Antibacterial solution (e.g., chlorhexidine) (requires a health care provider's order)
- Tongue blade
- Small oral airway (optional)
- Face towel
- Paper towels
- Emesis basin
- Water glass with cool water
- Water-soluble lip lubricant
- Small-bulb syringe or suction machine equipment (required for patients with poor or absent gag reflex)
- Clean gloves

STEP	RATIONALE

ASSESSMENT

1 Perform hand hygiene. Apply clean gloves.

Reduces transmission of microorganisms. Gloves prevent contact with microorganisms in blood or saliva.

2 Assess patient's risk for oral hygiene problems (see Table 28-6, p. 758).

Impaired level of consciousness increases the likelihood of alterations in integrity of oral cavity structures and requires more frequent care.

3 Test for presence of gag reflex by placing tongue blade on back half of tongue.

Reveals whether patient is at risk for aspiration.

- **Critical Decision Point:** Patients with impaired gag reflex require oral care as well. Determine the type of suction apparatus needed at the bedside to protect the patient's airway against aspiration.

---

4 Inspect condition of oral cavity (see Chapter 15).
5 Remove gloves. Perform hand hygiene.

Determines condition of oral cavity and need for hygiene.
Prevents transmission of microorganisms.

PLANNING

1 Explain procedure to patient, even if patient is unconscious.

Allows debilitated patient to anticipate procedure without anxiety. Unconscious patients sometimes retain the ability to hear.

PERFORMING MOUTH CARE FOR AN UNCONSCIOUS OR DEBILITATED PATIENT—cont'd

STEP	RATIONALE
2 Collect appropriate equipment.	Prevents interruptions during procedure.
3 Place paper towels on over-bed table, and arrange equipment. If needed, turn on suction machine, and connect tubing to suction catheter.	Prevents soiling of table top. Equipment prepared in advance ensures smooth, safe procedure.

IMPLEMENTATION

1 Unless contraindicated (e.g., head injury, neck trauma), raise bed, lower side rail, and position patient close to side of bed; turn patient's head toward mattress. Patient can also be placed on side in Sims' position. Raise side rail.	Allows secretions to drain from mouth instead of collecting in back of pharynx. Prevents aspiration. Moving the patient to the side of the bed facilitates proper body mechanics during the skill. Use of good body mechanics with bed in high position reduces risk for injury to nurse. Proper use of side rail protects caregiver from straining and provides for patient safety.
2 Apply clean gloves.	Reduces transfer of microorganisms.
3 Pull curtain around bed, or close room door.	Provides privacy.
4 Lower side rail.	Prevents straining to reach.
5 Place towel under patient's head and emesis basin under chin.	Prevents soiling of bed linen.
6 Remove dentures or partial plates if present.	Allows for thorough cleansing of prosthetics later. Provides clearer access to oral cavity.
7 If patient is unconscious, uncooperative, or having difficulty keeping mouth open, insert an oral airway. Insert upside down, then turn the airway sideways and then over tongue to keep teeth apart. Insert when patient is relaxed, if possible. Do not use force (see illustration).	Prevents patient from biting down on your fingers and provides access to oral cavity.

- **Critical Decision Point:** Never place fingers into the mouth of an unconscious or debilitated patient. The normal response is to bite down.

---

8 Clean mouth using brush moistened with dental cleansing agent, such as commercial diluted hydrogen peroxide and sodium bicarbonate solution or chlorhexidine, if prescribed. Clean chewing and inner tooth surfaces first. Clean outer tooth surfaces. Moisten brush with water to rinse. Use swab or toothette to clean roof of mouth, gums, and inside cheeks. Gently swab or brush tongue but avoid stimulating gag reflex (if present). Moisten clean swab or toothette with water to rinse. (Use bulb syringe to remove rinse.) Repeat rinse several times.	Brushing action removes food particles between teeth and along chewing surfaces. Swabbing helps remove secretions and crusts from mucosa and moistens mucosa. Repeated rinsing removes peroxide, which is irritating to mucosa, and debris. Hydrogen peroxide and sodium bicarbonate effectively remove debris, but if not diluted carefully may cause superficial burns (Munro and Grap, 2004).

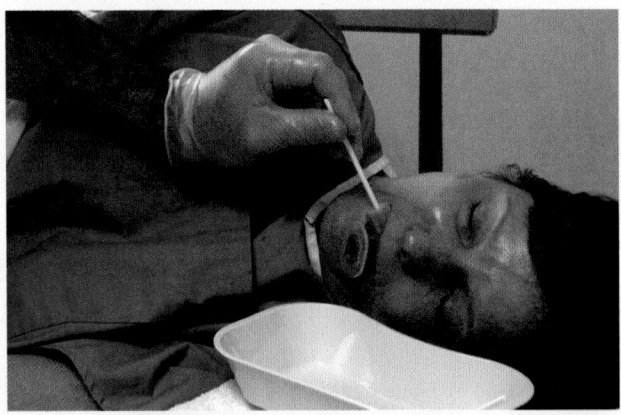

Step 7 ■ Insertion of oral airway.

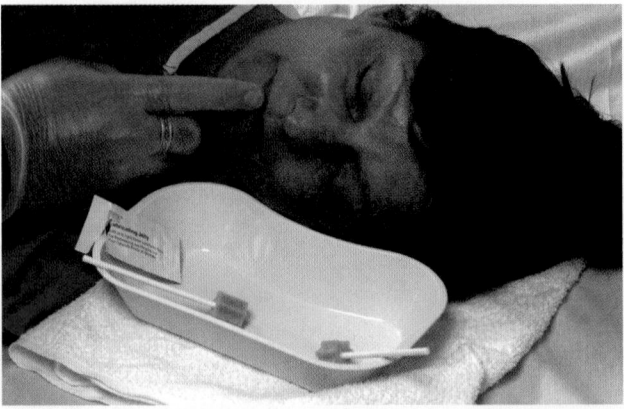

Step 11 ■ Application of water-soluble moisturizer to lips.

STEP	RATIONALE
9 For patients without teeth, use a toothette moistened in water or normal saline to clean oral cavity.	Less traumatic to mucosa of gums.
10 Suction oral secretions as they accumulate if needed.	Suction removes secretions and fluid that collect in posterior pharynx.
11 Apply thin layer of water-soluble jelly to lips (see illustration).	Lubricates lips to prevent drying and cracking.
12 Inform patient that procedure is completed.	Provides meaningful stimulation to unconscious or less-responsive patient.
13 Remove gloves, and dispose of in proper receptacle. Raise side rail. Perform hand hygiene.	Prevents transmission of microorganisms to environmental surfaces (e.g., side rails, patient's linens). Reduces risk for patient injury.
14 Reposition patient comfortably, raise side rail, and return bed to original position.	Maintains patient's comfort and safety. Raising all four side rails is considered a restraint; you will need a health care provider's order.
15 Apply clean gloves to cleanse equipment. Return supplies to proper place. Place soiled linen in proper receptacle.	Proper disposal of soiled equipment prevents spread of infection.
16 Remove soiled gloves and discard. Perform hand hygiene.	Reduces transmission of microorganisms.

EVALUATION

1 Apply gloves, and inspect oral cavity.	Determines efficacy of cleansing. Once you remove thick secretions, you will see if any underlying inflammation or lesions remain.
2 Remove gloves, and dispose of in proper receptacle. Perform hand hygiene.	Prevents transmission of microorganisms.
3 Ask debilitated patient if mouth feels clean.	Evaluates level of comfort.
4 Evaluate patient's respirations, and auscultate lung sounds on an ongoing basis.	Ensures early recognition of aspiration.

RECORDING AND REPORTING

- Record procedure, including pertinent observations (e.g., presence of bleeding gums, dry mucosa, ulcerations, crusts on tongue).

- Report any unusual findings to nurse in charge or health care provider.

UNEXPECTED OUTCOMES AND RELATED INTERVENTIONS

- Secretions or crusts remain on mucosa, tongue, or gums.
  - Increase frequency of oral hygiene care.
  - Use a pediatric-size toothbrush to provide better hygiene.
- Localized inflammation of gums or mucosa is present.
  - Increase frequency of oral hygiene care using a soft-bristled brush.
  - Apply water-soluble moisturizing gel to mucosa, and massage.

- Lips are cracked or inflamed.
  - Apply water soluble moisturizing gel or lubricant to lips.
- Patient aspirates secretions.
  - Suction oral airway as secretions accumulate to maintain patent airway (see Chapter 29).
  - Perform tracheal bronchial suctioning.
  - Notify health care provider immediately.
  - Elevate patient's head of bed to facilitate breathing.
  - Be prepared to have chest x-ray examination ordered by health care provider.

SKILL 28-4   MAKING AN OCCUPIED BED

DELEGATION CONSIDERATIONS

The skill of making an occupied bed can be delegated to nursing assistive personnel (NAP). Before delegating this skill the nurse will instruct NAP about:

- Any precautions or activity restrictions for the patient
- Looking for wound drainage, dressing material, drainage tubes, or IV tubing that becomes dislodged or is found in the linens
- What to do if patient becomes fatigued

EQUIPMENT (Figure 28-4)

- Linen bag(s)
- Mattress pad (*optional* depending on facility practice; changed only when soiled)
- Bottom sheet (flat or fitted)
- Drawsheet
- Top sheet
- Blanket
- Bedspread
- Waterproof pads and/or bath blankets (*optional*)
- Pillowcases
- Bedside chair or table
- Clean gloves (*optional*)
- Towel
- Disinfectant

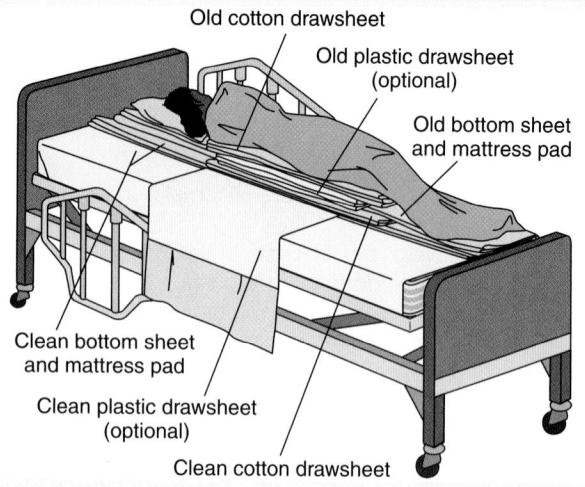

Old cotton drawsheet
Old plastic drawsheet (optional)
Old bottom sheet and mattress pad
Clean bottom sheet and mattress pad
Clean plastic drawsheet (optional)
Clean cotton drawsheet

Figure 28-4 ■ Equipment for making an occupied bed.

STEP	RATIONALE

ASSESSMENT

1 Assess potential for patient incontinence or for excess drainage on bed linen.

2 Check chart for orders or specific precautions concerning movement and positioning.

Determines need for protective waterproof pads or extra bath blankets on bed.

Ensures patient safety and use of proper body mechanics.

PLANNING

1 Explain procedure to the patient, noting that the patient will be asked to turn on side and roll over linen.

Minimizes anxiety and promotes cooperation.

IMPLEMENTATION

1 Perform hand hygiene, and apply clean gloves (wear gloves only if linen is soiled or there is risk for contact with body secretions).

Reduces transmission of microorganisms.

2 Assemble equipment, and arrange on clean bedside chair or table. Remove unnecessary equipment such as a dietary tray or items used for hygiene. Do not let clean linen touch your uniform.

Assembling all equipment provides for smooth procedure and assists in increasing patient's comfort. Placing linen on clean surface minimizes spread of infection. Uniform is less clean than clean linens.

3 Pull room curtain around bed and/or close door.

Maintains patient's privacy.

4 Adjust bed height to comfortable working position. Lower any raised side rail on one side of bed. Remove call light.

Minimizes strain on back. It is easier to remove and apply linen evenly to bed in flat position. Provides easy access to bed and linen.

5 Loosen top linen at foot of bed.

Makes linen easier to remove.

6 Remove bedspread and blanket separately. If spread and blanket are soiled, place them in linen bag. Keep soiled linen away from uniform.

Reduces transmission of microorganisms.

7 If blanket and spread are reused, fold them by bringing the top and bottom edges together. Fold farthest side over onto nearer bottom edge. Bring top and bottom edges together again. Place folded linen over back of chair.

Folding method facilitates replacement and prevents wrinkles.

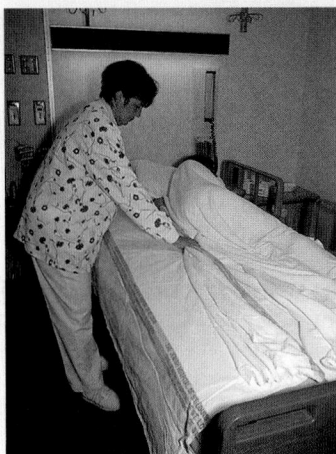

Step 11 ■ Old linen tucked under patient.   **Step 13b** ■ Clean linen applied to bed.

STEP	RATIONALE
8 Cover patient with bath blanket as follows: Unfold bath blanket over top sheet. Ask patient to hold top edge of bath blanket. If patient is unable to help, tuck top of bath blanket under shoulders. Grasp top sheet under bath blanket at patient's shoulders and bring sheet down to foot of bed. Remove sheet and discard in linen bag.	Bath blanket provides warmth and keeps body parts covered during linen removal.
9 With assistance, slide mattress toward head of bed.	If mattress slides toward foot of bed when head of bed is raised, it is difficult to tuck in linen. In addition, it is uncomfortable for the patient because the patient's feet will press against or hang over the foot of the bed.
10 Position patient on the far side of the bed, turned onto side and facing away from you. Be sure side rail in front of patient is up. Adjust pillow under patient's head.	Turning patient onto side provides space for placement of clean linen. Side rail ensures patient's safety by preventing forward falls from the bed surface and helps patient in moving.
11 Loosen bottom linens, moving from head to foot. With seam side down (facing the mattress), fanfold bottom sheet and drawsheet toward patient—first drawsheet, then bottom sheet. Tuck edges of linen just under buttocks, back, and shoulders. Do not fanfold mattress pad if it is to be reused (see illustration).	Prepares for removal of all bottom linen simultaneously. Provides maximum work space for placing clean linen. Later, when patient turns to the other side, you can remove soiled linen easily.
12 Wipe off any moisture on exposed mattress with towel and appropriate disinfectant. Make sure mattress surface is dry before applying clean linens.	Reduces transmission of microorganisms.
13 Apply clean linen to exposed half of bed:	
a Place clean mattress pad on bed by folding it lengthwise with center crease in middle of bed. Fanfold top layer over mattress. (If you reuse pad, simply smooth out any wrinkles.)	Applying linen over bed in successive layers minimizes energy and time used in bed making.
b Unfold clean bottom sheet lengthwise so that center crease is situated lengthwise along center of bed. Fanfold sheet's top layer toward center of bed alongside the patient. Smooth bottom layer of sheet over mattress, and bring edge over closest side of mattress. Pull fitted sheet smoothly over mattress ends. Allow edge of flat unfitted sheet to hang about 25 cm (10 inches) over mattress edge. Lower hem of bottom flat sheet lies seam down and even with bottom edge of mattress (see illustration).	Proper positioning of linen on one side ensures that adequate linen will be available to cover opposite side of bed. Keeping seam edges down eliminates irritation to patient's skin.
14 If flat sheet is used for bottom sheet, miter bottom flat sheet at head of bed:	Ensures secure flat sheet will not loosen easily.

| SKILL 28-4 | MAKING AN OCCUPIED BED—cont'd |

STEP	RATIONALE
a Face head of bed diagonally. Place hand away from head of bed under top corner of mattress, near mattress edge, and lift.	
b With other hand, tuck top edge of bottom sheet smoothly under mattress so that side edges of sheet above and below mattress meet when brought together.	
c Face side of bed and pick up top edge of sheet at approximately 45 cm (18 inches) from top end of mattress (see illustration).	
d Lift sheet, and lay it on top of mattress to form a neat triangular fold, with lower base of triangle even with mattress side edge (see illustration).	
e Tuck lower edge of sheet, which is hanging free below the mattress, under mattress. Tuck with palms down, without pulling triangular fold (see illustration).	
f Hold portion of sheet covering side of mattress in place with one hand. With the other hand, pick up top of triangular linen fold and bring it down over side of mattress (see illustrations). Tuck this portion under mattress (see illustration).	Mitered corners help sheet stay in place even if patient moves frequently in bed.
15 Tuck remaining portion of sheet under mattress, moving toward foot of bed. Keep linen smooth.	Folds of linen are source of irritation.
16 *Optional:* Open clean drawsheet so that it unfolds in half. Lay center fold along middle of bed lengthwise, and position sheet so that it will be under the patient's buttocks and torso (see illustration). Fanfold top layer toward patient, with edge along patient's back. Smooth bottom layer out over mattress, and tuck excess edge under mattress (keep palms down).	You will use drawsheet to lift and reposition patient. Placement under patient's torso distributes most of patient's body weight over sheet.
17 Place waterproof pad over drawsheet, with center fold against patient's side. Fanfold top layer toward patient.	Protects bed linen from being soiled.
18 Advise patient that he or she will be rolling over thick layer of linens and will feel a lump. Have patient roll slowly toward you, over the layers of linen. Raise side rail on working side, and go to other side.	Positions patient for removal of old linen and placement of new linens. Maintains patient's safety and body alignment during turning.

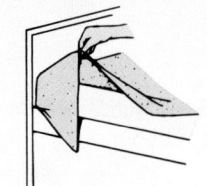

Step 14c ■ Top edge of sheet picked up.

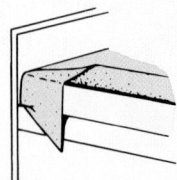

Step 14d ■ Sheet on top of mattress in a triangular fold.

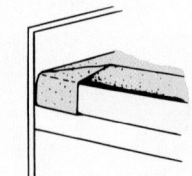

Step 14e ■ Lower edge of sheet tucked under mattress.

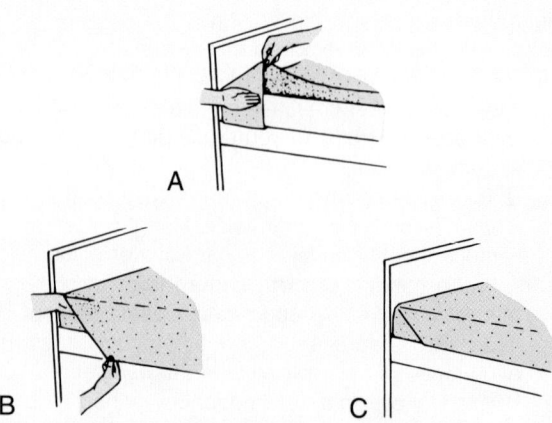

Step 14f ■ **A** and **B,** Triangular fold placed over side of mattress. **C,** Linen tucked under mattress.

STEP	RATIONALE
19 Lower side rail. Assist patient in positioning on other side, over folds of linen. Loosen edges of soiled linen from under mattress (see illustration).	Exposes opposite side of bed for removal of soiled linen and placement of clean linen. Makes linen easier to remove.
20 Remove soiled linen by folding it into a bundle or square, with soiled side turned in. Discard in linen bag. If necessary, wipe mattress with antiseptic solution, and dry mattress surface before applying new linen.	Reduces transmission of microorganisms.
21 Pull clean, fanfolded linen smoothly over edge of mattress from head to foot of bed.	Smooth linen will not irritate patient's skin.
22 Assist patient in rolling back into supine position. Reposition pillow.	Maintains patient's comfort.
23 Pull fitted sheet smoothly over mattress ends. Miter top corner of bottom sheet (see Step 14). When tucking corner, be sure that sheet is smooth and free of wrinkles.	Wrinkles and folds cause irritation to skin.
24 Facing side of bed, grasp remaining edge of bottom flat sheet. Lean back, keep back straight, and pull while tucking excess linen under mattress. Proceed from head to foot of bed. (Avoid lifting mattress during tucking to ensure fit.)	Proper use of body mechanics while tucking linen prevents injury.
25 Smooth fanfolded drawsheet out over bottom sheet. Grasp edge of sheet with palms down, lean back, and tuck sheet under mattress. Tuck from middle to top and then to bottom.	Tucking first at top or bottom pulls sheet sideways, causing poor fit.
26 Place top sheet over patient with center fold lengthwise down middle of bed. Open sheet from head to foot, and unfold over patient.	Correctly positioning center fold distributes sheet equally over bed.
27 Ask patient to hold clean top sheet, or tuck sheet around patient's shoulders. Remove bath blanket, and discard in linen bag.	Sheet prevents exposure of body parts. Having patient hold sheet encourages patient participation in care.
28 Place blanket on bed, unfolding it so that crease runs lengthwise along middle of bed. Unfold blanket to cover patient. Make sure top edge is parallel with edge of top sheet and 15 to 20 cm (6 to 8 inches) from top sheet's edge.	Place blanket to cover patient completely and provide adequate warmth.
29 Place spread over bed according to Step 28. Be sure that top edge of spread extends about 2.5 cm (1 inch) above blanket's edge. Tuck top edge of spread over and under top edge of blanket.	Gives bed neat appearance and provides extra warmth.
30 Make cuff by turning edge of top sheet down over top edge of blanket and spread.	Protect patient's face from rubbing against blanket or spread.

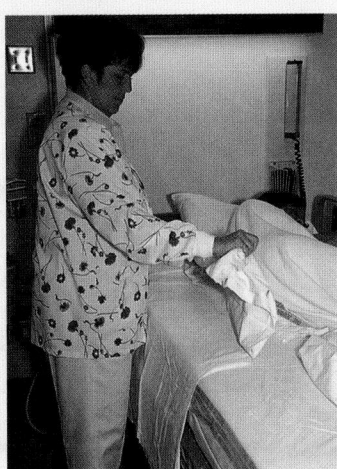

Step 16 ■ Optional drawsheet.

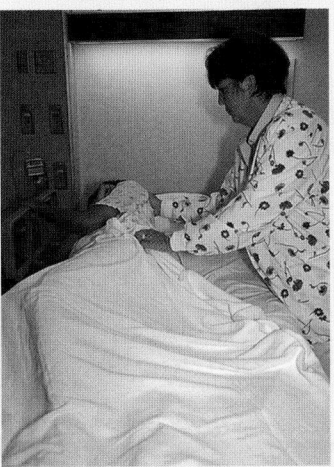

Step 19 ■ Assisting patient with rolling over folds of linen.

SKILL 28-4   MAKING AN OCCUPIED BED—cont'd

STEP	RATIONALE
31 Standing on one side at foot of bed, lift mattress corner slightly with one hand and tuck linens under mattress. Tuck top sheet, blanket, and spread under together. Be sure that linens are loose enough to allow movement of patient's feet. Making a horizontal toe pleat is an option.	Makes neat-appearing bed. Pressure ulcers develop on patient's toes and heels from feet rubbing against tight-fitting bed sheets.
32 Make modified mitered corner with top sheet, blanket, and spread (see illustration in Box 28-14, p. 775).	Ensures top covers will not loosen easily.
a Pick up side edge of top sheet, blanket, and spread approximately 45 cm (18 inches) from foot of mattress. Lift linen to form triangular fold, and lay it on bed.	
b Tuck lower edge of sheet, which is hanging free below mattress, under mattress. Do not pull triangular fold.	
c Pick up triangular fold, and bring it down over mattress while holding linen in place along side of mattress. Do not tuck tip of triangle.	Secures top linen but keeps even edge of blanket and top sheet draped over mattress.
33 Raise side rail. Make other side of bed; spread sheet, blanket, and bedspread out evenly. Fold top edge of spread over blanket and make cuff with top sheet (see Step 30); make modified mitered corner at foot of bed (see Step 32).	Side rail protects patient from accidental falls and aids patient's movement in bed.
34 Change pillowcase(s):	
a Have patient raise head. While supporting neck with one hand, remove pillow. Allow patient to lower head.	Support of neck muscles prevents injury during flexion and extension of neck.
b Remove soiled case by grasping pillow at open end with one hand and pulling case back over pillow with the other hand. Discard case in linen bag.	Pillows slide out easily, thus minimizing contact with soiled linen.
c Grasp clean pillowcase at center of closed end. Gather case, turning it inside out over the hand holding it. With the same hand, pick up middle of one end of the pillow. Pull pillowcase down over pillow with the other hand. Do not hold pillow against your uniform while changing the pillowcase.	Eases sliding of pillowcase over pillow. Prevents transfer of microorganisms from uniform to clean pillow case.
d Be sure pillow corners fit evenly into corners of pillowcase. Place pillow under patient's head.	Poorly fitting case constricts fluffing and expansion of pillow and interferes with patient comfort.
35 Place call light within patient's reach, and return bed to comfortable position and in low horizontal position.	Ensures patient safety and comfort.
36 Open room curtains, and rearrange furniture. Place personal items within easy reach on over-bed table or bedside stand.	Promotes sense of well-being.
37 Discard dirty linen bag in hamper or chute, and perform hand hygiene.	Prevents transmission of microorganisms.
38 Ask if patient feels comfortable.	Ensures bed linens are clean and smooth.

EVALUATION

1 Inspect skin for areas of irritation.	Folds in linen cause pressure on skin.
2 Observe patient for signs of fatigue, dyspnea, pain, or discomfort.	Provides you with data about patient's level of activity tolerance and ability to participate in other procedures.

RECORDING AND REPORTING

- It is not necessary to record the making of an occupied bed.

UNEXPECTED OUTCOMES AND RELATED INTERVENTIONS

- Patient feels discomfort from linen fold.
  - Tighten sheets.
  - Change patient's position frequently.

- Patient's skin shows signs of breakdown.
  - Institute skin care measures to reduce risk for pressure ulcer (see Chapter 36).
  - Change patient's position more frequently.

KEY POINTS

- Various personal, sociocultural, economic, and developmental factors influence patients' hygiene practices.
- Incorporate knowledge of the factors influencing the individual patient's hygiene practices into hygiene care.
- Assess the patient's physical and cognitive ability to perform hygiene self-care, and provide care according to the patient's needs and preferences.
- Integrate other activities such as physical assessment, wound care, teaching, and range-of-motion exercises while providing hygiene care.
- While providing daily hygiene needs, use communication skills and teaching to develop a caring relationship with the patient.
- Maintain privacy, comfort, and patient safety when providing hygiene care.
- Wear gloves during hygiene care when the risk for contacting body fluids or nonintact skin or mucosal surfaces

is present; always wear gloves during perineal care and when performing oral care.
- When providing oral care for a debilitated or unconscious patient, take precautions to prevent aspiration.
- Providing oral care for at-risk patients can help decrease the incidence of pneumonia.
- Patients who are immobilized and poorly nourished and who have reduced sensation or peripheral circulation are at risk for altered skin integrity; these patients require special nail, foot, and skin care.
- Administer symptom-relief therapies for complaints such as pain or nausea before hygiene care to enable the patient to better tolerate and participate in care.
- Base evaluation of hygiene care on the patient's sense of comfort, relaxation, well-being, and understanding of hygiene techniques.

CRITICAL THINKING EXERCISES

Mrs. Winkler's daughter is visiting her today at the nursing home. Jamie, the nursing student, enters the room and finds Carol, Mrs. Winkler's daughter, preparing a basin of water for her mother to soak her feet. Jamie introduces herself to Carol. Carol states, "Mom needs a good pedicure, so I'm going to soak her feet in hot water before I clip her nails. She likes for me to polish her nails."

1. Which response or action by Jamie is the appropriate initial response to Carol's statement?
   a. Sit down and help Mrs. Winkler and Carol pick out a nail polish color.
   b. "Oh my gosh! You shouldn't soak her feet."
   c. Explain why you should not soak the feet in hot water.
   d. Check with Mrs. Winkler's nurse to see if it is okay to soak her feet.
2. What assessment does Jamie need to do before helping Mrs. Winkler and Carol continue with foot care?
   a. Measure blood glucose level at the bedside.
   b. Observe condition of feet and nails.
   c. Ask Mrs. Winkler about her last bowel movement.
   d. Observe condition of oral mucosa

Jamie assesses Mrs. Winkler's feet and finds the following: dry skin, especially between toes and on heels; decreased touch and

temperature sensation in both feet; long, curving nails; and a tender area on the left little toe.

3. Which of the following points does Jamie need to include when teaching Mrs. Winkler and her daughter Carol about foot care? Select all that apply.
   a. Use nail clippers to trim nails.
   b. File nail edges smooth.
   c. Dry feet carefully after washing, especially between toes.
   d. Never walk barefoot.
   e. Report minor foot injuries immediately for treatment.
   f. Use over-the-counter treatments for corn removal.
4. Jamie helps wash Mrs. Winkler's feet and applies a lanolin cream. What approach should Jamie take regarding trimming Mrs. Winkler's toenails?
   a. Collaborate with Mrs. Winkler's nurse to obtain a podiatrist consultation order.
   b. Carefully cut the nails using nail scissors.
   c. File the long, curving nails.
   d. Ask Carol to trim the nails.

evolve *Answers to Critical Thinking Questions can be found on the Evolve website.*

REVIEW QUESTIONS

1. You are assisting a patient with rheumatoid arthritis to bathe at the sink. During the bath the patient complains of being tired; you notice the patient is breathing rapidly and the pulse is rapid. Select the most appropriate response.
   1. Hurry up and finish the bath quickly.
   2. Help the patient return to bed.

   3. Leave the patient to rest in the chair at the sink for a few minutes.
   4. Instruct the patient to take deep breaths and try to relax.
2. You are assigned to provide hygiene care for a cognitively impaired patient with dementia. You are told the patient often displays aggressive behavior such as screaming and hitting during the bath. What techniques do you select to

make the bathing experience less stressful for both you and the patient? Select all that apply.
1. Allow the patient to perform as much of the care as possible.
2. Start by washing the face.
3. Try an alternative to traditional bathing such as the "towel bath."
4. Use restraints to prevent the patient from injuring self or you.

3. What is the priority concern when providing oral hygiene for the unconscious patient?
1. Thoroughly brushing all tooth and oral surfaces
2. Preventing aspiration
3. Controlling mouth odor
4. Applying local antiseptic such as chlorhexidine

4. A male nurse is caring for a 32-year-old female Muslim patient who has an indwelling Foley catheter. After introducing himself to the patient, the nurse learns that the patient does not want him to help her with personal hygiene care. Which of the following are appropriate actions? Select all that apply.
1. Find out if a female nurse can help the patient.
2. Convince the patient he will work quickly and provide as much privacy as possible.
3. Skip hygiene care for the day except for the parts the patient can complete independently
4. Ask the patient if a family member can assist with the care.

5. You are helping a female patient bathe. As you are about to perform perineal care, the patient says, "I can finish my bath." The patient has been complaining of some discomfort and burning in the perineal area. What action do you need to take initially?
1. Explain to the patient that because of her symptoms you need to observe the area.
2. Insist that you are supposed to complete the care.
3. Honor the patient's request to complete her own perineal care to avoid any embarrassment.
4. Ask the patient if a family member can complete the care instead.

6. Your patient wears full dentures. His usual denture care includes taking the teeth out once a day to brush. He wears the dentures overnight. You are concerned that the patient might be at risk for developing denture stomatitis. Which points will you include in a teaching plan for denture care? Select all that apply.
1. Remove dentures overnight once a week while they soak in a cleansing bath.
2. Do not wear damaged or poorly fitting dentures.

3. Observe mouth for reddened areas under the dentures and for small red sores on the roof of the mouth.
4. See the dentist regularly.
5. Rinse dentures after meals.
6. Clean dentures every night with cleanser, rinsing well before replacing in mouth at bedtime.

7. You are caring for a patient who is receiving chemotherapy. The patient has inflamed gums and oral mucosa and has painful sores in the mouth. Which of the following oral care actions are appropriate? Select all that apply.
1. Decrease frequency of oral hygiene.
2. Apply water-soluble moisturizing gel on the oral mucosa.
3. Encourage intake of soft foods.
4. Use commercial mouthwash.
5. Apply topical anesthetic as prescribed.

8. You are caring for a group of four patients. As you plan your morning care, which of the following patients is the highest priority to receive his or her bath first?
1. A patient who just returned to the nursing unit from surgery and is experiencing pain at a level of 7 on a scale of 0 to 10.
2. A patient who prefers a bath in the evening when his wife visits and can help him.
3. A patient who is experiencing frequent incontinent diarrheal stools.
4. A patient who has just returned from diagnostic testing and complains of being very fatigued.

9. You have just finished giving your patient a complete bed bath and have changed his sheets with the patient in the bed. The patient has pneumonia and often experiences shortness of breath and labored breathing. The bed currently is in the flat position. Before you leave the room, it is important to change the bed position to:
1. Trendelenburg's
2. Reverse Trendelenburg's
3. Fowler's
4. Semi-Fowler's

10. As the nurse caring for a male patient, you observe the nursing assistive personnel (NAP) performing perineal care. Which of the following observed actions indicates a need for further teaching for the NAP?
1. Used clean gloves
2. Did not retract foreskin before cleansing
3. Used clean portion of washcloth for each cleansing wipe
4. Used a circular motion to cleanse from urinary meatus outward

Answers to Review Questions can be found on pages 1197-1198.

REFERENCES

American Academy of Dermatology: *Changes in skin care soothe aging skin*, 2008, http://www.skincarephysicians.com/agingskinnet/winter_skin.html.

American Dental Association: *Oral health topics A-Z: cleaning your teeth and gums (oral hygiene)*, 2008, http://www.ada.org/public/topics/cleansing.asp.

American Diabetes Association: Position statement on standards of medical care in diabetes—2007, *Diabetes Care* 30:S4, 2007.

Bauroth K and others: The efficacy of an essential oil antiseptic mouthwash vs dental flossing in controlling interproximal gingivitis: a comparative study, *J Am Dent Assoc* 144(3):359, 2003.

Berry AM and others: Systematic literature review of oral hygiene practices for intensive care patients receiving mechanical ventilation, *Am J Crit Care* 16(6):552, 2007.

Bulechek GM and others, editors: *Nursing interventions classification (NIC)*, ed 5, St. Louis, 2008, Mosby.

Columbia University College of Dental Medicine faculty: *Denture-induced stomatitis*, 2008, http://www.simplestepsdental.com/SS/ihtSS/r.WSIHW000/st.31862/t.25020/pr.3.html.

Ebersole P, Hess P: *Toward healthy aging: human needs and nursing response*, ed 7, St. Louis, 2008, Mosby.

El-Solh A and others: Colonization of dental plaques: a reservoir of respiratory pathogens for hospital-acquired pneumonia in institutionalized elders, *Chest* 126(5):1575, 2004.

Frykberg R and others: Diabetic foot disorders: a clinical practical guideline, *J Foot Ankle Surg* 45(5):S2, 2006.

Galanti GA: *Caring for patients from different cultures*, ed 3, Philadelphia, 2004, University of Pennsylvania Press.

Grap MJ and others: Oral care interventions in critical care: frequency and documentation, *Am J Crit Care* 12(2):114, 2003.

Grap MJ and others: Duration of action of a single, early oral application of chlorhexidine on oral microbial flora in mechanically ventilated patients: a pilot study, *Heart Lung* 33(2):83, 2004.

Hoeffer B and others: Assisting cognitively impaired nursing home residents with bathing: effects of two bathing interventions on caregiving, *Gerontologist* 46(4):524, 2006.

Martinez N, Tripp-Reimer T: Diabetes nurse educators' prioritized elder foot care behaviors, *Diabetes Educ* 31(6):858, 2005.

Meiner SE, Lueckenotte AG: *Gerontologic nursing*, ed 3, St. Louis, 2006, Mosby.

Moorhead S and others, editors: *Nursing outcomes classification (NOC)*, ed 4, St. Louis, 2008, Mosby.

Munro CL, Grap MJ: Oral health and care in the intensive care unit: state of the science, *Am J Crit Care* 13(1):25, 2004.

Munro CL and others: Oral health measurements in nursing research: state of the science, *Biol Res Nurs* 8(1):35, 2006.

National Center on Elder Abuse: *Fact sheet: elder abuse prevalence and incidence*, 2005, http://www.ncea.aoa.gov/ncearoot/main_Site/index.aspx.

National Institute on Deafness and Other Communication Disorders: *Hearing aids*, Pub No. 99-4340, Bethesda, Md, 2001, National Institutes of Health, http://www.nidcd.nih.gov/health/hearing/hearingaid.asp.

National Pediculosis Association: *Child care provider's guide to controlling head lice*, 2005, http://www.headlice.org.

Oncology Nursing Society: *Putting evidence into practice: mucositis*, 2007, http://www.ons.org/outcomes/volume2/mucositis.shtml.

Padilha DMP and others: Hand function and oral hygiene in older institutionalized Brazilians, *J Am Geriatr Soc* 55(9):1333, 2007.

Pender N, Murdaugh C, Parsons M: *Health promotion in nursing practice*, Upper Saddle River, NJ, 2002, Pearson Education.

Perlmutter JS, Camberg L: Better bathing for residents with Alzheimer's, *Nurs Homes Long Term Care Manage* 53(4):40, 2004.

Pinzur MS and others: Guidelines for diabetic foot care, The Diabetes Committee of the American Orthopaedic Foot and Ankle Society, *Foot Ankle Int* 26(1):113, 2005.

Piotrowski M and others: Massage as an adjuvant therapy in the management of acute postoperative pain: a preliminary study, *J Am Coll Surg* 197(6):1037, 2003.

Rader J and others: The bathing of older adults with dementia, *Am J Nurs* 106(4):40, 2006.

Sciubba JJ: *Denture stomatitis*, 2009, http://www.simplestepsdental.com/SS/ihtSS/r.WSIHW000/st.32219/t.25048/pr.3.html.

Scully C and others: Oral mucositis: a challenging complication of radiotherapy, chemotherapy, and radiochemotherapy. II. Diagnosis and management of mucositis, *Head Neck* 26(1):77, 2004.

Sloane PD and others: Effect of person-centered showering and the towel bath on bathing: associated aggression, agitation, and discomfort in nursing home residents with dementia: a randomized, controlled trial, *J Am Geriatr Soc* 52(11):1795, 2004.

Somboontanont W and others: Assaultive behavior in Alzheimer's disease: identifying immediate antecedents during bathing, *J Gerontol Nurs* 30(9):22, 2004.

The Joint Commission: *2009 National Patient Safety Goals Hospital Program*, Oakbrook Terrace, Ill, 2008, The Joint Commission, http://www.jointcommission.org, accessed July 2008.

Zullino DF and others: Local back massage with an automated massage chair: several muscle and psychophysiologic relaxing properties, *J Altern Complement Med* 11(6):1103, 2005.

29 Oxygenation

MEDIA RESOURCES

 CD COMPANION 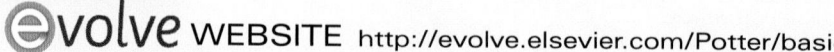 evolve WEBSITE http://evolve.elsevier.com/Potter/basic

- Video Clips
- Crossword Puzzle
- English/Spanish Audio Glossary

OBJECTIVES

- Describe the structure and function of the cardiopulmonary system.
- Identify the physiological processes of cardiac output, myocardial blood flow, coronary artery circulation, and respiratory gas exchange.
- Describe the relationship of cardiac output, preload, afterload, contractility, and heart rate.
- Diagram the electrical conduction system of the heart.
- Identify the physiological processes involved in ventilation, perfusion, and exchange of respiratory gases.
- Describe the impact of the patient's health status, age, lifestyle, and environment on tissue oxygenation.
- Identify and describe clinical outcomes as a result of disturbances in conduction, altered cardiac output, impaired valvular function, myocardial ischemia, and impaired tissue perfusion.
- Identify nursing interventions for promotion, maintenance, and restoration of cardiopulmonary function in the primary care, acute care, and restorative and continuing care settings.
- Identify and describe clinical outcomes for hyperventilation, hypoventilation, and hypoxemia.

KEY TERMS

afterload, p. 804
atelectasis, p. 809
atrioventricular (AV) node, p. 804
cardiac index, p. 804
cardiac output (CO), p. 804
cardiopulmonary rehabilitation, p. 830

cardiopulmonary resuscitation (CPR), p. 830
chest percussion, p. 826
chest physiotherapy (CPT), p. 826
chest tube, p. 828
depolarization, p. 805

diaphragmatic breathing, p. 831
diffusion, p. 801
dyspnea, p. 810
dysrhythmias, p. 806
hemoptysis, p. 814
hemothorax, p. 828
humidification, p. 822
hypercapnia, p. 809

hyperventilation, p. 803
hypoventilation, p. 803
hypoxemia, p. 809
hypoxia, p. 803
myocardial contractility, p. 804
myocardial infarction, p. 805

KEY TERMS, CONT.

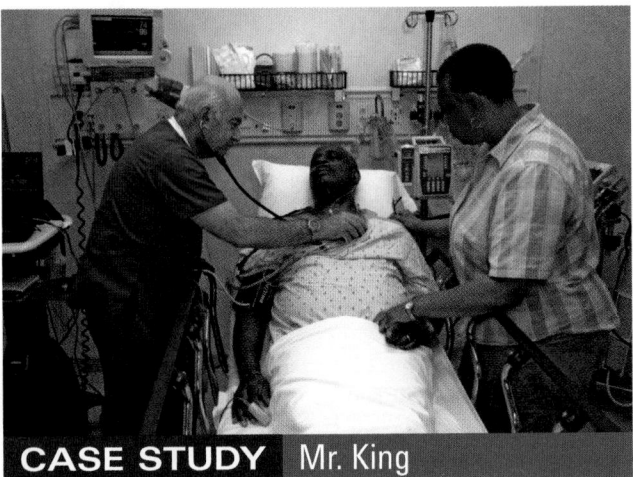

CASE STUDY   Mr. King

Mr. King, a 62-year-old man, entered the emergency department with a 6-day history of chest pain, shortness of breath, cough, and generalized malaise. His wife and son are with him. Mr. King works in sales and lives with his wife. He has a history of chronic obstructive pulmonary disease and alcohol abuse but at present is not drinking. Mr. and Mrs. King have been heavy smokers for more than 40 years. Mr. King used to help out with the housework and loves to tinker in the garden; however, lately he has been unable to participate in any of the activities. His wife states, "All he seems to be able to do is sit in his chair and watch TV."

John Smith is the nursing student assigned to his first hospital-based clinical experience. He has had some experience in health assessment and patient teaching related to health promotion activities from a recent clinical rotation in a clinic. In the previous clinical experience, patients were encouraged to adjust their at-risk health behaviors, such as smoking or poor diet. John feels confident when he arrives in the clinical area this morning because Mr. King has similar health needs to the clinical experiences he has had.

However, when John goes to meet Mr. King and performs his morning assessment, he is overwhelmed. This patient is in a great deal of respiratory distress. It seems that every breath is a struggle for him. Everything that John planned to do for Mr. King seems less important. The patient is extremely anxious. His wife is at his side, anticipating John's every move and demanding some action.

SCIENTIFIC KNOWLEDGE BASE

Oxygen is a basic human need. The heart and lungs supply the body with oxygen necessary for carrying out the respiratory and metabolic processes needed to sustain life. You will frequently meet patients who are unable to meet their oxygenation needs. This is often the result of ineffective gas exchange (lungs) or an ineffective pump (heart). Any condition that affects cardiopulmonary functioning directly affects the body's ability to meet oxygen demands.

Cardiopulmonary Physiology

The function of the cardiopulmonary system is to provide oxygen to the tissues and remove carbon dioxide and waste products from the body. The lungs assist with **ventilation,** the movement of air in and out of the lungs, and **diffusion,** the movement of gases between air spaces and the bloodstream. **Respiration** is the exchange of oxygen and carbon dioxide during cellular metabolism. The heart supports **perfusion,** the movement of blood into and out of the lungs to the body's organs and tissues.

Structure and Function of the Pulmonary System

The pulmonary system consists of two lungs, their airways, the chest walls, and the blood vessels that support them (Figure 29-1). The right lung is made up of three lobes, the upper, middle, and lower lobes. The left lung has two lobes, the upper and lower lobes. The trachea enters the thorax and bifurcates, or branches out, into the right and left mainstem bronchus. The bronchi branch into smaller and smaller bronchioles, similar to a tree. The last branch of the airways ends at the exchanging unit of the lung, the alveoli. With pulmonary surfactant, alveoli expand and contract, allowing for diffusion to occur.

REGULATION OF VENTILATION Successful ventilation depends upon neuroreceptors and chemoreceptors in the lungs and central nervous system (CNS), muscles that support inspiration and exhalation, and lung elasticity. Control of ventilation provides for adequate oxygen to meet metabolic demands, such as exercise, infection, or pregnancy. Ventilation promotes exhalation of metabolically produced carbon dioxide, which is a determinant of acid-base status (see Chapter 17).

Neural and chemical regulators control ventilation (Box 29-1). Neural regulation involves the central nervous system.

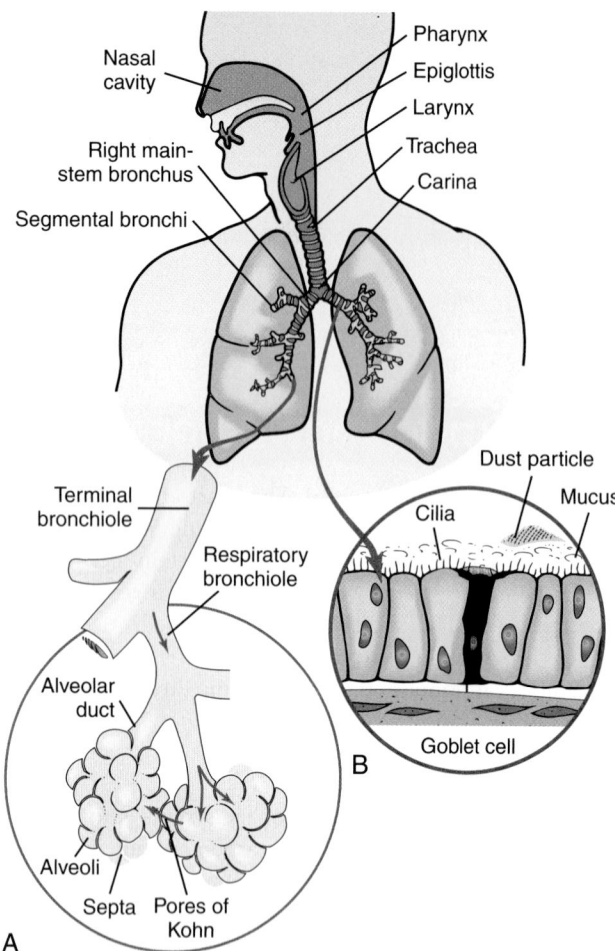

Figure 29-1 ■ Structures of the respiratory tract. **A,** Pulmonary functional unit. **B,** Ciliated mucous membrane. (From Lewis SM and others: *Medical surgical nursing: assessment and management of clinical problems,* ed 7, St. Louis, 2007, Mosby.)

The CNS sends signals to the chest wall musculature to control ventilation rate, depth, and rhythm. Chemical regulation involves the influence of chemicals, such as carbon dioxide and hydrogen ions, which affect the rate and depth of ventilation.

OXYGEN TRANSPORT The delivery of oxygen depends on the amount of oxygen entering the lungs (oxygenation) from the atmosphere. Ventilation allows for movement of oxygen and carbon dioxide into and out of the lungs. Once oxygen has reached the alveoli, diffusion occurs. Oxygen crosses the alveolocapillary membrane and is dissolved into the plasma (Figure 29-2). It then moves into the red blood cells (RBCs) and binds with hemoglobin molecules. Hemoglobin transports most oxygen and serves as a carrier for both oxygen and carbon dioxide. The hemoglobin molecule combines with oxygen to form oxyhemoglobin. The formation of oxyhemoglobin is easily reversible, allowing hemoglobin and oxygen to dissociate, which frees oxygen to enter tissues. The amount of dissolved oxygen in the plasma, the amount of hemoglobin, and the tendency of hemoglobin to bind with oxygen all influence the capacity of the blood to carry oxygen. Perfusion of oxygenated blood occurs in the capillary beds of the organs and tissues.

BOX 29-1 | Neural and Chemical Regulation of Respiration

NEURAL REGULATION
- Neural regulation maintains rhythm and depth of respiration, as well as the balance between inspiration and expiration.

CEREBRAL CORTEX
- Voluntary control of respiration delivers impulses to the respiratory motor neurons by way of the spinal cord. Voluntary control of respiration accommodates speaking, eating, and swimming.

MEDULLA OBLONGATA
- Automatic control of respiration occurs continuously.

CHEMICAL REGULATION
- Chemical regulation maintains appropriate rate and depth of respirations based on changes in the blood's carbon dioxide (CO_2), oxygen (O_2), and hydrogen ion (H^+) concentration.

CHEMORECEPTORS
- Chemoreceptors are located in the medulla, aortic body, and carotid body. Changes in chemical content of O_2, CO_2, and H^+ stimulate chemoreceptors, which in turn stimulate neural regulators to adjust the rate and depth of ventilation to maintain normal arterial blood gas levels. Chemical regulation occurs during physical exercise and in some illnesses. It is a short-term adaptive mechanism.

CARBON DIOXIDE TRANSPORT The blood carries CO_2 in three ways: (1) dissolved in plasma, (2) as carbamino compounds, and (3) as bicarbonate. At the capillary level, carbon dioxide diffuses from the cells into the plasma with 7% of CO_2 remaining dissolved in the plasma (PCO_2). The rest of the CO_2 rapidly moves into the red blood cells and is hydrated into carbonic acid (H_2CO_3). The carbonic acid dissociates into hydrogen (H^+) and bicarbonate (HCO_3^-) ions. The H^+ ion binds to hemoglobin, which has released its oxygen, to form HHb and deoxyhemoglobin ($HbCO_2$). Twenty-three percent of CO_2 is transported as $HbCO_2$. The HCO_3^- ion moves out of the RBCs and back into the plasma (see Chapter 17). Seventy percent of CO_2 is carried as HCO_3^-, helping to maintain an electroneutral state. Once the CO_2 is transported by the venous blood to the lungs, diffusion occurs again. The CO_2 is highly soluble, and it quickly crosses the gas membrane into the alveoli. Through ventilation the CO_2 is expelled from the lungs into the atmosphere.

Alterations of the Pulmonary System: Factors Affecting Ventilation and Oxygen Transport

Illnesses and conditions that affect ventilation or oxygen transport cause alterations in respiratory functioning. The three primary alterations are hypoxia, hypoventilation, and hyperventilation.

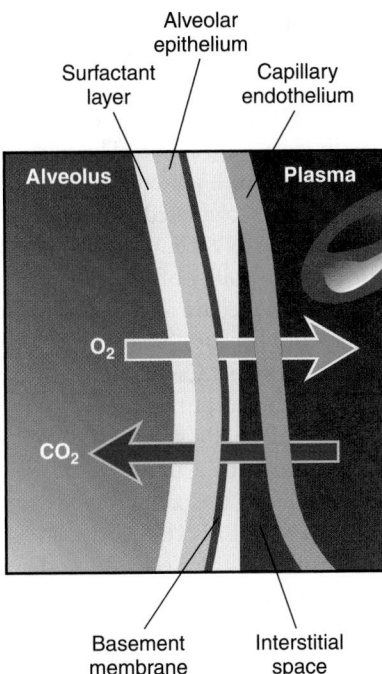

Figure 29-2 ■ Diffusion: The gas-exchange membrane. (Modified from McCance K, Huether S: *Pathophysiology: the biologic basis for disease in adults and children,* ed 5, St. Louis, 2006, Mosby.)

HYPOXIA **Hypoxia** is inadequate tissue oxygenation with a deficiency in oxygen delivery or oxygen utilization at the cellular level. Causes of hypoxia include the following:

- A lowered oxygen-carrying capacity, as in anemia or carbon monoxide poisoning
- Diminished concentrations of inspired oxygen, as in high altitudes and airway obstruction
- The inability of the tissues to extract oxygen from the blood, as in septic shock and cyanide poisoning
- Decreased diffusion of oxygen from the lung (alveoli) into the blood, as in pneumonia or atelectasis
- Poor tissue perfusion with oxygenated blood, as in hypovolemic shock, cardiogenic shock, or cardiomyopathy
- Impaired ventilation from multiple rib fractures, chest trauma, spinal cord injury, or head trauma
- Obstructive or restrictive diseases, such as chronic obstructive pulmonary disease (COPD), in which airways lose elasticity and become inflamed

When the partial pressure of oxygen (PaO_2) is low, your patient is hypoxic. Hypoxia is a life-threatening condition and if left untreated, will produce cardiac dysrhythmias and death. Treatment for hypoxia includes administration of oxygen and correction of the underlying cause.

HYPOVENTILATION **Hypoventilation** occurs when ventilation is inadequate to meet the body's oxygen demand or to eliminate carbon dioxide. This results in hypoxia or hypercapnia, an arterial carbon dioxide ($PaCO_2$) level greater than 45 mm Hg, and respiratory acidosis. Causes of hypoventilation include the following:

- Impaired ventilation related to trauma, pain, infection, obstructive diseases, or fluid volume overload
- Alterations in neurological regulation of breathing
- Alterations in chemical regulation of breathing
- Collapse of alveoli related to severe atelectasis

As ventilation decreases, $PaCO_2$ is elevated. Clinical signs and symptoms of hypoventilation include dizziness, occipital headache upon awakening, lethargy, disorientation, decreased ability to follow instructions, cardiac dysrhythmias, electrolyte imbalances, convulsions, and possible coma or cardiac arrest.

When caring for patients with COPD and chronically elevated $PaCO_2$ levels, remember that inappropriate administration of excessive oxygen will result in hypoventilation. Patients with COPD and hypercapnia (high carbon dioxide levels) have adapted to the higher carbon dioxide level. The carbon dioxide–sensitive chemoreceptors are essentially not functioning, and the stimulus to breathe is a decreased PaO_2.

When you administer excessive oxygen to patients with COPD, this satisfies the body's oxygen requirement and negates the stimulus to breathe. High concentrations of oxygen (e.g., greater than 24% to 28% [1 to 3 L/min]) prevent the PaO_2 from falling. As a result, this destroys the stimulus to breathe, resulting in hypoventilation. The excessive retention of carbon dioxide leads to respiratory arrest. If untreated, your patient's status will rapidly decline, and death is possible. Treatment for hypoventilation involves treating the underlying cause, improving tissue oxygenation, restoring ventilation, and achieving acid-base balance.

HYPERVENTILATION **Hyperventilation** is an increase in respiratory rate, resulting in excess amounts of carbon dioxide elimination. This results in a decrease in $PaCO_2$, or hypocapnia, and respiratory alkalosis. Causes of hyperventilation include severe anxiety, infection, head injury, medications, or acid-base imbalance. Acute anxiety and an increased respiratory rate may cause loss of consciousness from excess carbon dioxide exhalation. An increase of 1° F in body temperature causes a 7% increase in the metabolic rate, thereby increasing carbon dioxide production. The clinical response is increased rate and depth of respiration. Hypoxia associated with pulmonary embolus or shock also results in hyperventilation.

Hyperventilation produces signs and symptoms including tachycardia, shortness of breath, chest pain, dizziness, lightheadedness, decreased concentration, paresthesia, circumoral and/or extremity numbness, tinnitus, blurred vision, disorientation, and tetany (carpopedal spasm). Treatment for hyperventilation involves treating the underlying cause, improving tissue oxygenation, restoring ventilation, reducing respiratory rate, and achieving acid-base balance.

Structure and Function of the Circulatory System

The function of the circulatory system is to deliver oxygen, nutrients, and other substances to the body's tissues to support cellular life. Once cellular metabolism occurs, waste products accumulate. The system then removes waste products, such as carbon dioxide, and delivers them to the lungs and/or kidneys, where the wastes are eliminated. The pumping action of the heart is essential to support the circulatory system. The four heart valves (tricuspid, pulmonic, mitral, and aortic) ensure the one-way flow of blood through the heart (Figure 29-3).

REGULATION OF BLOOD FLOW There are multiple regulators of blood flow (Table 29-1). The heart muscle (myocardium) relaxes and contracts to support the regulation of blood flow. The contraction phase is called systole, in which blood is expelled from the ventricles into the systemic circulation. **Afterload** is the resistance of the ejection of blood from the left ventricle. The left ventricular pressure must exceed the aortic pressure in order to eject blood from the heart. The relaxation phase is called diastole, in which blood fills the ventricles. **Preload** is the amount of blood at the end of ventricular diastole, or measured as end-diastolic pressure. Each contraction and relaxation consists of one cardiac cycle.

The amount of blood ejected from the left ventricle each minute is termed **cardiac output (CO).** A normal cardiac output for a healthy adult is 4 to 6 L/min. The cardiac output is calculated as follows:

$$\text{Cardiac output (CO)} = \text{Stroke volume (SV)} \times \text{Heart rate (HR)}$$

Stroke volume (SV) is the amount of blood ejected from the ventricle with each contraction. The normal range for a healthy adult is 50 to 75 mL per contraction. The heart rate, or beats per minute, is regulated by the sympathetic and parasympathetic systems (WNL: 60 to 100 BPM). **Myocardial contractility** is the ability of the heart to squeeze blood from the ventricles and prepare for the next contraction. This is difficult to measure because preload, afterload, and heart rate must remain constant. **Cardiac index** is a measure of adequacy of the cardiac output. It equals the cardiac output divided by the patient's body surface area. This calculation provides the caregiver with a more accurate calculation of blood flow by considering the patient's body surface area.

CONDUCTION SYSTEM The conduction system generates impulses that initiate the electrical mechanical chain of events for a normal heartbeat. The rhythmic relaxation and contraction of the atria and ventricles depend on continuous, organized transmission of electrical impulses to the muscle. The conduction system generates, controls, and transmits these impulses (Figure 29-4). The autonomic nervous system influences the rate of impulse generation, the transmission speed through the conductive pathway, and the strength of contractions through sympathetic and parasympathetic (vagus nerve) nerve fibers in the atria and ventricles. The vagus nerve (parasympathetic) also innervates sinoatrial and atrioventricular nodes and is able to reduce the rate of impulse generation.

The conduction system originates with the **sinoatrial (SA) node,** the "pacemaker" of the heart. The SA node is in the right atrium next to the entrance of the superior vena cava. Impulses begin at the SA node at an intrinsic rate of 60 to 100 beats per minute. The resting adult rate ranges from 60 to 80 beats per minute. The older adult has a wide range from the 40s to more than 100 beats per minute (Seidel and others, 2006). Electrical impulses are then transmitted along intra-atrial pathways to the **atrioventricular (AV) node.** The AV node mediates impulse transmission between the atria and the ventricles. Delaying the impulse at the AV node before transmitting it through the bundle of His and ventricular Purkinje network assists atrial emptying.

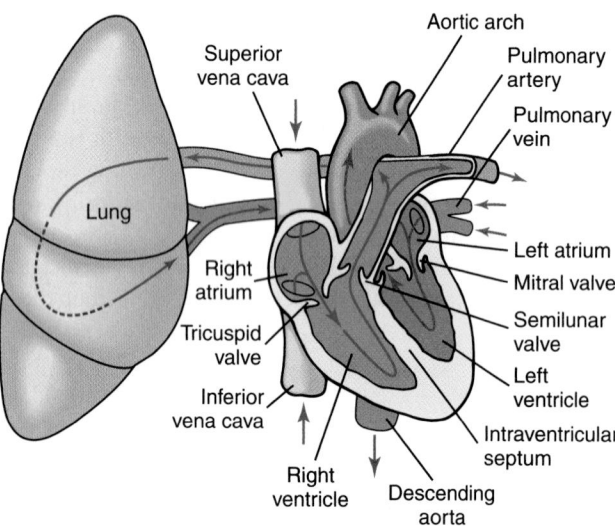

Figure 29-3 ▪ Schematic representation of blood flow through the heart. Arrows indicate direction of flow. (From Lewis SM and others: *Medical surgical nursing: assessment and management of clinical problems,* ed 7, St. Louis, 2007, Mosby.)

TABLE 29-1   Regulation of Blood Flow

REGULATOR	DEFINITION
Cardiac output	Amount of blood ejected from the left ventricle per minute Normal range (adult): 4-6 L/min
Cardiac index	Measure of adequacy of the cardiac output: cardiac index equals cardiac output divided by the patient's body surface area Normal range (adult): 2.5-4 L/min/m^3
Stroke volume	Amount of blood ejected from the ventricle with each contraction Normal range (adult): 50-75 mL per contraction
Preload	Amount of blood in the ventricles at end diastole
Afterload	Resistance of the ejection of blood from the left ventricle
Myocardial contractility	Ability of the heart to squeeze blood from the ventricles and prepare for the next contraction

An electrocardiogram (ECG) records the electrical activity of the conduction system as waves and complexes. An ECG monitors the regularity and path of the electrical impulse through the conduction system; however, it does not reflect the muscular work of the heart. The normal sequence of electrical impulses on the ECG is called **normal sinus rhythm (NSR)** (Figure 29-5). A normal ECG waveform consists of a P wave (atrial **depolarization**), QRS complex (ventricular depolarization), and T wave (ventricular **repolarization**). Care providers interpret the size, appearance, and sequence of waves to identify dysrhythmias and recognize the area of the heart affected.

Alterations of the Circulatory System

Illnesses and conditions that affect cardiac rate, rhythm, strength of contraction, blood flow through the chambers, myocardial blood flow, and peripheral circulation alter cardiac functioning.

DECREASED CARDIAC OUTPUT Failure of the myocardium to eject sufficient blood volume to the systemic and pulmonary circulations results in heart failure. Failure of the myocardial pump results from primary coronary artery disease (CAD), valvular disorders, cardiomyopathic conditions, and pulmonary disease.

MYOCARDIAL ISCHEMIA Myocardial ischemia happens when the coronary artery does not supply sufficient blood to the heart muscle (myocardium). Decreased perfusion to the myocardium results in chest pain, especially with activity. Angina or angina pectoris is the result of decreased blood flow to the myocardium as a result of coronary artery spasms or temporary constriction. When decreased myocardial blood perfusion is extensive or perfusion is completely blocked, the tissue becomes necrotic and a **myocardial infarction** occurs. Myocardial infarction presents clinically as severe or crushing chest pain, jaw pain, left arm pain, breathlessness, diaphoresis, and hypotension (a fall in blood pressure).

IMPAIRED VALVULAR FUNCTION Valvular heart disease is an acquired or congenital disorder of a cardiac valve characterized by stenosis resulting in obstructed blood flow or valvular degeneration and regurgitation resulting in backflow of blood. When stenosis occurs in the aortic and pulmonic valves, the adjacent ventricles work harder to move the ventricular volume beyond the stenotic valve. When regurgitation occurs, there is a backflow of blood into an adjacent chamber, which causes either pulmonary or systemic congestion.

LEFT-SIDED HEART FAILURE Left-sided heart failure is characterized by impaired functioning of the left ventricle. This is usually caused by increased preload (fluid volume overload) or afterload (increased systemic vascular resistance, such as hypertension). If left ventricular failure is significant, the amount of blood ejected from the left ventricle drops greatly, resulting in decreased cardiac output. Patients may present with pulmonary congestion, and, as a result, you note crackles on auscultation, and patient complaints of fatigue, dyspnea, and **orthopnea** (difficulty breathing while lying down).

RIGHT-SIDED HEART FAILURE Right-sided heart failure results from impaired functioning of the right ventricle. This is typically caused by pulmonary disease. When pressure increases in the pulmonary system, increased resistance occurs in the right ventricle. The right ventricle will fail as a result of this pressure. The patient has venous congestion in the systemic circulation and on assessment you will often identify distended jugular veins and peripheral edema. Right-sided heart failure may also result from untreated or end-stage left-sided heart failure.

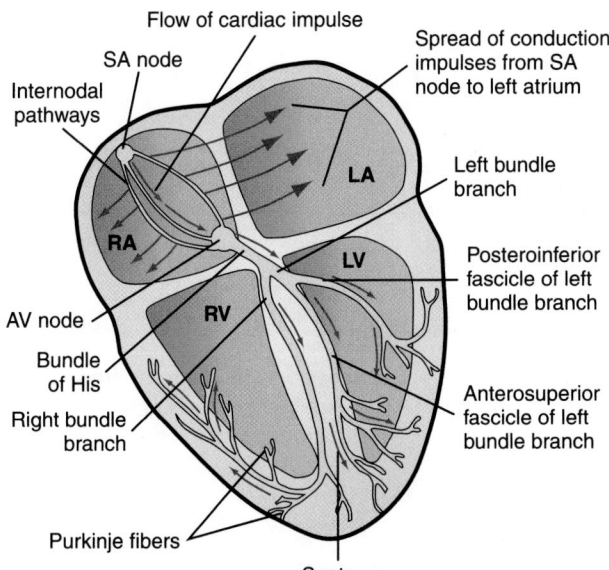

Figure 29-4 ■ Conduction system of the heart. *AV*, Atrioventricular; *LA*, left atrium; *LV*, left ventricle; *RA*, right atrium; *RV*, right ventricle; *SA*, sinoatrial. (From Lewis SM and others: *Medical surgical nursing: assessment and management of clinical problems,* ed 7, St. Louis, 2007, Mosby.)

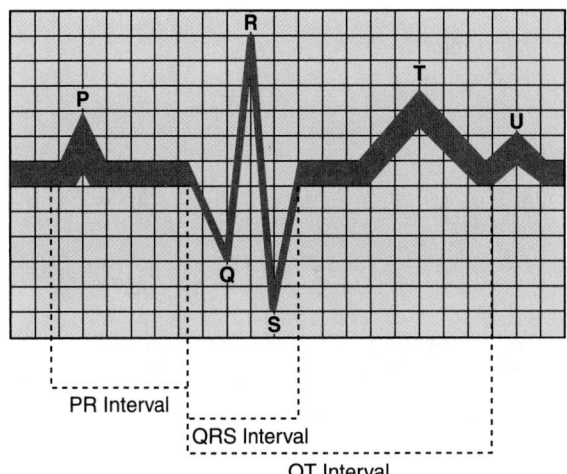

Figure 29-5 ■ Normal electrocardiogram (ECG) pattern. The P wave represents depolarization of the atria. The QRS complex indicates depolarization of the ventricles. The T wave represents repolarization of the ventricles. The U wave, if present, may represent repolarization of the Purkinje fibers, or it may be associated with hypokalemia. The PR, QRS, and QT intervals reflect the length of the time it takes for the impulse to travel from one area of the heart to another. (From Lewis SM and others: *Medical surgical nursing: assessment and management of clinical problems,* ed 7, St. Louis, 2007, Mosby.)

HYPOVOLEMIA Hypovolemia is a reduced circulating blood volume resulting from extracellular fluid losses that occurs in conditions such as shock and severe dehydration. If the fluid loss is significant, the body tries to adapt by increasing the heart rate and constricting peripheral vessels to increase the volume of blood returned to the heart and increase the cardiac output.

DISTURBANCES IN CONDUCTION A **dysrhythmia** is a disturbance in the electrical impulse of the heart rhythm. Any rhythm not generated at the SA node is classified as such. Dysrhythmias occur as primary conduction disturbances; as a response to ischemia, valvular abnormality, anxiety, and drug toxicity; as a result of caffeine, alcohol, or tobacco use; following cardiothoracic surgery; or as a complication of acid-base or electrolyte imbalance (see Chapter 17).

Dysrhythmias are classified by their site of origin and cardiac response (Table 29-2). The cardiac response can be an

TABLE 29-2   Common Basic Cardiac Dysrhythmias

RHYTHM CHARACTERISTICS	ETIOLOGY	CLINICAL SIGNIFICANCE	MANAGEMENT
SINUS TACHYCARDIA			

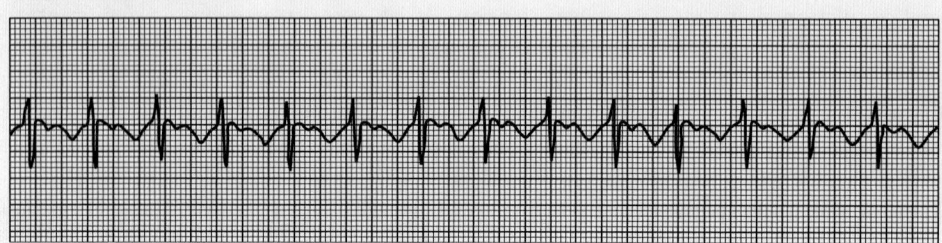

RHYTHM CHARACTERISTICS	ETIOLOGY	CLINICAL SIGNIFICANCE	MANAGEMENT
Regular rhythm, rate 100-180 beats/min (higher in infants), normal P wave, normal QRS complex	Rate increase is a normal response to exercise, emotion, or stressors, such as pain, fever, pump failure, hypovolemia, hyperthyroidism, and certain drugs (e.g., caffeine, nitrates, nicotine)	Patient with damaged heart may be unable to sustain increased workloads (increased myocardial oxygen consumption) brought on by persistent increases in heart rate; reduces myocardial perfusion	Assess and support ABCs Check vital signs Consult expert clinician Correct underlying factors; remove offending drugs Clinicians may attempt vagal maneuvers or administer adenosine IVP to temporarily stop the tachycardia, and the intrinsic NSR starts again

SINUS BRADYCARDIA

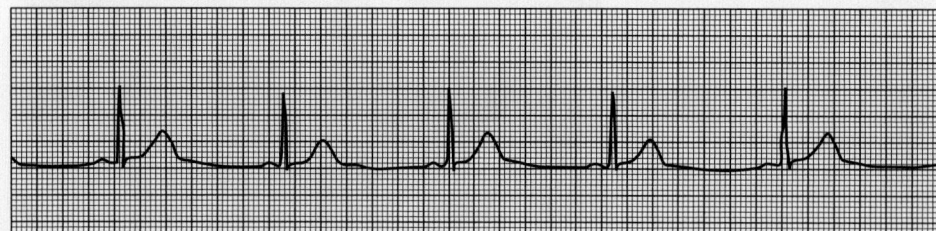

| Regular rhythm, rate <60 beats/min, normal P wave, normal PR interval, normal QRS complex | Rate decrease is a normal response to sleep or in well-conditioned athlete; abnormal drops in rate caused by diminished blood flow to SA node, vagal stimulation, hypothyroidism, increased intracranial pressure, or certain drugs (e.g., digoxin, propranolol, procainamide) | Has clinical significance when associated with signs of impaired cardiac output and symptoms of dizziness, hypotension, syncope, chest pain | Assess and support ABCs Check vital signs Consult expert clinician Correct underlying causes; prepare for transcutaneous pacing; consider atropine; consider epinephrine or dopamine, IV |

ABCs, Airway, breathing, circulation; *ABCDs,* airway, breathing, circulation, defibrillation; *AED,* automatic external defibrillator; *AV,* atrioventricular; *CPR,* cardiopulmonary resuscitation; *IO,* intraosseous; *IV,* intravenous; *IVP,* intravenous push; *NSR,* normal sinus rhythm; *SA,* sinoatrial.

TABLE 29-2 Common Basic Cardiac Dysrhythmias—cont'd

RHYTHM CHARACTERISTICS	ETIOLOGY	CLINICAL SIGNIFICANCE	MANAGEMENT

ATRIAL FIBRILLATION (A-FIB)

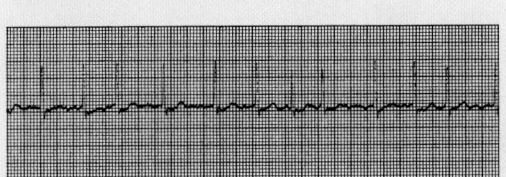

Irregular atrial activity resulting in an irregular ventricular response with resultant irregular cardiac rate and rhythm. No identifiable P wave. Rate is determined by the conduction of the multiple atrial impulses across the AV node	Caused by aging, calcification of the SA node, electrolyte imbalances, valvular disturbances, or changes in myocardial blood supply	Loss of the atrial kick (portion of the cardiac output squeezed in the ventricles with a coordinated atrial contraction), pooling of blood in the atria, and development of microemboli. Patients complain of fatigue, a fluttering in the chest, and shortness of breath if ventricular response is rapid. Patients may have hypotension	Assess and support ABCs Check vital signs Consult expert clinician Prepare for synchronized cardioversion (shock delivered during the relative refractory period of the cardiac cycle) Prepare for rate control medication therapy, such as diltiazem or beta-blockers Treat underlying cause Managed with blood thinners such as warfarin (Coumadin)

VENTRICULAR TACHYCARDIA

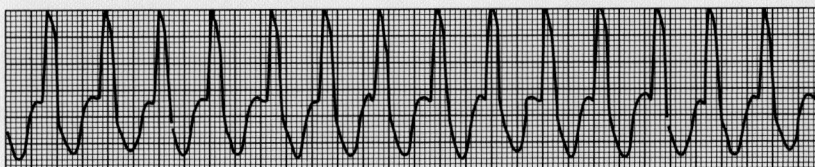

Rhythm slightly irregular, rate 100-200 beats/min, P wave absent, QRS complex wide and bizarre, >0.12 sec	Caused by irritable ventricular foci firing repetitively, commonly caused by myocardial infarction	Often a forerunner of ventricular fibrillation; if condition persistent and rapid, causes decreased cardiac output because of decreased ventricular filling time Patient may or may not have a pulse	Assess and support ABCDs Check vital signs Consult expert clinician Prepare for amiodarone IV over 10 min Prepare for synchronized cardioversion (patient with a pulse) Prepare for CPR and unsynchronized cardioversion/defibrillation (patient without a pulse)

ABCs, Airway, breathing, circulation; *ABCDs,* airway, breathing, circulation, defibrillation; *AED,* automatic external defibrillator; *AV,* atrioventricular; *CPR,* cardiopulmonary resuscitation; *IO,* intraosseous; *IV,* intravenous; *IVP,* intravenous push; *NSR,* normal sinus rhythm; *SA,* sinoatrial.

Continued

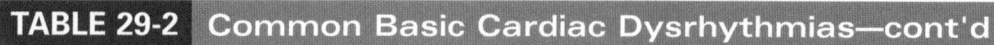

TABLE 29-2 Common Basic Cardiac Dysrhythmias—cont'd

RHYTHM CHARACTERISTICS	ETIOLOGY	CLINICAL SIGNIFICANCE	MANAGEMENT

VENTRICULAR FIBRILLATION

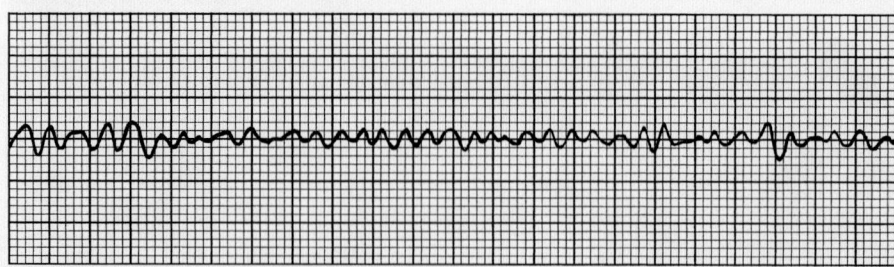

| Irregular and chaotic rhythm with no discernible waves or rate | Ventricles are quivering, not pumping | The patient is pulseless and apneic | Immediate resuscitation is required Begin ABCDs
In-hospital goals: Give rescue breaths, and begin CPR within 1 min. Apply AED or defibrillator within 3 min, and deliver unsynchronized shocks.
Prepare to administer epinephrine IV/IO every 3-5 min (or vasopressin to replace the first or second epinephrine dose)
Consider antiarrhythmics, such as amiodarone or lidocaine |

ASYSTOLE

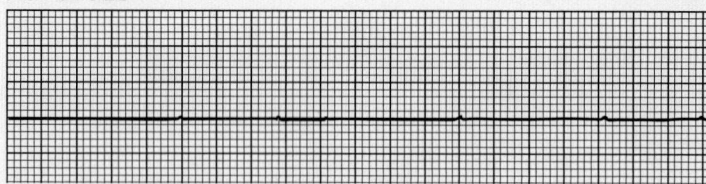

| Absence of electrical activity; no discernible rate or rhythm | Cardiac standstill | The patient is pulseless and apneic | Immediate resuscitation is required Begin ABCDs
Prepare to administer epinephrine IV/IO every 3-5 min (or vasopressin to replace the first or second epinephrine dose)
Prepare to administer atropine IV/IO every 3-5 min (up to three doses) |

Data from American Heart Association: *CPR*, 2005, http://www.Americanheart.org.
ABCs, Airway, breathing, circulation; *ABCDs*, airway, breathing, circulation, defibrillation; *AED*, automatic external defibrillator; *AV*, atrioventricular; *CPR*, cardiopulmonary resuscitation; *IO*, intraosseous; *IV*, intravenous; *IVP*, intravenous push; *NSR*, normal sinus rhythm; *SA*, sinoatrial.

increase in heart rate, tachycardia (a rate greater than 100 beats per minute or greater), a decrease in rate, bradycardia (a rate less than 60 beats per minute), premature (early beat) atrial or ventricular beats, or blocked (delayed or absent beat) atrial or ventricular beats. Dysrhythmias often affect the pumping mechanism of the heart.

Factors Affecting Oxygenation

Alterations in oxygenation result from a decrease in oxygen-carrying capacity of blood (e.g., anemia), an increase in the body's metabolic demands (e.g., fever or infection), and any alteration that affects the patient's chest wall movement or the central nervous system.

DECREASED OXYGEN-CARRYING CAPACITY Ninety-seven percent of oxygen is carried on the hemoglobin molecule. Any process that decreases or alters hemoglobin, such as anemia or inhalation of toxic substances, decreases the oxygen-carrying capacity of blood. Anemia is the reduction in RBCs or decrease in hemoglobin, the oxygen-carrying protein of RBCs. Acute blood loss or chronic disease may result in anemia.

Carbon monoxide is the most common toxic inhalant decreasing the oxygen-carrying capacity of blood. Hemoglobin tends to bind with carbon monoxide 210 times more readily than with oxygen, creating a functional hypoxemia (Thibodeau and Patton, 2004). Because of the bond's strength, it is not easy for carbon monoxide to dissociate (break away) from hemoglobin, making the hemoglobin unavailable for oxygen transport.

DECREASED INSPIRED OXYGEN CONCENTRATION When the concentration of inspired oxygen declines, the oxygen-carrying capacity of the blood decreases. An upper or lower airway obstruction limiting delivery of inspired oxygen to alveoli causes a decrease in the fraction of inspired oxygen concentration (FiO_2). Decreased environmental oxygen (as occurs at high altitudes) or decreased delivery of inspired oxygen, as the result of an incorrect oxygen concentration setting on respiratory therapy equipment, also results in a decreased FiO_2.

INCREASED METABOLIC RATE Increases in metabolic activity of the body increases oxygen demand. When the body is unable to meet the increased oxygen demand, the oxygen level falls. An increased metabolic rate is a normal response of the body to pregnancy, wound healing, and exercise because the body is building tissue. Most people are able to meet the increased oxygen demand and do not display signs of oxygen deprivation.

Fever increases the tissues' need for oxygen. As a result, carbon dioxide production also increases. If the fever lasts for a period of time, the metabolic rate remains high and the body begins to break down protein stores, resulting in muscle wasting and decreased muscle mass. Respiratory muscles, such as the diaphragm and intercostals, are also wasted. The body attempts to adapt to the increased carbon dioxide (**hypercapnia**) levels by increasing the rate and depth of respiration to eliminate the excess carbon dioxide. The patient's work of breathing increases, and the patient will eventually display signs and symptoms of **hypoxemia,** a decreased arterial oxygen level in the blood. Early clinical signs and symptoms of hypoxemia include the following:

* Anxiety
* Restlessness
* Inability to concentrate
* Increases in heart rate
* Increased respiratory rate and blood pressure
* Cardiac dysrhythmias, such as premature ventricular contractions, premature atrial contractions, and sinus tachycardia

As the hypoxemia worsens, some patients lose consciousness. Patients with pulmonary diseases are at greater risk for hypoxemia and hypercapnia, an elevated arterial carbon dioxide level. Patient assessments often show an increased rate and depth of respiration and the use of pursed-lip breathing and accessory muscles of respiration.

CONDITIONS AFFECTING CHEST WALL MOVEMENT Any condition that reduces chest wall movement will decrease ventilation. If the diaphragm is unable to fully descend with breathing, the volume of inspired air decreases, delivering less oxygen to the alveoli and subsequently to tissues.

Musculoskeletal Abnormalities Abnormalities in the thoracic region such as abnormal structural shapes and muscle disease contribute to decreased oxygenation and ventilation. Abnormal structural shapes impairing oxygenation include those that affect the rib cage, such as pectus excavatum, and those that affect the spinal column, such as kyphosis. The angle of curvature in kyphosis can progress with time, resulting in severe hypoventilation and hypoxemia.

Muscle diseases, such as muscular dystrophy, affect oxygenation by decreasing diaphragmatic movement, the patient's ability to expand and contract the chest. This impairs ventilation, and often causes **atelectasis,** hypercapnia, and hypoxemia.

Nervous System Diseases Myasthenia gravis, Guillain-Barré syndrome, and poliomyelitis are examples of nervous system diseases that result in hypoventilation. These diseases impair nervous and muscular control, causing reduced ventilation (hypoventilation).

Disease or trauma involving the medulla oblongata and spinal cord of the central nervous system has the ability to impair respiration. When the medulla oblongata is affected, neural regulation of respiration is damaged and abnormal breathing patterns develop. Damage to the spinal cord affects respiration in two ways. If the phrenic nerve is damaged, the diaphragm does not descend, thus reducing inspiratory lung volumes and causing hypoxemia. Cervical trauma at C3 to C5 level results in paralysis of the phrenic nerve. Spinal cord trauma below the fifth cervical vertebra usually leaves the phrenic nerve intact but damages nerves that innervate the intercostal muscles, preventing anteroposterior chest expansion.

Trauma Trauma to the chest wall also impairs inspiration. The person with multiple rib fractures sometimes develops a flail chest, a life-threatening condition in which fractures cause instability in part of the chest wall. This causes paradoxical breathing in which the lung underlying the injured area contracts on inspiration and expands on expiration, making ventilation ineffective.

Chest wall or upper abdominal incisions also decrease chest wall movement because incisional pain causes the patient to inhale shallowly, which decreases chest wall movement.

NURSING KNOWLEDGE BASE

Your nursing knowledge prepares you to anticipate a patient's oxygenation needs. Knowledge of the patient's lifestyle patterns and developmental status allows you to anticipate cardiopulmonary problems.

Developmental Factors

The developmental stage of the patient and the normal aging process affect tissue oxygenation.

PREMATURE INFANTS Premature infants are at risk for hyaline membrane disease, which is due to surfactant deficiency. **Surfactant** is a chemical in the lung that maintains the integrity of the alveoli, keeping the alveoli dry and preventing alveolar collapse. When surfactant is inadequate the alveoli become stiff, fluid filled, and impede the exchange of respiratory gases. The surfactant-synthesizing ability of the lung develops about the seventh month and is lacking in preterm infants born before or during the seventh month. Premature infants are at risk for development of respiratory illnesses, such as respiratory syncytial virus (RSV) infection as a result of the underdevelopment of the lung.

INFANTS AND TODDLERS Infants and toddlers are at risk for upper respiratory tract infections as a result of frequent exposure to other children and exposure to second-hand smoke. During the teething process some infants develop nasal congestion, which encourages bacterial growth and increases the risk for respiratory tract infection. Upper respiratory tract infections are usually not dangerous, and infants and toddlers recover with little difficulty. Infants and toddlers are also at risk for airway obstruction because of their tendency to place a foreign object in their mouth.

SCHOOL-AGE CHILDREN AND ADOLESCENTS School-age children and adolescents are exposed to respiratory infections and respiratory risk factors, such as secondhand smoke and beginning to smoke cigarettes. A healthy child usually does not have adverse pulmonary effects from respiratory infections. A person who starts smoking in adolescence and continues to smoke into middle age, however, has an increased risk for cardiopulmonary disease and lung cancer.

YOUNG AND MIDDLE-AGE ADULTS Young and middle-age adults are exposed to many cardiopulmonary risk factors: an unhealthy diet, lack of exercise, stress, and cigarette smoking. Reducing these modifiable factors will sometimes decrease the patient's risk for cardiac or pulmonary diseases.

Pregnancy causes changes in ventilation. As the fetus grows during pregnancy, the greater size of the uterus pushes abdominal contents up against the diaphragm. During the last trimester of pregnancy the inspiratory capacity declines, resulting in **dyspnea** on exertion and increased fatigue.

OLDER ADULTS The cardiac and pulmonary systems change throughout the aging process (Table 29-3). Normal changes of aging include alterations in the clinical state that

TABLE 29-3 Changes in the Aging Cardiopulmonary System

FUNCTION	PATHOPHYSIOLOGICAL CHANGE	KEY CLINICAL FINDINGS
HEART		
Muscle contraction	Thickening of the ventricular wall, increased collagen and decreased elastin in the heart muscle	Decreased cardiac output
Blood flow	Heart valves become thicker and stiffer, more often in the mitral and aortic valves	Systolic ejection murmur
Conduction system	The SA node becomes fibrotic from calcification; the number of pacemaker cells in the SA node decreases	Increased PR, QRS, and Q/T intervals, decreased amplitude of the QRS complex
Arterial vessel compliance	Vessels become calcified, loss of arterial distensibility, decreased elastin in the vessel walls, more tortuous vessels	Hypertension, with an increase in systolic blood pressure
LUNGS		
Breathing mechanics	Decreased chest wall compliance and loss of elastic recoil	Prolonged exhalation phase
	Decreased respiratory muscle mass and strength	Decreased vital capacity
Oxygenation	Increased ventilation-perfusion mismatch	Decreased PaO_2
	Decreased alveolar surface area and decreased carbon dioxide diffusion capacity	Decreased cardiac output
		Slightly increased PaO_2
Breathing control/ breathing pattern	Decreased responsiveness of central and peripheral chemoreceptors to hypoxemia and hypercapnia	Decreased tidal volume
		Increased respiratory rate
Lung defense mechanisms	Decreased number of cilia	Decreased airway clearance
	Decreased immunoglobulin A (IgA) production and humoral and cellular immunity	Increased risk for infection
Sleep and breathing	Decreased respiratory drive	Increased risk for arterial desaturation
	Decreased tone of upper airway muscles	Increased risk for aspiration and infection
		Snoring/obstructive sleep apnea

PaO_2, Partial pressure of oxygen; *SA*, sinoatrial.

are expected to occur gradually over time. Over time the ventricular wall thickens, and there is a decrease in elastin. This leads to a decreased cardiac output. Arterial vessels in the older adult become calcified and also lose elastin. This may lead to hypertension and a rise in systolic blood pressure. Both of these normal changes of aging place the older adult at risk for heart failure.

Ventilation and transfer of respiratory gases decline with age as a result of changes in the alveoli and a reduced surface area for gas exchange. Reduction of functional cilia in the airway causes a decrease in the effectiveness of the cough mechanism, putting the older adult at increased risk for respiratory infections. These and many other normal changes of aging place the older adult at risk for complications in oxygenation, particularly when these patients are hospitalized. The acute care setting increases the risk for serious complications in the older adult. Older adults are at increased risk for the development of influenza, community-acquired pneumonia, and RSV infection, which sometimes results in death (Centers for Disease Control and Prevention [CDC], 2005).

Lifestyle Factors

Lifestyle factors that influence cardiopulmonary function include nutrition, exercise, cigarette smoking, substance abuse, and anxiety and stress.

NUTRITION Nutrition affects cardiopulmonary function in several ways. Good nutritional status supports the normal metabolic functions. A poor diet leads to risk factors affecting the heart and lungs, such as obesity, hypertension, heart disease, and chronic lung disease.

Inadequate nutrition occurs when nutritional intake does not meet nutritional needs. Without essential nutrients the patient may experience respiratory muscle wasting, resulting in decreased muscle strength and respiratory excursion. Cough efficiency is reduced secondary to respiratory muscle weakness, putting the patient at risk for retention of pulmonary secretions. A patient with chronic lung disease usually requires a diet higher in calories because of the increased work of breathing. A moderate-carbohydrate diet is recommended to prevent an increase in carbon dioxide production. Calories from carbohydrates should be no more than 50% of the daily allowance.

Overnutrition, or the excess intake of nutrients, most commonly leads to obesity. This leads to a decrease in lung expansion and an increase in oxygen demand to meet metabolic needs. Diets high in fat increase cholesterol and development of plaque in the coronary arteries, putting your patient at risk for CAD. Calories from carbohydrates should be no more than 50% of the daily allowance. Patients who have alterations in nutrition are also at risk for anemia. If the diet does not supply iron needed for hemoglobin synthesis, red blood cell synthesis is reduced and oxygen-carrying capacity decreases.

HYDRATION Fluid intake is essential for cellular health. Fluid intake depends on the patient's diet and disease processes that would require more or less water. Fluid volume overload or hypervolemia may lead to vascular congestion in patients with heart, kidney, or lung diseases. Dehydration or fluid volume deficit may result in dizziness, fainting, hypotension, or a decrease in respiratory secretion production or a thickening of respiratory secretions, making it difficult for the patient to expectorate.

EXERCISE Exercise increases the body's metabolic activity and oxygen demand. The rate and depth of respiration increase, enabling the person to inhale more oxygen and exhale excess carbon dioxide. A physical exercise program has many benefits (see Chapter 26). People who exercise daily for 60 minutes have a lower heart rate, lower blood pressure, decreased cholesterol, increased blood flow, and greater oxygen extraction by working muscles. The addition of weight training has shown benefit in decreasing the work of the heart by increasing the efficiency of the other muscles of the body. Fully conditioned people are able to increase oxygen consumption by 10% to 20% because of increased cardiac output and increased efficiency of the myocardium.

CIGARETTE SMOKING Cigarette smoking is associated with a number of diseases, including heart disease, chronic obstructive lung disease, and lung cancer. Inhaled nicotine enables plaque to build up more quickly in the blood vessels, increases the risks for blood clots, and causes vasoconstriction in the coronary and peripheral vessels. The risk for lung cancer is 10 times greater for a person who smokes than for a nonsmoker. Exposure to secondhand smoke increases the risk for lung cancer in the nonsmoker and worsens other pulmonary problems, such as asthma or COPD.

SUBSTANCE ABUSE Excessive use of alcohol and other drugs impair tissue oxygenation. The patient who has chronic substance abuse usually has a poor nutritional intake. This often causes a decreased intake from iron-rich foods, leading to a decrease in hemoglobin production. Excessive use of alcohol and certain other drugs depresses the respiratory center, reducing the rate and depth of respiration and the amount of inhaled oxygen. Substance abuse by either smoking or inhaling causes direct injury to lung tissue that leads to permanent lung damage and impaired oxygenation. Intravenous drug use places the patient at risk for infections of the heart, (endocarditis or myocarditis), blood clots, and transmitted diseases, such as human immune deficiency virus (HIV).

STRESS Stress is the demand that exceeds the patient's coping ability, whether physically or emotionally. This can adversely affect the patient's health and well-being. A continuous state of stress increases the body's metabolic rate and the oxygen demand. The body responds to stress by an increased rate and depth of respiration and increased cardiac output. Stressors may alter the normal response to illness and pain. Patients with high levels of stress are at risk for CAD, hypertension, and asthma. Most people are able to adapt to physical or emotional stressors. Some patients, particularly those with chronic illnesses or acute life-threatening illnesses, cannot tolerate the oxygen demands associated with stress.

ENVIRONMENTAL FACTORS The environment also influences oxygenation. The incidence of pulmonary disease is higher in smoggy, urban areas than in rural areas. In addition, the patient's workplace sometimes increases the risks for cardiopulmonary disease. Occupational pollutants include asbestos, talcum powder, dust, and airborne fibers. For example tunnel workers exposed to dust from blasting, drilling, and rock transport have an increased risk for COPD. Construction workers may be at risk for asbestosis after exposure to asbestos. This leads to pulmonary fibrosis, a restrictive lung disease, and may also lead to lung cancer. Mesothelioma results from asbestos exposure, and the incidence is expected to rise.

CRITICAL THINKING

Synthesis

You will apply elements of critical thinking whenever you perform the nursing process with a patient. Consider the scientific knowledge you have learned, your experience, critical thinking attitudes, and standards to ensure an individualized approach to patient care (Box 29-2).

KNOWLEDGE When caring for patients with cardiopulmonary problems, you need to incorporate and apply knowledge from physiology and pathophysiology; pharmacology; nutrition; and fluid, electrolyte, and acid-base balance. Your knowledge about health promotion and disease prevention is essential. This prevents or helps to reduce at-risk behaviors and unhealthy lifestyles in your patients who are at risk for or have cardiopulmonary problems. Your knowledge also assists patients in attaining and maintaining optimal cardiopulmonary function.

EXPERIENCE In the acute care setting you will care for patients with acute aggravations of their disease. When your patients require nursing management in the community setting, they are usually stable, productive members of the community with little or no change in lifestyle. Use your experience with cardiopulmonary diseases to help you recognize clinical changes and select effective interventions. Most importantly, use the resources available in your work area to assist you in providing safe patient care.

ATTITUDES You will use critical thinking attitudes as you provide nursing care for patients with cardiopulmonary alterations. As the patient's advocate, take into account that the patient is aware of his or her risk factors, and then partner with the patient to find the best teaching approaches. Do not be judgmental. Use discipline when providing health care information to your patients. For example, when deciding on the approach for a patient who has respiratory disease and still smokes, use the best-known teaching approaches. On the other hand, it is unlikely that an older adult with end-stage disease will be willing or able to stop smoking. In this case it is better to acknowledge that your patients already know the risks of smoking and know why they should stop than to bombard them with literature.

Perseverance is also important to finding effective patient-centered solutions. For example, when a patient has severe

BOX 29-2 SYNTHESIS IN PRACTICE

 John's *knowledge* of the physiology of pulmonary conditions will assist him in caring for Mr. King. Mr. King's history reveals risk factors in addition to a 40-year history of smoking 2 packs per day. Also, he still continues to smoke. John knows that the shortness of breath is because the infection is obstructing his alveolocapillary membrane, preventing oxygenation of blood in some parts of his lung. He also is aware of his preexisting COPD and the effects of his smoking. With John's *experience* working with patients who are addicted to inhaled nicotine, John recognizes the difficulty in quitting. He knows that the most effective time to encourage a patient to stop smoking is when they are in an acute care setting with an illness exacerbated by smoking.

John's *attitude* about his nursing care reflects his respect for the patient's autonomy and balances this with continually educating Mr. King about the risk factors of smoking. John knows the impact of support systems in assisting patients with coping with chronic illnesses. He uses creativity and independent thinking to incorporate community and family resources into the plan of care for Mr. King. John will need to inquire about his social supports and the availability in his community of programs to help him quit smoking. John reviews the *standards* set by the American Cancer Society to identify that tobacco use accounts for at least 30% of all cancer deaths and 87% of lung cancer deaths. He uses this and the resources at http://www.cancer.org to assist in educating Mr. King and his wife about cancer statistics and methods to quit smoking.

COPD, Chronic obstructive pulmonary disease.

cardiac or pulmonary disease and has a limited income, your solutions for promoting health and maintaining patient independence are complex. Sometimes you will need to continue to provide the same information at each visit. Often patients with chronic hypoxemia have a decreased short-term memory, and you will need to reinforce information previously provided.

STANDARDS Regulatory bodies and nationally recognized organizations set forth best practices. The American Heart Association (AHA), American Lung Association (ALA), American Thoracic Society (ATS), American Cancer Society (ACS), and Agency for Healthcare Research and Quality (AHRQ) have specific guidelines for cardiopulmonary nursing care and disease management. The ANA also has guidelines and standards for patient care. Each of these organizations reviews best practice standards and publishes its findings. Knowledge of the evidence that supports your practice enables you to provide safe and effective nursing care.

You will use professional standards in the care of all patients. In the care of Mr. King, these standards assist in determining the appropriate medical and nursing interventions for the patient with pneumonia.

NURSING PROCESS

■■■ASSESSMENT

Make sure the nursing assessment of your patient's cardiopulmonary functioning includes data collected from the following areas:

- History of the patient's baseline and present cardiopulmonary function, past cardiopulmonary illnesses, and measures the patient uses to improve breathing or heart function (e.g., medications, treatments, exercises)
- Physical examination of the patient's cardiopulmonary status (see Chapter 15)
- Review of laboratory and diagnostic test results

NURSING HISTORY The nursing history focuses on your patient's ability to meet oxygen needs and control symptoms. Ask questions that assist the patient in describing symptoms. Box 29-3 gives examples of assessment questions for you to ask your patient with cardiopulmonary conditions.

Risk Factors Investigate familial and environmental risk factors, such as a family history of cardiovascular or lung disease or outdoor air quality. Document which blood relatives have cardiopulmonary disease and their present level of health or age at time of death. Ask the patient about other risk factors such as exercise, stress, family history, tobacco use, and diet. Other family risk factors to assess include the presence of infectious diseases, particularly tuberculosis (TB). Determine who in the patient's household has the disease and the status of the treatment.

Environmental exposure to many inhaled substances, such as smog, cotton fibers, silicon, secondhand smoke, and asbestos, is closely linked to respiratory disease. Investigate exposures in the patient's home and workplace. Ask the following:

- Are there environmental conditions that affect your breathing where you work?
- Have you recently traveled to countries or areas of the United States where you have been exposed to uncommon respiratory diseases?

Fatigue Fatigue is a subjective sensation reported as a loss of endurance. Fatigue is often an early sign of worsening of the chronic underlying cardiopulmonary disease. To provide a mechanism to objectively measure fatigue, use a visual analog scale (see Chapter 31) with a rating from 0 to 10, with 10 being the worst level of fatigue and 0 representing no fatigue. In addition, ask your patients questions about their perception of fatigue:

- When did you first notice the fatigue? What makes it get better or worse?
- Was the onset sudden or gradual? Is it related to any time of the day or constant throughout the day?
- Does it prevent you from doing what you want to do?

BOX 29-3   Nursing Assessment Questions

NATURE OF THE CARDIOPULMONARY PROBLEM
- What types of breathing problems are you having?
- Describe the problem you are having with your heart.
- Does it occur at a specific time of the day, during or after exercise, or all the time?

SIGNS AND SYMPTOMS
- How has your breathing pattern changed?
- Are you having sputum with coughing? Is this different?
- Is your sputum a different color?
- Are you having any chest pain? Does the pain occur with breathing?

ONSET AND DURATION
- If you are having chest pain, what causes the pain and how long does it last? Is this a different type of pain?
- When did you notice your sputum change in color and amount?
- When did your coughing increase? How does this differ from your usual pattern of coughing?

SEVERITY
- On a scale of 0 to 10, with 10 being the most severe, rate your shortness of breath.
- What helps your shortness of breath?
- On a scale of 0 to 10, with 0 being no pain and 10 the most severe pain, rate your chest pain. Is the severity of your pain different today?
- What do you do for this pain?

PREDISPOSING FACTORS
- Have you been exposed to another person who had a cold or the flu?
- Are you taking your prescribed medications?
- Do you smoke? Have you been exposed to secondhand smoke?
- Have you been doing any unusual exercises?

EFFECT OF SYMPTOMS ON PATIENT
- Do these symptoms affect your daily activities? If so, how?
- What impact do these symptoms have on your appetite, sleeping habits, activity status?

Pain Cardiac pain does not occur with respiratory variations. It is most often substernal and typically radiates to the left arm and jaw in males. Some women have epigastric pain, complaints of indigestion, or a choking feeling and dyspnea. Pericardial pain resulting from an inflammation of the pericardial sac is usually nonradiating and often occurs with inspiration. Use a visual analog scale to assist the patient in describing the pain (see Chapter 31).

Pleuritic chest pain is peripheral and usually radiates to the scapular regions. Inspiratory maneuvers, such as coughing, yawning, and sighing, aggravate pleuritic chest pain. An inflammation or infection in the pleural space usually causes pleuritic chest pain. Patients often describe it as knifelike, lasting from 1 minute to hours, and increasing with inspiration.

Musculoskeletal pain is often present following exercise, rib trauma, and prolonged coughing episodes. Inspiratory movements aggravate the pain and are easily confused with pleuritic chest pain.

When assessing pain in patients with cardiopulmonary disease, obtain information specific to cardiac or inspiratory pain. For example, ask your patient the following:

- Have you ever had pain in your chest? Explain.
- Where and when do you feel the pain? Does it radiate? Does it change with inspiration? Does this pain go away when you hold your breath?
- What does the pain feel like? Sharp, dull, stabbing?
- Does it occur at rest or with activity?
- How long does it last?
- What makes it better?

Breathing Patterns Dyspnea is the subjective sensation of breathlessness as perceived by the patient. It is a clinical sign of hypoxia. Dyspnea is associated with symptoms such as exaggerated respiratory effort, use of the accessory muscles of respiration, nasal flaring, and marked increases in the rate and depth of respirations. Use a visual analog scale to help patients objectively assess their dyspnea, with 0 being no dyspnea and 10 being the worst dyspnea the patient has experienced. Measurement of dyspnea on the analog scale helps to show change in the patient's perception of breathlessness. Chronic dyspnea has long-term physical, psychological, and sociocultural consequences.

Dyspnea that occurs when a patient is sleeping is called paroxysmal nocturnal dyspnea (PND). The patient awakens in a panic, feels as if they are suffocating and has a strong need to sit up to relieve the breathlessness. The cause of PND is probably reabsorption of fluid from dependent body areas when the patient is recumbent, or reclining (Lewis and others, 2007).

Orthopnea is an abnormal condition in which the patient uses multiple pillows when lying down or has to sit to breathe. The number of pillows required for sleep, such as two or three pillows, quantifies the presence and severity of orthopnea.

Wheezing is a high-pitched musical sound caused by high-velocity movement of air through a narrowed airway. Wheezing is present in asthma, acute bronchitis, or pneumonia. Wheezing occurs on inspiration, expiration, or both. Determine any precipitating factors, such as respiratory infection, allergens, exercise, or stress.

Cough Cough is a sudden, audible expulsion of air from the lungs. Coughing is a protective reflex to clear the trachea, bronchi, and lungs of irritants and secretions. Some patients with chronic sinusitis cough only in the early morning, while trying to sleep, or immediately after rising from sleep. This clears the airway of sputum resulting from sinus drainage. Patients with chronic bronchitis generally produce sputum

all day, although the body produces greater amounts after rising from a semirecumbent or flat position. A **productive cough** results in sputum production that is swallowed or expectorated. Carefully collect data about the type, amount, color, and quantity of sputum.

If a patient reports **hemoptysis** (bloody sputum), determine if it is associated with coughing and bleeding from the upper respiratory tract, from sinus drainage, or from the gastrointestinal tract (hematemesis). Describe the hemoptysis, including amount, color, duration of bleeding, and presence of sputum.

Respiratory Infections Determine if your patient has had a Pneumovax or flu vaccine in the past (CDC, 2008). Ask about any known exposure to tuberculosis and the results of the tuberculin skin test, including type of test and date. Determine the patient's risk for HIV infection. Some patients with a history of intravenous drug use, blood transfusions, multiple unprotected sex partners, or a homosexual lifestyle are at a higher risk for developing HIV infection. Some patients do not display any symptoms of HIV infection until they have an opportunistic infection or vague complaints of fatigue and malaise.

Medication Use Assess your patient's knowledge and ability to correctly take medication (see Chapter 16). Review the patient's understanding of medication side effects and what to report to the health care provider. Common drugs monitored by measuring blood levels include theophylline and digitalis preparations.

Many herbals and over-the-counter (OTC) medications affect the heart rate and blood pressure and promote blood thinning. For example, the herb ma huang, a naturally occurring ephedrine, increases blood pressure and heart rate. Patients with cardiopulmonary disease should not use this herb. Patients with asthma should not use ephedrine-containing products such as bronchodilators, because they cause increased bronchospasm and respiratory arrest. Ginseng, garlic capsules, and ginkgo biloba have properties similar to aspirin and decrease platelet aggregation.

Illicit drugs, particularly parenterally administered narcotics, often come diluted with talcum powder. This causes pulmonary disorders resulting from the irritant effect of talcum powder on lung tissues.

PATIENT EXPECTATIONS Knowing what the patient expects regarding his or her health and its maintenance assists in determining goals of care, interventions, and use of patient education and home care resources.

You need to assess the patient's willingness to follow a treatment schedule. In addition, determine what your patient expects from caregivers. Does the patient expect health to improve or expect supportive care? Does your patient want to be an active participant in care or for family members to make decisions and provide care?

PHYSICAL EXAMINATION The physical examination includes evaluation of the entire cardiopulmonary system (see Chapter 15) (Tables 29-4 to 29-6).

Be mindful of your patient's limitations, such as breathlessness or fatigue. In some cases you will have to complete

TABLE 29-4 Inspection of Cardiopulmonary Status

ABNORMALITY	CAUSE
EYES	
Xanthelasma (yellow lipid lesions on eyelids)	Hyperlipidemia
Corneal arcus (whitish opaque ring around junction of cornea and sclera)	Abnormal finding in young to middle-age adults associated with hyperlipidemia (normal finding in older adults with arcus senilis)
Pale conjunctivae	Anemia
Cyanotic conjunctivae	Hypoxemia
Petechiae on conjunctivae	Fat embolus or bacterial endocarditis
SKIN	
Peripheral cyanosis	Vasoconstriction and diminished blood flow
Central cyanosis	Hypoxemia
Decreased skin turgor	Dehydration (normal finding in older adults as a result of decreased skin elasticity)
Dependent edema	Right- and left-sided heart failure
Periorbital edema	Kidney disease
FINGERTIPS AND NAIL BEDS	
Cyanosis	Decreased cardiac output or hypoxia; sometimes the result of decreased circulation to the affected limb or vasoconstriction secondary to cold
Splinter hemorrhages	Bacterial endocarditis
Clubbing	Chronic hypoxemia
MOUTH AND LIPS	
Cyanotic mucous membranes	Decreased oxygenation (hypoxia)
Pursed-lip breathing	Chronic lung disease
NECK VEINS	
Distention	Right-sided heart failure
NOSE	
Flaring nares	Air hunger, dyspnea
CHEST	
Retractions	Increased work of breathing, dyspnea
Asymmetry	Chest wall injury

TABLE 29-5 Assessment of Abnormal Chest Wall Movement

ABNORMALITY	CAUSE
Retraction: Visible sinking in soft tissues of chest that lie between and around firmer tissue (e.g., cartilaginous and bony ribs); retractions have specific beginning point and worsening with need for increased inspiratory effort; possibly found at intercostal space, intraclavicular space, trachea, and substernally*	Any condition that causes increased inspiratory effort (e.g., airway obstruction, asthma, tracheobronchitis)
Paradoxical breathing: Asynchronous breathing; chest contraction during inspiration and expansion during expiration	Flail chest
Increased anteroposterior diameter	Senile emphysema or chronic obstructive pulmonary disease

*Infants can experience sternal and substernal retractions with only slight inspiratory effort because of chest pliability.

your assessment in short sections to allow the patient to rest and recover. If your patient is breathless or fatigued, you may ask closed-ended questions, with yes or no answers. Focus your initial assessment on your patient's immediate problems (Table 29-7).

DIAGNOSTIC TESTS Diagnostic tests determine adequacy of the cardiac conduction system, myocardial contraction, and blood flow. They also measure the adequacy of ventilation and oxygenation and visualize structures of the respiratory system. Some patients will need an ECG, chest

TABLE 29-6   Respiratory Patterns

TYPE/PATTERN	RATE (BREATHS PER MINUTE)	CLINICAL SIGNIFICANCE
Eupnea	12-20	Normal rate in the adult
Tachypnea	>35	Results from anxiety or response to pain or fever, respiratory failure, shortness of breath, or a respiratory infection; leads to respiratory alkalosis, paresthesia, tetany, and confusion
Bradypnea	<10	Results from sleep, respiratory depression, drug overdose, or central nervous system lesion
Apnea	Periods of no respiration lasting >15 seconds	Sometimes intermittent, such as in sleep apnea, or prolonged, as in a respiratory arrest
Kussmaul's	Usually >35, may be slow or normal	Tachypnea pattern associated with metabolic imbalances such as diabetic slow or normal ketoacidosis, metabolic acidosis, or renal failure
Cheyne-Stokes	Abnormal pattern of breathing, varying between apnea and tachypnea	Caused by damage to respiratory system; lungs are compensating for changing serum partial pressures of oxygen and carbon dioxide

TABLE 29-7   FOCUSED PATIENT ASSESSMENT

FACTORS TO ASSESS	QUESTIONS	PHYSICAL ASSESSMENT
Dependent edema	Do your legs swell every day? Are they swollen in the morning when you arise?	Palpate amount of edema: trace to 4+. Observe for neck vein distention.
	Do they get better if you put them up?	Observe for breathlessness at rest and on exertion. Assess pedal and popliteal pulses.
	Do you have trouble getting your socks and shoes on and off?	
	Does your belt or waistband feel tighter?	Observe for bilateral or unilateral edema.
Breathing pattern	When do you become short of breath?	
	Are you able to do your own personal hygiene?	Observe patient perform activities of daily living.
	How far can you walk without getting short of breath?	Observe ambulating. Determine distance walked without shortness of breath.
	How many pillows do you use to sleep at night?	
Airway patency	How often do you cough?	Observe for use of pursed-lip breathing.
	Do you bring up any mucus when coughing?	Observe patient in various positions.
	Is there anything that brings on your cough?	Monitor sputum for color, consistency, amount, and odor.

x-ray examination, pulse oximetry, laboratory tests (e.g., arterial blood gas levels, complete blood count, sputum analysis, cardiac enzyme levels), cardiac stress test, pulmonary function test, or cardiac catheterization.

Tuberculosis skin testing is important to determine exposure to TB (Box 29-4). Once a TB skin test is positive, the patient then has a chest x-ray examination.

■■■NURSING DIAGNOSIS

Your patient with an altered level of oxygenation may have nursing diagnoses that are primarily of cardiovascular or pulmonary origin. You will base each nursing diagnosis on specific defining characteristics and include the related etiology. The defining characteristics or signs and symptoms

BOX 29-4 Tuberculosis Skin Testing

- Skin testing determines the presence of *Mycobacterium tuberculosis*.
- Tuberculosis skin testing (TST) is performed by an intradermal injection of 0.1 mL of tuberculin purified protein derivative (PPD) on the inner surface of the forearm (see Chapter 16). The injection produces a pale elevation of the skin (a wheal) 6 to 10 mm in diameter. Afterward the injection site is circled and the patient is instructed not to wash off the circle.
- Tuberculin skin tests are read between 48 to 72 hours. If the site is not read within 72 hours, the patient must have another skin test.
- *Positive results:* A palpable, elevated, hardened area around the injection site, caused by edema and inflammation from the antigen-antibody reaction, measured in millimeters.
- A reddened flat area is **not** a positive reaction, and you do not need to measure it.
- TB testing in patients with altered immune function, such as an older adult, an HIV-positive patient, or someone receiving chemotherapy, is less reliable.

HIV, Human immune deficiency virus.

identified during your assessment validate the diagnostic label. Appropriate nursing diagnoses include but are not limited to the following:

- *Activity intolerance*
- *Ineffective airway clearance*
- *Ineffective breathing pattern*
- *Decreased cardiac output*
- *Fatigue*
- *Impaired gas exchange*
- *Risk for infection*
- *Acute pain*

During the assessment process, you collected data that accurately reflected the patient's needs. For example, your objective findings in a patient who comes to the clinic with a diagnosis of pneumonia include productive cough, breathlessness, crackles, tachypnea, changes in depth of respiration, and pleuritic pain. These findings support the diagnosis of *ineffective airway clearance related to the presence of tracheobronchial secretions*. The ability of your patient to bring up sputum is a crucial part of treatment for pneumonia. Pleuritic pain interferes with a patient's ability to rest and impairs the ability to cough and clear the airway, resulting in worsening infection.

Another example of a related nursing diagnosis is *activity intolerance related to imbalance between oxygen supply and demand*. The objective findings include an inability to move secretions, restlessness, tachycardia, breathlessness, use of accessory muscles, and hypoxia (PaO_2 less than 60 mm Hg). Patients will avoid physical effort because exercise often

brings on more breathlessness. Consequently their level of fitness decreases, they become weak, and they have difficulty with normal activities of daily living. As the patient increases the level of exercise tolerance, the degree of dyspnea and shortness of breath may diminish. Identifying the appropriate related factor will enable you to design nursing interventions to maximize the balance between the patient's oxygen supply and demand.

■■■PLANNING

GOALS AND OUTCOMES Patients with impaired oxygenation require a nursing care plan directed toward meeting the actual or potential oxygenation needs of the patient. Your individual goals come from your patient-centered needs. Oxygenation goals for your patient will include providing a patent airway, improving oxygenation, and increasing the level of independence and tolerance for activity (see Care Plan).

All goals need to have measurable outcomes for you to be able to determine whether they have been met. These include objective data, such as arterial blood gas levels, laboratory findings, chest radiographs, ECG patterns, blood pressure, and pulse. Quantify subjective findings, such as the reported degree of breathlessness or pain.

Patients have more than one nursing diagnosis and frequently these diagnoses have an impact on one another (Figure 29-6). It is important to include the family and patient in all care planning. Alterations in oxygenation are often chronic problems that affect the patient and the family. The patient remains a member of the community despite the illness. Planning with the family and using community resources help patients adapt to activities of daily living.

SETTING PRIORITIES Help the patient and family set priorities for care based on the patient's tolerance level. Ask the patient how he or she is feeling today, and then determine what aspects of care are most important. If the patient is having pain, relief of pain is the priority over getting up in the chair or completing personal hygiene. Ask patients what they want to accomplish. If they are diaphoretic, they will appreciate clean sheets and a bath after being medicated for pain.

Base your decision to delegate responsibility to nursing assistive personnel (NAP) on your assessment of the patient and the type of care the patient will receive. Consider what tasks are safe to delegate, within the skill set of the NAP, and how the patient will feel about the care that you have delegated. The priority is to maintain or improve the patient's oxygenation and meet the patient's needs. You are ultimately responsible for all total patient care.

COLLABORATIVE CARE Impaired levels of oxygenation affect all aspects of your patient's life, not just the physical component. Designing collaborative nursing interventions with physical and occupational therapy and social services will improve your patient's level of functioning. Respiratory therapy assists in designing measures to improve breathing and cough control. Social services are able to recommend support groups. When planning care for patients with impaired oxygenation, be sensitive to the needs of the

CARE PLAN   Oxygenation

 ASSESSMENT
John Smith begins his morning care for Mr. King. He finds Mr. King restless and anxious. As the day progresses, John notices that Mr. King's coughs are weaker, less sputum is produced, and Mr. King is becoming more fatigued.

ASSESSMENT ACTIVITIES

Ask Mr. King how long he has been short of breath.

Ask Mr. King how long he has had his cough and if it is a productive cough.

Auscultate Mr. King's lung fields.

Ask Mr. King to produce a sputum sample.

FINDINGS/DEFINING CHARACTERISTICS*

He replies, "I have been **short of breath for 1 week,** and it has **gotten worse.**" His vital signs are pulse rate, 120 beats per minute; temperature, 102° F; **increased respiratory rate, 36 breaths per minute;** blood pressure, 110/45 mm Hg, and **an SpO$_2$ of 82%.** Mr. King is **dyspneic** as he answers questions.

"I usually **cough** when I wake up in the mornings. Three days ago I noticed that I **was coughing up thick mucus** that has not stopped."

On auscultation there are **audible expiratory wheezes, crackles, and diminished breath sounds** over right lower lobe.

Sputum is thick and discolored (yellow-green).

NURSING DIAGNOSIS: Ineffective airway clearance related to pulmonary secretions.

PLANNING

GOAL

• Pulmonary secretions will return to baseline levels within 24 to 36 hours.

• Mr. King's oxygenation status will improve in 36 hours.

EXPECTED OUTCOMES (NOC)†

Respiratory Status: Gas Exchange
• Mr. King's sputum will be clear, white, and thinner in consistency within 36 hours.
• Mr. King's lung sounds will be at baseline within 36 hours.
• Mr. King's respiratory rate will be between 16 and 24 breaths per minute within 24 hours.
• Mr. King will be able to clear airway secretions by coughing in 24 hours.
• Mr. King's SpO$_2$ will be greater than 85% within 24 hours.
• Mr. King's perceptions of dyspnea will improve.

INTERVENTIONS (NIC)‡

Airway Management
• Have Mr. King deep breathe and cough every 2 hours while awake.

• Have Mr. King change position frequently if on bed rest. If able, have him ambulate 10 to 15 minutes every 8 hours, and encourage him to sit up in a chair as often as he is able to tolerate.
• Encourage Mr. King to increase his fluid intake to 2800 mL/24 hours if his cardiac condition does not contraindicate it. Avoid caffeinated beverages and alcohol; recommend water.

RATIONALE

A major complication of reduced mobility is retention of pulmonary secretions, which predisposes the patient to atelectasis and pneumonia.
Ambulation, sitting upright, and frequent position changes are consistent with normal activities and promote normal lung function and mucociliary clearance.

Fluid intake of 2800 mL/24 hours will help liquefy secretions for easier removal. Caffeinated and alcoholic beverages promote diuresis and dehydration. Water is an effective expectorant, easily available, and cost-effective.

***Defining characteristics** are shown in **bold** type.
†Outcomes classification label from Moorhead S and others, editors: *Nursing outcomes classification (NOC),* ed 4, St. Louis, 2008, Mosby.
‡Intervention classification labels from Bulechek GM and others, editors: *Nursing interventions classification (NIC),* ed 5, St. Louis, 2008, Mosby.

CARE PLAN Oxygenation—cont'd

EVALUATION

NURSING ACTIONS	PATIENT RESPONSE/FINDING	ACHIEVEMENT OF OUTCOME
Ask Mr. King to keep track of his fluid intake.	Mr. King has completed accurate intake list daily, averaging 2800 mL/hr. Coughing thin secretions.	Good daily fluid intake. Secretions are thin, white, and watery. Outcome met.
Ask Mr. King to ambulate for 10 minutes every 4 hours.	Mr. King ambulates once every 8 hours.	Mr. King ambulates for about 5 minutes. Outcome not completely achieved.
Auscultate the chest.	Lung sounds are clear.	Outcome met.
Ask Mr. King to keep track of deep breathing every 2 hours while awake.	Diary completed for each day. Mr. King has documented deep breathing every 2 hours while awake 85% of the time.	Secretions are thin, the lung is clear, and there is no evidence of infection. Outcome met.

patient as well as the family. Chronic illness changes the dynamics of family relationships. Sometimes roles need to change, and the patient and family have difficulty coping. Provide an empathic ear to the family as well as the patient. Help them develop solutions that maintain the dignity of both parties and continue to support the family unit.

■■■ IMPLEMENTATION

Nursing interventions for patients with oxygenation alterations are diverse. Cultural and religious beliefs of patients may affect the selection of interventions (Box 29-5). Health promotion activities may result in healthier lifestyle habits. Symptom management aids in reducing the severity of cardiopulmonary problems. Interventions aimed at improving respiration and ventilation make it easier for patients to breathe.

HEALTH PROMOTION Maintaining the patient's optimal level of health is important in reducing the number and severity of cardiopulmonary symptoms. Prevention of disease exacerbations and community-acquired infections is the goal of health promotion. Provide health education to help patients make choices for improving health practices (Box 29-6). Some patient education topics to consider include regular blood pressure checkups and taking blood pressure medication as prescribed; low-fat, low-salt, proper caloric diet; importance and benefits of pneumococcal vaccine and annual influenza vaccine; smoking cessation and avoiding secondhand smoke exposure. Be sure to individualize the patient teaching to meet the needs of the patient. Older adults have differing needs with educational material and respond differently than younger patients (Box 29-7, p. 822).

Influenza and Pneumococcal Vaccine Influenza is a viral infection that can cause serious complications in children, older adults, and those with cardiopulmonary diseases. Over 226,000 patients are admitted to the hospital each year because of influenza (CDC, 2008). The infection can lead to pneumo-

nia and critical conditions that require hospitalization. The Centers for Disease Control and Prevention (CDC) recommends annual influenza vaccines for all children 6 months of age and older and people over the age of 50 years. In addition, patients with chronic illnesses, women planning to be pregnant in the flu season, people with immune-compromised diseases, and anyone between the ages of 6 and 18 who is receiving aspirin therapy should receive the influenza vaccine (CDC, 2008). Persons with a known hypersensitivity to eggs should not receive the vaccine. Health care providers must assess all other allergies before administering the vaccine.

The pneumococcal vaccine protects high-risk patients from acquiring pneumococcal disease. It is recommended for all adults over the age of 65, those with chronic diseases, and people with immune-compromised diseases. Most people do not need a booster shot unless they received their first dose before the age of 65 and/or they have immune-compromised diseases, chronic kidney disease, or have received a transplant. Pregnant women should consult an obstetrician before receiving either vaccine (CDC, 2008).

Environmental Modifications Avoiding exposure to secondhand smoke is important for patients with cardiopulmonary illnesses. Most public places and businesses have now adopted a no-smoking policy or offer separate smoking areas. When a patient lives with secondhand smoke in the home, you need to provide counseling and support to help the smoker understand the effects of secondhand smoke on the patient. You must also assess environmental hazards in the workplace. Many health care institution dress codes prohibit the use of perfumes and colognes because they often affect patient breathing patterns and allergies. Discuss risk factors and ways to reduce exposure.

ACUTE CARE Patients with acute cardiopulmonary illnesses require nursing interventions directed toward halting the pathological process, such as a respiratory tract infection. Nursing interventions should also focus on shortening the

CONCEPT MAP

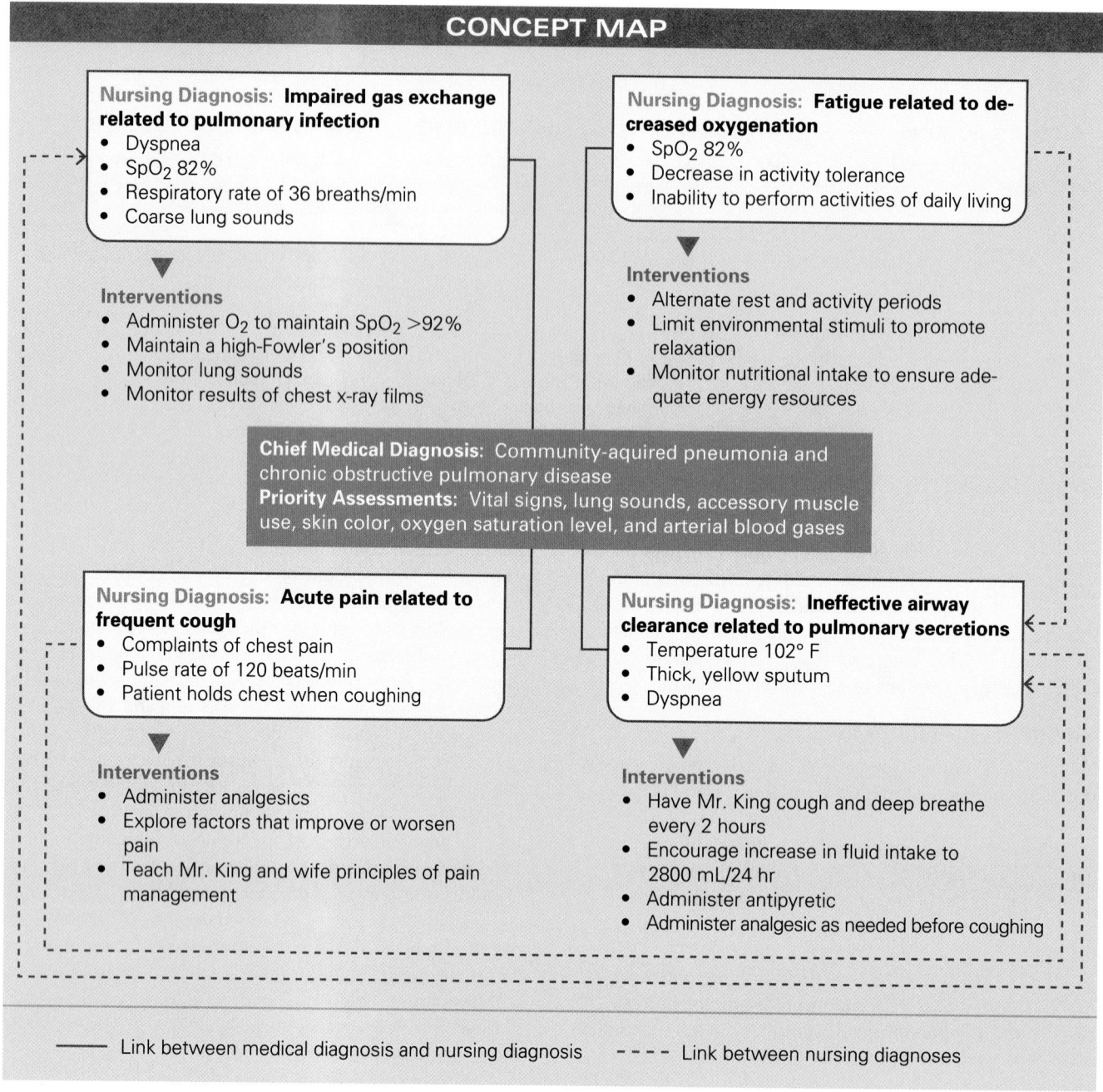

Nursing Diagnosis: Impaired gas exchange related to pulmonary infection
- Dyspnea
- SpO_2 82%
- Respiratory rate of 36 breaths/min
- Coarse lung sounds

Interventions
- Administer O_2 to maintain SpO_2 >92%
- Maintain a high-Fowler's position
- Monitor lung sounds
- Monitor results of chest x-ray films

Nursing Diagnosis: Fatigue related to decreased oxygenation
- SpO_2 82%
- Decrease in activity tolerance
- Inability to perform activities of daily living

Interventions
- Alternate rest and activity periods
- Limit environmental stimuli to promote relaxation
- Monitor nutritional intake to ensure adequate energy resources

Chief Medical Diagnosis: Community-aquired pneumonia and chronic obstructive pulmonary disease
Priority Assessments: Vital signs, lung sounds, accessory muscle use, skin color, oxygen saturation level, and arterial blood gases

Nursing Diagnosis: Acute pain related to frequent cough
- Complaints of chest pain
- Pulse rate of 120 beats/min
- Patient holds chest when coughing

Interventions
- Administer analgesics
- Explore factors that improve or worsen pain
- Teach Mr. King and wife principles of pain management

Nursing Diagnosis: Ineffective airway clearance related to pulmonary secretions
- Temperature 102° F
- Thick, yellow sputum
- Dyspnea

Interventions
- Have Mr. King cough and deep breathe every 2 hours
- Encourage increase in fluid intake to 2800 mL/24 hr
- Administer antipyretic
- Administer analgesic as needed before coughing

—— Link between medical diagnosis and nursing diagnosis   - - - - Link between nursing diagnoses

Figure 29-6 ■ Concept Map.

duration and severity of the illness, such as hospitalization with heart failure and preventing complications from illness or treatments, such as hospital-acquired infection resulting from invasive procedures.

Dyspnea Management Dyspnea is difficult to measure and treat, thus requiring individualized treatments for each patient. You will usually need to implement more than one therapy. Initially you will treat and stabilize the underlying processes that cause or worsen dyspnea, and then administer four additional therapies:

1. Medications (e.g., bronchodilators, steroids, mucolytics, antianxiety drugs)

2. Oxygen therapy as indicated
3. Physical techniques (e.g., cardiopulmonary reconditioning, breathing techniques, cough control)
4. Psychosocial techniques (e.g., relaxation techniques, biofeedback, meditation) to lessen the sensation of dyspnea

Maintenance and Promotion of Oxygenation Some patients require oxygen therapy to keep a healthy level of tissue oxygenation. The goal of **oxygen therapy** is to prevent or relieve hypoxia. Any patient with impaired tissue oxygenation will benefit from controlled oxygen administration. Oxygen is not a substitute for other treatments. Use it only when indicated. Oxygen is a drug. It is expensive and has dangerous

BOX 29-5   CULTURAL FOCUS

As a nursing student, you may encounter many different cultures and faiths. A patient's beliefs may affect how you care for your patient and his or her family. Jehovah's Witnesses is a religion in which the individual believes in God and Jesus. Jehovah's Witnesses adhere to the *New World Translation of the Holy Scriptures,* and all of their beliefs are based on the Bible. Patients of the Jehovah's Witnesses faith accept a great deal of health care practices. They do not believe in faith healing, and seeking medical care is a personal choice. A common ethical dilemma is the Jehovah Witnesses' avoidance of blood products, transfusions, and food that contains blood. Members quote, "It's blood—you must not eat" (Genesis 9:3-4) to support their choice not to receive blood. Our goal as nurses should be to understand and respect our patient's cultural and faith-based belief systems.

IMPLICATIONS FOR PRACTICE
- Inform patients who follow the Jehovah's Witnesses faith of their options, including alternatives to blood products, such as hetastarch and dextran.
- Ensure that patients know the risks of their choices and acknowledge the possible outcomes.

Data from Watchtower: official site of Jehovah's Witnesses, 2008, http://www.watchtower.org/.

BOX 29-6   PATIENT TEACHING

Health Maintenance

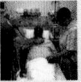 Mr. and Mrs. King are both interested in how to prevent hospitalizations in the future and what they can do to maintain their health. John Smith has developed the following teaching plan to help the Kings meet their goals:

OUTCOME
- Upon completion of the teaching session, Mr. and Mrs. King will be able to verbalize the steps they need to take to improve their health maintenance and reduce the risk for future hospitalizations.

TEACHING STRATEGIES
- Establish rapport with the Kings, and maintain eye contact during the teaching session.
- Use words the Kings will understand; avoid medical jargon when possible.
- Set goals in partnership with the Kings so that they are realistic, meaningful, and achievable.
- With each significant point, ask the Kings to repeat back the information you have given them.
- Provide an overview of chronic obstructive pulmonary disease and pneumonia, signs and symptoms of exacerbation, medications, and follow-up appointments.
- Encourage Mr. King to balance activity and rest. Report any changes in activity tolerance to his primary health care provider.
- Provide a written copy of the material taught for reinforcement and reference.
- Allow time for questions, and answer honestly.
- Summarize the material.

EVALUATION STRATEGIES
- Ask Mr. and Mrs. King to verbalize what they learned.
- Ask Mr. King to describe in simple terms what community-acquired pneumonia and chronic obstructive pulmonary disease are and signs and symptoms of exacerbation.
- Ask the Kings to verbalize understanding of each medication Mr. King will be taking.
- Ask Mr. and Mrs. King if they have any questions or need any additional information.

side effects. As with any drug, continuously monitor the dosage or concentration of oxygen. Routinely check the physician's or health care provider's orders to verify that the patient is receiving the prescribed oxygen concentration. The six rights of medication administration also apply to oxygen administration (see Chapter 16).

Safety Precautions With Oxygen Therapy. Oxygen is a highly combustible gas and fuels fire readily. Although it will not spontaneously burn or cause an explosion, it can easily cause a fire to ignite in a patient's room if it contacts a spark from a cigarette or electrical equipment.

With increasing use of home oxygen therapy, patients and health care professionals need to be aware of these dangers of combustion. Promote safety by using the following measures:

- Place "No smoking" signs on the patient's room door and over the bed. Inform the patient, visitors, roommates, and all personnel that smoking is not permitted in areas where oxygen is in use.
- Determine that all electrical equipment in the room is functioning correctly and is properly grounded (see Chapter 27).
- Know the fire procedures and the location of the closest fire extinguisher.
- Check the oxygen level of portable tanks before transporting to ensure there is enough oxygen in the tank.

Oxygen Supply. Oxygen tanks or a permanent wall-piped system supplies oxygen to the patient's bedside. Oxygen tanks are transported on wide-based carriers that allow the tank to be upright at the patient's bedside. Regulators control the amount of oxygen delivered. One common type of oxygen tank is an upright flowmeter with a flow-adjustment valve at the top. A second type is a cylinder indicator with a flow-adjustment handle.

Methods of Oxygen Delivery. Nasal cannula, nasal catheter, face mask, and the mechanical ventilator are all ways to deliver oxygen to the patient (Table 29-8).

Home Oxygen. Indications for home oxygen therapy include PaO_2 of 55 mm Hg or less or arterial oxygen saturation (SaO_2) of 88% or less on room air at rest, on exertion, or with exercise. When home oxygen is necessary, it is usually delivered by nasal cannula. If your patient has a permanent tra-

BOX 29-7   CARE OF THE OLDER ADULT

Oxygen Problem Manifestations

- Risk factor modification is important, including smoking cessation, weight reduction, a low-cholesterol and low-salt diet, management of hypertension, and exercise.
- Coronary artery disease is the leading cause of death and disability in women older than 40 years of age.
- Older adults have more atypical signs and symptoms of coronary artery disease.
- The incidence of atrial fibrillation increases with age and is the leading contributing factor for stroke in the older adult.
- Healthy behavior changes sometimes slow or halt the progression of the older adult's disease. However, it is often more difficult to get older adults to change long-term unhealthy habits.
- Mental status changes are often the first sign of respiratory problems in the older adult and include subtle increases in forgetfulness and irritability.
- The older adult often does not complain of dyspnea until it affects activities of daily living, and then only if the activities are important to the older adult.
- Use cough suppressants with caution because of changes in the older patient's cough mechanism. Cough suppression leads to retention of pulmonary secretions, plugged airways, and atelectasis.
- Chronic illness in the older adult sometimes results in unacceptable behavior patterns because of loss of control experienced with a chronic illness.

cheostomy, a T tube or tracheostomy collar is necessary to provide humidification to the airway.

Three types of oxygen systems are used: compressed oxygen, liquid oxygen, and oxygen concentrators. In the home the major consideration is the oxygen delivery source. Patients requiring home oxygen need extensive teaching to be able to continue oxygen therapy at home efficiently and safely. This includes oxygen safety, regulation of the amount of oxygen, and how to use the prescribed home oxygen delivery system. The case coordinator or social worker usually assists with arranging the home care nurse and oxygen vendor.

Mobilization of Pulmonary Secretions The ability of a patient to mobilize pulmonary secretions makes the difference between a short-term illness and a long recovery involving complications.

Hydration. Maintenance of adequate hydration promotes mucociliary clearance, the body's natural mechanism for removing mucus and cellular debris from the respiratory tract. In patients with adequate hydration, pulmonary secretions are thin, white, watery, and easily removable with minimal coughing. A fluid intake of 1500 to 2000 mL per day will help keep pulmonary secretions thin and easy to expectorate, unless contraindicated by cardiac condition.

Humidification. Humidification is necessary for patients receiving oxygen therapy at more than 4 L/min (AACR, 2007). You humidify a nasal catheter, nasal cannula, or face mask by

bubbling it through water. When using humidity, make sure to use sterile saline for inhalation. Also, make sure to change the solution according to agency procedures. Humidification is a source for hospital-acquired infections because the moist environment supports the growth of pathogens.

Nebulization. Nebulization uses the aerosol principle to suspend a maximum number of water drops or particles of the desired size in inspired air. The moisture added to the respiratory system through nebulization improves clearance and is often used for administration of bronchodilators and mucolytic agents.

Maintenance of a Patent Airway The airway is patent when the trachea, bronchi, and large airways are free from obstructions. You use three types of interventions to maintain a patent airway: coughing techniques, suctioning, and insertion of an artificial airway.

Coughing Techniques. Coughing maintains a patent airway by removing secretions from both the upper and lower airways. You evaluate cough effectiveness by sputum expectoration, the patient's report of swallowed sputum, or clearing of adventitious lung sounds. Encourage patients with chronic pulmonary diseases, upper respiratory tract infections, and lower respiratory tract infections to deep breathe and cough at least every 2 hours while awake. Encourage patients with a large amount of sputum to cough every hour while awake and to awaken to cough every 2 to 3 hours while asleep until the acute phase of sputum production has ended.

Cascade Cough. With the cascade cough, the patient takes a slow, deep breath and holds it for 2 seconds while contracting expiratory muscles. Then the patient opens the mouth and performs a series of coughs throughout exhalation, thereby coughing at progressively lowered lung volumes. This technique promotes airway clearance and a patent airway in patients with large volumes of sputum.

Huff Cough. The huff cough stimulates a natural cough reflex and is generally effective only for clearing central airways. While exhaling, the patient opens the glottis by saying the word *huff*. With practice the patient inhales more air and is able to progress to the cascade cough.

Quad Cough. The quad cough technique is for patients without abdominal muscle control, such as those with spinal cord injuries. While the patient breathes out with a maximal expiratory effort, the patient or you push inward and upward on the abdominal muscles toward the diaphragm, causing the cough.

Suctioning Techniques. When a patient is unable to effectively clear respiratory tract secretions with coughing, suctioning clears the airways. The primary suctioning techniques are oropharyngeal and nasopharyngeal suctioning, orotracheal and nasotracheal suctioning, and tracheal suctioning through an artificial airway (Skill 29-1).

These techniques are based on common principles. Because the nasotrachea and trachea are considered sterile, sterile technique is required for orotracheal and nasotracheal suctioning (Pedersen and others, 2009). The mouth is considered clean, and therefore the suctioning of oral and nasopharyngeal secretions requires only clean technique. Always suction oral secre-

TABLE 29-8 Oxygen Delivery Systems

DELIVERY SYSTEM	INDICATIONS	O_2 CONCENTRATION (FLOW RATE)	CONSIDERATIONS
Nasal cannula	Simple, comfortable device to deliver low-concentration O_2 (<6 L/min)	24% (1 L/min) 28% (2 L/min) 32% (3 L/min) 36% (4 L/min) 40% (5 L/min) 44% (6 L/min)	Flow rates more than 4 L/min often cause drying effect on mucosa; humidify oxygen; be alert for skin breakdown over ears and in nares; questionable efficiency in mouth breathers
Transtracheal O_2 (TTO) cannula	For chronic lung diseases; small, intravenous-size catheter inserted directly into trachea	Flow rates range from ¼ to 4 L/min and range from 22%-45% (AARC, 2007). This device is individualized to meet patient requirements.	TTO requires greater patient supervision and have an increased risk for complications. There is no O_2 lost to atmosphere; patients achieve adequate oxygenation at lower rates (more efficient, less expensive, and produces fewer side effects); patients more likely to use O_2 because of mobility, comfort, and cosmetic improvement
Oxygen masks	Administer O_2, humidity, or heated humidity		Be alert for skin breakdown around face and ears
Simple face mask	Short-term O_2 therapy	40%-60% (5-8 L/min)	Contraindicated for patients with carbon dioxide retention; effective for mouth breathers (Figure 29-7)
Partial non-rebreather mask with a reservoir bag	Delivers high concentrations of O_2	60%-95% (6-10 L/min)	Frequently inspect the bag to make sure it is inflated (Figure 29-8)
Venturi mask	Can deliver precise, high-flow rates of O_2; adapters can be applied to increase humidification	24%-28% (4 L/min) 35%-40% (8 L/min) 50%-60% (12 L/min)	Mask must be removed when patient eats (Figure 29-9)

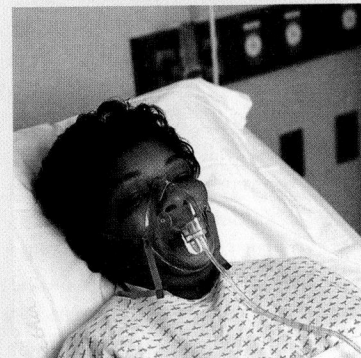

Figure 29-7 ■ Simple face mask.

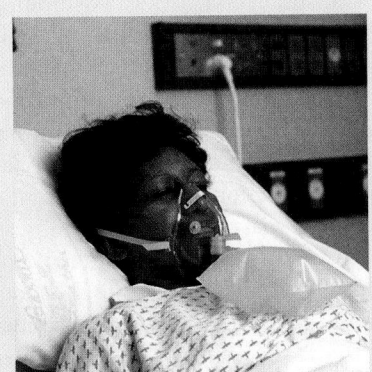

Figure 29-8 ■ Plastic face mask with inflated reservoir bag.

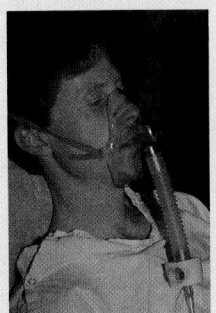

Figure 29-9 ■ Venturi mask.

tions after suctioning of the nasotrachea and trachea when combining suction techniques. Clinical assessment should determine the frequency of suctioning. When you notice secretions by inspection or auscultation techniques, suctioning is required. There is no evidence for routine suctioning every 1 to 2 hours (Pedersen and others, 2009).

Oropharyngeal and Nasopharyngeal Suctioning. Use oropharyngeal or nasopharyngeal suctioning to assist the patient who is able to cough effectively but is unable to clear secretions by expectorating or swallowing. Use a Yankauer or tonsillar tip suction device for oropharyngeal suctioning (Figure 29-10). A Yankauer suction catheter is a rigid plastic catheter with one

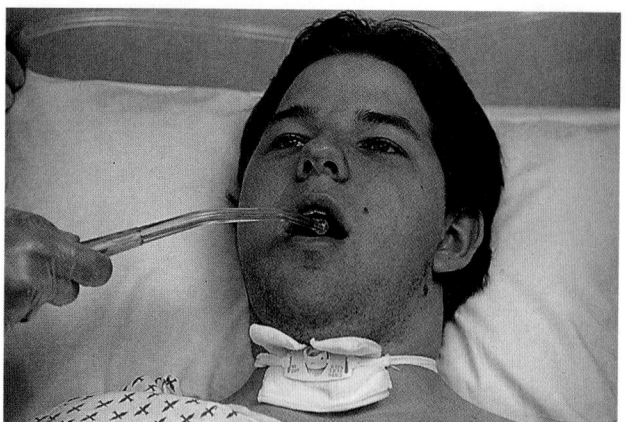

Figure 29-10 ■ Oropharyngeal suctioning. (From Perry AG, Potter PA: *Clinical nursing skills and techniques,* ed 7, St. Louis, 2010, Mosby.)

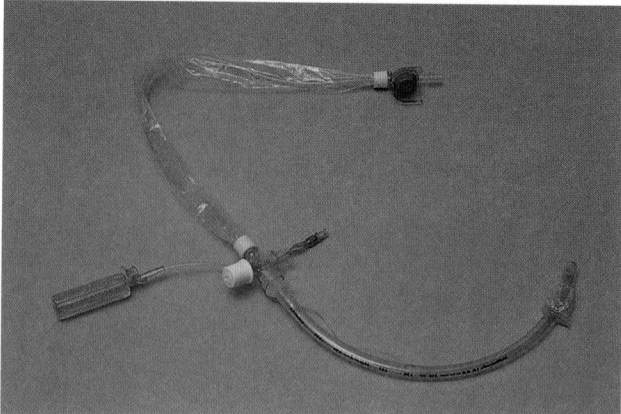

Figure 29-11 ■ Ballard tracheal care closed suction.

large and several small eyelets through which mucus is removed. The catheter is angled to facilitate removal of secretions from the mouth. Use the Yankauer suction catheter when oral secretions are thick and plentiful. Do not use the Yankauer suction catheter in the nares because of its size.

Orotracheal and Nasotracheal Suctioning. Orotracheal or nasotracheal suctioning is necessary when the patient is unable to cough and does not have an artificial airway (see Skill 29-1). You pass a catheter through the mouth or nose into the trachea. The nose is the preferred route because stimulation of the gag reflex is minimal. The procedure is similar to nasopharyngeal suctioning, but the catheter tip is in the trachea.

Tracheal Suctioning. Perform tracheal suctioning through the artificial airway, such as a tracheostomy tube or endotracheal tube (ET). Two suctioning methods currently used include use of a single catheter for one-time use and closed suctioning, including a multiple-use catheter. The suction catheter in closed suctioning is encased in a plastic sheath and used for 24 to 48 hours (Figure 29-11). You will use closed suctioning most often for patients who require mechanical ventilation because it continuously delivers oxygen during suctioning and keeps the delivery system sterile (Box 29-8).

Artificial Airways. An artificial airway is for a patient with decreased level of consciousness, airway obstruction, mechanical ventilation, and removal of tracheobronchial secretions (see Skill 29-1).

Oral Airway. The oral airway (Figure 29-12), the simplest type of artificial airway, prevents obstruction of the trachea by displacement of the tongue into the oropharynx. The oral airway extends from the teeth to the oropharynx, maintaining the tongue in the normal position. Determine proper oral airway size by measuring the distance from the corner of the mouth to the angle of the jaw just below the ear. The length is equal to the distance from the flange of the airway to the tip. You need to use the correct-size airway. If the airway is too small, the tongue will not stay in the anterior portion of the mouth; if too large, it will force the tongue toward the epiglottis and obstruct the airway.

Turning the curve of the airway toward the cheek and placing it over the tongue, insert the airway. When the airway

is in the oropharynx, turn it so the opening points downward. Correctly placed, the airway moves the tongue forward, away from the oropharynx and the flange. The flat portion of the airway rests against the patient's teeth. Incorrect insertion merely forces the tongue back into the oropharynx.

Tracheal Airway. Tracheal airways include endotracheal, nasotracheal, and tracheal tubes (Box 29-9). These allow easy access to the trachea for deep tracheal suctioning. Because of the artificial airway, the patient no longer has normal humidification of the tracheal mucosa. Ensure that nebulization or the oxygen delivery system is supplying humidity to the airway. This humidification is protective and helps reduce the risk for airway plugging.

Maintenance or Promotion of Lung Expansion Nursing interventions to maintain or promote lung expansion include positioning, incentive spirometry, chest physiotherapy, and chest tube management.

Positioning. Healthy people maintain adequate ventilation and oxygenation by frequent position changes. When a person has restricted mobility, this increases his or her risk for respiratory impairment. Frequent position changes are a simple and cost-effective method for reducing the patient's risk for pooled airway secretions and decreased chest wall expansion.

The most effective position for patients with cardiopulmonary diseases is the 45-degree semi-Fowler's position, using gravity to assist in lung expansion and reduce pressure from the abdomen on the diaphragm. Ensure that the patient does not slide down in bed, causing reduced lung expansion. Position patients with unilateral lung disease, such as a pneumothorax or atelectasis, with the healthy lung down. This promotes better perfusion of the healthy lung, improving oxygenation. In the presence of pulmonary abscess or hemorrhage, place the affected lung down to prevent drainage toward the healthy lung.

Incentive Spirometry. Incentive spirometry (IS) is a method of encouraging voluntary deep breathing by providing visual feedback to patients about inspiratory volume. IS promotes deep breathing to prevent or treat atelectasis in the postoperative patient. It encourages patients to breathe to their normal inspiratory capacities. A postoperative inspira-

BOX 29-8   PROCEDURAL GUIDELINES

Closed (In-Line) Suctioning

DELEGATION CONSIDERATIONS: Airway suctioning with a closed (in-line) suction catheter is not routinely delegated to nursing assistive personnel (NAP). In some situations, such as suctioning a patient with a permanent tracheostomy tube, this procedure may be delegated. The nurse is responsible for assessing the patient's cardiopulmonary status, and before delegation the nurse informs NAP about:

- Any individualized aspect of care that pertains to suctioning, such as position, duration of suction, and pressure settings
- Expected quality, quantity, and color of secretions and to immediately report any changes to the nurse
- Patient's anticipated response to suction, and to immediately report to the nurse any changes in vital signs, complaints of pain, and changes in patient's respiratory status, mental status, or restlessness,

EQUIPMENT: Closed system or in-line suction catheter (see Figure 29-11), suction machine; 6 feet of connecting tubing, clean gloves *(optional)*, mask *(optional)*, goggles *(optional)*, saline vial or syringe, face shield, clean towel, pulse oximeter and stethoscope

1 Perform assessment as in Skill 29-1.
2 Explain the procedure to the patient and the importance of coughing during the suctioning procedure.
3 Assist patient with assuming a position of comfort for both patient and nurse, usually semi-Fowler's or high-Fowler's position. Place towel across the patient's chest.
4 Perform hand hygiene, apply clean gloves and face shield, and attach suction. NOTE: If risk for splash is present or patient is on respiratory precautions, mask and goggles might also be needed.
   a In some settings, the catheter is attached to the closed ventilator circuit by a respiratory therapist. If catheter is not already in place, open the closed suction catheter package using aseptic technique, attach catheter to ventilator circuit by removing swivel adapter, and place catheter apparatus on ET or tracheostomy tube. Connect Y on mechanical ventilator circuit to closed suction catheter with flex tubing (see illustration).

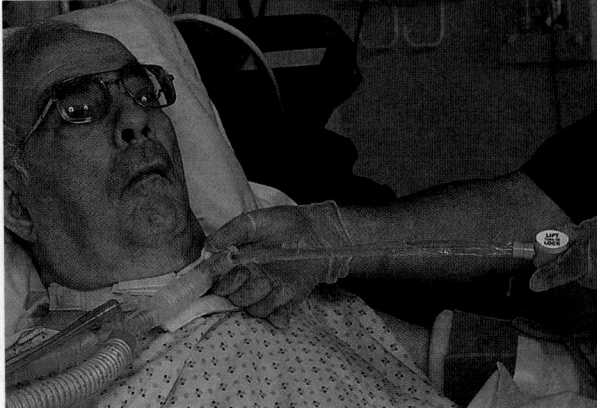

Step 4a ■ Suctioning tracheostomy with closed system suction catheter.

ET, Endotracheal tube.

   b Connect one end of connecting tubing to suction machine, and connect other to the end of a closed system or in-line suction catheter, if not already done. Turn suction device on, and set vacuum regulator to appropriate negative pressure (see manufacturer's directions). Many closed system suction catheters require slightly higher suction; consult manufacturer's guidelines.
5 Hyperinflate and/or hyperoxygenate patient with bag-valve-mask or manual breathing mechanism on mechanical ventilator according to institution protocol and clinical status (usually 100% oxygen).
6 Unlock suction control mechanism if required by manufacturer. Open saline port, and attach saline syringe or vial.
7 Pick up suction catheter enclosed in plastic sleeve with dominant hand.

Critical Decision Point: The instillation of normal saline into the airway before closed in-line suctioning may not be appropriate for all patients and needs further investigation. Normal saline instillation in conjunction with artificial airway suctioning may lead to dispersion of microorganisms into the lower respiratory tract (Celik and Kanan, 2006).

---

8 Insert catheter; use a repeating maneuver of pushing catheter and sliding (or pulling) plastic sleeve back between thumb and forefinger until you feel resistance or patient coughs.
9 Encourage patient to cough, and apply suction by squeezing on suction control mechanism while withdrawing catheter. It is difficult to apply intermittent pulses of suction and nearly impossible to rotate the catheter compared with a standard catheter. Be sure to withdraw catheter completely into plastic sheath so it does not obstruct airflow (AARC, 2004).
10 Reassess cardiopulmonary status, including pulse oximetry, to determine need for subsequent suctioning or complications. Repeat Steps 5 through 9 one or two more times to clear secretions. Allow adequate time (at least 1 full minute) between suction passes for ventilation and reoxygenation (AARC, 2004).
11 When airway is clear, withdraw catheter completely into sheath. Be sure that colored indicator line on catheter is visible in the sheath. Squeeze vial or push saline syringe while applying suction to rinse inner lumen of catheter. Use at least 5 to 10 mL of saline to rinse the catheter until you clear it of retained secretions, which cause bacterial growth and increase the risk for infection (AARC, 2004; Freytag and others, 2003). Lock suction mechanism, if applicable, and turn off suction.
12 If patient requires oral or nasal suctioning, perform Skill 29-1 with separate standard suction catheter.
13 Reposition patient.
14 Remove face shield and gloves and discard them, and perform hand hygiene.
15 Compare patient's cardiopulmonary assessments before and after suctioning, and observe airway secretions.

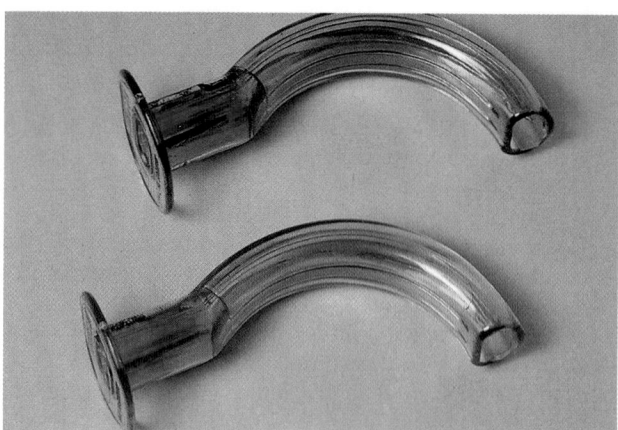

Figure 29-12 ■ Artificial oral airways.

BOX 29-9   BEST PRACTICES

Tracheostomy Care

SUMMARY OF EVIDENCE

Prevention of skin breakdown and tracheal occlusion is essential in the patient with a tracheostomy. The practice of tracheostomy care varies throughout health care facilities. Complications as a result of inconsistent practices have lead to poor patient outcomes, such as skin breakdown and site infections. Literature supports that evidence-based standards of care for tracheostomy sites and tubes reduces morbidity and mortality.

APPLICATION TO NURSING PRACTICE

- Assess and clean tracheostomy site with approved wound cleanser every 8 hours and as needed.
- Suction patient, based upon assessment, if there is shortness of breath, tachypnea, decrease in oxygenation, or increased secretions.
- Maintain sterile technique when suctioning a patient's airway.
- Place a drain sponge around the tracheostomy tube to prevent moisture-related skin irritation.
- Do NOT cut gauze to fit around the tube. Pieces of the gauze loosen and may enter the stoma.
- A Velcro tube holder is preferred to ties based on patient's comfort ratings and a decrease in skin tears on the neck.

REFERENCE
Dennis-Rouse M, Davidson J: An evidence-based evaluation of tracheostomy care practices, *Crit Care Nurs Q* 31(2):150, 2008.

BOX 29-10   Chest Physiotherapy

Nursing and respiratory therapy collaborate with the health care provider to determine if chest physiotherapy (CPT) is best for the patient. The following guidelines help you with physical assessment and subsequent decision making:

- Know the patient's normal range of vital signs. Conditions requiring CPT, such as atelectasis and pneumonia, affect vital signs. The degree of change is related to the level of hypoxia, overall cardiopulmonary status, and tolerance for activity.
- Know the patient's medications. Certain medications, particularly diuretics and antihypertensives, cause fluid and hemodynamic changes. These decrease the patient's tolerance for positional changes and postural drainage. Long-term steroid use increases the patient's risk for pathological rib fractures and often contraindicates vibration.
- Know the patient's medical history. Certain conditions, such as increased intracranial pressure, spinal cord injuries, and abdominal aneurysm resection, contraindicate the positional changes of postural drainage. Thoracic trauma or surgery also contraindicates percussion and vibration.
- Know the patient's level of cognitive function. Participation in controlled cough techniques requires the patient to follow instructions. Congenital or acquired cognitive limitations alter the patient's ability to learn and participate in these techniques.
- Be aware of the patient's exercise tolerance. CPT maneuvers are fatiguing. When the patient is not used to physical activity, usually the patient will have little tolerance for the maneuvers. However, with gradual increases in activity and planned CPT, patient tolerance for the procedure improves.

tory capacity one half to three fourths of the preoperative volume is acceptable because of postoperative pain. Administration of pain medications before IS helps the patient achieve deep breathing by reducing pain and splinting. There is no clinical benefit to using IS in place of early ambulation. Encourage your postoperative patients to ambulate as soon as possible.

Flow-oriented incentive spirometers consist of one or more plastic chambers that contain freely moving colored balls. The patient inhales slowly with an even flow to elevate the balls and keep them floating as long as possible. This will allow a maximally sustained inhalation.

Volume-oriented IS devices have a bellows that rises to a predetermined volume by an inhaled breath. An achievement light or counter is used to provide feedback. Some devices will not turn the light on unless the bellows is at a minimum desired volume for a specified period of time.

Chest Physiotherapy. Chest physiotherapy (CPT) is used to mobilize pulmonary secretions (Box 29-10). CPT includes postural drainage, chest percussion, and vibration, followed by productive coughing or suctioning. CPT is for patients who produce more than 30 mL of sputum per day or have evidence of atelectasis by chest x-ray film.

***Chest Percussion.* Chest percussion** involves striking the chest wall over the area being drained. You position the hand so that the fingers and thumb touch, cupping the hand (Figure 29-13). Percussion on the surface of the chest wall sends waves of varying amplitude and frequency through the chest, changing the consistency and location of the sputum. You perform chest percussion by alternating hand motion against the chest wall (Figure 29-14). Perform percussion over a single layer of clothing, not over buttons, snaps, or zippers. The single layer of

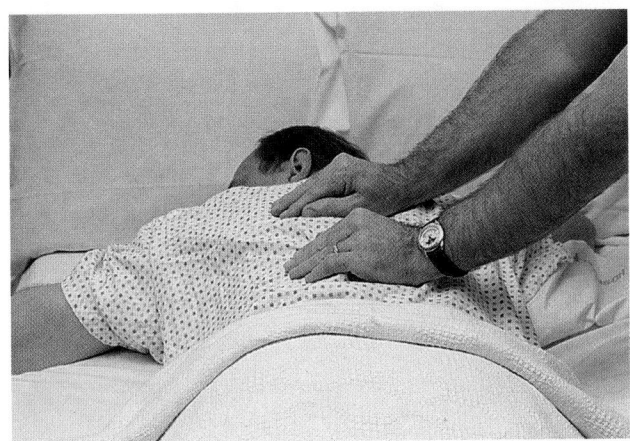

Figure 29-13 ■ Hand position for chest wall percussion during physiotherapy.

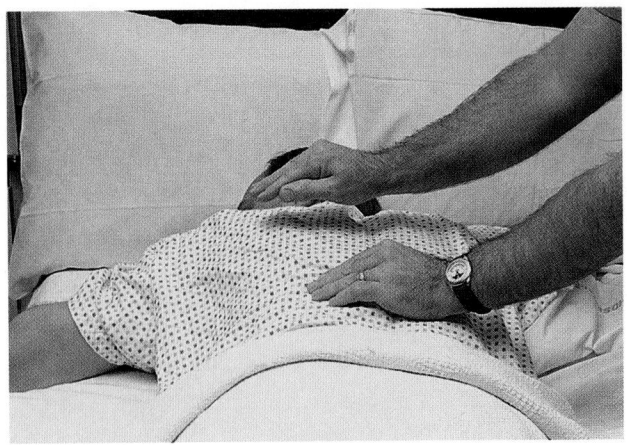

Figure 29-14 ■ Chest wall percussion, alternating hand motion against the patient's chest wall.

TABLE 29-9 Positions for Postural Drainage

LUNG SEGMENT	POSITION OF PATIENT	LUNG SEGMENT	POSITION OF PATIENT
ADULT Left and right upper lobes	High-Fowler's	Left and right middle lobes—anterior segment (right shown)	Three-fourths supine position with dependent lung in Trendelenburg's position
Apical Segments Right upper lobe—anterior segment	Supine with head elevated	Right middle lobe—posterior segment	Prone with thorax and abdomen elevated
Left upper lobe—anterior segment	Sitting on side of bed Supine with head elevated	Both lower lobes—anterior segments	Supine in Trendelenburg's position
Right upper lobe—posterior segment	Side-lying with right side of chest elevated on pillows	Left lower lobe—lateral segment	Right side-lying in Trendelenburg's position
Left upper lobe—posterior segment	Side-lying with left side of chest elevated on pillows		

Continued

TABLE 29-9   Positions for Postural Drainage—cont'd

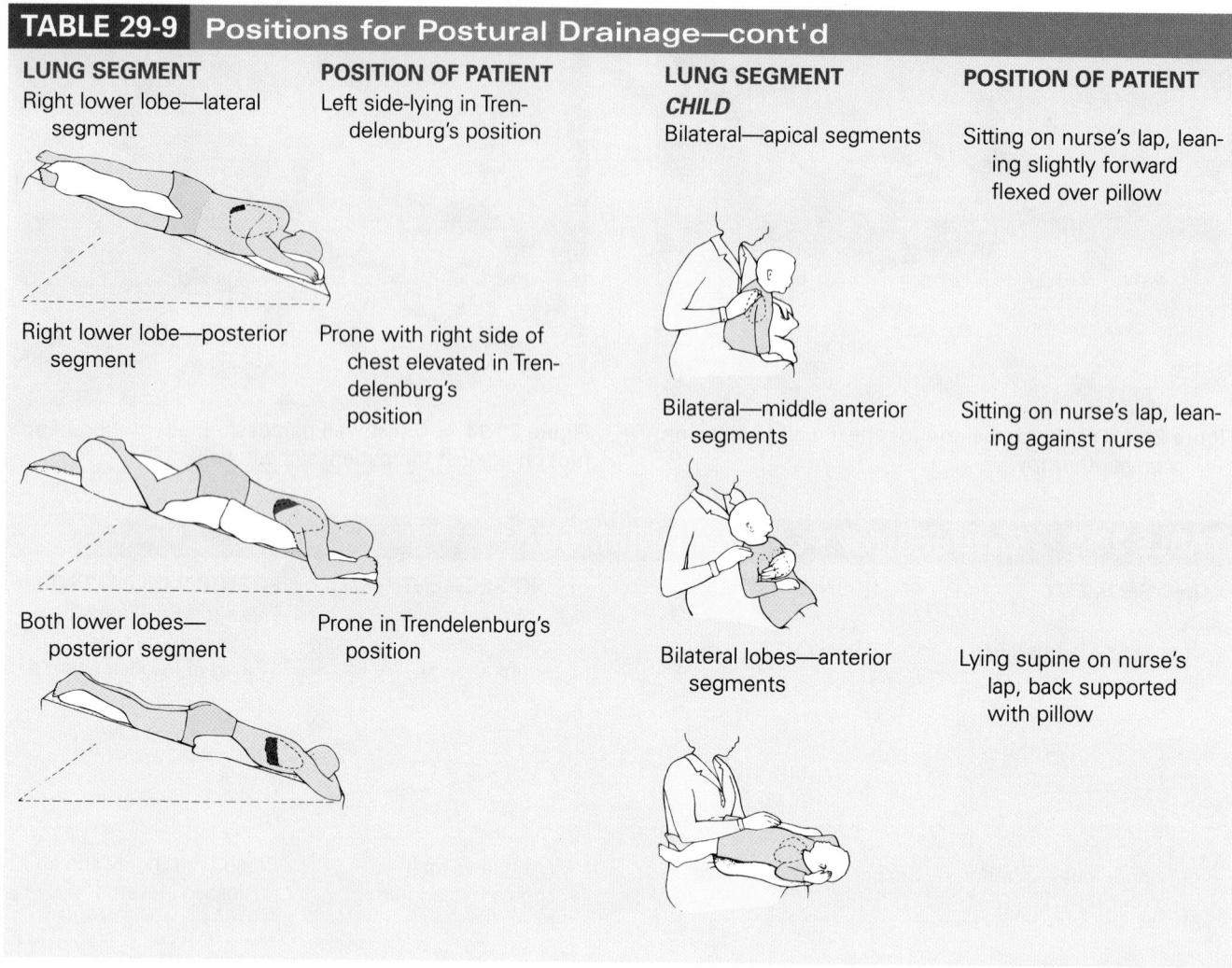

LUNG SEGMENT	POSITION OF PATIENT	LUNG SEGMENT CHILD	POSITION OF PATIENT
Right lower lobe—lateral segment	Left side-lying in Trendelenburg's position	Bilateral—apical segments	Sitting on nurse's lap, leaning slightly forward flexed over pillow
Right lower lobe—posterior segment	Prone with right side of chest elevated in Trendelenburg's position	Bilateral—middle anterior segments	Sitting on nurse's lap, leaning against nurse
Both lower lobes—posterior segment	Prone in Trendelenburg's position	Bilateral lobes—anterior segments	Lying supine on nurse's lap, back supported with pillow

clothing prevents slapping the patient's skin. Thicker or multiple layers of material dampen the vibrations.

Be cautious when percussing the lung fields not to percuss the scapular area, or trauma will occur to the skin and underlying musculoskeletal structures. Percussion is contraindicated in patients with bleeding disorders, osteoporosis, or fractured ribs.

Vibration. **Vibration** is a fine, shaking pressure applied to the chest wall only during exhalation. This technique increases the velocity and turbulence of exhaled air, facilitating secretion removal. Vibration increases the exhalation of trapped air, shakes mucus loose, and induces a cough. You will use vibration most often with patients with cystic fibrosis. It is not recommended for infants and young children.

Postural Drainage. **Postural drainage** is the use of positioning techniques that drain secretions from specific segments of the lungs and bronchi into the trachea. Table 29-9 includes some of the basic positions for postural drainage. Because some patients do not require postural drainage of all lung segments, base the procedure on clinical assessment findings. For example, some patients with left lower lobe bronchiectasis or pneumonia will require postural drainage of only the affected region, whereas a child with cystic fibrosis requires postural drainage of all segments.

Chest Tubes. A **chest tube** is a catheter inserted through the rib cage into the pleural space to remove air and fluids from the pleural space and to reestablish normal intrapleural and intrapulmonic pressures. Chest tubes are used after chest surgery and chest trauma and for pneumothorax or hemothorax to promote lung expansion (Skill 29-2).

A **pneumothorax** is a collection of air or other gas in the pleural space. The gas causes the lung to collapse because it destroys the negative intrapleural pressure. This exerts a counterpressure against the lung, making it unable to expand. There are a variety of mechanisms for a pneumothorax. It occurs spontaneously, from chest trauma, or secondary to chronic lung disease. The patient with a pneumothorax feels sharp pain as atmospheric air irritates the parietal pleura. Dyspnea is common and worsens as the size of the pneumothorax increases. A tension pneumothorax, a complete collapse of the lung, is a medical emergency resulting from a simple pneumothorax. Air is trapped in the pleural cavity between the chest wall and the lung, causing pressure on the lung. A large-bore cannula or chest tube must be placed immediately to release the pressure.

Hemothorax is an accumulation of blood and fluid in the pleural cavity between the parietal and visceral pleurae, usu-

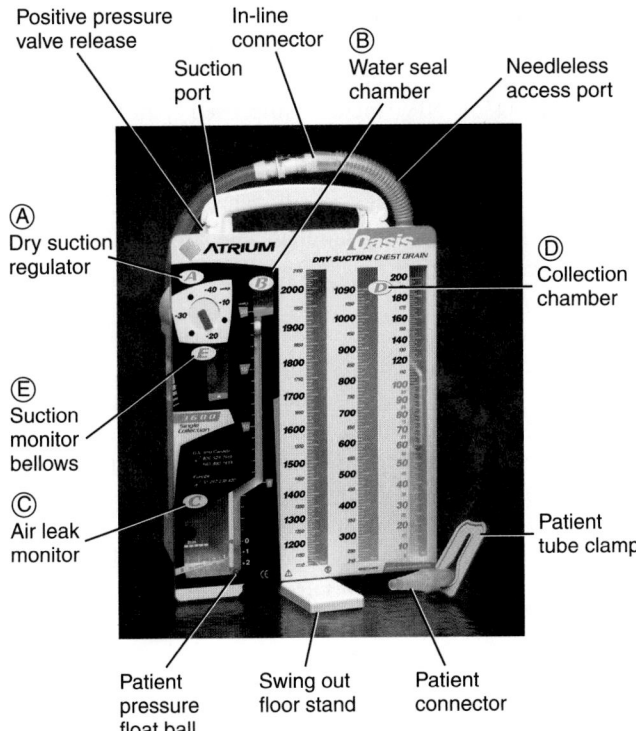

Positive pressure
valve release

In-line
connector

Ⓑ

Suction
port

Water seal
chamber

Needleless
access port

Ⓐ
Dry suction
regulator

Ⓓ
Collection
chamber

Ⓔ
Suction
monitor
bellows

Ⓒ
Air leak
monitor

Patient
tube clamp

Patient
pressure
float ball

Swing out
floor stand

Patient
connector

Figure 29-15 ■ Dry Suction chest drainage system. (Courtesy Atrium Medical Corp.)

ally as the result of trauma. It produces a counterpressure and prevents the lung from full expansion. In addition to pain and dyspnea, signs and symptoms of shock will develop if blood loss is severe.

Disposable chest drainage systems, such as Thora-Seal III or Pleur-Evac chest drainage system (DeKental), are one-piece molded plastic units that you use to evacuate any volume of air or fluid with controlled suction (Figure 29-15). The first chamber provides a water seal to prevent air from being drawn back into the pleural space. The second chamber collects fluid or blood. The third chamber is for suction, to facilitate removal of chest drainage. The suction pressure causes gentle, continuous bubbling in the third chamber. Suction pressure is measured in centimeters of water. You will usually set suction at −15 to −20 cm H_2O for adults. Children require lesser amounts of suction pressure.

The disposable units appear to be the system of choice because they are cost-effective and safe. Knowledge of the basics of chest tube management and troubleshooting maneuvers reduces the patient's risk for complications.

Special Considerations. Clamping the chest tubes is contraindicated when the patient is ambulating or being transported. Handle the chest drainage unit carefully, and maintain the drainage device below the patient's chest. The health care provider may choose to clamp the tube temporarily to determine if the patient has fluid accumulation. This requires an order, and the patient must be assessed frequently. If the tubing accidentally disconnects from the unit, instruct the patient to exhale as much as possible and cough. This maneuver rids the pleural space of as much air as possible. Quickly cleanse the tip

of the tubing and reconnect the tubing to the unit. Clamping the chest tube is not recommended because it may result in a tension pneumothorax, a life-threatening event.

Chest Tube Removal. Removal of a chest tube requires patient preparation. An analgesic administered before removal helps to minimize discomfort and anxiety. Generally the physician or health care provider removes the tube and places an occlusive petrolatum gauze dressing over the wound. Monitor the patient's vital signs and oxygen saturation (SpO_2). The most frequent sensations reported during removal of a chest tube include burning, pain, and a pulling sensation.

Noninvasive Ventilation. Noninvasive ventilation (NIV) maintains positive airway pressure and improves alveolar ventilation without the need for an artificial airway. In addition, this mechanical ventilator alternative reduces and reverses atelectasis, improves oxygenation, reduces pulmonary edema, and improves cardiac function (Woodrow, 2003a). Positive airway pressure keeps the terminal airways (alveoli) partially inflated, reducing the risk for atelectasis. If atelectasis has occurred, positive pressure assists in reinflation. Because the alveoli remain partially inflated, there is a continuous exchange of respiratory gases, and as a result the patient's oxygenation improves. In the cardiac patient, NIV reduces pulmonary edema because the increased alveolar pressure forces interstitial fluid out of the lungs and back into the pulmonary circulation. In patients with altered cardiac function secondary to sleep apnea, NIV provides improved myocardial oxygenation and improved function (Skill 29-3). Substantial reductions in mortality and the need for subsequent ventilation support are associated with noninvasive ventilation in acute respiratory failure, especially in patients with COPD (Peter and others, 2002).

Continuous positive airway pressure (CPAP) has been available for many years and maintains a steady stream of pressure throughout the patient's breathing cycle (Figure 29-16). It is very beneficial to the patient with sleep apnea. During sleep the upper airway collapses and prevents normal airflow. When the airflow is interrupted, there is a drop in the patient's oxygen saturation and frequent awakenings occur. CPAP uses continuous positive pressure to keep the airway open and prevent upper airway collapse (see Chapter 30). As a result the patient breathes more normally, sleeps better, and has markedly reduced snoring. A CPAP setting of 5 cm H_2O provides 5 cm of pressure during inspiration and expiration. The usual CPAP setting is 5 to 20 cm of water. There are disadvantages to this device (Table 29-10).

Bilevel positive airway pressure (BiPAP) works by providing assistance during inspiration and preventing airway closure during expiration. It provides two levels of pressure: inspiratory positive airway pressure (IPAP) and a lower expiratory positive airway pressure (EPAP). During inspiration BiPAP generates a preset positive-pressure support, which increases the patient's tidal volume and ultimately alveolar ventilation. This pressure support lowers when the patient begins exhaling, which allows for easier exhalation. As a result there is an increase in the functional residual capacity

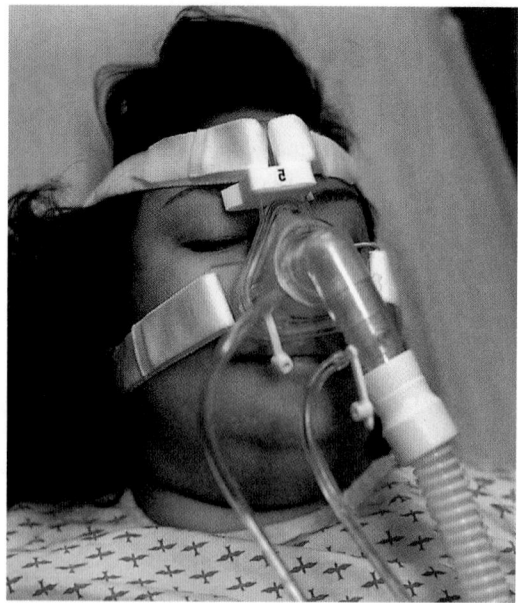

Figure 29-16 ■ Mask suitable for either continuous positive airway pressure (CPAP) or bilevel positive airway pressure (BiPAP) device.

TABLE 29-10	Problems Associated With CPAP
PROBLEM	**CAUSE**
Discomfort	Large tight-fitting mask that fits over patient's nose.
	Oxygen flow rate causes dry mucous membranes.
Risks to skin integrity	Tight fit of the mask causes pressure and diaphoresis. Patients need to remove the mask to relieve pressure.
Hypercapnia	Although CPAP improves alveolar function, which increases carbon dioxide clearance from the blood, it also causes air trapping. In some patients this causes a rise in carbon dioxide levels.
Gastric distention	CPAP forces more air into the stomach, which causes distention and discomfort in some patients. In addition, severe gastric distention impedes diaphragmatic motion and reduces lung volumes. It may be necessary to insert a nasogastric tube if this occurs.
Noise	Some patients find the machine very noisy. It interferes not only with sleep, but also with leisure activities.

Data from Peter J and others: Noninvasive ventilation in acute respiratory failure: a meta-analysis update, *Crit Care Med* 30(3):555, 2002; Woodrow P: Using non-invasive ventilation in acute wards, part I, *Nurs Stand* 18(1):39, 2003a.

CPAP, Continuous positive airway pressure.

(the amount of air remaining in the lungs at the end of expiration), reduced airway closure, reexpansion of atelectatic area, and improved oxygenation.

The goals of NIV include improved ventilation and sleep, enhanced quality of life, reduction of morbidity, improvement of physical and physiological function, and cost-effectiveness (Perkins and Shortall, 2000; Woodrow, 2003b). You prepare patients and families who are candidates for noninvasive ventilation for discharge by using a multidisciplinary team.

Restoration of Cardiopulmonary Functioning The AHA publishes guidelines for cardiopulmonary care and resuscitation every 5 years. These outline the standards for acute myocardial infarction (AMI), acute stroke, near fatal asthma, anaphylaxis, and cardiopulmonary arrest for children and adults (American Heart Association [AHA], 2005).

When hypoxia is severe and prolonged, cardiac arrest results. A cardiac arrest is a sudden cessation of cardiac output and circulation. When this occurs, the tissues do not receive oxygen, carbon dioxide is not transported from tissues, tissue metabolism becomes anaerobic, and metabolic and respiratory acidosis occurs. Permanent heart, brain, and other tissue damage occurs within 4 to 6 minutes.

Cardiopulmonary Resuscitation. An absence of pulse and respiration characterizes cardiac arrest. If you determine that the patient has experienced a cardiac arrest, begin **cardiopulmonary resuscitation (CPR)**. CPR is a basic emergency procedure of artificial respiration and manual external cardiac massage. The "ABCs" of CPR are to establish an airway, initiate breathing, and maintain circulation. When you cannot establish an airway, reassess proper head position and assess for airway obstruction. The 2005 guidelines for CPR **do not** recommend that lay rescuers perform blind sweeps of the mouth or abdominal thrusts (AHA, 2005). The recommendation is to begin standard CPR after calling 9-1-1 for adult victims, unless they have been involved in a drowning, drug overdose, or trauma. The rate of compression for an adult, child, or infant is more than 100 compressions per minute. The ratio of compressions to breaths in one- and two-rescuer CPR for persons 8 years or older and for one-rescuer child or infant is 30 compressions to 2 ventilations. You use a ratio of 15 compressions to 2 ventilations in infant and child two-rescuer CPR (AHA, 2005).

Defibrillation is recommended within 5 minutes for an out-of-hospital sudden cardiac arrest and within 3 minutes for an in-hospital victim. The recommendation further states that in addition to health care providers, specific lay individuals, police, firefighters, security personnel, ski patrol members, ferryboat crews, and airline flight attendants need training in CPR and the use of an automated external defibrillator (AED) (AHA, 2005) (Box 29-11).

RESTORATIVE AND CONTINUING CARE Restorative and continuing care emphasize cardiopulmonary reconditioning as a structured rehabilitation program. **Cardiopulmonary rehabilitation** is actively assisting the patient with achieving and maintaining an optimal level of health through controlled physical exercise, nutrition counseling, relaxation and stress management techniques, prescribed medications, and oxygen administration. As physical reconditioning occurs, the patient's physical symptoms, anxiety, depression, or somatic concerns decrease. The patient and the rehabilitation team define the goals of rehabilitation.

Respiratory Muscle Training Respiratory muscle training improves strength and endurance, resulting in improved activity tolerance. Respiratory muscle training will possibly prevent respiratory failure in patients with COPD.

Breathing Exercises. Breathing exercises include techniques to improve ventilation and oxygenation. The three basic techniques are deep breathing and coughing exercises, pursed-lip breathing, and diaphragmatic breathing. Review coughing techniques on p. 822.

Pursed-lip breathing involves deep inspiration and prolonged expiration through pursed lips to prevent alveolar collapse. While the patient is sitting up, instruct the patient to take a deep breath and to exhale slowly through pursed lips. Patients need to gain control of the exhalation phase so that exhalation is longer than inhalation. The patient is usually able to perfect this technique by counting inhalation time and gradually increasing the count during exhalation.

Diaphragmatic breathing is more difficult and requires the patient to relax intercostal and accessory respiratory muscles while taking deep inspirations. The patient concentrates on expanding the diaphragm during controlled inspiration. Teach the patient to place one hand flat below the breastbone above the waist and the other hand 2 to 3 cm below the first hand. Then ask the patient to inhale while the lower hand moves outward during inspiration. The patient observes for inward movement as the diaphragm ascends. Initially teach these exercises with the patient in the supine position and then practice while the patient sits and stands. The exercise is often used with the pursed-lip breathing technique.

■■■ EVALUATION

PATIENT CARE You evaluate nursing interventions and therapies by comparing the patient's progress to the goals and desired outcomes of the nursing care plan. When nursing measures directed to improve oxygenation are unsuccessful, modify the care plan by revising existing interventions or introducing new interventions. Do not hesitate to notify the physician or health care provider about a patient's decline in oxygenation status. Prompt notification will help to avoid an emergency situation or even the need for CPR.

Management of Mr. King, a patient with COPD, depends on achieving three major goals: reduction of airflow obstruction, prevention or management of complications, and improvement in the patient's quality of life (Box 29-12).

Patients with chronic cardiopulmonary disease present a nursing challenge. They require frequent nursing interventions when they are acutely ill. With chronic diseases, do not think in terms of recovery, but rather health maintenance. You are caring for patients with acute exacerbations of their chronic diseases. You will not see a dramatic cure, but our goal is to return the patient to his or her functional and cognitive status before this most recent exacerbation. You will be assisting patients with improving the quality of their lives in small but significant ways.

PATIENT EXPECTATIONS Individualize the goals that you set for the patient, and make sure they are realistic. Patients need to know how to cope with this chronic disease. Before any teaching program is effective, the patient must want to learn. Ask the patient if he or she would like to know more about COPD, vaccinations, and smoking cessation. Inform the patient that it is possible to gain greater independence, improve mobility, decrease dyspnea, and decrease the frequency of acute respiratory infections. Presenting an individualized education program, based on assessment data, helps to ensure the patient will comprehend, learn, use, and ultimately benefit from the education.

BOX 29-11   Automated External Defibrillator

- The AED is a device used to administer an electrical shock through the chest wall to the heart.
- The AED has a built-in computer that assesses the victim's heart rhythm and determines if defibrillation is needed.
- The rescuer delivers a shock to the victim after announcing, "Everyone stand back."
- The AED can be used by nonmedical personnel.
- Use of an AED will strengthen the chain of survival. Every minute of a sudden cardiac death without defibrillation decreases the survival rate by 7% to 10% (American Heart Association, 2005).

BOX 29-12   EVALUATION

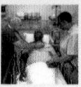

John cares for Mr. King throughout his hospital stay. Mr. King is afebrile, his white blood cells are within normal limits, and his sputum cultures are negative on day of discharge. He does not require supplemental oxygen use. He is able to describe ways to prevent respiratory infections, because they aggravate airways and precipitate an episode of acute respiratory failure. Because he now practices pursed-lip breathing, his breathing is more controlled, relieving his subsequent anxiety.

While John is observing Mr. King preparing for discharge, it is quite evident that Mr. King is using the various breathing techniques that they have worked on together. The patient is able to go home with improved activities of daily living. His wife even appears less anxious and states she feels as though for the first time they have taken a step (even though small) to improve the quality of their lives.

DOCUMENTATION NOTE

"Mr. King discharged to home. Able to state the purpose of breathing exercises and each medication, able to list causes and symptoms of respiratory tract infection. Has an appointment in 1 week with a community-based rehabilitation program. Scheduled to see his physician or health care provider in 2 weeks. Prescriptions explained and given to patient. Accompanied to the exit. Left with wife and son."

SAFETY GUIDELINES FOR NURSING SKILLS

Ensuring patient safety is an essential role of the professional nurse. To ensure patient safety, communicate clearly with members of the health care team, assess and incorporate the patient's priorities of care and preferences, and use the best evidence when making decisions about your patient's care. When performing the skills in this chapter, remember the following points to ensure safe, individualized care.

- Patients with sudden changes in their vital signs, level of consciousness, or behavior are *possibly experiencing profound hypoxia.* Patients who demonstrate subtle changes over time have worsening of a chronic or existing condition or a new medical condition (Jevon and Ewens, 2001).
- *Perform tracheal suctioning before pharyngeal suctioning whenever possible.* The mouth and pharynx contain more bacteria than the trachea does. If there is an abundance of oral secretions present before beginning the procedure, suction mouth with oral suction device.
- *Use caution when suctioning patients with a head injury.* The suction procedure causes elevations in intracranial pressure (ICP). Reduce this risk by presuctioning hyperventilation, which results in hypocarbia that in turn induces vasoconstriction. Vasoconstriction reduces the potential increase in ICP. It is recommended that you limit the introduction of a catheter to two times with each suctioning procedure (Moore, 2003).

- The routine use of normal saline instillation into the airway before endotracheal and tracheostomy suctioning is not recommended. Normal saline instillation in conjunction with endotracheal suction leads to the spread of microorganisms into the lower respiratory tract and decreases in oxygenation saturation (Pedersen and others, 2009; Rauen and others, 2008). Normal saline has not been shown to be effective in thinning secretions or improving removal of secretions (Rauen and others, 2008). In certain circumstances, if it is necessary to stimulate a cough, normal saline may be indicated (Halm and Krisko-Hagel, 2008). This requires collaboration with the health care team.
- *Check your institutional policy before stripping or milking chest tubes.* Most institutions have stopped this practice because stripping the tube greatly increases intrapleural pressure, which possibly damages the pleural tissue and will cause pneumothorax or worsen an existing pneumothorax. However, even though the literature is contradictory, you will perform stripping or milking in selected patients (e.g., fresh postoperative thoracic surgery or chest traumas). The rationale for selective use of stripping or milking is that the presence of clotted tube drainage decreases reexpansion and increases risk for tension pneumothorax (Allibone, 2003). Thus the benefits of stripping or milking outweigh the risks.

SKILL 29-1   SUCCESSIONING

DELEGATION CONSIDERATIONS

The skills of nasotracheal and artificial airway suctioning are not routinely delegated to nursing assistive personnel (NAP). However, when the patient is assessed by the nurse to be stable, oral and permanent tracheostomy tube suctioning may be delegated. Before delegation the nurse instructs the NAP about:

- Any individualized aspects of care that pertain to suctioning, such as position, duration of suction, and suction pressure settings
- Signs and symptoms of hypoxemia or respiratory distress, such as change in patient's respiratory status, confusion, and restlessness, and to immediately report these signs to the nurse
- Reporting changes in patient's secretion quality, quantity, and color

EQUIPMENT

- Appropriate-size suction catheter or closed-suction catheter (smallest diameter that will remove secretions effectively) or Yankauer catheter (oral suction)
- Nasal or oral airway (if indicated)
- Sterile gloves
- Clean gloves
- Pulse oximeter
- Stethoscope
- Clean towel or paper drape
- Portable or wall suction
- Mask, goggles, or face shield
- Connecting tube (6 feet)

If Not Using Closed-Suction Catheter

- Small Y-adapter (if catheter does not have a suction control port)
- Water-soluble lubricant
- Sterile basin
- Sterile normal saline solution or water (about 100 mL)

STEP	RATIONALE

ASSESSMENT

1. Assess for signs and symptoms of upper and lower airway obstruction, including abnormal respiratory rate, wheezes, crackles, or gurgling on inspiration or expiration; restlessness; ineffective coughing; unilateral, segmental, or lobar absent or diminished breath sounds (in absence of pneumonectomy or lobectomy); tachycardia; hypertension or hypotension; cyanosis; decreased level of consciousness, especially acute; or excess nasal secretions, drooling, or gastric secretions or vomitus in the mouth (Moore, 2003).

   Physical signs and symptoms result from decreased oxygen to tissues, as well as pooling of secretions in upper and lower airways. Complete assessment before and following the suction procedure (Moore, 2003).

2. Determine the presence of apprehension, anxiety, decreased ability to concentrate, lethargy, decreased level of consciousness (especially acute), increased fatigue, dizziness, behavioral changes (especially irritability), decreased oxygen saturation (from pulse oximetry), increased pulse rate, increased rate of breathing, decreased depth of breathing, elevated blood pressure, cardiac dysrhythmias, pallor, cyanosis, and dyspnea or use of accessory muscles.

   Signs and symptoms associated with hypoxia (low oxygen at the cellular or tissue level), hypoxemia (low oxygen tension in the blood), or hypercapnia (elevated carbon dioxide tension in the blood). Patients report sensations of pain and discomfort with the suctioning procedure; as a result, this increases their anxiety before suctioning. Anxiety and pain consume oxygen and in turn worsen the signs of hypoxia (Puntillo and others, 2003).

3. Assess for risk factors for upper or lower airway obstruction, including obstructive lung disease; pulmonary infections; impaired mobility; sedation; decreased level of consciousness; seizures; presence of feeding tube; anatomy of nasopharynx and oral pharynx; decreased gag or cough reflex; decreased swallowing ability; allergies; sinus drainage; and head, neck, or chest trauma.

   Presence of these risk factors impairs the patient's ability to clear secretions from the airway and necessitates nasopharyngeal or nasotracheal suctioning.

4. Determine additional factors that normally influence upper or lower airway function: recent surgery, ineffective or absent cough, chemical neuromuscular blockade, neuromuscular diseases, congestive heart failure, pulmonary edema, adult respiratory distress syndrome, hyaline membrane disease, or diaphragmatic weakness or paralysis (Moore, 2003).

   Allows nurse to identify patients at risk for airway obstruction needing endotracheal (ET) or tracheostomy tube suctioning.

SKILL 29-1	SUCTIONING—cont'd

STEP	**RATIONALE**

5 Assess the following factors that influence character of secretions:

   a Fluid status

         Fluid overload increases amount of secretions. Dehydration promotes thicker secretions.

   b Lack of humidity

         The environment influences secretion formation and gas exchange, necessitating airway suctioning when the patient cannot clear secretions effectively.

   c Infection (e.g., pneumonia)

         Patients with respiratory infections are likely to have increased secretions that are thicker and sometimes more difficult to expectorate.

6 Identify contraindications to nasotracheal suctioning:
   a Facial traumas/surgery
   b Bleeding disorders
   c Nasal bleeding
   d Epiglottitis or croup
   e Laryngospasm
   f Irritable airway
   g Gastric surgery with high anastomosis

         The passage of a catheter though the nasal route will cause additional trauma, increase nasal bleeding, or cause severe bleeding in the presence of bleeding disorders. In the presence of epiglottitis, croup, laryngospasm, or irritable airway, the entrance of a suction catheter via the nasal route causes intractable coughing, hypoxemia, and severe bronchospasm, necessitating emergency intubation or tracheostomy (Moore, 2003).

7 Examine sputum microbiology data.

         Certain bacteria are easy to transmit or require isolation because of virulence or antibiotic resistance.

8 Obtain patient's vital signs and oxygen saturation via pulse oximetry. Keep oximeter probe on during procedure.

         Establishes physiological baseline.

9 Assess patient's understanding of procedure.

         Reveals need for patient instruction and encourages cooperation.

PLANNING

1 Explain to patient how procedure will help clear airway and relieve breathing problems. Explain that temporary coughing, sneezing, gagging, or shortness of breath is normal during the procedure.

         Encourages cooperation and minimizes risks, anxiety, and pain of procedure.

2 Explain importance of coughing during procedure. Encourage patient to cough out secretions. Practice coughing, if able. Splint surgical incisions, if necessary.

         Facilitates secretion removal and reduces frequency and duration of future suctioning.

3 Assist patient with assuming position comfortable for nurse and patient (usually semi-Fowler's or sitting upright with head hyperextended, unless contraindicated).

         Reduces stimulation of gag reflex, promotes patient comfort and secretion drainage, and prevents aspiration and nurse strain.

4 Place towel or paper drape across patient's chest, if needed.

         Reduces transmission of microorganisms by protecting gown from secretions.

IMPLEMENTATION

1 Perform hand hygiene, and apply mask, goggles, or face shield if splashing is likely.

         Reduces transmission of microorganisms.

2 Connect one end of connecting tubing to suction machine, and place other end in convenient location near patient. Turn suction device on, and set vacuum regulator to appropriate negative pressure, 120 to 150 mm Hg (American Association of Respiratory Care [AARC], 2004).

         Negative pressure should not exceed 150 mm Hg because of increased risk for damage to pharyngeal and tracheal mucosa and suction-induced hypoxia (AARC, 2004).

3 If indicated, increase supplemental oxygen therapy to 100% or as ordered by physician or health care provider. Encourage patient to breathe deeply.

         Hyperoxygenation provides some protection from suction-induced decline in oxygenation. Hyperoxygenation is most effective in the presence of hyperinflation, such as encouraging the patient to deep breathe or increasing ventilator tidal volume (Pedersen and others, 2009).

STEP	RATIONALE

• **Critical Decision Point:** After suctioning is completed, readjust oxygen as ordered by physician or health care provider after procedure to avoid increased risk for oxygen toxicity and absorption, atelectasis from prolonged administration of high concentrations of oxygen, and increased carbon dioxide retention in patients with chronic obstructive lung diseases.

4 Prepare suction catheter.

  a One-time-use catheter

    (1) Open suction kit or catheter using aseptic technique. If sterile drape is available, place it across patient's chest or on the over-bed table. Do not allow the suction catheter to touch any nonsterile surfaces. | Maintains asepsis and reduces transmission of microorganisms.

    (2) Unwrap or open sterile basin, and place on bedside table. Be careful not to touch inside of basin. Fill with about 100 mL sterile normal saline solution or water (see illustration). | Use saline or water to clean tubing after each suction pass.

    (3) Open lubricant. Squeeze small amount onto open sterile catheter package without touching package. NOTE: Lubricant is not necessary for artificial airway suctioning. | Prepares lubricant while maintaining sterility. Use water-soluble lubricant to avoid lipoid aspiration pneumonia. Excessive lubricant occludes catheter.

  b Closed (in-line) suction catheter (see Box 29-8, p. 825)

5 Apply clean gloves for oropharyngeal suction. Apply sterile glove to each hand or clean glove to nondominant hand and sterile glove to dominant hand for all other suction techniques.

6 Pick up suction catheter with dominant hand without touching nonsterile surfaces. Pick up connecting tubing with nondominant hand. Secure catheter to tubing (see illustration). | Maintains catheter sterility. Connects catheter to suction.

7 Check that the equipment is functioning properly by suctioning small amount of normal saline solution from basin. | Ensures equipment function. Lubricates internal catheter and tubing.

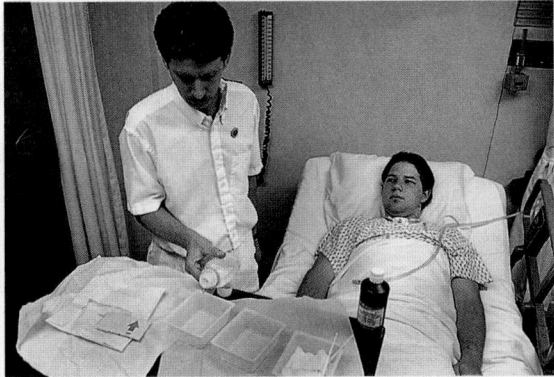

Step 4a(2) ■ Pouring sterile saline into tray.

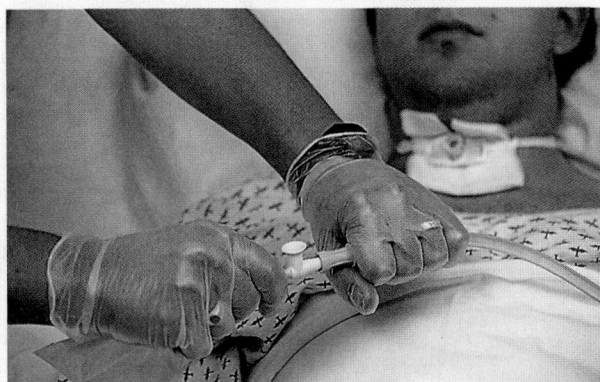

Step 6 ■ Attaching catheter to suction.

SKILL 29-1	SUCTIONING—cont'd

STEP	RATIONALE

8 Suction airway.

a Oropharyngeal suctioning

(1) Remove oxygen mask if present. Nasal cannula may remain in place. Keep oxygen mask near patient's face. Insert Yankauer catheter along gum line to pharynx. With suction applied, move catheter around mouth until the secretions are cleared. Encourage patient to cough. Replace oxygen mask, as appropriate.

Intermittent suction prevents invagination of oral mucosa into suction catheter. Invagination of mucosa causes trauma to the mucous membranes.

Coughing moves secretions from lower to upper airways into mouth.

(2) Rinse catheter with water in basin until catheter and connecting tube are cleared of secretions.

Clearing secretions before they dry reduces probability of transmission of microorganisms and enhances delivery of preset suction pressures.

(3) Place catheter or Yankauer in a clean, dry area for reuse with suction turned off. If patient able to suction self, place within patient's reach with suction on.

Facilitates prompt removal of airway secretions for future suctioning.

b Nasopharyngeal and nasotracheal suctioning

(1) Lightly coat distal 6 to 8 cm (2 to 3 inches) of catheter tip with water-soluble lubricant.

Lubricates catheter for easier insertion.

(2) Remove oxygen delivery device, if applicable, with nondominant hand. Without applying suction and using dominant thumb and forefinger, gently but quickly insert catheter into naris during inhalation. Following the natural course of the naris, slightly slant the catheter downward or through mouth. Do not force through naris (see illustration).

Application of suction pressure while introducing catheter into trachea increases risk for damage to mucosa and increases risk for hypoxia because of removal of entrained oxygen present in airways.

• *Critical Decision Point:* Be sure to insert catheter during patient inhalation, especially if inserting catheter into trachea, because epiglottis is open. Do not insert during swallowing or catheter will most likely enter esophagus. Never apply suction during insertion. Make sure patient coughs. If patient gags or becomes nauseated, the catheter is most likely in esophagus. Remove the catheter.

(a) *Nasopharyngeal suctioning:* In adults, insert catheter about 16 cm (6 to 7 inches); in older children, 8 to 12 cm (3 to 5 inches); in infants and young children, 4 to 8 cm (2 to 3 inches). Rule of thumb is to insert catheter distance from tip of nose (or mouth) to angle of mandible.

Ensures that you position catheter tip correctly in pharynx or trachea for suctioning.

(b) *Nasotracheal suctioning:* In adults, insert catheter about 20 cm (8 inches); in older children, 14 to 20 cm (5½ to 8 inches); and in young children and infants, 8 to 14 cm (3 to 5½ inches) (see Step 8b(2)).

• *Critical Decision Point:* When there is difficulty passing the catheter, ask patient to cough or say "ahh," or try to advance the catheter during inspiration. Both these measures assist in opening the glottis to permit passage of the catheter into the trachea.

(c) *Positioning for nasotracheal suctioning:* In some instances turning patient's head to right helps suction left mainstem bronchus; turning head to left helps suction right mainstem bronchus. If you feel resistance after insertion of catheter for maximum recommended distance, catheter has probably hit carina. Pull catheter back 1 to 2 cm before applying suction.

Turning the patient's head to the side elevates the bronchial passage on the opposite side.

STEP	RATIONALE

(3) With catheter tip in position, apply intermittent suction for no longer than 10 seconds (Moore, 2003) by placing and then releasing the nondominant thumb over vent of catheter and slowly withdrawing catheter while rotating it back and forth between dominant thumb and forefinger. Encourage patient to cough. Replace oxygen device, if applicable.

Intermittent suction and rotation of catheter when using a closed suctioning system reduce risk for injury to mucosa. If catheter "grabs" mucosa, remove thumb to release suction. Suctioning longer than 10 seconds causes cardiopulmonary compromise, usually from hypoxemia or vagal overload (Moore, 2003).

• **Critical Decision Point:** Monitor vital signs and oxygen saturation throughout suction procedure. If the pulse drops more than 20 beats per minute or increases more than 40 beats per minute, or if pulse oximetry falls below 90% or 5% from baseline, stop suctioning. Any deteriorating change in the patient's physiological status during suctioning requires termination of the procedure, hyperoxygenation, and other appropriate interventions (e.g., position change) (Moore, 2003).

(4) Rinse catheter and connecting tubing with normal saline or water until cleared.

Secretions that remain in suction catheter or connecting tubing decrease suctioning efficiency.

(5) Assess for need to repeat suctioning procedure. Observe for alte rations in cardiopulmonary status. Allow adequate time (1 to 2 minutes) between suction passes for ventilation and oxygenation. Do not perform more than two passes with the catheter (AARC, 2004). Ask patient to deep breathe and cough.

Suctioning sometimes induces hypoxemia, dysrhythmias, laryngospasm, and bronchospasm. Deep breathing reventilates and reoxygenates alveoli. Repeated passes clear the airway of excessive secretions but also remove oxygen and induce laryngospasm.

c Artificial airway suctioning

(1) Hyperinflate and/or hyperoxygenate patient before suctioning, using manual resuscitation bag-valve-mask connected to oxygen source or sigh mechanism on mechanical ventilator. Some mechanical ventilators have a button that when pushed delivers 100% oxygen for a few minutes and then resets to the previous value.

Hyperinflation along with hyperoxygenation decreases the risk for a decrease in oxygenation saturation. Routine use of hyperinflation is not recommended because of the possibility of trauma resulting from large volumes and high peak pressures (Pedersen and others, 2009).

(2) If patient is receiving mechanical ventilation, open swivel adapter, or if necessary remove oxygen or humidity delivery device with nondominant hand.

Exposes artificial airway.

(3) Without applying suction, gently but quickly insert catheter using dominant thumb and forefinger into artificial airway (it is best to try to insert catheter into the artificial airway while patient is inhaling) until you meet resistance or until patient coughs, then pull back 1 cm (½ inch) (see illustration).

Application of suction pressure while introducing catheter into trachea increases risk for damage to tracheal mucosa, as well as increased hypoxia related to removal of entrained oxygen present in airways. Pulling back stimulates cough and removes catheter from mucosal wall so that catheter is not resting against tracheal mucosa during suctioning.

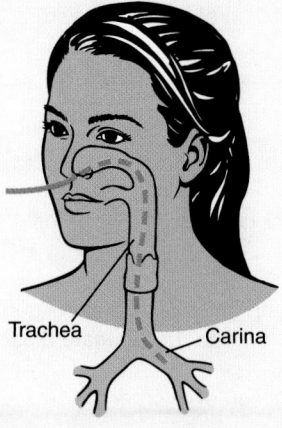

Step 8b(2) ■ Pathway for nasotracheal catheter progression.

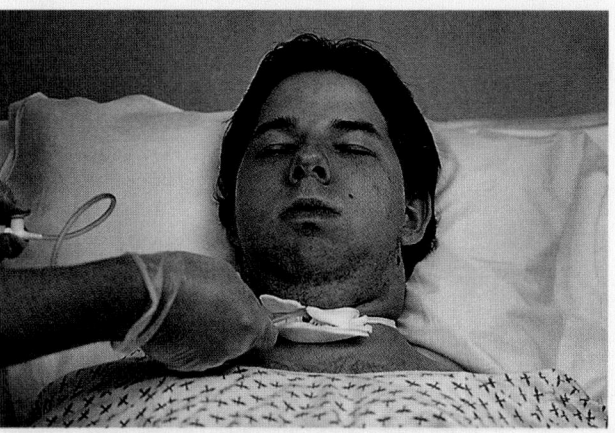

Step 8c(3) ■ Suctioning tracheostomy.

SKILL 29-1	SUCTIONING—cont'd

STEP	RATIONALE

- *Critical Decision Point:* If you are unable to insert catheter past the end of the ET tube, the catheter is probably caught in the Murphy eye (i.e., side hole at the distal end of the ET tube that allows for collateral airflow in the event of tracheal mainstem intubation). If so, rotate the catheter to reposition it away from the Murphy eye, or withdraw it slightly and reinsert with the next inhalation. Usually the catheter meets resistance at the carina. One indication that the catheter is at the carina is acute onset of coughing, because the carina contains many cough receptors. Pull the catheter back 1 cm (½ inch).

(4) Apply intermittent suction by placing and releasing nondominant thumb over vent of catheter; slowly withdraw catheter while rotating it back and forth between dominant thumb and forefinger. Encourage patient to cough. Watch for respiratory distress.	Intermittent suction and rotation of catheter prevent injury to tracheal mucosal lining. If catheter "grabs" mucosa, remove thumb to release suction.

- *Critical Decision Point:* If patient develops respiratory distress during the suction procedure, immediately withdraw catheter, and supply additional oxygen and breaths as needed. In an emergency, administer oxygen directly though the catheter. Disconnect suction, and attach oxygen at prescribed flow rate through the catheter.

(5) If patient is receiving mechanical ventilation, close swivel adapter, or replace oxygen delivery device.	Reestablishes artificial airway.
(6) Encourage patient to deep breathe, if able. Some patients respond well to several manual breaths from the mechanical ventilator or bag-valve-mask.	Reoxygenates and reexpands alveoli. Suctioning sometimes causes hypoxemia and atelectasis.
(7) Rinse catheter and connecting tubing with normal saline until clear. Use continuous suction.	Removes catheter secretions, which can decrease suctioning efficiency and provide environment for microorganism growth.
(8) Assess patient's cardiopulmonary status for secretion clearance. Repeat Steps (1) through (7) to clear secretions. Allow adequate time (1 to 2 minutes) between suction passes for ventilation and oxygenation. Do not perform more than two passes with the catheter (AARC, 2004).	Suctioning induces dysrhythmias, hypoxia, and bronchospasm and impairs cerebral circulation or adversely affects hemodynamic stability. A repeated pass with the suction catheter clears the airway of excessive secretions and promotes improved oxygenation (AARC, 2004).
(9) When you have cleared pharynx and trachea sufficiently of secretions, perform oropharyngeal suctioning to clear mouth of secretions. Do not suction nose again after suctioning mouth.	Removes upper airway secretions. More microorganisms are generally present in mouth. Upper airway is considered "clean" and lower airway is considered "sterile." Use the same catheter to suction from sterile to clean areas, but not from clean to sterile areas.
9 When you have completed suctioning, disconnect catheter from connecting tubing. Roll catheter around fingers of dominant hand. Pull glove off inside out so that catheter remains coiled in glove. Pull off other glove over first glove in same way to seal in contaminants. Discard in appropriate receptacle. Turn off suction device.	Reduces transmission of microorganisms.
10 Remove towel, place in laundry or appropriate receptacle, and reposition patient. Wear clean gloves if patient requires personal care.	Reduces transmission of microorganisms. Promotes comfort.
11 If indicated, readjust oxygen to original level because patient's blood oxygen level should have returned to baseline.	Prevents absorption atelectasis and oxygen toxicity while allowing patient time to reoxygenate blood.
12 Discard remainder of normal saline into appropriate receptacle. If basin is disposable, discard into appropriate receptacle. If basin is reusable, rinse it out and place it in storage area for soiled items in utility room.	Reduces transmission of microorganisms.

STEP	RATIONALE
13 Remove face shield and discard into appropriate receptacle. Perform hand hygiene.	Reduces transmission of microorganisms.
14 Place unopened suction kit on suction machine table or at head of bed.	Provides immediate access to suction catheter for next procedure.
15 Assist patient to a comfortable position, and provide oral hygiene as needed.	

EVALUATION

1 Compare patient's respiratory assessment before and after suctioning.	Provides subjective confirmation that you relieved airway obstruction during suctioning procedure.
2 Observe airway secretions.	Provides data to document presence or absence of respiratory tract infection.
3 Ask patient if breathing is easier and if there is less congestion.	Provides data to determine if you met patient expectations.

RECORDING AND REPORTING

- Record the amount, consistency, color, and odor of secretions.
- Record the patient's response to the suction procedure.

- Record and report the presuctioning and postsuctioning cardiopulmonary status.

UNEXPECTED OUTCOMES AND RELATED INTERVENTIONS

- Worsening cardiopulmonary status
  - Limit length of time suctioning.
  - Determine need for presuctioning hyperoxygenation and hyperinflation.
  - Determine need for more frequent, shorter-duration suctioning.
  - Notify physician or health care provider of changes.
- Return of bloody secretions
  - Determine amount of suction pressure used, and adjust accordingly.
  - Evaluate frequency of suctioning, and reduce if appropriate.
  - Determine other factors that lead to bloody secretions (e.g., prolonged bleeding time).
  - Provide more frequent oral hygiene.
- Unable to pass suction catheter through first naris attempted
  - Try other naris or oral route.
  - Insert nasal airway, especially if suctioning through patient's naris frequently.

- Guide catheter along naris floor to avoid turbinates.
- If obstruction is mucus, apply suction to relieve obstruction, but do not apply suction to mucosa. If you think the obstruction is a blood clot, consult physician or health care provider.
- Paroxysms of coughing
  - Administer supplemental oxygen.
  - Allow patient to rest between passes of suction catheter.
  - Consult physician or health care provider regarding need for inhaled bronchodilators or topical anesthetics.
- Unable to obtain secretions
  - Determine adequacy of humidification of oxygen delivery device.
  - Evaluate patient's fluid status.
  - Determine need for chest physiotherapy.
  - Assess for signs of infection.

SKILL 29-2   CARE OF PATIENTS WITH CHEST TUBES

DELEGATION CONSIDERATIONS

The skill of caring for a patient with chest tubes cannot be delegated to nursing assistive personnel (NAP). However, the nurse should inform NAP about:

- Proper positioning of the patient with chest tubes to facilitate chest tube drainage and optimal functioning of the system
- How to ambulate and transfer the patient with chest drainage
- Reporting any changes in vital signs, level of comfort, SpO$_2$, or excessive bubbling in water-seal chamber
- Immediately notifying the nurse if there is a disconnection of the system, change in type and amount of drainage, bleeding, or sudden cessation of bubbling

EQUIPMENT

- Disposable chest drainage system (see Figure 29-15, p. 829)
- Suction source and setup (wall canister or portable)
  - Water suction system: Add sterile water or normal saline solution to cover the lower 2.5 cm (1 inch) of water-seal U tube, sterile water or normal saline solution to put into the suction control chamber if suction is to be used (see manufacturer's directions)
  - Waterless system: Add vial of 30 mL injectable sodium chloride or water, 20-mL syringe, 21-gauge needle, and antiseptic swab
- Clean gloves
- 2-inch tape
- Sterile gauze sponges
- Two shodded hemostats

STEP	RATIONALE

ASSESSMENT

1 Perform hand hygiene.

2 Assess pulmonary status:

  a Assess for respiratory distress and chest pain, and breath sounds over affected lung area (see Chapters 14 and 15).

  b Signs and symptoms of increased respiratory distress and/or chest pain are decreased breath sounds over the affected and nonaffected lungs, marked cyanosis, asymmetrical chest movements, presence of subcutaneous emphysema around tube insertion site or neck, hypotension, and tachycardia.

  c Chest pain on inspiration.

3 Obtain vital signs, SpO$_2$, and level of cognition.

4 If possible, ask patient to rate level of comfort on a visual analog scale of 0 to 10.

5 Observe:

  a Chest tube dressing and site surrounding tube insertion.

  b Tubing for kinks, dependent loops, or clots.

  c Chest drainage system, to ensure it is upright and below level of tube insertion.

Signs and symptoms reflect improvement in respiratory distress and chest pain after insertion of chest tube. If respiratory distress is not relieved or worsens or if there is sharp stabbing chest pain with or without decreased blood pressure and increased heart rate, notify physician or health care provider immediately. These symptoms indicate a pneumothorax.

Changes in pulse SpO$_2$ and blood pressure indicate infection, respiratory distress, or pain. Cognitive changes indicate hypoxia.

Chest tubes are often painful and interfere with patient's mobility, coughing and deep breathing, and rehabilitation.

Ensures that dressing is intact, without air or fluid leaks, and that area surrounding insertion site is free of drainage or skin irritation.

Maintains a patent, freely draining system, preventing fluid accumulation in chest cavity. The presence of kinks, dependent loops, or clotted drainage increases the patient's risk for infection, atelectasis, and tension pneumothorax (Centre for Reviews and Dissemination, 2008).

Facilitates drainage. Ensures system is in position to function properly.

PLANNING

1 Provide two hemostats for each chest tube, attached to top of patient's bed with adhesive tape. Chest tubes are only clamped under specific circumstances per physician's or health care provider's order or nursing policy and procedure:

  a To assess air leak (Table 29-11).

  b To quickly empty or change disposable drainage system; performed by a nurse who has received education in the procedure.

Hemostats have a covering to prevent hemostat from penetrating chest tube once changed. The use of these hemostats or other clamp prevents air from reentering the pleural space.

TABLE 29-11 Emergency Care With Chest Tubes

ASSESSMENT	INTERVENTION
1. Air leak: can occur at insertion site, connection between tube and drainage, or within drainage device itself. Continuous bubbling occurs in water-seal chamber and water seal.	Locate leak by clamping tube at different intervals along the tube. Leaks are corrected when constant bubbling stops. Unclamp tube, reinforce chest dressing, and notify physician or health care provider immediately. Leaving chest tube clamped may cause collapse of lung, mediastinal shift, and eventual collapse of other lung from buildup of air pressure within the pleural cavity. If a leak is found in the drainage device, change it. Use adhesive tape at all connections.
2. Break in chest drainage device	Place the end of the chest tube in a bottle of sterile saline. Notify the health care provider immediately, and change the drainage device according to the manufacturer's instructions.
3. Chest tube dislodgment	Apply pressure to chest tube site wound using petroleum gauze, a dry gauze dressing, and adhesive tape. Notify the health care provider immediately, and obtain a STAT order for a chest x-ray examination. Prepare for the health care provider to insert another chest tube.
4. Tension pneumothorax Signs and symptoms include: • Severe respiratory distress • Low oxygen saturation • Chest pain • Absence of breath sounds on affected side • Tracheal shift to unaffected side • Tachycardia	Assess chest tube for any clamping or kinking of the tubing. Notify the health care provider immediately, and obtain a STAT order for a chest x-ray examination. Prepare for the health care provider to insert another chest tube. Have emergency equipment in the patient's room to prepare for resuscitation if needed.
5. Drainage suddenly stops	Assess chest tube for any clamping or kinking of the tubing. Notify the health care provider immediately, and obtain an order to gently milk the chest tube to reestablish chest drainage.

STEP	RATIONALE
c To assess if patient is ready to have chest tube removed (which is done by physician's or health care provider's order); monitor the patient for recurrent pneumothorax.	
2 Position the patient.	Permits optimal drainage of fluid and/or air.
a Semi-Fowler's position to evacuate air (pneumothorax).	Air rises to highest point in chest. Pneumothorax tubes are usually placed on the anterior aspect at midclavicular line, second or third intercostal space.
b High-Fowler's position to drain fluid (hemothorax).	Permits optimal drainage of fluid. Posterior tubes are placed on midaxillary line, eighth or ninth intercostal space.

IMPLEMENTATION

STEP	RATIONALE
1 Be sure tube connection between chest and drainage tube is intact and taped.	Secures chest tube to drainage system and reduces risk for air leak causing breaks in airtight system.
a Make sure water-seal vent is not occluded.	Permits displaced air to pass into atmosphere.
b Make sure suction control chamber vent is not occluded when using suction. Waterless systems have relief valves without caps.	Provides safety factor of releasing excess negative pressure into atmosphere.
2 Coil excess tubing on mattress next to patient. Secure with rubber band, safety pin, or plastic clamp.	Prevents excess tubing from hanging over edge of mattress in dependent loop. It is possible for drainage to collect in loop and occlude drainage system (Centre for Reviews and Dissemination, 2008).
3 Adjust tubing to hang in straight line from top of mattress to drainage chamber.	Promotes drainage and prevents fluid or blood from accumulating in pleural cavity (Halm, 2007).
4 If chest tube is draining fluid, indicate time (e.g., 0900) that you began drainage on drainage bottle's adhesive tape or on write-on surface of disposable commercial system.	Provides a baseline for continuous assessment of type and quality of drainage.

SKILL 29-2	CARE OF PATIENTS WITH CHEST TUBES—cont'd

STEP	RATIONALE

5 Strip or milk chest tube only if indicated (this means compressing along the tube to encourage clots to pass through the tube):

    Stripping: Compression along length of the tubing beginning at patient and continuing until reaching the drainage unit.

    Milking: Compressing and releasing the tube sequentially.

Stripping may cause complications because it can create excessive negative intrapleural pressure (over −100 cm H_2O). Milking causes less of a pressure change and is recommended (Halm, 2007).

    a Manipulate postoperative mediastinal chest tubes if nursing assessment indicates an obstruction or decreased drainage from clots or debris in the tubing.

Stripping is performed only if hospital policy permits and there is a physician's or health care provider's order. There is no evidence that stripping or milking increases output or causes significant complications (Centre for Reviews and Dissemination, 2008).

6 Perform hand hygiene.

Reduces transmission of microorganisms.

EVALUATION

1 Monitor vital signs, pulse oximetry as ordered.

Provides ongoing data regarding patient level of oxygenation.

2 Observe:

    a Chest tube dressing. Check the dressing carefully; it can come loose from the skin, although this is not always readily apparent.

Appearance of drainage is sometimes due to an occluded tube, causing drainage to exit around tube.

    b Make sure tubing is free of kinks and dependent loops.

Straight and coiled drainage tube positions are optimal for pleural drainage. However, when dependent loop is unavoidable, periodic lifting and draining of the tube will also promote pleural drainage.

    c Make sure the chest drainage system is upright and below level of tube insertion. Note presence of clots or debris in tubing. Monitor the position of the system relative to the chest tube carefully, especially during patient transport.

Ensures system is in position to function.

    d Water seal for fluctuations with patient's inspiration and expiration.

      (1) Waterless system: Diagnostic indicator for fluctuations with patient's inspirations and expirations.

In the non–mechanically ventilated patient, fluid rises in the water-seal chamber or diagnostic indicator with inspiration and falls with expiration. The opposite occurs in the patient who is mechanically ventilated. This indicates that the system is functioning properly (Lewis and others, 2007).

      (2) Water-seal system: Bubbling in the water-seal chamber.

When you initially connect system to the patient, expect bubbles from the chamber. These are from air that was present in the system and in the patient's intrapleural space. In many cases, the bubbling stops after a short time. Fluid continues to fluctuate in the water-seal chamber on inspiration and expiration until the lung reexpands or the system becomes occluded.

      (3) Water-seal system: Bubbling is in the suction control chamber (when suction is being used).

Suction control chamber has constant gentle bubbling. Tubing should be free of obstruction, and the suction source should be turned to the appropriate setting.

    e Waterless system: Bubbling is diagnostic indicator.

Mechanism to observe for presence of tidaling.

    f Type and amount of fluid drainage: Note color and amount of drainage, patient's vital signs, and skin color. What is the normal amount of drainage?

Character of drainage indicated if it is expected, or if infection or hemorrhage is developing.

      (1) In the adult, less than 50 to 200 mL/hr immediately after surgery in a mediastinal chest tube; approximately 500 mL in the first 24 hours.

Dark-red drainage is normal only in the postoperative period, turning serous with time (Lewis and others, 2007).

STEP	RATIONALE
(2) Between 100 and 300 mL of fluid drains in a pleural chest tube in an adult during the first 2 hours after insertion. This rate decreases after 2 hours; expect 500 to 1000 mL in the first 24 hours. Drainage is grossly bloody during the first several hours after surgery and then changes to serous (Lewis and others, 2007). A sudden gush of drainage is often retained blood and not active bleeding and is usually the result of patient repositioning.	Reexpansion of lungs forces drainage into the tube. Coughing also causes large gushes of drainage or air. Report excessive amounts and/or the continued presence of frank bloody drainage the first several hours after surgery to the physician or health care provider, along with patient's vital signs and respiratory status.

• ***Critical Decision Point:*** If drainage suddenly increases or if there is more than 100 mL/hr of bloody drainage (except for the first 3 hours postoperatively), inform the physician or health care provider and remain with the patient and assess vital signs, oxygen saturation by pulse oximetry, and cardiopulmonary status (Allibone, 2003). This may indicate hemorrhage or perforation of the lung.

STEP	RATIONALE
g Waterless system: The suction control (float ball) indicates the amount of suction the patient's intrapleural space is receiving.	The suction float ball dictates the amount of suction in the system. The float ball allows no more suction than dictated by its setting. If the suction source is set too low, the suction float ball cannot reach the prescribed setting. In this case, increase the suction for the float ball to reach the prescribed setting.
3 Evaluate patient for decreased respiratory distress and chest pain, breath sounds over affected lung area, and SpO$_2$.	Increase in respiratory distress, decrease in breath sounds, marked cyanosis, asymmetrical chest wall movements, presence of subcutaneous emphysema around insertion site or neck, hypotension, tachycardia, and/or mediastinal shift are critical and indicate a severe change in patient status, such as excessive blood loss or tension pneumothorax. Notify physician or health care provider immediately.
4 Ask patient to rate level of comfort on a scale of 0 to 10.	Indicates need for analgesia. Patient with chest tube discomfort hesitates to take deep breaths and as a result is at risk for pneumonia and atelectasis.

RECORDING AND REPORTING

• Record and report patency of chest tubes; presence, type, and amount of drainage; presence of fluctuations; patient's vital signs; chest dressing status; amount of suction and/or water seal; patient's level of comfort.

UNEXPECTED OUTCOMES AND RELATED INTERVENTIONS

• Air leak unrelated to patient respirations.
  • Locate source (see Table 29-11, p. 841).
  • Notify physician or health care provider.
  • Drain tubing contents into drainage bottle. Coil excess tubing on mattress and secure in place, or place in a straight line down the length of the bed.
• Tension pneumothorax is present.
  • Determine that chest tubes are not clamped, kinked, or occluded. Obstructed chest tubes trap air in intrapleural space when air leak originates within patient.
  • Notify physician or health care provider immediately.
  • Prepare immediately for another chest tube insertion. Obtain a flutter (Heimlich) valve or large-gauge needles for short-term emergency release of air in intrapleural space. Have emergency equipment (e.g., oxygen, code cart) near patient.

• Continuous bubbling is in water seal chamber, indicating that leak is between patient and water seal.
  • Tighten loose connections between patient and water-seal system.
  • Cross-clamp the chest tube closest to patient's chest. If bubbling stops, the air leak is inside patient's thorax or at chest tube insertion site. Unclamp tube, and notify physician or health care provider immediately. Reinforce chest dressing. Leaving chest tube clamped causes a tension pneumothorax and mediastinal shift.
  • Gradually move clamps down drainage tubing away from patient and toward drainage chamber, moving one clamp at a time. When bubbling stops, leak is in section of tubing or connection distal to the clamp. Replace tubing, or secure connections and release clamp.

SKILL 29-3   CARE OF THE PATIENT WITH NONINVASIVE VENTILATION

DELEGATION CONSIDERATIONS

The skill of caring for a patient with noninvasive ventilation (NIV) cannot be delegated to nursing assistive personnel (NAP). The nurse informs the NAP to report:

- Any changes in patient's vital signs or SpO_2, mental status, or change in skin color
- Any changes in patient's level of comfort
- Any difficulty in awakening patient

EQUIPMENT

NOTE: When device is used in the home, the home care equipment vendor provides the equipment.

- Nasal mask/full face mask (with quick-release straps) or nasal pillows
- Oxygen source and tubing
- CPAP/BiPAP per physician's or health care provider's order
- Humidification source, if needed
- Pressure generator (in institutional health care settings, the patient's room may have a pressure source)
- Delivery tubing
- Pulse oximeter
- Clean gloves
- Goggles (if splash risk exists)

STEP	RATIONALE

ASSESSMENT

1. Assess patient's respiratory status, including symmetry of chest wall expansion, respiratory rate and depth, SpO_2, sputum production, and lung sounds (see Chapters 14 and 15); when possible ask patient about dyspnea, and observe for signs and symptoms associated with hypoxia.

   Decreased chest wall movement, crackles or decreased lung sounds, increased respiratory rate, increased sputum production, or hypoxia can indicate the need for noninvasive ventilation to improve oxygenation.

2. Observe patient's ability to clear and remove airway secretions.

   Secretions plug the airway, decreasing the amount of oxygen that is available for gas exchange in the lung.

3. If available, note patient's most recent arterial blood gas (ABG) results or arterial oxygen saturation.

   Objectively documents the patient's pH, arterial oxygen, arterial CO_2, or arterial oxygen saturation.

- **Critical Decision Point:** If the patient is currently on NIV, evaluate if the therapy is meeting the patient's oxygenation and ventilation needs. Determine what factors have changed, resulting in the new assessment findings.

---

4. Obtain vital signs before initiation of therapy.

   Provides baseline data to compare desired or problematic vital sign changes resulting from the therapy.

5. Review patient's medical record for the medical order for CPAP/BiPAP and appropriate settings.

   Physician's or health care provider's order is necessary for this therapy.

PLANNING

1. Explain to patient and family the purpose and reasons for CPAP/BiPAP.

   Helps reduce the sense of claustrophobia from the mask. In addition, information reduces anxiety and increases cooperation and compliance with the therapy (Woodrow, 2003a).

IMPLEMENTATION

1. Perform hand hygiene; apply clean gloves and goggles. Apply barrier gown if secretions are projectile.

   Reduces transmission of microorganisms and exposure to pulmonary secretions.

2. Identify patient using two identifiers (e.g., name and birthday or name and account number, according to facility policy).

   Complies with The Joint Commission requirements and improves procedure safety.

3. Determine correct mask size. Use supplied masking charts to determine the correct size (S, M, L, and XL) (see illustration).

   Make sure the mask fits snugly over patient's nose (CPAP) or nose and mouth (BiPAP) because a tight seal is necessary to deliver the positive pressure. It is essential that the mask has quick-release straps so in the case of an emergency (e.g., vomiting, respiratory arrest) you can quickly remove the mask. This quick-release system also allows the patient to remove the mask quickly when needed (Preston, 2001).

STEP	RATIONALE

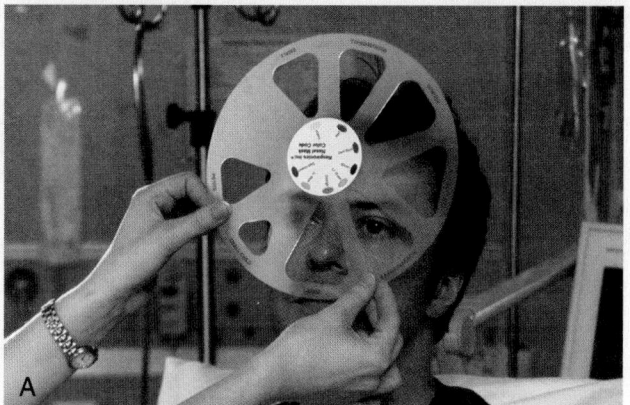 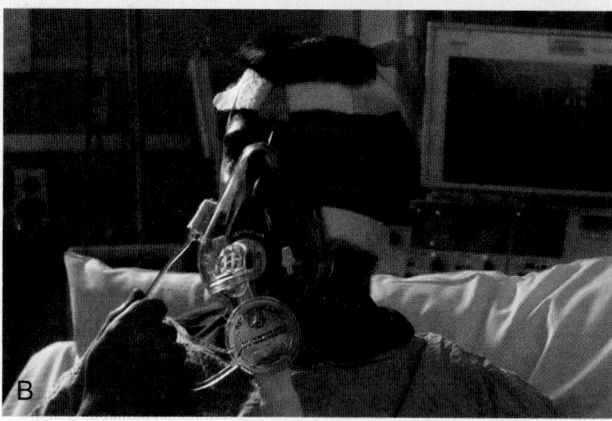

Step 2 ■ A, Mask sizing. **B,** Full face mask with quick-release restraining straps.

4 Connect CPAP/BiPAP device delivery tubing to pressure generator.	Ensures patient is receiving proper noninvasive ventilation as ordered.

• **Critical Decision Point:** In some patients it is also necessary to connect oxygen delivery source; however, you will frequently use this equipment without oxygen.

5 Monitor patient's to pulse oximetry readings.	It is important to continually monitor the patient's level of oxygenation when beginning NIV (Perkins and Shortall, 2000).

6 Set CPAP/BiPAP initial settings:
  a CPAP: 4 to 8 cm H_2O
  b BiPAP:
    (1) Inspiratory usually set at 8 cm H_2O
    (2) Expiratory usually set at 4 cm H_2O (Preston, 2001)
	These settings allow the health care team to determine initial patient response. CPAP provides single positive pressure at the end of exhalation, which helps to keep the alveoli open at end-expiration.
	
	BiPAP supplies pressures at both inhalation and exhalation. The inhalation pressure prevents airway closure and the expiratory pressure helps to keep the alveoli open at end-expiration (Preston, 2001).

7 Dispose of supplies as appropriate. Perform hand hygiene.	Reduces transmission of microorganisms.

EVALUATION

1 Evaluate patient's response to noninvasive ventilation. Observe for decreased anxiety; improved level of consciousness and cognitive abilities; decreased fatigue; absence of dizziness; decreased pulse, regular rhythm; decreased respiratory rate and work of breathing; return to normal blood pressure; improved color.	As hypoxia and hypercapnia are reduced or corrected, the patient's physical assessment parameters will improve.
2 Monitor ABG levels by pulse oximetry.	Documents patient's level of oxygenation. On first initiating NIV, especially in patients with underlying COPD, it is important to obtain ABGs after the first hour and every 2 to 6 hours during the first day. These patients often retain carbon dioxide (Perkins and Shortall, 2000).
3 Observe skin integrity over the bridge of the patient's nose.	A mask that is too tight causes skin breakdown over bridge of nose and around ears. Frequent skin assessment is necessary.
4 Monitor patient's and family's ability to manipulate device and face mask.	Determines patient's ability to perform self-care and to follow CPAP/BiPAP plan.

SKILL 29-3   CARE OF THE PATIENT WITH NONINVASIVE VENTILATION—cont'd

RECORDING AND REPORTING

- Record respiratory assessment findings, CPAP/BiPAP settings, SpO_2, and the patient's response to the noninvasive ventilation.
- Report any sudden change in patient's respiratory status or worsening ABG levels or pulse oximetry.

UNEXPECTED OUTCOMES AND RELATED INTERVENTIONS

- Patient experiences hypoxia.
  - Notify physician or health care provider.
  - Reassess patient.
  - Determine correct settings and integrity of noninvasive ventilation system.
- Patient experiences hypercapnia.
  - Notify physician or health care provider.
  - Reassess patient.
  - Determine correct settings and integrity of noninvasive ventilation system.
- Patient states a sense of smothering or claustrophobia.
  - Reexplain system to patient.
  - Demonstrate use of quick-release straps.
  - Have patient demonstrate use of quick-release straps.

KEY POINTS

- The primary function of the heart is to deliver deoxygenated blood to the lungs for oxygenation and to deliver oxygenated blood and nutrients to the tissues.
- Cardiac dysrhythmias are classified by cardiac activity and site of impulse origin.
- The primary function of the lungs is to transfer oxygen from the atmosphere into the alveoli and carbon dioxide out of the body as a waste product.
- Ventilation is the process of providing adequate oxygenation from the alveoli to the blood.
- The process of inspiration (active process) and expiration (passive process) is achieved with lung changes in pressures and volumes.
- The central nervous system and chemicals within the blood control respiration.
- Decreased hemoglobin levels alter the patient's ability to transport oxygen.
- Impaired chest wall movement reduces the level of tissue oxygenation.

- Hypoventilation causes carbon dioxide retention.
- Hypoxia occurs if the amount of oxygen delivered to tissues is too low.
- The nursing assessment includes information about the patient's respiratory symptoms, environmental exposures, respiratory and cardiopulmonary risk factors, use of medications, and physical functioning.
- Breathing exercises improve ventilation, oxygenation, and sensations of dyspnea.
- Chest physiotherapy includes postural drainage and percussion and vibration to mobilize pulmonary secretions.
- Coughing and suctioning techniques maintain a patent airway.
- Oxygen therapy improves levels of tissue oxygenation and is delivered by nasal cannula, nasal catheter, or oxygen mask.

CRITICAL THINKING EXERCISES

You are assigned to care for Mr. King, a 62-year-old salesman. He has a history of COPD and has been complaining of upper respiratory symptoms, including increasing shortness of breath, fever, nonproductive cough, nausea, and malaise. During your rounds you assess Mr. King. You observe he has labored breathing and is using the accessory muscles of respiration. His lungs have bibasilar crackles and diminished breath sounds. He is complaining of increasing shortness of breath and right-sided chest pain and is diaphoretic.

1. List two nursing assessments that you would perform immediately. Explain why.
2. What do the lungs sounds indicate?

The health care provider arrives at the patient's bedside. The patient's vital signs include the following: blood pressure, 152/90 mm Hg; pulse, 102 beats per minute; respiratory rate, 28 breaths per minute; temperature, 102.8° F; SpO_2, 78%. The health care provider orders a Venturi mask at 8 L/min to titrate to 92%, ABG determination, and a chest x-ray examination.

3. Why did the health care provider order a Venturi mask instead of a nonrebreather?
4. Why are Mr. King's blood pressure and heart rate elevated?
5. What preparations do you make in anticipation of acute respiratory failure? List possible nursing interventions.

ⓔvolve   *Answers to Critical Thinking Questions can be found on the Evolve website.*

REVIEW QUESTIONS

1. A priority assessment for the patient admitted complaining of a "rapid heart rate" is:
   1. Risk factors for CAD and family history of CAD
   2. Consumption of caffeine and herbal substances and sedentary lifestyle
   3. Heart rate, blood pressure, and respiratory rate
   4. Nutritional assessment for high-fat foods and poor nutrition
2. Which statement made by a patient newly diagnosed with COPD indicates a need for further teaching?
   1. "I will make sure that I rest between activities so I don't get short of breath."
   2. "I will rest for 30 minutes before eating my meals."
   3. "I will use two or three pillows at night if I have trouble breathing."
   4. "When I get short of breath, I will turn up my oxygen to 6 L/min."
3. The nurse finds a patient with labored breathing who is using the accessory muscles of respiration. The patient's lungs have bibasilar crackles and diminished breath sounds. The patient is complaining of increasing shortness of breath and right-sided chest pain. The nurse's next action is:
   1. Notify the charge nurse and health care provider of a change in condition
   2. Check pulse oximetry and blood pressure
   3. Force fluids and change the patient's position frequently
   4. Arrange for a chest x-ray examination
4. The health care provider has examined the above patient (in Question 3) and ordered ABG levels, chest x-ray examination, continuous pulse oximetry, vital signs every 2 hours, and oxygen via face mask at 40%. What signs does the nurse need to observe for in this patient? Select all that apply.
   1. Decreasing SpO_2 level
   2. Increased sputum production
   3. Respiratory rate and pattern
   4. Lower extremity pain

5. The nurse recognizes that which oxygen delivery system will provide a more precise oxygen concentration delivery to the patient?
   1. Nasal cannula
   2. Simple face mask without inflated reservoir bag
   3. Venturi mask system
   4. Plastic face mask with inflated reservoir bag
6. When caring for a patient with a decreased hemoglobin level, it is important to remember that:
   1. The patient is at risk for bleeding
   2. The patient has altered oxygen transport
   3. The patient is at risk for elevated carbon dioxide levels
   4. The patient has alterations in the chemical regulators of respiration
7. Which statement made by the nursing student indicates a need for further teaching related to suctioning a patient through an endotracheal tube?
   1. "Suctioning the patient will require use of sterile technique."
   2. "I will apply suction while rotating and withdrawing the suction catheter."
   3. "I will suction the mouth after I suction the endotracheal tube."
   4. "I will instill 5 mL normal saline into the tube before I hyperoxygenate the patient."
8. The nurse assesses a postoperative lung surgery patient 2 hours after insertion of a pleural chest tube. The nurse notes that there is 200 mL of drainage in the chest tube after surgery. What action should the nurse take?
   1. Record the amount and continue to monitor the drainage.
   2. Notify the physician.
   3. Strip the chest tube, starting at the chest.
   4. Increase the suction amount by 10 mm Hg.

9. The nurse is caring for a patient with severe atelectasis and recognizes the patient is experiencing hypoventilation. Select all of the signs of hypoventilation that were assessed by the nurse.
   1. Circumoral numbness
   2. Dizziness
   3. Headache in the early morning
   4. Lethargy
   5. Tetany (carpopedal spasm)
   6. Blurred vision

10. The nurse identifies the following characteristics on an ECG strip: regular rhythm, normal PR interval, normal QRS complex, and rate of 110 beats per minute. This rhythm is:
   1. Normal sinus rhythm
   2. Sinus bradycardia
   3. Sinus tachycardia
   4. Sinus arrhythmia

Answers to Review Questions can be found on pages 1197-1198.

REFERENCES

Allibone L: Nursing management of chest drains, *Nurs Stand* 17(22):45, 2003.

American Association of Respiratory Care : AARC clinical practice guideline: Oxygen therapy in the ahome or alternate site health care facility-2007 revion and update. *Respiratory Care*, 52(1): 1063, 2007.

American Association of Respiratory Care: AARC clinical practice guideline: nasotracheal suction—2004 revision and update, *Respir Care* 49:1080, 2004.

American Heart Association: *CPR*, 2005, http://www.Americanheart. org.

Bulechek GM and others, editors: *Nursing interventions classification (NIC)*, ed 5, St. Louis, 2008, Mosby.

Centers for Disease Control and Prevention: *Recommendations of the Advisory Committee on Immunization Practices for 2008-2009*, 2008, http://www.cdc.gov/flu/.

Centers for Disease Control and Prevention: *Respiratory syncytial virus*, 2005, http://www.cdc.gov/neidod/dyra/revb/resp/rsvfeat.htm.

Centre for Reviews and Dissemination: The nursing management of chest drains: a systematic review, *Joanna Briggs Institute for Evidence Based Nursing and Midwifery* 3:5, 2008.

Celik S, Kanan N: A current conflict: use of isotonic sodium chloride solution on endotracheal suctioning in critically ill patients, *Dimen Crit Care* 25(1): 11, 2008.

Dennis-Rouse M, Davidson J: An evidence-based evaluation of tracheostomy care practices, *Crit Care Nurs Q* 31(2):150, 2008.

Freytag CC and others: Prolonged application of closed in-line suction catheters increase microbial colonization of lower respiratory tract bacterial growth on catheter surface, *Infection* 31(1):31, 2003.

Halm MA: To strip or not to strip? Physiological effects of chest tube manipulation, *Am J Crit Care* 16(6):609, 2007.

Halm MA, Krisko-Hagel K: Instilling normal saline with suctioning: beneficial technique or potentially harmful sacred cow? *Am J Crit Care* 17(5):469, 2008.

Jevon P, Ewens B: Assessment of a breathless patient, *Nurs Stand* 15(16):48, 2001.

Lewis SM and others: *Medical surgical nursing: assessment and management of clinical problems*, ed 7, St. Louis, 2007, Mosby.

McCance K, Huether S: *Pathophysiology: the biologic basis for disease in adults and children*, ed 5, St. Louis, 2006, Mosby.

Moore T: Suctioning techniques for the removal of respiratory secretions, *Nurs Stand* 18(9):47, 2003.

Moorhead S and others, editors: *Nursing outcomes classification (NOC)*, ed 4, St. Louis, 2008, Mosby.

Pedersen CM and others: Endotracheal suctioning of the adult intubated patient: what is the evidence? *Intensive Crit Care Nurs* 25:21, 2009.

Perkins L, Shortall SP: Ventilation without intubation, *RN* 63(1):34, 2000.

Perry AG, Potter PA: *Clinical nursing skills and techniques*, ed 6, St. Louis, 2006, Mosby.

Peter J and others: Noninvasive ventilation in acute respiratory failure: a meta-analysis update, *Crit Care Med* 30(3):555, 2002.

Preston R: Introducing non-invasive positive pressure ventilation, *Nurs Stand* 15(26):42, 2001.

Puntillo KA and others: Pain assessment and management in the critically ill: wizardry or science? *Am J Crit Care* 12(4):10, 2003.

Rauen CA and others: Seven evidence-based practice habits: putting some sacred cows out to pasture, *Crit Care Nurse* 28(2):98, 2008.

Seidel HM and others: *Mosby's guide to physical examination*, ed 6, St. Louis, 2006, Mosby.

Thibodeau GA, Patton KT: *Structure and function of the body*, ed 12, St. Louis, Mosby, 2004.

Watchtower: official site of Jehovah's Witnesses, 2008, http://www.watchtower.org/.

Woodrow P: Using non-invasive ventilation in acute wards, part I, *Nurs Stand* 18(1):39, 2003a.

Woodrow P: Using non-invasive ventilation in acute wards, part II, *Nurs Stand* 18(1):41, 2003b.

Sleep

MEDIA RESOURCES

 CD COMPANION 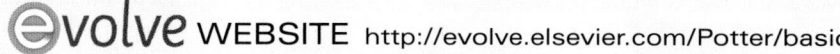 **WEBSITE** http://evolve.elsevier.com/Potter/basic

- Crossword Puzzle
- English/Spanish Audio Glossary

OBJECTIVES

- Compare the characteristics of rest and sleep.
- Explain the effect the 24-hour sleep-wake cycle has on biological function.
- Discuss mechanisms that regulate sleep.
- Describe the normal stages of sleep.
- Explain the functions of sleep.
- Compare and contrast the characteristics of sleep for different age-groups.
- Identify factors that promote or disrupt sleep.
- Discuss characteristics of common sleep disorders.

- Gather a patient's sleep history.
- Describe interventions appropriate in promoting sleep for patients with various sleep disorders.
- Discuss differences in sleep interventions for patients of different age-groups.
- Develop a teaching plan to improve a patient's sleep hygiene.
- Describe ways to evaluate the effectiveness of sleep therapies.

KEY TERMS

Biological clock, p. 850
Cataplexy, p. 856
Circadian rhythm, p. 850

Excessive daytime sleepiness (EDS), p. 852
Hypnotics, p. 866
Insomnia, p. 856
Narcolepsy, p. 856

Nocturia, p. 865
Nonrapid eye movement (NREM) sleep, p. 851
Rapid eye movement (REM) sleep, p. 851

Sedatives, p. 866
Sleep, p. 850
Sleep apnea, p. 856
Sleep deprivation, p. 856

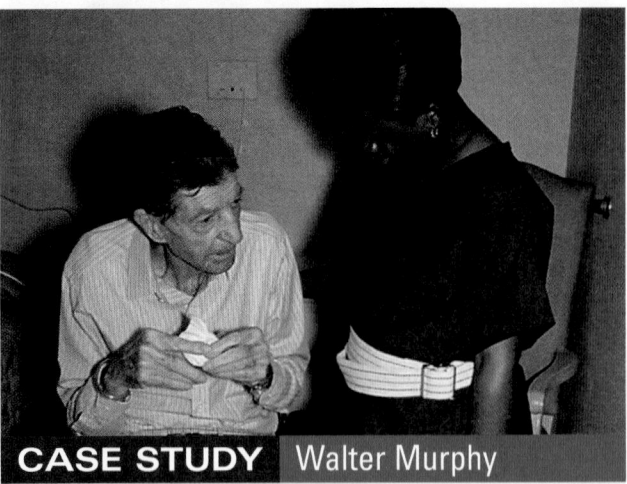

CASE STUDY Walter Murphy

Walter Murphy is 82 years old and has resided in the local nursing home for the last 3 months. His wife, Mary, still lives at home but visits Walter on a daily basis. Walter is confined to a wheelchair as a result of osteoarthritis and a mild stroke he experienced 1 year ago. Even though he has physical limitations, he is alert and oriented. Over the last several weeks, Mary found her husband to be very sleepy when visiting him just before lunchtime. Walter tells Mary that he has trouble falling asleep at night, and once he does fall asleep, he reawakens frequently during the night. Mary is concerned because her husband does not seem as alert or interested during her visit.

Anna is a 23-year-old nursing student assigned to the nursing home for her second semester in nursing school. She has had experience in nursing homes, having worked in one center as a nurse assistant during the last two summers. Anna's assignment is to care for Mr. Murphy over the next 4 weeks.

Physical and emotional health depend on adequate rest and sleep. Without proper amounts of rest and sleep, a person's ability to concentrate, make judgments, promote healing, and participate in daily activities decreases. To help a patient gain needed rest and sleep, you need to understand the nature of sleep, the factors influencing it, and the patient's sleep habits. Nurses care for patients who often have preexisting sleep disturbances and for patients who develop sleep problems as a result of illness or being in the health care environment. You will learn to use an individualized approach based on patients' personal sleep habits and patterns of sleep to provide effective sleep therapies.

SCIENTIFIC KNOWLEDGE BASE

Sleep and Rest

When people are at rest, they usually feel mentally relaxed, free from anxiety, and physically calm. They are in a state of mental and physical activity that leaves them feeling refreshed, rejuvenated, and ready to resume the activities of the day. Rest conserves and restores energy (Allison, 2007). Rest

does not imply inactivity, although everyone often thinks of it as settling down in a comfortable chair or taking a brief nap. Rest is also associated with activity or change in activity that expends energy but relieves stress and produces enjoyment and relaxation (Allison, 2007). All persons have their own preferences for obtaining rest. For example, reading a book, meditating, listening to music, practicing a relaxation exercise (see Chapter 31), or taking long walks are all restful habits.

Sleep is a recurrent, altered state of consciousness that occurs for sustained periods. When persons get proper sleep, they feel that their energy has been restored. Sleep provides time for the repair and recovery of body systems for the next period of wakefulness. Adequate quality and quantity of sleep contribute to optimum health.

Physiology of Sleep

Sleep is a cyclical physiological process that alternates with longer periods of wakefulness. The sleep-wake cycle influences and regulates body functions and behavioral responses.

CIRCADIAN RHYTHMS People experience cyclical rhythms as part of their everyday life. The most familiar rhythm is the 24-hour, day-night cycle known as the diurnal or **circadian rhythm.** Light and temperature affect all circadian rhythms, including the sleep-wake cycle. External factors such as social activities and environmental stressors also affect circadian rhythms. The natural secretion of melatonin supports circadian rhythm in the sleep-wake cycle by helping to ensure a smooth transition from wakefulness to sleep (Pandi-Perumal and others, 2007). Every person has a **biological clock** that is normally synchronized by exposure to light and activity. Some people fall asleep at 8 PM, whereas others go to bed at midnight or early in the morning. Different people also function best at different times of the day.

The normal rhythm of sleep is synchronized with other body functions. Normal variations in body temperature, for example, correlate with sleep-wake patterns (see Chapter 14). When the sleep-wake cycle becomes disrupted (e.g., by working rotating shifts), other physiological functions change as well. Failure to obtain sufficient sleep adversely affects a person's overall health. For example, a change in sleep patterns may lead to overeating or loss of appetite, depression or psychosis.

SLEEP-WAKE REGULATION Sleep-wake is a dual process that has two distinct states (Jones, 2005). It involves a series of physiological states maintained by highly integrated central nervous system (CNS) activity that is associated with changes in the peripheral nervous, endocrine, cardiovascular, respiratory, and muscular systems (McCance and Huether, 2006). Each series is identified by specific physiological responses and patterns of brain activity. The control and regulation of the sleep-wake state depend on the interrelationship between two cerebral mechanisms that intermittently activate and suppress the brain's higher centers to control sleep and wakefulness (Figure 30-1). The neurons in the brain stem reticular formation maintain a state of wakefulness, whereas

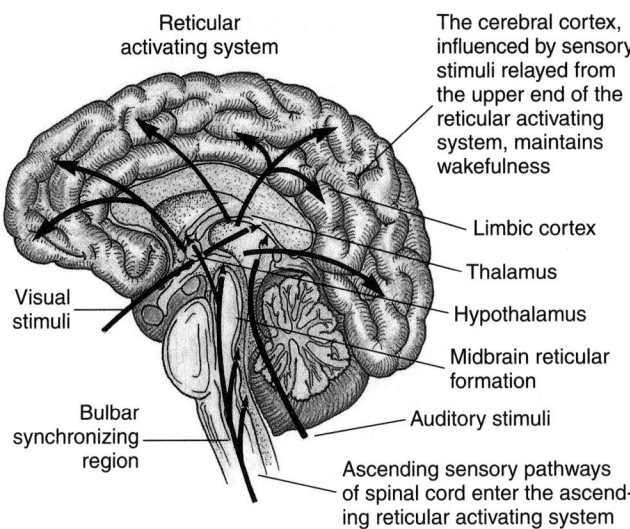

Figure 30-1 ■ The reticular activating system and bulbar synchronizing region control sensory input, intermittently activating and suppressing the brain's higher centers to control sleep and wakefulness.

the neurons in the parasympathetic control centers maintain a state of sleep.

When you try to fall asleep, you close your eyes, assume a relaxed position, and have the room dark, quiet, and at a comfortable temperature. Stimuli to the reticular activating system (RAS) in the upper brain stem decline. Gradually the bulbar synchronizing region (BSR) takes over, causing sleep. Evidence suggests that the neurotransmitter adenosine plays a role in the sleep-wake cycle (National Sleep Foundation, 2006). You will generally not reawaken until you finish your usual sleep cycle or stimuli in the environment (e.g., traffic outside or chirping of birds) stimulate the RAS to awaken.

Stages of Sleep   Normal sleep involves two phases: **non-rapid eye movement (NREM) sleep** and **rapid eye movement (REM) sleep** (Box 30-1). During NREM an individual progresses through four stages during a typical 90-minute sleep cycle. The quality of sleep from stage 1 through stage 4 becomes increasingly deep. Lighter sleep is characteristic of stages 1 and 2, when a person is more easily arousable. Stages 3 and 4 involve a deeper sleep called slow-wave sleep from which a person is more difficult to arouse. REM sleep is the phase at the end of each 90-minute sleep cycle. During REM sleep there is increased brain activity associated with rapid eye movements and muscle atonia. REM sleep is not divided into stages.

Sleep Cycle   Normally an adult's routine sleep pattern begins with a presleep period during which the person is aware only of a gradually developing sleepiness. This period normally lasts 10 to 30 minutes. Individuals experiencing difficulty falling asleep often remain in this stage for an hour or more.

Once asleep, the person usually passes through four to six complete sleep cycles, each consisting of four stages of NREM sleep and a period of REM sleep. Each cycle lasts approximately 90 to 110 minutes (National Sleep Foundation, 2006). The cyclical pattern usually progresses from stage 1 through

BOX 30-1   Stages of the Sleep Cycle

NREM STAGE 1
- Stage includes lightest level of sleep.
- Stage lasts a few minutes.
- Decreased physiological activity begins with gradual fall in vital signs and metabolism.
- Sensory stimuli, such as noise, easily arouse sleeper.
- If awakened, person feels as though daydreaming has occurred.

NREM STAGE 2
- Stage is period of sound sleep.
- Relaxation progresses.
- Arousal is still relatively easy.
- Stage lasts 10 to 20 minutes.
- Body functions continue to slow.

NREM STAGE 3
- It involves initial stages of deep sleep.
- Sleeper is difficult to arouse and rarely moves.
- Muscles are completely relaxed.
- Vital signs decline but remain regular.
- Stage lasts 15 to 30 minutes.

NREM STAGE 4
- It is deepest stage of sleep.
- It is very difficult to arouse sleeper.
- If sleep loss has occurred, sleeper will spend considerable portion of night in this stage.
- Vital signs are significantly lower than during waking hours.
- Stage lasts approximately 15 to 30 minutes.
- Sleepwalking and enuresis sometimes occur.

REM SLEEP
- Vivid, full-color dreaming occurs.
- Stage usually begins about 90 minutes after sleep has begun.
- Stage typified by autonomic response of rapidly moving eyes, fluctuating heart and respiratory rates, and increased or fluctuating blood pressure.
- Loss of skeletal muscle tone occurs.
- Gastric secretions increase.
- It is very difficult to arouse sleeper.
- Duration of REM sleep increases with each cycle and averages 20 minutes.

NREM, Nonrapid eye movement; *REM,* rapid eye movement.

stage 4 of NREM, followed by a reversal from stage 4 to 3 to 2, ending with a period of REM sleep (Figure 30-2).

With each successive cycle, stages 3 and 4 of NREM sleep shorten and the period of REM lengthens. REM sleep lasts up to 60 minutes during the last sleep cycle. Not all people progress consistently through the usual stages of sleep. For example, a sleeper fluctuates back and forth for short intervals between NREM stages 2, 3, and 4 before entering REM sleep. The amount of time spent in each stage varies. The number

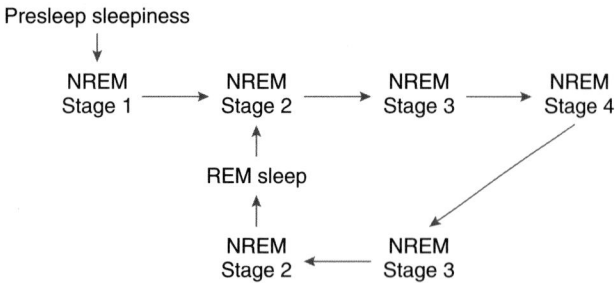

Figure 30-2 ■ The stages of the adult sleep cycle.

of sleep cycles depends on the total amount of time that the person spends sleeping.

Functions of Sleep

The purpose of sleep is still unclear. One theory suggests that sleep is a time of restoration and preparation for the next period of wakefulness (McCance and Huether, 2006). During NREM sleep, biological functions slow. A healthy adult's normal heart rate throughout the day averages 70 to 80 beats per minute. However, during sleep the heart rate normally falls to 60 beats per minute or less, thus preserving cardiac function.

Sleep helps maintain normal biological processes and optimal immune performance (Davis, Parker, and Montgomery, 2004). During NREM stage 4 sleep, the body releases human growth hormone for the repair and renewal of epithelial and specialized cells such as brain cells (Jones, 2005; McCance and Huether, 2006). Protein synthesis and cell division for the renewal of tissues also occur during rest and sleep. The basal metabolic rate is lowered during sleep, which conserves the body's energy supply (Izaac, 2006).

REM sleep appears to be important for brain tissue and cognitive restoration (Bussye, 2005). Researchers associate REM sleep with changes in cerebral blood flow, increased cortical activity, increased oxygen consumption, and epinephrine release. This association assists with memory storage and learning.

The benefits of sleep often go unnoticed until a person develops a problem resulting from sleep deprivation. Sleep deprivation affects immune functioning, metabolism, nitrogen balance, protein catabolism, and quality of life (Friese, 2008). A loss of REM sleep often leads to confusion and disorientation. Chronic sleep loss has been linked to decreased productivity, increased risk for development of health problems, increased risk for falls in older adults, and increased likelihood of accidents and work-related injuries. A relationship has been found between sleep loss and increased medical errors by health care workers (Institute of Medicine, 2006).

DREAMS The dreams of REM sleep are more vivid and elaborate than those of NREM sleep, and researchers believe them to be functionally important to learning, memory processing, and adaptation to stress (Stickgold, 2005). REM dreams progress in content throughout the night from dreams about current events to emotional dreams of childhood or the past. Personality influences the quality of dreams; for example, a creative person may have very vivid, unusual dreams, whereas a depressed person may have dreams of helplessness.

Dreams help people sort out immediate concerns or erase certain fantasies or nonsensical memories. Because most dreams are forgotten, many people have little dream recall and do not believe they dream at all. To remember a dream, a person must consciously think about it on awakening. People who recall dreams vividly usually awaken just after a period of REM sleep.

NURSING KNOWLEDGE BASE

Normal Sleep Requirements and Patterns

Sleep duration and quality vary among persons of all age-groups. The neonate and infant up to the age of 3 months average about 16 hours of sleep a day. Approximately 50% of this sleep is REM sleep, which stimulates the higher brain centers (Hockenberry and Wilson, 2007). Infants usually develop a nighttime pattern of sleep by 3 months of age. Infants sometimes take several naps during the day but usually sleep an average of 9 to 11 hours during the night. Infants spend about 30% of sleep time in the REM cycle. Awakening commonly occurs early in the morning, although infants sometimes awaken during the night.

By the age of 2 years, children usually sleep through the night and take daily naps. Total sleep averages 12 hours a day. Some children stop taking naps altogether at age 3. It is common for toddlers to awaken during the night. The percentage of REM sleep continues to fall. Toddlers are often unwilling to go to bed at night. A preschooler sleeps an average of 12 hours a night (about 20% is REM). By the age of 5, the preschooler rarely takes daytime naps (Hockenberry and Wilson, 2007) except in cultures in which a siesta is the custom. The preschooler usually has difficulty relaxing or quieting down after long, active days and often has problems with bedtime fears, waking during the night, and nightmares.

The school-age child usually does not require a nap. A 6-year-old averages 11 to 12 hours of sleep nightly, whereas an 11-year-old sleeps about 9 to 10 hours (Hockenberry and Wilson, 2007). Encouraging quiet activities usually persuades the 6- or 7-year-old to go to bed. The older child often resists sleeping because of an unawareness of fatigue or a need to be independent. Adolescents need between 8½ and 9½ hours of sleep each night. At a time when sleep needs actually increase, the typical adolescent is subject to a number of changes that often reduce the time spent sleeping (National Sleep Foundation, 2008b). The typical teenager gets about 7½ hours of sleep per night. Usually parents no longer set a specific bedtime. School demands, after-school social activities, and part-time jobs lessen time available for sleep. Teens often go to bed later and rise earlier during the high school years. Because of lifestyle demands that shorten the time available for sleep and physiological needs, teens often experience **excessive daytime sleepiness (EDS)**. Poor school performance, vulnerability to accidents, behavioral problems, primary headaches, and increased use of alcohol and stimulants are the result of

EDS due to insufficient sleep (Gilman and others, 2007; Walsh and others, 2005).

Most young adults average 6 to 8½ hours of sleep a night, but this varies. Young adults rarely take regular naps. Young adults spend approximately 20% of sleep time in REM sleep, which remains consistent throughout the remainder of life. Healthy young adults require adequate sleep to participate in the day's busy activities. However, lifestyle demands often interrupt usual sleep patterns, which results in insomnia. During middle adulthood the total time spent sleeping at night begins to decline. The amount of stage 4 sleep begins to fall, a decline that continues with advancing age. Health care workers often initially diagnose sleep disturbances among people in this age range even when the symptoms of a disorder have been present for several years. Members of this age-group sometimes rely on sleeping medications.

Complaints of sleeping difficulties increase with age. More than 50% of persons age 65 and older report regular problems with sleep (Cuellar and others, 2007). Older adults spend more time in stage 1 and have less stage 3 and stage 4 NREM sleep; some older adults have almost no NREM stage 4, or deep, sleep. Episodes of REM sleep tend to shorten. Older adults awaken more often during the night, and it takes more time for them to fall asleep. Their sleep efficiency (the amount of time asleep given the amount of time in bed) is reduced, and they increase the number of naps taken during the day (Cuellar and others, 2007). Tests show that older adults do not have an increased need for sleep, but have a reduction in the ability to sleep.

As people age, their circadian clock shifts, causing the person to "phase advance." This is common in older adults and often is the reason behind the complaint of waking early in the morning and being unable to get back to sleep. People with "phase advance" get sleepy early in the evening (e.g., 8 or 9 PM). If they go to bed at that time, they will sleep for about 8 hours and wake up around 4 or 5 AM. However, when people with advanced sleep phase syndrome stay up until their customary 10 or 11 PM, their bodies still awaken at 4 or 5 AM. Consequently, they receive only 5 to 6 hours of sleep, the amount of time they are in bed before their advanced sleep-wake cycle wakes them up (Cuellar and others, 2007).

Factors Affecting Sleep

A number of factors (physical, psychological, and environmental) affect the quantity and quality of sleep. Often more than one factor combine to cause a sleep problem.

PHYSICAL ILLNESS Any illness or condition that causes pain, difficulty breathing, nausea, or mood problems such as anxiety or depression can result in sleep problems. Individuals with such alterations have trouble falling or staying asleep. Illnesses also sometimes force patients to sleep in positions to which they are unaccustomed. Table 30-1 summarizes illnesses and conditions that have the potential for causing sleep alterations.

DRUGS AND SUBSTANCES A considerable number of drugs cause either sleepiness, insomnia, or fatigue as a side effect (Box 30-2). Medications prescribed for sleep often

TABLE 30-1	Illnesses and Conditions That Can Alter Sleep
ILLNESS/CONDITION	NATURE OF SLEEP ALTERATION
Respiratory disease (e.g., emphysema, asthma, bronchitis, allergic rhinitis, common cold)	Shortness of breath requires use of two to three pillows to raise head. Altered rhythm of breathing. Nasal congestion and sore throat impair breathing and ability to relax.
Coronary heart disease with episodes of chest pain and irregular heart rates	Frequent awakenings and sleep stage changes during sleep and significant alterations in all stages of sleep.
Hypertension	Reduced length and depth of NREM sleep and a shortened REM latency period cause arousals and early morning awakening, resulting in fatigue.
Hypothyroidism	Decreases in slow-wave sleep and REM sleep and increased movements during sleep contribute to daytime sleepiness.
Hyperthyroidism	Increase in metabolism causes insomnia due to increased time needed to fall asleep.
Nocturia (reduced bladder tone, diabetes, urethritis, prostate disease)	Awakenings at night to urinate; difficulty returning to sleep.
Gastric reflux	Burning pain in lower esophagus or nocturnal coughing; increases when lying flat in bed.
Depression	Awakenings in early morning with inability to return to sleep; worsened by anxiety or agitation.
Perimenopause	Awakenings at night caused by hot flashes and sweating.
Pain	Delay in sleep onset, increased sleep awakenings, and decreased slow-wave activity during sleep result in poor sleep quality. Worsened by increased sympathetic activity resulting in high cardiac heart rate.

NREM, Nonrapid eye movement; *REM,* rapid eye movement.

cause more problems than benefits. L-Tryptophan is a natural protein found in foods such as milk, cheese, and meats and sometimes helps a person sleep. It is a precursor, or forerunner, to the neurotransmitter serotonin, which has a role in the sleep-wake cycle.

<table>
<tr><td>

BOX 30-2   Effect of Medications and Other Substances on Sleep

HYPNOTICS
- Interfere with reaching deeper sleep stages
- Provide only temporary (1 week) increase in quantity of sleep
- Sometimes cause "hangover" feeling during day
- In some cases, worsens sleep apnea in older adults

DIURETICS (ADMINISTERED LATE IN THE DAY)
- Cause nocturia

ANTIDEPRESSANTS AND STIMULANTS
- Suppress REM sleep
- Decrease total sleep time

ALCOHOL
- Speeds onset of sleep and disrupts REM sleep
- Awakens person during night and causes difficulty returning to sleep

CAFFEINE
- Stimulant prevents person from falling asleep
- Causes person to awaken during night

BETA-ADRENERGIC BLOCKERS
- Cause nightmares and insomnia
- Cause awakening from sleep

BENZODIAZEPINES
- Increase sleep time
- Increase daytime sleepiness

NARCOTICS (OPIATES)
- Suppress REM sleep
- Cause increased daytime drowsiness

ANTIHISTAMINES
- Cause drowsiness
- Excess amounts cause insomnia

NASAL DECONGESTANTS
- Cause daytime sleepiness

REM, Rapid eye movement.

</td></tr>
</table>

LIFESTYLE A person's daily routine influences sleep patterns. For example, an individual who alternately works day and night shifts often has difficulty adjusting to the altered sleep schedule. Lifestyle changes that contribute to decreased quantity and quality of sleep include working an increased number of hours or at multiple jobs and spending more time watching television or being on the Internet (Institute of Medicine, 2006). Other alterations in routine that disrupt sleep patterns include performing unaccustomed heavy work or exercise, engaging in late-night social activities, and changing evening mealtime.

USUAL SLEEP PATTERNS AND EXCESSIVE DAYTIME SLEEPINESS On average, adults sleep 6 to 7 hours per night on weeknights and 7½ or more hours per night on weekends (National Sleep Foundation, 2008a). Many Americans suffer from sleep deprivation and experience EDS during the day. EDS often results in impairment of waking function, poor work or school performance, accidents while driving or using equipment, and behavioral or emotional problems. People usually feel sleepiest upon awakening from sleep or right before going to sleep and about 12 hours after the midsleep period.

Sleepiness becomes pathological when it occurs at times when persons need or want to be awake. Persons who temporarily experience sleep deprivation as a result of an active social evening or lengthened work schedule usually feel sleepy the next day. However, they are sometimes able to overcome these feelings even though they have difficulty performing tasks and remaining attentive. Chronic lack of sleep is much more serious than temporary sleep deprivation and causes serious alterations in the ability to perform daily activities. EDS is most difficult to overcome during sedentary tasks (e.g., driving).

EMOTIONAL STRESS Worry over personal problems or situations interferes with sleep. Emotional stress causes tension and often leads to frustration when sleep does not come. Stress also causes a person to try too hard to fall asleep, to awaken frequently during the sleep cycle, or to oversleep. Continued stress causes poor sleep habits in some cases.

ENVIRONMENT The physical environment in which a person sleeps has a significant influence on the ability to fall and remain asleep. Good ventilation, a comfortable temperature, and a darkened or softly lit room are essential for restful sleep. The size, firmness, and position of a bed also affect sleep quality. Hospital beds are often harder than those at home. If a person usually sleeps with another individual, sleeping alone during times of illness causes wakefulness. However, sleeping with a restless or snoring bed partner also disrupts sleep.

SOUND Noise affects sleep activity by causing arousal and sleep fragmentation (Cmiel and others, 2004). Noise easily disturbs older adults' sleep because most of their sleep is in lighter sleep stages. Some persons require silence to fall asleep, whereas others prefer background noise such as soft music or television.

In health care facilities, noise created by caregivers, equipment, and other patients causes a problem for patients. Noise in health care settings is usually new or strange to the patient. This problem is greatest the first night a patient stays in a hospital or other facility, when patients often experience increased total wake time, increased awakening, and decreased REM sleep and total sleep time. Nursing activities are a source of increased sound levels. The intensive care setting is one of the loudest, where close proximity of patients, noise from confused and ill patients, and ringing of alarm systems and telephones make the environment very disruptive.

EXERCISE AND FATIGUE A person who is moderately fatigued usually achieves restful sleep, especially if the fatigue results from enjoyable work or exercise. Completing vigorous exercise within 2 hours or more before bedtime allows the body to cool down and the drop in body temperature pro-

BOX 30-3   Classification of Select Sleep Disorders

INSOMNIAS
- Adjustment sleep disorder (acute insomnia)
- Inadequate sleep hygiene
- Paradoxical insomnia
- Insomnia due to mental disorder
- Behavioral insomnia of childhood
- Idiopathic insomnia
- Insomnia due to medical condition

SLEEP-RELATED BREATHING DISORDERS

Central Sleep Apnea Syndromes
- Primary central sleep apnea
- Central sleep apnea due to a drug or substance
- Central sleep apnea due to a medical condition

HYPERSOMNIAS NOT DUE TO A SLEEP-RELATED BREATHING DISORDER

Obstructive Sleep Apnea Syndromes
- Narcolepsy (four specified types)
- Menstrual-related hypersomnia
- Idiopathic hypersomnia with long sleep time
- Behaviorally induced insufficient sleep syndrome
- Hypersomnia due to a medical condition

PARASOMNIAS

Disorders of Arousal
- Sleepwalking
- Sleep terrors

Parasomnias Usually Associated With REM Sleep
- Nightmare disorder
- REM sleep behavior disorder
- Sleep paralysis

Other Parasomnias
- Sleep-related groaning
- Sleep-related hallucinations
- Sleep-related eating disorder
- Sleep-related enuresis (bed-wetting)

CIRCADIAN RHYTHM SLEEP DISORDERS

Primary Circadian Rhythm Sleep Disorders
- Delayed sleep phase type
- Advanced sleep phase type

Behaviorally Induced Circadian Rhythm Sleep Disorders
- Jet lag type
- Shift work type
- Delayed sleep phase type
- Due to a drug or substance

SLEEP-RELATED MOVEMENT DISORDERS
- Restless legs syndrome
- Periodic limb movements
- Sleep-related leg cramps
- Sleep-related bruxism (teeth grinding)

ISOLATED SYMPTOMS, APPARENTLY NORMAL VARIANTS, AND UNRESOLVED ISSUES
- Long sleeper
- Short sleeper
- Snoring
- Sleep talking
- Benign sleep myoclonus of infancy

OTHER SLEEP DISORDERS
- Physiological (organic) sleep disorders
- Environmental sleep disorder
- Sleep disorder not due to a substance or physiological condition

Modified from American Sleep Disorders Association, Diagnostic Classification Steering Committee: International classification of sleep disorders. Cited in Thorpy M: Classification of sleep disorders. In Kryger M and others, editors: *Principles and practice of sleep medicine,* ed 4, Philadelphia, 2005, Saunders.

motes sleep onset. A state of fatigue is maintained that promotes relaxation. Vigorous exercise before bedtime interferes with sleep onset because of increased body temperature. Also, excess fatigue resulting from exhausting or stressful work makes falling asleep difficult.

FOOD AND CALORIC INTAKE Following good eating habits is important for proper health, including sleep. Eating a large, heavy, and/or spicy meal within 3 to 4 hours of bedtime sometimes results in indigestion that interferes with sleep. Alcohol consumed in the evening has insomnia-producing and diuretic effects. Coffee, tea, cola, and chocolate contain caffeine and xanthines that cause sleeplessness as a result of CNS stimulation.

Weight loss or weight gain influences sleep patterns. Weight gain contributes to obstructive sleep apnea because of the increased size of the soft tissue structures in the upper airway (Schwab and others, 2005). Weight loss causes insomnia and decreased amounts of sleep (Benca and Schenck, 2005). Certain sleep disorders are the result of the semistarvation diets popular in a weight-conscious society.

Sleep Disorders

Sleep disorders are conditions that, if untreated, cause disturbed nighttime sleep that results in the problems of insomnia, movement disorders, sleep-related breathing disorders, or excessive daytime sleepiness (Malow, 2005). The occurrence of sleep disorders is becoming a significant health problem, especially for persons who are overweight or obese or who live in stressful environments. The American Academy of Sleep Medicine developed the International Classification of Sleep Disorders version 2 (ICSD-2), which classifies sleep disorders into eight major categories (Box 30-3).

In sleep-related movement disorders the person experiences simple stereotypical movements that disturb sleep. The isolated symptoms, apparently normal variants, and unresolved issues category includes sleep-related symptoms that fall between normal and abnormal sleep. The other sleep disorders category contains sleep problems that do not fit into other categories.

INSOMNIA **Insomnia** is a symptom experienced by patients who have chronic difficulty falling asleep, frequent awakenings from sleep, and/or a short sleep or nonrestorative sleep (Edinger and Means, 2005). The person with insomnia complains of EDS, as well as insufficient quantity and quality of sleep. Frequently, however, the patient gets more sleep than he or she realizes. Insomnia sometimes signals an underlying physical or psychological disorder. It is more common in older adults and females (Institute of Medicine, 2006). Shift work and the high demands of society contribute to the development of insomnia. Health care workers who work different shifts have an increased incidence of insomnia, which results in an increase in medication errors, charting errors, and falling asleep unintentionally at work (New Survey, 2008).

Often people experience transient or temporary insomnia as a result of situational stresses such as work or family problems. Insomnia sometimes recurs, but between episodes the patient is able to sleep well. However, a temporary case of insomnia caused by a stressful event has the ability to lead to chronic difficulty in obtaining sufficient sleep. Insomnia is often associated with poor sleep habits. If the condition continues, the fear of not being able to sleep is enough to cause wakefulness. During the day a person with chronic insomnia feels sleepy, fatigued, depressed, and anxious.

Direct treatments, such as improved sleep hygiene measures, biofeedback, and relaxation techniques, are aimed at the symptoms. It is important to treat underlying emotional or medical problems that cause the insomnia.

SLEEP APNEA **Sleep apnea** is a disorder in which the individual is unable to breathe and sleep at the same time. There is a lack of airflow through the nose and mouth for periods from 10 seconds to 1 to 2 minutes in length. There can be 10 or 15 to more than 100 respiratory events per hour of sleep (Mendez and Olson, 2006). There are three types of sleep apnea: obstructive, central, and mixed apnea, which has both an obstructive and a central component.

The most common form, obstructive sleep apnea (OSA), is a cessation or stopping of airflow despite the effort to breathe. It occurs when muscles or soft structures of the oral cavity or throat relax during sleep. The upper airway becomes partially or completely blocked and nasal airflow diminishes (hypopnea) or stops (apnea). The person tries to breathe because chest and abdominal movement continues, which often results in loud snoring sounds. When breathing is partially or completely diminished, the person becomes sufficiently hypoxic that he or she must awaken to breathe. Structural abnormalities such as a deviated septum, nasal polyps, narrow lower jaw, or enlarged tonsils sometimes predispose a patient to obstructive apnea.

Cessation of diaphragmatic and intercostal respiratory effort causes central sleep apnea. This cessation is a result of dysfunction of the brain's respiratory control center. The impulse to breathe temporarily fails. Nasal airflow and chest wall movement cease, with oxygen saturation of the blood also falling. You will see central sleep apnea in patients with congestive heart failure, brain stem injury, muscular dystrophy, and encephalitis, as well as in people who breathe normally during the day. It is the least common sleep apnea.

EDS is the most common complaint of people with obstructive sleep apnea. Patients with OSA are at risk for cardiac dysrhythmias, right heart failure, pulmonary hypertension, angina attacks, stroke, and hypertension. A serious decline in the arterial oxygen and cardiac arrhythmias occurs (see Chapter 29). The risk for life-threatening dysrhythmias is increased in patients experiencing sleep apnea (Lewis and others, 2007).

Treatment for sleep apnea includes therapy for underlying cardiac, respiratory, or emotional problems. The treatment of choice is use of a nasal continuous positive airway pressure (CPAP) device at night. The CPAP machine pushes positive air pressure into the airway in an attempt to reduce the apnea periods the patient experiences during sleep by serving as a splint for the airway. Improved sleep hygiene and a weight-loss program are also helpful to treat OSA.

NARCOLEPSY **Narcolepsy** is a rare CNS dysfunction of mechanisms that regulate sleep and wake states. EDS is the most common complaint associated with narcolepsy. During the day a person suddenly feels an overwhelming wave of sleepiness and falls asleep. It is possible for REM sleep to occur within 15 minutes of falling asleep. There are two narcolepsy states: with or without cataplexy. **Cataplexy** is a sudden muscle weakness during intense emotions such as anger or laughter that occurs at any time during the day. If the cataplectic attack is severe, the patient loses voluntary muscle control and falls to the floor.

A person with narcolepsy often falls asleep uncontrollably at inappropriate times. Unless you recognize this disorder, you will mistake someone who suddenly and inappropriately falls asleep as someone who is lazy, disinterested, or possibly drunk. Typically symptoms first occur in adolescence and are sometimes confused with EDS. You treat people who have narcolepsy with stimulants that sometimes only partially increase wakefulness and reduce inappropriate sleep. Medications, such as modafinil and sodium oxybate, that suppress cataplexy and the other REM-related symptoms are also effective (National Guidelines Clearinghouse, 2008).

SLEEP DEPRIVATION **Sleep deprivation** is a problem many patients have as a result of a sleep disorder. Sleep deprivation occurs from insufficient sleep or disrupted sleep. Causes include illness (e.g., fever, difficulty breathing, or pain), emotional stress, medications, environmental disturbances (e.g., frequent interruptions in sleep during nursing care), and variability in the timing of sleep as a result of shift work.

Hospitalization, especially in intensive care units, makes patients vulnerable to the circadian sleep disorders (Friese, 2008). Sleep deprivation involves decreases in the quantity and quality of sleep, as well as inconsistency in the timing of sleep. When sleep becomes interrupted or fragmented, changes in the normal sequencing of the sleep cycles occur. A cumulative sleep deprivation develops over time.

Individuals respond to sleep deprivation differently. Some patients experience a variety of physiological and psychological symptoms such as blurred vision, decreased reflexes, slow response time, confusion, and irritability. The severity of symptoms is often related to the duration of sleep deprivation. The most effective treatment for sleep deprivation is elimination or correction of environmental factors and patient care activities that disrupt the sleep pattern. Nurses play an important role in identifying treatable sleep deprivation problems. There is increasing evidence that suggests sleep deprivation contributes to development of obesity, diabetes mellitus, depressed mood, alcohol use, increased risk for infection, decreased immune response, hypertension, and cardiac dysrhythmias (Institute of Medicine, 2006; National Sleep Foundation, 2006).

PARASOMNIAS The parasomnias are sleep disorders that produce abnormal sleep movements, behaviors, emotions, perceptions, and dreaming as a result of autonomic nervous system changes and skeletal muscle activity during sleep (Thorpy, 2005). Disorders of arousal, partial arousal, and sleep transition are more common in children than in adults. An individual often experiences more than one parasomnia. Specific treatment for these disorders varies based on the underlying cause. However, in all cases it is important to support patients experiencing a disorder and to maintain their safety.

CRITICAL THINKING

You will apply elements of critical thinking whenever you perform the nursing process with a patient. Consider the scientific knowledge you have learned, your experience, critical thinking attitudes, and standards to ensure an individualized approach to patient care.

Synthesis

It is not uncommon for almost any patient to experience some type of sleep disorder, especially if sleeping in a new place. However, it is important not to overlook such a problem or consider it as normal. Use of a critical thinking approach helps you to correctly identify the nature of a sleep problem and then to initiate appropriate nursing care. Apply your knowledge, experience, and appropriate critical thinking attitudes and standards to make the correct clinical judgments for patients (Box 30-4).

KNOWLEDGE To make decisions about the nature and cause of a patient's sleep problems, it is important for you to synthesize knowledge regarding the physiology and functions of sleep and factors that affect sleep. Knowledge of the pathophysiology of select disease processes further helps in understanding the mechanisms for certain sleep problems. In addition, a good knowledge of pharmacological information is

BOX 30-4   SYNTHESIS IN PRACTICE

As Anna prepares to conduct an assessment of Mr. Murphy, she knows it is important to consider how sleep is altered in older adults. Because they typically have less deep sleep and more awakenings to begin with, it will be important to consider what factors in the nursing home environment disrupt sleep. In addition, she has learned that the pain of Mr. Murphy's osteoarthritis is a contributing factor to his sleep disturbances. His immobility resulting from the stroke adds discomfort. Anna also plans to assess Mr. Murphy's medications carefully to determine if any drugs are adding to a sleep alteration.

From Anna's experience in a nursing home, she knows that a resident's sleep is often fragmented. Furthermore, she has read in a journal article that multiple factors affect sleep in the nursing home patient, including physical illness, dementia, depression, high prevalence of sleep-disordered breathing, chronic bed rest, circadian rhythm disturbances, and the noise and lighting of the nursing home environment (Kryger and others, 2004). She wants to be sure that her assessment considers all potential factors influencing Mr. Murphy's sleep pattern. Because Mr. Murphy is in a nursing home, Anna determines whether there are environmental stimuli disrupting his sleep. Anna evaluates whether he has a roommate who stays up late or has multiple visitors, the presence of electrical equipment at Mr. Murphy's bedside, and the likelihood of noise coming from an outside hallway.

Anna plans to include Mr. Murphy's wife in the assessment to learn more about Mrs. Murphy's perceptions of changes in Mr. Murphy's behavior. A complete assessment needs to be clear and precise; thus Anna plans to talk with Mr. Murphy more than one time to gather the necessary information and to keep her patient from becoming fatigued.

important because many medications patients receive may contribute to sleeping difficulties.

Another important area of knowledge to synthesize is the patient's personal routine and cultural orientation. Infant care practices such as co-sleeping and the practice of regular siestas or naps are examples of cultural variations influencing sleep. Anticipate how such cultural factors ultimately influence an individual patient's ability to sleep.

EXPERIENCE You know of factors that have either disrupted or promoted your own ability to sleep. This personal experience is valuable when assessing patients' sleep problems or in selecting therapies for sleep promotion. Previous clinical experience with patients helps you to appreciate that environmental and lifestyle variations significantly affect the quality and quantity of sleep a patient receives.

ATTITUDES When dealing with sleep problems, it sometimes takes a long time to find effective therapies. For example, it is not easy to eliminate chronic insomnia in a short period. Perseverance and discipline are important critical thinking attitudes to use to help develop a plan of care with effective solutions to manage the sleep problems of the patient. The problems that result from sleep disruption also often require creative approaches. Sometimes an original idea is necessary to minimize or control environmental stressors in the patient's sleep environment.

STANDARDS   When learning about a patient's sleep problem, you will use numerous intellectual standards in conducting the nursing assessment. Always conduct a detailed sleep assessment to understand the nature of the sleep problem and potential causes and solutions. A clear, precise, specific, and accurate assessment is very important so that you establish an appropriate plan of care. Professional standards, such as *Nursing: Scope and Standards of Practice* (American Nurses Association, 2004) and sleep standards found in "Excessive Sleepiness" (Chasens and others, 2008), provide valuable guidelines and protocols to assess and address the needs of patients with sleep disorders. Nursing units often develop unit-based standards to promote sleep for patients.

NURSING PROCESS

■■■ ASSESSMENT

Assess a patient's sleep pattern to gather information about factors that usually influence sleep. Because sleep is a subjective experience, only the patient is able to report whether it is sufficient and restful. If a patient admits to or you suspect a sleep problem, you will need a more detailed history. Aim your assessment at understanding the characteristics of any sleep problem and the patient's usual sleep habits so that you incorporate ways for promoting sleep into nursing care.

SOURCES FOR SLEEP ASSESSMENT   Patients are your best resource for describing a sleep problem and any change from their usual sleep and waking patterns. Parents or bed partners offer information on patients' sleep patterns that reveal the nature of certain disorders.

Obtain a child's sleep history from the parents. Older children often are able to relate their fears or worries that prevent them from falling asleep. If a child frequently awakens in the middle of bad dreams, parents are usually able to identify the problem without necessarily knowing the meanings of the dreams. Parents can also describe typical behavior patterns that encourage or impair sleep. With chronic sleep problems, parents relate the duration of the problem, its progression, and the child's responses. It is a good idea for parents of an infant to keep a 24-hour log of their infant's waking and sleeping behavior over a period of several days.

SLEEP HISTORY   Obtain a brief sleep history from patients upon admission. Determine usual bedtime, normal bedtime rituals, preferred environment for sleeping, and what time the patient usually rises to plan care to support the patient's positive sleep habits and patterns. You need to assess the quality and characteristics of sleep in greater depth when you suspect a sleep problem.

Sleep Pattern   Begin the sleep history with the patient's self-report of his or her sleep pattern. Most patients will give a reasonably accurate estimate of their sleep patterns, particularly if any changes have occurred. An effective, subjective method for you to use for assessing sleep quality is the visual analog scale (Lashley, 2004). Draw a straight horizontal line about 100 mm (4 inches) long. Opposing statements such as "best night's sleep" and "worst night's sleep" are at each end of the line. Patients are asked to place a mark along the horizontal line at the point that best matches their perception of the previous night's sleep. The distance of the mark along the line in millimeters offers a numerical value for satisfaction with sleep. Use the scale with the same patient repeatedly to show change in sleep over time. Do not use the scale to compare the quality of sleep for different patients.

It is important to have patients describe their usual sleep pattern in case there are significant changes created by a sleep disorder. To assess the patient's sleep pattern, ask the following questions:

- What time do you usually get in bed?
- What time do you usually fall asleep? Do you do anything special to help you fall asleep?
- How many times do you awaken during sleep? Why do you think you awaken? What do you do about awakening?
- What time do you typically wake up?
- What time do you get out of bed, and how long do you stay up once you have awakened?
- What is the average number of hours you sleep?

Compare the assessment data with the pattern usually found for other patients of the same age, and look for patterns that suggest problems. Sometimes patients with sleep problems show patterns very different from their usual one, and sometimes the change is relatively minor. Hospitalized patients usually need or want more sleep as a result of illness. However, some will require less sleep because they are less active. Some patients who are ill think that it is important to try to sleep more than what is usual for them, eventually making sleeping difficult.

Description of Sleeping Problems   When a patient admits to or you suspect a sleep problem, ask open-ended questions to help a patient describe the problem more fully. A general description of the problem followed by more focused questions usually reveals specific sleep characteristics (Table 30-2). The Epworth Sleepiness scale is a screening tool to evaluate the severity of excessive daytime sleepiness (Chasens and others, 2008).

You need to understand the nature of the sleep problem, its signs and symptoms, its onset and duration, its severity, predisposing factors or causes, and the overall effect on the patient. Examples of assessment questions include the following:

1. *Nature of the problem:* Tell me what type of problem you have with your sleep. Tell me why you think you are not getting enough sleep. Describe for me a recent typical night's sleep. How is this sleep different from what you are used to?
2. *Signs and symptoms:* Have you been told that you snore loudly? Do you have headaches when awakening? Does

TABLE 30-2 FOCUSED PATIENT ASSESSMENT

FACTORS TO ASSESS	QUESTIONS	PHYSICAL ASSESSMENT
Bedtime routines	How do you prepare for bed? Do you go to bed at the same time each night? Do you eat before you go to bed?	Observe for dark circles under patient's eyes. Observe the number of times the patient yawns.
Bedtime environment	How much light is in your bedroom at night? What is the temperature of your room during the night? Do you listen to music to go to sleep?	Ask patient or sleeping partner about multiple patient position changes during sleep.
Current life events	What are your normal working hours? Have you experienced any recent changes in your job or home responsibilities? What activities do you do to relax outside of work? What hobbies do you have?	Observe the patient's ability to concentrate on the conversation.

your child awaken from nightmares? Ask bed partner or parents whether patient has restful sleep or problems such as going to the bathroom frequently.

3. *Onset and duration:* When did you notice the problem? How long has this problem lasted?

4. *Severity:* How long does it take you to fall asleep? How often during the week do you have trouble falling asleep or staying asleep?

5. *Predisposing factors:* Tell me what you do just before going to bed. Have you recently had any changes at work, school, or home? How would you describe your current mood, and have you noticed any recent changes? What medications or recreational drugs do you take regularly? Do you eat foods (e.g., spicy or greasy foods) or drink liquids (e.g., alcohol, caffeinated beverages) that disrupt your sleep? If so, how much do you eat or drink daily?

6. *Effect on patient:* How has the loss of sleep affected you? Do you feel excessively sleepy or irritable or have trouble concentrating? Do you have trouble staying awake? Have you fallen asleep at inappropriate times? Ask a family member or friend: Have you noticed any changes in the patient's behavior since the sleep problem started?

Sleep Log In addition to the sleep history, ask a patient and bed partner to keep a sleep-wake diary for 1 to 2 weeks (Cuellar and others, 2007). Have them complete the diary daily to provide information on day-to-day variations in sleep-wake patterns over time. Entries in the diary often include 24-hour information on waking and sleeping activities such as exercise, work activities, mealtimes, and alcohol and caffeine intake. They should also include time and length of daytime naps, evening and bed routines, the time the patient tries to fall asleep, time and number of awakenings, and the time of morning awakening. If necessary, have the partner help to complete the sleep-wake diary. The diary is most helpful if the patient is motivated to complete it thoroughly. Using a tape recorder is a helpful option for patients with visual impairment or who have difficulty writing. Do not use the diary with acutely ill patients who have short hospital stays.

Physical Illness Assess for any physical or psychological problems that affect a patient's sleep. Review of known medical conditions will reveal symptoms (e.g., pain, shortness of breath, or fear) that interfere with the patient's normal sleep pattern. Assess the patient's medication history, including over-the-counter and prescribed drugs. If a patient takes medications for sleep, gather information about the type and amount of medication the person uses. If a patient is scheduled for surgery, be sure to ask about a history of sleep apnea. Patients with sleep apnea who receive general anesthesia and pain medications after surgery have increased risk for developing airway obstruction during recovery (Cullen, 2001). If the patient has recently undergone surgery, expect the patient to experience some disturbance in sleep. The effect on sleep depends on the severity of pain experienced after surgery and the amount of care received during the night (Tranmer and others, 2003).

Current Life Events Changes in lifestyle disrupt a patient's sleep. A person's family situation or occupation offers clues to the nature of a sleep problem. Changes in job responsibilities, rotating shifts, or the recent birth of a child or loss of a family member sometimes contribute to a sleep disturbance. Questions about social activities, recent travel, or mealtime schedules also help clarify the sleep assessment.

Emotional and Mental Status If a patient is anxious, fearful, or angry, mental preoccupations seriously disrupt sleep. In this situation the patient experiences emotional stress related to illness or situational crises. Ask patients to explore feelings about family relationships, job, or other meaningful situations. When a sleep disturbance is related to an emotional problem, the key is to treat the primary problem, and its resolution often improves sleep (Ramakrishnan and Scheid, 2007).

Bedtime Routines Ask how the patient prepares for sleep. Assess habits that are beneficial compared with those that disturb sleep. You will need to point out that a particular habit is interfering with sleep and help patients find ways to change or eliminate their habits that disrupt sleep. A patient's activity or exercise pattern before bedtime offers additional information about sleep quality. Does the patient perform strenuous exercise within 2 hours of going to sleep? Does the patient usually spend 1 to 2 hours cooling down or relaxing before sleep?

Bedtime Environment Ask the patient to describe preferred bedroom conditions. For example, ask if the patient keeps the bedroom dark or softly lit and closes the door. Some patients listen to a radio or watch TV or prefer a quiet environment if noise prevents the patient from falling asleep. Also ask about room temperature and ventilation.

Assess the type of bed in which the person sleeps. Does the patient sleep in the same bed every night? Is the mattress comfortable? Does the patient need several pillows or cushions in bed to sit up during sleep? Does the patient use a lounge chair to sleep? Information about the sleeping environment helps you design better sleeping conditions.

Behaviors of Sleep Deprivation Some patients are unaware of how their sleep problems are affecting their behavior. Observe for behaviors such as irritability, disorientation (similar to a drunken state), and slurred speech. If sleep deprivation has lasted a long time, psychotic behavior such as delusions and paranoia develop. For example, a patient reports seeing strange objects or colors in the room or the patient acts afraid when you or other health personnel enter the room suddenly or without warning.

PATIENT EXPECTATIONS After assessing the patient's sleep history, determine the patient's expectations regarding nursing care. Use a caring and skilled approach to assess the patient's sleep needs and preferences. For example, ask, "Now that I understand more about your sleep habits and the recent problems you have had, what is it that you expect from us regarding your care?" or "In order to improve your sleep, what do you feel is most important that we do for you?" The patient sometimes has a different view on the relationship of sleep and health from your own. Examining patient expectations and preferences helps to clarify any misconceptions you have. Ask the patient what interventions he or she prefers and how to implement them. In the hospital setting some patients are more concerned about being sure you are checking their condition routinely than about whether you wake them and disturb sleep.

■■■NURSING DIAGNOSIS

Your assessment will reveal clusters of data that include defining characteristics for a sleep problem or other nursing diagnoses that result from disturbed sleep. If you identify a sleep pattern disturbance, it is helpful for you to specify the exact condition. By determining the nature of a sleep disturbance, you will design more effective interventions. The following is a list of potential nursing diagnoses that you may identify for a patient with a sleep problem:

- *Anxiety*
- *Ineffective breathing pattern*
- *Acute confusion*
- *Ineffective coping*
- *Fatigue*

- *Insomnia*
- *Disturbed sensory perception*
- *Sleep deprivation*
- *Readiness for enhanced sleep*
- *Disturbed sleep pattern*

Your assessment also needs to identify the probable cause or related factor for the sleep disturbance, such as a noisy environment, a high intake of caffeine, or stress involving work. The cause becomes the focus of interventions for minimizing or eliminating the problem. For example, a hospitalized patient who experiences insomnia as a result of a noisy sleeping environment will benefit from a reduction in hospital equipment noise or minimizing interruptions. If the insomnia is related to worry over a threatened marital separation, your interventions involve introducing coping strategies. If you define the probable cause or related factors incorrectly, the patient will not benefit from your care.

■■■PLANNING

GOALS AND OUTCOMES After identifying all relevant nursing diagnoses for a patient (Figure 30-3), you develop a plan of care (see Care Plan). You will develop an individualized care plan only after you understand how the nursing diagnosis relates to your patient's normal and current sleep pattern, your patient's perception of the sleep problem, and the factors disrupting sleep. Together you and the patient develop realistic goals and outcomes. For example, the goal of "Patient establishes a healthy sleep pattern" will include outcomes such as "Patient will fall asleep within a half hour of planned time" and "Patient will have less than two awakenings during the night." This will be realistic if you know from your assessment that it now takes the patient an hour to fall asleep and that awakenings occur three or four times a night. The outcomes will serve as measurable guidelines to determine goal achievement. An effective plan includes outcomes established over a realistic time frame that focus on the goal of improving the quality of sleep. This type of plan requires many weeks to accomplish.

SETTING PRIORITIES Using the data you gathered about the nature of the patient's problem, you need to identify priority strategies and interventions to promote sleep. Together, you and the patient identify and select the strategies and interventions that are most likely to be beneficial in the home or health care setting (see Figure 30-3). The plan of care includes priority strategies that support positive sleep habits and patterns that fit the patient's living environment, cultural orientation, and lifestyle. For example, the patient decides that purchasing a new mattress to increase comfort is the first step toward improving sleep. In a health care setting, you will plan treatments or routines to give the patient more time to rest. For example, you turn and reposition a patient at the same time you give him or her medication or perform a treatment such as suctioning, to limit the number of nurse-patient contacts. All staff caring for the patient need to know the plan so that they will cluster activities at times to reduce awakenings. In a nursing home some plan rest periods around the activities of other residents.

CONCEPT MAP

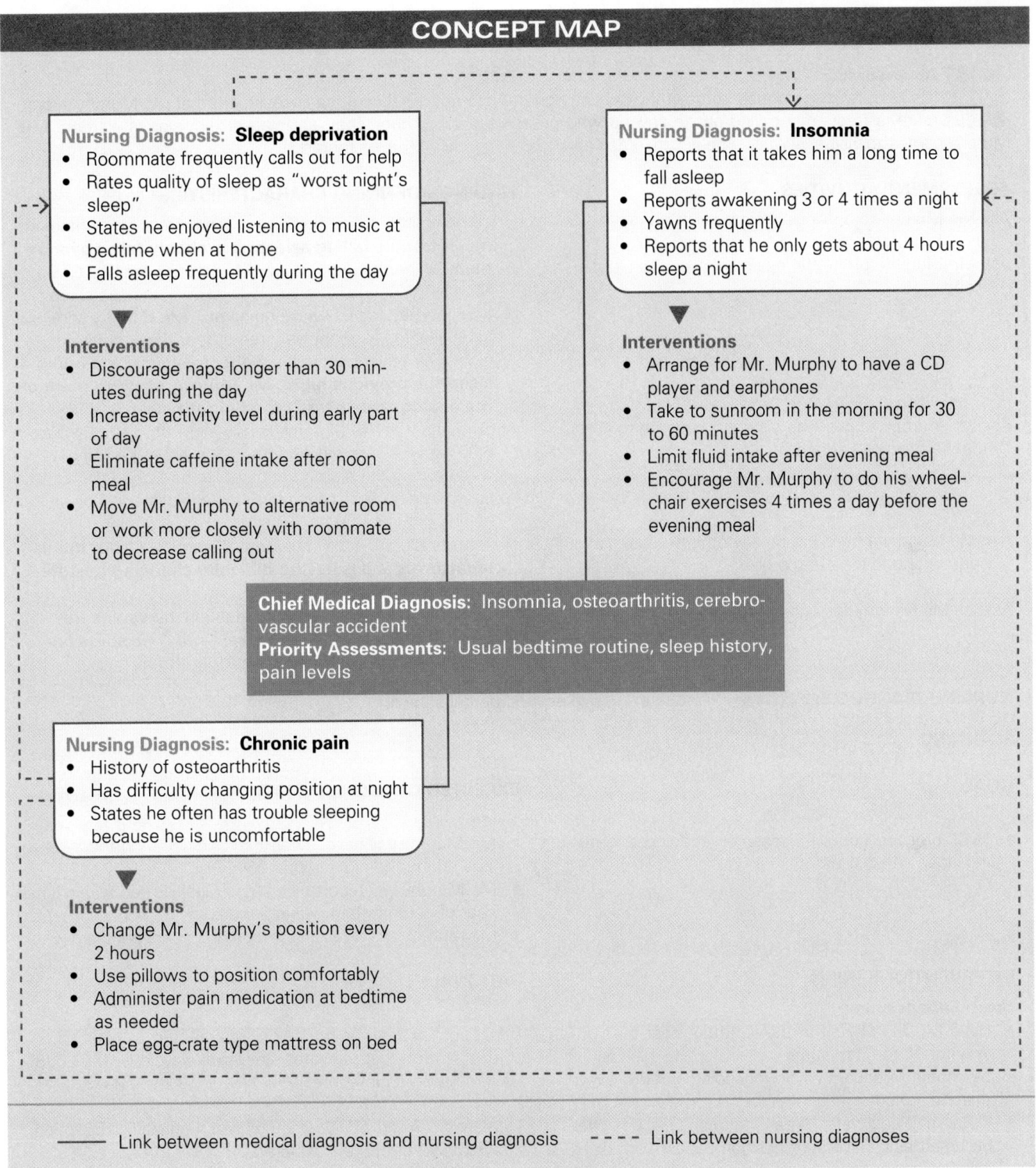

Nursing Diagnosis: Sleep deprivation
- Roommate frequently calls out for help
- Rates quality of sleep as "worst night's sleep"
- States he enjoyed listening to music at bedtime when at home
- Falls asleep frequently during the day

Interventions
- Discourage naps longer than 30 minutes during the day
- Increase activity level during early part of day
- Eliminate caffeine intake after noon meal
- Move Mr. Murphy to alternative room or work more closely with roommate to decrease calling out

Nursing Diagnosis: Insomnia
- Reports that it takes him a long time to fall asleep
- Reports awakening 3 or 4 times a night
- Yawns frequently
- Reports that he only gets about 4 hours sleep a night

Interventions
- Arrange for Mr. Murphy to have a CD player and earphones
- Take to sunroom in the morning for 30 to 60 minutes
- Limit fluid intake after evening meal
- Encourage Mr. Murphy to do his wheelchair exercises 4 times a day before the evening meal

Chief Medical Diagnosis: Insomnia, osteoarthritis, cerebrovascular accident
Priority Assessments: Usual bedtime routine, sleep history, pain levels

Nursing Diagnosis: Chronic pain
- History of osteoarthritis
- Has difficulty changing position at night
- States he often has trouble sleeping because he is uncomfortable

Interventions
- Change Mr. Murphy's position every 2 hours
- Use pillows to position comfortably
- Administer pain medication at bedtime as needed
- Place egg-crate type mattress on bed

——— Link between medical diagnosis and nursing diagnosis   - - - - Link between nursing diagnoses

Figure 30-3 ■ Concept Map.

COLLABORATIVE CARE The nature of a sleep disturbance determines whether referrals to additional health care providers are necessary. For example, if a sleep problem is related to a situational crisis or emotional problem, refer the patient to a psychiatric clinical nurse specialist, pastoral care professional, or clinical psychologist for counseling. This helps to ensure that you attend to the patient's problems not only in the health care setting but in the home as well. Sharing information with a home care nurse on patient discharge is useful in planning interventions to ensure the patient gets adequate sleep when home. When chronic insomnia is the problem, a medical referral or referral to a sleep center is beneficial.

CARE PLAN Insomnia

ASSESSMENT

Mr. Murphy is in a double room at the nursing home. Anna notices during the assessment that Mr. Murphy's roommate is frequently calling out to anyone who passes the room door. The roommate's television is also on. Mrs. Murphy comes to visit every day. She is concerned about how tired Mr. Murphy seems.

ASSESSMENT ACTIVITIES

Ask Mr. Murphy to describe the nature of his sleep problem.
Ask Mr. Murphy to rate the quality of previous night's sleep.

Ask Mr. Murphy to describe his usual bedtime routine that he practiced at home.

Ask Mr. Murphy if he is having any other trouble that is contributing to his sleep problem.

Assess Mr. Murphy for signs of sleep problems.

FINDINGS/DEFINING CHARACTERISTICS*

Since being in the nursing home, he now reports, **"I have so much trouble falling asleep; it probably takes over an hour."** When asked if he awakens during the night, Mr. Murphy responds, "Are you kidding? No one can sleep here; something is always going on." Mr. Murphy admits to awakening as many as three or four times during the night. The patient estimates he received maybe **4 hours of sleep the previous night. Mr. Murphy places a mark on the analog scale near "worst night's sleep."**

Anna learns that Mr. Murphy usually slept from 10:30 PM to 6:00 AM when he was at home, usually awakening once or twice during the night to urinate. He rarely had difficulty falling asleep, but according to his wife, listening to music helped him relax.

He reports that he is having **some discomfort from the osteoarthritis** and is **having difficulty changing positions** and **getting comfortable.**

While Mr. Murphy describes his situation, he **yawns frequently** and states, **"I really feel tired." He shifts his position in his wheelchair multiple times.**

NURSING DIAGNOSIS: Insomnia related to excessive environmental stimuli.

PLANNING

GOAL

- Mr. Murphy will obtain a sense of restfulness following sleep within 1 month.

EXPECTED OUTCOMES (NOC)†

Sleep
- Mr. Murphy will have fewer than two self-reported awakenings during the night within 2 weeks.
- Mr. Murphy will report being able to fall asleep within a half hour of going to bed within 2 weeks.
- Mr. Murphy will sleep an average of 7 hours per night within 4 weeks.

INTERVENTIONS (NIC)‡

Sleep Enhancement
- Have Mr. Murphy sit in the sunroom near the window for 30 to 60 minutes in the morning each day.
- Discourage frequent daytime napping or naps longer than 30 minutes.
- Have an egg-crate type mattress placed over bed mattress. Have staff position patient with extra pillows.
- Encourage Mr. Murphy to decrease his fluids 2 to 4 hours before sleep.

Simple Relaxation Therapy
- Arrange for Mr. Murphy to have a CD player with earphones to play music of his choice when first going to sleep.

RATIONALE

Bright light in the morning helps maintain the 24-hour circadian rhythm that regulates sleep-wake cycle (Joshi, 2008).
Daytime napping interferes with sleeping (Joshi, 2008).

Increases comfort of sleeping position, enhancing relaxation, which will promote a sleep state.

Decreases number of times patient awakens to urinate (Ebersole and others, 2008).

Soothing music blocks out sounds from the environment, promotes relaxation, and decreases the time to sleep onset (LaReau and others, 2008).

*Defining characteristics are shown in **bold** type.
†Outcomes classification labels from Moorhead S and others, editors: *Nursing outcomes classification (NOC)*, ed 4, St. Louis, 2008, Mosby.
‡Interventions classification label from Bulechek GM and others, editors: *Nursing interventions classification (NIC)*, ed 5, St. Louis, 2008, Mosby.

CARE PLAN Insomnia—cont'd

INTERVENTIONS (NIC)‡

Sleep Enhancement
- Arrange for Mr. Murphy to have some of his favorite reading material at his bedside.

Exercise Promotion
- Have Mr. Murphy get regular exercise (e.g., have Mr. Murphy propel down hallways in wheelchair for 5 minutes, 4 times a day before dinner).

RATIONALE

Reading before bedtime is a rest-promoting pre-bedtime activity.

Regular exercise improves sleep quality by slightly increasing the amount of stage 3 and stage 4 sleep (Tucker, 2007).

EVALUATION

NURSING ACTIONS	PATIENT RESPONSE/FINDING	ACHIEVEMENT OF OUTCOME
Ask Mr. Murphy to use a visual analog scale to rate the quality of his sleep at the end of each week.	At the end of the first week Mr. Murphy rates his quality of sleep as 6 out of 10. For the second week, Mr. Murphy rates his sleep at 8 out of 10.	Mr. Murphy is implementing sleep hygiene measures. His sleep is improving, because he rates his sleep as improving.
Ask Mrs. Murphy to evaluate her perceptions of Mr. Murphy's level of fatigue.	Mrs. Murphy states that her husband seems more awake, alert, and talkative when she visits. He does not nod off or nap in the early afternoon as he used to. She is also pleased that he enjoys doing the wheelchair exercises.	The sleep hygiene measures along with the exercises have contributed to improved sleep for Mr. Murphy, resulting in decreased daytime fatigue.
Ask Mr. Murphy at the end of 4 weeks to keep a record for a week of the length of time he estimates sleeping.	Mr. Murphy reports that he falls asleep within 30 minutes and generally wakes up 2 to 3 times a night. He reports that he is sleeping 6 hours a night.	Mr. Murphy's use of relaxation therapy and use of music has improved Mr. Murphy's sleep.

■■■IMPLEMENTATION

Your nursing interventions for improving the quality of a person's sleep will largely focus on health promotion. In an acute care setting, your focus becomes managing the environment in a way that supports the patient's normal sleep habits and keeps the patient safe. When patients enter long-term care or nursing home environments, you will need to make special considerations to promote adequate sleep and rest.

HEALTH PROMOTION Patients need adequate sleep and rest to maintain active and productive lifestyles. Your specific interventions will promote a person's normal sleep and rest pattern.

Environmental Controls All patients require a sleeping environment with a comfortable room temperature and proper ventilation, minimal noise, a comfortable bed, and proper lighting. Infants sleep best when the room temperature is 18° to 21° C (64° to 70° F) and covered with a light, warm blanket. Place healthy infants on their sides or backs when being put to sleep (American Academy of Pediatrics, 2000). The national "Back to Sleep" campaign has been very successful in teaching parents and infant caregivers to place infants on their backs for sleeping to reduce the incidence of sudden infant death syndrome (SIDS) (National Institute of Child Health and Human Development, 2005). Children and adults vary more in regard to comfortable room temperature but usually sleep best in cooler environments. Some prefer to sleep without covers. Older adults sometimes require extra blankets or covers or sleep wearing socks (Box 30-5).

Eliminate or reduce distracting noise so that the bedroom is as quiet as possible. In the home the TV or the ringing of the telephone disrupts a patient's sleep. Family members become important participants in care when each has a different schedule for going to sleep. It often requires the cooperation of several people living with the patient to reduce noise. Some patients sleep better with familiar inside noises, such as the hum of a ceiling fan.

BOX 30-5   CARE OF THE OLDER ADULT
Sleep Disturbances

SLEEP-WAKE PATTERN
- Maintain a regular rising time and bedtime.
- Eliminate naps unless they are a routine part of the schedule.
- If patient takes naps, limit to 20 minutes or less twice a day.
- Go to bed when sleepy.
- Use relaxation techniques and a regular bedtime routine to promote sleep.
- If unable to sleep in 15 to 30 minutes, get out of bed.

ENVIRONMENT
- Expose to natural light for 30 minutes to 2 hours daily, preferably soon after waking.
- Sleep where you sleep best.
- Keep noise to a minimum; use soft music to mask noise if necessary.
- Use night-light and keep path to bathroom free of obstacles.
- Set room temperature to preference; use blankets and socks to promote comfort.

MEDICATIONS
- Use sedatives and hypnotics as last resort and then only short-term use if needed.
- Adjust medications being taken for other conditions, and look for drug interactions that cause insomnia or EDS.

DIET
- Limit alcohol, caffeine, and nicotine in late afternoon and evening.
- Eat a light snack such as cereal and milk or cheese and crackers before bedtime.
- Decrease fluids 2 to 4 hours before sleep.

PHYSIOLOGICAL/ILLNESS FACTORS
- Elevate head of bed, and provide extra pillows as preferred.
- Use analgesics 30 minutes before bed to ease aches and pains.
- Use prescribed medications to control symptoms of chronic conditions.

EDS, Excessive daytime sleepiness.

Make sure the bed and mattress provide support and comfortable firmness. Place a bed board under the mattress to add support. Sometimes extra pillows help a person to position more comfortably in bed. The position of the bed in the room also makes a difference for some patients.

For any patient prone to confusion or falls, safety is critical. In the home a small night-light assists the patient in becoming oriented to the room environment before arising to go to the bathroom. Beds set lower to the floor will reduce the risk for falls when a person stands. Remove clutter from the path a patient uses to walk from the bed to the bathroom. If a patient needs help in ambulating from the bed to the bathroom, have a small bell at the bedside to call family members.

Patients vary in regard to the amount of light that they prefer at night. Infants and older adults sleep best in softly lit rooms. Do not have light shining directly on their eyes. Small table lamps or night-lights prevent total darkness. For older adults this reduces the chance of confusion when arising from bed. If streetlights shine through windows or when patients nap during the day, heavy shades, drapes, or slatted blinds are helpful.

Promoting Bedtime Routines Bedtime routines and sleep hygiene measures relax patients in preparation for sleep. It is important for persons to go to sleep when they feel fatigued or sleepy. To develop good sleep hygiene at home, patients and their bed partners need to learn techniques that promote sleep and conditions that interfere with sleep (Box 30-6).

Newborns and infants benefit from quiet activities such as holding them snugly in blankets, talking or singing softly, and gently rocking. A bedtime routine (e.g., same hour for bedtime or quiet activity) used consistently helps toddlers and preschool children avoid delaying sleep. Parents need to reinforce patterns of preparing for bedtime. Reading stories, allowing children to sit in a parent's lap while listening to music or praying, and coloring are routines associated with preparing for bed.

Adults need to avoid excessive mental stimulation just before bedtime. Reading a light novel, watching a relaxing television program, or listening to music helps a person relax. Relaxation exercises and praying often induce calm in patients (see Chapter 31).

Promoting Comfort People fall asleep only after feeling comfortable and relaxed. You will recommend and use several measures to promote comfort, such as encouraging the patient to wear loose-fitting nightwear and to void before bedtime. Have family members give a relaxing back rub. Minor irritants keep persons awake. Change diapers before placing infants in bed. An extra blanket prevents chilling when trying to fall asleep.

Have patients who suffer painful illnesses try a variety of measures at home to promote comfort. Application of dry or moist heat, use of supportive dressings or splints (see Chapter 36), and proper positioning with the use of extra pillows for support are very helpful. For patients with temporary acute pain (e.g., following surgery), it is sometimes advantageous to the patient and bed partner to let the patient sleep alone until the pain subsides. Also, encourage the patient to take pain medications 30 to 60 minutes before going to bed.

You will help patients with physical illness learn ways to control symptoms that disrupt sleep. For example, a patient

BOX 30-6   PATIENT TEACHING

Improving Sleep

 On one of her visits to the nursing home, Mary Murphy tells Anna, the nursing student, that she is having trouble sleeping and does not feel rested. Anna asks Mrs. Murphy to describe her current sleep habits. Using what she knows about sleep hygiene measures, Anna then develops a teaching plan to help Mrs. Murphy improve her sleeping.

OUTCOME

- At the end of the teaching session, Mrs. Murphy will develop a plan that includes effective sleep hygiene practices.

TEACHING STRATEGIES

- Discuss with Mrs. Murphy the need to practice sleep hygiene habits regularly.
- Caution Mrs. Murphy against delaying bedtime or sleeping long hours during weekends or holidays to maintain her normal sleep-wake cycle.
- Explain to her not to use the bedroom for watching television, snacking, or other nonsleep activity, besides sex.
- Encourage Mrs. Murphy to take a warm bath before bedtime.
- Encourage Mrs. Murphy to walk for 30 minutes every morning.
- Instruct Mrs. Murphy to play soft relaxing music at bedtime to help her fall asleep.
- Demonstrate relaxation techniques to Mrs. Murphy.
- Advise Mrs. Murphy that if she does not fall asleep within 20 minutes, she needs to get out of bed and do some quiet activity until feeling sleepy enough to go back to bed.
- Instruct Mrs. Murphy to avoid heavy meals for 3 hours before bedtime; a light snack including protein and carbohydrates helps.
- Answer questions that Mrs. Murphy has about sleep problems.

EVALUATION STRATEGIES

- Ask Mrs. Murphy to describe three sleep hygiene habits.
- Have Mrs. Murphy demonstrate a relaxation technique to use to promote sleep.
- Ask Mrs. Murphy to identify an appropriate bedtime snack.
- Ask Mrs. Murphy to identify soothing music to use at bedtime to help her relax.

with respiratory abnormalities needs to sleep with two pillows or in a semisitting position to ease the effort to breathe. The patient will often benefit from taking prescribed bronchodilators before sleep to prevent airway obstruction.

Promoting Activity In the home encourage patients to stay physically active during the day so that they are more likely to sleep at night. Increasing daytime activity lessens problems with falling asleep. Always plan rigorous exercise at least 2 to 3 hours before bedtime.

Research indicates that exercise is beneficial, particularly for older adults, to improve nighttime sleep. General recommendations often suggest increasing daytime activity or exercise (Tucker, 2007). However, older adults with chronic diseases that influence their functional abilities are likely to have limited activity (Ebersole and others, 2008). Recommend activities that are safe for older patients to perform. Walking, swimming, wheelchair propulsion, and cycling on a stationary bike are excellent for patients with limited physical impairment. Weight lifting using light weights (e. g., 2 to 5 lb) is also excellent to build upper body strength and endurance. Activity and exercise often prove to be beneficial by improving activity endurance, mobility, and sense of well-being.

Stress Reduction When patients feel emotionally upset, urge them to try not to force sleep. Otherwise, insomnia often develops, and soon they will associate bedtime with the inability to relax. Encourage a patient who has difficulty falling asleep to get up and pursue a relaxing activity rather than staying in bed and thinking about sleep. When the emotional problem is ongoing and the patient finds little relief, encourage referral to an appropriate counselor.

Children often have problems going to bed and falling asleep. After nightmares, have parents enter children's rooms immediately and talk to them briefly about their fears to provide a cooling-down period. Comforting children while they lie in their own bed is reassuring. Keeping a light on in the room also helps. Usually experts do not recommend that a child be allowed to sleep with parents; however, cultural traditions cause families to approach sleep practices differently. For example, Hispanic and Asian families often practice co-sleeping, in which parents allow children to sleep with them or siblings to lessen the child's anxiety and promote a sense of security (Box 30-7).

Bedtime Snacks Some persons enjoy bedtime snacks, whereas others cannot sleep after eating. A bedtime snack containing protein and carbohydrates, such as cereal and milk or cheese and crackers, which contain L-tryptophan, helps to promote sleep (National Sleep Foundation, 2007). A full meal before bedtime often causes gastrointestinal upset and interferes with the ability to fall asleep.

Make sure patients avoid drinking excess fluids or ingesting caffeine before bedtime. Coffee, tea, cola, and chocolate will cause a person to stay awake or awaken throughout the night. Alcohol interrupts sleep cycles and reduces the amount of deep sleep. Coffee, tea, colas, and alcohol act as diuretics, which cause **nocturia.**

Pharmacological Approaches to Promoting Sleep Many of the drugs patients take to manage their illnesses can cause insomnia. Make sure patients use CNS stimulants such as amphetamines, nicotine, terbutaline, theophylline, and pemoline sparingly and under medical management (McKenry, Tessier, and Hogan, 2006). Withdrawal from CNS depressants such as alcohol, barbiturates, and tricyclic antidepressants also causes insomnia and must be managed carefully.

BOX 30-7 CULTURAL FOCUS

Co-sleeping with children is a culturally preferred habit. Co-sleeping is more common in nonindustrialized countries. This practice is also common in the United States with Asian American and African American families. Health care personnel in the United States discourage this practice because of safety issues even though research does not show that the practice is unsafe. American culture promotes independence in childhood. Co-sleeping does not promote this independence, and thus health care workers discourage it. As a nurse you need to be culturally sensitive when discussing co-sleeping practices with parents and developing sleeping plans for children.

IMPLICATIONS FOR PRACTICE

- Complete a thorough sleep assessment of the child and family.
- Discuss the risks of co-sleeping with parents. During the discussion remain culturally sensitive and respectful of the parents' views.
- Co-sleeping affects the infant's normal sleep pattern by decreasing slow wave sleep and increasing the number of nighttime arousals.
- Co-sleeping has been linked to increased risk for sudden infant death syndrome (SIDS) under certain conditions such as parental smoking, alcohol or drug use.
- Instruct parents to avoid using alcohol or drugs that impair arousal. Decreased arousal prevents the parents from awakening if the child is having problems.
- Co-sleeping should only occur with parents and child and not another adult or child.
- Avoid soft bedding surfaces. Infants and children will become entangled or have their head covered if the bed contains loose coverings, pillows, or stuffed toys.
- Encourage the parents to use light sleeping clothes, keep the room temperature comfortable, and to not bundle the child tightly or in too many clothes.

Modified from Davis KF, Parker KP, Montgomery GL: Sleep in infants and young children. I. Normal sleep, *J Pediatr Health Care* 18(2):65, 2004.

Sleep medications help a patient if used correctly. **Sedatives** and **hypnotics** are groups of drugs that induce and/or maintain sleep. However, long-term use of these drugs disrupts sleep and leads to more serious problems. Benzodiazepines and nonbenzodiazepines are common classifications of drugs used to treat sleep problems. The nonbenzodiazepines have become the treatment of choice for insomnia because of improved effect and safety of use (Calamaro, 2008). Experts recommend a low dose of a short-acting medication such as zolpidem (Ambien) for short-term use (no longer than 2 to 3 weeks) (Cranwell-Bruce, 2007).

Short-acting benzodiazepines (e.g., oxazepam, lorazepam, or temazepam) at the lowest possible dose are recommended. Initial doses should be small, and increments are added gradually, based on patient response, for a limited time. The use of benzodiazepines in the older adult population is potentially dangerous because of the drugs' tendency to remain active in the body for a longer time. As a result of this tendency, the drugs also cause next-day sedation, amnesia, and rebound insomnia (Cranwell-Bruce, 2007).

Melatonin is a hormone produced in the brain that helps control circadian rhythms. It is a popular nutritional supplement in the United States used to aid sleep. Melatonin is usually sold in 3-mg tablets, but the body produces less than 0.5 mg. It has been found to be helpful in improving sleep efficiency and decrease nighttime awakenings (Pandi-Perumal and others, 2007). Ramelteon (Rozerem), a melatonin receptor agonist, is well tolerated and has been shown to be effective in improving sleep (Morin, Jarvis, and Lynch, 2007).

The use of nonprescription sleeping medications is not advisable. Over the long term, these drugs lead to further sleep disruption even when they initially seem effective. Caution older adults about using over-the-counter antihistamines because of their long duration of action that causes confusion, constipation, and urinary retention (Passarella and Duong, 2008). Help patients with interventions that do not require the use of drugs.

Regular use of any sleep medication leads to tolerance, and withdrawal causes rebound insomnia. Make sure all patients understand the possible side effects of sleep medications. In 2007 the Food and Drug Administration released a warning related to complex sleep-related behaviors, such as sleep driving or sleep eating, that have occurred with prescription sleep medications (U.S. Food and Drug Administration, 2007). Routine monitoring of patient response to sleeping medications is important.

Managing Specific Sleep Disturbances Patients who suffer specific sleep disturbances will likely benefit from the health promotion strategies discussed so far. Weight loss can be effective for the patient with obstructive sleep apnea. It is important for the patient to follow an appropriate weight reduction plan (see Chapter 32). In milder cases of obstructive sleep apnea, body position during sleep is effective. One suggestion is to elevate the head of the bed (Ebersole and others, 2008).

ACUTE CARE The nursing interventions described for health promotion are applicable to a patient requiring acute care. The nature of the acute care setting requires you to be creative in finding ways to maintain the patient's normal sleep pattern (Box 30-8).

Managing Environmental Stimuli A challenge in the hospital is controlling noise. Because many patients spend only a short time in hospitals, it is easy to forget the importance of establishing good sleep conditions.

In the hospital setting, plan nursing care activities to avoid awakening patients. Try to schedule assessments, treatments, procedures, and routines for times when patients are awake. Perform nursing activities before the patient receives sleeping medication or begins to fall asleep. For example, you have a patient who has had surgery. Before the patient gets ready for bed, change the surgical dressing, reposition the patient, administer pain medication, and check vital signs. Give medica-

BOX 30-8 BEST PRACTICES

SUMMARY OF EVIDENCE

Evidence suggests that using a combination of nonpharmacological measures is an effective way to manage sleep problems at home or in the hospital. Outcomes found to be associated with use of nonpharmacological sleep interventions include improvement in sleep quality, decreased awakenings, and decreased number of sleep medications used. Sleep hygiene measures and relaxation techniques are common behavioral strategies used to effectively manage insomnia in the home or health care setting. Environmental control measures such as reducing noise, keeping the room cool, and decreasing light levels are interventions that are helpful in promoting sleep particularly in a health care setting. It is also important to provide patients with adequate uninterrupted periods of sleep.

APPLICATION TO NURSING PRACTICE

- Teach patients effective sleep hygiene measures.
- Implement patients' sleep preferences and sleep hygiene practices in the health care setting when possible.
- Keep patient doors closed at night to minimize noise.
- Cluster patient care activities to provide uninterrupted periods of sleep.
- Post a sign on the patient door informing caregivers of patient's uninterrupted sleep periods.
- Discuss perception of sleep and sleep quality with patients in hospital.

REFERENCES

Carter PA: A brief behavioral sleep intervention for family caregivers of persons with cancer, *Cancer Nurs* 29(2):95, 2006.

Irwin MR, Cole JC, Nicassio PM: Comparative meta-analysis of behavioral interventions for insomnia and their efficacy in middle-aged adults and in older adults 55+ years of age, *Health Psychol* 25(1):3, 2006.

Friese RS: Sleep and recovery from critical illness and injury: a review of theory, current practice, and future directions, *Crit Care Med* 36(3):697, 2008.

LaReau R and others: Examining the feasibility of implementing specific nursing interventions to promote sleep in hospitalized elderly patients, *Geriatr Nurs* 29(3):197, 2008.

tions and draw blood during waking hours when possible. Plan with other departments and services to schedule therapies at intervals that give patients time to rest. Whenever it becomes necessary to awaken a patient, do it as quickly as possible so that the patient can fall back to sleep as soon as possible.

Safety Safety precautions are important for patients who awaken during the night to use the bathroom and for those with excessive daytime sleepiness. Set beds lower to the floor to lessen the chance of the patient falling when first standing. Remove clutter, and move equipment from the path a patient uses to walk from the bed to the bathroom. If a patient needs assistance in ambulating from the bed to the bathroom, make sure the call light is within the patient's reach. Be sure the patient knows how to turn the light on correctly.

If patients normally use a CPAP machine at home because of sleep apnea, it is important that they bring their home equipment with them to the hospital and use it every night. This is even more important for patients with sleep apnea who have surgery and receive general anesthesia. In these patients the anesthesia in combination with pain medications used after surgery reduces the patient's defenses against airway obstruction. After surgery the patient achieves very deep levels of REM sleep that lead to muscle relaxation and airway obstruction (Hwang and others, 2008). These patients need ventilatory support in the postoperative period because OSA is linked to increased postoperative respiratory complications. Make sure that the patients use their home CPAP equipment. Use pain medication carefully in these patients. Monitor the patient's breathing and oxygen levels regularly. Notify the health care provider right away if the patient is difficult to arouse or is having trouble breathing.

Patients who experience daytime sleepiness can fall asleep while sitting up in a chair or wheelchair. Position patients so that they will not fall out of the chair when sleeping. Elevating the patient's feet on an ottoman or small bench may assist in positioning the patient safely. A pillow placed in the patient's lap offers some support. If a patient enjoys leaning over an over-bed table while sitting in a chair, be sure the table is locked and secure. Avoid using safety belts because they are considered restraints (see Chapter 27).

Comfort Measures You will make the patient more comfortable in an acute care setting by providing personal hygiene before bedtime. A warm bath or shower is very relaxing. Offer patients restricted to bed the opportunity to wash their face and hands. Toothbrushing and care of dentures also help to prepare the patient for sleep. Have patients void before going to bed so they are not kept awake by a full bladder. While a patient prepares for bed, help to position the patient off any potential pressure sites. Offering a back rub or massage helps relax the patient.

Removal of irritating stimuli is another way to improve the patient's comfort for a restful sleep. Changing or removing moist dressings, repositioning drainage tubing, reapplying wrinkled thromboembolic hose, and changing tape on nasogastric tubes eliminate constant irritants to the patient's skin. When an intravenous (IV) site becomes irritated and painful, reinsertion of the IV is usually recommended (see Chapter 17). Cleanse the perineal or anal area thoroughly for patients who are incontinent. Diaphoretic patients will benefit from a cool bath and dry clothes or linens.

RESTORATIVE AND CONTINUING CARE The quality of sleep in a long-term care or nursing home environment is often fragmented. Residents of a nursing home often suffer chronic disease, incontinence, and dementia and take multiple medications, all of which can disrupt sleep. Noise, light, and repositioning of nursing home residents during linen changes are factors that cause patients to awaken. Besides care activities, nursing home residents themselves are very disruptive when they call out loudly to roommates or nursing staff.

In the long-term care environment many patients require rehabilitation or supportive care. The nature of their illnesses and treatment requirements disrupt sleep. For example, patients who are ventilator dependent will likely get brief periods of sleep throughout the day rather than prolonged sleep because of disruptions from ventilator alarm sounds and the need for occasional suctioning.

Maintaining Activity In the restorative care setting try to limit the time patients spend in bed. In the nursing home serve meals in the resident dining area. Otherwise patients should be up in a chair for meals and for personal hygiene activities. It is also important to keep the residents involved in social activities planned at the nursing home (e.g., card playing or arts and crafts). Regular exercise keeps the patients active and stimulated. It is also ideal to limit daytime napping to 30 minutes or less. Short naps taken in the midafternoon have been found to increase alertness and cognitive ability (Tucker, 2007).

Patients with dementia often have disrupted sleep-wake cycles. They often become easily fatigued and experience periods of insomnia (Ebersole and others, 2008). In this situation activities and visits need to be shortened to allow the patient to maintain an adequate energy level. If the patient awakens during the night, keeping the lights at a low level and using soothing techniques such as quiet music or a back rub will promote sleep.

Reducing Sleep Disruption Knowing the many factors that disrupt sleep in restorative care settings, you will find ways to make the environment more favorable to sleep. Noise control is critical. Often staff within a nursing home naturally speak louder because of residents' difficulties with hearing. Walking up close to a patient and talking in a normal but clear voice will likely improve the patient's hearing and reduce the chance of awakening a nearby roommate. Teach nursing assistive personnel to be more sensitive to the sources of noise that disrupt patients' sleep.

■■■ EVALUATION

PATIENT CARE You need to individualize evaluation of therapies designed to promote sleep and rest (Box 30-9). Patients in relatively good health often do not need as much sleep as patients whose physical condition is poor.

If you have established realistic goals of care, the expected outcomes become guidelines for evaluating the patient's progress and response to interventions. Use evaluative measures shortly after trying a therapy. Use other evaluative measures after a patient awakens from sleep (e.g., asking a patient to describe the number of awakenings during the night). Together the patient and bed partner can usually provide accurate information. If the patient lives or sleeps alone, the evaluation may be unreliable.

When the patient does not meet expected outcomes, revise the nursing measures based on the patient's needs or preferences. Document the patient's response to sleep therapies to maintain a continuum of care.

PATIENT EXPECTATIONS Review progress in the plan of care with your patient, and determine if your patient's expectations were met. Does the patient believe your interventions were helpful and useful? Did you incorporate the patient's typical sleep routine into the plan of care? For the hospitalized patient, did staff avoid unnecessary interruptions, giving the patient a chance to rest? The patient's perceptions are valuable sources of information regarding the overall success in improving the quality of the patient's sleep.

BOX 30-9   EVALUATION

After 4 weeks at the nursing home, Anna has been able to have Mr. Murphy transferred to a new room and has been monitoring his progress. He has been in the new room for 2 weeks. Anna asks Mr. Murphy, "Tell me how our plan to improve your sleep has been working. Have the music and headphones been helpful?" Mr. Murphy replies, "Well, it has helped to be down here at the end of the hall. It still is a bit noisy, especially if the nurses are working with people across the way. I have used the headphones the last 2 weeks, and they have helped me relax and fall asleep in about 20 or 30 minutes." Anna questions Mr. Murphy further and learns that he is awakening two or three times during the night. However, during the last week he estimated getting about 6 hours of sleep, an improvement from a month ago. Mr. Murphy also reports that the staff has usually been good about reminding him to do his daily exercises with the wheelchair. He dislikes staying in his room and has tried to exercise as much as possible.

Anna wants to know Mr. Murphy's level of satisfaction with her care. She asks, "Have I met your expectations so far? If not, tell me how I can better help you." Mr. Murphy replies, "You've been great. I know you can't make this place like home. There is so much to think about when you are here. I think about my wife a lot." Anna responds, "Tell me more. What do you mean, 'There is so much to think about'?" Anna recognizes that psychological and physical stressors alter sleep. She decides to reassess Mr. Murphy to determine if additional nursing interventions will be appropriate.

DOCUMENTATION NOTE
"Reports some improvement in overall sleep quality. Able to fall asleep within 20 to 30 minutes using headphones with music. Reports sleeping approximately 6 hours per night. Continues to experience awakenings, resulting from noise in outside hallway. Recommend closing room door at night to reduce noise further. Admits to thinking about his wife and other concerns. Will explore further with him."

KEY POINTS

- Researchers think that sleep provides physiological and psychological restoration.
- The 24-hour sleep-wake cycle is a circadian rhythm that affects physiological function and behavior.
- The control and regulation of sleep depends on a balance between CNS regulators.
- During a typical night's sleep a person fluctuates between NREM stages 2, 3, and 4 before entering REM sleep. The amount of time in each stage varies.
- The number of hours of sleep needed by each person to feel rested varies.
- Long-term use of sleeping pills leads to difficulty in initiating and maintaining sleep.
- The hectic pace of a person's lifestyle, emotional and psychological stress, and drug and alcohol ingestion disrupt the sleep pattern.
- An environment with a darkened room, reduced noise, comfortable bed, appropriate temperature, and good ventilation promotes sleep.

- The most common type of sleep disorder is insomnia. Characteristics of insomnia include the inability to fall asleep, to remain asleep during the night, or to go back to sleep after awakening earlier than desired.
- Use your patient's self-report to determine if sleep is restful.
- When using environmental controls to promote sleep, consider the usual characteristics of the patient's home environment and normal lifestyle.
- Noise can disrupt sleep and enhance pain perception.
- A bedtime routine of relaxing activities prepares a person physically and mentally for sleep.
- Pain or other symptom control is essential to promoting the ability to sleep.
- One of the most important nursing interventions for promoting sleep is establishing periods for uninterrupted sleep.

CRITICAL THINKING EXERCISES

On one of her visits, Mrs. Murphy tells Anna that her friends tell her she should start taking a sleeping pill at night. It will help her sleep better so as to be rested and able to help her husband during the day. Mrs. Murphy tells Anna that she is not sure about this and asks Anna about alternatives to sleeping pills.

1. How should Anna respond to Mrs. Murphy?
2. What recommendations can Anna make to Mrs. Murphy to improve her sleep?

Anna is required as part of her course requirements to present a health promotion program to the staff. She decides that she wants to do a health promotion program on sleep. She reviews the literature before the presentation.

3. What information should Anna include in the health promotion program?

During the program Donna, one of the staff, tells Anna that she is concerned about her 15-year-old daughter. Her grades in school are getting worse, and she says she is always tired.

4. What does Anna need to know about the daughter's sleep patterns?
5. List at least three suggestions for Donna, the staff nurse, to use to improve her daughter's sleep patterns.

ⓔvolve   *Answers to Critical Thinking Questions can be found on the Evolve website.*

REVIEW QUESTIONS

1. Which statement made by a patient during a preoperative assessment indicates an increased risk for respiratory complications following surgery?
   1. "I had two stents placed in my coronary arteries 6 months ago."
   2. "My dosage of morning insulin has decreased since I started exercising regularly."
   3. "I take a mild diuretic for my hypertension."
   4. "I brought my CPAP mask and machine to the hospital with me."
2. Which disease in the patient's history most likely contributes to the patient's concern about her early-morning awakenings?
   1. Hypertension
   2. Emphysema
   3. Gastric reflux
   4. Hyperthyroidism

3. When developing a plan of care for a patient newly admitted to a long-term care facility, which intervention will help promote sleep?
   1. Encourage the patient to continue to follow regular bedtime routines.
   2. Coordinate laboratory blood draws to be completed at 5:00 AM.
   3. Give the patient his or her prescribed sleeping medication by 11:00 PM.
   4. Turn the television on low during late-night programming.
4. Which is an appropriate nursing goal for a nursing care plan for a patient who has difficulty falling asleep? The patient will:
   1. Sleep for 7 hours each night
   2. Limit napping during the day to three or four naps
   3. Decrease awakenings to two or three a night
   4. Fall asleep within 20 minutes of getting in bed

5. A 68-year-old female patient tells you that she is having problems sleeping and does not feel rested in the morning. What is the **first** action you will take with the patient?
   1. Instruct her to start keeping a sleep diary.
   2. Ask her to describe a recent typical night's sleep.
   3. Discuss her sleep patterns with her husband.
   4. Talk to her about increasing her daytime activity.

6. Which snack selection by the patient is the best choice as a bedtime snack?
   1. Chocolate brownie and cup of tea
   2. Corn chips with salsa and diet cola
   3. Cheese and crackers with a glass of wine
   4. Bowl of oatmeal and glass of milk

7. Which interventions should be included in a care plan for an older patient who is having difficulty sleeping? Select all that apply.
   1. Encourage the patient to decrease fluids 2 to 4 hours before going to bed.
   2. Teach the patient relaxation techniques to use at night.
   3. Have the patient exercise in the evening to increase fatigue.
   4. Allow the patient to sleep as late as possible.
   5. Encourage the patient to nap during the day to make up lost sleep.
   6. Have the patient limit caffeine intake to early in the day.

8. A mother tells the nurse that her 4-year-old is having sleep problems. When you are gathering assessment data related to this problem, an important issue to question the mother about is:
   1. The age of other siblings in the home
   2. Usual bedtime practices for the child
   3. Growth and development patterns for the child
   4. The type of preschool the child attends during the day

9. A patient in the community clinic was just diagnosed with narcolepsy. Which statement made by the patient indicates an understanding of the disease?
   1. "Stress will increase the risk for having a sudden muscle weakness during periods of sleep."
   2. "I will stop breathing for a very short period while I am sleeping."
   3. "I can expect to wake up frequently during the night and have problems falling back asleep."
   4. "I understand now why I fall asleep at inappropriate times during the day."

10. Which sleep hygiene practice best promotes sleep in young children?
    1. Make sure the room is dark and quiet.
    2. Encourage reading a story just before bedtime.
    3. Increase the child's evening activities to promote fatigue.
    4. Allow the child to fall asleep in parents' bed.

Answers to Review Questions can be found on pages 1197-1198.

REFERENCES

Allison SE: Self-care requirements for activity and rest: an Orem nursing focus, *Nurs Sci Q* 20(1):68, 2007.

American Academy of Pediatrics: Changing concepts of sudden infant death syndrome: implications for infant sleeping environment and sleep position, *Pediatrics* 105:650, 2000.

American Nurses Association: *Nursing: scope and standards of practice*, Washington, DC, 2004, The Association.

American Sleep Disorders Association, Diagnostic Classification Steering Committee: International classification of sleep disorders. Cited in Thorpy M: Classification of sleep disorders. In Kryger M and others, editors: *Principles and practice of sleep medicine*, ed 4, Philadelphia, 2005, Elsevier Saunders.

Benca RM, Schenck CH: Sleep and eating disorders. In Kryger M and others, editors: *Principles and practice of sleep medicine*, ed 4, Philadelphia, 2005, Elsevier Saunders.

Bulechek GM and others, editors: *Nursing interventions classification (NIC)*, ed 5, St. Louis, 2008, Mosby.

Bussye DJ: Diagnosis and assessment of sleep and circadian rhythm disorders, *J Psychiatr Pract* 11(2):102, 2005.

Calamaro C: Sleeping through the night: are extended release formulations the answer? *J Am Acad Nurse Pract* 20:69, 2008.

Carter PA: A brief behavioral sleep intervention for family caregivers of persons with cancer, *Cancer Nurs* 29(2):95, 2006.

Chasens ER and others: Excessive sleepiness. In Capezuti E and others, editors: *Evidence-based geriatric nursing protocols for best practice*, ed 3, New York, 2008, Springer Publishing Co.

Cmiel CA and others: Noise control: a nursing team's approach to sleep promotion, *Am J Nurs* 104(2):40, 2004.

Cranwell-Bruce LA: Hypnotic sedative drugs, *Medsurg Nurs* 16(3):198, 2007.

Cuellar NG and others: Assessment and treatment of sleep disorders in the older adult, *Geriatr Nurs* 28(4):254, 2007.

Cullen DJ: Obstructive sleep apnea and postoperative analgesia: a potentially dangerous combination, *J Clin Anesth* 13:83, 2001.

Davis KF, Parker KP, Montgomery GL: Sleep in infants and young children. I. Normal sleep, *J Pediatr Health Care* 18(2):65, 2004.

Ebersole P and others: *Toward healthy aging: human needs and nursing response*, ed 7, St. Louis, 2008, Mosby.

Edinger JD, Means MK: Overview of insomnia: definitions, epidemiology, differential diagnosis, and assessment. In Kryger MH and others: *Principles and practice of sleep medicine*, ed 4, Philadelphia, 2005, Elsevier Saunders.

Friese RS: Sleep and recovery from critical illness and injury: a review of theory, current practice, and future directions, *Crit Care Med* 36(3):697, 2008.

Gilman DK and others: Primary headache and sleep disturbances in adolescents, *Headache* 47:1189, 2007.

Hockenberry MJ, Wilson D: *Wong's nursing care of infants and children*, ed 8, St. Louis, 2007, Mosby.

Hwang D and others: Association of sleep–disordered breathing with post-operative complications, *Chest* 133(5):1128, 2008.

Institute of Medicine: *Sleep disorders and sleep deprivation: an unmet public health problem*, Washington, DC, 2006, National Academies Press.

Irwin MR, Cole JC, Nicassio PM: Comparative meta-analysis of behavioral interventions for insomnia and their efficacy in middle-aged adults and in older adults 55+ years of age, *Health Psychol* 25(1):3, 2006.

Izaac SM: Basic anatomy and physiology of sleep, *Am J Electroneurodiagnostic Technol* 46:18, 2006.

Jones B: Basic mechanisms of sleep-wake states. In Kryger M and others, editors: *Principles and practice of sleep medicine*, ed 4, Philadelphia, 2005, Elsevier Saunders.

Joshi S: Nonpharmacologic therapy for insomnia in the elderly, *Clin Geriatr Med* 24:107, 2008.

Kryger M and others: Bridging the gap between science and clinical practice, *Geriatrics* 59(1):24, 2004.

LaReau R and others: Examining the feasibility of implementing specific nursing interventions to promote sleep in hospitalized elderly patients, *Geriatr Nurs* 29(3):197, 2008.

Lashley F: Measuring sleep. In Frank-Stromborg M, Olsen SJ, editors: *Instruments for clinical health-care research*, ed 3, Boston, 2004, Jones & Bartlett.

Lewis SM and others: *Medical-surgical nursing: assessment and management of clinical problems*, ed 7, St. Louis, 2007, Mosby.

Malow BA: Approach to the patient with disordered sleep. In Kryger M and others, editors: *Principles and practice of sleep medicine*, ed 4, Philadelphia, 2005, Elsevier Saunders.

McCance K, Huether S: *Pathophysiology: the biologic basis for disease in adults and children*, ed 5, St. Louis, 2006, Mosby.

McKenry LM, Tessier E, Hogan MA: *Mosby's pharmacology in nursing*, ed 22, St. Louis, 2006, Mosby.

Mendez JL, Olson EF: Obstructive sleep apnea syndrome. I. Identifying the problem, *J Respir Dis* 27(4):144, 2006.

Moorhead S and others, editors: *Nursing outcomes classification (NOC)*, ed 4, St. Louis, 2008, Mosby.

Morin AD, Jarvis CI, Lynch AM: Therapeutic options for sleep-maintenance and sleep-onset insomnias, *Pharmacotherapy* 27(1): 110, 2007.

National Guideline Clearing House: *EFNS guidelines on management of narcolepsy*, 2008, http://www.guideline.gov.

National Institute of Child Health and Human Development: *SIDS: "Back to Sleep" campaign*, 2005, http://www.nichd.nih.gov/sids/sids.cfm, accessed July 6, 2008.

National Sleep Foundation: *Sleep-wake cycle: its physiology and impact on health*, 2006, http://www.sleepfoundation.org/atf/cf/%7BF6BF2668-A1B4-4FE8-8D1A-A5D39340D9CB%7D/Sleep-Wake_Cycle.pdf.

National Sleep Foundation: Ingredients for slumber: how food and beverages may affect your sleep, *Sleep Matters*, winter 2007, http://www.sleepfoundation.org/site/c.huIXKjM0IxF/b.2453615/apps/nl/content3.asp?content_id={32BB1322-7AE9-425A-B9D9-5B43BF2FF9C9}&notoc=1.

National Sleep Foundation: *Sleep in teens*, 2008a, http://www.sleepfoundation.org/site/c.huIXKjM0IxF/b.2419127/k.9C6C/Sleep_and_Teens.htm.

National Sleep Foundation: *2008 Sleep in America poll*, 2008b, http://www.sleepfoundation.org/site/c.huIXKjM0IxF/b.3934129/k.31D9/Poll_Stats.htm.

New survey uncovers how insomnia affects job performance and safety: first study to show effects of insomnia on errors related to medication dispensing and charting practices, *Kans Nurse* 83(1):14, 2008.

Pandi-Perumal SR and others: Role of melatonin system in the control of sleep, *CNS Drugs 2007* 21(12): 995, 2007.

Passarella S, Duong M: Diagnosis and treatment of insomnia, *Am J Health Syst Pharm* 65:927, 2008.

Ramakrishnan K, Scheid DC: Treatment options for insomnia, *Am Fam Physician* 76(4):517, 2007.

Schwab RJ and others: Anatomy and physiology of upper airway obstruction. In Kryger MH and others: *Principles and practice of sleep medicine,* ed 4, Philadelphia, 2005, Elsevier Saunders.

Stickgold R: Why we dream. In Kryger M and others, editors: *Principles and practice of sleep medicine*, ed 4, Philadelphia, 2005, Saunders.

Thorpy M: Classification of sleep disorders. In Kryger M and others, editors: *Principles and practice of sleep medicine*, ed 4, Philadelphia, 2005, Saunders.

Tranmer JE and others: The sleep experience of medical and surgical patients, *Clin Nurs Res* 12(2):159, 2003.

Tucker AP: Sleep hygiene, *AARC Times* 31(8):12, 2007.

U.S. Food and Drug Administration: FDA requests label change for all sleep disorder drug products, 2007, http://www.fda.gov/bbs/topics/NEWS/2007/NEW01587.htm.

Walsh JK and others: Sleep medicine, public policy, and public health. In Kryger MH and others: *Principles and practice of sleep medicine*, ed 4, Philadelphia, 2005, Saunders.

Pain Management

 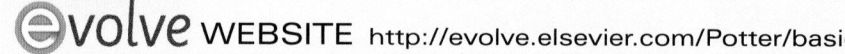
OBJECTIVES

- Discuss common misconceptions about pain.
- Describe the physiology of pain.
- Identify components of the pain experience.
- Explain how the gate control theory relates to the selection of nursing therapies for pain relief.
- Assess a patient experiencing pain.
- Develop appropriate nursing diagnoses for a patient in pain.
- Describe guidelines for selecting and individualizing pain therapies.
- Describe applications for use of nonpharmacological pain therapies.

- Discuss nursing implications for administering analgesics.
- Differentiate the nursing implications associated with managing cancer pain versus noncancer pain.
- Describe interventions for the relief of acute pain following operative or medical procedures.
- Describe the sequence of treatments recommended in pain management for cancer patients.
- Evaluate a patient's response to pain therapies.

KEY TERMS

analgesics, p. 892
cutaneous stimulation, p. 890
endorphins, p. 874
epidural infusion, p. 896
exacerbations, p. 876
guided imagery, p. 890
local anesthesia, p. 895

neurotransmitters, p. 874
nociceptors, p. 873
opioid, p. 892
pain, p. 873
patient-controlled analgesia (PCA), p. 879

perception, p. 874
placebos, p. 895
prostaglandins, p. 892
reaction, p. 880
reception, p. 874
relaxation, p. 890
remissions, p. 876

synapse, p. 874
threshold, p. 874
tolerance, p. 878
transcutaneous electrical nerve stimulation (TENS), p. 890

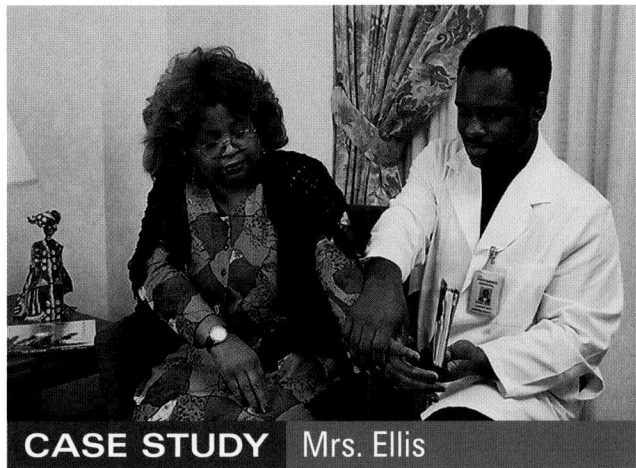

CASE STUDY Mrs. Ellis

Mrs. Ellis is a 70-year-old African American woman with hypertension, diabetes, and rheumatoid arthritis. She is receiving home visits following a recent hospitalization for the control of her diabetes. Her current health priority is the discomfort and disability associated with her rheumatoid arthritis. Arthritis has severely deformed her hands and feet. The pain in her feet is so severe that Mrs. Ellis often walks only short distances. The pain interferes with sleep and reduces her energy both physically and emotionally; as a result, she does not leave her home often. She has lived alone since her husband's death 6 years ago.

Jim is a 26-year-old nursing student assigned to do home visits with the community health nurse. Jim conducts assessments, performs procedures, and teaches health promotion to a variety of patients with various illnesses. This is Jim's first experience caring for a patient with severe chronic pain.

SCIENTIFIC KNOWLEDGE BASE

Comfort

Providing comfort is a concept central to the art of nursing. All patients bring physiological, sociocultural, spiritual, psychological, and environmental characteristics that influence how they interpret and experience comfort. An understanding of comfort gives you, as a nurse, a larger range of choices when selecting pain therapies. Pain management is more than administering analgesics. First you need to understand how the pain experience affects a patient's ability to function and then use therapies that meet the unique needs of patients (Pasero and McCaffery, 2004).

Nature of Pain

Pain is more than a single physiological sensation caused by a specific stimulus. It is subjective and highly individualized. The person having pain is the only authority on it. According to McCaffery (1979), "Pain is whatever the experiencing person says it is, existing whenever he says it does." Acute pain is a physiological mechanism that protects the individual from a harmful stimulus. Acute pain warns of tissue damage and alerts the body to protect itself (McCaffery and Pasero, 1999). However, if patients are unable to express their pain (e.g., patients with aphasia, who are intubated, or who have mental status changes), this does not necessarily mean that they do not have pain. Careful pain assessment is crucial. Some patients (e.g., some with spinal cord injuries) are unable to sense painful stimuli. You must take special precautions to protect them from additional injury.

Health care providers often have prejudices about patients in pain. Unless patients have objective signs of pain, nurses do not always believe all their patients are experiencing pain. These assumptions about patients in pain influence your nursing assessment and seriously limit your ability to offer pain relief. Too often, nurses allow misconceptions about pain (Box 31-1) to affect their willingness to provide pain relief (McCaffery and Pasero, 1999). Many nurses avoid acknowledging a patient's pain because of their own fear of contributing to addiction. These fears and beliefs lead to mistrust between the nurse and patient, increased patient recovery time, increased complications and mortality, increased psychological problems, and increased cost (Letizia and others, 2004).

The failure of health care providers to assess pain accurately and consistently results in poor pain management and increased patient suffering. National and international organizations have made efforts to correct this problem (Agency for Health Care Policy and Research [AHCPR], 1992; American Pain Society [APS], 2003). The Joint Commission (TJC) (2008) has a pain standard that requires health care workers to assess all patients for pain on a regular basis. Many health care institutions have adopted this standard by recommending pain as a "fifth vital sign" (APS, 2003). It is important that you develop a "pain conscience" when you care for patients. Assess for pain in every patient, select proper pain therapies, and evaluate the effects of your actions in relieving patients' pain.

Physiology of Pain

TRANSDUCTION Cellular damage from thermal (e.g., exposure to high or low temperatures), mechanical (e.g., edema distending body tissues), chemical (e.g., leakage of hydrochloric acid out of the stomach), or electrical (e.g., electrical burn) stimuli releases pain-producing substances such as histamine, bradykinin, and potassium. This stimulation causes an action potential on **nociceptors** (receptors that respond to harmful stimuli), thus converting the original stimuli into a pain impulse (McCaffery and Pasero, 1999). This conversion is known as transduction.

TRANSMISSION Painful stimuli produce nerve impulses that travel along afferent peripheral nerve fibers. There are primarily two types of peripheral nerve fibers that conduct painful stimuli: the fast, myelinated A-delta fibers and the small, slow unmyelinated C fibers. The A fibers send sharp, localized, and distinct sensations. The small C fibers relay slower impulses that are poorly localized, visceral, and persistent (Menefee-Pujol, Katz, and Zacharoff, 2007). For example, after stepping on a nail, a person initially feels a sharp localized

BOX 31-1 Common Biases and Misconceptions About Pain

- Patients who are knowledgeable about opioids and who make regular efforts to obtain them are drug seeking (addicted).
- There is no reason for patients to hurt when you cannot find a physical cause for pain.
- Administering analgesics regularly leads to patients' tolerance and drug dependence.
- The amount of tissue damage in an injury accurately indicates pain intensity.
- Health care personnel are the best judge of the existence and severity of pain.
- The pain **threshold** and tolerance are the same for everyone.
- Illness and its associated suffering are an inevitable part of aging.
- You use physical or behavioral signs of pain to verify the existence and severity of pain.
- Patients who fall asleep really do not have pain.

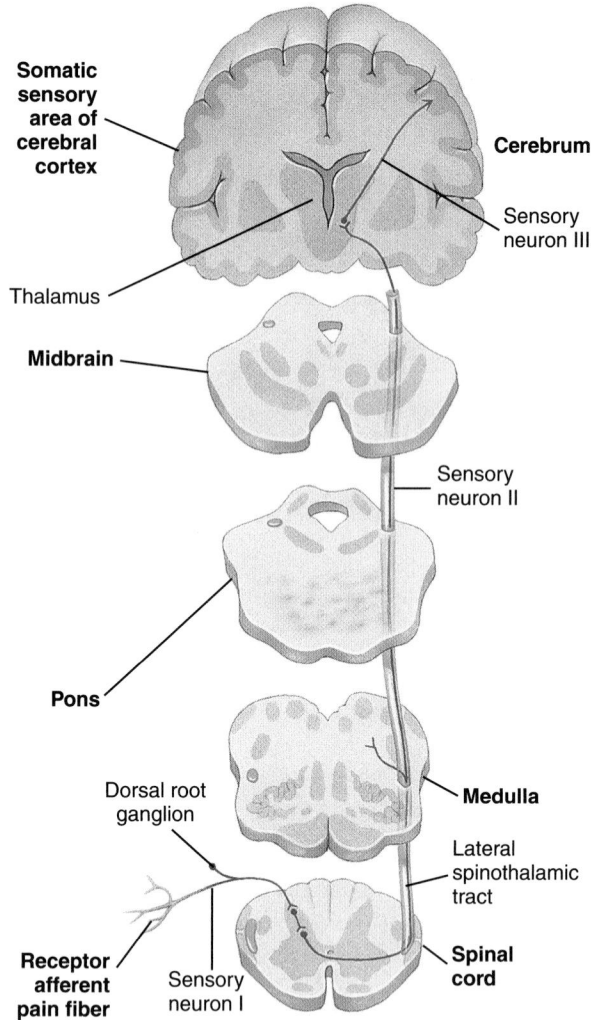

Figure 31-1 ■ Spinothalamic pathway that conducts pain stimuli to the brain.

pain, which is the result of A-fiber transmission. Within a few seconds, the whole foot aches from C-fiber stimulation.

A-delta and C fibers transmit impulses from the periphery to the dorsal horn of the spinal cord, where an excitatory neurotransmitter, substance P, is released. This causes a synaptic transmission from the afferent (sensory) peripheral nerve to spinothalamic tract nerves. Pain stimuli travel through nerve fibers in the spinothalamic tracts, cross to the opposite side of the spinal cord, and then travel up the spinal cord. Figure 31-1 shows the normal pain **reception** pathway. After the pain impulse ascends the spinal cord, information is sent quickly to higher centers in the brain.

PERCEPTION As the pain impulse ascends to the brain, the central nervous system extracts information, such as location, duration, and quality of the pain impulse. The thalamus is the first structure in the brain to process the impulse. It sends the impulse to many areas in the brain, including the cerebral cortex, hypothalamus, and limbic system. Thus the patient becomes aware of the experience of pain. There is no one "pain center" in the brain that supports the complex nature of pain. Any factor that interrupts or influences normal pain **perception,** such as normal fatigue, depression, or pain therapies, affects the patient's awareness and response to pain.

MODULATION When a person perceives a harmful impulse, the brain stimulates descending neurons. The neurons then inhibit nociceptors and interneurons in the ascending pathway. In addition, endogenous opioids and other neurotransmitters (serotonin and norepinephrine) further inhibit the transmission of the painful stimuli to the brain (Menefee-Pujol and others, 2007).

A protective reflex response also occurs with pain (Figure 31-2). When a person is injured, a noxious stimulus from the skin travels along sensory neurons to the dorsal horn of the

spinal cord where it synapses with spinal motor neurons. The impulse continues to travel along the spinal nerve to the skeletal muscle, causing the person to withdraw from the source of the pain.

Pain reception requires an intact peripheral nervous system and spinal cord. Common factors that disrupt pain reception include trauma, drugs, tumor growth, and metabolic disorders.

Neurotransmitters **Neurotransmitters** are substances that affect the sending of nerve stimuli (Box 31-2). They either excite or inhibit nerve transmission. Excitatory neurotransmitters, such as substance P, send electrical impulses across the synaptic cleft between two nerve fibers, enhancing the transmission of the painful impulse. Inhibitory neurotransmitters such as **endorphins** decrease neuron activity without directly transferring a nerve signal through a **synapse.** Researchers believe endorphins act indirectly by increasing or decreasing the effects of neurotransmitters. Pain perception is influenced by balancing neurotransmitters and

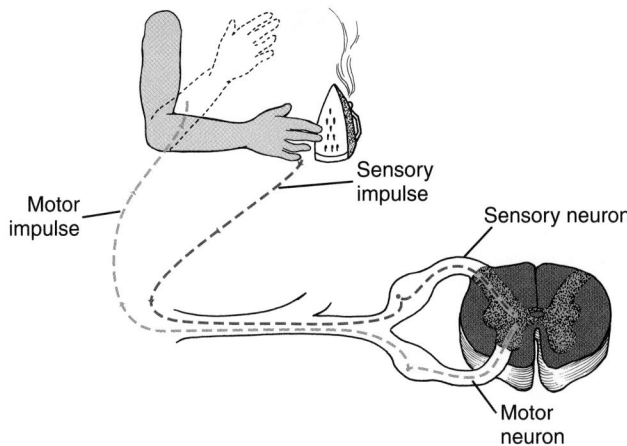

Figure 31-2 ■ Protective pain reflex. Sensory impulse directly stimulates motor nerves, bypassing the brain, causing withdrawal from pain stimulus.

BOX 31-2   Neurophysiology of Pain: Neurotransmitters

EXCITATORY NEUROTRANSMITTERS

Substance P
- Found in the pain neurons of the dorsal horn (excitatory peptide)
- Needed to transmit pain impulses from the periphery to higher brain centers
- Causes vasodilation and edema

Serotonin
- Released from the brain stem and dorsal horn to inhibit pain transmission

Prostaglandins
- Increase sensitivity to pain

INHIBITORY NEUROTRANSMITTERS

Endorphins, Enkephalins, and Dynorphins
- Body's natural supply of morphinelike substances
- Activated by stress and pain
- Located within the brain, spinal cord, and gastrointestinal tract
- Cause analgesia when they attach to opiate receptors in the brain

Bradykinin
- Released from plasma that leaks from surrounding blood vessels at the site of tissue injury
- Binds to receptors on peripheral nerves, increasing pain stimuli

---

by the descending pain-control fibers originating from the cerebral cortex.

Gate Control Theory of Pain   The gate control theory gives you a way to understand pain-relief measures. The gate control theory of Melzack and Wall (1996) suggests that gating mechanisms along the central nervous system can regulate and possibly block pain impulses. The gating mechanism occurs within the spinal cord, thalamus, reticular formation, and limbic system (Melzack and Wall, 1996). The brain determines whether the gate will be opened or closed, either increasing or decreasing the intensity of the ascending pain impulse (Menefee-Pujol and others, 2007). The theory suggests that pain impulses pass through when the gate is open and not while it is closed. In addition, the gate control theory suggests the importance of psychological variables (thoughts and feelings), as well as physiological sensations, in the perception of pain. Thus using psychological, physiological, and/or pharmacological interventions to close the gate lowers pain intensity (Freeman, 2006). For example, therapies such as exercise, heat, cold, massage, and transcutaneous electrical nerve stimulation (TENS) are thought to release endorphins, which close the gate (Barclay, 2007). This prevents or reduces the patient's perception of pain.

Physiological Responses   When acute pain impulses travel up the spinal cord toward the brain stem and thalamus, the autonomic nervous system is stimulated as part of the stress response. Acute pain of low-to-moderate intensity and superficial pain cause the fight-or-flight response of the general adaptation syndrome. Acute stimulation of the sympathetic branch of the autonomic nervous system results in transient physiological responses summarized in Table 31-1. If pain is unrelenting, severe, or deep, typically involving visceral organs, the parasympathetic nervous system goes into action. Most patients quickly adapt, with physical signs, such as vital signs, returning to normal. Thus a patient in pain, especially persistent pain, will not always have physical signs (McCaffery and Pasero, 1999).

It is important to understand that patients with chronic pain do not have the same physiological responses as those with acute pain. They do not demonstrate autonomic or sympathetic nervous system reactions. In addition, if you do not treat acute pain adequately, it can progress to chronic pain. It appears that unrelieved pain sensitizes and changes nerves (neuroplasticity), resulting in enhanced intensity, duration, and distribution of pain (Arnstein, 2003, 2007). These permanent neuroplastic changes contribute to the development of chronic pain syndromes. Chronic pain is not simply acute pain that lasts a long time.

Behavioral Responses   The response to pain is complex and variable. Responses integrate biological, social, and psychological characteristics of the individual. Whether the pain is acute or chronic also influences the behavioral response. Clenching the teeth, facial grimacing, holding or guarding the painful part, and bent posture are all indications of acute pain. Chronic pain affects the patient's activity (eating, sleeping, working, hygiene, social interactions), thinking (confusion, forgetfulness, helplessness), or emotions (anger, depression, irritability, frustration) (Arnstein, 2003, 2007). Recognizing the patient's unique response to pain is impor-

TABLE 31-1 Physiological Reactions to Acute Pain

RESPONSE	CAUSE OR EFFECT
SYMPATHETIC STIMULATION*	
Dilation of bronchial tubes and increased respiratory rate	Provides increased oxygen intake
Increased heart rate	Provides increased oxygen transport
Peripheral vasoconstriction (pallor, elevation in blood pressure)	Elevates blood pressure with shift of blood supply from periphery and viscera to skeletal muscles and brain
Increased blood glucose level	Provides additional energy
Diaphoresis	Controls body temperature during stress
Increased muscle tension	Prepares muscles for action
Dilation of pupils	Affords better vision
Decreased gastrointestinal motility	Frees energy for more immediate activity
PARASYMPATHETIC STIMULATION†	
Pallor	Causes blood supply to shift away from periphery
Muscle tension	Results from fatigue
Decreased heart rate and blood pressure	Results from vagal stimulation
Rapid, irregular breathing	Causes body defenses to fail under prolonged stress of pain
Nausea and vomiting	Causes return of gastrointestinal function
Weakness or exhaustion	Results from expenditure of physical energy

*Pain of low to moderate intensity and superficial pain.
†Severe or deep pain.

tant in assessing the success of the pain management plan. Improvement in the negative effects of chronic pain suggests successful pain relief because comfort usually results in improved function. However, lack of pain expression does not mean a patient is not having pain. Unless a patient openly reacts to pain, it is difficult to assess the nature and extent of the discomfort. You need to help a patient communicate the pain response effectively.

Acute and Chronic Pain

As a result of the physical, psychological, and financial toll of inadequate pain management, President Clinton declared 2001 to 2010 as the Decade of Pain Control and Research (Loeser, 2003). Chronic pain is emerging as a common and expensive twenty-first century health care problem. An estimated 10% of Americans are unable to work or perform activities of daily living independently because of severe pain (Arnstein, 2003). The most common types of pain you will observe in patients are acute/transient and chronic/persistent, which includes cancer and noncancer pain.

ACUTE PAIN Acute pain usually has an identifiable cause following acute injury, disease, or surgery. It begins rapidly, varies in intensity (mild to severe), and lasts briefly. Acute pain warns people of impending injury or disease; thus it is protective. It eventually resolves after a damaged area heals. Patients in acute pain are frightened, anxious, and expect relief quickly. Acute pain is self-limiting, and the patient therefore knows an end is in sight. Because acute pain usually has an identifiable cause and is usually of short duration, health team members are willing to treat it aggressively. However, conflict between you and the patient will arise if you do not provide quick relief.

Acute pain seriously threatens a patient's recovery by hampering the patient's ability to become active and involved in self-care. It causes complications such as physical and emotional exhaustion, immobility, sleep deprivation, delayed wound healing, and pulmonary complications (McCaffery and Pasero, 1999). If you are unable to control acute pain, it is likely that patient education and rehabilitation will be delayed and hospitalization will be prolonged. If not adequately controlled, acute pain progresses to chronic pain. When you relieve acute pain, the patient is able to direct full attention toward recovery.

CHRONIC PAIN Chronic pain is prolonged, varies in intensity, and usually lasts longer than is typically expected or predicted (Arnstein, 2003; McCaffery and Pasero, 1999). In chronic pain, endorphins either cease to function or are reduced. For example, chronic pain from cancer is sometimes a result of the tumor itself, the treatment (chemotherapy, radiation therapy, or surgery), or complications of the disease (fistulas).

Chronic noncancer pain such as low back pain often results from nonprogressive or healed tissue injury. Frequently there are no identifiable causes. The pain is ongoing and often does not respond to treatment. Health care workers are usually less willing to treat chronic pain as aggressively as acute pain. The Agency for Health Care Policy and Research (AHCPR) reported that up to 90% of the 8 million Americans who have cancer can have their pain managed effectively (Jacox and others, 1994). Too often health care workers undertreat these patients' pain.

Patients with chronic pain often have periods of **remissions** (partial or complete disappearance of symptoms) and **exacerbations** (increases in severity). This unpredictability frustrates the patient, often leading to depression. Chronic pain is a major cause of psychological and physical disability, leading to problems such as job loss, inability to perform simple daily activities, sexual dysfunction, and social isolation. The patient with chronic pain often does not show overt symptoms and does not adapt to the pain. But the patient seems to suffer more over time because of physical and mental exhaustion. Symptoms of chronic pain include fatigue, insomnia, anorexia, weight loss, withdrawal, depression, hopelessness, and anger.

Caring for the patient with chronic pain is a challenge. Do not become frustrated or offer false hope for a cure. Instead, help the patient identify ways to cope and to minimize the perception of pain. Providing care to the primary family caregiver is also important. The stress of caring for a loved one with persistent pain causes physical and emotional problems, especially true in older adult caregivers who may also suffer from chronic pain (Blyth and others, 2008; da Cruz and others, 2004). In addition, a family caregiver needs to understand and accept the pain plan in order to successfully implement it.

NURSING KNOWLEDGE BASE

Factors Influencing Pain

To accurately assess and then treat a patient's pain, you need to understand the various factors that influence the pain experience.

AGE Developmental differences influence how infants, children, and older adults react to pain. Infants demonstrate pain through crying, changes in vital signs, facial expression, and extremity movement (Schechter, Berde, and Yaster, 2003). Children have trouble understanding pain and nursing or medical care that causes pain. Children without full vocabularies have difficulty verbally describing and expressing pain to parents or caregivers. A child's temperament affects coping with pain. Children often describe treatments and procedures as the most difficult part of being sick or in the hospital.

Typically children are grossly undermedicated for pain. When comparing children with adults having the same medical diagnoses, children receive fewer medication doses (Schechter and others, 2003). Analgesic doses are often too small or given too infrequently to be effective. It is necessary for you to understand a child's response to pain. If a child is too young to speak, observe behavioral changes such as irritability, loss of appetite, unusual quietness, disturbed sleep patterns, restlessness, and rigid posturing as signs of pain (Jacox and others, 1994; Schechter and others, 2003). If a behavior such as crying changes after a child receives an analgesic, pain was probably the cause of the behavior.

Pain is not a natural part of aging. Likewise, pain perception does not decrease with age. However, older adults often suffer from acute and chronic painful diseases, which the person, the family, and health care providers frequently take for granted or underestimate. They use words such as *hurting* or *aching* instead of using the word *pain* to describe their pain. Older adults sometimes also have more than one painful site. They often hesitate to discuss their pain because of concerns of bothering their health care provider. Frequently older adults will adopt a fatalistic attitude toward pain and feel that they simply must endure it. These barriers contribute to the inadequate pain management of older adults (Herr and others, 2004). Older adults suffer serious loss of functional status as a result of pain. Pain reduces mobility, self-care activities, socialization, and activity tolerance (McCaffery and Pasero, 1999). A patient with cognitive impairment or who is nonverbal (aphasic, mental status changes, or not fluent in English) will have trouble communicating pain and providing a detailed description (Bruckenthal and D'Arcy, 2007; Hutt and others, 2007). Yet you will be able to assess pain accurately in most patients using physical and behavioral cues (American Geriatrics Society [AGS], 2002; Bruckenthal and D'Arcy, 2007; Hutt and others, 2007).

Multiple diseases and vague symptoms affecting similar parts of the body often complicate the ability of older adults to interpret pain. When older patients have more than one source of pain, you gather detailed assessments. Different diseases cause similar symptoms. For example, a patient who has had a below-knee amputation continues to perceive pain from the foot that has been amputated (phantom pain) and has suture-line pain from the surgery. A patient who has had a stroke sometimes has pain in the paralyzed arm and in areas of the body unaffected by the stroke (Jonsson and others, 2006).

GENDER Previously, researchers did not believe gender influenced pain perception or response. Recent research (Keogh, McCracken, and Eccleston, 2005; Logan and Gedney, 2004; Rustoen and others, 2004) on pain in men and women demonstrates a difference in responses to pain because of gender. Women appear to be more sensitive to pain, requiring less stimulation to evoke a pain response than men (Robinson and others, 2003). However, this topic needs further research.

CULTURE Culture influences how people perceive the causes of and learn to react to and express pain. Italian, Jewish, African American, and Spanish-speaking persons often smile readily and use facial expressions and gestures to communicate pain or displeasure (Taylor and Herr, 2003). In contrast, Irish, English, and Northern European persons tend to have less facial expression and are less responsive, especially to strangers such as professional caregivers. Understanding cultural background and personal characteristics will help you to more accurately assess pain and its meaning for patients (Hernandez and Sachs-Ericsson, 2006; Taylor and Herr, 2003) (Box 31-3). Even more important is recognizing how your own culture influences your attitude about pain. Understanding your values, personal biases, and assumptions will help you become culturally sensitive to others who are different from you.

MEANING OF PAIN The meaning a patient attributes to pain affects the pain experience. Patients perceive pain differently if it suggests a threat, loss, punishment, or challenge. The degree and quality of pain perceived by a patient are related to the meaning of pain (Feinberg, 2004).

ATTENTION The degree to which a patient focuses on pain influences pain perception. Increased attention has been associated with increased pain, whereas distraction has been associated with decreased pain. You will apply this concept when you use pain-relief therapies such as listening to music and rhythmical breathing. By focusing a patient's attention and concentration on other stimuli, you help turn the patient's focus away from the pain. Usually, increased **tolerance** for pain lasts only during the time of distraction (McCaffery and Pasero, 1999).

ANXIETY High anxiety levels increase pain perception. In addition, pain also causes anxiety. Autonomic arousal patterns are similar in pain and anxiety. Patients who worry about symptoms that are minor or do not exist have health anxiety. The presence of health anxiety in patients who have chronic pain negatively influences their response to pain and its associated treatments (Bruckenthal, 2008; Ferrell, 2005; Jann and Slade, 2007). Nurses act to reduce health anxiety levels to lower pain perception.

DEPRESSION The incidence of depression is very high in patients with chronic pain. They experience many losses, such as their ability to enjoy life, to be in control, to work, to socialize, and to be independent (Jann and Slade, 2007). Suicidal thoughts are relatively common; therefore you need to

routinely assess for suicidal tendencies (Menefee-Pujol and others, 2007). As a nurse, be aware of the possibility of depression in patients with persistent pain, and suggest a referral if symptoms of major depression emerge. *In the case study, Mrs. Ellis lives alone and has difficulty sleeping, washing dishes, and dressing. Jim wants to assess if family or friends who live nearby can offer assistance.*

FATIGUE Fatigue heightens pain perception. This intensifies pain and decreases coping abilities (Bursch, 2004). Patients are more likely to experience pain at the end of a tiring day than after restful sleep.

PREVIOUS EXPERIENCE Previous experience of pain includes pain the patient has experienced personally and pain the patient has heard about from someone else. Previous pain experience does not necessarily mean a patient will accept pain more easily in the future. Frequent episodes of pain without relief or bouts of severe pain produce anxiety or fear. In contrast, when the patient has experiences with the same type of pain that has successfully been relieved, it is easier for the patient to interpret the pain sensation. As a result, the patient is better prepared to take steps to relieve the pain. A patient who has had no experience with a particular type of pain sometimes has an impaired ability to cope with it. You prepare such a patient with a clear explanation of the type of

---

BOX 31-3   CULTURAL FOCUS

 Pain has both personal and cultural meanings. This influences the verbal expression of pain, individual reaction to pain, and pain treatment preferences. When researching pain in African Americans, Jim from the case study found that people of color, women, and older patients are at increased risk for inadequate pain management (Davidhizar and Giger, 2004). Disparities in pain perception, assessment, and treatment occur in all settings. In addition, he found that African American patients prefer a different pain intensity assessment tool than from 0 to 10 scale (Taylor and Herr, 2003; Ware and others, 2006). Jim plans to apply what he learns when assessing Mrs. Ellis further.

IMPLICATIONS FOR PRACTICE
- Because of the evidence available, Jim remains aware of the possibility of undertreating Mrs. Ellis' pain.
- Jim is attentive to Mrs. Ellis' reports of pain and informs her that he believes what she is telling him about her pain. He also asks her which word she prefers to use to describe pain. Many patients use *hurt* or *ache* to describe mild or moderate pain, reserving the word *pain* for severe discomfort.
- Jim explains several pain intensity tools and asks Mrs. Ellis which one she prefers.
- Cultural responses to pain are often divided into two categories: stoic and emotive. One is not better than the other. Health care providers need to appreciate cultural variations of verbal and nonverbal responses to pain in order to accurately assess pain. Jim asks Mrs. Ellis how she usually demonstrates pain.

- Health care providers are more likely to respond to communication about pain by an individual of the same cultural background and have less understanding of pain in patients from a different culture. Because Jim is of a different gender than Mrs. Ellis, he explores with her the possibility of miscommunication regarding her pain.
- Recognize that communicating pain is not always acceptable within a culture. Jim informs Mrs. Ellis that it is important to report her pain honestly.
- The meaning of pain differs among people of different cultures. Some people view pain as a punishment for the past, a part of life, or something to endure to enter heaven or progress to the next life. Jim gathers historical information about Mrs. Ellis, looking for possible meanings of pain for her.
- Biological variations of drug metabolism, dosing requirements, therapeutic response, and adverse effects are a function of race and ethnicity. It is important for Jim to reassess Mrs. Ellis' response to analgesics and not assume that an inadequate response is a nonadherence issue.
- Health care providers' beliefs about cultural groups and attitude toward pain influence pain management. Self-awareness of potential cultural bias is essential in order to provide adequate pain management. Jim attempts to gain insight into his potential cultural bias by learning more about the cultures of patients he cares for that are different from his.

Data from Davidhizar R, Giger J: A review of the literature on care of clients in pain who are culturally diverse, *Int Nurs Rev* 51:47, 2004.

pain that he or she will experience and the methods to reduce it (Vallerand and others, 2007).

COPING STYLE Pain can be lonely for some. Frequently patients feel a loss of control over their environments or the outcome of events. Coping style influences the ability to cope with pain. Patients with internal loci of control perceive themselves as having personal control over their environments and the outcome of events. They ask questions, desire information, and like choices of treatment. In contrast, patients with external loci of control perceive other factors in their environments, such as nurses, as being responsible for the outcome of events. These patients tend to be less demanding, follow directions, and are more passive in managing their pain. They want specific instructions but become anxious if you give them too much information (Vallerand and others, 2007). Frequently, those with internal loci of control report less severe pain than those with external loci. This concept is applied in the use of **patient-controlled analgesia (PCA).**

FAMILY AND SOCIAL SUPPORT Patients depend on the support and assistance of spouses, family, or friends when coping with pain. Family members sometimes have misconceptions about pain and pain management. Some think the patient should wait as long as possible before receiving pain medication and fear the possibility of addiction (Davidhizar and Giger, 2004). It is your responsibility to educate the patient, family, and public about the importance of early assessment and treatment of pain. The presence of a loved one usually minimizes loneliness and fear when a patient is experiencing pain. Patients of different sociocultural groups have different expectations of people to whom they report their pain. Absence of family or friends often makes the pain experience more stressful. The presence of parents is especially important for children in pain.

CRITICAL THINKING

Synthesis

You will apply elements of critical thinking whenever you perform the nursing process with a patient experiencing pain. Consider the scientific knowledge you have learned, your experience, critical thinking attitudes, and standards to ensure an individualized approach to patient care.

KNOWLEDGE It is important for you to apply knowledge regarding the physiology of pain, along with the physiology of any underlying disease processes, to understand the patient's pain response, type of pain, and interventions needed for pain management. Knowledge and application of communication skills enhance the thoroughness of a pain assessment. Once you have a clear picture of the physiological nature of a patient's condition, synthesis of knowledge regarding the patient's psychological and sociocultural perspective becomes critical for an individualized approach to care. In addition, an understanding of pharmacological and nonpharmacological therapies helps you to work with the patient and health care provider in selecting pain therapies (McCaffery and Pasero, 1999).

EXPERIENCE Caring for patients who have pain is an important part of a nurse's clinical experience. Because pain is so common, you soon learn that patients vary widely in their expressions of pain. The degree of pain affects their behaviors and the actions they take to find relief (Clark and others, 2006). Such experience will either positively or negatively affect your willingness to begin pain interventions. Furthermore, your own experience with pain emphasizes the importance of having someone who is supportive and understanding. Reflecting on the experiences of caring for those in pain helps you to search for better approaches for each new patient you meet.

ATTITUDES Critical thinking attitudes ensure that you make decisions that are fair and responsible. When a patient is in pain, you will need perseverance to find an approach that will offer the patient some degree of relief. Quick solutions, without follow-up, will aggravate a patient's discomfort. Learn as much as possible about the patient's pain, try various interventions, and continue different creative approaches until you discover an effective one. Accept the patient's report of pain (APS, 2003), even if you do not believe the severity of the pain reported. At times you will be concerned about patients trying to fool you. By acting according to your professional standards and guidelines and accepting the patient's self-report of pain, you are demonstrating integrity to your profession. You are also taking responsibility for providing optimal pain management to your patients by using these standards and guidelines.

STANDARDS The application of intellectual standards is particularly important when completing an accurate pain assessment. A clear, precise, and accurate description of the patient's pain is essential. Ensure that information related to factors influencing the patient's pain is relevant and complete. Also, have an open mind and listen to all sources affected by the patient's experience (patient, family, and friends) to gain a clear picture of what pain means for the patient. This ensures inclusion of all criteria needed for accurate evaluation of the patient's pain experience.

Professional standards, guidelines, and position statements such as those developed by the AHRQ, the American Pain Society (APS), the World Health Organization (WHO), the American Society of Pain Management Nurses (ASPMN), and The Joint Commission provide valuable guidelines for pain management. Experts have published these guidelines to improve the quality of care for those in pain. Apply these principles when making decisions about pain therapies.

NURSING PROCESS

■■■ ASSESSMENT

The assessment of pain aims to find the cause of a person's pain and to determine the effect of pain on the individual. Accurate and factual pain assessment is necessary for determining the patient's responses, arriving at proper nursing diagnoses, and selecting appropriate therapies (Table 31-2). Pain assessment is one of the most common and one of the most

TABLE 31-2	Focused Patient Assessment	
FACTORS TO ASSESS	**QUESTIONS**	**PHYSICAL ASSESSMENT**
Location of pain	Where is the pain located?	Depending on area of pain, use inspection to determine if body part is swollen, discolored, or warm to touch.
	Can you point to where the pain is?	Have patient use hand to locate area where pain originates and then spreads.
		Use light palpation over area identified by patient.
Aggravating factors	Does your pain get worse when you move?	When positioning of body part aggravates pain, determine if range of motion is altered.
	Are there other things that you do that make your pain worse?	Observe patient's facial expression and movement when patient attempts activity that typically aggravates pain.
	Is there anything that makes the pain better?	

TABLE 31-3	Implications of Pain Assessment for Nursing Interventions
ASSESSMENT CRITERIA (PQRSTU)	**NURSING INTERVENTIONS**
Precipitating or aggravating factors	Avoid activities that cause or aggravate pain. Teach patient or family to avoid same activities.
Quality	Suggest changing pharmacological interventions if the quality of pain (neuropathic versus nociceptive) changes.
Relief measures	Use measures that the patient uses to relieve pain, as long as they are safe and appropriate.
Region (location)	Position patient off affected area. Apply local treatments (e.g., elastic bandage, cold, heat, splinting) directly over painful site.
Severity	Change or revise interventions, depending on success of one intervention in reducing severity.
Timing (onset, duration, and pattern)	Administer analgesics so that peak action occurs when pain is most acute (e.g., during dressing change or exercise therapy).
U (effect of pain on patient)	Schedule activities that are important to the patient during the time of day when patient feels the pain least.

BOX 31-4 Routine Clinical Approach to Pain Assessment and Management (ABCDE)

- **A** *Ask* about pain regularly.
  - **Assess** pain systematically.
- **B** *Believe* the patient and family in their report of pain and what relieves it.
- **C** *Choose* pain control options appropriate for the patient, family, and setting.
- **D** *Deliver* interventions in a timely, logical, and coordinated fashion.
- **E** *Empower* patients and their families.
  Enable them to control their course to the greatest extent possible.

From Jacox A and others: *Management of cancer pain,* Clinical Practice Guideline No. 9, AHCPR Pub No. 94-0592, Rockville, Md, March 1994, Agency for Health Care Policy and Research, U.S. Department of Health and Human Services, Public Health Service.

difficult activities you will perform. It is important to carefully interpret pain cues and remember that psychological and physical components of pain influence the **reaction** to it.

The AHCPR (1992) established specific guidelines for assessing pain in patients having surgery or other procedures. The focus is preventing pain. The guidelines emphasize the importance of assessing the resources available for pain management, completing a preoperative patient assessment, and developing a collaborative plan for postoperative pain management with the physician or health care provider, patient, and family members. Patients need to understand that reporting their pain is valuable and necessary if the health care team is to manage pain in an individualized and effective way.

Be sensitive to a patient's level of discomfort. If pain is acutely severe, it is unlikely the patient will provide detailed information. During an episode of acute pain, assess how a patient feels, as well as the PQRSTU characteristics of the pain (Table 31-3). A more comprehensive pain assessment takes time; you do this when the patient becomes more alert and attentive.

BOX 31-5   SYNTHESIS IN PRACTICE

In the case study, Jim prepares for tomorrow's home care visit with Mrs. Ellis. He reviews what he has learned about pain physiology and the pathophysiology of rheumatoid arthritis. This allows him to anticipate the need to carefully assess to what extent pain limits Mrs. Ellis' ability to walk and perform activities of daily living.

Jim plans to assess the location, duration, and aggravating and relieving factors influencing Mrs. Ellis's pain, as well as any behavioral symptoms he observes. He plans to determine the pain scale Mrs. Ellis prefers, to assess a baseline for the severity of her pain. Because Mrs. Ellis is 70, Jim reviews gerontological principles and knows he needs to take time to establish a trusting relationship so as to encourage a complete description of the pain experience.

Jim recalls previous experiences with patients in chronic pain and interventions used to relieve pain. He remembers his own experiences with pain after suffering a broken arm during a soccer game. These experiences will make him sensitive to the personal and dynamic nature of each individual's pain experience.

Jim considers the AHCPR and AGS guidelines for the management of chronic pain. He wants to carefully clarify with Mrs. Ellis the extent to which the chronic arthritic pain and the acute exacerbations have affected her life. If Jim is to help her with pain relief and health promotion activities, he needs to learn as much as he can about Mrs. Ellis' lifestyle and the support systems that are available for her. Because Mrs. Ellis lives alone, Jim wants to assess if family or friends who can offer assistance live nearby.

For patients with chronic pain, focus assessment on the emotional impact and the meaning of the pain experience, as well as on its history and context (Arnstein, 2003). In addition, assessment includes level of function, because it is sometimes impossible to achieve complete pain relief. The AHCPR recommends that families of patients with cancer learn how to assess pain so they promote continuity of effective pain management (Box 31-4) (Jacox and others, 1994). In the home setting, family members' involvement in pain assessment offers the patient and family control over the pain experience. Be aware of possible errors in pain assessment. Bias (overestimating or underestimating level of pain), vague or unclear assessment questions, and use of unreliable or invalid pain-assessment tools will not provide accurate data (McCaffery and Pasero, 1999). Family estimates of a patient's pain are not always accurate (Vallerand and others, 2007). Therefore use these estimates only when the patient is unable to verbalize pain intensity (Box 31-5).

PATIENT'S EXPRESSION OF PAIN Patients often fail to report or discuss pain (McCaffery and Pasero, 1999). To complicate assessment, nurses frequently believe that patients will report pain if they have it; however, this is not always the case. Patients often feel that the health care providers know about the pain because that is their job. It is important to regularly *ask* patients about pain. Do not assume patients are pain-free if they do not volunteer their pain intensity. Also, pay attention to the nonverbal ways that patients communicate discomfort. In addition, refrain from using the phrase *complaining of pain* when discussing the patient's pain. Better to use words like *stating, telling,* or *reporting,* which is what the patient is doing.

Patients unable to communicate effectively often require special attention during assessment. Some examples are the following:

- Children
- People with developmental delays
- Patients with aphasia
- Patients who are psychotic
- Patients with dementia
- Patients receiving neurological-blocking medications
- People who do not speak English

These patients all require different approaches. Patients with cognitive impairments require simple assessment approaches involving close observation of behavior, especially changes in behavior. If a patient speaks a different language, you will need a family member or interpreter. Closely monitor patients receiving medications that paralyze their muscles, because these medications prevent patients from being able to communicate their pain verbally or behaviorally. Often proxy pain ratings, the rating of pain by family members, friends, or nurse's aides who care for patients or observe their behaviors, are useful (Clark and others, 2006; Vallerand and others, 2007).

CHARACTERISTICS OF PAIN Only the patient can describe pain characteristics. Patient self-report is the single most reliable indicator of the existence and intensity of pain and any related discomfort (APS, 2003; McCaffery and Pasero, 1999). Each pain characteristic presents implications for how you will help to manage patients' pain. The PQRSTU model is an effective tool for assessing pain in adults and determining interventions to relieve the pain (see Table 31-3).

Precipitating Factors It helps to assess specific events or conditions that precipitate or aggravate pain. Ask the patient to describe activities that cause pain, such as physical activity, coffee or alcohol ingestion, urination, swallowing, or emotional stress. Ask the patient to demonstrate actions that cause painful responses such as coughing or turning in a certain manner. After identifying specific factors, it is easier to plan interventions to avoid worsening the pain.

Quality Assessment of the quality of pain helps to differentiate nociceptive pain that is sometimes somatic or visceral from neuropathic pain (Table 31-4). Knowing the quality of pain assists in selecting medications to treat the pain. When assessing the quality of pain, do not provide descriptive words for the patient. Assessment is more accurate if a patient describes the sensation in his or her own words after

TABLE 31-4	Classification of Pain by Quality	
PAIN TYPE	**CHARACTERISTICS**	**EXAMPLE**
Somatic	Sharp Aching Throbbing Well localized	Osteoarthritis pain Myofascial pain

Visceral	Dull
	Cramping
	Colicky
	Poorly localized
		Myocardial
		  infarction
		Obstructed
		  bowel

Neuropathic	Shooting
	Burning
	Electric-like
		Trigeminal
		  neuralgia
		Postherpetic
		  neuropathy

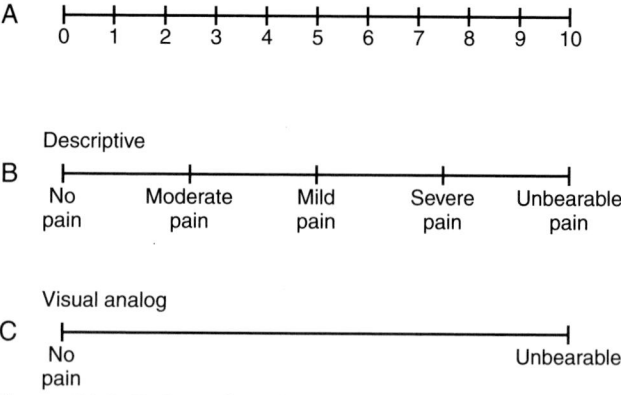

Figure 31-3 ■ Sample pain scales. **A,** Numerical. **B,** Descriptive. **C,** Visual analog.

open-ended questions. For example, say, "Tell me what your pain feels like." The only time you offer to list descriptive terms is when the patient is unable to describe pain.

There is some consistency in the way patients describe certain types of pain. People often describe the pain of a myocardial infarction (heart attack) as crushing or viselike. However, people describe the pain of a surgical incision as sharp and stabbing. When the descriptions fit the pattern forming in your assessment, you are able to make a clearer analysis of the nature and type of pain. If descriptions do not fit, it does not mean that the patient's pain is not real.

Relieving Factors Make sure you know if a patient has an effective way for relieving pain such as changing position, using ritualistic behavior (pacing, rocking, or rubbing), eating, or applying heat or cold to the painful site. In the home, determine if the patient uses relief measures safely. Assessment of relieving factors also includes identifying the patient's use of practitioners (e.g., internist, chiropractor, or faith healer). Patients with chronic pain are more likely to try alternative health care methods.

Region/Location To assess pain location, ask the patient to point to all areas of discomfort. To localize the pain more specifically, have the patient trace the area from the most severe point outward. This is difficult to do if pain is diffuse, involves several sites, or involves large parts of the body. Use a drawing showing the location of pain as a baseline if the pain changes. Use anatomical landmarks and descriptive terminology to record the pain location (e.g., "Pain is in the right upper abdominal quadrant"). Pain classified by location is superficial or cutaneous, deep or visceral, localized or diffuse, or referred or radiating.

Severity The most subjective characteristic of pain is its severity or intensity. Patients are often asked to describe pain as mild, moderate, or severe. However, the meaning of these terms differs for you and the patient. Descriptive scales attempt to measure pain severity objectively (Figure 31-3). Use a scale to measure the current severity of the patient's pain. In addition, ask the patient to rate the worst pain and least pain experienced in the past 12 hours. This helps to determine an average pain intensity that allows you to see trends.

A numerical rating scale (NRS) requires patients to rate pain on a line scale of 0 to 10, with 0 representing no pain and 10 representing the worst pain a patient can imagine. The scales work best when assessing an individual patient's pain intensity before and after therapeutic interventions to determine if relief is achieved. When you use scales to rate pain, a 10-cm (4-inch) baseline is recommended. However, new research findings suggest that culture influences a patient's choice of a pain intensity tool (Taylor and Herr, 2003). A verbal descriptor scale (VDS) consists of a line with three to six word descriptors equally spaced along the line. Show the patient the scale, and ask the patient to choose the descriptor that best represents the severity of pain.

A visual analog scale (VAS) consists of a straight line without labeled subdivisions. The straight line shows a continuum of intensity and has labeled endpoints. A patient indicates pain by marking the appropriate point on the VAS. This scale gives the patient total freedom to identify pain severity. The VAS is a more sensitive measure of pain severity but does not provide information on the emotional and sensory qualities of the patient's pain (Bruckenthal and D'Arcy, 2008; Hutt and others, 2007). Further research is needed to validate the usefulness of pain scales in clinical settings (Ware and others, 2006).

A good pain scale is easy to use, is understandable, and is not time consuming. If a patient is able to easily read and understand a scale, the description of pain is more accurate. If patients use a hearing aid or glasses, be sure they are using them when answering pain assessment questions or marking a pain scale. Descriptive scales are useful in assessing pain severity and in evaluating changes in a patient's condition. Do not use pain scale ratings to compare one patient with another. *In the case study, Jim wants to use the most reliable pain intensity scale to establish a baseline for the severity of the pain, as well as any behavioral symptoms he observes. Jim asks Mrs. Ellis what scale she would like to use to identify her pain intensity.*

Many patients cannot verbalize discomfort because of an inability to communicate or decreased levels of consciousness. In these cases, be alert for subtle behaviors that indicate pain (Box 31-6). When patients have pain, also assess their vocal response (e.g., moaning, crying, or gasping), facial movements

BOX 31-6   BEST PRACTICES

Pain Assessment in the Patient Who Is Nonverbal

SUMMARY OF EVIDENCE

An appointed task force of the American Society for Pain Management Nursing (ASPMN) has developed this position statement and clinical practice recommendations. No single assessment strategy, such as interpretation of behaviors, pathological condition, or estimates of pain by others, is sufficient by itself in determining the presence of pain in a patient who is nonverbal.

APPLICATION TO NURSING PRACTICE

- Recommended assessment considerations
  - Attempt a self-report of pain using simple yes/no response or vocalizations.
  - Explain why self-report cannot be used.
  - Search for potential causes of pain.
  - Assume pain is present (APP) after ruling out other problems (infection, constipation) that cause pain.
  - Identify pathological conditions or procedures that cause pain.
  - Observe patient behaviors, and list behaviors (e.g., facial expressions, vocalizations, body movements, changes in interactions or mental status) that indicate pain. These will vary depending on patient's developmental level.
  - Ask family members, parents, and caregivers for a surrogate report.

- Use behavioral pain assessment tool.
  - Use reliable and valid tools to ensure use of appropriate criteria in the pain assessment.
  - Appropriate scale is determined patient by patient; no one scale should be required for all specific groups of patients.
  - Vital signs are not sensitive indicators for the presence of pain.
- Attempt an analgesic trial.
  - Choose analgesic, dose, and titration based on estimated intensity of pain.
  - For mild to moderate pain, give nonopioid analgesics around the clock.
  - After 24 hours, reassess. If behaviors improve, assume pain was the cause.
  - If behaviors persist, consider giving a single, low-dose short-acting opioid (e.g., hydrocodone, oxycodone, morphine). Observe effect.
  - If behaviors continue, titrate dose upward by 25% to 50%, and observe effect.
  - Continue to titrate up until a therapeutic effect or bothersome adverse effects occur or there is no benefit.
  - If behaviors continue after a reasonable analgesic trial, explore other potential causes.
  - For severe pain, if may be appropriate to start the analgesic trial with an opioid.

REFERENCE

Data from Herr K and others: Pain assessment in the nonverbal patient: position statement with clinical practice recommendations, *Pain Manag Nurs* 7(2):44, 2006.

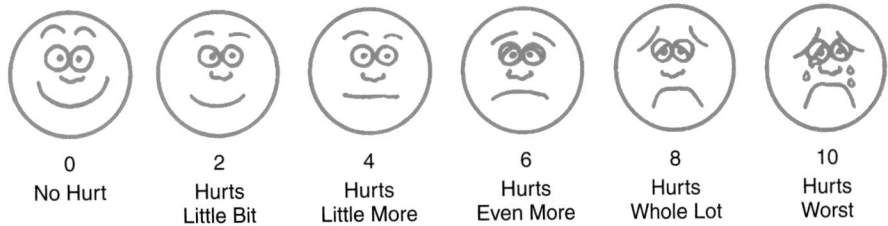

Figure 31-4 ■ Wong-Baker FACES Pain Rating Scale. (From Hockenberry ML and others: *Wong's nursing of infants and children,* ed 8, St. Louis, 2007, Copyrighted by Mosby. Reprinted by permission.)

(e.g., grimacing, clenched teeth, or tightly closed eyes), and body movements (e.g., restlessness, increased hand and finger movements, or pacing), or inactivity. Also assess social interaction. Does the patient avoid conversation or social contacts? Does the patient have a short attention span?

The critical care pain observation tool (CCPOT) attempts to quantify pain of patients in intensive care (Gelinas and others, 2004). Pasero and McCaffery (2004) proposed that nurses should "assume pain is present" and treat for pain in patients who are nonverbal if they have a condition or procedure that is usually considered painful.

Several pain scales are available to assess pain in children. Wong and Baker (1988) developed the FACES Pain Rating

Scale to assess pain in children (Figure 31-4). The scale consists of six cartoon faces ranging from a very happy, smiling face for "no pain" to increasingly less happy faces to a final sad, tearful face for "worst pain." Children as young as 3 years of age can use the scale. The advantage is that patients do not have to interpret the meaning of numbers or adjectives. The faces clearly and quickly depict the concept of pain or discomfort (Schechter and others, 2003).

Another tool designed to measure pain intensity in children is the Oucher pain scale (Beyer and others, 1992). The Oucher consists of two separate scales: a 0 to 100 scale on the left for older children and a six-picture photographic scale on the right for younger children (Figure 31-5). There are

OUCHER®

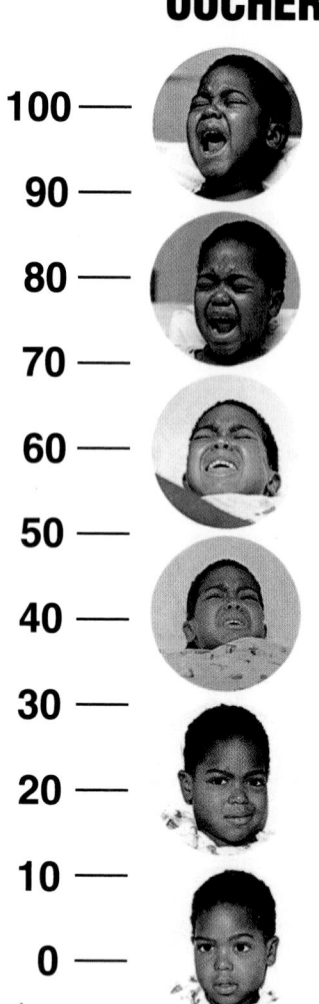

100 —

90 —

80 —

70 —

60 —

50 —

40 —

30 —

20 —

10 —

0 —

Figure 31-5 ■ Oucher pain scale. (© Beyer, Denyes, 1992. Used with permission.)

SLEEP
- Does the patient have difficulty falling asleep?
- Does pain awaken the patient at night?
- Are sleeping pills or other aids needed?

HYGIENE
- Does pain hinder the patient's ability to bathe, dress, or perform other hygiene measures independently?
- Are family members or friends available or needed to assist?

EATING
- Is the patient able to manipulate eating utensils?
- Can the patient chew and swallow without discomfort?

SEXUAL FUNCTIONING
- Do physical conditions such as arthritis or back pain prevent the patient from assuming usual positions during intercourse?
- Does pain or fatigue reduce the patient's desire for sex?
- Is the patient fearful that pain will increase as a result of intercourse?

HOME MANAGEMENT AND WORK ACTIVITIES
- Is the patient able to perform usual housework chores?
- Does the patient's job require physical activity, and does pain limit activity now?
- If pain is related to emotional stress, does the job involve tension-filled decision making?
- Does the patient need to stop activities momentarily to relieve pain?

SOCIAL ACTIVITIES
- Does the patient regularly socialize?
- To what extent has pain disrupted activities?

Oucher scales for whites, African Americans, and Hispanics. Photographs of the face of a child (in increasing levels of discomfort) are designed to cue children into understanding what pain is and its severity. A child merely points to the selection, simplifying the task of describing the pain. There are additional tools for children with verbal skills (Byers and Thornley, 2004; Herr and others, 2006; Merkel, 2002), as well as pain intensity scales for neonates (Herr and others, 2006; Pasero, 2002) and infants (Merkel and others, 2002) that you will implement in appropriate settings.

Timing (Onset, Duration, and Pattern) Ask questions to determine the start, duration, and time sequence of pain. When did the pain begin? How long has it lasted? Does it occur at the same time each day? How often does it recur? It is sometimes easier to diagnose the nature of pain by identifying time factors. The onset of sudden and severe pain is easier to assess then gradual, mild discomfort. Knowing the time cycle of a patient's pain helps you to intervene before the pain occurs or worsens. *In the case study, Mrs. Ellis has rheumatoid arthritis and always awakens in the morning with stiffness and pain in the*

joints. Consequently, part of Jim's recommendations will include having the patient use heat or warm baths upon awakening.

Effect of Pain on Patient Assessing the patient's ability to function is crucial to pain assessment and reassessment once you implement the pain management plan. First, ask patients what their pain prevents them from doing. Then, establish goals to provide sufficient pain relief to restore the ability to do those activities. Successful pain management results in improved function. It is important to remember that pain is not static but is dynamic and requires routine timely reassessment.

Pain is a stressful event that alters lifestyle and psychological well-being. By recognizing the effects of pain on patients, you will identify more clearly the nature and implications of the pain. Patients who live with daily pain are less able to participate in routine activities. Assessment reveals the extent of the disability and the adjustments that will be necessary for participation in self-care (Box 31-7).

CONCOMITANT SYMPTOMS Concomitant symptoms occur with pain and usually increase pain intensity. These include nausea, headache, dizziness, urge to urinate, constipation, depression, and restlessness. Certain types of pain have predictable symptoms. For example, severe rectal pain often causes constipation. These symptoms are as much a problem to a patient as the pain itself.

PATIENT EXPECTATIONS Patients rely on their caregivers to recognize and alleviate their physical discomfort. This may involve using a skilled and caring approach, trying a variety of comfort measures, and serving as an advocate for the patient. You demonstrate caring when you tailor care to the individual's needs. Always ask patients what they expect regarding their comfort needs. This includes asking not only what interventions they prefer but also how they think you should administer them. It is important to understand if patients expect full pain relief or if they simply hope to have their discomfort reduced. When your patients ask for assistance because of pain, they expect you to respond promptly.

DOCUMENTATION Carefully assess and routinely document your patient's report of pain and the effectiveness of interventions. Use the assessment tool that is appropriate for your patient, and always use the same tool to reassess the patient's pain.

■■■ NURSING DIAGNOSIS

You identify accurate nursing diagnoses for patients in pain by thorough data collection and analysis. You make an accurate diagnosis after reviewing all of the assessment data and identifying patterns of the defining characteristics. In the example of the diagnosis of *acute pain,* you might assess a patient's withdrawal from communication, rigid posturing, moaning, and verbalization of discomfort. In contrast, you make the diagnosis of *anxiety* by observing a patient's facial tension and appearance, poor eye contact, restlessness, and verbalization of feeling scared. The two diagnoses have similar defining characteristics, but you will sort out patterns to distinguish *acute pain* from *anxiety.*

The related factor for the diagnostic statement focuses on the specific nature of the patient's problem. *Acute pain related to physical trauma* and *acute pain related to natural childbirth processes* require very different nursing interventions. Successful identification of related factors ensures that you direct nursing therapies toward relieving the patient's discomfort.

The following nursing diagnoses are applicable for patients with acute or chronic pain:

- *Risk for caregiver role strain (caregiver)*
- *Ineffective coping*
- *Fatigue*
- *Impaired physical mobility*
- *Acute pain*
- *Chronic pain*
- *Bathing self-care deficit*
- *Dressing self-care deficit*

- *Risk for situational low self-esteem*
- *Social isolation*

■■■ PLANNING

GOALS AND OUTCOMES Develop an individualized plan of care for each nursing diagnosis identified (see Care Plan). Work with the patient and family to set realistic expectations for pain relief. Make sure the patient understands that complete pain relief is not guaranteed, but it will be attempted. You individualize realistic goals for pain relief and levels of function with measurable outcomes (Pasero and McCaffery, 2004). For example, if a patient's baseline assessment reveals a pain severity consistently between 7 and 8 on a VAS, a realistic goal is for the patient to achieve a level of comfort that permits the patient to function. A pain severity of 2 or 3 out of 10 usually allows for improved function or even full pain relief. Pain ratings of 4 or higher on a scale of 0 to 10 are unacceptable unless they are short term (McCaffery and Pasero, 1999). Pain ratings of 7 or higher on a 0 to 10 pain scale are a medical emergency and require immediate action (APS, 2005).

A concept map is a method that is useful in organizing patient care when patients have multiple problems (Figure 31-6). Links show the relationship between the nursing diagnoses and the medical diagnosis, as well as between the nursing diagnoses and associated interventions. This helps you learn how assessment findings and interventions can apply to more than one diagnosis.

In the home setting, plan to use the patient's remedies as long as the remedies are safe. Your assessment of the home environment should reveal if there are obvious risks to the patient. For example, a patient wishes to use a heating pad, but the electrical cord is frayed and damaged. Therefore instruct the patient not to use that heating pad, and help the patient locate a heating pad that is safer to use.

It is always important to remember that a successful plan of care requires development of a therapeutic relationship with the patient/family and a focus on education regarding pain. Helping patients learn how to manage their pain is an important goal of care. You will help best by seeing the patient as a total person, listening carefully to concerns, attending promptly to his or her needs, and respecting any response to pain. In a successful nurse-patient relationship, you recognize that the patient knows more about his or her own pain and is an important partner in identifying successful pain-relieving strategies.

SETTING PRIORITIES When developing the care plan, work with the patient to select priorities based on the patient's level of pain and its effect on the patient's condition. For acute severe pain, it is important to provide quick relief. Analgesics are very effective. Giving opioids to a patient in acute pain will *not* mask symptoms or deter diagnosis. In addition, early administration of opioids to patients with acute abdominal pain does not alter the treatment or outcome (Silka and others, 2004).

COLLABORATIVE CARE A comprehensive plan of care involves using the resources of a patient's family and friends. The family often gives care in the home and thus needs to be

CARE PLAN Chronic Pain

ASSESSMENT

When Jim enters Mrs. Ellis' four-room apartment, he finds the home to be in some disarray. Mrs. Ellis is sitting in a recliner in her living room, with clothing on the floor and soiled dishes on a nearby table. Mrs. Ellis reports that the pain she has been experiencing has made it very difficult to use her hands and walk between rooms. She is able to get to the bathroom, but it causes her to become fatigued. Her pain is constant and localized in the joints of her hands and knees.

ASSESSMENT ACTIVITIES

Ask Mrs. Ellis to select a pain scale she prefers and rate her current pain intensity.

Ask Mrs. Ellis to rate her pain intensity when it is most severe.

Ask Mrs. Ellis what she does to control her pain.

Ask Mrs. Ellis if the aspirin is causing any side effects.

Observe Mrs. Ellis standing and walking to the kitchen.

Ask Mrs. Ellis if she has friends or neighbors available to assist her.

FINDINGS/DEFINING CHARACTERISTICS*

She **rates the pain at the level of 3 on a FACES Pain Scale of 0 to 10.**

She **rates the pain at 4 on a FACES Pain Scale of 0 to 10.**

She currently takes aspirin for the pain, but the pain **prevents her from being able to fall asleep,** and when she does fall asleep, she **often reawakens at night.**

She reports "burning in the stomach" when she takes the aspirin.

She **has difficulty standing** and has an **unsteady gait.**

She states, "I hate to be a bother, although my next-door neighbor has offered to help in the past."

NURSING DIAGNOSIS: Chronic pain related to joint inflammation.

PLANNING

GOAL

• Mrs. Ellis will achieve a sense of pain relief within 1 week.

• Mrs. Ellis will ambulate with less discomfort on self-report within 14 days.

• Mrs. Ellis will be able to perform activities of daily living with less discomfort within 14 days.

EXPECTED OUTCOMES (NOC)†

Pain Level
• Mrs. Ellis will report pain at 2 on a FACES Pain Scale of 0 to 10 following relaxation therapy and heat application.

Pain: Disruptive Effects
• Mrs. Ellis will demonstrate ability to rise to standing position without assistance within 1 week.
• Mrs. Ellis will demonstrate ability to walk from room to room using a walker with steady gait in 2 weeks.
• Mrs. Ellis will be able to perform dishwashing and cleaning of the house in 2 weeks.

INTERVENTIONS (NIC)‡

Analgesic Administration
• Discuss the possibility of starting a disease-modifying antirheumatic drug (DMRAD) (e.g., methotrexate), a biological response modifier (BRM) (e.g., infliximab [Remicade]), a nonsteroidal antiinflammatory drug (NSAID) (e.g., ibuprofen), or an analgesic (e.g., acetaminophen) with Mrs. Ellis' primary health care provider.
• Have Mrs. Ellis take analgesics approximately 30 minutes before ambulating, performing self-care activities, or going to sleep. Instruct her to take medication with a light snack or meal and a full glass of water. During instruction, tell her the drug will relieve pain.

RATIONALE

Different medications are used to control the pain and symptoms of rheumatoid arthritis. DMRADs cause immunosuppression; DMRADs, NSAIDs, and BRMs decrease inflammation; and DMRADs, NSAIDs, and analgesics relieve pain (Arthritis Foundation, 2008).

Medication will exert peak effect when patient begins activities. Administration with meals and water reduces chance of gastrointestinal upset. An added positive effect occurs when the patient understands the action and purpose of the analgesic and believes the medication will relieve pain.

****Defining characteristics** are shown in **bold** type.

†Outcomes classification labels from Moorhead S and others, editors: *Nursing outcomes classification (NOC),* ed 4, St. Louis, 2008, Mosby.
‡Intervention classification labels from Bulechek GM and others, editors: *Nursing interventions classification (NIC),* ed 5, St. Louis, 2008, Mosby.

CARE PLAN Chronic Pain—cont'd

INTERVENTIONS (NIC)‡

Cutaneous Stimulation
- Have Mrs. Ellis place a sturdy stool in shower stall and run warm water continuously over joints of hands and feet.
- Have Mrs. Ellis apply moist, warm compresses to joints of hands 3 times a day.

Referral
- Refer Mrs. Ellis to a physical therapist to determine possible use of a walker or other assistive devices.

RATIONALE

Heat reduces pain by improving blood flow and reducing stiffness of inflamed tissues (Barclay, 2007).

Cutaneous stimulation activates mechanoreceptor A-beta fibers, thus inhibiting transmission of pain by releasing inhibitory neurotransmitters (Barclay, 2007).

Physical therapists teach effective exercise and ambulation techniques to reduce pain and conserve energy.

EVALUATION

NURSING ACTIONS	PATIENT RESPONSE/FINDING	ACHIEVEMENT OF OUTCOME
Observe Mrs. Ellis' ability to stand and walk from living room to kitchen.	Mrs. Ellis is able to ambulate with walker from living room to kitchen; gait is slow but steady.	Is successfully ambulating with steady gait.
Ask Mrs. Ellis if she experiences discomfort during dressing and bathing.	Mrs. Ellis has less discomfort from bathing after using warm water over joints. Dressing is still causing some discomfort when manipulating buttons on clothing.	Cutaneous stimulation is providing some pain relief. Consider referring to occupational therapy to adapt clothes fasteners requiring less hand mobility.
Ask Mrs. Ellis to rate pain on FACES Pain Scale 30 minutes after analgesic is administered.	Mrs. Ellis rates pain at a level of a 2 after receiving analgesic.	Continues to have discomfort, but less severe than preintervention level.

prepared to assess the patient's pain and administer therapies safely. Discharge teaching in an acute care setting prepares the patient and family to understand the nature and extent of the patient's pain, the choice of therapies, and how to safely administer therapies. Family members or friends who show a disinterest or prejudice toward pain will slow the patient's recovery. Additional resources in planning care include nurse and physician specialists, physical therapists, occupational therapists, medical social workers, and clergy. An oncology nurse specialist understands therapies for chronic cancer pain. Physician pain specialists are experts on invasive therapies. Physical therapists plan exercises that strengthen or relax muscle groups and lessen pain. Occupational therapists devise splints to support painful body parts. Clergy offer strategies to relieve spiritual pain. If an agency does not have the resources to manage the patient's pain, refer the patient to a health care provider or agency that will provide the care needed.

Because patients are often transferred between departments of the same institution and sometimes between different institutions, documentation of the pain management plan is crucial for continuity of care. You record all discharge teaching and referrals implemented. A notation of whom the patient or family member is to call if pain consistently exceeds the pain intensity goal is essential.

■■■ IMPLEMENTATION

The nature of pain and the extent to which it affects an individual's physical and psychosocial well-being determine the choice of pain-relief therapies. You are responsible for administering and monitoring therapies ordered by health care providers for pain relief and independently providing pain-relief measures that complement those prescribed. Implement any previously successful pain-relieving remedies used by the patient. Generally try the least invasive and safest therapy first. Do not delegate pain assessment and management to nursing assistive personnel (NAP). However, NAP may screen patients for the presence of pain by asking patients if they are having pain. If the patient is in pain, the NAP report this to the nurse for in-depth assessment and evaluation.

Regardless of the type of therapies used, your ability to show caring toward a patient will maximize pain control (see Chapter 18). You minimize pain through caring behaviors such as gentle handling and touch (Ferrell, 2005). Two types of touching, task-oriented and caring, will benefit patients. Task-oriented touching occurs when a nurse takes a patient's blood pressure or helps the patient walk. Caring touch successfully influences a patient's comfort. It shows concern, such as holding the patient's hand during a procedure. You will often combine task-oriented and affective touching (e.g.,

CONCEPT MAP

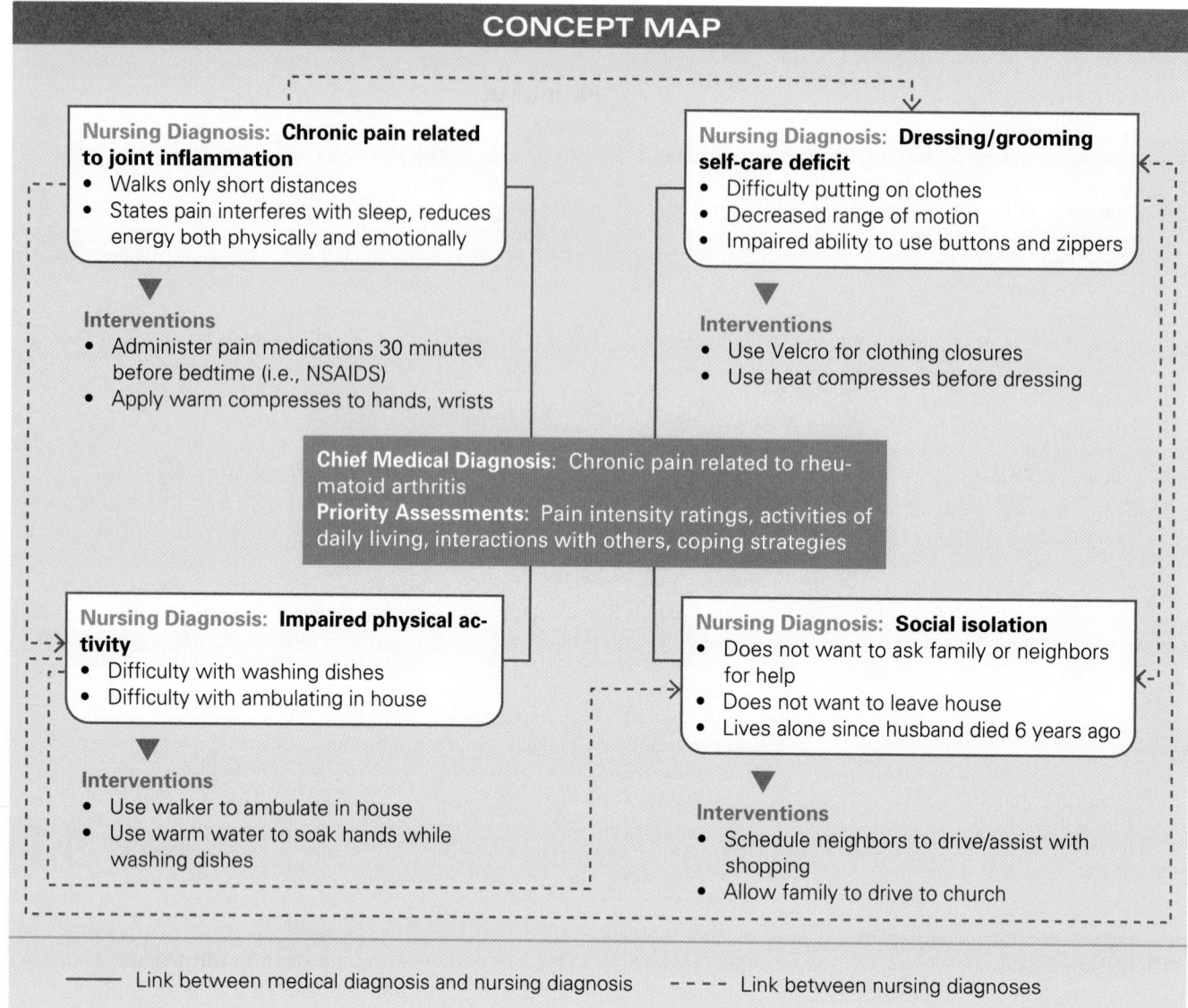

Nursing Diagnosis: Chronic pain related to joint inflammation
- Walks only short distances
- States pain interferes with sleep, reduces energy both physically and emotionally

Interventions
- Administer pain medications 30 minutes before bedtime (i.e., NSAIDS)
- Apply warm compresses to hands, wrists

Nursing Diagnosis: Dressing/grooming self-care deficit
- Difficulty putting on clothes
- Decreased range of motion
- Impaired ability to use buttons and zippers

Interventions
- Use Velcro for clothing closures
- Use heat compresses before dressing

Chief Medical Diagnosis: Chronic pain related to rheumatoid arthritis
Priority Assessments: Pain intensity ratings, activities of daily living, interactions with others, coping strategies

Nursing Diagnosis: Impaired physical activity
- Difficulty with washing dishes
- Difficulty with ambulating in house

Interventions
- Use walker to ambulate in house
- Use warm water to soak hands while washing dishes

Nursing Diagnosis: Social isolation
- Does not want to ask family or neighbors for help
- Does not want to leave house
- Lives alone since husband died 6 years ago

Interventions
- Schedule neighbors to drive/assist with shopping
- Allow family to drive to church

——— Link between medical diagnosis and nursing diagnosis   - - - - Link between nursing diagnoses

Figure 31-6 ■ Concept Map. *NSAIDs,* Nonsteroidal antiinflammatory drugs.

placing a hand on the patient's shoulder while administering a tablet). Chapter 18 explains forms of touch in detail. When you successfully convey compassion, maintain the patient's dignity, and consistently strive to minimize discomfort, pain-relieving measures will be more successful.

HEALTH PROMOTION When providing pain-relief measures, choose therapies suited to the patient's unique pain experience. Box 31-8 includes guidelines that are still applicable for individualizing pain therapy (McCaffery, 1979).

Maintaining Wellness Measures that promote a sense of well-being by minimizing or avoiding discomfort include warm baths, personal hygiene measures, and a schedule of adequate rest. Chapter 30 discusses the effect pain has on a patient's sleep pattern and ways to promote better sleep habits. Also help the patient find ways to plan rest periods before participating in exhausting activities. Patients with chronic pain need to rest before any social activities in the home.

Some pain disables and immobilizes a person enough to impair the ability to perform self-care activities. As a result,

the patient also experiences social isolation, depression, and changes in self-concept. Change in function means a significant loss to a patient. Help patients and families learn to discuss their feelings about the loss so as to find ways to cope with pain and the lifestyle it imposes (see Chapter 25).

Pain from an injury or disabling illness often limits a patient's mobility. In this case, you aim health promotion at retaining function. Instruct patients and families in the safe and proper use of elastic bandages, braces, and splints that protect body parts. When a patient has chronic, disabling pain, instruct family members in proper positioning techniques and ways to assist the patient with ambulation.

Refer patients who have difficulty eating, bathing, grooming, and dressing to an occupational therapist. Some agencies require a health care provider's order to begin occupational therapy. Devices designed to maintain function, even when finger movement or grasp is impaired, will help. The therapist attaches eating utensils, a comb, or a toothbrush to extension devices that have enlarged handles or splints for easy

BOX 31-8 Guidelines for Individualized Pain Therapy

- *Use different types of pain-relief measures.* This produces an additive effect in reducing pain and allows for changes in the character of pain.
- *Provide pain-relief measures before pain becomes severe.* It is easier to prevent severe pain than to try to relieve it after it occurs.
- *Use measures the patient believes are effective.* The patient's beliefs make pain therapy successful, so include those remedies unless they are harmful.
- *Some patients have ideas about measures to use and times to use them.* Consider the patient's ability or willingness to participate in pain-relief measures.
- *Suggest measures that require little physical effort for patients unable to actively assist with pain therapy because of fatigue or altered levels of consciousness.* Do not force participation.
- *Choose pain-relief measures on the basis of patient behavior that reflects the severity of pain.* Never administer a potent analgesic for mild pain. Only the patient can determine the potency of an effective therapy.
- *Depending on the therapy, ensure that you attempt a sufficient trial before abandoning it.* Pharmacological interventions, particularly, often need around-the-clock (ATC) administration for several days to attain and maintain therapeutic level and thus provide pain relief.
- *Keep an open mind about ways to relieve pain.* Rejecting nonconventional therapy leads to mistrust. Be sure all therapies are safe.
- *Keep trying.* When efforts at pain relief fail, do not abandon the patient but reassess the situation and consider alternative therapies.
- *Protect the patient.* Pain therapy does not cause more distress than the pain itself; you want to relieve pain without disabling the patient mentally, emotionally, or physically.
- *Educate the patient about pain.* Explain the cause of pain, times when you will give analgesics, and alternative therapies.

use. Velcro fasteners on clothing allow patients to remove or apply clothing by themselves.

Some patients with pain avoid sexual activity. However, pain does not negate the need for sexual warmth. Patients learn to express themselves sexually by assuming alternative positions during intercourse and learning more about ways to make their partner feel sexually stimulated. Caution patients that some pain medications decrease libido and often cause impotency.

Nonpharmacological Pain-Relief Measures There are a number of nonpharmacological or complementary therapies for pain relief: massage, imagery, music, biofeedback, meditation, hypnosis, prayer, journaling, exercise, therapeutic touch, acupuncture, and relaxation techniques (Barclay, 2007). Several of these therapies require special training to perform, including biofeedback and acupuncture. You will use other therapies, such as massage, imagery, and relaxation techniques that lessen the reception and perception of pain, in a variety of health care settings. Use these therapies in combination with pharmacological measures. The AHCPR guidelines for acute pain management (1992) cite nonpharmacological interventions to be appropriate for patients who:

- Find such interventions appealing
- Express anxiety or fear
- Will benefit from avoiding or reducing drug therapy
- Are likely to experience and need to cope with a prolonged interval of postoperative pain
- Have incomplete pain relief with use of pharmacological therapies

You are responsible for evaluating the effects of nonpharmacological measures to ensure pain relief. Do not exclude patients using nonpharmacological measures from use of pharmacological therapies.

Reducing Pain Reception and Perception. One of the most basic nursing responsibilities is protecting the patient from harm. A simple way to promote comfort is by removing or preventing painful stimuli. For example, tighten and smooth wrinkled bed linen, and be sure to position patients off tubing and other equipment. Change wet dressings or bed linen immediately. Do not allow tubing from a Foley catheter to become kinked, because bladder distention is uncomfortable. When repositioning patients, lift them in bed, using safe patient handling techniques, do not pull, and position them in correct anatomical alignment. Avoid exposing the skin to irritants such as diarrheal stool or wound drainage. Many of these measures are easy for family members to learn. Removing noxious stimuli is especially important for patients who are immobile. You prevent pain by anticipating painful activities (e.g., ambulation or turning). Before performing a procedure, consider the patient's condition, aspects of the procedure that are painful, and ways to avoid causing pain. It takes only simple consideration of the patient's comfort and a little extra time to avoid pain-producing situations.

Anticipatory Guidance. Modifying anxiety directly associated with pain relieves pain and adds to the effects of other pain-relief measures. The AHCPR (1992) reports that giving patients detailed descriptions of all medical procedures and expected postoperative discomfort and giving instruction for decreasing treatment- and mobility-related pain decrease self-reported pain, analgesic use, and postoperative length of stay. Provide patients sufficient procedural and sensory information (e.g., prick of a needle during blood draw or burning during urinary catheter insertion) to satisfy their interests and enable them to assess, evaluate, and communicate pain (McCaffery and Pasero, 1999).

Distraction. With meaningful sensory stimuli, a patient is able to ignore or become unaware of pain. Pleasurable sensory stimuli reduce pain perception by the release of endorphins. Distraction directs a patient's attention to something else, thus reducing the awareness of pain. Distraction works best for short, intense pain lasting a few minutes such as during an invasive procedure or while waiting for an analgesic to work. Useful forms of distraction include singing, praying, listening to music, describing photos out loud, telling jokes, and playing games.

Cutaneous Stimulation. Stimulation of the skin to relieve pain is called **cutaneous stimulation.** A massage, cold and heat applications, and **transcutaneous electrical nerve stimulation (TENS)** are simple ways to reduce pain perception. The mode of action for cutaneous stimulation is unclear, but it will often release endorphins. The gate control theory suggests that cutaneous stimulation activates larger, faster A-beta sensory nerve fibers that are sensitive to touch, pressure, and warmth. This decreases pain transmission through small diameter A-delta and C fibers. Synaptic gates thus close to pain transmission (Menefee-Pujol and others, 2007).

An advantage to cutaneous stimulation is that patients can use these measures in the home, giving them and their families some control over pain symptoms and treatment. The proper use of cutaneous stimulation reduces pain perception and helps to reduce muscle tension that will otherwise increase pain. When using cutaneous stimulation methods, eliminate environmental noise, help the patient to assume a comfortable position, and explain the purpose of the therapy. Do not use cutaneous stimulation directly on sensitive skin areas (e.g., burns, bruises, skin rashes, inflammation, or underlying bone fractures).

Nurses have used massage as a safe and effective way to produce physical and mental relaxation, reduce pain, and enhance the effectiveness of pain medication for many years. Massaging the back and shoulders or the hands and feet for 3 to 5 minutes helps relax muscles and promotes sleep (Cassileth and Vickers, 2004). The procedural guidelines (Box 31-9) summarize steps for administering a massage. Massage communicates caring, and family members are able to learn how to do this easily (McCaffery and Pasero, 1999).

Cold and heat applications relieve pain and promote healing (see Chapter 36). The choice to use heat or cold is based on the origin of the pain and the patient's past preferences and experiences with pain relief using these methods. The use of heat or cold applications in the acute care setting requires a health care provider's order. When using any form of heat or cold application, instruct the patient to avoid injury to the skin. For example, when using a heating pad for an extended period, set the control on a low temperature and wrap the pad in a towel to avoid injury. Never allow a patient to sleep lying on a heating pad. Patients with spinal cord or other neurological injuries, older adults, and confused patients are at risk for burns from heating pads or other devices.

TENS is a form of stimulation of the skin with a mild electrical current passed through external electrodes. TENS is useful in managing postoperative pain and in reducing pain caused by postoperative procedures (e.g., removing drains) (Barclay, 2007). TENS is safe, noninvasive, inexpensive, and easy to use. It requires a health care provider's order.

Relaxation. The ability to relax physically promotes mental relaxation. **Relaxation** techniques give patients self-control when pain occurs, reversing the physical and emotional stress of pain. Patients who use relaxation successfully go through physiological and behavioral changes (e.g., decreased pulse, blood pressure, and muscle tension). Relaxation strategies include simple relaxation, imagery, and music-assisted relaxation, which have been successful in reducing self-reported pain and analgesic use (McCaffery and Pasero, 1999). The techniques require periodic reinforcement through encouragement and coaching.

For effective relaxation, the patient needs to participate and cooperate. Teach relaxation techniques only when the patient is not in acute discomfort or severe pain and thus is able to concentrate. Explain the technique in detail. It sometimes takes several teaching sessions before patients effectively minimize pain. Patients can practice relaxation training indefinitely and usually with no side effects. Remove any noises or other irritating stimuli, such as bright lights, from the environment. Have the patient sit in a comfortable chair in good alignment or lie in bed. A light sheet or blanket keeps the patient warm and comfortable. Describe common sensations that the patient will experience (e.g., a decrease in temperature, a feeling of heaviness, or numbness of a body part). The patient uses these sensations as feedback. Acting as a coach, guide the patient slowly through the steps of the exercise. You perform relaxation alone or with guided imagery.

In **guided imagery,** the patient creates an image in the mind, concentrates on that image, and gradually becomes less aware of pain (Baird and Sands, 2004). Initially ask the patient to think of a pleasant scene or experience that promotes using all senses. The patient describes the image, and you record it for later use. Use only specific information given by the patient, and make no changes in the image. The following is an example of a portion of a guided imagery exercise:

Imagine yourself lying on a cool bed of grass with the sounds of water trickling over stones in a nearby stream. It's a warm day. You turn to see a patch of blue wildflowers in bloom, and you smell their fragrance.

Sit close enough so the patient can hear you, but not so close that you are intrusive. A calm, soft voice helps the patient to focus more completely on the suggested image. While relaxing, the patient focuses on the image, and you speak continuously. If the patient shows signs of agitation, restlessness, or discomfort, stop the exercise and begin later when the patient is more at ease.

Progressive relaxation exercises involve a combination of controlled breathing exercises and a series of contractions and relaxation of muscle groups (Dossey, Keegan, and Guzzetta, 2005). The patient begins by breathing slowly and diaphragmatically, allowing the abdomen to rise slowly and the chest to expand fully. Often a patient closes the eyes to focus on the exercise. When the patient establishes a regular breathing pattern, coach the patient to locate any area of

BOX 31-9   PROCEDURAL GUIDELINE

Massage

DELEGATION CONSIDERATIONS: The skill of a massage can be delegated to nursing assistive personnel (NAP). Direct the NAP by:

- Informing what massage techniques are effective with patient
- Explaining which body parts to massage
- Explaining the importance of not massaging reddened skin areas
- Clarifying the early signs of impaired skin integrity
- Instructing to report changes in skin appearance
- Instructing to report a worsening in patient's pain

EQUIPMENT: Lotion, bath towel, folded sheet

1 Based on patient assessment, decide on performing massage on one or more body parts.
2 Assess skin areas for reddened areas or impaired skin integrity.
3 Collect appropriate equipment.
4 Explain procedure to the patient.
5 Identify patient using two identifiers (e.g., name and birthday or name and account number, according to facility policy).
6 Perform hand hygiene.
7 Help patient to assume comfortable lying or sitting position.
8 Dim room lights, and/or turn on soft music.
9 Use warm body lotion as lubricant.
10 Massage each body part at least 10 minutes.

Hands: Make contact with the patient's skin, first with one hand and then the other. Using both hands, slowly open the patient's palm, gliding your fingers over the palmar surface. While supporting the hand, use both thumbs to apply friction to the palm, and use them in a circular motion to stretch the palm outward. Massage each finger outward and then separately, using a corkscrewlike motion from base of finger to the tip. With thumb and finger, knead each small muscle in the patient's fingers. Glide hands smoothly from fingertips to wrists. Repeat for other hand.

Arms: Use a gliding stroke to massage from the patient's wrist to forearm. With thumb and forefinger of both hands, knead muscles from forearm to shoulder. Continue kneading biceps, deltoid, and triceps muscles. Finish with gliding strokes from the wrist to the shoulder.

Neck: Support the neck at the hairline with one hand and starting at the base of the neck, massage upward with a gliding stroke. Knead muscles on one side. Switch hands to support neck, and knead other side. Stretch the neck slightly, with one hand at the top and the other at the bottom.

Back: Begin at sacral area, and massage in circular motion (Figure 31-7) while moving upward from buttocks to shoulders. Use a firm, smooth stroke over the scapula. Continue in one smooth stroke to upper arms and laterally along sides of back down to iliac crests. Use long, gliding strokes along muscles of spine. Knead any muscles that feel tense or tight.

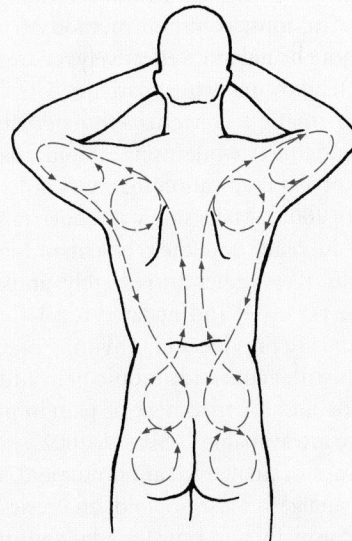

Figure 31-7 ■ Back massage pattern.

Critical Decision Point: Do not give back or neck massages to patients who have had neck or spinal trauma and/or surgery without an order by their primary health care provider.

---

11 At end of massage, have patient relax, taking slow, deep breaths.
12 Ask the patient to rate the level of pain.
13 Note any areas of muscle pain or tension.
14 Note any areas of redness or impairment.

---

muscular tension, think about how it feels, gently tense the muscles, and then completely relax them. This creates the sensation of removing all discomfort and stress. Gradually, the patient will relax the muscles without first tensing them. After the patient achieves full relaxation, pain perception is lowered, and anxiety toward the pain experience becomes minimal. If the patient becomes agitated or uncomfortable, stop the exercise. If the patient reports difficulty relaxing part of the body, slow the progression of the exercise and concentrate on the tensed body part. If the patient reports increased pain, focus on relaxing areas of muscle tension instead of consciously tensing the muscle. The patient may stop the exercise at any time. With practice, the patient will learn to perform relaxation exercises independently. Relaxation techniques are particularly effective for chronic pain, labor pains, and relief of procedure-related pain. The techniques are less effective for episodes of acute or severe pain.

ACUTE CARE In the acute care setting the additional effects of other symptoms and multiple treatments make pain management complex. Your ability to make appropriate decisions depends on a critical thinking approach.

Pharmacological Pain Therapy All pharmacological agents require a health care provider's order. Your judgment in the use of medications with or without other pain therapies ensures the best pain relief possible. A systematic approach to pain assessment and treatment choices ensures quick response on the part of caregivers to patient discomfort.

Analgesics. The most common method of pain relief is **analgesics.** Although analgesics effectively relieve pain, nurses and physicians tend to undertreat patients. This is due to incorrect drug information, concerns about addiction, anxiety over errors in judgment while using opioid analgesics, and administration of less medication than was ordered (D'Arcy, 2008; Nicholson, 2008). Make sure you understand the drugs available for pain relief and their pharmacological effects. Reassure patients that addiction is highly unlikely. Agency policies must be reviewed and updated regularly to support and guide health care providers in providing maximum pain relief to patients with acute and chronic pain and pain at the end of life. Guidelines for treatment of pain in patients with addictive disease are available (ASPMN, 2002).

The three types of analgesics are nonopioid, opioid, and adjuvant or coanalgesics. Nonopioid analgesics, including acetaminophen, aspirin, and nonsteroidal antiinflammatory drugs (NSAIDs), are effective in treating mild to moderate pain. Ketorolac (Toradol) is an injectable analgesic NSAID that is comparable to morphine in potency and used for severe pain. NSAIDs act by inhibiting the synthesis of **prostaglandins** and by inhibiting the cellular responses during inflammation. Most NSAIDs act on peripheral nerve receptors to diminish transmission and reception of pain stimuli. Acetaminophen acts on central nervous system prostaglandins.

You generally use **opioid** analgesics for severe pain. The term *opioid* is preferred to *narcotic* because the word *narcotic* generally infers illegal use of a variety of substances (McCaffery and Pasero, 1999). Opioids are natural, semisynthetic, or synthetic medications that relieve pain by binding to receptor sites in the nervous system. Opioid analgesics include codeine, morphine, hydromorphone (Dilaudid), fentanyl, oxycodone, propoxyphene (Darvon), and other natural and synthetic medications. Meperidine HCl (Demerol) is no longer a drug of choice because its metabolite, normeperidine, has the potential to cause seizures (APS, 2003; Raymo, Camejo, and Fudin, 2007). Opioids act on the central nervous system to produce a combination of depressing and stimulating effects. Opioid analgesics affect the higher centers of the brain and spinal cord by binding with opiate receptors (mu, kappa, and delta) to modify perception of and reaction to pain. Morphine is a derivative of opium that reduces the

perception of pain, reduces anxiety and fear (components of the reaction to pain), and induces sleep. Morphine and other opioids may depress vital nervous system functions such as respirations (rate and depth), although this is rare (McCaffery and Pasero, 1999). If severe respiratory depression develops, administer small doses of the opioid antagonist naloxone (Narcan) intravenously, according to policy, to increase respiratory rate and depth. Patients often have side effects such as nausea, vomiting, constipation, and altered mental processes when they take opioids (Palos and others, 2004). Traditionally opioids have been used to treat acute pain; however, their use to manage chronic pain is becoming acceptable (Vallerand and others, 2007).

When a patient uses opioids around-the-clock (ATC) for approximately a week or more, expect physical dependence. Physical dependence is the appearance of symptoms of withdrawal when the opioid is reduced or stopped abruptly or reversed with an opioid antagonist (naloxone). Addiction is psychological dependence. Physical dependence and addiction are not the same (APS, 2003). A patient may be physically dependent and addicted; however, a patient may also be physically dependent but not addicted. It is important to teach this distinction to patients and family members.

A variety of extended-release or controlled-release oral opioid formulations (dosing intervals of 8, 10, 12, or 24 hours) and transdermal patches (dosing interval of 72 hours) are available. These formulations maintain constant serum opioid concentration, minimizing toxic and subtherapeutic concentrations. They also lessen the severity of end-of-dose pain, allowing the patient to sleep through the night, and reduce "clock watching" by patients (APS, 2003).

When you convert a patient from an intravenous (IV) to an oral form of the same opioid, understand that the dose of the oral opioid is usually much higher than the IV dose because of the first-pass effect (McCaffery and Pasero, 1999). When a patient takes oral opioids, the opioids first go to the liver, where most (but not all) of the medication is inactivated. Thus the body needs larger doses of oral opioids to achieve the same level of pain relief as the same opioid given IV.

At times it is appropriate to switch a patient from one opioid to another. Sometimes a patient experiences intolerable side effects, is not able to swallow, or develops gastrointestinal problems. There are many opioid equianalgesic conversion charts available for determining equivalent doses of opioids (APS, 2003). If the health care provider switches the patient to a different opioid, it is important to reduce the new opioid dose by about 50% because of incomplete cross-tolerance (APS, 2003). Cross-tolerance is the development of tolerance to the therapeutic and adverse effects of pharmacologically related drugs (McCaffery and Pasero, 1999). Thus, although patients are tolerant to one opioid's effects, this does not mean they will be tolerant to a different opioid's effect.

Adjuvants or coanalgesics such as sedatives, anticonvulsants, steroids, antidepressants, antianxiety agents, and muscle relaxants have analgesic properties, enhance pain control, or relieve other symptoms associated with pain, such as anxiety, depression, and nausea. You give these alone or with analgesics (Bruckenthal and D'Arcy, 2007; Jann and Slade, 2007). Many of these agents are more effective than opioids in relieving neuropathic pain.

The proper use of analgesics requires careful assessment, application of pharmacological principles, and common sense (Box 31-10). Not all patients react the same way to analgesics. An NSAID is as effective as an opioid for some patients but not others. An orally administered analgesic usually brings the same relief as an injectable form. Remain familiar with comparative doses of different analgesics (equianalgesics). This information is readily available from your agency pharmacy. In addition, nurses on succeeding shifts will need to know the route of administration most effective for a patient so the patient will achieve controlled, sustained pain relief. Avoid repetitive intramuscular or subcutaneous injections of medications.

Children require careful calculation of drug doses. Equianalgesia charts that convert recommended adult doses to children's doses are available. These charts consider age and body size. Older adults also require special considerations (Box 31-11).

Patient-Controlled Analgesia. Patients benefit from having control over pain therapy. PCA is a safe method for a variety of painful conditions, including but not limited to postoperative, traumatic, labor and delivery, sickle cell crisis, cancer, and end-of-life pain management (Pasero, 2003d). It is a drug-delivery system that allows patients to administer pain medications when they want them, without repeated injections. It has been an effective form of pain management with older adults and with children as young as 5 years of age (Schechter and others, 2003). You administer PCA medications intravenously or subcutaneously. PCA uses portable infusion pumps containing a cassette or chamber for a syringe (Figure 31-8) that delivers a small preset dose of medication (usually morphine, fentanyl, or hydromorphone). To receive a dose, the patient pushes a button attached to the PCA device. The system is designed to deliver no more than a specified number of doses either every hour or every 4 hours (depending on the pump) to avoid overdoses. A typical PCA prescription relies on a series of "loading" doses (e.g., 3 to 5 mg of morphine, repeated every 5 to 10 minutes until initial pain diminishes). A low-dose basal infusion (0.5 to 1 mg/hr) at night allows uninterrupted sleep. Use continuous basal infusions with caution in opioid-naive patients (patients who have used opioids around the clock *less* than approximately 1 week) during the first 24 to 48 hours

---

BOX 31-10 Nursing Principles for Administering Analgesics

KNOW THE PATIENT'S PREVIOUS RESPONSE TO ANALGESICS
- Determine whether patient obtained relief.
- Ask whether a nonopioid was as effective as an opioid.
- Identify previous doses and routes of administration to avoid undertreatment.
- Determine whether the patient has allergies.

SELECT PROPER MEDICATIONS WHEN MORE THAN ONE IS ORDERED
- Use acetaminophen, NSAIDs, or combination drugs (e.g., oxycodone with acetaminophen) for mild to moderate pain.
- The concurrent use of opioids and NSAIDs often provides for more effective analgesia than either drug class alone.
- Use of NSAIDs helps reduce opioid dose and also opioid side effects.
- In older adults, avoid combinations of opioids.
- Remember that morphine, hydromorphone, and oxycodone are the opioids of choice for long-term management of severe pain.
- Know that injectable medications act quicker and relieve severe, acute pain within 1 hour and that oral medications take as long as 2 hours to relieve pain.
- For chronic pain, give oral extended-release formulations for longer, more sustained relief.

KNOW THE ACCURATE DOSAGE
- Remember that patients with severe pain generally need higher doses of analgesics.

- Adjust doses, as appropriate, for children and older patients.
- Dosage typically requires adjustment over time.
- Know the comparative potencies of analgesics (refer to drug manual or pharmacy) in oral and injectable form.

ASSESS THE RIGHT TIME AND INTERVAL FOR ADMINISTRATION
- Administer analgesics as soon as pain occurs and before it increases in severity.
- Do not give analgesics only on "as needed" (prn) schedules. An around-the-clock (ATC) administration schedule is best.
- Give analgesics *before* pain-producing procedures or activities.
- Know the average peak and duration of action for a drug so that you time drug administration to peak when pain is most intense.
- Give extended-release opioid formulations on an ATC basis and not prn.

CHOOSE THE RIGHT ROUTE
- Oral route is preferred; intravenous route preferred if patient is unable to swallow or has gastrointestinal problems.
- Avoid intramuscular and subcutaneous administration because those routes are painful and absorption is not reliable.

NSAIDs, Nonsteroidal antiinflammatory drugs.

BOX 31-11 CARE OF THE OLDER ADULT

Principles of Pain Management

- Pain is *not* a normal part of aging. Presence of pain requires aggressive assessment and management.
- Older adults are at high risk for pain-inducing situations.
- Several pain-producing conditions sometimes coexist.
- Older adults are often fearful that pain will result in loss of independence, making them a burden to their family.
- Age-related changes in pain perception are most likely not clinically significant (American Geriatrics Society [AGS], 2002).
- Older patients experience faster onset, longer duration of action, and adverse effects from analgesics because of lower serum protein levels and reduced liver, renal, and cardiac function.
- Older adults are more sensitive to the analgesic and adverse effects of opioid drugs because they experience a higher peak and longer duration of pain relief. Thus start with low doses of opioids, and increase the dose very slowly as needed (Bruckenthal and D'Arcy, 2007).
- When choosing an opioid, avoid propoxyphene (Darvon, Darvocet) in older patients because of possible cardiovascular and neurological adverse effects (AGS, 2002).
- There is an increased risk for gastric and renal toxicity from NSAIDs among older adults.

NSAIDs, Nonsteroidal antiinflammatory drugs.

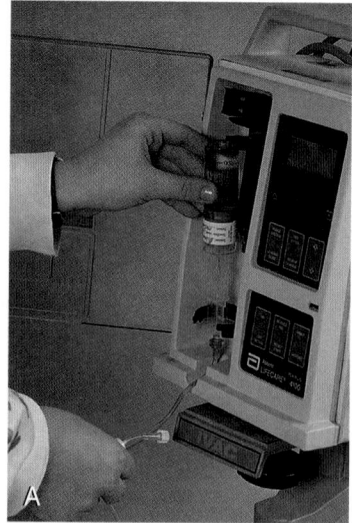

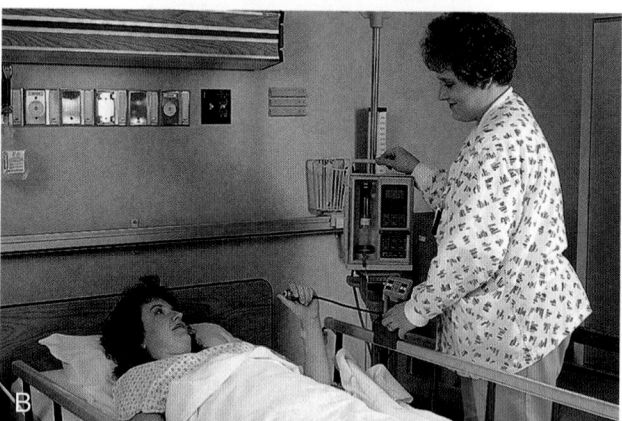

Figure 31-8 ■ **A,** PCA pump with syringe chamber. **B,** Patient learns to use PCA pump.

postoperatively because of the possibility of respiratory depression from the combination of anesthetics with opioids (McCaffery and Pasero, 1999). On-demand doses typically add 1 mg of morphine every 6 minutes, with a total hourly limit of 10 mg (APS, 2003). Most pumps have locked safety systems to prevent tampering.

Benefits of PCA include the following:

- Patients have control over pain.
- Pain relief does not depend on nurses' availability.
- Patients tend to take less medication.
- Small doses of opioids delivered at short intervals stabilize serum drug concentrations for sustained pain relief.

Patient preparation and teaching are critical to the safe and effective use of PCA (Box 31-12). Patients having surgery receive teaching and demonstration of the PCA pump before surgery if the health care provider orders PCA use. Patients need to understand the use of the equipment and be physically able to locate and press the button to deliver the dose (Pasero, 2003d; Wuhrman and others, 2006). Therefore PCA therapy is usually not appropriate for patients who are confused, have altered levels of consciousness, or are unable to understand how to use the equipment.

Check the patient's IV line or subcutaneous needle placement and PCA device regularly to ensure proper functioning. Certain pumps keep track of cumulative dosage and print out the information when needed. Document drug doses carefully, and record any wasted or unused opioid. Monitor the patient for adverse drug effects, as well as pain management effectiveness (Pasero, 2003d; Wuhrman and others, 2006). Use of PCA gives you and the patient more flexibility in pain management. Make sure to teach family members that only the patient can push the button to administer the medication. This will minimize the patient receiving too much medication. There are some situations (PCA use with children, nonverbal patients, patients with nonacute mental status changes, patients with paralysis) in which nurse-activated dosing (primary nurse) or family-controlled analgesia is appropriate. In such situations, family and nurse discussions are critical. With family-controlled analgesia, you select one family member or significant other to be the patient's primary pain manager (Pasero, 2003d). In addition, you place a sign on the PCA machine indicating the person responsible for pushing the button. The ASPMN is currently developing a position statement on proxy/other-than-patient–controlled analgesia (Arnstein, personal communication, 2005).

BOX 31-12 PATIENT TEACHING

Preparation for Patient-Controlled Analgesia

A female patient will be started on a subcutaneous patient-controlled analgesia (PCA) pump to manage her pain following a total knee replacement. The nurse develops the following teaching plan:

OUTCOME
- At the end of the teaching session, the patient will describe when and how to use the PCA machine and will demonstrate use of the equipment.

TEACHING STRATEGIES
- Teach the relationship among pain, pushing the PCA button, and pain relief (APS, 2003; Wuhrman and others, 2006).
- Instruct patient in the purpose of PCA, operating instructions, expected pain relief, precautions, and potential side effects (Pasero, 2003d), emphasizing that the patient controls medication therapy.
- Reinforce the principle of treating the pain *before* it becomes too severe.
- Remind patient to press the button before painful events (e.g., physical therapy).
- Explain that the pump minimizes risk for overdose.
- Tell family members or friends that they are *not* to operate the PCA device for the patient (Wuhrman and others, 2006).
- Demonstrate how to push the button and how to prevent pulling on PCA tubing to avoid dislodging catheter (Pasero, 2003d).

EVALUATION STRATEGIES
- Before activating the PCA system, have patient demonstrate use of the PCA delivery button.
- Ask patient and family to verbalize who is to push the button.
- Have patient state when to push the button.
- Ask patient to describe expected results of pushing the button and what to do if he or she does not get the expected results.

Placebo Effect. Dose forms that contain no pharmacologically active ingredients (e.g., normal saline injection or sugar pill) are called **placebos.** Use of placebos is considered highly unethical (Grace, 2006; McCaffery and Arnstein, 2006) and against policy in many hospitals even with a health care provider's order. However, you will use knowledge of the placebo response when administering analgesics by telling patients that the drug will act to reduce pain. Belief that a medication will work and trust in the nurse increase the likelihood of pain relief.

Local Anesthetics. The loss of sensation to a localized body part is termed **local anesthesia.** Health care providers provide local anesthesia by injecting a medication (e.g., lidocaine, bupivacaine [Marcaine], or ropivacaine [Naropin]) into tissues, near major nerves, or intraspinally before suturing a wound, moving a painful body part, delivering an infant, and performing some surgery. Local anesthetics have fewer risks than general anesthetics, which cause loss of consciousness and depress vital functions. The drugs produce temporary loss of sensation by inhibiting nerve conduction; they also block motor and autonomic functions when administered as nerve blocks. Typically, a patient loses sensation in small sensory nerves before losing motor function; conversely, motor activity returns before sensation.

After administration of a local anesthetic, you need to protect the patient from injury until full sensory and motor function return. Patients can easily injure themselves without knowing it. You need to educate patients receiving local anesthesia by explaining insertion sites and warning them that they will temporarily lose sensory function. Some patients also lose autonomic function (bowel and bladder control) temporarily. Further reassure patients by explaining the application of the anesthetic and the sensations that they will experience. Injection is painful unless the health care provider first numbs the injection site. Prepare patients for such discomfort. Before a patient receives an anesthetic, check the patient's medication allergies. To monitor systemic effects, assess vital signs.

Epidural Analgesia. Epidural analgesia is a form of local anesthesia and an effective therapy for the treatment of postoperative, traumatic, chronic noncancer, and cancer pain (Pasero, 2003b, 2003c; Roman and Cabaj, 2005). It permits control or reduction of severe pain without the sedative effects of opioids. Epidural analgesia is short or long term, depending on the patient's condition and life expectancy. Short-term epidural analgesia is especially effective for pain after intrathoracic, abdominal, and orthopedic surgery. Research has shown that epidural analgesia overall provides superior postoperative analgesia compared with intravenous patient-controlled analgesia (Wu and others, 2005). Long-term epidural therapy is effective for pain unresponsive to oral or parenteral medications. The advantages of epidural analgesia include the following:

- Production of excellent analgesia
- Occurrence of minimal sedation
- Longer-lasting pain relief with fewer opioid doses
- Facilitation of early ambulation
- Avoidance of repeated injections
- No significant effect on sensation
- Little effect on blood pressure or heart rate
- Fewer pulmonary complications or improved pulmonary function

Epidural analgesia is administered into the epidural space through a catheter, which is usually placed in the operating room, postanesthesia care unit, or intensive care unit. The patient lies in the fetal position (lateral decubitus) to open the space between the vertebrae. The health care provider administers a local anesthetic into the skin at the needle insertion site and then inserts the catheter and advances it to the level of the vertebral space (usually L4-L5) nearest to the area requiring analgesia. Once the physician or advanced practice nurse advances the catheter into the epidural space

(Figure 31-9) and removes the needle, the remainder of the catheter is secured with an occlusive dressing and taped up the back of the patient. A temporary catheter is sometimes connected to tubing positioned along the spine and over the patient's shoulder. You can then place the end of the catheter on the patient's chest for easier access. Permanent catheters are tunneled through the skin and exit at the patient's side. Assessment of the insertion site and patency of the tubing is an important nursing responsibility (Pasero, 2003b, 2003c).

The epidural catheter is connected to a continuous **epidural infusion** pump, a port, a reservoir, or it is capped off for bolus injections. In many hospitals only anesthesiologists or nurse anesthetists administer epidural anesthesia. However, registered nurses certified in this procedure also administer epidural anesthesia in some settings. In addition, some institutions allow patients to deliver the epidural analgesic (patient-controlled epidural analgesia) via a pump. To reduce the risk for accidental epidural injection of drugs intended for IV use, it helps to place a brightly colored intermittent injection cap on the catheter tubing. Labeling the catheter "epidural catheter" or using color coded catheters is recommended by The Joint Commission (2006) to prevent accidental connections of IV tubing to the epidural catheters. Hospitals use tubing that has no access ports in order to minimize accidental introduction of intravenous medications. Administer continuous infusions through electronic infusion devices for proper control. Because of the catheter location, follow strict surgical aseptic technique when handling tubing, to prevent a potentially fatal infection. Notify the health care provider immediately if any signs or symptoms of infection or pain at the insertion site develop (Pasero, 2003c).

Medications used commonly for epidural analgesia include preservative-free solutions of morphine sulfate, hydromorphone, fentanyl, sufentanil citrate, bupivacaine, ropivacaine, clonidine, and methadone. Sometimes your patient will receive a combination of two of these solutions. Morphine has a long-lasting effect but also causes more side effects. The medications block transmission of pain stimuli in the spinal cord by primarily blocking the release of the excitatory neurotransmitter substance P (Pasero, 2003a).

Nursing implications for managing epidural analgesia are numerous (Table 31-5). Monitoring for drug effects differs, depending on whether infusions are intermittent or continuous. Some complications of epidural opioid use are respiratory depression (rare), nausea and vomiting, urinary retention, constipation, orthostatic hypotension, and pruritus. Patients usually do not receive any other form of opioid, sedative, or hypnotic while receiving epidural analgesia. When you start patients on epidural analgesia, monitoring occurs as often as every 15 minutes, including assessment of respiratory rate, respiratory effort, and skin color. You may use pulse oximetry. If a patient remains stable, monitoring will take place every hour. Inform patients about the potential for respiratory depression, and instruct them to notify you if breathing difficulty develops. If respiratory depression develops, turn off the infusion immediately (Pasero, 2003a).

Invasive Pain-Relieving Devices. Advances in pain management continue to evolve. Patients with complex pain respond very effectively to invasive pain-relieving devices (D'Arcy, 2008). Continuous local anesthetic pumps used to manage primarily surgical pain have shortened hospitalization time and hastened patient recovery (D'Arcy, 2008). The surgeon places a catheter in the surgical site. The catheter exits the skin and connects to a pump with tubing secured to the external dressing. Some catheters have a "soaker hose" ending with multiple openings or a single opening at the end. Some pumps are programmed to deliver a preset, timed volume of local preservative-free anesthetic or allow patients to activate analgesic delivery when needed (demand mode). Patients often are discharged with the pump attached. Discharge teaching involves instructing patients in the signs and symptoms of anesthetic overdose and how to remove the catheter safely.

Patients With Cancer Pain Some cancer pain is stubborn and difficult to treat. It becomes so debilitating that patients will try anything to gain relief. Therefore AHCPR developed clinical practice guidelines for the management of cancer pain (Jacox and others, 1994). The guidelines treat cancer pain in a more comprehensive and aggressive manner, thus providing patients and families more options for pain relief. Figure 31-10 is a flowchart depicting cancer pain management from assessment to various treatment measures. The best choice of treat-

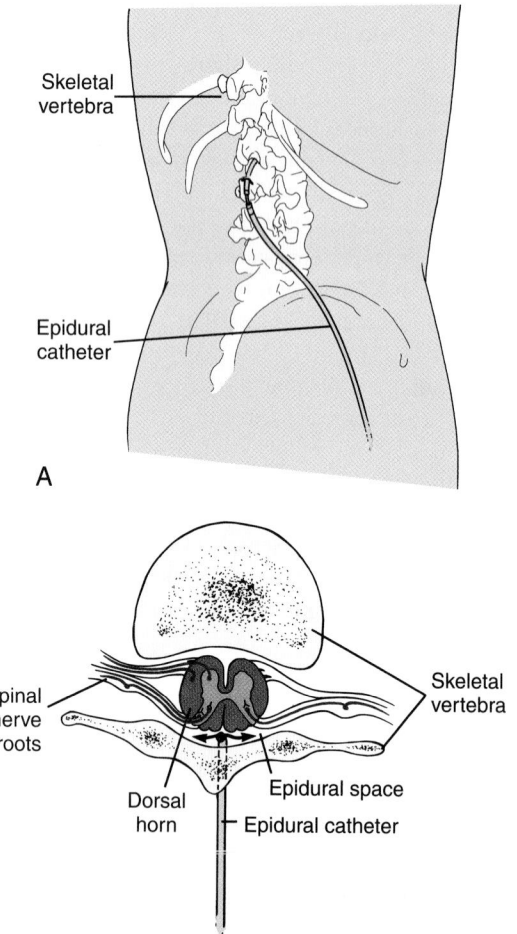

Figure 31-9 ■ **A,** Epidural catheter inserted into the L4-L5 space. **B,** Anatomical drawing of epidural space.

ment often changes when the patient's condition and the characteristics of pain change. Both nonpharmacological and pharmacological therapies are beneficial.

Administering analgesics to treat cancer-related pain requires applying principles different from those used to treat acute pain. WHO (1990) recommends a three-step approach to managing cancer pain (Figure 31-11). Therapy begins with NSAIDs and/or adjuvants and then progresses to strong opioids if pain persists. When a patient with cancer first has pain, it is best to begin with a higher dosage than what will be routinely needed. This provides the patient with immediate pain relief. The health care provider then slowly decreases the dosage to the amount that successfully controls pain. The health care provider treats side effects of analgesia aggressively so the patient is able to continue using analgesia. Patients receiving long-term opioids often develop a drug tolerance. Therefore they require higher dosages to attain pain relief. Higher dosages are not lethal, because most patients also develop tolerance to life-threatening side effects (McCaffery and Pasero, 1999). However, tolerance does not prevent the side effect of constipation. Unless this is contraindicated, patients

receiving long-term ATC opioids also receive ATC stimulant laxatives and not just stool softeners.

For patients with cancer the aim of drug therapy is to anticipate and prevent or minimize pain. Therefore it is necessary to give required analgesic dosages regularly, even when pain subsides. Regular administration maintains blood levels for ongoing pain control. However, patients still have flares of pain or "breakthrough pain" that requires additional bolus doses of medication (rescue doses). A decrease in the duration of pain relief or an increase in the intensity of pain relief provided by the regular analgesia therapy and the need for an increased number of rescue doses are indications that the patient needs a higher opioid dose (McCaffery and Pasero, 1999).

Transdermal drug systems administer drugs (e.g., fentanyl) via a patch placed on the skin. Patches are useful when patients are unable to take drugs orally. Self-adhesive patches deposit the opioid into the subcutaneous tissue. The subcutaneous tissue releases the drug slowly over time at predetermined rates for 48 to 72 hours. This results in effective analgesia throughout the day and night. Inform patients that it sometimes takes 12 to 16 hours for analgesia to take effect

TABLE 31-5   Nursing Care of Patients With Epidural Infusions

GOAL	ACTIONS
Prevent catheter displacement	Secure catheter (if not connected to implanted reservoir) carefully to skin.
Maintain catheter function	Check external dressing around catheter site for dampness or discharge. (Leak of cerebrospinal fluid may develop.)
	Use transparent, adhesive dressing to aid inspection.
	Inspect catheter for breaks.
Prevent infection	Use aseptic technique when caring for catheter.
	Do not routinely change dressing over site.
	Change tubing every 24 hours or per agency policy.
Monitor for respiratory depression	Monitor vital signs, especially respirations, per policy.
	Use pulse oximetry and apnea monitoring when necessary.
	Maintain head of bed at 30 to 45 degrees.
Prevent undesirable complications	Verify tubing is connected to epidural catheter; label appropriately.
	Verify with another RN correct preservative-free drug, dose, and volume as listed on medication order. Some institutions prohibit nurses from administering medications via the epidural catheter. Be sure to check your agency policy.
	Disinfect connection before removing port cap with only nonneurotoxic agent (povidone-iodine); do not use alcohol (Pasero, 2003a).
	Before injecting, aspirate catheter using a 5-mL syringe; allow time for fluid to travel up catheter. Less than 0.5 mL of fluid indicates catheter is in the epidural space. Return of cerebrospinal fluid or blood indicates catheter is in subarachnoid space or blood vessel. Do not administer analgesic, and notify physician or health care provider (Pasero, 2003a).
	Administer analgesic in at least a 5-mL syringe to reduce pressure on injection (Pasero, 2003a).
	If you meet strong resistance during injection, have patient flex the spine. If resistance continues, stop and notify the patient's health care provider.
	If patient reports pain during injection, stop and notify the health care provider.
	Do not flush catheter without a specific order.
Maintain urinary and bowel function	Monitor intake and output.
	Assess bladder and bowel for distention.
	Assess for discomfort, frequency, and urgency.
Monitor for adverse effects of analgesic	Assess for pruritus (itching) and nausea and vomiting.
	Administer antihistamines and antiemetics (as ordered) that cause minimal sedation.

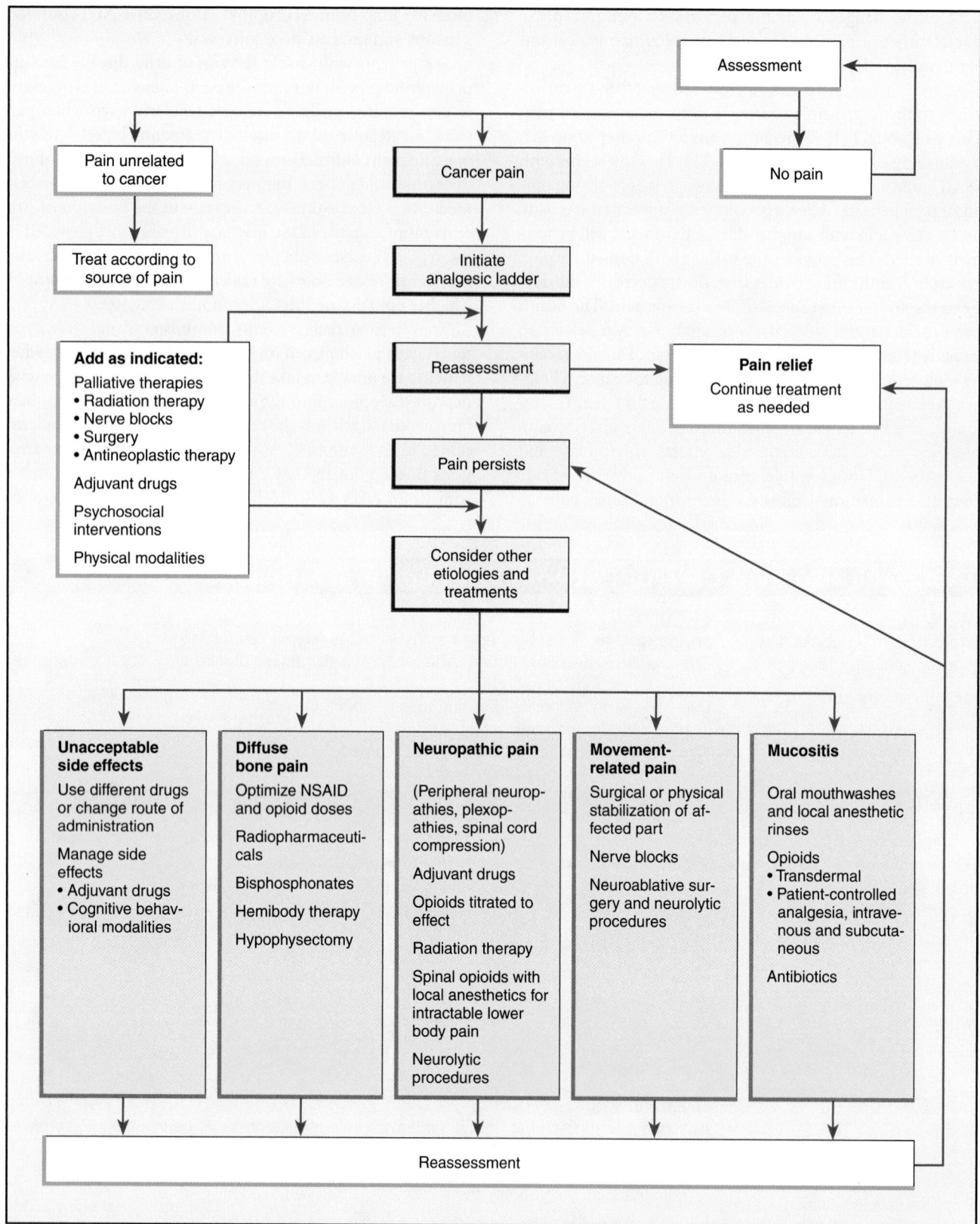

Figure 31-10 ■ Flowchart: continuing pain management in patients with cancer. *NSAID,* Nonsteroidal antiinflamma-tory drug. (From Jacox A and others: *Management of cancer pain,* Clinical Practice Guideline No. 9, AHCPR Pub No. 94-0592, Rockville Md, March 1994, Agency for Health Care Policy and Research, Public Health Service, U.S. Depart-ment of Health and Human Services.)

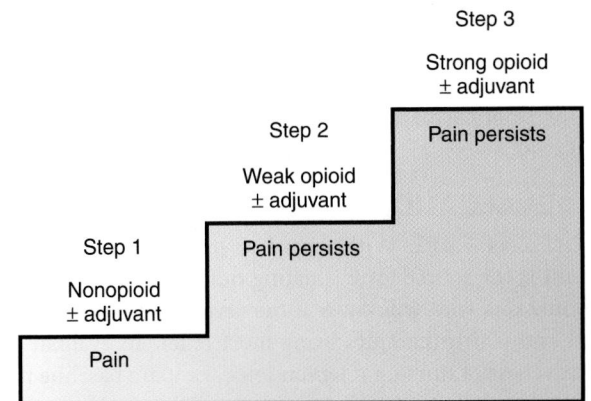

Figure 31-11 ■ WHO analgesic ladder is a three-step approach to using drugs in cancer pain management. ± *adjuvant,* With or without adjuvant medications. (From World Health Organization: *Cancer pain relief and palliative care,* Report of a WHO expert committee, WHO Technical Report Series No. 804, Geneva, Switzerland, 1990, WHO.)

when they first begin to use an analgesic patch (Argoff, 2007). Therefore it is important for you to obtain an order for an immediate-release opioid to be used for breakthrough pain. Heat causes more rapid drug absorption. For this reason, warn patients to avoid external heat such as heating pads, hot showers, and prolonged exposure to the sun while using a patch. Only patients who have chronic stable pain and who have routinely received 40 mg or more of morphine (or its equivalent) daily on an ATC basis for a week or more are candidates for a fentanyl patch.

Another measure to treat severe persistent cancer pain is morphine given by continuous IV drip or intermittently by a PCA pump. Continuous infusions provide uniform pain control at lower dosages. Thus there are fewer side effects. Continuous-drip morphine is given in acute care settings and the home. An infusion control pump delivers morphine intravenously to ensure safe and accurate administration. Each agency has guidelines for morphine dose and infusion rates.

When a patient receives continuous-drip morphine, assess the intravenous site to ensure it is patent and without complications (e.g., no redness, swelling, or drainage). When a patient starts on continuous IV morphine, you need to prevent overdose and central nervous system depression. Record baseline blood pressure and respiratory rates before the infusion begins. After the infusion starts, monitor vital signs as often as every 15 to 30 minutes for the first few hours until the patient gains relief at a constant dosage. If the patient's blood pressure or respirations decrease, reduce the infusion rate according to the health care provider's order or agency policy. For severe respiratory depression, administer small IV doses of the opioid antagonist naloxone (Narcan), according to policy, to increase respiratory rate and depth, but not reverse the pain relief.

RESTORATIVE AND CONTINUING CARE Patients in need of restorative care for pain usually have chronic persistent pain that is unrelenting. You will continue to use non-

pharmacological measures that are effective for individual patients. However, additional pharmacological measures designed to give a patient better long-term pain control are required. The focus in restorative care is to use a comprehensive approach in supporting the patient and family.

Opioid Infusions In the home or extended care settings, patients will use ambulatory infusion pumps for opioid infusions. The pumps are lightweight, compact, and allow free movement. The pump is battery powered and worn in a pouch attached to a belt or harness. The bag of medication and parenteral fluid fits inside the pump. A dose of opioid, delivered continuously over 24 hours, is usually slowly infused intravenously through a peripherally inserted central catheter (PICC) or a subclavian placed catheter (see Chapter 17). Both catheters are left in place for an extended period of time. Sometimes pain medication is infused subcutaneously using a small catheter that the patient inserts into subcutaneous tissue and replaces every 72 hours. The ambulatory pumps differ from PCA devices, which deliver only small, preset doses of medication. The patient and family learn to manage the pump, observe for drug side effects, and maintain function of the catheter that delivers the medication (Box 31-13). Because the patient is initially managed on the opioid in the hospital before going home, the risk for side effects is not as great. A home care nurse routinely visits to be sure patients or family members manage a pump correctly.

Palliative Care Palliative care offers treatments to help patients live, perhaps years, with a variety of incurable conditions, including persistent pain. The goal of palliative care is to relieve suffering and to support the best possible quality of life for patients with chronic and life-threatening conditions and their family members (National Consensus Project, 2004). Palliative care is not the same as end-of-life or hospice pain management.

Patients with chronic pain require a different approach to pain management than patients with acute pain. Unfortunately, physicians, nurses, and other health care providers cannot eliminate all pain, and learning to live with daily pain is not easy. It is important for patients with chronic pain to gain control of their pain versus allowing the pain to control them. Consider making a referral to a palliative care team when you care for patients diagnosed with incurable conditions that have persistent pain as a symptom. These teams are composed of a variety of health care professionals who help patients achieve a level of pain control that allows patients to function and enjoy life (National Consensus Project, 2004). The patient is an active participant in the management of the pain. Without patient involvement, adequate pain control will not be possible.

Hospice Hospice programs care for the terminally ill by helping patients continue to live at home in comfort and privacy with the help of a health care team. Pain control is a priority. Families learn to monitor the patient's symptoms and become primary caregivers. Chapter 25 discusses hospice in detail.

End-of-Life Care You will need to teach and reassure family members and patients about the use of analgesics at the end of life (EOL). Emphasize the need to provide maximum pain relief by increasing (titrating) the dosage of medication to meet the patient's pain-control needs (Ersek and others, 2004). It is acceptable to increase opioids by 25% to 100% depending on the patient's response and pain intensity (Curtiss, 2004). Titrating is based on percent change of a drug dose because the body does not recognize milligram or microgram changes. It is the concentration of the drug in the blood, not the number of milligrams or micrograms, that causes an effect. If the maximum dose ordered by the health care provider is ineffective, you are responsible for notifying the health care provider (ASPMN, 2002). The dosage needed to relieve the patient's pain sometimes exceeds the normal dosage range published in printed drug information. Explain that the opioid will *not* hasten the loved-one's death. In fact, appropriately dosed opioids will alleviate suffering and improve the quality of life as the end approaches (Arnold and others, 2004). You use the fastest route of medication administration until pain is under control. Once pain is controlled, use the least invasive route possible, including oral, rectal, transdermal, or sublingual routes. Remember, you will often need to use a combination of opioid, nonopioid, adjunct, and/or nonpharmacological therapies to provide adequate pain relief.

▪▪▪ EVALUATION

PATIENT CARE   With regard to pain management, the patient is the source for evaluating outcomes. The patient is the only one who will know if the severity of pain has lessened and which therapies bring most relief. To evaluate the effectiveness of nursing interventions, compare baseline pain assessments before treatments with ongoing assessment findings after treatment. Similarly, evaluate whether the patient's response to pain (e.g., positioning and body movements or ability to socialize or perform self-care) has changed (Box 31-14). Compare actual outcomes with expected outcomes (see Care Plan) to determine if your patient met his or her goal (McCaffery and Pasero, 1999). Is the patient able to per-

---

BOX 31-13   PATIENT TEACHING

Ambulatory Infusion Pumps

If your patient is discharged home with an opioid infusion pump, develop a teaching plan that will ensure adequate pain management with minimal adverse effects from the analgesic.

OUTCOMES
- At the end of the teaching session, the patient and/or family member will verbalize possible analgesic adverse effects and how to administer naloxone.
- The patient and/or family will demonstrate proper pump management and correct catheter maintenance.

TEACHING STRATEGIES
- Plan teaching session in a quiet environment at a time that is convenient for patient and family.
- Avoid teaching during times of moderate to severe pain.
- Teach patient and family the most frequent adverse effects associated with analgesic.
- Instruct family on administration of naloxone (Narcan) intramuscularly to reverse respiratory depression.
- Demonstrate how to assess the central venous catheter (CVC), peripherally inserted central catheter (PICC) line, or subcutaneous catheter insertion site and maintain or change pump flow rate.
- If the patient has a CVC or PICC, teach how to maintain the patency of the catheter by routinely flushing the catheter with saline or heparin (see agency policy or prescriber's orders to determine type, amount, and frequency of flush).
- Demonstrate how to prevent air from entering catheter and how to clamp catheter when infusion has stopped.
- Explain how to change medication bag and tubing, how to prevent infection at catheter site, and how to change the dressing per agency policy. Teach patients how frequently to change the medication bag and tubing and the

catheter dressing, and teach those with subcutaneous catheters how to change the catheter site and how frequently to change the site.
- Describe a preventive bowel routine using stool softeners, laxatives, dietary fiber, hydration, and routine exercise to prevent constipation.
- Warn patient against wearing pump in shower or submerging in bathtub. Instead have patient temporarily disconnect pump during shower or place in a plastic bag hung outside shower or tub.
- Suggest keeping the pump on the bed or on a nightstand when sleeping. During lovemaking, set pump to the side so it does not interfere with closeness and intimacy.
- Instruct the patient and family on the purpose of the pump alarms and what to do when they sound.
- Provide a 24-hour emergency telephone number.
- Answer questions honestly.
- Summarize what you taught, and clarify questions or concerns.

EVALUATION STRATEGIES
- Use open-ended questions (e.g., "Tell me some of the adverse effects that could occur that you would let your doctor or nurse know about.")
- Have patient/family demonstrate how to assess catheter insertion site and verify pump flow rate.
- If the patient has a CVC or PICC, have patient/family demonstrate how to flush the catheter.
- Have patient/family demonstrate cleaning/care of the catheter site and insertion of new subcutaneous catheter (if appropriate).
- Ask patient to explain what to do with the pump during bathing, sleeping, and lovemaking.
- Have patient verbalize what to do if the pump alarm sounds and the number to call for emergencies.

form those activities that pain had prevented? Continuous evaluation allows you to determine whether the patient needs new or revised therapies and if new nursing problems have developed. It is important to discuss the patient's ongoing pain management needs with family members and health care providers who will be involved in the patient's care upon discharge or transfer.

Part of the evaluation of the success of treatment involves consideration of abuse or misuse of opioids. Although addiction to opioids used to manage pain is rare, it is a concern that you need to evaluate (Argoff, 2007; Passik and Kirsh, 2004). You will reassess patients receiving long-term opioids for indicators of addiction such as worsening psychological well-being and social and vocational function despite aggressive attempts at pain management (Argoff, 2007). If you suspect an addiction, recommend a referral to a clinician who specializes in chemical dependency (Grant, Cordts, and Doberman, 2007).

PATIENT EXPECTATIONS Subtle behaviors such as a gentle smile or a sigh of relief indicate the level of a patient's satisfaction with pain relief. However, it is important for you to *ask* patients if you have met their expectations. Do not ask patients if they are satisfied with their pain management, because patients often answer "yes" even when their pain is severe (Whelan and others, 2004). Instead say to a patient, "Tell me how well you think your pain medicine is helping you" or "You agreed to try relaxation to lessen your abdominal pain. Tell me, how has this worked for you?" If a patient's expectations have not been met, then you need to spend more time understanding the patient's desires. Working closely with the patient will enable you to help the patient set realistic expectations that will be met within the limits of the patient's condition and treatment. It is also important to review the current pain management plan and suggest changes as appropriate.

BOX 31-14   EVALUATION

 Two weeks after his last visit, Jim returns to evaluate Mrs. Ellis' progress. Mrs. Ellis reports that she has gone to see a nurse practitioner, who prescribed an NSAID for her arthritic pain. She has not filled the prescription yet and is still taking her aspirin. Mrs. Ellis continues to have some gastrointestinal irritation after taking the aspirin. Jim gets the chance to observe Mrs. Ellis use a warm compress on her hands and wrists. She applies the heat correctly and afterward rates her pain on the FACES Pain Scale as a 3. She states that the heat is soothing. During the visit, Mrs. Ellis gets up to go to the kitchen using her walker, which she obtained from a physical therapist. Jim notes that although it takes her time to stand, her gait is steadier. Jim asks if Mrs. Ellis has found someone she can call when she needs help at home. The patient mentions that she has talked with her neighbor, who has offered help with shopping.

DOCUMENTATION NOTE

"Reports receiving some pain relief from using heat on hands. Rates pain at a level of 3 on a FACES Pain Scale after applying warm compresses. Appears less fatigued and is ambulating with steadier gait, using walker. Continues to have gastric irritation following use of aspirin. Identified a neighbor who can assist with shopping. Recommended she have neighbor pick up NSAID prescription at pharmacy as soon as possible. Explained need to replace aspirin with NSAID. Will evaluate effectiveness of NSAID at next visit in 2 weeks."

NSAID, Nonsteroidal antiinflammatory drug.

KEY POINTS

- Acute pain, a protective mechanism that warns a person of tissue injury, is completely subjective.
- Misconceptions about pain lead to undertreatment of the patient's pain.
- A patient's age, gender, anxiety, culture, previous experience, and meaning of pain influence the pain experience.
- A patient's pain tolerance influences your perceptions of the seriousness of the discomfort.
- The difference between acute and chronic pain involves the duration of discomfort, physical signs and symptoms, and the patient's perceptions regarding relief.
- Pain scales attempt to communicate the severity of pain and the effectiveness of pain therapies.
- The patient's family and friends are a key resource in pain assessment.
- You individualize pain therapy by collaborating closely with the patient, using assessment findings, trying a variety of therapies, and maintaining the patient's well-being.
- Eliminating sources of painful stimuli is a basic nursing measure for promoting comfort.

- Nonpharmacological therapies are effective in altering patient perception of pain, promoting muscle relaxation, and giving the patient control over pain experienced.
- Using a regular schedule for analgesic administration is more effective than an as-needed schedule.
- A PCA device gives patients pain control with a low risk for overdose.
- Your primary role in caring for a patient who receives local anesthesia is protecting the patient from injury.
- The aim of therapy for patients with chronic pain is to anticipate and prevent pain rather than to treat it.
- A serious but rare side effect of morphine infusions is respiratory depression, which you reverse with intravenous naloxone (Narcan).
- Evaluation of pain therapy requires consideration of the changing character of pain, response to therapy, ability to function, and the patient's perceptions of a therapy's effectiveness.

CRITICAL THINKING EXERCISES

Jim returns to evaluate Mrs. Ellis' progress over the past month. Jim asks her to rate her arthritic pain on a FACES Pain Scale of 0 to 10. Mrs. Ellis rates it as a 2. She states that although her joints are still stiff and tender when she awakens in the morning and after she sits for long periods, the pain is not as sharp in her hands and knees. Mrs. Ellis reports that she saw her nurse practitioner 2 weeks ago and has been referred to physical therapy for supportive hand splints. She is continuing to use the warm compresses three times a day. Mrs. Ellis reports that she has been having "stomach pains." Jim asks her to rate her stomach pain on the scale of 0 to 10. Mrs. Ellis rates it as a 3. She further states that she cannot point to the exact location of the stomach pain. Mrs. Ellis states that the nurse practitioner has prescribed an NSAID for pain control instead of the aspirin but she has not been to the pharmacy to pick up her prescription yet. When questioned about why she has not picked up the prescription, Mrs. Ellis states that she did not want to bother her neighbor again since he already takes her to the grocery store every 2 weeks. Mrs. Ellis further states that she plans to pick up the prescription when she goes to the grocery store next time. Jim asks her if any family members are able to assist her at home or with errands. Mrs. Ellis reports that her niece calls her several times a week, and her cousin takes her to church once a week. During the visit, Jim gets the chance to observe Mrs. Ellis walk to the kitchen. Jim notes that although it takes her time to stand, her gait is steadier. She is ambulating with a walker that the physical therapist recommended. When asked, Mrs. Ellis also states the she falls asleep more easily if she takes her medication 30 minutes before going to bed.

1. Based on the assessment findings, describe Mrs. Ellis' pain status using the PQRSTU model of pain assessment.
2. What kind of pain is Mrs. Ellis describing in reference to her "stomach pains"?

   a. Neuropathic
   b. Somatic
   c. Visceral
   d. Phantom
3. What is the priority nursing diagnosis for Mrs. Ellis?
   a. Social isolation
   b. Ineffective coping
   c. Impaired physical mobility
   d. Deficient knowledge related to pain medications
4. What plan would you recommend related to her aspirin and the new NSAID prescription?
   a. Continue using the aspirin until she picks up the NSAID prescription from the pharmacy when her neighbor takes her to the grocery store next week.
   b. Stop the aspirin, and call the health care provider for a different medication order.
   c. Stop the aspirin while she waits to pick up the NSAID prescription from the pharmacy when her neighbor takes her to the grocery store next week.
   d. Stop the aspirin, and call the pharmacy to arrange for the NSAID prescription to be delivered.
5. Given Mrs. Ellis' history and age, which nonpharmacological nursing intervention would Jim recommend she use to help alleviate the pain?
   a. Cutaneous stimulation
   b. Massage
   c. Distraction
   d. Progressive relaxation

ⓔvolve   *Answers to Critical Thinking Questions can be found on the Evolve website.*

REVIEW QUESTIONS

1. A patient has returned to the nursing unit after abdominal surgery and is reporting pain. What should be the first action taken by the nurse?
   1. Take the vital signs.
   2. Administer the ordered pain medication.
   3. Call the surgeon.
   4. Determine the pain characteristics.
2. A patient uses the call bell to notify you that he is in pain. The patient rates the pain as a 7 on the FPS of 0 to 10. The family member in the room states that the patient has been sleeping and does not need any pain medication at this time. As you assess the patient with pain, the most accurate assessment of the pain should be based on which of the following beliefs?
   1. The patient is the best resource for assessing the pain and thus should receive the pain medication.
   2. The patient is the best resource for assessing the pain but should not receive the pain medication because patients who are able to sleep cannot be in pain.
   3. The primary health care provider is the best resource for assessing the pain and should be called to determine if the pain medication should be administered.

4. The family member is the best resource for assessing the pain and thus the patient should not receive the pain medication because the family member reported the patient has been sleeping.
3. A Spanish-speaking patient arrives to the preoperative nursing unit before her knee replacement. When assessing this patient for pain, the nurse, who is fluent in English and Spanish, should anticipate which of the following?
   1. The patient will make no eye contact when being asked about her pain characteristics.
   2. The patient will use gestures and facial expressions while communicating her displeasure with the knee pain.
   3. The patient will offer no response when asked about her pain characteristics.
   4. The patient does not trust health care providers and will expect her family to answer questions.
4. A patient with a history of aphasia returns to the nursing unit after an appendectomy. The health care provider ordered an intravenous pain medication every 4 hours as needed (prn) for postoperative pain. The best nursing

intervention related to pain control postoperatively would be to:

1. Administer the intravenous pain medication every 4 hours
2. Wait until the patient verbalizes that he is experiencing pain
3. Ask the patient if he is having pain while conducting a full assessment
4. Administer the pain medication when the patient becomes restless

5. A patient with cancer was receiving 20 mg of immediate-release oxycodone every 4 hours around the clock for pain for the past 2 months. The patient has been allowed nothing by mouth (NPO) for the past 10 hours because of uncontrolled nausea. He begins to sweat and reports abdominal pains. These are symptoms of:

1. Addiction
2. Drug tolerance
3. Physical dependence
4. Pseudotolerance

6. A patient with terminal cancer is receiving around-the-clock pain medication but continues to report unrelieved pain. The physician increases the dosage of the prescribed pain medication. The nurse notes that this new order exceeds the upper limit of the normal range for this medication. What is the appropriate nursing intervention?

1. Hold the pain medication, and call the physician.
2. Administer the pain medication as ordered.
3. Ask the family if they are comfortable with the nurse's administering this increased dosage of the pain medication.
4. Administer the pain medication if the patient's respirations are above 8 breaths per minute.

7. A patient is receiving pain medication postoperatively via a PCA pump. The nurse observes that the family members are pushing the PCA pump button for the patient, who is capable of doing so. What action should the nurse take?

1. Encourage the family to continue pushing the PCA pump button for the patient as needed.
2. Inform the family that the nurse should be the only other person besides the patient to push the PCA pump button.

3. Explain that the patient should be the only person to push the PCA pump button.
4. Ask the family push the PCA pump button only when the patient begins to moan.

8. A patient is discharged with an order for hydrocodone/acetaminophen (Lortab) for pain control after a surgical procedure. The nurse has provided discharge instructions regarding this pain medication. Which statement by the patient demonstrates knowledge of the possible side effects of this medication?

1. "I will drink plenty of fluids and eat high-fiber foods while taking Lortab."
2. "I will report any muscle weakness, numbness, or tingling if it occurs."
3. "I can continue to drink alcoholic beverages while on Lortab."
4. "I will use a lubricating ointment if I start having itching of the skin."

9. A patient has received oral pain medication within the last hour. As the nurse is reassessing the patient's pain, the patient reports that although the pain is better her back continues to be painful. Based on her assessment, which actions implemented by the nurse may help with relieving the patient's continued pain? Select all that apply.

1. Assist the patient to a side-lying position.
2. Educate the patient regarding the frequency of the ordered pain medication.
3. Massage the back.
4. Apply a heating pad if not contraindicated.
5. Educate the patient on the symptoms of addiction.

10. A patient with chronic cancer pain received opioids around the clock (ATC) while hospitalized and is to continue taking opioids ATC at home to control pain. The patient's health care provider has also ordered medication for breakthrough pain. Which of the following primary complications should the nurse include in the discharge teaching? (Select all that apply.)

1. Constipation
2. Respiratory depression
3. Nausea
4. Uncontrolled pain

Answers to Review Questions can be found on pages 1197-1198.

REFERENCES

Agency for Health Care Policy and Research, Acute Pain Management Guideline Panel: *Acute pain management in infants,* children and adolescents: operative or medical procedures and trauma, Clinical Practice Guideline, AHCPR Pub No. 92-0032, Rockville, Md, February 1992, Agency for Health Care Policy and Research, Public Health Service, U.S. Department of Health and Human Services.

American Geriatrics Society: The management of persistent pain in older persons, *J Am Geriatr Soc* 50(6):S205, 2002.

American Pain Society: *Principles of analgesic use in the treatment of acute and cancer pain,* ed 5, Glenview, Ill, 2003, The Society.

American Pain Society: *Guideline for the management of cancer pain in adults and children,* Glenview, Ill, 2005, The Society.

American Society for Pain Management Nursing: *Pain management in patients with addictive disease,* 2002, http://www.aspmn.org/html/PSaddiction.htm.

Argoff C: Tailoring chronic pain treatment to the patient: long-acting, short-acting, and rapid-onset opioids, *Neurology & Neurosurgery,* 2007, http://www.medscape.com/viewarticle/554015.

Arnold E and others: Consideration of hastening death among hospice patients and their families, *J Pain Symptom Manage* 27(6):523, 2004.

Arnstein P: Comprehensive analysis and management of chronic pain, *Nurs Clin North Am* 38(3):403, 2003.

Arnstein P: Learning to "live with" chronic pain: lessons from Mrs. Tandy, *Advanced Practice Nursing eJournal,* 7(1), 2007, http://www.medscape.com/viewarticle/557719.

Arthritis Foundation: *Pain center: take medications wisely,* 2008, http://www.arthritis.org/taking-meds.php.

Baird C, Sands L: Pilot study of the effectiveness of guided imagery with progressive muscle relaxation to reduce chronic pain and mobility difficulties of osteoarthritis, *Pain Manag Nurs* 5(3):7, 2004.

Barclay L: Physical therapy modalities helpful for the family clinician to know, *Medscape Medical News*, 2007, http://www.medscape.com/viewarticle/567325.

Beyer J and others: The creation, validation, and continuing development of the Oucher: a measure of pain intensity in children, *J Pediatr Nurs* 7(5):335, 1992.

Blyth F and others: Caregiving in the presence of chronic pain, *J Gerontol A Biol Sci Med Sci* 63:399, 2008.

Bruckenthal P: Risk factors associated with the onset of persistent pain, *Highlights of the American Pain Society twenty-seventh annual scientific meeting*, 2008, http://www.medscape.com/viewprogram/14827.

Bruckenthal P, D'Arcy Y: Assessment and management of pain in older adults: a review of the basics, *Advanced Practice Nursing eJournal*, 7(1), 2007, http://www.medscape.com/viewarticle/556382.

Bulechek GM and others, editors: *Nursing interventions classification (NIC)*, ed 5, St. Louis, 2008, Mosby.

Bursch B: Physiological correlates of pain during sleep, *Program and abstracts of the twenty-third annual meeting of the American Pain Society*, 2004, http://www.medscape.com/viewarticle/480566.

Byers J, Thornley K: Cueing into infant pain, *MCN Am J Matern Child Nurs* 30(2):84, 2004.

Cassileth B, Vickers A: Massage therapy for symptom control: outcome study at a major cancer center, *J Pain Symptom Manag* 28(3):244, 2004.

Clark L and others: Nurses' reflections on pain management in a nursing home setting, *Pain Manag Nurs* 7(2):71, 2006.

Curtiss C: Consensus statements, positions, standards, and guidelines for pain and care at the end of life, *Semin Oncol Nurs* 20(2):121, 2004.

da Cruz Dde A and others: Caregivers of patients with chronic pain: responses to care, *Int J Nurs Terminol Classif* 15(1):5, 2004.

D'Arcy Y: Meeting the challenges of acute pain management, *Neurology & Neurosurgery*, 2008, http://www.medscape.com/viewarticle/574105.

Davidhizar R, Giger J: A review of the literature on care of patients in pain who are culturally diverse, *Int Nurs Rev* 51:47, 2004.

Dossey B, Keegan L, Guzzetta C: *Holistic nursing: a handbook for practice*, ed 4, Gaithersburg, Md, 2005, Aspen.

Ersek M and others: HPNA position paper: providing opioids at the end of life, *J Hospice Palliat Nurs* 6(4):244, 2004.

Feinberg S: Race, ethnicity, cultural factors and chronic pain, *Am Chronic Pain Assoc Chronicle* 21(2):6, 2004.

Ferrell B: Ethical perspectives on pain and suffering, *Pain Manag Nurs* 6(3):83, 2005.

Freeman S: Cognitive behavioral therapy in advanced practice nursing: an overview, *Advanced Practice Nursing eJournal*, 6(3), 2006, http://www.medscape.com/viewarticle/545336.

Gelinas G and others: Assessment in nonverbal populations (infants, mentally impaired, etc.): development of a critical care pain observation tool (CCPOT), *J Pain* 5(3, Suppl 1):S106, 2004.

Grace P: The clinical use of placebos, *Am J Nurs* 106(20):58, 2006.

Grant M, Cordts G, Doberman D: Acute pain management in hospitalized patients with current opioid abuse, *Advanced Practice Nursing eJournal*, 7(1), 2007, http://www.medscape.com/viewarticle/557043.

Hernandez A, Sachs-Ericsson N: Ethnic differences in pain reports and the moderating role of depression in a community sample of Hispanic and Caucasian participants with serious health problems, *Psychosom Med* 68:121, 2006.

Herr K and others: Evidence-based assessment of acute pain in older adults: current nursing practices and perceived barriers, *Clin J Pain* 20(5):331, 2004.

Herr K and others: Pain assessment in the nonverbal patient: position statement with clinical practice recommendations, *Pain Manag Nurs* 7(2):44, 2006.

Hutt E and others: Optimizing pain management in long-term care residents, *Geriatrics Aging* 10(8):523, 2007.

Jacox A and others: *Management of cancer pain*, Clinical Practice Guideline No. 9, AHCPR Pub No. 94-0592, Rockville, Md, March 1994, Agency for Health Care Policy and Research, U.S. Department of Health and Human Services, Public Health Service.

Jann M, Slade J: Antidepressant agents for the treatment of chronic pain and depression, *Pharmacotherapy* 27(11):1571, 2007.

Jonsson A and others: Prevalence and intensity of pain after stroke: a population based study focusing on patients' perspectives, *J Neurol Neurosurg Psychiatry* 77:590, 2006.

Keogh E, McCracken L, Eccleston C: Do men and women differ in their response to interdisciplinary chronic pain management? *Pain* 114(1-2):37, 2005.

Letizia M and others: Barriers to caregiver administration of pain medication in hospice care, *J Pain Symptom Manage* 27(2):114, 2004.

Loeser J: The decade of pain control and research, *Am Pain Soc Bull* 13(3):13, 2003.

Logan H, Gedney J: Sex differences in the long-term stability of forehead cold pressor pain, *J Pain* 5(7):406, 2004.

McCaffery M: *Nursing management of the patient with pain*, ed 2, Philadelphia, 1979, Lippincott.

McCaffery M, Arnstein P: The debate over placebos in pain management, *Am J Nurs* 106(2):62, 2006.

McCaffery M, Pasero C: *Pain: clinical manual*, ed 2, St. Louis, 1999, Mosby.

Melzack R, Wall P: *The challenge of pain*, ed 2, London, 1996, Penguin.

Menefee-Pujol L, Katz N, Zacharoff K: *The pain EDUmanual: a pocket guide to pain management*, Newton, Mass, 2007, Inflexxion.

Merkel S: Pain assessment in infants and young children: the finger span scale, *Am J Nurs* 102(11):55, 2002.

Merkel S and others: Pain assessment in infants and young children: the FLACC scale, *Am J Nurs* 102(10):55, 2002.

Moorhead S and others, editors: *Nursing outcomes classification (NOC)*, ed 4, St. Louis, 2008, Mosby.

National Consensus Project: *Clinical practice guidelines for quality palliative care*, 2004, http://www.nationalconsensusproject.org.

Nicholson B: *Acute pain management: overcoming barriers and enhancing treatment*, http://www.medscape.com/viewprogram/14826, accessed July 17, 2008.

Palos G and others: Perceptions of analgesic use and side effects: what the public values in pain management, *J Pain Symptom Manage* 28(5):460, 2004.

Pasero C: Pain assessment in infants and young children: neonates, *Am J Nurs* 102(8):61, 2002.

Pasero C: *Epidural analgesia for acute pain management in adults*, 2003a, http://www.baxter.com/doctors/iv_therapies/eduction/iv_therapy_ce/epidural/epidural.html.

Pasero C: Epidural analgesia for postoperative pain, *Am J Nurs* 103(10):62, 2003b.

Pasero C: Epidural analgesia for postoperative pain, part II, *Am J Nurs* 103(11):43, 2003c.

Pasero C: *Intravenous patient-controlled analgesia for acute pain management*, Pensacola, Fla, 2003d, American Society for Pain Management Nursing.

Pasero C, McCaffery M: Comfort-function goals, *Am J Nurs* 104(9):77, 2004.

Passik S, Kirsh K: Opioid therapy in patients with a history of substance abuse, *CNS Drugs* 18(1):13, 2004.

Raymo L, Camejo M, Fudin J: Eradicating analgesic use of meperidine in a hospital, *Am J Health Syst Pharm* 64(11):1148, 2007.

Robinson M and others: Altering gender role expectations: effects on pain tolerance, pain threshold, and pain ratings, *J Pain* 4(6):284, 2003.

Roman M, Cabaj T: Epidural analgesia, *Medsurg Nurs* 14(4):257, 2005.

Rustoen T and others: Gender differences in chronic pain: findings from a population-based study of Norwegian adults, *Pain Manag Nurs* 5(3):105, 2004.

Schechter N, Berde C, Yaster M: *Pain in infants, children, and adolescents*, ed 2, Philadelphia, 2003, Lippincott Williams & Wilkins.

Silka P and others: Pain scores improve analgesic administration patterns for trauma patients in the emergency department, *Acad Emerg Med* 11(3):264, 2004.

Taylor L, Herr K: Pain intensity assessment: a comparison of selected pain intensity scales for use in cognitively intact and cognitively impaired African American older adults, *Pain Manag Nurs* 4(2):87, 2003.

The Joint Commission: Tubing misconnection: a persistent and potentially deadly occurrence, *Sentinel Event Alert*, 36 (April 3, 2006), http://www.jointcommission.org/sentinelevents.

The Joint Commission: *Comprehensive accreditation manual for hospital standards: the official handbook*, Oak Brook, Ill, 2008, The Commission.

Vallerand A and others: Knowledge of and barriers to pain management in caregivers of cancer patients receiving homecare, *Cancer Nurs* 30(1):31, 2007.

Ware L and others: Evaluation of the revised faces pain scale, verbal descriptor scale, numeric rating scale, and Iowa pain thermometer in older minority adults, *Pain Manag Nurs* 7(3):117, 2006.

Whelan C and others: Pain and satisfaction with pain control in hospitalized medical patients, *Arch Intern Med* 164:175, 2004.

Wong DL, Baker CM: Pain in children: comparison of assessment scales, *Pediatr Nurs* 14(1):9, 1988.

Wong DL and others: *Wong's nursing of infants and children*, ed 8, St. Louis, 2007, Mosby.

World Health Organization: *Cancer pain relief and palliative care*, Report of a WHO expert committee, WHO Technical Report Series No. 804, Geneva, Switzerland, 1990, WHO.

Wu CL and others: Efficacy of postoperative patient-controlled and continuous infusion epidural analgesia versus intravenous patient controlled analgesia with opioids: a meta-analysis, *Anesthesiology* 103(5):1079, 2005.

Wuhrman E and others: Patient controlled analgesia (PCA), *Pain Manag Nurs* 7(4):134, 2006.

Nutrition

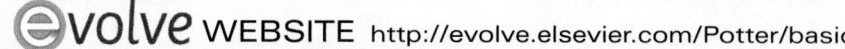
OBJECTIVES

- Explain the importance of a balance between energy intake and output.
- List the end products of carbohydrate, protein, and lipid metabolism.
- Explain the significance of saturated, unsaturated, and polyunsaturated lipids in nutrition.
- Describe the basic food groups (using the food guide pyramid) and their value in planning meals for good nutrition.
- Explain dietary guidelines.

- Discuss the major areas of nutritional assessment.
- Identify nutritional problems, and describe a patient at risk for these problems.
- Establish a plan of care to meet the nutritional needs of a patient.
- Discuss methods for feeding patients.
- Describe the procedure for initiating and maintaining tube feedings.
- Describe the procedure for initiating and maintaining total parenteral nutrition.

KEY TERMS

amino acids, p. 906
anabolism, p. 908
anthropometry, p. 916
basal metabolic rate (BMR), p. 908
body mass index (BMI), p. 914
carbohydrates, p. 906
catabolism, p. 908
dietary reference intakes (DRIs), p. 908

dysphagia, p. 918
enteral nutrition (EN), p. 924
gluconeogenesis, p. 908
glycogenesis, p. 908
hyperglycemia, p. 928
ideal body weight (IBW), p. 916
jejunostomy tube, p. 927
lipid, p. 907

medical nutrition therapy (MNT), p. 928
metabolism, p. 908
minerals, p. 907
monosaturated fatty acid, p. 907
nitrogen balance, p. 907
nutrients, p. 906
parenteral nutrition (PN), p. 927

polyunsaturated fatty acid, p. 907
saturated fatty acid, p. 907
unsaturated fatty acid, p. 907
vitamins, p. 907

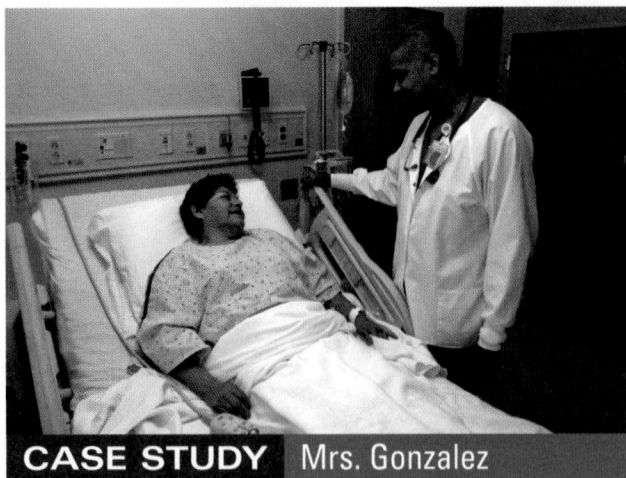

CASE STUDY   Mrs. Gonzalez

Mrs. Gonzalez is a 65-year-old Hispanic woman who comes to the emergency department with slurred speech, right facial droop, and weakness in her upper and lower right side extremities. She is admitted to the hospital with a diagnosis of acute stroke. Mrs. Gonzalez lives alone in a senior apartment complex. She has a daughter and two teenage grandchildren that live in another town nearby.

Mrs. Gonzalez is awake and alert in her hospital room but is drooling from the right side of her mouth. When she tries to drink water, she starts to cough. The physician has ordered nothing by mouth (NPO). The evaluation by the speech language pathologist (SLP) indicates inadequate clearance of food and liquid from the vocal folds and aspiration of thickened liquids. Mrs. Gonzalez has trouble swallowing with oropharyngeal dysphagia. The SLP recommends enteral feedings and speech and swallowing therapy to help her return to oral feedings.

Matt is a nursing student assigned to Mrs. Gonzalez. As Matt prepares to assess Mrs. Gonzalez, he recalls information about the effect of dysphagia on nutrition and rehabilitation. He will assess Mrs. Gonzalez's weight and weight history, diet history, and cultural customs. Matt knows to consult with a registered dietitian (RD) to assess Mrs. Gonzalez's nutritional status and to assist with nutritional interventions. Matt and the RD will work as team members along with the SLP and physician to assist Mrs. Gonzalez in her speech and swallowing rehabilitation.

Matt is responsible for inserting Mrs. Gonzalez's small-bore nasogastric feeding tube and starting her tube feedings. The RD has recommended a continuous tube feeding for 12 hours during the day to reduce the risk for aspiration.

Nutrition is a basic component of health and is essential for normal growth and development, tissue maintenance and repair, cellular metabolism, and organ function. The human body needs an adequate supply of nutrients for essential functions of cells.

Scientific principles regarding nutrition and the role of various nutrients in metabolism and health form a basis for the nutritional plan of care that you develop with your patients. Disease processes, age, gender, and activity all affect utilization of nutrients and nutritional requirements. Pharmaceutical agents prescribed to treat disease also interact with nutrients and foods.

SCIENTIFIC KNOWLEDGE BASE

Principles of Nutrition

The body requires food to provide energy for movement, maintenance of body temperature, growth and development, cellular metabolism, synthesis and repair of tissues, and organ function. The gastrointestinal (GI) system contains a number of organs and structures that enable the body to nourish itself through the ingestion of food. Each organ or structure in the GI tract has a specific function aimed toward preparing food for the digestion and absorption of its nutrients.

NUTRIENTS A **nutrient** is a chemical substance that provides nourishment and affects metabolic and nutritive processes. The essential nutrients include carbohydrates, proteins, lipids, vitamins, minerals, and water. Only carbohydrates, proteins, and lipids provide energy. Vitamins and minerals are catalysts for the use of nutrients for energy. Minerals and water regulate body processes.

Carbohydrates **Carbohydrates** are composed of carbon, hydrogen, and oxygen. They are starches and sugars obtained mainly from plant foods, with the exception of lactose, which is found in milk (milk sugar). Carbohydrates contribute as much as 90% of the total caloric intake in parts of the world where grains are a major food source. Carbohydrates are a source of energy, providing 4 kilocalories per gram (kcal/g).

Another type of carbohydrate is fiber. Fiber is the structural part of plants and is sometimes called nonstarch polysaccharides. Fiber also includes some nonpolysaccharides such as lignins and tannins. Human digestive enzymes cannot break down fiber. Therefore fiber does not contribute calorically to the diet. Each fiber has a different structure. Most contain monosaccharides; however, they differ in types of monosaccharides and types of bonds. Fiber is either soluble or insoluble. Soluble fiber becomes a gel in water and delays GI transit time; because of this, soluble fiber helps prevent diarrhea in tube-fed patients. Insoluble fiber does not change in water and accelerates intestinal transit; this is helpful in preventing constipation in patients taking pain medication.

Proteins Amino acids are the building blocks of proteins and are made of hydrogen, oxygen, carbon, and nitrogen. **Amino acids** are the most important components of proteins in the human body, and are essential for synthesis of body tissue in growth, maintenance, and repair. The body is unable to synthesize some amino acids, such as essential amino acids. The body can only obtain these from daily food sources. Proteins are a source of energy, providing 4 kcal/g.

The required daily intake of protein varies according to age. For example, infants under 6 months of age require 2.2 g/kg daily. Adolescents require 1 g/kg daily. Most healthy adults require only about 0.8 g/kg of body weight per day. In disease, protein requirements will double or triple, such as for patients with major burns. Pregnant women require an additional 30 g and lactating women an additional 20 g above the usual daily need.

The achievement of equal nitrogen input and output is called **nitrogen balance.** When intake of nitrogen is greater than output, the patient is in positive nitrogen balance. The body needs a positive nitrogen balance for growth, maintenance of lean muscle mass and vital organs and wound healing. The body uses nitrogen for building, repair, and replacement of body tissues. When output of nitrogen is greater than intake, then negative nitrogen balance occurs. Negative nitrogen balance occurs in infection, sepsis, fever, burns, starvation, and trauma. Protein provides energy, but because of the essential role of protein in growth, maintenance, and repair, a diet needs to provide adequate kilocalories from nonprotein sources. When there is insufficient carbohydrate in the diet to meet the energy needs of the body, protein stores are used as an energy source.

Fats Fats (**lipids**) are compounds that are insoluble in water but soluble in organic solvents such as ethanol and acetone. Fats are made up of triglycerides and fatty acids. Lipids are a source of energy, providing 9 kcal/g.

Triglycerides are made up of three fatty acids attached to a glycerol. Approximately 98% of the lipids in foods and 90% of the lipids in the human body are in the form of triglycerides. Triglycerides contribute to high blood levels of certain lipoproteins linked to cardiovascular diseases.

A **saturated fatty acid** contains as much hydrogen as it is able to hold. A **monounsaturated fatty acid** is able to take up another hydrogen atom, and a **polyunsaturated fatty acid** is able to take up many more hydrogen atoms and become hydrogenated or saturated fat. Ingestion of saturated fatty acids appears to increase blood cholesterol levels. Ingestion of **unsaturated fatty acids** has a minimal effect on blood cholesterol. Monounsaturated fatty acids appear to lower blood cholesterol levels. Fatty acids are usually not purely saturated, unsaturated, or polyunsaturated. Most animal fats have high proportions of saturated fatty acids; most vegetable fats have higher amounts of unsaturated and polyunsaturated fatty acids (e.g., safflower oil is about 75% polyunsaturated, olive oil about 25%).

There are also essential fatty acids (EFA). The two primary EFA are linoleic acid (an omega-6 fatty acid) and linolenic acid (an omega-3 fatty acid). EFA have many roles in the body, including the production of cell membranes and hormones, among others. The metabolism of EFA has effects on the regulation of blood pressure, blood clot formation, and immune response.

Vitamins **Vitamins** are organic substances present in small amounts in foods and are essential for normal metabolism. They serve as coenzymes or catalysts in cellular enzyme reactions. The body is unable to synthesize vitamins in the required amounts and depends on dietary intake. The exception to this is vitamin K, which the body synthesizes by bacteria in the intestine. Although vitamins are contained in many foods, processing, storage, and preparation all affect

them. Vitamin content is usually highest in foods that are fresh and used quickly after minimal exposure to heat, air, or water. Certain vitamins are being studied in their role as antioxidants. These vitamins neutralize substances called free radicals, which produce oxidative damage to body cells and tissues. These vitamins include beta-carotene and vitamins A, C, and E (Nix, 2005). Vitamins are water soluble and fat soluble.

Water-soluble vitamins (C and B complex) are stored in limited amounts for short periods of time, requiring daily consumption. Although water-soluble vitamins are not stored, toxicity can occur from excessive intake. Water-soluble vitamins are absorbed easily from the gastrointestinal tract.

Fat-soluble vitamins (A, D, E, and K) are able to be stored in the body for longer periods; however, dietary intake is still necessary, with some exceptions. Vitamin K is in dark leafy green vegetables, but the body also produces it within the large intestine. In addition, the body produces vitamin D as a response to sunlight exposure. Because the body has a high storage capacity for these vitamins, toxicity is possible when the patient takes large doses of them.

Minerals **Minerals** are inorganic elements that catalzye biochemical reactions. Minerals are classified as macrominerals when the daily requirement is 100 mg or more and microminerals or trace elements when the body needs less than 100 mg daily. Macrominerals help to balance the pH of the body, and specific amounts are necessary in the blood and cells to promote acid-base balance. Interactions occur among trace minerals. For example, excess of one trace mineral sometimes causes the deficiency of another. This deficiency then allows for toxicity of another or worsens the deficiency of another.

Water Water is an important nutrient because the function of cells depends on an aqueous environment. The roles of water in the body include transportation of nutrients and waste products; providing structure to large molecules (protein, glycogen); participation in metabolic reactions; serving as solvent, lubricant, and cushion; regulating body temperature; and maintaining blood volume.

Water makes up 60% to 70% of the total body weight. A lean person's body contains a higher percentage of water than an obese person's body. Infants have the greatest percentage of total body weight as water; older adults have the least. Infants and older adults are most vulnerable to water deprivation or water loss.

The human body requires 1.5 mL of water for every kilocalorie of energy used. The ingestion of liquids and solid foods, such as fresh fruits and vegetables, aids the body in meeting fluid needs. The body also produces water when food is oxidized during digestion.

Thirst is a protective mechanism that alerts the oriented person to the need for fluids. Thirst is a less reliable guide for infants and confused patients, who are usually unable to communicate that they are thirsty.

DIGESTION The process of digestion begins in the mouth, where mastication, or chewing, breaks down food into smaller particles, and amylase in saliva begins to break down starches. Mucus lubricates food particles for their passage through the esophagus into the stomach. Churning movements of the stomach mix food particles with hydrochloric acid in the stomach. The body produces gastric lipase and amylase to begin fat and starch digestion. Digestive proteins, or enzymes, in the GI system break food particles into a simpler form. The small intestine digests and absorbs most nutrients; the large intestine absorbs electrolytes and water, thus helping to maintain the body's electrolyte balance (see Chapter 17).

ABSORPTION The small intestine is the primary site of absorption of simple nutrients. It is lined with villi, which project into the lumen and greatly increase the surface area available for absorption. The upper duodenum absorbs cholesterol, vitamins E and K, folic acid, riboflavin, and thiamin. The lower duodenum and upper jejunum absorb glucose, amino acids, minerals, and fats, and the lower jejunum and ileum absorb sucrose, lactose, and maltose. Understanding sites of absorption explains the nature of diseases that might affect intestinal function.

Intestinal contents move by peristaltic action into the large intestine. Water and electrolytes are absorbed from the large intestine. The body excretes other nutrients remaining in the intestinal contents when they reach the large intestine as waste products. The body loses nutrients when intestinal motility is increased (i.e., diarrhea). This occurs because the diarrhea causes the nutrients to move through the small intestine too quickly for complete absorption.

METABOLISM **Metabolism** refers to all of the body's biochemical and physiological processes. Through metabolism, nutrients are converted into necessary substances for cell function. The two basic types of metabolism are anabolism and catabolism. **Anabolism** is the production of more-complex chemical substances by synthesis of nutrients needed to build or repair body tissue. **Catabolism** is the breakdown of body tissues into simpler substances. Although catabolism produces some energy, both processes require energy, which comes from food or stored sources.

Carbohydrates, protein, and fat produce chemical energy and maintain a dynamic balance of tissue buildup and breakdown. The chemical energy produced by metabolism is converted to other types of energy by different tissues. Muscle contraction involves mechanical energy, the nervous system involves electrical energy, and the mechanisms of heat production involve thermal energy. These forms of energy all begin in metabolism.

Absorbed nutrients are carried to the liver, where major metabolic processes occur. The liver also regulates energy through its control of glucose metabolism. Glucose is the primary fuel for the body. The liver and muscles store glucose in the form of glycogen via a process called **glycogenesis.** Lipogenesis converts glucose to fat for storage. Insulin and glucagon act as regulatory hormones to promote glucose storage or use. Insulin promotes glucose use, and glucagon promotes glucose storage. During states where energy needs exceed glycogen storage, the body breaks down fat and amino acids for conversion to glucose via a process called **gluconeogenesis.**

The **basal metabolic rate (BMR)** represents the energy needs of a person at rest after awakening. Energy needs are based on BMR along with activity level, energy required to break down food, and energy required for healing during illness. Energy balance occurs when energy requirements equal energy intake. In general, when a person exceeds his or her energy needs or his or her needs are insufficient, the person either gains or loses weight, respectively.

STORAGE The body stores energy as adipose tissue. Glycogen is stored in small reserves in liver and muscle tissue, and protein is stored in muscle mass. When the body's energy demands exceed dietary sources, the body uses stored (fat) energy. When the body has unused energy, it is stored principally in fat. Fat-soluble vitamins are also stored in limited reserves (6 to 8 months), and the body releases them to meet the needs when dietary intake is insufficient. Most water-soluble vitamins are stored for only 3 to 5 days.

ELIMINATION The intestinal contents move through the large intestine by peristalsis (see Chapter 34). As the contents move toward the rectum, water is reabsorbed through the mucosa. The end products of digestion include cellulose and similar fibrous substances the body is unable to digest. The body also eliminates sloughed cells from the intestinal walls, mucus, digestive secretions, water, and microorganisms.

Dietary Guidelines

A number of agencies and organizations in the United States regularly publish and update dietary guidelines. The guidelines change as nutritional researchers discover new knowledge.

FOOD GUIDELINES The food guide pyramid is designed as a part of the Food Guidance System of the U.S. Department of Agriculture (USDA) (Figure 32-1). It is designed to be used as part of a basic system for buying food and meal preparations for diets ranging from 1600 to 2800 kcal/day (USDA, 2005). In addition to the pyramid, the USDA also developed interactive educational tools that are accessible through CD-ROM, the Internet, and other venues. To provide additional dietary guidelines, the USDA and the U. S. Department of Health and Human Services (USDHHS) have published the *Dietary Guidelines for Americans, 2005* (Box 32-1). These guidelines are for Americans over the age of 2 years. You need to make sure to consider the food preferences of different racial and ethnic groups, vegetarians, and others when planning diets.

DIETARY REFERENCE INTAKES In 1997 the Food and Nutrition Board of the National Institute of Medicine/National Academy of Sciences, in partnership with Health Canada, initiated **dietary reference intakes (DRIs)** in response to the increased public use of nutritional supplements. The DRIs are nutrient reference values developed by the Institute of Medicine (IOM, 2009). The values are

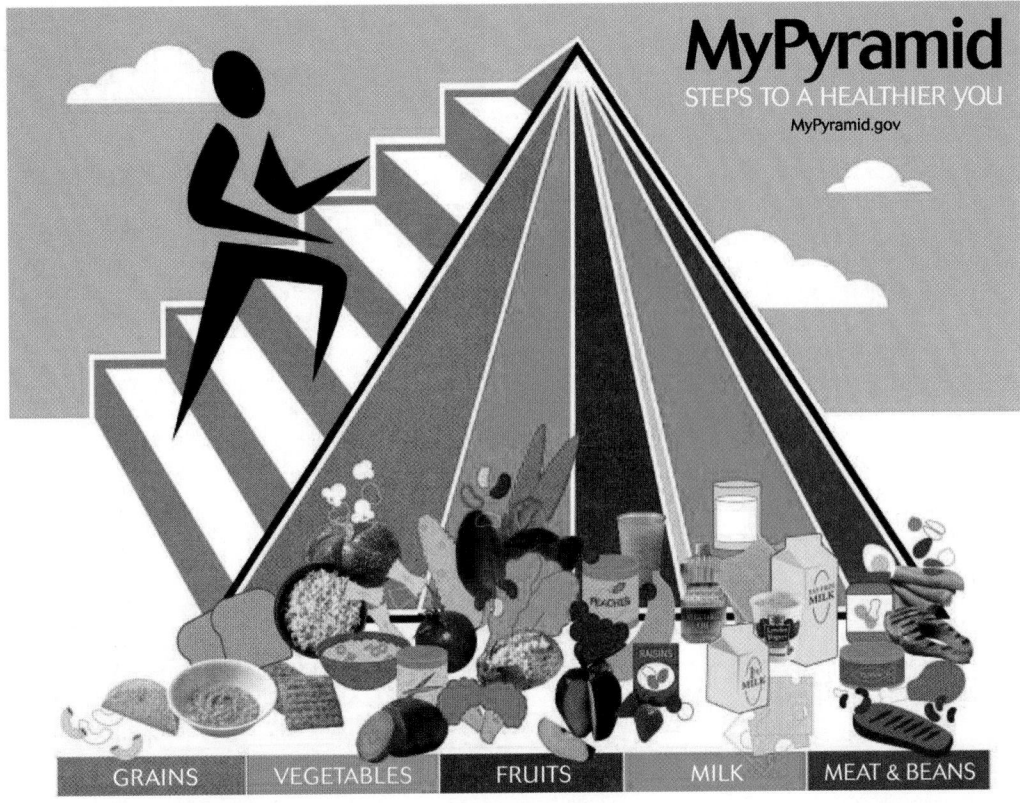

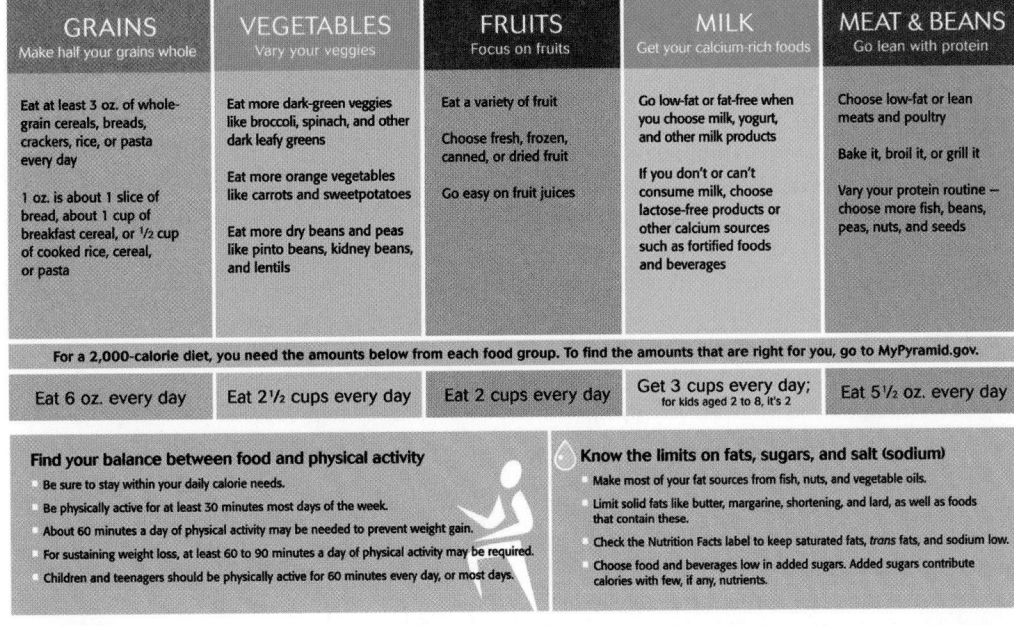

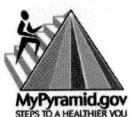

Figure 32-1 ■ Sample food guide pyramid for adults. (From U.S. Department of Agriculture Center for Nutrition Policy and Promotion: *USDA's food guide pyramid,* April 2005, http://www.MyPyramid.gov.)

BOX 32-1 | 2005 Dietary Guidelines for Americans: Key Recommendations for the General Population

- Adopt a balanced eating pattern with a variety of nutrient-dense food and beverages among the basic food groups.
- Maintain body weight in a healthy range.
- Encourage physical activity, and decrease sedentary activities.
- Encourage fruits, vegetables, whole-grain products, and fat-free or low-fat milk while staying within energy needs.
- Keep total fat intake between 20% and 35% of total calories with most fats coming from polyunsaturated or monounsaturated fatty acids.
- Choose and prepare foods and beverages with little added sugars or sweeteners.
- Choose and prepare foods with little salt while at the same time eating potassium-rich foods.
- Limit intake of alcohol.
- Practice food safety to prevent microbial food-borne illness.

Data from U.S. Department of Agriculture and U.S. Department of Health and Human Services: *Dietary guidelines for Americans, 2005,* ed 6, Washington, DC, 2005, U.S. Government Printing Office, http://www.healthierus.gov/dietaryguidelines.

intended to serve as a guide for good nutrition and provide the scientific basis for the development of food guidelines, such as recommended amounts of vitamins, in both the United States and Canada. There are four components to the DRIs: estimated average requirement (EAR), recommended dietary allowances (RDAs), adequate intakes (AIs), and tolerable upper intake levels (ULs). The EAR is the recommended amount of a nutrient that appears sufficient to maintain a specific body function for 50% of the population based on age and gender. The RDA is the average needs of 98% of the population, not the exact needs of an individual. The AI is the suggested intake for individuals based on observed or experimentally determined estimates of nutrient intakes by groups and is provided when there is insufficient evidence to set RDA. The tolerable UL is the highest level that likely poses no risk for adverse health events. It is not a recommended level of intake (Institute of Medicine, 2009).

OTHER DIETARY GUIDELINES Other professional organizations have published dietary guidelines. Examples of this are the American Cancer Society Guidelines for Cancer Prevention, American Diabetes Association, and the American Heart Association Guidelines for Heart Healthy Eating. These guidelines are similar to the Dietary Guidelines for Americans. Medical nutrition therapy (MNT) uses nutritional therapy and counseling to manage diseases (American Dietetic Association, 2006). Standards now exist that clearly designate the standard of care for promotion of optimal nutrition in all health care patients (American Heart Association, 2006; Kushi and others, 2006).

BOX 32-2 | Examples of Nutrition Objectives for *Healthy People 2010*

WEIGHT AND GROWTH
- Increase proportion of adults who are at a healthy weight (BMI 18.5 to 24.9).
- Reduce obesity in adults by 15%.
- Reduce obesity in children (6 to 11 years of age) and adolescents (12 to 19 years of age) by 15%.
- Reduce growth retardation in low-income children under 5 years of age.

FOOD AND NUTRIENT CONSUMPTION
- Decrease in fat intake to less than 30% daily intake and saturated fat intake to less than 10% of total calories daily.
- Increase vegetable and fruit intake to five daily servings in 75% of people.
- Increase grain products intake to six daily servings in 50% of people.
- Meet calcium DRI in 75% of people.
- Reduce sodium daily intake to no more than 2400 mg in 65% of people.

IRON DEFICIENCY AND ANEMIA
- Reduce prevalence of iron deficiency in children and childbearing women.
- Reduce prevalence of anemia in pregnant women in third trimester to 20%.

SCHOOLS, WORK SITES, AND NUTRITION COUNSELING
- Increase proportion of school-age children whose intake of meals and snacks at school contributes to good overall dietary quality.
- Increase work-site nutrition education and weight management program offerings.
- Offer nutritional assessment and individualized planning at primary care sites.

FOOD SECURITY
- Increase food security so that 94% of households have nutritionally adequate and safe food supplies.

Data from U.S. Department of Health and Human Services: *Healthy people 2010,* 2002, http://www.health.gov./healthypeople. *DRI,* Dietary reference intake.

In 1997 the USDHHS and the Public Health Service (PHS) began a consensus process that resulted in establishing nutritional goals and objectives for *Healthy People 2010: National Health Promotion and Disease Prevention Objectives* (see Chapter 1). *Healthy People 2010* continues the overall goal to promote health and reduce chronic disease related to diet and weight. The report defines national goals or objectives to be met to increase the proportion of Americans who live long, healthy lives (Box 32-2). The challenge is to motivate consumers to put these objectives into practice. Health professionals play a key role in promoting healthy dietary practices.

NURSING KNOWLEDGE BASE

There are sociological, cultural, psychological, and emotional aspects in eating and drinking in all societies. Holidays and events are celebrated with food, food is brought to those who are grieving, and food is used for medicinal purposes. We also recognize cultural and religious food differences (Box 32-3). Food is incorporated into family traditions and rituals, and appearance is often associated with eating behaviors. In attempting to affect eating patterns, you need to understand patients' values, beliefs, and attitudes about food and how those values affect food purchase, preparation, and intake.

Nutritional requirements depend upon many factors. Individual caloric and nutrient requirements vary by stage of development, body composition, activity levels, conditions such as pregnancy and lactation, and the presence of disease. Registered dietitians (RDs) use predictive equations that take into account some of those factors to estimate patient's nutritional requirements.

Alternative Food Patterns

Individuals follow special patterns of food intake based on religion, cultural background, ethics, health beliefs, personal preference, or concern about the environment. Such special diets do not necessarily provide more or less nutritional benefit than diets based on the food guide pyramid or other nutritional guidelines. Adequate nutritional intake depends on balanced consumption of all required nutrients. The vegetarian diet is an example of a dietary pattern that is commonly consumed because of religious or personal beliefs. The vegetarian diet is primarily plant based and includes the elimination of many animal-based foods. Vegetarians are grouped into several categories. Ovolactovegetarians avoid meat, fish, and poultry but eat eggs and milk. Lactovegetarians drink milk but avoid eggs and other animal-based foods. Vegans eat only foods of plant origin. Individuals consuming the vegan diet are susceptible to vitamin B_{12} and protein deficiency. Vegans supplement their diets with vitamin B_{12} and carefully choose foods to ensure ingestion of essential amino acids. Knowledge of high biological value protein versus low biological value protein sources ensures intake of all of the essential amino acids.

Developmental Needs

INFANTS THROUGH SCHOOL-AGE Infancy is marked by rapid growth and high protein, vitamin, mineral, and energy requirements. Infants need an energy intake of approximately 108 kcal/kg of body weight in the first half of infancy and 98 kcal/kg in the second half (USDA, 2005). Infants need about 100 to 120 mL/kg/day of fluid because a large portion of total body weight is water.

Breast-Feeding The American Academy of Pediatrics (2005) strongly supports breast-feeding. The benefits include reduced food allergies and intolerances, fewer infant infections, and easier digestion. In addition, breast milk is convenient, fresh, always the correct temperature, and economical,

---

BOX 32-3   CULTURAL FOCUS

Matt reads about the influence of culture on nutrition. He finds that culture influences food habits and eating patterns. Other factors influencing eating patterns include food availability, geography, economics, and personal meanings and beliefs about food. Foods in different cultures often have symbolic meanings and are associated with births, deaths, religion, and social occasions. Special ethnic dishes or foods are served at ceremonies, holidays, and family celebrations. Recipes for these special dishes or foods are passed from generation to generation. There has been an "Americanization" of some of the special dishes and eating patterns. Regular use of traditional foods is seen more frequently in older members of a family than in younger members. The younger family members generally use these foods more on holidays or for special events.

Matt wants to know more about Mrs. Gonzalez's eating patterns. Eventually the patient will return to oral feeding after rehabilitation. He finds that persons from a Mexican culture typically get their protein from dry beans, cheeses, meats, fish, and eggs. Their grain intake is generally corn made into tamales and tortillas, although many families still make these with flour. Rice and wheat products are other sources of fiber. Chili peppers and deep-green and yellow vegetables, along with a variety of fruits such as guava, papaya, mango, and other citrus fruits, are eaten. Matt must identify foods that the dietitian thinks the patient will be able to swallow on return home.

IMPLICATIONS FOR PRACTICE

- Matt helps Mrs. Gonzalez identify ways to increase vegetables and fruit in her daily meals.
- Matt asks Mrs. Gonzalez about food served at family gatherings.
- Matt helps Mrs. Gonzalez identify ways to decrease fat in food served.
- Matt works with the dietitian to incorporate some of Mrs. Gonzalez's favorite foods into her diet when she is eating again.
- Matt involves daughter in discussing food selection when mother returns home.

Data from Ebersole P and others: *Toward healthy aging: human needs and nursing response*, ed 7, St. Louis, 2008, Mosby; Giger JN, Davidhizer RE: *Transcultural nursing: assessment and interventions*, ed 5, St. Louis, 2008, Mosby; Nix S: *Williams' basic nutrition and diet therapy*, ed 12, St. Louis, 2005, Mosby.

---

because it is less expensive than formula. It also provides increased time for mother and infant interaction (Williams and Schlenker, 2003).

Formula Infant formulas contain the approximate nutrient composition of human milk. Infants should not have regular cow's milk during the first year of life. It causes GI bleeding and is too concentrated for the infant's kidneys to manage. It also increases the risk for milk product allergies and is a poor source of iron and vitamins C and E (Williams and Schlenker, 2003). The American Academy of Pediatrics recommends breast milk or formula as the major source of food for up to 1 year in age (Williams and Schlenker, 2003). Honey and corn syrup are potential sources of botulism toxin and should not be used in the infant's diet. The toxin is potentially fatal in children under 1 year of age (Nix, 2005).

Introduction to Solid Food Breast milk or formula provides sufficient nutrition for the first 4 to 6 months of life. Iron-fortified cereals are typically the first semisolid food to be introduced. For infants 4 to 11 months, cereals are the most important nonmilk source of protein (Fox and others, 2006). Caregivers introduce new foods one at a time, approximately 4 to 7 days apart to identify allergies. It is best to introduce new foods before milk or other foods to avoid satiety (Hockenberry and Wilson, 2006).

The growth rate slows during toddler years, requiring fewer kilocalories but an increased amount of protein in relation to body weight; consequently appetite often decreases at 18 months of age. Toddlers exhibit strong food preferences and become picky eaters. Small, frequent meals consisting of breakfast, lunch, and dinner with three interspersed high-nutrient-density snacks help improve nutritional intake (Hockenberry and Wilson, 2006). Calcium and phosphorus are important for healthy bone growth.

Toddlers need to drink whole milk until the age of 2 years to make sure there is adequate intake of fatty acids necessary for brain and neurological development. Certain foods such as hot dogs, candy, nuts, grapes, raw vegetables, and popcorn have been implicated in choking deaths and need to be avoided. Preschoolers' (3 to 5 years) dietary requirements are similar to those of toddlers. They consume slightly more than toddlers, and nutrient density is more important than quantity.

School-age children, 6 to 12 years old, grow at a slower and steadier rate, with a gradual decline in energy requirements per unit of body weight. Despite the better appetites and more varied food intake of school-age children, you need to assess their diets carefully for adequate protein and vitamins A and C. There has been a consistent decrease in physical activity level and increase in consumption of high-calorie readily available food, leading to an increase in childhood obesity (Edwards, 2005).

In the last 20 years the prevalence of overweight children has doubled for children age 6 to 11 years and tripled for adolescents (Budd and Hayman, 2008; National Center for Chronic Disease Prevention and Health Promotion, 2007). A combination of factors contributes to the problem, including a diet rich in high-calorie foods such as high-sugar-content beverages, inactivity, genetic predisposition, use of food as a coping mechanism for stress or boredom, and family and social factors (Wofford, 2008). Childhood obesity contributes to medical problems related to the cardiovascular system, endocrine system, and mental health (Budd and Hayman, 2008). Prevention of childhood obesity is critical because of the long-term effects. Family education is an important component of decreasing the prevalence of this problem. Promote healthy food choices and eating in moderation along with increased physical activity.

ADOLESCENTS During adolescence, energy needs increase to meet greater metabolic demands of growth. Daily requirement of protein also increases. Calcium is essential for the rapid bone growth of adolescence, and girls need a continuous source of iron to replace menstrual losses. Boys also need adequate iron for muscle development. Iodine supports increased thyroid activity, and use of iodized table salt ensures availability. B-complex vitamins are necessary to support heightened metabolic activity. Nutritional deficiencies often occur in adolescent girls as a result of dieting and use of oral contraceptives. Snacks provide approximately 25% of the teenager's total dietary intake. Fast food is common and adds extra salt, fat, and kilocalories. Skipping meals or eating meals with wrong choices of snacks contributes to nutrient deficiency and obesity (Hockenberry and Wilson, 2006).

YOUNG AND MIDDLE-AGE ADULTS The demands for most nutrients are reduced as the growth period ends. Mature adults need nutrients for energy, maintenance, and repair. Energy needs usually decline over the years. Obesity becomes a problem as a result of decreased physical exercise, dining out more often, and increased ability to afford more luxury foods. Adult women who use oral contraceptives often need extra vitamins. Iron and calcium intake continues to be important.

Pregnancy Poor nutrition during pregnancy causes low birth weight in infants and decreases chances of survival. The nutritional status of the mother at the time of conception is important. The energy requirements of pregnancy are related to the mother's body weight and activity. Protein intake throughout pregnancy needs to increase to 60 g daily. Calcium intake is especially critical in the third trimester, when fetal bones are mineralized. Supplemental iron provides for increased maternal blood volume, for fetal blood storage, and for blood loss during delivery.

Folic acid intake is particularly important for DNA synthesis and the growth of red blood cells. Inadequate intake will possibly lead to fetal abnormalities (Williams and Schlenker, 2003). It is now recommended that women of child-bearing age consume 400 mcg of folic acid daily, increasing to 600 mcg daily during pregnancy.

Lactation The lactating woman needs 500 kcal/day above the usual allowance because the production of milk increases energy requirements. Protein requirements during lactation are greater than the protein requirement during pregnancy. There is an increased need for vitamins A and C. Daily intake of water-soluble vitamins (B and C) is necessary to ensure adequate levels in breast milk. Fluid intake needs to be adequate but not excessive. Caffeine, alcohol, and drugs are excreted in breast milk and should be avoided.

OLDER ADULTS Adults 65 years and older have a decreased need for calories as metabolic rate slows with age. Numerous factors influence the nutritional status of the older adult. Income is significant because living on a fixed income often reduces the amount of money available to buy food. The older adult is often on a therapeutic diet or has difficulty eating because of physical symptoms, lack of teeth, or dentures or is at risk for drug-nutrient interactions. The diet of older adults needs to contain choices from all food groups and often requires a vitamin and mineral supplement (Box 32-4).

BOX 32-4 CARE OF THE OLDER ADULT

Dietary Teaching

- Eat a balanced diet that contains a variety of foods. Avoid too much fat, cholesterol, sugar, and sodium or salt.
- Eat foods that have adequate amounts of starch and fiber such as fruits and vegetables and whole-grain cereals and breads.
- Avoid grapefruit and grapefruit juice because these will decrease absorption of many drugs.
- Ask health care provider about medications and food interactions.
- Drink adequate fluids because thirst sensation diminishes, often leading to inadequate fluid intake or dehydration. Water requirements do not decrease with age.
- If unable to eat meat because of cost or difficulty chewing, find alternate sources of protein.
- Cream soups and meat-based vegetable soups are nutrient-dense sources of protein.
- Cheese, eggs, and peanut butter are also useful high-protein alternatives.
- Drink milk for calcium and vitamin D to protect against osteoporosis (a decrease of bone mass density). Provide calcium supplements if lactose intolerance is present.
- Vitamin and nutrient supplements are recommended for persons who experience nutritional deficits.

Data from Ebersole P and others: *Toward healthy aging: human needs and nursing response*, ed 7, St. Louis, 2008, Mosby; Nix S: *Williams' basic nutrition and diet therapy*, ed 12, St. Louis, 2005, Mosby.

The USDHHS's Administration on Aging (AOA) requires states to provide nutritional screening services to older adult patients who benefit from home-delivered or congregate meal services. An estimated 5% to 10% of community-dwelling older adults suffer from food inadequacies within any 6-month period (Furman, 2006). Homebound older adults with chronic illness have additional nutritional risks. Frequently this group lives alone with little or no social or financial resources to assist in obtaining or preparing nutritionally sound meals. Increased nutritional screening by the nurse results in early recognition of potential nutritional deficiencies and needed treatment of these deficiencies (Chen and others, 2005). Undernourishment of older adults often results in health problems that lead to admission to acute care hospitals or long-term care facilities.

CRITICAL THINKING

Synthesis

You will apply elements of critical thinking whenever you perform the nursing process with a patient. Consider the scientific knowledge you have learned, your experience, critical thinking attitudes, and standards to ensure an individualized approach to patient care (Box 32-5).

BOX 32-5 SYNTHESIS IN PRACTICE

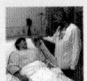 As Matt prepares to assess Mrs. Gonzalez, he recalls information about nutrition and its effect on rehabilitation, especially the importance of adequate caloric protein intake in patients who have had a stroke. He will focus assessment on Mrs. Gonzalez's weight, need for enteral nutrition, elimination patterns, and rehabilitation efforts. Matt knows that it is important to also assess for tolerance of tube feeding.

Matt knows that consulting with a dietitian to further assess Mrs. Gonzalez's nutritional status and assist with nutritional interventions will be beneficial. The dietitian will use data from Matt's initial nursing assessment and assist Matt in collecting further nutrition-related information.

Experience has taught Matt that economic and cultural preferences will also affect the acceptance of tube feeding. He is aware that Mrs. Gonzalez may perceive the initiation of enteral feedings as a loss of independence. Matt will reassure the patient that the tube feeding is necessary for her safety and to maintain nutritional intake. He also explains that the goal will be to restart oral feedings as soon as it is safe to do so.

KNOWLEDGE Application of knowledge from nutritional principles and the basic and social sciences form your knowledge base related to nutritional care. Information that comes from interviewing and observing the patient and the responses you obtain during nursing interventions will guide you toward application of knowledge. For example, your patient reports a dietary pattern of avoiding cabbage. This pattern could arise from physiological discomfort (gas-forming food), psychological issues (forced to eat cabbage as a child), sociological reasons (associated with lower socioeconomic class), ethnicity (not readily available in the country of origin), teaching- or learning-related reasons (never taught how to prepare cabbage), or mythology (a food that contains harmful chemicals). Consider these factors when planning a nutritious diet.

EXPERIENCE Just as multiple factors influence your patients' choices of dietary practices; multiple factors also influence your dietary patterns. Individuals who have nutritional or health problems change their long-standing dietary practices to enhance health. In assisting a patient in changing dietary patterns, draw on examples from your own experience. Perhaps you attempted to change a dietary practice or have a family member who requires a special diet. Previous experiences with therapeutic diets or behavioral changes will assist in the identification of nursing interventions that will be successful for the patient.

ATTITUDES Integrity and discipline are critical thinking skills that are beneficial during nutritional assessment and counseling. Although you will encounter patients whose dietary practices are dramatically different from yours, you assist those patients in attaining a nutritionally balanced diet.

In addition, you will care for patients whose dietary patterns are not healthful. Changes in dietary practices often occur over time. Perseverance will be necessary in educating patients to understand the impact of unhealthful food choices.

STANDARDS The use of professional standards, such as the DRIs, the USDA's food guide pyramid, dietary guidelines, and *Healthy People 2010* objectives provide guidelines for assessing and maintaining patients' nutritional status. Other professional standards by the American Heart Association (2006), the American Diabetes Association (2006), the American Cancer Society (Kushi and others, 2006), and the American Society for Parenteral and Enteral Nutrition (ASPEN) (2002) are available. These standards are evidence based and are regularly updated for optimal patient care.

NURSING PROCESS

■■■ASSESSMENT

SCREENING Nutritional screening is part of your initial assessment of the patient. The nutritional screening is a quick method of identifying malnutrition or risk for malnutrition (ASPEN, 2002). Nutritional screening tools commonly include objective measures such as height, weight, weight change, primary diagnosis, and the presence of comorbidities (ASPEN, 2002). Single objective measures alone are ineffective predictors of nutritional risk (Sarhill and others, 2003). You combine multiple objective measures with subjective measures related to nutrition to screen for nutritional risk. Health care institutions commonly use the initial nursing assessment as a nutritional screening. Certain nutritional risk factors, such as unintentional weight loss, the presence of a modified diet, or the presence of nutritional impact symptoms (i.e., nausea, vomiting, diarrhea, constipation), are triggers for nutritional consultation.

There are several standardized nutritional screening tools for you to use in the outpatient setting. The Subjective Global Assessment (SGA) is a validated clinical method that uses the patient history, weight, and physical assessment data to evaluate nutritional status (National Guideline Clearinghouse, 2006). The SGA is a simple, inexpensive technique that is able to predict nutrition-related complications. The Mini Nutritional Assessment (MNA) (Figure 32-2) was developed for the older adult population. This 18-item tool has two sections: screening and assessment. The screening contains 6 questions related to decline in food intake, weight loss, mobility, stress, and **body mass index (BMI).** The health care practitioner completes the assessment portion if the patient scores 11 or less (Guigoz and others, 1996). The 12-item assessment includes specific medical history and eating habits, as well as some anthropometric measurements. A score of less than 17 points indicates protein-energy malnutrition (PEM) (Guigoz and Vellas, 1999; Guigoz and others, 1996).

NUTRITIONAL ASSESSMENT If you find a patient is at risk for nutritional problems, refer the patient to an RD for a more in-depth nutritional assessment. Nutritional assessment is different from nutritional screening. The RD will complete a nutritional assessment, which includes an in-depth exploration of medical history, dietary history, physical examination, anthropometric measurements, and laboratory data (Table 32-1). This process often leads to the identification and diagnosis of nutritional issues. Nutritional assessment includes the determination of nutrient and protein needs. In an acute care setting the RD is available to make these calculations. In an outpatient setting, there is not always an RD to complete the nutritional assessment.

Diet History The diet history focuses on habitual intake of food and liquids and information about preferences, allergies, and digestive problems (Box 32-6). Open-ended questions encourage the patient to provide more information on food intake during the interview. For example, ask a patient who reports that she avoids dairy products, "Tell me what led you to avoid dairy products?" The patient's answer to this question will lead to physiological, psychological, sociological, religious, cultural, or food preference factors that you will further explore.

Ask a patient to keep a detailed record of food intake over 3 days, representing a typical eating pattern. Have the patient include a weekend day. This record allows you to calculate the patient's nutritional intake and to compare it with the DRIs. Instruct your patients to record the specific type of foods and the exact amounts ingested. This requires the use of measuring cups and scales. Information on patient's activity level and presence of disease will be necessary to estimate energy needs. For example, a patient who has a fever or has suffered severe trauma has high caloric demands even though the activity level is limited. You compare estimated energy need, as calculated through prediction equations, to actual caloric intake, through calorie counts. Calorie counts use records of exact amounts of food trays consumed as documented by the nursing or nutrition staff to calculate total calories and protein consumed daily. You will need to consult with an RD to determine an exact calorie count or requirements.

Medication History Prescribed and over-the-counter medications have the potential for drug-nutrient interactions. Knowing what medications your patients take is important when meeting nutritional needs. Consultation with a pharmacist will determine the specific risks for nutrient-drug interactions for your patients.

PATIENTS AT RISK FOR NUTRITIONAL PROBLEMS A patient with a condition that interferes with the ability to ingest, digest, or absorb adequate nutrients needs to be assessed for malnutrition. Use a standardized tool to assess nutritional risks when possible. Congenital anomalies and surgical revisions of the gastrointestinal tract interfere with normal function. Patients fed only by intravenous infusion of 5% to 10% dextrose are at risk for nutritional deficiencies. Older adults, infants, or the malnourished are at greatest risk.

PHYSICAL EXAMINATION Examine the patient for signs of actual or potential nutritional alterations (Table 32-2, p. 917). The skin and hair are primary areas that reflect nutrient and hydration deficiencies. Be alert for rashes, dry scaly skin, poor skin turgor, skin lesions, hair loss, easily pluckable hair, hair without luster, and an unhealthy scalp.

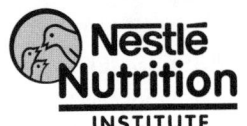

Mini Nutritional Assessment
MNA®

Last name:	First name:	Sex:	Date:
Age:	Weight, kg:	Height, cm:	I.D. Number:

Complete the screen by filling in the boxes with the appropriate numbers.
Add the numbers for the screen. If score is 11 or less, continue with the assessment to gain a Malnutrition Indicator Score.

Screening

A Has food intake declined over the past 3 months due to loss of appetite, digestive problems, chewing or swallowing difficulties?
0 = severe loss of appetite
1 = moderate loss of appetite
2 = no loss of appetite ☐

B Weight loss during the last 3 months
0 = weight loss greater than 3 kg (6.6 lbs)
1 = does not know
2 = weight loss between 1 and 3 kg (2.2 and 6.6 lbs)
3 = no weight loss ☐

C Mobility
0 = bed or chair bound
1 = able to get out of bed/chair but does not go out
2 = goes out ☐

D Has suffered psychological stress or acute disease in the past 3 months
0 = yes   2 = no ☐

E Neuropsychological problems
0 = severe dementia or depression
1 = mild dementia
2 = no psychological problems ☐

F Body Mass Index (BMI) (weight in kg) / (height in m²)
0 = BMI less than 19
1 = BMI 19 to less than 21
2 = BMI 21 to less than 23
3 = BMI 23 or greater ☐

Screening score (subtotal max. 14 points) ☐ ☐
12 points or greater   Normal – not at risk – no need to complete assessment
11 points or below   Possible malnutrition – continue assessment

Assessment

G Lives independently (not in a nursing home or hospital)
0 = no   1 = yes ☐

H Takes more than 3 prescription drugs per day
0 = yes   1 = no ☐

I Pressure sores or skin ulcers
0 = yes   1 = no ☐

Ref. Vellas B, Villars H, Abellan G, et al. Overview of the MNA® - Its History and Challenges. J Nut Health Aging 2006;10:456-465.
Rubenstein LZ, Harker JO, Salva A, Guigoz Y, Vellas B. Screening for Undernutrition in Geriatric Practice: Developing the Short-Form Mini Nutritional Assessment (MNA-SF). J. Geront 2001;56A: M366-377.
Guigoz Y. The Mini-Nutritional Assessment (MNA®) Review of the Literature - What does it tell us? J Nutr Health Aging 2006; 10:466-487.

J How many full meals does the patient eat daily?
0 = 1 meal
1 = 2 meals
2 = 3 meals ☐

K Selected consumption markers for protein intake
• At least one serving of dairy products (milk, cheese, yogurt) per day   yes ☐ no ☐
• Two or more servings of legumes or eggs per week   yes ☐ no ☐
• Meat, fish or poultry every day   yes ☐ no ☐
0.0 = if 0 or 1 yes
0.5 = if 2 yes
1.0 = if 3 yes ☐.☐

L Consumes two or more servings of fruits or vegetables per day?
0 = no   1 = yes ☐

M How much fluid (water, juice, coffee, tea, milk…) is consumed per day
0.0 = less than 3 cups
0.5 = 3 to 5 cups
1.0 = more than 5 cups ☐.☐

N Mode of feeding
0 = unable to eat without assistance
1 = self-fed with some difficulty
2 = self-fed without any problem ☐

O Self view of nutritional status
0 = views self as being malnourished
1 = is uncertain of nutritional state
2 = views self as having no nutritional problem ☐

P In comparison with other people of the same age, how does the patient consider his/her health status?
0.0 = not as good
0.5 = does not know
1.0 = as good
2.0 = better ☐.☐

Q Mid-arm circumference (MAC) in cm
0.0 = MAC less than 21
0.5 = MAC 21 to 22
1.0 = MAC 22 or greater ☐.☐

R Calf circumference (CC) in cm ☐
0 = CC less than 31   1 = CC 31 or greater

Assessment (max. 16 points)   ☐ ☐.☐

Screening score   ☐ ☐

Total Assessment (max. 30 points)   ☐ ☐.☐

Malnutrition Indicator Score
17 to 23.5 points   at risk of malnutrition ☐
Less than 17 points   malnourished ☐

Figure 32-2 ■ Mini Nutritional Assessment (MNA). (®Société des Produits Nestlé S.A., Vevey, Switzerland, Trademark Owners.)

TABLE 32-1   FOCUSED PATIENT ASSESSMENT

FACTORS TO ASSESS	QUESTIONS	PHYSICAL ASSESSMENT
Food and nutrient intake	How many meals a day do you eat? What times do you normally eat meals and snacks? What are the portion sizes that you eat at each meal? Are you on a special diet because of a health problem? Who purchases and prepares the food?	Inspect oral cavity for physical barriers to eating (e.g., tooth decay, poor-fitting dentures). Inspect condition of skin, hair, and nails. Assess skin turgor.
Patterns and dietary history	What types of food do you like? Are you allergic to any foods? What type of problems do you have with these foods? Have you noticed any changes in taste? Do you have any problems with chewing or swallowing?	Observe patient swallowing. Observe percentage of food consumed from meal tray.
Changes in weight	Have you had a change in your appetite? Have you noticed a change in your weight? Was this change an anticipated change (for example, were you on a weight-reduction diet)?	Weigh patient and analyze for changes. Observe patient's muscle tone. Inspect oral cavity for signs of malnutrition, such as cheilosis, stomatitis, and dry lesions at corners of mouth (see Table 32-2).
Skin	Have you noticed any changes in your skin such as scaliness, dryness, or bruising? Do you use skin moisturizers regularly?	Observe skin for color, moisture, changes in pigment, or bruising (see Table 32-2).

BOX 32-6   Information Contained in a Diet History

- Twenty-four-hour diet recall of the day
  - Use of enteral or parenteral nutrition
  - Food consumed for breakfast, lunch, dinner, and snacks
  - Number of meals and snacks a day
  - Timing of meals and snacks
  - Use of nutritional supplements
- Dietary restrictions
  - Medically prescribed diets
  - Modified-consistency diets
- Food preferences, allergies, and aversions
  - Foods that cause indigestion, diarrhea, or gas
- Chewing or swallowing difficulties (examine the mouth)
  - Use of dentures (have patient remove dentures to examine the mouth)
  - Presence of tooth decay
  - Presence of xerostomia, mucositis, or mouth sores
- Usual bowel movements
  - Presence of constipation or diarrhea
  - Duration of constipation or diarrhea
- Meal procurement and preparation responsibility
  - Appetite changes

Modified from Nix S: *Williams' basic nutrition and diet therapy*, ed 12, St. Louis, 2005, Mosby.

ANTHROPOMETRY **Anthropometry** is a systematic measurement of the size and makeup of the body using height and weight as the principal measures. You typically obtain height and weight measurements during a patient's admission to any health care setting. If the patient is unable to stand, you estimate height by measuring the patient's length with a tape measure while the patient lies supine. You can assess weight with bed scales. You then compare height and weight with usual measurements, called usual body weight (UBW) and standard norms for normal height-weight relationships, called **ideal body weight (IBW)**. Serial measures of weight over time provide more useful information than one measurement. When collecting serial measurements of weight, you weigh the patient about the same time each day, on the same scale, and with the same amount of clothing. In some patients, a weight change of 2 lb in 24 hours is significant because 1 lb is roughly equivalent to 500 mL of fluid.

BMI is an indicator of the relationship of height to weight. It is calculated it by dividing weight in kilograms (kg) by height in meters squared (m^2). A BMI range of 18.5 to 24.9 is recommended for optimal health. For example, a patient who weighs 75 kg (165 lb) is 1.8 m (5 feet 9 inches) tall has a BMI of 23.15 ($75 \div 1.8^2 = 23.15$). A patient is considered overweight if the BMI is 25 to 30. A BMI of greater than 30 is defined as obesity and places a patient at higher medical risk for coronary heart disease, some cancers, diabetes mellitus, and hypertension. Other factors such as lack of access to healthy food and inadequate health care also contribute to the development of these problems (Williams and Schlenker, 2003).

LABORATORY VALUES No single laboratory or biochemical test is diagnostic for malnutrition. Factors that frequently alter test results include fluid balance, liver function, kidney function, and the presence of disease. Laboratory values useful in nutritional assessment include complete blood count (CBC), albumin, prealbumin (transferrin), electrolytes, blood urea nitrogen, 24-hour urine urea nitrogen (UUN),

TABLE 32-2 Physical Signs of Nutritional Status

BODY AREA	NORMAL APPEARANCE	INDICATORS OF MALNUTRITION
General appearance	Alert, responsive	Listless, apathetic, cachectic
Weight	Normal for height, age, body build	Overweight, obesity, or underweight (special concern for underweight)
Posture	Erect, arms and legs straight	Sagging shoulders, sunken chest, humped back
Muscles	Well-developed, firm, good tone, some fat under skin	Flaccid, poor tone, undeveloped, tender, "wasted" appearance, impaired ability to walk
Nerve conduction and mental status	Good attention span, not irritable or restless, normal reflexes, psychological stability	Inattentive, irritable, confused, burning and tingling of hands and feet (paresthesia), loss of position and vibratory sense, weakness and tenderness of muscles (may result in inability to walk), decrease or loss of ankle and knee reflexes
Gastrointestinal function	Good appetite and digestion, normal regular elimination, no palpable (perceptible to touch) organs or masses	Anorexia, indigestion, constipation or diarrhea, liver or spleen enlargement
Cardiovascular function	Normal heart rate and rhythm, no murmurs, normal blood pressure for age	Rapid heart rate (above 100 beats per minute, tachycardia), enlarged heart, abnormal rhythm, elevated blood pressure
General vitality	Endurance, energetic, sleeps well, vigorous	Easily fatigued, no energy, falls asleep easily, looks tired, apathetic
Hair	Shiny, lustrous, firm, not easily plucked, healthy scalp	Stringy, dull, brittle, dry, thin and sparse, depigmented, easily plucked
Skin (general)	Smooth, slightly moist, good color	Rough, dry, scaly, pale, pigmented, irritated, bruises, petechiae
Face and neck	Skin color uniform; smooth, healthy appearance; not swollen	Greasy, discolored, scaly, swollen, skin dark over cheeks and under eyes, lumpiness or flakiness of skin around nose and mouth
Lips	Smooth, good color, moist, not chapped or swollen	Dry, scaly, swollen, redness and swelling (cheilosis), or angular lesions at corners of the mouth or fissures or scars (stomatitis)
Mouth, oral mucous membranes	Reddish pink mucous membranes in oral cavity	Swollen, deep red or magenta oral mucous membranes, oral lesions
Gums	Good pink color, healthy, red, no swelling or bleeding	Spongy, bleed easily, marginal redness, inflamed, receding
Tongue	Good pink color or deep reddish in appearance, not swollen or smooth, surface papillae present, no lesions	Swelling, scarlet and raw, magenta color, beefy (glossitis), hyperemic and hypertrophic papillae, atrophic papillae
Teeth	No pain, no sensitivity	Missing teeth, broken teeth
Eyes	Bright, clear, shiny, no sores at corner of eyelids, membranes moist and healthy pink color, no prominent blood vessels or mound of tissue or sclera, no fatigue circles beneath	Eye membranes pale (pale conjunctivae), redness of membrane (conjunctival injection), dryness or infection, Bitot's spots, redness and fissuring of eyelid corners (angular palpebritis), dryness of eye membrane (conjunctival xerosis), dull appearance of cornea (corneal xerosis), soft cornea (keratomalacia)
Neck (glands)	No enlargement	Thyroid or lymph nodes enlarged
Nails	Firm, pink	Spoon-shaped (koilonychia), brittle, ridged
Legs and feet	No tenderness, weakness, or swelling; good color	Edema, tender calf, tingling, weakness, lesions
Skeleton	No malformations	Bowlegs, knock-knees, chest deformity at diaphragm, beaded ribs, prominent scapulas

Data from Nix S: *Williams' basic nutrition and diet therapy,* ed 12, St. Louis, 2005, Mosby.

creatinine, glucose, cholesterol, and triglycerides. Individual laboratory measures alone are not specific enough to indicate nutritional risk, so they are combined with multiple objective measures to determine malnutrition. A low red blood cell count and depressed hemoglobin value indicates anemia. The hemoglobin, hematocrit, electrolyte, and blood urea nitrogen values also help to reflect the state of hydration. Researchers have linked decreased serum levels of albumin and prealbumin with malnutrition; however, disease state and metabolic stress highly affect these values (Fuhrman and others, 2004).

Nitrogen balance is important to establish serum protein status (see the discussion of protein in this chapter). The output of nitrogen is measured through laboratory analysis of a 24-hour UUN.

DYSPHAGIA **Dysphagia** refers to difficulty with swallowing. It occurs as a result of damage to muscles and nerves and obstructive causes (Box 32-7). The complications of dysphagia vary, including aspiration pneumonia, dehydration, decreased nutritional status, and weight loss. Dysphagia leads to disability or decreased functional status, increased length of stay and cost of care, increased likelihood of discharge to institutionalized care, and increased mortality (Ashley and others, 2006).

There are several indicators that warn you that your patient has dysphagia. Signs of dysphagia include cough; change in voice tone or quality after swallowing; abnormal movements of the mouth, tongue, or lips; and slow, weak, imprecise, or uncoordinated speech. Abnormal gag, delayed swallowing, incomplete oral clearance or pocketing, regurgitation, pharyngeal pooling, delayed or absent trigger of swallow, and inability to speak consistently are other signs of dysphagia. Patients with dysphagia do not usually exhibit overt signs such as coughing when food enters the airway. "Silent aspiration," or aspiration that occurs without a cough, is a common cause of complications (Nowlin, 2006). Silent aspiration accounts for 40% to 70% of cases of aspiration in patients with dysphagia after stroke (Kwon and others, 2006).

Dysphagia causes decreases in food intake, which often leads to malnutrition. Patients that experience dysphagia show changes in skin fold thickness and albumin. This malnutrition commonly occurs secondary to inability to consume an adequate volume of food caused by frustrations with the process of feeding and swallowing. The period of adjustment to new dietary restrictions and the rehabilitation period affect intake for long periods of time. Malnutrition resulting from inadequate protein, calorie, and micronutrient intake will significantly slow down recovery (Perry and Love, 2001). Early screening with a dysphagia screening protocol significantly decreases the risk for aspiration pneumonia in patients (Hinchey and others, 2005; Kwon and others, 2006).

Dysphagia Screening Dysphagia screening is done to quickly identify problems with swallowing and to refer at-risk patients for a more in-depth assessment (Skill 32-1).

There are many dysphagia screening tools. The Registered Dietitian Dysphagia Screening Tool includes medical record review, observation of a patient at a meal for change in voice quality, posture and head control, percentage of meal consumed, eating time, drooling of liquids and solids, cough during/after a swallow, facial or tongue weakness, difficulty with secretions, pocketing, and presence of voluntary and dry cough (Brody and others, 2000). Screening tools such as the Burke Dysphagia Screening Test and the Standardized Swallowing Assessment have also been validated in patients with dysphagia (Perry and Love, 2001). These tools evaluate holding, leakage, coughing, choking, breathlessness, and quality of voice. These tools are designed for multidisciplinary use by RNs, RDs, physicians, or speech-language pathologists (SLPs) (Brody and others, 2000; Daniels and others, 2000; Perry and Love, 2001).

PATIENT EXPECTATIONS Patients who require assistance with nutritional problems have a variety of expectations. It is important for you to learn what the patient expects in terms of resuming a normal diet or learning to adjust to a therapeutic diet. Patients with impairments in upper arm mobility expect assistance with activities such as preparing the meal, setting up the meal tray or plate, or being fed. Other patients expect information on the availability and use of assistive devices to increase independence with meals. A consultation with occupational therapy will help patients obtain these assistive devices and provide education on their proper use. You need to teach patients who have impaired vision how to feed themselves.

▪▪▪ NURSING DIAGNOSIS

Following nursing assessment, cluster relevant defining characteristics to determine whether actual or potential nutritional problems exist. An alteration occurs when the body does not ingest a nutrient in sufficient quantity, poorly digests or does not completely absorb nutrients, or when total daily caloric needs are deficient or excessive. The following are examples of nursing diagnoses appropriate for patients with nutritional alterations:

- *Risk for aspiration*
- *Diarrhea*
- *Adult failure to thrive*

BOX 32-7   Causes of Dysphagia

MYOGENIC (MUSCLE)	NEUROGENIC (NERVE)	OBSTRUCTIVE	OTHER
Myasthenia gravis	Stroke	Benign peptic stricture	Gastrointestinal or esophageal resection
Aging	Cerebral palsy	Lower esophageal ring	Rheumatological disorders
Muscular dystrophy	Guillain-Barré syndrome	Candidiasis	Connective tissue disorders
Polymyositis	Multiple sclerosis	Head and neck cancer	Vagotomy
	Amyotrophic lateral sclerosis (Lou Gehrig disease)	Inflammatory masses	
	Diabetic neuropathy	Trauma/surgical resection	
	Parkinson's disease	Anterior mediastinal masses	
		Cervical spondylosis	

- *Deficient knowledge (nutrition)*
- *Imbalanced nutrition: less than body requirements*
- *Imbalanced nutrition: more than body requirements*
- *Readiness for enhanced nutrition*
- *Risk for imbalanced nutrition: more than body requirements*
- *Feeding self-care deficit*

Your assessment also needs to identify the probable cause or related factor for the nutritional problem. Make sure the nursing diagnosis is as precise as possible. Related factors need to be accurate so that you select the appropriate interventions. For example, the overweight patient often has nutrient deficiencies and requires supplements or specialized nutritional support during episodes of acute illness. The nursing assessment identifies dietary patterns that have contributed to obesity. An assessment is needed that focuses on adequacy of all food groups. Patterns such as intake of high-fat foods and inadequate fruit and vegetable intake are examples of food habits that lead to nutrient deficiencies. In this situation you would use the nursing diagnosis *imbalanced nutrition: less than body requirements related to poor eating habits*. The Concept Map (Figure 32-3) shows the relationship of nursing diagnoses for Mrs. Gonzalez.

■■■PLANNING

During planning you will select nursing interventions intended to improve the patient's nutritional status and the monitoring and evaluation to determine the effectiveness of those interventions. The input of all disciplines involved in patient care is necessary for planning of the nutritional interventions. Reflect on the causes of the patient's malnutrition or risk for malnutrition. Individualize the intervention to the patient, and take into consideration the patient's comfort and wishes. Although there are variables between and among patients, common nutritional goals include symptom management, weight maintenance, and preservation of functional status. The use of modified diets, the addition of oral nutritional supplements, or the initiation of enteral or parenteral nutrition is sometimes required to improve nutritional status. Consider the cost of these modifications, as well as patient and caregiver burden, before beginning an intervention. The services of social workers are very beneficial in situations in which patients are not able to afford the intervention.

GOALS AND OUTCOMES The goal in caring for patients with nutritional alterations is to improve the patient's nutritional status. If the nutritional diagnosis is *imbalanced nutrition: less than body requirements,* the outcome will be for the patient to gain weight or to ingest adequate nutrients in a certain category. If a patient is obese, a goal of care will be to safely achieve weight reduction. You determine specific, individualized goals by identifying patient behaviors that have led to the nutritional alteration (see Care Plan). Correction of poor dietary patterns is a long-term rather than a short-term goal. Short-term goals usually involve achieving calorie or nutrient targets on a daily or weekly basis. It is important to explore patients' feelings about their weight and food and to help them

set realistic and achievable goals (Daniels, 2006). You achieve the goals through a prescribed diet, patient education, and assisting the patient in developing new behaviors that will enable the patient to achieve an adequate nutritional status.

Individualized planning for nutrition is critical. Mutually planned goals between the patient, registered dietitian, and nurse ensure success. Patients often have unrealistic expectations about nutritional repletion or dieting in reference to weight gain or loss. Help patients understand this concept by asking them to reflect on their rate of weight gain or loss. Changes in weight usually occur over months or years unless an acute illness has occurred. Patients become discouraged when they do not see rapid achievement of weight goals. Help the patient to be realistic in setting outcomes. For example, the following outcomes will assist in achieving a weight-loss goal:

- Patient loses ½ to 1 lb per week.
- Patient's daily fat intake is less than 30%.
- Patient eliminates sugared beverages from diet.
- Patient increases fruit and vegetable servings in diet to five servings per day.

SETTING PRIORITIES Patients at risk for nutritional problems have a plan of care aimed at improving nutritional status. However, many factors influence how you set priorities so that a patient receives proper nourishment. For example, if a patient is on oral intake, your priority involves symptom control (e.g., nausea or pain) before a patient feels comfortable to eat. Physiological factors such as fear or depression often influence a person's willingness to eat. If this is the situation, discussing a patient's concerns takes precedence over starting mealtime. Food is important for all persons, but when illness disrupts appetite or the ability to eat, you must anticipate what is most important to help your patient achieve good nutrition.

The development of the care plan requires collaboration of the health care team, the patient, and the family caregivers. Family and caregivers are often involved in food purchase and preparation. The nutritional plan of care will not succeed without their commitment to, involvement in, and understanding of nutritional goals.

COLLABORATIVE CARE Patient nutritional needs extend beyond the acute hospital setting and into the home or rehabilitation care setting, requiring collaboration of health care professionals. Professionals who assist in providing care include the registered dietitian, nutritional support clinical nurse specialist, pharmacists, and health care providers. Consult with a speech-language pathologist, RD, pharmacist, and/or occupational therapist when doing discharge planning that includes ongoing nutritional assessment and interventions to meet the nutritional needs of patients. Some patients with physiological conditions causing more severe cases of malnutrition require enteral tube feeding or parenteral nutrition to meet fluid, electrolyte, and nutritional needs.

Patients and family members need to learn the skills to administer nutritional therapies safely and effectively. Home care

CONCEPT MAP

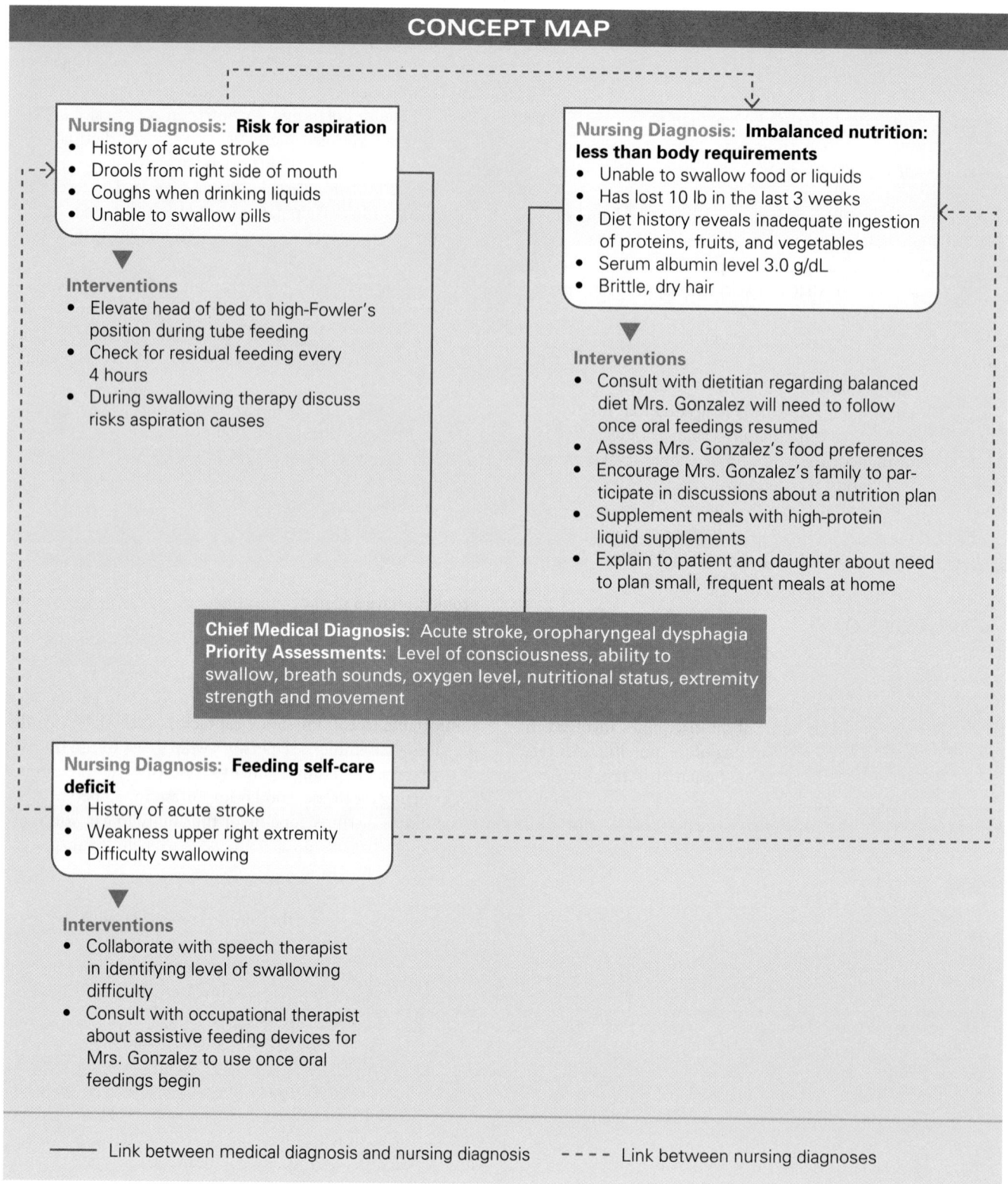

Nursing Diagnosis: Risk for aspiration
- History of acute stroke
- Drools from right side of mouth
- Coughs when drinking liquids
- Unable to swallow pills

Interventions
- Elevate head of bed to high-Fowler's position during tube feeding
- Check for residual feeding every 4 hours
- During swallowing therapy discuss risks aspiration causes

Nursing Diagnosis: Imbalanced nutrition: less than body requirements
- Unable to swallow food or liquids
- Has lost 10 lb in the last 3 weeks
- Diet history reveals inadequate ingestion of proteins, fruits, and vegetables
- Serum albumin level 3.0 g/dL
- Brittle, dry hair

Interventions
- Consult with dietitian regarding balanced diet Mrs. Gonzalez will need to follow once oral feedings resumed
- Assess Mrs. Gonzalez's food preferences
- Encourage Mrs. Gonzalez's family to participate in discussions about a nutrition plan
- Supplement meals with high-protein liquid supplements
- Explain to patient and daughter about need to plan small, frequent meals at home

Chief Medical Diagnosis: Acute stroke, oropharyngeal dysphagia
Priority Assessments: Level of consciousness, ability to swallow, breath sounds, oxygen level, nutritional status, extremity strength and movement

Nursing Diagnosis: Feeding self-care deficit
- History of acute stroke
- Weakness upper right extremity
- Difficulty swallowing

Interventions
- Collaborate with speech therapist in identifying level of swallowing difficulty
- Consult with occupational therapist about assistive feeding devices for Mrs. Gonzalez to use once oral feedings begin

——— Link between medical diagnosis and nursing diagnosis   - - - - Link between nursing diagnoses

Figure 32-3 ■ Concept Map.

nurses play an important role in initially establishing enteral and parenteral nutrition routes and then assisting patients and families with monitoring and supplement delivery. Long-term nutritional management is a challenge that requires collaboration among the patient, family, and health care team.

■■■ IMPLEMENTATION

HEALTH PROMOTION You play a major role in promoting healthy dietary practices. Using tools such as the food guide pyramid assists patients with food choices, menu planning, and dietary patterns. You will also educate

CARE PLAN Nutrition

ASSESSMENT

Mrs. Gonzalez has had a stroke. Matt knows that strokes often cause dysphagia, which increases the risk for aspiration. Mrs. Gonzale's diet history reveals that she ate balanced meals three times daily, including at least three servings of fruits and vegetables. A feeding tube is in place and enteral feedings are to be started. Mrs. Gonzalez states, "I just don't know about this tube. I wish my doctor would just let me eat."

ASSESSMENT ACTIVITIES	FINDINGS/DEFINING CHARACTERISTICS*
Assess Mrs. Gonzalez for risk for aspiration.	Mrs. Gonzalez has been diagnosed with **acute stroke.** She starts to **cough when she tries to drink water.**
Evaluate Mrs. Gonzalez's swallowing ability.	The speech-language pathologist's (SLP's) evaluation shows Mrs. Gonzalez is **unable to swallow and aspirates pills and thickened liquids.** The SLP has diagnosed her with **oropharyngeal dysphagia.**
Monitor Mrs. Gonzalez's respiratory status.	Lung sounds are clear. Respirations are regular at a rate of 12 breaths per minute. She has no shortness of breath. Oxygen saturation is 96% on room air.
Assess Mrs. Gonzalez's nutritional status.	**Enteral nutrition will begin at 60 mL/hr** to meet calculated caloric needs. Baseline prealbumin and albumin levels are within normal limits.

NURSING DIAGNOSIS: Risk for aspiration related to impaired swallowing.

PLANNING

GOAL

- Mrs. Gonzalez will receive adequate nutrients through enteral tube feeding without aspiration by discharge.
- Mrs. Gonzalez will regain swallowing ability from speech therapy by discharge.

EXPECTED OUTCOMES (NOC)†

Nutritional Status: Nutrient Intake
- Mrs. Gonzalez's weight at discharge will be within 2 lb of admission weight.
- Mrs. Gonzalez will not exhibit signs of aspiration before discharge.
- Mrs. Gonzalez's albumin and prealbumin levels will remain normal before discharge.
- Mrs. Gonzalez will progress to an oral diet before discharge to restorative care facility.

INTERVENTIONS (NIC)‡

Nutritional Management
- Insert feeding tube as ordered.

- Initiate enteral feeding as prescribed.

- Advance tube feeding as tolerated; monitor for tolerance.

Aspiration Precautions
- Position Mrs. Gonzalez with head of bed elevated a minimum of 30 degrees.

- Check tube placement every 4 to 6 hours.

- Check gastric residual volume every 4 hours.

RATIONALE

Enteral tube feeding will allow for safe provision of nutrients while swallowing is rehabilitated with the assistance of the SLP (Cirgin Ellett, 2006).

The tube feeding is initiated at a low rate of infusion and increased slowly to allow for maximum tolerance (Rolandelli and others, 2005).

Abdominal pain, large volume of gastric residuals, and diarrhea are signs of feeding intolerance and need to be evaluated promptly (Rolandelli and others, 2005).

Head of the bed elevated a minimum of 30 to 45 degrees decreases the risk for aspiration (Enteral Nutrition Practice Recommendations Task Force, 2009).

This confirms tube placement. Improperly positioned tubes increase the risk for aspiration (Bourgault and others, 2007).

Gastric residual volume indicates if gastric emptying is delayed. Delayed gastric emptying increases the risk for aspiration (Enteral Nutrition Practice Recommendations Task Force, 2009).

---

*__Defining characteristics__ are shown in **bold** type.
†Outcomes classification label from Moorhead S and others, editors: *Nursing outcomes classification (NOC)*, ed 4, St. Louis, 2008, Mosby.
‡Intervention classifications labels from Bulechek and others, editors: *Nursing interventions classification (NIC)*, ed 5, St. Louis, 2008, Mosby.

CARE PLAN   Nutrition—cont'd

INTERVENTIONS (NIC)‡

- Continue with speech therapy. Make sure the patient is properly positioned and supervised during trials.

RATIONALE

Regularly provided speech therapy will assist the patient in regaining the ability to swallow foods and liquids.

Speech therapy includes trials of various consistencies of foods and liquids. Aspiration of food and liquids lead to chest congestion and pneumonia (National Dysphagia Diet Task Force, 2002).

EVALUATION

NURSING ACTIONS	PATIENT RESPONSE/FINDING	ACHIEVEMENT OF OUTCOME
Ask Mrs. Gonzalez if she is experiencing any gastrointestinal discomfort.	Mrs. Gonzalez admits she has occasional constipation.	Mrs. Gonzalez is not experiencing diarrhea, but bowel movements need to be regular.
Weigh Mrs. Gonzalez weekly.	Mrs. Gonzalez's weight is ½ lb less than her admission weight.	Mrs. Gonzalez's weight is maintained.
Monitor the laboratory values.	Prealbumin remains 20 mg/dL, and albumin is 4 g/dL.	Prealbumin and albumin values are maintained within normal limits.
Ask SLP about Mrs. Gonzalez's swallowing rehabilitation.	Mrs. Gonzalez is able to tolerate ground diet and nectar-thickened liquids.	Calorie count indicates Mrs. Gonzalez's oral intake does currently meet her anticipated needs.

patients about food labels and their meanings. An area of particular importance is education about product claims that are misleading: some "reduced fat" foods still have significant amounts of fat, some "lite" foods still contain considerable calories, and "low cholesterol" does not always mean low fat.

Obesity is an epidemic in the United States. The prevalence of obesity is 35% (U.S. Department of Health and Human Services Centers for Disease Control and Prevention, 2008). Proposed contributing factors are sedentary lifestyle, work schedules, and poor meal choices often related to the increasing frequency of eating away from home and eating fast food (Kruskall, 2006). More patients are acknowledging their weight and seeking weight-loss strategies (Lee and others, 2004).

A high percentage of those who attempt to lose weight are unsuccessful, regaining lost weight over time. Diet and exercise compliance affects success with weight loss. Many individuals are willing to pay for weight-loss programs if the program meets individual needs (Roux and others, 2004). Information on weight-loss diets is available everywhere, from the bookstore to the Internet. However, there is a lack of good evidence evaluating the effectiveness of commercial weight-loss programs. A successful weight-loss plan must include awareness of portion sizes and knowledge of energy content of food (Kruskall, 2006).

Food safety is a commonly overlooked aspect of health promotion. Contaminated and undercooked food products, especially eggs and meats, often result in severe debilitating and even fatal illnesses (Table 32-3). Patient education is one method of improving safe food practices for patients and their families (Box 32-8).

ACUTE CARE It is common for oral intake to decrease during periods of stress. This occurs as a result of the anorexic effects of stress-induced hormones (Takeda and others, 2004). It is important that you monitor the patient's nutrient intake, identify influences that reduce appetite, and plan interventions to increase intake.

One disruptive influence on intake in acute care is diagnostic testing. Some blood and radiographic studies require the patient to receive nothing by mouth (NPO). Therefore the patient's food is withheld until the patient returns from the test or the testing is completed. This disrupts mealtimes, and sometimes patients are too fatigued to eat or experience discomfort related to the test. Emotional stress also influences intake. Patients who are worried about their families, finances, employment, or illness are not always able to eat or eat enough to compensate for the effect of stress on metabolism. Continue to assess the patient's nutritional status. Patients who are NPO and receive only standard intravenous fluids for more than 4 to 7 days are at nutritional risk.

Medications also affect intake and in some cases the use of nutrients. The use of certain medications is associated with anorexia, malabsorption, and increased metabolism. Medication-induced nausea, vomiting, and diarrhea also greatly affect intake. Taste changes occur with the use of medications such as chemotherapy, diuretics, and mineral preparations such as zinc. Work with the dietitian to help the

TABLE 32-3   Food Safety

FOOD-BORNE DISEASE	ORGANISM	FOOD SOURCE	SYMPTOMS*
Botulism	Clostridium botulinum	Improperly home-canned foods, smoked and salted fish, ham, sausage, shellfish	Symptoms are varied from mild discomfort to death in 24 hours, initially nausea and dizziness, progressing to motor (respiratory) paralysis
Escherichia coli	Escherichia E. coli O157:H7	Undercooked meat (ground beef)	Severe cramps, nausea, vomiting, diarrhea (may be bloody), renal failure. Appears 1-8 days after eating, lasts 1-7 days
Listeriosis	Listeria L. monocytogenes	Soft cheese, meat (hot dogs, pate, lunch meats), unpasteurized milk, poultry, seafood	Severe diarrhea, fever, headache, pneumonia, meningitis, endocarditis. Appears 3-21 days after infection
Perfringens enteritis	Clostridium C. perfringens	Cooked meats, meat dishes held at room or warm temperature	Mild diarrhea, vomiting. Appears 8-24 hours after eating, lasts 1-2 days
Salmonellosis	Salmonella S. typhi S. paratyphi	Milk, custards, egg dishes, salad dressings, sandwich fillings, polluted shellfish	Mild to severe diarrhea, cramps, vomiting. Appears 12-24 hours after ingestion, lasts 1-7 days
Shigellosis	Shigella S. dysenteriae	Milk, milk products, seafood, salads	Mild diarrhea to fatal dysentery. Appears 7-36 hours after ingestion; lasts 3-14 days
Staphylococcus	Staphylococcus S. aureus	Custards, cream fillings, processed meats, ham, cheese, ice cream, potato salad, sauces, casseroles	Severe abdominal cramps, pain, vomiting, diarrhea, perspiration, headache, fever, prostration. Appears 1-6 hours after ingestion, lasts 1-2 days

From Nix S: *Williams' basic nutrition and diet therapy*, ed 12, St. Louis, 2005, Mosby.
*Symptoms are generally most severe for youngest and oldest age-groups.

patient select foods that taste good or decrease the nausea. Sometimes medications need to be changed.

Symptoms associated with illness often have a major effect on appetite. Pain, nausea, and shortness of breath make it difficult for patients to chew, swallow, and tolerate stomach filling. Often patients refuse to eat to avoid the associated discomfort. Patients who are ill, had surgery, or have been NPO for a long period of time often have specialized dietary needs. The use of therapeutic diets has also been associated with the development of protein-energy malnutrition. The lack of taste of diets that are low in sodium and fat affect dietary intake. In this situation you need to weigh the benefits associated with the therapeutic diet against the detrimental effects of weight loss and malnutrition (Huffman, 2002). Table 32-4 describes commonly prescribed diets for patients in health care settings.

Food presentation is a factor in appetite. Hot foods that are cold or cold foods that are warm are not appetizing. Overcooked or undercooked foods are unappealing. A meal tray precariously balanced on a crowded, soiled over-bed table does not enhance the meal. Removal of the tray lid outside of the patient's room will help to decrease distress in those patients sensitive to odors, such as patients with nausea. Attention to details in food presentation, meal scheduling, and the patient's difficulties with food will enhance intake. You help to stimulate a patient's appetite through environmental adaptations, consultation with an RD, attention to food preferences, and patient and family counseling.

Providing a Comfortable Environment In the acute setting provide an environment conducive to eating. Make sure the patient's room is free of reminders of treatments and odors. Provide mouth care when necessary to remove unpleasant tastes. Plan to administer analgesics or antiemetics early enough so that patients are more comfortable to eat at mealtime. Position the patient comfortably so that the meal is more enjoyable. If a patient refuses a portion of the meal, make every effort to replace it with a suitable alternative.

Assisting Patients With Feeding Hospitalized patients may be unable to feed themselves adequately because of the severity of their illness or the fatigue and debilitation of the condition. You improve patient feeding by carefully protecting patients' dignity and actively involving them. Encourage the patient to eat a small amount of food at a comfortable pace when assisting patients with feeding. Provide independence through use of adaptive devices (Figure 32-4) or finger foods. Always position a patient in a chair or high-Fowler's position (if possible) to improve swallowing and digestion. Allow the patient time to empty the mouth after every spoonful, attempting to match the speed of feeding to the patient's readiness. Encourage patients to direct the order in which they wish to eat food items. Mealtime is a good time to instruct patients and their families about the selection of appropriate foods and the importance of a balanced diet.

Patients with visual deficits also need special assistance. Patients with decreased vision are able to independently feed themselves when they are given adequate information. Iden-

BOX 32-8   PATIENT TEACHING

Food Safety

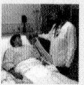Through his studies Matt learns that food safety is an important public health issue. The very young, older adults, patients with chronic illness, and those patients who are immunosuppressed are at risk for food-borne illnesses (see Table 32-3, p. 923). As Mrs. Gonzalez improves and begins to tolerate oral feeding, Matt consults with the dietitian, and together they develop a teaching plan regarding food safety for the foods that his patient's family will be preparing at home.

OUTCOME

- At the end of the teaching session Mrs. Gonzalez's family is able to state measures to reduce food-borne illnesses.

TEACHING STRATEGIES

- Instruct Mrs. Gonzalez's family on precautionary measures to avoid food-borne illnesses:
  - Wash hands, food preparation surfaces, and utensils with hot, soapy water.
  - Cook meat, poultry, fish, and eggs until well done (180° F).
  - Wash fresh fruits and vegetables thoroughly.
  - Do not eat raw meat or unpasteurized milk or juices.
  - Do not use food past expiration date.
  - Refrigerate foods at 40° F within 2 hours of cooking.
  - Keep foods properly refrigerated.
  - Thaw frozen foods in the refrigerator.
  - Discard food that you suspect is spoiled.
  - Do not use wooden cutting boards. Instead use plastic laminate or solid surface cutting boards that can be disinfected.
  - Wash dishrags, dishtowels, and sponges regularly with bleach, or use paper towels.
  - Clean inside of refrigerator and microwave regularly with bleach or soap.

EVALUATION STRATEGY

- Ask Mrs. Gonzalez's family to state six measures to prevent food-borne illnesses.
- Observe Mrs. Gonzalez's daughter at home for safe practices, if making a home visit.

Modified from Nix S: *Williams' basic nutrition and diet therapy*, ed 12, St. Louis, 2005, Mosby.

tify the food location on the plate as if it were a clock (e.g., meat at 9 o'clock and vegetable at 3 o'clock). Tell the patient where the beverages are located in relation to the plate. Be sure other care providers set the meal tray and plate in the same manner. Patients with impaired vision are more independent during mealtimes with the use of large-handled adaptive utensils. These are easier to grip and manipulate.

Dysphagia A certified SLP identifies patients at risk for dysphagia and makes recommendations for dysphagia therapy (Perry and Love, 2001). The assessment focuses on oral-motor and oral-sensory function, protective reflexes, respira-

tory status, level of arousal, cognitive-linguistic status, and perception. The SLP administers trials of several consistencies of foods and fluids to obtain a comprehensive description of the patient's phases of swallowing. Then the SLP determines the degree of dysfunction and aspiration risk (Perry and Love, 2001). Treatment recommendations focus on consistencies of foods and fluids and the use of swallowing therapies.

Dysphagia Diet Management. Patients with dysphagia are at risk for aspiration and need more assistance with feeding and swallowing. Provide a 30-minute rest period before eating (Palmer and Metheny, 2008). Position the patient in an upright, seated position in a chair, or raise the head of the bed to 90 degrees. Have the patient slightly flex the head to a chin-down position to help prevent aspiration. If the patient has unilateral weakness, teach the patient and caregiver to place food in the stronger side of the mouth. Determine the viscosity of foods that the patient tolerates best through the use of trials of different consistencies of foods and fluids. Thicker fluids are generally easier to swallow. The American Dietetic Association published the National Dysphagia Diet Task Force's (NDDTF's) National Dysphagia Diet in 2002 to provide uniformity of diets provided to patients with dysphagia (NDDTF, 2002). There are four levels of diet: dysphagia puree, dysphagia mechanically altered, dysphagia advanced, and regular. The four levels of liquid are thin liquids (low viscosity), nectarlike liquids (medium viscosity), honeylike liquids (viscosity of honey), and spoon-thick liquids (viscosity of pudding) (NDDTF, 2002).

Feed the patient with dysphagia slowly, providing smaller size bites and allow the patient to chew thoroughly and swallow the bite before taking another. More frequent chewing and swallowing assessments throughout the meal are necessary. Allow the patient time to empty the mouth after each spoonful, matching the speed of feeding to the patient's readiness. If the patient begins to cough or choke, remove the food immediately (Nowlin, 2006).

Patients With Disabilities Allow patients with disabilities that interfere with independent food intake to do as much as possible for themselves. When necessary, prepare the meal tray, cutting food into bite-size pieces, buttering bread, and pouring liquids. Use special eating utensils if necessary or as recommended by occupational therapy. Patients with decreased motor skills are more independent during mealtimes with the use of large-handled adaptive utensils. Some patients become fatigued during the course of the meal, leading to suboptimal intake. Provide assistance at the end of meals as needed. Evaluate the results of self-feeding on the basis of food intake. Recognize and commend any success the patient has.

Enteral Tube Feedings **Enteral nutrition (EN)** refers to nutrients given into the stomach or intestinal tract via a feeding tube. Nasogastric (NG) feedings are delivered through a feeding tube introduced through the nose and into the stomach. Nasointestinal feedings are delivered through a feeding tube inserted through the nose and into the jejunum. When patients have nasopharyngeal obstructions or are not candidates for nasal feeding tubes, physicians surgically insert

TABLE 32-4 Diet Progression and Therapeutic Diets

DIET	DESCRIPTION
Clear liquid	Broth, bouillon, coffee, tea, carbonated beverages, clear fruit juices, gelatin, Popsicles.
Full liquid	As above with addition of smooth-textured dairy products (e.g., ice cream, yogurt drinks, milk), custards, refined cooked cereals, vegetable juice, pureed vegetables, all fruit juices.
Dysphagia pureed	All of above with addition of scrambled eggs; pureed meats, vegetables, and fruits; mashed potatoes and gravy.
Mechanical soft	All of above with addition of ground or finely diced meats, flaked fish, cottage cheese, cheese, rice, potatoes, pancakes, light breads, cooked vegetables, cooked or canned fruits, bananas, soups, peanut butter.
Soft/low residue	Addition of low-fiber, easily digested foods such as pastas, casseroles, moist tender meats, and canned cooked fruits and vegetables. Desserts, cakes, and cookies without nuts or coconut.
High fiber	Addition of fresh uncooked fruits, steamed vegetables, bran, oatmeal, and dried fruits.
Low sodium	4-g (no added salt), 2-g, 1-g, or 500-mg sodium diets. These diets vary from no added salt to severe sodium restriction (500-mg sodium diet) that requires selective food purchases.
Low cholesterol	300 mg/day cholesterol, in keeping with American Heart Association guidelines for serum lipid reduction.
Diabetic	Recommended food exchanges by the American Diabetes Association. Usually the caloric recommendations are around 1800 calories. The diet needs to include a balanced intake of carbohydrates, fats, and proteins. Caloric recommendations vary to accommodate the patient's metabolic demands.
Regular	No restrictions, unless specified.

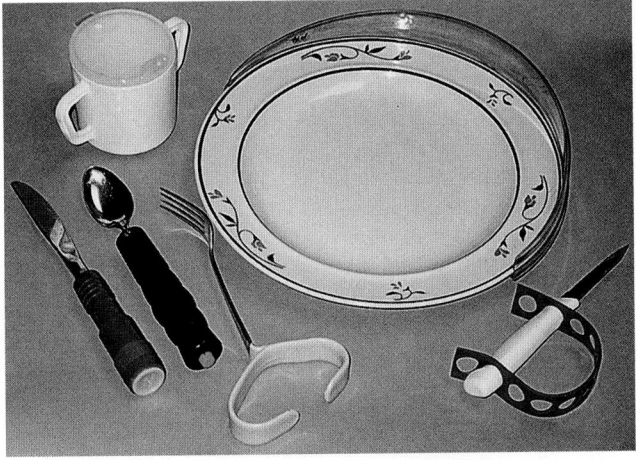

Figure 32-4 ■ Assist devices for self-feeding.

tubes directly into the stomach (gastrostomy) or jejunum (jejunostomy). The most desirable and appropriate method of providing nutrition is the oral route; unfortunately, this is not always possible. When oral feedings are not possible, yet the stomach or intestine is able to digest nutrients, enteral tube feeding is an alternative. Research has demonstrated a beneficial effect of EN over parenteral routes in patients with a functional GI tract. Therefore enteral feeding is preferred over parenteral nutrition (intravenous nutrition) because it improves utilization of nutrients, is generally safer for patients, maintains structure and function of the gut, decreases the risk for infection and sepsis, and is less expensive (ASPEN, 2002; Cirgin Ellett, 2006). A variety of enteral feeding formulas are available in whole protein or partially digested form. Special enteral formulas for renal disease, hepatic disease,

pulmonary disease, or diabetes are also available, as well as adult and pediatric formulas. The skills presented in this chapter focus on the administration of nutritional feedings directly into the gastrointestinal tract with the goal of restoring the patient's nutritional status.

Skill 32-2 describes insertion of a small-bore feeding tube. Feeding tubes are referred to as being nasally placed because that is the route most frequently used, primarily because the nose provides a natural stability for tubes. However, in the event of trauma to the nose, or in the event that the patient already has an endotracheal tube placed in the mouth, feeding tubes are sometimes placed orally. Avoid large-bore NG tubes for primary use as a feeding tube because they carry an increased risk for aspiration and are more irritating to the nasopharyngeal and esophageal mucosa (ASPEN, 2002). Occasionally you will use large-bore tubes inserted for gastric decompression to initiate enteral feeding because they are already in place. If the feeding continues for more than a few days, or if the patient is at high risk for aspiration, consult with the health care provider about placement of a small-bore feeding tube. Small-bore feeding tubes are used because they create less discomfort for the patient. For the adult, most of these tubes are 8 to 12 Fr and 36 to 44 inches long. A stylet is often used during insertion of a small-bore tube to stiffen it. The stylet is removed when the correct position of the tube is confirmed.

Feeding Tube Insertion. When the patient cannot ingest, chew, or swallow food but can digest and absorb nutrients, a small-bore feeding tube is placed nasally, laparoscopically, or surgically into the stomach or small intestine (Skills 32-2 and 32-3). When making the decision regarding enteral access, the health care provider considers rate of gastric emptying, GI anatomy, risk for gastric reflux and aspiration, and anticipated duration of requirement for enteral access. Nasal tubes are associated with sinusitis, otitis, vocal cord paralysis, and ulcers of the nose and sinuses. For this reason they are not used as long-term enteral access. Intestinal feedings require an infusion pump to allow for controlled slow administration. Surgically placed tubes such as a gastrostomy tube are preferred for long-term feeding (Rolandelli and others, 2005).

A serious complication associated with enteral feedings is aspiration of formula into the tracheobronchial tree, which irritates the bronchial mucosa (Box 32-9). This results in decreased blood supply to affected pulmonary tissue, often leading to necrotizing infection, pneumonia, and potential abscess formation. The high glucose content of a feeding serves as a bacterial medium for growth, promoting infection. Some of the common conditions that increase the risk for aspiration include coughing, nasotracheal suctioning, an

artificial airway, decreased level of consciousness, and lying flat. Prokinetic medications such as metoclopramide, erythromycin, or cisapride promote gastric emptying and decrease the risk for aspiration (Cirgin Ellett, 2006; Metheny, 2006b). To prevent aspiration, keep the head of the bed elevated at all times at a minimum of 30 degrees, preferably to 45 degrees, unless medically contraindicated (Enteral Nutrition Practice Recommendations Task Force, 2009). Measure the gastric residual volume (GRV) every 4 to 6 hours in patients receiving continuous feedings and immediately before the feeding in patients receiving intermittent feedings (Metheny, 2006). Delayed gastric emptying is a concern if 200 mL or more remains in the patient's stomach on two consecutive assessments (Metheny, 2006b). The North American Summit on Aspiration in the Critically Ill Patient made the following recommendations regarding gastric residual volumes: (1) stop feedings immediately if aspiration occurs; (2) withhold feed-

BOX 32-9 BEST PRACTICES

SUMMARY OF EVIDENCE

Two of the most frequent complications associated with tube feedings are pulmonary aspiration, potentially leading to pneumonia, and accidental placement of a nasoenteric feeding tube into the lung. Those at highest risk for aspiration are those with decreased level of consciousness, confusion, uncooperativeness, agitation, presence of an endotracheal tube and absent or poor gag reflex. Gastric residual volume is not consistently related to aspiration. A traditional bedside method used to assess for pulmonary aspiration of enteral feeding into the respiratory tract included the glucose method. The premise of the glucose method was that normal tracheal secretions contain minimal levels of glucose. Therefore, if glucose-rich enteral formula is aspirated into the airway, glucose levels of tracheal secretions increase. However, researchers have shown that the glucose levels of tracheal secretions vary widely, and this method is not sufficiently sensitive or specific to be useful to detect aspiration. Researchers are currently trying to develop new bedside methods for assessing for pulmonary aspiration, such as assessing for the presence of pepsin, a substance produced in the stomach, in tracheal secretions.

Routine assessment for placement of feeding tubes is a nursing responsibility. Traditionally nurses have used the auscultatory method of assessing placement. The auscultatory method to detect gastric or intestinal feeding tube placement has been shown to be unreliable. This method does not detect when a feeding tube has inadvertently been

placed into the respiratory tract and does not distinguish between placement in the stomach and the intestine. The most accurate method for checking feeding tube placement is x-ray examination. The most effective nonradiological methods include aspirating fluid from the feeding tube and measuring its pH and describing its appearance.

APPLICATION TO NURSING PRACTICE

- X-ray verification of feeding tube placement is the most reliable method available to confirm correct tube location. It is required in most acute care facilities after insertion of a small-bore tube.
- You should verify the placement of the feeding tube every 4 to 6 hours by aspirating gastric contents, observing the appearance of the aspirate, and testing pH. A properly obtained pH of 1 to 4 is a good indication of gastric placement. A pH of 6 or higher likely indicates placement in the lung, intestine, or even the stomach when gastric pH is unusually high. Intestinal fluid is usually bile stained (dark golden yellow). Gastric fluid is usually grassy green, off-white to tan, or clear and colorless.
- Do not use the auscultatory method to determine tube location.
- Do not use the glucose detection method to determine if aspiration has occurred.
- Check gastric residual volumes every 4 hours in patients at high risk for aspiration.

REFERENCES

Bourgault AN and others: Development of evidence-based guidelines and critical care nurses' knowledge of enteral feedings, *Crit Care Nurse* 27(4):17, 2007.

Metheny NA: Preventing respiratory complications of tube feedings: evidence-based practice, *Am J Crit Care* 15(4):360, 2006b.

Metheny NA and others: Indicators of tubesite during feedings, *J Neurosci Nurs* 37(6):320, 2005b.

Metheny NA and others: Verification of inefficacy of the glucose method in detecting aspiration associated with tube feedings, *Medsurg Nurs* 14(2):112, 2005c.

Metheny NA and others: Tracheobronchial aspiration of gastric contents in critically ill tube-fed patients: frequency, outcomes, and risk factors, *Crit Care Med* 34(4):1007, 2006.

Metheny NA and others: Gastric residual volume and aspiration in critically ill patients receiving gastric feedings, *Am J Crit Care* 17(6):512, 2008.

ings and reassess patient tolerance to feedings if GRV is over 500 mL; and (3) evaluate the patient for aspiration and use nursing measures to reduce the risk for aspiration if GRV is between 200 and 500 mL (Enteral Nutrition Practice Recommendations Task Force, 2009; Metheny, 2006b).

Traditional bedside methods of testing placement of feeding tubes, such as injection of air, are ineffective. The gold standard is radiographic confirmation of feeding tube location. pH testing is now also recommended to confirm the tube placement (Metheny and Meert, 2004; Serna and McCarthy, 2006). The use of pH measures for ongoing monitoring of tube placement is effective and less costly.

Gastrostomy/Jejunostomy Tube Feedings. When patients cannot tolerate nasally or orally placed tubes, there are other options. One is a gastrostomy tube (G-tube), surgically placed in the stomach and exiting through an incision in the upper left quadrant of the abdomen, where it is sutured in place. An alternative is a percutaneous endoscopic gastrostomy (PEG) tube. This tube also exits through a puncture wound in the upper left quadrant of the abdomen, but it is held securely in place by virtue of its design (Figure 32-5). When patients who cannot tolerate a nasal or oral tube have gastric ileus, delayed gastric emptying, gastric resections, or neurological impairments that place them at greater risk for aspiration, enteral nutrition is delivered via a **jejunostomy tube** (J-tube) (Skill 32-4). Jejunostomy feeding tubes, like gastrostomy tubes, are inserted during surgery (J-tube) or endoscopy (percutaneous endoscopic jejunostomy [PEJ]). Endoscopic insertion of a jejunostomy tube is also done through a PEG tube. After insertion of the large-bore PEG tube, the PEJ tube passes through the PEG and advances into the jejunum (Figure 32-6). A Y connector attached to the jejunostomy tube caps the PEG tube and closes the system. This Y connector labels the gastrostomy tube and designates the jejunostomy tube for feeding. You need to know which port is gastric and which port is jejunal.

Providing PN   **Parenteral nutrition (PN)** is the administration of a solution consisting of glucose, amino acids, lipids, minerals, electrolytes, trace elements, and vitamins provided through an indwelling peripheral or central venous catheter. Administration of PN is only for use when the GI tract is not functioning. PN is not appropriate for patients who are able to absorb adequate nutrients via EN or oral feeding. PN use is associated with increased risk for infection and cost (Heyland and Dhaliwal, 2005). PN is a specialized nutritional support that provides a specific amount of micronutrients and macronutrients intravenously. PN is selected when the gastrointestinal tract cannot be used or cannot absorb nutrients in sufficient amounts to provide adequate nutrition. A health care provider reevaluates the patient daily for continued need for PN. The goal is to move toward the use of the gastrointestinal tract for enteral nutrition and eventual normal oral intake (ASPEN, 2002).

You will reduce the complications of PN by meticulous aseptic care of the central venous access device (ASPEN, 2002), a gradual increase in the nutrient provision over several days, careful monitoring of laboratory results for metabolic or electrolyte abnormalities, and assessment of fluid balance.

PN solutions that contain 10% dextrose or greater are hyperosmolar (i.e., highly concentrated) and irritate small peripheral veins. As a result, you infuse PN at this concentration through central venous lines. This is called central PN. You administer solutions less than 900 mOsm through peripheral veins. This is referred to as peripheral PN. Each day the health care provider will prescribe PN, which is mixed in the pharmacy. This prescribed solution reflects the patient's most recent laboratory values and metabolic and nutritional status. The solution itself is made for the patient's specific

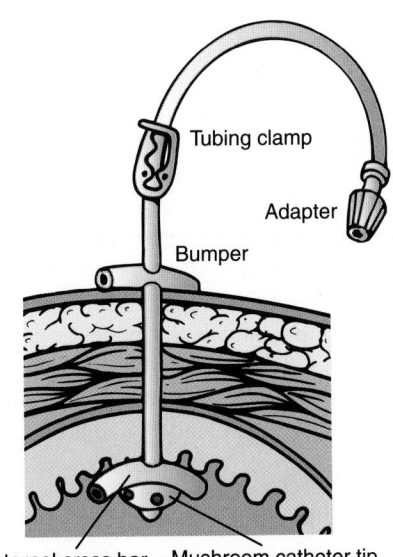

Tubing clamp

Adapter

Bumper

Internal cross bar   Mushroom catheter tip

Figure 32-5 ■ Percutaneous endoscopic gastrostomy tube.

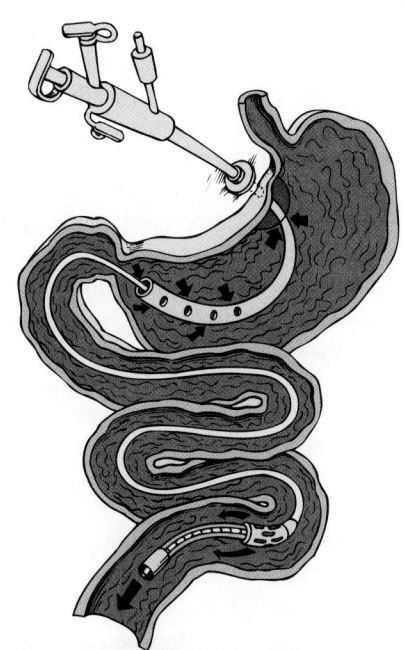

Figure 32-6 ■ Endoscopic insertion of jejunostomy tube.

nutritional needs, containing amino acids, dextrose, vitamins, minerals (electrolytes), and water. The solution may or may not contain lipid. Some patients receive no lipids or receive lipids only 2 or 3 times per week.

If the PN prescription includes lipid, it is sometimes combined with the other nutrients (total nutrient admixture [TNA]) or provided in a separate bag. Do not use TNA if you observe oil droplets or an oily or creamy layer on the surface of the solution. You co-infuse lipid emulsion peripherally or centrally using a Y connector, below an in-line filter. Infusion rate is 0.5 to 1 mL/min for the first 30 minutes. Reactions to lipid infusion include dyspnea, cyanosis, vomiting, headache, and/or chest pain. If reactions occur, stop the infusion, and notify the physician or health care provider. If the patient tolerates the slow lipid infusion, advance the rate as ordered by the physician or health care provider.

Initiating PN. PN therapy requires a central venous catheter (CVC) inserted into the jugular or subclavian vein (ASPEN, 2002). Nurses assist with this procedure for inserting a CVC. Specially trained nurses insert peripherally inserted central catheters (PICCs) (see Chapter 17). A chest x-ray film confirms the location of the CVC. Alternately, some patients have a long-term central venous access device, such as a tunneled catheter or an implanted port.

Before beginning an infusion, verify the health care provider's order. You always use an infusion pump. An initial rate of 40 to 60 mL/hr is recommended. The solution is provided at a specified rate over the course of the day to meet the patient's nutritional needs. Patients receiving PN at home frequently administer the entire daily solution over 12 hours at night. This allows the patient to disconnect from the infusion each morning, flush the central line, and have independent mobility during the day.

Caring for the Patient Receiving PN. Nursing care for the patient receiving PN is based on four major nursing goals: (1) preventing infection; (2) maintaining the PN system; (3) preventing metabolic, electrolyte, or fluid balance complications; and (4) assessing the patient's readiness for EN or discharge planning for home PN.

Primary methods to prevent infection include asepsis during insertion and care of the central venous catheter and dressing, use of an in-line intravenous filter, and maintaining secure, uncontaminated tubing connections. Make sure PN solutions do not exceed their 24-hour infusion limit. If you are using a CVC that has multiple lumens, use a port that is exclusively dedicated for the PN. Label the port for PN, and do not infuse other solutions or medications through the port (National Guideline Clearinghouse, 2003). During CVC dressing changes, always use a sterile mask and gloves and assess insertion sites for signs and symptoms of infection. Change the CVC dressing per institution policy and anytime it becomes wet or contaminated. Use either alcohol or chlorhexidine gluconate for skin asepsis and cleansing the injection port or catheter hub before and after each use (Hadaway, 2006). In some instances you will use an in-line 0.22-μm filter to remove bacteria.

Patients receiving PN have laboratory measurements monitored regularly. Capillary blood glucose testing or urine glucose testing occurs during the initiation of PN to assess for metabolic tolerance. In the hospital setting, this is usually done every 6 hours (check agency policy). Be alert for changes in vital signs or fluid balance and abnormal laboratory results that indicate osmotic diuresis and dehydration, infection, **hyperglycemia,** glucosuria, or electrolyte imbalance. Report any unusual symptoms to the health care provider. An increased temperature is an early sign of infection and needs to be reported to the health care provider immediately.

RESTORATIVE AND CONTINUING CARE

Diet Therapy in Disease Management. Patients discharged from a hospital with diet prescriptions often need dietary education to plan meals that meet specific therapeutic requirements. Restorative care includes immediate postsurgical care, posthospitalization care, and routine medical care. Therefore integrate preparation for the restorative aspect of patient care within the acute care setting.

Medical Nutrition Therapy. Optimal nutrition is important in health and illness, but the specific dietary intake pattern that results in optimal nutrition is modified for patients with particular diseases. **Medical nutrition therapy (MNT)** is the use of specific nutritional therapies to treat an illness, injury, or condition. MNT is necessary to assist the body's ability to metabolize certain nutrients, correct nutritional deficiencies related to the disease, and eliminate foods that may exacerbate disease symptoms. Patients with specific diseases often need modified dietary intake patterns in order to achieve good nutrition. These include gastrointestinal diseases, such as irritable bowel syndrome and malabsorption syndromes; metabolic disorders, such as diabetes mellitus and hypoglycemia; cardiovascular diseases; renal diseases; and cancers. Diet modifications are necessary to correspond with the body's ability to metabolize certain nutrients, to correct nutritional deficiencies, and to eliminate harmful foods from the diet. In all cases, work with the physician or health care provider and RD when planning and implementing modified diets.

Home Care Sometimes specialized nutritional therapies, such as EN and PN, need to be continued beyond the hospital setting to the home care setting. In home care you are often the only care provider who sees the patient on a regular basis. As a home care nurse you teach patients or caregivers how to do the following: administer PN or EN; check for feeding tube placement and flush the tube; assess the patient for tolerance of the nutrition through such measurements as weight, hydration, or blood capillary glucose level; when and how to order supplies; and evaluate the patient's progress toward nutritional goals. GRVs are typically not measured in adult patients at home because tolerance has likely been determined before discharge (Rolandelli and others, 2005).

▪▪▪EVALUATION

PATIENT CARE An ongoing evaluation will measure the value of your activities in meeting the patient's nutritional needs. Allow enough time to test a nursing approach to a problem, because nutritional improvement takes time.

Evaluation of clinical progress includes objective data, such as weight gain or improved laboratory parameters, or subjective data, such as the patient's reporting improvement in food choices or in self-reporting improved intake (Box 32-10). When clinical progress does not occur, determine whether the interventions were not effective, were not done or accepted by the patient, were not realistic or appropriate, or were affected by unanticipated or unidentified factors (see Care Plan, p. 921).

If outcomes are not met, reassess the patient to determine if you missed any important data. Some patients need reeducation if they have forgotten or misunderstood essential skills or knowledge. Also, attempt to validate that the patient is in agreement with the goals and is willing and able to follow the nutritional plan of care.

PATIENT EXPECTATIONS Nutritional interventions often depend on the patient's willingness and ability to change behavior patterns and learn new patterns. If the patient is not fully committed to the expected changes, the interventions will not always be successful. Some patients also find it difficult to change behavior and are less motivated with the passage of time. It is important to remember to individualize the nutrition care plan and focus on the patient.

Most patients respond well to the opportunity to make informed choices. Your explanations of the reasons for the behavioral change and providing the patient options for how to achieve the change will assist the patient in making the change. Provide education in several brief sessions, if necessary, to maximize the retention of information.

BOX 32-10   EVALUATION

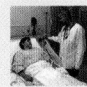 Matt sees Mrs. Gonzalez before discharge to a restorative care facility for rehabilitation before returning home. Mrs. Gonzalez is now able to consume all of her required nutrients with a ground diet and nectar-thickened liquids. Matt removes the feeding tube in preparation for her transport to the new facility. Before Mrs. Gonzalez regained her ability to orally consume adequate nutrients, her health care provider changed her enteral nutrition formula to a fiber-containing formula. This relieved her constipation and promoted daily bowel movements.

Matt advises Mrs. Gonzalez to continue the current plan of care and emphasizes that it is important to continue speech therapy. He discusses the importance of compliance with diet modifications until swallowing function returns completely.

DOCUMENTATION NOTE
"Swallows without aspirating. Daily regular bowel movements post initiation of fiber-containing formula. Oral intake of mechanically altered diet meets 100% of estimated needs. To be followed by restorative care facility."

SAFETY GUIDELINES FOR NURSING SKILLS

Ensuring patient safety is an essential role of the professional nurse. To ensure patient safety, communicate clearly with members of the health care team, assess and incorporate the patient's priorities of care and preferences, and use the best evidence when making decisions about your patient's care. When performing the skills in this chapter, remember the following points to ensure safe, individualized patient care:

- Use aseptic technique when preparing and delivering enteral feedings. Check agency policy for wearing of gloves when handling feedings (Enteral Nutrition Practice Recommendations Task Force, 2009).
- Label enteral equipment with patient name, room number, formula name, rate, date and time of initiation, and nurse initials (Enteral Nutrition Practice Recommendations Task Force, 2009).
- Practice "right patient, right formula, right tube" by matching formula and rate to feeding order and verifying enteral tubing set connects formula to feeding tube (Enteral Nutrition Practice Recommendations Task Force, 2009).
- Elevate the head of the bed a minimum of 30 to 45 degrees unless medically contraindicated for patients receiving enteral feedings (Enteral Nutrition Practice Recommendations Task Force, 2009).
- Trace all lines and tubing back to patient to ensure that you have only enteral-to-enteral connections (Enteral Nutrition Practice Recommendations Task Force, 2009).
- Do not add food coloring or dye to enteral nutrition. Use of dye has been linked to hypotension, metabolic acidosis, and death (Metheny, Meert, and Clouse, 2007).
- Refer to manufacturer's guidelines to determine hang time for enteral feedings. Maximum hang time for formula is 8 hours in an open system, 24 to 48 hours in closed, ready-to-hang system (if it remains closed). There is increased risk for bacterial growth in feedings that exceed the recommended hang time.
- Auscultation is not a reliable method for verification of nasogastric or nasointestinal tube placement because a tube inadvertently placed in the lungs, pharynx, or esophagus also transmits a sound similar to that of air entering the stomach (Metheny and others, 2007; Serna and McCarthy, 2006).
- Continuous enteral feedings and parenteral nutrition are always administered using an infusion pump.

SKILL 32-1	ASPIRATION PRECAUTIONS

DELEGATION CONSIDERATIONS

The assessment of a patient's risk for aspiration and determination of positioning cannot be delegated to nursing assistive personnel (NAP). However, NAP may feed patients after receiving instruction in aspiration precautions. The nurse instructs NAP to:

- Position patient with head elevated a minimum of 30 degrees to decrease aspiration risk
- Use aspiration precautions while feeding patients who need assistance
- Report to the nurse in charge any onset of coughing, gagging, a wet voice, or oral pocketing of food

EQUIPMENT

- Chair or electric bed (to allow patient to sit upright)
- Thickening agents as needed (rice, cereal, yogurt, gelatin, commercial thickening agent)
- Tongue blade
- Penlight
- Equipment for oral hygiene (see Chapter 28)
- Oral suction equipment (see Chapter 29)

STEP	RATIONALE

ASSESSMENT

1 Perform nutritional assessment.

Patients at risk for aspiration from dysphagia often alter their eating patterns or choose foods that do not provide adequate nutrition (Perry and McLaren, 2003; White and others, 2008).

2 Assess patients who are at increased risk for aspiration (see Box 32-7, p. 918) for signs and symptoms of dysphagia (e.g., cough, pharyngeal pooling, change in voice after swallowing). Use a dysphagia screening tool if available.

Patients at risk include those who have neurological or neuromuscular diseases and those who have had trauma to or surgical procedures of the oral cavity or throat.

3 Observe patient during mealtime for signs of dysphagia, and allow patient to attempt to feed self. Observe patient consume various consistencies of foods and liquids. Note at end of meal if patient fatigues.

Helps detect abnormal eating patterns such as frequent clearing of throat or prolonged eating time. Fatigue increases risk for aspiration.

4 Ask patient about any difficulties with chewing or swallowing various textures of food.

Patients are likely to aspirate certain foods more than others.

5 Report signs and symptoms of dysphagia to the health care provider.

Identifies patients who need to have an evaluation performed by a radiologist or speech language pathologist (Ramsey, Smithard, and Kaira, 2003).

6 Place identification on patient's chart or Kardex indicating that dysphagia is present.

Identifying patient as having dysphagia alerts the health care team to the problem to help the team develop and implement an individualized plan of care (Nowlin, 2006).

PLANNING

1 Instruct patient about what you are going to do and why.

Increases patient cooperation.

2 Explain to patient why you are observing him or her while he or she eats.

Signs or symptoms associated with aspiration indicate the need for further evaluation of swallowing, such as a fluoroscopic swallow study (Ashley and others, 2006).

3 Provide a 30-minute rest period before feeding time.

Swallowing difficulty is less likely in a well-rested patient (Palmer and Metheny, 2008).

IMPLEMENTATION

1 Perform hand hygiene.

Reduces transmission of microorganisms.

2 Provide thorough oral hygiene, including brushing of tongue, before meal.

Risk for aspiration pneumonia has been associated with poor oral hygiene (Palmer and Metheny, 2008).

3 Elevate head of patient's bed so that hips are flexed at a 90-degree angle, or help patient to same position in a chair. Have patient assume a chin-tuck position.

Chin-tuck or chin-down position helps reduce aspiration (Huang and others, 2006). A supine position increases the probability of aspiration (Palmer and Metheny, 2008).

4 Using penlight and tongue blade, gently inspect mouth for pockets of food.

Pockets of food in the mouth indicate difficulty swallowing (Ashley and others, 2006).

5 Add thickener to thin liquids to create the consistency of mashed potatoes, or serve patient pureed foods.

Thin liquids such as water and fruit juice are difficult to control in the mouth and are more easily aspirated (Ashley and others, 2006).

STEP	RATIONALE
6 Place ½ to 1 teaspoon of food on unaffected side of the mouth, allowing utensil to touch the mouth or tongue.	Placement of food in the mouth is varied based on the type of deficit (Metheny, 2007).
7 Place hand on throat to gently palpate swallowing event as it occurs. Swallowing twice is often necessary to clear the pharynx.	Assesses movement during swallowing (Ashley and others, 2006).
8 Observe patient consume various consistencies of foods and liquids.	Gradual increase in types and textures combined with constant monitoring ensures patient is able to eat safely (Ramsey and others, 2003). Referral to a dietitian is appropriate if a patient has difficulty with a particular consistency.

9 Provide verbal coaching and positive reinforcement while feeding patient.
  a Open your mouth.
  b Feel the food in your mouth.
  c Chew and taste the food.
  d Raise your tongue to the roof of your mouth.
  e Think about swallowing.
  f Close your mouth and swallow.
  g Swallow again.
  h Cough to clear airway.
	Verbal cueing keeps patient focused on swallowing. Positive reinforcement enhances patient's confidence in ability to swallow.

10 Observe for throat clearing, coughing, choking, gagging, and drooling of food; suction airway as necessary.	These are indications that suggest dysphagia and risk for aspiration (Ashley and others, 2006).
11 Provide rest periods as necessary during meal.	Avoiding fatigue decreases the risk for aspiration.
12 Ask patient to remain sitting upright for at least 30 minutes after the meal.	Reduces the risk for gastroesophageal reflux, which causes aspiration (Nowlin, 2006).
13 Help patient to perform hand hygiene and perform mouth care.	Mouth care after meals helps prevent dental caries.
14 Return patient's tray to appropriate place, and perform hand hygiene.	Reduces spread of microorganisms.

EVALUATION

1 Observe patient's ability to ingest foods of various textures and thickness.	Indicates whether aspiration risk is increased with thin liquids.
2 Monitor patient's food and fluid intake.	Patient needs to avoid certain types and textures of food that are difficult to swallow.
3 Weigh patient weekly.	Determines if weight is stable and reflects adequate caloric level.
4 Observe patient's oral cavity after meal to detect pockets of food.	Determines presence of pockets of food when meal has included foods of various textures.

RECORDING AND REPORTING

- Document the following in patient's chart: patient's tolerance of various food textures, amount of assistance required, position during meal, absence or presence of any symptoms of dysphagia, and amount eaten.

- Report any coughing, gagging, choking, or swallowing difficulties to nurse in charge or physician or health care provider.

UNEXPECTED OUTCOMES AND RELATED INTERVENTIONS

- Patient coughs, gags, complains of food "stuck in throat," or has pockets of food in mouth.
  - Patient needs to be evaluated for a swallowing study (see Box 32-7, p. 918).
  - Consider consultation with a speech therapist for swallowing exercises and techniques to improve swallowing and reduce risk for aspiration.
  - Notify health care provider of any symptoms of dysphagia or aspiration that occurred during meal and which foods caused the symptoms.

- Patient avoids certain textures of food.
  - Change consistency and texture of food.
- Patient experiences weight loss.
  - Discuss findings with health care provider and/or dietitian.

SKILL 32-2 INSERTING A NASOGASTRIC OR NASOINTESTINAL FEEDING TUBE

DELEGATION CONSIDERATIONS

The skill of inserting a nasogastric (NG) or nasointestinal (NI) feeding tube cannot be delegated to nursing assistive personnel (NAP). The nurse guides the NAP to:

- Assist with patient with positioning during tube insertion

EQUIPMENT

- NG tube or NI tube (8 to 12 Fr) with guide wire or stylet
- 60-mL or larger Luer-Lok or catheter-tip syringe
- Stethoscope
- Hypoallergenic tape and tincture of benzoin or tube fixation device

- pH indicator strip (scale 1 to 11)
- Glass of water and straw for patients able to swallow
- Emesis basin
- Towel
- Facial tissues
- Clean gloves
- Suction equipment in case of aspiration
- Penlight to check placement in nasopharynx
- Tongue blade
- Pulse oximeter

STEP	RATIONALE
ASSESSMENT	
1 Verify patient's identity and type of tube ordered with health care provider's order before beginning procedure	Complies with The Joint Commission requirements and improves procedure safety
2 Verify patient's need for enteral tube feedings: impaired swallowing, decreased level of consciousness, surgeries of the upper alimentary tract, need for long-term enteral nutrition. Also assess patient's height, weight, hydration status, electrolyte balance, and organ function.	Identifying patients who need tube feedings before they become nutritionally depleted helps to prevent complications related to malnutrition.
3 Assess patency of nares. Have patient close each nostril alternately and breathe. Examine each naris for patency and skin breakdown.	Nares are sometimes obstructed or irritated, or septal defect or facial fractures are present.
4 Assess patient's medical history: Nosebleeds, facial trauma, nasal surgery, deviated septum, anticoagulant therapy, coagulopathy.	Nasoenteric tubes are contraindicated in patients with recent nasal surgery, facial traumas, nosebleeds, and receiving anticoagulation. This includes patients with surgical procedures requiring a transsphenoidal approach used to remove pituitary tumors, because there is a risk for improper tube placement (Metheny, 2002).
5 Assess patient for gag reflex: Place tongue blade in patient's mouth, touching uvula.	Identifies patient's ability to swallow and determines if there is a greater risk for aspiration.
6 Assess patient's level of consciousness and ability to follow directions.	Alert patient is better able to cooperate with procedure. If vomiting occurs, an alert patient will usually expectorate vomitus, which will help to reduce the risk for aspiration.
7 Assess for bowel sounds.	Absence of bowel sounds indicates decreased or absent peristalsis and increased risk for aspiration.
8 Determine if health care provider wants a prokinetic agent administered before placement of tube.	Prokinetic agents, such as metoclopramide, given before tube placement help advance the tube into the intestine (Metheny, 2006a).
PLANNING	
1 Explain procedure to patient. Identify patient using at least two identifiers (e.g., name and birthday or name and account number according to agency policy).	Increases patient's cooperation. Ensures right patient receives right therapy.
2 Explain to patient how to communicate during intubation by raising index finger to indicate gagging or discomfort.	Reduces anxiety and provides a way of communicating during insertion.
3 Perform hand hygiene. Stand on same side of bed as naris for insertion. Position patient in sitting or high-Fowler's position, unless contraindicated. If patient is comatose, place in semi-Fowler's position with head propped forward using a pillow. An assistant is often necessary to help with positioning of confused or comatose patients.	Reduces transmission of microorganisms. Reduces risk for pulmonary aspiration if patient vomits. Assists with closure of airway and passage of the tube into the esophagus. The natural response to an object being inserted into the nose is to tip the head backward; avoid this because it opens the airway.
4 Place towel over patient chest. Keep facial tissues in reach.	Prevents soiling of gown. Insertion of tube often causes tearing.
5 Examine feeding tube for flaws: rough or sharp edges on distal end and closed or clogged outlet holes.	Flaws in feeding tube hamper tube intubation and will injure patient. Clogged outlets do not allow passage of feeding.

STEP	RATIONALE

6 Determine length of tube you will insert, and mark with tape or indelible ink (see illustration). Measure distance from tip of nose to earlobe to xyphoid process of sternum. Add additional 20 to 30 cm (8 to 12 inches) for NI tube.

Using appropriate measurement technique identifies depth of insertion of tube for proper placement.

7 Prepare NG or NI tube for intubation:

a If the tube has a guide wire or stylet, inject 10 mL of water from 60-mL Luer-Lok or catheter-tip syringe into the tube.

Aids in guide wire or stylet insertion.

b Make certain that you position guide wire securely against weighted tip and that both Luer-Lok connections are snugly fitted together.

Promotes smooth passage of tube into GI tract. Improperly positioned stylet will induce serious trauma.

8 Cut hypoallergenic tape 10 cm (4 inches) long, or prepare tube fixation device.

Anchors tube following insertion.

IMPLEMENTATION

1 Apply clean gloves.

Reduces transmission of microorganisms.

2 Dip tube with surface lubricant into glass of room temperature water, or apply water-soluble lubricant. Do not place plastic tubes in cold water or ice water.

Activates lubricant to facilitate passage of tube.
Tubes become stiff and inflexible, causing trauma to mucous membranes.

3 Hand the alert patient a glass of water with straw or glass with crushed ice (if able to swallow).

Asking patient to swallow water facilitates tube passage.

4 Gently insert tube through nostril to back of throat (posterior nasopharynx). May cause patient to gag. Aim back and down toward ear (see illustration).

Natural contours ease passage of tube into GI tract.

5 Check for position of tube in back of throat with penlight and tongue blade.

Checking ensures tube is not coiled, kinked, or entering trachea.

6 Have patient flex head toward chest after tube has passed through nasopharynx.

Closes off glottis and reduces risk for tube entering trachea.

7 Emphasize need to mouth breathe and swallow during insertion.

Helps facilitate passage of tube and alleviates patient's fears during the procedure.

8 When you insert the tube approximately 10 inches (in the adult), stop and listen for air exchange from the distal portion of the tube.

If air is heard, tube is in respiratory tract; remove tube and start over. **Never use this step for tube verification** (Metheny and Meert, 2004).

9 Encourage patient to swallow by giving small sips of water or ice chips. Advance tube as patient swallows. Rotate tube 180 degrees while inserting.

Swallowing facilitates passage of tube past oropharynx. Rotating decreases friction.

10 Advance tube each time patient swallows until it has passed the desired length.

Reduces discomfort and trauma to patient.

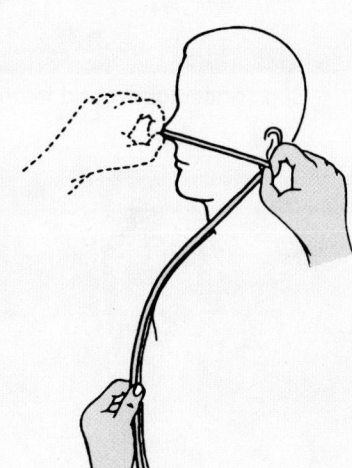

Step 6 ■ Determine length of tube you will insert.

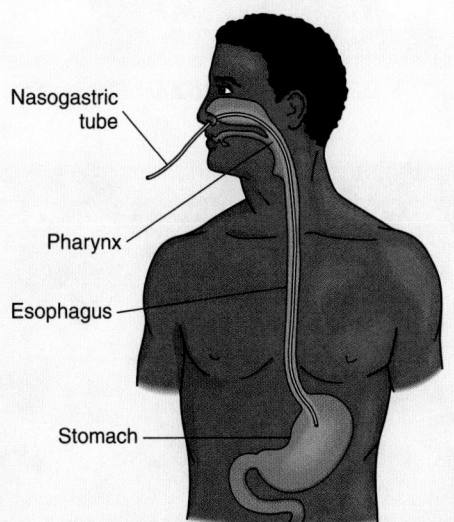

Nasogastric tube
Pharynx
Esophagus
Stomach

Step 4 ■ NG tube inserted through nose and esophagus into stomach.

SKILL 32-2	INSERTING A NASOGASTRIC OR NASOINTESTINAL FEEDING TUBE—cont'd

STEP	RATIONALE

• *Critical Decision Point:* Do not force tube. If you meet resistance or if patient starts to cough, choke, or become cyanotic, stop advancing the tube and pull tube back and start over.

STEP	RATIONALE
11 Check for position of tube in back of throat with penlight and tongue blade.	Tube may be coiled, kinked, or entering trachea.
12 Obtain gastric aspirate, and check placement of tube by measuring gastric pH (see Skill 32-3).	Properly obtained pH of 1 to 4 is a good indication of gastric placement (Metheny, 2006b).
13 After you obtain gastric aspirates, anchor tube to nose to avoid pressure on nares. Mark exit site with indelible ink. Use one of following options for anchoring:	A properly secured tube allows the patient more mobility and prevents trauma to nasal mucosa.
a Apply tape:	
(1) Apply tincture of benzoin or other skin adhesive on tip of patient's nose and allow it to become "tacky."	Helps tape adhere better. Protects skin.
(2) Split one end of the prepared tape strip lengthwise 5 cm (2 inches).	
(3) Wrap each of the 5-cm strips in opposite directions around tube as it exits nose (see illustration).	Securing tape to nares prevents tissue necrosis.

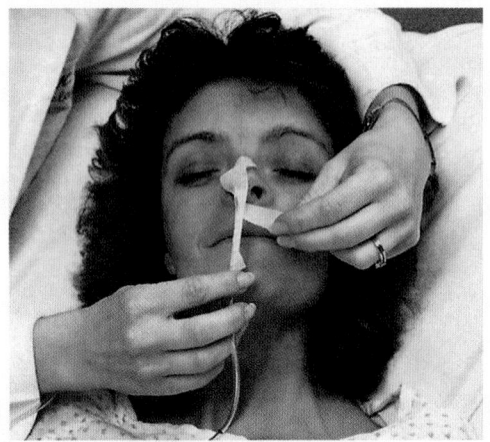

Step 13a(3) ■ Wrapping tape to anchor nasoenteral tube.

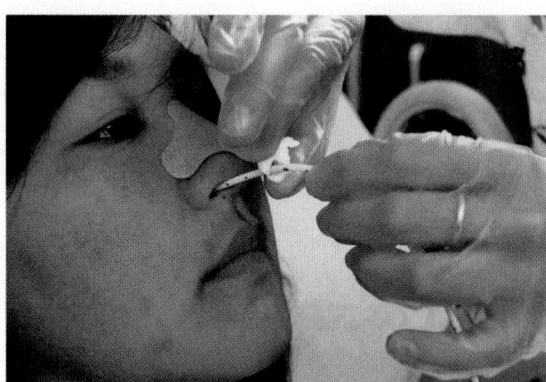

Step 13b(2) ■ Slip connector around feeding tube.

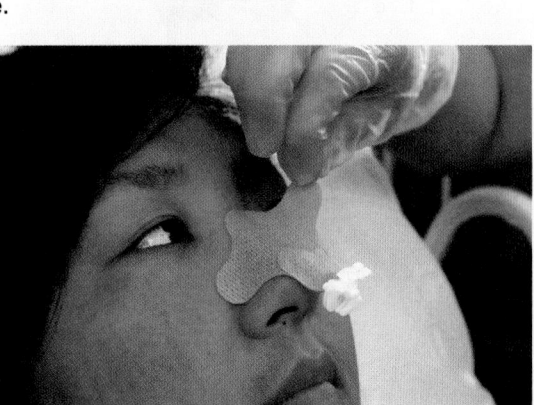

Step 13b(1) ■ Applying tube fixation patch to bridge of nose.

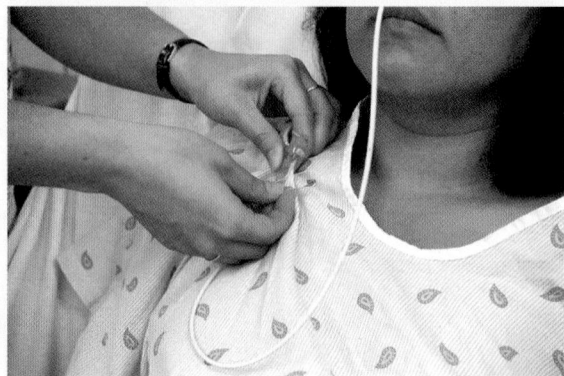

Step 14 ■ Fastening feeding tube to patient's gown.

STEP	RATIONALE
b Apply tube fixation device using shaped adhesive patch: **(1)** Apply wide end of patch to bridge of nose (see illustration). **(2)** Slip connector around feeding tube as it exits nose (see illustration).	Secures tube and reduces friction on naris.
14 Fasten end of NG tube to patient's gown using a piece of tape. Do not use safety pins to pin the tube to the patient's gown (see illustration).	Reduces traction on the nares if tube moves. Safety pins become unfastened and cause injury to the patient.
15 Assist patient with head of bed elevated at least 30 degrees unless contraindicated. For intestinal tube placement, position the patient on right side when possible until radiological confirmation of correct placement.	Promote patient comfort. Placing the patient on the right side promotes passage of the tube into the small intestine.

> • ***Critical Decision Point:*** Leave guide wire or stylet in place until you ensure correct position by x-ray film. Never attempt to reinsert a partially or fully removed guide wire or stylet while feeding tube is in place. This will cause perforation of the tube and injure the patient.

STEP	RATIONALE
16 Obtain x-ray film of chest/abdomen.	X-ray examination is currently the most accurate method to determine feeding tube placement.
17 Change gloves, and administer oral hygiene (see Chapter 28). Cleanse tubing at nostril with washcloth dampened in mild soap and water.	Promotes patient comfort and integrity of oral mucous membranes.
18 Remove gloves, dispose of equipment, and perform hand hygiene.	Reduces transmission of microorganisms.

EVALUATION

1 Observe patient to determine response to NG or NI tube intubation. Have the patient speak. Check vital signs and oxygen saturation.	A patient who is comfortable, is able to speak without difficulty, and has normal oxygen saturation is likely to have a correctly placed tube.
2 Confirm x-ray film results.	Proper position is essential before initiating feedings.
3 Remove the guide wire or stylet after x-ray verification of correct placement.	
4 Routinely assess location of external exit site marking on the tube, as well as color and pH of fluid withdrawn from the NG or NI tube.	Will reveal if end of tube has changed position. However, it is possible that the tube changed position inside the gastrointestinal tract with no external evidence of the change.

RECORDING AND REPORTING

- Record and report type and size of tube placed, location of distal tip of tube, patient's tolerance of procedure, and confirmation of tube position by x-ray examination. Documentation of nonrespiratory placement by x-ray examination is standard practice when you initially insert a small-bore tube. Record and report any type of unexpected outcome and the interventions performed.

UNEXPECTED OUTCOMES AND RELATED INTERVENTIONS

- Tube placed in the respiratory tract. Usually seen on x-ray film.
  - Remove the tube.
  - Report the incident to the health care provider; obtain order for reinsertion.
- Aspiration of stomach contents into respiratory tract (immediate response) in the alert patient evidenced by coughing, dyspnea, cyanosis, or decreases in oxygen saturation values during the procedure.
  - Position the patient on side to facilitate drainage of oral secretions.
  - Suction the patient nasotracheally or orotracheally to try to remove aspirated substance.

- Report the event immediately to the health care provider.
- Aspiration of stomach contents into respiratory tract (delayed response or small-volume aspiration), evidenced by auscultation of crackles or wheezes, dyspnea, or fever.
  - Report change in patient condition to the health care provider to obtain order for chest x-ray examination.
  - Prepare for possible initiation of antibiotics.
- Nasal mucosa becomes inflamed, tender, and/or eroded.
  - Retape the tube in a different position to relieve pressure on mucosa.
  - If the tube has been in the same site for an extended period, consider reinsertion of the tube in the opposite naris (health care provider's order required).

SKILL 32-3   VERIFYING FEEDING TUBE PLACEMENT

DELEGATION CONSIDERATIONS

This skill of verifying feeding tube placement cannot be delegated to nursing assistive personnel (NAP). The nurse directs NAP to immediately inform the nurse if:

- The patient's respirations change or the patient complains of being short of breath, coughing, or choking
- The patient vomits or NAP notices vomitus in patient's mouth during oral hygiene
- Nasal irritation is present
- Displacement of the feeding tube occurs

EQUIPMENT

- 60-mL Luer-Lok or catheter-tip syringe
- Clean gloves
- Medicine cup
- pH indicator strip (scale 1 to 11)
- Normal saline or tap water
- Paper towel

STEP	RATIONALE

ASSESSMENT

1 Know the policy and procedures for frequency and method of checking tube placement in your facility.

Verifies agency procedure for checking placement of feeding tube. Regardless of the method, make sure you obtain x-ray confirmation at the time of placement.

2 Identify signs and symptoms of coughing, choking, or cyanosis.

Indicates accidental migration of feeding tube into the airway. However, their absence does not ensure that respiratory migration has not occurred, especially in the patient with altered level of consciousness and/or altered gag and cough reflexes.

3 Identify conditions that increase the risk for spontaneous tube dislocation from the intended position:
  a Retching/vomiting
  b Nasotracheal suctioning
  c Severe bouts of coughing

Increased intraabdominal pressure dislocates tube (e.g., stomach to esophagus, intestine to stomach).

4 Observe the external portion of the tube for movement of the ink mark away from the mouth or nares (see Skill 32-2).

Increased external length of a tube indicates that the distal tip is no longer in the correct position.

5 Review patient's medication record: is patient receiving a gastric acid inhibitor (e.g., cimetidine, ranitidine, famotidine, nizatidine) or a proton pump inhibitor (e.g., omeprazole)?

Histamine-2 receptor antagonists reduce volume of gastric acid secretion and the acid content of secretions, possibly causing the pH value to be higher, that is, more basic (Metheny and Meert, 2004).

6 Review patient's record for history of prior tube displacement.

Patients who have a history of tube displacement are at increased risk.

PLANNING

1 Explain procedure to patient. Check patient's identity using at least two identifiers.

Improves patient cooperation. Ensures right patient receives right therapy.

IMPLEMENTATION

1 Perform hand hygiene, and apply clean gloves.

Reduces transmission of microorganisms.

2 Measures to verify placement of tube should be conducted at the following times:
  a For intermittently tube-fed patients, test placement immediately before each feeding and before medications (usually a period of at least 4 hours will have elapsed since previous feeding).

More frequent checking has been associated with increased clogging of small-bore tubes. To avoid clogging, flush tubes with a minimum of 30 mL water (Bourgault and others, 2007).

  b For continuously tube-fed patients, test placement every 4 to 6 hours and before medication administration.

Verifies tube placement and decreases risk for aspiration (Metheny, 2006b).

  c Wait at least 1 hour after medication administration by tube or mouth.

Premature aspiration of contents will remove unabsorbed medication, reducing dose delivered to patient. Medication also interferes with pH testing and appearance of aspirate (Metheny and Meert, 2004).

STEP	RATIONALE
3 Draw up 30 mL of air into 60-mL syringe, then attach to end of feeding tube. Flush tube with 30 mL of air before attempting to aspirate fluid. Repositioning the patient from side to side is helpful. Flushing more than one bolus of air through the tube is necessary in some cases.	Burst of air aids in aspirating fluid more easily (Metheny and others, 1993). Smaller syringes generate unnecessarily high pressures inside the tube. It is sometimes more difficult to aspirate fluid from the small intestine than from the stomach.
4 Draw back on syringe slowly, and obtain 5 to 10 mL of gastric aspirate (see illustration *A*). Observe appearance of aspirate to help assess the position of the tube (see illustration *B*).	Drawing back quickly, or with a smaller syringe, increases intratubular pressure and causes the tube to collapse. Aspirates from NG tubes of continuously tube-fed patients often have appearance of curdled enteral formula. Aspirates from NI tubes are often stained yellow from bile. Gastric aspirates from intermittently tube-fed patients are not typically bile stained (unless intestinal fluid has refluxed into the stomach).
5 Gently mix aspirate in syringe, and expel into medicine cup. Dip the pH strip into the fluid, or apply a few drops of the fluid to the strip. Compare the color of the strip with the color on the chart provided by the manufacturer (see illustration).	Mixing ensures equal distribution of contents for testing. pH paper covering a minimum range of 1 to 11 provides an appropriate pH range to be sufficiently sensitive (Metheny and Meert, 2004).
a Gastric fluid from patient who has fasted for at least 4 hours usually has pH range of 1 to 4.	Range of 1 to 4 is a reliable indicator of stomach placement, especially when a gastric acid inhibitor is *not* being used.
b Fluid from NI tube of fasting patient usually has pH greater than 6.	Intestinal contents are less acidic than stomach contents (Cirgin Ellett, 2006).
c Patient with continuous tube feeding may have pH of 5 or higher.	Formulas contain solutions that are basic.

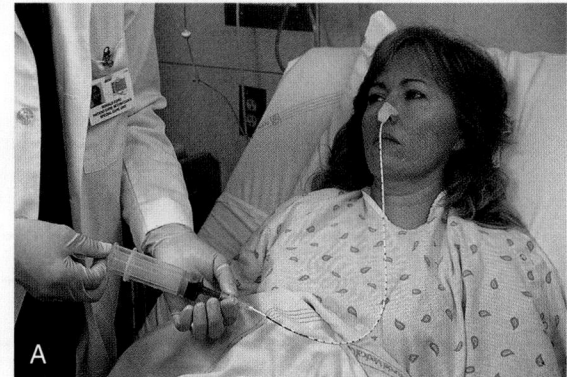

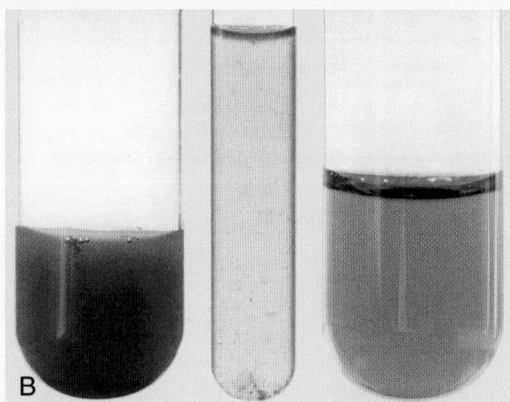

Step 4 ■ **A,** Obtaining gastric aspirate. **B,** Typical color of aspirates from stomach, intestine, and airway. (Used with permission from Metheny NA and others: pH, color, and feeding tubes, *RN* 61(1):25, 1998.)

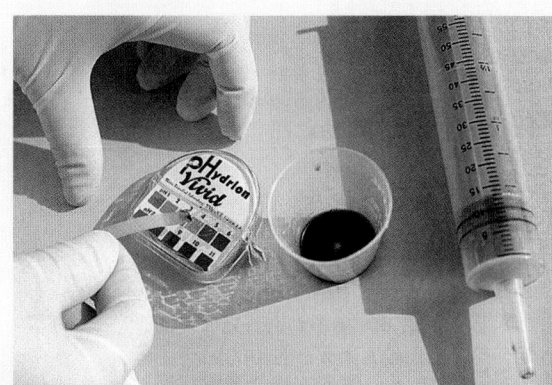

Step 5 ■ Compare color on test strip with color on pH chart.

SKILL 32-3 VERIFYING FEEDING TUBE PLACEMENT—cont'd

STEP	RATIONALE
d pH of pleural fluid from the tracheobronchial tree is generally greater than 6.	The pH of pleural fluid makes it difficult to differentiate between respiratory and intestinal placement (Metheny and Meert, 2004).
e Patient who takes acid inhibitor medication will usually have an acidic pH (4 to 6).	
6 If after repeated attempts, it is not possible to aspirate fluid from a tube that you originally established by x-ray examination to be in desired position, and (a) there are no risk factors for tube dislocation, (b) tube has remained in original taped position, and (c) patient is not experiencing respiratory distress, assume tube is correctly placed (Metheny and Meert, 2004; Metheny and others, 2005b).	It is reasonable to assume you correctly placed the tube. When you obtain abdominal x-ray films for clinical reasons, take advantage of the reports to monitor tube location.
7 Irrigate tube.	Keeps tube patent.
a Draw up 30 mL normal saline or tap water in syringe.	Flushes full length of tube.
b Kink feeding tube, and then insert tip of syringe into end of feeding tube.	Prevents leakage of gastric secretions.
c Release kink, and slowly instill irrigation solution.	Irrigation clears tubing.
d If unable to irrigate, reposition patient on left side, then try again.	Tip of tubing may be against stomach wall. Repositioning moves tip.
e When irrigant is instilled, remove syringe. Reinstitute continuous tube feeding, or replug end of tube.	Tube is clear and patent.
8 Remove and dispose of gloves. Perform hand hygiene.	Reduces transmission of microorganisms.
EVALUATION	
1 Observe patient for respiratory distress:	Feeding entered airway.
a Persistent gagging	
b Paroxysms of coughing	
c Respiratory patterns (e.g., rate and depth) that are inconsistent with patient's baseline measures	
2 Verify that color, pH, and appearance of aspirate are consistent with the initial tube placement according to x-ray results.	Indicates that the tip of the tube is likely to be in the same place as it was following x-ray confirmation.

RECORDING AND REPORTING

- Record and report pH and appearance of aspirate.

UNEXPECTED OUTCOMES AND RELATED INTERVENTIONS

- Red or brown coloring (coffee grounds in appearance) of fluid aspirated from a feeding.
  - If the color is not related to medications recently administered, notify the physician or health care provider. Red or brown coloring is an indicator of new or old blood, respectively.

SKILL 32-4   ADMINISTERING ENTERAL NUTRITION VIA NASOENTERIC, GASTROSTOMY, OR JEJUNOSTOMY TUBES

DELEGATION CONSIDERATIONS

Administration of enteral tube feeding may be delegated to nursing assistive personnel (NAP). However, the nurse must first verify tube placement and patency. The nurse is responsible for patient assessment. Instruct NAP to:

- Elevate head of bed a minimum of 30 degrees or sit patient up in bed or a chair
- Infuse feeding slowly
- Report any difficulty infusing the feeding or any discomfort voiced by the patient
- Report any gagging, paroxysms of coughing, or choking

EQUIPMENT

- Disposable feeding bag and tubing or ready-to-hang system
- 60-mL Luer-Lok or catheter-tip syringe
- Stethoscope
- pH indicator strip (scale of 1 to 11)
- Infusion pump (required for continuous or intestinal feedings): Use pump designed for tube feedings
- Prescribed enteral feeding
- Normal saline or tap water
- Clean gloves
- Equipment to obtain blood glucose by fingerstick

STEP	RATIONALE

ASSESSMENT

1. Assess patient's need for enteral tube feedings (see Skill 32-2).

   Identify patients who need tube feedings before they become nutritionally depleted.

2. Assess patient for food allergies.

   Prevents patient from developing localized or systemic allergic responses.

3. Auscultate for bowel sounds.

   Absent bowel sounds indicate decreased ability of GI tract to digest or absorb nutrients.

4. Obtain baseline weight, and review laboratory values. Assess patient for fluid volume excess or deficit, electrolyte abnormalities, and metabolic abnormalities such as hyperglycemia.

   Provides objective data to measure responses to and effectiveness of feedings.

5. Verify health care provider's order for formula, rate, route, and frequency.

   Ensures you will administer correct formula in appropriate volume.

6. For feeding tubes placed through the abdominal wall, assess stoma site for breakdown, irritation, or drainage.

   Infection, pressure from gastrostomy tube, or drainage of gastric secretions cause skin breakdown.

PLANNING

1. Explain procedure to patient.

   Decreases patient anxiety.

2. Perform hand hygiene.

   Reduces transmission of microorganisms.

3. Prepare feeding container to administer formula continuously:

   a. Identify patient using two identifiers (e.g., name and birthday or name and account number, according to facility policy). Verify tube and feeding with health care provider's order.

   Complies with The Joint Commission requirements and improves procedure safety.

   b. Check expiration date on formula and integrity of container.

   Tube feedings administered within the designated shelf life from a container without cracks or breaks reduces the patient's risk for obtaining tube feeding–borne GI infections. Prevents leakage of tube feeding.

   c. Have tube feeding at room temperature.

   Cold formula causes gastric cramping and discomfort because the mouth and esophagus did not warm the liquid.

   d. Connect tubing to container, or prepare ready-to-hang container. Use aseptic technique, and avoid handling the feeding system, touching the can tops, container openings, spike, and spike port. If you need to handle the system, perform hand hygiene and wear gloves.

   Ensures the feeding system, including the bag, connections, and tubing, is free of contamination to prevent bacterial growth (Enteral Nutrition Practice Recommendations Task Force, 2009; Matlow and others, 2006).

   e. Shake formula container well, and fill container with formula (see illustration, p. 940). Open stopcock on tubing, and fill tubing with formula to remove air (prime tubing). Hang on feeding pump pole.

   Filling the tubing with formula prevents excess air from entering gastrointestinal tract once infusion begins.

SKILL 32-4   ADMINISTERING ENTERAL NUTRITION VIA NASOENTERIC, GASTROSTOMY, OR JEJUNOSTOMY TUBES—cont'd

STEP	RATIONALE
4 For intermittent feeding, measure formula in container and have syringe ready. Be sure formula is at room temperature.	Cold formula causes gastric cramping.
5 Place patient in high-Fowler's position, or elevate head of bed at least 30 degrees.	Elevated head helps prevent aspiration (Bourgault and others, 2007).

IMPLEMENTATION

1 Perform hand hygiene. Apply clean gloves.

Reduces transmission of microorganisms.

2 Verify tube placement (see Skill 32-3).

Feedings instilled into a misplaced tube sometimes cause serious injury or death.

   A Nasoenteric (see Skill 32-2).

   B Gastrostomy tube: Attach syringe, and aspirate gastric secretions; observe their appearance, and check pH. Return aspirated contents to stomach unless the volume exceeds 200 mL.

Fluid from gastric tube of patient who has fasted for at least 4 hours usually has a pH of 1 to 4, especially when patient is not receiving a gastric acid inhibitor. Continuous administration of tube feedings elevates pH (Metheny and Meert, 2004; Metheny and Titler 2001).

   C Jejunostomy tube: Aspirate intestinal secretions, observe their appearance and check pH.

Presence of intestinal fluid indicates that the end of the tube is in the small intestine (i.e., duodenum or jejunum). If fluid tests acidic on pH test, looks like gastric fluid, or the residual volume is large (more than 10 mL), displacement of the tube into the stomach has possibly occurred.

3 Check gastric residual (see illustration).

Residual volume indicates if gastric emptying is delayed. Delayed gastric emptying is a concern if 200 mL or more remains in the patient's stomach on two consecutive assessments (Metheny, 2006b). Return of aspirate prevents fluid and electrolyte imbalance.

   a Draw up 10 to 30 mL of air, and connect syringe to end of feeding tube. Flush tube with air. Pull back slowly, and aspirate the total amount of gastric contents that you can aspirate.

   b Return aspirated contents to stomach unless volume is greater than 200 mL (check agency policy). If the volume is greater than 200 mL on two consecutive assessments, hold feeding and notify health care provider (Metheny, 2006b).

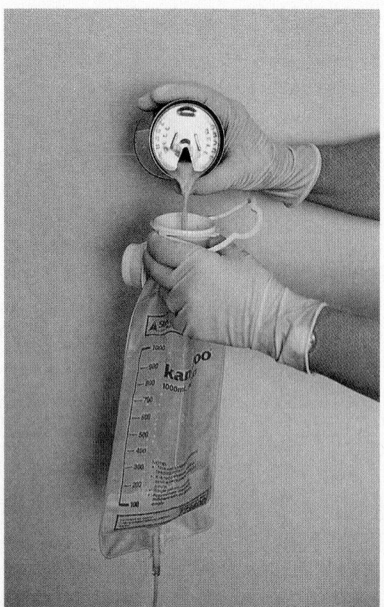

Step 3e ■ Pour formula into feeding container.

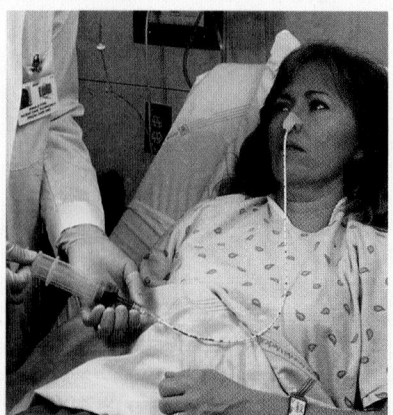

Step 3 ■ Check for gastric residual (small-bore tube).

STEP	RATIONALE
c Assess residual volume before each feeding for intermittent feedings. Assess residual volume every 4 hours for continuous feedings.	
4 Flush tube with 30 mL of water (see Skill 32-3).	Ensures tube is clear and decreases risk for occlusion (Bourgault and others, 2007).
5 Initiate feeding.	Usually patients receive enteral feedings continuously to ensure proper absorption. However, patients often receive initial feedings by bolus to assess patients' tolerance to formula. See Box 32-11 (p. 942) for guidelines to advance enteral feedings.
a Syringe for intermittent feeding	
(1) Pinch proximal end of feeding tube.	Prevents air from entering patient's stomach or intestine or leaking of contents.
(2) Remove plunger from syringe, and attach barrel of syringe to end of tube.	Barrel receives formula for instillation.
(3) Fill syringe with measured amount of formula (see illustration). Release tube, elevate syringe to no more than 18 inches (45 cm) above insertion site, and allow it to empty gradually by gravity. Repeat Steps 1 to 3 until you have delivered prescribed amount to patient.	Height of syringe allows for safe, slow, gravity drainage of formula. Total delivery of bolus feedings take several minutes, depending on the amount of the bolus. Administering the feeding too quickly will cause abdominal discomfort to the patient or increase the risk for aspiration.
b Feeding bag for intermittent feeding	
(1) Prime feeding bag tubing, and attach it to end of feeding tube. Set rate by adjusting roller clamp on tubing or placing on a feeding pump.	Reduces air introduced to stomach.
(2) Allow bag to empty gradually over 30 to 60 minutes (see illustration). Label bag with tube-feeding type, strength, and amount. Include date, time, and initials. Change bag every 24 hours.	Gradual emptying of tube feeding by gravity from syringe or feeding bag reduces risk for abdominal discomfort, vomiting, or diarrhea induced by bolus or too-rapid infusion of tube feedings. Helps decrease bacterial colonization.
c Continuous-drip method	
(1) Prime and hang feeding bag and tubing on feeding pump pole.	Continuous-feeding method delivers prescribed hourly rate of feeding with less risk for abdominal discomfort.
(2) Connect distal end of tubing to proximal end of feeding tube.	
(3) Connect tubing through infusion pump for enteral feedings, and set rate (see illustration).	Delivers continuous feeding at a steady rate and pressure. Alarms for increased resistance.

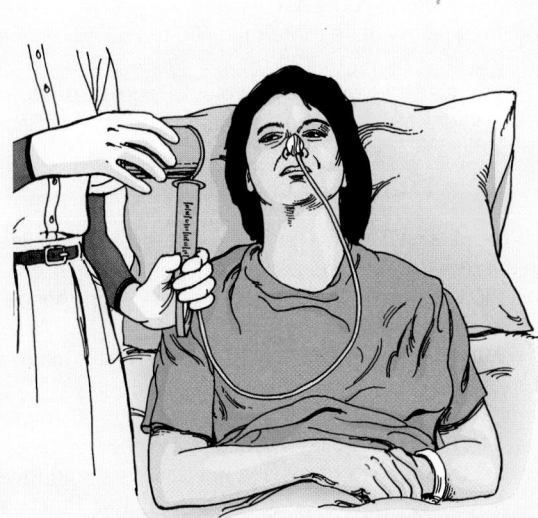

Step 5a(3) ■ Fill syringe with formula.

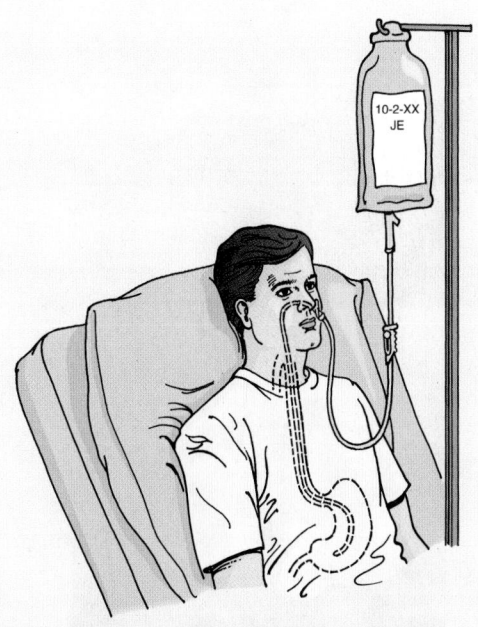

Step 5b(2) ■ Administer feeding.

SKILL 32-4   ADMINISTERING ENTERAL NUTRITION VIA NASOENTERIC, GASTROSTOMY, OR JEJUNOSTOMY TUBES—cont'd

STEP	RATIONALE
6 Advance rate of concentration of tube feeding gradually (Box 32-11).	Helps to prevent diarrhea and gastric intolerance to formula.
7 Flush with 30 mL of water every 4 hours during continuous feeding, before and after intermittent feeding, and after residual volume measurement. Have registered dietitian recommend total free water requirement per day, and obtain a health care provider's order.	Clears tubing of formula and prevents clogging of tube (Enteral Nutrition Practice Recommendations Task Force, 2009). Provides patient with source of water to help maintain fluid and electrolyte balance.

- *Critical Decision Point:* Flush tube with 30 mL sterile water in immunocompromised or critically ill patients (Enteral Nutrition Practice Recommendations Task Force, 2009).

STEP	RATIONALE
8 When you are not administering tube feedings, cap or clamp the proximal end of the feeding tube.	Prevents air from entering stomach between feedings.
9 Rinse bag and tubing with warm water whenever feedings are interrupted. Use a new administration set every 24 hours.	Rinsing bag and tubing with warm water clears old tube feedings and reduces bacterial growth.

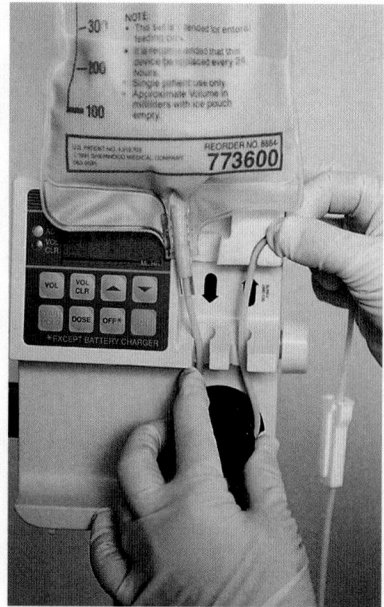

Step 5c(3) ■ Connect tubing through infusion pump.

BOX 32-11 Advancing the Rate of Tube Feeding

Protocols for advancing tube feedings are commonly facility specific. Most of these protocols are untested for validity. There does not appear to be a benefit to slow initiation of enteral nutrition over days. Most patients can tolerate feedings 2 to 3 days after initiation (ASPEN, 2002; Parrish and McCray, 2002).

INTERMITTENT
1. Start formula at full strength. Do not dilute formulas with water; this increases the risk for bacterial contamination (Enteral Nutrition Practice Recommendations Task Force, 2009).
2. Infuse intermittent feedings over 30 to 45 minutes via syringe or feeding container.
3. Begin feedings with no more than 150 to 250 mL at one time. Increase by 60 to 120 mL per feeding every 8 to 12 hours to achieve needed volume and calories in three to eight feedings (Enteral Nutrition Practice Recommendations Task Force, 2009).

CONTINUOUS
1. Start formula at full strength. Do not dilute formulas with water; this increases the risk for bacterial contamination (Enteral Nutrition Practice Recommendations Task Force, 2009).
2. Begin infusion rate at designated initiation rate, usually at 10 to 40 mL/hr.
3. Advance rate slowly in increments of 10 to 20 mL/hr every 8 to 12 hours to target rate as tolerated (tolerance indicated by absence of nausea and diarrhea, and low-volume gastric residuals) (Enteral Nutrition Practice Recommendations Task Force, 2009).

STEP	**RATIONALE**
10 For tubes placed through the abdominal wall, the insertion site of the tube is usually left open to air. Cleanse insertion site per agency policy.	Provides visualization of site. Decreases risk for infection.

EVALUATION

1 Measure residual volume per policy.	Evaluates tolerance of tube feeding.
2 Monitor finger-stick blood glucose (usually at least every 6 hours until maximum administration rate is reached and maintained for 24 hours).	Requires a health care provider order. Alerts nurse to patient's tolerance of enteral nutrition. Changes in blood glucose levels require physician or health care provider to revise type of formula administered.
3 Monitor intake and output at least every 8 hours.	Intake and output are indications of fluid balance or fluid volume excess or deficit.
4 Weigh patient daily until patient reaches and maintains maximum administration rate for 24 hours, then weigh patient 3 times per week.	Weight gain is indicator of improved nutritional status; however, sudden gain of more than 2 lb in 24 hours usually indicates fluid retention.
5 Monitor laboratory values (e.g., albumin, transferrin, prealbumin).	Laboratory values are indicators of patient's nutritional status.
6 Observe patient's respiratory status.	Change in respiratory status may indicate aspiration of tube feeding.
7 Observe patient's level of comfort.	Reduced gastric emptying will lead to abdominal discomfort.
8 Auscultate bowel sounds.	Assess gastric peristalsis.
9 For tubes placed through the abdominal wall, observe insertion site for skin integrity, symptoms of infection, injury, or necrosis.	Gastric or intestinal secretions cause injury and necrosis at insertion site.

RECORDING AND REPORTING

- Record amount and type of feeding, patient's response to tube feeding and patency of tube.
- Record volume of formula and any additional water on intake and output form.

- Report type of feeding, status of feeding tube, patient's tolerance, and adverse effects.

UNEXPECTED OUTCOMES AND RELATED INTERVENTIONS

- The feeding tube becomes clogged.
  - To avoid this problem, flush the tube with 30 mL water every 4 hours after checking the residual volume (Bourgault and others, 2007). Do not use cranberry juice to unclog feeding tubes; water works better than cranberry juice.
- Gastric residual exceeds 200 mL (check agency policy).
  - Notify health care provider to determine if you need to hold feedings.
  - Maintain patient in semi-Fowler's position; have head of bed elevated at least 30 degrees.
  - Reassess residual volume 1 hour after you stop the feeding to determine if volume has lessened or increased. If it has increased, make sure the health care provider is aware.
- Patient vomits and aspirates formula when gastric emptying is delayed or formula is administered too rapidly and produces vomiting.
  - Position patient in side-lying position.
  - Suction airway.
  - Notify health care provider.
  - Obtain chest x-ray film.
- Patient develops diarrhea three times or more in 24 hours; indicates possible intolerance.
  - Notify health care provider.

- Confer with RD to determine need to modify type of formula, concentration, or rate of infusion.
- Consider other causes (e.g., bacterial contamination of the feeding, patient infection).
- Determine if patient is receiving antibiotics or medications (e.g., those containing sorbitol) that will induce diarrhea.
- Provide skin care measures.
- Patient develops nausea and vomiting.
  - Withhold tube feeding, and notify physician or health care provider.
  - Check patency of tube.
  - Aspirate for gastric residual.
- Skin breakdown is noted around the abdominal insertion site of a gastrostomy or jejunostomy.
  - Institute skin care practices per agency policy.
  - Notify health care provider.
  - Provide wound care per health care provider's orders (see Chapter 36).
- There is a foul odor or unusual appearance of the aspirated fluid.
  - Notify the health care provider, and document the findings.
  - Do not return aspirated material of unusual odor or appearance without first consulting the physician or health care provider.

KEY POINTS

- Eating a balanced diet of carbohydrates, protein, lipids, vitamins, microminerals, and macrominerals provides the essential nutrients to carry out the body's normal physiological functioning.
- You maintain body weight when energy intake as food or fluids equals energy requirements.
- Digestion is the mechanical and chemical process by which food is broken down into its simplest form for absorption. Digestion and absorption occur mainly in the small intestine.
- Dietary reference intakes (DRIs), basis for diet selection, were formulated for population groups, not individuals.
- Guidelines for dietary change advocate reduced intake of fat, saturated fat, salt, refined sugar, and cholesterol and increased intake of complex carbohydrates and fiber.
- Age affects the requirements for essential nutrients. Periods of rapid growth increase the need for protein, vitamins, and minerals.

- Because improper nutrition affects all body systems, nutritional assessment includes a review of the total physical assessment.
- Special hospital diets alter the composition, texture, digestibility, and residue of foods to suit the patient's particular needs.
- Enteral nutrition is for patients who are unable to ingest food but are able to digest and absorb foods.
- Enteral nutrition protects intestinal structure and function and enhances immunity.
- Total parenteral nutrition supplies essential nutrients in appropriate amounts through a concentrated nutrient solution administered into the superior vena cava.
- Medical nutrition therapy is a recognized treatment modality for both acute and chronic disease states.

CRITICAL THINKING EXERCISES

While Matt is caring for Mrs. Gonzalez, he meets Mrs. Gonzalez's daughter, Martina. Martina tells Matt that Martina's physician just told her that she has high blood pressure. Martina's physician wants her to lose 50 lb to decrease her risk for developing diabetes mellitus. Martina also expresses concern about her teenage daughter, Lisa, who is underweight.

1. **a.** What information about Lisa's diet do you need to determine whether it is adequate in calories and protein?
   b. What laboratory tests would determine Lisa's protein status?
   c. What physical assessment findings might suggest inadequate protein intake in Lisa?

2. Martina asks Matt to help her develop a plan for losing weight as her physician has prescribed. What points should Matt include in the weight-loss plan for Martina?

3. As part of his clinical assignment, Matt is doing a presentation for his classmates on preventing aspiration during feeding in older adults with dysphagia. Develop an outline of key points for Matt to include in his presentation.

ℯvolve *Answers to Critical Thinking Questions can be found on the Evolve website.*

REVIEW QUESTIONS

1. You receive an order to place a nasogastric tube. Number the steps in the correct order for the placement.
   ___ **1.** Document the tube placement and patient response.
   ___ **2.** Encourage the patient to swallow as tube is being gently advanced.
   ___ **3.** Verify health care provider order for tube insertion.
   ___ **4.** Secure tube to nose to avoid pressure on nares.
   ___ **5.** Mark tube to visualize length of tube to insert.
   ___ **6.** Position patient in high-Fowler's position.
   ___ **7.** Verify tube placement.

2. You are developing a nursing care plan to reduce the risk for aspiration in a patient. Which interventions will help to reduce the risk? Select all that apply.
   1. Check gastric residual volume every 4 hours.
   2. Infuse enteral feeding no faster than 50 mL/hr.
   3. Elevate head of bed at least 30 degrees.
   4. Administer 60 mL of water every 4 hours.
   5. Check tube placement per protocol.

3. The nurse is checking the placement of a tube just inserted in a patient before initiating enteral feedings.

Which pH would lead the nurse to suspect that the tube is in the tracheobronchial tree?
   1. 1
   2. 3
   3. 5
   4. 7

4. Which statement made by the patient during a health history requires follow-up by the nurse?
   1. "I eat three meals a day with a bedtime snack."
   2. "I try to eat five or six servings of fruits and vegetables a day."
   3. "I have begun a walking program to build up my strength and lose weight."
   4. "I have lost 5 lb in the last 2 weeks without being on a diet."

5. Which statement made by the patient receiving a clear liquid diet indicates the need for further teaching?
   1. "I am glad that I can continue to have water to drink."
   2. "I plan on ordering two apple juices for tomorrow morning."
   3. "I am going to order milk to put in my coffee."
   4. "I hope that I can get my favorite orange Popsicles."

6. Which intervention is a priority in decreasing the risk for infection in a patient receiving parenteral nutrition?
   1. Check the patient's temperature every 4 hours.
   2. Ambulate patient 4 times per day.
   3. Change dressing per protocol using aseptic technique.
   4. Monitor serum glucose level every 6 hours.

7. You begin working with an overweight patient to achieve weight reduction. What is an ideal weight-loss goal to establish with the patient?
   1. ½ to 1 lb per week
   2. 1 to 2 lb per week
   3. 2 to 3 lb per week
   4. More than 3 lb per week

8. Which finding in a patient receiving enteral feedings at 80 mL/hr through a nasointestinal tube needs further follow-up?
   1. Gastric residual volume is 100 mL for the last 4 hours.
   2. Gastric aspirate is dark brown with a foul odor.
   3. Patient had two formed stools during the previous 24-hour period.
   4. Patient has active bowel sounds during morning assessment.

9. You are caring for a patient newly diagnosed with diabetes mellitus who states that he needs to make changes in his eating habits and patterns. Which nursing diagnosis is most appropriate to include on the nursing care plan?
   1. *Readiness for enhanced nutrition*
   2. *Feeding self-care deficit*
   3. *Risk for aspiration*
   4. *Imbalanced nutrition: less than body requirements*

10. Which finding assessed on physical examination of a patient is a possible indicator of malnutrition?
    1. Heart rate of 88 beats per minute
    2. Shiny hair
    3. Spoon-shaped nails
    4. Pinkish red oral mucous membranes

Answers to Review Questions can be found on pages 1197-1198.

REFERENCES

American Academy of Pediatrics: Policy statement: breastfeeding and the use of human milk, *Pediatrics* 115(2):496, 2005.

American Diabetes Association: Position statement: nutrition recommendations and interventions for diabetes—2006, *Diabetes Care* 29(9):2140, 2006.

American Dietetic Association: Position of the American Dietetic Association: food and nutrition misinformation, *J Am Diet Assoc* 106(4):601, 2006.

American Heart Association: AHA scientific statement: diet and lifestyle recommendations revision 2006, *Circulation* 114:82, 2006.

Ashley J and others: Speech, language, and swallowing disorders in the older adult, *Clin Geriatr Med* 22:291, 2006.

ASPEN Board of Directors and the Clinical Guidelines Task Force: Guidelines for the use of parenteral and enteral nutrition in adult and pediatric patients, *JPEN J Parenter Enteral Nutr* 26(1 Suppl):1SA, 2002.

Bourgault AN and others: Development of evidence-based guidelines and critical care nurses' knowledge of enteral feedings, *Crit Care Nurse* 27(4):17, 2007.

Brody RR and others: Role of registered dietitians in dysphagia screening, *J Am Diet Assoc* 100(9):1029, 2000.

Budd GM, Hayman LL: Addressing the childhood obesity crisis: a call to action, *MCN Am J Matern Child Nurs* 33(2):111, 2008.

Bulechek GM and others, editors: *Nursing interventions classification (NIC)*, ed 5, St. Louis, 2008, Mosby.

Chen CC and others: Dynamics of nutritional health in a community sample of American elders, *Adv Nurs Sci* 28(4):376, 2005.

Cirgin Ellett ML: Important facts about intestinal feeding tube placement, *Gastroenterol Nurs* 29(2):112, 2006.

Daniels J: Obesity: America's epidemic, *Am J Nurs* 106(1):40, 2006.

Daniels S and others: Clinical predictors of dysphagia and aspiration risk: outcome measures in acute stroke patients, *Arch Phys Med Rehabil* 81:1030, 2000.

Ebersole P and others: *Toward healthy aging: human needs and nursing response*, ed 7, St. Louis, 2008, Mosby.

Edwards B: Childhood obesity: a school-based approach to increase nutritional knowledge and activity levels, *Nurs Clin North Am* 40:661, 2005.

Enteral Nutrition Practice Recommendations Task Force: ASPEN Enteral nutrition practice recommendations, *JPEN OnlineFirst*, doi:10.1177/0148607108330314, published January 27, 2009.

Fox MK and others: Sources of energy and nutrients in the diets of infants and toddlers, *J Am Diet Assoc* 106(1 Suppl 1):S28e1, 2006.

Fuhrman MP and others: Hepatic proteins and nutrition assessment, *J Am Diet Assoc* 104(8):1258, 2004.

Furman EF: Undernutrition in older adults across the continuum of care: nutritional assessment, barriers, and interventions, *J Gerontol Nurs* 32(1):22, 2006.

Giger JN, Davidhizer RE: *Transcultural nursing: assessment and interventions*, ed 5, St. Louis, 2008, Mosby.

Guigoz Y, Vellas B: The Mini Nutritional Assessment (MNA) for grading the nutritional state of elderly patients: presentation of the MNA, history and validation, *Nestle Nutr Workshop Ser Clin Perform Programme* 1:3, 1999.

Guigoz YB and others: Assessing the nutritional status of the elderly: the Mini Nutritional Assessment as part of the geriatric evaluation, *Nutr Rev* 54(1 Pt 2):S59, 1996.

Hadaway LC: Keeping central line infection at bay, *Nursing* 36(4):58, 2006.

Heyland DK, Dhaliwal R: Early enteral nutrition vs. early parenteral nutrition: an irrelevant question for the critically ill? *Crit Care Med* 33(1):260-1, 2005.

Hinchey JA and others: Formal dysphagia screening protocols prevent pneumonia, *Stroke* 36:1972, 2005.

Hockenberry MJ, Wilson D: *Wong's nursing care of infants and children*, ed 8, St. Louis, 2006, Mosby.

Huang and others: Training in swallowing prevents aspiration pneumonia in stroke patients with dysphagia, *J Int Med Res* 34(3):303, 2006.

Huffman GB: Evaluating and treating unintentional weight loss in the elderly, *Am Fam Physician* 65(4):640, 2002.

Institute of Medicine: *Dietary reference intakes*, 2009, http://www.iom.edu/CMS/54133.aspx, accessed September 22, 2009.

Kruskall LJ: Portion distortion: sizing up food servings, *ACSM's Health Fitness J* 10(3):8, 2006.

Kushi LH and others: American Cancer Society guidelines on nutrition and physical activity for cancer prevention: reducing the risk for cancer with health food choices and physical activity, *CA Cancer J Clin* 56:254, 2006.

Kwon HM and others: The pneumonia score: a simple grading scale for prediction of pneumonia after acute stroke, *Am J Infect Control* 34(2):64, 2006.

Lee JS and others: Weight-loss intention in the well-functioning, community-dwelling elderly: associations with diet quality, physical activity, and weight change, *Am J Clin Nutr* 80(2):466, 2004.

Matlow A and others: Enteral tube hub as a reservoir for the transmissible enteric bacteria, *Am J Infect Control* 34(3):131, 2006.

Metheny N and others: How to aspirate fluid from small-bore feeding tubes, *Am J Nurs* 93(5):86, 1993.

Metheny NA: Inadvertent intracranial nasogastric tube placement, *Am J Nurs* 102(8):25, 2002.

Metheny NA: Preventing respiratory complications of tube feedings: evidence-based practice, *Am J Crit Care* 15(4):360, 2006.

Metheny NA, Meert KL, Clouse R: Complications related to feeding tube placement, *Curr Opin Gastroenterol*, 23(2): 178-82, 2007.

Metheny NA: Preventing aspiration in older adults with dysphagia, *Am J Nurs* 108(2):45, 2007.

Metheny NA, Meert KL: Monitoring feeding tube placement, *Nutr Clin Pract* 19(5):487, 2004.

Metheny NA, Titler MG: Assessing placement of feeding tubes, *Am J Nurs* 101:36, 2001.

Metheny NA and others: pH, color, and feeding tubes, *RN* 61(1):25, 1998.

Metheny NA and others: Effect of feeding-tube properties on residual volumes measurements in tube-fed patients, *JPEN* 29(3):192, 2005a.

Metheny NA and others: Indicators of tubesite during feedings, *J Neurosci Nurs* 37(6):320, 2005b.

Metheny NA and others: Verification of inefficacy of the glucose method in detecting aspiration associated with tube feedings, *Medsurg Nurs* 14(2):112, 2005c.

Metheny NA: Preventing respiratory complications of tube feeding: evidence-based practice, *Am J Crit Care* 15:360, 2006a.

Metheny NA and others: Tracheobronchial aspiration of gastric contents in critically ill tube-fed patients: frequency, outcomes, and risk factors, *Crit Care Med* 34(4):1007, 2006b.

Metheny NA and others: Gastric residual volume and aspiration in critically ill patients receiving gastric feedings, *Am J Crit Care* 17(6):512, 2008.

Moorhead S and others, editors: *Nursing outcomes classification (NOC)*, ed 4, St. Louis, 2008, Mosby.

National Center for Chronic Disease Prevention and Health Promotion. *Health topics: childhood overweight*, 2007, http://www.cdc.gov/HealthyYouth/overweight/index.htm, accessed July 10, 2007.

National Dysphagia Diet Task Force: *National Dysphagia Diet: standardization for optimal care*, Chicago, 2002, American Dietetic Association.

National Guideline Clearinghouse: *Infection control: prevention of healthcare-associated infection in primary and community care*, 2003, http://www.guideline.gov/summary/summary.aspx?doc_id=5069&nbr=003553&string=Prevention+AND+healthcare-associated+AND+infection, accessed December 19, 2006.

National Guideline Clearinghouse: *Nutrition assessment: adults guideline*, 2006, http://www.guideline.gov/summary/summary.aspx?ss=15&doc_id=3625&nbr=002851&string=nutrition+AND+assessment, accessed December 14, 2006.

Nix S: *Williams' basic nutrition and diet therapy*, ed 12, St. Louis, 2005, Mosby.

Nowlin A: The dysphagia dilemma: how you can help, *RN* 69(6):44, 2006.

Palmer JL, Metheny NA: Preventing aspiration in older adults with dysphagia, *Am J Nurs* 108(2):40, 2008.

Parrish C, McCray S: Enteral feeding: dispelling myths, *Pract Gastroenterol* 9:33, 2003.

Perry L, Love C: Screening for dysphagia and aspiration in acute stroke: a systematic review, *Dysphagia* 16:7, 2001.

Perry L, McLaren S: Eating difficulties after stroke, *J Adv Nurs* 43(4):360, 2003.

Ramsey D, Smithard D, Kaira L: Silent aspiration: what do we know? *Dysphagia* 20(3):218, 2003.

Rolandelli RH and others: *Clinical nutrition: enteral feeding and tube feeding*, Philadelphia, 2005, Saunders.

Roux L and others: Valuing the benefits of weight loss programs: an application of the discrete choice experiment, *Obes Res* 12(8):1342, 2004.

Sarhill N and others: Evaluation of nutritional status in advanced metastatic cancer, *Support Care Cancer* 11(10):652, 2003.

Serna ED, McCarthy MS: Heads up to prevent aspiration during enteral feeding, *Nursing* 36(1):76, 2006.

Takeda EJ and others: Stress control and human nutrition, *J Med Invest* 51(3-4):139, 2004.

U.S. Department of Agriculture Center for Nutrition Policy and Promotion: *USDA's food guide pyramid*, April 2005, http://www.MyPyramid.gov.

U.S. Department of Agriculture and U.S. Department of Health and Human Services: *Dietary guidelines for Americans, 2005*, ed 6, Washington, DC, 2005, U.S. Government Printing Office, http://www.healthierus.gov/dietaryguidelines.

U.S. Department of Health and Human Services: *Healthy people 2010*, 2002, http://www.health.gov/healthypeople.

U.S. Department of Health and Human Services Centers for Disease Control and Prevention: *Overweight and obesity*, 2008, http://www.cdc.gov/nccdphp/dnpa/obesity/.

White G and others: Dysphagia: cause, assessment, and management, *Geriatrics* 63(5):15, 2008.

Williams SD, Schlenker ED: *Essentials of nutrition and diet therapy*, ed 8, St. Louis, 2003, Mosby.

Wofford LG: Systematic review of childhood obesity prevention, *J Pediatr Nurs* 23(1):5, 2008.

Urinary Elimination

MEDIA RESOURCES

 CD COMPANION 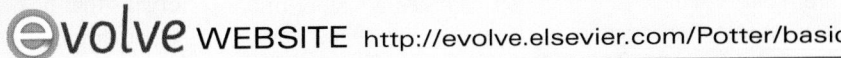 **WEBSITE** http://evolve.elsevier.com/Potter/basic

- Crossword Puzzle
- English/Spanish Audio Glossary

OBJECTIVES

- Explain the structures of the urinary system, including function and role in urine formation and elimination.
- Identify factors that commonly influence urinary elimination.
- Discuss common alterations associated with urinary elimination.
- Obtain a nursing history from a patient with an alteration in urination.
- Perform a beginning physical assessment related to urinary elimination.
- Describe characteristics of normal and abnormal urine.

- Describe nursing implications of common diagnostic tests of the urinary system.
- Identify nursing diagnoses associated with alterations in urinary elimination.
- Discuss nursing measures to promote normal urination and to control incontinence.
- Discuss nursing measures to reduce urinary tract infections.
- Apply an external catheter and insert a urinary catheter.

KEY TERMS

bacteremia, p. 949
bacteriuria, p. 949
catheterization, p. 967
dysuria, p. 961
graduated measuring
    container, p. 957
hematuria, p. 958

micturition, p. 949
proteinuria, p. 948
residual urine, p. 949
stoma, p. 951
suprapubic catheter,
    p. 969
ureterostomy, p. 972

urinal, p. 964
urinary diversion,
    p. 949
urinary incontinence
    (UI), p. 949
urinary reflux, p. 972

urinary retention,
    p. 949
urine hat, p. 958
urometer, p. 958
urosepsis, p. 949
voiding, p. 949

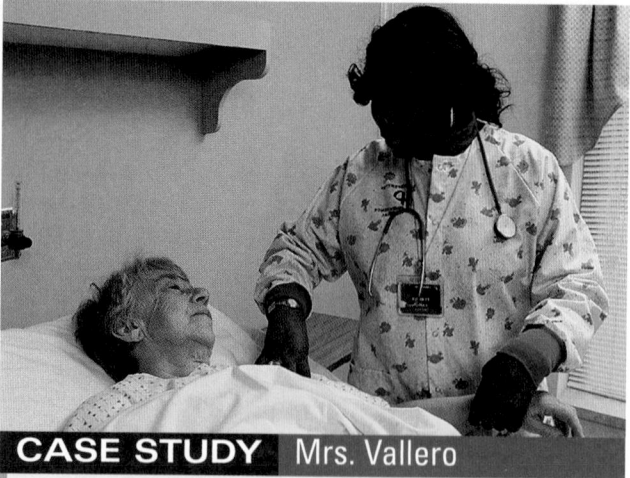

CASE STUDY   Mrs. Vallero

Mrs. Vallero is a 65-year-old woman. She has been in the hospital for 4 days with problems related to heart failure, fluid retention, and diabetes. She has a history of urinary retention secondary to neuropathy caused by her diabetes. At the 3 PM shift report, Sandy, the nursing student, learns that the Mrs. Vallero's indwelling urinary catheter was removed 2 days ago and subsequently replaced yesterday at 6 AM because of her inability to urinate more than 100 mL at a time, being incontinent of small amounts of urine, complaints of urinary urgency, and lower abdominal pain. Sandy notes the urinary catheter was removed at 7 AM this morning and the patient has no recorded urine output for the day. Mrs. Vallero verifies she has only "dribbled" urine. While making rounds, Sandy talks with Mrs. Vallero, who says she is worried because "I thought this was all under control." The health care provider was notified, and an order was obtained for an intermittent catheterization. The registered nurse on the day shift catheterized Mrs. Vallero at 3 PM with a return of 600 mL of pale, clear yellow urine.

Normal elimination of urinary wastes is a function most people take for granted. When the urinary system fails to function properly, it affects virtually all body systems. Patients with alterations in urinary elimination may also have body image problems as a result. To meet elimination needs, patients frequently rely on interventions from health professionals. Your role as a nurse involves being sensitive to these needs as you critically think and use the nursing process to provide care to patients with altered urinary elimination.

SCIENTIFIC KNOWLEDGE BASE

Knowledge from the biological and social sciences helps you to identify actual and potential urinary tract problems that patients develop. A thorough understanding of related information helps you to provide complete and competent care to patients with altered elimination. Your role in helping a patient with urinary elimination involves applying the nursing process to provide an appropriate plan of care so that you can

intervene both independently and in collaboration with others to meet the patient's urinary elimination needs.

Urinary Elimination

Urinary elimination depends on the function of the kidneys, ureters, bladder, and urethra (Figure 33-1). The kidneys remove wastes from the blood. The ureters transport urine from the kidneys to the bladder. The bladder holds urine until the urge to urinate develops and urine leaves the body through the urethra. All of these organs must be intact and functional for the successful removal of urinary wastes. The normal range of urine production is 1 to 2 L/day (Huether and McCance, 2008). Fluid intake and body temperature affect urine production. Urine is usually 95% water and 5% solutes. These solutes include electrolytes and organic solutes such as urea, uric acid, creatinine, and ammonia.

KIDNEYS   The kidneys are reddish-brown, bean-shaped organs that lie on either side of the vertebral column behind the abdominal peritoneum and against the deep muscles of the back. The kidneys are level with the twelfth thoracic and third lumbar vertebrae. The functional units of the kidney are the nephrons. Nephrons remove waste products from the blood and regulate water and electrolyte concentrations in body fluids. The kidneys efficiently filter the blood of waste products in part because of their high blood flow, which represents approximately 25% of the cardiac output.

A cluster of capillaries forms the glomerulus, which is the initial site of urine formation. These capillaries filter water and glucose, amino acids, urea, uric acid, creatinine, and major electrolytes. Protein does not normally filter through the glomerulus. Therefore **proteinuria,** protein in the urine, is a sign of glomerular injury.

However, not all glomerular filtrate is excreted as urine. The body reabsorbs approximately 99% of the filtrate into the plasma. When the filtrate leaves the glomerulus, it passes through a system of tubules in which water and glucose, amino acids, uric acid, sodium, potassium, and bicarbonate ions are selectively reabsorbed into plasma. Hydrogen and potassium ions and ammonia are secreted into the tubules and become a part of the urine.

URETERS   A ureter is attached to each kidney pelvis and carries urinary wastes into the bladder. Urine draining from the ureters to the bladder is sterile. Peristaltic waves cause the urine to enter the bladder in spurts rather than steadily. Contractions of the bladder during urination compress the lower portion of the ureters to prevent urine from returning to the ureters (Huether and McCance, 2008).

BLADDER   The urinary bladder is a hollow, distensible, muscular organ that is a reservoir for urine. When empty, the bladder lies in the pelvic cavity behind the symphysis pubis. In the male the bladder rests against the rectum posteriorly, and in the female it rests against the anterior wall of the uterus and vagina. The bladder's shape changes as it fills with urine. When the bladder is full, its superior surface expands up into a dome and pushes above the symphysis pubis. A greatly distended bladder may reach the umbilicus. In a pregnant woman the fetus pushes against the bladder, causing a feeling of fullness and reducing its capacity.

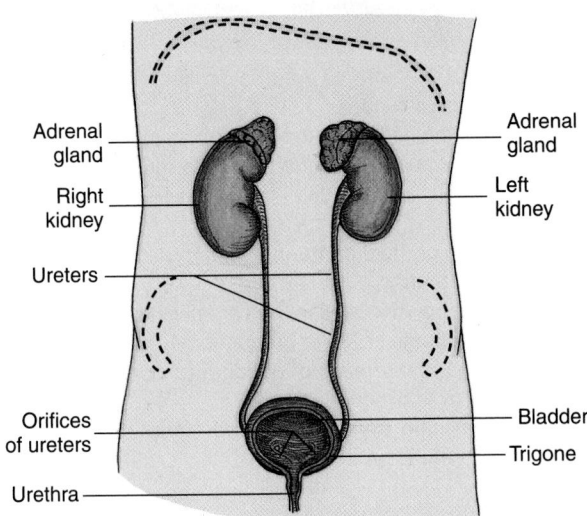

Figure 33-1 ■ Organs of the urinary system.

URETHRA Urine travels from the bladder through the urethra and passes to the outside of the body through the urethral meatus. Mucous membrane lines the urethra, and urethral glands secrete mucus into the urethral canal. The external urethral sphincter, made up of striated muscles, permits voluntary flow of urine (Huether and McCance, 2008).

Act of Urination

Urination, **micturition,** and **voiding** are all terms for expelling urine from the urinary bladder. A person senses a desire to urinate when the bladder contains only a small amount of urine (150 to 200 mL in an adult and 50 to 100 mL in a child). As the volume of urine increases, the bladder wall stretches. Normally a person is conscious of the need to urinate. If the person chooses not to void, the external urinary sphincter remains contracted, inhibiting the reflex. When a person is ready to void, the external sphincter relaxes, the micturition reflex stimulates the detrusor muscle to contract, and urination occurs.

Factors Influencing Urination

Physiological factors, psychosocial conditions, and diagnostic or treatment-induced factors all affect normal urinary elimination (Box 33-1). Knowledge of these factors enables you to anticipate possible elimination problems and how to intervene when problems develop.

Common Urinary Elimination Problems

The most common urinary elimination problems involve the inability to store or fully empty urine from the bladder. These problems result from impaired bladder function, obstruction to urine outflow, or an inability to voluntarily control micturition. Some patients have permanent or temporary changes in the normal pathway of urination. For example, the patient with a **urinary diversion** has special needs because urine drains through an artificial opening (stoma) on the abdominal wall.

URINARY RETENTION **Urinary retention** is an accumulation of urine in the bladder because the bladder is unable to partially or completely empty. The patient who retains at least 25% of total bladder capacity is experiencing urinary retention. Urine collects in the bladder, stretching its walls and causing feelings of pressure, discomfort, tenderness over the symphysis pubis, restlessness, and diaphoresis. These findings along with an absence of urinary output over several hours and a distended bladder may indicate urinary retention. In urinary retention, the bladder sometimes holds more than 1000 mL of urine. *In the case study, Mrs. Vallero has shown signs of urinary retention. She has had diabetes for over 35 years, and it is likely neuropathy has contributed to her bladder problem.*

In retention the pressure in the bladder builds so that the external urethral sphincter is unable to hold back urine. The sphincter opens to allow a small volume of urine (25 to 60 mL) to escape, after which the bladder pressure falls enough to allow the sphincter to close. The patient may develop overflow incontinence, that is, the patient will void small amounts of urine two or three times an hour with no relief of distention or discomfort (Milne, 2004). Decreased urine production causes retention by filling the bladder gradually, thus preventing activation of the stretch receptors. After distending beyond a certain point, the bladder cannot contract. Retention also occurs because of many other factors (Table 33-1).

URINARY TRACT INFECTIONS Urinary tract infections (UTIs) account for more than 8.3 million health care provider visits a year (Mehnert-Kay, 2005). They also account for 80% of health care–acquired infections (HAIs) and are most commonly associated with indwelling urinary catheter use (Gokula and others, 2004). Approximately 15% to 25% of all patients admitted to the hospital are catheterized (Ritin and others, 2006). *Escherichia coli,* a bacterium commonly found in the colon, is responsible for 75% to 95% of uncomplicated urinary tract infections (Mehnert-Kay, 2005). Poor perineal hygiene, that is, failure to wipe from front to back after voiding or defecating, is a common cause of UTI developing in women.

Bacteria inhabit the vagina in women and the distal urethra and external genitalia in men and women. Organisms enter the urethral meatus easily and travel up the inner mucosal lining of the urethra to the bladder. Women are more susceptible to UTIs. The length of the urethra and an antibacterial substance in prostatic secretions reduce the risk for UTI in males. Normally the body flushes out organisms during voiding. However, bladder distention reduces blood flow to the mucosal and submucosal layer, and tissues become more susceptible to bacteria. **Residual urine** is urine that remains in the bladder after urination. The urine becomes alkaline and promotes bacterial growth. Bacteria in bladder urine (**bacteriuria**) may ascend into the kidneys and result in bacteria entering the bloodstream (**bacteremia** or **urosepsis**).

URINARY INCONTINENCE **Urinary incontinence (UI)** is the temporary or permanent loss of control over voiding. There are numerous types of UI (Table 33-2, p. 952). The patient is unable to control the external urethral sphincter, and

BOX 33-1   Factors Influencing Urinary Elimination

GROWTH AND DEVELOPMENT

- Infants and young children are unable to concentrate urine and reabsorb water effectively.
- Children cannot control urination voluntarily until 18 to 24 months.
- A child must be able to recognize the feeling of bladder fullness, to hold urine for 1 to 2 hours, and to communicate the sense of urgency.
- With age, the ability to concentrate urine declines and the frequency of urination increases.
- The process of aging impairs micturition by interfering with mobility, sometimes making it difficult for older adults to reach the toilet or bedside commode in time (Figure 33-2).

SOCIOCULTURAL FACTORS

- Cultural and gender norms vary on the privacy or publicness of urination. North Americans expect toilet facilities to be private, whereas some European cultures accept communal toilet facilities. Religious or cultural norms dictate who is acceptable to assist in elimination practices.
- Social expectations (e.g., school recesses) influence the time of urination.

PSYCHOLOGICAL FACTORS

- Anxiety and stress do not affect the characteristics of urine but sometimes affect a sense of urgency and increase the frequency of urination.
- Anxiety prevents complete urination because tension makes it difficult to relax abdominal muscles.

PERSONAL HABITS

- Privacy and adequate time to urinate are usually important to most people. Some people need distractions to relax.

MUSCLE TONE

- Weak abdominal and pelvic floor muscles impair bladder contraction and control of the external sphincter.

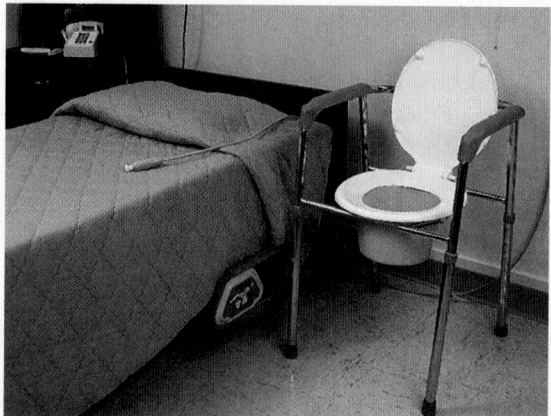

Figure 33-2 ■ Bedside commode. (From Sorrentino S: *Mosby's textbook for nursing assistants*, St. Louis, 2004, Mosby.)

- Immobility, childbirth, or trauma sometimes cause decreased muscle tone.
- Continuous drainage of urine through an indwelling catheter often causes loss of the bladder's muscle tone.

FLUID INTAKE

- Foods with high fluid content, such as fruits and vegetables, increase urine production.
- If fluids, electrolytes, and solutes are balanced, increased fluid intake increases urine production.
- Alcohol stops the release of antidiuretic hormones, thus promoting urine production.
- Fluids containing caffeine increase urinary output frequency and urgency.

PATHOLOGICAL CONDITIONS

- Diabetes mellitus and multiple sclerosis cause neuropathies that alter bladder function.
- Rheumatoid arthritis, degenerative joint disease, and Parkinson's disease slow or hinder physical activity and interfere with urination.
- Chronic diseases, such as stroke, alter urinary patterns by interfering with mobility or bladder sensation.
- Acute renal disease reduces urine volume; chronic renal disease initially increases volume of poorly concentrated urine.
- Febrile conditions reduce the amount of urine but increase the concentration.
- Spinal cord injuries interrupt voluntary bladder emptying.

SURGICAL PROCEDURES

- The stress response to surgery reduces the amount of urinary output to increase circulatory fluid volume.
- Anesthetics and pain-killing drugs slow the filtration rate and reduce urinary output.
- Local trauma during lower abdominal and pelvic surgery sometimes obstructs urine flow, making indwelling catheters necessary.

MEDICATIONS

- Diuretics prevent reabsorption of water and certain electrolytes, thus increasing urinary output.
- Some drugs also change the color of urine (e.g., amitriptyline turns it blue-green, methyldopa turns it red, warfarin sodium turns it orange, indomethacin turns it green).
- Some medications affect the ability to relax and empty the bladder.

DIAGNOSTIC EXAMINATIONS

- Following an intravenous pyelogram, patient may have complications such as hypersensitivity reactions to the injected dye and acute renal failure.
- Cystoscopy causes localized edema of the urethral passageway and bladder sphincter spasm, resulting in urinary retention and the passing of red or pink urine.

TABLE 33-1 Urinary Disorders

DISORDER	CAUSES
URINARY RETENTION Urine flow is obstructed; urine accumulates in bladder.	Prostate gland enlargement, fecal impaction, pregnancy in third trimester, urethral stricture or edema after childbirth, and urethral edema after surgery or diagnostic examination obstruct urine flow. Spinal cord and peripheral nerve trauma and degeneration of peripheral nerves (e.g., diabetic neuropathy) alter sensory and motor innervation. Emotional anxiety and muscle tension alter ability to relax sphincters. Medications (anesthetics and opioid analgesics) dull bladder sensations.
LOWER URINARY TRACT INFECTION Microorganisms enter urethra, resulting in bacterial spread, causing inflammation of bladder muscle.	Kinked or blocked urethral catheter and urinary retention cause obstruction of urine flow. Poor perineal hygiene, frequent sexual intercourse, ingredients in bubble baths, improperly handled diagnostic instruments, improperly sterilized instruments, and contaminated urine receptacles cause spread of bacteria.
URINARY INCONTINENCE Incontinence involves incompetent or weakened sphincter and loss of control of voiding.	Multiple childbirths, pelvic organ surgery, and removal of prostate gland weaken sphincter. Mental confusion, sedatives or analgesics, spinal cord injury, bladder spasm, and bladder atrophy cause loss of voiding control.

urinary leakage is continuous or intermittent. It is a myth that incontinence is part of the aging process; however, UI affects approximately 30% of older adults living at home and about 50% of older adults in nursing homes (Mauk, 2005). The highest incidence (55%) in women is in those who are 80 to 90 years of age and in men over the age of 60 (Specht, 2005). An older person with restricted mobility has a greater chance of being incontinent because of the inability to reach toilet facilities in time. Low-set chairs and high beds are additional obstacles for the older adult who needs to get up to reach a toilet. An older adult who has difficulty undoing buttons or manipulating zippers faces another obstacle. Some older adults with chronic health problems lack the energy to walk very far at one time, and if there is only one toilet in the home, the distance is sometimes too far for the patient with urge incontinence. Besides skin breakdown, continued episodes of incontinence can create a variety of emotional problems, including frustration, depression, and embarrassment, leading to social isolation and loss of independence (Mauk, 2005).

Urinary Diversions

It may be necessary in some patients who have conditions such as bladder cancer, radiation injury to the bladder, or chronic UTIs to surgically divert the drainage of urine from a diseased or dysfunctional bladder through an opening in the abdominal wall. The opening is called a **stoma** and is constructed from a section of small intestine. Urinary diversions are either temporary or permanent, and continent or incontinent.

There are two types of continent urinary diversions. One is a continent urinary reservoir (Figure 33-3, *A*), which is created from a distal portion of the ileum and proximal portion of the colon. The ureters are imbedded in the reservoir. This reservoir is situated under the abdominal wall and has a narrow ileal segment brought out through the abdominal wall to form a small stoma. The ileocecal valve creates a one-way valve in the pouch through which a catheter is inserted through the stoma to empty the urine from the pouch. Patients must be willing and able to catheterize the pouch 4 to 6 times a day for the rest of their lives.

The other type of continent urinary diversion is an orthotopic neobladder, which also uses an ileal pouch to replace the bladder. Anatomically, the pouch is in the same position as the bladder was before removal, allowing a patient to void normally.

Incontinent urinary diversions are less commonly performed. The surgery involves connecting the ureters to a section of the intestinal ileum with formation of a stoma on the abdominal wall (Figure 33-3, *B*). Urine drains continuously because the patient has no sensation or control over urinary output, requiring the application of a collection pouch at all times.

NURSING KNOWLEDGE BASE

Urinary elimination is a natural and often private process that requires physiological and psychological health. Therefore providing nursing care for a patient with potential or actual urinary problems requires an understanding beyond anatomy and physiology. Be knowledgeable about concepts such as infection control, hygiene measures, growth and development, and be sensitive to the patient's psychosocial needs when a urinary problem develops.

TABLE 33-2 Types of Urinary Incontinence

DESCRIPTION	CAUSES	SYMPTOMS
TOTAL Total uncontrollable and continuous loss of urine	Neuropathy of sensory nerves Trauma or disease of spinal nerves or urethral sphincter	Constant flow of urine at unpredictable times Nocturia Lack of awareness of bladder filling or incontinence
FUNCTIONAL Involuntary unpredictable passage of urine in patient who has a mental or physical disability and intact urinary and nervous systems	Fistula between bladder and vagina Change in environment Sensory, cognitive, or mobility deficits	Strong urge to void with loss of urine before reaching appropriate receptacle
STRESS Increased intraabdominal pressure causing leakage of small amount of urine	Coughing, laughing, vomiting, or lifting with full bladder Obesity Full uterus pressing against bladder during third trimester of pregnancy Incompetent bladder outlet Weak pelvic musculature	Dribbling of urine with increased intraabdominal pressure Urinary urgency Frequency
URGE Involuntary passage of urine after strong sense of urgency to void	Decreased bladder capacity Irritation of bladder stretch receptors Alcohol or caffeine ingestion Increased fluid intake Interstitial cystitis	Urinary urgency Abnormal frequency (more often than every 2 hours) Bladder contracture or spasm Nocturia Voiding in small (less than 100 mL) or in large (more than 550 mL) amounts
REFLEX Involuntary loss of urine occurring at somewhat predictable intervals when patient reaches specific bladder volume	Upper spinal cord injury or disease involving area above reflex arc, blocking cerebral awareness Lower spinal cord injury blocking impulses to reflex arc	Lack of awareness of bladder filling No urge to void Uninhibited bladder contraction or spasm at regular intervals

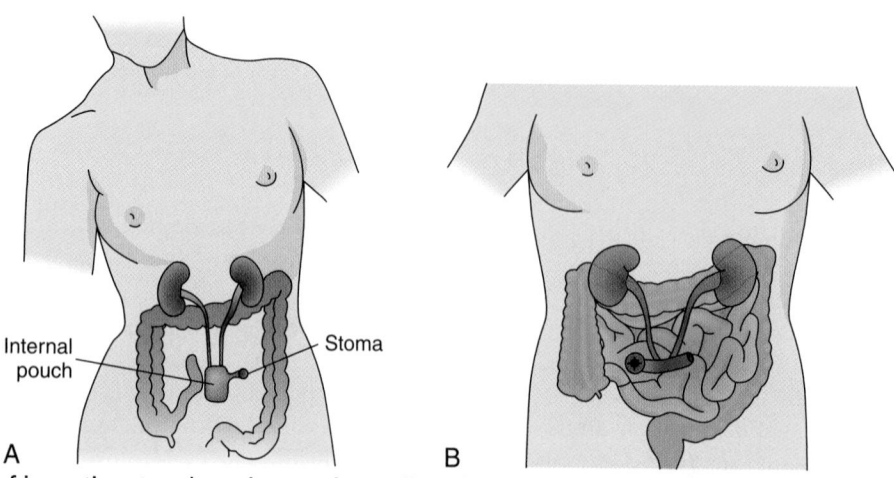

Figure 33-3 ■ Types of incontinent and continent urinary diversions. **A,** Continent urinary reservoir. **B,** Urostomy (ileal conduit).

Infection Control and Hygiene

The urinary tract is a common site for infection. Therefore you will follow the principles of infection control to prevent the onset and spread of UTIs and to promote the treatment of infections that do occur (see Chapter 13). *E. coli* often causes urinary tract infections because of the spread of organisms from fecal soiling to the urethra. Infections occur anywhere along the urinary tract from the urethra to the kidneys.

You will need to follow the principles of medical and surgical asepsis meticulously when carrying out procedures involving the urinary tract or external genitalia. Procedures that involve manipulation of the perineum, such as perineal care or examination of the genitalia, require the use of medical asepsis.

Any instrumentation used on or in the urinary tract, such as catheterization, requires the use of sterile technique. Urinary catheterization is a common procedure in all care settings. It is an invasive procedure that commonly results in catheter-associated UTIs (CAUTIs). Gokula and others (2004) indicate that 80% of HAIs are associated with indwelling catheter use. CAUTI is associated with significant morbidity, prolonged hospitalization, and mortality (Toughill, 2005). Current evidence supports the insertion of antibiotic-impregnated and silver-coated indwelling catheters, which have been shown to reduce the risk for CAUTI for up to 7 days and 2 weeks, respectively (Parker and others, 2009).

Developmental Considerations

Throughout the life span, normal growth and development processes affect a person's ability to void. Normally neonates void within 24 hours after birth. In the neonate and infant, urination is a voiding response and produced by a full bladder. As the child reaches the age of 2 or 3 years, the neuromuscular and cognitive functions develop to the point where the child begins to control voiding (see Chapter 21).

As we age, changes occur in both the male and female that contribute to the development of voiding problems. In the male it is possible for prostate enlargement to start after age 40 and continue until the 80s, causing partial obstruction of the urethra and resulting in inadequate emptying of the bladder. This change produces increased urinary frequency. In the female, childbearing and hormonal levels influence urination. Changes associated with pregnancy often produce urinary frequency and urgency. With repeated deliveries or hormone changes after menopause, temporary or permanent changes can occur that result in decreased perineal muscle tone. These changes may lead to urgency and stress incontinence (see Table 33-2). Hormonal changes may also contribute to an increased susceptibility to infection. Decreased levels of estrogen tend to cause the urethral mucosa to become thinner and more fragile and consequently more easily traumatized and infected (Huether and McCance, 2008).

Psychosocial Implications

Self-concept, culture, and sexuality are all closely related concepts that are affected when a patient has elimination problems. Self-concept changes over one's life span and includes one's body image, self-esteem, roles, and identity (see Chapter 22).

When children begin to achieve bladder control and learn the appropriate skills, they sometimes resist urinating on the toilet. Children often associate their urine and feces as extensions of self, and they do not want to flush part of themselves away.

Gender influences the position we use to urinate. Males tend to stand to urinate, and females assume a sitting position. Culture influences how people talk about urination and how much privacy a person needs. It is improper in some cultures for a male to ask a female patient about private matters such as urination (Box 33-2).

BOX 33-2   CULTURAL FOCUS

Urinary elimination is an activity that is personal and private. Culture influences how people talk about urination and how much privacy a person needs. It is important to remember to provide privacy during procedures by using adequate draping and bedside screens. Being a skilled practitioner will help prevent prolonged exposure of the patient. There are often gender-congruent care needs among cultures that emphasize separate gender roles and female modesty, such as in African, Hispanic, Asian, Islamic, Arabic, Hindu, Jewish Orthodox, and Amish cultures. It is important to be knowledgeable about a culture's impact on patient care. Be open to and respect practices different from your own.

Implications for Practice

- Recognize and accommodate the need for gender-congruent care. Explain the procedure you will perform, and ask the patient how he or she wants this done. Assign female caregivers to catheterize females and male caregivers for male patients. Allow presence of a family member at the bedside if requested by the patient. Prevent entrance of the opposite sex during the procedure.
- Control verbal and nonverbal communication when performing catheterization of a circumcised female. Avoid judgmental comments, and assess for landmarks in a professional manner. Use a smaller catheter when scarring constricts the area. Explain the procedure you will perform.
- Use simple and clear sentences when communicating with patients for whom English is a second language. Use an interpreter as needed. Repeat explanations if the patient's anxiety about the loss of privacy creates distraction. Explain measures to protect the patient's privacy.
- Provide for patients' hygiene needs. Certain cultures, such as Hindus and Muslims, observe meticulous hygiene practices that designate the left hand to perform unclean procedures such as catheterization. Perform hand hygiene before touching the patient, and use your right hand when possible. However, to insert a catheter, use your dominant hand to hold the catheter and use your nondominant hand to retract the labia. Use the left hand to handle the urinal and/or urinary secretions.
- Change the bed linens and gown of the patient promptly if contaminated with urine. Do not place the urinal or soiled bed linens on top of the bedside table or surface used for praying or eating.
- Provide the patient with the equipment and supplies for cleansing after elimination.

CRITICAL THINKING

Synthesis

You will apply elements of critical thinking whenever you perform the nursing process with a patient. Consider the scientific knowledge you have learned, your experience, critical thinking attitudes, and standards to ensure an individualized approach to patient care (Box 33-3).

KNOWLEDGE The knowledge that you have about the elimination process, the conditions that create alterations in elimination, and a comprehensive view of your patient's situation will allow you to make the most accurate decisions about patient care. Information about fluid and electrolyte balance and knowledge of medications will further complement your knowledge base. When patients have changes in their fluid balance, this affects elimination patterns. In addition, these changes increase the patients' risks for problems in urination such as infection, incontinence, or retention. You also need to have an understanding of the effects of the aging process on

urinary elimination, as well as skills and procedures used for patients with alterations in urinary elimination, in order to intervene in a competent manner. Finally, your ability to refer to what you have learned about cultural sensitivity and concepts of self-concept and body image will help you provide an individualized and compassionate approach to care.

EXPERIENCE Previous and personal experiences provide a basis for determining a patient's elimination needs. Perhaps you cared for a previous patient who was incontinent. Perhaps you or a close friend has had the experience of an indwelling catheter or a UTI and experienced frequency, burning, urgency, and frequency. As you care for patients, you will find that self-care abilities related to urinary elimination differ based on age and functional and cognitive ability. As you care for patients, reflect on your previous experiences involving individuals with alterations in elimination patterns.

ATTITUDES Critical thinking attitudes allow you to design an approach to care that is relevant and meaningful for patients. Be curious about your patients so you can learn more about them and provide individualized care. Being creative is important when working with individuals with different types of urinary diversions to meet their unique elimination needs. Similarly, you will need perseverance to assist patients in finding solutions to urinary problems such as incontinence and retention.

STANDARDS Because urination is a private matter, follow the standard of protecting the patient's privacy. In addition, it is important that you adhere to the standards of care for asepsis. Some of the interventions you implement to promote urinary elimination will be invasive. Follow the standards of asepsis to reduce the risk for infection (see Chapter 13). When patients are in an acute care or long-term care setting, sterile insertion technique is required when catheterizing a patient because of the high risk for HAIs (Newman, 2004). When assessing a patient's urinary symptoms, apply intellectual standards and make sure your findings are specific, clear, precise, and accurate so an appropriate nursing diagnosis can be identified. Advocating for your patient is a component of the standard of professional responsibility. You are in a key position to serve as a patient advocate by suggesting noninvasive alternatives to catheterization use. For example, you may decrease the risk for a UTI by suggesting the use of a bladder scanner to evaluate bladder urine volume without invasive instrumentation or implement a toileting schedule for the incontinent patient.

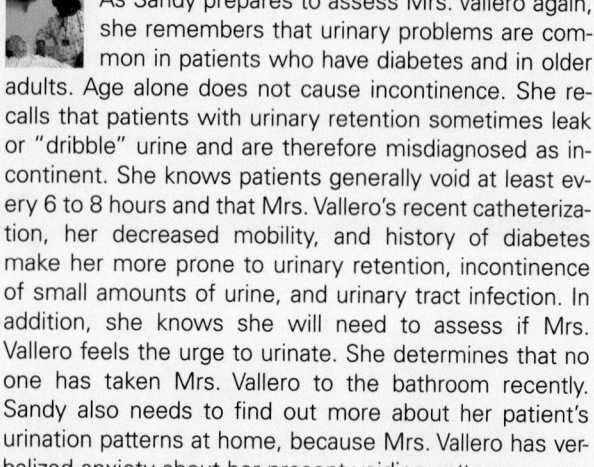

BOX 33-3	SYNTHESIS IN PRACTICE

As Sandy prepares to assess Mrs. Vallero again, she remembers that urinary problems are common in patients who have diabetes and in older adults. Age alone does not cause incontinence. She recalls that patients with urinary retention sometimes leak or "dribble" urine and are therefore misdiagnosed as incontinent. She knows patients generally void at least every 6 to 8 hours and that Mrs. Vallero's recent catheterization, her decreased mobility, and history of diabetes make her more prone to urinary retention, incontinence of small amounts of urine, and urinary tract infection. In addition, she knows she will need to assess if Mrs. Vallero feels the urge to urinate. She determines that no one has taken Mrs. Vallero to the bathroom recently. Sandy also needs to find out more about her patient's urination patterns at home, because Mrs. Vallero has verbalized anxiety about her present voiding patterns.

Previous clinical experience has taught Sandy that palpation of the abdomen over a distended bladder causes some discomfort and the patient often experiences an urge to urinate. Mrs. Vallero grimaces slightly when her abdomen is palpated and says she has a little *dolor* (pain).

Because the heart failure and bed rest have left Mrs. Vallero in a weakened state, Sandy is flexible and creative in designing a plan of care to meet the patient's elimination needs. The plan incorporates scheduled voiding, oral fluids, increased physical activity, and giving Mrs. Vallero as much assistance as needed. She understands the need to establish a relationship with the patient that allows discussion and intervention. Sandy realizes she has an ethical responsibility to provide culturally sensitive care and teaching for Mrs. Vallero.

NURSING PROCESS

■■■ASSESSMENT

You need to complete a nursing history, perform a physical assessment, assess the patient's urine, and review information from laboratory and diagnostic tests to identify a urinary elimination problem.

NURSING HISTORY Information from the scientific and nursing knowledge bases assists you in completing a nursing history. The nursing history includes a review of the patient's elimination patterns, symptoms of urinary alterations, and assessment of factors that are affecting the ability to urinate normally.

Pattern of Urination Ask the patient about daily voiding patterns, including frequency and times of day, normal volume at each voiding, and history of recent changes. Frequency varies among individuals. Most people void an average of 5 or more times a day. The patient who voids frequently during the night often has renal or cardiovascular disease or cystitis. Information about the pattern of urination is necessary to establish a baseline for comparison.

Symptoms of Urinary Alterations Certain symptoms of alterations occur in more than one type of urinary disorder. During assessment ask the patient about the presence of symptoms listed in Table 33-3. Also determine whether the patient is aware of conditions or factors that precipitate or aggravate the symptoms.

Factors Affecting Urination Focused assessment enables you to gather data relevant to your patient's elimination pattern (Table 33-4). In addition, there are important factors in the patient's history that normally affect urination. These factors include the following:

1. *Medication usage:* Ask the patient to identify any prescription, over-the-counter, and herbal supplements in use because they sometimes affect fluid and electrolyte balance. Diuretics are used to regulate fluid balance; however, side effects can include fluid and electrolyte imbalances. Opioid analgesics cause urinary retention. Some anesthetics temporarily depress renal or bladder function.

2. *Mobility status:* Assess patients' use of walking aids, the ability to remove clothing, or the ability to get in and out of the bathroom or on and off the toilet.

3. *Environmental barriers:* Assess both home and health care setting for barriers that prevent the patient from accessing the toilet. Some patients need an elevated toilet seat, grab bars, or a portable commode. Also consider the lack of lighting and distance to the toilet (Lekan-Rutledge and Colling, 2003).

4. *Sensory restrictions:* Assess for those sensory changes that obstruct self-toileting (e.g., patients with visual problems who have trouble reaching toilet facilities safely). If the patient has difficulty with hand coordination, assess the type of clothing and the patient's ease in using clothing fasteners.

5. *Past illness:* Assess for history of UTI or bladder surgery that may increase the risk for recurrent problems. Chronic diseases (e.g., multiple sclerosis) that impair bladder function require you to consider preventive care measures. Patients returning from surgery often have difficulty voiding the first few hours until the effects of anesthesia diminish.

6. *Major surgery:* Patients recovering from major surgery and suffering critical illness or disability often have an indwelling catheter to aid urinary drainage and provide a measurement of urinary output. A catheter places a patient at risk for infection.

7. *Urinary diversion:* If the patient has a urinary diversion, assess its type, location, and function. Also assess the condition of surrounding skin and usual methods for management (presence of appliance or pouch, type of skin care products and application). If the patient has an incontinent diversion, assess the methods and frequency of appliance changes and the type of nighttime drainage system. In addition, in the patient with a continent urinary diversion determine the frequency and type of catheters used to drain urine.

8. *Personal habits:* Some personal habits may inhibit urination or put the patient at risk for infection (i.e., poor hand or perineal hygiene). If a patient is hospitalized, assess how this alters his or her personal habits. Privacy is often difficult to accomplish in a health care setting, particularly if a patient uses a bedpan (see Chapter 34) or a urinal. Determine the patient's knowledge and practices of perineal hygiene.

9. *Fluid intake:* A patient's physical condition affects the frequency with which you monitor fluid intake (see Chapter 17). Regular intake and output (I&O) measurements help to assess a patient's overall fluid balance. Patients who have UTIs with urgency, burning, and frequency often mistakenly decrease their fluid intake to try to fix the symptoms.

10. *Age:* Toilet training and enuresis are concerns that arise in the toddler and preschooler. In the adult, increasing age sometimes brings disease and physiological changes that predispose to incontinence.

PATIENT EXPECTATIONS Note the patient's responses to questions about urination. Does the patient seem hesitant or embarrassed? Psychosocial factors such as culture or sexuality sometimes influence the patient's response. In addition, ask the patient what he or she expects from care. Does the patient expect the infection to be resolved? Does the woman who has stress incontinence expect this condition to be relieved?

Because urination is often considered a private matter, some patients find it difficult to talk about their voiding habits. Postoperative patients or patients taking medications that affect urination become concerned that something is wrong when you ask them every couple of hours if they have voided. Also, patients receiving intravenous (IV) fluids do not always realize that they have an increased need for urination. Urinary catheters indicate to some that the patient is very ill; they do not know that urinary catheters are used for diagnosis and monitoring for a variety of patients.

PHYSICAL ASSESSMENT When conducting a physical assessment, particularly when you suspect a patient has a urinary alteration, consider how you would assess for typical signs and symptoms. For example, patients with UTIs often have an irritated bladder, so you would want to palpate the bladder for discomfort. Patients with retention cannot empty their bladder, so you would palpate to determine bladder emptying. If an infection spreads to the kidneys (pyelonephritis), the patient will have fever, flank pain and tenderness.

TABLE 33-3 Common Symptoms of Urinary Alterations

DESCRIPTION	CAUSES OR ASSOCIATED FACTORS
URGENCY Feeling of the need to void immediately	Full bladder Inflammation or irritation to bladder mucosa from infection Incompetent urethral sphincter Psychological stress
DYSURIA Painful or difficult urination	Bladder inflammation Trauma or inflammation of urethra
FREQUENCY Voiding at frequent intervals	Increased fluid intake, intake of caffeine or alcohol Bladder inflammation Increased pressure on bladder (e.g., pregnancy, psychological stress)
HESITANCY Difficulty in initiating urination	Prostate enlargement Anxiety Urethral edema
POLYURIA Voiding large amount of urine	Excess fluid intake Diabetes mellitus or insipidus Use of diuretics
OLIGURIA Diminished urinary output in relation to fluid intake	Dehydration Renal failure Urinary tract obstruction Increased secretion of antidiuretic hormone (ADH)
NOCTURIA Urination, particularly excessive, at night	Excess intake of fluids (especially coffee or alcohol before bedtime) Renal disease Cardiovascular disease
DRIBBLING Leakage of urine despite voluntary control of micturition	Urine retention from incomplete bladder emptying Stress incontinence
HEMATURIA Presence of blood in urine	Neoplasms of kidney, certain glomerular diseases, infections of kidneys or bladder, traumatic injury to urinary structure, calculi, blood dyscrasia
RETENTION Accumulation of urine in bladder, with inability of bladder to empty	Urethral obstruction, bladder inflammation, decreases in sensory activity, neurogenic bladder, prostate enlargement after anesthesia, side effects of certain medications (e.g., anticholinergics, antispasmodics, antidepressants)
RESIDUAL URINE Volume of urine remaining in bladder after voiding (volumes of 100 mL or more)	Inflammation or irritation of bladder mucosa from infection, neurogenic bladder, prostatic enlargement, trauma, or inflammation of urethra

TABLE 33-4   FOCUSED PATIENT ASSESSMENT

FACTORS TO ASSESS	QUESTIONS	PHYSICAL ASSESSMENT
Fluid intake	Do you have any fluid restrictions? Are you able to obtain fluids by yourself? What is your usual 24-hour oral intake?	Observe skin and mucous membranes. Obtain intake and output over 24 hours. Observe patient's ability to reach toilet facilities.

Urinary elimination	In ambulatory patients:
	    Are you able to easily use toileting facilities?
	For patients with restricted mobility:
	    Do you need help in getting to the toileting facility?
	    How often do you need this help?
	    What type of assistance do you use at home?
		Observe if assistance needed with transfer and ambulation to and from the toilet area.

Bladder function	When did you last urinate? Do you have any difficulty feeling the urge to void? Do you feel like you have completely emptied your bladder after you have urinated?	Palpate bladder.

In this situation, you would conduct an abdominal assessment. Older adult with UTIs will often have an accompanying fever and exhibit alterations in mental status such as acute confusion, requiring a neurological assessment (Lewis and others, 2007). Here are additional assessment tips.

Skin and Mucosa Assess the skin's hydration status by noting texture and turgor. Observe the skin around periurethral tissues and stomas for excoriation, drainage, and tenderness. Urinary incontinence, fluid imbalance, and electrolyte disturbances increase the risk for skin breakdown. Observation of the oral mucosa also reveals whether hydration is adequate.

Kidneys If the kidneys become infected or inflamed, flank pain typically develops. You assess for tenderness early in the disease by gently percussing the costovertebral angle (the angle formed by the spine and twelfth rib). Inflammation of the kidney results in pain on percussion.

Bladder Normally the bladder rests below the symphysis pubis, and you are unable to palpate it. When distended, the bladder rises above the symphysis pubis at the midline of the abdomen and just below the umbilicus. Then, when you apply light pressure to the bladder, the patient feels tenderness or even pain. Palpation also causes the urge to urinate.

Urethral Meatus The female patient assumes a dorsal recumbent position to provide full exposure of the genitalia. Using the gloved nondominant hand, retract the labial folds to observe the urethral meatus. Look for drainage and lesions, and ask the patient if there is discomfort. There is normally no discharge from the meatus. Drainage indicates infection. Be sure you note the color and consistency of drainage.

The male's urethral meatus is normally a small opening at the tip of the penis. To inspect the meatus for discharge, lesions, and inflammation, it is necessary for you to retract the foreskin in uncircumcised males. Following inspection of the meatus, return foreskin over the meatus.

The assessment of urine involves measuring the patient's fluid intake and urinary output and observing the characteristics of the urine.

Intake and Output. When patients have altered or impaired urinary elimination, you measure I&O to monitor their fluid and electrolyte balance. Although often written as part of a health care provider's order, placing a patient on I&O is often a nursing judgment. Obtaining an accurate I&O measurement requires cooperation and assistance from the patient and family. Intake measurements need to include all oral liquids and semi-liquids (including those given with oral medications); all enteral feedings through nasogastric, gastrostomy, or jejunostomy tubes; and all parenteral fluids such as intravenous solutions, blood components, and parenteral nutrition (see Chapter 17).

You are responsible for accurate recording. Measurements are kept throughout the day and totaled every 8 hours, but sometimes you will decide that you need more frequent measurements. Recording I&O when the patient has voided or eaten is often a task that you delegate. Before delegating this task, inform the care provider what the metric conversions are for common liquid-holding containers such as a coffee cup or milk carton, and ensure that the care provider knows aseptic principles relating to body fluids. In addition, caution the care provider to be sensitive to the privacy needs of the patients, and clarify what he or she needs to report to you about I&O, such as changes in color, amount, or odor of urine or presence and frequency of incontinence. If the patient needs assistance, inform the care provider about the amount of assistance the patient requires. Also inform the care provider if the patient needs to use a urinal or bedpan or if the patient has bathroom privileges.

Urinary output is a key indicator of kidney function. A change in urine volume is a significant indicator of fluid imbalance, kidney dysfunction, or decreased blood volume. For example, hourly urinary output in a patient who is catheterized postoperatively, hourly urinary output provides an indirect measure of circulating blood volume. If the urinary output falls below 30 mL/hr, notify the health care provider immediately and assess for other signs of blood loss.

Assess urine volume by measuring with a **graduated measuring container** (receptacle for volume measurement) the output collected in a bedpan, urinal, **urine hat** (a receptacle that fits inside the commode) (Figure 33-4), or catheter bag. It is critical that each patient have an individual measuring container with name and room number marked on it and that you use only one container for each patient. Transmission of microorganisms occurs when you use equipment that belongs to other patients. If you need a precise measurement of fluid intake from a patient who is at home, show the patient or family caregiver the type of commonly used glass or cup on which to base measurement of intake.

Special **urometers** attach to catheter drainage tubing and are a convenient means of measuring small urine volume on a regular basis (Figure 33-5). A urometer holds 100 to 200 mL

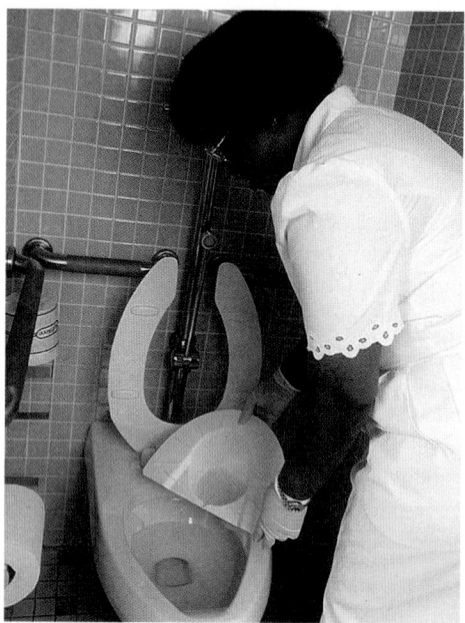

Figure 33-4 ■ Urine hat.

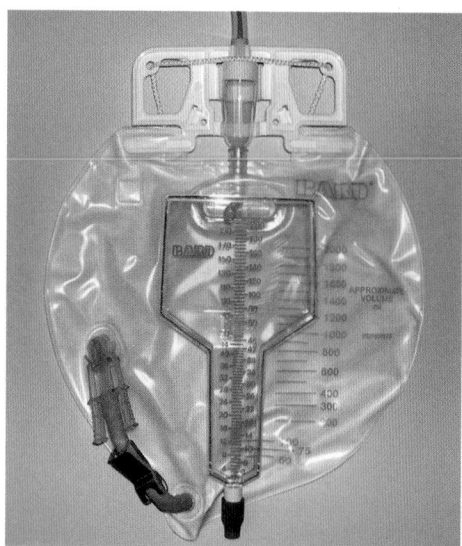

Figure 33-5 ■ Urometer. (Courtesy Michael Gallager, RN, BSN, MSN, OSF Saint Francis Medical Center, Peoria, Ill.)

of urine. After measuring urine from the urometer, drain the cylinder into the urinary drainage bag or into a receptacle for disposal.

Characteristics. Inspect the patient's urine for color, clarity, and odor. Monitor and document any changes. You monitor and record unusual characteristics, such as sediment in the urine, for improvement.

Color. Normal urine ranges in color from a pale straw color to amber, depending on its concentration. Urine is usually more concentrated in the morning. As the person drinks more fluids, it becomes less concentrated.

Unexpected changes such as the appearance of blood in the urine (**hematuria**) alert you to assess for associated signs and symptoms and report the information to the health care provider. Bleeding from the kidneys or ureters usually causes urine to become dark red; bleeding from the bladder or urethra usually causes bright red urine.

Drugs also change the urine's color. For example, patients taking metronidazole or docusate sodium will pass urine that is reddish brown in color. Beets, rhubarb, and blackberries cause red urine. The kidneys excrete special dyes used in intravenous diagnostic studies, and this discolors the urine. Dark amber urine is the result of high concentrations of bilirubin (urobilinogen) in patients with liver disease. Report unexpected color changes to the health care provider.

Clarity. Normal urine appears transparent at the time of voiding. Urine that stands several minutes in a container becomes cloudy. In patients with renal disease, freshly voided urine appears cloudy because of protein concentration. Urine also appears thick and cloudy as a result of bacteria.

Odor. Urine has a characteristic ammonia odor. The more concentrated the urine, the stronger the odor. As urine remains standing (e.g., in a collection device), more ammonia breakdown occurs, and the odor becomes stronger.

LABORATORY AND DIAGNOSTIC TESTING You are responsible for collecting urine specimens for laboratory testing. The type of test determines the method of collection. Label all specimens with the patient's name, date, time, and type of collection. Table 33-5 lists routine urinary analysis values and specific nursing interpretations for each type of measurement.

Specimen Collection You will sometimes collect several types of urine specimens for testing. Always collect specimens in appropriate containers, at the correct time, and in the correct manner. Also, label all specimens properly with the patient's identification, and complete the laboratory requisition with the necessary information. Urine specimens need to reach the laboratory within 1 hour of collection or be refrigerated. Urine that stands in a container at room temperature will grow bacteria.

Urinalysis Sample. A simple urinalysis does not require a sterile urine specimen or sample. The laboratory performs urinalysis on a routine or clean-voided specimen or on a specimen obtained from a catheter. The urinalysis is a screening test for renal disease, metabolic disorders, lower urinary tract alterations, and fluid imbalances (see Table 33-5). For a quick screening, you perform certain portions of the urinalysis with special reagent strips. Dip the strip into the urine, and watch for a color change, which indicates the presence of protein, blood, sugar, ketones, and other solutes. You will also perform a specific gravity test in the clinic or hospital unit.

The patient voids into a clean urine cup, a urinal, or a bedpan. The patient needs to void before defecating so feces do not contaminate the specimen. If a woman is menstruating, make note of this on the specimen requisition in case red blood cells appear. Wear clean gloves and transfer the urine to the proper container, and send it to the laboratory. Do not allow a specimen to sit unrefrigerated.

Clean-Voided or Midstream Specimen. To obtain a specimen relatively free of the microorganisms growing in the lower urethra, you need to instruct the patient in the method for obtaining a clean-voided specimen. Anxiety, difficulty or inability to read, or language barriers will prevent the patient from fully comprehending the instructions independently. Give the patient a sterile urine cup and sterile disinfectant wipes. The cup and disinfectant wipes are often prepackaged together. The package usually contains instructions, but explain to the patient how to wash the perineum and how to collect the specimen. Instruct female patients to use the disinfectant wipes to clean from the meatus toward the rectum, using a separate clean wipe or clean section of a wipe for each cleansing swipe. Instruct men to clean the meatus in a circular motion moving from the center of the meatus to the outside. Caution patients against wiping repeatedly with the contaminated wipe. After cleansing have the patient open the sterile urine cup. Tell your patient to start and discard the initial stream into a toilet or bedpan. This cleans or flushes the urethral orifice and meatus of resident bacteria. During the midstream, or middle portion of voiding, have the patient place the cup in the urine stream to collect the specimen. Immediately after obtaining the specimen, place a sterile top securely over the labeled container and send it to the laboratory for testing.

Sterile Specimen. Another method for collecting a sterile urine specimen for culture is by catheterizing a patient or by obtaining the specimen from an existing indwelling catheter. During straight catheterization collect the specimen as soon as urine flows from the catheter's end. After filling the sample container, you withdraw the straight catheter (Skill 33-1). Do not collect urine specimens for culture from urine drainage bags unless the specimen is the first urine drained into a new sterile bag. Bacteria grow rapidly in drainage bags, giving the specimen a false measurement of bacteria.

If a patient already has an indwelling catheter, use a sterile syringe to withdraw urine. Most urine drainage tubes have special ports referred to as sampling ports to withdraw specimens. Some companies have catheters with a sampling port that accepts most plastic or blunt cannulas (needleless) to reduce the risk for needle stick. Read the manufacturer's instructions to determine if the catheter tubing in use accepts blunt cannulas.

First, clamp the tubing about 3 inches below the sampling port, allowing fresh sterile urine to collect in the tube (10 to 15 minutes). Then wipe the port with a disinfectant swab. Using the agency-recommended procedure, withdraw 3 mL for a culture. While aspirating urine, be careful not to raise the tubing, which causes urine to return (backflow) to the bladder.

After obtaining the specimen, transfer the urine into a sterile container using sterile aseptic technique, label the specimen, and place it in a plastic pouch or bag per agency

TABLE 33-5 Routine Urinalysis Values

MEASUREMENT (NORMAL VALUE)	INTERPRETATION
pH (4.6 to 8.0)	pH level indicates acid-base balance. Urine that stands for several hours becomes alkaline from bacterial growth.
Protein (up to 8 mg/100 mL)	Protein is normally not present in urine. It is seen in renal disease because damage to glomerular membrane allows protein to enter urine. However, temporary presence of protein occurs after strenuous exercise, exposure to cold or psychological stress.
Glucose (not normally present)	Patients with diabetes have glucose in urine because of inability of tubules to reabsorb high serum glucose concentrations (over 180 mg/100 mL). Ingestion of high concentrations of glucose causes some to appear in urine of healthy persons.
Ketones (not normally present)	With poor control of diabetes, patients experience breakdown of fatty acids. End product of fatty acid metabolism is ketones. Patients with dehydration, starvation, or excessive aspirin ingestion also have ketonuria.
Blood (up to two red blood cells)	Damage to glomerulus or tubules causes blood cells to enter urine. Trauma or disease of lower urinary tract also causes hematuria.
Specific gravity (1.01 to 1.03)	Specific gravity tests measure concentration of particles in urine. High specific gravity reflects concentrated urine, and low specific gravity reflects diluted urine. Dehydration, reduced renal blood flow, and increase in ADH secretion elevate specific gravity. Overhydration and inadequate ADH secretion reduce it.

ADH, Antidiuretic hormone.

policy for transportation to the laboratory. The laboratory requisition will indicate the way you collected the specimen. Inspect the site from which you obtained the specimen periodically to check that the catheter is not leaking.

Twenty-Four–Hour Urine Specimen. Some tests of renal function and urine composition require a 24-hour collection of urine. You indicate the starting time on the gallon container and on the laboratory requisition. **Always discard the first sample at the beginning of the collection period.** The 24-hour collection period begins after you throw away the first specimen. The patient then collects all urine voided in 24 hours. Any missed specimens make the results inaccurate and require you to restart the test. Remind the patient to void before defecating, so feces do not contaminate urine. If there is fecal contamination, consult the laboratory for instructions. Have the patient void the last specimen as close as possible to the end of the 24-hour period.

Common Urine Tests. In addition to urinalysis, other tests that you will perform are measurement of specific gravity, urine culture, and glucose and ketone levels. Your role in collecting specimens is that of teaching. Explain the purpose of all tests; identify what preparation (if any) the patient needs before the test, what you expect of the patient during the test, and any posttest care.

Urine Culture. A urine culture simply requires a sterile sample of urine. It takes approximately 72 hours before the laboratory is able to report significant findings of bacterial growth. If bacteria are present, an additional test for sensitivity determines the antibiotics that will be effective or ineffective.

Diagnostic Examinations The urinary system is one of the few organ systems accessible to accurate diagnostic study by radiographic techniques. The two approaches for visualizing urinary structures, namely direct and indirect techniques, are either quite simple or very complex, requiring extensive nursing interventions. These procedures are further subdivided into invasive and noninvasive categories.

Noninvasive Procedures

Abdominal Roentgenogram. An abdominal roentgenogram, also called a plain film, KUB (kidneys, ureter, bladder), or flat plate of the abdomen, assesses the gross structures of the urinary tract for abnormalities. Health care providers use the x-ray examination to determine the size, shape, and location of the kidneys, ureters, and bladder structures. It is also useful in visualizing calculi (stones) or tumors in these organs.

Intravenous Pyelogram. The health care provider performs an excretory urogram or intravenous pyelogram (IVP) to view the entire urinary system and to assess some renal functions. Although these procedures are noninvasive, the IVP does require that the patient receive an IV injection of a radiopaque dye. Because the kidneys and ureters lie behind the intestines, it is necessary that the patient receive a bowel preparation before the procedure.

Nursing implications before the test include recognizing patients at risk for complications caused by the contrast material. The contrast material is toxic to the kidney tissue if the patient is dehydrated. Any patient with preexisting renal insufficiency is at risk. Older adults in particular are

prone to problems because of their risk for volume depletion during bowel preparation. It is important to appropriately assess fluid volume status before this procedure (see Chapter 17).

Additional nursing implications before the test are as follows:

1. Obtain a signed consent (if agency policy)
2. Assess the patient for allergy: IV contrast materials; shellfish or iodine allergy, which sometimes predicts allergies to the IVP dye.
3. If ordered, have the patient complete bowel preparation the evening before the test.
4. If ordered, explain that the patient is allowed nothing by mouth (NPO) after midnight.
5. Explain that you will start an IV infusion for dye injection before the test.
6. Explain that facial flushing is normal during dye injection and that the patient may feel dizzy, warm, or nauseous.
7. Explain that the test involves x-ray studies taken at several intervals and that the patient will void near the end of the test.

Nursing implications after the test are as follows:

1. Ensure that the patient resumes a normal diet.
2. Encourage fluid intake to minimize dehydration caused by fasting and to avoid the potential nephrotoxic effects of the contrast material.
3. Remind the patient to report itching, rash, or hives, which indicate delayed hypersensitivity to IVP dye.
4. Monitor I&O, or explain to the patient to report decreased or absent urination.

Computerized Axial Tomography. Computerized axial tomography visualizes abnormal pathological conditions such as tumors, obstructions, retroperitoneal masses, and lymph node enlargement. The computer enhances the x-ray examination to show "slices" of the body part. Although this procedure is noninvasive, in some examinations oral and/or IV contrast material enhances the areas under study.

Invasive Procedures

Endoscopy. Endoscopy is the visualization of organs with the aid of a telescope or fiberoptic imaging. To view the interior of the bladder and urethra, the radiologist performs a cystoscopy. The cytoscope looks like a urinary catheter, although it is not as flexible. It is inserted through the urethra. The procedure is painful during instrument insertion. Unless the patient lies still, the bladder may be perforated. Cystoscopy is performed under general or local anesthesia with sedation. A patient's age and general health and the expected duration of the procedure affect the choice of anesthesia. Because the test requires insertion of a foreign object into a sterile cavity, the patient receives large amounts of fluids (intravenously or orally) before and during the procedure to maintain a continuous urine flow and to flush out bacteria. It is common to administer antibiotics intravenously. During the test, you collect some urine and tissue specimens.

Nursing implications before the test include the following:

1. Verify that the patient signed an informed consent form.
2. Perform a bowel preparation or enema or administer a cathartic on the evening before the test.
3. If local anesthetic will be used, encourage intake of oral fluids.
4. If general anesthetic will be used, ensure that the patient is NPO after midnight.
5. Because this procedure is considered a minor surgical procedure, you will need to complete a preoperative checklist in some cases (see Chapter 38).
6. Explain that insertion of the cystoscope is similar to insertion of a urethral catheter.
7. Explain the importance of lying still during the test, if local anesthesia is used.
8. Explain that an IV line will be started to give fluids during the test.
9. Administer a sedative or analgesic per the health care provider's orders.

Nursing implications after the test include the following:

1. Instruct the patient to remain in bed as ordered.
2. Assess for signs of urinary retention and first voiding.
3. Observe characteristics of urine, noting bloody or cloudy urine.
4. Encourage increased fluid intake, and monitor I&O.
5. Observe for fever, **dysuria,** or a change in blood pressure.
6. Administer medications to calm bladder spasms and/or lower back pain.

In addition to complete visual inspection of the bladder and urethra through the cystoscope, the radiologist sometimes performs a retrograde pyelography. During this procedure the radiologist passes a small catheter through the cystoscope into the bladder that allows catheterizing of the ureters and renal pelvis. Urine specimens are then collected separately from each ureter.

Invasive examinations to visualize the bladder and urethra include retrograde cystograms, voiding cystourethrogram, and cystourethrogram. All of these studies involve the instillation of a radiopaque fluid into the bladder via a catheter (urethral or suprapubic). Serial x-ray films taken during this procedure will provide information regarding abnormalities. Nursing implications for this procedure are the same as those for the cystoscopy procedure.

Urodynamic Testing. Urodynamic testing is the gold standard for assessing bladder function or dysfunction by reproducing the patient's urinary symptoms (McKertich, 2008). Urodynamic tests study the storage of urine within the bladder and the flow of urine through the urinary tract to the outside of the body. The patient does not need to fast before the procedure because the patient is not sedated during the testing. The patient lies on a tilt table to obtain x-ray (fluoroscopic urodynamics) or ultrasound images and assumes a

sitting position to help produce urinary symptoms. Specialized computerized equipment is required to perform urodynamic testing. Steps in the procedure include the following:

1. Having the patient urinate into a commode to measure urine flow and volume
2. Inserting urodynamic catheters into the bladder and rectum for pressure measurement
3. Inserting a urethral catheter and filling the bladder at a fixed rate while recording bladder pressures at the same time the patient reports symptoms
4. Having the patient cough and strain during the procedure at fixed bladder volumes to check for stress urinary incontinence

Explain the procedure to the patient. Depending on the type of study, the patient starts the test with a full bladder. Measure residual urine volume (amount of urine left in the bladder) immediately after a urine flow study to determine urinary retention (Lewis and others, 2007). Nursing care after the procedures includes teaching the patient the signs and symptoms of infection, including pain, chills, and fever. Stress to the patient the importance of reporting these signs and symptoms to the health care provider. It is normal for mild discomfort to occur for a few hours posttest when the patient urinates. Increasing fluids for a few hours posttest may help relieve the discomfort (Urodynamic Testing, 2008).

■■■NURSING DIAGNOSIS

Following assessment of the patient's urinary function, you identify defining characteristics that support actual or at-risk nursing diagnoses for urinary elimination problems. Identification of the defining characteristics leads you to select an appropriate NANDA International nursing diagnostic label. It is very helpful to read the definition of the diagnosis and to examine whether there is a match between the data you collected and the defining characteristics (see Chapter 8).

For example, there are five recognized diagnoses for incontinence, and it is not easy for a beginning student to select the correct one without looking for a match between data and defining characteristics. The differentiation between stress and urge incontinence is a common problem. In both, the patient has an involuntary loss of urine, but the accuracy of data collection helps to identify the correct diagnosis. If the patient loses urine after sneezing or coughing, then the diagnosis is stress incontinence. If the patient reports that there was a strong urge to urinate just before the incontinence occurred, then the diagnosis is urge incontinence. Other nursing diagnoses are appropriate when the urinary problem affects other patient functions. A selected list of possible nursing diagnoses includes the following:

- *Disturbed body image*
- *Functional urinary incontinence*
- *Reflex urinary incontinence*
- *Stress urinary incontinence*
- *Urge urinary incontinence*

- *Risk for infection*
- *Deficient knowledge*
- *Toileting self-care deficit*
- *Impaired skin integrity*
- *Impaired urinary elimination*
- *Urinary retention*

Associated problems require interventions that often have no direct effect on urinary elimination. For example, when the patient has the diagnosis *toileting self-care deficit related to limited lower extremity mobility,* appropriate nursing interventions provide the patient a means of easy access to toileting facilities. When forming a nursing diagnosis, select ap-propriate related factors to ensure that you select the relevant interventions. If you identify the related factor in the example as a loss of voluntary control of micturition, you would select interventions to prevent incontinence. It is important to identify the correct related factors for a given nursing diagnosis; otherwise, your nursing interventions will be ineffective.

■■■**PLANNING**

GOALS AND OUTCOMES Patients often have more than one nursing diagnosis (Figure 33-6). Evaluate the relationships between these diagnoses and establish patient-centered goals and outcomes in collaboration with the patient and family. For example, a realistic patient goal is that the patient has normal

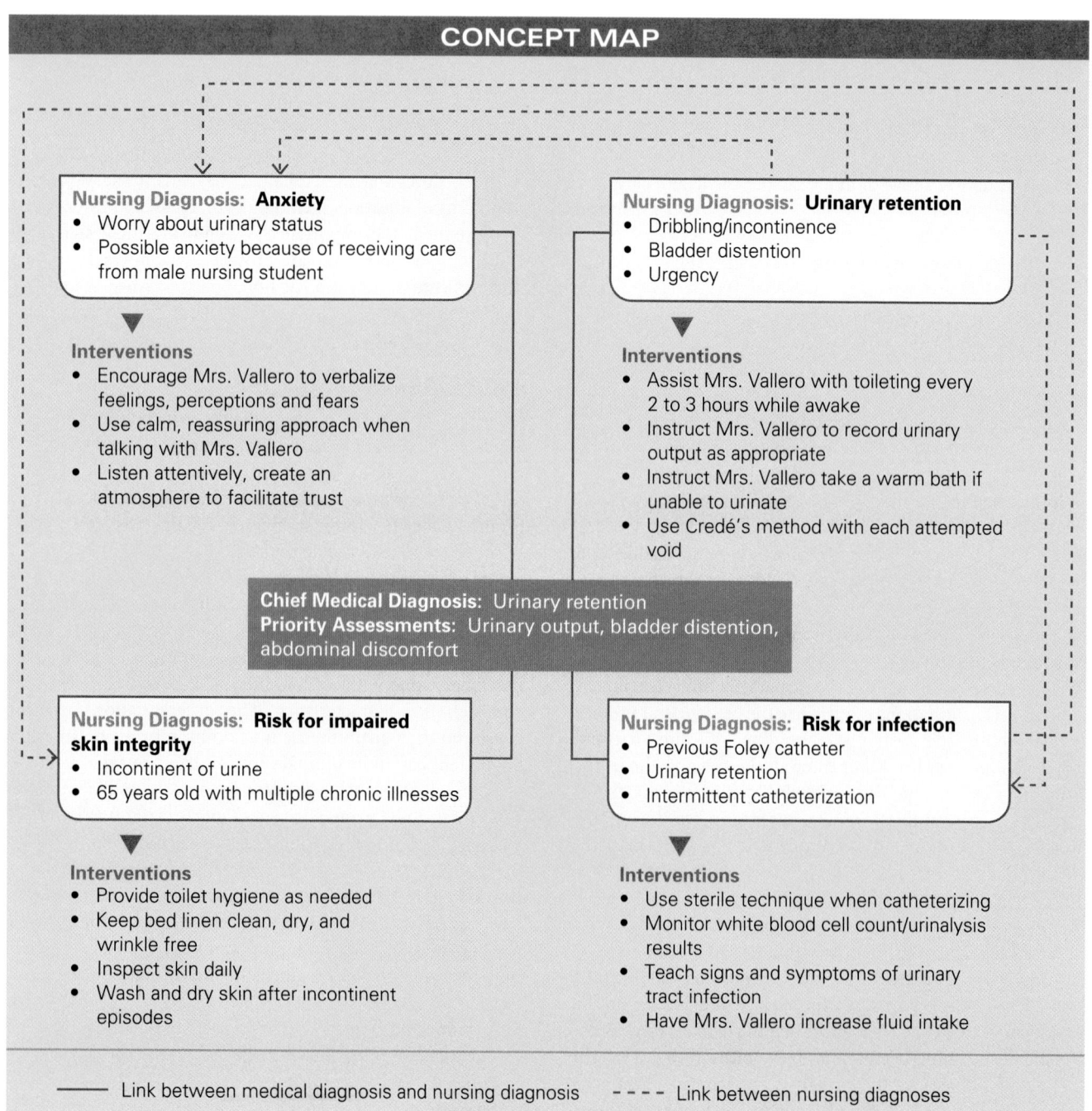

CONCEPT MAP

Nursing Diagnosis: Anxiety
- Worry about urinary status
- Possible anxiety because of receiving care from male nursing student

Interventions
- Encourage Mrs. Vallero to verbalize feelings, perceptions and fears
- Use calm, reassuring approach when talking with Mrs. Vallero
- Listen attentively, create an atmosphere to facilitate trust

Nursing Diagnosis: Urinary retention
- Dribbling/incontinence
- Bladder distention
- Urgency

Interventions
- Assist Mrs. Vallero with toileting every 2 to 3 hours while awake
- Instruct Mrs. Vallero to record urinary output as appropriate
- Instruct Mrs. Vallero take a warm bath if unable to urinate
- Use Credé's method with each attempted void

Chief Medical Diagnosis: Urinary retention
Priority Assessments: Urinary output, bladder distention, abdominal discomfort

Nursing Diagnosis: Risk for impaired skin integrity
- Incontinent of urine
- 65 years old with multiple chronic illnesses

Interventions
- Provide toilet hygiene as needed
- Keep bed linen clean, dry, and wrinkle free
- Inspect skin daily
- Wash and dry skin after incontinent episodes

Nursing Diagnosis: Risk for infection
- Previous Foley catheter
- Urinary retention
- Intermittent catheterization

Interventions
- Use sterile technique when catheterizing
- Monitor white blood cell count/urinalysis results
- Teach signs and symptoms of urinary tract infection
- Have Mrs. Vallero increase fluid intake

—— Link between medical diagnosis and nursing diagnosis   - - - - Link between nursing diagnoses

Figure 33-6 ■ Concept Map.

micturition with complete bladder emptying within 1 month. To achieve this goal you identify a number of outcomes; for example, the patient will ingest at least 2000 mL of fluids per day, empty the bladder within 2 hours of drinking, and have less than 50 mL of residual urine. Problems develop when you make goals and outcomes without adequate assessment and collaboration with the patient.

You and the patient work together to maintain patient involvement in care and to maintain normal elimination patterns when possible (see Care Plan). If you reinforce good health habits that the patient already follows, the patient will be more likely to comply with the plan of care. Determine the patient's educational needs. Return demonstrations of psychomotor and self-care skills by the patient will verify learning of procedures and accuracy in their performance.

SETTING PRIORITIES It is important to establish priorities of care based on the patient's immediate physical and safety needs, patient expectations, and readiness to perform some self-care activities. For example, a patient with a long-term continent urinary diversion admitted with a severe

---

CARE PLAN Urinary Retention

 ASSESSMENT

Mrs. Vallero was unable to void 8 hours after catheter removal. She was straight catheterized, and 600 mL of urine was obtained. It is now 4 hours since the catheterization. She has been drinking fluids, including hot tea and water, to increase her chances of urinating on her own. She complains of a feeling of pressure over her lower abdomen.

ASSESSMENT ACTIVITIES

Palpate for bladder distention every 2 hours on the even hours.

Assess the patient's voiding pattern, including volume at each voiding, frequency, times of day, and history of any changes.

FINDINGS/DEFINING CHARACTERISTICS*

Able to palpate bladder, indicating **bladder distention.** During palpation, patient states she has the **sensation of bladder fullness.**

She complains of **dribbling frequently** and being **unable to urinate.**

NURSING DIAGNOSIS: Urinary retention related to weakened detrusor muscle and recent removal of indwelling urinary catheter.

PLANNING

GOAL

• Mrs. Vallero will have normal micturition within 1 month.

EXPECTED OUTCOMES (NOC)†

Urinary Elimination
• Mrs. Vallero will void greater than 150 mL each time.

Urinary Continence
• Mrs. Vallero will verbalize no episodes of dribbling or incontinence.

Symptom Severity
• Mrs. Vallero will verbalize relief of lower abdominal discomfort.

INTERVENTIONS (NIC)‡

Urinary Retention Care
• Assist with toileting every 2 to 3 hours while awake.

• Instruct the patient/family to record urinary output as appropriate.

• Have Mrs. Vallero take a warm bath if unable to urinate.
• Use Credé's method with each attempted void.

RATIONALE

Scheduled toileting is the primary behavioral intervention used for chronic retention and is used to reduce bladder capacity (Lewis and others, 2007).
Keeping a record of urinary output is important to confirm voiding in small amounts. Also, it is important to note amount urinated before obtaining residual urine (Newman and others, 2005).
Relaxing in a bath eases discomfort and induces micturition (Wareing, 2003).
Credé's method involves putting pressure on the suprapubic area and is used for the relief of urinary retention (Madineh, 2008).

---

*Defining characteristics** are shown in **bold** type.
†Outcomes classification label from Moorhead S and others, editors: *Nursing outcomes classification (NOC)*, ed 4, St. Louis, 2008, Mosby.
‡Intervention classification labels from Bulechek GM and others, editors: *Nursing interventions classifications (NIC)*, ed 5, St. Louis, 2008, Mosby.

CARE PLAN Urinary Retention—cont'd

EVALUATION

NURSING ACTIONS	PATIENT RESPONSE/FINDING	ACHIEVEMENT OF OUTCOME
Ask Mrs. Vallero about her urge to void, sensation of bladder fullness, and dribbling episodes.	Mrs. Vallero denies dribbling episodes, and she has a decreased urgency to urinate.	Dribbling episodes and sense of urgency relieved.
Have Mrs. Vallero keep a log of her pattern of elimination, including urine output volumes with each voiding, during the 1-month period.	Mrs. Vallero states she and her family have measured her urine, and most output is greater than150 mL.	Urinary output is greater than 150 mL with each void.
Ask Mrs. Vallero if she continues to have lower abdominal pain.	Mrs. Vallero denies lower abdominal pain at this time. States since she has urinated more at a time, she no longer has discomfort.	Lower abdominal discomfort is absent.

UTI expects to resume his or her self-care routine. However, due to the severity of the infection, you perform all care for the patient's urinary diversion with sterile technique. In this case the priorities are to treat the infection, prevent reinfection, and teach the patient how to perform sterile technique.

COLLABORATIVE CARE In the hospital, planning for care also includes preparations for discharge. Explore the patient's need for home care services, and make appropriate referrals. Planning includes consideration of the patient's home environment and normal elimination routines. Determine if there is a need to collaborate with other disciplines in this planning process (e.g., social services) to explore family financial resources or other influences that may affect the discharge process. Use community resources as well, such as ostomy support groups for patients with incontinent urinary diversions (urostomy or ileal conduit) and continent urinary diversions.

Family and significant others are also included in discharge planning and in teaching sessions. Identify who will be involved with the care of the patient at home. Your active and thoughtful role in planning these interventions will result in the patient's progress toward improved urinary elimination.

■■■IMPLEMENTATION

Your care of patients with elimination alterations will focus on three general areas: health promotion, acute care, and restorative and continuing care. The specific interventions include patient education, promoting normal micturition and complete bladder emptying, prevention of infection, and promotion of skin integrity and comfort.

HEALTH PROMOTION Success of therapies aimed at optimizing normal urinary elimination depends in part on successful patient education (Box 33-4). Instruct patients in their specific elimination problems. For example, a patient who practices poor hygiene will benefit from learning about normal sterility of the urinary tract and ways to prevent bacterial invasion of the urinary tract. It is also useful to discuss the

basic mechanism for urine production and voiding for patients with elimination alterations. Knowledge of factors that affect urine production and voiding will also help. Health promotion skills are always the initial focal point of teaching.

Incorporate teaching during delivery of care (Box 33-5). For example, if you are attempting to increase the patient's fluid intake, a good time to discuss benefits is while giving fluids with medications or meals. You will possibly be more successful in teaching about perineal hygiene during a bath or while giving catheter care. When possible, include family members in these discussions.

Normal Micturition

Stimulating the Micturition Reflex. The patient's ability to void depends on feeling the urge to urinate, on being able to control the urethral sphincter, and on being able to relax. You promote relaxation and stimulate the reflex to void by helping patients to assume the normal position for voiding.

Females are better able to void in a squatting position. If the patient cannot use a toilet, position her on a bedpan or bedside commode (see Chapter 34).

The male patient voids more easily in the standing position. At times it is necessary for one or more nurses to assist a male patient in standing. If the patient is unable to reach a toilet, have him stand at the bedside and void into a urinal (a plastic or metal receptacle for urine) (Figure 33-7). Always assess the patient's mobility status and determine if he feels dizzy when standing before having him stand to void. If dizziness develops, have the patient sit back down until it subsides.

If the patient is unable to stand at the bedside, you will need to assist him in using the urinal in bed. When possible, the patient holds the urinal and positions the penis in the urinal. If the patient needs assistance, position the penis completely within the urinal and hold the urinal in place or assist the patient in holding the urinal. Make sure you place the penis completely within the urinal to avoid urine spills. Once the patient has finished voiding, remove the urinal and wash and dry the penis to prevent growth of microorganisms

BOX 33-4   Urinary Elimination Health Promotion/Restoration Activities

ADEQUATE HYDRATION
- A patient with normal renal function who does not have heart disease or alterations requiring fluid restriction should drink six to eight glasses of fluid daily (Huether and McCance, 2008).

MICTURITION HABITS
- Ensure patient comfort and privacy.
- Allow sufficient time to void (at least 15 minutes).
- Integrate the patient's habits into the care plan to foster a more normal voiding pattern.
- Offer the patient use of toilet facilities if possible, avoiding bedpans.
- Ensure access to toilet facilities.
- Assist the patient in the appropriate position for voiding if possible (i.e., females—sitting, males—standing).

PERSONAL HYGIENE
- Instruct female patients to cleanse the perineum and urethra from front to back after each voiding and bowel movement.
- Encourage patients prone to urinary tract infections to shower instead of tub bathing.

COMPLETE BLADDER EMPTYING
- Patients who have difficulty starting or stopping the urine stream benefit from exercises to strengthen pelvic muscles (Milne, 2004).

- Credé's method of manual bladder compression helps to stimulate urination and manually expels urine when bladder tone is reduced.
- Drug therapy alone or in conjunction with other therapies is useful for treating problems of incontinence and retention.

INFECTION PREVENTION
- Ensure adequate fluid intake of 2000 mL daily.
- Encourage good hand washing technique.
- Prevent breaks in closed catheter drainage systems.
- Follow tips for preventing infection in catheterized patients.
- Teach patient how to keep urine acidic. Acid urine tends to inhibit growth of microorganisms. Meats, eggs, whole-grain breads, cranberries, and prunes increase urine acidity.

SKIN INTEGRITY
- Cleanse the skin with warm soap and water following contact with urine because the normal acidity of urine is irritating to the skin.
- After performing hygiene, apply dry clothing immediately on incontinent patient.
- Patients with external urinary devices need to receive assistance in selecting appliances that fit appropriately. Also, teach them preventive skin care measures.

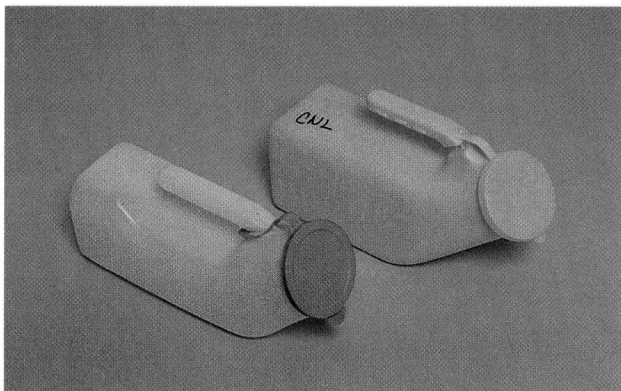

Figure 33-7 ■ Types of male urinals.

and prevent skin breakdown. For the female patient, remove the bedpan and wash and dry the perineum from pubis to the anus.

Other measures to promote normal micturition include the use of sensory stimuli (e.g., turning on running water, putting a patient's hand in a pan of warm water, or stroking the female patient's inner thigh). Each tends to promote relaxation and the reflex to void.

Maintaining Elimination Habits. Many patients follow their set routines of normal voiding. Unfortunately, in a hospital or long-term care facility, institutional routines often conflict with those of the patient. Integrating the patient's

habits into the care plan fosters a more normal voiding pattern.

Make sure you give the patient privacy, and do not rush him or her. Privacy is essential for normal voiding. If the patient is unable to reach the bathroom, make sure the bedside area is private for use of a bedpan or bedside commode. In the home, some debilitated patients may prefer using a bedside commode enclosed behind a partition or room divider. Some patients are embarrassed by the sound of voiding. Running water or flushing the toilet masks the sound effectively. Young children are often unable to void in the presence of persons other than parents.

Assess the times when a patient normally voids, and offer the opportunity to use a toilet at those times. Respond in a timely manner to the patient's urge to urinate. Delay in assisting the patient to the bathroom may interfere with normal micturition. Research has shown that promptly assisting patients to toileting facilities reduces incontinence when the patients are able to perceive the urge to void (Palmer and Newman, 2004). Older adults may also require other special interventions (Box 33-6).

Comfort is an important factor in facilitating voiding. Therefore activities that increase patient comfort will aid urination. If the patient typically uses special measures to void (e.g., reading or listening to music), encourage continued use at home and, when possible, in the health care setting. Use toilet seat extenders for patients with arthritis or

BOX 33-5   PATIENT TEACHING

Urinary Retention Care

 Mrs. Vallero is concerned about regaining her urinary function. Sandy develops the following teaching plan for her regarding her urinary retention.

OUTCOME
- At the end of the teaching session Mrs. Vallero will be able to describe approaches to promote normal urinary elimination habits.

TEACHING STRATEGIES
- Establish rapport with Mrs. Vallero.
- Find out what Mrs. Vallero already knows about good practices for urinary health.
- Use the correct terms for the anatomy that you will discuss, but explain them so Mrs. Vallero knows what they are.
- Provide appropriate visual diagrams and written materials for Mrs. Vallero.
- Instruct her in observations to make regarding urinary output.
- Instruct her in adequate fluid intake, incorporating her fluid preferences.
- Discuss how to do intake and output measurement at home.
- Reinforce correct perineal hygiene measures to reduce the risk for urinary tract infection.
- Provide Mrs. Vallero with pertinent signs and symptoms of infection to report to her health care provider.

EVALUATION STRATEGIES
- Use open-ended questions to determine level of learning.
- Ask Mrs. Vallero to verbalize her understanding of normal urinary function.
- Ask Mrs. Vallero to verbalize the abnormal signs and symptoms to report to her health care provider.
- Have Mrs. Vallero measure water in a container to simulate intake and output measures.

BOX 33-6   CARE OF THE OLDER ADULT

Urinary Elimination Problems

- The older patient sometimes experiences urinary elimination problems as a result of mobility problems or neurological impairments. Be aware of these problems, and arrange scheduled toileting and promote access to toileting facilities.
- Older patients are prone to physiological urinary retention as a result of diminished bladder muscle tone, capacity, and contractility. This increases their risk for large postvoid residuals with an associated risk for frequent infections. Teaching sessions include techniques to stimulate the voiding reflex and to provide for complete bladder emptying and prevention of infections (Wyman, 2003).
- Older patients also experience delayed sensations to void, resulting in urgency. Educate the patient regarding any factor that interferes with the patient's perceptions of sensation to void (e.g., medications, emotional disturbances, decreased fluid intake).
- Older adults experience physiological changes that make them more prone to incontinence. During teaching sessions, consider these normal physiological changes to plan appropriate interventions:
  - Decreased renal blood flow secondary to decreased cardiac output (make sure patient takes ordered medications that increase cardiac output, such as digoxin and diuretics)
  - Decreased ability to concentrate urine secondary to decrease in nephron mass (unless patient is fluid restricted, ensure adequate intake to prevent dehydration)
  - Decreased tone of the pelvic floor muscles (Huether and McCance, 2008) (encourage strengthening of pelvic floor muscles by teaching Kegel exercises)
- Older adults in institutionalized settings (e.g., hospitals, nursing homes) are at the greatest risk for experiencing incontinence problems because of sensory and physical mobility losses (Lekan-Rutledge and Colling, 2003).
- Older adults also experience sensory alterations, such as diminished vision, which delay attempts to locate toilet facilities. In care settings, orient patients to their environment with special emphasis on the location of toileting facilities, bedpans or urinals, and assistive devices (e.g., walkers, call light).

after a total hip replacement to aid the patient in sitting on and rising off the toilet.

Encourage and provide appropriate personal hygiene, including hand washing and perineal care (see Chapter 28) as needed. Health care–acquired genitourinary infections are second only to respiratory infections. Bacteria are the most common cause of these infections, and *E. coli* invasion through the urethra is the most frequent organism and route.

Maintaining Adequate Fluid Intake. A simple method of promoting normal micturition is maintenance of fluid intake. A patient with normal renal function who does not have heart disease or alterations requiring fluid restriction needs to drink six to eight glasses of fluid daily. When a person increases fluid intake, excreted urine flushes out solutes or particles that collect in the urinary system. Because a patient probably is not accustomed to drinking eight glasses of water

daily, offer fluids the patient prefers. At home it helps to set a schedule for drinking fluids (e.g., with meals or medications). A simple trick is to encourage the patient to drink a cup of water after voiding. Voiding becomes a natural cue to drinking fluids. The patient will not need a rigid schedule. To prevent nocturia, suggest that the patient avoid drinking fluids 2 hours before bedtime.

Promotion of Bladder Emptying Patients with urinary retention and incontinence are frequently unable to empty the bladder. Incontinence is a major nursing challenge.

TABLE 33-6 Treatment Options for Incontinence

TYPE	TREATMENTS TO ATTAIN CONTINENCE
Functional	Toileting programs/bladder training Environmental alterations
Stress	Conditioning (Kegel) exercises Alpha-adrenergic agonists Intravaginal electrical stimulation Bladder neck suspension surgery Artificial sphincter Penile clamp
Urge	Anticholinergic drug therapy Biofeedback Treatment of associated UTI Treatment of associated vaginitis or interstitial cystitis Diet modification to minimize bladder irritants
Reflex (upper motoneuron lesion)	Intermittent self-catheterization Bladder training Electrical stimulation Credé's method

UTI, Urinary tract infection.

Choosing from a variety of treatment options, you and the patient will work together to design interventions that promote continence (Table 33-6). The use of indwelling catheters is a last resort because infection is always a threat.

Strengthening Pelvic Floor Muscles. Patients who have difficulty starting and stopping the urine stream benefit from exercises to strengthen pelvic muscles (Sampselle, 2003). This technique is helpful for both men and women with urinary problems, such as stress incontinence. The patient is able to practice the Kegel exercises anytime and anywhere. No one will be aware that the patient is doing this exercise. Simple steps will show gradual improvement in urinary control. The patient follows these instructions:

1. Squeeze and hold the muscles around the vagina and/or anus for 10 seconds without tensing leg, buttock, or abdominal muscles. Then relax the muscles for 10 seconds. This maneuver allows the patient to identify the posterior muscles of the pelvic floor.
2. Do this exercise 15 times in the morning; 15 times in the afternoon, and 20 times at night. Work up to 25 times each time period. If done consistently, the patient will see improvement in urinary control (Wyman, 2003).

Manual Bladder Compression. By manually compressing the walls of the bladder, a person improves bladder emptying. Credé's method helps to stimulate micturition and manually expels urine when bladder tone is reduced. Instruct the patient to place both hands flat on the abdomen below the umbilicus and above the symphysis pubis with the fingers pointed down toward the bladder's dome. Have the patient compress the hands downward against the bladder's walls while tightening the perineum, contracting the abdominal wall, and holding the breath. When urine is in the bladder, Credé's method causes the sensation of bladder fullness. The maneuver also promotes bladder emptying by relaxing the urethral sphincter.

Drug Therapy. Drug therapy alone or along with other therapies is useful for treating problems of incontinence and retention. Drugs increase bladder emptying (e.g., retention), bladder capacity (e.g., urge incontinence), and sphincter tone (e.g., stress incontinence).

When the bladder empties, the detrusor muscle contracts in response to stimulation. Incomplete bladder emptying results from impaired innervation or weakness of the detrusor muscle. As a result, the patient experiences retention and overflow incontinence. Therapy with cholinergic drugs increases bladder contraction and improves emptying. Bethanechol (Urecholine) stimulates nerves to increase bladder wall contraction and relax the sphincter. You administer this drug subcutaneously or orally. Alpha-adrenergic agents such as phenoxybenzamine are also used to improve bladder emptying. Using Credé's method or other measures for stimulating micturition increases the effect of the drug.

If urine is in the bladder, urge incontinence sometimes occurs as a result of hyperactivity of the bladder muscle that suddenly increases pressure. Local irritants such as stones or infection cause uncontrolled bladder contractions. The elimination of caffeine, carbonated drinks, and alcohol is useful in reducing urge incontinence. Anticholinergic drugs (e.g., propantheline) reduce incontinence by blocking contractility of the bladder. Patients with heart disease, glaucoma, high blood pressure, kidney and liver disease, and urinary retention must use these drugs with caution. Direct smooth-muscle relaxants (e.g., oxybutynin) are also effective. These drugs work by decreasing the contractility of the bladder. Patient instructions are similar to those for propantheline (McKenry and others, 2005).

To treat stress incontinence, anticholinergic agents, antimuscarinic drugs, imipramine (a tricyclic antidepressant), and alpha-adrenergic drugs are often used (McKenry and others, 2005). Combining medications with pelvic strengthening exercises helps many women. Some have used estrogen therapy to decrease stress incontinence.

ACUTE CARE. Often patients need care in hospitals, clinics, or their homes for urinary conditions of sudden onset and/or severity that require the expertise of the health care team.

Catheterization Catheterization of the bladder involves introducing a rubber or plastic tube through the urethra and into the bladder. The catheter provides a continuous flow of urine in patients unable to control micturition or in patients with obstructions. Because bladder catheterization carries a high risk for a UTI, first try other interventions to empty the bladder. Holroyd-Leduc and others (2008) reported evidence regarding factors most likely to contribute to infection from catheterization (Box 33-7).

Types of Catheterization. Intermittent and indwelling catheterizations are the two types of catheter insertion. With the intermittent technique, you introduce a straight single-use catheter (Figure 33-8) long enough to drain the bladder (5 to 10 minutes). When the bladder is empty, you remove the catheter immediately. You repeat intermittent catheterization as needed, but each insertion increases risk for trauma and infection. An indwelling or Foley catheter remains in place until a patient is able to void completely and voluntarily or continuous accurate measurements are no longer needed. It is sometimes necessary to change indwelling catheters periodically.

The single-use straight catheter has a single lumen with a small opening approximately 1.3 cm (1½ inch) from the tip. Urine drains from the tip, through the lumen, and to a receptacle. An indwelling Foley catheter has a small inflatable balloon that encircles the catheter just below the tip (see Figure 33-8). When inflated, the balloon rests against the bladder outlet to anchor the catheter in place. The indwelling catheter also has as many as two or three separate lumens within the body of the catheter. One lumen drains urine through the

catheter to a collecting tube. A second lumen carries sterile water to and from the balloon when it is inflated or deflated. A third (optional) lumen is used to instill fluids or drugs into the bladder. You insert a three-lumen catheter when you anticipate irrigations of the catheter. Usually you use three-way catheters with male patients who have had a transurethral resection of the prostate.

Indications for Use. Intermittent catheterization is preferred for short-term use or to minimize infection in patients who are chronically unable to void. Intermittent catheterization is indicated in the following situations:

1. For immediate relief of acute bladder distention
2. For long-term management of patients with incompetent bladders
3. To obtain a sterile urine specimen
4. To assess for residual urine after voiding
5. To instill a medication

Done correctly, intermittent catheterization has a lower risk for infection than indwelling catheterization. Indwelling catheterization is indicated in the following situations:

1. Obstruction to urine outflow
2. Patients undergoing surgical procedures involving the urinary tract or surrounding structures
3. To prevent urethral obstruction from blood clots
4. To accurately record output in critically ill or comatose patients
5. To provide continuous or intermittent bladder irrigations

Catheter Insertion. Urethral catheterization requires a health care provider's order. Insert the catheter using strict sterile technique. The steps for inserting an indwelling and a single-use straight catheter are the same. The difference lies in the procedure taken to inflate the indwelling catheter balloon and secure the catheter. You collect needed specimens while inserting either catheter. Skill 33-1 lists steps for performing female and male urethral catheterization.

Closed Drainage Systems. After you insert an indwelling catheter, it is necessary to maintain a closed urinary drainage system to minimize the risk for infection. Urinary drainage bags are plastic and hold approximately 2000 mL of urine.

BOX 33-7   BEST PRACTICES

Appropriate Use of Indwelling Catheterization

SUMMARY OF EVIDENCE
Holroyd-Leduc and others (2007) designed a research study to determine the association between indwelling urinary catheterization without a specific medical indication and adverse outcomes, specifically, longer hospital stay or greater risk for death. Specific medical indications are surgery, urinary retention, or need for accurate urine output measurement. The researchers found that older adult patients (greater than 70 years of age) with limited functional ability were often catheterized to facilitate their care. For example, patients are often catheterized to reduce the need for toileting and to reduce the need for changing incontinent patients rather than for medical indications.

APPLICATION TO NURSING PRACTICE
- Nonmedical use of indwelling catheters in older adults may result in longer hospital stays and greater risk for death secondary to development of urinary tract infection (UTI) and subsequent bacteremia (urosepsis).
- You need to understand the reason for the patients being catheterized.
- Collaborate with health care providers to remove catheters when medical indications no longer exist.
- Suggest noninvasive continent devices such as condom catheters to reduce risk for UTI and urosepsis.

REFERENCE
Holroyd-Leduc JM and others: The relationship of indwelling urinary catheters to death, length of hospital stay, functional decline, and nursing home admission in hospitalized older medical patients, *J Am Geriatr Soc* 55(2):227, 2008.

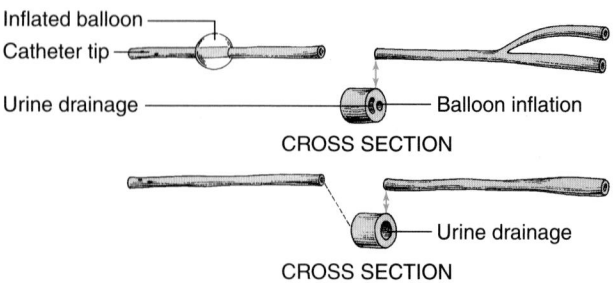

Figure 33-8 ■ Indwelling and straight urinary catheters.

The bag hangs on the lower bed frame without touching the floor. Some urinary drainage bags have special urometers between the collection tubing and bag. When the patient ambulates, instruct patient or caregiver to carry the bag below the level of the patient's bladder. Never raise a drainage bag and tubing above the level of the patient's bladder. Urine in the bag and tubing is a medium for bacterial growth, and infection will develop if urine is allowed to reflux (return to the bladder).

Most drainage bags contain an antireflux valve to prevent urine from reentering the drainage tubing and contaminating the bladder. A spigot at the base of the bag provides a means to empty the bag. Make sure the spigot is always clamped, except during emptying, and tucked into the protective pouch at the bag's side. To keep the drainage system patent, check for kinks or bends in the tubing, avoid positioning the patient on drainage tubing, prevent tubing from becoming dependent, and observe for clots or sediment that block the tubing.

Routine Catheter Care. Patients with indwelling catheters require specific perineal hygiene care to reduce the risk for urinary tract infection. In most institutions, patients receive catheter care every 8 hours as the minimal standard of care. In addition, provide catheter care each time the patient defecates or has bowel incontinence. Proper care involves removal of any secretions or encrustation at the catheter insertion site and cleansing of the first 4 inches of the catheter.

Provide thorough perineal care (see Chapter 28), and observe the urethral meatus and surrounding tissues for inflammation, swelling, and discharge. Note the amount, color, odor, and consistency of discharge to determine local infection and status of hygiene. Use soap and water to cleanse along the length of the catheter for 10 cm (4 inches) (Figure 33-9). Hold the catheter firmly as you cleanse away from the urethra down toward the end of the catheter. Cleansing away from the urethra reduces microorganisms around the meatus. The use of powders or lotions on the perineum is contraindicated because of the risk for growth of microorganisms, which travel up the urinary tract.

Replace, as necessary, the adhesive tape or multipurpose tube holder that anchors the catheter to the patient's leg or abdomen, and remove adhesive residue from the skin. Secure the catheter, thus reducing the risk for the catheter being pulled on and exposing the portion that was in the urethra. This also prevents drag on the catheter and avoids pressure from the balloon on the bladder neck. Check the drainage tubing and bag to ensure that no tubing loops hang below the level of the bladder. Make sure that the tube is coiled and secured onto the bed linen, the tube is not kinked or clamped, and the drainage bag is positioned on the bed frame. If it is necessary to change the urinary tubing and collection bag, use principles of surgical asepsis. Change the tubing and bag if signs of leakage develop.

Catheter Removal. The procedure for removal of an indwelling catheter requires a nurse to promote normal bladder function and prevent urethral trauma. Follow medical asepsis when removing a catheter (see Skill 33-1). It is

normal for a patient to experience some dysuria, especially if the catheter has been in place several days or weeks. Until the bladder regains full tone, some patients also have frequency or urinary retention. Assess the patient's urinary function by noting the first voiding after catheter removal. If 6 to 8 hours elapse without voiding or the patient experiences discomfort, it often becomes necessary to reinsert the catheter.

Alternatives to Urethral Catheterization To avoid the risks associated with catheters inserted through the urethra, alternatives for urinary drainage exist. A **suprapubic catheter** is inserted surgically into the bladder through the lower abdomen above the symphysis pubis (Figure 33-10). Although most successfully used for short periods with patients who have had gynecological and bladder surgery, the suprapubic catheter is sometimes used in older adult males who require a long-term alternative to urinary catheterization. As with indwelling urinary catheters, the suprapubic catheter predisposes the patient to UTIs, but the incidence is lower. Spread of infection to the kidneys requires removing the catheter. Suprapubic catheters have the advantages of allowing patients to void naturally when the catheter is clamped and the catheters are more comfortable. Daily care will depend on policy, but the cleaning and dressing of the site are similar to care of any surgical drain (see Chapter 36).

The condom catheter is suitable for incontinent or comatose male patients who still have complete and spontaneous bladder emptying (Box 33-8). The condom catheter poses little risk for infection. Local infections, however, result from buildup of secretions around the urethra, trauma to the urethral meatus, or buildup of pressure in the outflow tubing.

It is necessary to remove the condom catheter daily to check for skin irritation. Clean the urethral meatus and penis thor-

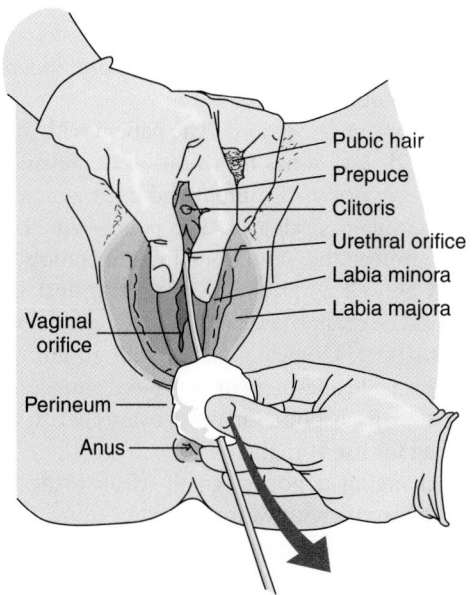

Figure 33-9 ■ Cleansing the catheter during catheter care. (From Sorrentino S: *Mosby's textbook for nursing assistants*, St. Louis, 2004, Mosby.)

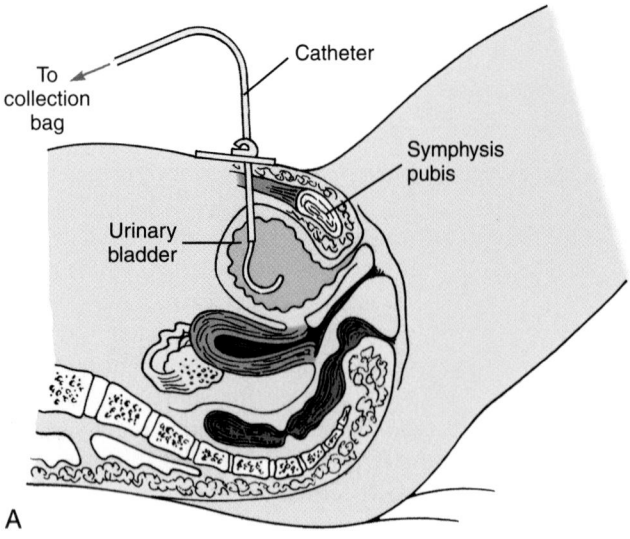

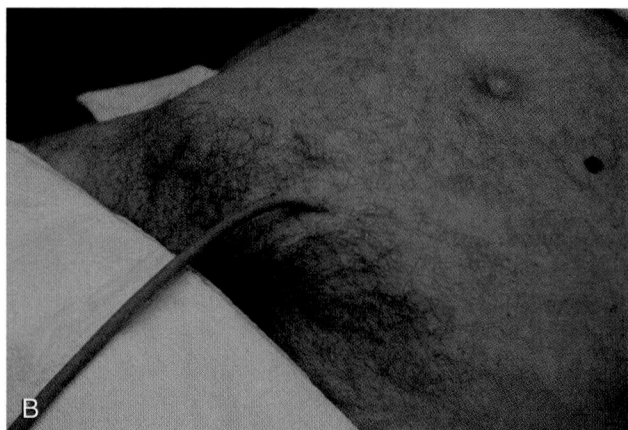

Figure 33-10 ■ A, Placement of suprapubic catheter above the symphysis pubis. **B,** Suprapubic catheter without a dressing.

oughly with each condom catheter change. Twisting of the condom at the drainage tube attachment irritates the skin and obstructs urine outflow. Check the drainage tubing frequently for patency. For a man with a retracted foreskin, maintaining the intactness of a conventional condom catheter is difficult. Special devices are available to help with the problem. Review manufacturer's guidelines for product application.

There is a lack of a full spectrum of devices and appliances for incontinent adults, particularly women (Mason and others, 2003). Some women wear the newer absorbent pads and adult disposable undergarments. However, wearers of these disposable undergarments report skin irritation, odor, and increased infection rate. For the active incontinent woman, behavioral treatment options such as pelvic floor exercises and diet management will promote more independence (Macaulay and others, 2004).

Care of Urinary Diversions The patient with an incontinent urinary diversion has no sensation or control over the time or frequency of urine output and must wear a pouch to collect the effluent (drainage). The pouch will contain the urine and protect the skin from local irritation and skin breakdown as well as provide a barrier against odor. The pouch should be changed every 3 to 7 days, not daily (Colwell and others, 2004). Urinary pouches with an antireflux flap are clear, drainable one-piece or two-piece pouches, cut to fit or precut size. Each pouch may be connected to a bedside drainage bag for use at night.

When changing a pouch, gently cleanse the skin surrounding the stoma with warm tap water using a washcloth and pat dry. Measure the stoma, and cut the opening in the pouch. Then apply the pouch after removing the protective backing from the adhesive surface. Press firmly into place over the stoma. Observe the appearance of the stoma and surrounding skin. The stoma is normally red and moist and originates from a portion of the ileum. The stoma protrudes

above the skin and is located in the right lower quadrant of the abdomen.

Patients with continent urinary diversions do not have to wear an external pouch. However, if the patient has a continent urinary reservoir, you must teach the patient how to intermittently catheterize the pouch. Patients will need to be able and willing to do this 4 to 6 times a day for the rest of their lives. Patients will have frequent episodes of incontinence of urine after creation of an orthotopic neobladder and will need to follow a bladder-training schedule and perform pelvic muscle exercises until continence is achieved.

Specially trained surgeons perform both of these continent urinary diversion surgeries, which require long operating times. Smaller community hospitals do not often perform these procedures. The postoperative care of patients having continent urinary diversions varies widely with the surgical techniques used, and it is important to learn the surgeon's preferred routine or health care facility's procedures before caring for these patients.

RESTORATIVE AND CONTINUING CARE Returning to normal micturition often means preventing complications from treatment. Many restorative functions are related to preventing infection after catheterization, promoting comfort and habit training, and preventing skin breakdown if the patient is incontinent.

Preventing Infection Maintaining a closed urinary drainage system is important in infection control. A break in the system leads to introduction of microorganisms. Sites at risk are at the place of catheter insertion, drainage bag, spigot, tube junction, and junction of tube and bag (Figure 33-11). In addition, monitor the patency of the system to prevent pooling of urine. Urine in the drainage bag is an excellent medium for microorganism growth. Bacteria travel up drainage tubing to grow in pools of urine. Therefore it is important to prevent the abnormal backward flow of urine

BOX 33-8 PROCEDURAL GUIDELINES

Applying a Condom Catheter

DELEGATION CONSIDERATIONS: After assessing patient for latex allergy, you can delegate the skill of applying a condom catheter to nursing assistive personnel (NAP). The nurse instructs NAP to:

- Be sensitive to privacy needs of patients
- Be sure the skin of penile shaft is intact and free from swelling, redness, or open lesions before applying the condom catheter
- Ask for assistance if the NAP is uncertain how to apply the adhesive strip that secures the condom catheter

EQUIPMENT: Condom catheter (sometimes comes with self-adhesive or an elastic adhesive), collection bag, skin prep, basin with warm water, towel and washcloth, clean gloves, scissors or hair guard, bath blanket and sheet

1. Check health care provider's order. Identify patient using two identifiers (e.g., name and birthday or name and account number, according to facility policy).
2. Perform hand hygiene.
3. Assess urinary elimination patterns, patient's ability to voluntarily urinate, and continence.
4. Assess mental status of patient, and explain procedure.
5. Provide for privacy by closing room door or bedside curtain. Raise bed to working height, and lower side rail on working side.
6. Prepare condom catheter and drainage bag and tubing (see manufacturer's directions).
7. Assist patient to a supine or sitting position. Place bath blanket over upper torso, fold a sheet over lower torso so that only penis is exposed.
8. Apply clean gloves; provide perineal care (see Chapter 28), and dry thoroughly. If patient is uncircumcised, return foreskin to normal position.
9. If needed, clip hair at base of penile shaft. Do not shave the pubic area. An alternative to trimming pubic hair is placement of a hair guard (see manufacturer's directions) over the penis before applying the catheter.
10. Assess condition of penis and scrotum. Use the manufacturer's measuring guide to measure the diameter of penis in a flaccid state. The penile shaft should be at least 2 cm in length to ensure successful application.
11. *Option:* Apply skin-cleansing preparation to penile shaft, and allow to dry.
12. Hold penis along shaft in nondominant hand. With dominant hand, hold condom sheath at tip of penis and smoothly roll sheath onto penis. Allow 2.5 to 5 cm (1 to 2 inches) of space between tip of penis and end of catheter (see illustration).
13. Secure condom catheter according to manufacturer's directions:
    a. If using elastic adhesive, wrap the strip of adhesive over the condom to secure it in place by using a spiral technique (see illustration). **NOTE: Never use adhesive tape.**
    b. For self-adhesive catheter, apply catheter as in Steps 11 and 12, then apply gentle pressure on penile shaft for 10 to 15 seconds to secure.
14. Connect drainage tubing to end of condom catheter. Be sure condom is not twisted. Connect catheter to large-volume drainage bag or leg bag (see illustration). Attach large-volume drainage bag to lower bed frame. Coil excess tubing on bed.
15. Make patient comfortable, lower bed, and place side rails as appropriate.
16. Dispose of contaminated supplies, remove gloves, and perform hand hygiene.
17. Observe urinary drainage, drainage tube patency, condition of penis, and tape placement.

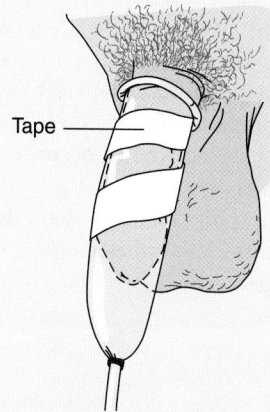

Tape

Step 13 ■ Apply elastic tape in a spiral fashion to secure the condom catheter to the penis.

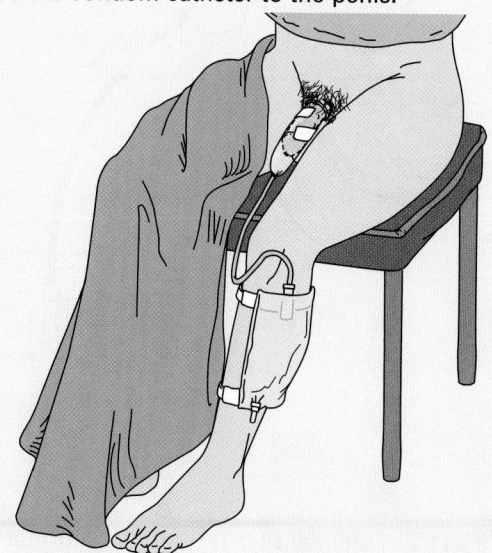

Step 14 ■ Attach condom catheter tubing to leg bag.

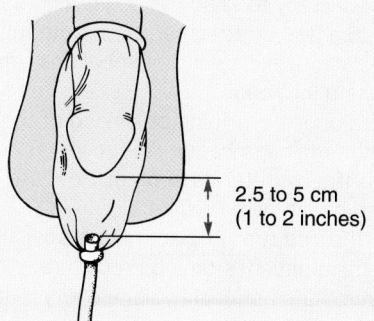

2.5 to 5 cm (1 to 2 inches)

Step 12 ■ Distance between end of penis and tip of condom.

(**urinary reflux**). If this urine flows back into the bladder, an infection will probably develop. Box 33-9 lists ways to prevent infections in catheterized patients.

Promotion of Comfort Patients with urinary alterations are often uncomfortable as a result of the symptoms of urinary problems. Frequent or unpredictable voiding, dysuria, and painful distention are sources of discomfort.

The incontinent patient gains comfort from having clean, dry clothing. When incontinence is the problem, a protective pad or sanitary belt protects against soiling. Wet clothing sticks to the skin and can cause rubbing and irritation. Check pads frequently, and change them as needed.

Giving urinary analgesics that act on the urethral and bladder mucosa sometimes relieve dysuria. Phenazopyridine (Pyridium) helps to relieve dysuria, burning, and itching. It is available in combination with sulfonamide antibiotics in preparations such as Azo Gantanol and Azo Gantrisin. The sulfonamide provides additional antibacterial action. Make patients taking drugs with phenazopyridine aware that their urine will appear orange and possibly stain their clothing. They need to drink large amounts of fluids to prevent toxicity from the sulfonamides and to maintain optimal flow through the urinary system. Always ask patients about allergies to sulfa before giving these drugs.

If the patient has local discomfort from an inflamed urethra, a warm sitz bath will provide pain relief (see Chapter 36). The warm water soothes inflamed tissues near the urethral meatus by improving blood supply. The patient is often relaxed after a sitz bath, so voiding occurs easily.

The pain of distention cannot be relieved unless the patient is able to empty the bladder. Methods for stimulating micturition or intermittent catheterization are often the only sources of pain relief.

Maintenance of Skin Integrity Acidic urine is irritating to the skin. When urine becomes alkaline, encrustation or precipitate collects on the skin, causing breakdown. Continuous exposure of the skin to urine leads to gradual maceration and excoriation. Washing with mild soap and warm water is the best way to remove urine from the skin. Special no-rinse cleansers are useful because they avoid the problem of skin irritation that results from incomplete removal of cleansers from the skin (Gray, 2004). Body lotion keeps the skin moisturized and provides a barrier to the urine. Patients who wet their clothing need a clean set of clothes after each voiding.

When the skin becomes irritated or inflamed, the health care provider often prescribes a cream or spray containing steroids to reduce inflammation (e.g., triamcinolone [Kenalog]). If fungal growth develops, the antifungal drug nystatin (Mycostatin), available in cream or powder form, is effective (McKenry and others, 2005; Wound, Ostomy and Continence Nurses Society [WOCN], 2005).

The patient with a **ureterostomy** has a special hygiene problem because urine drains from the ostomy site continuously. The drainage pouch or appliance frequently becomes moist and slips from the skin (WOCN, 2005). Continual oozing of urine around the stoma causes skin breakdown. Skin barriers provide a layer of protection between the skin and ostomy pouch. When urine leaks, it frequently covers the outer skin barrier. An enterostomal therapist helps the pa-

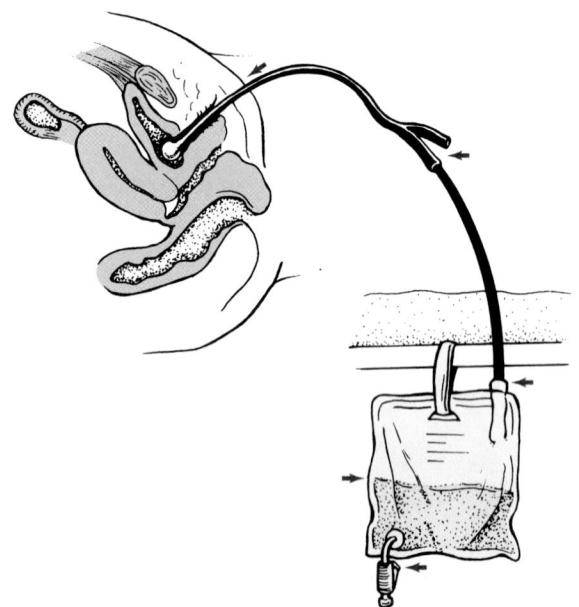

Figure 33-11 ■ Potential sites *(arrows)* for introduction of infection.

BOX 33-9	Tips for Preventing Infection in Catheterized Patients

- Follow good hand hygiene techniques.
- Do not allow the spigot on the drainage bag to touch a contaminated surface.
- Do not open the drainage system at connection points to obtain specimens or measure urine.
- If the drainage tubing becomes disconnected, do not touch the ends of the catheter or tubing. Wipe the ends of the tube with antiseptic solution before reconnecting.
- Each patient needs to have a separate receptacle for measuring urine to prevent cross contamination.
- Prevent pooling of urine and reflux of urine into the bladder. Avoid raising the drainage bag above the level of the bladder.
- Avoid allowing any dependent loops of tubing.
- If it is necessary to raise the bag during transfer of the patient to a bed or stretcher, clamp the tubing.
- Before patient exercises or ambulates, drain all urine from tubing into bag.
- Avoid prolonged clamping or kinking of the tubing.
- Empty the drainage bag at least every 8 hours.
- Remove the catheter as soon as possible after conferring with health care provider.
- Secure the catheter in place. Note specific guidelines for the male patient's taping procedure.
- Perform routine perineal hygiene every 8-hour shift and after defecation.

tient select an ostomy appliance that fits snugly against the skin's surface around the stoma (see Chapter 34).

Habit Training A patient with functional incontinence benefits from habit training, which improves the voluntary control over urination. The patient establishes a flexible toileting schedule based on his or her pattern. Have the patient establish the pattern by documenting episodes of incontinence and then schedule voiding opportunities just before the urge time interval. The goal is to keep the patient dry. Help the patient to the bathroom before the urge usually occurs. Time fluids and medications to prevent interference with the toileting schedule.

■■■EVALUATION

PATIENT CARE To evaluate the care plan use the expected outcomes developed during planning to determine whether interventions were effective (Box 33-10). This evaluation process is a dynamic one. You use this information to monitor the patient's progress and to direct future interventions. The optimal goal is the patient's ability to urinate voluntarily without dysuria, urgency, or frequency. The patient's urine needs to be an amber color, clear, without abnormal constituents, and within the normal range of pH and specific gravity.

You also evaluate specific outcomes designed to demonstrate normal urinary function and prevent complications of urinary alterations. Has the patient's intake been at least 2000 mL? Is the bladder distended? Is there less than 50 mL of residual urine on the second voiding? Is urinary output in proportion to fluid intake? Are there a reduced number of incontinent episodes? Does the patient use correct hand hygiene? Are there any areas of skin breakdown around the perineum, stoma, or condom? Be systematic in evaluating the patient's response to care. Nursing research is being conducted to validate the effectiveness of nursing interventions. Evidence-based practice will improve the quality of care you provide (see Chapter 6).

PATIENT EXPECTATIONS Many take control over urination for granted until it is lost. Patients report that it is degrading and they feel like a baby when they lose control over voiding. Therefore evaluation of care from the incontinent patient's standpoint centers around maintaining a level of dryness that is personally satisfactory. Patients want to have control, and to achieve that outcome they need to have confidence in utilizing triggering mechanisms to initiate voiding.

Patients who have a UTI find that pain, urgency, and frequency rule their lives. Patients who have an infection will be satisfied with their care if they are able to report an absence or decrease in their symptoms. Does the patient void without dysuria? Does the patient sleep and carry out activities of daily living with lessened or no discomfort?

For all patients with urinary problems, lack of privacy is a potential issue. Did they feel that staff were considerate, and did the staff protect their privacy? Patients will also evaluate whether you include them in the planning of their care. Were they able to tell you the important information about their habits? Did you consider that information when you suggested a plan of care or implemented an intervention?

BOX 33-10   EVALUATION

Sandy talks with Mrs. Vallero the next evening. The patient's care plan incorporates scheduled voiding, oral fluids, and use of Credé's method of manual compression during voiding. She palpates Mrs. Vallero's bladder and then assists her to the toilet. After being sure she is comfortable and leaving the call light in place, Sandy instructs her to use Credé's method of manual compression. She returns to measure Mrs. Vallero's urinary output and evaluates for bladder residual using ultrasound bladder scan.

DOCUMENTATION NOTE

"Moved slowly to the bathroom with assistance. Gait was slightly unsteady and slow. Stated she was 'weak.' Breathing was even and nonlabored. While sitting on the toilet, stated, 'I'm ready.' Used manual bladder compression and turned the water on in the sink. Voided 400 mL of clear, pale yellow urine. Stated, 'I don't feel so full now.' Returned to bed. No evidence of residual urine in bladder using portable ultrasound."

SAFETY GUIDELINES FOR NURSING SKILLS

SAFETY CONSIDERATIONS
Ensuring patient safety is an essential role of the professional nurse. To ensure patient safety, communicate clearly with members of the health care team, assess and incorporate the patient's priorities of care and preferences, and use the best evidence when making decisions about your patient's care. When performing the skill in this chapter, remember the following points to ensure safe, individualized patient care:

- Follow principles of surgical asepsis when performing catheterizations.
- Follow principles of medical asepsis when handling urine specimens or assisting patients with their toileting needs.

SKILL 33-1   INSERTING AND REMOVING STRAIGHT OR INDWELLING CATHETERS

DELEGATION CONSIDERATIONS

The skill of inserting a straight or indwelling catheter cannot be delegated; however, the nursing assistive personnel (NAP) can assist the nurse. In long-term care settings, these skills are often delegated (check agency policy). The nurse evaluates possible alternatives to catheter use. The nurse directs the NAP to:

- Assist with patient positioning
- Focus lighting for the procedure
- Aid in the patient's comfort during the procedure by measures such as holding the patient's hand or keeping the patient warm

EQUIPMENT

Catheter Insertion

- Bladder scanner (if available)
- Foley catheter kit containing the following sterile items:
  - Urinary catheter with drainage tubing and collection bag that is usually connected (for indwelling catheter only)
  - Sterile gloves (extra pair optional)
  - Waterproof drapes (one fenestrated—has an opening in the center of drape)
  - Lubricant
  - Antiseptic cleansing agent (povidone-iodine) or alternative such as Hibiclens or Shur-Clens

- Cotton balls or sterile antiseptic swabs
- Forceps
- Prefilled syringe with sterile water (for indwelling catheter only)
- Specimen container
- Sterile drainage tubing and collection bag (if not included in the kit)
- A urethral catheterization tray for straight/intermittent catheterization will contain a single-use catheter, receptacle for urine, and will have the supplies in the equipment list except as noted
- Multipurpose Velcro tube holder or nonallergic/paper tape
- Bath blanket
- Waterproof absorbent pad
- Clean gloves, basin with warm water, soap, washcloth, and towel
- Appropriate additional lighting as needed (such as a flashlight or procedure light)

Catheter Removal

- Sterile Luer-Lok syringe at least as large as the size of the retention balloon (printed on the inflation port
- Washcloth, soap, and towels
- Trash receptacle
- Graduated container

STEPS	RATIONALE

ASSESSMENT

1 Review patient's medical record, including prescriber's order and nurses' notes. Assess for time of previous catheterization, if applicable, including catheter size and response of patient.

Data explains purpose of inserting catheter, such as preparation for surgery, urinary irrigations, collection of sterile urine specimen, or measurement of residual urine.

2 Assess status of patient:

a Ask patient when was time of last urination. Check I&O flow sheet.

Determines time of last voiding and indicates likelihood of bladder fullness.

b Level of awareness or developmental stage.

Reveals patient's ability to cooperate during procedure, level of explanation needed, and ability to perform self-catheterization.

c Patient's mobility and physical limitations.

Determines how you will position patient.

d Patient's gender and age.

Determines catheter size: 5 to 6 Fr is generally for an infant; 8 to 10 Fr with 3-mL balloon is generally for children; 14 to 16 Fr is indicated for adult women; 12 Fr may be considered for young girls; 16 to 18 Fr is used for male patients. The prescriber may order a larger size.

- *Critical Decision Point:* Large catheters (greater than 16 Fr) can distend the urethra and permanently damage the urethra and bladder neck, as well as cause bladder spasms and leaking around the catheter (Hart, 2008). Use the smallest-size catheter possible, to minimize trauma and promote adequate drainage of the periurethral glands. This will decrease the risk for infection (Emr and Ryan, 2004; Hart, 2008; Senese and others, 2006a).

---

e Allergies.

Procedure risks exposure to allergies associated with antiseptic, tape, latex, and lubricant. Allergy to povidone-iodine is common. If patient is unaware of allergy, ask if allergic to shellfish. Alternatives to povidone-iodine include Hibiclens or Shur-Clens (Senese and others, 2006 b, c).

STEPS	RATIONALE
3 Assess bladder for fullness (distended bladder is palpable above symphysis pubis), or apply bladder scanner (if available). 　**a** Using a bladder scanner: 　　**(1)** Assist the patient into a supine position with head elevated on a pillow. Expose the lower abdomen. 　　**(2)** After turning on the scanner, indicate gender, using "female" only if the patient has not had a hysterectomy and selecting "male" for men and for women who have had a hysterectomy. 　　**(3)** Wipe the scanner head with an alcohol pad. 　　**(4)** Palpate the patient's symphysis pubis, and apply ultrasound gel to the scan head or to the midline on the abdomen about 1 to 1½ inches above the symphysis pubis. 　　**(5)** Aim the scan head toward the patient's bladder. Watch the bladder image on the scanner screen. This image should be centered. If not centered, reposition the scanner head and repeat the procedure until the bladder is in the center of the graph. 　　**(6)** Press and hold the scan button until a beep is heard. The volume measurement will appear on the screen.	Full bladder with inability to void indicates need to insert catheter. A bladder scan noninvasively determines the amount of urine in the bladder.
4 Perform hand hygiene, apply clean gloves, and assess for perineal anatomical landmarks, erythema, drainage, and odor. Remove gloves, and perform hand hygiene.	Determines condition of perineum.
5 Review medical record for any pathological condition that will impair passage of catheter (e.g., enlarged prostate gland in men).	Obstruction prevents passage of catheter through urethra into bladder.
6 Assess patient's knowledge of the purpose for catheterization, whether patient has had catheter placed previously, and patient's reaction.	Reveals need for patient instruction and/or support.

PLANNING

1 Collect appropriate equipment.	
2 Arrange for extra nursing personnel to assist as necessary.	Patient may need assistance to assume positioning for procedure.
3 Identify patient using two identifiers (e.g., name and birthday or name and account number, according to facility policy).	Complies with The Joint Commission requirements and improves procedure safety. In most acute care settings you will use the patient's name and identification number on armband and MAR to identify patients (The Joint Commission, 2009).

IMPLEMENTATION

1 Perform hand hygiene.	Reduces transmission of microorganisms.
2 Close curtain or door.	Provides privacy and reduces embarrassment to patient, thus promoting relaxation.
3 Raise bed to appropriate working height. Facing patient, stand on left side of bed if right-handed and on right side if left-handed. If side rails in use, raise side rail on opposite side of bed and lower side rail on working side.	Successful catheter insertion requires a comfortable position with all equipment easily accessible.
4 Place waterproof pad under patient.	Prevents soiling of bed linen.

• ***Critical Decision Point:*** Obtain assistance to position and to support weak, frail, or confused patients.

SKILL 33-1	INSERTING AND REMOVING STRAIGHT OR INDWELLING CATHETERS—cont'd

STEPS

5 Position patient:

  A Female Patient

    (1) Assist to dorsal recumbent position (supine with knees flexed). Ask patient to relax thighs to externally rotate the hip joints.

    (2) *Optional:* Position female patient in side-lying (Sims') position with upper leg flexed at knee and hip if unable to be supine.

    (3) Take extra precautions to cover rectal area with drape during procedure. Support patient with pillows if necessary to maintain position.

  B Male Patient

    (1) Assist to supine or sitting position with thighs slightly abducted.

6 Drape patient:

  A Female Patient

    (1) Drape with bath blanket. Place blanket diamond fashion over patient, with one corner at patient's neck, side corners over each arm and side, and last corner over perineum (see illustration).

  B Male Patient

    (1) Drape upper trunk with bath blanket, and cover lower extremities with bed sheet, exposing only genitalia (see illustration).

7 Apply clean gloves. Wash perineal area with soap and water as needed; dry. Locate urinary meatus in female patients while performing perineal hygiene. Have NAP hold flashlight or light source to illuminate perineum as needed. Remove and discard gloves; perform hand hygiene.

RATIONALE

Provides good visualization of perineal structures. This position is optimal because it minimizes the risk for contamination by fecal material (Cochran, 2007).

Use this alternate position if patient cannot abduct leg at hip joint (e.g., if patient has arthritic joints). In addition, this position is often more comfortable for patient.

Reduces chance of cross contamination.

Comfortable position for patient that aids in visualization of penis.

Avoids unnecessary exposure of body parts and maintains patient's comfort.

Keeps legs and lower abdomen covered as nurse exposes genitalia during procedure.

Washing ensures area is not contaminated before catheter insertion (Leaver, 2007).

It is sometimes difficult to visualize the urinary meatus of a female patient because of individual anatomical differences (Senese and others, 2006a). Additional lighting improves visualization of meatus.

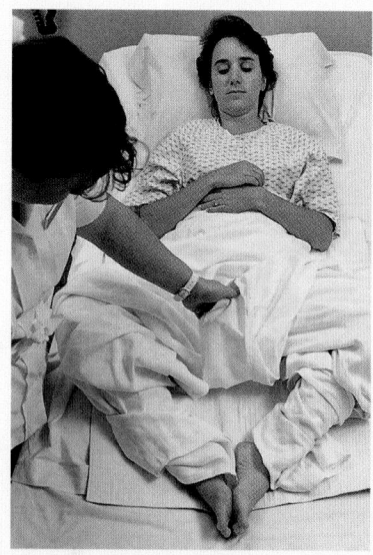

Step 6A(1) ■ Draping female for catheterization.

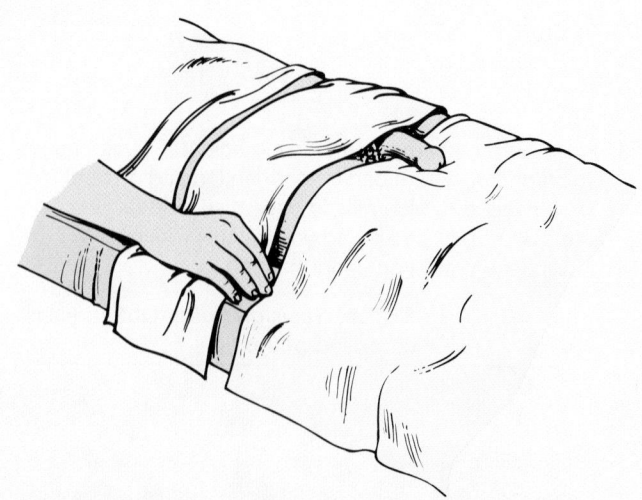

Step 6B(1) ■ Draping male for catheterization.

STEPS	RATIONALE
8 Open outer wrapping of either an indwelling Foley catheterization kit or urethral catheterization kit (for intermittent catheterization) by tearing package on paper-lined edge of plastic wrap. Place inner wrapped box on easily accessible, clean bedside table, or set it in between patient's legs. Patient's size and positioning will dictate exact placement. Place empty package (outer plastic wrap) near end of bed and use for waste disposal.	Provides easy access to supplies during catheter insertion. Maintains aseptic technique during procedure. This method works best with flexible, average-size patients.
9 Open sterile wrap covering box containing catheter supplies: Use sterile technique (see Chapter 13); fold back each flap of the sterile package one at a time, with the last flap opened toward patient.	The tray is now open and sitting on its own sterile field.
A The supplies in an intermittent catheterization tray are located in a sterile receptacle used to collect urine. There is no drainage bag in the tray.	Minimizes chance of contaminating supplies.
B The supplies in an indwelling catheter kit are arranged in sequence of use.	Designed to facilitate procedure preparation, minimizes handling of supplies.
10 Apply sterile gloves and then apply sterile drape:	
A Female Patient	
(1) While maintaining sterility of square drape, let drape unfold after removing from tray. Allow top edge of drape to form a cuff over both gloved hands.	Outer surface of drape covering hands remains sterile.
(2) Have patient lift hips (if unable to lift hips, get assistance) as you place sterile drape with the plastic (shiny) side down under the patient's buttocks.	Sterile drape against sterile gloves is sterile. Drape creates sterile work field.
(3) Pick up fenestrated sterile drape out of tray. Allow it to unfold without touching a nonsterile surface. Form cuff from edges to protect sterile gloves. Apply drape over perineum exposing only labia. Be sure not to touch contaminated surface (see illustration).	Drape creates sterile field for nurse to insert catheter.
B Male Patient: There are two methods for draping, depending on preference.	
(1) Apply fenestrated sterile drape over thighs and below penis without completely opening drape. Use this technique when you choose not to apply square sterile drape.	Creates sterile work field.
(2) Apply sterile drape with plastic (shiny) surface over thighs just below penis (instead of under buttocks). Pick up fenestrated sterile drape, allow it to unfold, form cuff from edges to protect sterile gloves; drape it over penis with fenestrated slit resting over penis (see illustration).	Drape creates sterile field for nurse to insert catheter.

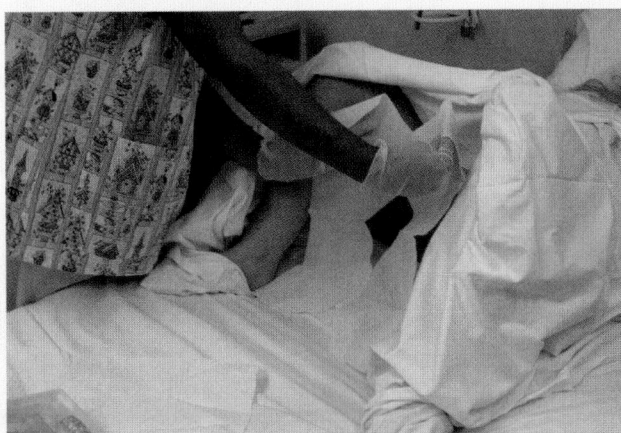

Step 10A(3) ■ Place sterile fenestrated drape (with opening in center) over perineum with labia exposed.

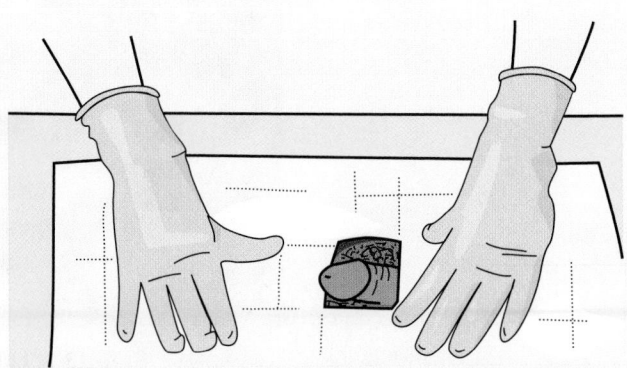

Step 10B(2) ■ Draping male with fenestrated drape.

SKILL 33-1 INSERTING AND REMOVING STRAIGHT
OR INDWELLING CATHETERS—cont'd

STEPS	RATIONALE
11 Move box on sterile field closer to patient, so sterile wrap under tray and drape under patient form a continuous field.	Provides sterile work area to handle equipment.
a Organize remaining supplies on sterile field. Take top tray out of box, and place it on sterile field. (Sterile catheter and drainage bag are under the top tray in the box.) Make sure clamp on drainage port of bag is closed. If drainage bag is preconnected to the catheter, leave the bag on the sterile field until the catheter is inserted. If drainage bag is not connected to catheter, open package containing sterile collection bag and drainage tubing. Keep cover on tip of drainage tubing until ready to connect to catheter.	Maintains principles of surgical asepsis and organizes work area, minimizing need to handle equipment once you are ready to insert catheter. Keeping cover on tip of sterile drainage tubing prevents contamination.
b Loosen lid on sterile specimen container if urine specimen required. Otherwise, discard into waste disposal bag.	
c Open package of sterile antiseptic solution. Pour solution over sterile cotton balls. NOTE: Sometimes there are sterile antiseptic swabs instead of solution. If swabs are available, open package with "stick" ends up for access.	
d Open packet containing lubricant. NOTE: Lubricant is sometimes in a prefilled syringe. If in a prefilled syringe, remove protective cap. Spread lubricant into sterile tray.	Prepares lubricant for catheter.
12 Remove plastic covering from catheter (usually on indwelling catheter only). Take care to coil length of catheter in palm.	Prevents contamination of catheter.

- **Critical Decision Point:** Testing the balloon of an indwelling catheter by injecting fluid from the prefilled sterile water syringe into the balloon port is no longer common practice. Testing the balloon may stretch it and lead to damage, causing increased trauma on insertion (Smith, 2006).

---

13 Place length of catheter in lubricant: Lubricate catheter 2.5 to 5 cm (1 to 2 inches) for women and 12.5 to 17.5 cm (5 to 7 inches) for men (see illustration).	Lubricating catheter will minimize urethral trauma and discomfort when inserting catheter.

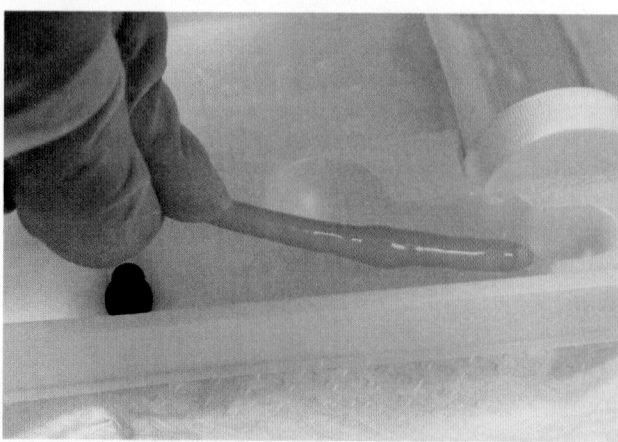

Step 13 ■ Lubricating catheter.

STEPS	RATIONALE

14 Cleanse urethral meatus:

A Female Patient

(1) With nondominant hand, fully expose urethral meatus by spreading labia. Have NAP focus flashlight if unable to visualize meatus with available lighting. Maintain position of nondominant hand throughout catheter insertion.

Optimal visualization of urethral meatus is possible. Fully spreading labia prevents contamination of urethral meatus during cleansing.

- ***Critical Decision Point:*** If unable to visualize urethra, place one finger of sterile gloved hand inside the vagina and apply gentle pressure upward to support and straighten the urethra. This may open the urethral meatus, creating better visualization. Insert the catheter just above the finger and below the clitoris (Senese and others, 2006b). Ensure that the patient understands what you are doing.

(2) Using forceps in sterile dominant hand, pick up cotton ball saturated with antiseptic solution or antiseptic swab sticks and clean perineal area, wiping front to back from clitoris toward anus. Using a new cotton ball or swab for each area, wipe along the far labial fold, near labial fold, and last, directly over center of urethral meatus (see illustration).

Cleansing reduces number of microorganisms at urethral meatus. Follows principles of medical asepsis. Dominant gloved hand remains sterile.

- ***Critical Decision Point:*** Closure of labia during cleansing requires that the cleaning procedure be repeated because the area now is contaminated.

B Male Patient

(1) If patient is not circumcised, retract foreskin with nondominant hand. Grasp penis at shaft just below glans. Gently spread urethral meatus so opening is more visible. Keep nondominant hand in this position throughout procedure.

Exposes urethral meatus.
Accidental release of foreskin or dropping of penis during cleansing requires repeating the process because area becomes contaminated.

(2) With dominant hand, pick up antiseptic-soaked cotton ball with forceps or swab stick and clean penis. Move cotton ball or swab in circular motion from urethral meatus down to base of glans. Repeat cleansing three more times, using clean cotton ball/stick each time (see illustration).

Reduces number of microorganisms at urethral meatus. Follows principles of medical aseptic technique. Dominant gloved hand remains sterile.

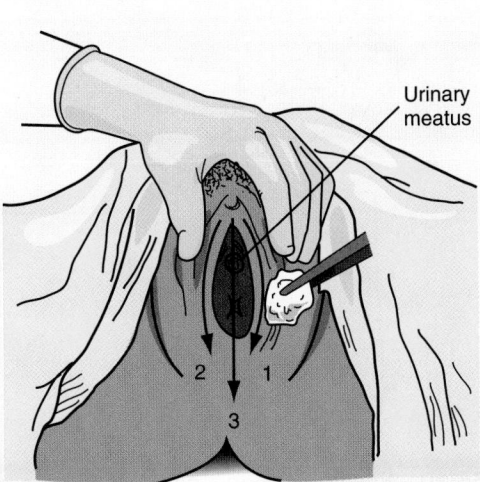

Urinary meatus

Step 14A(2) ■ Cleansing female perineum.

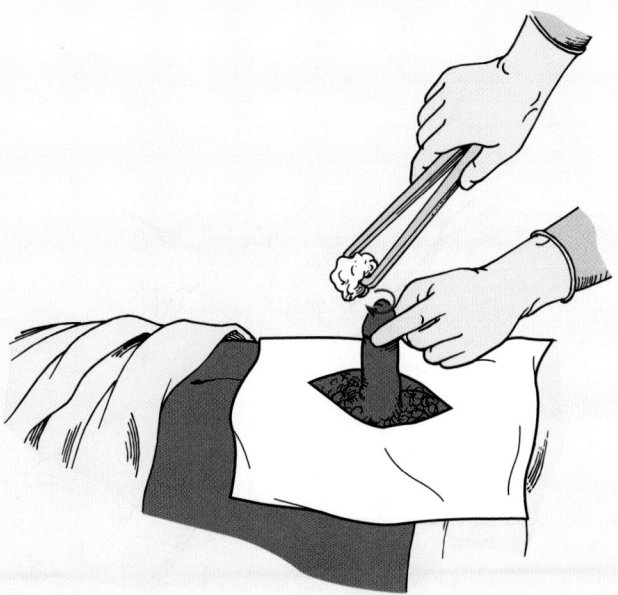

Step 14B(2) ■ Cleansing male urinary meatus.

SKILL 33-1   INSERTING AND REMOVING STRAIGHT OR INDWELLING CATHETERS—cont'd

STEPS	RATIONALE
15 Pick up catheter with gloved dominant hand, holding the catheter 2.5 to 5 cm (1 to 2 inches) from catheter tip, and **hold end of catheter loosely coiled in palm of dominant hand.**	Hold catheter near tip to allow easier manipulation during insertion into urethral meatus and prevent distal end from striking contaminated surface.
16 Insert catheter:	
A Female Patient	
(1) Ask patient to bear down gently as if to void, and slowly insert catheter through urethral meatus (see illustration).	Relaxation of external sphincter aids in insertion of catheter.
(2) Advance catheter a total of 5 to 7.5 cm (2 to 3 inches) in an adult **or until urine flows out catheter's end.** As soon as urine appears, advance the indwelling catheter another 2.5 to 5 cm (1 to 2 inches). Further insertion of a straight catheter is not necessary. Do not force against resistance.	Female urethra is short. Appearance of urine indicates that catheter tip is in bladder or lower urethra. Advancement of catheter ensures that the inflation balloon is in the bladder and not the urethra (Senese and others, 2006b).

- *Critical Decision Point:* If no urine appears, catheter may be in vagina. If misplaced, leave catheter in vagina as landmark indicating where not to insert, and insert another sterile catheter. Have the NAP get a new catheter without your having to break sterile technique.

STEPS	RATIONALE
(3) Release labia, and hold catheter securely with nondominant hand.	Bladder or sphincter contraction will cause accidental expulsion of catheter.
B Male Patient	
(1) Lift penis to position perpendicular to patient's body, and apply light traction (see illustration).	Straightens urethral canal to ease catheter insertion.
(2) Ask patient to bear down as if to void, and slowly insert catheter through urethral meatus.	Relaxation of external sphincter aids in insertion of catheter.
(3) In the adult, advance a straight catheter in an adult until urine flows out catheter's end. For an indwelling catheter, advance to the bifurcation of the drainage and balloon inflation port. If you meet resistance, do not attempt forceful catheter insertion (see illustration).	There is natural resistance as the catheter enters the external sphincter. However, do not use force to insert the catheter inward. Advancement of catheter to the bifurcation of the drainage and balloon inflation port ensures proper placement of indwelling catheter through the longer urethra for male patient (Daneshgari and others, 2002; Senese and others, 2006c).

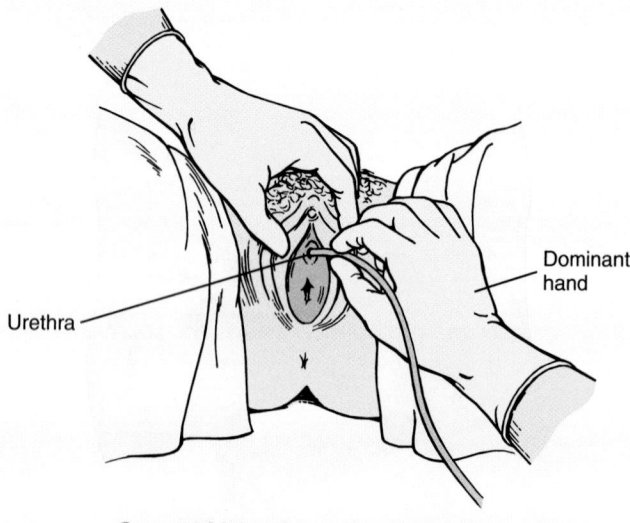

Urethra — | Dominant hand

Step 16A(1) ■ Inserting the catheter.

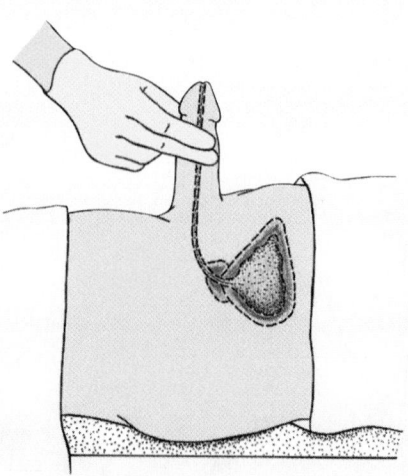

Step 16B(1) ■ Position of penis perpendicular to body for catheter insertion.

STEPS	RATIONALE

- ***Critical Decision Point:*** If there is resistance to catheter insertion, have the patient take slow, deep breaths while you insert the catheter slowly to promote relaxation (Senese and others, 2006c). Another technique is to rest your arm against the patient's leg, and ask him to relax. When the leg muscles begin to relax, continue the insertion process (Senese, 2004). NOTE: If there is persistent resistance to insertion, the patient may have an enlarged prostate. Notify the health care provider; you may need to use a Coudé catheter, with a slightly curved end, to facilitate insertion (Senese, 2004).

STEPS	RATIONALE
(4) Lower penis, and hold catheter securely in nondominant hand. Reposition foreskin if necessary.	Prevents accidental dislodgment of catheter.
17 Collect uring specimen as needed by holding end of catheter over cup. A residual volume requires all urine to be drained. A test for culture requires 20 to 30 mL of urine.	Holding catheter stabilizes it. Prevents accidental removal of an indwelling catheter.
18 Remove the straight catheter at this time. Withdraw slowly while gently palpating over patient's bladder. Check the amount of urine collected by placing in graduated cylinder.	Determines residual volume.
19 Balloon inflation, for **indwelling Foley catheter only:**	Balloon inflation anchors catheter tip above bladder outlet.
a While holding catheter with nondominant hand at urethral meatus, take end of catheter by dominant hand and place catheter between first two fingers of nondominant hand. Maintain a secure hold on the catheter with nondominant hand.	Holding on to catheter before inflating balloon will prevent expulsion of catheter from urethra.
b With free dominant hand, connect syringe with saline to end of catheter at inflation valve, and then slowly inject total amount of solution (see illustration). Follow manufacturer's instructions regarding amount of fluid used for balloon inflation. In general, a 5-mL balloon requires approximately 10 mL of fluid for symmetrical inflation. If patient complains of sudden pain, aspirate solution, and advance catheter further.	Inflation of balloon anchors catheter tip in place above bladder outlet to prevent removal of catheter. Underinflation or overinflation can result in an asymmetrical balloon, which may deflect the catheter tip to one side of the bladder, resulting in irritation of the bladder wall, occlusion of drainage, and bladder spasms (Mercer Smith, 2003).
c After inflating balloon, pull ***gently*** on the catheter tubing until resistance is felt.	Ensures catheter tip is anchored.

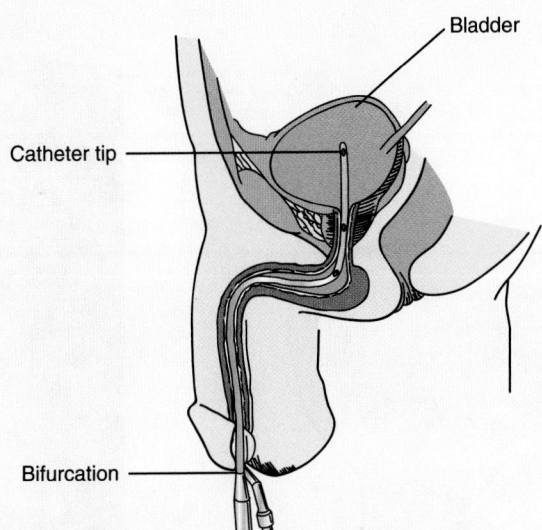

Step 16B(3) ■ Male anatomy with correct catheter insertion to the bifurcation of the drainage and balloon inflation port.

SKILL 33-1	INSERTING AND REMOVING STRAIGHT OR INDWELLING CATHETERS—cont'd

STEPS	RATIONALE
d Connect drainage tubing to catheter if it is not already preconnected. Place drainage bag below level of bladder (see illustration); **do not** place bag on side rails of bed.	Ensures proper drainage by gravity. Placement on side rails increases risk for tension applied to catheter, and bag can be raised above level of bladder.

• *Critical Decision Point:* If resistance occurs when inflating balloon or the patient verbalizes or shows nonverbal signs of pain, the balloon may not be entirely within the bladder. Stop inflation; allow fluid to flow back into syringe, and advance the catheter a little more before reattempting to inflate.

STEPS	RATIONALE
20 Allow bladder to empty fully unless institution policy restricts maximal volume of urine drained with catheterization (about 500 to 1000 mL).	Relieves bladder distention. There is no definitive evidence regarding whether there is benefit in limiting maximal volume drained.
21 Anchor indwelling catheter:	
A Female Patient	
(1) Secure catheter tubing to inner thigh with strip of nonallergic tape (use paper tape if allergic to silk tape), or use a commercial multipurpose tube holder with a Velcro strap, if available. Allow for slack so movement of thigh does not create tension on catheter (see illustration). Clip drainage tubing to edge of mattress.	Securing the catheter will minimize the accidental dislodgment of the catheter (Gray, 2006). Also minimizes the risk for bleeding, trauma, meatal necrosis, and bladder spasms from pressure and traction (Senese and others, 2006a).
B Male Patient	
(1) Secure catheter tubing to top of thigh or lower abdomen (with penis directed toward chest). Allow slack in catheter so movement does not create tension on catheter (see illustration). Clip drainage tubing to edge of mattress.	Anchoring catheter to lower abdomen reduces pressure on urethra at junction of penis and scrotum, thus reducing possibility of tissue injury in this area (Senese and others, 2006a).
22 Be sure there are no obstructions in tubing. Coil excess tubing on bed, and fasten it to bottom sheet with clip from kit or with rubber band and safety pin.	Obstruction will prevent free flow of urine, leading to bladder retention.

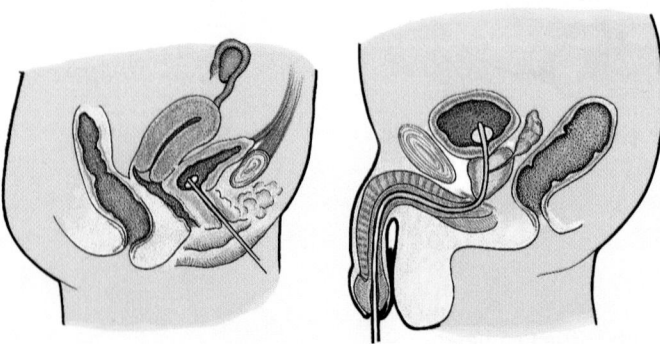

Step 19b ■ Placement of inflated balloon in bladder.

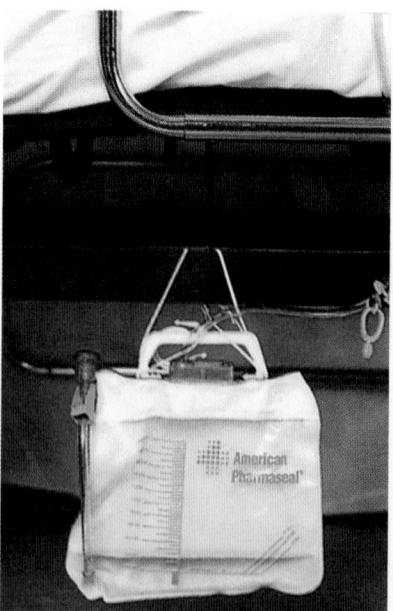

Step 19d ■ Drainage bag below level of bladder, connected to bed frame.

STEPS	RATIONALE
23 Assist patient to comfortable position. Perform perineal catheter care routinely (each shift) and when secretions build up in perineum (see Chapter 28). In male patient always replace foreskin (if retracted before procedure) in original position covering glans.	Regular hygiene reduces incidence of catheter-related UTI. Paraphimosis (retraction and constriction of the foreskin behind the glans penis) secondary to catheterization may occur if foreskin is not placed in original position.
24 Dispose of used equipment in appropriate receptacles. Remove gloves, and perform hand hygiene.	Reduces transmission of microorganisms.
25 Label specimen container for culture and send to laboratory.	Ensures prompt diagnostic analysis.
26 Record on I&O form amount of urine drained or collected for specimen.	Determines urine output.
27 Removal of indwelling Foley catheter:	
a Perform hand hygiene, put on clean gloves, and provide privacy.	Procedure requires use of medical asepsis.
b Prepare the patient:	
(1) Provide an explanation of procedure.	Will be able to visualize the urethra easily in women.
(2) Position the patient in the same position as during catheterization (see Step 5).	
(3) Remove the tape or Velcro strap securing the catheter tubing.	
c Place a towel between a female patient's thighs or over a male patient's thighs.	Prevents soiling of patient and bed linen
d Insert the syringe tip into the balloon injection port. Slowly and completely withdraw all the solution to deflate the balloon completely.	If a portion of solution remains, the partially inflated balloon will traumatize the urethral canal as the catheter is removed (Robinson, 2003).
e Gently withdraw the catheter, and gather it in the towel. Discard supplies. Wash and dry perineal area, and position patient to comfort.	Restores patient's comfort.
f Empty urine collection bag into graduated container, and measure amount for I&O. Discard items into trash receptacle. Perform hand hygiene.	Prevents transmission of microorganisms.

EVALUATION

1 Palpate bladder for distention.	Determines if distention is relieved.
2 Ask patient to describe level of comfort.	Determines if patient's sensation of discomfort or bladder fullness has been relieved.
3 Observe character and amount of urine in drainage system or collection container.	Determines if urine is flowing adequately and whether urine shows signs of infection.
4 Determine that there is no urine leaking from catheter or tubing connections and that all connections are secure.	Prevents injury to patient's skin and ensures a closed sterile system.

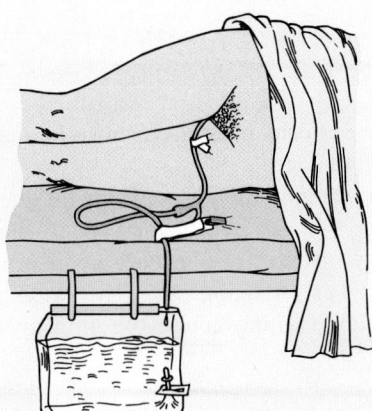

Step 21A(1) ■ Securing the female indwelling catheter.

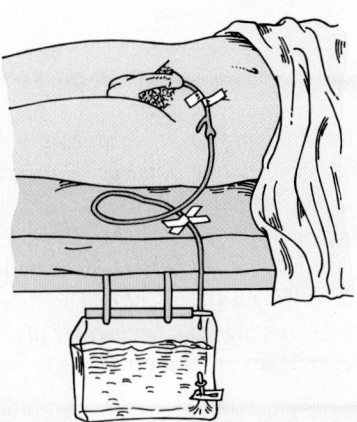

Step 21B(1) ■ Securing the male indwelling catheter.

| SKILL 33-1 | INSERTING AND REMOVING STRAIGHT OR INDWELLING CATHETERS—cont'd |

RECORDING AND REPORTING

- Report and record type and size of catheter inserted, amount of fluid used to inflate balloon, characteristics of urine, amount of urine, reasons for catheterization, specimen or residual collection, and if appropriate, patient's response to procedure and teaching topics.

- Initiate I&O records (see Chapter 17).
- Record removal of retention catheter, assessment of urethral meatus, and character and amount of urine in drainage bag. Record patient's next voiding.

UNEXPECTED OUTCOMES AND RELATED INTERVENTIONS

- Urethral or perineal irritation is present.
  - Observe for leaking, and replace catheter if necessary.
  - If catheter is present, ensure that indwelling catheter is anchored.
  - If securing catheter does not help irritation, or if irritation persists after catheter has been removed, notify health care provider.
- Patient has fever and/or odor in urine, or patient experiences small, frequent voidings or burning or bleeding.
  - Monitor vital signs and urine, but report findings to health care provider because any of these symptoms/signs may indicate a UTI.

- Patient experiences urinary retention and is unable to void after catheter removal.
  - Ensure adequate oral intake.
  - Provide privacy and facilitate urination by relaxation.
  - If patient unable to void within 6 to 8 hours of catheter removal, notify health care provider and anticipate order for straight catheterization.

KEY POINTS

- Voluntary control from higher brain centers and involuntary control from the spinal cord influence voiding.
- Symptoms common to urinary disturbances include urgency, dysuria, frequency, polyuria, oliguria, and difficulty in starting the urinary stream.
- When collected properly, a clean-voided urine specimen does not contain bacteria from the urethral meatus.
- A patient will better understand the importance of perineal hygiene by knowing that the urinary tract is normally sterile.
- An increased fluid intake results in urine formation that flushes particles and solutes from the urinary system.

- Incontinence is classified as total, urge, stress, reflex, or functional. Each type of incontinence has specific nursing interventions.
- An indwelling urinary catheter remains in the bladder for an extended period, making the risk for infection greater than with intermittent catheterization.
- Strict asepsis is necessary when caring for a patient with a closed bladder drainage system.
- Because urine drains almost continuously from a ureterostomy, there is risk for skin breakdown around a stoma site.
- A primary function of the elimination process is fluid balance.

CRITICAL THINKING EXERCISES

Even though her dribbling has lessened, Mrs. Vallero indicates that she is afraid of urinating in the bed during the night. She tells Sandy that she has fallen numerous times in the past and that "I had to go so quickly last night I almost fell." She also indicates that she has limited her outside activities because of being afraid of "having an accident and wetting myself." She says that nothing can be done for her because the "dribbling and falling are a normal part of getting old."

1. Formulate a priority nursing diagnosis for the patient and a corresponding goal.
2. Develop a corresponding plan of care for question 1.
3. How would you respond to the patient's statement that the urinary incontinence, urinary frequency, and falling are a normal part of aging?
4. What health teaching could you implement for Mrs. Vallero?

ⓔvolve   *Answers to Critical Thinking Questions can be found on the Evolve website.*

REVIEW QUESTIONS

1. The nurse notes that the patient's Foley catheter bag has remained empty for 3 hours. The nurse would first:
   1. Notify the health care provider
   2. Increase the patient's fluid intake
   3. Make sure the balloon is inflated
   4. Check for kinks in the tubing

2. The nurse is instructing nursing assistive personnel (NAP) about procedures related to Foley catheters on the clinical unit. The nurse evaluates that the NAP understands catheter-related procedures when the NAP states:
   1. "Collection bags should be emptied at least every 8 hours."
   2. "Perineal and catheter care is given daily as a part of AM care."
   3. "A urine specimen for culture and sensitivity is routinely obtained from the drainage bag."
   4. "Urinary drainage bags should be waist level when the patient ambulates."

3. A 75-year-old man is comatose and frequently incontinent following a stroke. Which would be the most appropriate action to promote continence?
   1. Place a urinal in between his legs when in bed.
   2. Perform intermittent catheterizations.
   3. Decrease fluid intake at night.
   4. Place a condom catheter.

4. Credé's method would be beneficial for the patient who:
   1. Complains the bladder is full, but cannot void
   2. Is incontinent associated with laughing or coughing
   3. Has unpredictable, involuntary passage of urine
   4. Has a sudden overwhelming urge to urinate

5. Which is a nursing priority when caring for a patient with a condom catheter?
   1. Changing the condom catheter every 2 days
   2. Keeping the tubing from kinking to promote urinary drainage
   3. Using sterile technique when placing the condom
   4. Making sure the securing adhesive is tight to prevent condom from falling off

6. An older adult male patient states he is having problems starting and stopping his stream of urine and he feels an urgency to void. The best way to assist this patient is to:
   1. Get a bedside commode
   2. Provide a condom catheter
   3. Teach him Credé's method
   4. Reinforce the use of Kegel exercises

7. A male patient returned from the operating room 6 hours ago with a cast on his right arm. He has not yet voided. Which action would be the most beneficial in assisting the patient to void?
   1. Suggest he stand at the bedside to void.
   2. Stay with the patient while he attempts to urinate.
   3. Give him the urinal to use in bed.
   4. Tell him if he does not urinate, he will be catheterized.

8. The nurse directs a NAP to remove a Foley catheter at 1000. The nurse would notify the health care provider if the patient is unable to void by:
   1. 1100
   2. 1300
   3. 1500
   4. 1800

9. The patient verbalizes being "uncomfortable." The nurse palpates the bladder and notes it is distended. There is an order to catheterize the patient as necessary and an order to administer pain medication. The best action by the nurse would be to first:
   1. Implement measures to stimulate voiding
   2. Catheterize the patient and record the amount of urine obtained
   3. Administer pain medication
   4. Notify the health care provider to verify the order

Answers to Review Questions can be found on pages 1197-1198.

REFERENCES

Bulechek GM and others, editors: *Nursing interventions classifications (NIC)*, ed 5, 2008, Mosby

Cochran S: Care of the indwelling urinary catheter: Is it evidenced based? *J Wound Ostomy Continence Nurs* 34(3):282, 2007.

Colwell J and others: *Fecal and urinary diversions: management principles*, St. Louis, 2004, Mosby.

Daneshgari F and others: Evidence-based multidisciplinary practice: improving the safety and standards of male bladder catheterization, *Medsurg Nurs* 11(5):236, 2002.

Emr K, Ryan R: Best practices for indwelling catheter in the home setting, *Home Heathc Nurse* 22(12):820, 2004.

Gokula RR and others: Inappropriate use of urinary catheters in elderly patients at a Midwestern community hospital, *Am J Infect Control* 32:196, 2004.

Gray M: What nursing interventions reduce the risk of symptomatic urinary tract infection in the patient with an indwelling catheter, *J Wound Ostomy Continence Nurs* 31(1):3, 2004.

Gray M: Expert review: best practices in managing the indwelling catheter, *Perspectives* 25(1):1, 2006.

Hart S: Urinary catheterization, *Nurs Stand* 22(27):44, 2008.

Holroyd-Leduc JM and others: The relationship of indwelling urinary catheters to death, length of hospital stay, functional decline, and nursing home admission in hospitalized older medical patients, *J Am Geriatr Soc* 55(2):227, 2007.

Huether SE, McCance KL: *Understanding pathophysiology*, ed 4, St. Louis, 2008, Mosby.

Leaver R: The evidence for urethral meatal cleansing, *Nurs Stand* 21(41):39, 2007.

Lekan-Rutledge D, Colling J: Urinary incontinence in the frail elderly, *Am J Nurs* 103(Suppl 3):36S, 2003.

Lewis SM and others: *Medical-surgical nursing*, ed 7, St. Louis, 2007, Mosby.

Macaulay M and others: A pilot study to evaluate reusable absorbent body-worn products for adults with moderate/heavy urinary incontinence, *J Wound Ostomy Continence Nurs* 31(6):357, 2004.

Madineh SMA: Avicenna's cannon of medicine and modern urology, *Urol J* 5(4):284, 2008.

Mason DJ and others: Changing UI practice, *Am J Nurs* 103(Suppl 3):2S, 2003.

Mauk KL: Conservative therapy for urinary incontinence can help older adults, *Nursing* 35(8):20, 2005.

McKenry LM and others: *Mosby's pharmacology in nursing*, ed 22, St. Louis, 2005, Mosby.

McKertich K: Urinary incontinence, *Aust Fam Physician* 37(3):112, 2008.

Mehnert-Kay S: Diagnosis and management of uncomplicated urinary tract infection, *Am Fam Physician* 72(3):451, 2005.

Mercer Smith J: Indwelling catheter management: from habit-based to evidence-based practice, *Ostomy Wound Mange* 49(12):34, 2003.

Milne JL: Behavioral therapies at the primary care level: the current state of knowledge, *J Wound Ostomy Continence Nurs* 31(6):367, 2004.

Moorhead S and others, editors: *Nursing outcomes classification (NOC)*, ed 4, St. Louis, 2008, Mosby.

Newman D: Incontinence products and devices for the elderly, *Urol Nurs* 24(4):316, 2004.

Newman DK and others: Innovation in bladder assessment: use of technology in extended care, *J Gerontol Nurs* 12:33, 2005.

Palmer MH, Newman DK: Bladder matters: urinary incontinence in nursing homes, *Am J Nurs* 104(11):57, 2004.

Parker D and others: Nursing interventions to reduce the risk of catheter-associated urinary tract infection, *J Wound Ostomy Continence Nurs* 36(1):23, 2009.

Ritin F and others: Duration of short-term indwelling catheters: a systematic review of the evidence, *J Wound Ostomy Continence Nurs* 33(2):145, 2006.

Robinson J: Deflation of a Foley catheter balloon, *Nurs Standard* 17(27):33-38, 2003.

Sampselle CM: Behavioral interventions in young and middle-aged women, *Am J Nurs* 103(Suppl 3):9S, 2003.

Senese V: Secrets revealed for male catheterization, *Urol Nurs* 24(2):78, 2004.

Senese V and others: SUNA clinical practice guidelines: care of the patient with an indwelling catheter, *Urol Nurs* 26(1):80, 2006a.

Senese V and others: SUNA clinical practice guidelines: female urethral catheterization, *Urol Nurs* 26(4):314, 2006b.

Senese V and others: SUNA clinical practice guidelines: male urethral catheterization, *Urol Nurs* 26(4):315, 2006c.

Smith JM: Current concepts in catheter management. In Doughty DB: *Urinary and fecal incontinence: current management concepts*, ed 3, St. Louis, 2006, Mosby.

Sorrentino S: *Mosby's textbook for nursing assistants*, St. Louis, 2004, Mosby.

Specht JKP: Nine myths of incontinence in older adults, *Am J Nurs* 105(6):58, 2005.

The Joint Commission: *National Patient Safety Goals*, 2009, http://www.jointcommission.org/PatientSafety/NationalPatientSafetyGoals.

Toughill E: Indwelling urinary catheters: common mechanical and pathogenic problems, *Am J Nurs* 105(5):35, 2005.

Urodynamic testing, October 10, 2008, htpp://www.kidney.niddk.nih.gov/kudiseases/pdf/UrodynamicTesting.pdf, accessed December 23, 2008.

Wareing M: Urinary retention: issues of management and care, *Emerg Nurse* 11(8):24, 2003.

Wound, Ostomy and Continence Nurses Society: *Stoma complications: best practice for clinicians*, Glenview, Ill, 2005, The Society.

Wyman JF: Treatment of urinary incontinence in men and older women, *Am J Nurs* 103(Suppl 3):26S, 2003.

Bowel Elimination

MEDIA RESOURCES

 CD COMPANION 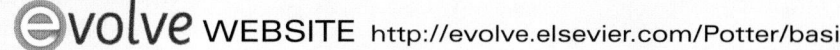 **WEBSITE** http://evolve.elsevier.com/Potter/basic

- Video Clips
- Crossword Puzzle
- English/Spanish Audio Glossary

OBJECTIVES

- Explain the physiology of digestion, absorption, and bowel elimination.
- Discuss physiological and psychological factors that influence bowel elimination.
- Describe common physiological alterations in bowel elimination.
- Assess a patient's bowel elimination pattern.
- Perform a fecal occult blood test.
- List nursing diagnoses related to alterations in bowel elimination.

- Describe nursing implications for common diagnostic examinations of the gastrointestinal tract.
- Administer an enema.
- List nursing measures aimed at promoting normal elimination and defecation.
- Describe nursing care required to maintain structure and function of a bowel diversion.
- Insert a nasogastric tube.

KEY TERMS

cathartics, p. 1007
chyme, p. 988
colon, p. 989
constipation, p. 990
defecation, p. 990
diarrhea, p. 992
enema, p. 1008

fecal impaction, p. 990
fecal incontinence, p. 992
fecal occult blood test (FOBT), p. 1000

feces, p. 990
flatus, p. 989
hemorrhoids, p. 992
laxatives, p. 1007
melena, p. 1000
ostomy, p. 993

peristalsis, p. 988
segmentation, p. 988
stoma, p. 992
Valsalva maneuver, p. 990

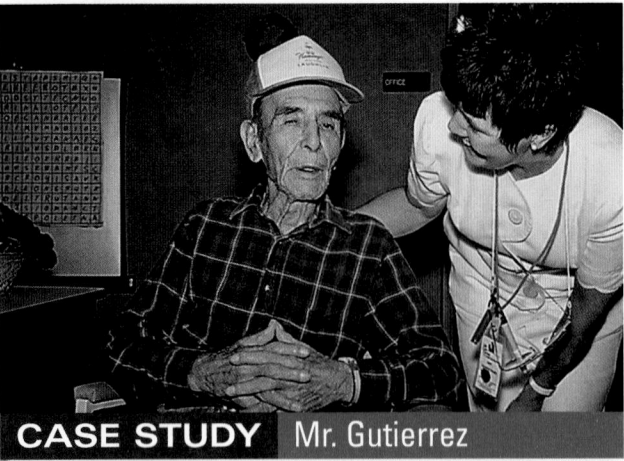

CASE STUDY   Mr. Gutierrez

Mr. Gutierrez resides in an assisted living apartment of a long-term care center. He keeps busy in his small garden plot and enjoys other activities of the center, such as nightly card/bingo games and outings to major league baseball games and local museums. He is 82 years old and widowed and has lived in this area of the care center for over 3 years. His family, with whom he is quite close, is scattered across the country. He has one niece who lives in the same town. Mr. Gutierrez feels he is in good health. As long as he eats green chili peppers every day, he believes he will remain healthy. Because he has a small kitchen in his apartment, he is able to make some of his favorite foods. His diet consists of flour and corn tortillas, beans, and rice. He likes most meats, but he prefers chicken and *asado* (made with pork). For breakfast, he usually has huevos rancheros. He has been hospitalized only twice, once for the flu and once for placement of a pacemaker. He presently takes three medications: digoxin, Zestril, and Metamucil.

This afternoon Mr. Gutierrez has telephoned his niece for the fourth time. Mr. Gutierrez reports, "My bowels are locked up and haven't moved in the last 2 days." He ate a big meal the previous evening and now reports feeling "all gassed up." His niece tried to explain about eating foods containing fiber and more vegetables. She reminded Mr. Gutierrez that the nursing student was coming later this afternoon and he could talk to the student about his problem.

Vickie is the nursing student assigned to Mr. Gutierrez. She has been seeing Mr. Gutierrez once a week for 5 weeks as a portion of a home health care clinical experience. They have developed a good rapport. Mr. Gutierrez's self-identified problems with his bowels are a frequent topic of conversation.

Regular bowel elimination is essential to maintain a healthy body. Alterations in bowel elimination are often early signs or symptoms of problems within either the gastrointestinal (GI) or other body systems. Because bowel function depends on the balance of several factors, elimination patterns and habits vary among individuals.

Although such drugs are often considered a common and expected occurrence in the older adult, individuals of any age sometimes experience changes in intestinal elimination. These changes are often the result of illness, diagnostic testing, the aging process, or surgical intervention. Alterations in intestinal elimination respond to both preventive and supportive nursing care.

SCIENTIFIC KNOWLEDGE BASE

Anatomy and Physiology of the Gastrointestinal Tract

The GI tract is a series of hollow mucous membrane–lined muscular organs that begin at the mouth and end at the anal orifice. The functions of the GI tract are to break down ingested food for use by the body's cells and to promote the absorption of fluid and nutrients. The GI tract is a complex system, and changes in any one area alter total body functioning.

MOUTH   The mouth mechanically and chemically breaks down nutrients into usable size and form. The teeth chew food, breaking it down into a size suitable for swallowing. Saliva, produced by the salivary glands in the mouth, dilutes and softens the food in the mouth for easier swallowing. Digestion begins in the mouth and ends in the small intestine.

ESOPHAGUS   As food enters the upper esophagus, it passes through the upper esophageal sphincter, a circular muscle that prevents air from entering the esophagus and food from refluxing into the throat. The bolus of food travels down the esophagus and **peristalsis,** contractions that propel food through the length of the GI tract, pushes the food.

The food moves down the esophagus and reaches the cardiac sphincter, which lies between the esophagus and the upper end of the stomach. The sphincter prevents reflux of stomach contents back into the esophagus.

STOMACH   The stomach performs three tasks: the storage of the swallowed food and liquid; the mixing of food, liquid, and digestive juices; and the emptying of its contents into the small intestine. The stomach produces and secretes hydrochloric acid (HCl), mucus, the enzyme pepsin, and intrinsic factor. Pepsin and HCl facilitate the digestion of protein. Mucus protects the stomach mucosa from acidity and enzyme activity. Intrinsic factor is essential in the absorption of vitamin B_{12}.

SMALL INTESTINE   Movement within the small intestine, occurring by both **segmentation** and peristalsis (Figure 34-1), facilitates both digestion and absorption. **Chyme**, a semifluid material, mixes with digestive juices. Reabsorption in the small intestine is so efficient that by the time the chyme reaches the end of the small intestine, it is pastelike in consistency. The small intestine is divided into three sections: the duodenum, the jejunum, and the ileum.

The duodenum is approximately 8 to 11 inches long and continues to process the chyme from the stomach. The second section, the jejunum, is approximately 8 feet long and absorbs carbohydrates and proteins. The ileum is approximately 12 feet long and absorbs water, fats, and bile salts. The duodenum and jejunum absorb most nutrients and electrolytes in the small intestine. The ileum absorbs certain vitamins, iron, and bile salts.

When small intestine function is impaired, this greatly alters the digestive process. Conditions such as inflammation, surgical resection, or obstruction disrupt peristalsis, reduce the area of absorption, or block the passage of chyme. Electrolyte and nutrient deficiencies then develop.

LARGE INTESTINE   The lower GI tract is called the large intestine (**colon**) because it is larger in diameter than the small intestine. However, its length (1.5 to 1.8 m [5 to 6 feet]) is much shorter. The large intestine is divided into the cecum, colon, and rectum (Figure 34-2). The large intestine is the primary organ of bowel elimination.

Chyme enters the large intestine by waves of peristalsis through the ileocecal valve, a circular muscle layer that prevents regurgitation. The colon is divided into the ascending, transverse, descending, and sigmoid colons. The colon's muscular tissue allows it to accommodate and eliminate large quantities of waste and gas (**flatus**). The colon has three functions: absorption, secretion, and elimination. The colon absorbs a large volume of water (up to 1.5 L) and significant amounts of sodium and chloride daily (Doughty, 2006). The amount of water absorbed from chyme depends on the speed at which colonic contents move. Chyme is normally a soft, formed mass. If peristalsis is abnormally fast, there is less time for water to be absorbed and the stool will be watery. If peristaltic contractions slow down, water continues to be absorbed and a hard mass of stool forms, resulting in constipation.

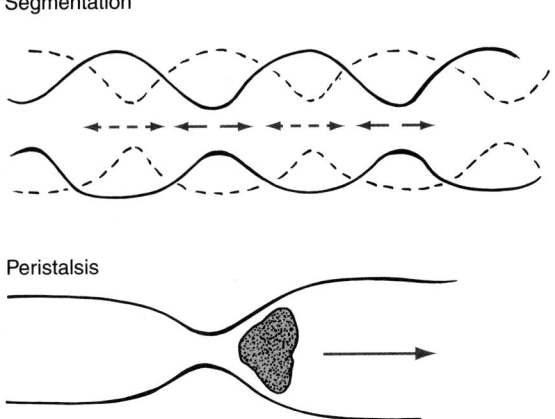

Segmentation

Peristalsis

Figure 34-1 ■ Segmented and peristaltic waves.

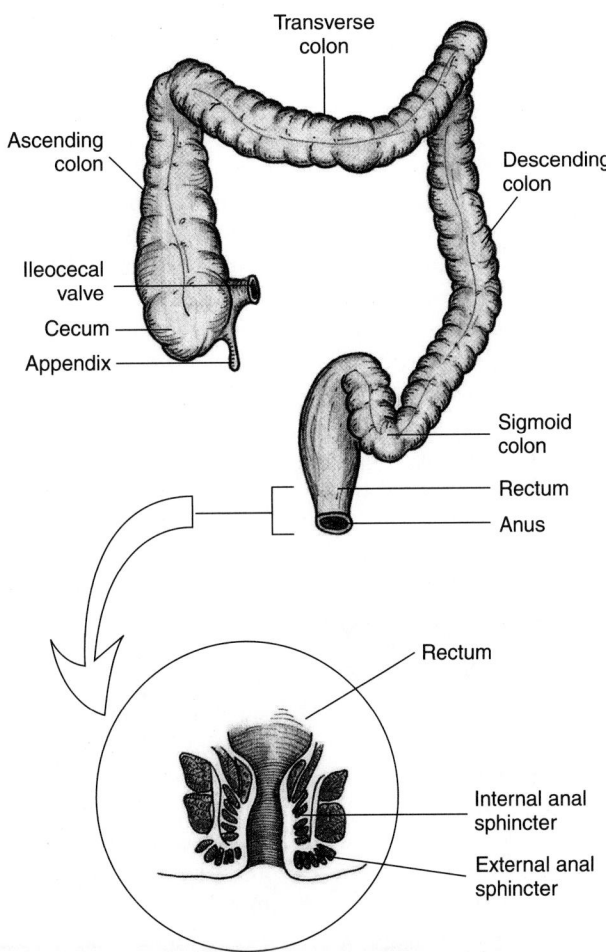

Transverse colon

Ascending colon

Descending colon

Ileocecal valve

Cecum

Appendix

Sigmoid colon

Rectum

Anus

Rectum

Internal anal sphincter

External anal sphincter

Figure 34-2 ■ Divisions of the large intestine.

The secretory function of the colon aids in electrolyte balance. Bicarbonate is secreted in exchange for chloride. About 4 to 9 mEq of potassium is also excreted daily. Serious alterations in colon function (e.g., diarrhea) cause severe electrolyte disturbances.

Slow peristaltic contractions move contents through the colon. Intestinal content is the main stimulus for contraction. Mass peristalsis pushes undigested food toward the rectum. These mass movements occur only three or four times daily, with the strongest during the hour after mealtime.

The rectum is the final portion of the large intestine. Normally, the rectum is empty of waste products (**feces**) until just before defecation. The rectum contains vertical and transverse folds of tissue that help to temporarily hold fecal contents during **defecation.** Each fold contains an artery and veins that can become distended from pressure during straining. This distention results in hemorrhoid formation.

ANUS The body expels feces and flatus (gas) from the rectum through the anal canal and anus. Contraction and relaxation of the internal and external sphincters, innervated by sympathetic and parasympathetic stimuli, aid in the control of defecation. The anal canal contains a rich supply of sensory nerves that help to control continence.

DEFECATION The physiological factors critical to bowel function and defecation include normal GI tract function, sensory awareness of rectal distention and rectal contents, voluntary sphincter control, and adequate rectal capacity and compliance (Doughty, 2006). Normal defecation begins with movement in the left colon, moving stool toward the anus. When stool reaches the rectum, the distention causes relaxation of the internal sphincter and an awareness of the need to defecate. At the time of defecation, the external sphincter relaxes and abdominal muscles contract, increasing intrarectal pressure and forcing the stool out (Doughty, 2006). Normally defecation is painless, resulting in passage of soft, formed stool. However, at times pressure is exerted to expel feces through voluntary contractions of the abdominal muscles while maintaining forced expiration against a closed airway. This is termed the **Valsalva maneuver,** and it assists in stool passage. When a person strains, this maneuver traps the blood in veins within the chest, and upon relaxing the venous blood rushes to the heart. The Valsalva maneuver also traps blood in the veins of the abdomen, causing increases in intraabdominal pressure.

NURSING KNOWLEDGE BASE

To manage your patient's elimination problems, you need to understand normal elimination and factors that promote, impede, or cause alterations in elimination, such as constipation, diarrhea, and fecal incontinence (Box 34-1). Supportive nursing care respects the patient's privacy and emotional needs. In addition, interventions designed to promote normal bowel elimination will also minimize discomfort.

Any alteration in bowel elimination is embarrassing for a patient. Because of the sensitivity many patients experience regarding bowel elimination with its associated sounds and odors, be very sensitive to how you communicate, especially nonverbally. The patient may perceive changes in facial expression as disgust. Also, be aware of the patient's need for privacy during elimination.

Patients with chronic diseases of the GI system often have numerous hospitalizations, perhaps multiple surgeries, and significant changes in eating habits and lifestyles. They are often on complicated medication schedules that are taxing both physically and financially. Their desire for wellness sometimes leads them to consider alternative forms of medical treatment, such as vitamin or herbal supplements. Always remain accepting of a patient's health care choices.

Some patients with chronic GI diseases require an ostomy, which involves the surgical creation of a stoma on the abdomen for the passage of stool. An ostomy results in body image changes, with patients losing control over a very basic body function. Even though clothing conceals an ostomy, the patient feels different. The idea of being different or not a whole person affects the patient's social interaction with others, resulting in isolation. Some patients have difficulty maintaining or initiating normal sexual relations. One important factor in the patient's acceptance of this change in body functioning is the ability to control fecal secretions. Foul odors, spillage, leakage of liquid stools, and the inability to regulate bowel movements further place the patient at risk for loss of self-esteem.

Common Bowel Elimination Problems

Alteration in bowel elimination results from a variety of factors. Below is a discussion of some of the more common alterations.

CONSTIPATION Constipation is a symptom, not a disease (Box 34-2). Common causes of constipation include changes in diet, medications, inflammation, environmental factors (e.g., unavailability of toilet facilities or lack of privacy), and lack of knowledge about regular bowel habits. Regardless of etiology, intestinal motility slows, causing prolonged exposure of the fecal mass to the intestinal walls. Fecal water continues to be absorbed, leaving the stool hard and underlubricated.

Constipation is a significant health hazard. Straining during defecation causes problems for patients with recent abdominal, gynecological, or rectal surgery. An effort to pass a stool can cause sutures to separate, reopening a wound. In addition, patients with cardiovascular disease, diseases causing elevated intraocular pressure (glaucoma), and increased intracranial pressure need to prevent constipation and avoid using the Valsalva maneuver.

IMPACTION Fecal impaction results from unrelieved constipation. The patient is unable to expel the hardened feces wedged in the rectum. In severe impaction, the hardened fecal mass extends up into the sigmoid colon. Patients at greatest risk for impaction include those who are confused or unconscious, weak, or unaware of the need to defecate or those who have experienced an interruption in nerve supply to the bowel.

BOX 34-1   Factors Influencing Bowel Elimination

AGE

- Infants have a smaller stomach capacity, less secretion of digestive enzymes, and more rapid intestinal peristalsis. The ability to control defecation does not occur until 2 to 3 years of age.
- Adolescents experience rapid growth and increased metabolic rate. There is also rapid growth of the large intestine and increased secretion of gastric acids to dissolve food fibers and act as a bactericide against swallowed organisms.
- Older adults have decreased chewing ability. Partially chewed food is not digested as easily. Peristalsis declines, and esophageal emptying slows. This impairs absorption by the intestinal mucosa. Muscle tone in the perineal floor and anal sphincter weakens, causing difficulty in controlling defecation (see Box 34-2) (Hall and others, 2007).

DIET

- Regular daily food intake promotes peristalsis.
- High-fiber foods such as raw fruits, cooked fruits, greens, raw vegetables, and whole grains (cereals and breads) promote peristalsis and defecation by creating bulk.
- Low-fiber foods (e.g., pasta, lean meats, milk) slow peristalsis.
- Gas-producing foods (e.g., broccoli, cauliflower, onions, dried beans) stimulate peristalsis.
- Persons with lactose intolerance lack the enzyme lactase, which is needed to digest the simple sugars in milk. Such intolerance leads to diarrhea and cramping.

POSITION DURING DEFECATION

- Squatting allows a person to lean forward, exert intraabdominal pressure, and contract thigh muscles for normal defecation.
- Older adults or those with arthritis are sometimes unable to rise from a toilet seat.
- Immobilized patients, required to use a bedpan while lying down, cannot contract muscles to defecate.

PREGNANCY

- As pregnancy advances and the fetus enlarges, this exerts pressure on the rectum. Constipation commonly occurs.

DIAGNOSTIC TESTS

- Certain examinations involving visualization of GI structures require the emptying of bowel contents. Patients receive nothing by mouth (NPO), bowel evacuants, and enema administration to cleanse the bowel before a test. These factors interfere with normal elimination.
- Barium examinations require ingestion of barium, a mixture that hardens and causes serious constipation unless eliminated soon after a test.

FLUID INTAKE

- The body absorbs fluid into the fecal mass and increases bulk for easier passage.
- Warm beverages and fruit juices soften stool and increase peristalsis.
- Large quantities of milk slow peristalsis and cause constipation.

ACTIVITY

- Immobilization depresses colon motility.
- Regular physical exercise promotes peristalsis.

PSYCHOLOGICAL FACTORS

- Stress, anxiety, or fear initiates parasympathetic impulses, causing the acceleration of digestion and peristalsis. Diarrhea and gaseous distention will result.
- Emotional depression decreases peristalsis and leads to constipation.

PERSONAL HABITS

- Personal habits such as failing to respond to the need to defecate and lack of privacy interfere with normal elimination patterns and lead to constipation.
- Hospitalized patients often share toilet facilities or use bedpans or bedside commodes. The resulting embarrassment causes them to ignore the urge to defecate.

PAIN

- Hemorrhoids, rectal surgery, and abdominal surgery cause a patient to suppress defecation because of pain; constipation develops.

MEDICATIONS

- Laxatives and cathartics soften stool and promote peristalsis.
- Antidiarrheal agents inhibit peristalsis.
- Narcotic analgesics, opiates, and anticholinergic drugs depress peristalsis and cause constipation.
- Antibiotics alter normal bowel flora and often produce diarrhea.
- Drugs that contain iron sometimes turn the stool black. Antacids cause a white discoloration. Anticoagulants can cause frank or occult blood in the stool.

SURGERY AND ANESTHESIA

- General anesthetics cause slowing or halting of peristalsis.
- Surgery involving bowel manipulation temporarily stops peristalsis (paralytic ileus) for 24 to 48 hours.

BOX 34-2 | Common Causes of Constipation

- Irregular bowel habits and ignoring the urge to defecate.
- Chronic illnesses (e.g., Parkinson's disease, multiple sclerosis, rheumatoid arthritis, chronic bowel diseases, depression, eating disorders) (Davis and others, 2007).
- Low-fiber diet high in animal fats (e.g., meats, dairy products, eggs) and refined sugars (rich desserts). Also, low fluid intake slows peristalsis (Amerine and Keirsey, 2006).
- Stress (e.g., illness of a family member, death of a loved one, divorce) (Davis and others, 2007).
- Lengthy bed rest or physical inactivity (Kyle, 2006).
- Heavy laxative use causes loss of normal defecation reflex. In addition, the lower colon is completely emptied, requiring time to refill with bulk (Heitkemper and Wolff, 2007).
- Older adults experience slowed peristalsis, loss of abdominal muscle elasticity, and reduced intestinal mucus secretion. Older adults often eat low-fiber foods (Kyle, 2006).
- Neurological conditions that block nerve impulses to the colon (e.g., spinal cord injury, tumor) (Hocevar and Gray, 2008).
- Organic illnesses such as hypothyroidism, hypocalcemia, or hypokalemia (Hill, 2007).

An obvious sign of impaction is the inability to pass a stool for several days, despite a repeated urge to defecate. When a continuous oozing of diarrhea stool develops, this indicates impaction. This diarrhea is liquid stool seeping around the fecal mass. Loss of appetite, abdominal distention and cramping, nausea and/or vomiting, and rectal pain also occur.

DIARRHEA **Diarrhea** is an increase in the number of stools and the passage of liquid, unformed stools (Table 34-1). It is associated with disorders affecting digestion, absorption, and secretion in the GI tract. Intestinal contents pass too quickly through the small intestine and colon to allow for the usual absorption of fluid and nutrients. Serious fluid and electrolyte and acid-base imbalances can result from diarrhea. Older adults and the very young are at the greatest risk for electrolyte imbalance. Because of the irritating effects of the intestinal contents, persistent diarrhea readily leads to skin breakdown in the perianal region.

A common cause of diarrhea in health care facilities is *Clostridium difficile*, in which symptoms range from mild to severe diarrhea. This infection is acquired in one of two ways, by factors that cause an overgrowth of *C. difficile* and by contact with the *C. difficile* organism (Harris, 2006). The organism is most commonly transmitted in hospitals and nursing homes through contact with infected surfaces. In addition, antibiotic therapy depresses natural intestinal flora, causing an overgrowth of *C. difficile*. The bacterium releases a toxin, which causes colonic epithelium necrosis resulting in severe diarrhea (Ignatavicius and Workman, 2006).

Communicable food-borne pathogens also cause diarrhea. Simple hand washing following the use of the bathroom, before and after meal preparation, and cleansing and storing fresh produce and meats helps reduce food-borne illnesses.

Fecal incontinence is the inability to control the passage of feces and gas from the anus. Incontinence harms a person's body image. Often a person is mentally alert but physically unable to avoid defecation. Some patients have little or no warning before the incontinence episode of loose, watery diarrhea presents itself. Physical conditions that impair anal sphincter function or control cause incontinence. Conditions that create frequent, loose, large-volume, watery stools also predispose to incontinence. Management of fecal incontinence requires a complete understanding of the causes. Incontinence affects patients in many ways. Because of the associated embarrassment, incontinence leads to social isolation, changes in body image and sexuality (see Chapter 22), and feelings of inadequacy or guilt. Like diarrhea, incontinence predisposes the patient to skin breakdown.

FLATULENCE Flatulence (gas) is one of the most common GI disorders. It refers to a sensation of bloating and abdominal distention accompanied by excess gas. As gas accumulates in the lumen of the intestines, the bowel wall stretches and distends. Normally, intestinal gas escapes through the mouth (belching) or the anus. However, when intestinal motility is reduced as a result of opiates, general anesthetics, abdominal surgery, or immobilization, flatulence becomes severe, causing abdominal distention and severe sharp pain.

HEMORRHOIDS **Hemorrhoids** are dilated, engorged veins in the lining of the rectum. Increased venous pressure resulting from straining at defecation, pregnancy, and chronic illnesses, such as congestive heart failure and chronic liver disease, are problems that lead to hemorrhoids. A hemorrhoid forms either within the anal canal (called internal) or through the opening of the anus (called external). Passage of hard stool causes hemorrhoid tissue to stretch and bleed. Hemorrhoid tissue becomes inflamed and tender, and patients complain of itching and burning. Because pain worsens during defecation, the patient sometimes ignores the urge to defecate, resulting in constipation.

BOWEL DIVERSIONS Certain diseases prevent the normal passage of intestinal contents throughout the small and large bowel. The treatment for these disorders results in the need for a temporary or permanent artificial opening (**stoma**) in the abdominal wall. Surgical openings are created in the ileum (ileostomy) or colon (colostomy) by bringing the end of the intestine through the abdominal wall to create the stoma.

The standard bowel diversion creates a stoma, or the patient has reconstructive bowel surgery that uses the native sphincter for continence. The reconstructive surgery that is most common is the ileoanal pouch anastomosis, which is described in a later section.

TABLE 34-1 Conditions That Cause Diarrhea

CONDITION	PHYSIOLOGICAL EFFECTS
Emotional stress (anxiety)	Increased intestinal motility
Intestinal infection (streptococcal or staphylococcal enteritis)	Inflammation of intestinal mucosa, increased mucus secretion in colon
Food allergies	Reduced digestion of food elements
Food intolerance (greasy foods, coffee, alcohol, spicy foods)	Increased intestinal motility, increased mucus secretion in colon
Tube feedings	Hyperosmolarity of some enteral solutions results in diarrhea, because hyperosmolar fluids draw fluids into the gastrointestinal tract
Medications	
Iron	Irritation of intestinal mucosa
Antibiotics	Superinfection allowing overgrowth of normal flora, inflammation and irritation of mucosa
Laxatives (short term)	Increased intestinal motility
Inflammatory bowel disease (colitis, Crohn's disease)	Inflammation and ulceration of intestinal walls, reduced absorption of fluids, increased intestinal motility
Surgical alterations	
Gastrectomy	Loss of reservoir function of stomach, improper absorption because food moves into duodenum too quickly
Colon resection	Reduced size of colon, reduced amount of absorptive surface

Ostomies The location of an **ostomy** determines stool consistency. The more intestine remaining, the more formed and normal the stool. For example, an ileostomy bypasses the entire large intestine, creating frequent, liquid stools. The sigmoid colostomy emits near-normal stool. The location of an ostomy depends on the patient's medical problem and general condition.

Loop colostomies are frequently performed on an emergency basis and are temporary large stomas constructed in the transverse colon (Figure 34-3). The surgeon pulls a loop of bowel onto the abdomen and places a plastic rod, bridge, or rubber catheter temporarily under the bowel loop to keep it from slipping back. The surgeon then opens the bowel and sutures it to the skin of the abdomen. The loop ostomy has two openings through the stoma. The proximal end drains stool, and the distal portion drains mucus.

The end colostomy consists of one stoma formed from the proximal end of the bowel with the distal portion of the GI tract either removed or sewn closed (called Hartmann's pouch) and left in the abdominal cavity. End colostomies are a surgical treatment for colorectal cancer. In such cases, the rectum is sometimes removed. Patients with diverticulitis often have a temporary end colostomy constructed with a Hartmann's pouch (Figure 34-4).

Unlike the loop colostomy, surgeons surgically sever the bowel in a double-barrel colostomy (Figure 34-5) and bring the two ends out onto the abdomen. The double-barrel colostomy consists of two distinct stomas: the proximal functioning stoma and the distal nonfunctioning stoma (mucous fistula).

Managing a stoma that produces frequent passage of liquid stool (e.g., an ileostomy) can be challenging. Skin protection is important because of the liquid and caustic nature of the output, which may cause contact dermatitis, fungal infec-

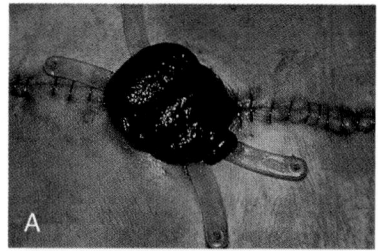

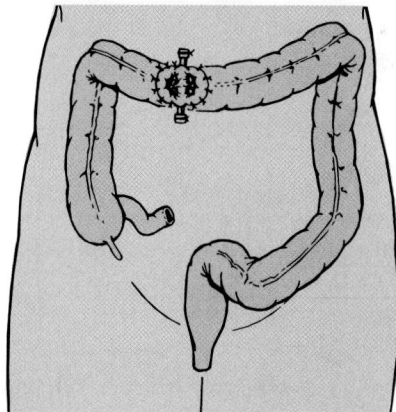

Figure 34-3 ■ **A,** A temporary transverse loop colostomy supported by a loop ostomy bridge. **B,** Abdominal view of loop colostomy in transverse colon. (**A** courtesy Hollister Incorporated, Libertyville, Ill. Permission to use this copyrighted material has been granted by the owner, Hollister Incorporated. **B** from Hampton BG, Bryant RA: *Ostomies and continent diversions: nursing management,* St. Louis, 1992, Mosby.)

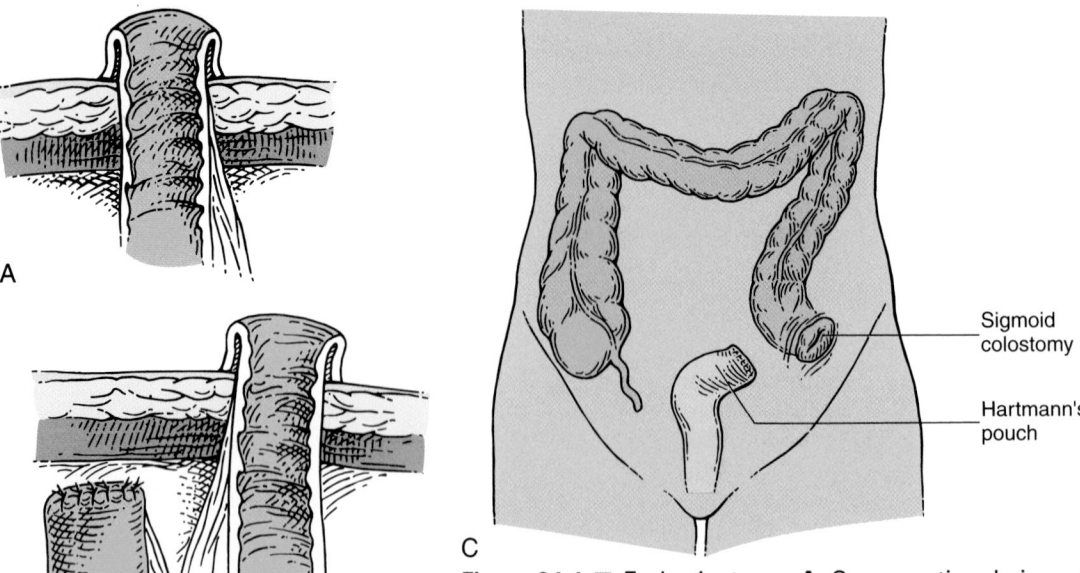

C

Figure 34-4 ■ End colostomy. **A,** Cross-sectional view of end stoma. **B,** Cross-sectional view of end stoma with distal bowel oversewn and secured to anterior peritoneum at stoma site. **C,** Sigmoid colostomy. Distal bowel is oversewn and left in place to create Hartmann's pouch. (From Hampton BG, Bryant RA: *Ostomies and continent diversions: nursing management,* St. Louis, 1992, Mosby.)

Sigmoid colostomy

Hartmann's pouch

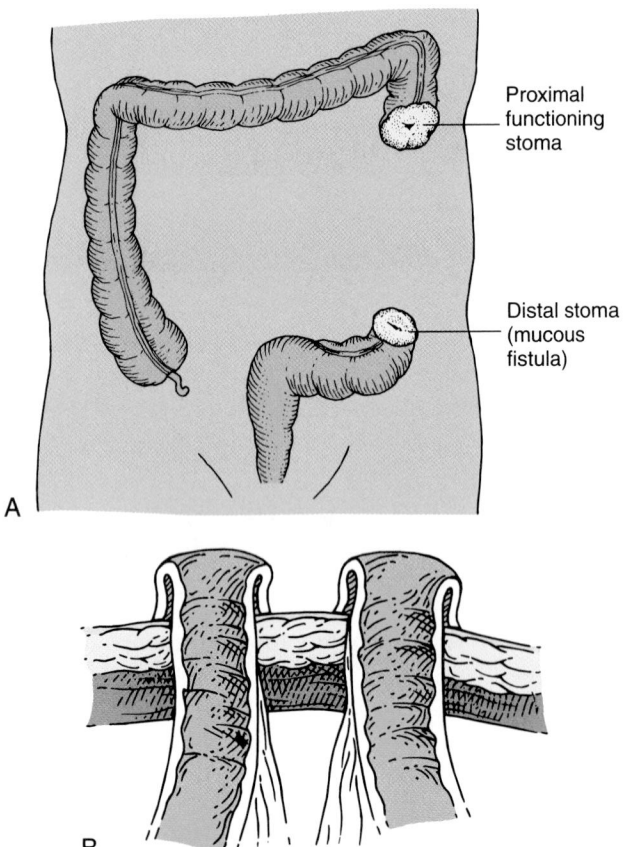

Proximal functioning stoma

Distal stoma (mucous fistula)

Figure 34-5 ■ Double-barrel colostomy. **A,** Double-barrel colostomy in the descending colon. **B,** Cross-sectional view of double-barrel stoma. (From Hampton BG, Bryant RA: *Ostomies and continent diversions: nursing management,* St. Louis, 1992, Mosby.)

tions, or folliculitis (Wound, Ostomy and Continence Nurses Society [WOCN], 2005). A pouch with a skin barrier surrounds the stoma. Empty the pouch several times a day. Change the pouching system approximately every 3 to 5 days, depending upon the type of system utilized.

Alternative Procedures The ileoanal pouch anastomosis is a surgical procedure that is an option for some patients who need to undergo a colectomy, removal of the colon, for treatment of ulcerative colitis or familial polyps. In this procedure the colon is removed, a pouch is created from the end of the small intestine, and the pouch is attached to the anus (Figure 34-6). The ileoanal pouch provides for collection of waste material in a fashion similar to the rectum. The patient is continent of stool because stool evacuates via the anus. When surgeons create the ileal pouch, they also make a temporary ileostomy to allow the pouch anastomosis to heal.

The Kock continent ileostomy involves creating a pouch from the small intestine (Figure 34-7). The Kock continent ileostomy is occasionally indicated for the treatment of ulcerative colitis. The pouch has a continent stoma, a type of nipple valve that drains only when the patient places an external catheter intermittently into the stoma. The patient empties the pouch several times a day.

The Macedo-Malone antegrade continence enema (MACE) procedure was developed to improve continence in patients with fecal soiling associated with neuropathic or structural abnormalities of the anal sphincter. This procedure isolates a 3-cm flap on the left colon. A Foley catheter placed on the surface of the flap creates a tubular passage. This produces a continence valve mechanism. The distal end of the tube is made into a V shape to the skin flap (Figure 34-8). Enema ad-

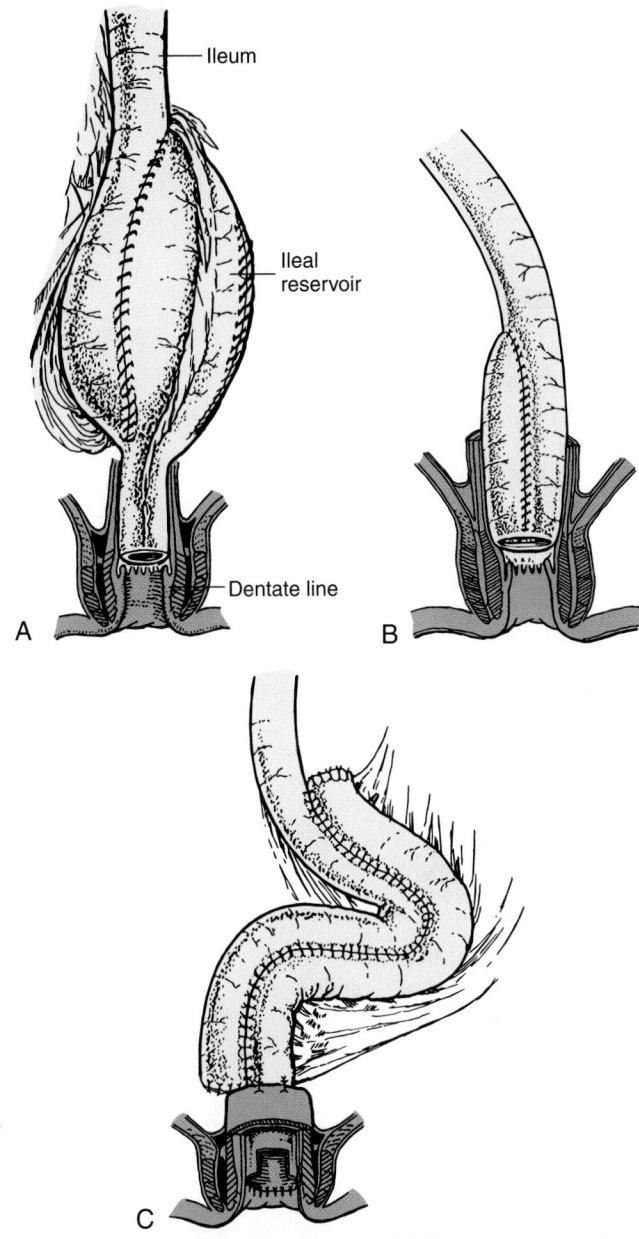

Figure 34-6 ■ Ileoanal reservoirs (IARs). **A,** S-shaped configuration. **B,** J-shaped configuration. **C,** Lateral or side-by-side ileoanal pouch configuration. (From Hampton BG, Bryant RA: *Ostomies and continent diversions: nursing management,* St. Louis, 1992, Mosby.)

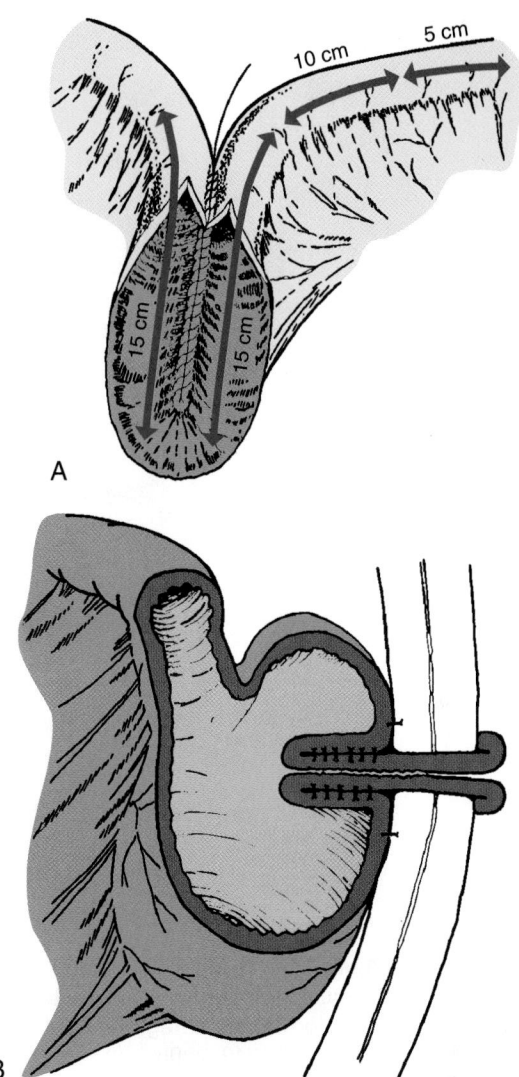

Figure 34-7 ■ Construction of Kock continent ileostomy—Kock pouch. **A,** Two 15-cm limbs are used to create pouch, and one 15-cm limb is used to fashion a nipple valve and stoma. **B,** Distal limb is intussuscepted into reservoir to create a one-way valve and accomplish continence. Sutures or staples or both are placed to stabilize and maintain nipple. Anterior surface of reservoir is anchored to anterior peritoneal wall. (From Hampton BG, Bryant RA: *Ostomies and continent diversions: nursing management,* St. Louis, 1992, Mosby.)

ministration begins 7 to 10 days after surgery. Colonic evacuation occurs within 60 minutes after the patient receives 250 to 800 mL of enema fluid (Calado and others, 2005).

CRITICAL THINKING

Synthesis

You will apply elements of critical thinking whenever you perform the nursing process with a patient. Consider the scientific knowledge you have learned, your experience, critical thinking attitudes, and standards to ensure an individualized approach to patient care (Box 34-3).

KNOWLEDGE Reflect on knowledge regarding normal anatomy and physiology of the GI tract, as well as knowledge regarding specific GI alterations. This information will help you more accurately focus your nursing assessment and identify alterations when they exist. Even insignificant alterations in bowel elimination produce significant health problems for the patient. For example, diarrhea leads to electrolyte imbalances, dehydration, and rectal soreness.

Abdominal pain is one of the most common complaints of patients who seek health care. Apply knowledge of the nature of pain (see Chapter 31) and pain assessment to analyze elimination problems. This helps in determining if the pain causes the symptoms associated with altered bowel

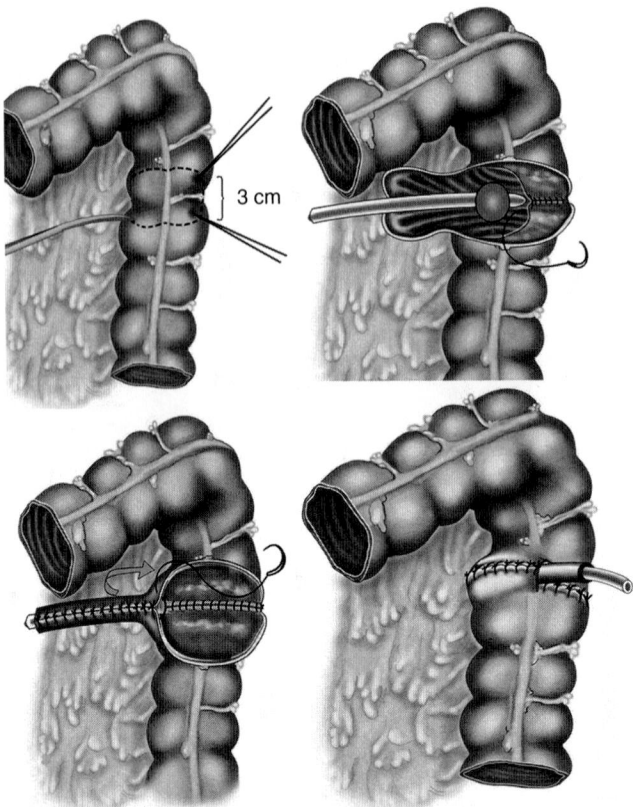

Figure 34-8 ■ Macedo-Malone antegrade continence enema (MACE) procedure. Surgical techniques. (Used with permission. From Calado A and others: The Macedo-Malone antegrade continence enema procedure: early experience, *J Urol* 173:1340, 2005.)

elimination or conversely if the bowel elimination problem results in pain or discomfort.

Functional bowel disorders make up the most frequently reported GI complaints. It is important that you have the knowledge from anatomy and physiology, as well as information from the psychosocial sciences, to understand and consider the psychological aspects associated with these diseases to provide appropriate care.

The intake of certain foods also reflects the patient's culture or beliefs. Foods in various cultures have different status relating to religion, availability, cost, and tradition. For example, some Hispanic Americans like Mr. Gutierrez use certain hot foods (e.g., chocolate, cheese, and eggs) for conditions producing fever, and cold foods (e.g., fresh vegetables, dairy foods, and honey) are for disorders such as cancer or headaches. Understand the patient's cultural heritage and the role diet plays in health promotion and maintenance (see Chapter 19).

When caring for patients from other cultures and ethnic groups, modifications of care are frequent. This is particu-

larly important when you care for patients' elimination needs (Box 34-4).

A final area of knowledge is an understanding of the changes that occur because of the aging process. Far too often nurses discount an older adult's problems with intestinal elimination as an everyday complaint. Remember that what appears at the outset to be quite insignificant is sometimes a major problem to the patient physically and psychologically.

EXPERIENCE Elimination alterations are common for many patients who seek health care. In the acute care environment numerous variables, including diet changes, medications, fluid restrictions, decreased activity, and diagnostic tests, cause major alterations to bowel function. You will provide better care to patients by reflecting on your previous experiences involving patients with similar alterations and similar lifestyle habits affecting elimination.

ATTITUDES Apply all of the attitudes of critical thinking when caring for a patient with elimination problems (see Chapter 7). Creativity comes into play, especially when patients need adjustments in their diet and exercise planning or

BOX 34-3   SYNTHESIS IN PRACTICE

As Vickie prepares to assess Mr. Gutierrez, she reflects back on experiences with other patients in the home setting. She recalled one patient in particular who had elimination problems resulting from a diet consisting mainly of high-fat and high-carbohydrate foods. She believes that her involvement with that patient is likely to help in the care of Mr. Gutierrez.

Vickie also reviews her class notes on the anatomy and physiology of the GI system. Given Mr. Gutierrez's age, Vickie reviews the physiological changes that aging produces within the GI system. These changes include loss of teeth, taste bud atrophy, decreased secretion of gastric acid, and a slight decrease in small intestine motility.

Vickie will thoroughly assess Mr. Gutierrez's dietary intake by using a 24-hour diet recall. Being familiar with Mr. Gutierrez's Hispanic heritage, Vickie anticipates certain food preferences and will need to assess these. Vickie knows Mr. Gutierrez does not like the food served at the long-term care center and frequently requests "home-cooked" tortillas and green chili peppers from his niece.

The symptoms Mr. Gutierrez exhibits, no bowel movement in 2 days and a feeling of bloating, are associated with several different problems. Vickie plans a thorough and precise assessment, being sure to rule out any abdominal discomfort or other symptoms expected from elimination problems. Because problems with bowel elimination have been an ongoing concern for Mr. Gutierrez, Vickie will persevere as she begins to identify nursing diagnoses and outline goals of care. Vickie will need to avoid preconceived ideas regarding constipation in older adults. She will remain open to all of the possibilities concerning changes in GI functioning.

BOX 34-4   CULTURAL FOCUS

As Vickie prepares to care for Mr. Gutierrez, she learns that people from different cultures have different beliefs and practices. She knows that Mr. Gutierrez keeps many of his cultural practices, and it is important that she understand early in his care how his culture and customs may impact her care plan. Elimination needs are very personal, and Vickie knows she needs to respect and be sensitive to her patient's elimination practices.

IMPLICATIONS FOR PRACTICE
- Accommodate need for gender-congruent care among cultures emphasizing separate gender roles and female modesty such as African, Hispanic, Asian, Islamic, Arabic, Hindu, Jewish Orthodox, and Amish cultures.
- In any culture the presence and care of an ostomy presents unique challenges. New ostomies require monitoring and observation, and patients from other cultures may find this more invasive and embarrassing.
- Most cultures consider bowel and urinary secretions as not fit for public display. However, exposure of the lower torso, which is needed for ostomy care, is generally avoided among Asians, Africans, Hispanics, Hindus, Muslims, Arabic, Orthodox Jewish, and Amish groups.
- When caring for patients with ostomies from these cultures, it is helpful to assign gender-congruent caregivers if possible and to allow presence of a family member if requested by the patient.
- Provide for hygiene needs of patients.
- Distinct hygienic practices are observed by certain cultures such as Hindus and Muslims that designate the left hand to perform unclean procedures such as bowel elimination. Wash your hands thoroughly before touching the patient, and use your left hand when possible.
- Promote patients' understanding of the procedure to be done.
- Use an interpreter if needed.
- Repeat explanations because patient's anxiety about the loss of privacy can pose a distraction.

when caring for patients with a bowel diversion. Similarly, perseverance is important in selecting effective diet therapies and in finding the best appliances for patients with ostomies. Confidence is an important factor in providing care to patients with bowel diversions or resections. Often these patients are very ill and in significant pain. Your confidence with moving and positioning the patient, handling stoma supplies, and managing pain will place the patient at ease and facilitate the recovery process.

STANDARDS To establish regular bowel habits, patients require consistency in bowel care and training. It is possible to establish regular bowel habits by setting standards for appropriate nutritional and elimination support. For example, the Association for Parenteral and Enteral Nutrition (ASPEN) has specific guidelines for nutritional support (see Chapter 32). The Wound, Ostomy and Continence Nurses Society (2005) has specific standards for ostomy care. Regardless of age or disease state, maintenance of bowel function and integrity is essential to well-being.

When assessing a patient's abdominal pain, make sure your findings are specific, clear, precise, and accurate. Although the intellectual standards for critical thinking apply to all symptoms, thorough pain assessment is critical. Multitudes of problems are detectable based on the nature of abdominal pain. Collaborate with health care providers as you assess your patients and identify appropriate plans of care.

Patients with alterations in bowel elimination, especially incontinence, are at risk for ridicule and shame on the part of some health care providers. This is especially true for providers with limited educational experience, to whom the task of patient hygiene is often delegated. It is your responsibility to make certain such individuals understand the needs of your patients and attend to their needs in a respectful way.

NURSING PROCESS

The needs and problems of patients experiencing alterations in bowel elimination are distinct and numerous. Incorporate a caring approach and use appropriate communication techniques throughout the nursing process.

■■■ASSESSMENT

Assessment of bowel elimination requires you to focus on any problems the patient has affecting the GI system. Because the patient's chewing ability, recent intake of both solids and liquids, personal eating habits, and level of stress all influence bowel function, include this information in your assessment (Davis and others, 2007).

HEALTH HISTORY In determining the patient's bowel habits, remember "normal" is unique to each individual. Apply this knowledge in preparing questions for the patient interview to determine the presence and extent of GI alterations. Family members are usually helpful if the patient is unable to provide necessary information. Organize much of the nursing history around factors that affect bowel elimination (Davis and others, 2007):

1. Determine your patient's usual pattern of bowel elimination. Usual frequency and time of day are important, but also determine if any changes in elimination patterns have occurred. Ask the patient to make suggestions about the reason for any change.
2. Get the patient's description of usual characteristics of stool. Determine if the stool is normally watery or formed, soft or hard, and the typical color. Ask the patient to describe a normal stool's shape and the number of stools per day. Use a scale such as the Bristol Stool

Form Scale to get an objective measure of stool characteristics (Figure 34-9).

3. Identify specific routines followed to promote normal elimination. Examples are drinking warm liquids, laxatives, eating specific foods, or taking time to defecate during a certain part of the day. If your patient uses a specific routine that is appropriate, consider incorporating the routine in your plan of care.
4. Assess the use of artificial aids at home, for example, the use of enemas, laxatives, or special foods before having a bowel movement. Ask how often the patient uses them.
5. Determine the presence of any bowel diversions. If the patient has an ostomy, assess the frequency of fecal drainage, character of feces, type of appliance used, and methods used to maintain the ostomy function.
6. Identify changes in appetite. Include changes in your patient's eating patterns and a change in weight, either loss or gain. If a change in weight is present, inquire if the patient planned the weight change, such as weight loss with a diet.
7. Ask about diet history, including the patient's dietary preferences. Is mealtime regular or irregular, and does the patient eat certain foods infrequently? This enables you to determine the intake of grains, fruits, meats, and vegetables.
8. Get a description of daily fluid intake. This includes the type and amount of fluid. Have the patient estimate the amount using common household measurements. You can ask the patient to give you a 24-hour diet recall during your assessment. You may also want to ask the patient to complete a 72-hour food intake diary for the next visit.

The Bristol Stool Form Scale

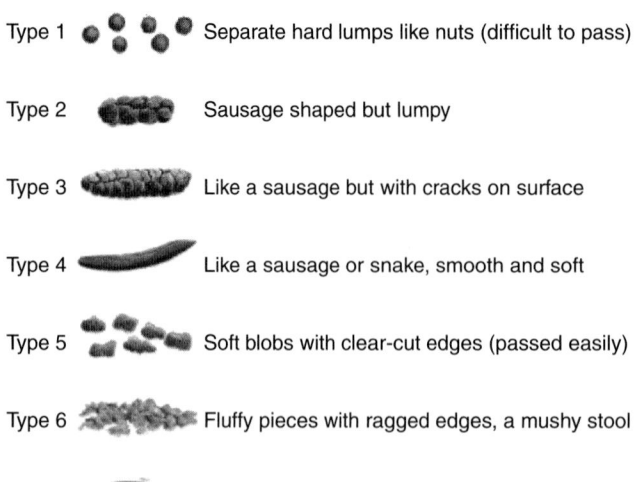

Type 1		Separate hard lumps like nuts (difficult to pass)
Type 2		Sausage shaped but lumpy
Type 3		Like a sausage but with cracks on surface
Type 4		Like a sausage or snake, smooth and soft
Type 5		Soft blobs with clear-cut edges (passed easily)
Type 6		Fluffy pieces with ragged edges, a mushy stool
Type 7		Watery, no solid pieces (entirely liquid)

Figure 34-9 ■ The Bristol Stool Form Scale. (Used with permission. *Bristol Stool Form Scale guideline,* http://about-constipation.org/site/about-constipation/treatment/stool-form-guide, accessed April 24, 2009.)

9. Obtain a history of surgery or illnesses affecting the GI tract. This information often helps to explain if a patient has the ability to maintain or restore normal elimination patterns and if there is a family history of cancer involving the GI tract.

10. Ask about medication history. Determine whether the patient takes medications that alter defecation or fecal characteristics.

11. Assess the patient's emotional state, including tone of voice and mannerisms, which will reveal significant behaviors indicating stress.

12. Assess the patient's exercise history. Obtain a description of the type, frequency, and amount of daily exercise.

13. Gather a history of pain or discomfort. Ask the patient whether there is a history of abdominal or anal pain. The location and nature of pain helps to locate the source of a problem (see Chapter 31).

14. Assess patient's mobility and dexterity. Determine your patient's ability to toilet independently or if the patient needs assistive devices. Does the patient rely on a family caregiver in the home?

15. Assess use of alternative therapies such as herbal supplements, because there is lack of standardization in alternative products.

PHYSICAL ASSESSMENT Assess the status of GI function to detect factors that affect elimination. Focus your patient assessment to identify problems associated with bowel elimination (Table 34-2). You will need to conduct an examination of the oral cavity, abdomen, and anus and rectal canal (see Chapter 15).

When a digital examination is necessary, inspect the fecal material on the glove for several characteristics (Table 34-3). If there are no feces on the glove, ask the patient to describe a typical stool, noting recent changes. The patient or family caregiver is the most knowledgeable about changes. You also determine whether the patient passes an unusual amount of gas or little gas.

LABORATORY AND DIAGNOSTIC EXAMINATIONS

Laboratory Tests Several laboratory tests are available to assist in diagnosing problems with the GI system, including the following blood tests:

Total bilirubin: A degraded product of hemoglobin excreted in the bile. Elevated in hepatobiliary diseases.

Alkaline phosphatase: An enzyme found in many tissues. Elevated in obstructive hepatobiliary diseases and carcinomas, bone tumors, and healing fractures.

TABLE 34-2 FOCUSED PATIENT ASSESSMENT

FACTORS TO ASSESS	QUESTIONS	PHYSICAL ASSESSMENT
Chewing	Do you have difficulty chewing? Do you wear dentures?	Inspect condition of teeth, tongue, gums, and mouth. Observe for fit of dentures, observing for sores or pressure areas from dentures. Observe patient eating meal, determine patient's ability to eat all types of foods.
Mobility	**In Ambulatory Patients** Do you exercise regularly? How often do you exercise? What type of exercise do you do? How active are you? **For Patients With Restricted Mobility** Are you able to use the toilet independently? How much assistance do you need for toileting?	Observe patient's gait. Observe patient's ability to assist with transfer, positioning, and activity.
Abdomen	Do you have gas, feel bloated, or have any pain or discomfort? Can you point to the area of pain or discomfort on your abdomen? Is the pain or discomfort always in the same place?	Observe all four abdominal quadrants, noting the presence of scars, masses, venous patterns, stomas, lesions, and peristaltic waves. Auscultate all four quadrants for the presence of bowel sounds; note if sounds are normal (5 to 30 high-pitched, gurgling sounds per minute). Do not bother to count them, but judge whether they are normal, hypoactive or hyperactive. Listen for 5 minutes before deciding sounds are absent (Jarvis, 2008) Gently palpate all four quadrants, noting areas of distention, masses, or pain. When pain is present, note the location.
Anal sphincter function	Can you feel if you are distended?	Inspect anal sphincter at rest, and perform digital examination while asking patient to contract and relax sphincter. NOTE: A small amount of stool is normal; large amount of stool or hard stool indicates impaired emptying of bowel.

TABLE 34-3	Fecal Characteristics		
CHARACTERISTIC	**NORMAL**	**ABNORMAL**	**ABNORMAL CAUSE**
Color	Infant: Yellow; adult: brown	White or clay	Absence of bile
		Black or tarry (melena)	Iron ingestion or upper GI bleeding
		Red	Lower GI bleeding, hemorrhoids, ingestion of beets
		Pale with fat	Malabsorption of fat
		Translucent mucus	Spastic constipation, colitis, excess straining
		Bloody mucus	Blood in feces, inflammation, infection
Odor	Pungent; affected by food type	Noxious change	Blood in feces or infection
Consistency	Soft, formed	Liquid	Diarrhea, reduced absorption
		Hard	Constipation
Frequency	Varies: Infant 4 to 6 times daily (breast-fed) or 1 to 3 times daily (bottle-fed); adult daily or 2 to 3 times a week	Infant more than 6 times daily or less than once every 1 to 2 days; adult more than 3 times a day or less than once a week	Hypomotility or hypermotility
Amount	150 g per day (adult)		
Shape	Resembles diameter of rectum	Narrow, pencil shaped	Obstruction, rapid peristalsis
Constituents	Undigested food, dead bacteria, fat, bile pigment, cells lining intestinal mucosa, water	Blood, pus, foreign bodies, mucus, worms	Internal bleeding, infection, swallowed objects, irritation, inflammation
		Excess fat	Malabsorption syndrome, enteritis, pancreatic disease, surgical resection of intestine

GI, Gastrointestinal.

Amylase: An enzyme secreted by the pancreas. Elevated in conditions of the pancreas, such as inflammation or tumors. Also elevated in cholecystitis, necrotic bowel, and diabetic ketoacidosis.

Carcinoembryonic antigen (CEA): A protein. Typically elevated in persons with cancers of the GI tract or hepatobiliary organs.

Fecal Specimens. Analysis of fecal contents will also detect alterations in GI functioning. Careful handling of a specimen is important to prevent exposure to infectious microorganisms. Follow standard precautions (Chapter 13) when collecting and sending specimens to the laboratory. The patient is often capable of obtaining the specimen without assistance, if properly instructed. Make sure the patient understands not to mix feces with urine or water. The patient defecates into a clean, dry bedpan or special container placed under the toilet seat.

Laboratory tests for blood in the stool, ova and parasites, and stool cultures require only a small sample. Blood loss of over 50 mL causes stool to turn black, the sign of **melena.** To detect quantities less than 50 mL of blood, you will need a laboratory analysis. Collect approximately an inch of formed stool or 15 to 30 mL of liquid diarrhea stool. Tests for measuring the output of fecal fat require the patient to collect stools for 3 to 5 days. You need to save all fecal material throughout the test period. Stool specimen tests for ova and parasites require a chemical preservative. Fresh specimens are best for revealing parasites or larvae; therefore collected specimens should be taken directly to the laboratory for immediate examination.

After obtaining a specimen, tightly seal the container, place in the proper biohazard bag, complete laboratory requisition forms, and record all specimen collections in the patient's medical record. Avoid delays in sending specimens to the laboratory. Some tests require the stool to be warm. When stool specimens stand at room temperature, bacteriological changes occur that alter test results.

A common test is the **fecal occult blood test (FOBT),** or guaiac test, which measures microscopic amounts of blood in the feces (Box 34-5). It is a useful screening test for colon cancer (Box 34-6). The noninvasive FOBT is one colorectal screening tool recommended by the American Cancer Society (ACS, 2009). There are three types of FOBT available to date. They include the most commonly used guaiac fecal occult blood test (gFOBT), the fecal immunochemical test (FIT), and the stool deoxyribonucleic acid (DNA) test (Greenwald, 2005). One positive result does not confirm GI bleeding. You need to repeat the test at least three times while the patient refrains from ingesting foods and medications that cause a false-positive result. The FOBT is done in the patient's home or health care provider's office. FOBT is a screening tool, not a diagnostic tool (American Cancer Society [ACS], 2009). All positive tests should be

BOX 34-5   PROCEDURAL GUIDELINES

Measuring Fecal Occult Blood

DELEGATION CONSIDERATIONS: The skill of guaiac fecal occult blood test (gFOBT) can be delegated to nursing assistive personnel (NAP). However, the nurse is responsible for assessing the significance of the findings. You may need to send the specimen to the laboratory. Refer to your facility policies. The nurse instructs the NAP to:

• Notify the nurse if frank bleeding occurs after obtaining the sample

EQUIPMENT: Hemoccult test paper, Hemoccult developer, wooden applicator, and clean gloves. (Check the expiration dates on the developer and the test paper before using.)

1 Identify patient using two identifiers (e.g., name and birthday or name and account number, according to facility policy). Compare identifiers with information on patient's MAR or medical record.

2 Explain purpose of test and ways patient can assist. Patient can collect own specimen, if possible.

3 Perform hand hygiene, and apply clean gloves.

4 Use tip of wooden applicator (see illustration) to obtain a small portion of uncontaminated stool specimen. Be sure specimen is free of toilet paper.

5 Perform Hemoccult slide test:

   a Open flap of slide, and using a wooden applicator, thinly smear stool in first box of the guaiac paper. Apply a second fecal specimen from a different portion of the stool to slide's second box (see illustration).

   b Close slide cover, and turn the packet over to reverse side (see illustration). After waiting 3 to 5 minutes, open cardboard flap and apply two drops of developing solu-

tion on each box of guaiac paper. A blue color indicates a positive guaiac, or presence of fecal occult blood.

   c Interpret the color of the guaiac paper after 30 to 60 seconds.

   d After determining if the patient's specimen is positive or negative, apply one drop of developer to the quality control section and interpret within 10 seconds.

   e Dispose of test slide in proper receptacle.

6 Wrap wooden applicator in paper towel, remove gloves, and discard in proper receptacle.

7 Perform hand hygiene.

8 Record results of test; note any unusual fecal characteristics. (Submit only one sample per day.)

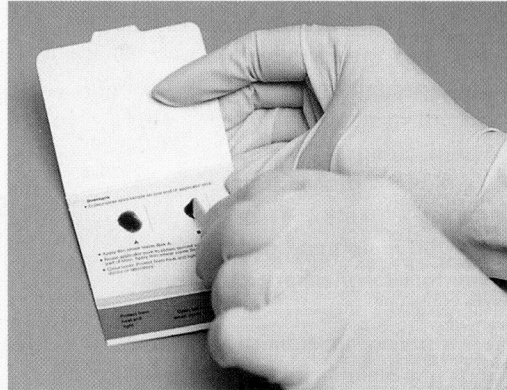

Step 5a ■ Application of fecal specimen on guaiac paper.

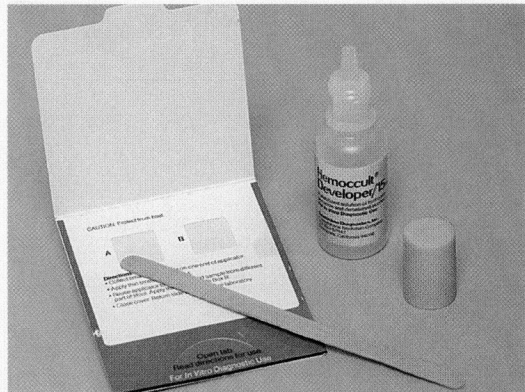

Step 4 ■ Equipment needed for fecal occult blood testing.

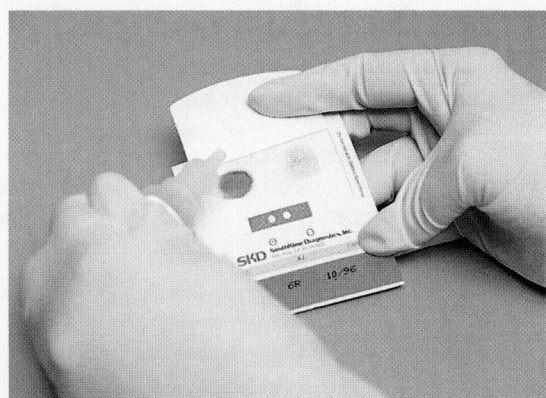

Step 5b ■ Application of Hemoccult developing solution on the guaiac paper on the reverse side of test kit.

followed up with flexible sigmoidoscopy or colonoscopy (ACS, 2009).

When your patients are going to have an FBOT, it is important to instruct them in which foods to avoid, because some foods cause a false-positive test result. Examples of these foods and medications include red meat, poultry, fish, some raw vegetables, vitamin C, and aspirin (ACS, 2009). Patients on anticoagulants are at risk for developing GI bleeding and are regularly screened with this test.

Diagnostic Examinations For patients experiencing alterations in the GI system, there are various radiological and diagnostic tests. The preparation and the test itself are often quite unpleasant for the patient. See Box 34-7 for an explanation of these tests.

PATIENT EXPECTATIONS When you assess the patient's expectations of care, it is helpful to anticipate the patient's need for privacy and respect. Bowel elimination problems are embarrassing for some. Ask the patient what

BOX 34-6 Screening for Colorectal Cancer

RISK FACTORS
- Age: Over 50
- Personal or family history: Colorectal cancer, polyps, inflammatory bowel disease (IBD)
- Race: African Americans have highest colon cancer rates
- Diet: High intake of animal fats or red meat and low intake of fruits and vegetables
- Obesity and physical inactivity
- Smoking and alcohol consumption
- Diabetes

WARNING SIGNS
- Change in bowel habits (e.g., diarrhea, constipation, narrowing of stool lasting more than few days)
- Rectal bleeding or blood in stool
- A sensation of incomplete evacuation
- Cramping or gnawing stomach pain

AMERICAN CANCER SOCIETY SCREENING GUIDELINES FOR THE EARLY DETECTION OF COLORECTAL CANCER IN AVERAGE-RISK ASYMPTOMATIC PEOPLE

Men and women Age 50+	Fecal occult blood test (FOBT) with at least 50% test sensitivity for cancer, or fecal immunochemical test (FIT) with at least 50% test sensitivity, or	Annual, starting at age 50
	Stool DNA test	Interval uncertain, starting at age 50
	Flexible sigmoidoscopy, or	Every 5 years, starting at age 50
	FOBT and flexible sigmoidoscopy, or	Annual FOBT and flexible sigmoidoscopy every 5 years starting at age 50
	Double-contrast barium enema, or	Every 5 years, starting at age 50
	Colonoscopy	Every 10 years, starting at age 50
	Computed tomography colonography	Every 5 years, starting at age 50

BOX 34-7 Radiological and Diagnostic Tests

DIRECT VISUALIZATION

Endoscopy
- Routine examination, such as a sigmoidoscopy or colonoscopy, uses a lighted fiberoptic tube to gain direct visualization of the upper GI tract (upper endoscopy) or large intestine (colonoscopy). The fiberoptic tube contains a lens, forceps, and brushes for biopsy. If an endoscopy identifies a lesion, such as a polyp, a biopsy can be obtained. Normally the GI tract is free of polyps, tumors, inflammation, ulcerations, obstructions, or hernias.

INDIRECT VISUALIZATION

Anorectal Manometry
- Measures the pressure activity of internal and external anal sphincters, and reflexes during rectal distention, relaxation during straining, and rectal sensation (Davis and others, 2007).

Plain Film of Abdomen/Kidneys, Ureter, Bladder
- A simple x-ray film of the abdomen requiring no preparation.

Barium Swallow/Enema
- An x-ray examination using an opaque contrast medium (barium, which is swallowed) to examine the structure and motility of the upper GI tract, including pharynx, esophagus, and stomach. The barium enema provides visualization of the structures of the lower GI tract.

Ultrasound Imaging
- A technique that uses high-frequency sound waves to echo off body organs, creating a picture of the GI tract.

Computed Tomography Scan or CT Colonoscopy (Virtual Colonoscopy)
- An x-ray examination of the body from many angles utilizing a scanner analyzed by a computer.

Colonic Transit Study
- The patient swallows a capsule containing radiopaque markers. The patient maintains a high-fiber diet for 5 days and refrains from medications that affect bowel function. On the fifth day, x-ray examination is performed (Davis and others, 2007).

Magnetic Resonance Imaging
- A noninvasive examination that uses magnet and radio waves to produce a picture of the inside of the body.

CT, Computed tomography; *GI,* gastrointestinal.

is important to ensure that you give care in a personal and professional way.

Because there is a direct link between nutrition and bowel elimination, consider the patient's cultural choices of foods and fluids. Sometimes the patient will have to make concessions on certain food selections. Methods of preparation are also a concern, especially if tradition and cost are deciding factors.

When determining the patient's expectations, consider his or her normal bowel pattern. Some patients wish to have activities planned in order to maintain their normal routines. If what is "normal" to a patient is unhealthy or promotes negative health practices, you must educate the patient and work with him or her to adopt healthier routines.

■■■ NURSING DIAGNOSIS

Gather data from the nursing assessment, validate the data, and analyze clusters of defining characteristics to identify relevant nursing diagnoses. Reflecting on each of your data sources is necessary in determining the correct diagnosis. Defining characteristics identified during your assessment sometimes apply to more than one diagnosis, so be clinically skillful in determining patterns that reveal the diagnosis that best fits the patient's situation.

In another example, a patient reports not having a bowel movement for several days. This defining characteristic applies to the diagnosis of *constipation* and *perceived constipation*. The difference is that on examination the patient with *constipation* has a dry, hard stool with abdominal or rectal fullness. In contrast, the patient with *perceived constipation* has expectation of having a stool daily, when in fact the stools are quite normal. There are a variety of nursing diagnoses that are relevant for patients with altered bowel elimination. Below are some examples (NANDA International, 2009):

- *Disturbed body image*
- *Bowel incontinence*
- *Constipation*
- *Perceived constipation*
- *Risk for constipation*
- *Diarrhea*
- *Nausea*
- *Imbalanced nutrition*
- *Acute pain*
- *Toileting self-care deficit*

It is important to establish the correct "related to" factor for a diagnosis. For example, with the diagnosis of *constipation* you distinguish between related factors of nutritional imbalance, exercise, medications, and emotional problems. Selection of the correct related factors for each diagnosis ensures that you will implement the appropriate nursing interventions.

■■■ PLANNING

GOALS AND OUTCOMES After you identify nursing diagnoses, determine how they are related (Figure 34-10). Then, you and the patient set goals and expected outcomes to direct interventions. When possible, these goals and outcomes incorporate the patient's elimination routines or habits as much as possible and reinforce those that promote health. In addition, consider the patient's preexisting health concerns. For example, one method of reducing the risk for constipation is to achieve the goal of "establishing a normal defecation pattern" by increasing fluids and bulk to the patient's diet. An outcome would be the patient "will pass a soft, formed stool within 48 hours." However, if your patient is at risk for the development of congestive heart failure, you need to tailor the intervention of increasing fluid intake to the patient's cardiac function. For this reason it might take longer to achieve the outcome.

The goals and expected outcomes you establish need to be realistic. The outcomes provide measurable behaviors or physiological responses that indicate progress toward the goal of a normal bowel elimination pattern. Design nursing interventions to achieve the outcomes of care.

SETTING PRIORITIES Defecation patterns vary among individuals. For this reason, you and the patient work together to plan effective interventions to meet the patient's elimination needs and priorities (see Care Plan). A realistic time frame to establish a normal defecation pattern for one patient is sometimes very different for another. In addition, if the patient has a new ostomy resulting from cancer, the priority of coping with cancer and its treatment precedes the patient's need to become independent in managing the care of the bowel diversion. In addition, when a bowel diversion is necessary, coping with changes in body image is a high priority for both the patient and family.

COLLABORATIVE CARE Other health care team members are important resources for the patient and family. You will sometimes refer a patient with chronic constipation to a dietitian to plan a nutritionally balanced diet that incorporates the patient's food preferences and lifestyle.

Involvement of the family in the plan of care is important. When patients are disabled or debilitated, family members often become the primary caregivers. Patient and family education is important to promote understanding of ways to establish normal bowel function. If access to proper nutrition is a concern, community organizations that deliver meals to the home (e.g., Meals on Wheels and church groups) or that provide transportation for patients will be beneficial.

A clinical nurse specialist or wound, ostomy, and continence nurse specialist will provide guidance in the care and management of ostomy sites and problems involving incontinence or skin breakdown. In many institutions, members of the health care team work together in developing a critical pathway for patient care.

■■■ IMPLEMENTATION

HEALTH PROMOTION Factors that normally promote bowel elimination are appropriate interventions for helping patients develop normal bowel habits. It is important to teach your patient about the benefits and effects of a balanced diet, regular exercise, and stress management and how to integrate each into a bowel routine. Teach your patients to try to develop a routine time for bowel evacuation. A good time is

CONCEPT MAP

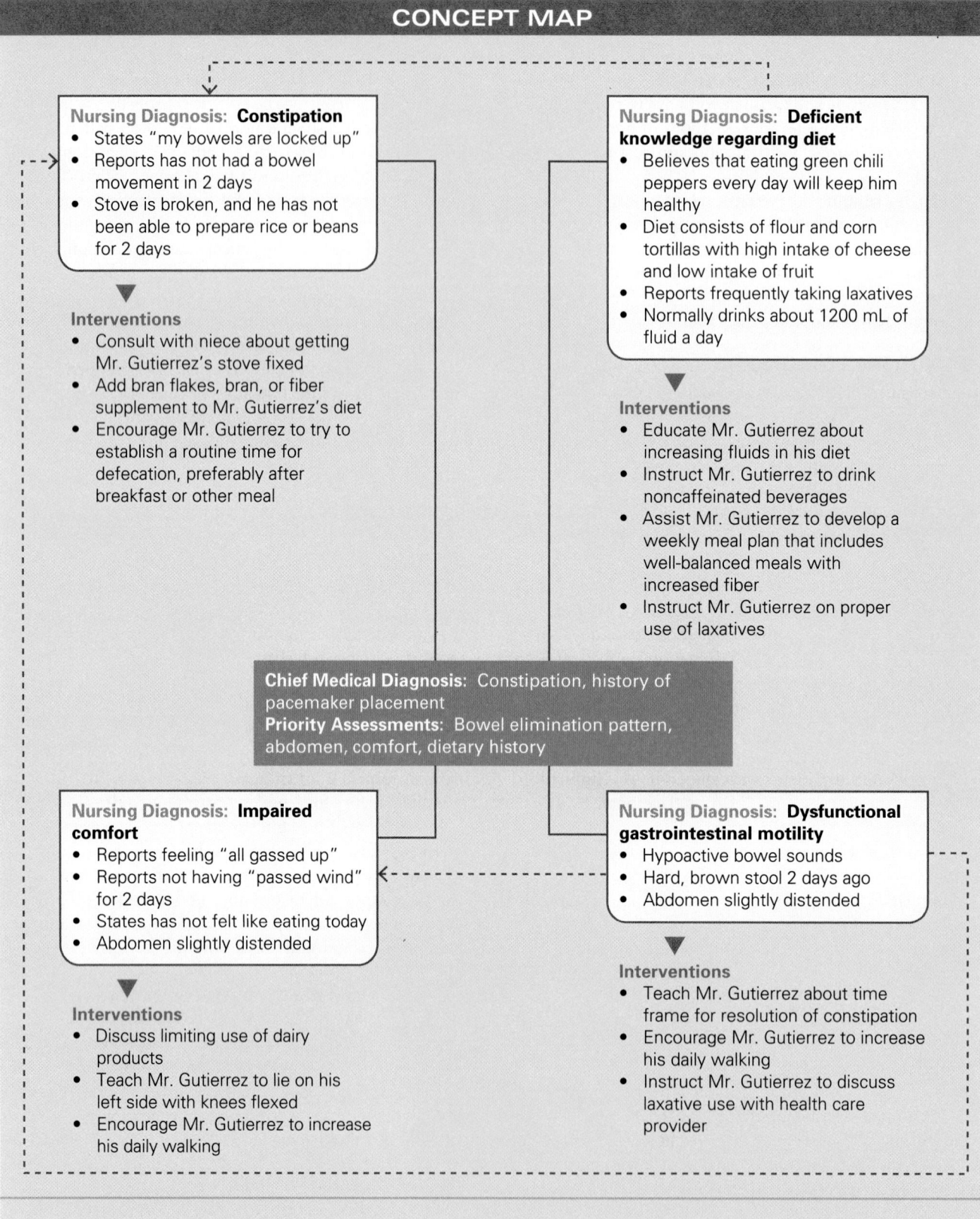

Nursing Diagnosis: Constipation
- States "my bowels are locked up"
- Reports has not had a bowel movement in 2 days
- Stove is broken, and he has not been able to prepare rice or beans for 2 days

Interventions
- Consult with niece about getting Mr. Gutierrez's stove fixed
- Add bran flakes, bran, or fiber supplement to Mr. Gutierrez's diet
- Encourage Mr. Gutierrez to try to establish a routine time for defecation, preferably after breakfast or other meal

Nursing Diagnosis: Deficient knowledge regarding diet
- Believes that eating green chili peppers every day will keep him healthy
- Diet consists of flour and corn tortillas with high intake of cheese and low intake of fruit
- Reports frequently taking laxatives
- Normally drinks about 1200 mL of fluid a day

Interventions
- Educate Mr. Gutierrez about increasing fluids in his diet
- Instruct Mr. Gutierrez to drink noncaffeinated beverages
- Assist Mr. Gutierrez to develop a weekly meal plan that includes well-balanced meals with increased fiber
- Instruct Mr. Gutierrez on proper use of laxatives

Chief Medical Diagnosis: Constipation, history of pacemaker placement
Priority Assessments: Bowel elimination pattern, abdomen, comfort, dietary history

Nursing Diagnosis: Impaired comfort
- Reports feeling "all gassed up"
- Reports not having "passed wind" for 2 days
- States has not felt like eating today
- Abdomen slightly distended

Interventions
- Discuss limiting use of dairy products
- Teach Mr. Gutierrez to lie on his left side with knees flexed
- Encourage Mr. Gutierrez to increase his daily walking

Nursing Diagnosis: Dysfunctional gastrointestinal motility
- Hypoactive bowel sounds
- Hard, brown stool 2 days ago
- Abdomen slightly distended

Interventions
- Teach Mr. Gutierrez about time frame for resolution of constipation
- Encourage Mr. Gutierrez to increase his daily walking
- Instruct Mr. Gutierrez to discuss laxative use with health care provider

—— Link between medical diagnosis and nursing diagnosis   - - - - Link between nursing diagnoses

Figure 34-10 ■ Concept Map.

CARE PLAN   Constipation

ASSESSMENT

From their first visit, Vickie and Mr. Gutierrez have been able to communicate without difficulty. Mr. Gutierrez complains of feeling "full of gas" but has not "passed any wind," in the last 2 days. His stove has not been working well, and he has been unable to prepare rice and beans. Based on the nursing history, Vickie estimates Mr. Gutierrez normally drinks about 1200 mL of fluid daily.

ASSESSMENT ACTIVITIES

Determine when Mr. Gutierrez had his last bowel movement.

Determine Mr. Gutierrez's medication history.

Establish Mr. Gutierrez's dietary habits.

Assess Mr. Gutierrez's abdomen.

FINDINGS/DEFINING CHARACTERISTICS*

Mr. Gutierrez had his **last bowel movement 2 days ago. The stool was brown in color and hard.** "I took a laxative last night, and I think I need an enema."

A medication history shows that Mr. Gutierrez **frequently resorts to taking laxatives.**

Mr. Gutierrez' eats a **high intake of corn tortillas and cheese and a low intake of fruits**. Mr. Gutierrez also states, "I really **haven't felt like eating today and have not eaten much for the last 4 days**, and I need to move my bowels."

Hypoactive bowel sounds in all four quadrants. Abdomen is soft but **slightly distended.**

NURSING DIAGNOSIS: Constipation related to less than adequate fluid and dietary intake and chronic laxative use.

PLANNING

GOAL

- Mr. Gutierrez will establish and maintain a normal defecation pattern within 1 month.

- Mr. Gutierrez will identify practices that reduce the risk for or prevent constipation within 2 weeks.

EXPECTED OUTCOMES (NOC)†

Bowel Elimination
- Mr. Gutierrez will have a bowel movement within 48 hours.
- Mr. Gutierrez's abdomen will be soft, nondistended, and nontender within 24 hours.
- Mr. Gutierrez will pass soft, formed stools at least every 3 days.

Nutritional Status: Food and Fluid Intake
- Mr. Gutierrez will identify need to increase the fiber content of his diet within 1 week.
- Mr. Gutierrez will immediately discontinue laxative use and will use fiber supplements when needed.
- Mr. Gutierrez will identify need to drink eight 8-ounce glasses of noncaffeinated beverages within 3 days (Amerine and Keirsey, 2006).

INTERVENTIONS (NIC)‡

Constipation/Impaction Management
- Instruct Mr. Gutierrez in a weekly menu plan, including foods high in fiber: brown rice, beans and rice, tomatoes, and wheat tortillas.

- Add bran flakes, bran, or fiber supplement to Mr. Gutierrez's diet.

- Consult with Mr. Gutierrez's niece and long-term care center to have patient's stove repaired.

RATIONALE

High-fiber foods increase the bulk of the fecal contents, which in turn increases peristalsis and improves the movement of intestinal contents through the GI tract (Doughty, 2006; Hill, 2007).

Bran as flakes or fiber supplements add bulk to the feces and increase the number of soft-formed stools. Dietary fiber, either through diet or supplement, reduces the need for laxatives (Doughty, 2006; McKenry and others, 2006).

Cooking facilities are necessary for preparation of selected food preferences.

---

*__Defining characteristics__ are shown in **bold** type.
†Outcomes classification labels from Moorhead S and others, editors: *Nursing outcomes classification (NOC)*, ed 4, St. Louis, 2008, Mosby.
‡Intervention classification labels from Bulechek GM and others, editors: *Nursing interventions classification (NIC)*, ed 5, St. Louis, 2008, Mosby.

CARE PLAN   Constipation—cont'd

INTERVENTIONS (NIC)‡

Constipation/Impaction Management

- Educate Mr. Gutierrez about use of liquids to promote softening of stool and defecation; have patient drink noncaffeinated beverage of choice.

- Encourage Mr. Gutierrez to try to establish a routine time for defecation, establishing a routine after breakfast or other meal.

RATIONALE

Caffeinated beverages cause the body to increase excretion of fluids and dehydrate the patient. Fluids help to keep fecal mass soft and increase stool bulk, causing increase in colon peristalsis (Amerine and Keirsey, 2006).

With aging there are some normal changes in rectal sensation, and the body needs larger volumes to elicit the sensation to defecate. Using the normal gastrocolic reflex, which results in movement of colon contents approximately 1 hour after a meal, assists in establishing routine bowel habits (Amerine and Keirsey, 2006).

EVALUATION

NURSING ACTIONS	PATIENT RESPONSE/FINDING	ACHIEVEMENT OF OUTCOME
Review Mr. Gutierrez's diary of foods, and ask him about his intake as well.	Mr. Gutierrez described likes and dislikes, but admits to eating high-fat foods and few fruits and vegetables. Fluid intake averaged 1400 mL daily for a week.	Mr. Gutierrez's intake of high-fiber foods is still limited. Fluid intake improving.
Ask Mr. Gutierrez about his pattern of elimination over the last 2 weeks and laxative use.	Mr. Gutierrez says, "I still go about the same," but states that he thinks he now goes about every 2 days. Mr. Gutierrez has not used any laxatives for a week.	He has bowel movements approximately every 2 days. He is successfully avoiding use of laxatives.
During follow-up visit examine patient's abdomen and observe stool (if possible).	Patient reports stool is formed but is "not hard like before." Bowel sounds are normal. Abdomen is soft and nontender with no distention.	Stool is more soft in character. His abdomen is less distended.

after a morning or evening meal when your patient does not feel rushed. Establishing a consistent time for bowel hygiene is just one practice to avoid constipation (Box 34-8).

Diet Depending on the patient's elimination problem, specific foods ensure proper nutrient intake and normal defecation (see Boxes 34-1, p. 991, and 34-8). When your patient has an ostomy, the location of the ostomy determines the type of diet needed for regular evacuation. Initially place patients with ostomies on low-fiber diets to avoid stoma obstruction. Slowly add high-fiber foods one at a time over a period of several weeks. Maintain a high fluid intake. Teach your patient to avoid foods that cause blockage, such as oranges, apples with tough skins, corn, and popcorn.

Exercise An age-specific exercise program also assists patients in maintaining a healthy bowel pattern. Regular exercise, such as walking, biking, or swimming 30 minutes daily, promotes normal GI motility. Regular activity keeps the intestines working well (Hill, 2007). Have a patient who experiences a period of immobilization from illness ambulate as soon as possible. Ambulation promotes peristalsis and a return to normal bowel function.

Timing and Privacy One of the most important habits you will teach your patients regarding bowel habits is to take time for defecation. Ignoring the urge to defecate and not taking time to defecate completely are common causes of constipation. To establish regular bowel habits, a patient needs to respond to the urge to defecate. Prompt response will help the patient to reduce episodes of constipation.

Defecation is most likely to occur an hour after meals. If the patient attempts to defecate during the time when mass colonic peristalsis occurs, the chances of success are great. If a patient is restricted to bed or requires assistance in ambulating, recommend use of a bedside commode or a bedpan or have a caregiver help the patient reach the bathroom. Patients need prompt assistance before the urge disappears.

Some patients have previously established routines to assist them with defecation. When patients are hospitalized, health promotion habits become disrupted. Encourage patients to maintain as many of these regular practices as possible. Privacy is often a concern for patients. Health care providers often walk in and out of rooms without knocking, and many patients reside in semiprivate rooms or living ar-

BOX 34-8   BEST PRACTICES

Bowel Hygiene

SUMMARY OF EVIDENCE

Multiple areas of research support the increasing evidence that low fat intake and increases in dietary fiber and bulk-forming foods reduce the patient's risk for colorectal cancers, digestive diseases, and other cancers. Assisting patients and their families in different food selection and preparation practices helps to reduce the risks of GI disease. Give consideration to whether a patient is able to afford the foods recommended. In addition to solid foods, the patient with elimination problems needs to drink 2000 to 3000 mL of fluids daily, if not contraindicated by other medical conditions.

APPLICATION TO NURSING PRACTICE*

- Recommend fluid intake of at least 1.5 L per day. Preferred fluid is water because it is sodium-, caffeine-, and calorie-free. Patient will benefit from one or two glasses of fruit juice as well (Amerine and Keirsey, 2006).
- Teach patients to avoid coffee, tea, and alcohol because of their diuretic properties.
- Suggest a high-fiber diet (25 to 30 g per day) to reduce constipation; as fiber passes though the colon, it acts as

a sponge. As a result, bulkier and softer stools develop. In addition, the waste moves through the body more easily and results in more regular bowel movements. High-fiber diet is not for individuals who are immobile or who do not consume at least 1.5 L of fluid per day (Hall and others, 2007).

- Teach patients to use a combination of insoluble and soluble fiber (e.g., bran, fruits, and vegetables) to prevent constipation.
- Assess the patient's ability to afford foods.
- Encourage physical activity in combination with adequate fluid intake and high-fiber diet to manage constipation. Walking once or twice a day for 15 to 20 minutes is sufficient.
- Suggest chair or bed exercises such as pelvic tilt, low trunk rotation, and single leg lifts for individuals who are unable to walk.
- Explain need to use laxatives with caution. A stepwise progression of laxatives is recommended: first bulk-forming laxatives, followed by stool softeners, osmotic stimulants, suppositories, and enemas as a last resort.

*Modified from Hinrichs M, Huseboe J: *Evidence-based protocol: management of constipation.* In Titler MG, series editor: Series on evidence based practice for older adults, Iowa City, 1998, The University of Iowa, Gerontological Nursing Interventions Research Center, Research Dissemination Core. For more information, visit http://www.nursing.uiowa.edu/center/gnirc/disseminatecore.htm.

---

eas. Remain acutely aware of the patient's need for modesty and privacy.

Promotion of Normal Defecation To help patients evacuate contents normally and without discomfort, recommend interventions that stimulate the defecation reflex or increase peristalsis. One way to promote defecation is by having the patient assume a squatting position during defecation. Squatting increases pressure on the rectum and facilitates use of intraabdominal muscles. Patients who have difficulty in squatting because of muscular weakness or mobility limitations benefit from the use of elevated toilet seats. Regular toilets are too low for patients unable to lower themselves to a squatting position because of joint or muscle-wasting diseases or for those who have had abdominal surgery. With an elevated seat, the patient exerts less effort to sit or stand.

ACUTE CARE When patients become acutely ill, this often affects the GI system first. Simple changes in activity levels, sleeping patterns, diet, and medications directly affect regular bowel habits. Surgical intervention creates additional elimination problems for the patient in acute care (e.g., discomfort from an abdominal incision, absent or decreased gastrointestinal peristalsis, or increased accumulation of intestinal gas following surgery). Sensitivity to the patient's need to provide as much self-care as possible will assist the patient in coping with the changes.

Positioning on Bedpan A patient restricted to use of a bedpan for defecation will usually need assistance. Sitting on a bedpan is uncomfortable and awkward. Help position the

patient comfortably. Two types of bedpans are available (Figure 34-11). The regular bedpan, made of hard plastic, has a curved smooth upper end and a sharp-edged lower end and is about 5 cm (2 inches) deep. A fracture pan is used for patients with lower extremity fractures. It has a shallow upper end about 1.3 cm (½ inch) deep. The shallow end of the pan fits under the buttocks toward the sacrum, and the handled deeper end goes just under the upper thighs. The pan needs to be high enough so the stool can enter the pan.

The most important element for you to consider in positioning the patient is preventing muscle strain and discomfort. Never place a patient on a bedpan and then leave the bed flat unless activity restrictions demand it. This forces the patient to hyperextend the back to lift the hips onto the pan (Figure 34-12, *A*). It is often necessary to have the bed flat when placing the patient on a bedpan. In this case you then raise the head of the bed 30 to 45 degrees (Figure 34-12, *B*). Patients who have overhead trapeze frames are able to lift themselves by grasping the trapeze bar. Box 34-9 describes steps in assisting a patient with a bedpan.

For the more mobile patient, a bedside commode is a safe, effective alternative to a bedpan. Its use is less exhausting and allows the patient to assume a more "normal" or "familiar" position for defecation.

Medications Some medications initiate and facilitate stool passage. **Cathartics** and **laxatives** have the short-term action of emptying the bowel. These agents are also used in bowel evacuation for patients undergoing GI tests and

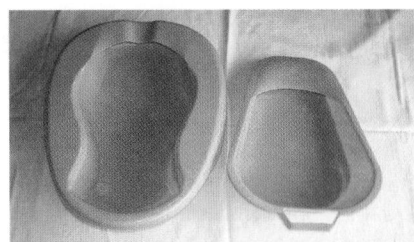

Figure 34-11 ■ Types of bedpans. *From left:* Regular bedpan and fracture pan.

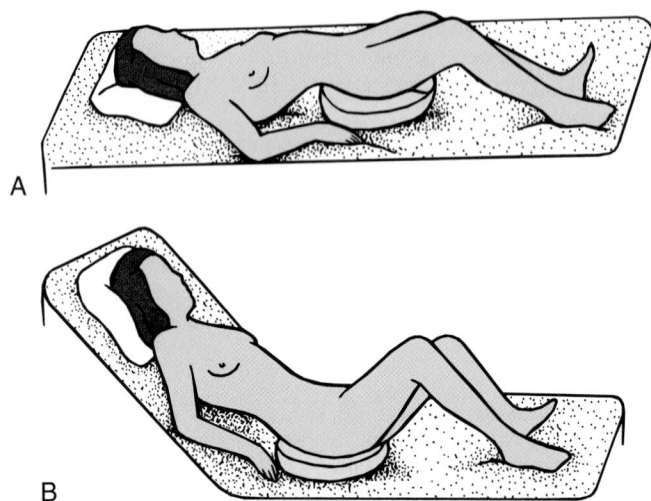

Figure 34-12 ■ Positions on a bedpan. **A,** Improper positioning of a patient. **B,** Proper position reduces patient's back strain.

abdominal surgery. Although the terms *cathartic* and *laxative* are often used interchangeably, cathartics have a stronger and more rapid effect on the intestines.

Although patients usually take medications orally, cathartics prepared as suppositories are more effective because of their stimulant effect on the rectal mucosa. Cathartic suppositories such as bisacodyl (Dulcolax) act within 30 minutes. Give the suppository shortly before the patient's usual time to defecate or immediately after a meal. Teach patients about the potential harmful effects of repeated use of laxatives, such as permanent bowel damage, osteomalacia, and electrolyte imbalances (McKenry, Tessier, and Hogan, 2006). Make sure the patient understands that laxatives and cathartics are not for long-term maintenance of bowel function.

Cathartics are classified by the method by which the agent promotes defecation. Stimulant cathartics cause local irritation to the intestinal mucosa, increase intestinal motility, and inhibit reabsorption of water in the large intestine. The rapid movement of feces causes retention of water in the stool. The drugs cause formation of a soft to fluid stool in 6 to 8 hours.

Saline or osmotic agents contain a salt preparation that the intestines do not absorb. The cathartic draws water into the fecal mass. This osmotic action increases the bulk of the intestinal contents and enhances lubrication. Rapid bowel evacuation occurs in 1 to 3 hours.

Emollient or wetting agents are detergents and act as stool softeners to lower the surface tension of feces, allowing water and fat to penetrate the fecal material. These drugs also block absorption of water by the intestines. The fecal mass becomes large and soft, preventing the patient from straining during defecation. A bowel movement occurs within 12 to 24 hours.

Bulk-forming cathartics absorb water and increase solid intestinal bulk. The fecal bulk stretches the intestinal walls, stimulating peristalsis. Passage of stool will occur in 12 to 24 hours. Bulk-forming laxatives are the least irritating and safest of all cathartics. Encourage patients to take bulk cathartics with plenty of liquids.

Lubricants soften the fecal mass, thus easing the strain of defecation. Patients with painful hemorrhoids particularly benefit from a lubricant. The only lubricant laxative available is mineral oil. However, teach patients that the regular use of mineral oil interferes with absorption of the fat-soluble vitamins A, D, E, and K. In addition, because this medication is an oil-based preparation, it causes a dangerous form of pneumonia when aspirated. Therefore warn patients with nausea and vomiting not to take the medication.

For patients with diarrhea, the most effective antidiarrheal agents are opiates. Antidiarrheal agents decrease intestinal muscle tone to slow the passage of feces. As a result, the body absorbs more water through the intestinal walls. Use antidiarrheal agents with caution because opiates are habit forming.

Enemas   An **enema** is an instillation of a preparation into the rectum and sigmoid colon. An enema is given primarily to promote defecation by stimulating peristalsis. The volume of fluid instilled breaks up the fecal mass, stretches the rectal wall, and begins the defecation reflex. Enemas are also a vehicle for drugs that exert a local effect on rectal mucosa.

The most common use for an enema is temporary relief of constipation. Other indications include removing impacted feces; emptying the bowel before diagnostic tests, surgery, or childbirth; and beginning a program of bowel training. Discourage patients from relying on enemas to maintain bowel regularity. Enemas do not treat the cause of constipation. As with laxative abuse, frequent use will destroy normal defecation reflexes.

Cleansing enemas promote complete evacuation of feces from the colon. They act by stimulating peristalsis through the infusion of a large volume of solution or through local irritation of the colon's mucosa. Cleansing enemas include tap water, normal saline, low-volume hypertonic saline, and soapsuds solution. Each solution exerts a different osmotic effect, causing the movement of fluids between the colon and interstitial spaces beyond the intestinal wall. Infants and children will tolerate only normal saline because they are at risk for fluid imbalance (see Chapter 17).

Tap water is hypotonic and exerts a lower osmotic pressure than fluid in interstitial spaces. After infusion into the colon, tap water escapes from the bowel lumen into interstitial spaces. The net movement of water is low; the infused

BOX 34-9   PROCEDURAL GUIDELINES

Assisting Patient On and Off a Bedpan

DELEGATION CONSIDERATIONS: The skill of assisting a patient onto a bedpan can be delegated to nursing assistive personnel (NAP). The nurse guides and assists the NAP in the proper way to position patients who have mobility restrictions. Also, instruct the NAP in how to position patients who also have therapeutic equipment present, such as drains, intravenous catheters, or traction.

EQUIPMENT: Appropriate type of clean bedpan; toilet tissue; specimen container (if necessary); washbasin; washcloths; towels; soap; waterproof, absorbent pads; clean drawsheet *(optional)*; clean gloves

1 Assess the patient's level of mobility, strength, ability to help, and presence of any condition (e.g., orthopedic) that interferes with the use of a bedpan.
2 Explain the technique you will use in turning and positioning to the patient.
3 Offer the bedpan at a time that coincides with the peristaltic reflex.
4 Perform hand hygiene, and apply clean gloves.
5 Close the room curtain for privacy.
6 Raise the bed to a comfortable working height. Position the patient high in bed with head elevated 30 degrees (unless contraindicated). Raise the side rail opposite the side where you are standing.
7 Fold back top linen to patient's knees.
8 Assist with positioning an independent patient: Instruct patient to bend knees and place weight on heels. Place your hand, palm up, under patient's sacrum, resting elbow on mattress. Then have patient lift hips while you slip bedpan into place with other hand.
9 Dependent patient: Lower head of bed flat, and roll the patient onto side opposite nurse. Apply powder lightly to lower back and buttocks *(optional)*. Place bedpan firmly against buttocks (see illustration A). Push bedpan down into mattress with open rim toward patient's feet (see illustration B). Keeping one hand against bedpan, place other hand around patient's fore hip (see illustration C). Ask patient to roll onto pan, flat on bed. With patient positioned comfortably, raise head of bed 30 degrees.
10 Place rolled towel under lumbar curve of patient's back.
11 Place call light and toilet tissue within patient's reach, and keep side rails up as needed. Give patient time to defecate.
12 Remove bedpan as patient lifts hips up or as patient carefully rolls off pan and to side. Hold pan firmly as patient moves.
13 Assist in cleansing anal area. Wipe from pubic area toward anus. Replace top covers.
14 If you collect a specimen or intake and output, do not dispose of tissue in bedpan.
15 Have patient wash and dry hands.
16 Empty pan's contents, dispose of gloves, and perform hand hygiene.
17 Inspect stool for color, amount, consistency, odor, or presence of abnormal substances. Document findings.

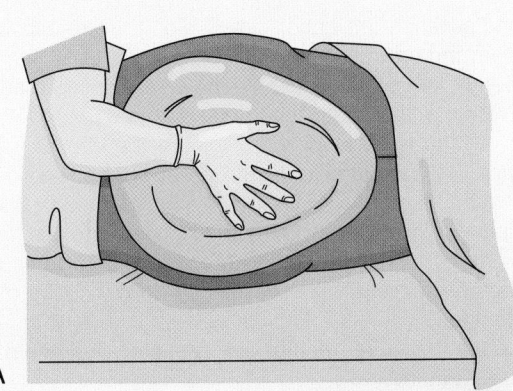

A

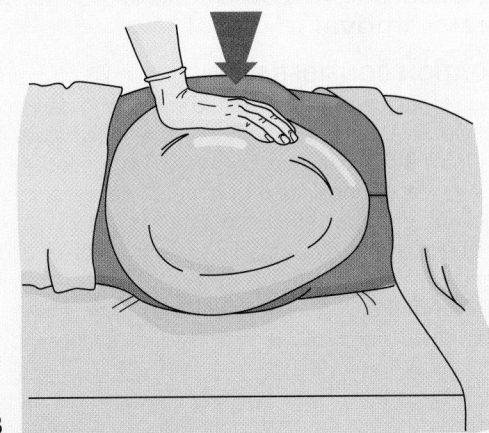

B

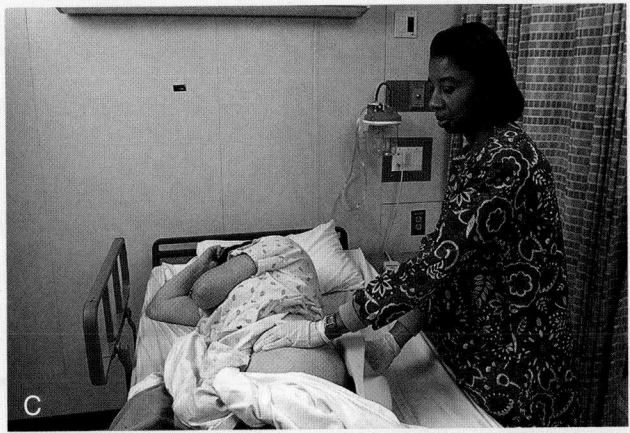

C

Step 9 ■ Place one hand against bedpan; place other hand around patient's fore hip.

volume stimulates defecation before large amounts of water leave the bowel. Do not repeat tap water enemas, because water toxicity or circulatory overload will develop if the body absorbs large amounts of water.

Physiologically, normal saline is the safest solution to use because it exerts the same osmotic pressure as fluids in interstitial spaces around the bowel. The volume of infused saline stimulates peristalsis. Giving saline enemas does not create the danger of excess fluid absorption. Add soap solution to tap water or saline to create the additional effect of intestinal irritation. Only pure castile soap is safe. Harsh soaps or detergents cause serious bowel inflammation.

Hypertonic solutions infused into the bowel exert osmotic pressure that pulls fluids out of interstitial spaces. The colon fills with fluid, and the resultant distention promotes defecation. Patients unable to tolerate large volumes of fluid benefit most from this type of enema. A hypertonic solution of 120 to 180 mL (4 to 6 oz) is usually effective. The Fleet enema is the most common.

A health care provider will sometimes order a high or low cleansing enema. The terms *high* and *low* refer to the height and the pressure with which you deliver the fluid. You give high enemas to cleanse the entire colon. A low enema cleans only the rectum and sigmoid colon. After you infuse the enema, ask the patient to turn from the left lateral to the dorsal recumbent, then over to the right lateral position. The position changes help fluid to reach the large intestine.

Oil-retention enemas lubricate the rectum and colon. The feces absorb the oil and become softer and easier to pass. To enhance action of the oil, the patient retains the enema for several hours if possible.

Certain enemas or enema administrations contain drugs. An example is sodium polystyrene sulfonate (Kayexalate), used to treat patients with dangerously high serum potassium levels. Skill 34-1 outlines the steps for enema administration.

Digital Removal of Stool For patients with an impaction, the fecal mass is sometimes too large for the patient to pass voluntarily. If enemas fail, the mass needs to be broken up digitally. Patients with an impaction frequently have a continuous oozing of liquid stool because liquid passes around the impacted feces. This procedure is practiced only when all other measures have failed.

The procedure is very uncomfortable for the patient. Excess rectal manipulation causes irritation to the mucosa and bleeding. There is also risk of stimulation of the vagus nerve which can result in a reflex slowing of the heart rate. Because of the procedure's potential complications, some institutions restrict nurses from removing impactions digitally. Before you perform the procedure, check your agency's policy regarding a health care provider's order (Box 34-10).

BOX 34-10   PROCEDURAL GUIDELINES

Digital Removal of Stool

DELEGATION CONSIDERATIONS: The skill of digitally removing stool cannot be delegated to nursing assistive personnel (NAP). In some institutions, only health care providers perform this procedure. The nurse instructs the NAP:

- To provide perineal care and other necessary hygiene following each bowel movement
- To observe any evacuated stool for color and consistency

EQUIPMENT: Bedpan, waterproof pad, stethoscope, water-soluble lubricant, washcloths, towels, soap, and clean gloves

1 Identify patient using two identifiers (e.g., name and birthday or name and account number, according to facility policy).
2 Perform hand hygiene, pull curtains around bed, obtain patient's baseline vital signs and assess level of comfort, auscultate for bowel sounds and palpate for abdominal distention before the procedure.
3 Explain the procedure, and help the patient to lie on the left side in Sims' position with knees flexed and back toward you.
4 Drape the trunk and lower extremities with a bath blanket, and place a waterproof pad under the buttocks. Keep a bedpan next to the patient.
5 Apply clean gloves; lubricate the index finger of dominant hand with water-soluble lubricant.
6 Instruct the patient to take slow, deep breaths. Gradually and gently insert the index finger into the rectum, and advance the finger slowly along the rectal wall toward the umbilicus.
7 Gently loosen the fecal mass by massaging around it. Work the finger into the hardened mass.
8 Work the feces downward toward the end of the rectum. Remove small pieces one at a time, and discard into bedpan.
9 Periodically reassess the patient's heart rate and look for signs of fatigue. Stop the procedure if the heart rate drops significantly (check agency policy) or the rhythm changes.
10 Continue to clear rectum of feces, and allow the patient to rest at intervals.
11 After completion, wash and dry the buttocks and anal area.
12 Remove bedpan; inspect feces for color and consistency. Dispose of feces. Remove gloves by turning them inside out, and then discard.
13 Assist patient to toilet or clean bedpan if urge to defecate develops.
14 Perform hand hygiene. Record results of procedure by describing fecal characteristics and amount.
15 Follow procedure with enemas or cathartics as ordered by health care provider.
16 Reassess patient's vital signs and level of comfort, auscultate bowel sounds and observe status of abdominal distention.

Inserting and Maintaining a Nasogastric Tube for Gastric Decompression There are times following major surgery or because of conditions affecting the gastrointestinal tract when normal peristalsis is temporarily altered. A patient cannot eat or drink fluids without causing abdominal distention if peristalsis slows or is absent. The temporary insertion of a nasogastric (NG) tube into the stomach serves to decompress the stomach, keeping it empty until normal peristalsis returns (Skill 34-2).

An NG tube is a pliable tube that is inserted through the patient's nasopharynx into the stomach. The tube has a hollow lumen that allows the removal of gastric secretions and the introduction of solutions into the stomach. A nasogastric tube can be also be used for enteral feedings, but a softer small-bore feeding tube is preferred for feeding purposes (see Chapter 32). The Levin and Salem sump tubes are most commonly used for stomach decompression. The Levin tube is a single-lumen tube with holes near the tip. You connect the tube to a drainage bag or an intermittent suction device to drain stomach secretions. The Salem sump tube is preferable for stomach decompression. The tube has two lumina: one for removal of gastric contents and one to provide an air vent. A blue "pigtail" is the air vent that connects with the second lumen. When you connect the sump tube's main lumen to suction, the air vent permits free, continuous drainage of secretions. *Never clamp the air vent if connected to suction or use for irrigation.*

Nasogastric tube insertion does not require sterile technique. Clean technique is adequate. The procedure is uncomfortable, with patients experiencing a burning sensation as the tube passes through the sensitive nasal mucosa. One of the greatest nursing care challenges is keeping the patient comfortable because the tube is a constant irritation to mucosa. Routinely assess the condition of the nares and mucosa for inflammation and excoriation. Supportive care includes changing soiled tape or fixation devices daily when they become soiled, keeping the nares lubricated and clean, and providing frequent mouth care to minimize dehydration from mouth breathing.

CONTINUING AND RESTORATIVE CARE Before the patient is able to return home or is transferred to an extended care facility, you need to assist with the establishment of regular elimination patterns. Bowel retraining is one essential step in regaining independence.

Bowel Training A bowel-training program will help patients who still have some neuromuscular control to achieve normal defecation. The training program involves setting up a daily routine. By attempting to defecate at the same time each day and using measures that promote defecation, the patient gains control of bowel reflexes. The program requires time, patience, and consistency. The health care provider determines the patient's physical readiness and ability to benefit from bowel training.

Ostomy Care Immediately after surgical diversion or removal of a portion of bowel, it is necessary to place a pouch over the newly created stoma because in some ostomies effluent, or discharge, begins immediately. The pouch collects all effluent and protects the skin from irritating drainage. A proper pouch fits comfortably with its skin barrier, covers the skin surface around the stoma, and creates a good seal. The postoperative pouch allows visibility of the stoma.

The technique of pouching a newly formed stoma differs from techniques used to pouch a stoma several days or weeks old. In the case of a new stoma there is usually an incision line from the bowel resection that lies close to or around the stoma. Care is taken to avoid disrupting the suture line.

For up to 6 weeks, the new stoma is edematous, or swollen. The stoma itself often has a series of small stitches around its perimeter. Apply a pouch and skin barrier that do not constrict the stoma or traumatize healing tissues. Initially some patients will not need to empty the pouch over a postoperative colostomy frequently because drainage is diminished or lacking. Several days will pass before a patient's normal elimination pattern returns. In the case of an ileostomy, the patient will have frequent liquid stools when peristalsis returns (Pontieri-Lewis, 2006).

Many types of pouches and skin barriers are available (Pontieri-Lewis, 2006). Some pouches have skin barriers directly preattached and are one-piece pouching systems (Figure 34-13). Some of these one-piece pouches already are precut to size by the manufacturer, whereas others you will custom cut to size for the patient's stoma measurement. Other systems are two separate pieces. Attach the pouch to the skin barrier by attaching it to the flange (a plastic ring) on the barrier. Often you will have to custom cut the skin barrier to the patient's specific stoma size. For two-piece systems, use the skin barrier with flange with the corresponding-size pouch that fits that flange *from the same manufacturer* to use

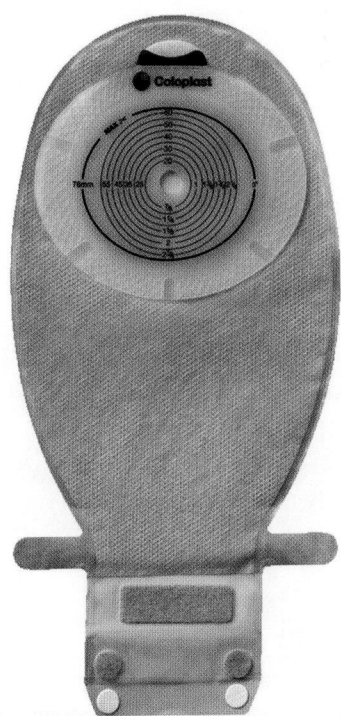

Figure 34-13 ■ One-piece pouch with Velcro closure. (Courtesy Coloplast, Minneapolis, Minn.)

the system correctly without leakage. Understand how to use each of these different pouching systems (Figure 34-14). Modifications for preventing complications related to leakage of feces or urine are essential (Pontieri-Lewis, 2006). Perform meticulous skin care to prevent liquid stool from irritating skin around a stoma (Box 34-11).

Change the pouch when there is little drainage from the ostomy, usually before meals or at bedtime. Have the patient participate in the procedure as much as possible. The patient needs to learn to recognize the normal appearance of a stoma. Skill 34-3 describes the steps for pouching an ostomy.

A patient with an ostomy suffers a change in body image. The appearance of the stoma and accompanying body odors cause psychological stress. For the patient with a new ostomy, it is important for you to promote independence and acceptance of the ostomy. Early involvement in self-care promotes the patient's independence. Even simple tasks such as holding pieces of equipment during stoma pouching help the patient begin to adjust to bodily changes. Many patients benefit from the information and encouragement from ostomy support groups.

Care of Hemorrhoids   Many patients experience discomfort from alterations in elimination. The patient with hemorrhoids has pain when hemorrhoidal tissues are directly irritated from passage of hard stool. The primary goal for the patient with hemorrhoids is soft-formed stools. Treatment includes proper diet, fluids, and regular exercise. Local heat provides temporary relief to swollen hemorrhoids. A sitz bath is the most effective means of heat application (see Chapter 36).

When hemorrhoids are present, it is important to prevent trauma to tissues. Use caution when inserting rectal thermometers, suppositories, or rectal tubes. A generous amount of lubricating jelly reduces friction. Often the patient is better able to insert an object safely into the rectum. You never attempt to force a thermometer or suppository into the rectum without full view of the anus.

Maintenance of Skin Integrity   The patient with diarrhea or fecal incontinence is at risk for skin breakdown when fecal contents remain on the skin (see Chapter 36). The same problem exists for the patient with an ostomy that drains liquid stool. Liquid stool is usually acidic and contains digestive enzymes. Irritation from repeated wiping with toilet tissue aggravates skin breakdown. To prevent skin irritation, cleanse and dry the skin immediately after soiling occurs.

Instruct the patient about cleansing the anal area with mild soap and water after each passage of stool. When caring for a patient who is debilitated, incontinent, and unable to ask for assistance, check frequently for defecation. Protect the skin around anal areas with barrier ointments that hold moisture in the skin and protect the skin from irritation. Yeast infections of the skin develop easily. Do not use baby powder or cornstarch because they have no medicinal properties and they frequently cake on the skin and become difficult to remove.

BOX 34-11   PATIENT TEACHING

The Patient With an Ostomy

OUTCOME
- Patient/caregiver will be able to demonstrate changing an ostomy pouch.

TEACHING STRATEGIES
- Provide a comprehensive list of the products needed to care for the ostomy.
- Provide the patient/caregiver with supplies to last 1 to 2 weeks and the contact number of the closest medical supply store.
- Show patient/caregiver the step-by-step approach for changing an ostomy pouch.
- Provide at least one opportunity for patient/caregiver to change the ostomy pouch while patient is in hospital.
- Set up visits from a stoma care nurse or home care nurse, and provide contact numbers.
- Provide detailed discharge instructions for skin care, driving, lifting, resuming exercise, and when to contact the health care provider.

EVALUATION STRATEGIES
- Observe patient/caregiver change ostomy pouch.
- Ask patient/caregiver to state signs of stoma irritation and how to relieve it.
- Ask patient/caregiver about expected output from stoma and when to call health care provider.

REEFERENCE
Cronin E: Best practice in discharging patients with a stoma, *Nurs Times* 101(47):67, 2005.

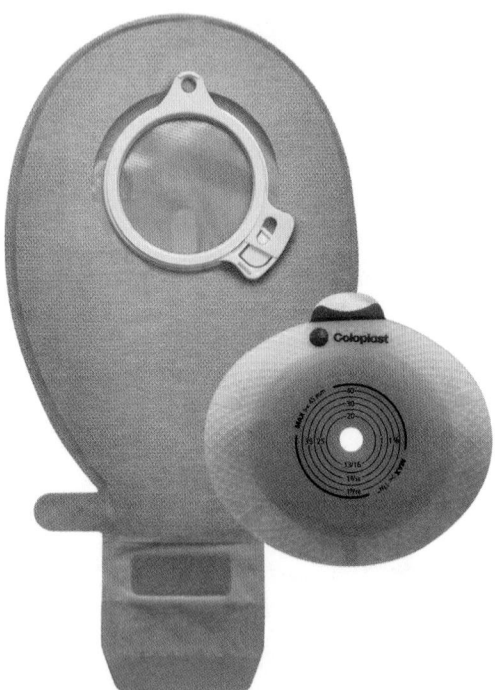

Figure 34-14 ■ Two-piece pouching system with separate skin barrier and attachable pouch. (Courtesy Coloplast, Minneapolis, Minn.)

■■■EVALUATION

PATIENT CARE Evaluate the effectiveness of nursing interventions for the patient with alterations in bowel elimination by determining success in meeting the patient's expected outcomes and goals of care. Optimally the patient will be able to eliminate soft-formed stools regularly. In addition, the patient will gain the information necessary to establish a normal elimination pattern.

Evaluate success of the plan by having the patient describe his or her elimination pattern following therapy. Also make it a point to evaluate the character of the patient's stool. A return to a more normal, regular elimination pattern can take time. Periodically reevaluate the patient (Box 34-12). A patient who defecates every 2 to 3 days and who has a soft, nondistended abdomen, with soft formed stool is a desirable finding.

Evaluate the success of a patient with an ostomy during self-care. Inspect the patient's peristomal skin, looking for impairment in skin integrity. Your evaluation will also include observing the patient change and empty an ostomy pouch. Evaluate the output or functioning of the ostomy or reservoir as well. In addition, consider the patient's self-esteem, and evaluate it by the patient's response to and willingness to care for the ostomy.

PATIENT EXPECTATIONS Using patient expectations identified during assessment, determine the patient's level of satisfaction with nursing care. Does the patient feel that you provided care respectfully, offering privacy and support when necessary? Is the patient satisfied with the elimination pattern established? Are stools easier to manage?

Your goal for the patient with an ostomy is to achieve a realistic level of self-care and to maintain or reinforce a healthy body image. When discussing these issues with the patient, determine if the patient's participation in care helped the patient accept the ostomy. Were expectations of the patient unrealistic? Did the patient feel like a partner in care? Learning about the patient's level of satisfaction with care will go a long way toward helping future patients.

BOX 34-12   EVALUATION

Vickie returns to see Mr. Gutierrez 2 weeks later. Vickie is eager to determine if Mr. Gutierrez has made changes in his diet and if his problems with bowel elimination have been progressing. Vickie is also eager to learn if the niece has assisted in having Mr. Gutierrez's stove repaired.

Mr. Gutierrez tells Vickie that he has been eating bran cereal in the morning, has been eating rice and/or beans for dinner, and has added one fruit each day to his diet. He has been walking twice a day through the long-term care center. Although he does not have a bowel movement each day, his stools are much softer and easier to pass and he says he is less concerned. He has not taken a laxative for a stool since last talking with Vickie.

DOCUMENTATION NOTE

"Bowel elimination is improving. Abdomen is soft and nondistended; bowel sounds normal and audible in all quadrants. After discussing the teaching plan, has agreed to alter his eating habits to include more fiber, fruit, and fluids. Although concern over bowel habits has not ceased, does state he feels 'in better control' and has decreased laxative use. Niece assisted in having stove repaired."

SAFETY GUIDELINES FOR NURSING SKILLS

Ensuring patient safety is an essential role of the professional nurse. To ensure patient safety, communicate clearly with the members of the health care team, assess and incorporate the patient's priorities of care and preferences, and use the best evidence when making decisions about your patient's care. When performing the skills in this chapter, remember the following points to ensure safe, individualized patient care:

- If a patient has cardiac disease or is on cardiac or hypertensive medication, obtain preprocedural pulse rate because manipulation of rectal tissue stimulates the vagus nerve and can cause a sudden decline in pulse rate, which can increase patient's risk for fainting while on the bedpan, commode, or toilet.
- Instruct patients who self-administer enemas to use the side-lying position. Administering an enema with the patient sitting on the toilet is unsafe because the curved rectal tubing will scrape the rectal wall.

SKILL 34-1   ADMINISTERING A CLEANSING ENEMA

DELEGATION CONSIDERATIONS

The skill of administering an enema can be delegated to nursing assistive personnel (NAP). It is the nurse's responsibility to assess the patient for specific considerations such as need for alternative positioning, comfort, and stable vital signs before the procedure. Instruct NAP about:

- Proper ways to position patients who have mobility restrictions

- Positioning of patients with therapeutic equipment present, such as drains, intravenous catheters, or traction
- Signs and symptoms of patient not tolerating the procedure, and when to stop it, including abdominal pain more than a pressure sensation, abdominal cramping, abdominal distention, or rectal bleeding
- The expected outcome of the enema and to immediately inform the nurse about the presence of blood in the stool

or around the rectal area, any change in patient vital signs, or new symptoms so the nurse is able to further assess the patient

EQUIPMENT
- Clean gloves
- Water-soluble lubricant
- Waterproof, absorbent pads
- Bath blanket
- Toilet tissue
- Bedpan, bedside commode, or access to toilet
- Basin, washcloths, towel, and soap
- Intravenous (IV) pole

Enema Bag Administration
- Clean gloves
- Enema container with tubing and clamp attachment
- Appropriate-size rectal tube:
  - Adult: 22 to 30 Fr
  - Child: 12 to 18 Fr
- Correct volume of warmed solution:
  - Adult: 750 to 1000 mL
  - Child:
    - 150 to 250 mL, infant
    - 250 to 350 mL, toddler

- 300 to 500 mL, school-age child
- 500 to 700 mL, adolescent

Prepackaged Enema
- Prepackaged enema container with rectal tip (Figure 34-15).

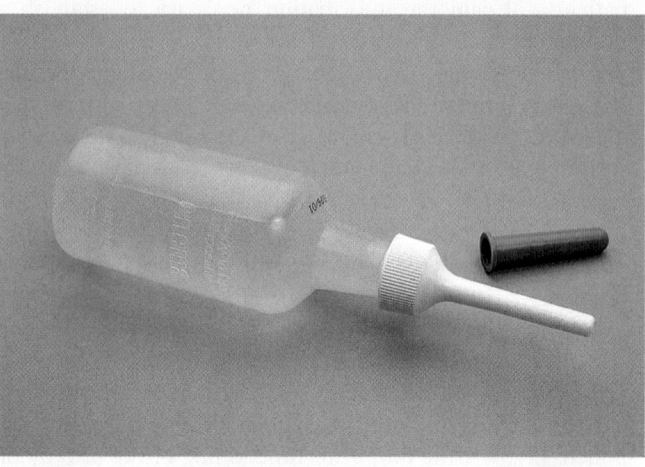

Figure 34-15 ■ Prepackaged enema container with rectal tip.

STEP	RATIONALE

ASSESSMENT

1 Assess status of patient: last bowel movement, normal versus most recent bowel pattern, bowel sounds, hemorrhoids, mobility, external sphincter control, presence of abdominal pain.

Determines factors indicating need for enema and influencing the type of enema used. Also establishes a baseline for bowel function.

2 Review medical record for presence of increased intracranial pressure, glaucoma, or recent abdominal, rectal or prostate surgery.

These conditions contraindicate use of enemas.

3 Inspect abdomen for presence of distention and auscultate for bowel sounds.

Provides a baseline for determining effectiveness of the enema.

4 Determine patient's level of understanding of purpose of enema.

Allows you to plan for appropriate teaching measures.

5 Review the health care provider's order for type of enema and number to administer.

Enemas require a health care provider's order. Determines number and type of enema you will give.

- **Critical Decision Point:** "Enemas until clear" order means that you repeat enemas until patient passes fluid that is clear of fecal matter. Check agency policy, but usually patients receive no more than three consecutive enemas, to avoid disruption of fluid and electrolyte balance. It is essential to observe contents of solution passed. Consider the results "clear" when no solid fecal material exists, but the solution is sometimes colored.

PLANNING

1 Collect appropriate equipment.
2 Identify patient using two identifiers (e.g., name and birthday or name and account number, according to facility policy).

Complies with The Joint Commission requirements and improves procedure safety. In most acute care settings you will use the patient's name and identification number on armband and MAR to identify patients (The Joint Commission, 2009). Information promotes patient cooperation and reduces anxiety.

STEP	RATIONALE

3 Assemble enema bag with appropriate solution and rectal tube.

IMPLEMENTATION

1 Perform hand hygiene, and apply clean gloves.

Reduces transmission of microorganisms.

2 Provide privacy by closing curtains around bed or closing door.

Reduces embarrassment for patient.

3 Raise bed to appropriate working height for nurse: Stand on right side of bed, and raise side rail on opposite side.

Promotes good body mechanics and patient safety.

4 Assist patient into left side-lying (Sims') position with right knee flexed. Children may also be placed in dorsal recumbent position.

Positioning allows enema solution to flow downward by gravity along natural curve of sigmoid colon and rectum, thus improving retention of solution.

• **Critical Decision Point:** If you suspect patient of having poor sphincter control, position on bedpan in a comfortable dorsal recumbent position. Patients with poor sphincter control are unable to retain all of the enema solution. Administering an enema with the patient sitting on the toilet is unsafe because the curved rectal tubing will scrape the rectal wall.

---

5 Place waterproof pad under hips and buttocks.

Prevents soiling of linen.

6 Cover patient with bath blanket, exposing only rectal area, clearly visualizing anus. Separate buttocks, and examine perianal region for abnormalities, including hemorrhoids, anal fissure, and rectal prolapse.

Provides warmth, reduces exposure of body parts, and allows patient to feel more relaxed and comfortable.

Findings will influence approach to insert enema tip. Prolapse contraindicates an enema.

7 Place bedpan or commode in easily accessible position. If patient will be expelling contents in toilet, ensure that toilet is free. (If patient will be getting up to bathroom to expel enema, place patient's slippers and bathrobe in easily accessible position.)

Used in case patient is unable to retain enema solution.

8 Administer enema:

A Enema Bag

   (1) Add warmed solution to enema bag: warm tap water as it flows from faucet, place saline container in basin of hot water before adding saline to enema bag, and check temperature of solution by pouring small amount of solution over inner wrist. If soap suds enema is ordered, add castile soap.

Hot water will burn intestinal mucosa. Cold water causes abdominal cramping and is difficult to retain.

   (2) Raise container, release clamp, and allow solution to flow long enough to fill tubing.

Removes air from tubing.

   (3) Reclamp tubing.

Prevents further loss of solution.

   (4) Lubricate 6 to 8 cm (2½ to 3 inches) of tip of rectal tube with lubricating jelly.

Allows smooth insertion of rectal tube without risk for irritation or trauma to mucosa.

   (5) Gently separate buttocks, and locate anus. Instruct patient to relax by breathing out slowly through mouth.

Breathing out promotes relaxation of external anal sphincter.

   (6) Insert tip of enema tube slowly by pointing tip in direction of patient's umbilicus (see illustration). Length of insertion varies: Adult and adolescent: 7.5 to 10 cm (3 to 4 inches); child: 5 to 7.5 cm (2 to 3 inches); infant: 2.5 to 3.75 cm (1 to 1½ inches).

Careful insertion prevents trauma to rectal mucosa from accidental lodging of tube against rectal wall. Insertion beyond proper limit causes bowel damage.

• **Critical Decision Point:** If pain occurs or resistance is felt during the procedure, stop and confer with health care provider. Do not force tube into rectum.

---

   (7) Hold tubing in rectum constantly until end of fluid instillation.

Bowel contraction causes expulsion of rectal tube.

   (8) Open regulating clamp, and allow solution to enter slowly while holding container at patient's hip level.

Rapid instillation stimulates evacuation of rectal tube.

SKILL 34-1 **ADMINISTERING A CLEANSING ENEMA—cont'd**

STEP	RATIONALE
(9) Raise height of enema container slowly to appropriate level above anus: 30 to 45 cm (12 to 18 inches) for high enema, 30 cm (12 inches) for regular enema, 7.5 cm (3 inches) for low enema. Installation time varies depending on the volume of solution you administer (e.g., 1 L/10 min) (see illustration).	Allows for continuous, slow instillation of solution; raising container too high causes rapid instillation and possible painful distention of colon. High pressure causes rupture of bowel in infant.
(10) Lower container or clamp tubing if patient complains of cramping or if fluid escapes around rectal tube.	Temporarily stopping instillation prevents cramping, which prevents patient from retaining all fluid, altering the effectiveness of the enema.
(11) Clamp tubing after you instill all solution.	Prevents air from entering the rectum.
B Prepackaged Disposable Container	
(1) Remove plastic cap from rectal tip. Apply more jelly as needed to the prelubricated tip.	Lubrication provides for smooth insertion of rectal tube without causing rectal irritation or trauma.
(2) Gently separate buttocks, and locate rectum. Instruct patient to relax by breathing out slowly through mouth.	Breathing out promotes relaxation of external rectal sphincter.
(3) Expel any air from the enema container.	Introducing air into the colon causes further distention and discomfort.
(4) Insert tip of bottle gently into rectum toward the umbilicus. *Adult/adolescent:* 7.5 to 10 cm (3 to 4 inches) *Child:* 5 to 7.5 cm (2 to 3 inches) *Infant:* 2.5 to 3.75 cm (1 to 1½ inches)	Gentle insertion prevents trauma to rectal mucosa.
(5) Squeeze bottle until all of solution has entered rectum and colon. Instruct patient to retain solution until the urge to defecate occurs, usually 2 to 5 minutes.	Hypertonic solutions require only small volumes to stimulate defecation.
9 Place layers of toilet tissue around tube at anus, and gently withdraw rectal tube.	Provides for patient's comfort and cleanliness.
10 Explain to patient that a feeling of distention is normal, as well as some abdominal cramping. Ask patient to retain solution as long as possible while lying quietly in bed. (For infant or young child, gently hold buttocks together for few minutes.)	Solution distends bowel. Length of retention varies with type of enema and patient's ability to contract rectal sphincter. Longer retention promotes more effective stimulation of peristalsis and defecation.

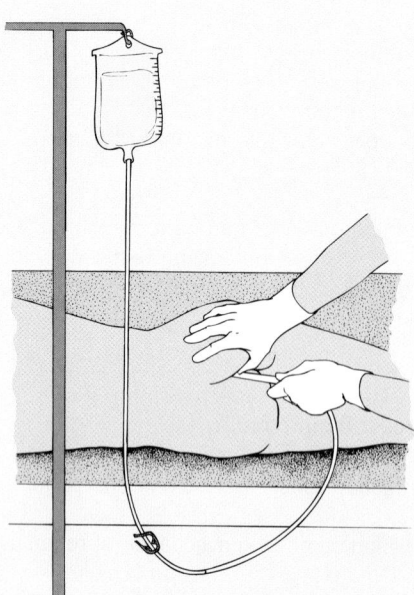

Step 8A(6) ■ Insertion of enema tube into rectum.

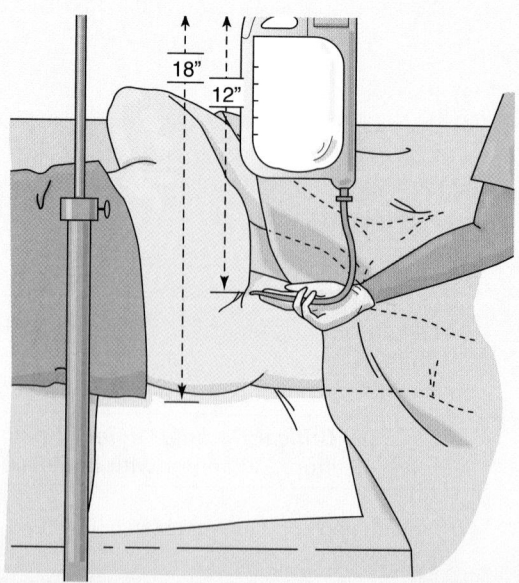

Step 8A(9) ■ An enema is given in teh Sims' position. The IV pole is positioned so that the enema bag is 12 inches above the anus and approximately 18 inches above the mattress (depending on the patient's size). (From Sorrentino SA: Mosby's textbook for nursing assistants, ed 6, St. Louis, 2006, Mosby.)

STEP	RATIONALE
11 Discard enema container and tubing in proper receptacle, or rinse bag out thoroughly with warm soap and water if container is reusable.	Reduces transmission and growth of microorganisms.
12 Assist patient to bathroom or help to position patient on bedpan.	Normal squatting position promotes defecation.
13 Assist patient as needed in washing anal area with warm soap and water (if you administer perineal care, use clean gloves).	Fecal contents irritate skin. Hygiene promotes patient's comfort.
14 Remove and discard gloves, and perform hand hygiene.	Reduces transmission of microorganisms.

EVALUATION

1 Observe character of feces and solution evacuated (caution patient against flushing toilet before inspection). Inspect color, consistency, amount of stool, odor, and fluid passed.	Determines if stool is evacuated or fluid is retained. Note abnormalities such as presence of blood or mucus.
2 **Auscultate bowel sounds.** Assess condition of abdomen; cramping, rigidity, or distention indicates a serious problem.	Determines if distention is relieved. Excess volume distends or damages the bowel.

RECORDING AND REPORTING

- Record type and volume of enema given, time administered, characteristics of results, and patient's tolerance to the procedure in nurses' notes.

- Report failure of patient to defecate and any adverse effects to the health care provider.

UNEXPECTED OUTCOMES AND RELATED INTERVENTIONS

- Abdomen becomes rigid and distended.
  - Stop enema.
  - Notify health care provider.
  - Obtain vital signs.

- Abdominal pain or cramping develops.
  - Slow rate of instillation; have patient take slow, deep breaths.
- Bleeding develops.
  - Stop enema.
  - Notify health care provider.
  - Remain with patient, and obtain vital signs.

SKILL 34-2 INSERTING AND MAINTAINING A NASOGASTRIC TUBE FOR GASTRIC DECOMPRESSION

DELEGATION CONSIDERATIONS

The skill of inserting and maintaining a nasogastric (NG) tube cannot be delegated to nursing assistive personnel (NAP). The nurse is responsible for the proper function and drainage of the NG tube, all relevant assessments, and determining the patient's level of comfort. The nurse directs the NAP to:
- Measure and record the drainage from an NG tube
- Provide oral and nasal hygiene measures
- Perform selected comfort measures, such as positioning, ice chips if allowed
- Use the correct technique to anchor the tube to the patient's gown during routine care to prevent accidental displacement

EQUIPMENT

- 14 or 16 Fr NG tube (smaller-lumen catheters are not used for decompression in adults because they must be able to remove thick secretions)
- Water-soluble lubricating jelly
- Clean gloves
- pH test strips (measure gastric aspirate acidity)
- Tongue blade
- Flashlight
- Emesis basin
- Asepto bulb or catheter-tipped syringe
- 2.5-cm (1-inch)-wide hypoallergenic tape or commercial fixation device
- Safety pin and rubber band
- Clamp, suction machine, or pressure gauge if wall suction is to be used
- Towel
- Glass of water with straw
- Normal saline
- Tincture of benzoin *(optional)*
- Suction equipment

| SKILL 34-2 | INSERTING AND MAINTAINING A NASOGASTRIC TUBE FOR GASTRIC DECOMPRESSION—cont'd |

STEP	RATIONALE

ASSESSMENT

1 Perform hand hygiene.

2 Inspect condition of patient's nasal and oral cavity.

3 Ask if patient has had history of nasal surgery, and note if deviated nasal septum is present.

4 Auscultate for bowel sounds. Palpate patient's abdomen for distention, pain, and rigidity.

5 Assess patient's level of consciousness and ability to follow instructions.

6 Determine if patient has had an NG tube insertion in the past and which nares was used.

7 Check medical record for health care provider's order, type of NG tube to be placed, and whether tube is to be attached to suction.

Rationale (Assessment):

Reduces transmission of microorganisms.

Baseline condition of nasal and oral cavity determines need for special nursing hygiene measures after tube placement.

Alerts nurse to possible obstruction. Insert tube into *__uninvolved__* nasal passage. Procedure may be contraindicated if surgery is recent.

In the presence of diminished or absent bowel sounds, auscultate the abdomen for 5 minutes in all four quadrants to make sure you do not miss any sounds and to localize specific sounds (Jarvis, 2008). Baseline determination of level of abdominal distention and function later serves as comparison once tube is inserted. Decreased bowel sounds occur with peritonitis and paralytic ileus.

Determines patient's ability to assist in procedure.

Patient's previous experience will complement any explanations.

Procedure requires health care provider's order. Adequate decompression depends on NG suction.

PLANNING

1 Prepare equipment at the bedside. Have a 10-cm (4-inch) piece of tape ready with one end split in half to form a V, or have NG tube fixation device available.

2 Identify patient using two identifiers (e.g., name and birthday or name and account number, according to facility policy).

3 Position patient in high-Fowler's position with pillows behind head and shoulders. Raise bed to a horizontal level comfortable for the nurse.

Rationale (Planning):

Ensures well-organized procedure. Tape will be used to initially hold tube in place after insertion.

Complies with The Joint Commission requirements and improves procedure safety. In most acute care settings you will use the patient's name and identification number on armband and medical record to identify patients (The Joint Commission, 2009). Identification prevents error of placing tube in wrong patient. Explanation gains patient's cooperation and ability to anticipate nurse's action.

Promotes patient's ability to swallow during procedure. Good body mechanics prevents injury to nurse.

IMPLEMENTATION

1 Peform hand hygiene. Apply clean gloves.

2 Place bath towel over patient's chest; give facial tissues to patient. Place emesis basin within reach.

3 Pull curtain around the bed, or close room door. Wash bridge of nose with soap and water or alcohol swab.

4 Stand on patient's right side if right-handed, left side if left-handed.

5 Instruct patient to relax and breathe normally while occluding one naris. Then repeat this action for other naris. Select nostril with greater airflow.

Rationale (Implementation):

Reduces transmission of microorganisms.

Prevents soiling of patient's gown. Tube insertion through nasal passages may cause tearing and coughing with increased salivation.

Provides privacy. Removes oils from nose to allow tape to adhere.

Allows easiest manipulation of tubing.

Tube passes more easily through naris that has more airflow.

STEP	RATIONALE

6 Measure distance to insert tube:

a *Traditional method:* Measure distance from tip of nose to earlobe to xiphoid process (see illustration).

Tube should extend from naris to stomach; distance varies with each patient.

b *Hanson method:* First mark 50-cm point on tube; then do traditional measurement. Tube insertion should be to midway point between 50 cm (20 inches) and traditional mark.

7 Mark length of tube to be inserted with small piece of tape placed around tube so it can be easily removed.

Marks amount of tube to be inserted from naris to stomach.

8 Curve 10 to 15 cm (4 to 6 inches) of end of tube tightly around index finger, then release.

Curving tube tip aids insertion and decreases stiffness of tube.

9 Lubricate 7.5 to 10 cm (3 to 4 inches) of end of tube with water-soluble lubricating gel.

Minimizes friction against nasal mucosa and aids insertion of tube. Water-soluble lubricant is less toxic if aspirated.

10 Alert patient that procedure is to begin.

Decreases patient anxiety and increases patient cooperation.

11 Initially instruct patient to extend neck back against pillow; insert tube slowly through naris with curved end pointing downward (see illustration).

Facilitates initial passage of tube through naris and maintains clear airway for open naris.

12 Continue to pass tube along floor of nasal passage, aiming down toward ear. When you feel resistance, apply gentle downward pressure to advance tube (do not force past resistance).

Minimizes discomfort of tube rubbing against upper nasal turbinates. Resistance is caused by posterior nasopharynx. Downward pressure helps tube curl around corner of nasopharynx.

13 If resistance is met, try to rotate the tube and see if it advances. If still resistant, withdraw tube, allow patient to rest, relubricate tube, and insert into other naris.

Forcing against resistance can cause trauma to mucosa. Helps relieve patient's anxiety.

• *Critical Decision Point:* If unable to insert tube in either naris, stop procedure and notify health care provider.

---

14 Continue insertion of tube until just past nasopharynx by gently rotating tube toward opposite naris.

a Once past nasopharynx, stop tube advancement, allow patient to relax, and provide tissues.

Relieves patient's anxiety; tearing is natural response to mucosal irritation, and excessive salivation may occur because of oral stimulation.

b Explain to patient that next step requires that patient swallow. Give patient glass of water unless contraindicated.

Sipping of water aids passage of NG tube into esophagus.

15 With tube just above oropharynx, instruct patient to flex head forward, take a small sip of water, and swallow. Advance tube 2.5 to 5 cm (1 to 2 inches) with each swallow of water. If patient is not allowed fluids, instruct to dry swallow or suck air through straw. Advance tube with each swallow.

Flexed position closes off upper airway to trachea and opens esophagus. Swallowing closes epiglottis over trachea and helps move the tube into the esophagus. Swallowing water reduces gagging or choking. Water can be removed later from stomach by suction.

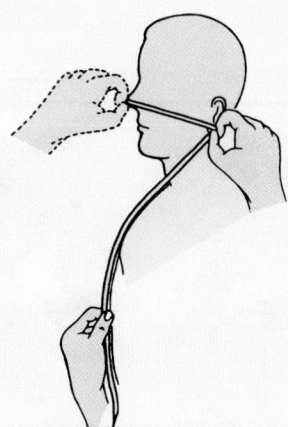

Step 6a ■ Technique for measuring distance to insert NG tube.

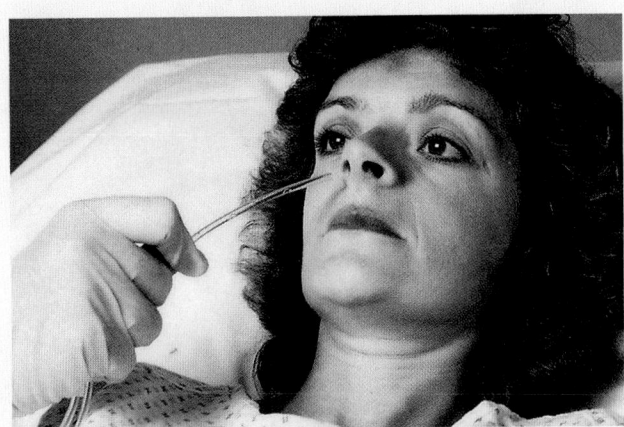

Step 11 ■ Insert NG tube with curved end pointing downward.

SKILL 34-2	INSERTING AND MAINTAINING A NASOGASTRIC TUBE FOR GASTRIC DECOMPRESSION—cont'd

STEP	RATIONALE
16 If patient begins to cough, gag, or choke, withdraw slightly and stop tube advancement. Instruct patient to breathe easily and take sips of water.	Tubing may accidentally enter larynx and initiate cough reflex, and withdrawal of the tube reduces risk for laryngeal entry. Swallowing water eases gagging, which you must give cautiously to reduce the risk for aspiration.

• **Critical Decision Point:** If vomiting occurs, assist patient in clearing airway; oral suctioning may be needed. Do not proceed until airway is cleared.

STEP	RATIONALE
17 If patient continues to cough during insertion, pull tube back slightly.	Tube may enter larynx and obstruct airway.
18 If patient continues to gag and cough or complains that the tube feels as though it is coiling in the back of the throat, check back of oropharynx using flashlight and tongue blade. If tube is coiled, withdraw it until the tip is back in the oropharynx. Then reinsert with the patient swallowing.	Tube may coil around itself in back of throat and stimulate gag reflex.
19 After patient relaxes, continue to advance tube with swallowing until you reach the tape or mark on tube, which signifies the tube is at the desired distance. Temporarily anchor tube to patient's cheek with a piece of tape until tube placement is verified.	Tip of tube should be within stomach to decompress properly. Anchoring of tube prevents accidental displacement while the tube placement is verified.
20 Verify tube placement: Check agency policy for preferred methods for checking tube placement.	
a Ask patient to talk.	Patient is unable to talk if NG tube has passed through vocal cords.
b Inspect posterior pharynx for presence of coiled tube.	Tube is pliable and can coil up in back of pharynx instead of advancing into esophagus.
c Attach Asepto or catheter-tipped syringe to end of tube and aspirate by gently pulling back on syringe to obtain gastric contents. Observe color (see illustration).	Gastric contents are usually cloudy and green, but may be off-white, tan, bloody, or brown in color. Aspiration of contents provides means to measure fluid pH and thus determine tube tip placement in gastrointestinal tract. Other common aspirate colors include duodenal placement (yellow or bile stained) and esophagus (may or may not have saliva-appearing aspirate).
d Measure pH of aspirate with color-coded pH paper with range of whole numbers from 1 to 11 (see illustration).	Gastric aspirates have decidedly acidic pH values, preferably 4 or less, compared with intestinal aspirates, which are usually have a pH greater than 4, or respiratory secretions, which usually have a pH greater than 6.

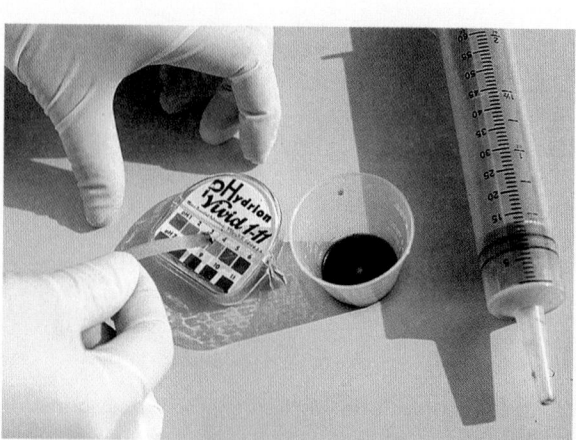

Step 20c ■ Aspiration of gastric contents.   **Step 20d** ■ Checking pH of gastric aspirate.

STEP	RATIONALE

• **Critical Decision Point:** Be sure to use gastric (Gastroccult) pH test and not Hemoccult test.

e Have ordered x-ray examination of chest/abdomen performed.

f If tube is not in stomach, advance another 2.5 to 5 cm (1 to 2 inches) and repeat Steps 20a to d to check tube position.

X-ray examination is best method to verify initial placement of the tube.

Tube must be in stomach to provide decompression.

21 Anchoring tube:

a After tube is properly inserted and positioned, either clamp end or connect it to suction machine.

Drainage bag is used for gravity drainage. Intermittent suction is most effective for decompression. Patient going to the operating room or for diagnostic tests often has tube clamped.

b Tape tube to nose; avoid putting pressure on nares.

(1) Take prepared 4-inch strip of tape and split halfway.

Prevents tissue necrosis. Tape anchors tube securely.

(2) Before taping tube to nose, apply small amount of tincture of benzoin to lower end of nose and allow to dry *(optional)*. Apply tape to nose, leaving the split end free. Be sure top end of tape over nose is secure.

Benzoin prevents loosening of tape if patient perspires.

(3) Carefully wrap two split ends of tape around tube (see illustration).

(4) *Alternative:* Apply tube fixation device using shaped adhesive patch (see illustration).

c Fasten end of NG tube to patient's gown by looping rubber band around tube in slipknot. Pin rubber band to gown (provides slack for movement). Do not attach pin to NG tube itself.

Reduces pressure on naris if tube moves.

d Unless health care provider orders otherwise, head of bed should be elevated 30 degrees. When using a Salem sump tube, keep pigtail above level of stomach

Helps prevent esophageal reflux and minimizes irritation of tube against posterior pharynx.

Prevents siphoning action that clogs the tube.

e Explain to patient that sensation of tube should decrease somewhat with time.

Adaptation to continued sensory stimulus.

f Remove gloves, discard, and perform hand hygiene.

Reduces transmission of microorganisms.

22 Once placement is confirmed:

a Place a mark, either a red mark or tape, on the tube to indicate where the tube exits the nose.

The mark or tube length is to be used as a guide to indicate whether displacement may have occurred.

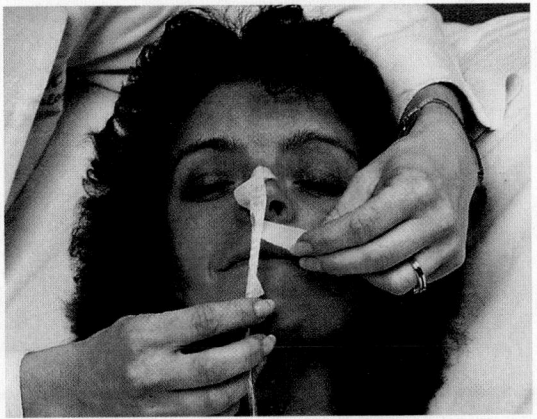

Step 21b(3) ■ Tape is crossed over and around NG tube.

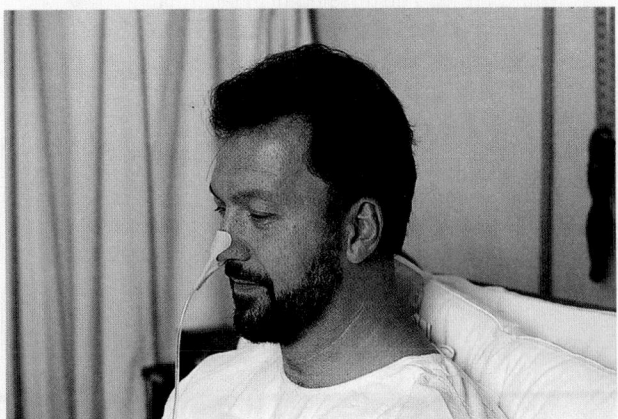

Step 21b(4) ■ Patient with tube fixation device.

SKILL 34-2	INSERTING AND MAINTAINING A NASOGASTRIC TUBE FOR GASTRIC DECOMPRESSION—cont'd

STEP	RATIONALE
b *Option:* Measure the tube length from naris to connector as an alternative method.	
c Document the tube length in the patient record.	
23 Attach NG tube to suction as ordered. Usual setting is low intermittent.	Suction creates gastric decompression.
24 Tube irrigation:	
a Perform hand hygiene, and apply clean gloves.	Reduces transmission of microorganisms.
b Check for tube placement in stomach (see Step 20). Then, temporarily clamp tube or reconnect to connecting tube and remove syringe.	Prevents accidental entrance of irrigating solution into lungs.
c Draw up 30 mL of normal saline into Asepto or catheter-tip syringe.	Use of saline minimizes loss of electrolytes from stomach fluids.
d Clamp NG tube. Disconnect from connecting tubing, and lay end of connection tubing on towel.	Reduces soiling of patient's gown and bed linen.
e Insert tip of irrigating syringe into end of NG tube. Remove clamp. Hold syringe with tip pointed at floor, and inject saline slowly and evenly. Do not force solution.	Position of syringe prevents introduction of air into vent tubing, which could cause gastric distention. Solution introduced under pressure can cause gastric trauma.

* ***Critical Decision Point:*** Do not introduce saline through blue "pigtail" air vent of Salem sump tube.

STEP	RATIONALE
f If resistance occurs, check for kinks in tubing. Turn patient onto left side. Report repeated resistance to health care provider.	Tip of tube may lie against stomach lining. Repositioning on left side may dislodge tube away from the stomach lining. Buildup of secretions will cause distention.
g After instilling saline, immediately aspirate by pulling back slowly on syringe to withdraw fluid. If amount aspirated is greater than amount instilled, record the difference as output. If amount aspirated is less than amount instilled, record the difference as intake.	Irrigation clears tubing, so stomach should remain empty. Fluid remaining in stomach is measured as intake.
h Reconnect NG tube to drainage or suction. (If solution does not return, repeat irrigation.)	Reestablishes drainage collection; may repeat irrigation or repositioning of tube until NG tube drains properly.
i Remove gloves, and perform hand hygiene.	Reduces transmission of microorganisms.
25 Discontinuation of NG tube:	
a Verify order to discontinue NG tube.	Health care provider's order required for procedure.

* ***Critical Decision Point:*** Immediately before removing the nasogastric tube, verify the presence of bowel sounds.

STEP	RATIONALE
b Explain procedure to patient, and reassure that removal is less distressing than insertion.	Minimizes anxiety and increases cooperation. Tube passes out smoothly.
c Perform hand hygiene, and apply clean gloves.	Reduces transmission of microorganisms.
d Turn off suction, and disconnect NG tube from drainage bag or suction. Remove tape or fixation device from bridge of nose, and unpin tube from gown.	Have tube free of connections before removal.
e Stand on patient's right side if right-handed, left side if left-handed.	Allows easiest manipulation of tube.
f Hand the patient facial tissue; place clean towel across chest. Instruct patient to take and hold a deep breath.	Patient may wish to blow nose after tube is removed. Towel may keep gown from getting soiled. Airway will be temporarily obstructed during tube removal.
g Clamp or kink tubing securely, and then pull tube out steadily and smoothly into towel held in other hand while patient holds breath.	Clamping prevents tube contents from draining into oropharynx. Reduces trauma to mucosa and minimizes patient's discomfort. Towel covers tube, which is an unpleasant sight. Holding breath helps to prevent aspiration.

STEP	**RATIONALE**
h Measure amount of drainage, and note character of content. Dispose of tube and drainage equipment into proper container.	Provides accurate measure of fluid output. Reduces transfer of microorganisms.
i Clean nares, and provide mouth care.	Promotes comfort.
j Position patient comfortably, and explain procedure for drinking fluids, if not contraindicated.	Depends on health care provider's order. Sometimes patients are allowed nothing by mouth (NPO) for up to 24 hours. When fluids are allowed, oral intake usually begins with a small amount of ice chips each hour and increases as patient is able to tolerate more.
26 Clean equipment, and return to proper place. Place soiled linen in utility room or proper receptacle.	Proper disposal of equipment prevents spread of microorganisms and ensures proper exchange procedures.
27 Remove gloves, and perform hand hygiene.	Reduces transmission of microorganisms.

EVALUATION

1 Observe amount and character of contents draining from NG tube. Ask if patient feels nauseated.	Determines if tube is decompressing stomach of contents.
2 Auscultate for the presence of bowel sounds. Turn off suction while auscultating. Then, palpate patient's abdomen periodically, noting any distention, pain, and rigidity.	Always auscultate before palpation of the abdomen. Determines success of abdominal decompression and the return of peristalsis. The sound of the suction apparatus may be transmitted to abdomen and be misinterpreted as bowel sounds.
3 Inspect condition of nares and nose.	Evaluates onset of skin and tissue irritation.
4 Observe position of tubing.	Determines if tension is being applied to nasal structures.
5 Ask if patient feels sore throat or irritation in pharynx.	Evaluates level of patient's discomfort.

RECORDING AND REPORTING

- Record length, size, and type of gastric tube inserted, time of insertion, and through which nostril it was inserted. Also record patient's tolerance to procedure, confirmation of tube placement, character of gastric contents, pH value, whether the tube is clamped or connected to suction, and the amount of suction supplied.

- Record amount of normal saline instilled and amount of gastric aspirate removed on intake and output (I&O) sheet. Record in nurses' notes or flow sheet amount and character of contents draining from NG tube every shift.
- Record removal of tube as "intact," the patient's tolerance of procedure, and final amount and character of NG drainage.

UNEXPECTED OUTCOMES AND RELATED INTERVENTIONS

- Patient's abdomen is distended or painful.
  - Assess patency of the tube.
  - Irrigate tube.
  - Verify that suction is on as ordered.
- Patient complains of sore throat from dry, irritated mucous membranes.
  - Perform oral hygiene more frequently.
  - Ask health care provider whether patient can suck on ice chips or throat lozenges.

- Patient develops irritation or erosion of skin around nares.
  - Provide frequent skin care to area.
  - Retape tube to avoid pressure on naris.
  - Consider re-insertion and switching tube to other naris. Consult with health care provider.
- Patient develops signs and symptoms of pulmonary aspiration: fever, shortness of breath, or pulmonary congestion.
  - Perform complete respiratory assessment.
  - Notify health care provider.
  - Obtain chest x-ray examination as ordered.
  - Clamp tubing, and do not flush it or put any medications or feedings through it until tube placement is verified.

| SKILL 34-3 | POUCHING AN OSTOMY |

DELEGATION CONSIDERATIONS

The skill of pouching the ostomy cannot be delegated to nursing assistive personnel (NAP). The one exception in some agencies is care of an enterostomy (4 weeks or more postoperatively). The nurse informs the NAP about:

- The expected amount, color, and consistency of drainage from the enterostomy
- The expected appearance of the stoma
- Special equipment needed to complete procedure
- When to report changes in the patient's stoma and surrounding skin integrity

EQUIPMENT

- Clear drainable colostomy/ileostomy/urostomy pouch in correct size for two-piece system (see Figure 34-14, p. 1012) or custom cut-to-fit, one-piece type with attached skin barrier (see Figure 34-13, p. 1011)
- Ostomy measuring guide
- Pouch closure device, such as a clamp or pouch valve
- Adhesive remover *(optional)*
- Clean gloves
- Ostomy deodorant, if needed
- Gauze pads or washcloth
- Towel or disposable waterproof barrier
- Basin with warm tap water
- Scissors/pen
- Skin barrier such as sealant wipes or wafer
- Tape or ostomy belt *(optional)*
- Stethoscope

| STEP | RATIONALE |

ASSESSMENT

1 Perform hand hygiene, and apply clean gloves. Auscultate for bowel sounds.

Reduces transmission of microorganisms. Documents presence of peristalsis. Absence of sounds indicates a problem.

2 Observe existing skin barrier and pouch for leakage and length of time in place. Depending on type of pouching system used (such as opaque pouch), remove the pouch to fully observe the stoma. Clear pouches permit the viewing of the stoma without their removal.

Determines likelihood of pouch loosening from stoma and failing to collect effluent. Routine observation allows for early detection of potential problems (Turnbull, 2007). Leaking indicates the need for a different pouch or sealant.

3 Observe stoma for color, swelling, trauma, and healing; make sure stoma is moist and reddish pink. Assess type of stoma. Stomas are flush with the skin or are a budlike protrusion on the abdomen (see illustration).

Stoma characteristics are one of the factors to consider when selecting an appropriate pouching system (WOCN, 2005).

- **Critical Decision Point:** When a new ostomy is present, it is important to measure the stoma with each pouching system change to determine correct size of equipment needed. The system may need modifications as the stoma size changes (WOCN, 2005). Follow each ostomy pouch manufacturer's directions and measuring guide to determine which size ostomy pouch to use based on patient's actual stoma measurement size.

---

4 Observe abdominal contour and abdominal incision (if present).

Relationship of abdominal contour to stoma determines proper placement of pouch. The presence of pressure areas from the pouching system may necessitate the use of a new pouching system (WOCN, 2005).

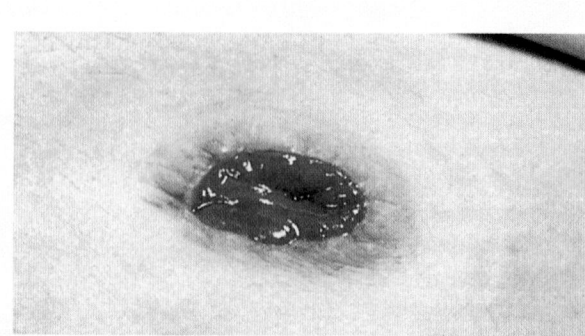

Step 3 ■ Normal bud stoma. (Courtesy Hollister, Incorporated, Libertyville, Ill. Permission to use this copyrighted material has been granted by the owner, Hollister International.)

STEP	RATIONALE
5 Observe effluent from stoma, and keep a record of intake and output. Ask patient about skin tenderness.	Plan on routine changing of skin barrier pouch at times of less effluent output. Generally avoid changing after meals, when gastrocolic reflux increases chance of fecal effluent output.
6 Assess condition of peristomal skin; check that pouching system is not leaking.	Irritation suggests pouch leaking. Leaking indicates the need for a different type of pouch or sealant.

> • ***Critical Decision Point:*** Because of stoma and abdominal characteristics, some patients need their ostomy pouching system to curve outward to avoid leakage.

STEP	RATIONALE
7 To minimize skin irritation, avoid unnecessary changing of entire pouching system. You change a one-piece pouch with attached skin barriers or the skin barrier of a two-piece pouching system every 3 to 5 days, *not* daily (Colwell and others, 2004).	Empty pouches when one-third to one-half full because weight of contents will dislodge skin seal, and ostomy drainage is irritating to the skin. Also, pouches collect flatus (gas), which will disrupt skin seal if it is not expelled.
8 Assess abdomen for best type of pouching system to use. Consider: **a** Contour and peristomal plane	Determines pouching system selection and need for other equipment. A firm/flat and round/hard abdomen usually needs a flexible or soft pouching system, whereas a flabby or soft abdomen usually needs a firmer system (see illustration for Step 3). Stomas that are retracted or in skin folds need convexity (curving outward), and different pouching systems are necessary to prevent leaking.

b Presence of scars, incisions
  c Location and type of stoma
9 Select appropriate pouching system:
  a One-piece pouch with skin barrier already attached; precut pouch and skin barrier; or two-piece pouch system, which consists of pouch that detaches from skin barrier and remains around patient's stoma for several days.	

b Two-piece pouches give patient choice of using either an open-ended or closed-ended pouch.	Patient is able to remove the pouch from skin barrier to empty effluent. For some patients, accessory products, such as karaya paste or careful use of a pouch belt, will enhance the seal and prevent leakage.
c Determine the need for the patient to switch to a pouch with a vent or filter if excessive gas accumulation is present.	Allows for patient comfort.
10 Assess the patient's self-care ability to determine the best type of pouching system to use. Assess the patient's vision, dexterity or mobility, and cognitive function.	Patients with poor vision will benefit by using yellow-tinted sunglasses to reduce glare and improve contrast and by using magnification mirrors. Patients who also have mobility problems or spinal cord injuries will benefit by using equipment that has a longer pouch, which is easier to empty independently when sitting (Hocevar and Gray, 2008). Patients who have difficulty using their hands or who have limited vision will find a one-piece system or a precut pouch and skin barrier more desirable to use; others prefer being able to keep the skin barrier in place for several days and changing just the pouch. For these patients the two-piece system is preferable.
11 Remove existing pouch, if any, by gently pushing skin from adhesive barrier; properly dispose of soiled pouch (save clamp if attached to pouch). After skin barrier and pouch removal, assess skin around stoma, noting scars, folds, skin breakdown, and peristomal suture line, if present.	Prevents skin irritation and controls odor. Determines need for barrier paste to increase adherence of pouch to skin or to fill in irregularities. Many enterostomal pouch systems have a flexible adhesive, a pectin, karaya or synthetic wafer flange that assists in leak prevention. Karaya is a natural gum product that softens with body heat and conforms to the contours around the stoma. A deeper skin crease will need a paste to fill in the defect and prevent leakage (Turnbull, 2007).

SKILL 34-3   POUCHING AN OSTOMY—cont'd

STEP	RATIONALE
12 Remove gloves, and perform hand hygiene.	Reduces transmission of microorganisms.
13 Determine patient's emotional response, knowledge, and understanding of an ostomy and its care.	Assists in determining how able the patient is to participate in care and determines the need for teaching and information clarification (Pontieri-Lewis, 2006).

PLANNING

1 Identify patient using two identifiers (e.g., name and birthday or name and account number, according to facility policy).	Complies with The Joint Commission requirements and improves procedure safety. In most acute care settings you will use the patient's name and identification number on armband and MAR to identify patients (The Joint Commission, 2009).
2 Explain procedure to patient; encourage patient's interaction and questions.	Lessens anxiety and promotes patient's participation.
3 Assemble equipment, and close room curtains or door.	Organization saves time, optimizes use of time, and conserves the patient's energy. Provides privacy.

IMPLEMENTATION

1 Position patient either standing or supine, and drape, leaving area around stoma exposed. If seated, position patient either on or in front of toilet.	When patient is supine, there are fewer skin wrinkles, which allows for ease of application of pouching system; maintains patient's dignity.
2 Perform hand hygiene, and apply clean gloves.	Reduces transmission of microorganisms.
3 Place towel or disposable waterproof barrier under patient.	Protects bed linen.
4 Cleanse peristomal skin gently with warm tap water using gauze pads or clean washcloth; do not scrub skin; dry completely by patting skin with gauze or towel.	Avoid use of soap because it leaves a residue on skin that interferes with pouch adhesion. Skin needs to be dry as skin barrier; pouch does not adhere to wet skin, and moisture increases patient's risk for fungal infections. If blood appears on gauze pad, do not be alarmed. If rubbed, stomas ooze some blood as a result of cleaning process. Stoma's surface is highly vascular mucous membrane. Bleeding into pouch is abnormal (Pontieri-Lewis, 2006).
5 If portions of the skin barrier remain, use an adhesive remover to gently remove them.	Improper removal of barrier will irritate patient's skin, cause skin tears, and result in poor adhering of the new pouch.

> • *Critical Decision Point:* Adhesive removers should not be routinely used. However, adhesive removers may be necessary when the patient's skin tears easily or there is a buildup of sticky residue over the peristomal skin. When adhesive removers are used, follow up with washing the skin with water and a mild soap to remove the oily coating on the skin from the adhesive remover (Pontieri-Lewis, 2006).

6 Measure stoma for correct size of pouching system needed using the manufacturer's measuring guide (see illustration).	Ensures accuracy in determining correct pouch size needed. Stoma shrinks and does not reach usual size for 6 to 8 weeks.
7 Select appropriate pouch for patient based on patient assessment. With a custom cut-to-fit pouch, use an ostomy guide to cut opening on the pouch $1/16$ to $1/8$ inch larger than stoma before removing backing. Prepare pouch by removing backing from barrier and adhesive. With ileostomy, apply thin circle of barrier paste around opening in pouch; allow to dry (see illustrations).	Size of pouch opening keeps drainage off skin and lessens risk for damage to stoma during peristalsis or activity. Change pouch and skin barrier whenever leaking. Change when patient is comfortable; before a meal is better because this avoids increased peristalsis and chance of evacuation during pouch change. Also, change pouch before or after tub bath or shower. Paste facilitates seal and protects skin. Stool is alkaline and contains enzymes, and this irritates skin; fecal bacteria colonize on skin and increase risk for infection.

> • *Critical Decision Point:* If patient has large amount of liquid stool from an ileostomy, consider using a "high-output" pouch that will contain this effluent and reduce frequency of pouch emptying.

STEP	RATIONALE

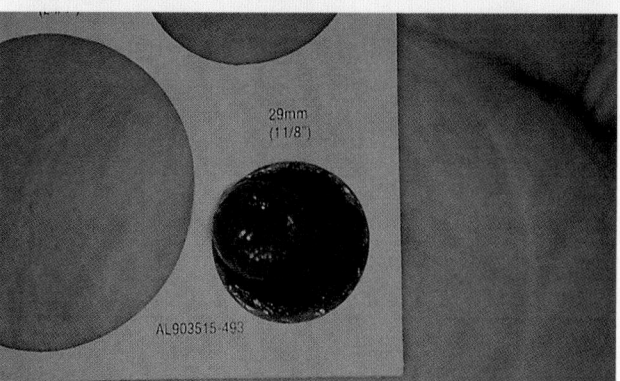

Step 6 ■ Measuring a stoma.

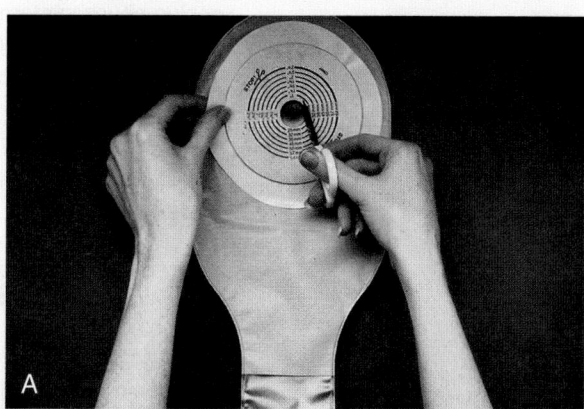

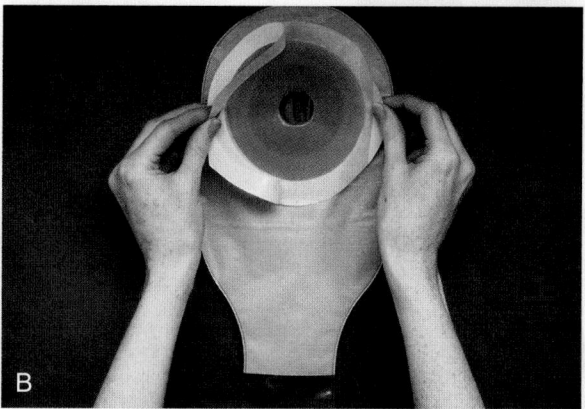

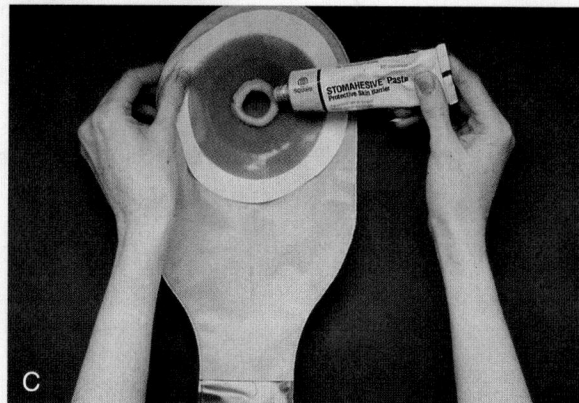

Step 7 ■ **A,** Cut-to-fit, one-piece drainable ostomy pouch. **B,** Removing the backing paper for the barrier of a one-piece pouch. **C,** Applying barrier paste to a one-piece ostomy pouch. (Courtesy ConvaTec, Princeton, NJ.)

8 Apply skin barrier and pouch. If creases next to stoma occur, use barrier paste to fill in; let dry 1 to 2 minutes.

Paste creates flat surface for pouch application.

9 Trim the skin barrier to fit when applying skin barrier to stoma that is close to patient's abdominal incision.

Allows for a better fit.

A For One-Piece Pouching System

   (1) Use skin sealant wipes on skin directly under adhesive skin barrier or pouch; allow to dry. Press adhesive backing of pouch and/or skin barrier smoothly against skin, starting from the bottom and working up and around sides.

Ensures smooth, wrinkle-free seal. Be aware of any irritated or open areas because the skin sealant wipes often contain alcohol (Pontieri-Lewis, 2006).

SKILL 34-3	POUCHING AN OSTOMY—cont'd

STEP	RATIONALE
(2) Hold pouch by barrier, center over stoma, and press down gently on barrier; bottom of pouch points toward patient's knees (see illustration).	A different positioning of the pouch is sometimes necessary to allow better gravity flow. For example, a patient confined to bed needs to have pouch positioned horizontally over the side of the abdomen.
(3) Maintain gentle finger pressure around barrier for 1 to 2 minutes.	Gentle pressure and body heat assist in adhesion.
B If Using Two-Piece Pouching System	
(1) Apply barrier-paste flange (barrier with adhesive) as in previous steps for one-piece system. Then snap on pouch, and maintain finger pressure (see illustration).	Creates wrinkle-free, secure seal; decreases irritation from adhesive on skin. Some two-piece pouching systems have a snapping or clicking sound that occurs when attaching pouch to skin barrier.
C For both pouching systems gently tug on pouch in a downward direction.	Determines that you have securely attached the pouch.
10 Gently press on the pectin or karaya flange to facilitate adhesion.	A pectin, karaya, or synthetic skin barrier adds to security of keeping pouch system attached securely (Turnbull, 2007). Some patients prefer a belt attached to the pouch for extra security.

- ***Critical Decision Point:*** Make sure patient who chooses to wear an ostomy belt does not have the belt too tight. To check for appropriate tightness, make sure two fingers fit comfortably between the belt and the patient's skin.

---

11 Although many ostomy pouches are odor proof, explain to patient not to use "home remedies," which will harm the stoma, to control ostomy odor. Do not make a hole in pouch to release flatus.	Causes damage to pouch and defeats purpose of odor-proof pouch. A hole for flatus will also allow effluent to leak. **Never add aspirin to an ostomy pouch.** It will cause stoma bleeding.
12 Fold bottom of drainable open-ended pouches up once, and close using a closure device such as a clamp (or follow manufacturer's instructions for closure).	Maintains secure seal to prevent leaking.
13 Properly dispose of old pouch and soiled equipment. Some patients will also request you to spray the room with air freshener.	Lessens odors in room.
14 Remove gloves, and perform hand hygiene.	Reduces transmission of microorganisms.
15 Change one- or two-piece pouch every 3 to 7 days unless leaking. Pouch remains in place for tub bath or shower. After bath, pat adhesive dry.	Avoids unnecessary trauma to skin from too-frequent changes. If patient removes pouch for bathing, have the patient use a mild soap without oils or deodorants. Make sure patient rinses all soap residue off. Drying ensures adhesion of pouch and prevention of skin irritation under pouch.

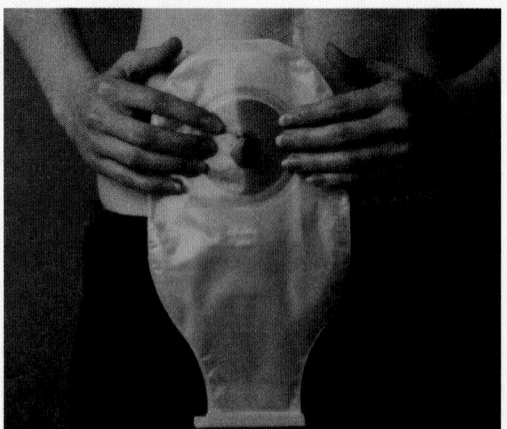

Step 9A(2) ■ Applying a one-piece pouch. (Courtesy ConvaTec, Princeton, NJ.)

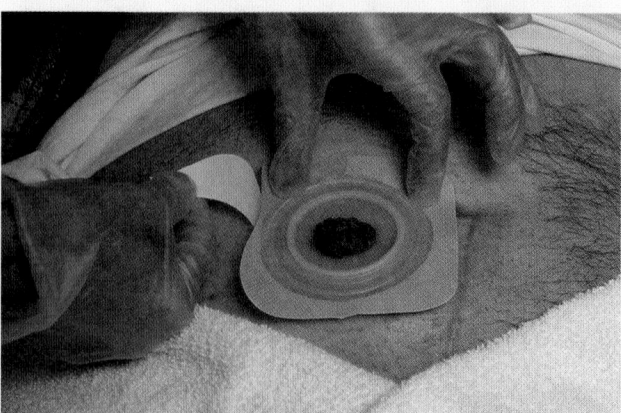

Step 9B(1) ■ Application of a barrier-paste flange. (Courtesy ConvaTec, Princeton, NJ.)

STEP	RATIONALE

EVALUATION

1 Ask if patient feels discomfort around stoma.

2 Note appearance of stoma, peristomal skin and existing incision (if present) while removing pouch and cleansing skin. Inspect condition of skin barrier and adhesive. Inspect edges of pouch for "tracking" of effluent under edges. This indicates a potential leak resulting from skin fold or wrinkles.

3 Auscultate bowel sounds, and observe characteristics of stool.

4 Observe patient's nonverbal behaviors as you apply pouch. Ask if patient has any questions about pouching.

Determines presence of skin irritation.

Determines condition of tissues and progress of healing. Determines presence of leaks.

Determines status of peristalsis and bowel elimination.

Indicates emotional response to stoma and readiness for teaching. Determines level of understanding of procedure.

RECORDING AND REPORTING

- Document type of pouch and skin barrier applied.
- Record amount and appearance of stool or drainage in pouch, size of stoma, color of stool, texture, condition of peristomal skin, and sutures.
- Document abdominal distention and excessive tenderness.
- Document nature and location of bowel sounds.

- Record patient's level of participation and need for teaching.
- Report any of the following to nurse in charge and/or health care provider:
  - Abnormal appearance of stoma, suture line, peristomal skin, character of output, absence of bowel sounds
  - No flatus in 24 to 36 hours and no stool by third day

UNEXPECTED OUTCOMES AND RELATED INTERVENTIONS

- Skin around stoma is irritated; a rash with red papules or white pustules may be present. The patient may complain of burning or itching sensations. May indicate an allergic reaction, evident by erythema and blistering, usually confined to one area immediately under allergen (Turnbull, 2007).
  - Assess stoma for separation of mucosal layer of stoma from skin.
  - Cleanse the area with normal saline, tap water, or noncytotoxic wound cleanser. Fill the separation to absorb drainage and provide healing (WOCN, 2005).
  - Determine if there is an undermining of pouch seal by fecal contents.
  - Increase frequency of pouching system changes to provide wound care. Use a pouching system that allows access to the separation so the entire system does not need to be changed (WOCN, 2005).
- Stoma is necrotic (purple or black color, has dry instead of moist texture, fails to bleed when washed gently, or has the presence of tissue sloughing).
  - Assess circulation to stoma.
  - Determine presence of excessive edema or excessive tension on bowel suture line.
  - Use transparent pouching system (WOCN, 2005).
  - Report finding to health care provider.

- Patient complains of irritation and burning around stoma.
  - Assess skin for breaks in integrity, skin inflammation, maceration, or infection.
  - Eliminate exposure of underlying skin to moisture or effluent.
  - If topical fungal infection is present, apply antifungal powder (WOCN, 2005).
  - If the patient has diabetes, assess serum glucose levels and determine the need for tighter controls to control risk for fungal infections (WOCN, 2005).
- Patient refuses to view stoma or participate in care.
  - Obtain information about ostomy support groups in community.
  - Refer patient and family to other volunteer patients with an ostomy in community for individual support.

KEY POINTS

- Mechanical breakdown of food elements, GI motility, and selective absorption and secretion of substances by the large intestine influence the character of feces.
- Food high in fiber content and an increased fluid intake keep feces soft.
- The greatest danger from diarrhea is fluid and electrolyte imbalance.
- The location of an ostomy influences the consistency of stool.
- Assessment of an elimination pattern focuses on bowel habits, an analysis of factors that normally influence defecation, a review of recent changes in elimination, and a physical examination.
- A fecal occult blood test is for patients who are over 50 years of age, take anticoagulants, have a bleeding disorder or GI disorder causing bleeding, or are at risk for colon cancer.

- Consider frequency of defecation, fecal characteristics, and effect of foods on GI function when selecting a diet promoting normal elimination.
- Consider the patient's usual time of defecation in the administration of cathartics or laxatives.
- Proper administration of an enema requires the slow instillation of the correct volume of a warm solution.
- A continent ostomy provides control over when fecal material exits.
- Dangers during digital removal of stool include traumatizing the rectal mucosa and promoting vagal stimulation.
- Skin breakdown occurs after repeated exposure to liquid stool. This is especially true in patients with a stoma.

CRITICAL THINKING EXERCISES

You are now caring for Mr. Gutierrez in the hospital. He had a colon resection for cancer 2 days ago and has a temporary colostomy.

1. What further data do you need to gather?
2. Describe what you would expect in assessing the stoma.

3. Mr. Gutierrez has not looked at the ostomy. What effect will this have on his independence? What are some strategies that you will use to help him with this adjustment?

ⓔvolve   *Answers to Critical Thinking Questions can be found on the Evolve website.*

REVIEW QUESTIONS

1. The nurse is placing a bedpan under a frail, underweight female patient. The nurse's actions are appropriate if what method is used?
   1. Slide the bedpan under the patient.
   2. Roll the patient onto a fracture bedpan.
   3. Shove the bedpan under the patient.
   4. Keep the patient flat after rolling her on the bedpan.
2. The nurse is assessing a 55-year-old patient who is in the clinic for a routine physical. The nurse plans on having the patient obtain a fecal occult blood test at home and then return the specimen. The nurse tells the patient to avoid eating fish, and certain raw vegetables. This precaution prevents:
   1. Development of diarrhea prior to the test
   2. Abdominal pain
   3. False positive test results
   4. Need to repeat FBOT
3. Diarrhea that occurs with a fecal impaction is the result of:
   1. A clear liquid diet
   2. Irritation of the intestinal mucosa
   3. Seepage of stool around the impaction
   4. Inability of the patient to form a stool
4. The nurse is caring for a patient with an established ostomy. The patient manages her colostomy on her own. However, she is now complaining of peristomal irrita-

tion. To determine the cause of this irritation, the nurse identifies the factors to assess. Select all that apply.
   1. Circulation to stoma and fit of pouch
   2. Quantity and consistency of fecal drainage in pouch
   3. Presence of signs of infection at the stoma or peristomal skin
   4. The use of an opaque pouching system
5. The nurse is to give a cleansing enema to a 55-year-old patient before intestinal surgery. The maximum amount given is:
   1. 150 to 200 mL
   2. 200 to 400 mL
   3. 400 to 750 mL
   4. 750 to 1000 mL
6. During an enema, the patient begins to complain of pain. The nurse notes blood in the return fluid and rectal bleeding. The first action by the nurse is:
   1. Stop the instillation
   2. Slow down the rate of instillation
   3. Obtain vital signs
   4. Tell the patient to breathe slowly and relax
7. The nursing assistive personnel (NAP) is preparing to administer a soapsuds enema to an adult patient. Which statement made by the NAP shows understanding of the correct technique to administer the enema?

1. "I will insert the tip of the tube 2 inches."
2. "I will administer the enema over 10 minutes."
3. "I will lubricate the tip of the enema tubing 1 to 1½ inches."
4. "I will raise the enema container to 24 inches above the anus."

8. Which of the following tasks can the nurse delegate to nursing assistive personnel?
   1. Insert a nasogastric tube.
   2. Administer a soapsuds enema.
   3. Assess for bowel sounds.
   4. Select the best ostomy pouch system for a stoma.

9. After caring for a first-day postoperative surgical patient with a new colostomy, which of the following would be expected in the documentation? Select all that apply.

1. Type of pouch applied
2. The appearance of the stoma
3. Presence/absence of bowel sounds
4. Small amount of semiformed stool

10. During insertion of a nasogastric tube, the nurse has the patient flex the head forward. What is the rationale for having the patient assume this position?
    1. It closes off the epiglottis over airway so the tube enters the esophagus.
    2. It facilitates the tube passing through the nasal passage.
    3. It prevents stimulation of the gag reflex.
    4. It helps to distract the patient during the procedure.

Answers to Review Questions can be found on pages 1197-1198.

REFERENCES

American Cancer Society: Cancer Facts and Figures 2009, Atlanta Ga, 2009.

Amerine E, Keirsey M: How should you respond to constipation? *Hosp Nurs* 36(10):64, 2006.

Bristol stool form guideline, http://aboutconstipation.org/site/about-constipation/treatment/stool-form-guide, accessed April 24, 2009.

Bulechek GM and others, editors: *Nursing interventions classification (NIC),* ed 5, St. Louis, 2008, Mosby.

Calado A and others: The Macedo-Malone antegrade continence enema procedure: early experience, *J Urol* 173:1340, 2005.

Colwell J and others: *Fecal and urinary diversions: management principles,* St. Louis, 2004, Mosby.

Cronin, E: Best practice in discharging patients with a stoma, *Nurs Times* 101(47):67, 2005.

Davis RH and others: Managing the chronically constipated adult: emerging approaches to diagnosis and treatment, *Clin Advisor* (Suppl):4, 2007.

Doughty D: *Urinary and fecal incontinence nursing,* ed 2, St. Louis, 2006, Mosby.

Greenwald B: A comparison of three stool tests for colorectal cancer screening, *Medsurg Nurs* 14(5): 292, 2005.

Hall K and others: Managing constipation in the elderly, *Geriatrics* (Suppl):3, 2007.

Hampton BG, Bryant RA: *Ostomies and continent diversions: nursing management,* St. Louis, 1992, Mosby.

Harris H: *C. difficile* attack of the killer diarrhea, *Nursing Made Incredibly Easy* 4(3):12, 2006.

Heitkemper M, Wolff J: Challenges in chronic constipation, *Nurse Pract* 32(4):36, 2007.

Hill R: Don't let constipation stop you up, *Nursing Made Incredibly Easy* 5(5):40, 2007.

Hinrichs M, Huseboe J: *Evidence-based protocol: management of constipation.* In Titler MG, series editor: Series on evidence based practice for older adults, Iowa City, 1998, The University of Iowa, Gerontological Nursing Interventions Research Center, Research Dissemination Core. For more information, http://www.nursing.uiowa.edu/center/gnirc/disseminatecore.htm.

Hocevar B, Gray M: Intestinal diversion (colostomy or ileostomy) in patients with severe bowel dysfunction following spinal cord injury, *J WOCN* 35(2):159, 2008.

Ignatavicius D, Workman L: *Medical-surgical nursing: critical thinking for collaborative care,* ed 5, St. Louis, 2006, Saunders.

Jarvis C: Physical examination & health assessment. Ed 5, Philadelphia, 2008, Saunders.

Kyle G: Assessment and treatment of older patients with constipation, *Nurs Stand* 21(8):41, 2006.

McKenry LM, Tessier E, Hogan MA: *Mosby's pharmacology in nursing,* ed 22, St. Louis, 2006, Mosby.

Moorhead S and others, editors: *Nursing outcomes classification (NOC),* ed 4, St. Louis, 2008, Mosby.

NANDA International: *NANDA International nursing diagnoses: definitions and classifications, 2009-2011,* Oxford, UK, 2009, Wiley-Blackwell.

Pontieri-Lewis V: Basics of ostomy care, *Medsurg Nurs* 15(4):199, 2006.

The Joint Commission: *2009 National Patient Safety Goals Hospital Program,* Oakbrook Terrace, Ill, 2009, The Joint Commission, http://www.jointcommission.org, accessed August 2009.

Turnbull G: An alternative solution for difficult-to-manage colostomies in the descending and sigmoid colon, *Ostomy Wound Manage* 21(6):12, 2007.

Wound, Ostomy and Continence Nurses Society: *Stoma complications: best practice for clinicians,* Glenview, Ill, 2005, The Society.

MEDIA RESOURCES

 CD COMPANION 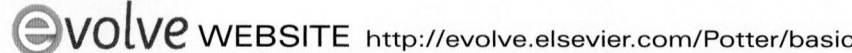 WEBSITE http://evolve.elsevier.com/Potter/basic

- Crossword Puzzle
- Audio Glossary
- English/Spanish Audio Glossary

OBJECTIVES

- Describe mobility and immobility.
- Discuss the benefits and hazards of bed rest.
- Identify changes in metabolic rate associated with immobility.
- Describe physical and physiological changes associated with immobility.
- Discuss factors that contribute to pressure ulcer formation.
- Describe psychosocial and developmental effects of immobilization.

- Complete a nursing assessment of an immobilized patient.
- Develop a nursing care plan for an immobilized patient.
- List appropriate nursing interventions for an immobilized patient.
- Evaluate nursing care for the immobilized patient.

KEY TERMS

activities of daily living (ADLs), p. 1033
anthropometric measurements, p. 1037
bed rest, p. 1033
bone resorption, p. 1035
disuse osteoporosis, p. 1035

diuresis, p. 1034
footdrop, p. 1035
hypercalcemia, p. 1034
hypostatic pneumonia, p. 1033
immobility, p. 1033
instrumental activities of daily living (IADLs), p. 1052

ischemia, p. 1035
isometric exercises, p. 1049
joint contracture, p. 1035
mobility, p. 1033
negative nitrogen balance, p. 1033

orthostatic hypotension, p. 1034
osteoporosis, p. 1035
pathological fractures, p. 1035
renal calculi, p. 1035
thrombus, p. 1034

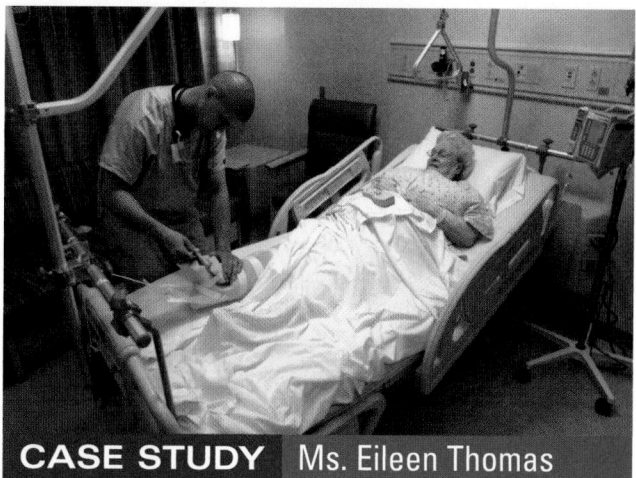

CASE STUDY   Ms. Eileen Thomas

Ms. Eileen Thomas, an 82-year-old widow, is admitted to the orthopedic unit for a fractured right hip. She is on complete bed rest in Buck's traction. She is waiting to receive medical clearance for surgery from her cardiologist because she has been on anticoagulants since her mitral valve was replaced a few months ago. She has had type 2 diabetes mellitus for the past 10 years and is a smoker. She lives by herself but has a son and two daughters who live within 5 miles of her home. She says, "I have no complaints. Just this thing with my heart, but it is OK now. But my goodness, now this fall!" She attends mass daily. Her weight is 195 lb, and she is 5 feet 7 inches tall. She cooks for herself, "using very little salt, but I do like to make cakes for the family." Her son takes her shopping.

Sergio Louis is a 19-year-old nursing student assigned to Ms. Thomas. It is his first day on the orthopedic unit; he spent the evening before caring for Ms. Thomas reviewing hip fractures and nursing care, Buck's traction, special needs of patients on anticoagulant therapy, and possible hazards Ms. Thomas may face because of her age and being immobilized in bed.

SCIENTIFIC KNOWLEDGE BASE

Mobility

Mobility is the capacity to move around freely in the environment. It serves many purposes, including expressing emotion, self-defense, attaining basic needs, participating in recreational activities, and completing **activities of daily living (ADLs)** such as bathing, dressing, and eating. Mobility through normal exercise assists in maintaining the body's normal physiological activities and requires the functioning of the nervous and musculoskeletal systems.

Immobility

Immobility occurs when a patient is unable to move independently or is restricted for therapeutic reasons, such as bed rest. **Bed rest** is an intervention in which a patient is restricted to bed for therapeutic reasons. Advantages of bed rest

include decreasing the body's oxygen needs, reducing pain, and allowing the debilitated or ill patient to rest. The duration of bed rest depends on the type and nature of the illness or injury and the patient's prior state of health. Another example in which immobilization is used therapeutically to limit movement is in the application of a cast or restrictive bandage.

When restricted mobility is not initiated for therapeutic reasons, but is the result of a patient's health condition, numerous types of health problems can develop. Patients with certain illnesses, injuries, or surgeries experience a period of immobilization. Factors that further contribute to the extent of a patient's immobility include length and severity of illness, presence of pain, cognitive and emotional status such as depression, and physical condition. No body system is immune to the hazardous effects of immobility (McCance and Huether, 2006). The greater the extent and longer the duration of immobility, the more pronounced the effects.

PHYSIOLOGICAL EFFECTS Each body system is at risk for impairment from immobility (Box 35-1). The severity of impairment depends on the patient's age, overall mental and physical health, and the extent of immobility. Despite a patient's age, impairment as a result of immobility affects the respiratory system, metabolism, fluid and electrolyte balance, gastrointestinal tract, cardiovascular system, musculoskeletal system, integument, and urinary elimination.

RESPIRATORY CHANGES Decreased lung expansion, generalized respiratory muscle weakness, and stasis of secretions occur with immobility. These conditions often contribute to the development of atelectasis (collapse of alveoli) and **hypostatic pneumonia** (inflammation of the lung from stasis or pooling of secretions).

With decreased lung expansion and weakened respiratory muscles, secretions stagnate or pool in the dependent lung regions. In atelectasis, secretions block a bronchiole or a bronchus and the distal lung tissue (alveoli) collapses. General muscle weakness reduces the patient's ability to cough. Mucus accumulates, particularly when the patient lies supine, providing an excellent medium for bacterial growth. The result may be hypostatic pneumonia.

CHANGES IN METABOLISM Immobility disrupts normal metabolic functioning, decreasing the metabolic rate and altering the metabolism of carbohydrates, proteins, and fats. A patient's basal metabolic rate (BMR) decreases in response to reduced cellular energy and oxygen demands. However, in the presence of an infection, immobilized patients have an increased BMR. Fever and wound repair increase cellular oxygen requirements (McCance and Huether, 2006).

Prolonged bed rest decreases the body's ability to produce insulin and metabolize glucose. When the body is unable to metabolize glucose, it begins to break down its protein stores for energy. Nitrogen is the end product of protein metabolism. Nitrogen balance therefore provides a reliable indicator of protein use by the body. A **negative nitrogen balance** exists when the excretion of nitrogen from the breakdown of protein exceeds intake. A negative nitrogen balance predisposes the patient to problems with wound healing and nor-

BOX 35-1 Pathophysiology of Immobility

PHYSIOLOGICAL OUTCOMES
- ↓ Basal metabolic rate
- ↓ Gastrointestinal motility
  - ↓ Nutrients/fluids
  - ↓ Appetite
- Shift in electrolyte balance
- ↓ O_2 availability/ischemia
  - ↓ O_2/CO_2 exchange
  - ↑ Respiratory muscle weakness
  - ↓ Lung expansion
  - ↑ Atelectasis/hypostatic pneumonia
- ↓ Cardiac output
  - ↑ Cardiac workload
  - ↑ Oxygen demand
  - ↑ Dependent edema
  - ↑ Clot formation (deep vein thrombosis)
- ↑ Muscle atrophy
  - ↓ Strength/flexibility/endurance
  - ↑ Joint contractures
- ↑ Disuse osteoporosis
- ↑ Bone resorption

PSYCHOLOGICAL OUTCOMES
- ↑ Stressors
- ↑ Depression
  - ↓ Self-identity
  - ↓ Self-esteem
- ↑ Behavioral changes
- ↑ Changes in sleep-wake cycles
- ↓ Coping successes
- ↑ Isolation
- ↑ Passive behaviors
- ↑ Sensory deprivation/overload

DEVELOPMENTAL OUTCOMES
- ↑ Dependence
- ↑ Regression in development

mal tissue growth. Immobility thus results in a loss of lean body mass and an increased percentage of body fat.

FLUID AND ELECTROLYTE BALANCES Major shifts in blood volume occur in immobile patients. **Diuresis** (increased urine excretion) occurs as a result of increased blood flow to the kidneys and expanded circulating blood volume. Diuresis causes the body to lose electrolytes, such as potassium and sodium. Diuresis also affects serum calcium levels. Immobility increases calcium resorption (loss) from bones, causing a release of excess calcium into circulation. This leads to **hypercalcemia** if the kidneys are unable to respond appropriately and the danger of pathological fractures if the immobility continues. (Copstead-Kirkhorn and Banasik, 2005).

GASTROINTESTINAL CHANGES Activity stimulates peristalsis. The immobile patient is at risk for constipation from lack of activity and from hypercalcemia, which de-

presses peristalsis. Constipation is sometimes so severe that fecal impaction occurs (see Chapter 34). Left untreated, a partial or complete bowel obstruction will occur.

CARDIOVASCULAR CHANGES Orthostatic hypotension occurs in patients on bed rest and after prolonged sitting. **Orthostatic hypotension** is a drop of 20 mm Hg or more in systolic blood pressure or a decrease in diastolic blood pressure of more than 10 mm Hg when the patient rises from a lying or sitting position to a standing position (Jarvis, 2008). In the immobilized patient decreased circulating fluid volume, pooling of blood in the lower extremities, and a decreased autonomic response occur. These factors result in decreased venous return, decreased central venous pressure and stroke volume, and a drop in systolic blood pressure when the patient stands (McCance and Huether, 2006).

Prolonged bed rest increases the heart's workload, producing a need for more oxygen. Bed rest also increases the resting heart rate 4 to 15 beats per minute. When the immobilized patient performs physical activity such as range-of-joint-motion (ROJM) exercises or ADLs, this increased rate is more pronounced).

Immobilized patients are at risk for deep vein thrombosis (DVT). A **thrombus** is an accumulation of platelets, fibrin, clotting factors, and cellular elements of the blood attached to the interior wall of a vein or artery, sometimes occluding the lumen of the vessel. Three factors contribute to venous thrombus formation: (1) loss of integrity of the vessel wall (e.g., injury), (2) abnormalities of blood flow (e.g., slow blood flow in calf veins associated with bed rest), and (3) alterations in blood constituents (e.g., a change in clotting factors or increased platelet activity). These three factors are referred to as Virchow's triad (McCance and Huether, 2006). Two additional problems predispose the immobilized patient to DVTs: (1) the weight of the legs on the bed compresses the blood vessels of the calves, causing stasis and injury to vessel linings, and (2) the skeletal muscles in the legs lose their pumping action, leading to stasis and less blood returning to the heart.

Venous thrombi place the patient at risk for pulmonary emboli, a life-threatening complication. Pulmonary emboli are clots that move to the lung and block a portion of the pulmonary artery, which disrupts the blood flow to the lungs. Immobilized surgical and older adult patients are at high risk for developing pulmonary emboli (Bartley, 2006).

MUSCULOSKELETAL CHANGES Immobility leads to loss of strength and endurance, decreased muscle mass, and decreased balance or stability. The body loses muscle strength when muscles are inactive. The rate of muscle decline varies with the degree of immobility, but it is rapid while mobility and weight bearing are restricted. These effects are devastating to patients who are marginally functional with their ADLs.

Reduced endurance develops when patients are immobile from changes in muscle strength and altered cardiovascular functioning. Muscle endurance decreases as a result of the inability of the cardiopulmonary system to meet the oxygen needs of the body. Reduced metabolism leads to a loss of muscle and body mass, causing fatigue with prolonged activity.

As immobility progresses and muscles are not exercised, muscle mass continues to decrease. The muscle atrophies, and the size of the muscle decreases. Immobility affects the leg muscles the most, which explains the difficulty older patients have in getting up out of a chair after periods of bed rest.

Immobility causes two skeletal changes: a joint contracture and disuse osteoporosis. A **joint contracture** is an abnormal and possibly permanent condition characterized by fixation of the joint. Disuse, atrophy, and shortening of muscle fibers and surrounding joint tissues cause joint contracture. When a contracture occurs, the joint cannot maintain full ROJM (Figure 35-1). Contractures leave joints in nonfunctional positions, as seen in patients who are permanently curled in a fetal position.

One common and debilitating contracture is **footdrop** (Figure 35-2). When footdrop occurs, the foot is permanently in plantar flexion. Ambulation is difficult with the foot in this position because the patient cannot dorsiflex.

Disuse osteoporosis is a disorder characterized by **bone resorption.** Immobilization increases the rate of bone resorption, which results in reduced bone tissue density. This increases the patient's risk for **pathological fractures.**

Osteoporosis is a major health concern in this country. This disease frequently affects women, whereas only 20% of men are diagnosed with the disease. The National Osteoporosis Foundation (2007) reports that 44 million Americans (55% of those over the age of 50) either have osteoporosis or are at risk for developing it. Although primary osteoporosis is different in origin from the osteoporosis that results from immobility, it is imperative to recognize that immobilized patients are at high risk for accelerated bone loss if they have primary osteoporosis.

INTEGUMENT CHANGES The direct effect of pressure on the skin by immobility is compounded by metabolic changes. Older adult patients and patients with paralysis have a greater risk for developing pressure ulcers (see Chapter 36). Pressure affects cellular metabolism by decreasing or obliterating tissue circulation. When a patient lies in bed or sits in a chair, the weight of the body is on bony prominences. The longer the pressure is applied, the longer the period of **ischemia** (temporary decrease of blood flow to an organ or tissue) and therefore the greater the risk for skin breakdown. Because of the change of circulation, any break in the skin's integrity is difficult to heal in the immobilized patient.

URINARY ELIMINATION CHANGES Urine flows out of the renal pelvis into the ureter and then the bladder because of gravitational forces when a patient is upright. When the patient is reclining or flat, the kidneys and ureters move toward a more level plane, and urine formed by the kidney enters the bladder against gravity. Because the peristaltic contractions of the ureters are not strong enough to overcome gravity, the renal pelvis fills before urine enters the ureters. This condition, called urinary stasis, increases the patient's risk for urinary tract infection (UTI) and renal calculi. **Renal calculi** are calcium stones that lodge in the renal pelvis and pass through the ureters. Immobilized patients are at risk for calculi because of altered calcium metabolism and the resulting hypercalcemia (see Chapter 33).

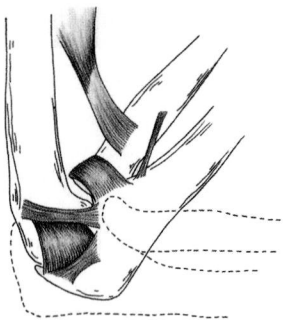

Figure 35-1 ■ Flexion contracture of elbow resulting in permanent flexion of joint. Normally the elbow is able to extend to a 90-degree angle *(dotted line)* and to a 180-degree angle *(not shown).*

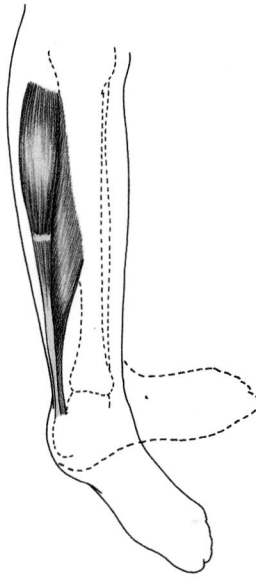

Figure 35-2 ■ Footdrop. Ankle is fixed in plantar flexion.

NURSING KNOWLEDGE BASE

Monitoring or assisting patients with mobility is basic to nursing. Concepts that relate to mobility such as movement, exercise and rest, and posture are soundly grounded in nursing research and nursing theories. Immobilization leads to a variety of psychosocial responses. Nurses must use assessment skills to fully understand the patient's initial condition and to monitor and evaluate care.

Psychosocial Effects

Immobilization reduces a patient's independence and creates a sense of loss. As a result, emotional, intellectual, sensory, and socio-cultural responses occur. The most common emotional changes are depression, sleep-wake disturbances, and impaired coping.

Some immobilized patients become depressed because of changes in self-concept (see Chapter 22). Depression is an affective disorder characterized by exaggerated feelings of sadness, melancholy, dejection, worthlessness, emptiness, helplessness, and hopelessness. Depression often reduces a person's willingness to take part in activity, thereby aggravating any immobile condition.

Immobilized patients require vigilant nursing care, such as repositioning at least every 2 hours or more often, to avoid physical complications. Because of the need for frequent repositioning, it is important to organize care activities together, including nursing and medical interventions to ensure the patient receives sufficient sleep (see Chapter 30). Disruption of normal sleeping patterns causes further behavioral changes and affects coping patterns.

Long-term immobility or bed rest affects usual coping patterns. Some immobilized patients withdraw and become passive. The passive patient demonstrates little interest in achieving independence or participating in care. Assess the patient's normal coping mechanisms, and develop a nursing care plan based on patient strengths.

Developmental Effects

Developmental effects of immobility more commonly affect the very young and the older adult. The immobilized young or middle-age adult experiences few, if any, developmental changes.

When the infant, toddler, or preschooler is immobilized, it is usually because of trauma or the need to correct a congenital skeletal abnormality. Prolonged immobilization delays the child's motor skill and intellectual development. When caring for immobilized children, plan activities that provide physical and psychosocial stimuli (Hockenberry and Wilson, 2007).

Immobilization in older adult patients increases their physical dependence on others and accelerates functional losses in physiological systems (Ebersole and others, 2008). Immobilization in older adults usually results from a degenerative disease, neurological trauma, or a chronic illness. For some patients immobilization occurs gradually and progressively, whereas for others—especially those who have had a cerebrovascular accident (CVA)—immobilization is sudden. Develop nursing care plans that encourage patient independence in as many self-care activities as possible.

CRITICAL THINKING

Synthesis

You will apply elements of critical thinking whenever you perform the nursing process with a patient. Consider the scientific knowledge you have learned, your experience, critical thinking attitudes, and standards to ensure an individualized approach to patient care. Gather information from a variety of sources when caring for patients. Integrating knowledge and experience makes it possible to determine physical, psychosocial, and developmental needs of immobilized patients.

KNOWLEDGE   Knowledge of pathophysiology helps you anticipate how patients will be affected by limitations in mobility. These limitations are sometimes the direct result of musculoskeletal alteration, such as a broken ankle, or deconditioning

from a chronic health problem, such as poor activity tolerance associated with cardiac problems. Your assessment of any limitation should focus on the pathophysiological changes you expect. For example, if you understand how a stroke affects the motor cortex, you know to assess for motor function on the side opposite the stroke. Conduct an assessment to determine the full extent of any limitations.

Also apply knowledge of patients' developmental stages to determine their current functional and mobility status and health care needs. Application of knowledge gained from the study of human growth and development is essential for accurately assessing patient needs and then selecting interventions for mobility alterations.

Knowledge of the physiological changes associated with immobility enables you to identify complications and intervene appropriately. Also knowledge of patient teaching is essential to prepare patients for rehabilitation following immobilization.

EXPERIENCE   Taking care of patients who had mobility restrictions in the past allows you to anticipate patients' needs for comfort, pain control, positioning, and support of ADLs. Experiential learning also occurs during visits to a physical therapy unit in the hospital or in a community. Your experience with a variety of exercise strategies helps develop health promotion activities or rehabilitation plans for assigned patients.

ATTITUDES   Design creative solutions to improve a patient's mobility status. Speak with other health care providers to determine the best setting to provide care. Collaboration and creativity help to establish an individualized rehabilitation program. The attitude of perseverance is essential for coordinating patient care and working with patients experiencing psychological and developmental changes resulting from immobilization. Use discipline and be thorough in your approach, considering patients' needs once they return home and how family caregivers can become involved.

STANDARDS   Promote a patient's independence while adhering to the prescribed rehabilitation plan and maintaining safety. Since 2003 in the *Position Statement on Elimination of Manual Patient Handling to Prevent Work-Related Musculoskeletal Disorders,* the American Nurses Association (2003) has prompted the use of evidence-based research upon which to develop policies for safe patient handling. Nursing policies and procedures offer standards for the safe use of transfer and positioning equipment with the result of decreased injuries to nurses and patients. Discharge instructions must be clear and explicit. Always use the ethical standard of autonomy in supporting patients in making decisions about their discharge needs. To evaluate discharge teachings, have patients demonstrate required actions to ensure that they understand them completely, can perform them correctly, and therefore validate the quality of the teaching sessions.

Synthesis of knowledge, experience, attitudes, and standards is important in developing an individualized care plan for the immobilized patient. This plan of care will help to prevent complications, promote rehabilitation, and expedite discharge.

NURSING PROCESS

■■■ ASSESSMENT

Mobility assessment focuses on patients' past and present mobility and the potential effects of immobility. Table 35-1 presents a focused patient assessment of immobility, pain associated with movement, and activity tolerance.

MOBILITY Assessment of the patient's mobility focuses on the musculoskeletal system and includes range of motion, muscle strength, activity tolerance, gait, and posture. Table 35-2 describes the ROJM for all joints in the body. Observing the patient's posture while sitting and standing and assessing gait helps to determine the type of assistance the patient requires for ambulation or transfer (see Chapter 26). Assess the patient for stiffness, muscle strength, pain and swelling of joints, and unequal or limited movement. These data provide baseline information to assess the patient's overall level of mobility and coordination and to then determine the extent of assistance needed to help the client maintain self-care skills. Patient immobility leads to physical, psychosocial, and developmental changes.

The major musculoskeletal changes expected during assessment of an immobilized patient include decreased muscle strength, loss of muscle tone and mass, and contractures. Patients with musculoskeletal injuries or chronic conditions require careful palpation of joints and extremities to minimize discomfort. Because immobilized patients are weakened, determine if difficulty in moving joints is the result of fatigue or decreased range of joint motion.

RESPIRATORY SYSTEM Perform a respiratory assessment at least every 2 hours for acutely ill patients with restricted activity. Monitor the patient's respiratory rate and oxygen saturation. Inspect chest wall movements, and auscultate the lungs to identify regions of diminished breath sounds. Focus auscultation for adventitious lung sounds on the dependent lung field because pulmonary secretions tend to accumulate in the lower lobes. If a patient has an atelectatic area (an area of collapsed alveoli), breath sounds will be asymmetrical. A complete respiratory assessment identifies the presence of secretions and is used to determine nursing interventions necessary to maintain optimal respiratory function.

METABOLIC SYSTEM When assessing the patient's metabolic functioning, measure intake and output and review laboratory data to evaluate fluid and electrolyte status. Assess the patient's nutritional status to determine the risk for nitrogen imbalance. A patient whose mobility is restricted often has a reduced appetite, altered gastrointestinal function, and a reduced capacity to self-feed.

Anorexia commonly occurs in immobilized patients. Assess food intake and the environment for unpleasant odors or noises that interfere with appetite. You can avoid nutritional imbalances if you learn the patient's previous dietary patterns and food preferences early in the immobilization (see Chapter 32).

Anthropometric measurements include height, weight, mid upper-arm circumference, and triceps skinfold measurements. Ideally, perform these assessments early in the period of immobilization, and repeat them at regular intervals.

TABLE 35-1 FOCUSED PATIENT ASSESSMENT

FACTORS TO ASSESS	QUESTIONS	PHYSICAL ASSESSMENT
Range of joint motion (ROJM)	Do you have any limited movement in your joints? Do you have a history of connective tissue disorders, fractures, or have had damage to your ligaments or tendons?	Observe patient's gait. Observe patient's ROJM for all joints. Inspect joints for deformity. Observe patient while performing self-care activities.
Pain	Do you have any pain or discomfort on movement? Ask patient to rate pain on a 0-10 pain scale. Please tell me about your pain, including its onset, duration, location, precipitating factors, and relief measures. Would you like your pain medication before I assist you with walking?	Observe for objective signs of pain such as grimacing, moaning, increasing respiratory rate, pulse, and blood pressure. Inspect joints for redness or swelling, indicating potential inflammatory process.
Endurance and activity	Are you feeling fatigued now? Are you having difficulty with bathing or washing yourself, getting to the bathroom, or dressing yourself because of muscle weakness? Are you experiencing shortness of breath or shortness of breath when you move about, palpitations, light-headedness, or dizziness?	Observe for signs of fatigue. Observe patient's performance of ADLs. Observe patient for pallor; obtain baseline vital signs. Monitor oxygen saturation before and following activity.

ADLs, Activities of daily living.

TABLE 35-2 Range-of-Motion Exercises

BODY PART	TYPE OF JOINT	TYPE OF MOVEMENT	RANGE (DEGREES)	PRIMARY MUSCLES
Neck, cervical spine	Pivotal	*Flexion:* Bring chin to rest on chest	45	Sternocleidomastoid
		Extension: Return head to erect position	45	Trapezius
		Hyperextension: Bend head back as far as possible	10	Trapezius
		Lateral flexion: Tilt head as far as possible toward each shoulder	40-45	Sternocleidomastoid
		Rotation: Turn head as far as possible in circular movement	180	Sternocleidomastoid, trapezius
Shoulder	Ball and socket	*Flexion:* Raise arm from side position forward to position above head	45-60	Coracobrachialis, deltoid
		Extension: Return arm to position at side of body	180	Latissimus dorsi, teres major, triceps brachii
		Hyperextension: Move arm behind body, keeping elbow straight	45-60	Latissimus dorsi, teres major, deltoid
		Abduction: Raise arm to side to position above head with palm away from head	180	Deltoid, supraspinatus
		Adduction: Lower arm sideways and across body as far as possible	320	Pectoralis major
		Internal rotation: With elbow flexed, rotate shoulder by moving arm until thumb is turned inward and toward back	90	Pectoralis major, latissimus dorsi, teres major, subscapularis
		External rotation: With elbow in full circle, move arm until thumb is upward and lateral to head	90	Infraspinatus, teres major
		Circumduction: Move arm in full circle (Circumduction is combination of all movements of ball-and-socket joint.)	360	Deltoid, coracobrachialis, latissimus dorsi, teres major
Elbow	Hinge	*Flexion:* Bend elbow so that lower arm moves toward its shoulder joint and hand is level with shoulder	150	Biceps brachii, brachialis, brachioradialis
		Extension: Straighten elbow by lowering hand	150	Triceps brachii
Forearm	Pivotal	*Supination:* Turn lower arm and hand so that palm is up	70-90	Supinator, biceps brachii
		Pronation: Turn lower arm so that palm is down	70-90	Pronator teres, pronator quadratus
Wrist	Condyloid	*Flexion:* Move palm toward inner aspect of forearm	80-90	Flexor carpi ulnaris, flexor carpi radialis
		Extension: Move fingers and hand posterior to midline	80-90	Extensor carpi radialis brevis, extensor carpi radialis longus, extensor carpi ulnaris
		Hyperextension: Bring dorsal surface of hand back as far as possible	80-90	Extensor carpi radialis brevis, extensor carpi radialis longus, extensor carpi ulnaris
		Abduction (radial deviation): Bend wrist laterally toward fifth finger	Up to 30	Flexor carpi radialis, extensor carpi radialis brevis, extensor carpi radialis longus
		Adduction (ulnar deviation): Bend wrist medially toward thumb	30-50	Flexor carpi ulnaris, extensor carpi ulnaris
Fingers	Condyloid hinge	*Flexion:* Make fist	90	Lumbricales, interosseus volaris, interosseus dorsalis

TABLE 35-2   Range-of-Motion Exercises—cont'd

BODY PART	TYPE OF JOINT	TYPE OF MOVEMENT	RANGE (DEGREES)	PRIMARY MUSCLES
Fingers— cont'd		*Extension:* Straighten fingers	90	Extensor digiti quinti proprius, extensor digitorum communis, extensor indicis proprius
		Hyperextension: Bend fingers back as far as possible	30-60	Extensor digitorum
		Abduction: Spread fingers apart laterally	30	Interosseus dorsalis
		Adduction: Bring fingers together laterally	30	Interosseus volaris
Thumb	Saddle	*Flexion:* Move thumb across palmar surface of hand	90	Flexor pollicis brevis
		Extension: Move thumb straight away from hand	90	Extensor pollicis longus, extensor pollicis brevis
		Abduction: Extend thumb laterally (usually done when placing fingers in abduction and adduction)	30	Abductor pollicis brevis and longus
		Adduction: Move thumb back toward hand	30	Adductor pollicis obliquus, adductor pollicis transversus
		Opposition: Touch thumb to each finger of same hand		Opponens pollicis, opponens digiti minimi
Hip	Ball and socket	*Flexion:* Move leg forward and up	90-120	Psoas major, iliacus, sartorius
		Extension: Move leg behind body	90-120	Gluteus maximus, semitendinosus, semimembranosus
		Hyperextension: Move leg behind body	30-50	Gluteus maximus, semitendinosus, semimembranosus
Knee	Hinge	*Abduction:* Move leg laterally away from body	30-50	Gluteus medius, gluteus minimus
		Adduction: Move leg back toward medial position and beyond if possible	30-50	Adductor longus, adductor brevis, adductor magnus
		Internal rotation: Turn foot and leg toward other leg	90	Gluteus medius, gluteus minimus, tensor fasciae latae
		External rotation: Turn foot and leg away from other leg	90	Obturatorius internus, obturatorius externus, quadratus femoris, piriformis, gemellus superior and inferior, gluteus maximus
		Circumduction: Move leg in circle	120-130	Psoas major, gluteus maximus, gluteus medius, adductor magnus
		Flexion: Bring heel back toward back of thigh	120-130	Biceps femoris, semitendinosus, semimembranosus, sartorius
		Extension: Return leg to floor	120-130	Rectus femoris, vastus lateralis, vastus medialis, vastus intermedius
Ankle	Hinge	*Dorsal flexion:* Move foot so that toes are pointed upward	20-30	Tibialis anterior
		Plantar flexion: Move foot so that toes are pointed downward	45-50	Gastrocnemius, soleus
Foot	Gliding	*Inversion:* Turn sole of foot medially	10 or less	Tibialis anterior, tibialis posterior
		Eversion: Turn sole of foot laterally	10 or less	Peroneus longus, peroneus brevis
Toes	Condyloid	*Flexion:* Curl toes downward	30-60	Flexor digitorum, lumbricalis pedis, flexor hallucis brevis
		Extension: Straighten toes	30-60	Extensor digitorum longus, extensor digitorum brevis, extensor hallucis longus
		Abduction: Spread toes apart	15 or less	Abductor hallucis, interosseus dorsalis
		Adduction: Bring toes together	15 or less	Adductor hallucis, interosseus plantaris

Chapter 32 discusses assessment of height and weight. A decrease in mid upper-arm circumference, measured in centimeters, or triceps skinfold, measured in millimeters, indicates a decline in muscle mass. After the initial assessment, take this measurement every 2 to 4 weeks, depending on the patient's age, previous physical condition, and the amount of immobility.

If an immobilized patient has a wound, the speed of healing indicates how well the body delivers nutrients to the tissues for use (see Chapter 36). The normal progression of wound healing indicates that the metabolic needs of the injured tissues are met.

CARDIOVASCULAR SYSTEM Cardiovascular assessment of the immobilized patient includes monitoring blood pressure, apical and peripheral pulses, and observing the venous system. Because of the risk for orthostatic hypotension, measure blood pressure when the patient moves from lying to a sitting or standing position. This assesses the patient's ability to tolerate postural changes and is important to know during transferring (see Chapter 26).

Recumbency increases the cardiac workload and results in an increased heart rate. In some patients, particularly the older adult, the heart is not able to tolerate the increased workload, and a form of cardiac failure develops. Assessing heart rate at rest and during exercise, such as getting up to a chair or walking in a hallway determines the patient's exercise tolerance.

To determine the status of peripheral circulation, assess peripheral pulses. If a patient is immobilized as a result of an external cast or bandage, assess for the presence of pulses below the affected area. Document and report the absence of a peripheral pulse, particularly one that was previously present, after the completion of the circulatory assessment (see Chapter 15).

Peripheral edema is one indicator of the heart's inability to handle the increased workload. Because fluid moves to dependent body regions, focus your assessment on the sacrum, legs, feet, and hips. If the heart is unable to tolerate the increased cardiac workload, the peripheral body regions such as the hands, feet, nose, and earlobes will be colder than the central body regions. This is a result of the body trying to compensate because of the heart having a problem tolerating the increased workload. One of the compensatory mechanisms is peripheral vasoconstriction, which results in more blood being directed back to the heart and less to the peripheral areas, so hands, feet, and other peripheral areas become cool to touch.

Assess the venous system for DVT. To assess for DVT, remove the patient's antiembolic stockings or sequential compression device (SCD) once every 8 hours, and observe the calves and thighs for unilateral leg swelling, redness, warmth, and tenderness. Ask the patient about calf pain. Assessing for Homans' sign, discomfort in the upper calf during forced dorsiflexion of the foot, is no longer considered an accurate predictor of DVT (Black and Hawks, 2009). Approximately half of all patients with DVTs are asymptomatic.

SKIN INTEGRITY Continually assess the skin for signs of pressure ulcer formation, especially over bony prominences. When you identify areas of redness, palpate the skin to determine if it blanches, which is normal. Skin that does not blanch is an early sign of skin injury. All immobilized patients are at high risk for developing pressure ulcers. Use of scales such as the Braden Scale (see Chapter 36) or the Gosnell Scale (Box 35-2) assesses a patient's risk for pressure ulcer formation. The type of risks then directs the interventions most appropriate to treat ulcers.

ELIMINATION SYSTEM Assess the patient's elimination status during each shift and the total intake and output every 24 hours (see Chapter 33). Assessment of elimination also includes auscultation for bowel sounds, the frequency and consis-

---

BOX 35-2 BEST PRACTICES

Selecting Clinical Tools to Determine Pressure Ulcer Risk Related to Immobility

SUMMARY OF EVIDENCE

When patients are immobile in bed, one of the possible complications is the development of pressure ulcers. Over the years, several tools have been developed to assess patients at the time of admission to predict those at risk for developing these painful and costly complications. However, there has been little evidence for choosing one tool over the others.

The purposes of these studies were to compare the predictive validity of four pressure ulcer risk assessment scales: Braden, Gosnell, Norton, and Waterlow. At the time of admission, 230 patients, free of any pressure ulcers, were assessed using the four scales and were reassessed once every 24 hours for a minimum of 14 weeks to identify any signs of skin breakdown.

The Gosnell Scale was most predictive in one study, whereas the Braden Scale was most predictive for a specific population. More studies must be conducted to provide more evidence to support which scale will work best for which population of patients.

APPLICATION TO NURSING PRACTICE

- Look at the evidence in research before using a particular tool or scale for all patients.
- Make sure that the evidence is adequate before implementing a broad change.
- The correct scale will save the patient needless pain and possible risk for infection.
- Prevention is much more cost-effective than treatment.
- Making an informed clinical decision at the beginning will result in the best patient outcomes.

REFERENCES

Ayello E: Predicting pressure ulcer risk, *Try This: Best Practices in Nursing Care to Older Adults*, issue 5, revised 2007, New York University College of Nursing, The Hartford Institute for Geriatric Nursing, http://www.ConsultGeriRN.org, accessed February 1, 2009.

Jalali R, Rezaie M: Predicting pressure ulcer risk: comparing the predictive validity of 4 scales, *Adv Skin Wound Care* 18(2):92, 2005.

tency of bowel movements, and the patient's typical urine and bowel elimination patterns (see Chapter 34). Accurate assessment and identification of patient problems enables you to intervene before fecal impaction and urinary incontinence occur.

PSYCHOSOCIAL CONDITION Changes in psychosocial status usually occur slowly. Observe for changes in emotional status (e.g., depression) and behavioral changes (e.g., cooperative patients who become argumentative or modest patients who begin to expose themselves repeatedly). Continual communication with family members is vital because they will identify and report changes in a patient's personality that the nurse or other caregiving team members may not recognize.

Evaluate patients' readiness to improve their level of independence. Be prepared to adapt teaching and motivational strategies to meet their expectations and needs.

Identify and correct any changes in the patient's sleep-wake cycle, such as difficulty falling asleep or frequent awakenings (see Chapter 30). Many sleep disruptions are preventable with an assessment of prior sleep habits and early intervention when you suspect problems. Observe for changes in the use of normal coping mechanisms to adapt to immobilization. Decreasing coping ability causes the patient to become disoriented, confused, or depressed.

DEVELOPMENT Assessment of the immobilized patient includes developmental considerations. Assess a young child's developmental stage before immobilization. Developmental delays or regression occur with prolonged bed rest. Reassure parents that these developmental changes are usually temporary.

Meeting the developmental needs of patients, especially older adults, with altered immobility is very important. Assess developmental needs of older adults to determine the patient's ability to meet needs independently. A decline in developmental functioning prompts investigation to determine the reasons the change occurred and the interventions necessary to restore the patient to an optimal level of functioning (see Chapter 21).

■■■NURSING DIAGNOSIS

Assessment reveals clusters of data that indicate whether a patient is at risk or if a mobility problem exists. The clusters of data include pertinent defining characteristics that support the nursing diagnosis and probable cause of the nursing diagnosis.

Locating the probable cause of the diagnosis is important to planning patient-centered goals and selecting nursing interventions that will best help the patient (Box 35-3).

An immobilized or partially immobilized patient will possibly have one or more of the following nursing diagnoses:

- *Ineffective airway clearance*
- *Risk for constipation*
- *Risk for disuse syndrome*
- *Risk for falls*
- *Impaired bed mobility*
- *Impaired physical mobility*
- *Risk for impaired skin integrity*
- *Ineffective peripheral tissue perfusion*
- *Impaired urinary elimination*

The two diagnoses most directly related to mobility problems are *impaired physical mobility* and *risk for disuse syndrome. Impaired physical mobility* is for the patient who demonstrates functional limitations but is not completely immobile. For the patient who is immobile and at risk for multisystem complications, the more pertinent nursing diagnosis is *risk for disuse syndrome.* The list of potential nursing diagnoses related to immobility is more extensive when alterations in physical, psychosocial, or developmental functioning occur. Often these problems are interrelated, and it is imperative that nursing care focus on all dimensions.

■■■PLANNING

Active care planning focused on prevention of physical, psychosocial, and developmental complications is essential. For example, encouraging or providing for range of joint motion and patient repositioning is a first step in preventing serious complications such as pneumonia or pulmonary emboli. In addition, routine monitoring of patients' skin condition using the Braden Scale helps avoid deterioration leading to infection or sepsis. Attention to detail in care planning is critical.

GOALS AND OUTCOMES Patients at risk for hazards of immobility require nursing care plans directed at meeting their actual and potential needs (see Care Plan). It is important to develop patient-centered goals aimed at preventing or reducing the hazards of immobility. Set realistic goals and

---

BOX 35-3   SYNTHESIS IN PRACTICE

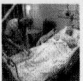

As Sergio prepares for the assessment on Ms. Thomas, he reviews the pathophysiology regarding the hazards of immobility. He gathers knowledge about fractures, hip surgery, and the expected postoperative physical therapy and rehabilitative measures. During a previous clinical experience, Sergio cared for a patient who received a cardiac valve and was given anticoagulant therapy. He knows that the medication will affect Ms. Thomas' postoperative status in several ways. Bleeding may be a problem during surgery. But after surgery, Ms. Thomas' bleeding times must be monitored very closely to prevent clots in the veins and in the chambers of the heart.

Sergio knows that he needs to respect Ms. Thomas' need to be independent and desire to participate in her care as much as possible. Sergio realizes he and his patient are far apart in age and knows that Ms. Thomas probably has her own rate at which to do things. He approaches this clinical experience with patience and creativity; he plans to implement individualized care to increase Ms. Thomas' activity level, help to keep her as independent as possible, prevent hazards of immobility, and assist her progression through the acute phase of her care.

CARE PLAN Impaired Bed Mobility

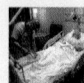

ASSESSMENT

As Ms. Thomas awaits surgery, Sergio knows that patients who smoke, have type 2 diabetes mellitus, are on anti-coagulants because of valve replacement surgery, and have a fractured hip are at risk for complications related to the hazards of immobility.

ASSESSMENT ACTIVITIES

Assess Ms. Thomas' skin for potential breakdown using the Braden Scale for a baseline.

Auscultate lungs sounds bilaterally.

Assess color, temperature, and capillary refill of lower extremities bilaterally.

Assess lower extremities at ankle, mid calf, and mid thigh bilaterally for edema.

Ask Ms. Thomas if she is having pain. Ask how she rates her pain right now on a scale of 0 to 10.

Ask Ms. Thomas if she is having any trouble taking a deep breath.

FINDINGS/DEFINING CHARACTERISTICS*

Ms. Thomas' score on the Braden Scale is **14.**

Ms. Thomas' **lungs are clear bilaterally.**

Right leg is cooler and 2 cm greater than left leg at mid-thigh. Capillary refill is equal bilaterally.

Unable to measure mid-calf of right leg at this time. No edema palpated.

Ms. Thomas said, "My leg **hurts like a 6,** but it is a little better now that it is in this thing."

Patient denies **having problems taking a deep breath.** Patient denies any chest pain.

NURSING DIAGNOSIS: Impaired bed mobility related to hip fracture/traction as evidenced by activity restrictions and pain.

PLANNING

GOAL

- Ms. Thomas will achieve pain control following analgesic administration.

- Ms. Thomas will maintain proper alignment in traction while in acute care facility.

EXPECTED OUTCOMES (NOC)†

Pain Control
- Ms. Thomas will rate her pain level as 3 or less on a scale of 0 to 10 within 30 minutes after receiving her pain medication.
- By the time of discharge to the rehabilitation facility, Ms. Thomas will verbalize her pain is successfully managed using pharmacological and nonpharmacological modalities.

Traction/Immobilization Care
- Right hip is aligned without evidence of joint displacement.

INTERVENTIONS (NIC)‡

Pain Management
- Assure Ms. Thomas that pain medication is available for her, and administer it on schedule rather than prn.

- Observe for nonverbal cues of discomfort, such as grimacing or clenching of fists.

- Teach use of nonpharmacological techniques for Ms. Thomas' pain reduction in conjunction with her pain medication. Demonstrate use of massage for relaxation and distraction to reduce Ms. Thomas' awareness of pain.

RATIONALE

- Administering pain medication on a schedule provides better control of pain and better patient outcome (Paice and others, 2005).
- Ms. Thomas may exhibit nonverbal signs of being in pain, as well as telling you she is experiencing pain. Therefore you must observe for such nonverbal cues.
- Massage produces physical and mental relaxation and reduces pain perception related to the gate control theory (McCance and Huether, 2006).

---

*Defining characteristics** are shown in **bold** type.

†Outcomes classification labels from Moorhead S and others, editors: *Nursing outcomes classification (NOC),* ed 4, St. Louis, 2008, Mosby.

‡Interventions classification label from Bulechek GM and others, editors: *Nursing interventions classification (NIC),* ed 5, St. Louis, 2008, Mosby.

CARE PLAN   Impaired Physical Mobility—cont'd

INTERVENTIONS (NIC)‡	RATIONALE

INTERVENTIONS (NIC)‡

Pain Management

- Monitor Ms. Thomas' satisfaction with pain management at specified intervals. Document her response to prescribed pain medication and nonpharmacological interventions.

Positioning

- Position Ms. Thomas in proper body alignment.
- Maintain proper position in bed to enhance traction.

- Ensure proper weights (15 lb) are applied to Ms. Thomas' right leg.
- Maintain the Buck's traction at all times.

- Monitor skin and bony prominences for signs of skin breakdown.

- Monitor circulation, movement, and sensation of affected extremity every 2 hours or more often if necessary. Observe the color of the toes and the nail beds, perform capillary refill, and feel for the pedal pulse and the temperature of the right foot compared to the left foot.

- Monitor Ms. Thomas for complications of immobility because of her high risk level.

- Arrange for a special bed for her on the orthopedic unit and at the rehabilitation center to reduce skin breakdown.

Self-Care Assistance: Bathing/Hygiene

- Determine type and amount of assistance Ms. Thomas will need to perform a partial bath, mouth care, brushing her hair, applying makeup if desired, etc.

- Provide an environment for Ms. Thomas that is therapeutic, warm, private, and conducive to performing personal care activities, and assist her as needed.

RATIONALE

- Continuous evaluation and documentation of pain relief is necessary to determine if Ms. Thomas requires new or revised therapies (see Chapter 31).

- Proper body alignment and maintaining proper position in bed enhances the action of the traction, thereby reducing the spasms of the muscles.
- The prescribed weight added to the Buck's traction is sufficient to reduce the muscle spasms, but should not cause an increase in pain. Applying the ordered weight to the Buck's traction maintains traction.

Meticulous skin care must be a priority for Ms. Thomas, especially over bony prominences, because she will be immobile in bed as a result of the fractured hip and the use of traction because she was not a candidate for surgery.

Comparing the affected extremity to the unaffected extremity provides a baseline. Capillary refill and palpation of the pedal pulses provide information about the quality of the circulation to the foot and the toes. Ms. Thomas has diabetes, which puts her at additional risk for skin breakdown, infection, circulatory problems, and neuropathy (McCance and Huether, 2006).

Her history reveals several factors that put her at high risk for complications:

- Smoker (decreased airway clearance at risk for hypostatic pneumonia)
- Fracture of head of femur (long bone fracture increases risk for fat embolism)
- Cardiac problem
- Advanced age
- Complete bed rest
- Traction limits movement in bed
- All physiological changes associated with diabetes (McCance and Huether, 2006)

Independence is very important for older adult patients, and having Ms. Thomas participate in her care as much as possible affords her "control" over her situation, thereby contributing to her sense of self-esteem (Ebersole and others, 2008).

Assist Ms. Thomas as needed, and assess her skin for any signs of impaired circulation or pressure. This is also a good time to perform a psychosocial assessment.

Continued

CARE PLAN Impaired Physical Mobility—cont'd

EVALUATION

NURSING ACTIONS	PATIENT RESPONSE/FINDING	ACHIEVEMENT OF OUTCOME
Ask Ms. Thomas about how often she will receive pain medication.	Ms. Thomas explained to the nurse her understanding of the pain medication schedule and how to use the pain scale to let the staff know her level of pain.	Ms. Thomas is knowledgeable about pain-control measures.
Ask Ms. Thomas to rate her pain on a scale of 0 to 10.	Ms. Thomas rated her pain as a 2 or 3 with medication and eventually with nonpharmacological methods.	Pain control is satisfactory.
Observe Ms. Thomas for nonverbal signs of pain.	There are no nonverbal signs of pain.	Pain control is satisfactory.
Observe Buck's traction each shift for proper weights, free hanging of weights, and safety of lines and pulleys.	Ms. Thomas maintained proper alignment and could explain the importance of "keeping my body in a straight line with the thing on my leg." She did not report any abnormal circulatory sensations or neurological symptoms. Pulses and capillary refill are equal bilaterally.	Interventions are successful at preventing adverse effects of immobility.
Observe Ms. Thomas' sacral region and affected leg for impaired skin integrity.	Skin is dry and intact without any redness or blistering.	Ms. Thomas' skin integrity is maintained, and no hazards of immobility are manifested.

outcomes mutually with the patient and family. A family who does too much or too little in an attempt to help the patient will seriously impede the patient's progress. Watching a family member walk slowly and using effort seems cruel, and some families excessively perform tasks that patients need to learn how to do for themselves. Patients often suffer immobility for a long time. Thus setting sequential outcomes helps ensure progressive improvement over time.

SETTING PRIORITIES Prioritize care by taking into consideration the patient's most immediate needs. Patients with impaired mobility often have multiple diagnoses that affect mental and physical health (Figure 35-3). For example, relieve a patient's pain first before implementing aggressive mobility activities. Because you can delegate many of the skills associated with care of the immobile patient, such as turning and applying antiembolic stockings, it is easy to overlook the potential complications of immobility until they occur. Therefore be vigilant in assessing and monitoring patients, reinforcing prevention techniques, and supervising nursing assistive personnel in carrying out activities aimed at preventing complications of immobility.

COLLABORATIVE CARE You often need the help of another health team member, such as a physical or occupational therapist, when considering mobility needs. Collaboration of health care providers is important for patients in institutional and home settings. Begin discharge planning when a patient enters the health care system. Anticipating the patient's discharge from an institution, a referral is necessary to help the patient remain mobile or regain mobility at home.

■■■ IMPLEMENTATION

Nursing interventions for the completely or partially immobilized patient focus on health promotion and prevention of complications. Many patients with limited mobility function in the home or assisted living settings, thus they require active intervention to prevent complications that might necessitate hospitalization. Specific interventions, in the acute care setting, focus on reducing severity of complications that have developed, for example by positioning and transferring patients correctly. In restorative and continuing care, direct your interventions at regaining and maximizing functional mobility and independence.

HEALTH PROMOTION Structured exercise programs for immobile patients improve their endurance, strength, overall health, and feelings of well-being. Exercise is recommended preoperatively for patients expected to have mobility restrictions after surgery. Consult with a physical therapist to determine if patients have adequate exercise programs.

Disuse and disease account for much of the functional decline in the older adult population. The older adult patient need not accept muscle deterioration as inevitable (Box 35-4). It is important to be alert to prevent further disuse while the older adult is ill.

CONCEPT MAP

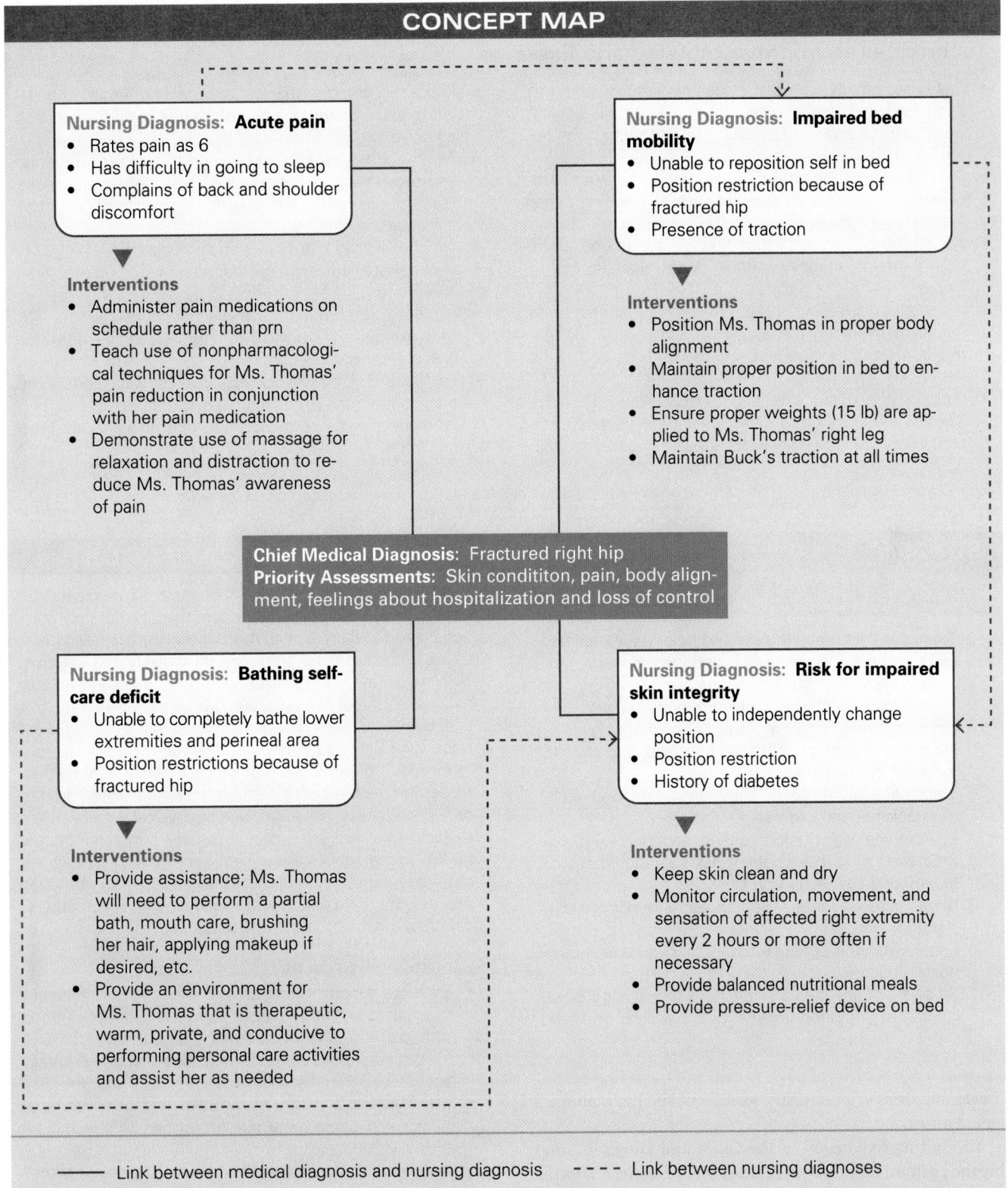

Nursing Diagnosis: Acute pain
- Rates pain as 6
- Has difficulty in going to sleep
- Complains of back and shoulder discomfort

▼

Interventions
- Administer pain medications on schedule rather than prn
- Teach use of nonpharmacological techniques for Ms. Thomas' pain reduction in conjunction with her pain medication
- Demonstrate use of massage for relaxation and distraction to reduce Ms. Thomas' awareness of pain

Nursing Diagnosis: Impaired bed mobility
- Unable to reposition self in bed
- Position restriction because of fractured hip
- Presence of traction

▼

Interventions
- Position Ms. Thomas in proper body alignment
- Maintain proper position in bed to enhance traction
- Ensure proper weights (15 lb) are applied to Ms. Thomas' right leg
- Maintain Buck's traction at all times

Chief Medical Diagnosis: Fractured right hip
Priority Assessments: Skin conditition, pain, body alignment, feelings about hospitalization and loss of control

Nursing Diagnosis: Bathing self-care deficit
- Unable to completely bathe lower extremities and perineal area
- Position restrictions because of fractured hip

▼

Interventions
- Provide assistance; Ms. Thomas will need to perform a partial bath, mouth care, brushing her hair, applying makeup if desired, etc.
- Provide an environment for Ms. Thomas that is therapeutic, warm, private, and conducive to performing personal care activities and assist her as needed

Nursing Diagnosis: Risk for impaired skin integrity
- Unable to independently change position
- Position restriction
- History of diabetes

▼

Interventions
- Keep skin clean and dry
- Monitor circulation, movement, and sensation of affected right extremity every 2 hours or more often if necessary
- Provide balanced nutritional meals
- Provide pressure-relief device on bed

——— Link between medical diagnosis and nursing diagnosis   - - - - Link between nursing diagnoses

Figure 35-3 ■ Concept Map.

Contribute to promoting health for patients by encouraging or starting managed exercise programs (Box 35-5). Encourage patients to do stretching, ROJM, and light walking, depending on their physical capabilities. Measure distances walked in feet and yards instead of "walked to the nurses' station and back to room," Or "Walked from dining room to bedroom twice". Adults also enjoy and benefit from exercise postoperatively. Activities other than traditional Western exercises, such as walking or swimming, are beneficial when patients return home (Box 35-6).

Respiratory System Aim interventions for the respiratory system at promoting expansion of the chest and lungs,

BOX 35-4 CARE OF THE OLDER ADULT

Techniques to Improve Mobility and Exercise

- Base program on individual assessment data (underlying conditions, medications, present activity level). Consult health care provider for specific exercise restrictions before starting exercise program.
- Provide information on the benefits of exercise and emphasize the short-term benefits such as sleeping better and a feeling of well-being.
- Assess for barriers and then how to get around them. Use them as stepping-stones rather than stumbling blocks.
- Appropriate clothing, exercise-specific shoes, and sufficient hydration are all important, as well as self-monitoring methods so progress can be visualized by the individual.
- Perform a gradual, extended exercise warm-up (e.g., 15 minutes) to maximize flexibility and decrease muscle injury, and cool-down sessions are also important.

- Make the program fun and entertaining—walking to favorite tunes or with a group of friends gives the exercise a festive and social element.
- Avoid sudden twisting movements, rapid movements, and rapid transitions from one movement to the next. Fluid movements are much more appropriate and enjoyable.
- Avoid exercises that tax vision and balance.
- Avoid sustained isometric contractions of greater than 10 seconds.
- Avoid exercise during acute viral infections.
- Stop exercising if cardiac dysrhythmias, angina, or excessive breathlessness occurs.
- Each exercise plan is as individual as each participant. Exercise comes in many forms: gardening, walking or swimming. The most important thing is to keep moving.

Modified from Ebersole P and others: *Toward healthy aging: human needs and nursing response,* ed 7, St. Louis, 2008, Mosby.

BOX 35-5 Guidelines for Assisting Patients With Exercising

1 Teach patients breathing skills to help reduce anxiety and to fully oxygenate tissues and expand lungs.
2 Always know patients' limitations.
3 Do not force a muscle or a joint during exercise.
4 Let each patient move at his or her own pace.
5 Keep a record of the patient's progress, and provide feedback as the patient exercises.
6 Maintain posture, body alignment, and good body mechanics during exercise.
7 Monitor vital signs before, during, and after exercise.
8 Stop exercising if the patient has pain, shortness of breath, or a change in vital signs.
9 Make sure patients wear shoes and comfortable clothing.
10 Know what the patient's mobility skills were before hospitalization.
11 Be aware of any medical limitations (e.g., weight-bearing status, untreated fracture, cardiovascular disease).

BOX 35-6 CULTURAL FOCUS

Culture and ethnic traditions influence many aspects of patients' lives, including time orientation, health care practices, and nutrition. Not as much attention has been given to the impact of these traditions on mobility and exercise. However, they do influence health care behaviors and play an important role in exercise and physical activity.

Exercise is often described based on white, middle-class values. For example, not everyone has access to a tennis court or golf course at a local country club. Furthermore, the patient's ethnic group may determine whether or not the patient will participate in physical activity after a medical intervention such as surgery (Lim and others, 2009). Young African American women who have given birth may resist getting out of bed because it is believed that new mothers need to rest because they are at greater risk than the newborns (Purnell, 2009).

IMPLICATIONS FOR PRACTICE

- Evaluate patient's patterns of daily living and culturally prescribed activities before suggesting specific forms of exercise to patients (Purnell and Paulanka, 2008).
- Help patients plan physical activities that are culturally acceptable (Purnell, 2009).
- Make exercise programs flexible, and accommodate family and community responsibilities of the culture (Purnell, 2009).
- Incorporate cultural beliefs and desired patient outcomes when designing the plan of care (Lim and others, 2009).

preventing stasis of pulmonary secretions, and maintaining a patent airway.

Promoting Expansion of the Chest and Lungs. Changing the position of the patient at least every 2 hours allows the dependent lung regions to reexpand. Reexpansion maintains the elastic recoil property of the lungs and clears the dependent lung regions of pulmonary secretions (see Chapter 29). Your assessment will determine if patients need more frequent position changes. You can also promote lung expansion through regular deep breathing exercises.

Preventing Stasis of Pulmonary Secretions. Stagnant secretions accumulating in the bronchi and lungs of the im-

mobilized patient lead to the growth of bacteria and the subsequent development of pneumonia. Changing the patient's position every 2 hours or more often reduces stagnation of secretions. This change rotates the dependent lung, mobilizing secretions.

Make sure the immobile patient has a fluid intake of at least 2000 mL per day, if not contraindicated, to help keep muco-ciliary clearance intact. In patients free from infection and with adequate hydration, pulmonary secretions will appear thin, watery, and clear. It is easy for the patient to remove these se-cretions with coughing. Without adequate hydration, secre-tions become thick, tenacious, and difficult to remove. One method for removing pulmonary secretions is chest physio-therapy (CPT). The use of this technique drains secretions from specific segments of the bronchi and lungs into the tra-chea and helps the patient expel the secretions by coughing (see Chapter 29). Combine coughing with the deep breathing exercises, and have the patient do these on a regular schedule.

Metabolic System Design a dietary plan of carbohydrates, proteins, and fats to combat the effects of immobility. Carbo-hydrates are necessary to meet energy requirements. Proteins are necessary for tissue repair and to counter negative nitrogen balance. Fats prevent further breakdown of nutritional stores. Determine the patient's specific caloric and diet prescription from the nutritional assessment. In the home setting, involve family caregivers in developing meal plans. Collaborate with a registered dietitian if a patient has any dietary restrictions re-lated to other medical conditions (see Chapter 32).

Cardiovascular System Design health promotion nurs-ing therapies to minimize or prevent thrombus formation.

Preventing Thrombus Formation. Proper positioning used with other therapies (e.g., anticoagulants and antiembolic stockings) helps reduce thrombus formation. When position-ing patients, use caution to prevent pressure on the posterior knee and deep veins in the lower extremities. Teach patients to avoid crossing the legs, sitting for prolonged periods of time, wearing tight clothing that constricts the legs or waist, putting pillows under the knees, and massaging the legs.

ROJM exercises reduce the risk for contractures and also aid in preventing thrombi (Box 35-7). Activity causes con-traction of the skeletal muscles, which exerts pressure on the veins to promote venous return. An increase in venous return reduces venous stasis. Specific exercises that help prevent thrombophlebitis are ankle pumps, foot circles, hip rotation, and knee flexion. Ankle pumps, sometimes called calf pumps, include alternating plantar flexion and dorsiflexion. Foot circles require the patient to rotate the ankle. While the pa-tient is supine (lying on back) or sitting, he or she rotates the hip joint by rotating the entire leg and pointing the toes in-ward and outward. Knee flexion involves alternately extend-ing and flexing the knee. These exercises aimed at preventing thrombi are sometimes called antiembolic exercises. Patients should do these exercises hourly while awake.

Musculoskeletal System The immobilized or partially immobilized patient needs to exercise to prevent excessive muscle atrophy, decreased endurance, and joint contractures. The amount of activity required to prevent physical disuse syndromes is only about 2 hours in a 24-hour period, so schedule this regularly throughout the day based on individ-ual patient needs and tolerance.

If the patient is unable to move any part or all of the body, perform passive ROJM exercises for all immobilized joints at

---

BOX 35-7 Incorporating Active Range-of-Joint-Motion Exercises Into Activities of Daily Living

- Nodding head "yes" exercises *neck* (flexion).
- Shaking head "no" exercises *neck* (rotation).
- Moving right ear to right shoulder exercises *neck* (lat-eral flexion).
- Moving left ear to left shoulder exercises *neck* (lateral flexion).
- Reaching to turn on overhead light exercises *shoulder* (extension).
- Reaching to bedside stand for book exercises *shoulder* (extension).
- Scratching back exercises *shoulder* (hyperextension).
- Rotating shoulders toward chest exercises *shoulder* (abduction).
- Rotating shoulders toward back exercises *shoulder* (ad-duction).
- Eating, bathing, shaving, and grooming exercise *elbow* (flexion and extension).
- All activities requiring fine motor coordination, such as writing and eating, exercise *fingers* and *thumb* (flexion, extension, abduction, adduction, and opposition).
- Walking exercises *hip* (flexion, extension, and hyperex-tension).
- Moving to side-lying position exercises *hip* (flexion, ex-tension, and abduction).
- Moving from side-lying position exercises *hip* (exten-sion and adduction).
- Rolling feet inward exercises *hip* (internal rotation).
- Rolling feet outward exercises *hip* (external rotation).
- Walking exercises *knee* (flexion and extension).
- Moving to and from a side-lying position exercises *knee* (flexion and extension).
- Walking exercises *ankle* (dorsiflexion and plantar flexion).
- Moving toe toward head of bed exercises *ankle* (dorsi-flexion).
- Moving toe toward foot of bed exercises *ankle* (plantar flexion).
- Walking exercises *toes* (extension and hyperextension).
- Wiggling toes exercises *toes* (abduction and adduction).

---

least 3 or 4 times a day unless contraindicated. Teach family caregivers how to provide these exercises in the home. If one extremity is paralyzed, teach the patient to perform passive ROJM on the paralyzed limb, and encourage the patient to engage in active ROJM with all other extremities. For patients on bed rest, incorporate active ROJM exercises into their ADL schedule (see Box 35-7). The bath is an excellent time to do ROJM.

The best nursing intervention is establishing an individu-alized progressive exercise program. A progressive exercise program gradually increases the patient's physical activity to reverse the deconditioning associated with immobility. Teach-ing is an important aspect for patients with limited mobility (Box 35-8). Depending on the setting and resources available,

Increasing Mobility and Independence

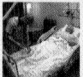 Ms. Thomas is interested in knowing what she can do to make herself stronger and heal faster once her surgery is completed. She wants to learn about an exercise plan that will make her become more mobile and independent. Sergio has developed a teaching plan that includes components that will allow her to have some control over activities that will meet her physical and psychosocial needs.

OUTCOME

At the end of the teaching session Ms. Thomas will verbalize essential elements of her care that she will perform and have some control over.

TEACHING STRATEGIES

- Apply demonstration and offer an instructional DVD on rehab exercises based on Ms. Thomas' interest and cognitive ability.
- Use common terminology to describe Ms. Thomas' nutrition, healing, and mobility needs postoperatively.
- During her postoperative stay, begin isometric exercises of her uninvolved extremities and provide adequate pain control before beginning the teaching session.
- Explain mobility restrictions to the involved hip in collaboration with physical therapist.
- Include instruction in and demonstration of activities such as use of isometric exercises, self-care activities, and importance of keeping arms and legs toned.

EVALUATION STRATEGIES

- Use focused questions to evaluate Ms. Thomas' understanding of isometric exercise regimen.
- Observe Ms. Thomas demonstrating self-care activities while in bed: hygiene, hair, makeup, etc.
- Ask Ms. Thomas to explain the rationale for the use of analgesics and anticoagulants.
- Observe Ms. Thomas during exercises to strengthen upper body and legs.
- Ask Ms. Thomas to identify foods with decreased fat and increased protein that will promote weight loss and wound healing.

refer the patient for physical therapy to assist in setting up the exercise program.

Skin Integrity The major risk to the skin from restricted mobility is the formation of pressure ulcers. Early identification of high-risk patients (e.g., wheelchair-bound patients, stroke patients) assists in preventing pressure ulcers. Interventions aimed at prevention are positioning, skin care, and the use of pressure-relief devices. Change the immobilized patient's position according to the patient's activity level, perceptual ability, status of peripheral circulation, treatment protocols, and daily routines (see Chapter 36). For example, a person in a wheelchair learns to move the buttocks and hips up and off of the wheelchair seat every 15 to 20 minutes. Turning at least every 1 to 2 hours is recommended for pre-

venting ulcers in patients restricted to bed. Although turning is essential, it is sometimes necessary to use devices for relieving pressure. Normally, the time a mobile patient sits uninterrupted in a chair is 1 hour or less, but make sure to individualize this time interval. Reposition the patient frequently because uninterrupted pressure will cause skin breakdown. Teach patients who are able to move to shift their weight every 15 to 20 minutes. Make sure chair-bound patients have a pressure-reducing device for the chair (Agency for Healthcare Research and Quality [AHRQ], 2003).

Elimination System Direct interventions for maintaining optimal urinary functioning to keep the patient well hydrated without causing bladder distention and the reflux of urine into the ureters and renal pelvis. Adequate hydration helps to prevent renal calculi and urinary tract infections. Timely toileting prevents bladder distention. Make sure the patient's urine is light yellow and comparable in amount to the fluid intake by monitoring total fluid intake and output each shift or each day when in the home.

Monitoring the frequency and amount of urinary output also helps to prevent bladder distention. A patient who continually dribbles urine and whose bladder is distended likely has reflex incontinence. If the immobilized patient does not have voluntary control of bladder elimination, bladder retraining is necessary. It may become necessary to insert a straight or indwelling Foley catheter (see Chapter 33) if the patient experiences ongoing bladder distention.

Record the frequency and consistency of bowel movements. A diet rich in fruits and vegetables helps to facilitate normal peristalsis. If a patient is unable to maintain normal bowel patterns, initiate a bowel training program, and the health care provider may order stool softeners, cathartics, or enemas (see Chapter 34).

Psychosocial Problems Health promotion for the immobilized patient requires anticipation of changes in psychosocial status and intervention with preventive measures. Provide routine and informal socialization for the patient. Help family caregivers to learn the importance of keeping patients involved in decisions about their care and to engage them in conversation and self-help activities. Plan activities to give patients in health care settings the opportunity to interact with the staff. If possible, place these patient in a room with other mobile patients. If the patient remains in a private room, ask staff members to visit periodically throughout waking hours. Provide stimuli to maintain orientation and to entertain the patient.

Encourage patients to wear their glasses or dentures and to shave or apply makeup. These are normal activities to enhance body image. Encourage the patient to perform as much self-care as possible. Make sure hygiene and grooming articles are within easy reach so the patient can attend to personal needs.

Developmental Changes Plan care to stimulate the patient mentally, as well as physically, particularly with a young child. Incorporate play activities into the nursing care plan. Puzzles, for example, help patients develop fine motor skills. Place an immobilized child in a room with children of the same age who are mobile, unless a contagious disease is present (Hockenberry and Wilson, 2007). Health promotion for older adults requires matching mobility needs with the patient's developmental limitations. Older adults benefit when exercise routines are mildly progressive. Walking, aquatic exercise, swimming, and gardening are good ways to promote range of joint motion and endurance.

ACUTE CARE Patients in acute care settings demonstrate more rapid and pronounced complications of immobility because of the presence of multisystem involvement. In these patients design nursing interventions to reduce the impact of immobility on body systems, and prepare the patient for restorative and continuing care. Use interventions in combination with those outlined in the health promotion section to return the patient to an optimal level of function.

Respiratory System Encourage the patient to cough and deep breathe every 1 to 2 hours while awake. This action expands all lobes of the lungs and prevents atelectasis. Coughing reduces the stasis of pulmonary secretions. Some immobile patients, particularly after surgery, will need to use an incentive spirometer to aid in deep breathing (see Chapter 29).

Postoperative patients who have undergone general anesthesia especially need to cough and deep breathe to prevent atelectasis and stasis of secretions. Timely pain management for incision discomfort is essential. Patients cough more effectively when their pain is under control. If a patient becomes drowsy from medication, actively reinforce coughing and deep breathing. Encouraging early ambulation helps prevent multiple pulmonary complications.

Maintaining a Patent Airway. Immobilized patients and those on bed rest are generally weakened. The cough reflex gradually becomes inefficient as the weakness progresses. If the patient is too weak or unable to cough up secretions, maintain the patient's airway by using suctioning techniques (see Chapter 29). This usually involves oral or nasotracheal suctioning and suctioning of artificial airways. Suspect hypostatic bronchopneumonia if the patient develops a productive cough with greenish-yellow sputum, fever, and pain on breathing.

Cardiovascular System After prolonged bed rest, patients usually have an increased heart rate, a decrease in pulse pressure, and a drop in blood pressure with an increase in fainting when arising to a sitting or standing position (Black and Hawks, 2009). Attempt to get the patient moving as soon as the physical condition allows, even if this only involves dangling at the bedside or moving to a chair. This activity maintains muscle tone and increases venous return. **Isometric exercises,** those activities that involve muscle tension without muscle shortening, do not have any beneficial effect on preventing orthostatic hypotension but improve activity tolerance (see Chapter 26).

When transferring from a supine position into a chair, move the patient gradually. First obtain a baseline blood pressure and pulse with the patient in the supine position. Then raise the patient to a high-Fowler's position, and measure blood pressure and pulse again to detect decreases in blood pressure or elevations in pulse. Leave the patient in this position for 2 minutes to allow the body to adapt. Monitor

the patient for dizziness or light-headedness. The patient is now ready to sit at the side of the bed with the feet on the floor. If there is no dizziness, assist the patient to a chair. When transferring an immobile patient for the first time, make sure the appropriate safe patient handling and movement algorithm is used (Figure 35-4) (Nelson, 2006).

It is also important to direct nursing interventions at reducing cardiac workload. When a patient moves up in bed or strains on defecation, a Valsalva maneuver occurs. During a Valsalva maneuver the patient holds his or her breath and strains, increasing intrathoracic pressure, which decreases venous return and cardiac output. When the strain is released, venous return and cardiac output immediately increase, and systolic blood pressure and pulse pressure rise. These pressure changes produce a reflex bradycardia that can be associated with sudden cardiac death, particularly in patients with heart disease. Teach the patient to breathe out while moving or being lifted up in bed to avoid straining.

Interventions that reduce the risk for thrombus formation in the immobilized patient include leg exercises, encouraging fluids, and position changes. Instruct preoperative patients in exercise before surgery (see Chapter 38). Other interventions, such as antiembolic elastic stockings and SCDs, require a health care provider's order.

Elastic stockings aid in maintaining pressure on the muscles of the lower extremities and therefore promote venous return. Make sure to measure the patient's lower extremities correctly to ensure proper pressure, and to apply the stockings properly (Box 35-9). Remove and reapply them at least every 8 hours. Improper application of stockings can lead to decreased circulation in the lower extremities. Always observe the status of circulation to the extremities (see Chapter 15), and check to be sure stockings are properly fitted. Patients are usually discharged home with these stockings. Be sure they learn how to apply the stockings correctly and how to observe the status of circulation to the extremities. Instruct patients on the signs of allergic reactions, thrombophlebitis, or skin irritation so that they can report changes to their health care provider.

SCDs consist of inflatable plastic sleeves wrapped around the legs and secured with Velcro. The sleeves are connected to an air pump that alternately inflates and deflates, providing rhythmic, external extremity compression (Box 35-10). Use of SCDs on the legs decreases venous stasis by increasing venous return. In postoperative patients, keep these compression devices in place until the patient is ambulatory.

Immobilized patients are frequently on prophylactic (preventive) low-dose heparin therapy to minimize the risk for venous thromboembolism. Heparin is an anticoagulant that suppresses clot formation. This therapy requires a health care provider's order. Newer low-molecular-weight (LMW) heparins such as ardeparin and enoxaparin are being prescribed in place of older forms of unfractionated heparin. The LMW heparins have a more predictable anticoagulant effect (McKenry and others, 2006). The drugs are given subcutaneously, usually every 12 hours until the risk for DVT declines. LMW heparin compared with unfractionated heparin re-

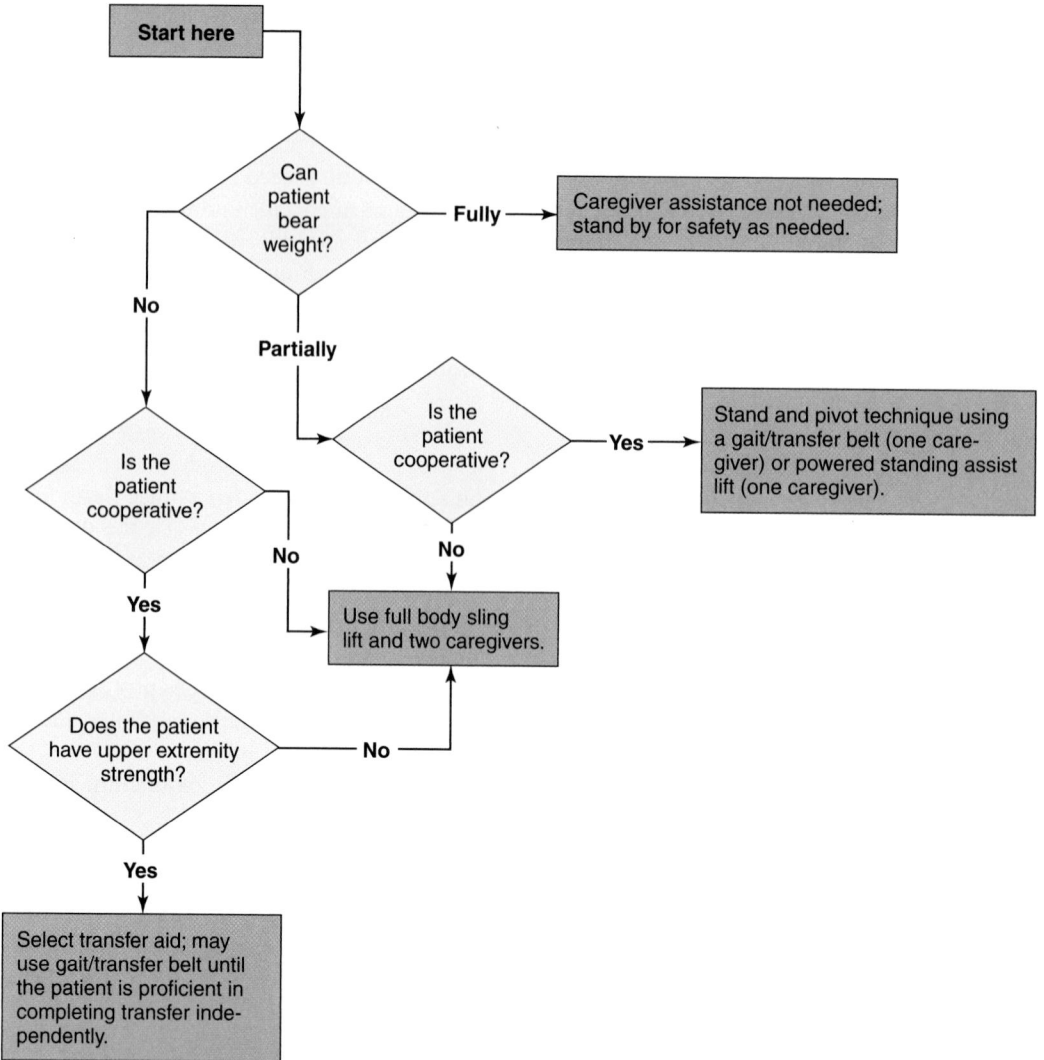

Figure 35-4 ■ Algorithm used to transfer patient to and from the bed to chair, chair to toilet, chair to chair, or car to chair. (From Nelson A: *Safe patient handling and movement algorithms,* 2006, VISN8 Patient Safety Center, http://www.visn8.med.va. gov/patientsafetycenter/SafePtHandling/default.asp.)

duces the occurrence of major hemorrhage as a side effect (van Dongen and others, 2005). Local irritation such as erythema, hematoma, and urticaria at injection sites is common. However, it is still wise to monitor the patient for signs of bleeding (e.g., increased bruising, guaiac-positive stools, and bleeding gums). Report any occurrence of hemorrhage immediately.

When you suspect DVT, do not massage the area. Report assessment findings to the health care provider immediately. Elevate the leg, with no pressure on the area of the leg with

the suspected thrombus. If the patient complains of shortness of breath or severe chest pain, suspect a pulmonary embolus. Immediately place the patient in high-Fowler's position, and check the patient's oxygen saturation. This complication is life threatening and requires prompt medical attention.

Musculoskeletal System The immobilized patient needs to receive some exercise to prevent excessive muscle atrophy and joint contractures. For patients on bed rest, incorporate active ROJM exercises into their daily schedules. Patients with

BOX 35-9   PROCEDURAL GUIDELINES

Applying Antiembolic Elastic Stockings

DELEGATION CONSIDERATIONS: You can delegate the skill of applying antiembolic elastic stockings to nursing assistive personnel (NAP). Before delegation, instruct the NAP to inform the nurse:

- If patient complains of leg pain or leg swelling
- If patient has any skin irritation

Also, instruct the NAP to inform the patient:

- To avoid activities that promote venous stasis (e.g., crossing legs, wearing garters)
- To elevate legs while sitting and before applying stockings to improve venous return
- Not to massage legs
- To avoid wrinkles in the stockings

EQUIPMENT: Tape measure, elastic support stockings

1 Identify patient using two identifiers (e.g., name and birthday or name and account number, according to agency policy). Assess patient for risk factors in Virchow's triad:
   a *Hypercoagulability:* All patients with clotting disorders, fever, dehydration, pregnancy and first 6 weeks' postpartum if the woman was confined to bed, and oral contraceptive use (especially if patient smokes)
   b *Venous wall abnormalities:* Local trauma, orthopedic surgeries, major abdominal surgery, varicose veins, atherosclerosis
   c *Blood stasis:* Immobility, obesity, pregnancy
2 Observe for signs, symptoms, and conditions that contraindicate use of antiembolic elastic stockings. Signs and symptoms include:
   a Dermatitis or open skin lesion
   b Recent skin graft
   c Decreased circulation in lower extremities as evidenced by cyanotic, cool extremities, gangrenous conditions affecting the lower limb(s)
3 Assess and document the condition of the patient's skin and circulation to the legs (i.e., presence of pedal pulses, edema, and discoloration of the skin, temperature, lesions, or abrasions).
4 Obtain physician's or health care provider's order.
5 Assess patient's or caregiver's understanding of application of antiembolic elastic stockings.
6 Assess the condition of the patient's skin and circulation to the leg and foot (e.g., presence of popliteal and pedal pulses, edema, and discoloration of the skin, skin temperature, lesions, or cuts).

Critical Decision Point: Clinical signs of thrombophlebitis vary according to the size and location of the thrombus. Signs and symptoms of superficial thrombosis include palpable veins and the surrounding area's being tender to the touch, reddened, and warm. Temperature elevation and edema may or may not be present. Signs and symptoms of deep vein thrombosis (DVT) include swollen extremity; pain; warm, cyanotic skin; and temperature elevation. However, up to 80% of patients are asymptomatic. Homans' sign (pain in the calf on dorsiflexion of the foot) is no longer considered a reliable assessment. Less than 20% of patients have a positive Homans' sign (Black and Hawks, 2009).

7 Use a tape measure to measure patient's legs to determine proper stocking size.
8 Explain procedure and reasons for applying stockings.
9 Perform hand hygiene. Provide hygiene to patient's lower extremities as needed.
10 Position patient in supine position.
11 Apply elastic stockings:
   a Turn elastic stocking inside out up to the heel. Place one hand into stocking, holding heel. Pull top of stocking with the other hand inside out over foot of stocking.
   b Place patient's toes into foot of elastic stocking, making sure that stocking is smooth (see illustration).
   c Slide remaining portion of stocking over patient's foot, being sure that the toes are covered. Make sure the foot fits into the toe and heel position of the stocking (see illustration).

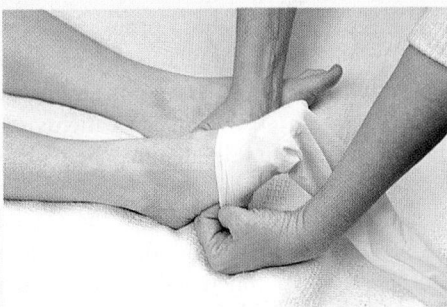

Step 11b ■ Place toes into foot of stocking.

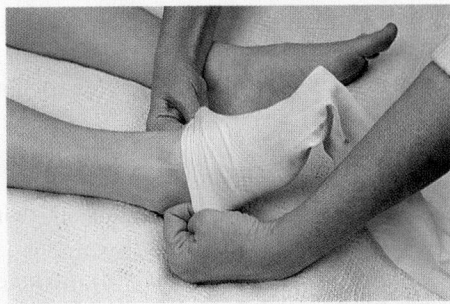

Step 11c ■ Slide heel of stocking over foot.

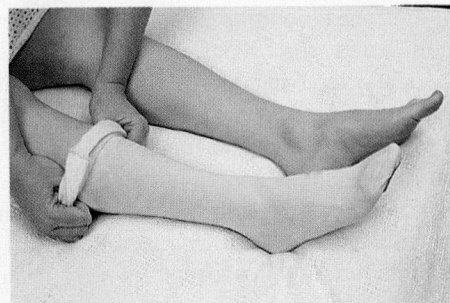

Step 11d ■ Slide stocking up leg until completely extended.

BOX 35-9   PROCEDURAL GUIDELINES—cont'd

 d Slide top of stocking up over patient's calf until stocking is completely extended. Be sure stocking is smooth and no ridges or wrinkles are present, particularly behind the knee (see illustration).

 e Instruct patient not to roll stockings partially down.

12 Reposition patient for comfort, and perform hand hygiene.

13 Remove stockings at least once per shift.

14 Inspect stockings for wrinkles or constriction.

15 Inspect elastic stockings to determine that there are no wrinkles, rolls, or binding.

16 Observe circulatory status of lower extremities. Observe color, temperature, and condition of skin. Palpate pedal pulses.

17 Observe the patient's response to wearing the antiembolic elastic stockings.

18 Observe patient or caregiver applying stockings.

impaired nervous, skeletal, or muscular system functioning and significant weakness often require help to attain and maintain body alignment.

Several devices are available for maintaining proper patient positioning (Table 35-3). Pillows are commonly used to support body alignment. Before using a pillow, determine whether it is the proper size. A thick pillow under a patient's head causes excessive cervical flexion. A thin pillow under bony prominences is inadequate to protect skin and tissue from damage. When additional pillows are unavailable, use folded sheets, blankets, or towels as positioning aids. The 30-degree semi-Fowler's position is for patients at risk for pressure ulcer development. Elevate the patient's calves on a pillow to avoid pressure on the heels. A trochanter roll prevents external rotation of the hips when the patient is in a supine position (Figure 35-5). Hand rolls maintain the hand, thumb, and fingers in a functional position. Hand-wrist splints are individually molded for the patient to maintain proper alignment of the thumb. A trapeze bar is a triangular device that hangs from a securely fastened overhead bar that is attached to the patient's bed frame (Figure 35-6). It is a useful device for helping to increase patient independence, maintain upper body strength, and reduce friction from movement in bed.

Some orthopedic and neurological conditions require more frequent passive ROJM exercises to restore the injured joint or extremity to maximal function. Patients with such conditions use automatic equipment for passive ROJM exercises. The continuous passive motion (CPM) machine moves the extremity within a prescribed range for a specific period. This method is beneficial when the patient gradually increases ROJM of a particular joint. For example, it is used for patients who have had total knee replacement surgery. It is applied immediately postoperatively and is only removed when the patient is receiving physical therapy. Over time, the patient progresses from its use to flexion and extension of the joint without the aid of the CPM (Figure 35-7).

Psychosocial Problems Establish a balance between rest and the physiological effects of bed rest. Keep assessments to a minimum in a stable patient who is able to turn in bed unassisted. More seriously ill patients will need medications, assessments, and skin care during the night. Coordinate nursing care to prevent as many interruptions as possible between 10 PM and 7 AM.

Finally, observe the patient for failure to cope with restricted mobility. If the nursing care plan is not improving the patient's coping patterns, outside assistance is necessary. Incorporate referrals to community resources into the care plan.

Developmental Changes Immobilization or restricted mobility of an older adult requires complex care and innovative approaches. Inactive older adults are at risk for cognitive changes and depression as a result of immobilization, chronic illnesses, and medications. It is important to focus on activities to promote cognitive awareness of the patient's surroundings (see Chapter 21). Give explanations before starting care, and encourage the patient to make decisions about care. Plan nursing care to allow the older adult patient to perform as many ADLs as possible. Not only are older adults more susceptible to the hazards of immobility, but also the consequences of immobility appear more quickly and become severe more rapidly.

RESTORATIVE AND CONTINUING CARE The goal of restorative and continuing care for the immobilized patient is to maximize independence, increase endurance, and prevent injury. Restorative interventions focus on **instrumental activities of daily living (IADLs)** such as shopping, preparing meals, banking, and taking medications, in addition to ADLs. Often, patients with mobility issues are transferred to rehabilitation centers to work on improving IADLs. Make sure to provide the rehabilitation center with a complete report to ensure patient safety and continuity of care (The Joint Commission, 2009).

Use many of the same interventions as described in the health promotion and acute care sections, but the emphasis now is on working collaboratively with patients, family caregivers, and other health care professionals. Sometimes occupational or physical therapy is ordered. Work collaboratively with these professionals, and reinforce exercises and teaching. Common items used to help the patient adapt to mobility limitations include walkers, canes, wheelchairs, and assistive devices such as toilet seat extenders, reaching sticks, special silverware, and clothing with Velcro closures.

■■■EVALUATION

PATIENT CARE Evaluate interventions for reducing the risks of immobility by comparing the patient's actual response to the expected outcomes for each goal. If expected outcomes are not achieved, revise the care plan. Base the suc-

BOX 35-10　PROCEDURAL GUIDELINES

Applying Sequential Compression Devices

DELEGATION CONSIDERATIONS: You can delegate the skill of applying SCDs to NAP. The nurse is responsible for assessing circulation in the extremities. Instruct the NAP to notify nurse:

- If patient complains of leg pain
- If discoloration develops in extremities

EQUIPMENT: Sequential compression device (SCD) insufflator with air hoses attached, adjustable Velcro compression stockings/SCD sleeve, hygiene supplies

1. Assess patient for need for sequential compression stockings (see Box 35-9, p. 1051).
2. Obtain baseline assessment data about the status of circulation, pulse, and skin integrity on patient's lower extremities before initiating sequential compression stockings.
3. Identify patient using two identifiers (e.g. name and birthday or name and account number, according to agency policy). Ask patient to state name.
4. Perform hand hygiene. Provide hygiene to patient's lower extremities, as needed.
5. Assemble and prepare equipment.
6. Arrange SCD sleeve under the patient's leg according to the leg position indicated on the inner lining of the sleeve (see illustration).
   a. Back of patient's ankle should line up with the ankle on inner lining of the sleeve.
   b. Position back of knee with the popliteal opening (see illustration).
7. Wrap SCD sleeve securely around patient's leg.
8. Verify fit of SCD sleeves by placing two fingers between patient's leg and sleeve (see illustration).
9. Attach SCD sleeve's connector to plug on mechanical unit. Arrows on compressor line up with arrows on plug from mechanical unit (see illustration).
10. Turn mechanical unit on. Green light indicates unit is functioning.
11. Observe functioning of unit for one complete cycle.
12. Reposition patient for comfort, and perform hand hygiene.
13. Remove compression stockings at least once per shift.
14. Monitor skin integrity and circulation to patient's lower extremities as ordered or as recommended by SCD manufacturer.

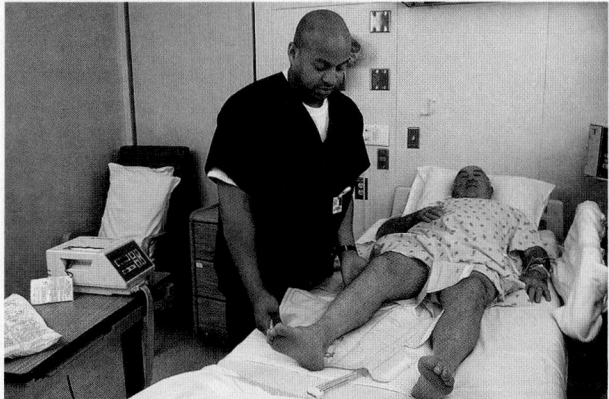

Step 6 ■ Correct leg position on inner lining.

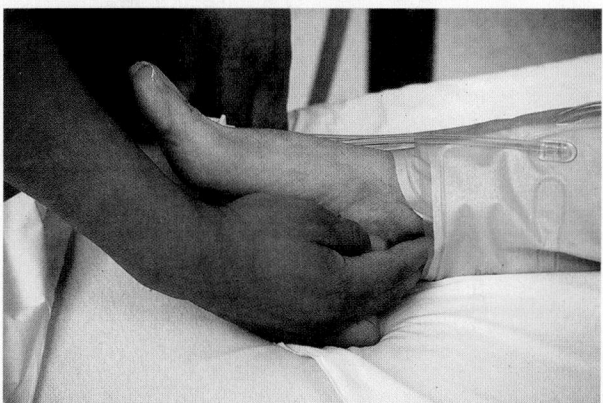

Step 8 ■ Check fit of SCD sleeve.

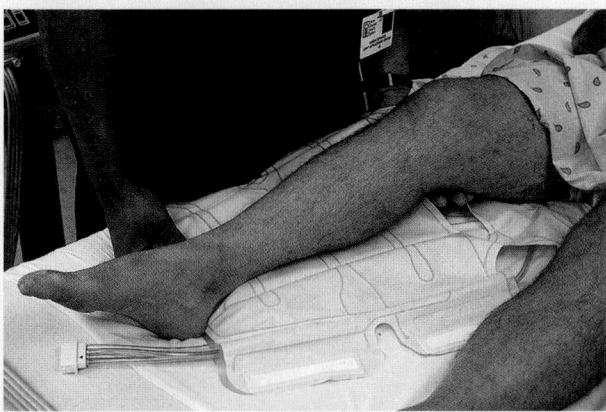

Step 6b ■ Position back of patient's knee with the popliteal opening.

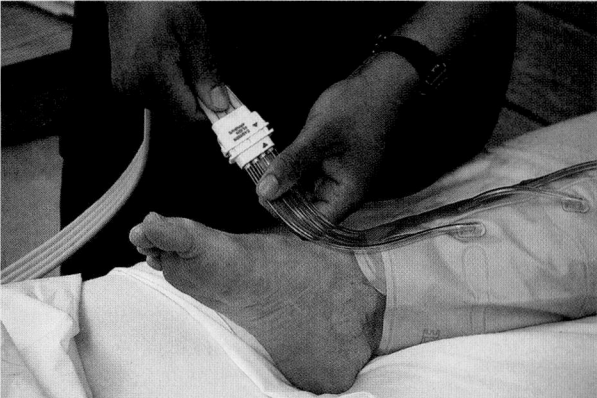

Step 9 ■ Align arrows when connecting to mechanical unit.

TABLE 35-3 Devices Used for Proper Positioning

DEVICES	USES AND DESCRIPTIONS
Pillows	Pillows are readily available in most health care facilities, including the home. Make sure they are the appropriate size for the body part you will position. Pillows provide support, elevate body parts, and splint incisional areas, reducing postoperative pain during activity or coughing and deep breathing.
Foot boots	Foot boots maintain feet in dorsiflexion. Boots are made of rigid plastic or heavy foam and keep the foot flexed at the proper angle. Remove the foot boots at least every 4 hours to assess skin integrity and joint mobility.
Trochanter rolls	Trochanter rolls prevent external rotation of legs when patients are in the supine position. To form a trochanter roll, fold a cotton bath blanket or a sheet lengthwise to a width extending from the greater trochanter of the femur to the lower border of the popliteal space (see Figure 35-5). Place the blanket under the buttocks and then rolled away from the patient until the thigh is in the neutral position or an inward position with the patella facing upward.
Sandbags	Sandbags provide support and shape to body contours; they immobilize extremities and maintain specific body alignment. Sandbags are filled plastic tubes that you shape to body contours. They are used in place of, or in addition to, trochanter rolls.
Hand rolls	Hand rolls maintain the thumb slightly adducted and in opposition to the fingers; they maintain fingers in a slightly flexed position. The nurse evaluates the position of the hand roll to make certain the hand is indeed in a functional position.
Hand-wrist splints	Hand-wrist splints are individually molded for the patient to maintain proper alignment of the thumb in slight adduction and the wrist in slight dorsiflexion. Use these splints only for the patient for whom the splint was made.
Trapeze bar	The trapeze bar descends from a securely fastened overhead bar attached to the bed frame (see Figure 35-6). The trapeze allows the patient to use upper extremities to raise the trunk off the bed, to assist in transfer from bed to wheelchair, or to perform upper arm strengthening exercises.
Wedge pillow	A wedge or abductor pillow is a triangular-shaped pillow made of heavy foam. It is used to maintain the legs in abduction following total hip replacement surgery.

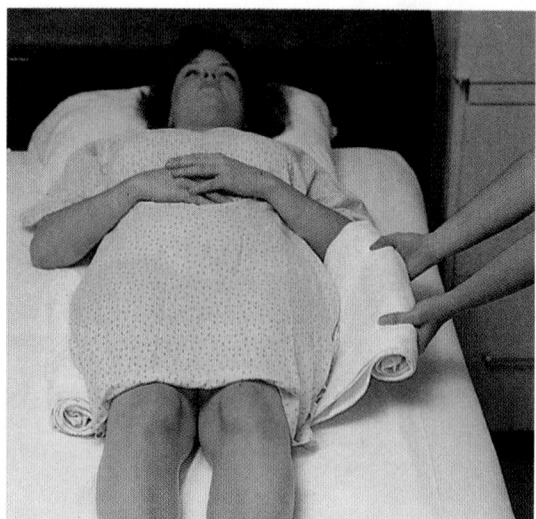

Figure 35-5 ■ Trochanter roll.

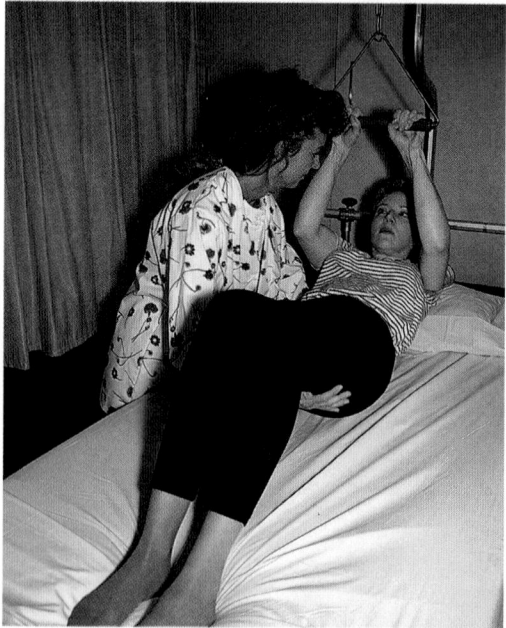

Figure 35-6 ■ Patient using a trapeze bar.

cess in meeting each outcome on the use of evaluative measures such as ROJM status, exercise tolerance, and fluid intake.

Evaluate outcomes designed to demonstrate normal function of specific systems and to prevent complications (Box 35-11). For example, are the lungs clear; are there any areas of skin showing signs of skin breakdown; is the patient regularly performing leg exercises? Evaluation provides evidence if you are meeting the outcomes set with the patient during the planning phase of care. If the answers to the questions indicate the outcomes are being met, the plan is working; if not, you need to reassess and revise the plan with input from the patient.

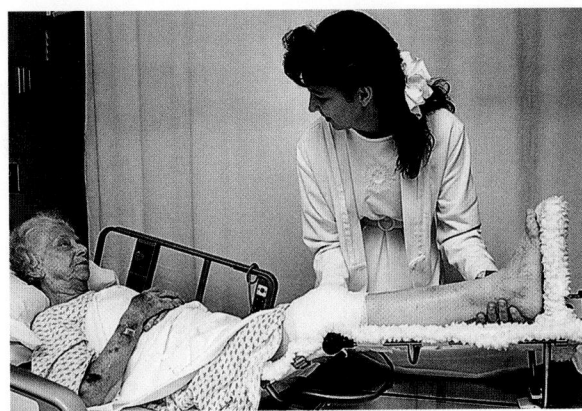

Figure 35-7 ■ Continuous passive range-of-motion machine.

PATIENT EXPECTATIONS People often take movement for granted. Patients who are immobile and dependent on others for some or all of their needs sometimes become overly dependent or try to do too much themselves too early. It is a difficult task finding the balance between independence and dependence. Patients will want control over their mobility that is personally satisfactory. For patients who are completely dependent on others for care, control over how and when things are done is very important. Do they feel they are treated with dignity? Do caregivers treat them as adults? Patients who are dependent on others for care sometimes see their demands as the only control they have over their lives.

For most patients with mobility problems, lack of control is often a major issue. Do they feel staff are considerate, and do staff protect their privacy? Are patients' preferences taken into consideration when planning care? Do caregivers talk to them or ignore them? It is helpful to remember that lack of movement is often associated with punishment in our society. We give children "time-outs," teens are "grounded," and people who do not receive promotions are seen as failures. It

is therefore important to recognize that immobility possibly leads to fear, anger, grief, withdrawal, or hostility. If you are sensitive to these reactions and help the patient work through them, instead of responding negatively to the patient, you will make a big difference in the patient's outcome.

BOX 35-11   EVALUATION

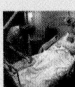 It has been 3 days since Ms. Thomas' surgery for repair of her hip fracture. Ms. Thomas is becoming more independent. She can bathe the upper part of her body, complete oral hygiene, apply some makeup, and fix her hair. She is reporting her pain at a level 3 on the pain scale following the administration of her pain medication. Transport to the rehabilitation center is scheduled for 10 AM tomorrow.

During her stay in the acute care agency, Sergio taught Ms. Thomas the importance of following the American Diabetes Association (ADA) diet. In addition, Sergio worked with the patient and her physical therapist in deciding what exercises she will perform in rehabilitation and eventually at home. Ms. Thomas will concentrate on increasing the strength of her upper extremities, reducing her weight by following an ADA diet as prescribed by her primary health care provider, and strengthening her leg muscles as her right hip heals.

DOCUMENTATION NOTE

"Ms. Thomas discharged via ambulance to rehabilitation center. Dressing on right hip is dry and intact. Patient presently reports pain at a level of 3 on a scale of 0 to 10. Has been able to describe restrictions in mobility involving right leg. A complete report was given to receiving caregiver at rehabilitation center to ensure safety of Ms. Thomas and continuity of her care. Her son and daughters were notified via phone call of the discharge and transfer to rehabilitation center."

KEY POINTS

- Normal physical mobility depends on intact and functioning nervous and musculoskeletal systems.
- The risk for disabilities related to immobilization depends on the extent and duration of the immobilization.
- Immobility results from illness or trauma or is prescribed for therapeutic reasons; it presents hazards in the physical, psychological, and developmental dimensions.
- Pressure ulcers, although often preventable, are one of the most common physical hazards of immobility.
- Effects of immobility include depression, behavioral changes, changes in the sleep-wake cycle, decreased coping abilities, and developmental delays.
- Assessment focuses on range of joint motion, musculoskeletal status, and complete physical examination for

potential adverse effects in all body systems, as well as psychosocial and developmental effects.
- Adequate hydration measures reduce immobility-related complications in the respiratory and elimination systems.
- Elastic antiembolic stockings and sequential compression devices both improve venous return and help prevent the potentially life-threatening complication of DVT.
- The primary evaluation criterion for nursing care in the developmental dimension for immobilized patients is the prevention of any measurable decline in functioning or delay in development.
- Early mobilization helps to decrease the effects of bed rest.

CRITICAL THINKING EXERCISES

1. Based on Eileen Thomas' medical history of type 2 diabetes mellitus, heart valve replacement surgery a few months ago, and being an active smoker, list three nursing interventions that you will initiate to prevent respiratory complications related to her immobility.
2. The health care provider has ordered a daily stool softener. This medication will help to prevent what potentially life-threatening complication of constipation in an immobilized patient with heart disease?
3. Eileen Thomas asks, "I know I had to take blood thinners because of my heart valve surgery, but why did my doctor order special medication for me after my hip surgery?" How will you explain the purpose of the anticoagulant therapy ordered for Ms. Thomas?
4. Identify four additional actions that will reduce the risk for clot formation in Ms. Thomas' condition.

ⓔvolve   *Answers to Critical Thinking Questions can be found on the Evolve website.*

REVIEW QUESTIONS

1. When a patient has an order for complete bed rest it is important to:
   1. Complete all care at one time to minimize disruptions
   2. Design a plan of care to meet the patient's physical, psychosocial, and developmental needs
   3. Arrange for a private room to reduce excessive stimulation from roommates
   4. Limit visitors so the patient's sleep-wake cycle will not be disturbed
2. Which patient is at greatest risk for developing the adverse effects of immobility?
   1. 5-year-old following an adenoidectomy
   2. 76-year-old following an appendectomy
   3. 79-year-old following surgery for a broken femur
   4. 51-year-old following liposuction surgery
3. When assisting a patient to stand following a prolonged period of bed rest, a drop in which assessments are important to reduce the risk for falling? Select all that apply.
   1. Steadiness of gait
   2. Respiratory rate
   3. Orthostatic hypotension
   4. Edema
4. Which of the following nursing assessments indicate a possible deep vein thrombosis (DVT)? Select all that apply.
   1. Swollen calf
   2. Reddened warm calf
   3. Calf pain when dorsiflexing the foot
   4. Painful calf
5. The family of the patient asks the nurse, "Are people on bed rest the only ones who have to worry about osteoporosis?" The best answer would be which of the following?
   1. "Actually yes. They are not walking like you and me, so we don't have to worry about it."
   2. "You should ask your doctor if you think you may have a problem with your bones."
   3. "Being on best rest can increase one's chances, and both men and women can develop it if they have the risk factors. Do you have specific concerns about it?"
   4. "There are risk factors associated with osteoporosis, but you are young and don't look like you have anything to worry about. So don't worry about it until you get older."
6. The nurse is supervising nursing assistive personnel (NAP) on the unit. To make sure that the NAP understand the importance of using the appropriate assistive device when moving patients, the nurse emphasizes that:
   1. Prolonged bed rest affects the legs muscles the most, so as a patient begins to stand or transfer there is an increased risk for falling.
   2. Arm muscles atrophy most rapidly, so patients cannot hold on to canes or walkers.
   3. Nonstriated muscles are affected most rapidly, so patients need at least one helper to rise from a bed.
   4. Prolonged bed rest affects the cardiac muscles most, so all patients must have a tilt board ordered.
7. The nurse has multiple patient assignments, and each patient has various mobility limits. Which patient care responsibility can be safely delegated?
   1. Repositioning a patient who is unstable after a cerebral vascular accident and who has left-sided paralysis
   2. Teaching a postoperative patient who has undergone hip arthroplasty to perform range-of-motion exercises
   3. Applying antiembolic stockings for a patient with dehydration and anemia
   4. Assessing a stage I sacral pressure ulcer
8. What population's self-esteem is most affected by prolonged dependency on others for care?
   1. Infants
   2. Children
   3. Adults
   4. Older adults
9. What is the best nursing strategy to implement with an immobilized patient to avoid joint contractures?
   1. Early ambulation
   2. Occupational therapy
   3. Continuous passive motion
   4. Passive and active range of joint motion
10. Once an older adult patient is medically cleared to participate in an exercise program, which of the following should be taken into consideration? Select all that apply.
    1. The attitude the patient has toward exercise
    2. Cost of gym memberships
    3. Preferences for types of activities
    4. Scheduled times for warm-up and cool-down
    5. Whether there is transportation to and from the activity

Answers to Review Questions can be found on pages 1197-1198.

REFERENCES

Agency for Healthcare Research and Quality: *Pressure ulcer prevention and treatment*, 2003, http://hstat.nlm.nih.gov/hq/Hquest/screen/TestBrowse/t/1049658066834/s/40521, accessed January 29, 2009.

American Nurses Association: *Position statement on elimination of manual patient handling to prevent work-related musculoskeletal disorders*, 2003, http://www.unap.org/files/Safe%20Patient%Handling%-%20ANA%20position.pdf, accessed January 29, 2009.

Ayello E: Predicting pressure ulcer risk, *Try This: Best Practices in Nursing Care to Older Adults,* issue 5, revised 2007, New York University College of Nursing, The Hartford Institute for Geriatric Nursing, http://www.ConsultGeriRN.org, accessed February 1, 2009.

Bartley M: Keeping venous thromboembolism at bay, *Nursing* 36(10):36, 2006.

Black J, Hawks J: *Medical-surgical nursing: clinical management for positive outcomes*, ed 7, Philadelphia, 2009, Elsevier.

Bulechek and others, editors: *Nursing interventions classification (NIC)*, ed 5, St. Louis, 2008, Mosby.

Copstead-Kirkhorn LEC, Banasik JL: *Pathophysiology*, ed 3, Philadelphia, 2005, Saunders.

Ebersole P and others: *Toward healthy aging: human needs and nursing response*, ed 7, St. Louis, 2008, Mosby.

Hockenberry M, Wilson D: *Wong's nursing care of infants and children*, ed 7, St. Louis, 2007, Mosby.

Jalali R, Rezaie M: Predicting pressure ulcer risk: comparing the predictive validity of 4 scales, *Adv Skin Wound Care* 18(2):92, 2005.

Jarvis C: *Physical examination and health assessment*, ed 5, St. Louis, 2008, Saunders/Elsevier.

Lim J and others: *A cultural health belief model to understand health behaviors and health-related quality of life between Latina and Asian-American breast cancer survivors.* Paper presented at the 13th annual conference for the Society for Social Work and Research, Washington, DC, January 16-18, 2009, http://sswr.confex.com/sswr/2009/webprogram/Paper10556.html, abstract accessed February 1, 2009.

McCance K, Huether S: *Pathophysiology: the biologic basis for disease in adults and children*, ed 5, St. Louis, 2006, Mosby.

McKenry LM and others. *Pharmacology in nursing*, ed 22, St. Louis, 2006, Mosby.

Moorhead S and others, editors: *Nursing outcomes classification (NOC)*, ed 4, 2008, Mosby.

National Osteoporosis Foundation: *American's bone health: the state of osteoporosis and low bone mass in our nation*, Washington, DC, 2007, The Foundation.

Nelson A: Safe patient handling and movement algorithms, 2006, VISN8 Patient Safety Center, http://www.visn8.med.va.gov/patientsafetycenter/SafePtHandling/default.asp.

Nelson A, Baptiste A: Evidence-based practices for safe patient handling and movement, *Orthrop Nurs* 25(6):366, 2006.

Paice JA and others: Efficacy and safety of scheduled dosing of opioid analgesics: a quality improvement study, *J Pain* 6(10):639, 2005.

Purnell L: *Guide to culturally competent health care*, ed 2, Philadelphia, 2009, FA Davis.

Purnell L, Paulanka B: *Transcultural health care*, ed 3, Philadelphia, 2008, FA Davis.

The Joint Commission: *2009 National Patient Safety Goals Hospital Program*, Oakbrook Terrace, Ill, 2008, The Joint Commission, http://www.jointcommission.org, accessed July 2008.

van Dongen CJJ and others: Fixed dose subcutaneous low molecular weight heparins versus adjusted dose of unfractionated heparin for venous thromboembolism, *Cochrane Database Syst Rev* 2005(4), http://www.cochrane.org/reviews/en/ab001100.html.

36 Skin Integrity and Wound Care

 CD COMPANION 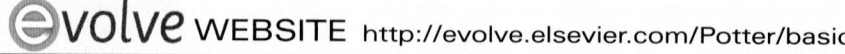 WEBSITE http://evolve.elsevier.com/Potter/basic

- Video Clips
- Crossword Puzzle
- English/Spanish Audio Glossary

OBJECTIVES

- Describe risk factors for pressure ulcer development.
- List the National Pressure Ulcer Advisory Panel (NPUAP) classification of pressure ulcer staging.
- Discuss the body's response during each phase of the wound healing process.
- Describe wound assessment criteria: anatomical location, size, type and percentage of wound tissue, volume and color of wound drainage, and condition of surrounding skin.
- Differentiate healing by primary and secondary intention.
- Discuss common complications of wound healing.
- Explain factors that impair or promote normal wound healing.

- Describe the purposes of and precautions taken with applying dressings and binders.
- Describe the mechanism of action of wound care dressings.
- Describe the differences in therapeutic effects of heat and cold.
- Complete an assessment for a patient with impaired skin integrity.
- List nursing diagnoses associated with impaired skin integrity.
- Develop a nursing care plan for a patient with impaired skin integrity.
- State evaluation criteria for a patient with impaired skin integrity.

KEY TERMS

abrasion, p. 1070
binders. p. 1082
blanchable hyperemia, p. 1059
cachexia, p. 1061
compress, p. 1088
debride, p. 1078
dehiscence, p. 1064

ecchymosis, p. 1071
eschar, p. 1061
evisceration, p. 1064
fistula, p. 1064
friction, p. 1059
granulation tissue, p. 1062
hematoma, p. 1064

hemostasis, p. 1064
induration, p. 1069
laceration, p. 1062
maceration, p. 1075
nonblanchable hyperemia, p. 1059
pressure ulcer, p. 1059
primary intention, p. 1062

reactive hyperemia, p. 1059
secondary intention, p. 1062
shear, p. 1059
sitz bath, p. 1088
tissue ischemia, p. 1059

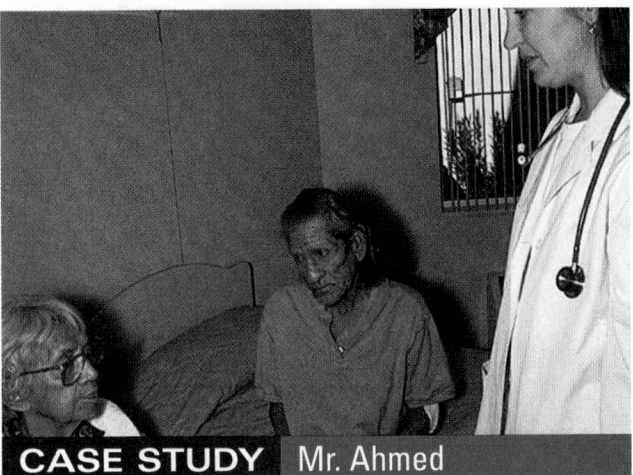

CASE STUDY   Mr. Ahmed

Mr. Omar Ahmed, a 76-year-old accountant, has come to the hospital again, this time for treatment of pneumonia. Before admission he was unable to eat and had lost more than 20 lb over the last 2 months. Three years ago he had coronary artery bypass surgery. As a precaution, he is placed on telemetry monitoring. He also has hypertension and type 2 diabetes mellitus. His mobility is limited because of his weakness, difficulty breathing, and acutely ill state. Mr. Ahmed is retired. He lives in a one-family home with his wife, Natalie. Their children and grandchildren live nearby and visit often. He complains that his "bottom hurts" from lying in bed.

Lynda Abraham is the nursing student who is assigned to the medical nursing unit. This is her first hospital-based clinical practice.

▌ SCIENTIFIC KNOWLEDGE BASE

Pressure Ulcers

Pressure ulcer (formerly called *pressure sore, decubitus ulcer,* or *bedsore*) is the term that describes impaired skin integrity resulting from pressure (Wound, Ostomy and Continence Nurses Society [WOCN], 2003) (Figure 36-1). The National Pressure Ulcer Advisory Panel (NPUAP) (2008) defines a pressure ulcer as a localized injury to the skin and/or underlying tissue, usually over a bony prominence, as a result of pressure or pressure in combination with shear and/or friction. A number of contributing factors are also associated with pressure ulcers; the significance of these factors is yet to be determined. A patient with decreased mobility, inadequate nutrition, excessive skin moisture, decreased sensory perception, or decreased activity is at risk for pressure ulcer development. More than 1 million individuals develop pressure ulcers each year. Because pressure ulcers can develop quickly when a patient is hospitalized, it is important to identify high-risk groups to target interventions (Box 36-1).

Tissue ischemia, decreased blood flow to tissue resulting in tissue death, occurs when capillary blood flow is obstructed, as in the case of pressure. When pressure is relieved in a relatively short time, a phenomenon called reactive hy-

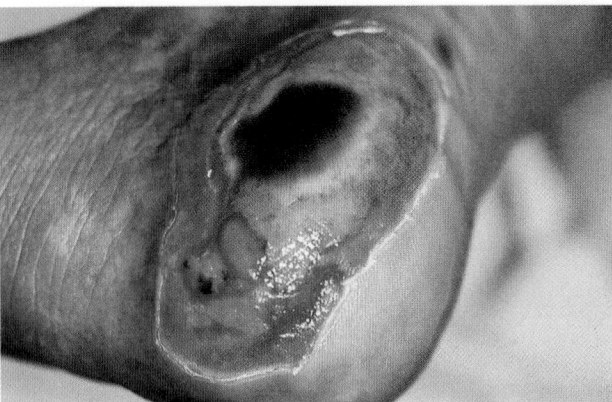

Figure 36-1 ■ Pressure ulcer with tissue necrosis.

peremia occurs. **Reactive hyperemia** is a redness of the skin resulting from dilation of the superficial capillaries (WOCN, 2003). You can determine if reactive hyperemia is present by checking for blanching. In **blanchable hyperemia,** the area that appears red and warm will blanch (turn lighter in color) following fingertip palpation (Figure 36-2). This hyperemia usually resolves without tissue loss if pressure is reduced or relieved. Blanchable hyperemia is harder to assess in patients with dark skin. The discoloration or redness appears as a deepening of normal ethnic color or a purple hue to the skin (Ayello and Lyder, 2001).

Nonblanchable hyperemia is redness that persists after palpation and indicates tissue damage (Figure 36-3). When you press a finger against the red or purple area, it does not turn lighter in color. Deep tissue damage is present and is commonly the first stage of pressure ulcer development. This stage of skin injury is also reversible if the pressure is relieved and the tissue protected.

FACTORS CONTRIBUTING TO PRESSURE ULCER FORMATION   In addition to pressure, other factors increase the patient's risk for developing pressure ulcers. External factors include shear, friction, and moisture, and internal factors include nutrition, infection, and age.

Shear   The force exerted against the skin while the skin remains stationary and the bony structures move is called **shear.** For example, when the head of the bed is elevated, gravity causes the bony skeleton to pull toward the foot of the bed, while the skin remains against the sheets (Figure 36-4). The underlying tissue blood vessels are stretched and angulated, and blood flow is impeded to the deep tissue. Ulcers occur with large areas of undermined damage and less damage at the skin surface.

Friction   Friction is an injury to the skin that has the appearance of an abrasion. An abrasion is the loss of the top layer of the skin, the epidermis. **Friction** results from two surfaces rubbing against one another. The body surfaces most at risk for friction are the elbows and heels because abrasion of these surfaces occurs when they are rubbed against the sheets during repositioning. A skin insult caused by friction looks like an abrasion (Bryant and Clark, 2007).

BOX 36-1   BEST PRACTICES

Reducing Hospital-Acquired Pressure Ulcer Incidence

SUMMARY OF EVIDENCE

The development of pressure ulcers is a serious quality of care issue in all health care settings. A patient with a pressure ulcer has an increased mortality risk when compared with a patient with intact skin. The development of a pressure ulcer interferes with recovery, causes pain and infection, and often contributes to a prolonged hospital stay. Recently the Centers for Medicare and Medicaid Services (CMS) announced a change that will reward hospitals for quality care and avoids payment for unnecessary and preventable costs. CMS will no longer reimburse an acute care facility if a patient is admitted with intact skin and develops a pressure ulcer. From a quality and fiscal standpoint it is key to adopt prevalence- and incidence-monitoring programs for prevention and intervention of pressure ulcers. Pressure ulcers may be preventable in many cases when a comprehensive program is developed. A comprehensive program should include skin and risk assessment upon admission to the health care facility and on an ongoing basis, quarterly collection of prevalence and incidence data, prevention and intervention protocols based upon evidence-based guidelines, and a multidisciplinary team focused on prevention and early intervention.

APPLICATION TO NURSING PRACTICE

- Complete a thorough skin and risk assessment on all patients upon admission to the health care setting, and continue on an ongoing defined basis.
- Use the results of the skin and risk assessment to plan topical therapy; risk reduction interventions are based on evidence-based guidelines.
- Collect nursing unit prevalence and incidence data to focus on areas of practice that require attention.
- A multidisciplinary team is valuable for preventing pressure ulcers and promoting early intervention of pressure ulcers.

REFERENCES

Dibsie LG: Implementing evidence-based practice to prevent skin breakdown, *Crit Care Nurs Q* 31(2):140, 2008.

McInerney JA: Reducing hospital-acquired pressure ulcer prevalence through a focused prevention program, *Adv Skin Wound Care* 21(2):175, 2008.

Reddy M, Gill SS, Rochon PA: Preventing pressure ulcers: a systematic review, *JAMA* 296(8):974, 2006.

Moisture Moisture on the skin increases the risk for ulcer formation. Moisture reduces the skin's resistance to other physical factors such as pressure or shear. Moisture originates from wound drainage, perspiration, and/or fecal and urinary incontinence. Skin moisture and wetness from incontinence can cause skin breakdown (Fader, Bain, and Cottenden, 2004).

Nutrition Poor nutrition, specifically severe protein deficiency, causes soft tissue to become susceptible to breakdown. Low protein levels cause edema or swelling, which contributes to problems with oxygen transport and the transport of nutrients (Pieper, 2007).

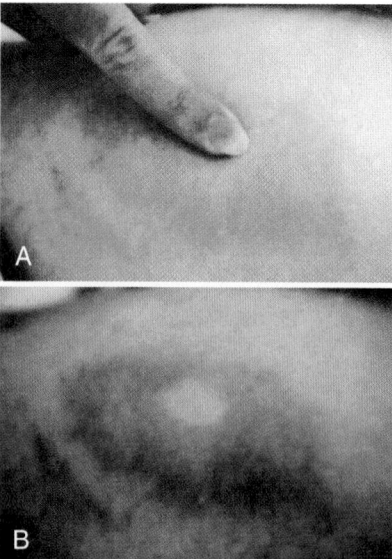

Figure 36-2 ■ **A,** Check for blanching by applying fingertip pressure. **B,** Area of blanchable hyperemia.

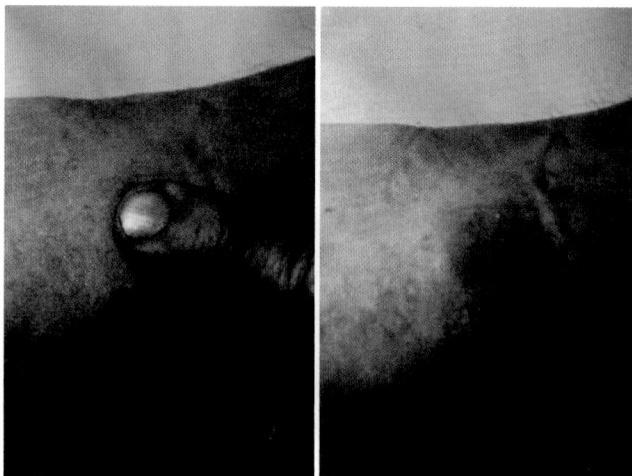

Figure 36-3 ■ Nonblanchable hyperemia: The area is darker than the surrounding skin and does not blanch with fingertip pressure.

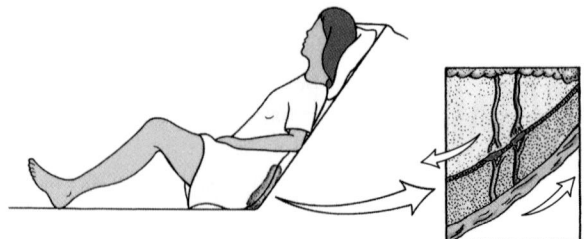

Figure 36-4 ■ Shear exerted in the sacral area.

Poor nutrition alters fluid and electrolyte balance. In patients with severe protein loss, hypoalbuminemia (serum albumin level below 3 g/100 mL) leads to a shift of fluid from the extracellular fluid volume to the tissues, resulting in edema (Mathus-Vliegen, 2004). Edema increases the affected tissue's risk for pressure ulcer formation. The blood supply to the edematous tissue is decreased, and waste products remain because of the changing pressures in the capillary circulation and capillary bed.

Cachexia is generalized ill health and malnutrition, marked by weakness and emaciation, or extreme thinness. Basically the cachectic patient has lost the adipose tissue necessary to protect bony prominences from pressure and suffers from poor nutrition.

Infection Infection results from the presence of pathogens in the body. A patient with an infection usually has a fever. Infection and fever increase the metabolic needs of the body, making already hypoxic tissue more susceptible to ischemic injury. In addition, fever results in diaphoresis and increased skin moisture, which further predispose the patient to skin breakdown.

Age Skin structure changes with age, causing a loss of dermal thickness and an increase in the risk for skin tears. Older adults are at highest risk for development of pressure ulcers; 60% to 90% of all pressure ulcers occur in patients over 65 years of age (Stotts and Wu, 2007). Neonates and young children (i.e., younger than 5 years old) are also at high risk for pressure ulcer occurrence (Noonan, Quigley and Curley, 2006; WOCN, 2003).

Origins of Pressure Ulcers

Pressure exerted against the skin surface causes pressure ulcers; usually a bone and the surface of the bed compress the skin. However, pressure ulcers also occur on any skin surface where pressure applied against the skin exceeds capillary closure pressure. Classic research identified that normal capillary pressure, the amount of pressure needed to keep the capillary open, is in the range of 12 to 32 mm Hg, depending on the location in the capillary (Landis, 1930). When the intensity of the pressure exerted on the capillary exceeds 12 to 32 mm Hg, this occludes the vessel, causing ischemic injury to the tissues it normally feeds. However, pressure to the tissue will not routinely result in pressure ulceration. Two other concepts, duration of the pressure and tissue tolerance, play a role.

High pressure over a short time and low pressure over a long time cause skin breakdown. Thus duration influences the effects of pressure; the longer the pressure is applied, the more likely tissue loss will occur. Tissue tolerance also plays an important role in pressure ulcer development. The integrity of the skin and the supporting structures influence the skin's ability to redistribute the pressure. The factors mentioned above—shear, friction, moisture, and the internal factors such as nutrition, infection, and age—alter the ability of the skin and supporting tissue to respond to the pressure (Ayello and others, 2004).

Pressure Ulcer Classification

One method to classify pressure ulcers is to stage the ulcer according to tissue layer involvement. The National Pressure Ulcer Advisory Panel (2008) supports the following staging system:

Stage I: Intact skin with nonblanchable redness of a localized area, usually over a bony prominence. Darkly pigmented skin may not have visible blanching; its color may differ from that of the surrounding area (Figure 36-5, *A*).

Further description: The area may be painful, firm, soft, warmer or cooler compared with adjacent tissue. Stage I may be difficult to detect in individuals with dark skin tones. May indicate "at-risk" persons (a heralding sign of risk).

Stage II: Partial-thickness loss of dermis presenting as a shallow open ulcer with a red-pink wound bed, without slough. May also present as an intact or open/ruptured serum-filled blister (Figure 36-5, *B*).

Further description: Presents as a shiny or dry shallow ulcer without slough or bruising.* This stage should not be used to describe skin tears, tape burns, perineal dermatitis, maceration, or excoriation.

Stage III: Full-thickness tissue loss. Subcutaneous fat may be visible, but bone, tendon, or muscle is not exposed. Slough may be present but does not obscure the depth of tissue loss. May include undermining and tunneling (Figure 36-5, *C*).

Further description: The depth of a stage III pressure ulcer varies by anatomical location. The bridge of the nose, ear, occiput, and malleolus do not have subcutaneous tissue, and stage III ulcers can be shallow. In contrast, areas of significant adiposity can develop extremely deep stage III pressure ulcers. Bone/tendon is not visible or directly palpable.

Stage IV: Full-thickness tissue loss with exposed bone, tendon, or muscle. Slough or **eschar** may be present on some parts of the wound bed. Often includes undermining and tunneling (Figure 36-5, *D*).

Further description: The depth of a stage IV pressure ulcer varies by anatomical location. The bridge of the nose, ear, occiput, and malleolus do not have subcutaneous tissue, and these ulcers can be shallow. Stage IV ulcers can extend into muscle and/or supporting structures (e.g., fascia, tendon, or joint capsule), making osteomyelitis possible. Exposed bone/tendon is visible or directly palpable.

Unstageable: Full-thickness tissue loss in which the base of the ulcer is covered by slough (yellow, tan, gray, green, or brown) and/or eschar (tan, brown, or black) in the wound bed.

Further description: Until enough slough and/or eschar is removed to expose the base of the wound, the true depth, and therefore stage, cannot be determined. Stable (dry, adherent, intact without erythema or fluctance) eschar on the heels serves as "the body's natural (biological) cover" and should not be removed.

Wound assessment (regardless of cause) includes the following parameters: anatomical location, size (dimensions and depth of wound), type (viable or nonviable) and percentage of wound tissue (the proportion of tissue type), volume and color of wound drainage, and condition of surrounding skin (Nix, 2007a). These measures assist in evaluating the progress of the wound, drive decision making, and provide evaluation of wound healing.

Wound Healing Process

All wounds heal through an orderly series of integrated physiological responses. Multiple factors promote or impede wound healing (Box 36-2). A wound with little or no tissue

---

*Bruising indicates suspected deep tissue injury.

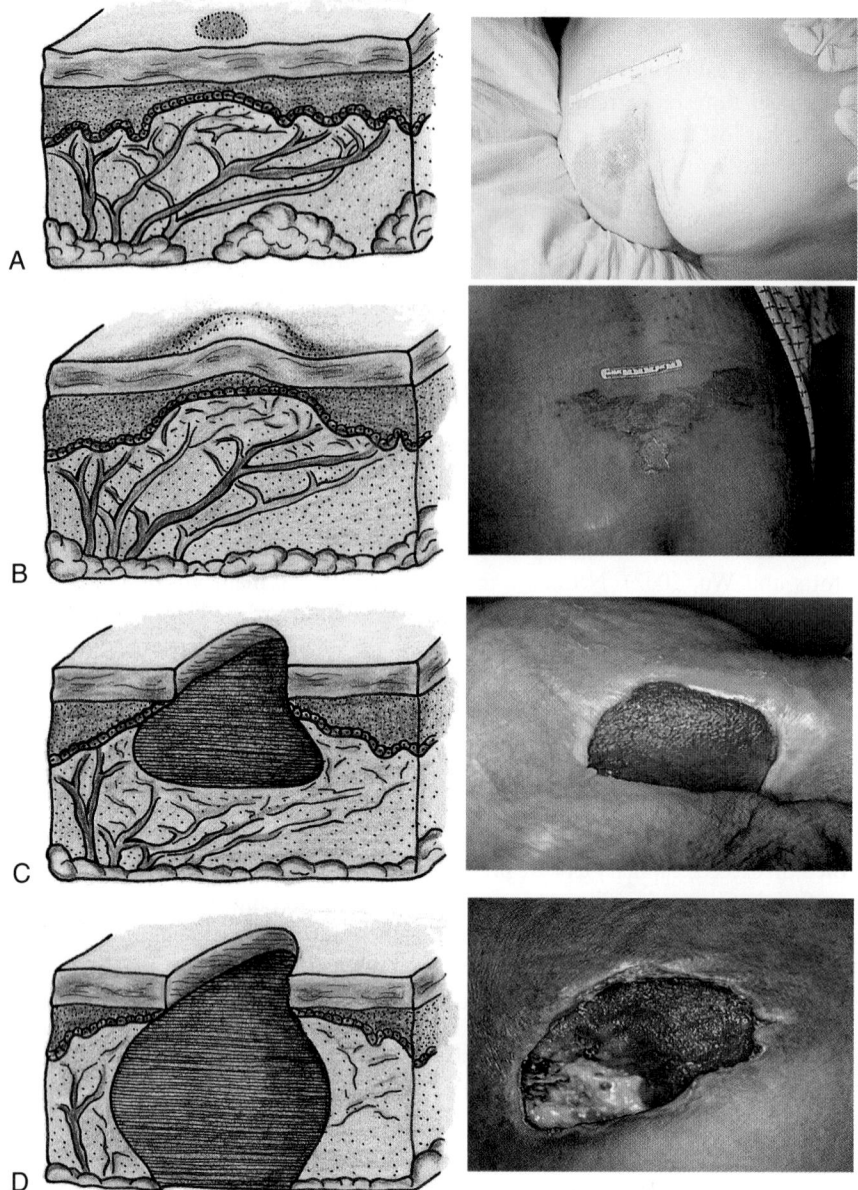

Figure 36-5 ■ **A,** Stage I pressure ulcer. **B,** Stage II pressure ulcer. **C,** Stage III pressure ulcer. **D,** Stage IV pressure ulcer. (Courtesy Laurel Wiersma-Bryant, RN, MSN, Clinical Nurse Specialist, Barnes Hospital, St. Louis.)

loss, such as a clean surgical incision, heals by **primary intention.** The skin edges approximate, or close together, and the risk for infection developing is slight. In contrast, a wound involving loss of tissue such as a severe **laceration** or a chronic wound such as a pressure ulcer heals by **secondary intention.** The skin edges cannot come together, and healing occurs gradually. A layer of **granulation tissue,** which is red, moist tissue consisting of blood vessels and connective tissue, covers the wound; wound contraction brings the wound edges together; and the wound closes with a scar. There are also instances in which a surgical wound is initially closed in the deep tissue layers; however, the subcutaneous fat and skin layers are left open. This method of wound closure is called tertiary intention or delayed primary closure. The wound heals with a layer of granulation tissue at the edges and base,

and several days after the initial wounding the wound edges are brought together with sutures or adhesive closures. An example of a wound closure by delayed primary closure occurs when a patient has a ruptured appendix. In some cases the surgeon is unsure if the appendix had microperforations and subsequent spilling of the intestinal contents into the abdomen and wound. Thus the surgeon will leave the incision open for up to 4 to 5 days following surgery. Then the surgeon evaluates the wound, and, if after 4 to 5 days the surgeon does not note any clinical signs of infection, the wound is closed with either adhesive strips or sutures.

Wounds heal by one of two mechanisms: partial-thickness wound repair or full-thickness wound repair. Partial-thickness wound repair is necessary when there is loss of the epidermis and/or part of the dermis, such as wound healing

BOX 36-2　Factors Influencing Wound Healing

AGE
- Blood circulation and oxygen delivery to the wound, clotting, inflammatory response, and phagocytosis are sometimes impaired in the very young and older adults. Risk for infection is greater.
- Cell growth and differentiation in reconstruction are slower with advancing age.
- Scar tissue never regains the tensile strength of noninjured skin, increasing the risk for altered body part function in older adults.
- Age affects all phases of wound healing. A decline in the number of white blood cells places older adults at greater risk for a wound infection. A slowdown is common in the deposition of collagen in re-epithelialization.

NUTRITION
- Tissue repair and infection resistance depend on a balanced diet. Surgery, severe wounds, serious infections, and preoperative nutritional deficits increase nutritional requirements.
- Nutrients provide raw materials needed for cellular activities that contribute to wound healing.

INFECTION
- Wound infection prolongs the inflammatory phase, delays collagen synthesis, and prevents epithelialization.

OBESITY
- The less abundant supply of blood vessels in fatty tissue impairs delivery of nutrients and cellular elements needed for healing.

EXTENT OF WOUND
- Wounds with extensive tissue loss heal by secondary intention and remain open for a prolonged period of time to heal.

TISSUE PERFUSION
- Oxygen fuels the cellular function essential to the repair process. Chronic tissue hypoxia is associated with impaired collagen synthesis and reduced tissue resistance to infection.

SMOKING
- Nicotine causes vasoconstriction and functional hemoglobin levels decrease, impairing oxygen release to tissues.

IMMUNOSUPPRESSION
- Cortisone suppresses the inflammatory response, increasing the wound's vulnerability to infection.
- Because steroids decrease the inflammatory response, detection of early signs of inflammation or infection is difficult.
- Chemotherapeutic drugs and certain cancerous diseases interfere with leukocyte production and the immune response.
- Immunosuppressive therapy impairs wound healing by preventing normal progression of the phases of wound healing.

DIABETES MELLITUS
- The patient with diabetes has small vessel disease that impairs tissue perfusion; thus oxygen delivery is poor.
- An elevated blood glucose level (hyperglycemia) impairs macrophage function. Risk for infection is increased because of hyperglycemia and poor wound healing.
- Patients with diabetes demonstrate the following problems with wound healing: reduced collagen synthesis, decreased wound strength, and impaired white blood cell functioning. These adverse effects are at least in part due to poor glycemic control.

RADIATION
- Radiation therapy, which eventually results in fibrosis and vascular scarring, interferes with postoperative wound healing when surgery is delayed more than 4 to 6 weeks and irradiated tissues have become fragile and poorly perfused.

WOUND STRESS
- Sustained stress (e.g., vomiting, abdominal distention, coughing) disrupts wound layers and tissue repair.

Modified from Doughty DL, Defriese Sparkes B: Wound healing physiology in acute and chronic wounds. In Bryant RA, Nix DP, editors: *Acute and chronic wounds: current management concepts*, ed 3, St. Louis, 2007, Mosby.

by primary intention. Full-thickness wound repair is necessary when there is loss of the epidermis, dermis, and possible extension into subcutaneous layers, bone, and/or muscle.

PARTIAL-THICKNESS WOUND REPAIR The body repairs wounds that heal by primary intention and shallow wounds that involve loss of only the epidermis and perhaps some of the dermis by resurfacing of the wound with new epidermal cells. The wounds go through several phases of wound healing.

Inflammatory Response Erythema and edema are the first response, bringing white blood cells to the site. The wounded area appears red and swollen. If the exudate, or discharge, that brings the white blood cells to the area is allowed to dry, a scab will form. This response is limited and usually subsides in less than 24 hours (Doughty and Sparks-Defriese, 2007).

Epidermal Repair Epidermal cells begin migration across the wound, originating from the epidermal cells at the wound edges or the epidermal appendages. Peak epithelial proliferation occurs within 24 to 72 hours after injury. Wounds kept in a moist environment will heal in approximately 4 days (as opposed to 7 days when kept dry) because new epithelial cells migrate across a moist surface. If a wound is dry, the cells have to find moisture below the skin surface (Doughty and Sparks-Defriese, 2007).

Dermal Repair The epidermis thickens, anchors to adjacent cells, and resumes normal function. The new epidermis is pink, dry, and fragile. If dermal repair is necessary, dermal repair occurs concurrently with epidermal repair.

FULL-THICKNESS WOUND REPAIR Full-thickness wounds involve tissue loss and extend to at least the subcutaneous layer. A full-thickness wound may be either acute (a surgical wound) or chronic (a pressure ulcer). Healing of a full-thickness acute wound such as a surgical incision proceeds by primary intention; healing of a full-thickness chronic wound such as a pressure ulcer proceeds by secondary intention. The key events differ between a chronic wound healing by secondary intention and an acute wound healing by primary intention.

Hemostasis Phase The first event in the hemostasis phase involving a full-thickness wound healing by primary intention is hemostasis, the control of bleeding. Platelets cause coagulation and vasoconstriction. The platelets break down and release growth factors, which appear to initiate the entire wound-healing process (Jones, Bale, and Harding, 2004). Bleeding and hemostasis do not occur in wounds healing by secondary intention, thus compromising the repair process (Doughty and Sparks-Defriese, 2007).

Inflammation Phase The goal of this phase is to establish a clean wound bed and to obtain bacterial balance. The inflammatory response brings white blood cells to the area, cleaning up the site and releasing additional growth factors. This phase lasts approximately 3 days in an acute clean wound, such as a surgical incision. However, in a chronic wound healing by secondary intention this phase is prolonged and may last longer than 3 days.

Proliferative Phase The key events in the proliferative phase are production of new tissue, epithelialization, and contraction. In a wound healing by primary intention, new capillary networks form to provide oxygen and nutrients for new tissue and contribute to the synthesis of collagen. As collagen fibers and capillary networks continue to synthesize and increase in size, the wound begins to contract. The last component of this phase is epithelialization, in which the epithelial cells migrate and cover the defect. It is important to note that epithelialization occurs faster in a moist environment, supporting the role of moist wound dressings in wound care. In healing by secondary intention in a chronic wound such as a pressure ulcer, the proliferative phase is prolonged. As granulation tissue forms to fill in the defect, it is followed by contraction and epithelialization, the final phase. Contraction is much more important in secondary intention wounds because it reduces the amount of granulation tissue needed to fill the defect (Doughty and Sparks-Defriese, 2007).

Remodeling Phase The remodeling phase, which lasts up to 1 year, reorganizes the collagen to produce a more elastic, stronger collagen for the scar tissue. The tensile strength of the scar tissue is never more than 80% of the tensile strength in nonwounded tissue (Jones and others, 2004). The remodeling process is the same for wounds healing by primary and secondary intention.

Complications of Wound Healing

Wound healing is not without complications. When caring for patients with wounds, you will observe the healing process while observing for complications.

HEMORRHAGE Bleeding from an acute wound is normal during and immediately after initial trauma, but **hemostasis,** which is cessation of bleeding by vasoconstriction and coagulation, usually occurs within several minutes. Hemorrhage occurring later could indicate a slipped surgical suture, a dislodged clot, infection, or the erosion of a blood vessel by a foreign object (e.g., a drain). Hemorrhage is external or internal. Symptoms of internal bleeding are hypovolemic shock and swelling of the affected body part. A **hematoma,** a collection of clotted blood, is a localized collection of blood underneath tissues, often appearing as a bluish swelling or mass. External hemorrhaging is usually more obvious because dressings covering the wound soon become saturated with blood. Surgical drains also drain blood. You will note a decrease in the patient's hemoglobin level and hematocrit.

INFECTION Bacterial wound infection prevents healing by increasing tissue damage and altering the healing process. The chances of wound infection are greater when the wound contains dead or necrotic tissues, when foreign bodies are in or near the wound, and when the blood supply and local tissue defenses are lower than normal.

A contaminated or traumatic wound infection develops within 2 to 3 days; a surgical wound infection develops within 4 to 5 days. Locally, drainage is often yellow, green, or brown and odorous, depending on the causative organism. The wound edges will appear tense, swollen, and painful, with redness extending beyond the immediate wound edge. Systemic signs include fever, general malaise, and an elevated white blood cell count.

DEHISCENCE When an acute wound fails to heal properly, the layers of skin and tissue separate. This most commonly occurs before collagen formation (3 to 11 days after injury). **Dehiscence** is the partial or total separation of layers of skin and tissue above the fascia in a wound that is not healing properly. Obese patients have a high risk for dehiscence because of constant strain on their wounds and the poor vascularity of fatty tissue. Dehiscence occurs most often in abdominal surgical wounds after a sudden strain such as coughing, vomiting, or sitting up in bed. Patients often report feeling as though something has given way. When serosanguineous drainage increases from a wound, be alert for dehiscence.

EVISCERATION **Evisceration** occurs when wound layers separate below the fascial layer, and visceral organs protrude through the wound opening. It is a medical emergency requiring placement of sterile towels soaked in sterile saline over the extruding tissues to reduce chances of bacterial invasion and drying before surgical repair occurs.

FISTULA A **fistula** is an abnormal opening between two organs or between an organ and the skin. Fistulas result from wound-healing problems associated with trauma, infection, radiation exposure, or disease such as cancer. Fistulas increase the risks of infection, fluid and electrolyte imbalances, and skin breakdown from chronic drainage.

NURSING KNOWLEDGE BASE

A major aspect of nursing care is the maintenance of skin integrity and wound care. Nursing research has an important role in developing guidelines for pressure ulcer care and prevention.

Prediction and Prevention

In 2003 the Wound, Ostomy and Continence Nurses Society (WOCN) developed the *Guideline for Prevention and Management of Pressure Ulcers*. A panel of nurse experts performed extensive searches on available literature on pressure ulcers and established a level of evidence rating that provides the best available evidence in the prevention and manage-

ment of pressure ulcers. This guideline was accepted by the guideline resource component of the Agency for Healthcare Research and Quality. Included in these guidelines are predictive tools for pressure ulcer development that identify those patients at highest risk for development of pressure ulcers. Patients identified to be at risk need a care plan that addresses and reduces the identified risk factors. Patients with little risk for pressure ulcer development do not have the unnecessary expense of preventive treatments.

One reliable predictive tool is the Braden Scale. The Braden Scale is made of six subscales: sensory perception, moisture, activity, mobility, nutrition, and friction and shear (Table 36-1). A hospitalized adult with a score of 16 or below and an older adult at 18 or below are at risk for pressure ulcer development (Ayello and Braden, 2002; Bergstrom and others, 1998). This instrument is highly reliable in the identification of patients at greatest risk for pressure ulcers (Ayello and others, 2004; Bergstrom and others, 1987a, 1987b, 1998).

TABLE 36-1 Braden Scale for Predicting Pressure Sore Risk

SENSORY PERCEPTION

| Ability to respond meaningfully to pressure-related discomfort | 1. **Completely limited:** Unresponsive (does not moan, flinch, or grasp) to painful stimuli because of diminished level of consciousness or sedation. **or** Limited ability to feel pain over most of body surface. | 2. **Very limited:** Responds only to painful stimuli. Cannot communicate discomfort except by moaning or restlessness. **or** Has a sensory impairment that limits the ability to feel pain or discomfort over half of body. | 3. **Slightly limited:** Responds to verbal commands but cannot always communicate discomfort or need to be turned. **or** Has some sensory impairment, which limits ability to feel pain or discomfort in 1 or 2 extremities. | 4. **No impairment:** Responds to verbal commands. Has no sensory deficit that limits ability to feel or voice pain or discomfort. |

MOISTURE

| Degree to which skin is exposed to moisture | 1. **Constantly moist:** Perspiration, urine, etc. keep skin moist almost constantly. Dampness is detected every time patient is moved or turned. | 2. **Often moist:** Skin is often, but not always, moist. Linen must be changed at least once a shift. | 3. **Occasionally moist:** Skin is occasionally moist, requiring an extra linen change approximately once per day. | 4. **Rarely moist:** Skin is usually dry; linen requires changing only at routine intervals. |

ACTIVITY

| Degree of physical activity | 1. **Bedfast:** Confined to bed. | 2. **Confined to chair:** Ability to walk severely limited or nonexistent. Cannot bear own weight and/or must be assisted into chair or wheelchair. | 3. **Walks occasionally:** Walks occasionally during day, but for very short distances, with or without assistance. Spends majority of each shift in bed or chair. | 4. **Walks frequently:** Walks outside the room at least twice a day and inside room at least once every 2 hours during waking hours. |

Continued

TABLE 36-1 Braden Scale for Predicting Pressure Sore Risk—cont'd

MOBILITY
Ability to change and control body position

1. Completely immobile: Does not make even slight changes in body or extremity position without assistance.

2. Very limited: Makes occasional slight changes in body or extremity position but unable to make frequent or significant changes independently.

3. Slightly limited: Makes frequent though slight changes in body or extremity position independently.

4. No limitations: Makes major and frequent changes in position without assistance.

NUTRITION
Usual food intake pattern

1. Very poor: Never eats a complete meal. Rarely eats more than one third of any food offered. Eats 2 servings or less of protein (meat or dairy products) per day. Takes fluids poorly. Does not take a liquid dietary supplement.
or
Is NPO and/or maintained on clear liquids or IVs for more than 5 days.

2. Probably inadequate: Rarely eats a complete meal and generally eats only about half of any food offered. Protein intake includes only 3 servings of meat or dairy products per day. Occasionally will take a dietary supplement.
or
Receives less than optimal amount of liquid diet or tube feeding.

3. Adequate: Eats over half of most meals. Eats a total of 4 servings of protein (meat, dairy products) each day. Occasionally will refuse a meal, but will usually take a supplement if offered.
or
Is on a tube-feeding or TPN regimen that probably meets most nutritional needs.

4. Excellent: Eats most of every meal. Never refuses a meal. Usually eats a total of 4 or more servings of meat and dairy products. Occasionally eats between meals. Does not require supplements.

FRICTION AND SHEAR

1. Problem: Requires moderate to maximal assistance in moving. Complete lifting without sliding against sheets is impossible. Frequently slides down in bed or chair, requiring frequent repositioning with maximal assistance. Spasticity, contractions, or agitation leads to almost constant friction.

2. Potential problem: Moves feebly or requires minimal assistance. During a move skin probably slides to some extent against sheets, chair, restraints, or other devices. Maintains relatively good position in chair or bed most of the time but occasionally slides down.

3. No apparent problem: Moves in bed and in chair independently and has sufficient muscle strength to sit up completely during move. Maintains good position in bed or chair at all times.

Copyright 1988. Used with permission of Barbara Braden, PhD, RN, Professor, Creighton University School of Nursing, Omaha, Nebraska and Nancy Bergstrom, Professor, University of Texas–Houston, School of Nursing, Houston, Texas.
IV, Intravenous; *NPO,* nothing by mouth; *TPN,* total parenteral nutrition.
Instructions: Score patient in each of the six subscales. Maximum score is 23, indicating little or no risk. A score of 16 indicates "at risk"; ≤9 indicates high risk.

CRITICAL THINKING

Synthesis

You will apply elements of critical thinking whenever you perform the nursing process with a patient. Consider the scientific knowledge you have learned, your experience, critical thinking attitudes, and standards to ensure an individualized approach to patient care. When you care for patients who have pressure ulcers or chronic wounds, integrate information from all health-related sciences, as well as knowledge from courses, experiences, and appropriate standards of practice into the management of your patient's wounds (Box 36-3).

KNOWLEDGE Performing a pressure ulcer risk assessment requires you to use a validated risk assessment tool. Knowing normal physiology of wound healing enables you to practice protective and preventive nursing measures. In addition, knowledge of the normal healing process helps you to recognize complications requiring intervention. In choosing interventions, consider the type of wound, the pain associated with it, conditions that affect healing, and the patient's psychological well-being.

EXPERIENCE By observing the normal characteristics of a healing wound, you assess how your patient's wound is healing. This is especially important when your patient has some factors that impede wound healing, such as peripheral vascular disease, poor nutrition, or reduced mobility.

You are better able to assess a patient's wound by being able to draw from experience and recognize normal characteristics of wound healing. When caring for a patient who develops problems with wound healing, learn the clinical signs of complications. This is especially important when caring for a patient with darkly pigmented skin (Box 36-4). Reflecting on such experience prepares you to assess wounds more accurately.

ATTITUDES Be perseverant when caring for an acutely ill patient. At times assessment of skin or wound integrity or for skin breakdown is overlooked because of other perceived priorities, such as respiratory or cardiac status. Assume responsibility for ensuring that meticulous skin assessment and pressure ulcer prevention measures are incorporated in the plan of care. Skin assessment is important whenever a patient's health status changes (WOCN, 2003). Be aware that skin breakdown is sometimes unavoidable. However, the sooner you assess for and identify the risk factors for skin breakdown and plan interventions, the less severe the impaired skin integrity should be.

In the immediate postoperative period, some patients require well-thought-out modifications of wound care techniques. The dressing may not be changed, but you are responsible for ensuring that the dressing remains dry and intact. With knowledge about pressure ulcers, wounds, and normal wound healing, use creative measures to reduce the risks of impaired skin integrity and promote wound healing.

BOX 36-4   CULTURAL FOCUS

Skin Assessment for the Patient With Intact Darkly Pigmented Skin

ASSESS LOCALIZED SKIN COLOR CHANGES
Any of the following may appear:
- Skin color changes are different from usual skin tone.
- Skin appears darker than surrounding skin—purplish, bluish, eggplant.

IMPORTANCE OF LIGHTING SOURCE
- Use natural or halogen light.
- Avoid fluorescent lamps.
- Avoid wearing tinted lenses when assessing skin color.

TISSUE CONSISTENCY
- Skin is taut, shiny, or indurated; edema occurs with induration of more than 15 mm in diameter.
- Assess for edema/swelling.
- Assess for firm or boggy feel.

SENSATION
- Assess for pain or changes in skin sensation, such as burning or itching.

ASSESS SKIN TEMPERATURE
- Initially skin in the area of pressure may feel warmer than the surrounding skin.
- Subsequently skin may feel cooler than the surrounding skin.
- Feel areas of skin that are not involved in or around a pressure point to serve as a point of temperature reference.

Data from Bennett MA: Report of the task force on the implications for darkly pigmented intact skin in the prediction and prevention of pressure ulcers, *Adv Wound Care* 8(6):34, 1995; Henderson CT and others: Draft definition of stage I pressure ulcers: inclusion of persons with darkly pigmented skin, *Adv Wound Care* 10(5):16, 1997.

BOX 36-3   SYNTHESIS IN PRACTICE

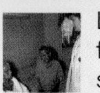

Lynda reviews the nursing assessment and she finds that Mr. Ahmed was admitted with a pressure ulcer. The ulcer is a stage II, 1- × 2-inch (2.5 × 3.5 cm) × ⅛-inch-deep partial-thickness wound over his sacral area. There is no necrotic tissue, and the wound bed has red, moist tissue. When Lynda prepares to conduct a skin assessment on Mr. Ahmed, she recalls information about the pathogenesis of pressure ulcers and guidelines for skin assessment for patients with darkly pigmented skin. She will focus on determining changes in Mr. Ahmed's skin integrity.

Lynda observed care of a stage IV pressure ulcer during an experience in an extended care facility. From that experience she increased her knowledge about the debilitating effects of pressure ulcers. In addition, she was able to practice skin assessment techniques during her clinical experience in the extended care facility.

STANDARDS WOCN wrote the 2003 pressure ulcer guidelines to support clinical practice by providing consistent research-based clinical decisions (Box 36-5). In addition, wound care protocols such as surgical wound management vary by agency policy. Know your agency's policy and practices regarding the use of skin care products, dressing materials, and frequency of dressing change.

NURSING PROCESS

■■■ ASSESSMENT

Baseline and continual focused assessment data provide critical information about the patient's skin integrity and the increased risk for pressure ulcer development or impaired wound healing (Table 36-2). Although there are multiple factors that affect skin integrity, it is important that you identify and assess those factors relevant for your patient.

PRESSURE ULCERS Perform assessment of the patient for risk for development of pressure ulcers using one of the established predictive tools, such as the Braden Scale. Do this on admission to the agency, 24 to 48 hours after admission, at regular intervals, and when there is a significant change in the patient's condition. Ongoing assessment is important because the patient's condition may change; continual assessments help identify changes that increase the patient's risk for pressure ulcer development. In addition to assessing the patient for potential risk factors, perform a thorough skin assessment on a daily basis. The skin assessment provides for prompt problem identification and development of individualized interventions (Skill 36-1). Prompt identification of such patients enables nurses to individualize costly resources to appropriate patients and reduce their risk. When patients are identified as being at risk for pressure ulcers, specific prevention and ulcer treatment strategies are included in the plan of care.

Skin Assessment for tissue pressure indicators includes visual and tactile inspection of the skin. Baseline assessment determines the patient's normal skin characteristics and any actual or potential areas of breakdown. This is especially important with high-risk patients such as those with diabetes, stroke, or serious malnutrition. The skin of an older adult patient is more fragile and has an increased risk for skin breakdown (Box 36-6). Pay particular attention to areas exposed to casts, traction, or splints.

BOX 36-5   Pressure Ulcer Prevention Points

ASSESSMENT

1 Assess individual risk for developing pressure ulcers.
2 Perform a risk assessment (using a tool such as the Braden Scale) on entry to a health care setting, and repeat on a regularly scheduled basis or when there is a significant change in the patient's condition.
3 Assess for cognition, sensation, immobility, shear, friction, and incontinence.
4 Identify high-risk settings and groups to target prevention efforts to minimize risk.
5 Inspect skin and bony prominences at least daily.

SKIN CARE AND EARLY TREATMENT

1 Continue preventive measures even when a patient has a pressure ulcer to prevent additional pressure areas from developing.
2 Clean and dry skin after each incontinent episode.
3 Use incontinence skin barriers such as creams, ointments, pastes, and film-forming skin protectants as needed to protect and maintain intact skin.
4 Use turning or lift sheets or devices to turn or transfer patients.
5 Maintain head of bed at or below 30 degrees or at the lowest level of elevation consistent with the patient's medical condition.
6 Avoid vigorous massage over bony prominences.

SUPPORT SURFACES/PRESSURE REDUCTION

1 Place at-risk individuals on a pressure-reduction surface and not on an ordinary hospital mattress.

2 Schedule regular and frequent turning and repositioning for bed- and chair-bound individuals. Turn at least every 2 to 4 hours on a pressure-reducing mattress or at least every 2 hours on a non–pressure-reducing mattress.
3 Reposition chair-bound individuals every hour if they are unable to perform pressure-relief exercises every 15 minutes.

NUTRITION

1 Maintain adequate nutrition that is compatible with the individuals' wishes or condition.
2 Consult a registered dietitian in cases of suspected or identified nutritional deficiencies or when nutrition supplementation is necessary to prevent malnutrition.

PATIENT/CAREGIVER EDUCATION

1 Educate patient/caregiver about the causes and risk factors for pressure ulcer development and ways to minimize risk.
2 Include information on the following:
   a Etiology of and risk factors for pressure ulcers
   b Risk assessment tools and their application
   c Skin assessment
   d Selection/use of support surfaces
   e Development with implementation of individualized programs of skin care
   f Demonstration of positioning to decrease risk for tissue breakdown
   g Accurate documentation of pertinent data

Data from Wound, Ostomy and Continence Nurses Society: *Guideline for prevention and management of pressure ulcers,* WOCN Clinical Practice Guidelines Series, Glenview, Ill, 2003, The Society.

Assess all areas of the skin, from head to toe, paying attention to any reddened areas or breaks in skin integrity. Document the assessment. When you notice hyperemia, document location, size, and color, and reassess the area after 1 hour. If you suspect nonblanchable hyperemia, outlining the affected area with a marker makes reassessment easier. Nonblanchable hyperemia is an early indicator of impaired skin integrity, but damage to the underlying tissue is sometimes more progressive. Palpate the tissues next to the observed area to acquire further data about **induration** (red warm area) and the damage to the skin and underlying tissues.

Assess patients with lightly pigmented skin for blanching with return to normal skin tones. Also note changes in color, temperature, and hardness of the surrounding skin and tissues. Use visual and tactile inspection over the body areas most frequently at risk for pressure ulcer development (Figure 36-6). When a patient lies in bed or sits in a chair, the body places weight heavily on certain bony prominences. Body surfaces subjected to the greatest weight or pressure are at greatest risk for pressure ulcer formation.

Mobility Assessment includes documenting level of mobility, the potential effects of impaired mobility on skin integrity, and data regarding the quality of muscle tone and strength. For example, determine whether the patient is able to lift the weight off the ischial tuberosities and roll the body to a side-lying position. Some patients have adequate range of motion (ROM) to independently move into a more protective position. Finally, assess the patient's activity tolerance (see Chapter 26).

Nutritional Status Malnutrition is associated with overall morbidity and mortality. Best practice involves monitoring the nutritional status as part of the total assessment (WOCN, 2003) (Box 36-7) (see also Chapter 32). Inadequate caloric intake causes weight loss and a decrease in subcutaneous tissue, allowing bony prominences to compress and restrict circulation.

WOUNDS The assessment of a patient's wound varies from one health care setting to another. It is important for you to be thorough in this assessment and accurately collect relevant data. Accurate and regular assessments of the patient's wounds drive treatment decisions and provide a baseline to evaluate the wounds' status (WOCN, 2003).

Emergency Setting In an emergency the type of wound determines the criteria for inspection. After you stabilize a

TABLE 36-2   FOCUSED PATIENT ASSESSMENT

FACTORS TO ASSESS	QUESTIONS	PHYSICAL ASSESSMENT
Adequacy of the patient's sensory perception	Do you feel me pinching the skin on your left hip? Can you feel me rubbing your left lower leg?	Apply painful stimuli to various body locations. If patient is unable to respond by affirming that he or she feels the stimuli, the patient has limited sensory perception.
Moisture	Does the bedsheet under your buttocks feel moist?	Routinely observe patient's bed linens for moisture. Observe patient's skin, noting if it is dry (rarely moist) or seldom damp (occasionally moist) or if skin is often but not always wet (moist). Observe for wound drainage. Check whether the patient is incontinent of urine and stool.
Activity	Can you get out of bed by yourself to use the toilet? Are you able to get out of the bed or chair by yourself? Are you able to change your position in bed by yourself?	Assess patient's ability to walk at least once every 2 hours while awake (walks frequently) or whether patient is only able to ambulate short distances. Observe if patient is able to independently change positions in bed.
Nutrition	Were you able to eat the entire tray of food at breakfast? Are you hungry at mealtime? How much of your tray of food were you able to eat at the last meal?	Observe patient eating: Does patient need assistance? Determine if patient takes most of the meal and if intake is balanced (excellent nutrition). Assess the amount of food the patient eats at meals for adequate nutrition, such as if patient finishes over half of meals, or whether patient is on tube feedings or TPN.
Friction and shear	When you are sitting up in the bed, do you find that you slide down toward the foot of the bed? Do you need assistance in moving up in bed or chair?	Assess if patient moves in bed and chair independently and if patient maintains a good position at all times (no apparent problem). Determine if patient requires moderate to maximum assistance in moving, and if the patient slides down in the bed and/or chair, which indicates a problem.

NPO, Nothing by mouth; *TPN,* total parenteral nutrition.

patient's cardiopulmonary status (see Chapter 29), inspect the wound for bleeding. An **abrasion,** or loss of the dermis, is usually superficial with little bleeding but some weeping (plasma leakage from damaged capillaries). A laceration is damage to the dermis and epidermis and is a torn, jagged wound. The depth and location of the laceration affect the extent of bleeding, with serious bleeding possible in lacera-

---

BOX 36-6   CARE OF THE OLDER ADULT

Issues Related to Skin Integrity

- The older adult's skin loses the ability to retain moisture within the dermis, resulting in less-pliable tissue vulnerable to minor trauma.
- Aging skin experiences decreased epidermal turnover, so healing requires more time.
- The thinning of the dermis and flattening of the dermal-epidermal junction that occur in aging predispose the older adult's skin to tearing.
- A flattening of the dermal-epidermal junction occurs, so there is less nutrient exchange and less resistance to shear force.
- Risk factors for skin tears include sensory loss, impaired nutritional status, impaired cognition, dependency on staff for activities of daily living, and the need for mechanical devices (e.g., lifts, wheelchairs).

Data from Pieper B: Mechanical forces: pressure, shear, friction. In Bryant RA, Nix DP, editors: *Acute and chronic wounds: current management concepts,* ed 3, St. Louis, 2007, Mosby.

---

tions greater than 5 cm (2 inches) long or 2.5 cm (1 inch) deep.

Puncture wounds bleed in relation to the depth and size of the wound; internal bleeding and infection are the primary dangers. Inspect the wound for contaminant material such as soil, broken glass, shreds of cloth, and foreign substances clinging to penetrating objects. Next, assess the size of the wound and the need for suturing or surface protection. When the injury is the result of trauma from a dirty penetrating object, determine if the patient has received a tetanus toxoid injection within the last year.

Stable Setting Once an acute wound is stable after surgery or treatment, assess its progress toward healing. If a dressing covers the wound and there are written orders not to change it, inspect only the dressing and any external drains. If a dressing appears saturated with drainage, reinforce the secondary dressing pending a definitive response and orders from the health care provider. Saturated dressings provide an excellent environment for bacterial growth, and you will need to inform the health care provider of the color, odor, and estimate of drainage amount.

When you plan a dressing change, consider giving the patient an analgesic at least 30 minutes before exposing a wound. Refer to notes documenting pain levels at previous dressing changes. Discuss with the patient his or her pain levels at previous dressing changes to decide upon the appropriate intervention to manage the patient's pain. Avoid accidentally removing or displacing underlying drains.

First, inspect the appearance of the wound, noting the anatomical location, size, approximation of wound edges, the

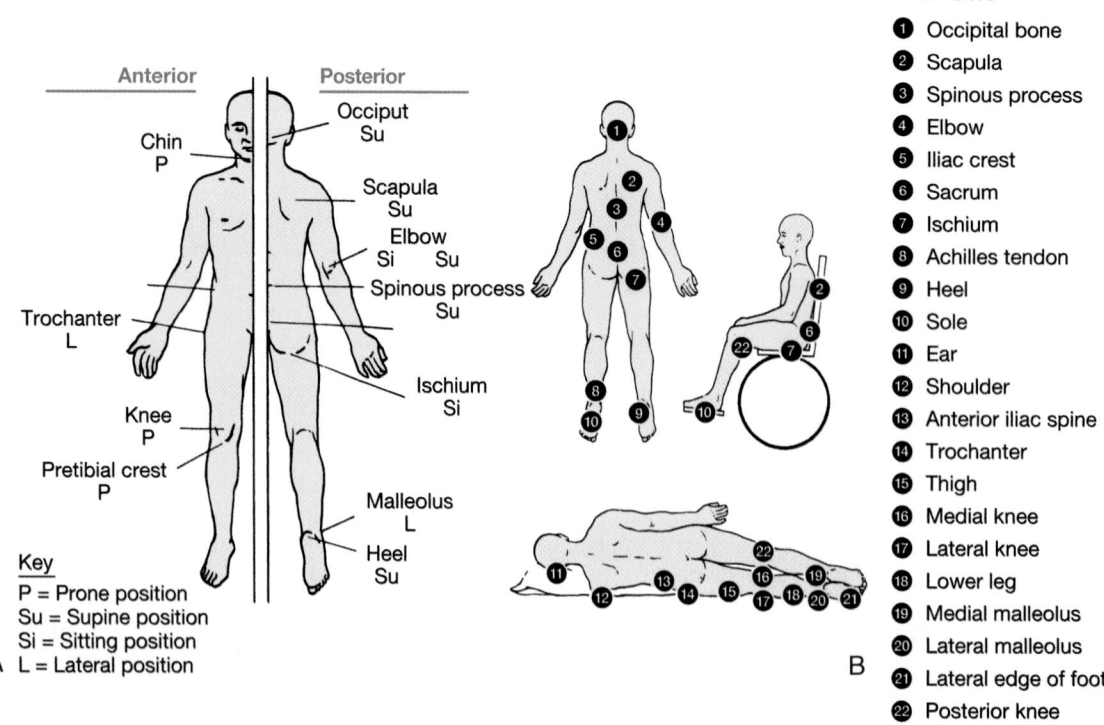

Figure 36-6 ■ **A,** Bony prominences most frequently underlying pressure ulcers. **B,** Pressure ulcer sites. (From Trelease CC: Developing standards for wound care, *Ostomy Wound Manage* 20:46, 1988.)

presence of exudate, the condition of the tissue in an open wound, the skin around the wound, and signs of dehiscence, evisceration, or infection. Measure the length, diameter, or depth of wound using a centimeter measuring guide. Note any **ecchymosis,** skin discoloration, or bruising caused by blood leakage into subcutaneous tissues after trauma to underlying vessels. The outer edges of a wound normally appear inflamed for the first 2 to 3 days, but this slowly disappears. When an infection develops, the wound edges are usually brightly inflamed, warm, tender, and swollen.

Next, assess the character of wound drainage by noting the amount, color, odor, and consistency. The amount of drainage depends on the location and extent of the wound. A simple method for estimating the volume of wound drainage is to report the number and type of dressings used and saturated over an interval of time. The color and consistency of drainage vary, depending on its components. Types of drainage include the following:

1. *Serous:* Clear, watery plasma
2. *Sanguineous:* Fresh bleeding
3. *Serosanguineous:* Pale, more watery, a combination of plasma and red cells, may be blood streaked

---

BOX 36-7	Nutritional Assessment and Management of Pressure Ulcers: WOCN 2003 Guideline Recommendations

Perform nutritional assessment on entry to a new health care setting and whenever there is a change in an individual's condition that will increase the risk for malnutrition (see Chapter 32). **Include the following parameters in the assessment:**

- Current and usual weight
- History of involuntary weight loss or gain
- Nutritional intake versus needs, incorporating protein, calorie, and fluid needs
- Appetite
- Dental health
- Medical/surgical history or interventions that influence nutritional intake or absorption of nutrients.
- Drug/nutrient interaction

Assess laboratory parameters for nutritional status:

a Standard measurements of protein status include albumin, transferrin, and prealbumin
b Nutritional assessments, including protein markers, should be repeated to measure effectiveness of any interventions
c Risks for malnutrition include the following:
- *Age:* Younger than 18 years or older than 64 years
- *Weight:* 5% to 10% loss in 1 to 6 months
- *Albumin:* Less than 2.1 mg/dL (severe risk)
- *Transferrin:* Less than 100 mg/dL (severe risk)
- *Prealbumin:* Less than 7 mg/dL (severe risk)

WOCN, Wound, Ostomy and Continence Nurses Society.

4. *Purulent:* Thick, yellow, green, or brown, indicating the presence of dead or living organisms and white blood cells

If the drainage has a pungent or strong odor, an infection is likely. Objectively document the integrity of the wound and the character of drainage, describing the appearance by observable characteristics.

The presence of drains is another important assessment. A drain is used in a surgical wound if the health care provider expects a large amount of drainage and if keeping wound layers closed is especially important, because accumulated fluid under the tissues prevents closure. Drains lie under a dressing, extend through a dressing, or are connected to a drainage bag or suction apparatus. A pin or clip through a Penrose drain prevents it from slipping farther into a wound (Figure 36-7). As wound drainage decreases, the health care provider slowly withdraws the drain or leaves orders for you to withdraw the drain a specified length over several days. First, observe the security of the drain and its location with respect to the wound. Next, note the character and amount of drainage if there is a collecting device. You need to pay particular attention to the flow of drainage through the tubing and notify the health care provider of any sudden decrease that indicates a blocked drain or an increase indicating bleeding or infection.

In the case of a surgical wound, inspect the staples, sutures, or wound closures for irritation, and note whether the closures are intact. You may choose to count sutures when the health care provider has removed a portion of them. After the first few days when normal swelling around closures usually has subsided, continued swelling sometimes indicates overly tight closures, which will cause wound separation or dehiscence.

When a wound exhibits swelling, separation of its edges, or redness in the periwound area, it is important to evaluate for the presence of cellulitis. Use light palpation to detect localized areas of tenderness or collection of drainage. Wearing gloves, gently place your fingertips along the wound edges. If pressure causes fluid to be expressed from the wound, note the character of the drainage and collect a wound culture if needed. Sensitivity to such palpation is normal, but extreme tenderness indicates infection.

Pain assessment is an important component of wound assessment for detecting complications and planning for future wound care (see Chapter 31). Serious discomfort during in-

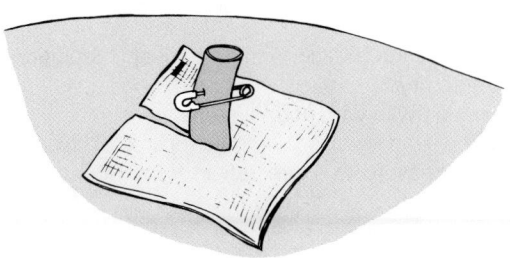

Figure 36-7 ■ Penrose drain.

spection or palpation of the wound suggests underlying problems, whereas discomfort related to dressing removal or application calls for administration of analgesics before future dressing changes.

Wound Cultures If you detect purulent (pus) or suspicious-looking drainage, this indicates the probable need for a wound culture. Never collect a wound culture sample from old drainage, because resident colonies of bacteria grow in exudate. First clean the wound to remove skin flora. Aerobic organisms grow in superficial wounds exposed to the air, and anaerobic organisms tend to grow within body cavities. To collect an aerobic specimen, wipe a sterile swab from a Culturette tube onto clean, healthy-appearing tissue, place the specimen in an appropriate container, and transport to the laboratory to keep the organisms viable (Stotts, 2007).

To collect an anaerobic specimen deep in a body cavity, use a sterile syringe tip to aspirate visible drainage from the inner wound, expel any air from the syringe, and inject contents into a special vacuum container with culture medium. In some institutions you place a cork over the needle to prevent entrance of air and send the syringe to the laboratory. Box 36-8 defines the procedure for a needle aspiration technique and the quantitative swab technique.

PATIENT EXPECTATIONS When your patient has a pressure ulcer or a chronic wound, the course of treatment is usually costly and lengthy. Because your patient needs to be involved with wound care management, it is important to know the patient's expectations. A patient who unrealistically expects rapid wound healing will be easily discouraged and

---

BOX 36-8 Recommendations for Standardized Techniques for Wound Cultures

NEEDLE ASPIRATION PROCEDURE (ANAEROBIC CULTURE)
- Use a sterile 10-mL syringe with a 22-gauge needle.
- Aspirate 5 mL of air into the syringe.
- Clean intact skin with a disinfectant. Allow to dry.
- Insert needle into interior of the wound.
- Aspirate wound drainage, moving needle back and forth in two to four areas of the wound.
- Withdraw needle from wound; expel any remaining air from syringe.

QUANTITATIVE SWAB PROCEDURE (AEROBIC CULTURE)
- Obtain a sterile swab, sterile normal saline, and antiseptic solution.
- Clean wound surface with an antiseptic solution, and allow to dry.
- Moisten swab with normal saline.
- Swab wound in a 1 × 1 cm (4 cm²) area of clean tissue.
- Apply pressure to express fluid from wound onto the sterile swab.

Modified from Stotts NS: Wound infection: diagnosis and management. In Bryant RA, Nix DP, editors: *Acute and chronic wounds: current management concepts*, ed 3, St. Louis, 2007, Mosby.

---

not follow the treatment plan. Likewise, a patient who knows that the process is lengthy may unrealistically expect the area to heal without scarring. Knowing these expectations assists you in providing individualized care and helping the patient modify expectations when needed.

■■■NURSING DIAGNOSIS

A patient with actual or high risk for *impaired skin integrity* usually has one or more nursing diagnoses related to the condition. Assessment reveals clusters of data that indicate whether an actual or a risk for *impaired skin integrity* exists. After gathering appropriate assessment data, cluster defining characteristics to establish nursing diagnoses. For example, the destruction of the skin's surface clearly allows you to diagnose *impaired skin integrity*. The identification of nursing diagnoses related to wound healing helps you to anticipate the need for supportive or preventive care. There are many nursing diagnoses that are potentially relevant to your patient who requires wound care:

- *Risk for infection*
- *Impaired bed mobility*
- *Impaired physical mobility*
- *Imbalanced nutrition: less than body requirements*
- *Acute pain*
- *Chronic pain*
- *Situational low self-esteem*
- *Impaired skin integrity*
- *Risk for impaired skin integrity*
- *Ineffective peripheral tissue perfusion*

Assess for related factors that contribute to each diagnostic statement. These related factors become the focus of your interventions. For example, the patient with *impaired skin integrity related to a surgical incision* requires a different set of interventions than the patient with *impaired skin integrity related to pressure and nutritional deficiency*. The patient whose surgical incision has increased drainage will require different and perhaps more frequent skin cleansing and dressings chosen to contain additional drainage.

■■■PLANNING

Plan therapeutic interventions for your patients with actual or potential risks to skin integrity (see Care Plan and Concept Map, Figure 36-8). Design your therapies according to severity of risks to the patient. Individualize the plan according to the patient's developmental stage and level of health.

GOALS AND OUTCOMES You need to develop patient-centered goals aimed at preventing or reducing impaired skin integrity or promoting wound healing. Individualize care planning for the patient, taking into consideration the patient's most immediate needs. Assess all patients for risk for skin breakdown, and have skin and wound assessments performed at least daily. Integrate the information from the pressure ulcer risk and skin assessments into the plan of care, and write reasonable goals, such as "Patient will not develop further skin breakdown" and "Patient's wounds will demonstrate healing." Include the patient and the family in the assessment process so they will begin to see their contribution to reducing risk factors.

CARE PLAN   Health-Seeking Behaviors

ASSESSMENT

Mr. Ahmed has limited activity tolerance. He does not tolerate position changes or sitting out of bed; he wants to stay in a semi-Fowler's position at all times. He complains of a painful, burning sensation in his sacral region. An ulcer is present that measures 1 × 2 inches with a depth of ⅛ inch.

ASSESSMENT ACTIVITIES

Identify the support surface that would be appropriate to decrease pressure on Mr. Ahmed's skin.

Inspect and palpate wound.

Conduct a calorie count.

FINDINGS/DEFINING CHARACTERISTICS*

Mr. Ahmed **cannot tolerate positions that might relieve or reduce pressure to his skin.** Mr. Ahmed says, "I am uncomfortable in any position except in a sitting position in bed."

The wound: 1 × 2 inches, full-thickness ulcer over sacral area with a red, moist base. Reddened periwound skin.
On palpation, underlying skin is soft and indurated.
Mr. Ahmed is eating fewer than 1600 calories daily.

NURSING DIAGNOSIS: Impaired skin integrity related to pressure over bony prominence in sacral region.

PLANNING

GOAL

- Pressure will be reduced to the sacral area, and the wound will show movement toward healing in 1 week.

INTERVENTIONS (NIC)‡

Pressure Management
- Post and implement a turning schedule.

- Obtain and place over the patient's mattress a low-air-loss overlay.

Wound Care
- Cleanse wound and periwound skin; dry periwound skin.

- Apply a hydrocolloid dressing to wound, as per order; extend the dressing 1½ inches beyond the wound edges.

Nutrition Management
- Determine in collaboration with dietitian appropriate number of calories and type of nutrients needed to promote wound healing.

EXPECTED OUTCOMES (NOC)†

Tissue Integrity: Skin, Mucous Membranes
- Wound will decrease in diameter in 7 days.
- There will be no evidence of further wound formation in 3 days.

RATIONALE

Repositioning redistributes pressure (Pieper, 2007; WOCN, 2003).
Redistributes the amount of pressure on the bony prominences (Nix, 2007b).

Removes debris and old drainage from wound site, preventing further wound progression and/or skin breakdown (Ayello and others, 2004).
The use of hydrocolloid dressing will support moist wound healing and protect the wound (Rolstad and Ovington, 2007).

Adequate nutrition such as increased calorie count, protein intake, and vitamins aid in wound healing (WOCN, 2003).

EVALUATION

NURSING ACTIONS

Observe wound to determine healing progress: measure wound diameter and depth; note the condition of periwound skin; observe the appearance of the wound drainage and tissue at each dressing change.

PATIENT RESPONSE/FINDING

- Ulcer is 1 × 1 inch.
- Serous drainage is present.
- Wound color remains red.

ACHIEVEMENT OF OUTCOME

- Improved tissue type.
- Reduction in wound size.

---

*Defining characteristics are shown in **bold** type.
†Outcomes classification label from Moorhead S and others, editors: *Nursing outcomes classification (NOC)*, ed 4, St. Louis, 2008, Mosby.
‡Intervention classification labels from Bulechek GM and others, editors: *Nursing interventions classification (NIC)*, ed 5, St. Louis, 2008, Mosby.

CARE PLAN Health-Seeking Behaviors—cont'd

NURSING ACTIONS	PATIENT RESPONSE/FINDING	ACHIEVEMENT OF OUTCOME
Palpate underlying skin around wound.	Underlying skin around wound remains intact with no palpable tissue change.	No evidence of advancing pressure ulcer or tissue damage.
Ask Mr. Ahmed about any discomfort or sensations of tingling or burning at the wound site.	Mr. Ahmed denies any new sensations at the wound site.	No evidence of new tissue damage
Ask Mr. Ahmed about his food intake.	Mr. Ahmed reports that his appetite is increasing and he is eating most of his meals.	Improved nutritional intake
Review calorie count over last week.	Calorie count denotes a steady increase in daily calorie consumption.	

SETTING PRIORITIES When planning care, establish priorities based on your comprehensive assessment, goals, and expected outcomes. Acute needs are immediate; however, also prioritize preventive interventions, and institute them in a timely manner. Maintenance of skin integrity and promotion of wound healing prevent additional health care issues. Skin and wound priorities include ongoing assessment of pressure ulcer risk and wound status and providing interventions to control or eliminate contributing factors of pressure, shear, friction, moisture, and infection.

Consider other patient factors when setting priorities, including everyday activities and family factors. Sometimes you will need the help of another health care team member, such as a physical or occupational therapist, when considering mobility needs. These factors are important for patients in institutional and home settings.

COLLABORATIVE CARE With the trend toward earlier discharge from health care settings, it is important to consider the patient's plan for discharge. Discharge planning begins when a patient enters the health care system. Anticipating the patient's discharge from an institution, a referral to a skilled nursing care facility or home care agency is necessary to help the patient remain mobile or regain mobility at home.

Patients and their families need to continue the objectives of wound management after discharge. Thus they will need to discuss the likelihood of the patient's returning home, returning home with the assistance of home nursing, or transferring to a skilled nursing facility for more care and observation.

Use the case manager to plan for the necessary resources for support once the patient is discharged. Include the physical therapist for evaluation of the patients' ability to transfer and walk up stairs (if there are stairs in the patient's home.) Consult with a registered dietician to assess the patient's nutritional status and to assist with nutrition interventions.

■■■**IMPLEMENTATION**

HEALTH PROMOTION Health promotion for a surgical patient involves instruction on increasing protein intake preoperatively and learning ways to reduce strain on surgical incision postoperatively (see Chapter 38). Early identification of high-risk patients aids in the prevention of pressure ulcers. Prevention minimizes the impact of risk factors and contributing factors on pressure ulcer development (see Box 36-5, p. 1068). Nursing interventions for prevention of pressure ulcers include topical skin care, positioning and use of the 30-degree lateral position, and the use of support surfaces.

Topical Skin Care Perform skin assessment daily, paying special attention to the bony prominences. Do not massage reddened areas because reddened areas indicate tissue injury (Ayello and others, 2004). Massage to these areas further injures the tissue by causing breaks in the tissue capillaries. Examine skin for signs of dryness, cracking, edema, or excessive moisture. When cleansing the skin, use a mild cleansing agent. Soaps alter the skin's acid mantle, causing dryness and increasing the risk for skin infection. Skin lubrication will help keep the skin intact; consider using a moisturizer on a routine basis (WOCN, 2003). Keep the patient's skin clean and dry because this is an initial line of defense for preventing skin breakdown. The types of products available for skin care are numerous, and you need to match their uses to the specific needs of the patient.

For a patient who is incontinent of stool or urine, use a specialized incontinence cleanser. To protect the skin you apply a moisture-barrier product (generally petrolatum or dimethicone based) liberally to the exposed area. The moisture barrier will provide skin protection from the irritating effects of stool or urine and will allow you to clean the next incontinent episode easily. Apply the moisture-barrier ointment after each cleansing. For skin that has become denuded or stripped from incontinence, use a barrier paste that will stick to the irritated area and not be removed with each cleansing. You can contain fecal incontinence with a fecal incontinence collector (Figure 36-9), in which an adhesive skin barrier is attached to a drainable pouch applied around the anus to collect liquid stool. A fecal incontinence collector is used when the patient is experiencing frequent liquid bowel movements and has intact perianal skin. Other external collection devices include male external catheters applied to the shaft of the penis to collect urine. Underpads and briefs are used to protect skin in patients incontinent of stool and urine. Most underpads

CONCEPT MAP

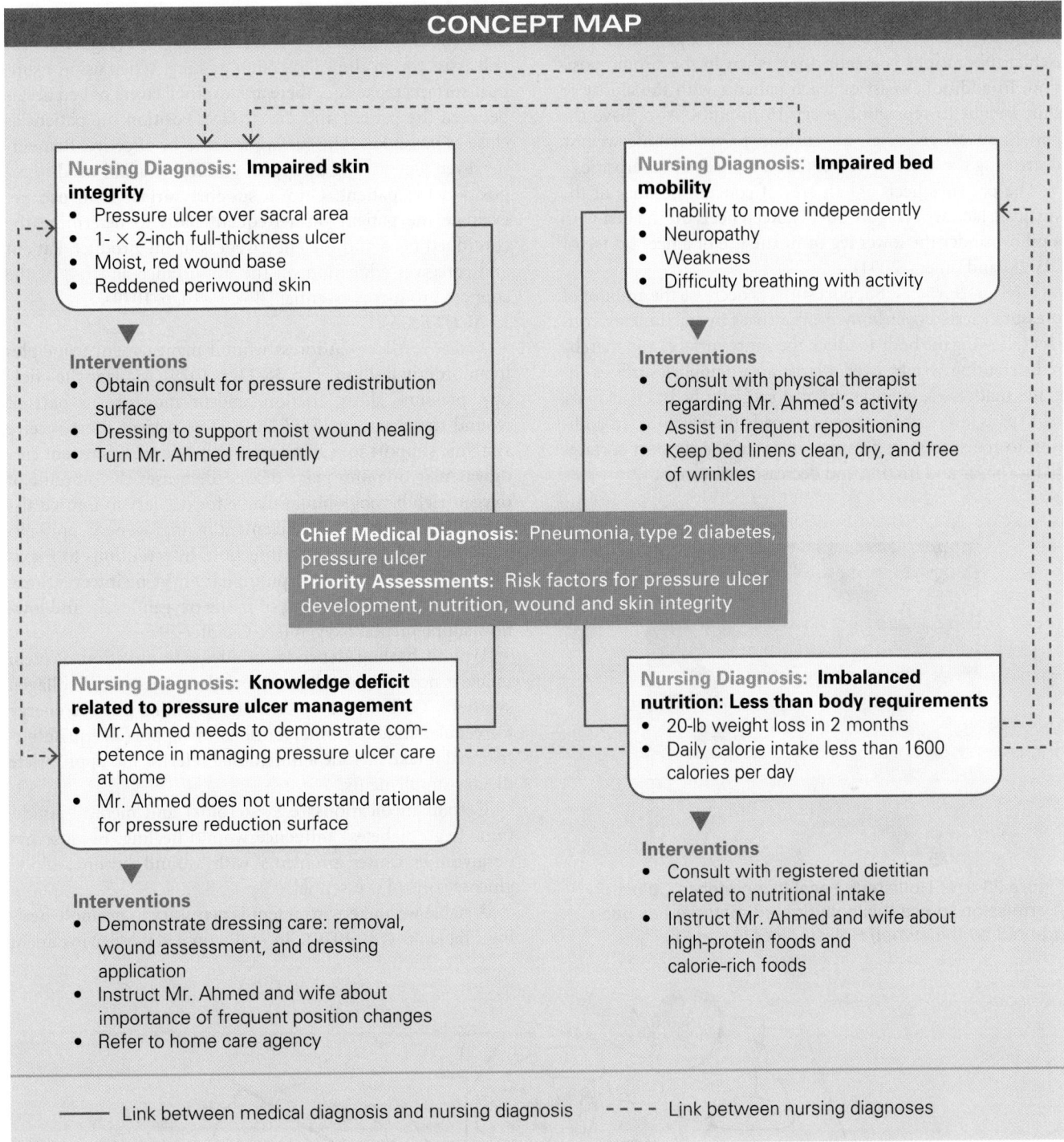

Nursing Diagnosis: Impaired skin integrity
- Pressure ulcer over sacral area
- 1- × 2-inch full-thickness ulcer
- Moist, red wound base
- Reddened periwound skin

Interventions
- Obtain consult for pressure redistribution surface
- Dressing to support moist wound healing
- Turn Mr. Ahmed frequently

Nursing Diagnosis: Impaired bed mobility
- Inability to move independently
- Neuropathy
- Weakness
- Difficulty breathing with activity

Interventions
- Consult with physical therapist regarding Mr. Ahmed's activity
- Assist in frequent repositioning
- Keep bed linens clean, dry, and free of wrinkles

Chief Medical Diagnosis: Pneumonia, type 2 diabetes, pressure ulcer
Priority Assessments: Risk factors for pressure ulcer development, nutrition, wound and skin integrity

Nursing Diagnosis: Knowledge deficit related to pressure ulcer management
- Mr. Ahmed needs to demonstrate competence in managing pressure ulcer care at home
- Mr. Ahmed does not understand rationale for pressure reduction surface

Interventions
- Demonstrate dressing care: removal, wound assessment, and dressing application
- Instruct Mr. Ahmed and wife about importance of frequent position changes
- Refer to home care agency

Nursing Diagnosis: Imbalanced nutrition: Less than body requirements
- 20-lb weight loss in 2 months
- Daily calorie intake less than 1600 calories per day

Interventions
- Consult with registered dietitian related to nutritional intake
- Instruct Mr. Ahmed and wife about high-protein foods and calorie-rich foods

——— Link between medical diagnosis and nursing diagnosis   - - - - Link between nursing diagnoses

Figure 36-8 ■ Concept Map.

and briefs have a plastic outer lining that holds moisture against skin. Diapers and underpads will irritate the skin if left under patients for prolonged periods of time. Select underpads, diapers, or briefs that are absorbent to wick incontinence moisture away from the skin versus trapping the moisture against the skin, which causes **maceration** (softening of the skin due to moisture) (WOCN, 2003). When providing skin care to the incontinent patient, the health care team first assesses and treats the cause of the incontinence, then decides upon protection and/or collection interventions.

Positioning Positioning interventions reduce pressure and shear to the skin. You change the immobilized patient's position according to activity level, perceptual ability, and daily routines (Bergstrom and others, 1987a, 1987b). Therefore a standard turning interval of 1 to 2 hours will not prevent pressure sore development in some patients. The WOCN (2003) recommends reducing shear by keeping the patient's head of bed below the 30-degree angle, using assistive devices when turning or transferring patients, using the bed gatch or footboard, and using the 30-degree lateral position (Figure 36-10).

When the patient is able to sit in the chair, reposition the patient every hour. In the sitting position, the pressure on the ischial tuberosities is greater than when in the supine position. In addition, assist or teach patients with the ability to shift weight to reposition every 15 minutes. Also, have the patient sit on gel or an air cushion to redistribute weight, decreasing the amount of weight on the ischial tuberosities.

The patient's heels are an area of concern because of the small surface area (Figure 36-11). Keep heels off the bed with a pillow under the lower leg or by the use of a heel protector (Ayello and others, 2004).

Support Surfaces   Support surfaces decrease the amount of pressure exerted over bony prominences by maximizing contact (allowing the body to touch the entire surface) and thereby redistributing weight over a large area. Support surfaces include mattresses, overlays, framed specialty beds, chair pads, table pads, and crib mattresses or pads (Table 36-3). In addition to redistributing pressure, many of the support surfaces reduce shear and friction and decrease moisture.

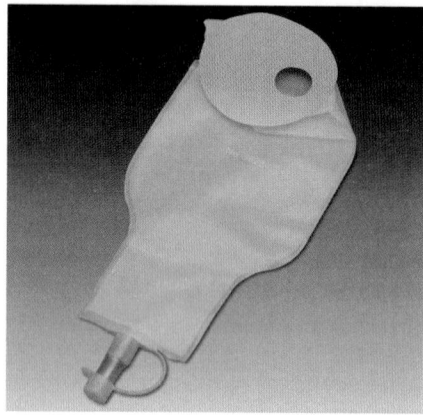

Figure 36-9 ■ Hollister® Fecal Incontinence Collector. (Permission to use this copyrighted material has been granted by the owner, Hollister Incorporated.)

Select an appropriate support surface based on your assessment findings (Box 36-9). A flow diagram (Figure 36-12) will assist you in clinical decision making. When using a support surface, make sure there are minimal layers of bed linens between the patient and the surface. Position the patient as close as possible to the surface for it to be effective. Remember, even when using a support surface, you still need to reposition the patient. Once a support surface is in use, reevaluate the patient on a frequent basis to determine the continued need and the effectiveness of the product. Patient and caregiver education on the importance and use of the support product is essential (Box 36-10, p. 1079).

ACUTE CARE

Pressure Ulcers   Address wound management principles in an orderly fashion (Box 36-11, p 1079). Manage the etiology, pressure, shear, friction, and/or moisture as part of wound management (Skill 36-2). The patient must receive systemic support to achieve wound healing. Concurrent cardiovascular or pulmonary disease decreases the amount of oxygen-rich hemoglobin available for delivery to injured tissue. Oxygen is an essential element in angiogenesis, epithelialization, and resistance to infection. Interventions to maximize oxygen levels include pulmonary hygiene interventions, assessment and monitoring of tissue oxygen levels, and low-flow supplemental oxygen (see Chapter 29).

Wound healing depends on adequate nutrition. Protein intake is necessary to support new blood vessels and collagen synthesis. Carbohydrates, fats, and vitamins provide energy for cellular function. Interventions to support adequate nutritional intake include a nutritional referral and appropriate dietary supplements.

Certain medications (e.g., steroids) and medical conditions (e.g., diabetes) influence wound healing. Because hyperglycemia causes problems with wound healing, blood glucose control is essential.

A stable wound environment is necessary to promote healing (Table 36-4, p. 1079). To maintain a stable environment

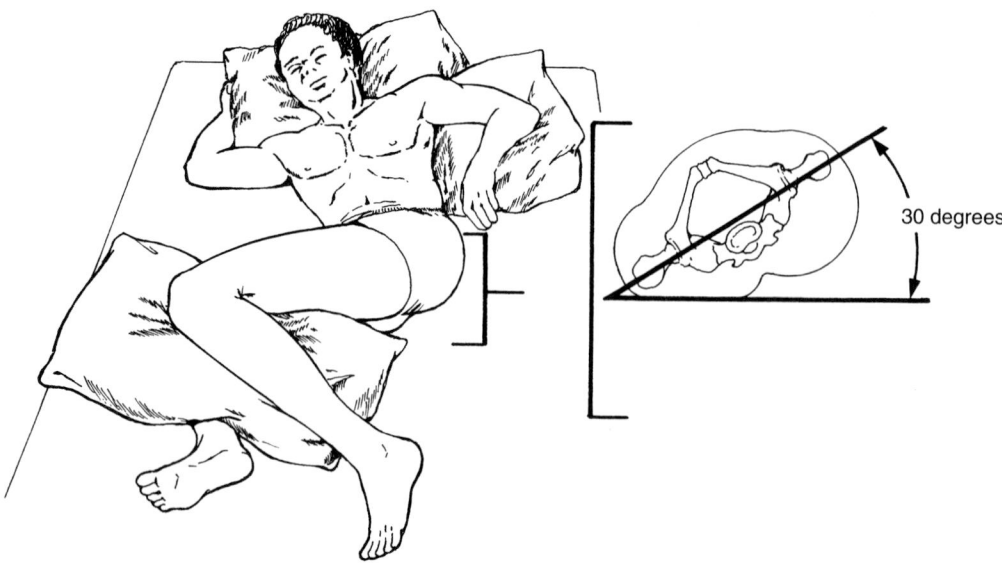

30 degrees

Figure 36-10 ■ Thirty-degree lateral position. (From Pieper B: Mechanical forces: pressure, shear, friction. In Bryant RA, Nix DP, editors: *Acute and chronic wounds: current management concepts*, ed 3, St. Louis, 2007, Mosby.)

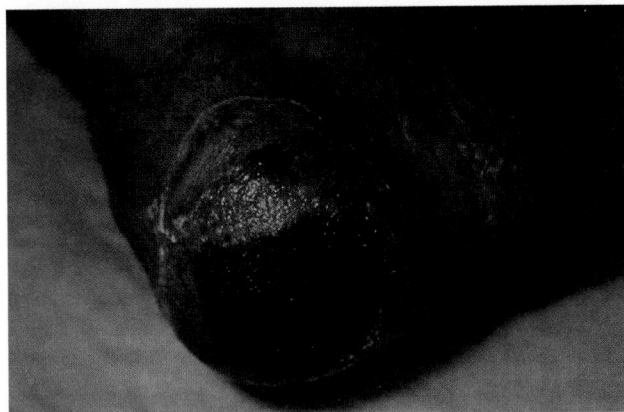

Figure 36-11 ■ Formation of pressure ulcer on heel resulting from external pressure from mattress of bed. (Courtesy Janice Colwell, RN, MS, CWOCN, FAAN, Clinical Nurse Specialist, University of Chicago Medical Center.)

BOX 36-9	WOCN 2003 Pressure Reduction/Relief Recommendations

- Place at-risk individuals on a pressure-reduction/relief surface and not on an ordinary hospital mattress.
- Pressure reducing or relief devices work by redistributing pressure over the bony prominences (see Table 36-3).
- Avoid using foam rings, donuts, and sheepskin for pressure reduction. Foam rings or donuts concentrate the pressure to the surrounding tissue.
- Use pressure-relief devices in the operating room for individuals assessed to be at high risk for pressure ulcer development.
- Refer to professional health care specialists to select appropriate pressure-reduction/relief devices for chairs, wheelchairs, and beds.

Data from Wound, Ostomy and Continence Nurses Society: *Guideline for prevention and management of pressure ulcers*, WOCN Clinical Practice Guidelines Series, Glenview, Ill, 2003, The Society.

TABLE 36-3 Support Surfaces

CATEGORIES	MECHANISM OF ACTION	INDICATIONS	EXAMPLES OF MANUFACTURERS/ PRODUCT NAMES
LOW-AIR-LOSS SYSTEM Available in a full bed or as an overlay	Pressure redistribution device Bed: The entire surface is a powered, inflated surface with air loss Overlay: Powered surface, constant inflation and air loss at the surface; place over the bed mattress	Prevention of skin breakdown in patients who cannot be turned or have existing skin breakdown	Hill-Rom/Flexicair Eclipse Kinetic Concepts, Inc/First Step Select Crown Therapeutics/ Select-Air Mattress
FOAM Available as an overlay or in a full mattress	Redistributes pressure and the cover (top) can reduce friction and shear Overlay: Placed on top of bed mattress Full mattress: Used in place of the usual mattress	Pressure redistribution for high-risk patients	Bio Clinic/Bio Guard BG Industries/MaxiFloat
STATIC AIR-FILLED OVERLAY Available as an overlay	Interconnected air-filled cells, inflated to appropriate level Pressure redistribution	High-risk patients	Crown Therapeutics/RoHo mattress Gaymar Industries/Sof-Care
AIR-FLUIDIZED BED Available as a bed	Bed frame with silicone-coated beads that become fluidized when air is pumped through the beads Pressure redistribution, antishear, antifriction surface	For patients with burns or multiple stage III or stage IV pressure ulcers, protection of new grafts and flaps	Kinetic Concepts, Inc/Fluid-Air Hill-Rom/Clinitron
KINETIC THERAPY Available as a bed	Provides continuous passive motion to promote mobilization of respiratory secretions; also provides low-air-loss therapy	Patients who are at risk for or have developed atelectasis and/or pneumonia	Hill-Rom/Total Care Sport Kinetic Concepts, Inc/ TriaDyne II

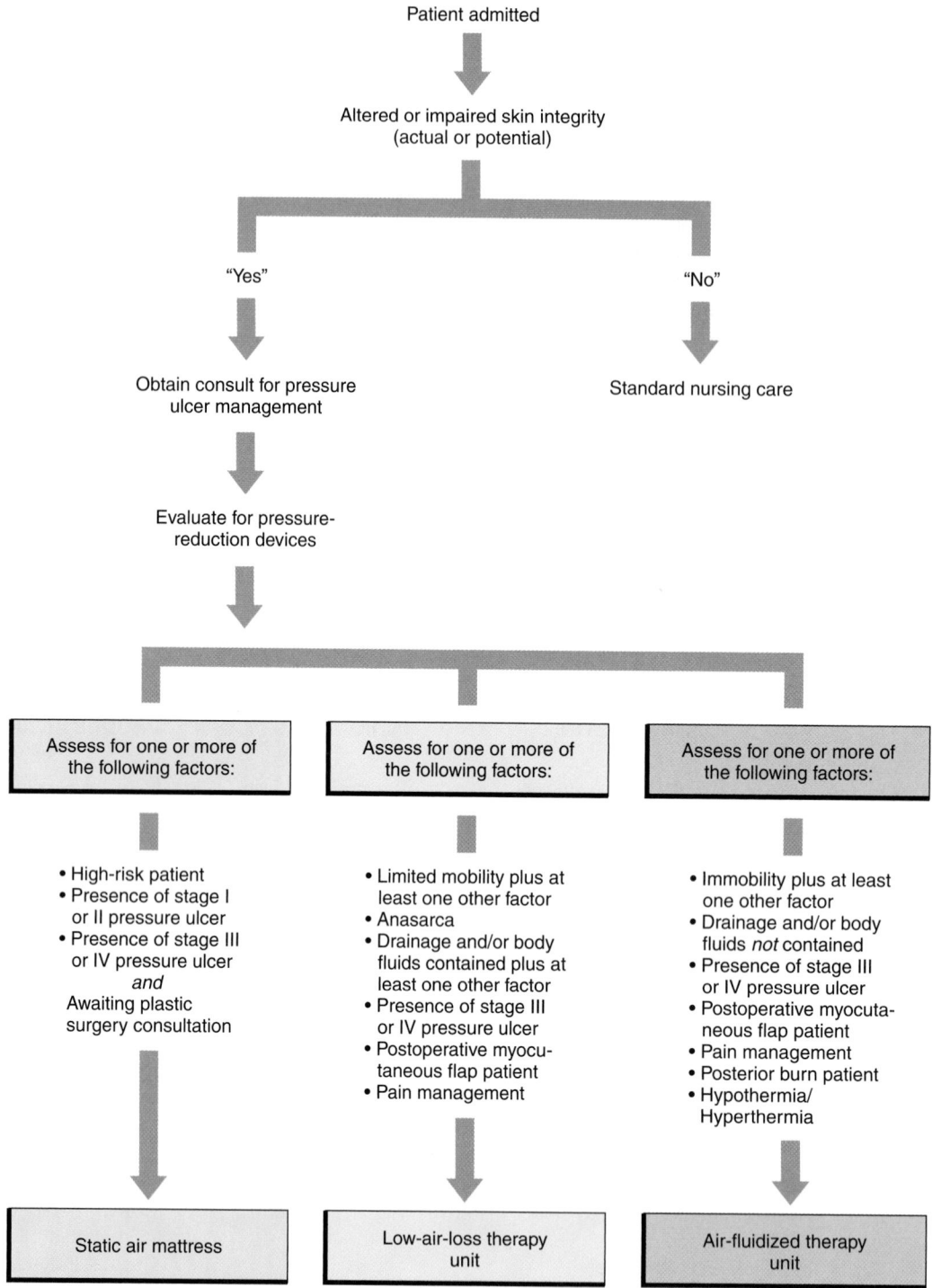

Figure 36-12 ■ Flow diagram for ordering specialty surfaces. (Modified from Thomas C: Specialty beds: decision making made easy, *Ostomy Wound Manage* 23:51, 1989.)

it is important to control infection and promote cleansing, **debride** (remove) necrotic tissue, provide exudate management, control dead space, and provide wound protection. Assess the patient with a pressure ulcer for signs and symptoms of a wound infection: redness, warmth of surrounding tissue, odor, and the presence of exudate. If any of these signs are present, consult with the health care team to determine if you should culture the wound and if systemic or topical antibiotics are indicated.

Cleanse pressure ulcers at each dressing change to promote removal of wound debris and bacteria from the wound surface (WOCN, 2003). Cleanse dirty wounds by irrigation. Clean wounds require only gentle flushing with normal saline solution.

Necrotic tissue slows wound healing because it becomes a source for infection and a barrier for epithelialization (Schultz and others, 2003). After consulting with the physician or wound care specialist, plan a method of debridement. Types

BOX 36-10 Guidelines for Patient Education Regarding Therapeutic Surfaces

- Explain the rationale for utilization of support surfaces. Be sure the patient and family know that this will reduce pressure on the bony prominences by redistributing the pressure between the surface and the patient's skin.
- Teach patient and family the importance of minimal layers of linen or absorbent pads between patient and surface.
- Instruct in the importance of frequent position changes, demonstrating small shifts of weight.
- Demonstrate to patient and caregiver the procedure for lateral positioning at a 30-degree angle and the use of pillows to support various positions.

BOX 36-11 Wound Healing Principles

1 Control or eliminate causative factors
   a Pressure
   b Shear
   c Friction
   d Moisture
2 Provide systemic support to reduce existing and potential cofactors
   a Nutritional and fluid support
   b Control of systemic conditions affecting wound healing
3 Maintain physiological wound environment
   a Prevent and manage infection
   b Cleanse wound
   c Remove nonviable tissue (debridement)
   d Manage exudates
   e Eliminate dead space
   f Control odor
   g Protect wound
   h Provide a moist environment

From Rolstad BS, Ovington LG: Principles of wound management. In Bryant RA, Nix, DP, editors: *Acute and chronic wounds: current management concepts*, ed 3, St. Louis, 2007.

TABLE 36-4 Treatment Options by Ulcer Stage

ULCER STAGE	ULCER STATUS	DRESSING	COMMENTS*	EXPECTED CHANGE	ADJUVANTS
I	Intact	None	Allows visual assessment.	Resolves slowly without epidermal loss over 7 to 14 days.	Turning schedule. Support hydration. Nutritional support.
		Transparent dressing	Protects from shear. Do not use in the presence of excessive moisture. May not allow visual assessment.		
II	Clean	Hydrocolloid Composite film	Limits shear.	Heals through reepithelialization.	Pressure redistribution mattress or chair cushion.
		Hydrocolloid	Change when seal of dressing breaks, maximal wear time 7 days.		See previous stage. Manage incontinence.
		Hydrogel	Provides a moist environment.		
III	Clean	Hydrocolloid	See stage II.	Heals through granulation and reepithelialization.	See previous stages. Evaluate pressure redistribution needs.
		Hydrogel Foam	Apply over wound to protect and absorb moisture.		
		Calcium alginate	Use when there is significant exudate. Cover with secondary dressing.		
		Gauze	Use with normal saline or other prescribed solution. Wring out excess solution, unfold to make contact with wound.		
			Use with gauze per manufacturer's instructions.		
IV	Clean Eschar	Hydrogel	See stage III, clean.	Heals through granulation and reepithelialization.	Surgical consult may be necessary for closure. See stages I, II, and III.
		Calcium alginate	See stage III, clean.		
		Gauze	See stage III, clean. Fill all dead space with gauze.		
		Hydrocolloid	Will facilitate softening of eschar.	Eschar will lift at the edges as healing progresses.	See previous stages. Surgical consult may be considered for debridement.
		Gauze plus ordered solution	Will deliver solution and wick wound drainage.		
			Will facilitate debridement.		
		Enzymes		Eschar will soften.	May be considered for slow debridement.
		None	Rarely, if eschar is dry and intact, no dressing is used, allowing eschar to act as physiological cover.		

*As with *all* occlusive dressings, wounds should *not* be clinically infected.

of debridement include mechanical, chemical, sharp, and autolytic (Ramundo, 2007).

A moist wound environment supports wound healing; however, excessive wound moisture will macerate the wound edges and interfere with wound healing. Select a dressing that absorbs excessive moisture while providing the wound with the necessary hydration. Eliminate dead space by loosely filling all cavities with dressings. You need to fill wound cavities to support the growth of granulation tissue and to discourage infection.

It is important to involve the patient's family or other caregiver in management of pressure ulcers and their treatment. Frequently patients are discharged home and still require dressing changes. The patient's family or caregiver are

---

BOX 36-12   PATIENT TEACHING

Pressure Ulcer Dressing Change

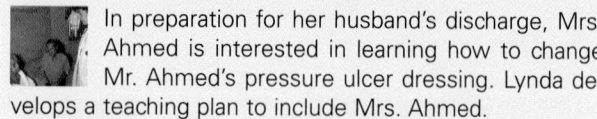 In preparation for her husband's discharge, Mrs. Ahmed is interested in learning how to change Mr. Ahmed's pressure ulcer dressing. Lynda develops a teaching plan to include Mrs. Ahmed.

OUTCOME
- At the end of the teaching session Mrs. Ahmed will perform an acceptable return demonstration of dressing application.

TEACHING STRATEGIES
- Plan time Mrs. Ahmed is present and prepared to spend 30 minutes in two separate teaching sessions.
- Avoid using words that Mrs. Ahmed will not understand.
- Provide a brief description of what will be taught to both the patient and wife. Include the patient in all of the teaching even though he is unable to see the wound.
- Bring an extra dressing to the bedside to show Mrs. Ahmed what the dressing looks like and how to apply it.
- Use a pictorial guide of a pressure ulcer to help Mrs. Ahmed understand what the wound looks like and how it will progress if it shows signs of healing.
- Plan one session in which Mrs. Ahmed will watch a demonstration of the wound being cleansed and the dressing applied. Plan a second session where she will do a return demonstration.
- At the end of each session ask Mrs. Ahmed how she felt doing the dressing, and include Mr. Ahmed in this evaluation.

EVALUATION STRATEGIES
- Ask Mrs. Ahmed questions as she does the procedure to evaluate her understanding of each step.
- Ask Mrs. Ahmed what she will evaluate at each dressing change.
- Observe Ms. Ahmed changing the dressing and cleansing the wound. Observe any body language that indicates how she is feeling while doing the procedure.

---

excellent sources for dressing support and identification of possible wound-healing complications (Box 36-12).

Wounds

First Aid for Wounds. In an emergency setting use first aid measures for wound care. Under more stable conditions you are able to use a variety of interventions for wound healing. When a patient suffers a traumatic wound, first aid interventions include promoting hemostasis, cleansing the wound, and protecting the wound from further injury.

Hemostasis. After assessing the type and extent of the wound, control bleeding from a laceration with application of direct pressure to the wound with a sterile or clean dressing. After bleeding subsides, an adhesive dressing strip or gauze dressing taped over the laceration allows skin edges to close and a blood clot to form. If a dressing becomes saturated with blood, add another layer of dressing, continue to apply pressure, and elevate the affected part. A health care provider will suture serious lacerations in an emergency clinic or hospital.

Allow a puncture wound to bleed to remove dirt and other contaminants. If a penetrating object such as a knife blade is in a patient's body, do not remove the object. Removal will cause massive, uncontrolled bleeding. You apply pressure around the object but not on it or on surrounding tissues.

Cleansing. Gentle cleansing of a wound removes contaminants that serve as sources of infection. However, vigorous cleaning causes bleeding or further injury. For abrasions, minor lacerations, and small puncture wounds, rinse the wound in running water, gently cleanse with mild soap and water, rinse, and apply an over-the-counter antiseptic. When a laceration is bleeding profusely, only brush away surface contaminants and concentrate on hemostasis until the patient reaches a clinic or hospital.

Protection. Regardless of whether bleeding has stopped, protect the wound by applying a sterile or clean dressing, and immobilize the body part. A light dressing applied over minor wounds prevents entrance of microorganisms. In the case of small abrasions, it is acceptable to leave the wound open to air so that a scab will form.

The more extensive the wound, the larger the dressing required. In the home a clean towel or diaper is often the best dressing. A bulky dressing applied with pressure minimizes movement of underlying tissues and helps to immobilize the entire body part. A dressing or cloth wrapped around a penetrating object will immobilize it adequately.

Dressings The use of dressings requires an understanding of wound healing and factors influencing healing. A variety of dressing materials are commercially available. Unless a dressing is suited to the characteristics of a wound, the dressing will impede wound repair.

The choice of dressing and the method of dressing a wound influence healing. The proper dressing does not allow a full-thickness wound to become dry with scab formation. When this occurs, the dermis dehydrates and crusts. As a result, a barrier forms against normal epidermal cell growth, slowing wound healing. Furthermore, dryness will increase discomfort. Ideally, a dressing provides a moist environment to promote normal epidermal cell migration. The proper dressing also absorbs drainage to prevent pooling of exudate that promotes bacterial growth and prevents wound drainage from coming into contact with intact skin.

For surgical wounds that heal by primary intention, dressings are commonly removed as soon as drainage stops. Frequently the health care provider removes the dressing 24 to 48 hours postoperatively. This coincides with initial epithelialization, so when the health care provider removes the primary dressing, it reduces the risk for infection.

Purposes. A dressing serves several purposes. It discourages wound exposure to microorganisms. However, if a wound has minimal drainage, the natural formation of a fibrin seal eliminates the need for a dressing. A pressure dressing promotes hemostasis by exerting localized, downward pressure over an actual or potential bleeding site and fosters normal healing by eliminating dead space in underlying tissues. Assess skin color, pulses in distal extremities, patient comfort, and any changes in sensation to ensure pressure dressings do not interfere with circulation.

A dry dressing promotes healing by allowing the wound to heal by primary intention and absorbing minimal oozing of wound drainage. When a wound is healing by secondary intention, you use a dressing to provide a moist environment. You moisten the gauze with a solution, usually normal saline, wring it out, unfold it, and lightly pack it into the wound. The purpose of a moist gauze dressing is to act as a sponge, absorbing excessive wound drainage, while providing a moist environment. You change the dressing when it is saturated or if it begins to dry out. You always cover a moist dressing with a dry, secondary dressing.

A firmly taped or wrapped dressing supports or immobilizes a body part, minimizing movement of the underlying incision and traumatized tissues. Finally, a dressing promotes thermal insulation to the wound surface and protects it from the dehydrating effects of air.

Types. Dressings vary by type of material and mode of application (dry or moist). They are easy to apply, comfortable, and made of materials that promote wound healing.

Gauze is the most common dressing type. Gauze does not interact with wound tissues and thus causes little wound irritation. Gauze is available in different textures and in squares, rectangles, and rolls of various lengths and widths. Gauze dressings are best for wounds with moderate drainage, deep wounds, undermining, and tunnels. You apply gauze either moist or dry. A moist gauze dressing is saturated with the prescribed solution, wrung out, opened up and placed onto the wound tissue. The moistened gauze increases the absorptive ability of the dressing to collect exudate. Then cover the moist gauze with a secondary layer of dry gauze. Be sure the moist gauze does not cover the normal skin to prevent maceration. The moist dressing is changed on a scheduled basis to prevent drying of the gauze.

Transparent film dressings are clear sheets coated on one side with an adhesive. The adhesive side will not stick to the wound because of the moisture and will trap moisture over the wound bed, providing a moist environment. The film is impermeable to fluid but semipermeable to oxygen. This type of dressing is used as a primary dressing in wounds with minimal tissue loss that have very little wound drainage. You change the dressing when the seal is broken.

Hydrocolloid dressings are made of gelling agents and have an adhesive wound surface. They come in a variety of sizes and shapes and are used to cover wounds, extending the hydrocolloid dressing at least 1½ inches beyond the wound margin. Hydrocolloids form a gel as they interact with the wound surface. Because hydrocolloids are occlusive, they protect the wound from surface contaminants and you can leave them over a wound for several days. When removed, you will note a gel over the wound base; the gel maintains a moist environment to support healing and washes away during wound cleansing.

Hydrogel dressings are available in sheets or in a gel in a tube (amorphous). They contain a high percentage of water and are indicated for wounds that require moisture, either a wound with granulation (maintaining the moist wound environment needed for healing) or a wound that has a high percentage of necrotic tissue (the hydrogel facilitates debridement by softening the dead tissue). Hydrogels maintain moisture in some wounds for 1 to 3 days.

Negative pressure wound therapy (NPWT) uses negative pressure to assist wound healing (Figure 36-13). NPWT supports wound healing by evacuating wound fluids, stimulating granulation tissue formation, reducing the bacterial burden of a wound, and maintaining a moist wound environment (Frantz and others, 2007). The foam is cut to fit the shape of the wound, and a drainage/suction tube is placed in the interior or on top of the foam dressing. Then seal the foam and the tube with a transparent dressing, and connect the tube to a prescribed amount of negative pressure, which creates suction. The suction pulls all air out of the wound and creates an airtight seal. This therapy provides removal of excess wound fluid to stimulate granulation tissue and to decrease wound

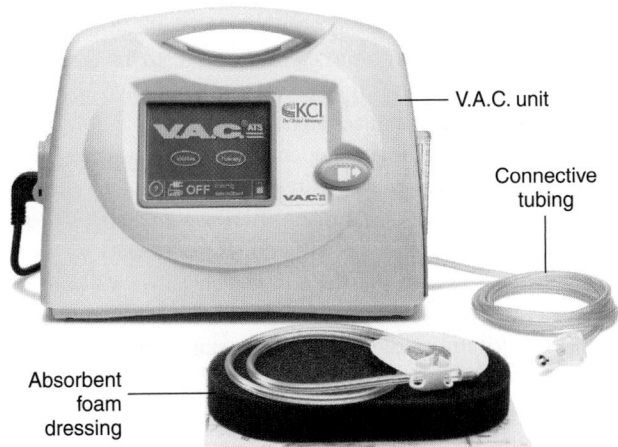

Figure 36-13 ■ The V.A.C. ATS® Therapy System. *Top to bottom:* V.A.C. system itself, connective tubing to go between V.A.C. system and dressing, absorbent foam dressing. (Courtesy KCI Licensing, Inc., San Antonio, Tex.)

bacteria (Skill 36-3). The suction tubing is connected to a container that collects the wound fluid. NPWT is changed on a scheduled basis, usually every 48 hours. This therapy has reduced healing time in chronic wounds and has resulted in early grafting of wounds (Frantz and others, 2007).

Changing Dressings. To prepare for changing a dressing, you need to know the type of dressing, any underlying drains used, and the type of supplies needed for wound care. You can adjust the type and amount of dressings if the amount of drainage changes or if a wound becomes deeper. Notifying the health care provider of any change is essential.

The order for changing a dressing usually indicates the dressing type, frequency of changing, and solutions or ointments you will apply. An order to "reinforce dressing prn" (add dressings without removing existing ones as needed) is common immediately after surgery, when the health care provider does not want accidental disruption of the suture line or loss of hemostasis. A patient's medical or operating room record usually reveals whether drains are present. After the initial dressing change, communicate on the care plan the type of dressing materials and solutions to use and the type and location of drains.

Use aseptic technique during dressing change procedures (see Chapter 13). It is also essential for the patient to understand the steps of the procedure beforehand so he or she experiences less anxiety. Describe normal signs of the healing process, and offer to answer questions about the procedure or wound.

If a patient needs to care for a wound at home, you will demonstrate dressing changes to the patient and family and then provide an opportunity for practice. In the home, wound healing stabilizes so that sterile technique is usually unnecessary. However, patients need to learn clean technique. Make sure the patient is able to change a dressing independently or with assistance from a family member before discharge unless home care will be provided. Skill 36-4 outlines the steps for applying moist saline dressings.

Securing Dressings. Use tape, ties, or dressings and cloth binders to secure a dressing over a wound site. **Binders** are dressings made of large pieces of material to fit a specific body part. An arm sling and a breast binder are two examples of binders. A binder reduces stress on a wound.

The choice of anchoring depends on the wound size, location, drainage, frequency of dressing changes, and the patient's level of activity. You most often use tape strips to secure dressings if the patient does not react to tape. Hypoallergenic paper, plastic, and woven fabric tapes minimize skin reactions. Adhesive tape, the most likely anchor to cause skin irritation, adheres well to the skin's surface, whereas elastic adhesive tape compresses closely around pressure dressings and permits more movement of a body part (O'Brien and Reilly, 1995).

Tape is available in various widths. Choose a size that sufficiently secures the dressing. Make sure the tape crosses the dressing and adheres to several inches of skin on each side. When securing the dressing, gently press the tape, exerting pressure away from the wound. Never apply tape over irri-

tated skin. Apply a skin barrier to the skin around the wound so that the tape is secured to the skin barrier rather than to sensitive skin. To remove tape safely, loosen the tape end and gently release the tape from the patient's skin by pressing the skin away from the tape.

To avoid repeated removal of tape from sensitive skin, secure dressings with reusable Montgomery ties (see Skill 36-4, Step 16). Each tie consists of a long strip; half contains an adhesive backing to apply to the skin, and the other half folds back and contains a cloth tie that you tie across a dressing and untie at dressing changes. A large, bulky dressing requires two or more sets of Montgomery ties. To provide even support to a wound and immobilize a body part, apply elastic gauze or cloth dressings and binders over a dressing.

Comfort Measures. Any wound can be painful, depending on the extent of tissue injury. You will use several techniques to minimize discomfort. Careful removal of tape, gentle cleansing of wound edges, and gentle manipulation of dressings and drains minimize stress on sensitive tissues. Proper turning and positioning of the patient also reduce strain on the wound. Administration of analgesic medications 30 to 60 minutes before dressing changes (depending on a drug's time of peak action) also reduces discomfort (Rook, 1996) (see Chapter 31).

Wound Cleansing Wound cleansing removes surface bacteria, preventing the invasion of healthy tissue. Normal saline effectively cleanses when delivered to the wound site with adequate force to agitate and wash away bacteria (Rolstad and Ovington, 2007). Do not use povidone-iodine (e.g., Betadine), hydrogen peroxide, and acetic acid to irrigate a clean, granular wound. These solutions are toxic to fibroblasts, a key cellular component in wound healing. Apply the following concepts when cleaning wounds:

1. Cleanse in a direction from the least contaminated area to the most contaminated, such as from the wound or incision to the surrounding skin (Figure 36-14) or from an isolated drain site to the surrounding skin (Figure 36-15).
2. Use light friction when applying antiseptics locally to the skin.
3. When irrigating, allow the solution to flow from the least contaminated to the most contaminated area.

Wound Irrigation. Irrigation is a way of cleansing wounds of exudate and debris. You use an irrigating syringe to flush the area with a constant flow of solution. Irrigations are useful for cleaning open deep wounds or sensitive or inaccessible body parts. Administer the prescribed solution (usually normal saline) at body temperature to enhance comfort and provide local cleansing application.

When irrigating a clean wound, use sterile technique and an irrigation system with a safe level of pressure (4 to 15 psi) to prevent trauma to the newly formed granulation tissue (WOCN, 2003). An example of a safe wound cleansing and irrigation system is a 35-mL syringe and a 19-gauge needle, which has a psi of 8. This method provides an ideal solution pressure for cleansing wounds while minimizing tissue

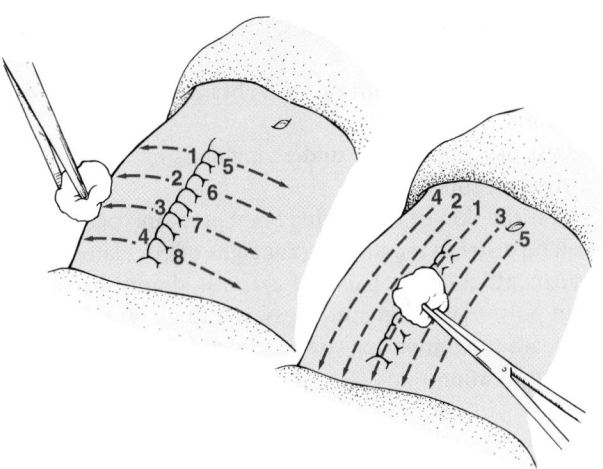

Figure 36-14 ■ Methods for cleansing wound site.

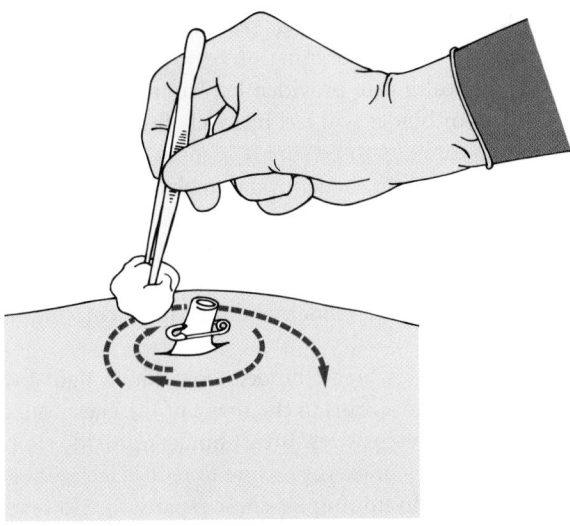

Figure 36-15 ■ Cleansing of drain site.

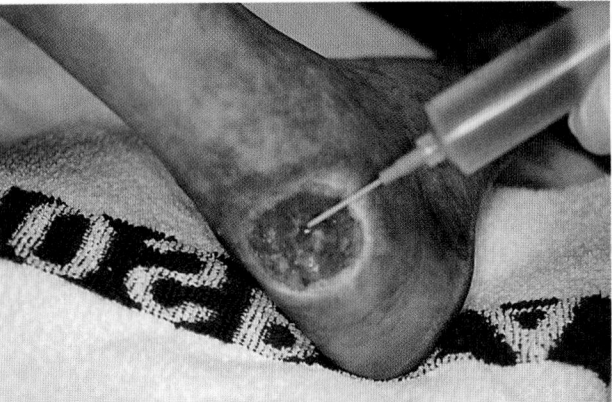

Figure 36-16 ■ Wound irrigation using 35-mL syringe to facilitate removal of necrotic tissue.

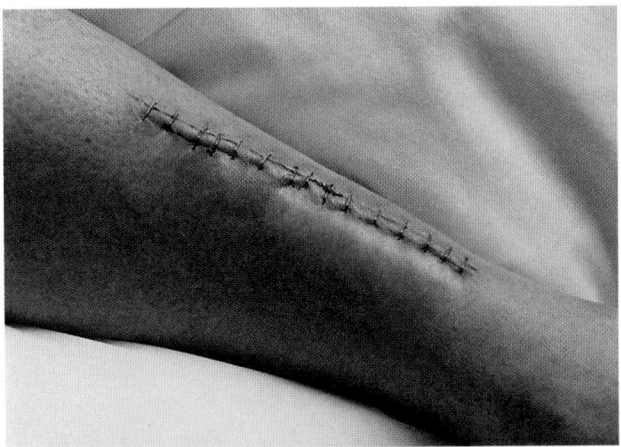

Figure 36-17 ■ Wound closed with staples.

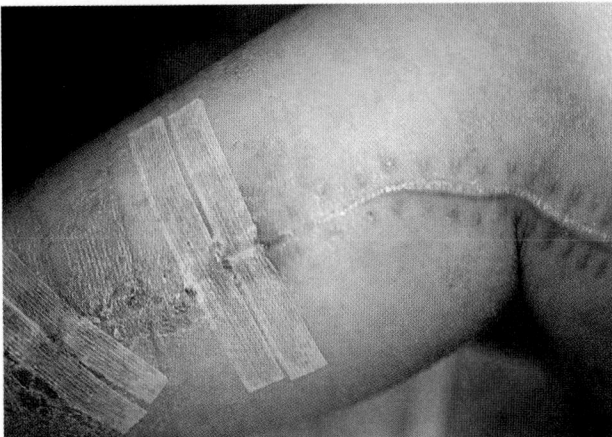

Figure 36-18 ■ Steri-Strips placed over incision for closure.

trauma (Figure 36-16). Make sure the syringe tip is over but not sticking into the wound. Skill 36-5 lists steps for wound irrigation.

Suture Care. A surgeon closes a wound by bringing the edges as close together as possible to reduce the formation of scar tissue while minimizing trauma and tension and controlling bleeding. Sutures are threads or wires made of silk, steel, cotton, nylon, and polyester (Dacron) and are used to sew body tissues together. Dacron sutures minimize scar formation. Surgeons frequently use steel staples, a type of outer skin closure, because they result in less tissue trauma while providing extra strength (Figure 36-17). Wounds can also be closed with Steri-Strips, a sterile tape applied along both sides of a wound to keep the edges closed (Figure 36-18).

Policies vary among institutions as to who removes sutures. If you remove sutures, a health care provider's order is necessary. Be familiar with the types of suture methods (Figure 36-19).

Drainage Evacuation. When drainage interferes with healing, drainage evacuation is achieved by using a drain or a drainage tube with continuous suction. Drainage evacuators are convenient, portable units that connect to tubular drains within a wound bed and exert a safe, constant, low-pressure vacuum to remove and collect drainage (Figure 36-20). Ensure that suction is exerted and that all connection points between the evacuator and tubing are intact. The evacuator collects drainage that is assessed for volume and character. When the evacuator fills, measure output by emptying the

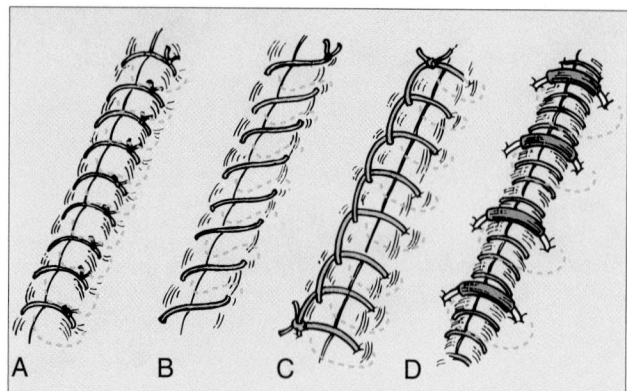

Figure 36-19 ■ Examples of suturing methods. **A,** Intermittent. **B,** Continuous. **C,** Blanket continuous. **D,** Retention.

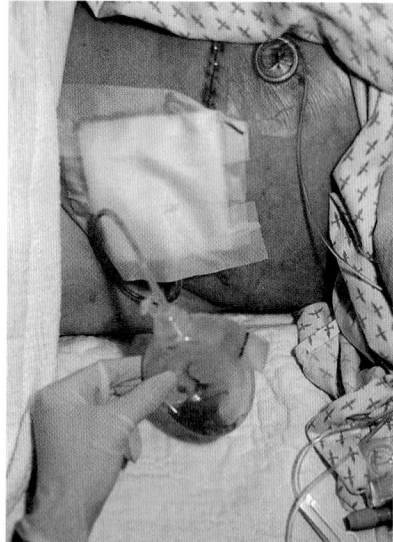

Figure 36-20 ■ Jackson-Pratt drain and reservoir.

contents into a graduated cylinder, and immediately reset the evacuator to apply suction.

Bandages and Binders A simple gauze dressing is often not enough to immobilize or provide support to a wound. Bandages and binders applied over or around dressings will provide extra protection and therapeutic benefits by creating pressure over a body part, immobilizing a body part, supporting a wound, reducing or preventing edema, securing a splint, or securing dressings.

Dressings are available in rolls of various widths and materials, including gauze, elasticized knit, elastic webbing, flannel, and muslin. Gauze dressings are lightweight and inexpensive, mold easily around contours of the body, and permit air circulation to underlying skin to prevent maceration. Elastic dressings conform well to body parts but are also used to exert pressure over a body part.

Principles for Application of Bandages and Binders. Correctly applied dressings and binders do not cause injury to underlying or nearby body parts or create discomfort for the patient. Before applying a dressing or binder, perform the following steps:

1. Inspect the skin for abrasions, edema, discoloration, or exposed wound edges.
2. Cover exposed wounds or open abrasions with a sterile dressing.
3. Assess the condition of underlying dressings, and change if they are soiled.
4. Assess the skin of underlying body parts and parts that will be distal to the dressing for signs of circulatory impairment (coolness, pallor or cyanosis, diminished or absent pulses, swelling, numbness, and tingling) to provide a means for comparing changes in circulation after dressing application.

Table 36-5 outlines the principles of dressing and binder application. After you apply a dressing, assess, document, and immediately report any changes in circulation, comfort level, body function such as ventilation, and skin integrity. After you apply a dressing, loosen or readjust it as necessary, but seek an order before loosening or removing a dressing applied by the health care provider. Explain to the patient that any dressing or binder will feel relatively firm or tight; assess the dressing carefully to be sure it is applied properly and is providing therapeutic benefit, and replace dressings when they become soiled.

Binder Application. Binders are especially designed for the body part to be supported. The most common types of binders are the breast binder, abdominal binder, and sling (Box 36-13).

Breast Binder. A breast binder looks like a tight-fitting sleeveless vest. It conforms to the shape of the chest wall and is available in different sizes. Breast binders provide support after breast surgery or exert pressure to reduce lactation after childbirth. They do not impair chest expansion. However, if a patient develops pulmonary secretions, encourage active pulmonary hygiene exercises.

Abdominal Binder. An abdominal binder supports large incisions that are vulnerable to stress when the patient moves or coughs. It is a rectangular piece of cotton or elasticized material with many tails attached to the two longer sides or long extensions on each side to surround the abdomen (Figure 36-21).

Slings. Slings support arms with muscular sprains or fractures. A commercially made sling consists of a long sleeve that extends to the elbow and a strap that fits around the neck. In the home, patients can use a large triangular piece of cloth as a sling. The patient sits or lies supine for a sling application (Figure 36-22). Instruct the patient to bend the affected arm, bringing the forearm straight across the chest. The open sling fits under the patient's arm and over the chest, with the base of the triangle under the wrist and the triangle's point at the elbow. One end of the sling fits around the back of the neck. Bring the other end up over the affected arm while supporting the extremity. Tie the two ends at the side of the neck so that the knot does not press against the cervical spine. You can fold the loose fold at the elbow evenly around the elbow and pin it. To prevent the formation of dependent edema, make sure the lower arm is always supported at a level above the elbow.

TABLE 36-5   Principles for Bandage and Binder Application

PRINCIPLE	RATIONALE
Position body part you will be dressing in comfortable position of normal anatomical alignment.	Dressings cause restriction in movement. Immobilization in normal functioning position reduces risks of deformity or injury.
Prevent friction between and against skin surfaces by applying gauze or cotton padding.	Skin surfaces in contact with each other (e.g., between toes, under breasts) rub against each other to cause abrasion or chafing. Dressings over bony prominences rub against skin to cause breakdown.
Apply dressings securely to prevent slippage during movement.	Friction between dressing and skin causes skin breakdown.
When bandaging extremities, apply dressing first at distal end and progress toward trunk.	Gradual application of pressure from distal toward proximal portion of extremity promotes venous return and minimizes risk for edema or circulatory impairment.
Apply dressings firmly, with equal tension exerted over each turn or layer. Avoid excess overlapping of dressing layers.	Equal tension prevents unequal pressure distribution over dressing body part. Localized pressure causes circulatory impairment.
Position pins, knots, or ties away from wound or sensitive skin areas.	Pins and ties used to secure dressings and binders exert localized pressure and irritation.

BOX 36-13   PROCEDURAL GUIDELINES

Applying Abdominal or Breast Binders

DELEGATION CONSIDERATIONS: You can delegate the application of an abdominal or breast binder to others. It is the responsibility of the nurse to assess the area where the binder will be applied and to assess the patient's comfort level after application.

EQUIPMENT: Abdominal binder/breast binder; clean gloves; pins, metal fasteners as indicated by type of binder used

1 Observe patient with need for support of thorax or abdomen. Observe ability to breathe deeply and cough effectively.
2 Identify patient using two identifiers (e.g., name and birthday or name and account number, according to facility policy). Review medical record if medical prescription for particular binder is necessary and reasons for application.
3 Inspect skin for actual or potential alterations in integrity. Observe for irritation, abrasion, skin surfaces that rub against each other, or allergic response to adhesive tape used to secure dressing.
4 Inspect any surgical dressing for drainage.
5 Assess patient's comfort level, using analog scale of 0 to 10 (see Chapter 31) and noting any objective signs and symptoms.
6 Gather necessary data regarding size of patient and appropriate binder.
7 Explain procedure to patient.
8 Perform hand hygiene, and apply gloves (if likely to contact wound drainage).
9 Close curtains or room door.
10 Apply binder.
  a **Abdominal binder:**
    (1) Position patient in supine position with head slightly elevated and knees slightly flexed.
    (2) Fanfold far side of binder toward midline of binder.
    (3) Instruct and assist patient in rolling away from you toward raised side rail while firmly supporting abdominal incision and dressing with hands.
    (4) Place fanfolded ends of binder under patient.

    (5) Instruct or assist patient in rolling over folded ends toward you.
    (6) Unfold and stretch ends out smoothly on far side of bed.
    (7) Instruct patient to roll back into supine position.
    (8) Adjust binder so that supine patient is centered over binder using symphysis pubis and costal margins as lower and upper landmarks.
    (9) Close binder. Pull one end of binder over center of patient's abdomen. While maintaining tension on that end of binder, pull opposite end of binder over center and secure with Velcro closure tabs, metal fasteners, or horizontally placed safety pins (see Figure 36-21, p. 1086).
    (10) Assess patient's comfort level.
    (11) Adjust binder as necessary.
  b **Breast binder:**
    (1) Assist patient in placing arms through binder's armholes.
    (2) Assist patient to supine position in bed.
    (3) Pad area under breasts if necessary.
    (4) Using Velcro closure tabs or horizontally placed safety pins, secure binder at nipple level first. Continue closure process above and then below nipple line until entire binder is closed.
    (5) Make appropriate adjustments, including individualizing fit of shoulder straps and pinning waistline darts to reduce binder size.
    (6) Instruct and observe skill development in self-care related to reapplying breast binder.
11 Remove gloves, and perform hand hygiene.
12 Observe site for skin integrity, circulation, and characteristics of the wound. (Periodically remove binder and surgical dressing to assess wound characteristics.)
13 Evaluate comfort level of patient, using analog scale of 0 to 10 and noting any objective signs and symptoms.
14 Evaluate patient's ability to ventilate properly, including deep breathing and coughing.

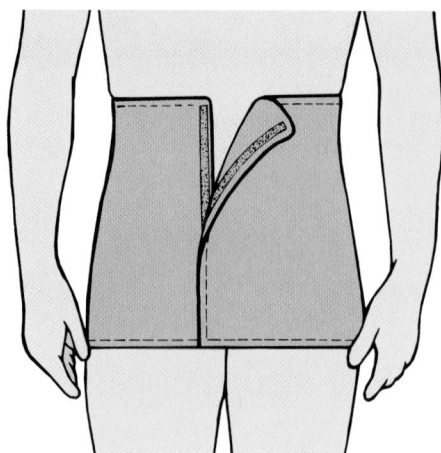

Figure 36-21 ■ Abdominal binder secured with Velcro.

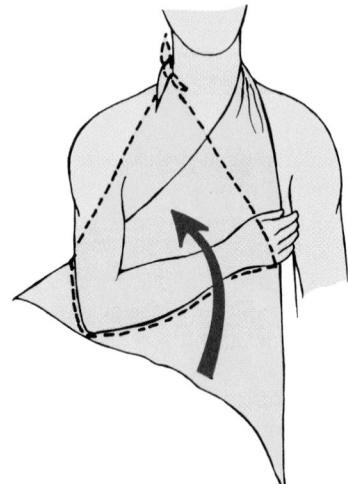

Figure 36-22 ■ Application of a sling.

Bandage Application. Rolls of dressing secure or support dressings over irregularly shaped body parts. Each roll has a free outer end and a terminal end at the center. The rolled portion of the dressing is its body, and you place its outer surface against the patient's skin or dressing. Box 36-14 describes essential points when applying an elastic bandage.

Heat and Cold Therapy The local application of heat and cold to an injured body part provides therapeutic benefits. Before using these therapies, however, understand normal body responses to local temperature variations, assess the integrity of the body part, determine the patient's ability to sense temperature variations, and ensure proper operation of equipment. You are legally responsible for the safe administration of all heat and cold applications.

Body Responses to Heat and Cold. Exposure to heat and cold will cause systemic and local responses. Systemic responses occur through heat loss mechanisms (sweating or vasodilation) or mechanisms promoting heat conservation (vasoconstriction or piloerection) and heat production (shivering) (see Chapter 14). Local responses to heat and cold occur through stimulation of temperature-sensitive nerve endings within the skin.

The body's adaptive ability creates the major problem in protecting patients from injury resulting from temperature extremes. A person initially feels an extreme change in temperature, but within a short time hardly notices the temperature variation. This phenomenon is dangerous because a person insensitive to heat and cold extremes is at risk for serious tissue injury. Recognize patients most at risk for injuries from heat and cold applications (Table 36-6).

Local Effects of Heat and Cold. Heat and cold stimuli create different physiological responses. The choice of heat or cold therapy depends on the local responses desired for wound healing (Table 36-7).

Heat generally is therapeutic. If heat is applied for 1 hour or more, however, a reflex vasoconstriction reduces blood flow as the body attempts to control heat loss from the area. The periodic removal and reapplication of local heat will restore vasodilation. Continuous exposure to heat damages epithelial cells, causing redness, localized tenderness, and even blistering of the skin.

Prolonged exposure of the skin to cold results in a reflex vasodilation. The cell's inability to receive adequate blood flow and nutrients results in tissue ischemia. The skin initially takes on a reddened appearance, followed by a bluish-purple mottling with numbness and a burning type of pain. Tissues will actually freeze from exposure to extreme cold.

Factors Influencing Heat and Cold Tolerance. The body's response to heat and cold therapies depends on the following factors:

1. *Duration of application:* A person is better able to tolerate short exposures to any temperature extremes.
2. *Body part:* The neck, inner aspect of the wrist and forearm, and perineal regions are more sensitive to temperature variations. The foot and the palm of the hand are less sensitive.
3. *Damage to body surface:* Exposed skin layers are more sensitive to temperature variations.
4. *Prior skin temperature:* The body responds best to minor temperature adjustments.
5. *Body surface area:* A person is less tolerant of temperature changes over a large area of the body.
6. *Age and physical condition:* The very young and old are most sensitive to heat and cold. If a patient's physical condition reduces the reception or perception of sensory stimuli, the tolerance to temperature extremes is high, but the risk for injury is also high.

Assessment for Temperature Tolerance. Before applying heat or cold therapies, first observe the area you will treat so that you are able to later evaluate therapy-related skin changes. Alterations in skin integrity, such as abrasions, open wounds, edema, bruising, bleeding, or localized areas of inflammation, increase the risk for thermal injury. Identify conditions that contraindicate heat or cold therapy. *Do not* apply heat over an active area of bleeding (risk for continued bleeding) or an acute localized inflammation such as appendicitis (risk for rupture). If the patient has cardiovascular problems, it is

BOX 36-14 PROCEDURAL GUIDELINES

Applying Elastic Bandages

DELEGATION CONSIDERATIONS: The application of elastic bandages cannot be delegated to nursing assistive personnel (NAP). The nurse is responsible to assess the area, apply the wrap, and then again assess the area for signs of circulatory occlusion (coolness of area wrapped, pain in the area, change in color of tissue in area).

EQUIPMENT: Correct width and number of elastic dressings; clips, adhesive tape, or mesh dressing to secure elastic dressing; gloves if wound drainage is present

1 Identify patient using two identifiers (e.g., name and birthday or name and account number, according to facility policy). Review patient's medical record and order for application of elastic dressing.
2 Inspect areas to be dressed for the following:
   a Intact skin
   b Abrasions
   c Draining wounds
   d Skin discoloration
3 Note circulation to the area requiring an elastic bandage.
   a Palpate skin, noting temperature, color.
   b Palpate pulse, noting pulse quality.
   c Observe extremity for edema or dehydration.
4 Determine level of function of affected extremity.
5 Assess level of pain severity to area (scale 0 to 10).
6 Explain procedure to patient.
7 Perform hand hygiene, and apply gloves, if indicated.
8 Close curtains or room door.
9 Hold roll of elastic bandage in dominant hand, and use other hand to tightly hold the beginning of bandage at distal body part.
10 Apply bandage from distal point toward proximal boundary, stretching the dressing slightly, using a variety of bandage turns to cover various body shapes. Prevent uneven dressing tension or circulatory impairment by overlapping turns by one-half to two-thirds width of dressing roll. NOTE: Be sure bandage is smooth (without creases).
11 Secure each roll with clip or tape before applying additional roll(s).
12 When finished with application, secure last elastic roll with clip, adhesive tape, or mesh to prevent wrap from becoming dislodged and thus decreasing extremity support.
13 Remove gloves, and perform hand hygiene.
14 Evaluate circulation to dressing area every 4 hours.
   a Palpate distal pulse.
   b Palpate skin, noting temperature every 4 hours.
   c Observe skin color.
15 Determine patient's level of comfort, using analog scale of 0 to 10 and noting any objective signs and symptoms.
16 Observe for changes from baseline assessment in level of extremity function.

TABLE 36-6 Conditions That Increase Risk for Injury From Heat and Cold Application

CONDITION	RISK FACTORS
Very young; older adults	Thinner skin layers in children and older adults increase risk for burns; older adults have reduced sensitivity to pain.
Open wounds, broken skin	Subcutaneous tissue is more sensitive to temperature variations.
Areas of edema or scar formation	There is reduced sensation to temperature stimuli because of scar formation.
Peripheral vascular disease (e.g., diabetes, arteriosclerosis)	Body's extremities are less sensitive to temperature and pain stimuli because of circulatory impairment and local tissue injury; cold application further compromises blood flow.
Confusion or unconsciousness	There is reduced perception of sensory or painful stimuli.
Spinal cord injury	Alterations in nerve pathways prevent reception of sensory or painful stimuli.

unwise to apply heat to large portions of the body because massive vasodilation will disrupt blood supply to vital organs. Cold is contraindicated if the site of injury is edematous or the patient has impaired circulation or is shivering (may intensify shivering and reduce blood flow).

Also assess the patient's sensory function and ability to recognize when heat or cold becomes excessive. If a patient has peripheral vascular disease, observe circulation to the extremities. If a patient is confused or unresponsive, observe skin temperature, circulation, and integrity frequently after therapy begins. Finally, assess the condition of all equipment used, checking for cracked cords, frayed wires, damaged insulation, exposed heating components, leaks, and evenness of temperature distribution.

Patient Education and Safety. Before application of heat or cold therapy, make sure the patient understands its purpose, the symptoms of temperature exposure, and the precautions taken to prevent injury. Box 36-15 provides hints for safely applying heat and cold therapy.

Applying Heat and Cold. A prerequisite to using heat or cold application is a health care provider's order, which includes the body site to be treated and the type, frequency, and duration of application. The correct temperature to use for heat and cold applications varies according to agency policy.

TABLE 36-7 Therapeutic Effects of Heat and Cold Applications

PHYSIOLOGICAL RESPONSE	THERAPEUTIC BENEFIT	EXAMPLES OF CONDITIONS TREATED
HEAT THERAPY		
Vasodilation	Improves blood flow to injured body part	Arthritis or degenerative joint disease
Reduced blood viscosity	Promotes delivery of nutrients and removal	Localized joint pain or muscle strains
Reduced muscle tension	of wastes	Low back pain
Increased tissue metabolism	Improves delivery of leukocytes and antibiot-	Menstrual cramping
Increased capillary permeability	ics to wound site	Hemorrhoidal, perianal, and vaginal
	Promotes muscle relaxation	inflammation
	Reduces pain from spasm or stiffness	Local abscesses
	Increases blood flow	
	Provides local warmth	
	Promotes movement of waste products and nutrients	
COLD THERAPY		
Vasoconstriction	Reduces blood flow to injured site, prevent-	Immediately after direct trauma (e.g.,
Local anesthesia	ing edema formation	sprains, strains, fractures, muscle
Reduced cell metabolism	Reduces inflammation	spasms)
Increased blood viscosity	Reduces localized pain	Superficial laceration or puncture
Decreased muscle tension	Reduces oxygen needs of tissues	wound
	Promotes blood coagulation at injury site	Minor burn
	Relieves pain	After injections
		Arthritis or joint trauma

BOX 36-15 Safety Suggestions for Applying Heat or Cold Therapy

- Explain to the patient the sensations he or she will feel during the procedure.
- Instruct the patient to report changes in sensation or discomfort immediately.
- Provide a timer, clock, or watch so that the patient is able to help you to time the application.
- Keep the call light within the patient's reach.
- Refer to the institution's policy and procedure manual for safe temperatures.
- Do not allow the patient to adjust temperature settings.
- Do not allow the patient to move an application or place his or her hands on the wound site.
- Do not place the patient in a position that prevents movement away from the temperature source.
- Do not leave unattended a patient who is unable to sense temperature changes or move from the temperature source.

Choice of Moist or Dry. You administer heat and cold applications in dry or moist forms. Consider the type of wound or injury, location of the body part, and presence of drainage or inflammation when selecting dry or moist applications.

Warm Moist Compresses. A warm moist compress improves circulation, relieves edema, and promotes concentration of pus and drainage. A **compress** is a piece of gauze dressing moistened in a prescribed warmed solution. A pack is a larger cloth or dressing applied to a larger body area.

Heat from warm compresses evaporates quickly. To maintain a constant temperature, change the compress frequently or apply a warm aquathermia pad or waterproof heating pad over the compress. Because moisture conducts heat, make sure any device's temperature setting is lower for a moist compress than for a dry application. A layer of plastic wrap or a dry towel will insulate the compress and retain heat. Moist heat promotes vasodilation and evaporation of heat from the skin's surface. For this reason a patient feels chilly. Control drafts, and keep the patient covered with a blanket or robe.

Warm Soaks. Immersion of a body part in a warmed solution promotes circulation, lessens edema, increases muscle relaxation, and allows application of medicated solution. You also accomplish a soak by wrapping the body part in dressings and saturating them with the warmed solution.

Position the patient comfortably, place waterproof pads under the area you will treat, and heat the solution to the patient's tolerance. Check the temperature by placing a small amount of solution on the inside of the forearm. After immersing the body part, cover the container and extremity with a towel to reduce heat loss. It is usually necessary to remove the cooled solution and the body part and add heated solution after about 10 minutes. The problem is to keep the solution at a constant temperature. Never add a hotter solution while the body part remains immersed. After any soak, dry the body part thoroughly to prevent maceration.

Sitz Bath. The patient who has had rectal surgery or an episiotomy during childbirth or who has painful hemorrhoids or vaginal inflammation will benefit from a **sitz bath,** a bath in which only the pelvic area is immersed in warm fluid. The patient sits in a special tub or chair or in a basin that fits on the toilet so that the legs and feet remain out of the water. Immersing the entire body causes widespread vasodilation and negates the effect of local heat to the pelvic area.

The desired temperature for a sitz bath depends on whether the purpose is to promote relaxation or to clean a wound. It is often necessary to carefully add warm water during the procedure, which usually lasts 20 minutes. A disposable basin contains an attachment that resembles an enema bag and allows the gradual introduction of warmer water.

Prevent overexposure by draping bath blankets around the patient's shoulders and thighs and controlling drafts. Make sure the patient is able to sit in the basin or tub with feet flat on the floor and without pressure on the sacrum or thighs. Because exposure of a large portion of the body to heat causes extensive vasodilation, assess the patient's pulse and facial color and ask whether the patient feels light-headed or nauseated.

Aquathermia (Water-Flow) Pads. The aquathermia pad is useful for treating muscle sprains and areas of mild inflammation or edema (Figure 36-23). The unit consists of a waterproof plastic or rubber pad connected by two hoses to an electrical control unit that has a heating element and motor. Distilled water circulates through hollowed channels within the pad to the control unit where water is heated or cooled (depending on temperature setting). Although the units are safer than the conventional heating pad, you still check for equipment malfunctions. You fix the temperature setting by inserting a plastic key into the temperature regulator. If the water in the unit runs low, simply add distilled water to the reservoir at the top of the control unit.

To avoid burning the patient's skin, fold a thin cloth or pillowcase over the heating pad; use tape, ties, or a gauze roll to hold the pad in place. Never use pins. Observe the skin frequently for signs of burning. An application lasts only 20 to 30 minutes, and the patient does not lie on the pad.

Commercial Hot Packs. Commercially prepared, disposable hot packs apply warm, dry heat to an injured area. Striking, kneading, or squeezing the pack mixes chemicals that release heat. Package directions recommend the time for heat application.

Hot-Water Bottles. The hot-water bottle is an economical means of applying heat to an injured body part. Many patients use them in the home. Give patients and family members the following instructions about the safe use of water bottles:

1. Ensure that there are no leaks. Fill the bottle with warm tap water, secure the cap, and turn the bottle upside down.
2. Fill the bag only two-thirds full, expel air at the top, and secure the cap. The bag is then easier to mold over a body part.
3. Wipe off moisture on the outside of the bag.
4. Never apply a water bottle directly to the skin surface. Cover it with a towel or pillowcase.
5. Keep the bottle in place for 20 to 30 minutes.

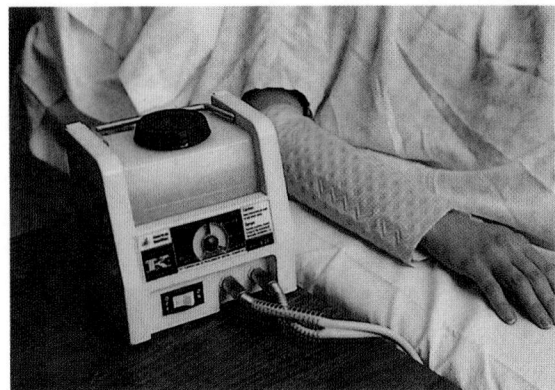

Figure 36-23 ■ Aquathermia pad.

Electric Heating Pads. Another conventional form of heat therapy is the heating pad, an electric coil enclosed within a waterproof pad covered with cotton or flannel cloth. The pad is connected to an electric cord that has a temperature-regulating unit for a high, medium, or low setting. Advise patients to avoid using the high setting and to never lie on the pad. Another precaution to note is that a safety pin inserted through a pad will result in an electrical shock.

Cold Moist Compresses. The procedure for applying cold moist compresses is the same as that for warm compresses. Apply cold compresses for 20 minutes at a temperature of 15° C (59° F) to relieve inflammation and swelling. Compresses are clean or sterile. Observe for adverse reactions such as burning or numbness, mottling of the skin, redness, extreme paleness, or a bluish skin discoloration.

Cold Soaks. The procedure for preparing cold soaks and immersing a body part is the same as for warm soaks. The desired temperature for a 20-minute soak is 15° C (59° F). Take precautions to protect the patient from chilling.

Ice Bag or Collar. For a patient who has a muscle sprain, localized hemorrhage, or hematoma or has undergone dental surgery, an ice bag is ideal to prevent edema formation, control bleeding, and anesthetize the body part. Proper use of the bag requires the following:

1. Fill the bag with water, secure the cap, invert to check for leaks, and pour out the water.
2. Fill the bag two-thirds full with crushed ice so that the bag molds easily over a body part.
3. Release air from the bag by squeezing its sides before securing the cap (because excess air interferes with conduction of cold).
4. Wipe off excess moisture.
5. Cover the bag with a flannel cover, towel, or pillowcase.
6. Apply the bag to the injury site for 20 to 30 minutes; you may reapply the bag in an hour.

Commercial Cold Packs. Commercially prepared single-use ice packs come in various sizes and shapes. When you squeeze or knead the pack, an alcohol-based solution is released inside to create the cold temperature. The soft outer coverings are usually safe to apply directly to the skin surface.

RESTORATIVE AND CONTINUING CARE Some chronic wounds are the result of underlying pathological conditions that continue long after wound healing occurs. Healing for a pressure ulcer or a chronic wound is lengthy and requires continuity of care from the acute care setting to the restorative care setting. In this setting, you use many of the principles and interventions detailed in the acute care section. Continue diligent assessment to identify those patients at risk for impaired skin integrity, and institute preventive measures as needed.

Despite efforts with wound care, wound healing will not occur if the patient is malnourished. Tissue repair requires more protein, carbohydrates, fats, vitamins, minerals, water, and oxygen than normal tissue metabolism (see Chapter 32). In addition, the delivery of nutritional substances to tissues depends on a healthy circulatory system. Malnutrition causes an insufficient supply of the necessary nutritional elements and alterations in blood vessel integrity. Therefore work closely with registered dietitians to provide a well-balanced diet, and educate the patient about the importance of good dietary habits. For patients weakened or debilitated by illness, supportive nutritional therapies will become necessary. The surgical patient who is well nourished and has no complications requires at least 0.8 g of protein per kilogram daily for nutritional maintenance. Supplemental tube feedings (enteral feedings) introduce nutrients directly into the gastrointestinal tract. If a patient is unable to tolerate enteral feedings, the health care provider will often order parenteral (intravenously administered) nutrition.

The patient with a wound that restricts mobility or has the potential to compromise the function of a joint sometimes requires additional physical and/or occupational therapy. Work closely with the physical therapist in monitoring the patient's activity and tolerance for exercise. It is important to optimize activity within the patient's physical limitations and return function as rapidly as possible.

■■■EVALUATION

PATIENT CARE You evaluate nursing interventions for reducing and treating pressure ulcers by determining the patient's response to nursing therapies and determining whether you achieved each goal (Box 36-16). The primary

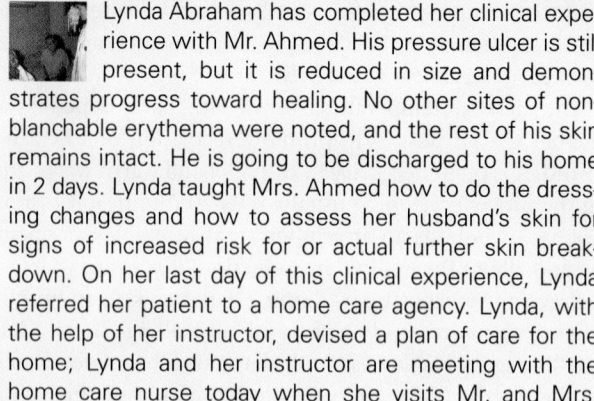

BOX 36-16   EVALUATION

Lynda Abraham has completed her clinical experience with Mr. Ahmed. His pressure ulcer is still present, but it is reduced in size and demonstrates progress toward healing. No other sites of non-blanchable erythema were noted, and the rest of his skin remains intact. He is going to be discharged to his home in 2 days. Lynda taught Mrs. Ahmed how to do the dressing changes and how to assess her husband's skin for signs of increased risk for or actual further skin breakdown. On her last day of this clinical experience, Lynda referred her patient to a home care agency. Lynda, with the help of her instructor, devised a plan of care for the home; Lynda and her instructor are meeting with the home care nurse today when she visits Mr. and Mrs. Ahmed in the hospital.

DOCUMENTATION NOTE
"Small amount of serous drainage from stage II pressure ulcer on his sacrum. Wound is 1 × 1 inch × ½ inch deep, with red tissue. Mrs. Ahmed cleansed the wound with normal saline and applied a hydrocolloid dressing. Maintained aseptic technique and correctly assessed skin. She reminds her husband to change his position every 1½ to 2 hours. Awaiting visit from home care nurse."

goals are to prevent injury or further injury to the skin and tissues, to reduce injury to the skin and underlying tissues, and to restore skin integrity. Also evaluate specific interventions designed to promote skin integrity and to teach the patient and family to reduce future threats to skin integrity. In addition, evaluate the patient's and family's need for additional support services, and initiate the referral process.

PATIENT EXPECTATIONS The patient and caregiver need to understand how to prevent or treat pressure ulcers. Some patients enter into the wound-healing phase with unrealistic expectations regarding duration of care. Collect evaluation data about the patient's perception of wound care management. Patients with chronic wounds receive care in their home settings and have certain expectations about their level of comfort, lifestyle, independence, and privacy. Therefore you determine from the patient whether you respected and met his or her expectations.

SAFETY GUIDELINES FOR NURSING SKILLS

Ensuring patient safety is an essential role of the professional nurse. To ensure patient safety, communicate clearly with members of the health care team, assess and incorporate the patient's priorities of care and preferences, and use the best evidence when making decisions about your patient's care. When performing the skills in this chapter, remember the following points to ensure safe, individualized patient care.

• When assessing the patient's skin, reposition the patient to view all areas of the patient's skin. Depending upon the patient's mobility, condition and size, consider asking a member of the health care team to assist in repositioning the patient to avoid trauma or harm to the patient or the caregiver.
• Understand that unwounded skin is always stronger that healed skin. When a patient has a previous history of pres-

sure ulcer or skin damage, the healed skin and tissue present a greater risk for skin breakdown than healthy nonwounded skin.
• Modify the frequency and type of skin assessment to match the patient's risk.
• Modify the frequency of wound assessment based on wound condition.
• Modify skin care and pressure ulcer prevention interventions to match the patient's risk.
• Chronic diseases, especially cardiopulmonary and vascular diseases and diabetes increase the patient's risk for pressure ulcer development and impede healing of wounds.
• When the potential for contamination from spray exists when cleansing a wound, use goggles and moisture-proof gowns.

SKILL 36-1   ASSESSMENT OF PATIENT FOR PRESSURE ULCER: RISK AND SKIN ASSESSMENT

View Video!

DELEGATION CONSIDERATIONS

The skill of assessment of adults for risk for pressure ulcers cannot be delegated to nursing assistive personnel (NAP). The nurse informs NAP to report:

• Any redness or break in the patient's skin
• Any abrasion from assistive devices
• Changes in patient's frequency of incontinence

EQUIPMENT

• Risk assessment tool (e.g., Braden Scale)
• Skin assessment tool
• Documentation record
• Clean gloves

STEP	RATIONALE
ASSESSMENT	
1 Explain procedure.	Information promotes patient cooperation and reduces anxiety.
2 Perform hand hygiene. Close door or bedside curtains.	Reduces transmission of microorganisms. Maintains patient privacy.
3 Identify patient's risk for pressure ulcer formation using the Braden Scale; assign a score for each of the six subscales (see Table 36-1, p. 1065).	Identifies patients at risk for developing pressure ulcers, allowing you to initiate individualized preventive interventions (Ayello and Braden, 2002).
4 Obtain the risk score, and evaluate based on patient's overall condition.	The score will predict the need for interventions to prevent skin breakdown (see Table 36-1).
5 Conduct a systematic skin assessment of bony prominences. Apply clean gloves because you will be pressing on reddened areas and draining wound may be present. Look for at-risk areas of skin breakdown, including (see Figure 36-6, p. 1070): back of head, shoulders, ribs, hips, sacral region, ischium, inner and outer knees, inner and outer ankles, heels, and feet (see Figure 36-6)	Bony prominences are at high risk for skin breakdown because of high pressures exerted on these areas when patient is immobile. A finding of redness or impairment in skin integrity necessitates planning appropriate interventions.
6 Assess the following potential sites for skin breakdown:	
a Ears and nares	Cartilage that nasal cannulas or tubing compresses will develop pressure necrosis.
b Lips	Oral airway and endotracheal tubes exert pressure if left in place for prolonged time periods.

SKILL 36-1	ASSESSMENT OF PATIENT FOR PRESSURE ULCER: RISK AND SKIN ASSESSMENT—cont'd

STEP	RATIONALE
c Tube sites (e.g., gastrostomy or nasogastric tubes, Foley catheters, Jackson-Pratt drains)	Tubes exert pressure if taped snugly against skin or if there is stress at the insertion site. If moisture is present around tube insertion sites, leakage of bodily fluids will compromise skin integrity.
d Orthopedic and positioning devices (e.g., casts, braces, cervical collar)	Improperly fitted or applied devices have the potential to cause pressure on adjacent skin and underlying tissue.
7 Assess all skin surfaces for the following:	
a Absence of superficial skin layers	Damage of superficial skin layers is indicative of injury from friction or moisture. The area will be moist and sore to the touch.
b Blisters	Suggest skin damage from friction and/or inappropriate tape removal. Blisters occur when the top layer of skin is pulled or rubbed, separating the epidermis from the dermis.
c Any loss of epidermis and dermis	Indicates damage to skin. Determine the cause of this damage, and begin interventions to prevent further damage.
8 Determine the patient's ability to sense or report pressure-related discomfort (sensory perception).	Patient with complete or partial limited ability to respond to pressure-related discomfort cannot communicate discomfort or has a limitation in the ability to feel pain, and thus is at risk for developing pressure ulcers.
9 Assess the degree to which the patient's skin is exposed to moisture.	A patient whose skin is exposed to excessive moisture has an increased risk for developing skin breakdown (Pieper, 2007).
10 Evaluate the patient's activity level.	The patient who is bedfast, chairfast, or only walks occasionally is at risk for developing pressure areas because of the degree of physical inactivity (WOCN, 2003).

IMPLEMENTATION

1 If any of the risk factors receive low scores on the risk assessment tool, consider one or more of the interventions listed in Box 36-5 (p. 1068).	The identified risk factors can be eliminated or reduced by instituting appropriate interventions.
2 Assist patient when changing positions during the assessment.	Different positions (e.g., prone, supine, side-lying) are used when completing skin assessment.
3 When you note a reddened area, check for the following:	
a Skin discoloration (e.g., redness in light-tone skin; purplish or bluish in darkly pigmented skin) (see Box 36-4, p. 1067)	May indicate that tissue was under pressure.
b Blanchable erythema	Indicates pressure damage that will resolve. If the redness lightens under the application of pressure, make sure the vessels are intact and that there is no tissue damage present.
c Nonblanchable erythema	Indicates potential damage to blood vessels and tissue damage. Once the blood vessels are damaged, the red area will not lighten in color because the tissue and blood vessels are inflamed.
d Pallor or mottling	Persistent hypoxia in tissues alters circulation, and pallor or mottling may occur.
4 Remove gloves, perform hand hygiene, and reposition patient.	Reduces transmission of microorganisms.

EVALUATION

1 Evaluate patient's skin daily, especially those areas at high risk for breakdown (check agency policy).	Helps you determine success of prevention measures.
2 Compare current risk score with previous scores.	Allows you to provide individualized plan of care.

RECORDING AND REPORTING

- Record risk score, frequency of risk assessment, and appearance of skin, especially pressure points; describe positioning and turning schedule; describe preventive skin interventions; report changes in skin care protocol; document consultation from skin/wound care specialists.

UNEXPECTED OUTCOMES AND RELATED INTERVENTIONS

- Skin becomes mottled, reddened, or blistered.
  - Position patient off affected area, keeping head of bed below 30-degree angle.
  - Obtain health care provider's order for skin care or pressure-reduction or pressure-relieving mattresses.

- Pressure areas become discolored or indurated or exhibit temperature changes.
  - Consult nurse specialist to revise skin care regimen for patient.
  - Consider supportive mattresses.

| SKILL 36-2 | TREATING PRESSURE ULCERS | |

DELEGATION CONSIDERATIONS

The skill of pressure ulcer treatment cannot be delegated to nursing assistive personnel (NAP). The nurse instructs the NAP to:

- Position patient off affected area, keeping head of bed below 30-degree angle.

EQUIPMENT

- Clean gloves (check agency policy regarding use of sterile gloves)
- Goggles and cover gown (optional)
- Plastic bag for dressing disposal
- Measuring device
- Cotton-tipped applicators
- Topical agent (as ordered)
- Cleansing agent (as ordered)
- Sterile solution container
- Washbasin, washcloths, towels
- Dressing of choice
- Hypoallergenic tape (if needed)
- Documentation records

STEP	RATIONALE

ASSESSMENT

1 Identify patient using two identifiers (e.g., name and birthday or name and account number, according to facility policy).

Complies with The Joint Commission requirements and improves procedure safety. In most acute care settings you will use the patient's name and identification number on armband and medical record to identify patients (The Joint Commission, 2009). Information promotes patient cooperation and reduces anxiety.

2 Assess the patient's level of comfort and need for pain medication (Dallan and others, 2004). Administer analgesic as needed.

The dressing change should not be a traumatic event for the patient; the majority of patients with pressure ulcers report pain at dressing change (Krasner, Shapshak, and Hopf, 2007).

3 Determine if patient has allergies to latex or topical agents.

Latex gloves and topical agents contain elements that may cause localized skin reactions.

4 Review the order for topical agent or dressing. Follow six rights of medication administration for a topical agent.

Ensures that proper medication and treatment are administered to right patient.

5 Assess each of the patient's pressure ulcer(s) and surrounding skin to determine ulcer characteristics, including the stage (see Figure 36-5, p. 1062).

Staging is a way of assessing a pressure ulcer, based on the depth of tissue destruction.

SKILL 36-2	TREATING PRESSURE ULCERS—cont'd

STEP	**RATIONALE**

• ***Critical Decision Point:*** To correctly stage a pressure ulcer, you need to be able to see the base of the wound. Therefore pressure ulcers that are covered with necrotic tissue cannot be staged until the eschar is debrided (NPUAP, 2008; WOCN, 2003). Document that the ulcer is unstageable.

6 Assess the type of tissue in the wound bed. Color type indicates the type of tissue. Black tissue is necrotic tissue, yellow tissue is slough, and red tissue is granulation tissue. Chart the approximate amount of each tissue found in the wound bed.

The approximate percentage of each type of tissue in the wound provides critical information on the progress of wound healing and the choice of dressing. A wound with a high percentage of black tissue requires debridement, yellow tissue or slough tissue indicates the presence of an infection, and granulation tissue indicates a wound is beginning to heal.

7 Assess need for revisions to therapy during each dressing change (WOCN, 2003).

Changes in the appearance of a wound can indicate that the topical therapy or type of dressing should be adjusted to continue to promote wound healing.

a Note color, temperature, edema, moisture, and condition of skin around the ulcer. Modify the assessment technique based on the patient's individual skin color (see Box 36-4, p. 1067).

Skin condition at the ulcer edge may indicate progressive tissue damage. Maceration on the periwound skin may show the need to alter the choice of the wound dressing.

b Measure the wound's length and width per agency protocol.

Consistency in how the wound is measured is important for determining wound progress.

c Measure the depth of the pressure ulcer using a sterile cotton-tipped applicator or other device that will allow measurement of wound depth. Place the applicator *gently* into the pressure ulcer until it touches the bottom. Mark the place on the applicator where it reaches the top of the wound, and then remove the applicator from the ulcer. Measure the distance from the tip of the applicator to the mark using a measuring tape or ruler to determine the depth of the pressure ulcer.

Depth measure is important for determining the amount of tissue loss.

d Measure depth of undermining tissue. Use a cotton-tipped applicator, and gently probe under skin edges (see illustration).

Represents the loss of the underlying tissue and may indicate progressive tissue necrosis or ongoing injury from shearing.

8 Remove gloves, discard appropriately, and perform hand hygiene.

Reduces transmission of microorganisms. Different wounds may be contaminated by different organisms. Failure to repeatedly perform hand hygiene can cause cross-wound contamination.

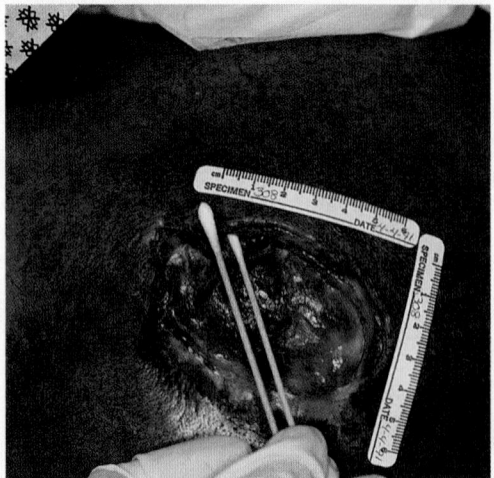

Step 7b-d ■ Measuring length, width, and depth of pressure ulcer.

STEP	RATIONALE

PLANNING

1 Explain procedure to patient and family. Individualize the teaching plan for older adult patients, taking into account the normal aging changes that affect learning.

Preparatory explanations relieve anxiety, correct any misconceptions about the ulcer and its treatment, and offer an opportunity for patient and family education.

2 Prepare the following necessary equipment and supplies:

a Washbasin, warm water, soap, washcloth, and bath towel.

Used to bathe surrounding skin.

b Normal saline or other wound-cleansing agent in sterile solution container.

Ulcer surface must be cleansed before the application of topical agents and a new dressing.

• *Critical Decision Point:* Use only noncytotoxic agents to clean ulcers.

c Prescribed topical agent (e.g., enzymatic agents, topical antibiotic). Follow manufacturer's instructions on the package insert carefully.

Enzymes debride dead tissue to clean ulcer surface. Topical antibiotics are used to decrease the bioburden of the wound and should be considered for use if no healing is noted after 2 to 4 weeks of optimal care (WOCN, 2003).

• *Critical Decision Point:* If using an enzymatic debriding agent, do not use wound-cleansing agents with metals.

d Select an appropriate dressing and tape based on the pressure ulcer characteristics, purpose for which the dressing is intended, and patient care setting (see Table 36-4, p. 1079).

The dressing should maintain a moist environment for the wound while keeping the surrounding skin dry.

3 Position patient to allow dressing removal, and position plastic bag for dressing disposal.

Area should be accessible for dressing change. Proper disposal of old dressing promotes proper handling of contaminated waste.

IMPLEMENTATION

1 Close room door or bedside curtains. Perform hand hygiene and apply clean gloves. Open sterile packages and topical solution containers.

Maintains patient privacy. Have supplies for easy application so that you can use supplies without contaminating them; reduces transmission of microorganisms.

2 Remove bed linen and patient's gown to expose ulcer and surrounding skin. Keep remaining body parts draped.

Prevents unnecessary exposure of body parts.

3 Gently wash skin surrounding ulcer with warm water and soap.

Cleansing of skin surface reduces bacteria.

4 Rinse area thoroughly with water.

Soap can be irritating to skin.

5 Gently dry skin thoroughly by patting lightly with towel.

Retained moisture causes maceration of skin layers.

6 Remove gloves, perform hand hygiene, and apply a new pair of gloves.

Aseptic technique must be maintained during cleansing, measuring, and application of dressings. Refer to institutional policy regarding use of clean or sterile gloves.

7 Cleanse ulcer thoroughly with normal saline or prescribed wound-cleansing agent.

Cleansing wound at each dressing change minimizes the trauma to the wound (WOCN, 2003).

8 Use whirlpool treatments if needed to assist with wound debridement. Keep the wound directly away from the water jets.

Removes wound debris. Previously applied enzymes may require soaking for removal. Do not use whirlpool on clean granulating wounds.

9 Apply topical agents, if prescribed.

a Enzymes:

Follow manufacturer's directions for frequency of application. Be aware of what solutions inactivate the enzymes, and avoid their use in wound cleaning.

SKILL 36-2	TREATING PRESSURE ULCERS—cont'd

STEP	RATIONALE
(1) Using a wooden tongue blade, apply a small amount of enzyme debridement ointment directly to the necrotic areas on the base of pressure ulcer. Avoid getting the enzyme on the surrounding skin. The amount of enzyme should be the same as the amount of butter you would spread on bread. A thick layer of ointment is not necessary; a thin layer absorbs and acts more effectively. Do not apply enzyme to surrounding skin.	Proper distribution of ointment ensures effective action. Some enzymes can cause transient erythema and irritation when in contact with intact skin (Ramundo, 2007).
(2) Place gauze dressing directly over ulcer, and tape it in place. Follow specific manufacturer's recommendation for type of dressing material to use to cover a pressure ulcer when using enzymatic agent.	Protects wound and prevents removal of ointment during turning or repositioning.
(3) If using an antibiotic solution, apply per order and cover with gauze pad. Generally, solution is applied every 12 hours.	
b Hydrogel agents:	
(1) Cover surface of ulcer with hydrogel using applicator or gloved hand.	Provides a moist environment.
(2) Apply a secondary dressing, such as dry gauze, hydrocolloid, or transparent dressing over gel to completely cover ulcer.	Holds hydrogel against wound surface because hydrogel amorphous form (in tube) or sheet form does not adhere to the wound and requires a secondary dressing to hold it in place.
c Calcium alginates:	Use in heavily draining wounds.
(1) Pack wound with alginate using applicator or gloved hand.	
(2) Apply a secondary dressing, such as dry gauze, foam, or hydrocolloid over alginate.	Holds alginate against wound surface.
10 Reposition patient comfortably off pressure ulcer.	Avoids accidental removal of dressings.
11 Remove gloves, and dispose of soiled supplies. Perform hand hygiene.	Reduces transmission of microorganisms.

EVALUATION

1 Observe skin surrounding ulcer for inflammation, edema, and tenderness.	A clean pressure ulcer should show evidence of healing within 2 to 4 weeks.
2 Inspect dressings and exposed ulcers, observing for drainage, foul odor, and tissue necrosis. Monitor patient for signs and symptoms of infection, including fever and elevated white blood cell (WBC) count.	Ulcers can become infected.
3 Compare subsequent ulcer measurements.	Allows comparison of serial measurements to assess wound healing.
4 Use one of the scales designed to measure wound healing, such as the PUSH Scale (Nix, 2007a) or the PSST (Bates-Jensen, 1990).	Provides a standard method of data collection that will demonstrate wound progress, or lack thereof.

RECORDING AND REPORTING

- Record appearance of ulcer in patient's record; describe type of topical agent used, dressing applied, and patient's response; report any deterioration in ulcer appearance to nurse in charge or health care provider.

UNEXPECTED OUTCOMES AND RELATED INTERVENTIONS

- Skin surrounding ulcer becomes macerated.
  - Reduce exposure of surrounding skin to topical agents and moisture.
  - Select a dressing that has increased moisture-absorbing capacity.
- Ulcer becomes deeper with increased drainage and/or development of necrotic tissue.
  - Review current wound care management.
  - Consult with multidisciplinary team regarding changes in wound care regimen.
  - Obtain wound cultures.

- Pressure ulcer extends beyond original margins.
  - Monitor for systemic signs and symptoms of poor wound healing, such as abnormal laboratory results (WBC, hemoglobin/hematocrit, serum albumin, serum prealbumin, total proteins), weight loss, and fluid imbalance.
  - Assess and revise current turning schedule.
  - Consider different pressure-relieving devices (see Table 36-3, p. 1077).

SKILL 36-3	NEGATIVE PRESSURE WOUND THERAPY

DELEGATION CONSIDERATIONS
The skill of negative pressure wound therapy cannot be delegated to nursing assistive personnel (NAP). The nurse instructs NAP to report to the nurse any change in the patient's temperature or level of comfort, the pressure of the negative pressure wound therapy unit, or the dressing.

EQUIPMENT
- Negative pressure wound therapy (NPWT) system (requires health care provider's order) (see Figure 36-13, p. 1081)
- (NPWT) foam dressing

- NPWT tubing for connection between unit and dressing
- Gloves, clean and sterile
- Scissors, sterile
- Waterproof bag for disposal
- Skin preparation/skin barrier
- Moist washcloth
- Linen bag
- Protective gown, mask, goggles (used when spray from wound is a risk)

STEP	RATIONALE

ASSESSMENT

1 Identify patient using two identifiers (e.g., name and birthday or name and account number, according to facility policy).

Complies with The Joint Commission requirements and improves procedure safety. In most acute care settings you will use the patient's name and identification number on armband and medical record to identify patients (The Joint Commission, 2009). Information promotes patient cooperation and reduces anxiety.

2 Assess location, appearance, and size of wound to be dressed.

Allows you to gather information regarding status of wound healing, presence of complications, and type of supplies and assistance needed to apply the NPWT dressing.

3 Review health care provider's orders for frequency of dressing change, type of foam to use, and amount of negative pressure to be used.

Health care provider orders frequency of dressing changes and special instructions.

4 Assess patient's level of comfort using a scale of 0 to 10.

Patient who is comfortable during procedure is less likely to move suddenly, causing wound or supply contamination.

5 Assess patient's and family member's knowledge of purpose of dressing.

Identifies patient's learning needs. Prepares patient and family if dressing will need to be changed at home.

PLANNING

1 Collect equipment and arrange at bedside.

Organizes procedure.

2 Explain procedure to patient.

Relieves anxiety and promotes understanding of healing process.

3 Position patient to allow access to wound site.

Facilitates application of dressing.

4 Plan dressing change to occur 30 minutes after any analgesic is administered.

Provides time for pain medication to reduce or relieve patient's pain at the wound site.

STEP	RATIONALE

IMPLEMENTATION

1 Close room door or cubicle curtains.

2 Position patient, expose wound site, and cover patient.

3 Cuff top of disposable waterproof bag, and place within reach of work area.

4 Perform hand hygiene, and put on clean gloves. If risk for spray exists, apply protective gown, goggles, and mask.

5 Push therapy on/off button on the NPWT system.

6 Raise the tubing connectors above the level of the NPWT unit. Engage clamp on the dressing tubing.

7 Separate canister and dressing tubing at the connection junctions.

8 Allow the therapy unit to pull any drainage in the canister tubing into the canister; then engage the clamp on the canister tubing (Frantz and others, 2007).

9 Gently stretch transparent film horizontally, and slowly pull up from the skin.

10 Remove the foam dressing. Observe the appearance of drainage on dressing. Use caution to remove dressing around drains. Dispose of soiled dressings in waterproof bag. Remove gloves by pulling them inside out, and dispose of them in waterproof bag. Avoid having patient see old dressing. Perform hand hygiene.

11 Apply sterile or clean gloves. Irrigate the wound with normal saline or other solution ordered by the health care provider. Gently blot to dry (see Skill 36-5).

12 Measure wound as ordered: At baseline, first dressing change, weekly, and discharge from therapy. Remove and discard gloves. Perform hand hygiene.

RATIONALE

Provides for patient privacy and reduces transmission of organisms.

Draping provides access to wound while minimizing exposure. Positioning ensures patient comfort during procedure.

Cuff prevents accidental contamination of top of outer bag.

Reduces transmission of infectious organisms from soiled dressings to nurse's hands.

Deactivates therapy.

Allows for proper drainage of fluid in drainage tubing.

Reduces stress on suture line or wound edges and reduces irritation and discomfort.

Determines dressings needed for replacement. Avoids accidental removal of drains. Sight of wound drainage may be upsetting to the patient. Reduces transmission of microorganisms.

Irrigation removes wound debris and cleanses wound bed.

Provides objective measure of wound healing progress.

• *Critical Decision Point:* Wound cultures may be ordered on a routine basis. Obtain cultures during the dressing change if there are local signs of infection: pus, change in odor or character of exudate, redness, induration or change in wound odor (Stotts, 2007).

---

13 Depending on the type of wound, apply new sterile or clean gloves.

Fresh sterile wounds require sterile gloves. Chronic wounds may require clean technique. Do not use the same gloves worn to remove old dressing because cross contamination may occur.

14 Prepare wound edges with a skin preparation product to enhance dressing seal and to protect the periwound skin.

15 Select appropriate foam dressing depending on wound type and stage of healing. Use sterile scissors to cut foam to exact wound size, making sure to fit the size and shape of the wound, including tunnels and undermined areas.

Black polyurethane (PU) foam has larger pores and is most effective in stimulating granulation tissue and wound contraction. Hydrophobic properties of this foam repel moisture, which enhances exudate removal. White polyvinyl alcohol (PVA) soft foam is denser with smaller pores and is used when the growth of granulation tissue must be controlled (Frantz and others, 2007).

• *Critical Decision Point:* Use of black foam may cause patients to experience more pain because of excessive wound contraction. Patients may need to be switched to the white foam.

STEP	RATIONALE
16 Gently place foam in wound, ensuring that the foam is in contact with entire wound base, margins, and tunneled and undermined areas (see illustration). Multiple pieces of foam can be used to adequately fill the wound providing the pieces of foam are in direct contact with each other.	Maintains negative pressure to entire wound. Achieves even distribution of negative pressure (Frantz and others, 2007).
17 Size and trim the transparent dressing to cover wound, and overlap onto intact healthy surrounding skin.	Ensures that the wound is properly covered and a negative pressure seal can be achieved.
18 Secure tubing to the unit to transparent film, aligning drainage hole to ensure an occlusive seal. Do not apply tension to drape and tubing (see illustrations).	Tubing will connect to negative pressure from the NPWT unit to the wound foam. Excessive tension compresses foam dressing and impedes wound healing and produces a shear force on periwound area (KCI, 2004),

---

- *Critical Decision Point:* The wound must stay sealed to avoid wound desiccation. Wounds around joints and near the sacrum are problem areas to seal. An airtight seal can be assisted by clipping hair around wound, cutting transparent film to extend 3 to 5 cm beyond wound perimeter, avoiding wrinkles in transparent film, patching leaks with transparent film, and using multiple small strips of transparent film to hold dressing in place before covering dressing with large piece of transparent film (Chua and others, 2000).

---

19 Secure tubing several centimeters away from the dressing.	Prevents pull on the primary dressing, which can cause leaks in the NPWT system.
20 After the wound is completely covered, connect the tubing from the dressing to the tubing from the NPWT canister (see illustration). **a** Remove new canister from sterile packaging, and push into the negative pressure wound therapy unit until a click is heard. **An alarm will sound if the canister is not properly engaged.**	The target pressures for NPWT vary from 75 mm Hg to 175 mm Hg, depending on the characteristics of the individual wound (Frantz and others, 2007).

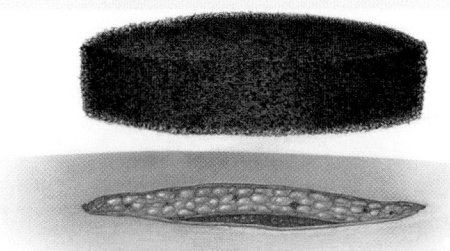

Step 16 ■ Dressing application. Properly sized foam to cover wound.

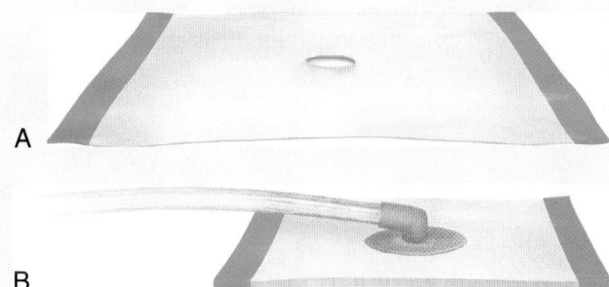

Step 18 ■ **A,** The V.A.C.® GranuFoam™ Dressing. **B,** Secure tubing to the foam and transparent dressing unit. (Courtesy KCI Licensing, Inc., San Antonio, Tex.)

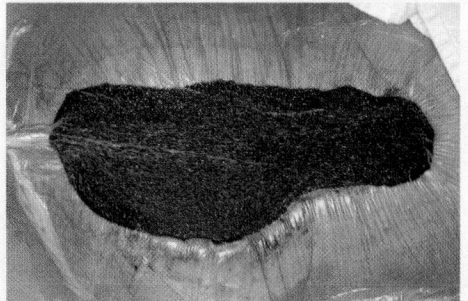

Step 20 ■ Foam dressing, transparent dressing, and V.A.C.® Drape. (Courtesy KCI Licensing, Inc., San Antonio, Tex.)

SKILL 36-3   NEGATIVE PRESSURE WOUND THERAPY—cont'd

STEP	RATIONALE
b Connect the dressing tubing to the canister tubing. Make sure both clamps are open.	
c Place the NPWT unit on a level surface, or hang from the foot of the bed. **The unit will alarm and deactivate therapy if the unit is tilted beyond 45 degrees.**	
d Power the system on using green-lit power button and set negative pressure as ordered.	
21 Discard soiled dressing change materials properly. Remove gloves. Perform hand hygiene.	Reduces transmission of microorganisms.
22 Inspect the NPWT unit to verify that negative pressure is achieved.	Negative pressure is reached when an airtight seal is achieved.
a Verify that display screen reads THERAPY ON.	
b Be sure clamps are open and tubing is patent.	
c If a leak is present, use strips of transparent film to patch areas around the edges of the wound.	
23 Assist patient to a comfortable position.	Enhances patient comfort and relaxation.

EVALUATION

1 Inspect condition of wound on ongoing basis; note drainage and odor.	Determines status of wound healing.
2 Ask patient to rate pain using a scale of 0 to 10.	Determines patient's level of comfort following the procedure.
3 Verify airtight dressing seal and correct negative pressure setting.	Determines patient's level of comfort following the procedure.
4 Measure wound drainage output in canister on a regular basis.	Monitors fluid balance and wound drainage.
5 Observe patient's or family member's ability to perform dressing change.	Indicates patient and family learning has occurred.

RECORDING AND REPORTING

- Record wound appearance, color and characteristics of any drainage, presence of wound healing, and patient tolerance to procedure. Record date and time of new dressing on the dressing as per agency policy.

- Report any brisk, bright red bleeding, evidence of poor wound healing, evisceration or dehiscence, and possible wound infection.

UNEXPECTED OUTCOMES AND RELATED INTERVENTIONS

- Wound appears inflamed and tender, drainage has increased, and an odor is present.
  - Notify health care provider.
  - Obtain wound culture.
- Patient reports increase in pain.
  - If using black foam, switch to white foam.
- Patient needs more analgesic support when negative pressure wound therapy unit is initiated.
  - Reduce negative pressure.

- Negative pressure seal has broken.
  - Take preventive measures; before applying the transparent dressing, clip hair around wound; avoid wrinkles in transparent dressing; and avoid use of adhesive remover because it will leave a residue that interferes with adherence.
  - Reinforce with transparent dressing strips.

SKILL 36-4   APPLYING DRESSINGS: DRY, MOIST, AND TRANSPARENT

DELEGATION CONSIDERATIONS

The care of acute new wounds and those that require sterile technique or a moist dressing cannot be delegated to nursing assistive personnel (NAP). In some states, you can delegate certain aspects of wound care. This sometimes includes the changing of a dry dressing or changing the top dressing. The *assessment* of the wound must be completed by the nurse. The nurse instructs the NAP about:

- Any unique modifications of the skill, such as the need for special tape or methods to secure the dressing
- The need to immediately report to the nurse: increased erythema, drainage, redness in the skin around the wound, or increased pain in the area, which may indicate signs of infection or poor wound healing

EQUIPMENT

- Clean and sterile gloves (check agency policy regarding use of sterile gloves)
- Sterile dressing set (scissors, forceps) (may be *optional;* check agency policy)
- Sterile drape *(optional)*
- Dressings: Sterile fine mesh 4 × 4 gauze flats, abdominal (ABD) pads, roll gauze, and transparent dressing
- Sterile basin *(optional)*
- Antiseptic ointment (as prescribed)
- Cleansing solution (as prescribed)
- Sterile normal saline or prescribed solution
- Tape, ties, or dressing as needed (include nonallergenic tape if necessary)
- Protective waterproof underpad
- Waterproof bag
- Adhesive remover *(optional)*
- Measurement device (optional): tape measure, camera *(optional)*
- Protective gown, mask, goggles (used when spray from wound is a risk)
- Additional lighting if needed (e.g., flashlight, treatment light)

STEP	RATIONALE
ASSESSMENT	
1 Identify patient using two identifiers (e.g., name and birthday or name and account number, according to facility policy). Explain procedure.	Complies with The Joint Commission requirements and improves procedure safety. In most acute care settings you will use the patient's name and identification number on armband and medical record to identify patients (The Joint Commission, 2009). Information promotes patient cooperation and reduces anxiety.
2 Assess size of wound to be dressed (see Skill 36-2).	Assists in planning for proper type and amount of supplies needed.
3 Assess location of wound.	Determines dressing type needed and if assistance is needed to hold dressings in place.
4 Ask patient to rate pain using a scale of 0 to 10.	Removal of dressing can be painful; patient may require pain medication before dressing change to allow drug's peak effect during procedure.
5 Assess patient's knowledge of purpose of dressing change.	Determines level of support and explanation required by patient.
6 Assess need and readiness for patient or family member to participate in dressing wound.	Prepares patient or family member if dressing must be changed at home.
7 Review medical orders for dressing change procedure.	Indicates type of dressing or applications to use.
8 Identify patients with risk factors for wound-healing problems (e.g., aging, prematurity, obesity, diabetes, compromised circulation, poor nutritional status, immunosuppressive drugs, irradiation in area of wound, high levels of stress, steroids).	Risk factors have the potential to affect wound healing and resistance to pathogens (Doughty and Sparks-Defriese, 2007).
PLANNING	
1 Explain procedure to patient.	Decreases patient's anxiety.
2 Position patient to allow access to area to be dressed.	Facilitates application of dressing.
3 Plan dressing change to occur 30 to 60 minutes following administration of analgesic.	Dressing change is better tolerated by patient if pain medication has been administered at least 30 minutes before dressing change.
IMPLEMENTATION	
1 Close room or cubicle curtains. Perform hand hygiene. Apply gown, goggles, and mask if risk for spray exists.	Provides for privacy and reduces transmission of microorganisms.

SKILL 36-4 APPLYING DRESSINGS: DRY, MOIST, AND TRANSPARENT—cont'd

STEP	RATIONALE
2 Position patient comfortably, and drape to expose only wound site. Instruct patient not to touch wound or sterile supplies.	Draping provides access to the wound yet minimizes unnecessary exposure.
3 Place disposable bag within reach of work area. Fold top of bag to make cuff. Put on clean gloves.	Ensures easy disposal of soiled dressings. Prevents contamination of bag's outer surface. Prevents transmission of microorganisms.
4 Remove tape: Pull parallel to skin, toward dressing, and hold down uninjured skin. If over hairy areas, remove in the direction of hair growth. Remove remaining adhesive from skin.	Pulling tape toward dressing reduces stress on suture line or wound edges and reduces irritation and discomfort (Nelson and Dilloway, 2002).
5 With clean-gloved hand or forceps; remove dressings. Carefully remove outer secondary dressing first, and then remove inner primary dressing that is in contact with the wound bed. If drains are present, slowly and carefully remove dressings one layer at a time. Keep soiled undersurface from patient's sight.	The purpose of the primary dressing is to remove necrotic tissue and exudate. Avoids accidental removal of drain. Appearance of drainage may be upsetting to patient.

- *Critical Decision Point:* In a moist dressing, the inner primary dressing if applied properly will have dried and will adhere to underlying tissues; do not moisten it. It is incorrect technique and a common error by some clinicians to moisten the dried gauze before removing it so it does not stick to the wound. This defeats the purpose of using this type of dressing and reduces the amount of debris the dressing will remove (Ramundo, 2007).

6 Inspect wound for color, edema, drains, exudate, and integrity (see illustration). Observe appearance of drainage on dressing. Assess for odor. Gently palpate the wound edges for drainage, bogginess, or patient report of increased pain. Measure wound size (length, width, and depth [if indicated]) (see Skill 36-2).	Provides assessment of drainage and of wound's condition. Indicates movement toward healing (Nix, 2007a).

- *Critical Decision Point:* Dressings that are heavily saturated with exudate indicate a need to add more absorbent gauze dressing to the wound. Assess the wound for any changes in color, drainage, odor, or edema.

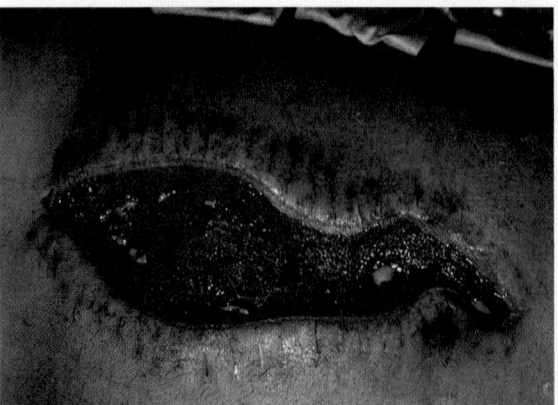

Step 6 ■ Abdominal wound, with beefy red granulation tissue present and attached wound edges. (From Bryant RA, Dix NP, editors: *Acute and chronic wounds: current management concepts,* ed 3, St. Louis, 2007, Mosby.)

STEP	RATIONALE
7 Describe the appearance of the wound and any indicators of wound healing to the patient.	Wounds may appear unsettling and frightening to patients; it is helpful for the patient to know that the wound appearance is as expected and that healing is taking place.
8 Dispose of soiled dressings in disposable bag. Remove gloves by pulling them inside out. Dispose of gloves in bag. Perform hand hygiene.	Reduces transmission of microorganisms.
9 Open sterile dressing tray or individually wrapped sterile supplies. Place on bedside table.	Sterile dressings remain sterile while on or within sterile surface. Preparation of all supplies prevents break in technique during dressing change.
10 Open prescribed cleansing solution, and pour over sterile gauze.	Keeps supplies sterile. Solution may be packaged to spray or pour directly on wound. Microorganisms move from non-sterile environment through dressing package to dressing itself by capillary action.

• **Critical Decision Point:** If sterile drape or gauze packages become wet from solution, repeat preparation of supplies.

STEP	RATIONALE
11 Put on gloves, clean or sterile depending on institution policy.	Sterile gloves allow handling of sterile supplies without contamination. Follow the guidelines of the health care institution related to clean versus sterile gloves. There is insufficient research to support either sterile or clean gloves as being more effective in decreasing infection and improving wound healing (Gray and Doughty, 2001).
12 Cleanse wound:	
a Use separate swab for each cleansing stroke, or spray wound surface.	Prevents contaminating previously cleaned area.
b Clean from least contaminated area to most contaminated, with center of wound least contaminated.	Cleansing in this direction prevents introduction of organisms into wound.
c Cleanse around the drain (if present), using circular stroke starting near drain and moving outward and away from the insertion site.	Correct aseptic technique in cleansing prevents contamination of wound.
13 Use dry gauze to blot in same manner as in Step 12 to dry wound. Dry thoroughly.	Drying reduces excess moisture, which could eventually harbor microorganisms. Transparent dressings do not adhere to damp surfaces.
14 Apply antiseptic ointment if ordered, using same technique as for cleansing.	Helps reduce growth of microorganisms.
15 Apply dressings to incision or wound site:	A dressing protects wound, prevents infection, and provides comfort.
a Dry Dressing	
(1) Apply loose woven gauze as contact layer.	Promotes proper absorption of drainage.
(2) Cut 4 × 4 gauze flat to fit around drain if present, or use precut split drain flat.	Secures drain and promotes drainage absorption at site.
(3) Apply additional layers of gauze as needed.	Layering ensures proper coverage and optimal absorption.
(4) Apply thicker woven pad (e.g., Surgipad, abdominal dressing [ABD]).	This type of dressing is often used for postoperative wounds.
b Moist Dressing	
(1) Moisten gauze dressing with prescribed solution.	

• **Critical Decision Point:** Open or unfold the gauze that will be placed directly against the wound bed. Sometimes "packing strip" may be used to pack the wound (see illustration A for Step 15b(2)). When using packing strip, with sterile scissors cut the amount of dressing that is anticipated to be used to pack the wound. Do not let the packing strip touch the side of the bottle. Pour prescribed solution over the gauze or strip to moisten it, wring out excess fluid. Contact layer must be moist to increase dressing's absorptive abilities.

STEP	RATIONALE
(2) Wring out excess fluid, and apply moist fluffed gauze or packing strip directly onto wound surface without having the gauze touch the surrounding skin (see illustration A).	Moist gauze absorbs drainage and wicks wound debris (Rolstad and Ovington, 2007).

STEP	RATIONALE

- *Critical Decision Point:* If wound is deep, gently lay moistened woven gauze over wound surface with forceps until all surfaces are in contact with moist gauze and the wound is loosely filled. Fill the wound, but avoid packing the wound too tightly or having the gauze extend beyond the top of the wound (see illustration *B* for Step 15b(2)*B*).

(3) Make sure any dead space from sinus tracts, undermining, or tunneling is loosely packed with gauze.	Do not overpack the wound too tightly; it can cause wound trauma (Rolstad and Ovington, 2007).
(4) Apply dry sterile gauze over moistened gauze.	Dry layer absorbs excessive moisture from wound.
(5) Cover the packed wound with a secondary dressing such as an ABD pad, Surgipad, or gauze.	Protects wound from entrance of microorganisms.
c **Transparent Dressing**	
(1) Apply dressing according to manufacturer's directions. Do not stretch film during application. Avoid wrinkles in film.	Wrinkles provide a tunnel for exudate to accumulate.
16 Secure dressing with roll gauze (for circumferential dressings) (see illustration *A*), tape, Montgomery ties or straps (which are applied perpendicular to the wound) (see illustration *B*), or binder.	Supports wound and ensures placement and stability of dressing.

- *Critical Decision Point:* If areas of redness appear from tape, paper tape or alternatives such as elastic dressing, Kerlix, or a binder may be used to secure dressing. Sometimes strips of a hydrocolloid dressing are placed on the skin under the Montgomery ties to further protect the skin.

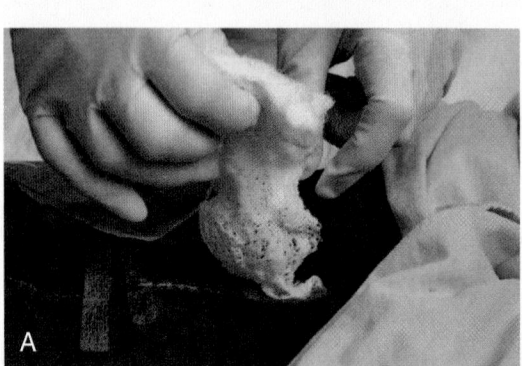

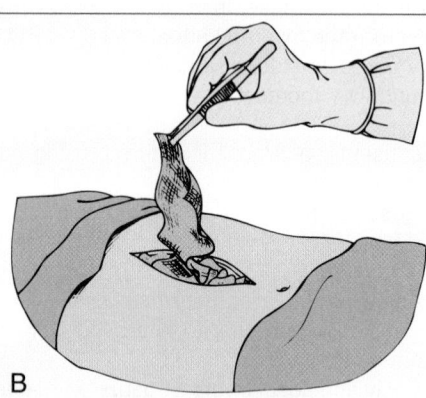

Step 15b(2) ■ **A,** Packing wound. **B,** Wound packed loosely, until wound is filled.

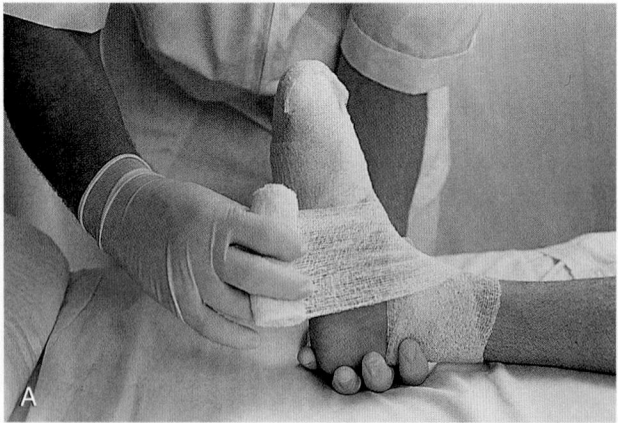

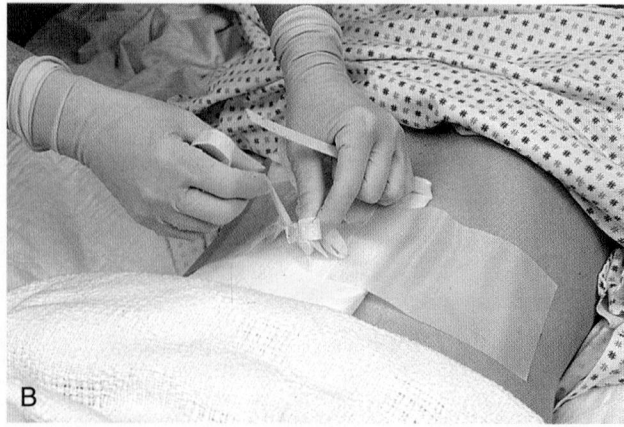

Step 16 ■ **A,** Application of roll gauze. **B,** Securing Montgomery ties.

STEP	RATIONALE
17 Remove gloves, gown (if worn), and dispose of them in bag. Dispose of all supplies. Remove goggles if worn.	Reduces transmission of microorganisms. Clean environment enhances patient comfort.
18 Assist patient to comfortable position.	Promotes patient's sense of well-being.
19 Perform hand hygiene.	Reduces transmission of microorganisms.

EVALUATION

1 Inspect condition of wound and presence of any drainage.	Determines rate of healing.
2 Have patient rate level of pain during procedure.	Pain is often an early indication of wound complication or result of dressing pulling tissue.
3 Inspect condition of dressing at least every shift.	Determines status of wound drainage.
4 Ask patient to describe steps and techniques of dressing change.	Evaluates patient's learning.

RECORDING AND REPORTING

- Record appearance of wound, color, presence and characteristics of exudate, change in wound characteristics, especially drainage amount, type and amount of dressings applied, and tolerance of patient to dressing change.

- Report unexpected appearance of wound drainage or accidental removal of drain, bright red bleeding, or evidence of wound dehiscence or evisceration.
- Write your initials, date, and time of dressing change on a piece of tape in ink (not marker), and place on dressing.

UNEXPECTED OUTCOMES AND RELATED INTERVENTIONS

- Wound drainage increases.
  - Increase frequency of dressing changes.
  - Notify health care provider, who may consider drain placement or alternative dressing method.
- Wound bleeds during dressing change.
  - Assess patient medication history and history of bleeding disorder.
  - If excessive, may need to apply pressure.
  - Observe color and amount of drainage.
  - Notify health care provider.

- Patient reports sensation that "something has given way under the dressing."
  - Remove dressing, and inspect wound for dehiscence or evisceration.
  - Protect wound. Cover with sterile moist dressing.
  - Instruct patient to lie still.
  - Remain with patient to monitor vital signs.
  - Notify health care provider.
- Skin around wound margins becomes red, macerated, or excoriated.
  - Avoid allowing outer layer of wet-to-dry dressing to become too moist.
  - Notify health care provider.
  - Consult with wound care specialist on the appropriate dressing to use.
  - Securing method for dressing is causing irritation.
  - Change to paper tape.

| **SKILL 36-5** | PERFORMING WOUND IRRIGATION | |

DELEGATION CONSIDERATIONS

The skill of wound irrigation cannot be delegated to nursing assistive personnel (NAP). In some settings you can delegate the cleansing of chronic wounds using clean technique to NAP. It is the responsibility of the nurse to assess the wound and evaluate wound care interventions before any delegation. The nurse instructs the NAP to:
- Report any changes in the patient's comfort level or wound drainage, increase in temperature, or any bright red drainage.
- Report when a wound is cleansed the wound color, presence of bleeding, or drainage.

EQUIPMENT
- Irrigant/cleansing solution (volume one to two times the estimated wound volume)
- Irrigation delivery system depending on amount of pressure desired:
- Sterile 35-mL irrigation syringe with sterile soft angiocatheter or 19-gauge needle (WOCN, 2003)
- Clean and sterile gloves
- Waterproof underpad, if needed
- Dressing supplies
- Disposable waterproof bag
- Gown, goggles, mask for risk for spray
- Wound assessment supplies

| SKILL 36-5 | PERFORMING WOUND IRRIGATION—cont'd |

STEP	RATIONALE

ASSESSMENT

1　Identify patient using two identifiers (e.g., name and birthday or name and account number, according to facility policy). Explain procedure.

Complies with The Joint Commission requirements and improves procedure safety. In most acute care settings you will use the patient's name and identification number on armband and medical record to identify patients (The Joint Commission, 2009). Information promotes patient cooperation and reduces anxiety.

2　Review health care provider's order for irrigation of open wound and type of solution to be used.

Open wound irrigation requires medical order including type of solution(s) to use.

3　Assess recent recording of signs and symptoms related to patient's open wound:

  a　Extent of impairment of skin integrity, including size of wound (measure length, width, and depth). Wounds should be measured in centimeters and in the following order: length, width, and depth.

This assesses volume of irrigation solution needed. Data also used as baseline to indicate change in condition of wound.

  b　Drainage from wound (amount and color). Amount can be measured by part of dressing saturated or in terms of quantity (e.g., scant, moderate, copious).

Expect amount to decrease as healing takes place. Serous drainage is clear like plasma; sanguineous or bright red drainage indicates fresh bleeding; serosanguineous drainage is pink; purulent drainage is thick and yellow, pale green, or white.

  c　Odor. Must state whether or not there is odor.

Strong odor indicates infectious process.

  d　Wound color.

Color represents a balance between necrotic tissue and new scar tissue. Proper selection of wound products, based on the color of the wound, facilitates removal of necrotic tissue and promotes new tissue growth (Rolstad and Ovington, 2007).

  e　Consistency of drainage.

Type and color of drainage is dependent on moisture of the wound and type of organisms present.

  f　Culture reports.

Chronic wounds heal by secondary intention, and they are often colonized with bacteria.

  g　Dressing: dry and clean; evidence of bleeding, profuse drainage.

Provides an initial assessment of present wound drainage.

4　Assess comfort level or pain on a scale of 0 to 10, and identify symptoms of anxiety.

Discomfort may be related directly to wound or indirectly to muscle tension or immobility. Anxiety results from multiple factors (e.g., surgery, diagnosis, awaiting pathology reports) and anticipation of unknown nursing interventions (e.g., first wound irrigation).

5　Assess patient for history of allergies to antiseptics, tapes, or dressing material.

Known allergies suggest application of a sample of prescribed antiseptic as skin test before flushing wound with large volume of solution or selection of different tape or dressing material.

PLANNING

1　Explain procedure of wound irrigation and cleansing.

Information will reduce patient's anxiety.

2　Administer prescribed analgesic 30 to 60 minutes before starting wound irrigation procedure.

Promotes pain control and permits patient to move more easily and be positioned to facilitate wound irrigation.

3　Position patient.

  a　Position comfortably to permit gravitational flow of irrigating solution through wound and into collection receptacle (see illustration).

Directing solution from top to bottom of wound and from clean to contaminated area prevents further infection. Position patient during planning stage, keeping in mind the bed surfaces needed for later preparation of equipment.

  b　Position patient so that wound is vertical to collection basin. Place container of irrigant/cleaning solution in basin of hot water to warm solution to body temperature.

Warmed solution increases comfort and reduces vascular constriction response in tissues.

  c　Place padding or extra towel in the bed.

Protects bedding.

  d　Expose only wound.

Prevents chilling of patient.

STEP	RATIONALE

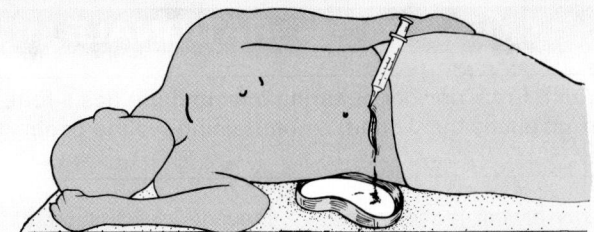

Step 3a ■ Position of patient for abdominal wound irrigation.

IMPLEMENTATION

STEP	RATIONALE
1 Perform hand hygiene.	Reduces transmission of microorganisms.
2 Form cuff on waterproof biohazard bag, and place it near bed.	Cuffing helps to maintain large opening, thereby permitting placement of contaminated dressing without touching refuse bag itself.
3 Close room door or bed curtains.	Maintains privacy.
4 Apply gown, goggles, and mask.	Protects nurse from splashes or sprays of blood and body fluids.
5 Apply clean gloves, and remove soiled dressing and discard in waterproof bag. Discard gloves. Perform hand hygiene.	Reduces transmission of microorganisms.
6 Prepare equipment; open sterile supplies.	
7 Apply sterile gloves.	Prevents transfer of microorganisms to wound surface.
8 To irrigate wound with wide opening:	
a Fill 35-mL syringe with irrigation solution.	Flushing wound helps remove debris and facilitates healing by secondary intention.
b Attach 19-gauge angiocatheter.	Provides ideal pressure for cleansing and removal of debris (Rolstad and Ovington, 2007).
c Hold syringe tip 2.5 cm (1 inch) above upper end of wound and over area being cleansed.	Prevents syringe contamination. Careful placement of the syringe prevents unsafe pressure of the flowing solution.
d Using continuous pressure, flush wound; repeat Steps 8a, b, and c until solution draining into basin is clear.	Clear solution indicates all debris has been removed.
9 To irrigate deep wound with very small opening:	
a Attach angiocatheter to filled irrigating syringe.	Catheter permits direct flow of irrigant into wound. Expect wound to take longer to empty when opening is small.
b Lubricate tip of catheter with irrigating solution; then gently insert tip of catheter, and pull out about 1 cm (½ inch).	Removes tip from fragile inner wall of wound.

   • *Critical Decision Point:* Do not force catheter into the wound, because this could cause tissue damage.

---

c Using slow, continuous pressure, flush wound.	Provides adequate force to remove debris without damaging healthy tissue (Ramundo, 2007).

   • *Critical Decision Point:* CAUTION: Splashing may occur during this step.

---

  d Remove and refill syringe. Reconnect to catheter, and repeat until solution draining into basin is clear.

   • *Critical Decision Point:* Pulsatile high-pressure lavage may be the irrigation of choice for necrotic wounds. The amount of irrigant is wound-size dependent. Pressure settings on the device should remain between 8 and 15 psi. Do not use pulsatile high-pressure lavage on exposed blood vessels, muscle, tendon, and bone. This type of irrigation should not be used with graft sites and should be used with caution in patients receiving anticoagulant therapy (Ramundo, 2007).

---

10 When indicated, obtain cultures after cleansing with non-bacteriostatic saline.

| SKILL 36-5 | PERFORMING WOUND IRRIGATION—cont'd |

STEP	RATIONALE

- **Critical Decision Point:** Consider culturing a wound if it has a foul, purulent odor; inflammation surrounds the wound; a nondraining wound begins to drain; or patient is febrile.

STEP	RATIONALE
11 Dry wound edges with gauze; dry patient if shower or whirlpool is used.	Prevents maceration of surrounding tissue from excess moisture.
12 Apply appropriate dressing (see Skill 36-4).	Maintains protective barrier and healing environment for wound.
13 Remove gloves, mask, goggles, and gown.	Prevents transfer of microorganisms.
14 Assist patient to comfortable position.	
15 Dispose of equipment and soiled supplies, and perform hand hygiene.	Reduces transmission of microorganisms.

EVALUATION

1 Observe type of tissue in wound bed.	Identifies wound healing progress and determines type of wound cleansing and dressing needed.
2 Inspect dressing periodically.	Determines patient's response to wound irrigation and need to modify plan of care.
3 Evaluate skin integrity.	Determines if extension of wound has occurred.
4 Observe patient for signs of discomfort.	Patient's pain should not increase as a result of wound irrigation.
5 Observe for presence of retained irrigant.	Retained irrigant is a medium for bacterial growth and subsequent infection.

RECORDING AND REPORTING

- Record wound irrigation and patient response in progress notes.
- Immediately report any evidence of fresh bleeding, sharp increase in pain, retention of irrigant, or signs of shock to attending health care provider.

UNEXPECTED OUTCOMES AND RELATED INTERVENTIONS

- Bleeding or serosanguineous drainage appears.
  - Flush wound during next irrigation using less pressure.
  - Notify health care provider of bleeding.
- Opening in suture line extends.
  - Notify health care provider.
  - Reevaluate amount of pressure to use for next wound irrigation.

- Retained fluid and debris appear.
  - Increase amount of fluid used during irrigation.
  - Increase amount of pressure when flushing wound.
  - Make sure wound is clear of retained fluid and debris before applying dressing.

KEY POINTS

- Wounds with partial-thickness tissue loss heal by epidermal repair, and full-thickness wounds heal by forming scar tissue.
- A clean surgical incision with little tissue loss heals by primary intention.
- When there is extensive tissue loss, a wound heals by secondary intention.
- Healing of full-thickness wounds proceeds through four overlapping phases: hemostasis, inflammation, proliferation, and remodeling.
- The chances of wound infection are greater when the wound contains dead or necrotic tissue, when foreign bodies lie on or near the wound, and when blood supply and tissue defenses are reduced.

- Physical stress from vomiting, coughing, or sudden muscular contraction causes separation of wound edges, dehiscence.
- Wound assessment includes anatomical location, size (dimensions and depth of wound), type and percentage of wound tissue, volume and color of wound drainage, and condition of surrounding skin.
- Wound drains remove secretions within tissue layers to promote wound closure.
- Never collect a wound culture from old drainage.
- Principles of wound management include controlling or eliminating the cause, providing systemic support to reduce existing and potential cofactors, and maintaining a physiological local wound environment.

- A moist environment supports wound healing.
- When cleaning wounds or drain sites, clean from the least to most contaminated area.
- Apply a dressing or binder in a manner that does not impair circulation or irritate the skin.
- The safe use of heat or cold therapy requires an assessment of the patient's sensory function, identification of risk factors, and understanding of the physiological effects of heat and cold.
- An acute sprain, fracture, or bruise responds best to cold applications.
- Warm applications are effective for improving circulation to wound sites and promoting muscle relaxation.

CRITICAL THINKING EXERCISES

1. Mr. Ahmed has a pressure ulcer over his sacral area. After reviewing his case study what is the major contributing factor to the development of this pressure ulcer? Name two interventions that would be appropriate for reducing the contributing factor. Explain the rationale for your answer.

2. Mr. Ahmed has a stage II pressure ulcer. What information does the assessment of a stage II pressure ulcer provide, what other assessments are important when assessing the pressure ulcer, and why are these assessments important?

3. On assessing the patient for risk of development of a pressure ulcer using the Braden Scale, you note that Mr. Ahmed scores very low on the moisture subscale. You determine that the patient has had frequent bowel movements and is incontinent of liquid stool at least two times in 24 hours. What are some of the possible interventions that you will plan for Mr. Ahmed to protect his skin from fecal incontinence?

℮volve   *Answers to Critical Thinking Questions can be found on the Evolve website.*

REVIEW QUESTIONS

1. When repositioning an immobile patient, the nurse notices redness over a bony prominence. When the area is assessed, the red spot blanches with fingertip pressure, indicating:
   1. A local skin infection requiring antibiotics
   2. This patient has sensitive skin and requires special bed linen
   3. A stage III pressure ulcer, needing the appropriate dressing
   4. Pressure damage that will resolve upon redistribution of the pressure

2. Pressure injury to the skin results from:
   1. Blood vessel damage from repeated injections
   2. Continual exposure of the skin to fecal or urinary incontinence
   3. Compression of the skin by two surfaces for a prolonged period of time
   4. Excessive dryness of the epidermis, allowing damage to the dermis

3. The topical management of a clean, granular wound healing by secondary intention requires:
   1. A moist wound dressing
   2. An antibiotic cream applied twice a day
   3. Whirlpool treatments to stimulate granulation tissue
   4. A treatment plan that allows the wound to be exposed to air for 15 minutes twice a day

4. When obtaining a wound culture specimen to determine the presence of a wound infection, the nurse correctly collects the specimen from:
   1. The necrotic tissue
   2. The wound drainage
   3. The drainage on the dressing
   4. Clean, healthy-looking tissue

5. Postoperatively the patient with a closed abdominal wound reports a sudden "pop" after coughing. When the nurse examines the surgical wound site, the sutures are open and pieces of small bowel are noted at the bottom of the now opened wound. The correct intervention is:
   1. Allow the area to be exposed to air until all drainage has stopped
   2. Pace several cold packs over the area, protecting the skin around the wound
   3. Cover the area with sterile saline–soaked towels and immediately notify the surgical team
   4. Cover the area with sterile gauze, place a tight binder over the area, and ask the patient to remain in bed for 30 minutes

6. The nurse recognizes that serous drainage from a wound is defined as:
   1. Fresh bleeding
   2. Thick and yellow
   3. Clear, watery plasma
   4. Beige to brown and foul smelling

7. Nursing interventions to manage a patient who is experiencing fecal and urinary incontinence include which of the following? Select all that apply.
   1. Using a large absorbent diaper, changing when saturated
   2. Keeping the buttocks exposed to air at all times
   3. Using an incontinence cleanser, followed by application of a moisture-barrier ointment
   4. Offering of frequent ambulation and assistance to the toilet

8. The patient asks the nurse what a hydrocolloid dressing is. The best description provided by the nurse is that a hydrocolloid dressing is:
   1. A seaweed derivative that is highly absorptive
   2. Premoistened gauze, placed over a granulating wound
   3. A debriding enzyme that is used to remove necrotic tissue
   4. A dressing that forms a gel that interacts with the wound surface

9. The nurse recognizes that a binder placed around a surgical patient with a new abdominal wound is indicated for:
   1. Collection of wound drainage
   2. Reduction of abdominal swelling
   3. Reduction of stress on the abdominal incision
   4. Stimulation of peristalsis (return of bowel function) from direct pressure

10. A patient undergoes emergency surgery for a ruptured diverticulum. At the time of surgery it is determined to allow the wound to heal by secondary intention because there was fecal spillage into the abdominal cavity. It is determined that negative pressure wound therapy would be the appropriate wound intervention because:
    1. It provides wound protection from bacteria or other contaminants, preventing overgrowth of bacteria in the wound base
    2. It is a system that provides continuous irrigant under negative pressure in the wound bed, stimulating granulation tissue
    3. It is a wound management system that uses negative pressure to the wound to promote and accelerate healing
    4. It is a method to clean the wound bed of necrotic tissue without the use of toxic solutions

Answers to Review Questions can be found on pages 1197-1198.

REFERENCES

Ayello EA, Braden B: How and why do pressure ulcer risk assessment, *Adv Skin Wound Care* 15(3):125, 2002.

Ayello EA, Lyder CH: Pressure ulcers in person of color: race and ethnicity. In Cuddigan J, editor: *Pressure ulcers in America: prevalence, incidence, and implications for the future,* Reston, VA, 2001, National Pressure Ulcer Advisory Panel.

Ayello EA and others: Pressure ulcers. In Baranoski S, Ayello EA: *Wound care essentials: practice principles,* Philadelphia, 2004, Lippincott Williams & Wilkins.

Bates-Jensen B: New pressure ulcer status tool, *Decubitus* 3(3):14, 1990.

Bennett MA: Report of the task force on the implications for darkly pigmented intact skin in the prediction and prevention of pressure ulcers, *Adv Wound Care* 8(6):34, 1995.

Bergstrom N and others: A clinical trial of the Braden Scale for predicting pressure sore risk, *Nurs Clin North Am* 22(2):417, 1987a.

Bergstrom N and others: The Braden Scale for predicting pressure sore risk, *Nur Res* 36:205, 1987b.

Bergstrom NL and others: Predicting pressure ulcer risk: a multisite study of the predictive validity of the Braden Scale, *Nurs Res* 47(5):261, 1998.

Bulechek GM and others, editors: *Nursing interventions classification (NIC),* ed 5, St. Louis, 2008, Mosby.

Bryant RA, Clark RAF: Skin pathology and types of damage. In Bryant RA, Nix DP, editors: *Acute and chronic wounds: current management concepts,* ed 3, St. Louis, 2007, Mosby.

Chua PC and others: Vacuum Assisted Closure, *Am J Nurs* 100(12):45, 2000.

Dallan LE and others: Pain management and wounds. In Baranoski S, Ayello EA: *Wound care essentials: practice principles,* Philadelphia, 2004, Lippincott Williams & Wilkins.

Dibsie LG: Implementing evidence-based practice to prevent skin breakdown, *Crit Care Nurs Q* 31(2):140, 2008.

Doughty DL, Sparks-Defriese B: Wound healing physiology in acute and chronic wounds. In Bryant RA, Nix DP, editors: *Acute and chronic wounds: current management concepts,* ed 3, St. Louis, 2007, Mosby.

Fader M, Bain D, Cottenden A: Effects of absorbent incontinence pads on pressure management mattresses, *J Adv Nurs* 48(6):569, 2004.

Frantz RA and others: Devices and technology in wound care. In Bryant RA, Nix DP, editors: *Acute and chronic wounds: current management concepts,* ed 3, St. Louis, 2007, Mosby.

Gray M, Doughty DB: Clean versus sterile technique when changing wound dressings, *J Wound Ostomy Continence Nurs* 28(3):125, 2001.

Henderson CT and others: Draft definition of stage I pressure ulcers: inclusion of persons with darkly pigmented skin, *Adv Wound Care* 10(5):16, 1997.

Jones V, Bale S, Harding K: Acute and chronic wound healing. In Baranoski S, Ayello EA: *Wound care essentials: practice principles,* Philadelphia, 2004, Lippincott Williams & Wilkins.

Kinetic Concepts Inc (KCI): *The V.A.C.: Vacuum Assisted Closure—V.A.C. therapy clinical guidelines: a reference source for clinicians,* Product information, San Antonio, Tex, 2004, Kinetic Concepts, Inc.

Krasner DL, Shapshak D, Hopf HW: Managing wound pain. In Bryant RA, Nix DP, editors: *Acute and chronic wounds: current management concepts,* ed 3, St. Louis, 2007, Mosby.

Landis EM: Micro-injection studies of capillary blood pressure in human skin, *Heart* 15:209, 1930.

Mathus-Vliegen EMH: Old age, malnutrition and pressure sores: an ill fated alliance, *J Gerontol A Biol Sci Med Sci* 59(4):355, 2004.

McInerney JA: Reducing hospital-acquired pressure ulcer prevalence through a focused prevention program, *Adv Skin Wound Care* 21(2):75, 2008.

Moorhead S and others, editors: *Nursing outcomes classification (NOC),* ed 4, St. Louis, 2008, Mosby.

National Pressure Ulcer Advisory Panel (NPUAP): *Pressure ulcer staging,* 2008, http://www.npuap.org.

Nelson DB, Dilloway MA: Principles, products, and practical aspects of wound care, *Crit Care Nurs Q* 25(1):33, 2002.

Nix DP: Patient assessment and evaluation of healing. In Bryant RA, Nix DP, editors: *Acute and chronic wounds: current management concepts,* ed 3, St. Louis, 2007a, Mosby.

Nix DP: Support surfaces. In Bryant RA, Nix DP, editors: *Acute and chronic wounds: current management concepts,* ed 3, St. Louis, 2007b, Mosby.

Noonan C, Quigley SM, Curley MAQ: Skin integrity in hospitalized infants and children: a prevalence survey, *J Pediatr Nurs* 21(6):445, 2006.

O'Brien JM, Reilly NJ: Comparison of tape products on skin integrity, *Adv Wound Care* 8(6):26, 1995.

Pieper B: Mechanical forces: pressure, shear, friction. In Bryant RA, Nix DP, editors: *Acute and chronic wounds: current management concepts,* ed 3, St. Louis, 2007, Mosby.

Ramundo JM: Wound debridement. In Bryant RA, Nix DP, editors: *Acute and chronic wounds: current management concepts,* ed 3, St. Louis, 2007, Mosby.

Reddy M, Gill SS, Rochon PA: Preventing pressure ulcers: a systematic review, *JAMA* 296(8):974, 2006.

Rolstad BS, Ovington LG: Principles of wound management. In Bryant RA, Nix DP, editors: *Acute and chronic wounds: current management concepts,* ed 3, St. Louis, 2007, Mosby.

Rook JL: Wound care pain management, *Adv Wound Care* 9(6):24, 1996.

Schultz GS and others: Wound bed preparation: a systematic approach to wound management, *Wound Repair Regen* 11(suppl 1):S1, 2003.

Stotts NA: Wound infection: diagnosis and management. In Bryant RA, Nix DP, editors: *Acute and chronic wounds: current management concepts,* ed 3, St. Louis, 2007, Mosby.

Stotts NA, Wu HS: Hospital recovery is facilitated by prevention of pressure ulcers in older adults, *Crit Care Nurs Clin North Am* 19(3):269, 2007.

Thomas C: Specialty beds: decision making made easy, *Ostomy Wound Manage* 23:51, 1989.

Trelease CC: Developing standards for wound care, *Ostomy Wound Manage* 20:46, 1988.

Wound, Ostomy and Continence Nurses Society (WOCN): *Guideline for prevention and management of pressure ulcers,* WOCN Clinical Practice Guidelines Series, Glenview, Ill, 2003, The Society.

Sensory Alterations 37

MEDIA RESOURCES

 CD COMPANION   evolve **WEBSITE** http://evolve.elsevier.com/Potter/basic

- Crossword Puzzle
- English/Spanish Audio Glossary

OBJECTIVES

- Differentiate the processes of reception, perception, and reaction to sensory stimuli.
- Discuss common causes and effects of sensory alterations.
- Discuss common sensory changes that occur with aging.
- Identify factors to assess in determining a patient's sensory status.
- Describe behaviors indicating sensory alterations.
- Develop a nursing care plan for patients with visual, auditory, tactile, gustatory, and olfactory alterations.

- Describe nursing interventions with rationale that promote effective communication with patients who have sensory alterations.
- Describe conditions in the health care agency or patient's home that you will adjust to promote meaningful sensory stimulation.
- Discuss ways to maintain a safe environment for patients with sensory alterations.

KEY TERMS

accommodation, p. 1113
age-related macular degeneration, p. 1112
auditory, p. 1112
cataracts, p. 1112
diabetic retinopathy, p. 1112

glaucoma, p. 1112
gustatory, p. 1112
Meniere's disease, p. 1114
olfactory, p. 1112
ototoxic, p. 1113
presbycusis, p. 1113

presbyopia, p. 1114
proprioception, p. 1112
refractive errors, p. 1122
sensory deficits, p. 1112
sensory deprivation, p. 1112

sensory overload, p. 1112
tactile, p. 1112
tinnitus, p. 1113
visual, p. 1112

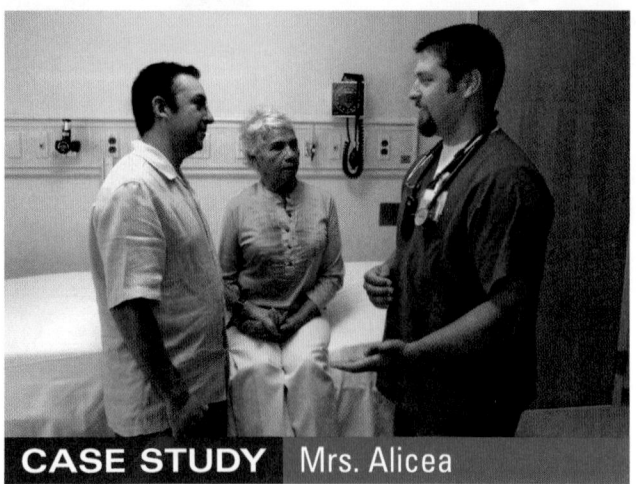

CASE STUDY Mrs. Alicea

Mrs. Alicea is a 73-year-old woman who is at the senior health center for her routine 6-month checkup. She has been visiting the senior center on a regular basis for the past 8 years. Mrs. Alicea has lived alone since her husband died 1 year ago. She lives in a single-story, four-room home a few miles away from the health center. Her son, Rico, lives 5 minutes away. Rico drives Mrs. Alicea to her health care visits. Six months ago Mrs. Alicea reported progressive hearing loss. Today when she enters the clinic she reports "having trouble seeing."

Peter Morris, a 33-year-old nursing student assigned to the senior health center, is learning to conduct assessments and to develop health promotion plans for visiting patients. For the past month, Peter has been attending his clinical rotation at the center and participating in teaching health promotion activities. He is enjoying this rotation because he is learning more about geriatric patients and is finding that they are very independent and capable of having productive lifestyles.

People are unique because they are able to sense a variety of stimuli in their environment. Stimulation comes from many sources in and outside the body, particularly through the senses of sight (**visual**), hearing (**auditory**), touch (**tactile**), smell (**olfactory**), and taste (**gustatory**). Additional senses include the senses of pressure, pain, temperature, vibration, and position sense (**proprioception**) (Meiner and Lueckenotte, 2006). People learn about the environment from healthy sensory organs. The patient's ability to relate to and function within the environment changes when sensory function is altered. As a nurse, you need to recognize when patients are at risk for developing sensory problems. Furthermore, you need to understand and help to meet the needs of patients when they have sensory alterations. Your nursing care helps patients learn to alter their environment for improved safety.

SCIENTIFIC KNOWLEDGE BASE

Normal Sensation

People feel and react to sensations when the nervous system is intact. Perception or awareness of sensations depends on a region of the cerebral cortex where specialized brain cells interpret the quality and nature of each sensory stimulus. Sensory experiences include reception, perception, and reaction. People react to stimuli that are most meaningful to them. When people attempt to react to every stimulus within their environment or when stimuli are lacking, sensory alterations occur.

Types of Sensory Alterations

Many factors influence the capacity to receive or perceive sensations (Box 37-1). In your nursing experience you will care for patients with **sensory deficits, sensory deprivation,** and **sensory overload.** When patients suffer from more than one sensory alteration, their ability to function and relate within the environment becomes impaired.

SENSORY DEFICITS Four major diseases frequently cause impaired vision in Americans age 40 and over. They are **age-related macular degeneration, glaucoma, cataracts,** and **diabetic retinopathy** (Ebersole and others, 2008). The National Eye Institute (2008) predicts that by 2020 age-related macular degeneration will affect 2.9 million people; glaucoma, 3.3 million people; cataracts, 30.1 million people; and diabetic retinopathy, 7.2 million people.

A sensory deficit occurs when problems with sensory reception or perception exist (Box 37-2). Patients are not able to receive certain stimuli (e.g., light and sound), or stimuli are distorted (e.g., blurred vision from cataracts and abnormal taste sensation from xerostomia). A sudden sensory loss caused by injury or as a side effect to medications (Box 37-3) causes fear, anger, and feelings of helplessness. Some patients withdraw socially to cope with the loss (Ebersole and others, 2005). In addition, the patient's safety is threatened because the person is unable to respond normally to stimuli. When a deficit is chronic or develops gradually, the patient learns to rely on unaffected senses. Some senses even become more acute to compensate for an alteration. For example, a patient who is blind often develops an acute sense of hearing. Changes in sensory deficits cause patients to change their behaviors in adaptive or maladaptive ways.

SENSORY DEPRIVATION Sensory deprivation occurs when inadequate quality or quantity of stimuli impairs perception. Reduced sensory input (hearing loss), confusion, and a restricted environment (bed rest) are three types of sensory deprivation. These effects sometimes produce cognitive changes such as the inability to solve problems, poor task performance, and disorientation. Second, affective changes, which include boredom, restlessness, increased anxiety, or emotional lability, occur. Finally, perceptual changes such as reduced attention span, disorganized visual and motor coordination, and confusion of sleeping and waking states also occur.

BOX 37-1   Factors That Influence Sensory Function

AGE

Infants

Binocular vision begins at 6 weeks and is well established by 4 months. During the second year of life, infants discriminate shapes, objects, and colors.

Neonates respond to loud noises. Within a year infants visually locate the source of noises.

Newborns react to strong odors such as alcohol and vinegar by turning their heads. Newborns can identify their own mother's milk.

Children

Refractive errors are the most common types of visual disorders in children and are treated with corrective lenses. Serious visual impairment affects a child's ability to play and socialize. Children are usually frightened and confused by a sudden or progressive loss of sight. Parents and children need support to help them adjust to the disability (Hockenberry and Wilson, 2007).

Adults

Visual changes include presbyopia and the need for glasses for reading (ages 40 to 50). Also, the cornea, which assists with light refraction to the retina, becomes flatter and thicker. These aging changes lead to astigmatism. Pigment is lost from the iris and collagen fibers build up in the anterior chamber, which increases the risk for glaucoma by decreasing the reabsorption of intraocular fluid.

Older Adults

Hearing changes often associated with aging include decreased hearing acuity, speech intelligibility, and pitch discrimination, which is referred to as **presbycusis.** Low-pitched sounds are easiest to hear, but it is difficult to hear conversation over background noise. It is also difficult to discriminate consonants (*f, z, s, th, ch, p, k, t,* and *g*). Vowels that have a low pitch are easier to hear. Speech sounds are distorted, and there is a delayed reception and reaction to speech. A decrease in active sebaceous glands causes the cerumen to become dry and completely obstruct the external auditory canal (Ebersole and others, 2008).

Visual changes often include reduced visual fields, increased glare sensitivity, impaired night vision, reduced **accommodation,** reduced depth perception, and reduced color discrimination. Many of these symptoms occur because the pupils in the older adult take longer to dilate and constrict secondary to weaker iris muscles. Color vision decreases because the retina is duller and the lens yellows. Nearly everyone between ages 40 and 45 requires glasses for close vision acuity (Ebersole and others, 2005).

Olfactory changes begin around age 50 and include a loss of cells in the olfactory bulb of the brain and a decrease in the number of sensory cells in the nasal lining. Reduced sensitivity to odors is common. A small decrease in the number of taste cells occurs with aging, beginning around age 60. Reduced sour, salty, and bitter taste discrimination is common. The ability to detect sweet tastes seems to remain intact (Ebersole and others, 2005).

Proprioceptive changes in some older adults include an increased difficulty with balance, spatial orientation, and coordination. These older adults cannot avoid obstacles as quickly nor are they able to prevent an accident from happening to themselves when fast action is necessary. The automatic response to protect and brace oneself when falling is slower.

Older adults sometimes experience tactile changes, including declining sensitivity to pain, pressure, and temperature secondary to peripheral vascular disease and neuropathies.

MEDICATIONS

Ototoxic medications (see Box 37-3), such as analgesics, antibiotics, or diuretics, affect hearing acuity, balance, or both, with the most common symptom being **tinnitus** (ringing in the ears). Ototoxicity causes a progressive or continuing hearing loss that in many patients goes unnoticed (McKenry and others, 2005). Hearing loss is not always permanent depending upon the extent of damage and the length of time that the drug is given. Patients with renal failure have an increased sensitivity to ototoxic drugs (McKenry and others, 2005).

ENVIRONMENT

Excessive environmental stimuli result in sensory overload, marked by confusion, disorientation, and inability to make decisions. Restricted environmental stimulation leads to sensory deprivation. Poor quality of environment worsens sensory impairment.

PREEXISTING ILLNESSES

Peripheral vascular disease causes reduced sensation in the extremities and impaired cognition. Diabetes often causes reduced vision or blindness or peripheral neuropathy. Some neurological disorders, such as stroke, impair sensory reception (Meiner and Lueckenotte, 2006).

SMOKING

Chronic tobacco use atrophies the taste buds and affects olfactory function.

NOISE LEVELS

Constant exposure to high noise levels causes hearing loss.

Children often demonstrate behaviors related to sensory deprivation by a higher-than-normal level of anxiety that causes restlessness, difficulty with problem solving, and depression (Hockenberry and Wilson, 2007). In adults the symptoms of sensory deprivation are similar to psychological illness, confusion, symptoms of severe electrolyte imbalance, or the influence of psychotropic drugs. Accurate diagnosis of a problem is crucial.

SENSORY OVERLOAD When a person receives multiple sensory stimuli, the brain has difficulty distinguishing the stimuli, which cause a sensory overload to occur. The person no longer perceives the environment in a way that makes

BOX 37-2 | Common Sensory Deficits

VISUAL

- **Presbyopia:** Gradual decline in ability of the lens to accommodate or to focus on close objects. Reduces ability to see near objects clearly.
- *Cataract:* Cloudy or opaque areas in part of the lens or the entire lens. Interferes with passage of light through the lens and reduces the light that reaches the retina. Cataracts usually develop gradually and result in cloudy or blurry vision, glare, and poor night vision (National Eye Institute, 2008).
- *Dry eyes:* Result when tear glands produce too few tears, resulting in itching, burning, or even reduced vision.
- *Glaucoma:* A slowly progressive increase in intraocular pressure that causes progressive pressure against the optic nerve. At first, vision stays normal, and there is no pain. If left untreated, there will be a loss of peripheral (side vision), and straight-ahead vision may decrease until no vision remains (National Eye Institute, 2006a).
- *Diabetic retinopathy:* Pathological changes of the blood vessels of the retina secondary to increased pressure resulting in hemorrhage, macular edema, and reduced vision or vision loss (Mohamed and others, 2007).
- *Age-related macular degeneration:* Occurs when the macula (specialized portion of the retina responsible for central vision) degenerates as a result of aging and loses its ability to function efficiently. An early sign includes distortion that causes edges or lines to appear wavy. In later stages, patients may see dark or empty spaces that block the center of vision (Ebersole and others, 2005).

HEARING

- *Presbycusis:* A common progressive hearing disorder in older adults.

- *Cerumen accumulation:* Buildup and hardening of earwax in the external auditory canal causes conduction deafness.

BALANCE

- *Dizziness and disequilibrium:* Common condition in older adulthood, usually resulting from vestibular dysfunction and precipitated by change in position of the head to the rest of the body.
- **Meniere's disease:** Cause is unknown but diagnosis is based on medical history interview, physical examination, and clinical symptoms of intermittent hearing loss, vertigo, tinnitus, and a full feeling or pressure in the affected ear (American Hearing Research Foundation, 2006).

TASTE

- *Xerostomia:* Decrease in salivary production that leads to thicker mucus and a dry mouth. Interferes with the ability to eat and leads to appetite and nutritional problems.

NEUROLOGICAL

- *Peripheral neuropathy:* Most commonly associated with diabetes. Other causes include alcoholism, peripheral vascular disease, traumatic injury, medication effects, infections, and immune system diseases (Torpy, 2008). Characterized by symptoms that include numbness and tingling of the affected area and stumbling gait.
- *Hemiplegia:* Caused by a thrombus, hemorrhage, or embolus affecting a blood vessel leading to or within the brain. Creates altered proprioception with marked incoordination and imbalance. Loss of sensation and motor function in extremities controlled by the affected area of the brain also occurs.

BOX 37-3 | Examples of Medications Reported to Cause Ototoxicity

ANTIBIOTICS
- Aminoglycosides
- Vancomycin

SALICYLATES
- Aspirin

NSAIDS
- Ibuprofen

DIURETICS
- Ethacrynic acid
- Furosemide
- Bumetanide

ANTINEOPLASTIC AGENTS
- Cisplatin

From Monahan FD: Assessment of the auditory system. In Monahan F and others: *Phipps' medical-surgical nursing: health and illness perspectives*, ed 8, St. Louis, 2007, Mosby.

sense. Overload prevents a meaningful response to a stimulus by the brain. As a result, thoughts race, attention moves in many directions, and restlessness occurs. The patient demonstrates panic, confusion, and aggressiveness. Sleep loss is common. Sensory overload causes a state similar to sensory deprivation.

Patients who are acutely ill easily develop sensory overload in the health care environment. Constant pain, noise from equipment, and the nursing activities of turning, repositioning, and administering treatments bombard patients with stimuli. Some patients are more sensitive to sensory overload than others. Behavioral changes are easily confused with mood swings or disorientation. Constant reorientation and control of excessive stimuli become an important part of the patient's care.

NURSING KNOWLEDGE BASE

An estimated 28 million Americans suffer from some type of hearing loss (National Institute on Deafness and Other Communication Disorders, 2008). Eighty million Americans have

BOX 37-4 BEST PRACTICES

Risk Factors for Self-Reported Visual Impairment

SUMMARY OF EVIDENCE

Visual impairment is a risk factor for a variety of negative health-related outcomes. A better understanding of the prevalence of and risk factors for visual impairment will help nurses plan appropriate interventions to meet the needs of persons with impaired vision. One group of researchers asked middle-age and older American adults about their vision status and risk factors for visual impairment during telephone interviews. The evidence indicated that self-reported visual impairment is an extremely prevalent condition. Advanced age, ethnicity, poorer self-rated health, and low availability of informal social support were significant risk factors associated with visual impairment. Vision rehabilitation interventions are needed to reduce the functional limitations that can result from visual impairment.

APPLICATION TO NURSING PRACTICE
- Assess all patients for signs of visual impairment.
- Share with patients the signs and behaviors that may indicate vision problems.
- Encourage patients to notify their health care provider of pain in the eyes, difficulty seeing in darkened areas, double or distorted vision, and flashes of light or halos surrounding light.
- Be aware that cultural influences may affect your patient's willingness to self-report a visual impairment.
- Ask patients who have visual impairments what they think is important in their care and what goals are important to them.
- Inquire about the patient's perceived availability of social support and informal assistance.
- Work with patients and families to determine how to make the environment safe while promoting the patients' independence and meeting their individualized health care needs.
- Inform patients and caregivers of resources available in the community that can influence the patient's functional and emotional well-being.

REFERENCE

Horowitz A, Brennan M, Reinhardt JP: Prevalence and risk factors for self-reported visual impairment among middle-aged and older adults, *Res Aging* 27(3):307, 2005.

---

eye diseases that will lead to blindness, while 14 million will have low vision (American Federation for the Blind, 2004). By 2020, 5.5 million Americans over the age of 40 will have a diagnosis of blindness or low vision (National Eye Institute, 2004). It is estimated that the United States population of older adults age 65 and over will double by 2030 (Ebersole and others, 2005). Therefore age-related declines in sensory function will continue to increase and will contribute to sensory alterations in many older adults. The loss of major sensory input can have profound consequences on patients' functioning and everyday life. As a nurse, stay informed of new health care and nursing knowledge as it pertains to the older adult population and the effects of diverse sensory changes.

Vision and hearing alterations often have profound consequences for function and quality of life of older adults (Ebersole and others, 2005). There is a relationship between sensory impairments, self-esteem, and communication. Patients with sensory impairments may feel a loss of control or independence. Feelings of grief, anger, isolation, depression, and loneliness are also common. To promote healthy aging, you must be knowledgeable about the effects of sensory loss on your patients. Assess how a sensory impairment influences a patient's self-concept and ability to communicate and function in the everyday world.

Older adults who experience sensory deficits often withdraw from social activities. The risk for social isolation, depression, fear, and low self-esteem interferes with their ability to care for themselves and interact with others. According to research, reduced visual acuity is also negatively associated with quality of life in individuals with type 2 diabetes who are

40 to 75 years of age (Clarke and others, 2006). Education by the nurse about disease process, available social services, assistive devices, and the need for annual physical examinations helps provide the older patient with better coping abilities and health maintenance.

Managing patients with sensory alterations challenges you to apply nursing research and information from your practice to help patients participate in their environment, remain socially interactive, and continue to be productive. In addition, your application of critical thinking principles helps you to promote patients' sensory function and to protect them from possible injury (Box 37-4).

CRITICAL THINKING

Synthesis

You will apply elements of critical thinking whenever you perform the nursing process with a patient. Consider the scientific knowledge you have learned, your experience, critical thinking attitudes, and standards to ensure an individualized approach to patient care (Box 37-5). As you apply the nursing process for patients with sensory alterations, anticipate the kind of information necessary to form good clinical judgments. A combination of past patient care experiences and the application of scientific and nursing knowledge help you select an individualized plan of care for the patient.

KNOWLEDGE A number of factors cause sensory alterations. Knowledge of those factors as well as anatomy and physiology, and the normal components of a sensory experi-

BOX 37-5   SYNTHESIS IN PRACTICE

 While Peter prepares to assess Mrs. Alicea, he recalls what he has learned about the pathophysiology of eye disorders. Peter will focus on the "warning signs" of eye problems, determining which, if any, of the signs Mrs. Alicea has experienced. Because Mrs. Alicea reportedly has hearing and visual losses, Peter will consider the communication approaches best suited for conducting a successful assessment. It will be helpful for Peter to position himself so that Mrs. Alicea is able to see his face clearly. Peter also needs to speak slowly and enunciate words clearly, giving time for Mrs. Alicea to respond to questions. Avoidance of questions answered by "yes" or "no" will require Mrs. Alicea to provide more detailed answers, ensuring that she has heard the questions correctly.

Peter respects Mrs. Alicea's cultural background and explores the role Rico plays in supporting his mother. The Hispanic culture often shows respect for elders and authority figures by not maintaining direct eye contact. They also often engage in "small talk" before discussing the serious aspects of the interview, because being direct is considered rude, and self-disclosure is for those whom the indi-

vidual knows well (Gonzalez and others, 2008). It will thus be important for Peter to express caring and respect for Mrs. Alicea and provide time for small talk to be successful in gathering a complete assessment. Hispanic patients frequently value health practitioners who are informal and friendly and who include family members in the interactions. Taking time to listen is also important. Family interdependence is valued in the Mexican American culture (Gonzalez and others, 2008). Rico will play a key role in Mrs. Alicea's ability to maintain self-care. Peter needs to determine if Rico is the primary individual who offers assistance with Mrs. Alicea's instrumental activities of daily living (IADLs) or other activities.

Peter's own grandmother has bilateral cataracts. He reflects on how his grandmother adjusted to her visual loss in order to continue activities she enjoys. Peter learned in class that you can make a variety of adaptations to maximize the sensory functions a patient still has. Peter will plan to discover if Mrs. Alicea has made any adaptations in her home environment. Creativity will be an important attitude to exercise.

ence help you understand how a particular alteration affects a patient's function. Knowing the pathophysiological changes of sensory organ disorders will also help you anticipate how sensory changes affect a patient. When you identify characteristics of sensory alterations and the interventions to minimize them, you are able to implement a comprehensive and individualized plan of care.

Depending on the patient's problem, use your knowledge of communication principles (see Chapter 10) to select the best method to communicate with the patient. Patients with hearing impairments require different communication approaches to obtain a complete and accurate nursing assessment and to deliver interventions effectively. You also need to have a good knowledge of pharmacology because a variety of medications affect sensory function. Being able to anticipate the side effects of medications allows you to prepare patients for possible sensory changes.

EXPERIENCE Many of us have experienced altered sensory function personally or while interacting with family, friends, or patients. Previous personal or clinical experiences with sensory changes help you to anticipate the patient's care needs. How do individuals adapt to hearing aids and glasses? What adjustments do they make to function safely in their homes? What communication techniques are necessary when speaking to individuals with hearing impairment? Such experiences will help you to choose successful nursing interventions when caring for patients in a variety of health care settings.

ATTITUDES Critical thinking attitudes lead you to become a more disciplined thinker. Creativity is often necessary to find the right solutions for your patient's problems. For example, living in a nonstimulating home environment can cause your patient's sensory deprivation. Working with the

patient, suggest changes to the environment that improve the quality of stimulation and reduce the patient's risk for injury. Curiosity applies when a patient shows unexplained behavioral changes. Asking why and being curious help you to assess a less obvious sensory problem.

STANDARDS An important ethical standard to follow when assisting patients with sensory alterations is preservation of autonomy (see Chapter 5). For the patient to regain independence, do not override autonomy with the principle of beneficence. You need to remember that although professionals believe they know what is best, patients have to live with the sensory alteration and adapt to the consequences of their own choices. The Joint Commission, along with the Americans with Disabilities Act (ADA), requires health care institutions to address the needs of patients with sensory alterations and to provide interpretation services as necessary to establish understanding and to maintain confidentiality (The Joint Commission [TJC], 2008).

NURSING PROCESS

■■■ ASSESSMENT

When assessing your patients, consider age and other factors that influence sensory function. Collect a complete nursing history by examining how a sensory deficit affects your patient's lifestyle, self-care ability, psychosocial adjustment, health promotion habits, and safety. Also, focus the assessment on the quality and quantity of stimuli within the patient's environment.

PATIENTS AT RISK Conduct a sensory assessment for any patient at risk for sensory alterations. Older adults are a high-risk group because of normal physiological changes associated

BOX 37-6   CULTURAL FOCUS

 Peter is aware that Hispanic/Latino people are the largest minority group in the United States. However, he is uncertain if disparities in sensory alteration exist across ethnicities. Therefore, before he meets with Mrs. Alicea on his next clinical day, Peter takes some time to read about sensory alterations in the Latino population.

Peter learns that Hispanic/Latino individuals in the United States have higher rates of visual impairment and blindness than members of other ethnic groups. Visual field loss has a negative impact on health-related quality of life. Areas of health-related quality of life most affected include difficulties related to driving, distance and peripheral vision activities, and a sense of dependency. Peter uses this information to develop a culturally competent plan that focuses on Mrs. Alicea's visual impairment.

IMPLICATIONS FOR PRACTICE

- Review with Mrs. Alicea at each visit the importance of early intervention through regular vision examinations.
- Provide information about side effects of the visual impairment and encourage the use of visual and adaptive devices whenever possible.
- Ask Mrs. Alicea how she is coping with visual alterations.
- Ask Mrs. Alicea about her social networks and supportive relationships.
- Assess for changes in mood and depression.
- Determine if Mrs. Alicea has experienced new limitations of activities of daily living or a change in participation in leisure activities.
- Refer to community resources and activities.

Data from McKean-Cowdin R and others: Severity of visual field loss and health-related quality of life, *Am J Ophthalmol* 143:1013, 2007; National Eye Institute: *Statement on the prevalence of visual impairment and how it affects quality of life among Hispanic/Latino Americans*, 2006b, http://www.nei.nih.gov.

with aging. Older patients may be unaware of sensory changes or be sensitive about admitting sensory losses (Ebersole and others, 2005). Patients who are immobilized by bedrest, physical impediments (e.g., casts or traction), or chronic disability are unable to experience all the normal sensations of free movement. Such conditions lead to sensory deprivation. Always remain alert for any behavioral changes common to sensory deprivation. Patients isolated in a health care setting or at home because of conditions such as active tuberculosis or severe immune system depression are often isolated in a private room and frequently experience sensory deprivation.

Hospital environments are full of sensory stimuli. When ill or hospitalized, patients are often confined to an unfamiliar and unresponsive environment. This does not mean that all hospitalized patients experience sensory overload. Carefully assess patients subjected to high stress levels (e.g., intensive care unit [ICU] environment, long-term hospitalization, and multiple therapies). Be aware that patients can have a combination of a sensory deficit and overload simultaneously.

Certain sensory alterations occur more commonly in select ethnic groups. Data from the National Health Interview Survey (NHIS) showed that Aleuts, Eskimos, and American Indians have three times the rate of simultaneous hearing and visual impairment relative to Asian/Pacific Islander Americans (Caban and others, 2005). Be aware of sensory alterations that are associated with a patient's cultural heritage (Box 37-6).

SENSORY STATUS Include in the nursing history an assessment of the nature and characteristics of sensory alterations. Assessment categories include the type and extent of sensory impairment, the onset and duration of symptoms, and whether there are factors that aggravate or relieve symptoms. Often you will observe such characteristics by watching the patient perform routine activities of daily living (ADLs) in the home or health care setting. Table 37-1 provides examples of factors to assess, relevant questions to address with your patient, and appropriate physical assessment strategies.

PATIENT'S LIFESTYLE Learn about a patient's perception of a sensory loss to find out how the patient's quality of life has been influenced. Ask patients to describe any problems the sensory alteration creates for their normal daily routines and lifestyle (see Table 37-1). Does a sensory alteration change your patient's ability to retain social relationships, continue performing at work or school, or function within the home?

SOCIALIZATION The amount and quality of contact with family members or friends determines whether a patient with sensory alterations becomes isolated. Assess if a patient lives alone and whether family, friends, or neighbors frequently visit. The absence of visitors at home or to a health care setting creates a sense of monotony that contributes to social isolation. Also assess the patient's social skills and level of satisfaction in the support given by family and friends.

SELF-CARE MANAGEMENT A patient's functional ability incorporates ADLs (e.g., grooming, bathing, dressing, and toileting) and instrumental activities of daily living (IADLs) (e.g., grocery shopping, writing a check, and using a phone). If a sensory alteration impairs your patient's functional ability, planning for discharge from a health care setting and providing resources within the home become necessary. You need to consider the activities patients normally do for themselves and how the sensory alteration impairs their functioning (see Table 37-1).

PSYCHOSOCIAL ADJUSTMENT Because some patients are unaware of or are unwilling to discuss behavioral changes, family and friends are often the best resources when determining if sensory changes have altered a patient's behavior. Assess if the patient has shown any recent mood swings such as outbursts of anger, depression, or fear. Does the patient avoid interactions with others? Sensory alterations also often cause changes in the patient's orientation and ability to concentrate.

HEALTH PROMOTION PRACTICES Assess the daily routines patients follow in maintaining sensory function. The information will determine the patient's need for education or referral to appropriate resources (see Table 37-1).

TABLE 37-1 FOCUSED PATIENT ASSESSMENT

FACTORS TO ASSESS	QUESTIONS	PHYSICAL ASSESSMENT
Sensory status	Do you have problems with your ears, hearing, balance, vision, or sensing touch? If so, when did the difficulty begin? Did it begin gradually or suddenly? Is it constant, or does it come and go? How would you describe it? What are your preferences for treatment? If appropriate, would you wear glasses to improve your vision or hearing aids to improve communication?	Assess patient's hearing, balance, vision, and sense of touch (see Chapter 15). Observe patient behaviors during conversation and while watching the patient perform IADLs and ADLs.
Self-care management in home and community care settings	Are you able to prepare a meal or write a check (for patients with visual alterations)? Is there a certain pitch that you have trouble hearing, such as conversation on the telephone or the telephone ringing (for patients with hearing impairments)? Are you able to dress or bathe safely using warm water (for patients with decreased tactile sensation)?	Observe patient in the home, in the kitchen while preparing a meal. Observe the patient's ability to communicate effectively. Observe patient during dressing and bathing.
Health promotion practices	How do you clean your ears? Do you have difficulty caring for your glasses, hearing aids, or contact lenses? Do you wear safety glasses, eye shields, or ear noise protective gear when appropriate?	Find out when the patient last had an eye or ear screening. Observe ear/eye routine care. Check for appropriate eye protection with eye shields and safety glasses or face shields.

ADLs, Activities of daily living; *IADLs,* instrumental activities of daily living.

HAZARDS Make sure the home environment is healthy, comfortable, and safe. A thorough home assessment will help you provide options for ways to make the home safe. First assess the home setting, including the outdoors and all rooms in the home, for any hazards that increase the risk for injury (e.g., poorly lit stairs, obstacles in walking paths, uneven sidewalks). A home safety checklist is usually available in most home care agencies. The type of sensory alteration makes certain home features more hazardous than others. Patients with impaired vision will require more light. Patients who are blind often need information written in braille. Patients with hearing deficits sometimes require safety alarms with visual signals. Those with severe hearing impairments need to have a telecommunication device for the deaf (TDD). The TDD has a keyboard and displays numbers and letters that provide messages to the hearing impaired from another TDD. The Americans with Disabilities Act requires any health care facility that receives financial aid from Medicare to have TDDs for the hearing impaired (Ebersole and others, 2005).

In a health care setting, assess for any factors that will be dangerous to the patient. Assess a patient's hospital room for clutter, unnecessary equipment, and obstacles in the path leading to the bathroom. Also ask the patient about barriers or obstacles the patient perceives as potentially dangerous.

MEANINGFUL STIMULI Meaningful stimuli reduce the incidence of sensory deprivation. In the home, check for the use of bright colors, comfortable furnishings, adequate lighting, good ventilation, and clean surroundings. Also observe for presence of pets, family pictures, television, a clock, or calendar.

In a health care setting, note if patients have roommates, visitors, or any personal items such as pictures. A patient will become disoriented in a barren environment that gives few signals for normal sensory perception. Meaningful stimuli influence the patient's alertness and the ability to participate in self-care.

ENVIRONMENT Excessive environmental stimuli causes sensory overload. In an acute care setting the frequency of observations, tests, and procedures is often stressful to the patient. The location of a patient's room near repetitive or loud noises (e.g., nurses' station or supply room) contributes to sensory overload. In addition, explore a loud television or roommate or a bright room light as possible contributing factors. Patients who are in pain, traction, or restricted by a cast are also at risk for excessive stimulation. Your responsibility as a nurse is to reduce or eliminate excessive stimuli.

COMMUNICATION METHODS To understand the quality of patients' communication, assess whether they have trouble speaking, understanding, reading, or writing. Next, ask patients what communication method they prefer. Patients with existing sensory deficits often develop alternative ways of communicating. Some patients with hearing impairments read lips, use sign language, wear a hearing aid, or read and write notes. Patients with visual impairments learn to detect voice tones and inflections to identify the emotional tone of a conversation. To assess communication methods, sit facing the patient, speaking in a normal tone. Disorganized speech, long periods of silence, or a patient who continually asks you to repeat your sentence indicates a sensory deficit in the patient. Some patients also exhibit signs and symptoms of

TABLE 37-2 Behaviors Indicating Sensory Deficits

BEHAVIOR INDICATING DEFICIT (CHILDREN)	BEHAVIOR INDICATING DEFICIT (ADULTS)
VISION	
Self-stimulation, including eye rubbing, body rocking, sniffing, arm twirling; hitching (using legs to propel while in sitting position) instead of crawling	Poor coordination, squinting, underreaching or overreaching for objects, persistent repositioning of objects, impaired night vision, accidental falls
HEARING	
Frightened when unfamiliar people approach, no reflex or purposeful response to sounds, failure to be awakened by loud noise, slow or absent development of speech, greater response to movement than to sound, avoidance of social interaction with others	Blank looks, decreased attention span, lack of reaction to loud noises, increased volume of speech, positioning of head toward sound, smiling and nodding of head in approval when someone speaks, use of other means of communication such as lip reading or writing, complaints of ringing in ears
TOUCH	
Inability to perform developmental tasks related to grasping objects or drawing, repeated injury from handling of harmful objects (e.g., hot stove, sharp knife)	Clumsiness, overreaction or underreaction to painful stimulus, failure to respond when touched, avoidance of touch, sensation of pins and needles, numbness
SMELL	
Difficult to assess until child is 6 or 7 years old, difficulty discriminating unpleasant odors	Failure to react to noxious or strong odors, increased body odor, decreased sensitivity to odors
TASTE	
Inability to tell whether food is salty or sweet, possible ingestion of strange-tasting things	Change in appetite, excessive use of seasoning and sugar, complaints about taste of food, weight change
POSITION SENSE	
Clumsiness, extraneous movement, excessive arm swinging in those with hyperactivity or learning difficulty	Poor balance and spatial orientation, shuffling gait, reduced response to brace self when falling, more precise and deliberate movements

confusion or respond in an inappropriate manner secondary to their hearing impairment.

PHYSICAL EXAMINATION Patients with known or suspected sensory deficits resulting from visual and hearing losses, spinal cord injury, or peripheral neuropathies require complete and detailed sensory examinations (see Chapter 15). Assessing the extent of sensory loss allows you to focus your review on behaviors of sensory deficits (Table 37-2). If your examination suggests a sensory deprivation, observation during history taking, physical examination, or care will provide additional information about the person's condition. Also observe the patient's physical appearance, measure cognitive ability, and assess emotional stability. At this time, also remember that factors other than sensory deprivation or overload cause impaired perception (e.g., medications, pain, or electrolyte imbalances).

PATIENT EXPECTATIONS When conducting an assessment, review the patient's expectations. Some patients enter the health care system willingly, whereas others experience confusion or unfamiliarity in that environment. Many patients have a definite plan as to how they want their care delivered. Some patients expect you to either perform care or provide equipment for them so they will properly care for their sensory aids (glasses or hearing aids). Asking patients what they expect helps you to know if you need special communication methods.

Some patients request that family members or friends help with their care. Begin by asking, "What do you expect from the nursing staff to feel you are being well cared for?" and "Now that I better understand what affects your ability to see/hear, what do you expect in the care we will be providing you?"

■■■ NURSING DIAGNOSIS

After assessment, review all available data and look for patterns of defining characteristics that represent nursing diagnoses relating to sensory alterations. For example, asking others to repeat spoken words, inappropriate response to questions, head tilting, social avoidance, irritability, ear pain, and withdrawal are defining characteristics for the nursing diagnosis *disturbed sensory perception: auditory*. Validate your findings by collaborating with a colleague or asking the patient to self-rate his or her hearing on a scale of 1 to 10, 1 representing perfect hearing and 10 representing deafness. The same approach can be used with vision. The following are examples of nursing diagnoses you can use for patients with sensory alterations:

- *Anxiety*
- *Disturbed body image*
- *Fear*
- *Hopelessness*
- *Risk for injury*

- *Deficient knowledge*
- *Risk for loneliness*
- *Bathing self-care deficit*
- *Disturbed sensory perception*
- *Impaired social interaction*

Next, determine the likely related factor for the nursing diagnosis to ensure that you select appropriate interventions. For example, impacted cerumen is the cause of a patient's hearing alteration. In this case, irrigation of the canal with 2 to 3 ounces of tepid water in a 60-mL syringe will improve auditory percep-

tion (Barnett, 2007). If the patient's auditory alteration is related to altered sensory reception from nerve deafness, nursing interventions of alternative communication methods will be more successful in minimizing the patient's hearing impairment.

■ ■ ■ PLANNING

Patients with sensory alterations will have many needs (Figure 37-1). The plan of care you develop depends on your assessment of the patient's sensory perception and acceptance of the sensory alteration and how well the patient has adjusted to the loss (see Care Plan).

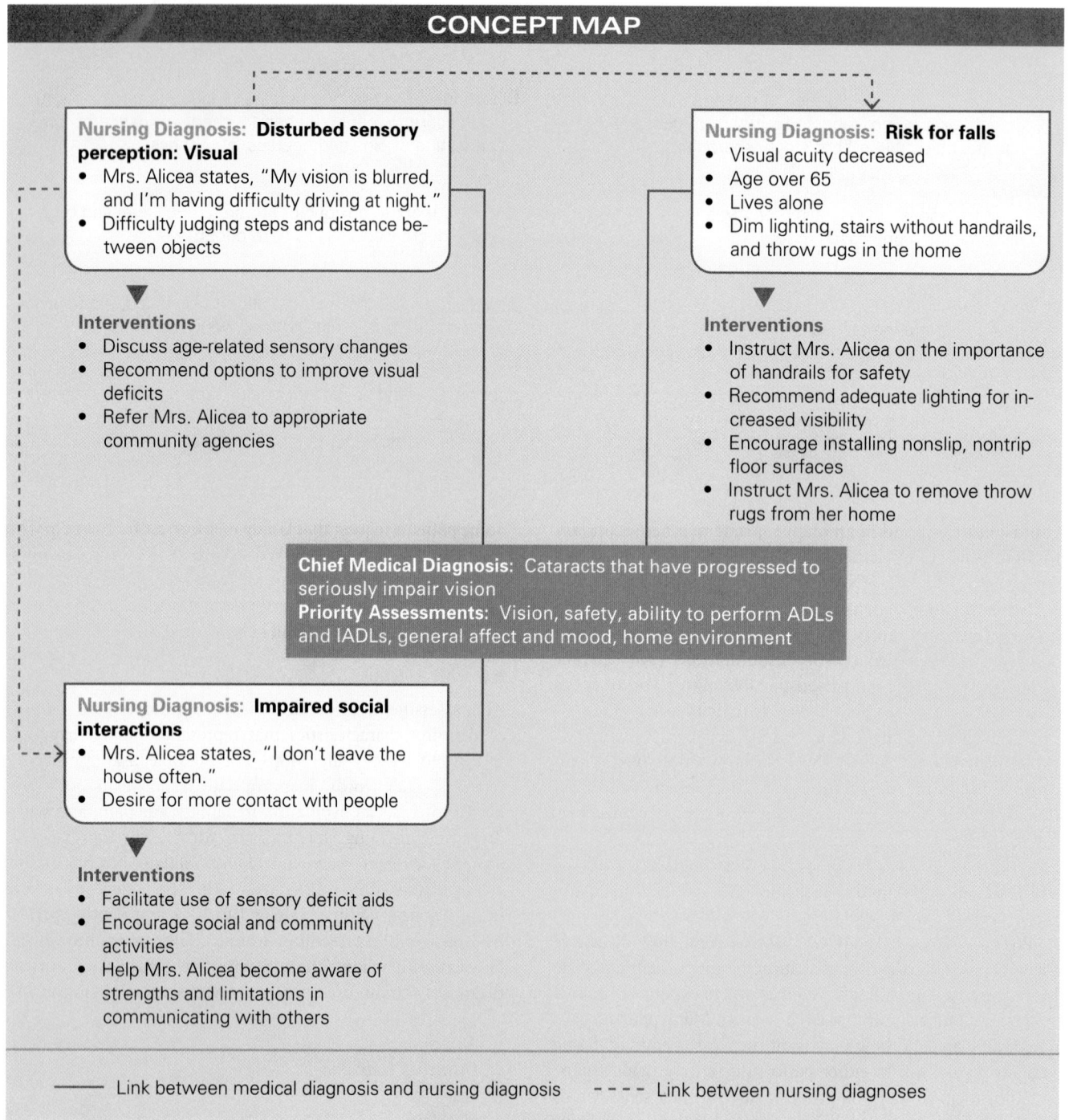

CONCEPT MAP

Nursing Diagnosis: Disturbed sensory perception: Visual
- Mrs. Alicea states, "My vision is blurred, and I'm having difficulty driving at night."
- Difficulty judging steps and distance between objects

▼

Interventions
- Discuss age-related sensory changes
- Recommend options to improve visual deficits
- Refer Mrs. Alicea to appropriate community agencies

Nursing Diagnosis: Risk for falls
- Visual acuity decreased
- Age over 65
- Lives alone
- Dim lighting, stairs without handrails, and throw rugs in the home

▼

Interventions
- Instruct Mrs. Alicea on the importance of handrails for safety
- Recommend adequate lighting for increased visibility
- Encourage installing nonslip, nontrip floor surfaces
- Instruct Mrs. Alicea to remove throw rugs from her home

Chief Medical Diagnosis: Cataracts that have progressed to seriously impair vision
Priority Assessments: Vision, safety, ability to perform ADLs and IADLs, general affect and mood, home environment

Nursing Diagnosis: Impaired social interactions
- Mrs. Alicea states, "I don't leave the house often."
- Desire for more contact with people

▼

Interventions
- Facilitate use of sensory deficit aids
- Encourage social and community activities
- Help Mrs. Alicea become aware of strengths and limitations in communicating with others

——— Link between medical diagnosis and nursing diagnosis   - - - - Link between nursing diagnoses

Figure 37-1 ■ Concept Map. *ADLs,* Activities of daily living; *IADLs,* instrumental activities of daily living.

CARE PLAN Risk for Falls

ASSESSMENT

Mrs. Alicea comes to the clinic reporting "having trouble seeing." Peter notes that Mrs. Alicea appears unsteady when standing. Peter knows that people with vision impairments are at risk for impaired balance and slow reaction time, contributing to a greater fall risk. Peter plans to assess Mrs. Alicea's changes in vision more closely in order to identify interventions to decrease her risk for injury related to visual alterations.

ASSESSMENT ACTIVITIES

Ask Mrs. Alicea to describe her vision changes.

Ask Mrs. Alicea to describe any life changes that have occurred since the changes in vision.

Assess Mrs. Alicea's visual acuity.

Ask Mrs. Alicea the results of her last visit with the ophthalmologist.

Conduct a home hazard assessment.

FINDINGS/DEFINING CHARACTERISTICS*

Mrs. Alicea states, "When I try to read or sew, my **vision is blurred** even with my glasses. I have **difficulty judging distances between objects, which is worse at night.**"

Mrs. Alicea states, "I'm having **difficulty reading** and moving around the house. **I cannot judge the steps clearly,** and my son has been helping me more with household chores."

Mrs. Alicea's corneas appear opaque, and there is a reduction in accommodation.

Mrs. Alicea reports that it has been about 2 years since she has been to an eye doctor. Mrs. Alicea states, "At my last visit, I was told I had a cataract."

The home has **dim lighting, stairs without handrails,** and **numerous throw rugs on floors.**

NURSING DIAGNOSIS: Risk for falls related to visual alterations from cataracts.

PLANNING

GOAL

- Mrs. Alicea's home environment is safe and free of hazards within 4 weeks.

EXPECTED OUTCOMES (NOC)†

Risk Control: Visual Impairment
- Mrs. Alicea will report an increased sense of home safety and independence within 2 weeks.
- Mrs. Alicea and her son will make recommended changes to home environment within 4 weeks.

INTERVENTIONS (NIC)‡

Environmental Management: Safety
- Recommend Rico install a nonglare work surface in the kitchen area.

- Recommend Rico install incandescent lights in the home.

- Help Rico identify potential trip hazards, such as throw rugs, and suggest they either be modified or removed.

Fall Prevention
- Teach Rico methods to improve environmental safety such as installation of handrails along stairs, securing carpeting, removal of throw rugs, and painting of stairs.
- Suggest that Rico place a nonslip surface such as a nonskid mat in the bathtub and shower.

RATIONALE

Sensitivity to glare increases because of clouding of the lens and vitreous, which result in scattering of light that passes through the lens.

The intensity of lighting needs to be three times as powerful for older adults to produce the same visual acuity as for younger people (Ebersole and others, 2005).

Removal of trip hazards prevents falls and promotes a safe environment.

A decrease in visual acuity and depth perception places the patient at risk for falls in the presence of environmental hazards (Ebersole and others, 2005).

Mrs. Alicea is at a higher risk for falling in the shower and bathtub because of visual impairments and difficulties with depth perception. Nonskid surfaces prevent falling in bathtubs and showers.

---

*Defining characteristics are shown in **bold** type.

†Outcomes classification labels from Moorhead S and others, editors: *Nursing outcomes classification (NOC),* ed 4, St. Louis, 2008, Mosby.

‡Interventions classification label from Bulechek GM and others, editors: *Nursing interventions classification (NIC),* ed 5, St. Louis, 2008, Mosby.

Continued

CARE PLAN Risk for Falls—cont'd

EVALUATION

NURSING ACTIONS	PATIENT RESPONSE/FINDING	ACHIEVEMENT OF OUTCOME
During her next visit to the health center, ask Mrs. Alicea if she has experienced any trips or falls since modifications to her home were made. Ask Rico if his mother is having any difficulties moving through her home.	Mrs. Alicea states she has not fallen or tripped since Rico made the suggested modifications to her home. Rico states his mother is able to walk through her home with steady, purposeful gait.	Outcome met.
Conduct a home visit, and reassess the home environment.	Rico has changed all light bulbs in the halls and stairways. He removed all throw rugs and painted edges of stairs bright white. Kitchen work surface has not changed yet.	Home environment has improved. Rico needs help identifying contractors to help him change the work surface in the kitchen to decrease glare.

GOALS AND OUTCOMES The patient will be able to work with you in adapting to the environment and remaining safe and productive if the plan includes clear goals and attainable outcomes. Make sure goals not only meet the immediate needs of the patient, but also strive toward rehabilitation. Goals and outcomes need to be realistic and measurable. Some sensory alterations are short term, requiring only temporary interventions. Permanent sensory alterations require long-term goals, with a series of outcomes that the patient reaches over time. For example, if a patient suffers an injury causing blindness, the long-term goal of "managing self-care within the home" will require numerous short-term outcomes and outcomes that require progressive advancement. Examples of outcomes include "Patient will ambulate safely within the home in 2 weeks" and "Patient will perform ADLs with minimal assistance within 4 weeks."

SETTING PRIORITIES After selecting nursing diagnoses and mutually agreed-upon goals and outcomes, work with the patient in setting priorities. Generally you will rank diagnoses in order of importance based on the patient's safety, personal desires, and needs. When setting priorities, safety is always a top priority. Sometimes it becomes necessary for the patient to make major changes in self-care activities, communication, and socialization. Helping patients learn about ways to communicate more effectively or use adaptive equipment promotes safety and allows patients to participate in favorite activities.

COLLABORATIVE CARE Review all resources available to patients when you develop a plan of care, and make appropriate referrals to other health care professionals. Referrals to occupational or speech therapists and social service ensure a multidisciplinary approach. Referral to home care is another option. The family plays a key role in providing meaningful stimulation and learning ways to help a patient adjust to any limitations once the patient returns home. Teach hospitalized patients and their families how to adapt interventions to their lifestyles. Community resources, such as the American Foundation for the Blind, American Red Cross, and the Lions Club, provide information to assist patients and families with discharge planning and home needs.

■■■ IMPLEMENTATION

Nursing interventions involve the patient and family in order to maintain a safe, pleasant, and stimulating sensory environment. Effective interventions help the patient with sensory alterations to function safely with existing deficits and to continue a normal lifestyle.

HEALTH PROMOTION Good sensory function begins with promoting the health of sensory organs and maximizing existing sensory function. When a patient seeks health care, provide interventions that reduce risk for sensory losses.

Screening and Prevention Visual screening in children is important because the occurrence of blindness and serious visual impairment is estimated to be between 30 and 64 children per 100,000 in the pediatric population (Hockenberry and Wilson, 2007). Children need appropriate visual screenings to help detect problems early. Three interventions to help prevent visual impairment in children include screening women considering pregnancy for rubella and syphilis; advocating adequate prenatal care to prevent premature birth, which results in infants' being exposed to excessive oxygen during care; and periodic screening of all children for congenital blindness and visual impairment caused by **refractive errors** and strabismus.

Nearsightedness is common during childhood. School nurses usually conduct routine vision testing of school-age and adolescent children. Your role as a nurse is one of detection, education, and referral. Parents need to know the signs of visual impairment such as failure to react to light and reduced eye contact from the infant. Parents need to report any signs of visual impairments to their health care provider.

Trauma is a common cause of blindness in children. Examples include injury from flying objects or penetrating wounds. Parents and children need education on ways to avoid eye trauma, for example, wearing safety devices and buying only "safe" toys. Safety equipment worn to avoid sports-related trauma is available in sport and department stores.

Adults also need routine visual screenings. If left undetected and untreated, glaucoma leads to permanent visual loss. The American Academy of Ophthalmology (2007) recommends regular medical eye examinations every 2 to 4 years for those over 40 years old. Adults 65 years and older need examinations every 1 to 2 years. Patients with risk factors for disease, including a family history of glaucoma or serious eye injury, often need additional evaluations during this time. Individuals of African descent also need closer follow-up because they are at risk for an earlier onset, higher incidence, and more rapid progression of glaucoma.

Adults are at risk for eye injury when playing sports and working in jobs involving exposure to chemicals or flying objects. The Occupational Safety and Health Administration (OSHA) (2006) has guidelines for workplace safety. Employers must have employees wear eye goggles and/or use equipment that reduces risk for injury. Reinforce eye safety at work and in activities that place the adult at risk for eye injury when appropriate.

In the United States, hearing impairments are common. At-risk children include those with a family history of childhood hearing impairment, perinatal infection (rubella, herpes, or cytomegalovirus), low birth weight, chronic ear infections, and Down syndrome. Advise pregnant women to seek early prenatal care and to avoid ototoxic drugs.

Chronic middle ear infections are a common cause of hearing impairment in children. These children need periodic auditory testing. Exposure to loud or high-intensity noise is a risk factor for hearing loss. Advise both children and parents to take precautions and use earplugs or earphones to block high-decibel sounds.

In adults, guidelines for hearing screening are variable. If a patient works or lives in a high noise level environment, an annual screening is recommended. The most important concept for adults to understand is hearing loss is not a natural part of aging. Once a patient reports a hearing loss, regular testing becomes necessary.

Use of Assistive Aids   Patients with sensory deficits often require use of assistive aids. Patients who wear corrective lenses, eyeglasses, or hearing aids need to keep them accessible, functional, and clean (Box 37-7) (see Chapter 28). A family member or friend may also need to know how to clean and care for the aids. Contact lens wearers who do not clean their lenses appropriately, use contaminated lens storage cases or contact lens solutions, or who use homemade saline are at risk for serious eye infections. Reinforce proper lens care in any health maintenance discussions.

A wide variety of cosmetically acceptable hearing aids that enhance a person's hearing ability are currently available. Patients will often need encouragement and support to explore assistive devices. Because hearing aids are expensive, explore potential financial resources with your patients. Offer patients printed information on hearing loss, the benefits of hearing aid use, and how to use the hearing aid (Meiner and Lueckenotte, 2006). Family members or friends who support the use of the

---

BOX 37-7 | Care of Hearing Aids

- Place battery in hearing aid when it is turned off.
- Remove hearing aid battery when not in use.
- Batteries are toxic if swallowed; keep them away from pets and children.
- Protect hearing aids from water and excessive heat or cold.
- Clean batteries as needed with a sharpened pencil eraser and gently scrape.

Modified from Ebersole P and others: *Toward healthy aging: human needs and nursing response*, ed 7, St. Louis, 2008, Mosby.

BOX 37-8 | Promoting Sensory Stimulation

- Reduce glare by eliminating waxed floors and shiny surfaces exposed to bright sunlight, installing tinted glass or sheer curtains over large windows, and using soft and diffused lighting.
- Teach use of assistive devices to improve visual acuity (e.g., pocket magnifiers, telescopic lens eyeglasses, large-print books, clocks, watches).
- Recommend introducing brighter colors (e.g., red, orange, yellow) into the home environment so that patients are able to differentiate between surfaces and room objects.
- Explain how to maximize hearing reception or minimize effects of hearing loss by increasing amplification on TVs or radios and using recorded music in low-frequency sound.
- Promote sense of taste through good oral hygiene, serving well-seasoned and differently textured foods, chewing food thoroughly, and avoiding blending or mixing foods.
- Enhance the sense of smell by removing unpleasant odors from the environment and introducing pleasant smells such as mild room deodorizers or fragrant flowers.

---

aid will often influence the patient to use the aid as instructed. However, some patients are reluctant to wear hearing aids for a variety of reasons. When patients report that they have hearing aids but do not wear them, investigate potential reasons such as the appearance of the hearing aid, poor fit, difficulty in seeing or working with a small object, and lack of patient education about the hearing aid. When a patient has a new hearing aid, provide adequate patient education. Patients usually begin wearing the hearing aid for 15 to 20 minutes and gradually increase the time until they can wear the hearing aid for 10 to 12 hours. If your patient is having problems tolerating a hearing aid, refer your patient to an audiologist and suggest that the patient explore other types of hearing aids.

Promoting Meaningful Stimulation   You will help patients make their environments more stimulating by making adaptations that incorporate the normal physiological changes that accompany sensory deficits (Box 37-8). For example, the pupils lose the ability to adjust to light as patients age. You reduce this sensitivity to glare by having family members install non glare surfaces in the home.

Some patients experience reduced tactile sensations in a limited portion of their body. Touch therapy helps to stimulate existing function. If the patient is willing, your brushing and combing of the patient's hair, giving a back rub, and touching of the arms or shoulders increase tactile contact. Turning and positioning also improve the quality of tactile sensation.

Creating a Safe Environment Patients become less secure within their home and workplace when they have a sensory alteration. An actual or potential sensory loss determines the type of safety precautions necessary. Security is necessary for a person to feel independent. Make recommendations for improving safety within a patient's living environment without restricting the patient's independence. Inform patients that organizing informal network agreements with neighbors can have a positive effect on home safety and security concerns (Ebersole and others, 2008).

Visual Adaptations. Safety is a concern when patients experience decreases in visual acuity, peripheral vision, adaptation to the dark, or depth perception. With reduced peripheral vision a patient cannot see panoramically. With reduced depth perception, a person is unable to judge how far away objects are located. The home safety assessment helps you identify hazards in the patient's living environment. Remove clutter such as footstools or electrical cords. Install thresholds over uneven floor surfaces between rooms. Arrange furniture so that a patient is able to move about easily without fear of tripping or running into objects. Make sure all flooring is in good repair, and remove all throw rugs. Stairwells need to be well lighted and have securely fastened handrails extending the full length of the stairs. Handrails on both sides of stairs is preferable.

Front and back entrances to the home and work areas need good lighting. Light fixtures need high-wattage bulbs with wider illumination. A light switch located at the top and bottom of stairwells adds an additional safety element. Replace fluorescent lighting with incandescent lights.

Driving is sometimes a safety hazard for older adults. A sensitivity to glare creates a problem for driving at night with headlights. Reduced peripheral vision prevents a driver from seeing cars in the next lane. Reduced vision, complicated by a decrease in reaction time, reduced hearing, and decreased strength in the legs and arms frequently limits the older adult's driving skills. To minimize risk, encourage older patients to drive only in familiar areas and not during rush hour. Urge patients to drive defensively and to avoid driving at night or at dusk. Older adults need to drive slowly but not so slowly that they create a safety problem for other drivers.

Some patients have problems seeing dials or controls on electrical appliances and equipment when they are unable to contrast colors. Use color contrasts such as tape, paint, or fingernail enamel to highlight dials. Have patients describe their usual daily activities to find opportunities for color coding to prevent accidents related to visual impairments.

Hearing Adaptations. Individuals need to hear environmental sounds such as fire alarms, alarm clocks, phones, or doorbells. Change or amplify the sound of these devices to a more low-pitched, buzzerlike quality. Signaling devices, such as a flashing light on a phone, allow patients with hearing impairments greater independence. Sound lamps that respond with light to the sounds of babies crying, smoke detectors, and burglar alarms are also available. Advise family and friends who call the patient regularly to let the phone ring for a longer period.

Smell and Tactile Adaptations. The patient with a reduced sensitivity to odors is often unable to smell leaking gas, a smoldering cigarette, fire, or tainted food. Make sure the patient uses smoke detectors and takes precautions such as checking ashtrays or placing cigarette butts in water. Also advise the patient to check food package dates and inspect the appearance of food. Patients with reduced tactile sensation need to use hot and cold water bottles or heating pads cautiously and **never** use the high setting. Make sure the temperature on the home water heater is no higher than 120° F.

Communication Individuals need to interact with people around them. The type of sensory loss influences the methods and styles of communication you use during interactions with patients. Some patients with hearing impairments are able to speak normally. To more clearly hear what a person communicates, family and friends need to learn to move away from background noise, rephrase rather than repeat sentences, be positive, and have patience. On the other hand, some deaf patients have serious speech alterations. Deaf patients use sign language, read lips, write with pad and pencil, or learn to use a computer for communication (Box 37-9).

ACUTE CARE Some hospitalized patients are treated for sensory deficits (e.g., acute eye infection), and some have preexisting sensory problems. You need to know the patient's health history to appropriately support self-care activities while promoting a safe environment.

Orientation to the Environment Completely orient patients with sensory impairments to a health care setting. Always keep your name tag visible, address the patient by name, explain the patient's location, and frequently include the time and date in conversations. Repeating explanations in short and simple terms reduces confusion. Encourage family and friends not to argue with or contradict a confused patient but to explain calmly their location, identity, and time of day.

Patients with serious visual impairments need to feel comfortable in knowing the boundaries of their environment. The patient needs to walk through a room and feel the walls to establish a sense of direction. Remember to approach the blind patient from the front. Explain the location of objects within the room, such as chairs or equipment. It is important to keep all objects in the same place and position. Moving an object, even a short distance, creates a safety hazard. You will need to reorient the patient frequently by describing the location of key items. Place necessary objects such as the call light, patient-controlled analgesia (PCA) button, glasses, water, or facial tissue in front of patients to prevent falls caused by reaching. Also, ask the patient how to arrange objects so ambulation is easier. Remove clutter and unnecessary equipment. Always keep the path to the bathroom clear.

Safety Measures You will need to assist patients with acute visual impairments with walking (Figure 37-2). Stand on the patient's dominant, stronger or uninjured side. The patient grasps your elbow or upper arm. You then walk one-half step ahead and slightly to the patient's side. The patient's shoulder is directly behind your shoulder. Relax, and walk at a comfortable pace. Warn the patient when approaching doorways, and tell the patient whether the door opens in or out. Do not leave a patient with visual impairment alone in an unfamiliar area. If the patient has unstable mobility, use a gait belt during walking (see Chapter 26).

Strategies to enhance communication include the provision of adequate lighting and rearrangement of furniture so that you can face the patient while talking. When communicating with patients, always actively listen and provide adequate time for patients with sensory deficits to respond (Wallhagen, Pettengill, and Whiteside, 2006). Alert the entire multidisciplinary team when a patient has a sensory alteration. Note the most effective way to communicate with the patient in the patient's medical record (Ebersole and others, 2005).

Controlling Sensory Stimuli Reduce sensory overload by organizing the patient's care to control for excessive stimuli. Combining activities such as dressing changes, bathing, and vital sign assessment in one visit prevents the patient from becoming overly fatigued. Coordination with other departments will reduce the time needed for tests and examinations. The patient needs time for rest and quiet. Perform routine nursing procedures as quietly as possible. Encourage a family member to sit quietly with a patient or involve the patient in an undemanding repetitive activity such as combing hair.

Try to control extraneous noise in and around a patient's room, such as television volume and visitors. Turn off bedside equipment not in use. Close the patient's room door if necessary. Hospital staff need to control loud laughter or conversation at the nurses' station. In addition to controlling excess stimuli, try to introduce meaningful stimulation that makes the environment pleasing and comfortable (Box 37-10).

RESTORATIVE AND CONTINUING CARE After patients have experienced a sensory loss, they need to adjust to continue a normal lifestyle. Many of the interventions previously discussed under health promotion are adaptable for the home setting. The home environment needs to be healthy, comfortable, and safe. Suggest changes in a person's home environment after you assess the home setting for any hazards that increase the risk for injury.

Promoting Self-Care Patients who have had surgery related to a sensory deficit need a plan of care that allows them to return safely to their home environment. Most patients have same-day surgical procedures (see Chapter 38). Family members or friends need to understand how the patient's sensory impairment will affect the ability to perform ADLs and IADLs and the factors that lessen or worsen sensory problems. IADLs require a higher level of cognitive and physical functioning than ADLs and include such tasks as

---

BOX 37-9 PATIENT TEACHING

Communication Strategies for Interacting With Patients Who Have Hearing Impairments

 Rico tells Peter that he is concerned about communicating well with his mother now that she has both hearing and vision deficits. Peter understands that hearing impairment is a debilitating problem for many older adults, but interventions by health care providers, family, and friends help patients maintain communication. Peter investigates strategies for interacting with hearing impaired patients. Using this information, Peter develops the following teaching plan for Rico:

OUTCOME
- At the end of the teaching session, Rico will be able to verbalize understanding of four strategies he will use to improve communication with his mother.

TEACHING STRATEGIES
- Teach Rico to approach his mother from the front and to lightly place a hand on her shoulder or forearm to avoid startling her (Austen, 2005).
- Explain to Rico that he needs to face his mother directly and maintain good eye contact throughout the interaction (Lieu and others, 2007).
- Explain to Rico that communication is improved when there is good lighting and there is no glare in his mother's visual field. His mother should be positioned to avoid looking into a brightly lit background (Lieu and others, 2007).
- Inform Rico to speak in a normal tone and articulate clearly without using exaggerated lip movements (Wallhagen and others, 2006).
- Tell Rico to avoid covering his mouth with his hand when speaking (Wallhagen and others, 2006).
- Explain to Rico that when he is not understood he should rephrase sentences rather than repeat them (Wallhagen and others, 2006).
- Teach Rico to make sure that his mother's hearing aids are in place and her glasses are worn when needed (Wallhagen and others, 2006).
- Explain to Rico that comprehension is enhanced when background noise is minimized or eliminated (Wallhagen and others, 2006).
- Teach Rico to talk toward his mother's best or normal ear and speak with his hands, face, and eyes.
- Tell Rico that written information will enhance the spoken word. He should write legibly and make sure that his mother can read the writing (Lieu and others, 2007).

EVALUATION STRATEGIES
- Ask Rico to verbalize at least four communication approaches to use with his mother.
- Have Rico role-play and use some of the communication strategies that you discussed.

cleaning, yard maintenance, shopping, and money management (Ebersole and others, 2008). Community resources discussed in the planning section will be useful.

Patients with sensory impairments are often able to continue independent self-care activities. In the case of eating meals, you arrange food on the plate and condiments, salad, or drinks around the plate according to numbers on the face of a

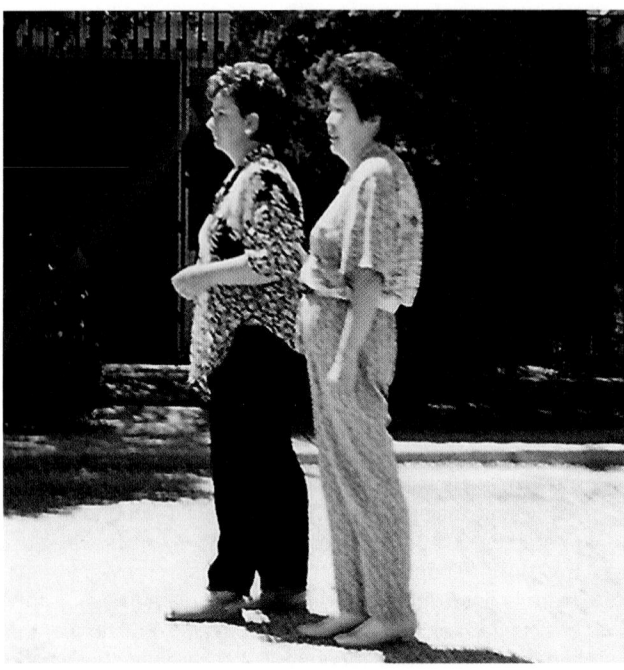

Figure 37-2 ■ Nurse assists visually impaired patient with ambulation.

BOX 37-10	Introducing Stimuli Into the Care Setting

VISUAL
- Open the drapes to the patient's room.
- Raise the head of the bed, and draw back dividing curtains or partitions.
- Provide attractive decorations on tables or cabinets, such as fresh flowers, plants, a picture, or greeting cards.
- Provide talking books and large-print reading material.

AUDITORY
- Sit down and speak with the patient. Make the conversation meaningful.
- Turn on a radio with the type of music the patient enjoys. A favorite radio or television program is stimulating.

TASTE AND SMELL
- Provide attractive, taste-appealing meals. Be sure tableware and glasses are clean. Make sure warm foods are served warm and cold foods are served cold.
- Provide a variety of textures, aromas, and flavors to enhance the patient's appetite.

clock (Figure 37-3). The patient will become oriented to the items after the family member explains each item's location. Patients will need assistance in arranging self-care items, such as clothing, hygiene, food supplies, and utensils in a consistent location to continue managing daily care activities.

The patient with visual impairments will also need assistance in reaching the bathroom safely. Safety bars need to be installed near the toilet. A bar that is a different color from the wall is easier to see. Never place towels on safety bars because this interferes with a person's grasp.

If tactile sense is decreased, zippers or Velcro strips, pullover sweaters or blouses, and elasticized waists are easier for the patient to use. If the patient has a partial paralysis, you dress the affected side first. Some patients also need assistance with basic grooming such as brushing, combing, shaving, and shampooing hair.

Socialization Interacting with others is difficult for many patients with vision and hearing impairments. Patients often lose the motivation to engage in social activities and withdraw from interaction. A patient with a hearing loss will become embarrassed and exhausted after asking people to continuously repeat what they say. Introduce therapies to reduce loneliness, particularly for older adult patients (Box 37-11). Family members need to learn to focus on a person's ability rather than his or her disability. Never assume that a person with a hearing or visual impairment does not wish to speak.

■■■EVALUATION

PATIENT CARE It is important to evaluate whether care measures maintain or improve a patient's ability to interact and function within the environment (see Care Plan and Box 37-12). Adapt evaluation measures to determine whether actual outcomes are the same as expected outcomes. For example, be sure a patient with a hearing deficit hears your questions about responses to treatment. Be sure the patient with a visual alterations is able to walk in the home without the risk of running into barriers. When expected outcomes have not been achieved, there is a need to change interventions or add new ones.

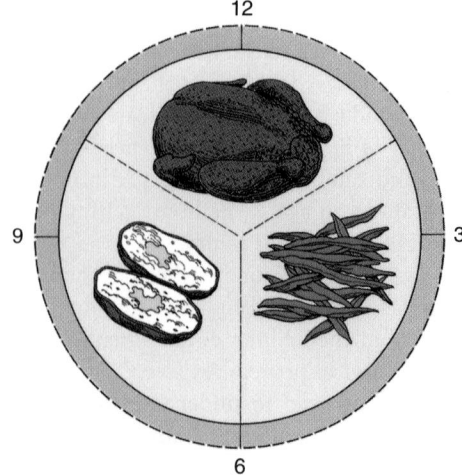

Figure 37-3 ■ Arrange food on a plate and orient patient to placement based on numbers on a clock face.

For all patients it is important to evaluate the integrity of the sensory organs and the patient's ability to perceive stimuli. This often involves a simple vision or hearing evaluation by asking the patient to perform a self-care skill. Be sure to determine if patients are following recommended therapies and meeting mutually set goals. If nursing care has been directed at improving or maintaining sensory acuity, asking the patient to explain or demonstrate a newly learned self-care skill is an effective evaluative measure.

PATIENT EXPECTATIONS It is important to learn if patients think they are receiving appropriate care. A sensory deficit is potentially embarrassing and threatens a person's self-image. Does the patient feel comfortable relating to you? Was the patient able to maintain the plan of care for assistive devices? Did the patient think you were exhibiting a caring, professional approach? Asking patients if nursing care successfully met their expectations will provide valuable knowledge when you care for other patients with similar sensory problems.

BOX 37-11   CARE OF THE OLDER ADULT

Therapies to Reduce Loneliness

- Recommend alterations in living arrangements such as living with a family caregiver if physical isolation is a factor.
- Give older adults extra time to communicate.
- Assist patients in keeping contact with people important to them (Ebersole and others, 2005).
- Encourage and facilitate socialization.
- Provide information about support groups.
- Link patients with religious organizations attuned to the social needs of older adults.
- Introduce the idea of bringing a companion, such as a pet, into the home when appropriate (Ebersole and others, 2005).

BOX 37-12   EVALUATION

One month has passed since Mrs. Alicea's last visit to the senior health care center. Today Peter sits down and talks with both Mrs. Alicea and Rico. He learns that Mrs. Alicea is no longer having problems with glare because Rico changed the lights in the house to incandescent bulbs. Rico also reports that he plans to install sheer curtains Mrs. Alicea chose last week in the living room. Mrs. Alicea also tells Peter that Rico has made a "few changes around the house" including rearranging furniture, securing some throw rugs while removing others, and removing the extension cords. After purchasing a magnifier at a local drug store, Mrs. Alicea is able to read the newspaper and medication labels more easily.

On examination, Mrs. Alicea's visual acuity continues to reveal blurring when she tried to read an informational pamphlet. Her pupils continue to respond slowly to accommodation. Peter asks if Mrs. Alicea has made an appointment with her ophthalmologist. She confirms the appointment is within the next 2 weeks.

Mrs. Alicea confides, "Overall, I think I have been helped with the ideas we talked about last time. I feel a little better about getting around the house and doing the things I like to do." When asked if he has noticed any changes in his mother's actions, Rico states, "She seems less fearful of falling."

DOCUMENTATION NOTE

"Visited clinic this morning as scheduled. Implemented measures at home to improve visual acuity and sensitivity to glare. Son supportive in making necessary home environment changes. Plans to make additional ones. Appointment with ophthalmologist in 2 weeks."

KEY POINTS

- Sensory perception depends on a region in the cerebral cortex where specialized brain cells interpret the quality and nature of sensory stimuli.
- Because a patient learns to rely on unaffected senses after a sensory loss, you design interventions to preserve function of these senses.
- Aging results in a gradual decline of acuity in all senses.
- Environmental stimuli in a hospital, such as an intensive care unit, place a patient at risk for sensory overload.
- The extent of support from family members and significant others influences the quality of sensory experiences.
- Assessment of sensory function includes a physical examination and measurement of functional abilities.
- The presence of cerumen in the external auditory canal is a common cause of hearing loss in older adults.
- Sensory losses create loneliness and impair the ability to socialize.
- An assessment of environment includes identifying hazards, sources of meaningful stimulation, and the amount of stimuli.

- Prenatal screening and childhood immunizations prevent sensory alterations in the newborn and child.
- The care plan for patients with sensory alterations includes participation by family members.
- Patients with visual impairments need to learn boundaries within the environment to ambulate safely.
- Patients with existing hearing deficits are able to learn alternative ways to communicate.
- Nursing care for patients with sensory alterations includes using stronger sensory stimuli, compensating with other senses, and modifying the environment to maximize remaining sensory function.
- To prevent sensory overload, control stimuli, orient the patient to the environment, and promote rest by minimizing interruptions.
- Safety is a top concern when setting priorities for patients who experience sensory deprivation.

CRITICAL THINKING EXERCISES

At Mrs. Alicea's last visit to the senior center, she reported that she feels more comfortable moving around the house, but Peter also learns that she does not leave the house often. She reports feeling alone much of the time. She tells Peter that she is having more problems hearing. Peter knows that Mrs. Alicea has hearing aids. He also knows that hearing aids are essential for communication and safety, so Peter decides to ask Mrs. Alicea if she wears her hearing aids. She reports that she does not wear her hearing aids every day.

1. Discuss reasons why Mrs. Alicea may be reluctant to wear her hearing aids.

2. Identify some suggestions that Peter could share with Mrs. Alicea that might influence her adaption to hearing aid use.

3. Discuss how loss of sensory function may affect Mrs. Alicea's independence and health, related quality of life.

4. Based on these data, Peter develops a nursing diagnosis of *impaired social interaction related to hearing deficits.* Identify one goal, two expected outcomes, and three related nursing interventions that will help the patient meet the identified goals and outcome.

evolve   Answers to Critical Thinking Questions can be found on the Evolve website.

REVIEW QUESTIONS

1. The nurse has completed an assessment on a 60-year-old man who is visiting the clinic for the first time. During the examination, the patient appeared distracted and he frequently asked for questions to be repeated. At one point, the patient responded inappropriately to a question. Assessment data most likely indicate:
   1. A hearing deficit
   2. A visual deficit
   3. Sensory deprivation
   4. Patient is normal

2. The nurse is reviewing the health history of a 33-year-old woman. The patient reports that she is planning a pregnancy in the next year. The nurse understands that to help prevent visual impairments in infants before and after birth, the following intervention(s) need to be implemented. Select all that apply.
   1. Screen the patient for rubella and syphilis.
   2. Advocate adequate prenatal care to prevent premature birth.
   3. Monitor the infant's oxygen therapy.
   4. Recommend avoidance of infant and childhood immunizations.

3. An 80-year-old man with a history of cataract surgery comes to the clinic today for a routine checkup. He reports that he is having trouble hearing in his left ear. Strategies to improve communication include which of the following? Select all that apply.
   1. Speak at a normal rate and louder tone.
   2. Ask how the nursing staff can help the patient to communicate.
   3. Avoid situations in which there is a glare in the patient's line of vision.
   4. Speak directly into the patient's left ear.

4. When a nurse performs a home assessment, the observation that would be most significant for the safety of a patient with peripheral neuropathy is:
   1. Cluttered walkways
   2. Absence of smoke detectors
   3. Lack of bathroom safety bars
   4. Improper water heater setting

5. An occupational health nurse is providing hearing and vision conservation classes to employees of an industrial factory. Which of the following statements by an employee indicates that teaching was effective?
   1. "The Occupational Safety and Health Act outlines employer responsibilities to provide a safe workplace. However, I can make an individual choice whether to use safety gear."
   2. "Repeated exposures to loud noise will result in a temporary loss of hearing."
   3. "Because I already have hearing loss, hearing prevention measures will not work for me."
   4. "My employer has a duty to provide a workplace free from serious recognized hazards and to comply with occupational safety and health standards."

6. A nurse is performing a home care assessment on a patient suspected of having a visual impairment. Which assessment finding(s) may indicate a visually impaired person? Select all that apply.
   1. Mismatched clothes
   2. Minimal eye contact
   3. Eating small, frequent meals
   4. Stumbling in the room

7. A 72-year-old woman has been in the intensive care unit for 1 week because of a respiratory infection. Her private room is directly across from a busy central nurses' station. The patient is on a cardiac monitor and undergoes repeated tests daily. The staff nurse reports that she has noticed a change in the patient's behavior. The patient has been restless and disoriented and has had difficulty concentrating. Nursing measures to reduce sensory overload include which of the following? Select all that apply.
   1. Frequently orient the patient to the environment and to reality.
   2. Arrange for the patient to have a roommate.
   3. Explain unusual sounds, and prepare the patient for procedures in advance.
   4. Encourage the patient's family to visit frequently and throughout the day.
   5. Reestablish normal sleep-wake cycle, and encourage frequent rest periods.

8. Because trauma is a common cause of blindness in children, a priority nursing intervention is to:
   1. Reinforce education on preventive safety strategies to avoid eye trauma
   2. Advise parents not to have their children participate in contact sports
   3. Have the child demonstrate how to walk with a pointed object
   4. Discourage the use of safety equipment because it contributes to a false reassurance of safety

9. A nurse is conducting discharge teaching for a patient with a visual deficit and diminished tactile sensation. Which of the following statements by the patient would indicate that teaching was ineffective?
   1. "It is important to label water faucets 'hot' or 'cold' or use color codes."
   2. "I can use cold water bottles to comfort my back, but I should avoid heating pads."
   3. "I should test my bathwater with a thermometer."
   4. "I should inspect my skin daily."

10. A 75-year-old woman has macular degeneration. The home care nurse is conducting a home environment screening. Which of the following interventions will assist the patient in functioning safely with existing deficits and maintaining a normal lifestyle?
    1. Advise the patient to share her home with a roommate.
    2. Discourage the use of bright lighting, which may be a sign that the patient is not coping with her chronic, gradual vision loss.
    3. Encourage the use of brightly colored throw rugs throughout the home.
    4. Work closely with the patient to identify ways to modify her environment, and as appropriate, refer to community-based resources.

Answers to Review Questions can be found on pages 1197-1198.

REFERENCES

American Academy of Ophthalmology: *Preferred practice pattern guidelines: comprehensive adult medical eye evaluation,* San Francisco, 2007, The Academy.
American Federation for the Blind: *Quick facts and figures on blindness and low vision,* 2004, http://www.afb.org.
American Hearing Research Foundation: *Meniere's disease,* 2006, http://www.american-hearing.org.
Austen JD: Adapting de-escalation techniques with deaf service users, *Nurs Stand* 19(49):41, 2005.
Barnett TO: Problems of the ear. In Monahan F and others: *Phipps' medical-surgical nursing: health and illness perspectives,* ed 8, St. Louis, 2007, Mosby.
Bulecheck GM and others, editors: *Nursing interventions classification (NIC),* ed 5, St. Louis, 2008, Mosby.
Caban AJ and others: Prevalence of concurrent hearing and visual impairment in US adults: the national health interview survey, 1997-2002, *Am J Public Health* 95(11):1940, 2005.
Clarke PM and others: Assessing the impact of visual acuity on quality of life in individuals with type 2 diabetes using the short form 36, *Diabetes Care* 29(7):1506, 2006.
Ebersole P and others: *Gerontological nursing and healthy aging,* ed 2, St. Louis, 2005, Mosby.
Ebersole P and others: *Toward healthy aging: human needs and nursing response,* ed 7, St. Louis, 2008, Mosby.
Gonzalez EW and others: Mexican Americans. In Giger JN, Davidhizar RE: *Transcultural nursing,* ed 5, St. Louis, 2008, Mosby.
Hockenberry MC, Wilson D: *Wong's nursing care of infants and children,* ed 8, St. Louis, 2007, Mosby.
Horowitz A, Brennan M, Reinhardt JP: Prevalence and risk factors for self-reported visual impairment among middle-aged and older adults, *Res Aging* 27(3):307, 2005.
Lieu CC and others: Communication strategies for nurses interacting with patients who are deaf, *Dermatol Nurs* 19(6):541, 2007.
McKean-Cowdin R and others: Severity of visual field loss and health-related quality of life, *Am J Ophthalmol* 143:1013, 2007.
McKenry L and others: *Mosby's pharmacology in nursing,* ed 22, St. Louis, 2005, Mosby.
Meiner SE, Lueckenotte AG: *Gerontologic nursing,* ed 3, St. Louis, 2006, Mosby.
Mohamed Q and others: Management of diabetic retinopathy: a systematic review, *JAMA* 298(8):902, 2007.
Monahan FD: Assessment of the auditory system. In Monahan F and others: *Phipps' medical-surgical nursing: health and illness perspectives,* ed 8, St. Louis, 2007, Mosby.
Moorhead S and others, editors: *Nursing outcomes classification (NOC),* ed 4, St. Louis, 2008, Mosby.
National Eye Institute: *Vision loss from eye diseases will increase as Americans age,* 2004, http://www.nei.nih.gov.
National Eye Institute: *Facts about glaucoma,* 2006a, http://www.nei.nih.gov/.
National Eye Institute: *Statement on the prevalence of visual impairment and how it affects quality of life among Hispanic/Latino Americans,* 2006b, http://www.nei.nih.gov.
National Eye Institute: *Facts about cataract,* 2008, http://www.nei.nih.gov.
National Institute on Deafness and Other Communication Disorders: *Healthy hearing 2010: where are we now,* 2008, http://www.nidcd.nih.gov.
Occupational Safety and Health Administration: *Eye and face protection,* 2006, U.S. Department of Labor, http://www.osha.gov.
The Joint Commission: *The Joint Commission 2008 requirements related to the provision of culturally and linguistically appropriate healthcare,* 2008, http://www.jointcommission.org.
Torpy JM: Peripheral neuropathy, *JAMA* 299(9):1096, 2008.
Wallhagen MI, Pettengill E, Whiteside M: Hearing impairment is a significant, often debilitating, problem for many older adults, but assessment and intervention by nurses can help, *Am J Nurs* 106(10):40, 2006.

CHAPTER 38

Surgical Patient

MEDIA RESOURCES

 CD COMPANION 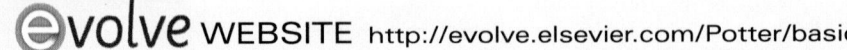 **evolve WEBSITE** http://evolve.elsevier.com/Potter/basic

- Video Clip
- Crossword Puzzle
- English/Spanish Audio Glossary

OBJECTIVES

- Explain the concept of perioperative nursing care.
- Differentiate among classifications of surgery and types of anesthesia.
- List factors to include in the preoperative assessment of a surgical patient.
- Design a preoperative teaching plan.
- Prepare a patient for surgery.
- Explain the differences in caring for the patient undergoing outpatient surgery versus the patient undergoing inpatient surgery.

- Describe intraoperative factors that affect a patient's postoperative course.
- Identify factors to assess in a patient in postoperative recovery.
- Describe the rationale for nursing interventions designed to prevent postoperative complications.

KEY TERMS

antiembolic stockings, p. 1149
atelectasis, p. 1131
bronchospasm, p. 1137
circulating nurse, p. 1151
conscious sedation, p. 1154
embolism, p. 1132
general anesthesia, p. 1153

laryngospasm, p. 1137
malignant hyperthermia, p. 1138
moderate sedation/ analgesia, p. 1154
nasogastric (NG) tube, p. 1147
operating room, p. 1150
outpatient, p. 1131

paralytic ileus, p. 1159
perioperative nursing, p. 1131
postanesthesia care unit (PACU), p. 1154
preanesthesia care unit, p. 1150
preoperative teaching, p. 1144

presurgical care unit (PSCU), p. 1150
pulmonary hygiene, p. 1137
regional anesthesia, p. 1153
scrub nurse, p. 1151
sequential compression stockings, p. 1149

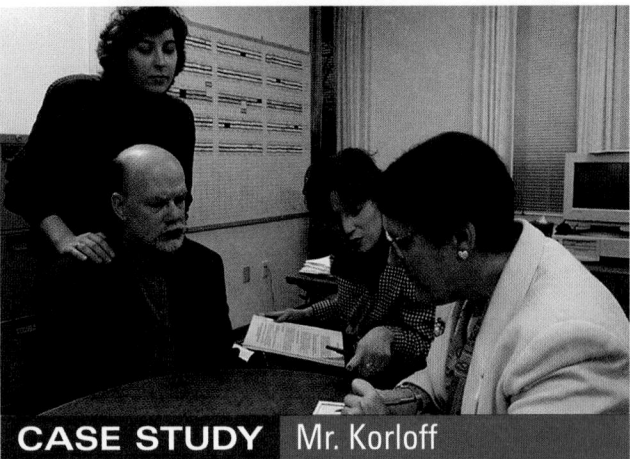

CASE STUDY   Mr. Korloff

Mr. Korloff is a 53-year-old man who has been experiencing abdominal pain for 2 months. Following a series of diagnostic tests, he is now scheduled for elective laparoscopic gallbladder surgery. Mr. Korloff is originally from Russia and has lived in the United States for 10 years. He speaks English relatively well but still speaks in Russian when family is present. He is a vice president for an international business firm. He is widowed and has two adult daughters, both born in Russia before coming to the United States. The daughters are married and live in the same neighborhood as Mr. Korloff. However, both have full-time jobs.

Sue Collins is a nursing student assigned to the preadmission center at the local hospital where she has been working for 2 weeks. She is completing her last clinical rotation and will graduate in 1 month. Sue is 30 years old, is married, and has no children. She plans to seek employment in a hospital on a general surgery floor after graduation. Sue's father recently had surgery for prostate cancer.

This chapter synthesizes many concepts and skills previously presented in this text. You will recognize these previously learned areas such as patient education, oxygenation, and elimination and apply this information when caring for the surgical patient in the preoperative and postoperative phases.

Perioperative nursing care includes nursing care given before (preoperative), during (intraoperative), and after (postoperative) surgery. Surgery takes place in a variety of settings, including hospitals, ambulatory surgery centers, clinics, health care providers' offices, and even mobile units. Minor surgeries are performed on an **outpatient** basis, with the patient entering the setting, undergoing surgery, and being discharged the same day. Many surgical patients enter the setting as outpatients for preoperative screening and testing and are admitted to the hospital after surgery. Patients requiring extensive preoperative care are admitted to the hospital before surgery. The principles of caring for perioperative patients are the same regardless of the setting.

SCIENTIFIC KNOWLEDGE BASE

Classification of Surgery

Surgical procedures are classified according to the seriousness, urgency, and purpose of surgery (Table 38-1). For example, a breast biopsy, done for diagnostic purposes, is classified as urgent and done on an outpatient basis. Knowing the classification will help you to plan appropriate preoperative and postoperative care for each patient.

Surgical Risk Factors

There are numerous factors that create risks for a person undergoing surgery. Knowledge regarding the physiology of the stress response (see Chapter 24) and factors that affect a patient's response to the stress of surgery is necessary to anticipate patient needs for preoperative preparation, teaching, and postoperative care.

SMOKING There is a significant association between smoking and postoperative pulmonary complications, specifically pneumonia and **atelectasis.** Chronic smoking increases the amount and thickness of mucous secretions in the lungs. After surgery a patient who smokes has greater difficulty clearing the airways of mucus and needs to practice deep breathing and coughing exercises (see Chapter 29). Smoking also increases the risk for circulatory and infectious complications (Warner, 2005).

AGE Very young and older patients are at greater surgical risk as a result of an immature or a declining physiological status. Maintaining the patient's normal body temperature is a concern during surgery. When compared with adults, infants have a proportionately greater surface area and less subcutaneous fat, placing them at risk for wide temperature variations. In addition, general anesthetics inhibit shivering, a protective reflex to maintain body temperature, and anesthetics cause vasodilation, which results in heat loss. During surgery an infant also has difficulty in maintaining a normal circulatory blood volume. The total blood volume of infants is considerably less than that of older children and adults, creating a risk for both dehydration and overhydration. With advancing age a patient's physical capacity to adapt to the stress of surgery lessens because of deterioration of certain body functions. Table 38-2 summarizes physiological factors that place older adult patients at risk during surgery.

NUTRITION Normal tissue repair and resistance to infection depend on adequate nutrition. Surgery increases the need for nutrients. Postoperatively a patient requires at least 1500 kilocalories per day to maintain energy reserves. Additional protein, carbohydrates, zinc, and vitamins A, B, C, and K are necessary for proper wound healing (see Chapters 32 and 36). Malnourished patients are more likely to have poor tolerance of anesthesia, negative nitrogen balance, delayed postoperative recovery, infection, and delayed wound healing (Black and Hawks, 2005).

OBESITY A patient who is obese usually has reduced ventilatory capacity because of the upward pressure against the diaphragm caused by an enlarged abdomen. There is also

TABLE 38-1   Classification for Surgical Procedures

TYPE	DESCRIPTION	EXAMPLE
SERIOUSNESS		
Major	Involves extensive reconstruction or alteration in body parts; poses great risks to well-being	Coronary artery bypass, colon resection, removal of larynx, resection of lung lobe
Minor	Involves minimal alteration in body parts; often designed to correct deformities; involves minimal risks compared with major procedures	Cataract extraction, facial plastic surgery, tooth extraction
URGENCY		
Elective	Performed on basis of patient's choice; not essential and is not always necessary for health	Bunionectomy, facial plastic surgery, breast reconstruction
Urgent	Necessary for patient's health, will possibly prevent additional problems from developing (e.g., tissue destruction, impaired organ function); not necessarily an emergency	Excision of cancerous tumor, removal of gallbladder for stones, vascular repair for obstructed artery (e.g., coronary artery bypass)
Emergency	Must be done immediately to save life or preserve function of body part	Repair of perforated appendix, repair of traumatic amputation, control of internal hemorrhaging
PURPOSE		
Diagnostic	Surgical exploration that allows physician or health care provider to confirm diagnosis; sometimes involves removal of tissue for further diagnostic testing	Exploratory laparotomy (incision into peritoneal cavity to inspect abdominal organs), breast mass biopsy
Ablative	Amputation or removal of diseased body part	Amputation, removal of appendix, cholecystectomy
Palliative	Relieves or reduces intensity of disease symptoms; will not produce cure	Colostomy, removal of necrotic tissue, resection of nerve roots
Reconstructive/ restorative	Restores function or appearance to traumatized or malfunctioning tissues	Internal fixation of fractures, scar revision
Procurement for transplant	Removal of organs and/or tissues from a person pronounced brain dead for transplantation into another person	Kidney, cornea, or liver transplant
Constructive	Restores function lost or reduced as result of congenital anomalies	Repair of cleft palate, closure of atrial septal defect in heart
Cosmetic	Performed to improve personal appearance	Blepharoplasty to correct eyelid deformities; rhinoplasty to reshape nose

an increased risk for aspiration during the administration of anesthesia (Scales and Master, 2003). The recumbent and supine positions required on the operating bed (table) for surgery further limit the patient's ventilation. The increased workload of the heart and atherosclerotic blood vessels often results in compromised cardiovascular function. Because of these physiological changes, patients who are obese often have difficulty in resuming normal physical activity after surgery. Hypertension, coronary artery disease, type 2 diabetes mellitus, and heart failure are common in this population. Patients who are obese are more susceptible to developing **embolism** (see Table 38-11, p. 1158), atelectasis, and pneumonia postoperatively than patients who are not obese (Black and Hawks, 2005).

In addition, excess weight placed on skin over bony prominences restricts blood flow and poses risk for impaired skin integrity. Obesity increases the risk of poor wound healing and wound infection because fatty tissue contains a poor blood supply, which slows the delivery of essential nutrients and antibodies needed for healing. It is often difficult to close the surgical wound of when a patient is obese because of the thick adipose layer. The risk for wound dehiscence and evisceration is increased because of these factors (see Chapter 36).

OBSTRUCTIVE SLEEP APNEA Obstructive sleep apnea (OSA) increases the risk for perioperative respiratory complications such as oxygen desaturation and apnea. OSA is a syndrome of periodic complete or partial obstruction of the upper airway during sleep. Many patients diagnosed with OSA need to be instructed to bring their continuous positive airway pressure machine for use postoperatively. However, many patients have undiagnosed OSA and can be screened preoperatively with simple questions regarding snoring, apnea during sleep, frequents arousals during sleep, morning headaches, daytime somnolence, and chronic fatigue (American Society of Anesthesiologists [ASA], 2006; Blouin and Magro, 2005).

TABLE 38-2   Physiological Factors That Place the Older Adult at Risk During Surgery

ALTERATIONS	RISKS	NURSING IMPLICATIONS
CARDIOVASCULAR SYSTEM		
Degeneration of myocardium and valves	Reduces cardiac reserve.	Assess baseline vital signs and patient's fluid volume status.
Rigid arteries and reduction in sympathetic and parasympathetic innervation to heart	Predisposes patient to postoperative hemorrhage and hypertension.	Instruct patient in techniques for performing leg exercises and proper turning.
Increase in calcium and cholesterol deposits within small arteries; thickened arterial walls	Increases risk for clot formation in lower extremities.	Apply antiembolism stockings, sequential compression devices.
INTEGUMENTARY SYSTEM		
Decreased subcutaneous tissue and increased fragility of skin	Patient is prone to pressure ulcers and skin tears.	Assess skin every 2 hours or more often; pad all bony prominences during surgery. Turn or reposition every 2 hours if possible.
PULMONARY SYSTEM		
Rib cage stiffened and reduced in size	Reduces vital capacity.	Instruct patient in proper technique for coughing, deep breathing, splinting incision, and use of incentive spirometer.
Reduced range of movement in diaphragm	Greater residual capacity or volume of air left in lung after normal breath, reducing amount of new air brought into lungs with each inspiration.	When possible, have patient ambulate and sit in chair frequently.
Stiffened lung tissue and enlarged air spaces	Reduces blood oxygenation levels.	Provide supplemental oxygen when ordered.
Decreased ability to cough and clear upper airway	Increases the risk for postoperative pulmonary infection.	Have patient cough, deep breathe, and use incentive spirometer every 2 hours.
RENAL SYSTEM		
Reduced blood flow to kidneys	Increases risk for damage to renal tissues.	For patients hospitalized before surgery, determine baseline urinary output for 24 hours.
Reduced glomerular filtration rate and excretory times	Limits ability to eliminate drugs or toxic substances.	Maintain adequate hydration.
Reduced bladder capacity	Voiding frequency increases, and larger amount of urine stays in bladder after voiding.	Instruct patient to notify nurse immediately when sensation of bladder fullness develops.
	Sensation of need to void sometimes does not occur until bladder is full.	Keep call light and bedpan within easy reach.
NEUROLOGICAL SYSTEM		
Sensory losses, including reduced tactile sense and increased pain tolerance	Patient is less able to respond to early warning signs of surgical complications.	Orient patient to surrounding environment. Observe for nonverbal signs of pain.
Decreased reaction time	Patient becomes easily confused after anesthesia.	Reorient frequently. Keep side rails up and room free from clutter.
METABOLIC SYSTEM		
Reduced number of red blood cells and hemoglobin levels	Reduces ability to carry adequate oxygen to tissues.	Administer necessary blood products. Monitor blood test results.
Change in total amounts of body potassium and water volume	Increases risk for fluid or electrolyte imbalance.	Monitor fluid and electrolyte levels.

IMMUNOCOMPETENCE Radiation and chemotherapeutic drugs used to treat cancer, immunosuppressive agents used to prevent rejection after organ transplantation, and steroids used to treat inflammatory conditions make the body vulnerable to infection. All of these therapies suppress the body's immune system. In addition, disorders affecting the immune system such as acquired immunodeficiency syndrome (AIDS) suppress the immune system. Patients with immunosuppression have an increased risk for infection following surgery. For example, the patient with cancer may have radiotherapy before surgery to reduce the size of a cancerous tumor in order to remove it surgically. Radiation causes fibrosis and vascular scarring in the radiated area. This causes tissues to become fragile and poorly oxygenated, increasing the risk for wound infection. Ideally surgery takes place 4 to 6 weeks after the completion of radiation treatments to avoid wound-healing problems.

FLUID AND ELECTROLYTE BALANCE The body responds to surgery as a form of trauma. As a result of the adrenocortical stress response, hormonal reactions cause sodium and water retention and potassium loss within the first 2 to 5 days after surgery. Severe protein breakdown creates a negative nitrogen balance. The severity of the stress response influences the degree of fluid and electrolyte imbalance. More extensive surgery is associated with more severe physiological stress. Patients with preexisting renal, fluid and electrolyte, gastrointestinal, respiratory, or cardiovascular problems are at greatest risk for operative complications. For example, a patient who is dehydrated from vomiting preoperatively is at greater risk for hypovolemic shock (see Chapter 17).

PREGNANCY When dealing with a pregnant patient, consider the needs of both the pregnant woman and her unborn fetus. Surgery is only for urgent or emergent reasons, such as appendicitis or trauma. The enlarged uterus displaces abdominal organs and distorts landmarks, making surgery more complex. Anesthetics and medications cause fetal abnormalities during the first trimester.

During pregnancy the following maternal physiological changes occur that make monitoring this surgical patient very difficult (Rothrock, 2007):

1. Cardiac output and respiratory tidal volume increase to keep up with the increase in metabolic rate and blood pressure decreases, making interpretation of vital signs and recognition of hypovolemic shock more difficult.
2. The high level of progesterone relaxes the lower esophageal sphincter (LES) and decreases gastrointestinal motility, which slows gastric emptying, resulting in an increased risk for aspiration of stomach contents.
3. Near term there is an increase in white blood cells beyond the normal range for that of nonpregnant women who have no infection.
4. There is an increased risk for deep vein thrombosis as a result of increased fibrinogen levels and decreased clotting time.

In addition, the pregnant patient and her family experience increased psychological stress because of fear of fetal loss or deformity. The perioperative team addresses these concerns.

NURSING KNOWLEDGE BASE

Perioperative Communication

Perioperative nurses recognize the importance of providing continuity of care for the surgical patient using the nursing process. In some settings, perioperative nurses assess a patient's health status preoperatively, identify specific patient needs, teach and counsel, attend to the patient's needs in the operating room (OR), and then follow the patient's recovery. In other words, one nurse follows a patient throughout the operative experience. However, in other institutions, different nurses care for the patient during each phase of the surgical experience. Therefore verbal and written communication between perioperative nurses is essential to ensure continuity of care. Transitions from one care provider to another place patients at risk for injuries and errors. A standardized approach to hand-off communication between perioperative nurses minimizes these risks. One recognized approach to addressing this concern is using the SBAR (i.e., situation, background, assessment, and recommendation) communication technique (Amato-Vealey, Barba, and Vealey, 2008) (see Chapter 10).

Complication Prevention

Patients are at high risk for a variety of complications following surgery. Prevention of respiratory and cardiac complications requires skill at assessment and knowledge of the pulmonary and cardiovascular system. Assessment begins in the preoperative area and continues through the postoperative period. Detection of breathing difficulties or airway issues requires you to anticipate problems, know a patient's risk, and have excellent assessment skills. Quick intervention prevents significant problems. Prevent cardiac complications through monitoring of vital signs, fluid and electrolytes, and tissue perfusion. Quick detection of subtle changes will prevent potentially dangerous complications.

Infection Prevention

Evidence has shown that there is a relationship between wound and tissue infection and blood glucose levels. Poor control of blood glucose levels (specifically hyperglycemia) during surgery and afterwards increases the risk for wound infection and patient mortality in certain types of surgery (Patel, 2008; Ramos and others, 2008). Perioperative nurses work with their medical colleagues to maintain normal glucose levels in the postoperative period to reduce the risk for wound and tissue infection.

Pressure Ulcer Prevention

Surgical patients pose a unique challenge in preventing pressure ulcers. Patients are at risk for pressure ulcer formation intraoperatively as a result of sustained pressure from positioning on OR tables. Pressure compresses skin and muscle between bones and the OR bed, resulting in tissue ischemia. Anesthetic agents lower blood pressure, altering tissue perfusion. Factors such as shear force, negativity from multiple layers of drapes, and moisture on the OR bed add to the risk for ulcer formation. The incidence of pressure ulcers in postoperative patients ranges between 4.7% and 45% (Schoonhoven and others, 2002). Operating room nurses work to prevent pressure ulcers intraoperatively by careful positioning and use of pressure-relieving surfaces. Postoperatively, nurses perform careful skin assessment and intervene by using low-air-loss or pressure-reduction beds and mattresses and frequent repositioning for those unable to move themselves.

CRITICAL THINKING

Synthesis

Apply elements of critical thinking whenever you perform the nursing process with a patient. Consider the scientific knowledge you have learned, your experience, critical thinking attitudes, and standards to ensure an individualized approach to patient care.

KNOWLEDGE It is essential to have a strong knowledge base in anatomy and physiology, principles of aseptic technique (see Chapter 13), pharmacology (see Chapter 16), and teaching-learning principles (see Chapter 11). In addition, understanding the effect surgical procedures and medications will have on different body systems is essential. It is also important to understand the normal stress response in order to anticipate potential complications during the perioperative experience. Effective preoperative teaching requires a knowledge base of teaching and communication principles and the planned surgical procedure.

EXPERIENCE Any personal experience with surgery helps you to understand the anxiety of the patient and family, as well as to explain some of the physical sensations that patients experience. Past experiences with surgical patients enable you to anticipate questions that the patient and family will ask and to focus preoperative teaching. In addition, past experiences will help you recognize physiological changes in patients more quickly so that you are able to initiate preventive and corrective measures early.

ATTITUDES A key attitude for a perioperative nurse is responsibility. As a perioperative nurse, you are responsible for following perioperative care standards and being a patient advocate. When a patient consents to surgery and receives an anesthetic agent that alters the level of consciousness, health care providers have the responsibility to protect the patient. You are responsible for maintaining the rights of the patient when the patient cannot speak on his or her own behalf.

Perioperative nurses who are creative apply evidence in the plan of care to deal with individual patient differences. For example, to promote venous return, position pregnant patients on the operating table with a positioning wedge under the right hip to displace the uterus to the left. Assess each patient, and use the most appropriate padding and positioning techniques possible to prevent injury.

Your attitude about the discipline of nursing is also important when caring for surgical patients. The patient will experience numerous routines necessary both for preparation for surgery and for an efficient and optimal recovery. Systematically follow the current standards of practice to ensure high-quality care for each patient.

STANDARDS The application of critical thinking intellectual standards is important for the patient having surgery, particularly if the patient has preexisting physical or psychological factors that will influence the outcomes of surgery. Be very precise, accurate, and complete in gathering assessment data, and use a logical, relevant, and well-thought-out approach in making clinical decisions because the patient's condition can change quickly.

The Association of periOperative Registered Nurses (AORN) established standards and recommended practice for nurses in perioperative clinical practice. The standards and position statements cover practices that ensure patient safety, appropriate monitoring and evaluation, infection control practices, and timely and effective nursing interventions. As a perioperative nurse, you are responsible for following these standards (AORN, 2009). The Joint Commission (2009) has a Universal Protocol guideline and a national patient safety goal related to prevention of surgical site infections.

PREOPERATIVE SURGICAL PHASE

Patients having surgery enter the health care setting in different stages of health. Some patients enter the facility feeling relatively healthy while awaiting elective surgery. Other patients enter in great distress when facing emergency surgery. Many tests and procedures are often necessary to ensure that surgery is indicated and that the patient is in optimum condition for surgery. During these tests and procedures, the patient meets many health care personnel who play a role in the patient's care and recovery. Family members or friends also play an important role by providing support and education reinforcement, but they also face many of the same stressors as the patient.

Some patients have preoperative preparation several days before the day of surgery. Preadmission testing is often done in the hospital, surgeon's office, or outpatient laboratory. With this testing completed, the patient usually enters the hospital the day surgery is performed. Many hospitals have special outpatient or "ambulatory" surgery centers for elective surgery, where patients come to the center, have surgery, and return home on the same day. Outpatient surgery is also performed in freestanding clinics. At times, the patient will enter the hospital the day before surgery. Be able to properly prepare the patient for surgery regardless of where the patient enters the health care setting.

NURSING PROCESS

▪▪▪ ASSESSMENT

Your preoperative assessment of the patient establishes a normal baseline for the patient before surgery and alerts you to special needs and potential intraoperative and postoperative complications. You will need good communication skills to gather information and screen patients for potential risk factors for surgery (Scales and Master, 2003).

NURSING HISTORY The preoperative history includes key elements that are relevant to the patient's risks and needs (Box 38-1). In the ambulatory surgical setting the history is often less detailed than when the patient is hospitalized the evening before surgery; however, the basic information outlined below is necessary for competent care in each setting. Interview family members or significant others if a patient is unable to relate all needed information. As with any admission to a health care facility, include information concerning advance directives. Ask if the patient has a durable power of attorney for health care and a living will (see Chapter 4), and include a copy in the chart. The law requires advance directive identification for patients of all ages and for all surgical procedures. Often directives are modified during the perioperative period but are reestablished after postoperative stabilization.

Medical History A review of the patient's medical history includes past illnesses and the primary reason for seeking medical care. Candidates for surgery are screened for major medical conditions that will increase the risk for complications (Table 38-3). If a patient is at increased risk, surgery as an outpatient may not be advisable. Ask women of childbearing age about the date of their last menstrual period (LMP), if their last period was "typical" for them, and if they have had unprotected sex in the last month. Because many women do not know they are pregnant early in the first trimester, many institutions require a pregnancy test when a patient of childbearing age is scheduled for surgery and has not had surgical sterilization. Inquire about family history for anesthetic complications because an adverse reaction called **malignant hyperthermia** is an inherited disorder. Malignant hyperthermia is a life-threatening complication resulting in high carbon dioxide levels, tachypnea, tachycardia, heart rhythm irregularities, and muscular rigidity with elevated temperature in the late stages.

Previous Surgeries Review of the patient's past experience with surgery reveals physical and psychological responses that potentially could occur during the current planned procedure. Complications such as anaphylaxis or malignant hyperthermia during previous surgery alert you to the need for preventive measures and availability of emergency equipment. A history of postoperative complications, such as persistent vomiting or uncontrolled pain, also alerts you to the possible need for different medications. Reports of severe anxiety before a previous surgery identify the need for additional emotional support, medications, and preoperative teaching. Inform the sur-

BOX 38-1	SYNTHESIS IN PRACTICE

 As Sue prepares to conduct the preadmission assessment of Mr. Korloff, she recalls what she has learned regarding risk factors for patients undergoing surgery. Mr. Korloff has a history of heart disease. Five years ago he was treated for a cardiac rhythm irregularity but has had no further problems. Sue will plan to question Mr. Korloff thoroughly about any potential cardiac symptoms. She plans to have his daughters present during the discussion.

Sue's knowledge of laparoscopic surgery will help her anticipate the types of postoperative problems Mr. Korloff is likely to develop, such as food intolerance and abdominal or referred pain from the carbon dioxide gas used during laparoscopy. Sue's experience with her own father after surgery will help her to explain some of the sensations that Mr. Korloff will experience, such as a sore throat from the breathing tube used for administering anesthesia. She will also need to draw on her experiences with patients she cared for after laparoscopic surgeries during her previous rotation on a general surgery floor. She will inform Mr. Korloff and his daughters that he will have intravenous (IV) fluids infusing until he tolerates oral fluids and that he will likely experience mild discomfort. Mr. Korloff will be able to get out of bed the evening of surgery, and if all goes well he will likely be discharged the next day.

geon of your findings when you believe medications are indicated.

Medication History Review whether the patient is taking any medications that predispose him or her to surgical complications (Table 38-4). Many medications interact unpredictably with anesthetic agents during surgery (McKenry and Salerno, 2003). If a patient regularly uses prescription or over-the-counter (OTC) medications, or herbal supplements, some surgeons will temporarily discontinue the medications before surgery or adjust the dosages. Instruct patients to ask the surgeon whether they should take their usual medications the morning of surgery. If the patient is having inpatient surgery, all prescription drugs taken before surgery are automatically discontinued after surgery unless reordered. Be vigilant in reviewing the surgeon's preoperative orders so that you do not forget any medication the patient needs to take before the operation. It is very important that as the patient moves through the different areas during the surgical procedure that a complete list of the patient's medications is accurately communicated from nurse to nurse (The Joint Commission, 2009).

Allergies Allergies to medications, topical agents used to prepare the skin for surgery, and latex create significant risks for the surgical patient. An allergic response to any agent is potentially fatal, depending on its severity. Latex allergies are on the rise (see Chapter 13). A latex allergy manifests as contact dermatitis with redness, inflammation, and blisters; as

TABLE 38-3 Medical Conditions That Increase the Risks of Surgery

TYPE OF CONDITION	REASON FOR RISK
Bleeding disorders (thrombocytopenia, hemophilia)	Disorders increase risk for hemorrhaging during and after surgery.
Diabetes mellitus	Diabetes increases susceptibility to infection and impairs wound healing from altered glucose metabolism and associated circulatory impairment. Fluctuating blood glucose levels cause central nervous system alterations during anesthesia. Stress of surgery causes increases in blood glucose levels.
Heart disease (recent myocardial infarction, dysrhythmias, congestive heart failure) and peripheral vascular disease	Stress of surgery causes increased demands on myocardium to maintain cardiac output. General anesthetic agents depress cardiac function.
Hypertension	Hypertension increases the risk for cardiovascular complications during anesthesia (e.g., stroke, inadequate tissue oxygenation).
Upper respiratory infection	Infection increases risk for respiratory complications during anesthesia (e.g., pneumonia, spasm of laryngeal muscles).
Renal disease	Renal disease alters the excretion of anesthetic drugs and their metabolites and alters acid-base balance, increasing risk for surgical complications.
Liver disease	Liver disease alters metabolism and elimination of drugs administered during surgery and impairs wound healing and clotting time because of alterations in protein metabolism.
Fever	Fever predisposes patient to fluid and electrolyte imbalances and often indicates underlying infection.
Chronic respiratory disease (emphysema, bronchitis, asthma)	Respiratory disease reduces patient's means to compensate for acid-base alterations. Anesthetic agents reduce respiratory function, increasing risk for severe hypoventilation.
Immunological disorders (leukemia, acquired immunodeficiency syndrome [AIDS], bone marrow depression, organ transplantation, and use of chemotherapeutic drugs)	Immunological disorders increase risk for infection and delay wound healing after surgery.
Abuse of alcohol and street drugs	Patients who abuse drugs sometimes have underlying disease (human immune deficiency virus [HIV], hepatitis) and altered wellness, which affect healing. Alcohol addiction causes unpredictable reactions to anesthesia. Persons go into withdrawal during and after surgery.
Chronic pain	Regular use of pain medications can result in higher tolerance. Increased doses of opioids are frequently necessary to achieve postoperative pain control.

contact urticaria with pruritus, redness, and swelling; or as hay fever–like symptoms and anaphylaxis.

All health care workers need to know about their patient's allergies. In most agencies, patients who have allergies receive an allergy identification band at the time of admission. It remains until discharge. Allergies are also listed on the front of the patient's chart, on the medical order sheet, and on the patient's medication administration record. Verify your patient's allergies before, during, and after surgery.

Smoking Habits The patient who smokes is at a greater risk for postoperative pulmonary complications than a patient who does not smoke. Smoking decreases ciliary movement of mucus from the lower airways upward, increases mucus production, and causes bronchial constriction, thus increasing airway obstruction. After surgery patients have greater difficulty clearing the airways of mucous secretions and are at increased risk for **bronchospasm** and **laryngo-**

spasm. Use this information to plan aggressive postoperative **pulmonary hygiene,** including more frequent turning, deep breathing, coughing, use of incentive spirometry, and chest physical therapy (PT) if ordered. Smoking causes hypercoagulability of the blood and increased risk for clot formation (Black and Hawks, 2005). Provide measures to decrease the risk for clot formation such as pneumatic compression stockings, deep breathing, leg exercises, and early ambulation.

Alcohol and Controlled Substance Use and Abuse The surgical team needs to be aware of the use of alcohol and controlled substances by patients to prepare for adverse reactions, such as withdrawal, that may occur during surgery. Increased tolerance to opioids occurs with chronic opioid use, resulting in an increased need for anesthesia and postoperative analgesics (Black and Hawks, 2005).

Family Support Determine if and to what extent the patient will have support from family members or friends. Sur-

TABLE 38-4   Drugs With Special Implications for the Surgical Patient

DRUG CLASS	EFFECTS DURING SURGERY
Antibiotics	Antibiotics potentiate action of anesthetic agents. If taken within 2 weeks before surgery, aminoglycosides (gentamicin, tobramycin, neomycin) cause mild respiratory depression from depressed neuromuscular transmission.
Antidysrhythmics	Antidysrhythmics reduce cardiac contractility and heart rate and impair cardiac conduction during anesthesia.
Anticoagulants	Anticoagulants alter normal clotting factors, increasing risk for hemorrhage during and after surgery. Discontinue them at least 48 hours before surgery. Aspirin is a common medication that alters clotting mechanisms.
Anticonvulsants	Long-term use of certain anticonvulsants (e.g., phenytoin [Dilantin], phenobarbital) alters metabolism of anesthetic agents.
Antihypertensives	Antihypertensives interact with anesthetic agents and cause bradycardia, hypotension, and impaired circulation. They inhibit synthesis and storage of norepinephrine in sympathetic nerve endings.
Corticosteroids	With prolonged use, corticosteroids cause adrenal atrophy, which reduces the body's ability to withstand stress and results in hypotension during surgery. Dosages are sometimes temporarily increased before and during surgery.
Insulin	Patients with diabetes often need less insulin after surgery because their nutritional intake is decreased. However, stress response and intravenous administration of glucose solutions increase insulin dosage requirements after surgery.
Diuretics	Diuretics potentiate electrolyte imbalances (particularly potassium), increasing the risk for dysrhythmias during and after surgery.
Nonsteroidal antiinflammatory drugs (NSAIDs)	NSAIDs inhibit platelet aggregation and prolong bleeding time, increasing susceptibility to bleeding during and after surgery.

gery often results in temporary disability that requires direct care and assistance from significant others during recovery. The patient does not always immediately assume the same level of physical activity and often returns home with dressings to change or exercises to perform. Ask questions to determine the condition of the patient's home environment and factors that will interfere with postoperative restrictions or care activities. For example, a patient receives discharge instructions that state no stair climbing due to limited mobility. When talking with the patient and family, you discover that the bathroom in the home is on the second floor. In this case, you make sure that the patient has a commode to use on the first level of the home until normal activity can be resumed.

Occupation Surgery often results in physical alterations that hinder or prevent a person from returning to work. Assess the patient's occupational history to anticipate the effect surgery will have on convalescence and eventual work performance. Explain any restrictions the patient will have when returning to work.

Feelings Surgery causes anxiety and a feeling of loss of control for most patients. Many families are concerned about the ability of the patient to return to a productive life and the impact recovery will have on the family. Assess the patient's feelings about having surgery from both verbal and nonverbal cues. A patient who is fearful may ask many questions or be very quiet, will seem uneasy when strangers enter the room, or will actively seek the company of friends and relatives.

It is difficult to assess patients' feelings thoroughly before ambulatory surgery is scheduled. You will have limited time to spend with the patient. As the nurse in an outpatient surgi-

cal program, telephone the patient at home before surgery or interview the patient during a preadmission testing visit. For patients in the hospital, choose a time for discussion after preliminary admitting or diagnostic tests are complete. The patient's ability to share feelings depends in part on your willingness to ask questions, listen, be supportive, and clarify misconceptions.

Cultural and Spiritual Factors Cultural differences in the use of both verbal and nonverbal communication require you to validate interpretation of cues with the patient and family (Box 38-2). This is especially important after you conduct the initial preoperative assessment and then look for changes in the patient's status after surgery. For example, patients from Asian cultures often remain silent out of respect, not fear. Individuals from Central America usually prefer the presence of many family members and friends, who help to express the patient's needs. In some cultures, women follow what the significant male member of the family dictates; therefore it is very important to explain everything to your female patient's husband, father, or brother for her to participate in the plan of care (Giger and Davidhizar, 2004). When doing this, make sure to have permission from the patient to share personal health information. Many cultural and religious taboos exist concerning the body, who cares for the physical needs of others, and treatments appropriate for healing, so it is important to explore these issues with the patient and/or family. Although it is important to recognize and plan for differences based on culture, remember that not all members of one family always hold the beliefs of a particular religion or culture. Asking relevant questions of each patient concerning cultural and spiritual beliefs and expectations will further individualize your nursing care (see Chapters 19 and 20). Patients' spiritual beliefs help in coping with fears and anxieties related to the upcoming surgery. Help the patient obtain the spiritual help requested before surgery. For example, contact the hospital chaplain per patient request before going to surgery.

Coping Resources Assessment of patients' feelings and self-concept reveals whether they have the ability to cope with the stress of surgery. It is also valuable to ask patients about stress management. If a patient has had previous surgery, discuss the behaviors that helped to resolve past tension or nervousness. You may instruct a patient in relaxation exercises (see Chapter 31), which help control anxiety.

Body Image Surgical removal of a diseased tissue or organ often leaves permanent disfigurement or alteration in body function. Concern over mutilation, change in sexuality, or loss of a body part adds to a patient's fears. Individuals react differently, depending on age, culture, occupation, self-image, and self-esteem. Encourage patients to express these concerns so you can offer support (see Chapter 22).

Patient Expectations It is important to identify the patient's and family's perceptions and expectations regarding surgery, recovery, and health care providers. This information allows you to plan interventions for teaching and emotional preparation and provides the basis for evaluation of care. For example, some patients have expectations regarding pain control and the use of pain medications that are unrealistic. Patients who are prepared to experience pain and know the proper use of pharmacological and nonpharmacological pain-relief measures tend to require less medication (Rothrock, 2007).

Patients and family members often have misconceptions about surgery. It is important to discuss with them their understanding of the purpose of the tests, the possible outcomes, and the persons responsible for informing them of results and providing follow-up care. When a patient is well prepared and knows what to expect, reinforce the patient's knowledge.

You will face an ethical dilemma when a patient is unaware of the actual reason for surgery. In such a case, speak with the surgeon before revealing specific information related to the medical diagnosis to prevent confusion and identify the need for clarification.

PHYSICAL EXAMINATION You will conduct a partial or complete physical examination (see Chapter 15), depending on the setting and nature of the surgery. The assessment focuses on findings related to the patient's medical history and on body systems that surgery or anesthesia will affect (Table 38-5).

General Survey Gestures and body movements often reflect decreased energy or weakness caused by illness. Height and body weight are important indicators of nutritional status and are used to calculate medication dosages. Preoperative vital signs provide a baseline for intraoperative and postoperative comparison. Anesthetic agents and medications produce vital sign changes. Preoperative assessment of

---

BOX 38-2   CULTURAL FOCUS

In preparing her preoperative teaching, Sue discovers that Russian Americans, such as Mr. Korloff, expect the nurse to be warm and caring. Nurses are expected to help patients cope with their health problems. Russian Americans expect the nurse to be friendly, using open inviting nonverbal postures and a friendly smile. They freely share health problems with nurses conveying this friendly, caring behavior. Russian Americans are also willing to follow teaching provided by nurses who they feel are sincere, competent, and trustworthy. They value receiving immediate information and answers from health care workers and follow up on health care instructions when they fully understand them. Russian Americans typically have strong family ties and values. The father usually plays a primary role in the function of the family. Using the knowledge of Russian Americans Sue gained from her reading and past experience, she developed a culturally competent plan of care for Mr. Korloff.

IMPLICATIONS FOR PRACTICE
- Assess Mr. Korloff's opinions about surgery first and then include his family.
- Assess the level of involvement of Mr. Korloff's family in his surgical preparation and care.
- Provide preoperative teaching in a warm, caring, open manner using frequent smiles and hand gestures.
- Speak slowly and clearly in a low, calm voice using simple words.
- Provide an explanation of the importance of postoperative exercises so Mr. Korloff will understand why the exercises are important and will be more willing to do them after surgery.
- Determine if family members are close to Mr. Korloff and include them in the teaching session.

From Giger JN, Davidhizar RE: *Transcultural nursing: assessment and intervention*, ed 4, St. Louis, 2004, Mosby.

---

vital signs is also important to detect fluid and electrolyte abnormalities (see Chapter 17).

An elevated temperature is cause for concern. If the patient has an underlying infection, elective surgery will often be postponed until the infection is treated or resolved. An elevated body temperature also alters drug metabolism and increases the risk for fluid and electrolyte imbalances.

Head and Neck Assessment of oral mucous membranes reveals the level of hydration. Dehydration increases the risk for the development of serious fluid and electrolyte imbalances during surgery. During the oral examination, identify loose or capped teeth because they often become dislodged during endotracheal intubation. Note any dentures or partial plates your patient uses. When necessary, remove them and give to family member to protect them from loss or damage.

Inspection of the soft palate and nasal sinuses sometimes reveals sinus drainage indicative of respiratory or sinus infection. To rule out the possibility of local or systemic infection,

TABLE 38-5 FOCUSED PATIENT ASSESSMENT

FACTORS TO ASSESS	QUESTIONS	PHYSICAL ASSESSMENT
Significant medical history and previous surgeries	Do you have any bleeding disorders, diabetes, heart, lung, renal, or liver disease or any immune disorder?	Monitor vital signs, and note any abnormalities. Inspect neck for jugular vein distention (cardiac disease, fluid overload). Palpate heart, vascular system, abdomen for abnormalities (thrill, masses).
	Have you had a recent fever or upper respiratory infection?	Inspect skin for turgor, dryness, rashes, skin breakdown. Auscultate heart and lungs for abnormal sounds (murmurs, congestion, bruits).
	Do you experience chronic pain?	Perform pain assessment with pain tool, including severity, location, description, measures used to relieve.
Medication history and allergies	What prescription, over-the-counter, and herbal medications are you currently taking?	Assess extremities for decreased sensation, hair loss, clubbed fingers, deformed nails, sluggish capillary reflex, color.
	What instructions were you given from your surgeon concerning taking or omitting medications preoperatively?	Inspect any medication containers brought in by patient or family.
	Do you have any personal and/or family history of allergic responses to medications (including anesthetics) or environmental factors (e.g., latex, foods)?	Monitor laboratory values for any evidence of side effects of medications or drug levels, if ordered.
	What allergic reaction did you have after exposure?	Observe skin and mucous membranes for any evidence of allergic response.

palpate for cervical lymph node enlargement. Also inspect the jugular veins for distention. Excess fluid within the circulatory system or failure of the heart to contract efficiently frequently leads to jugular vein distention. A patient with heart disease or fluid overload is at risk for cardiovascular complications during surgery.

Skin   Thoroughly inspect the patient's skin overlying all body parts, especially bony prominences. During surgery a patient lies in a fixed position, often for several hours. Avoid positioning a patient over an area where the skin shows signs of pressure over bony prominences. A patient is susceptible to skin breakdown if the skin is thin or dry or has poor turgor (see Chapter 36).

Thorax and Lungs   A decline in ventilatory function, assessed through breathing pattern and chest excursion, indicates a patient's risk for respiratory complications. Serious pulmonary congestion often causes postponement of surgery. For example, narrowing of the airways, as occurs with chronic lung disease (CLD, formerly known as chronic obstructive pulmonary disease [COPD]), increases the risk for airway obstruction because of bronchospasm related to endotracheal intubation and anesthesia.

Heart and Vascular System   If the patient has heart disease, assess the apical pulse. After surgery compare the rate and rhythm of the patient's pulse with preoperative baseline values. Assessment of peripheral pulses, color, and temperature of extremities is particularly important for the patient undergoing vascular or orthopedic surgery and when applying constricting bandages or casts to an extremity after surgery. Postoperative color changes, change in sensation, or

development of a weak or absent pulse in a patient who had adequate circulation before surgery indicates impaired circulation.

Abdomen   Alterations in gastrointestinal function after surgery often result in decreased or absent bowel sounds and abdominal distention. Assess the patient's usual abdominal anatomy to assess for distention. Assessment of preoperative bowel sounds and normal elimination pattern is useful as a baseline. If surgery requires manipulation of portions of the gastrointestinal tract or if a general anesthetic is used, normal peristalsis sometimes does not return and bowel sounds are absent or diminished for hours to several days.

Neurological Status   A patient's level of consciousness will change as a result of general anesthesia. However, after the effects of anesthesia disappear, the patient will return to the preoperative level of responsiveness. Spinal or epidural anesthesia causes temporary paralysis of the lower extremities. Be aware of preexisting weakness or impaired mobility of the lower extremities to avoid becoming alarmed when full motor function does not return immediately after a procedure.

RISK FACTORS   Knowledge of preoperative risk factors discussed earlier will enable you to take necessary precautions in planning care.

DIAGNOSTIC SCREENING   Before a patient has surgery, diagnostic tests screen for preexisting abnormalities. Patients scheduled for elective surgery take these tests as an outpatient on or before the morning of surgery. If tests reveal severe problems, the surgeon or anesthesiologist will cancel surgery until the condition stabilizes. As the preoperative nurse, coordinate the completion of tests and verify that the

TABLE 38-6   Common Laboratory Blood Tests

TEST	NORMAL VALUES*	SIGNIFICANCE	
		LOW	HIGH
COMPLETE BLOOD COUNT (CBC)			
Hemoglobin (Hgb)	Female: 12-16 g/dL; male: 14-18 g/dL	Anemia	Polycythemia (elevated red blood cell count)
Hematocrit (Hct)	Female: 37%-47%; male: 42%-52%	Fluid overload	Dehydration
Platelet count	150,000-400,000/mm^3	Decreased clotting	Increased risk of blood clot
White blood cell count	5,000-10,000/mm^3	Decreased ability to fight infection	Infection
BLOOD CHEMISTRY			
Sodium (Na)	136-145 mEq/L	Fluid overload	Dehydration
Potassium (K)	3.5-5.0 mEq/L	Cardiac rhythm irregularities	Cardiac rhythm irregularities
Chloride (Cl)	98-106 mEq/L	Follows shifts in sodium blood levels	Follows shifts in sodium blood levels
Carbon dioxide (CO_2)	23-30 mEq/L	Affects acid base balance in blood	Affects acid base balance in blood
Blood urea nitrogen (BUN)	10-20 mg/dL	Liver disease/fluid overload	Renal disease/ dehydration
Glucose	70-110 mg/dL fasting	Insulin reaction, inadequate glucose intake	Diabetes mellitus and stress of surgery
Creatinine	Female: 0.5-1.1 mg/dL; male: 0.6-1.2 mg/dL	Malnutrition	Renal disease
COAGULATION STUDIES			
Prothrombin time (PT)	11-12.5 sec; 85%-100%	Risk of clot	Risk of bleeding
Partial thromboplastin time (PTT)	60-70 sec	Risk of clot	Risk of bleeding
Activated PTT (APTT)	30-40 sec		Excess heparin; risk of spontaneous bleeding

From Pagana KD, Pagana TJ: *Mosby's diagnostic and laboratory test reference,* ed 9, St. Louis, 2009, Mosby.
*Normal ranges vary slightly among laboratories.

patient is prepared properly. Review diagnostic results when available, and alert the surgeon and/or anesthesiologist to findings and intervene as appropriate.

Screening tests depend on the condition of the patient and the nature of the surgery. Table 38-6 summarizes routine screening tests. In addition, the patient will need a blood type and screen if transfusions are anticipated. Additional preoperative tests include a urinalysis screen for urinary tract infections, renal disease, or diabetes mellitus; and a 12-lead electrocardiogram to analyze heart rate and rhythm. A chest x-ray study to assess the size and shape of the heart, presence of lung lesions and chest wall abnormalities, and position of the diaphragm and the aorta is also a common preoperative test for the older adult patient and those with cardiovascular or pulmonary abnormalities.

■■■NURSING DIAGNOSIS

After you obtain assessment data, cluster defining characteristics to identify appropriate nursing diagnoses and related factors. The nature and type of surgery, as well as the patient's age and health status, suggest defining characteristics for many nursing diagnoses. The diagnoses establish direction for care during one or all of the surgical phases. For example,

a patient's restlessness, poor eye contact, and expressed concern about the results of surgery point to the diagnosis of *anxiety.* However, you need to validate the assessment to avoid misdiagnosis. In the foregoing assessment, restlessness may also indicate pain. Therefore you need to ensure that you identify the nursing diagnosis that best fits your patient's problem. Nursing diagnoses for the preoperative patient may include the following:

- *Anxiety*
- *Compromised family coping*
- *Ineffective coping*
- *Fear*
- *Risk for imbalanced fluid volume*
- *Deficient knowledge*
- *Risk for imbalanced nutrition: more than (or less than) body requirements*
- *Powerlessness*
- *Ineffective role performance*
- *Risk for spiritual distress*

A diagnosis and its related factors offer direction to the most effective nursing interventions. Ensure the related factors are accurate to avoid inappropriate interventions. For example, *anxiety related to deficient knowledge of perioperative routines* will require you to offer thorough instruction preoperatively and immediately postoperatively. However, *anxiety related to threat of ineffective role performance* will require counseling and coaching during postoperative recovery.

■■■ PLANNING

Always include the patient and family in any discussions before surgery. Involving the patient early minimizes surgical risks and postoperative complications. Structured preoperative teaching reduces the amount of anesthesia and postoperative pain medication needed, decreases the occurrence of postoperative urinary retention, promotes an earlier return to normal oral intake, and decreases length of hospital stay (Rothrock, 2007). Patients informed about the surgical experience are less likely to be fearful and are better prepared for expected outcomes.

GOALS AND OUTCOMES   The plan of care begins in the preoperative phase and is modified during the intraoperative and postoperative phases (see Care Plan). The goals of care for the surgical patient include the following:

- Understanding the physiological and psychological responses to surgery
- Understanding intraoperative and postoperative events
- Achieving emotional and physiological comfort and rest
- Achieving return of normal physiological function after surgery (e.g., return of normal vital signs, fluid and electrolyte balance, muscle function)
- Remaining free of surgical wound infection
- Remaining safe from harm during the perioperative period

Outcomes established for each goal of care provide measurable evidence to determine the patient's progress toward meeting stated goals. For example, in the case of "understanding intraoperative and postoperative events," outcomes would include the patient being able to describe postoperative exercises to follow or the patient being able to explain positioning during surgery.

SETTING PRIORITIES   Establish individualized care by prioritizing nursing diagnoses and interventions based on the assessed needs of each patient. Setting priorities requires clinical judgment. For example, if a patient has *anxiety* and *deficient knowledge*, the patient's priority is deficient knowledge. In this case, instruction of the patient will likely relieve the anxiety. Your approach to each patient needs to be thorough and reflect your understanding of the implications of

---

CARE PLAN   Surgery

ASSESSMENT

As Mr. Korloff enters the preadmission center for testing, Sue greets him and his daughters. She explains the need to gather a history and asks Mr. Korloff if he wishes to have his daughters join him. He smiles and says, "Yes, my daughters will be my nurses for a few days." The nursing staff report that Mr. Korloff's daughters have been calling on the phone and asking many questions about intraoperative and postoperative events. Mr. Korloff is alert and appropriate. His vision and hearing are normal. This will be his first experience having surgery.

ASSESSMENT ACTIVITIES	FINDINGS/DEFINING CHARACTERISTICS*
Ask Mr. Korloff what he has been told regarding surgery by his surgeon.	He states that **he knows very little about the surgery.**
Ask Mr. Korloff what he understands about preoperative preparation and what to expect postoperatively.	**He says he knows few specifics and asks if he will have an IV.**
Ask Mr. Korloff what concerns him about having surgery.	He repeatedly says, "Oh, I'm not worried," but then **asks many questions, often repeatedly.**

NURSING DIAGNOSIS: Deficient knowledge regarding implications of surgery (cholecystectomy) related to first surgical experience and inadequate preparation.

PLANNING

GOAL	EXPECTED OUTCOMES (NOC)†
• Mr. Korloff will understand preoperative, intraoperative, and postoperative events before the day of surgery.	*Knowledge: Treatment Procedures* • Patient and his daughters will describe events that commonly occur in the holding area and operating room on the day before surgery. • Patient and his daughters will describe routine postoperative nursing procedures on the day of admission. • Patient and his daughters will describe ways to participate in postoperative care on the day of admission.

---

*Defining characteristics** are in **bold** type.

†Outcomes classification label from Moorhead S and others, editors: *Nursing outcomes classification (NOC)*, ed 4, St. Louis, 2008, Mosby.

CARE PLAN Surgery—cont'd

INTERVENTIONS (NIC)‡

Teaching: Procedure/Treatment

- Give Mr. Korloff a copy of the teaching booklet *Your Surgical Experience.* Arrange time to call at home to reinforce information and answer any questions on booklet's content.
- Provide planned teaching session for Mr. Korloff and his daughters after preadmission testing. Explain events that will occur in holding area (e.g., insertion of IV catheter, vital sign check) and in operating room (e.g., positioning, anesthesia). Use visual aids to assist Mr. Korloff's understanding of the laparoscopic procedure.
- Allow Mr. Korloff to express his feelings and fears related to surgery.

- Provide planned teaching session on day of admission with Mr. Korloff and his daughters to explain common events that occur after surgery and demonstrate postoperative exercises included in the teaching booklet.
- Have Mr. Korloff perform return demonstration of postoperative exercises.

RATIONALE

Patients who are prepared for surgery experience less anxiety and report a greater sense of psychological well-being and satisfaction (Mordiffi and others, 2003; Prouty and others, 2006).

Teaching focused on information patient will need to know on morning of admission will decrease anxiety and allow patient and family to better participate in care (Prouty and others, 2006).

Expressing feelings and fears decreases anxiety related to the surgical experience in order for patient teaching to be more effective.

Preoperative teaching improves patient's ability to ambulate, participate in care activities, and resume activities of daily living after surgery. Demonstration is an effective method in teaching psychomotor skills.

Return demonstration of exercises verifies that learning has occurred and patient is able to correctly perform exercises to reduce postoperative complications.

EVALUATION

NURSING ACTIONS	PATIENT RESPONSE/FINDING	ACHIEVEMENT OF OUTCOME
Ask Mr. Korloff and his daughters to identify the basic purpose of the surgery and changes to expect afterward.	Mr. Korloff describes the surgical procedure and explains why he needs the surgery.	Mr. Korloff demonstrates a good understanding of the surgery.
Ask Mr. Korloff and his daughters to identify routine types of postoperative monitoring and treatment.	He describes postoperative exercises to perform after surgery but is not able to discuss monitoring activities.	Mr. Korloff describes postoperative exercises, requires further instruction on monitoring activities.
Ask Mr. Korloff to state the most frightening aspect of surgery for him.	Mr. Korloff says he is most afraid of being put to sleep not knowing if he'll wake up.	Mr. Korloff verbalized his concern; support provided by his daughters.
Observe Mr. Korloff perform postoperative exercises.	Mr. Korloff demonstrated coughing, deep breathing, and use of leg exercises. Has difficulty using incentive spirometer. Mr. Korloff's daughters remind him to hold his breath for 2 to 3 seconds with use of incentive spirometer.	Mr. Korloff demonstrated coughing, deep breathing, and leg exercises appropriately. Requires further demonstration and assistance from his daughters in use of incentive spirometer.

‡Intervention classification label from Bulechek GM and others, editors: *Nursing interventions classification (NIC),* ed 5, St. Louis, 2008, Mosby.

the patient's age, physical and psychological health, educational level, cultural and religious practices, and stated and/or written wishes concerning advance directives.

COLLABORATIVE CARE For the ambulatory surgical patient the preoperative planning phase usually occurs in the outpatient surgery setting before or on the morning of surgery. Ideally, it begins in the surgeon's office and continues in

the home. This gives the patient time to reflect on the surgical experience, make necessary physical preparations, and ask questions about postoperative procedures. Well-planned preoperative care ensures that the patient is well informed and actively participates during recovery. The family or significant others also play an active supportive role for the patient.

BOX 38-3   PATIENT TEACHING

Perioperative Patient Preparation

 Sue plans time after completing Mr. Korloff's assessment to discuss the planned surgery with the patient and his daughters. She begins by asking Mr. Korloff to describe what he thinks the procedure will involve and the type of information he wants to understand. This shows Sue's cultural sensitivity, which will make teaching more appropriate.

OUTCOME

- At the end of the teaching session Mr Korloff will (1) describe preoperative, intraoperative, and postoperative procedures to anticipate for a laparoscopic procedure and (2) demonstrate postoperative exercises.

TEACHING STRATEGIES

1 Preoperative Procedures
   - State time to arrive at facility and time of surgery (approximate time or to follow).
   - Explain extent and purpose of food and fluid restrictions.
   - Explain or review informed consent.
   - Teach about physical preparation required (e.g., bowel or skin preparation).
   - Explain about procedures just before transport to operating room (IV line, catheterization or void, preoperative medications). These are often done in the preanesthesia care unit.

2 Intraoperative Procedures
   - Describe preanesthesia care environment and activities.
   - Describe operating room environment.
   - Explain about the roles of circulating nurse, scrub nurse, and anesthesia care provider.

3 Postoperative Procedures
   - Describe postanesthesia care environment and activities.
   - Teach about pain control and other comfort measures.
   - Explain purpose of any anticipated tubes, drains, or IV lines.
   - Emphasize importance of postoperative exercises (see Skill 38-1).
   - Demonstrate exercises, and have patient perform return demonstration.
   - Encourage Mr. Korloff and family to verbalize any concerns.
   - Assess Mr. Korloff and his family's understanding of perioperative preparation, and respond appropriately.

EVALUATION STRATEGIES

- Have Mr. Korloff describe his understanding of select preoperative, intraoperative, and postoperative procedures.
- Have Mr. Korloff demonstrate coughing, deep breathing, and turning exercises.

IV, Intravenous.

Planning also requires referral to other members of the health care team. Patients who will require aggressive pulmonary rehabilitation, such as those having thoracic surgery, are referred to a respiratory therapist. Many patients and their families benefit from referral to pastoral care, especially if the procedure is an emergency or is life threatening.

■■■ IMPLEMENTATION

Preoperative nursing interventions focus on patient education and physical preparation of the patient for surgery.

INFORMED CONSENT A surgeon cannot legally perform surgery nor can an anesthesia care provider administer an anesthetic until a patient understands the need for the procedure and the steps involved, as well as the risks, expected results, and alternative treatments. Chapter 4 summarizes issues and guidelines for informed consent. Patients need to sign all consent forms before you administer any preoperative medications that alter the patient's consciousness. The primary responsibility for informing the patient rests with the surgeon and anesthesia care personnel. However, if the patient is confused or uncertain about a procedure, you are ethically obligated to contact the surgeon and/or anesthesia care provider so that further discussion and clarification are provided to meet the patient's needs. The patient always has the right to refuse surgery or treatment even after giving written consent.

HEALTH PROMOTION Health promotion activities during the preoperative phase focus on prevention of complications, health maintenance, and support of possible rehabilitation needs postoperatively.

Preoperative Teaching Patient education relieves anxiety, increases patient satisfaction, speeds up the recovery process, decreases the amount of perceived pain, and facilitates a more rapid return to work or normal functioning (Lewis and others, 2002). **Preoperative teaching** provided in a systematic, structured, and interactive format has a positive influence on patients' recovery. Structured teaching often influences the following postoperative factors:

1. *Ventilatory function:* Teaching improves the ability and willingness to deep breathe and cough effectively.
2. *Physical functional capacity:* Teaching increases understanding and willingness to ambulate and resume activities of daily living.
3. *Sense of well-being:* Patients who are prepared for surgery experience less anxiety and report a greater sense of psychological well-being (Prouty and others, 2006).
4. *Length of hospital stay:* Teaching frequently reduces the patient's length of hospital stay by preventing or minimizing postoperative complications.
5. *Anxiety about pain and amount of pain medication needed for comfort:* Patients who learn about pain and ways to relieve it are less anxious about the pain, ask for what they need, and actually require less pain medication.

The most effective type of teaching program for surgical patients covers the entire surgical experience. Box 38-3 outlines the parameters for perioperative preparation. Today, because many patients are not admitted to the hospital before surgery, preoperative teaching often occurs in the home, surgeon's office, or preadmission unit. Offer printed literature, DVDs, or videotapes to patients. Call patients before surgery to provide education and clarify questions (Black and Hawks, 2005).

Always include family members and significant others in preoperative preparation. They are frequently the coaches for postoperative exercises when the patient returns from surgery. If family members and significant others do not understand routine postoperative events, their anxiety will heighten the patient's fears or concerns. Reduce misunderstanding and anxiety with thoughtful preparation. However, if the patient does not wish to include them, respect the request for privacy.

Timing. Preoperative teaching is most useful when started the week before admission and reinforced immediately before surgery. Teaching performed when the patient is less anxious will result in more effective learning. Anxiety and fear are barriers to learning. Assess the surgical patient's readiness and ability to learn (see Chapter 11). Always present information in a logical sequence beginning with preoperative events and advancing to intraoperative and postoperative routines. Preoperative teaching checklists offer helpful guidelines for presenting patients with a comprehensive set of instructions.

Content. Preoperative teaching includes information to assist the patient, family, and significant others in preparing for the surgical experience and participating in the plan of care (Bernier and others, 2003). Always assess their level of understanding about the surgery, perioperative routines, and expectations first. Then reinforce or teach information, based on the patient's and family's prior knowledge (Box 38-4).

Surgical Procedure. After the surgeon has explained the basic purpose of the surgical procedure and its steps, the patient will ask you additional questions. Avoid saying anything that contradicts the surgeon's explanation. One way to avoid contradictions is to first ask what the surgeon has told the patient. If the patient has little or no understanding about the surgery, refer the patient back to the surgeon for additional information.

Preoperative Routines. Explain the preoperative routines a patient will undergo. For example, if your patient needs an enema, explain why it is necessary. Knowing what tests and procedures are planned and why will increase the patient's sense of control.

The anesthesiologist will visit with the patient to complete a preanesthesia assessment either during the preoperative admission process or in the presurgical care unit. The patient

---

BOX 38-4 BEST PRACTICES

SUMMARY OF EVIDENCE

An increased number of surgeries are performed in ambulatory surgery centers. Patients arrive the morning of surgery and are discharged the same day. This type of surgery challenges nurses to provide effective and thorough preoperative teaching to patients in shorter time frames. Research demonstrates that meeting all of the patient's perceived educational needs in the preoperative period is challenging. In a study of same-day surgery patients, researchers found that patients reported the highest ratings for information regarding situational/procedural information, patient role information, and psychosocial support; however, patients gave low ratings regarding information received on sensation/discomfort (Bernier and others, 2003). Heikkinen and others (2007) studied patients having ambulatory orthopedic surgery and found that patients perceived receiving the greatest knowledge in the biophysical sphere and the least knowledge about experiential, ethical, social, and financial dimensions of perioperative care.

An alternative method of preoperative preparation was studied in an adolescent population undergoing outpatient tonsillectomy-adenoidectomy. O'Conner-Von (2008) compared an Internet-based method of preoperative preparation to the traditional method of an outpatient class before scheduled surgery. The adolescents using the Internet method had a significantly higher level of knowledge acquisition and satisfaction with the method than those in the traditional method. In addition, participation in the educational format was higher with the Internet group. Some of the identified benefits of the Internet program include viewing the program in privacy, at the patient's own pace, and the ability to view the program more than one time.

APPLICATION TO NURSING PRACTICE

The results of these studies will help nurses in ambulatory surgery centers provide thorough and effective preoperative teaching to patients.

- Nurses in ambulatory surgical centers need to have structured preoperative teaching programs to make sure patients of all ages have information related to surgery that they need.
- Nurses need to make sure that they give equal emphasis to all areas of preoperative teaching.
- All patients having surgery require information about psychosocial support.
- New methods of teaching such as Internet programs provide an alternative and may provide certain patient populations with a more satisfying preoperative education experience.

REFERENCES
Bernier MR and others: Preoperative teaching received and valued in a day surgery setting, *AORN J* 77(3):563, 2003.
Heikkinen K and others: Ambulatory orthopaedic surgery patients' knowledge expectations and perceptions of received knowledge, *J Adv Nurs* 60(3):270, 2007.
O'Conner-Von S: Preparation of adolescents for outpatient surgery: using an Internet program, *AORN J* 87(2):374, 2008.

and family need to know about this visit, so they can ask any questions and be prepared to provide necessary information, such as previous experience with anesthesia.

Explain to the patient and family the importance of the patient's following oral intake instructions for food and liquids as provided by the surgeon and anesthesiologist. The American Society of Anesthesiologists (ASA) provides recommendations on fluid and food intake before procedures requiring general anesthesia, regional anesthesia, or sedation/analgesia. The ASA recommendations include fasting from intake of clear liquids for 2 or more hours, breast milk for 4 hours, formula and nonhuman milk for 6 hours, and a light meal of toast and clear liquids for 6 hours. The patient also cannot have any meat or fried foods 8 hours before surgery, unless explicitly specified by the anesthesiologist or surgeon (American Society of Anesthesiologists Task Force on Perioperative Fast, 1999). During the use of general anesthesia, the muscles relax and gastric contents can reflux into the esophagus. The anesthetic eliminates the patient's ability to gag. Therefore the patient is at risk for aspiration of food or fluids from the stomach into the lungs. The surgeon's orders provide additional guidance for routines to explain to the patient (e.g., intravenous [IV] therapy, preoperative medications, or insertion of a urinary catheter or a nasogastric tube).

Intraoperative Routines. The scheduled operative time is only an anticipated time. Unanticipated delays occur for many reasons that have nothing to do with your patient. Emphasize that the scheduled time is a rough estimate and the actual time will possibly be sooner or later than the scheduled time. Tell family members where to wait, and inform them that the surgeon will speak to them when the surgery is completed. Communicate excessive delays to the family if they occur.

Postoperative Routines. The patient and family want to know about postoperative events. If they understand routine postoperative vital sign monitoring, they are less likely to worry when nurses perform these assessments. Also explain if the patient is to have IV lines, dressings, or drainage tubes. It is important to neither overprepare nor underprepare the patient and family. You cannot predict all the patient's requirements, and a patient may be misinformed about a therapy that may not be initiated. Contradictions between your explanations and reality cause anxiety.

Sensory Preparation. Provide the patient with information about sensations typically experienced before, during, and after surgery. Preparatory information helps patients anticipate the steps of a procedure and form a realistic image of the surgical experience. When sensations occur as predicted, the patient is better at coping with the experiences. For example, the OR room is very bright and cool. Also explain that you will apply a cuff for a noninvasive blood pressure monitor to the patient's arm. This monitor makes a hum and a beep, and the cuff tightens around the patient's arm. Informing the patient about these and other sensations in the OR will reduce anxiety before the patient is anesthetized, which will help decrease the amount of anesthetic needed for induction. Other postoperative sensations to describe include

blurred vision from ophthalmic ointment, dryness of the mouth or the sensation of a sore throat resulting from an endotracheal tube, pain at the incision site, tightness of the dressings, and feeling cold.

Pain Relief. One of the surgical patient's greatest fears is pain. The family is also concerned about the patient's comfort. Preoperative preparation regarding pain and pain control measures helps the patient to cope with the pain. Patient-controlled analgesia (PCA) is common and provides the patient with control over pain. Explain to the patient how to operate a pump and the importance of administering medication as soon as pain becomes persistent (see Chapter 31). Epidural analgesia is becoming more common and is effective. Patients need a thorough understanding of how this affects movement and sensation (see Chapter 31).

Analgesics will not provide adequate pain relief if the patient waits until the pain becomes excruciating before using or requesting an analgesic. Even though around-the-clock (ATC) analgesia is more effective, most patients still have analgesics ordered prn (as needed). Pain control is essential for a surgical patient to recover quickly. Encourage the patient to use analgesics as needed and not be fearful of any dependence on pain medications following surgery. Explain the schedule for administration of epidural, intramuscular, and oral analgesics. If analgesics are not ordered ATC, encourage the patient to inform nurses as soon as pain becomes a persistent discomfort. The patient also needs to know it takes time for a drug to act and that the drug will rarely eliminate all the discomfort. In addition, inform the patient and family of other therapies available for pain relief, such as focused breathing and relaxation, distraction, and the use of heat or cold compresses.

Postoperative Exercises Every preoperative teaching program includes explanation and demonstration of postoperative exercises: diaphragmatic breathing, incentive spirometry, controlled coughing, turning, and leg exercises (Skill 38-1). Diaphragmatic breathing improves lung expansion and oxygen delivery without using excess energy. The patient learns to use the diaphragm during deep breathing to take slow, deep, and relaxed breaths. Eventually the patient's lung volume improves. Deep breathing also helps to clear any anesthetic gases from the airways.

To facilitate deep breathing the health care provider often orders an incentive spirometer for the patient (see Chapter 29). Incentive spirometry encourages forced inspiration. The therapy is effective in preventing atelectasis postoperatively.

Coughing assists in removing retained mucus in the airways. A deep, productive cough is more beneficial than merely clearing the throat. The patient needs to anticipate postoperative discomfort and understand the importance of coughing, even when it is difficult. Teach the patient to splint an abdominal or thoracic incision to minimize pain during coughing. Pain control is essential for effective deep breathing and coughing; educate the patient to ask for pain medications as needed.

Leg exercises and turning improve blood flow to the extremities and thus reduce venous stasis, reducing the risk for clot formation and subsequent pulmonary emboli. Contractions of lower leg muscles promote venous return, making it difficult for clots to form. Turning also helps to mobilize pulmonary secretions and increases ventilation and perfusion of the lungs. After explaining each exercise, demonstrate it. Then, while acting as a coach, ask the patient to demonstrate each exercise.

Activity Resumption The type of surgery affects how quickly a patient is able to resume normal physical activity and regular eating habits. Explain that it is normal for a patient to progress gradually in activity and eating. If the patient tolerates activity and diet well, activity levels will progress more quickly. For example, if the patient is not nauseated following cholecystectomy, encourage ambulation the night of surgery.

Promotion of Nutrition The surgical patient is vulnerable to fluid and electrolyte imbalances as a result of inadequate preoperative intake, excessive fluid loss during surgery, and the stress response. A patient usually takes nothing by mouth for several hours before surgery to reduce risks for vomiting and aspirating emesis during surgery. Instruct the patient to eat and drink sufficient amounts before fasting to ensure adequate fluid and nutrient intake. Make sure the patient's diet includes foods high in protein, with sufficient amounts of carbohydrates, fat, and vitamins. Instruct the patient and family members regarding preoperative fasting requirements and oral medication use. Notify the surgeon and anesthesiologist as soon as possible if the patient eats or drinks during the fasting period.

For patients who are hospitalized, remove all fluids and solid foods from the bedside and post a sign over the bed to alert hospital personnel and family members about fasting restrictions. Instruct the patient to rinse the mouth with water or mouthwash and brush the teeth, but instruct the patient not to swallow anything, even clear liquids. Patients may take oral medications with sips of water if ordered by the health care provider. Notify the dietary department to cancel meals. A patient who is at home the evening before surgery needs to understand the importance of not taking food or fluids and be willing to follow restrictions.

Promotion of Rest Rest is essential for normal healing. Anxiety about surgery interferes with the ability to relax or sleep. The underlying conditions requiring surgery are often painful, further impairing rest. Frequent visits by staff members, diagnostic testing, and physical preparation for surgery take a long time, and the patient has few opportunities to reflect on events. Make sure that the patient's individual needs are met. The patient and family need time to express feelings about surgery, either together or separately. The patient's level of anxiety influences the frequency of discussions, and you will need to encourage expression of these concerns.

Attempt to make the patient's environment quiet and comfortable. The surgeon occasionally orders a sedative-hypnotic or antianxiety agent for the night before surgery. Sedative-hypnotics affect and promote sleep. Antianxiety agents act on the cerebral cortex and limbic system to relieve anxiety. An advantage to ambulatory surgery or same-day surgical admissions is that the patient is able to sleep at home the night before surgery.

ACUTE CARE The degree of preoperative physical preparation depends on the patient's health status, the surgery, and the surgeon's preferences. A seriously ill patient will receive more supportive care than the patient facing a less serious elective procedure.

Minimize Risk for Surgical Wound Infection The risk for developing a surgical wound infection depends on the amount and type of microorganisms contaminating a wound, the susceptibility of the host, and the condition of the wound at the end of the operation. All three factors interact, determining the risk for infection (see Chapter 13).

The skin is a favorite site for microorganisms to grow and multiply. Without proper skin preparation, the risk for postoperative wound infection is high. Many surgeons have patients bathe or shower with an antimicrobial soap the evening before surgery. Often patients have to bathe or shower more than once, whereas others give special attention to cleansing the proposed operative site. If the surgical procedure involves the head, neck, or upper chest area, the patient also is required to shampoo the hair. Surgeons generally order hair removal only if the hair has the potential to interfere with exposure, closure, or dressing of the surgical site. Hair removal is done as close to the time of surgery as possible (AORN, 2009). Instruct patients not to shave the surgical area.

Prevention of Bowel Incontinence and Contamination The patient will often receive a bowel preparation (e.g., a cathartic or an enema) if surgery involves the lower gastrointestinal system. Manipulation of portions of the gastrointestinal tract during surgery results in absence of peristalsis for 24 hours and sometimes longer. Enemas and cathartics cleanse the gastrointestinal tract to prevent problems with incontinence or constipation. An empty bowel reduces risk for injury to the intestines and minimizes contamination of the operative wound in case a portion of the bowel is incised or opened. Chapter 34 summarizes enema administration.

Interventions on Day of Surgery On the morning of surgery, complete the routine procedures discussed in the following sections before releasing the patient for surgery.

Documentation. Before the patient goes to the OR, check the medical record to be sure all relevant laboratory and test results are present. Check all consent forms for completeness and accuracy of information. A preoperative checklist (Figure 38-1) provides guidelines for ensuring completion of all nursing interventions. Check the nurses' notes to be sure documentation is current, especially if the patient experienced unpredicted problems the night before surgery.

Assessment of Vital Signs. Make a final assessment of vital signs, and document them on the preoperative checklist and in the nurses' notes. If the vital signs are abnormal, notify the surgeon.

Hygiene. Basic hygiene measures remove skin contamination and increase the patient's comfort. If the patient is unwilling or unable to take a complete bath, a partial bath is refreshing and removes irritating secretions or drainage from

BARNES JEWISH Hospital
BJC HealthCare™

SURGICAL/PROCEDURE CHECKLIST
**Complete this side for inpatients and outpatients
having any invasive procedure**
Please check (✔) the appropriate box (☐) and fill in the blank(s) as needed.

ADDRESSOGRAPH

Date of Procedure: _____   Type of Procedure: _____

Off Floor Reports printed and placed in chart: ☐ Yes   ☐ No   ☐ N/A: _____

ITEM	Yes/Initials	NA	COMMENT	Date
Face sheet in chart				
Consent to Surgery or Other Procedure signed			☐ To be signed in treatment area.	
SPECIALTY Consent signed			☐ To be signed in treatment area. (Specify)	
Transfusion consent signed				
ID Band on				
Allergies Noted: ☐ Armband ☐ Medication Record ☐ Allergies/Sensitivities Record/Override Order Form				
Height & Weight documented				
Dentures, eyeglasses, contact lenses, nail polish, hairpins, prosthesis, jewelry removed				
Surgical/Procedural skin prep done				
Patient in hospital gown/pajamas				
Patient has been NPO since: _____				
Voided or catheterized				
Vital Signs taken and documented				
Patient is on isolation			(Specify)	
History & physical in chart				
Lab work in chart (Printed Off Floor reports)				
Urinalysis in chart				
EKG in chart				
Chest X-ray (done if ordered)				
Change in condition/VS reported to:				
Valuables/Inventory checklist done				
Pre-Operative meds given:				
Addressograph plate in chart				
Patient transferred to Surgical/Procedure area in HIS				
Mode of travel: ☐ Amb ☐ W/C ☐ Stretcher ☐ Bed				
Operative Site Marked			☐ Site to be marked in holding area	
Case Cancelled				

Family contact during surgery:

Name: _____   Location: _____   Phone: _____

INITIALS	SIGNATURES	INITIALS	SIGNATURES

BJ 2-3343-465 (10/12/05) Page 1 of 2 TAB: TREATMENT   **DO NOT WRITE BELOW THIS LINE**

BJ 2-3343-465

Figure 38-1 ■ Surgical/procedure checklist. (Courtesy Barnes-Jewish Hospital, St. Louis, Mo.)

the skin. Because the patient cannot wear personal nightwear to the OR, provide a clean hospital gown and instruct the patient to remove all other articles of clothing, including undergarments. After having nothing by mouth throughout the night, the patient usually has a very dry mouth. Offer mouthwash and toothpaste and caution the patient not to swallow anything.

Preparation of Hair and Removal of Cosmetics. During major surgery the anesthesiologist positions the patient's head to put an endotracheal tube into the airway (see Chapter 29). This involves manipulation of the hair and scalp. To avoid injury, ask the patient to remove hairpins or clips. Also, have patients remove hairpieces or wigs. Patients can braid long hair. The patient will wear a disposable hat to contain hair before entering the operating room.

During and after surgery the anesthesia care provider and nurses assess skin and mucous membranes to determine the patient's level of oxygenation, circulation, and fluid balance. A pulse oximeter is applied to a finger to monitor oxygen saturation of the blood (see Chapter 14). For these reasons, have patients remove all makeup (lipstick, powder, blush, nail polish) and at least one artificial fingernail to expose normal skin and nail coloring. Anything in or around the eye will irritate or injure the eye during surgery. Have patients remove contact lenses, false eyelashes, and eye makeup. Eyeglasses usually remain in the room, or you can give them to the family immediately before the patient enters the OR.

Removal of Prostheses. It is easy for any type of prosthetic device to become lost or damaged during surgery. The patient removes all removable prosthetics for safekeeping. If the patient has a brace or splint, check with the surgeon to determine whether it should remain with the patient, to be reapplied after surgery. Although patients need to remove hearing aids, eyeglasses, and contact lenses, do not have them do this until just before the surgery. Allowing the patient to wear these aids facilitates communication and increases the patient's sense of control. Refer to the institution's policies for clarification.

For many patients, removing dentures is embarrassing. If the patient removes the dentures before surgery, provide privacy. Place dentures in special containers, and label with the patient's name for safekeeping to prevent breakage. Assess the patient for loose teeth. A broken tooth can become dislodged during insertion of an endotracheal tube and obstruct the airway.

Inventory and secure all prosthetic devices. Give prosthetics to family members or significant others, or keep the devices at the patient's bedside. Follow agency policy, and document the devices' location.

Preparation of Bowel and Bladder. Some patients receive an enema or cathartic the morning of surgery. If so, give it at least 1 hour before the patient leaves for surgery, allowing time for the patient to defecate without rushing.

Instruct the patient to void just before leaving for the operating room. If the patient is unable to void, enter a notation on the preoperative checklist. An empty bladder minimizes incontinence and injury to the bladder during surgery. An empty bladder also makes abdominal organs more accessible during surgery. The surgeon will order an indwelling catheter if the surgery is long or the incision is in the lower abdomen (see Chapter 33).

Application of Antiembolism Devices. Many health care providers order antiembolic stockings or sequential compression stockings to be worn during surgery. When correctly sized and properly applied, these devices reduce the risk for thrombi (see Chapter 35). **Antiembolic stockings** maintain compression of small veins and capillaries of the lower ex-

tremities. The constant compression forces blood into larger vessels, thus promoting venous return and preventing venous stasis. **Sequential compression stockings** are attached to an air pump that inflates and deflates the stockings, applying intermittent pressure sequentially from the ankle to the knee and alternating calves, mimicking the venous return process of walking.

Promotion of Patient's Dignity. During preoperative preparations, care will become depersonalized unless you maintain the patient's privacy and reduce sources of anxiety. Ambulatory and same-day surgical admission patients often sit in a waiting room before surgery. To protect patients' modesty, allow patients to wear underclothes when possible and provide cover robes. Ensure hospitalized patients their privacy by closing room curtains or doors during preoperative preparation. Allow family to stay until the patient goes to the operating room.

Performing Special Procedures. Sometimes a patient's condition requires special interventions before surgery. Upon the surgeon's order start IV infusions, insert a Foley catheter, and insert a **nasogastric (NG) tube** for gastric decompression (see Chapter 34) or the administration of medications (see Chapter 16).

Safeguarding Valuables. If a patient has valuables, turn them over to family members or secure them for safekeeping in a designated location. Many facilities require patients to sign a release to free the institution of responsibility for lost valuables. Prepare a list with a description of items, place a copy with the patient's chart, and give a copy to a designated family member. Patients are often reluctant to remove wedding rings or religious medals. Tape a wedding band in place; however, do not create a tourniquet with the tape. If there is a risk that the patient will experience swelling of the hand or fingers, remove the band. Many hospitals allow patients to pin religious medals to their gowns, although the risk for loss increases (Phillips, 2004).

Administering Preoperative Medications. Typically, the surgeon or anesthesia provider orders preoperative drugs for you to give before the patient leaves for the OR. Complete all nursing care measures before giving the preoperative medication. Preoperative drugs such as benzodiazepines, opioids, antiemetics, and anticholinergics usually do not induce sleep, but they can cause dry mouth, drowsiness, and dizziness. If the drug causes drowsiness or dizziness, keep the side rails in the up position, the bed in the low position, and the call bell within easy reach for the patient. Instruct the patient to remain in bed until the surgical nursing assistant or transporter arrives to take the patient to the OR and to call for assistance if there is a need to get out of bed. A patient can easily fall, thinking that nothing is wrong, only to realize the medications have seriously hampered the ability to walk steadily.

■■■**EVALUATION**

Evaluation of the preoperative goals and outcomes of the plan of care begins before surgery and extends into the postoperative period, providing direction for future interventions. For some patients, surgery is an emergency. Others will require procedures up until surgery. This leaves little time for evaluation. For some measures, such as those to prevent infection, perform evaluation postoperatively when you are able to determine the outcome.

PATIENT CARE Determine if the patient and family have adequate preoperative preparation by asking the patient to describe the surgical procedure, its purpose, and the postoperative care (Box 38-5). By having the patient and family describe the reasons for postoperative exercises and incentive spirometry, for example, you evaluate the patient's understanding of the physiological and psychological responses to surgery. Evaluate adequacy of preoperative teaching by asking the patient to demonstrate exercises. Evaluate anxiety by monitoring pulse and blood pressure, facial expressions, and verbal interactions. In addition, ask the patient if he or she remains anxious or fearful of any aspect of the surgery.

PATIENT EXPECTATIONS Determine if the patient's and family's expectations have been met up to this point. Spend time talking with the patient and family to learn if they are satisfied with their preparation. Knowing this information allows you to help the patient to redefine realistic expectations. In emergency situations this becomes more difficult to evaluate. The family often becomes the focus of the evaluation if the patient is unable to respond or is in a condition that prevents a meaningful discussion.

Transport to the Operating Room

Personnel in the **operating room (OR)** notify the nursing unit or preoperative surgery holding area when it is time for surgery. In many hospitals a nursing assistant or a transporter brings a wheelchair or stretcher for transporting the patient. The transporter checks the patient's identification bracelet against the patient's medical record to be sure the correct person is going to surgery. When using a stretcher to transport a patient, the nurses and transporter assist the patient with safely transferring from bed to stretcher. The ambulatory surgery patient, if able and not medicated, often walks to the OR, providing more control over the event.

Give the family the opportunity to visit before the patient goes to the OR. Then direct the family to the appropriate waiting area. If the patient has been hospitalized before surgery and will be returning to the same nursing unit, prepare the bed and room for the patient's return. You will be better prepared for postoperative care if the room is ready before the patient's return. Include the following in a postoperative bedside unit:

1. Sphygmomanometer, stethoscope, and thermometer
2. Emesis basin
3. Clean gown
4. Washcloth, towel, and facial tissues
5. IV pole and pump
6. Suction equipment (if needed)
7. Oxygen equipment (if ordered)
8. Extra pillows for positioning the patient comfortably
9. Bed pads to protect bed linen from drainage
10. Patient-controlled analgesia (see Chapter 31) pump and tubing if ordered
11. Bed raised to stretcher height, bed linen turned back, and furniture moved to accommodate the stretcher

PREANESTHESIA CARE UNIT In most hospitals the patient enters a **preanesthesia care unit** or **presurgical care unit (PSCU)** (sometimes called a holding area) outside the OR, where preoperative preparations are completed. Nurses in the PSCU are usually part of the OR room staff and wear surgical scrub suits. In the PSCU, if an IV catheter is not already present, a nurse, nurse anesthetist, or anesthesiologist will insert an IV catheter into the patient's vein to establish a route for fluid replacement, IV drugs, and blood or blood products if needed. He or she will also administer preoperative medications and/or conscious sedation at this time.

If a patient needs to have hair removed around the surgical site, perform this procedure in a private area near the OR immediately before surgery. AORN-recommended practices include the use of electric or battery-operated clippers for preoperative hair removal. Clippers minimize the risk for irritation and small cuts, which predispose the patient to infec-

---

BOX 38-5   EVALUATION

It is the morning of Mr. Korloff's surgery, and Sue admits him to the hospital with the help of one of his daughters. She checks that the informed consent has been signed and witnessed. She completes his physical assessment, which focuses on assessing breath sounds, condition of his skin, and vital signs. Sue also completes the preoperative checklist. She asks Mr. Korloff if he has any questions about the nature or purpose of the surgery. At times he still seems a bit anxious about what to expect. Sue also reviews with Mr. Korloff and his daughter the events that will occur in the holding area and the postanesthesia care unit. She asks if they are frightened about any aspect of the procedure or routine, and she addresses their concerns. Sue then reviews with Mr. Korloff the exercises that were in the booklet he received in the preadmission testing center. Sue has Mr. Korloff demonstrate coughing and deep breathing, while reinforcing its importance once surgery is over. She then gives Mr. Korloff a hospital gown and cover-up and shows him to the changing area. After he has removed his clothes and put on the hospital gown, Sue accompanies Mr. Korloff and his daughter to the holding area.

DOCUMENTATION NOTE

"Admitted for scheduled laparoscopic cholecystectomy. Blood pressure, 142/84 mm Hg; pulse, 88 beats per minute; respirations, 18 breaths per minute; temperature, 98.9° F. Lungs clear to auscultation bilaterally with normal excursion. Skin warm and dry; no evidence of lesions. Remained NPO during the night. Reviewed instructions on postoperative exercises, and is able to demonstrate coughing and deep breathing. Has some difficulty holding incentive spirometer in mouth. Daughters will be in waiting area during procedure."

tion. Follow the manufacturer's guidelines if you use a depilatory to remove hair (AORN, 2009).

INTRAOPERATIVE SURGICAL PHASE

Care of the patient during surgery requires careful preparation and knowledge of the events that will occur during the surgical procedure.

Nurse's Role During Surgery

A nurse usually assumes one of two roles in the OR: **circulating nurse** or **scrub nurse** (Figure 38-2). The circulating nurse, who is a licensed registered nurse (RN), cares for the patient while in the operating room by completing a preoperative assessment, establishing and implementing the intraoperative plan of care, evaluating the care, and providing for the continuity of care postoperatively. The circulating nurse assists the anesthesia provider with endotracheal intubation, calculating blood loss and urinary output, and administering blood. This nurse monitors sterile technique of all members of the team and a safe OR environment. The nurse also assists the surgeon and scrub nurse by operating nonsterile equipment, providing additional instruments and supplies, maintaining accurate and complete documentation, and tracking sponge, needle, and instrument counts.

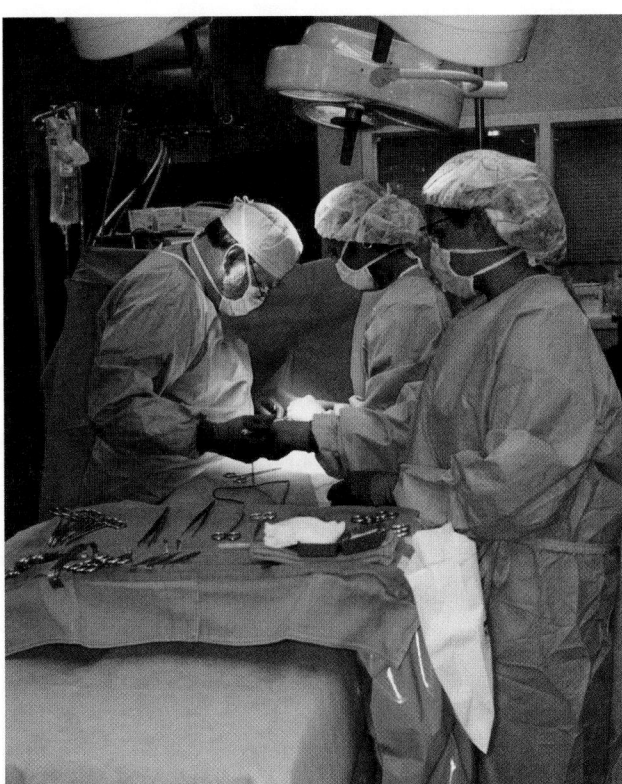

Figure 38-2 ■ Nurses in the operating room. (Courtesy OFS Healthcare.)

The scrub nurse is an RN, a licensed practical nurse (LPN), or a surgical technician. Like the surgeon, the scrub nurse performs a hand scrub and applies sterile gown and gloves for the procedure. The scrub nurse is responsible for maintaining a sterile field during the surgical procedure and adhering to strict surgical asepsis. This nurse assists with applying surgical drapes and hands the surgeon instruments, sponges, sutures, and other supplies.

NURSING PROCESS

■■■ ASSESSMENT

As a circulating nurse in the PSCU and OR, conduct a special preoperative assessment to verify the patient is ready for surgery and to plan intraoperative care. Ask the patient his or her name and date of birth and compare the response with the identification band and medical record. Review consent forms, allergies, medical history, physical assessment findings, and test results. Verify with the patient the type of surgery and the surgical site (Table 38-7). Pay special attention to the patient's psychological comfort of the patient. Also perform a brief assessment of key body systems (see Table 38-5, p. 1140).

■■■ NURSING DIAGNOSIS

Review preoperative nursing diagnoses, and modify them to individualize the care plan in the OR. Add additional diagnoses and related factors based on the patient's condition, specific surgical intervention, and method and type of anesthesia. Nursing diagnoses for the intraoperative patient often include the following:

- *Risk for latex allergy response*
- *Risk for aspiration*
- *Decreased cardiac output*
- *Risk for deficient fluid volume*
- *Impaired gas exchange*
- *Risk for infection*
- *Risk for perioperative-positioning injury*
- *Impaired skin integrity*
- *Ineffective thermoregulation*
- *Ineffective peripheral tissue perfusion*

Nursing care in the operating room routinely includes monitoring for *latex allergy response* and prevention of *risk for perioperative-positioning injury*. These diagnoses provide direction for both intraoperative and postoperative care for this patient.

■■■ PLANNING

GOALS AND OUTCOMES Some patient-centered outcomes of preoperative care extend into the intraoperative phase. These include remaining free of infection and achieving psychological and physical comfort. Additional goals include maintaining skin integrity, therapeutic body temperature, and fluid and electrolyte balance. Measure goal

TABLE 38-7 FOCUSED PATIENT ASSESSMENT

Intraoperative Assessment

FACTORS TO ASSESS	QUESTIONS	PHYSICAL ASSESSMENT
The right patient	What is your full name?	Ask patient to state name. Inspect patient identification band for patient name and date of birth and compare with medical record.
The right surgical procedure on the right body part	What surgery are you here for? Compare answer with operative permit.	Inspect and palpate body part to add any physical evidence of need for surgery (redness, edema, pain). Sometimes there is none, depending on the nature of the surgery. Observe for surgical site marking if laterality of body part involved (i.e., right ankle marked with "yes"). Marking often performed in presurgical care unit by surgeon.
The right set of data in chart	Verify and clarify with patient any medical, surgical, medication, and allergy history found in preoperative assessment. Review findings from laboratory reports, diagnostic tests, x-ray films, and electrocardiogram.	Inspect skin for stated surgical scars. Observe for the presence and patency of ordered tubes and lines (NG, Foley, IV).
The right frame of mind of patient	What do you expect as an outcome of surgery? How do you feel about surgery? If patient changes mind about surgery, notify surgeon. Surgery will be canceled or postponed.	Observe for signs of fear and anxiety. Monitor vital signs for indications of excessive anxiety. Compare vital signs to baseline.

IV, Intravenous; *NG,* nasogastric.

achievement through outcome criteria, such as the presence of intact skin, without redness or irritation; body temperature within the patient's normal range; stable vital signs; and adequate urinary output.

Priority setting and continuity of care come from the plan of care and any additional information from oral and written reports of the preadmission area and/or the presurgical care unit.

■■■ IMPLEMENTATION

A major focus of intraoperative care is to prevent injury and complications related to anesthesia, surgery, positioning, and equipment used. As the perioperative nurse, act as an advocate for the patient during surgery. Protect the patient's dignity and rights at all times.

ACUTE CARE

Admission to the Operating Room After assessing the patient, the circulating nurse transfers the patient into the OR. The patient is usually still awake and will notice nurses and health care providers wearing surgical masks, protective eyewear, and gowns. Carefully transfer the patient to the operating bed, being sure the stretcher and bed are locked in place. After being transferred to the operating bed, the OR team will secure the patient with safety straps. Just before starting the surgical procedure, the surgical team takes a "time out" for a final verification of the right patient, right procedure, and right site. This final "time out" is part of The Joint Commission's Universal Protocol for Eliminating Wrong

Site, Wrong Procedure, and Wrong Person Surgery (The Joint Commission, 2009).

Physical Preparation After securing the patient safely, first apply small plastic electrodes on the chest and extremities for continuous electrocardiographic monitoring during surgery. A monitor displays the heart's electrical activity. Next, apply a blood pressure cuff around the patient's arm for the anesthesiologist to measure the blood pressure. Attach a pulse oximeter sensor to the patient's finger or earlobe for measurement of the oxygen saturation of the blood and an evaluation of ventilation.

Psychological Support Entering the OR room is stressful for most patients. Reassure the patient, and remain at the patient's side until after anesthesia is induced. Offering a hand to hold is often helpful. If the patient is awake during surgery, give support throughout the surgical procedure.

Positioning Positioning typically occurs after relaxation from anesthesia has been achieved. For example, when using general anesthesia, the nursing personnel and surgeon usually do not position the patient until the anesthesia care provider notifies them that the patient is intubated and has entered the stage of complete relaxation. Proper positioning of the patient provides good access to and exposure of the operative site and promotes adequate circulatory and respiratory function. Ensure positioning does not impair neuromuscular structures or skin integrity. Most ORs now use a variety of pressure-relieving surfaces to reduce the incidence of pressure ulcers intraoperatively (see Chapter 36).

TABLE 38-8 Intraoperative Nursing Care

OUTCOMES	INTERVENTIONS
Patient will be free of infection.	Maintain standard precautions.
	Monitor surgical asepsis.
	Perform surgical skin scrub.
Patient will be free of pressure ulcer.	Use appropriate pressure-relieving overlays on operating room bed, especially for high-risk patients (e.g., very obese, nutritionally depleted, long surgical procedure). Overlays on the operating table have been shown to reduce postoperative pressure ulcer incidence (Cullum and others, 2004).
Patient will be free of injury.	Apply sterile surgical drapes.
	Perform accurate sponge, needle, and instrument counts.
	Provide grounding for electrosurgical cautery.
	Provide eye protection when using a laser.
Patient will maintain body temperature.	Monitor body temperature
	Warm irrigating solutions.
	Apply warming blanket intraoperatively if possible or immediately after surgery.
Patient will maintain fluid and electrolyte balance.	Monitor blood loss, NG drainage, and urinary output.
	Provide blood products as ordered.
	Monitor type and flow rate of IV fluids.

IV, Intravenous; *NG,* nasogastric.

Consider the patient's comfort and safety. It is sometimes difficult for the patient to understand why he or she feels a wide range of discomfort after surgery. If a joint is extended too far in an alert person, pain stimuli warn the individual that muscle and joint strain is too great and the individual changes position. In an anesthetized patient, normal defense mechanisms do not guard against joint damage and muscle stretch and strain. The patient's muscles are so relaxed that it is relatively easy to place the patient in a position he or she normally does not assume while awake. The patient often remains in a given position for several hours. Once the patient awakens, musculoskeletal pain is significant. Intraoperative nursing care also includes interventions to prevent infection and injury to the patient, to maintain fluid and electrolyte balance, and to control the patient's temperature (Table 38-8).

Introduction of Anesthesia The nature and extent of a patient's surgery and current physical status influence the type of anesthesia administered in surgery. It is especially important postoperatively that you know the complications to anticipate after a patient receives anesthesia (Table 38-9).

General Anesthesia. Under **general anesthesia** the patient loses all sensations, consciousness, and reflexes, including gag and blink reflexes. The patient's muscles relax, and he or she experiences amnesia. General anesthesia is administered during major procedures requiring extensive tissue manipulation or any time analgesia, muscle relaxation, immobility, and control of the autonomic nervous system are required. This includes minor procedures, especially with children.

Regional Anesthesia. Regional anesthesia results in loss of sensation in an area of the body by anesthetizing sensory pathways. This type of anesthesia is accomplished by injecting a local anesthetic along the pathway of a nerve from the spinal cord (Rothrock, 2007). Administration techniques include peripheral nerve blocks and spinal, epidural, and caudal blocks. The patient requires careful monitoring during

TABLE 38-9 Examples of Complications of Anesthesia

TYPE	COMPLICATIONS
General anesthesia	Aspiration of vomitus
	Cardiac irregularities
	Decreased cardiac output
	Hypotension
	Hypothermia
	Hypoxemia
	Laryngospasm
	Malignant hyperthermia
	Nephrotoxicity
	Respiratory depression
Regional anesthesia	Hypotension
Epidural	Hypothermia
Spinal	Injury to spinal cord
	Injury to numb legs
	Respiratory paralysis
	Spinal headache
Local anesthesia	Anaphylactic shock
	Hives
	Rash
Conscious sedation	Aspiration
	Decreased level of consciousness
	Hypoxemia
	Respiratory depression

and immediately after regional anesthesia for return of sensation and movement distal to the regional anesthesia.

Local Anesthesia. Local anesthesia involves loss of sensation at the desired site by inhibiting peripheral nerve conduction. It is used during minor procedures performed in ambulatory surgery. Local anesthetics are also used in addition to general or regional anesthesia. Long-acting local anesthetics are sometimes injected into the incision at the end of the patient's surgery for postoperative pain relief (see Chapter 31).

Moderate Sedation (Conscious Sedation). IV **moderate sedation/analgesia** or **conscious sedation** is routinely used for diagnostic or therapeutic procedures (e.g., colonoscopy or certain laparoscopies) that do not require complete anesthesia but simply a decreased level of consciousness. The patient needs to maintain respirations and respond appropriately to physical and verbal stimuli. Advantages to IV conscious sedation include adequate sedation, diminished anxiety, amnesia, pain relief, mood alteration, enhanced patient cooperation, stable vital signs, and rapid recovery with minimal risk (ASA, 2004).

The administration of conscious sedation generally requires facility certification to care for these patients. The ability to assess, diagnose, and intervene if a complication arises is essential, including skills in airway management, oxygen delivery, and use of resuscitation equipment (AORN, 2009). Document vital signs, oxygen saturation, assessment of breath sounds and heart rhythm, and level of consciousness every 15 minutes during the procedure and during the immediate recovery period (AORN, 2009; ASA, 2002).

Support any patient who remains awake by explaining procedures, encouraging questions, and warning the patient when unpleasant sensations will be experienced. Some settings provide music to mask unpleasant sounds and to promote relaxation.

Documentation of Intraoperative Care During the intraoperative phase, continue the established plan of care and modify it as needed. Throughout the surgical procedure, keep an accurate record of patient care activities and procedures performed by operating room personnel. This record provides useful data for the nurse who cares for the patient postoperatively.

■■■EVALUATION

Evaluation of many interventions implemented during the intraoperative phase occurs in the postoperative phase because complications (e.g., infection) often arise days after surgery.

PATIENT CARE After surgery, perform a postoperative evaluation of the patient before the patient leaves the operating room. Inspect the skin under the grounding pad and areas of the skin where equipment or positioning has exerted pressure. Monitor body temperature immediately postoperatively to assess thermoregulation. Obtain vital signs and auscultate lung sounds to assess pulmonary and fluid and electrolyte status (Box 38-6).

PATIENT EXPECTATIONS Frequently ask questions about pain, numbness, and perceived room temperature to patients who are not receiving general anesthesia during the procedure. This determines if the analgesia is adequate and if the patient is comfortable in regard to position and temperature.

When the patient is having major surgery, it is very important to keep the family informed. Typically, family members want to know if surgery is progressing without problems. Most hospitals provide phones within waiting areas that al-

BOX 38-6   EVALUATION

 Mr. Korloff's surgery is complete, and he is transferred to the PACU. Sue accompanies Mr. Korloff into the PACU. Sue reviews the operative record. Mr. Korloff received general anesthesia, and the procedure was uneventful. Mr. Korloff did not receive any blood or blood products. He received Ringer's lactate solution intravenously via a catheter in the left lower forearm. Sue examines the IV site, and it is without signs of phlebitis or infiltration. Small gauze dressings were applied to the four small abdominal puncture wounds, with no drainage at this time. Sue positions Mr. Korloff to maintain a patent airway and notes his respirations are 12 breaths per minute and unlabored. Airway is clear of secretions. There are no signs of pressure over bony prominences.

PACU, Postanesthesia care unit.

low nursing staff to reach families and to explain the progress of the surgery. If you are on the surgical nursing unit, give the families updates and support in the waiting areas.

POSTOPERATIVE SURGICAL PHASE

Following surgery, a patient's postoperative course involves two phases: the immediate recovery period and convalescence. For a patient following ambulatory surgery, the immediate recovery period normally lasts only 1 to 2 hours, and convalescence will occur at home. For a hospitalized patient the immediate postoperative period often lasts a few hours, with convalescence taking 1 or more days, depending on the extent of surgery and the patient's response.

Recovery

During recovery it is important to be very conscientious in monitoring the patient and making the clinical judgments necessary to determine if the patient is progressing as expected. This is a time when the patient's condition will change very quickly. Immediately after surgery the patient goes to the **postanesthesia care unit (PACU)** for close monitoring (Figure 38-3). Before the patient arrives, the PACU nurse will receive a report from the surgical team in the OR to relay the patient's most current status, nursing care priorities, and the need for special equipment. The report will include information about anesthetic agents given during surgery; IV fluids and blood products administered; status of the wound, including the presence of drainage devices; and whether the patient has had any surgical complications, such as excessive blood loss. While the patient is in the PACU, conduct ongoing assessments every 15 minutes or more often.

POSTANESTHESIA CARE IN AMBULATORY SURGERY The postanesthesia care of patients having ambulatory surgery occurs in two phases. Phase 1 is essentially the

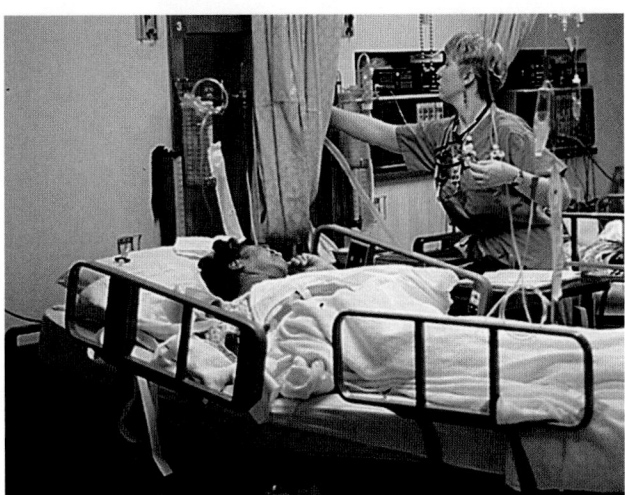

Figure 38-3 ■ Nurse in the postanesthesia care unit (PACU).

BOX 38-7	Information Given to Ambulatory Surgical Patients

- Health care provider's office telephone number (24-hour answer)
- Surgery center's telephone number
- Follow-up appointment date and time
- Review of prescribed medications
- Guidelines related to specific surgery and surgeon's preference: dressing and wound care, activity restrictions
- Guidelines related to anesthesia: diet resumption, activity restrictions
- Warning signs of complications

same as described for hospitalized patients in the PACU. Phase 2, however, prepares the patient for discharge and self-care. The patient receiving only local anesthesia is usually admitted directly to the phase 2 area. In phase 2, encourage the patient to gradually sit up on the stretcher or recliner and begin to take ice chips or sips of water or other clear liquids after regaining full alertness.

Phase 2 postanesthesia care occurs in a room equipped with medical recliner chairs, side tables, and footrests. Kitchen facilities for preparing light snacks and beverages are in the area, along with bathrooms. The phase 2 environment promotes the patient's and family's comfort and well-being until discharge. Continue to monitor the patient but not at the same intensity as in phase 1. In phase 2, initiate postoperative teaching with the patient and family members (Box 38-7). When the patient's condition remains stable in the sitting position, and there is no nausea or dizziness, he or she is discharged.

Convalescence

Once the patient is stable, usually within 2 to 3 hours, the anesthesia provider or surgeon transfers the hospitalized patient to a postoperative nursing unit, whereas the ambulatory

surgical patient will return home. Unstable patients remain in the PACU or go to an intensive care unit for more intense monitoring and care. During convalescence, consider the goals of care established during the preoperative and intraoperative phases, to support the patient in returning to normal physiological function. In addition, direct your nursing care toward facilitating a patient's smooth transition home. Encourage family participation in the patient's plan of care. The family provides coaching during postoperative exercises and important psychosocial support to the patient.

NURSING PROCESS

■■■ASSESSMENT

The parameters you assess for a patient following surgery are basically the same during recovery and convalescence. When patients enter the PACU, perform a rapid assessment of the respiratory and circulatory status and attach electronic monitors. Conduct assessments while considering patients' surgical risks and the type of surgery performed. For example, if a patient has a history of smoking and underwent abdominal surgery involving a high abdominal incision, focus on the patient's respiratory status. The patient's pain could potentially reduce ventilation, leading to the development of atelectasis.

Once a patient reaches a postoperative nursing unit, perform vital sign measurements and assessments less often, usually every 15 to 30 minutes initially, then hourly, and then less often per surgeon's or health care provider's orders. Check the institution's policy on vital signs following surgery. Table 38-10 summarizes a focused postoperative assessment.

RESPIRATION Assess the quality of the patient's respirations and the patency of the airway. A patient receiving a general anesthetic often has an artificial airway still in place when arriving in the PACU. Certain anesthetic agents and opioids often continue to cause respiratory depression. Thus be especially alert for slow, shallow breathing. Assess respiratory rate, rhythm, and depth and quality of ventilatory movement. Auscultate the lungs for adventitious sounds such as crackles, which do not clear with coughing and for wheezing, which results from air squeezed through passageways narrowed almost to closure from secretions (Jarvis, 2008). If breathing is unusually shallow, place your hand over the patient's face or mouth to feel exhaled air. Pulse oximetry reflecting 92% to 100% saturation is within normal limits unless the surgeon or anesthesia care provider orders other limits (see Chapter 14).

Once a patient is on a surgical nursing unit, respirations have usually stabilized. Frequent auscultation of lung sounds is still important because the patient is still at risk for developing pneumonia unless he or she follows postoperative exercises routinely. Remember that pain control will be important during convalescence so that the patient is able to cough and deep breathe with relative ease.

CIRCULATION The patient is at risk for cardiovascular complications from actual or potential blood loss at the

TABLE 38-10 FOCUSED PATIENT ASSESSMENT

FACTORS TO ASSESS	QUESTIONS/RECORD REVIEW	PHYSICAL ASSESSMENT
Respirations	Ask if patient feels short of breath or has discomfort during breathing.	Monitor respiratory rate, rhythm, and depth every 15 min × 4 or until stable, then every 30 min × 2, and then every hour × 4. Compare with baseline findings.
	Review history for medical conditions involving respiratory system, medications taken, and any allergies.	Observe for symmetry of chest wall movements, color of skin and mucous membranes.
	Review report of type of anesthesia and agents used during surgery.	Auscultate breath sounds for rales, wheezing, decreased or absent sounds.
	Review report of any medications given during surgery or in postanesthesia care unit that affect respiratory function (analgesics, antianxiety agents).	Apply pulse oximeter to detect oxygen saturation.
Circulation	Review baseline heart rate for current comparison.	Monitor pulse rate and rhythm as well as blood pressure at same frequency as respiratory rate or more often as patient's condition warrants. Maintain continuous ECG monitoring if ordered
	Review report of amount of blood loss and any replacement blood or blood products in the OR and PACU.	Assess level of consciousness and symptoms of restlessness or altered mental status.
	Review current IV orders as to type of fluid and infusion rate.	Observe skin, nail beds, and mucous membranes for color and hydration.
	Ask if patient is having any dizziness or visual disturbances when changing positions.	Palpate peripheral pulses distal to surgical site, tight dressing, or cast if present.
		Inspect for amount of bleeding on dressing, in drainage systems (NG suction, Hemovac, Jackson-Pratt drain, Foley catheter) and underneath patient.
Infection control	Review patient history for risk factors for infection and poor wound healing (contaminated surgical site, history of diabetes mellitus, HIV, or use of immunosuppressing drugs [prednisone]).	Monitor patient temperature and white blood cell count as indicated.
	Ask if patient is having any burning or pain with urination.	Inspect any urine output, note color, consistency, and odor.
	Ask if patient is having extreme tenderness at wound site.	Observe surgical wound for redness, edema, warmth, drainage, and dehiscence. What does drainage look like?
Gastrointestinal function	Review report for history of problems with gastrointestinal function.	Inspect for abdominal distention.
	Are you having any nausea, abdominal cramping? How's your appetite?	Auscultate for bowel sounds in all four quadrants at least every shift until discharge.
	Have you passed any gas or had a bowel movement today? How was the stool compared to your normal?	Palpate abdomen for firmness.
		Monitor NG tube for patency and NG tube output for color and amount of drainage if present.
		Observe patient's ability and willingness to tolerate fluids and food.
Comfort	Review symptoms of pain before surgery, type of anesthesia, location of surgery, and expected level of pain associated with this type of surgery.	Observe for signs and symptoms of discomfort (restlessness; elevated pulse, respirations and blood pressure; grimaces; guarding).
	Review any history of alcohol or illicit drug use.	Assess for any side effects of pain medication (altered mental status, depressed respirations, bradycardia, orthostatic hypotension, nausea or vomiting, urinary retention, constipation).
	Ask patient to rate pain on a 0-10 scale. Inquire about pain level before and after each administration of pain medication.	Observe patient's expressions, body position, ability to rest or sleep.

ECG, Electrocardiogram; *HIV,* human immune deficiency virus; *NG,* nasogastric; *OR,* operating room; *PACU,* postanesthesia care unit.

surgical site, side effects of anesthesia, electrolyte imbalances, and depression of normal circulatory regulating mechanisms. Continuous electrocardiographic (ECG) monitoring is routine in the PACU to detect rhythm and rate disturbances. Assessment of heart rate and rhythm and blood pressure monitors the patient's cardiovascular status. Compare preoperative vital signs with postoperative values to determine the patient's status.

Assess circulatory perfusion, especially for patients who have had procedures that impair circulation, such as vascular surgery, use of a tourniquet, or application of casts or tight dressings. Always be alert to the amount of bleeding that occurs after surgery and the possibility of hemorrhage. The risk for hemorrhage continues for several days postoperatively. Blood loss occurs externally through a drain or incision or internally within the surgical site. Either type of hemorrhage is indicated by a fall in blood pressure; elevated heart and respiratory rates; thready pulse; cool, clammy, pale skin; and restlessness.

TEMPERATURE CONTROL The OR environment is cool, and the patient's depressed level of body function results in a lowering of metabolism and fall in body temperature. When patients begin to awaken in the PACU, they often complain of feeling cold and uncomfortable. Shivering is not always a sign of hypothermia, but rather a side effect of certain anesthetic agents. Measure body temperature to plan for interventions. On a surgical unit, monitoring of body temperature is important for detecting early occurrence of infection, for example, wound or lung. If a patient develops a fever, report it to the surgeon immediately.

NEUROLOGICAL FUNCTION In the PACU the patient is usually drowsy but reacts to verbal commands. However, drugs, electrolyte and metabolic changes, pain, reduced oxygen saturation, and emotional factors influence level of consciousness. Normally as anesthetic agents are metabolized, the patient's reflexes return, he or she regains muscle strength, and a normal level of orientation returns. Check for pupillary and gag reflexes, hand grasp, and movements of the extremities (see Chapter 15). If a patient has had surgery involving a portion of the neurological system, conduct a more thorough neurological assessment.

Once a patient returns to a surgical nursing unit, a sudden change in consciousness is not normal. However, routine detailed neurological assessment is unnecessary unless a patient is slow to awaken fully or has had surgery involving the neurological system.

FLUID AND ELECTROLYTE BALANCE Because of the surgical patient's risk for fluid and electrolyte abnormalities, assess hydration status and monitor cardiac and neurological function for signs of electrolyte alterations (see Chapter 17). Routinely inspect the IV catheter and insertion site to verify patency, absence of signs of phlebitis and infiltration, and proper infusion of IV fluids. It is important that a good venous access is available in case the patient requires fluid and/or blood replacement. IV fluids will continue on the surgical nursing unit, sometimes for several days. Duration of IV catheter use depends on the type of surgery, the medications

the patient receives, and how well the patient tolerates resumption of oral fluids and food.

Monitor and accurately record intake and output to assess fluid balance, as well as renal and cardiac function. Measure all sources of input (e.g., IV fluids and oral intake) and output (e.g., NG tubes, drains, diarrhea, and urine), and consult with the health care provider if appropriate.

SKIN INTEGRITY AND CONDITION OF THE WOUND Thoroughly assess the condition of the patient's skin. A rash often indicates a drug sensitivity or allergy. Abrasions or petechiae result from inadequate padding during positioning or securing on the operating bed. If a patient has burns or serious injury to the skin, communicate this information by completing an incident or occurrence report (see Chapter 4).

The surgical wound sometimes has no dressing, or it is covered with gauze or transparent dressing that protects the wound site. For open wounds or during the changing of a dressing, observe the appearance of the suture line and note the color, odor, and consistency of any drainage (see Chapter 36). Estimate the amount of drainage by noting the extent and area of the dressing covered (e.g., lower half of dressing saturated with sanguineous drainage). If a patient has a wound drainage system, monitor the output routinely and note the character of drainage. Keep the drainage tubes patent. A sudden increase in drainage indicates possible hemorrhage.

A critical time for wound healing is 24 to 72 hours after surgery (see Chapter 36). A patient exerts physical stress on a wound from coughing, vomiting, or movement in bed. Inadequate nutrition, impaired circulation, and metabolic alterations further impair healing. Observe the incision for signs of dehiscence and evisceration (Table 38-11). Notify the surgeon of any area of dehiscence. Evisceration is a medical emergency. In the event of evisceration, cover any exposed abdominal contents with gauze soaked with sterile normal saline. Prepare an IV infusion set for rapid infusion of IV fluids.

If a wound becomes infected, it usually occurs 3 to 6 days after surgery, when the patient is at home. Ongoing observation of the wound includes inspection for redness, increased warmth, edema, and purulent drainage. Instruct the patient or family caregiver to assess the wound and immediately report any signs and symptoms of wound infection to the surgeon.

GENITOURINARY FUNCTION Spinal anesthesia often prevents the patient from feeling bladder fullness or distention and may cause urinary retention for up to 6 to 8 hours. Palpate the lower abdomen just above the symphysis pubis for bladder distention. You might also choose to use a bladder scanner to determine if urine has accumulated in the bladder (see Chapter 33). A full bladder is painful and is often the cause of a patient's restlessness, agitation, or high blood pressure. If the patient has an indwelling urinary catheter (see Chapter 33), monitor urine output and expect at least 30 mL/hr in adults or 1 to 2 mL/kg/hr in infants and children. Observe the color and odor of urine. Surgery involving portions of the urinary tract normally causes bloody urine for at least 12 to 24 hours.

TABLE 38-11 Common Postoperative Complications

COMPLICATION	CAUSE
RESPIRATORY SYSTEM	
Atelectasis: Collapse of alveoli with retained mucous secretions. Signs and symptoms: elevated respiratory rate, dyspnea, fever, crackles over involved lobes of lungs, productive cough.	Caused by inadequate lung expansion. Greater risk in patients with upper abdominal surgery who have pain during inspiration and repress deep breathing.
Pneumonia: Inflammation of alveoli caused by infectious process. Usually develops in lower dependent lobes of lung if patient is immobilized. Signs and symptoms: fever, chills, productive cough, chest pain, purulent mucus, dyspnea.	Caused by poor lung expansion with retained secretions. *Streptococcus pneumoniae,* a resident bacterium in the respiratory tract, causes most cases of pneumonia.
Hypoxemia: Inadequate concentration of oxygen in arterial blood. Signs and symptoms: restlessness, dyspnea, hypertension, tachycardia, diaphoresis, cyanosis.	Respirations depressed by anesthetics or analgesics. Increased retention of mucus with impaired ventilation occurs from pain, poor positioning, or poor coughing and deep breathing.
Pulmonary embolism: Clot blocks pulmonary artery and disrupts blood flow to one or more lobes of lung. Signs and symptoms: dyspnea, sudden chest pain, cyanosis, tachycardia, hypotension.	Immobilized patient with preexisting circulatory or coagulation disorders is at high risk. Patients with pelvic and abdominal cancer surgeries are at higher risk.
CIRCULATORY SYSTEM	
Hemorrhage: Loss of large amount of blood externally or internally in short period of time. Signs and symptoms: same as for hypovolemic shock.	Slipping of suture or dislodged clot at incisional site. Patients with coagulation disorders are at greater risk.
Hypovolemic shock: Reduced perfusion of tissues and cells from loss of circulatory fluid volume. Signs and symptoms: hypotension, weak and rapid pulse, cool and clammy skin, rapid breathing, restlessness, reduced urine output.	Hemorrhage usually causes hypovolemic shock following surgery.
Thrombophlebitis: Inflammation of vein (usually in leg), often accompanied by clot formation. Signs and symptoms: swelling and inflammation of involved site, aching or cramping pain. Vein feels hard, cordlike, and sensitive to touch.	Venous stasis is aggravated by prolonged sitting or immobilization, trauma to vessel wall, and hypercoagulability of blood.
Thrombus: Formation of clot attached to interior wall of vein or artery, which occludes vessel lumen. Symptoms include localized tenderness along vein, swollen calf or thigh in affected leg. Decreased pulse below thrombus (if arterial).	Venous stasis and vessel trauma. Venous injury is usually common after surgery of legs, abdomen, pelvis, and major vessels. Patients with major surgery or trauma to these areas are at risk for thrombus formation.
Embolus: Piece of thrombus that has dislodged and circulates in bloodstream until it lodges in another vessel, commonly lungs, heart, or brain.	Thrombi also form from increased coagulability of blood.
GASTROINTESTINAL SYSTEM	
Paralytic ileus: Nonmechanical obstruction of the bowel caused by physiological, neurogenic, or chemical imbalance; it may be associated with decreased peristalsis. Common in initial hours following surgery.	Handling of intestines during surgery can lead to loss of peristalsis for a few hours to several days.
Abdominal distention: Retention of air within intestines. Signs and symptoms: increased abdominal girth, complaint of fullness and "gas pains."	Caused by slowed peristalsis from anesthesia, bowel manipulation, or immobilization.
Nausea and vomiting: Symptoms of improper gastric emptying or chemical stimulation of vomiting center. Patient complains of gagging or feeling full or sick to stomach.	Caused by severe pain, abdominal distention, fear, medications, eating or drinking before peristalsis returns, and initiation of gag reflex.
GENITOURINARY SYSTEM	
Urinary retention: Involuntary accumulation of urine in bladder as result of loss of muscle tone. Signs and symptoms: inability to void, restlessness, and bladder distention occurring 6-8 hours postoperatively.	Caused by effects of anesthesia, opioid analgesics, local manipulation of tissues surrounding bladder, and poor positioning of patient, which impairs voiding reflex.

TABLE 38-11 Common Postoperative Complications—cont'd

COMPLICATION	CAUSE
Urinary tract infection caused by bacteria or yeast entering through urethra. Possible symptoms: pain, itching, burning, urgency, and frequency.	A health care–acquired urinary tract infection can occur after bladder catheterization and poor adherence to catheter care.

INTEGUMENTARY SYSTEM

Wound infection: An invasion of deep or superficial wound tissues by pathogenic microorganisms. Signs and symptoms: warm, red, and tender skin around incision, fever and chills, purulent drainage. It usually appears 3-6 days postoperatively.	Caused by poor aseptic technique intraoperatively or during postoperative dressing changes, contaminated wound before surgical exploration. Chronically ill, obese, or immunosuppressed patients are at high risk.
Wound dehiscence: Separation of wound edges at suture line. Signs and symptoms: increased drainage and appearance of underlying tissues occurring 6-8 days after surgery.	Caused by malnutrition, obesity, preoperative radiation to surgical site, old age, poor circulation to tissues, and unusual strain on suture line from coughing.
Wound evisceration: Protrusion of internal organs and tissues through incision. It usually occurs 6-8 days after surgery.	Develops following dehiscence (see above).

NERVOUS SYSTEM

Intractable pain: Pain that is not amenable to analgesia or pain-relief measures.	Related to wound healing, type of dressing, anxiety, or patient positioning.

GASTROINTESTINAL FUNCTION Anesthetic agents slow gastrointestinal motility and cause nausea. In addition, manipulation of the intestines during abdominal surgery further impairs peristalsis. Faint or absent bowel sounds are typical during the immediate recovery phase. Normal bowel sounds usually return in about 24 hours, unless major abdominal surgery was performed. **Paralytic ileus,** loss of function of the intestine that causes abdominal distention, is always a possibility after abdominal surgery. On the surgical nursing unit ask whether the patient is passing flatus, an important sign indicating return of normal bowel function that may be more indicative of postoperative gastrointestinal function return in patients undergoing abdominal surgery than presence of bowel sounds (Madsen and others, 2005). Inspect the abdomen for distention caused by gas. Distention also develops if internal bleeding occurs in a patient who has had abdominal surgery. If an NG tube is in place for decompression, assess the patency of the tube (see Chapter 34) and the color and amount of drainage.

COMFORT As a patient awakens from general anesthesia, the sensation of discomfort often becomes prominent. Some patients perceive pain before regaining full consciousness. Acute incisional pain causes patients to become restless and frequently causes changes in vital signs. Pain management is perhaps one of the most important priorities in postoperative care. Appropriate pain management will enable patients to deep breathe and cough more effectively and to initiate ambulation. If a patient has PCA or is receiving patient-controlled epidural analgesia (PCEA), have the patient begin using the device as soon as possible. The American Pain Society suggests that if you anticipate pain for the majority of the day, the patient should receive analgesics ATC and not prn.

The patient who had regional or local anesthesia usually does not experience pain initially, because the incisional area is still anesthetized. You need to be skilled at assessing levels of pain and be alert to the patient's need for pain medication. Pain scales are an effective method of assessing pain, evaluating the response to analgesics, and objectively documenting the severity of a patient's pain (see Chapter 31).

■■■NURSING DIAGNOSIS

Based on your assessment and information gathered from the reports of members of the surgical team, identify nursing diagnoses that apply to your patient. Nursing diagnoses that give direction to the continuing care of the patient in the PACU and on the surgical nursing unit include the following:

- *Ineffective airway clearance*
- *Anxiety*
- *Disturbed body image*
- *Ineffective breathing pattern*
- *Risk for deficient fluid volume*
- *Risk for infection*
- *Impaired physical mobility*
- *Nausea*
- *Acute pain*
- *Delayed surgical recovery*

Analyze and validate assessment data, and cluster defining characteristics to identify correct nursing diagnoses. For example, a finding of *anxiety* manifested by restlessness could be related to *acute pain, urinary retention,* or *ineffective peripheral tissue perfusion.* Further assessment and clustering of findings will lead to the correct diagnosis.

■■■ PLANNING

Because of the critical nature of the immediate postoperative period, the plan of care in the PACU involves close monitoring of the patient and frequent assessments to ensure stable physiological function. On the surgical nursing unit, care will be focused on facilitating the patient's recovery (Box 38-8). Nursing care will be based on your nursing assessment and the surgeon's postoperative orders. Typical postoperative orders include the following:

1. Frequency of vital signs monitoring and special assessments
2. Types of IV fluids and rate of infusion
3. Postoperative medications (including those for pain, nausea, and antibiotic prophylaxis)
4. Oxygen therapy or incentive spirometry
5. Fluids and food allowed by mouth
6. Level of activity the patient is allowed to resume
7. Position that patient is to maintain while in bed
8. Intake and output measures
9. Laboratory tests and x-ray studies

GOALS AND OUTCOMES During recovery in the PACU, goals of care include returning the patient to normal physiological functioning without complications and maintaining physical and psychological comfort. Examples of outcomes include stable vital signs within the patient's normal range, patent airway, palpable peripheral pulses, oxygen saturation over 95%, an intact incision with minimal wound drainage, and balanced intake and output. Another outcome is for the patient to be awake and oriented to the PACU environment with the ability to move all extremities and to verbalize pain relief and decreased anxiety.

Once the patient is on the surgical nursing unit, goals are more long term. Maintenance of pain control with improvement in physiological function is still a priority. Adequate wound healing without the presence of infection, restoration of nutrition, the patient's return to a functional state of health, and maintenance of self-concept and body image are additional goals. Examples of measurable outcomes include the following: patient states level of pain relief is acceptable, appetite and nutritional intake return to previous or improved state, and patient states willingness to participate in discharge instruction.

SETTING PRIORITIES While in the PACU, a patient's priorities usually center on physiological needs. As you review preoperative and intraoperative data, as well as your ongoing assessments in the PACU, you will determine how a patient is progressing and set priorities on developing needs. For example, if a patient begins to awaken without complications but urinary output is less than normal, consult with the surgeon or anesthesia care provider to determine if IV fluids need to be increased to prevent dehydration. Data indicating any immediate postoperative complications such as hemorrhage require alteration in the plan of care and implementation of necessary emergency measures.

The patient's physical status often changes on the surgical nursing unit, so it remains important to be alert for developing complications. Focus priorities on returning the patient to preoperative functioning or better. Patients will generally have many nursing diagnoses (Figure 38-4). However, management of acute pain will often be the priority of postoperative nursing care. If a surgical patient's pain is properly managed, ambulation will begin earlier, deep breathing and coughing will be less difficult, and the patient will have a better sense of well-being. In addition, begin to prepare the patient for discharge by providing the patient and family necessary instruction and ensuring that adequate resources are available in the home. Monitoring the patient for any psychosocial problems such as body image disturbance or altered coping will also be important during convalescence.

CONTINUITY OF CARE Continuity of nursing care between the OR, the PACU, and the surgical nursing unit depends on good communication among all members of the nursing and surgical team. Nursing staff within each area must be able to convey clear and accurate information about the patient's status and medications to the next nurse who assumes care for the patient. For example, you need to thoroughly describe the condition of a wound so that each nurse knows what to anticipate during wound assessment and care. In that way you will be able to detect any signs of poor wound healing early.

BOX 38-8   SYNTHESIS IN PRACTICE

Postoperative Assessment and Planning

Mr. Korloff's stay in the PACU is uneventful except for pain in the right shoulder. Sue explains to Mr. Korloff that air is put into the abdominal cavity during a laparoscopy. The air causes referred pain. In the PACU Mr. Korloff's pain was a 7 on a scale of 0 to 10.

It is the evening of the day of Mr. Korloff's surgery. Mr. Korloff is in the nursing division for an overnight stay because of his previous cardiac history. He performs deep breathing and coughing exercises and after a few demonstrations by Sue, uses the incentive spirometer as ordered. Because he is ambulating frequently in the hall, with the assistance of his daughters, he is not performing postoperative leg exercises. The IV fluids were discontinued just before he left the PACU. Mr. Korloff was able to tolerate a clear liquid diet and is passing flatus. He rates his pain as 5 on a scale of 0 to 10, continuing to note some discomfort in the shoulder area. His pain has been controlled with an oral pain medication, acetaminophen with codeine, which he receives every 3 to 4 hours around the clock. His vital signs are within normal limits compared with preoperative values, and his lungs are clear on auscultation. The four small abdominal puncture wounds are without drainage or redness.

IV, Intravenous; *PACU,* postanesthesia care unit.

The ambulatory surgical patient will likely be discharged home with family members or friends. It is essential that the patient and family understand continuing care needs of the patient. Usually the ambulatory surgery nursing staff has discharge instruction sheets available. When caring for patients on surgical nursing units, consider the patient's continuing care needs in the home. Referral to home care services or a clinical nurse specialist in wound care or ostomy care, for example, will provide valuable assistance.

CONCEPT MAP

Nursing Diagnosis: Deficient knowledge
- First experience with surgery
- Primary language of Russian affects ability to understand medical terms
- Has questions about procedure

Interventions
- Provide planned teaching sessions (including daughters) in preadmission
- Use visual teaching aids showing laparoscopy method and positioning in surgery
- Provide reinstruction morning of surgery, focusing on areas about which Mr. Korloff and daughters remain uncertain

Nursing Diagnosis: Anxiety
- Expresses concerns about surgery
- States, "I am just worried about how this will affect me over the next few weeks."
- Requires repeat explanations on aspects of preoperative instruction

Interventions
- After preadmission tests, sit down with Mr. Korloff and daughters and discuss their specific concerns
- Teach relaxation exercise to Mr. Korloff and have him demonstrate
- Suggest to daughters use of distraction through conservation and bringing business magazines for Mr. Korloff to read after surgery

Chief Medical Diagnosis: Elective laparoscopic surgery—cholecystectomy
Priority Assessments: Readiness to learn, level of knowledge, coping strategies, ability to understand questions

Nursing Diagnosis: Impaired verbal communication
- Sometimes looks away from nurse during discussion and turns to daughters instead
- Ability to speak in English reduced when discussing medical terms
- Hesitates to find words when asking questions

Interventions
- Have daughters present when explaining medical procedures
- Ask Mr. Korloff if there is anything about his culture that will influence his acceptance of postoperative care
- Incorporate Mr. Korloff's values into way postoperative care is delivered: when to involve daughters, how to manage pain

———— Link between medical diagnosis and nursing diagnosis   - - - - Link between nursing diagnoses

Figure 38-4 ■ Concept Map.

■■■IMPLEMENTATION

Critical thinking is important in the postoperative care of the patient. Consider the interrelationship of all body systems and the effect of the therapies. The patient remains at risk for a variety of postoperative complications (see Table 38-11, p. •••) unless aggressive care is provided and unless the patient becomes actively involved in recovery and convalescence. Review the patient's perioperative teaching, and reinforce as needed (Box 38-9). If the patient is an older adult, the gerontological nursing practice guidelines in Box 38-10 will be helpful.

RESPIRATION Following general anesthesia, a patient in the PACU often has an oral or nasal airway present from the OR to maintain a patent airway until regular breathing at a normal rate resumes. This airway is not taped in place. As respiratory function returns, the patient will spit out the airway. The patient's ability to do so signifies a return of a normal gag reflex.

One of the greatest concerns following surgery is airway obstruction resulting from weakness of pharyngeal or laryngeal muscle tone (from the effects of anesthetics); aspiration of emesis; accumulation of secretions in the pharynx, tra-

---

BOX 38-9	PATIENT TEACHING

Postoperative Teaching

 Mr. Korloff tells Sue that the plan is for discharge tomorrow. In their conversation he says to Sue that he hopes he will remember all of the care she taught him before surgery. Sue develops the following teaching plan for Mr. Korloff:

OUTCOME
- At the end of the teaching session, Mr. Korloff is able to verbalize understanding of pain-relief approaches and wound care practices.

TEACHING STRATEGIES
- Explain the rationale for postoperative exercises so Mr. Korloff will know how the exercises will benefit him.
- Encourage Mr. Korloff to practice postoperative exercises every 1 to 2 hours.
- Reinforce the need to ask for pain medication before pain becomes severe.
- Encourage to avoid smoking because nicotine accelerates the metabolism of pain medication, resulting in shorter duration of effect.
- Teach nonpharmacological means of pain control, such as slow deep breathing, progressive relaxation, and use of tactile stimulation, such as back rubs (see Chapter 31).
- Teach the names, purpose, and timing of medications that Mr. Korloff will continue at home.
- Teach signs and symptoms of hemorrhage and wound infection.
- Instruct in proper hand hygiene.
- Demonstrate wound care techniques that are necessary after discharge (see Chapter 36).
- Review high-protein foods needed for wound healing.

EVALUATION STRATEGIES
- Use open-ended questions.
- Have Mr. Korloff provide return demonstration of the coughing, deep breathing, and leg exercises, hand hygiene, and wound care techniques.
- Ask Mr. Korloff to identify foods to include in his diet.
- Have Mr. Korloff verbalize wound care and signs and symptoms of abnormal wound healing to report to the physician or health care provider.

BOX 38-10	CARE OF THE OLDER ADULT

Principles of Postoperative Care

- Discuss cognitive and sensory functioning, such as decision-making processes, vision, and hearing in the preoperative phase of education (Swan, 2008), then design appropriate strategies postoperatively.
- Increase preoperative teaching time to ensure thorough understanding after surgery
- If the patient will be on bed rest for more than 24 hours, an order for subcutaneous heparin or enoxaparin is necessary to prevent deep vein thrombosis.
- Intake and output is maintained longer postoperatively because perfusion of kidneys is compromised and the older adult frequently decreases oral intake of fluids to minimize voiding frequency.
- Any fluid, electrolyte, or acid-base imbalance will quickly alter mental status. Older adults often need to be closer to the nurses' station and be monitored more frequently for confusion, disorientation, or decreased level of consciousness. Fall precautions are necessary.
- Patients with increased pain tolerance need to be appropriately medicated when they indicate they have pain. Ask patients often to rate their pain, and give them treatment options. Offer pain medications before painful procedures (e.g., dressing changes, walking in the hallway, getting up in a chair).
- Pain medication is more likely to cause altered mental status in older adults, increasing the need to monitor for confusion and disorientation.
- Metabolism of drugs is slowed in older patients, so the effects of medication persist for a longer period of time.
- Nutritional deficits are common, and diets high in protein, calcium, and vitamins B and C are necessary for wound healing and positive nitrogen balance. Carbohydrate intake is essential for energy and to spare protein use for wound healing. Increase iron intake if the patient is anemic.
- Older adults have more difficulty with constipation because of decreased peristalsis, decreased activity, weakening of abdominal muscles, and the risk for dehydration. Orders for a stool softener and/or extra fiber are accompanied by increased fluid intake despite the resulting increased need to void.

chea, or bronchial tree; or laryngeal or subglottic edema. Often the tongue causes airway obstruction. The following measures maintain airway patency:

1. *Position the patient on one side with the face downward and the neck slightly extended* (Figure 38-5). A small, folded towel supports the head. Neck extension prevents occlusion of the airway at the pharynx. When the face is angled downward, the tongue moves forward and mucous secretions flow out of the mouth instead of accumulating in the pharynx. If the nature of the surgery prevents turning the patient on one side, elevate the head of the bed and slightly extend the patient's neck, with the head turned to the side. Never position the patient with arms over or across the chest, because this reduces maximum chest expansion.
2. *Suction the artificial airway and oral cavity for mucous secretions as necessary* (see Chapter 29). Avoid continually eliciting the gag reflex, which will cause vomiting. Before removing an airway, suction the back of the airway to remove any mucous plugs or secretions.
3. *Begin deep breathing and coughing exercises* as soon as the patient responds to instructions.
4. *Administer oxygen as ordered,* and monitor oxygen saturation with a pulse oximeter.

Once a patient reaches a surgical nursing unit, begin aggressive pulmonary hygiene. The patient will participate actively if preoperative instruction was effective. Remember, have the family help coach patients in completing their exercises. Encourage diaphragmatic breathing exercises every hour while the patient is awake. Follow diaphragmatic breathing by having the patient use the incentive spirometer. Encourage the patient to reach the inspiratory volume achieved preoperatively on the spirometer. Proper use of the spirometer will ensure a maximum inspiration. Encourage regular turning and early ambulation. Walking stimulates an increased respiratory rate and improves circulation. Assist patients who are restricted to bed to turn side-to-side every 1 to 2 hours while awake and to sit when possible. If a patient develops pulmonary secretions, encourage coughing exercises followed by deep breathing at least once an hour. Maintain pain control so that the patient achieves a full, productive cough. Provide frequent oral hygiene to help the patient expectorate mucus easily. If the patient is not allowed to have anything by mouth (NPO) or is on a limited fluid intake, the mouth easily becomes dry. Initiate postural drainage and suctioning if the patient is too weak or unable to cough secretions (see Chapter 29).

CIRCULATION In the PACU it is important to monitor for changes in blood pressure or heart rate. The surgeon usually writes an order indicating which changes to report. However, use critical thinking and notify the surgeon when there is a significant change or a continuous negative trend in vital signs. If hemorrhage is external, observe for increased bloody drainage on dressings or through drains. If a dressing becomes saturated, the blood will ooze down the patient's sides and collect in a pool under bedclothes. Always check under the patient for drainage whether or not the dressing is saturated. When hemorrhage is internal, the operative site becomes swollen and tight, and a hematoma develops. Report the first signs of suspected hemorrhaging to the surgeon immediately. Maintain the IV infusion, monitor vital signs continuously, continue oxygen, and raise the patient's legs in a modified Trendelenburg's position to promote venous return until the patient's condition stabilizes.

Early measures directed at preventing venous stasis are aimed at preventing deep vein thrombosis during convalescence. On the surgical nursing unit, begin these interventions as soon as possible:

1. Encourage the patient to perform leg exercises at least every hour while awake unless contraindicated by surgery.
2. *Apply elastic antiembolism stockings or sequential compression stockings as ordered by the surgeon* (see Chapter 35). Often you will apply these devices on the patient in the OR. Remove the stockings every 8 hours and leave off for 1 hour. Thoroughly assess the skin of the legs at this time.
3. *Encourage early ambulation.* Most patients are ordered to ambulate the evening of surgery, depending on the severity of surgery and the patient's condition. The degree of activity allowed progresses as the patient's condition improves. Before ambulation, assess vital signs. Abnormalities often contraindicate ambulation. If vital signs are normal, first assist the patient with sitting on the side of the bed. Dizziness is a sign of postural hypotension (see Chapter 14). Check the patient's blood pressure again and ensure that the patient is not dizzy to determine if ambulation is safe. Assist with ambulation by standing at the patient's side and helping to either hold or move equipment. During the first few times out of bed, the patient often walks only a few feet. Tolerance improves each time. Evaluate the patient's tolerance to activity by periodically assessing pulse rate.
4. *Avoid positioning the patient in a manner that interrupts blood flow to the extremities.* While the patient is in bed, do not place pillows or rolled blankets directly under the knees. Compression of the popliteal vessels causes a thrombus to form. When sitting in a chair, have the patient elevate the legs on a footstool, avoiding hyperextension of the knee. Never allow the patient to sit with one leg crossed over the other.

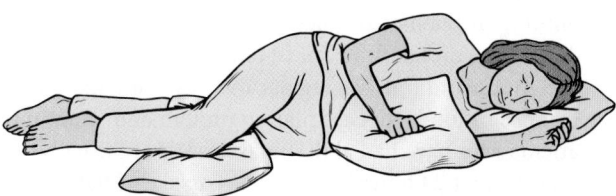

Figure 38-5 ■ Position of patient during recovery from general anesthesia. (From Lewis S and others: *Medical-surgical nursing: assessment and management of clinical problems,* ed 7, St. Louis, 2007, Mosby.)

5. *Administer anticoagulant drugs if ordered.* Small doses of anticoagulants, such as low-molecular-weight heparin given subcutaneously, reduce risk for thrombus formation.

6. *Promote adequate fluid intake orally or intravenously.* Adequate hydration prevents the concentration of platelets and red blood cells and thus prevents formation of small clots within blood vessels. Adequate hydration also promotes tissue healing and liquefies respiratory secretions.

TEMPERATURE CONTROL As a result of the cool temperature in the OR and evaporative heat loss, the patient is usually cool when arriving in the PACU. Provide specially warmed blankets or other warming devices (e.g., heated air blankets). Increasing body warmth causes the patient's metabolism to rise and circulatory and respiratory functions to improve. Patients often still feel cold when reaching a surgical nursing unit. Offer extra blankets or apply a loose-fitting pair of socks to the feet.

NEUROLOGICAL FUNCTION Deep breathing and coughing help to expel retained anesthetic gases and increase the patient's level of consciousness. Try to arouse the patient by calling his or her name in a moderate tone of voice, noting whether the patient responds appropriately. If the patient remains asleep or is unresponsive, waken them through touch or by gently moving a body part. If you need a painful stimulus to wake the patient, then notify the anesthesia care provider. Orientation to the environment is important in maintaining alertness. Explain that surgery is complete, and describe all procedures and nursing measures performed.

FLUID AND ELECTROLYTE BALANCE The patient's only source of fluid intake immediately after surgery is intravenous; therefore it is important to maintain patency of the IV catheter (see Chapter 17). You will typically remove the IV catheter once a patient awakens after ambulatory surgery and is able to tolerate water without gastrointestinal upset. A more seriously ill patient will require an IV catheter to receive blood products, depending on the amount of blood lost during surgery. The surgeon orders a prescribed solution and rate for each IV infusion. Infuse IV solutions through an infusion pump to ensure correct volume delivery.

GENITOURINARY FUNCTION A full bladder is painful and causes a patient awakening from surgery to become restless or agitated. Patients who have abdominal surgery or surgery of the urinary system frequently have indwelling catheters inserted until voluntary control of urination returns. If a catheter is in place and urinary output is less than 30 mL/hr in an adult patient and 1 to 2 mL/kg/hr in infants and children, check for catheter occlusion or kinking. Notify the surgeon if measured output does not improve. During convalescence the following measures promote normal urinary elimination (see Chapter 33):

1. Assist the patient in assuming normal positions for voiding.
2. Check the patient frequently for the need to void when a catheter is not in place. The feeling of bladder fullness and urgency to void is often sudden, and you need to respond promptly when the patient calls for assistance.

3. Assess for bladder distention. The patient's surgeon usually orders a straight urinary catheter to be inserted if a patient does not void within 8 hours of surgery or sooner if the bladder is distended. Even if the patient has been NPO for hours, IV fluids give the renal system sufficient fluid to excrete urine. Continued difficulty in voiding requires an indwelling catheter, although the risk for urinary tract infection increases (see Chapter 33).

4. Monitor intake and output. If the patient's urine is dark and concentrated, notify the surgeon. A patient easily becomes dehydrated. Remember, the minimum urine output is 30 mL/hr in adults or 1 to 2 mL/kg/hr in infants and children. Notify the surgeon if output is less than those ranges.

GASTROINTESTINAL FUNCTION Minimize a patient's nausea during recovery in the PACU by avoiding sudden movement of the patient. If the patient has an NG tube, maintain tube patency with normal saline irrigations as ordered (see Chapter 34). Occlusion of an NG tube causes the accumulation of gastric contents in the stomach. Because stomach emptying slows under anesthesia, the accumulated contents cannot escape, and nausea and vomiting develop. Normally a patient does not receive fluids to drink in the PACU because of the risk for vomiting and altered mental status from general anesthesia. Use a moist swab to relieve dryness of the patient's lips and mouth. If the patient is nauseated, give prescribed medication to prevent vomiting and aspiration.

Interventions for preventing gastrointestinal complications during convalescence promote the return of normal elimination and faster resumption of normal nutritional intake. It takes several days for a patient who has had surgery on gastrointestinal structures to resume a normal dietary intake. Normal peristalsis does not usually return for 24 to 48 hours. In contrast, the patient whose gastrointestinal tract is unaffected directly by surgery simply recovers from the effects of anesthesia before resuming dietary intake. Follow these guidelines:

1. *Maintain a gradual progression in dietary intake.* Patients undergoing ambulatory surgery can generally resume their diet immediately postoperatively. Patients requiring an intraoperative IV receive only IV fluids initially. Once the surgeon orders resumption of oral intake, first provide clear liquids, such as water, apple juice, or decaffeinated tea or coffee, after nausea subsides. Overloading with large amounts of fluids leads to distention and vomiting. If the patient tolerates liquids without nausea, advance the diet to full liquids, followed by a light diet of solid foods, and finally a regular diet, stressing the importance of foods that are high in protein and vitamin C. Patients who have had abdominal surgery are usually NPO the first 24 hours or until the passage of flatus.

2. *Promote ambulation and exercise.* Physical activity stimulates a return of peristalsis. The patient who suffers abdominal distention and "gas pain" will often obtain relief while walking.

3. *Maintain an adequate fluid intake.* Fluids keep fecal material soft for easy passage.

4. *Administer fiber supplements, stool softeners, enemas, and rectal suppositories as ordered.* Constipation or distention often develops postoperatively related to side effects of anesthetic agents and pain medication, and dehydration.

5. *Stimulate the patient's appetite* by removing sources of noxious odors and providing small servings of nonspicy foods.

6. *Assist the patient in sitting* (if possible) during mealtime to minimize pressure on the abdomen.

7. *Provide frequent oral hygiene.*

8. *Provide meals when the patient is rested and free from pain.* A patient will often lose interest in eating if he or she is exhausted by activities such as ambulation before mealtime.

COMFORT The anesthesiologist or nurse anesthetist orders medications for pain management in the PACU. IV opioid analgesics, such as morphine sulfate, are the drugs of choice for the immediate postoperative period. Titrate IV morphine as ordered until pain relief is achieved. Morphine can depress level of consciousness and vital signs, but at appropriate doses this is rare. Assess the patient for the proper dose of analgesic, and monitor for possible side effects. Once a patient is awake, a PCA pump or a PCEA pump may be initiated as ordered. If the patient has an epidural catheter, caution is needed if additional analgesics are ordered (see Chapter 31).

A patient's pain increases as the effects of anesthesia wear off; this often occurs once the patient reaches the surgical nursing unit. The patient becomes more aware of surroundings and more perceptive of discomfort. The incisional area is only one source of pain. Irritation from drainage tubes, tight dressings, or casts and the muscular strains caused from positioning on the operating bed also cause discomfort. Air insufflation during laparoscopic surgery can cause significant discomfort, especially in the shoulder area.

Pain significantly slows recovery. Assess the patient's pain thoroughly. Do not assume that the pain is incisional in origin. When the patient requests pain medication, determine the nature and character of the pain. Patients have the most surgical pain during the first 24 to 48 hours after surgery. Provide analgesics as often as allowed. Intravenous or epidural PCA systems allow the patient to administer analgesics from specially prepared pumps (see Chapter 31). A PCA device is attached to the IV line, or the analgesic is given via an epidural catheter, as with fentanyl or morphine. The patient controls the amount of analgesia received within set doses and times ordered by the surgeon or anesthesia care provider. Program the doses and frequencies of pain medication into the pump. PCA medication is delivered at a preprogrammed basal rate, a bolus dose at specified intervals as needed, or both. Continuous epidural analgesia is frequently used postoperatively for thoracic and abdominal surgical procedures. Several research studies have shown continuous epidural analgesia to provide superior pain relief compared with IV PCA (Gupta and others, 2006; Taqi and others, 2007; Wu and others, 2005).

When a patient is receiving pain medications through a PCA pump or through an epidural catheter, document respirations and level of consciousness. Documentation of frequent objective pain assessment using a pain scale, appropriate nursing interventions, and evaluation of the patient's response must be in every patient's medical record; this standard was set in January 2001 by The Joint Commission 2000 standards, and they continue today (The Joint Commission, 2009).

PROMOTING WOUND HEALING Surgical dressings remain in place the first 24 hours after surgery to reduce the risk for infection. During this time, add an extra layer of gauze on top of the original dressing if drainage develops. Mark or draw around the drainage on the dressing and date and time the marking. This will provide a means to monitor increasing amounts of drainage. Notify the surgeon if bleeding is excessive. In certain types of surgery the surgeon will choose to use no dressing at all.

During convalescence continue close observation of the surgical wound. If a wound becomes infected, it usually occurs 3 to 6 days after surgery. Always use aseptic technique during dressing changes and wound care. Surgical drains need to remain patent so that accumulated secretions are removed from the incision site. Observation of the wound identifies early signs and symptoms of infection (see Chapter 36).

To ensure continuity of care be sure that all staff are aware of the proper materials to use in a dressing change. It is not uncommon for patients to feel discomfort during an extensive dressing change, so offer pain medication 5 to 30 minutes before the procedure. Time the procedure to begin when the pain medication begins to work. For example, oral pain medications take about 30 minutes to begin working; therefore give oral pain medication 30 minutes before the procedure. Pain medications given by IV push usually only take 5 to 10 minutes to work. In this case give the IV pain medication about 5 to 10 minutes before the dressing change.

If you anticipate that the patient will need to continue dressing changes in the home, plan instruction at a time when the patient is alert and comfortable, and family caregivers are present. Before discharge, ensure that the patient knows how to obtain the materials needed for the dressing change.

MAINTAINING SELF-CONCEPT During a patient's convalescence, the appearance of wounds, bulky dressings, and extruding drains and tubes threaten the self-concept. The nature of the surgery often also creates a permanent change in body image. If surgery leads to impairment in body function, the patient's role within the family and community often changes significantly. Observe the patient for alterations in self-concept (see Chapter 22). Some patients show revulsion toward their appearance by refusing to look at an incision or carefully covering dressings with bedclothes. The fear of not being able to return to a functional role in the family or at a previously held job even causes the patient to avoid participating in the care plan.

The family or significant other frequently plays an important role in efforts to improve the patient's self-concept. Help the family to accept the patient's needs and still encourage independence. The following measures maintain the patient's self-concept:

1. *Provide privacy* during dressing changes or wound inspection by closing room curtains and draping the patient so that only the dressing and incisional area are exposed.
2. *Maintain the patient's hygiene.* A complete bath the first day after surgery usually makes the patient feel renewed. Offer a clean gown and washcloth if the gown becomes soiled. Keep the patient's hair neatly combed, and offer frequent, every 2 hours while awake, oral hygiene, especially for the patient who is NPO.
3. *Prevent drains from overflowing.* Measure the drainage sets every 8 hours for output recording, but sometimes drains will need to be emptied and measured more often if drainage is excessive.
4. *Maintain a pleasant environment.* Store or remove all unused supplies, and keep the bedside orderly and clean.
5. *Offer opportunities for the patient to discuss feelings about appearance.* Patients worry about permanent scarring. When the patient chooses to look at an incision for the first time, make sure the area is clean. Eventually the patient will care for the incision site by applying simple dressings or bathing.
6. *Give the family opportunities to discuss ways to promote the patient's self-concept.* Encouraging independence is difficult for a family member who has a strong desire to assist the patient in any way. By knowing about the appearance of a wound or incision, family members will be supportive during dressing changes.

RESTORATIVE AND CONTINUING CARE There are other postoperative care activities that promote a patient's return to a functional state of health. Throughout the postoperative convalescent period promote the patient's independence and active participation in care. When a patient is in pain or suffers from postoperative complications, motivation for self-care could be low. The goals set for a patient's involvement need to be realistic. It is unrealistic to involve the patient if movement is highly restricted or if participation increases the patient's discomfort.

Keep the patient and family informed of progress made toward recovery. Many patients become depressed if they think recovery is slow. Explain the length of time expected to reach a level of maximal recovery. For some patients, surgery also causes permanent physical limitations that require time to accept.

Plan care daily, keeping in mind the ultimate goals for recovery. From the moment the patient enters the hospital, anticipate and plan for the patient's return home.

Involvement of family members in the care plan facilitates early discharge and adequate care at home. Instruct family members in care activities such as dressing changes, how to

assist with ambulation, and medication management. If family members are unable to assist the patient, work with the surgeon, social worker, and/or discharge planner for referrals to home care agencies to provide services at home.

■■■**EVALUATION**

PATIENT CARE In the PACU continuously evaluate the effectiveness of interventions and the patient's response. The patient's condition can change quickly. Evaluation of the patient's status involves ongoing measurement of vital signs, pulse oximetry, wound drainage, intake and output, and other physical assessments. The modified Aldretti score evaluates the patient's level of consciousness and return of motor function. Determine frequency of assessments based on the patient's response to anesthesia. If evaluation reveals the patient is recovering from anesthesia, the surgeon or anesthesia care provider will discharge the patient from the PACU.

On the surgical nursing unit evaluate the effectiveness of care on the basis of expected outcomes resulting from nursing interventions). Evaluation will occur over several days. It is important to evaluate the patient's clinical progress and readiness for discharge by observing the patient's participation in postoperative exercises, self-care activities, and ambulation (Box 38-11). Evaluate the ambulatory surgical patient's outcomes by making a postoperative telephone call to the patient's home. The call, usually placed 24 hours after surgery, reassures the patient and allows for evaluation of recov-

---

BOX 38-11   EVALUATION

  Mr. Korloff progressed well and is ready for discharge the day after surgery. He expresses relief that everything went well and that he will be able to return to work, hopefully by next week. Sue continues to care for him on the surgical patient care unit. Sue explains how to remove the gauze on the puncture sites and tells Mr. Korloff to bathe and shower tomorrow. Symptoms the patient and family need to watch for include redness, swelling, bile-colored drainage or pus from the abdominal wounds, severe abdominal pain, nausea, vomiting, and fever with a temperature greater than 100° F (37.7° C) or chills. Any of these symptoms need to be reported to Mr. Korloff's surgeon immediately. His daughters observed the puncture sites and are able to identify symptoms of complications. Mr. Korloff is ready for discharge and plans to stay with one of his daughters over the weekend. Sue makes a follow-up surgical appointment for Mr. Korloff and gives him the surgeon's phone number in case he has any questions or concerns once he returns home.

DOCUMENTATION NOTE
"Abdominal puncture site dry and intact, without redness. Discharge teaching provided to patient and daughters. Repeated signs and symptoms of complications; wound care instructions; activity restrictions; and follow-up appointment time, date, and place. Patient and daughters verbalize understanding of all discharge instruction."

ery progress and the opportunity to answer any questions from the patient or family.

PATIENT EXPECTATIONS In the PACU some patients are not able to voice expectations. However, evaluation of pain is critical. Because pain is subjective, validate it by frequently asking the patient how he or she feels. If possible, use a pain assessment scale. Note the patient's movement and positioning, because nonverbal behaviors indicate if a patient is comfortable. If pain is not adequately relieved, change the dosage or type of medication. Also, evaluate the patient's level of anxiety by assessing presence of any concerns or fears.

Further explanation of postoperative progress and procedures reduces anxiety.

As the patient progresses through convalescence, physical and psychological comfort continues to be a typical expectation of patients and families. Also evaluate if the patient feels prepared for discharge from the acute care facility. Is the patient able to explain the required care to continue following discharge? Have the patient demonstrate any procedures such as wound care or medication administration. Give the patient and family numerous opportunities to ask questions about what to anticipate once the patient returns home.

SAFETY GUIDELINES FOR NURSING SKILLS

Ensuring patient safety is an essential role of the professional nurse. To ensure patient safety, communicate clearly with members of the health care team, assess and incorporate the patient's priorities of care and preferences, and use the best evidence when making decisions about your patient's care. When performing intraoperative skills, remember the following points to ensure safe, individualized patient care (The Joint Commission, 2009):

- Use the Universal Protocol before any surgical procedure and when providing any care or treatment: verify patient's name verbally whenever possible and compare to chart and armband, and patient's expectation of planned procedure and site are verified with consent.
- For all procedures involving incision or percutaneous puncture or insertion the intended site is marked with the patient's involvement whenever possible.

- A time-out is performed immediately before starting the surgery and includes correct patient identity, confirmation of marked site, accurate procedure consent, agreement by all on the procedure to be done, correct patient position, relevant images and results properly labeled and appropriately displayed, need to administer antibiotics or fluids for irrigation purposes, and safety precautions based on patient history or medication use.
- Perform standardized hand-off communications between care providers in the holding area, OR, and postanesthesia care unit and nursing unit, allowing an opportunity to ask and respond to questions.
- Implement best practices to prevent surgical site infections.

SKILL 38-1   TEACHING POSTOPERATIVE EXERCISES

DELEGATION CONSIDERATIONS

Postoperative exercise teaching cannot be delegated. Nursing assistive personnel reinforce and assist patients in performing postoperative exercises.

EQUIPMENT

- Pillow (*optional;* used to splint surgical incision when coughing)
- Incentive spirometer (IS)
- Positive expiratory pressure device

STEP	RATIONALE

ASSESSMENT

1 Verify patient's identity by using at least two patient identifiers. Compare patient's name and one other identifier, such as hospital identification number, with medical record. Ask patient to state name as a third identifier, and explain procedure.

Complies with The Joint Commission requirements and improves procedure safety. In most acute care settings you will use the patient's name and identification number on armband and medical record as identifiers (The Joint Commission, 2009). Information promotes patient cooperation and reduces anxiety.

2 Assess patient's risk for postoperative respiratory complications: Review medical history to identify presence of chronic pulmonary condition (e.g., emphysema, asthma), any condition that affects chest wall movement, history of smoking, and presence of reduced hemoglobin (low red blood cell [RBC] count).

General anesthesia predisposes patient to respiratory problems because lungs do not fully inflate during surgery, cough reflex is suppressed, and mucus collects within airway passages. After surgery patient will have reduced lung volume and require greater effort to deep breathe and cough; inadequate lung expansion leads to atelectasis and pneumonia. Patient is at greater risk for developing respiratory complications if chronic lung conditions are present (Kaw and Stoller, 2008). Smoking damages ciliary clearance and increases mucus secretion. A reduced hemoglobin level leads to inadequate oxygenation.

SKILL 38-1	TEACHING POSTOPERATIVE EXERCISES—cont'd

STEP	RATIONALE
3 Auscultate lungs.	Establishes a baseline for postoperative comparison.
4 Assess patient's ability to cough and deep breathe by having patient take a deep breath and observing movement of shoulders, chest wall, and abdomen. Observe chest excursion during a deep breath. Ask patient to cough after taking a deep breath.	Reveals maximum potential for chest expansion and ability to cough forcefully; serves as baseline to measure patient's ability to perform exercises postoperatively. Diaphragmatic breathing allows for greater lung expansion, improved ventilation, and increased blood oxygenation. Coughing loosens and removes secretions from the pulmonary alveoli.
5 Assess patient's risk for postoperative thrombus formation (e.g., older patients, those with active cancer, immobilized patients, those with personal or family history of clots, women over 35 years who smoke and are taking oral contraceptives). Observe the calves for redness, warmth, and tenderness, swollen calf or thigh, calf swelling more than 3 cm compared with asymptomatic leg, pitting edema in symptomatic leg, and collateral superficial veins. Compare legs for bilateral equality.	Determines baseline for circulation status. Thrombus forms when venous stasis, hypercoagulability, and vein trauma exist simultaneously (Lewis and others, 2007). Following general anesthesia, circulation slows, resulting in a greater tendency for clot formation. Immobilization results in decreased muscular contraction in lower extremities, which promotes venous stasis. The physical stress of surgery creates a hypercoagulable state in most individuals. Manipulation and positioning during surgery sometimes cause trauma to leg veins.

- *Critical Decision Point:* If you suspect a thrombus, notify surgeon and refrain from manipulating extremity any further. Surgery will usually be postponed. Graduated compression stockings or intermittent pneumatic compression stockings may be ordered for patients at risk for thrombus formation.

STEP	RATIONALE
6 Assess patient's ability to move independently while in bed.	Patients confined to bed rest, even for limited periods, will need to turn regularly. Determines existence of any mobility restrictions.
7 Assess patient's willingness and capability to learn exercises; note attention span, anxiety, level of consciousness, and language level.	Ability to learn depends on readiness, ability, and learning environment.
8 Assess family members' or significant other's willingness to learn and to support patient postoperatively.	Encourage family member or significant other to coach patient on exercise performance.
9 Assess patient's medical orders preoperatively and postoperatively.	Some patients will require adaptations in way to perform exercises.

PLANNING

STEP	RATIONALE
1 Prepare equipment as needed.	
2 Plan teaching sessions to occur when patient is not in pain.	Decreased levels of pain enhance patient learning.
3 Explain the postoperative exercises to patient, including importance to recovery and physiological benefits.	Information allows patient to understand significance of exercises and motivates learning. Promotes patient cooperation and decreases anxiety.
4 Prepare the room for teaching.	Environment needs to be conducive to learning (see Chapter 11).

IMPLEMENTATION

STEP	RATIONALE
1 Demonstrate Exercises	
A Diaphragmatic Breathing	
(1) Assist patient to a comfortable semi-Fowler's position in bed or in a sitting position on side of bed or in chair.	Upright position facilitates diaphragmatic excursion.
(2) Stand or sit facing patient.	Allows patient to observe breathing exercises performed by nurse.
(3) Instruct patient to place palms of hands across from each other, down, and along lower borders of anterior rib cage; place fingers lightly together on upper abdomen (see illustration). Demonstrate for patient.	Position of hands allows patient to feel movement of chest and abdomen as diaphragm descends and lungs expand.

STEP	RATIONALE

(4) Instruct patient to take slow, deep breaths, inhaling through nose, and pushing abdomen against hands. Tell patient to feel middle fingers separate during inhalation. Explain that patient will feel normal downward movement of diaphragm while inhaling and that abdominal organs descend and chest wall expands. Demonstrate for patient.

Slow, deep breaths prevent panting or hyperventilation. Inhaling through nose warms, humidifies, and filters air. Diaphragmatic breathing allows air to pass by partially obstructing mucous plug, thus increasing the force to expel the mucus. Explanation and demonstration focus on normal ventilatory movement of chest wall. Patient learns how diaphragmatic breathing feels.

(5) Instruct the patient to avoid using chest and shoulders while inhaling.

Using auxiliary chest and shoulder muscles during breathing wastes energy and does not promote full lung expansion.

(6) Instruct patient to hold a slow, deep breath, for count of three, and then slowly exhale through mouth as if blowing out a candle (through pursed lips). Demonstrate for patient. Tell patient middle fingertips will touch as chest wall contracts during exhalation.

Pursed-lip exhalation allows for gradual expulsion of air.

(7) Repeat complete breathing exercise 3 to 5 times.

Allows patient to observe slow, rhythmical breathing pattern. Repetition reinforces learning

(8) Have patient practice exercise. Instruct patient to take 10 slow, deep breaths every hour while awake during postoperative period.

Regular deep breathing prevents postoperative complications.

B Incentive Spirometry

(1) Perform hand hygiene.

Reduces transmission of microorganisms.

(2) Instruct patient to assume semi-Fowler's or high-Fowler's position.

Promotes optimal lung expansion during spirometry.

(3) For a patient who is obese, consider the reverse Trendelenburg's position.

Patients who are obese are often able to move their diaphragm better in this position.

(4) Indicate to patient on the IS device the volume level to obtain with each inhalation. Use the manufacturer's guidelines to set the volume for the patient.

Establishes goal of volume level necessary for adequate lung expansion.

(5) Demonstrate and then have patient place mouthpiece of incentive spirometer so that lips completely cover mouthpiece (see illustration).

Demonstration is a reliable technique for teaching psychomotor skill and enables patient to ask questions.

(6) Instruct patient to inhale slowly and maintain constant flow through unit, while attempting to reach goal volume. When patient reaches maximal inspiration, have patient hold his or her breath for 3 to 5 seconds (see illustration) and then exhale slowly (Pruitt, 2006). Make sure the number of breaths does not exceed 10 to 12 per minute.

Maintains maximal inspiration and reduces risk for progressive collapse of individual alveoli. Slow breathing (less than 12 breaths per minute) prevents or minimizes pain from sudden pressure changes in chest.

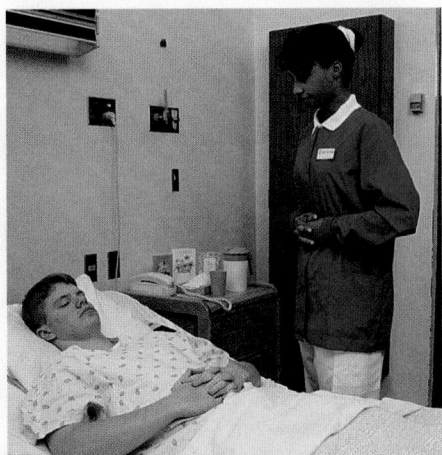

Step 1A(3) ■ Deep breathing exercise: placement of hands during inhalation.

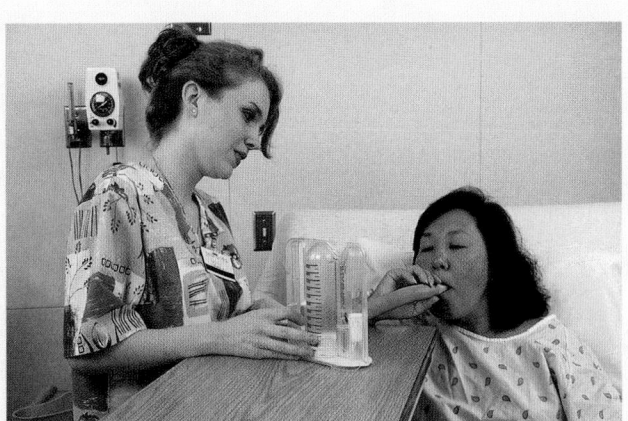

Step 1B(5) ■ Patient demonstrating incentive spirometry.

SKILL 38-1	TEACHING POSTOPERATIVE EXERCISES—cont'd

STEP	RATIONALE
(7) Instruct patient to breathe normally for short period between the 10 breaths on spirometer.	Prevents hyperventilation and fatigue.
(8) Have patient repeat maneuver until goals are achieved.	Ensures correct use of spirometer.
(9) Perform hand hygiene.	Reduces transmission of microorganisms.
C Positive Expiratory Pressure Therapy and "Huff" Coughing	
(1) Perform hand hygiene.	Reduces transmission of microorganisms.
(2) Set positive expiratory pressure (PEP) device for setting ordered.	Higher settings require more ventilatory effort.
(3) Instruct patient to assume semi-Fowler's or high-Fowler's position, and place nose clip on patient's nose (see illustration).	Promotes optimum lung expansion, enabling patient to expectorate mucus.
(4) Have patient place lips around mouthpiece, or demonstrate placement. Instruct patient to take a full breath and then exhale two or three times longer than inhalation. Repeat pattern for 10 to 20 breaths.	Ensures that patient does all breathing through mouth and that patient uses the device properly.
(5) Remove device from mouth, and have patient take a slow, deep breath and hold for 3 seconds.	Promotes lung expansion before coughing.
(6) Then have patient exhale in quick, short, forced "huffs."	"Huff" coughing, or forced expiratory technique, promotes bronchial hygiene by increasing expectoration of secretions (Fink, 2007).
D Controlled Coughing	
(1) Explain importance of maintaining an upright position.	Facilitates diaphragm excursion and enhances thorax expansion.
(2) If surgical incision will be either abdominal or thoracic, teach patient to place pillow or bath blanket over incisional area and place hands over pillow to splint incision. During breathing and coughing exercises, have patient press gently against incisional area for splinting or support (see illustrations).	Surgical incision cuts through muscles, tissues, and nerve endings. Deep breathing and coughing exercises place additional stress on suture line and cause discomfort. Splinting incision with hands or pillow provides firm support and reduces incisional pulling.
(3) Demonstrate coughing. Instruct patient to take two slow, deep breaths, inhaling through nose and exhaling through mouth.	Deep breaths expand lungs fully so that air moves behind mucus and facilitates effects of coughing.
(4) Instruct patient to inhale deeply a third time and hold breath to count of three. Instruct patient to cough fully for two or three consecutive coughs without inhaling between coughs. (Tell patient to push all air out of lungs.)	Consecutive coughs help remove mucus more effectively and completely than one forceful cough.

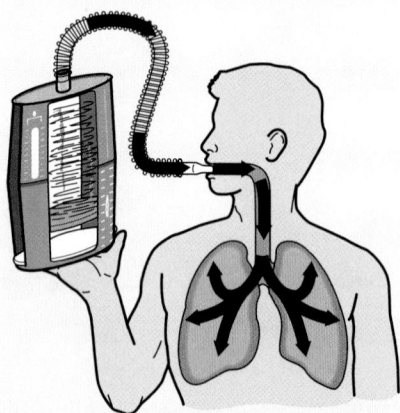

Step 1B(6) ■ Diagram of use of incentive spirometer.

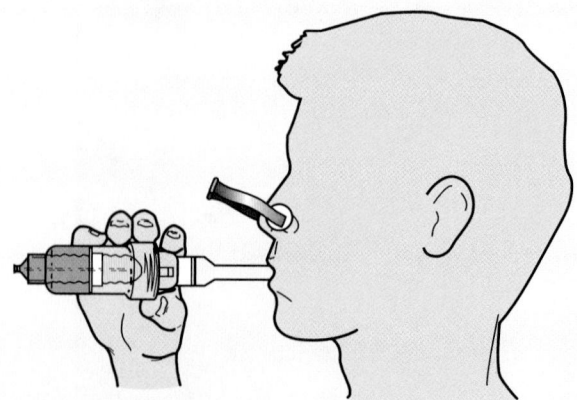

Step 1C(3) ■ Diagram of use of positive expiratory pressure device.

STEP	**RATIONALE**

> • *Critical Decision Point:* Coughing is often contraindicated after brain, spinal, head, neck, or eye surgery because of a potential increase in intracranial or intraocular pressure.

STEP	**RATIONALE**
(5) Caution patient against just clearing throat instead of coughing. Explain that coughing will not cause injury to incision.	Clearing throat does not remove mucus from deeper airways. Postoperative incisional pain makes it harder to cough effectively.
(6) Have patient continue to practice coughing exercises, splinting imaginary incision. Instruct the patient to cough 2 to 3 times every 2 hours while awake.	Stresses value of deep coughing with splinting to effectively expectorate mucus with minimal discomfort.
(7) Instruct patient to examine sputum for consistency, odor, amount, and color changes.	Sputum characteristics indicate the presence of a pulmonary complication, such as pneumonia.
E Turning	
(1) Instruct patient to assume supine position and move to side of bed (left side in this example) by bending knees and pressing heels against the mattress to raise and move buttocks (see illustration).	Positioning begins on one side of bed so that turning to other side will not cause patient to roll toward bed's edge. Buttocks lift prevents shearing force from body movement against sheets.

> • *Critical Decision Point:* If patient has decreased strength or mobility on one side, have patient assume position on the other side of the bed. Also, use safe patient handling to turn patient.

STEP	**RATIONALE**
(2) Instruct patient to place the right hand over incisional area to splint it *(optional)*.	Splinting incision supports and minimizes pulling on suture line during turning.
(3) Instruct patient to keep right leg straight and flex left knee up (see illustration).	Straight leg stabilizes the patient's position. Flexed left leg shifts weight for easier turning.

> • *Critical Decision Point:* Patients who have had back surgery, brain surgery, or vascular repair are often restricted from flexing their legs. They will need to logroll or require assistance for positioning.

STEP	**RATIONALE**
(4) Have patient grab right side rail with left hand, pull toward right, and roll onto right side.	Pulling toward side rail reduces effort needed for turning.
(5) Instruct patient to turn every 2 hours while awake.	Reduces risk for vascular and pulmonary complications.
F Leg Exercises	
(1) Have patient assume supine position in bed. Demonstrate leg exercises by performing passive range-of-motion exercises and simultaneously explaining exercise.	Provides normal anatomical position of lower extremities.

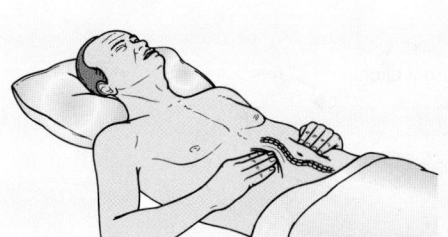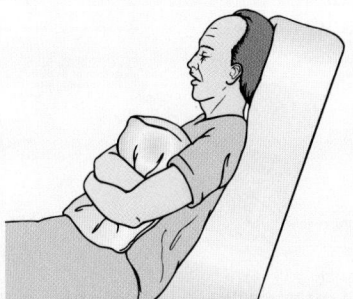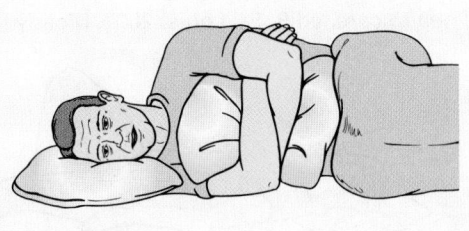

Step 1D(2) ■ Techniques for splinting incision. (From Lewis S and others: *Medical-surgical nursing: assessment and management of clinical problems,* ed 7, St. Louis, 2007, Mosby.)

SKILL 38-1	TEACHING POSTOPERATIVE EXERCISES—cont'd

STEP	RATIONALE

• *Critical Decision Point:* If patient's surgery involves one or both lower extremities, surgeon must order leg exercises in postoperative period. Leg unaffected by surgery can be safely exercised unless the patient has preexisting thrombosis (blood clot formation) or thrombophlebitis (inflammation of the vein wall).

(2) Rotate each ankle in complete circle. Instruct patient to draw imaginary circles with big toe. Repeat 5 times (see illustration).	Maintains joint mobility and promotes venous return.
(3) Alternate dorsiflexion and plantar flexion of both feet. Direct patient to feel calf muscles contract and relax alternately (see illustrations *A* and *B*). Repeat 5 times.	Stretches and contracts gastrocnemius muscles, improving venous return.
(4) Perform quadriceps setting by tightening thigh and bringing knee down toward mattress, then relaxing (see illustration). Repeat 5 times.	Contracts muscles of upper legs, maintains knee mobility, and enhances venous return.
(5) Have patient alternately raise each leg up from bed surface, keeping legs straight, and then have patient bend leg at hip and knee (see illustration). Repeat 5 times.	Contracts and relaxes quadriceps muscles and prevents venous pooling. Bending leg reduces strain on back.
2 Have patient continue to practice exercises at least every 2 hours while awake. Instruct patient to coordinate turning and leg exercises with diaphragmatic breathing, incentive spirometry, and coughing exercises.	Repetition of exercise sequence reinforces learning. Establishes routine for exercises that develops habit for performance. Sequence of exercises is leg exercises, turning, breathing, and coughing.

EVALUATION

1 Observe patient performing all four exercises independently.	Provides opportunity for practice and return demonstration of exercises. Ensures patient has learned correct technique.
2 Observe family members or significant others' ability to coach patient.	Family members or significant others can assist positively or interfere with correct technique.
3 Observe patient's chest excursion.	Determines extent of lung expansion.
4 Auscultate patient's lungs.	Reveals presence of abnormal lung sounds.
5 Palpate calves gently for redness, warmth, and tenderness. Assess pedal pulses.	Absent signs and normal pulses usually indicate that no venous thrombosis is present.

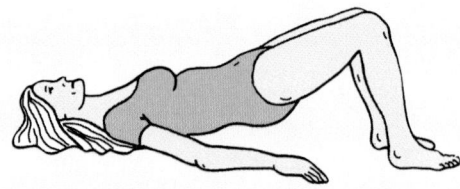

Step 1E(1) ■ Buttocks lift for moving to side of bed. (From Lowdermilk D, Perry SE: *Maternity and women's health care,* ed 9, St. Louis, 2007, Mosby.)

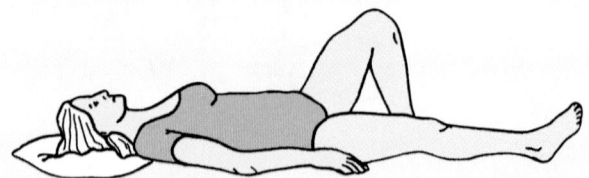

Step 1E(3) ■ Leg position for turning. (From Lowdermilk D, Perry SE: *Maternity and women's health care,* ed 9, St. Louis, 2007, Mosby.)

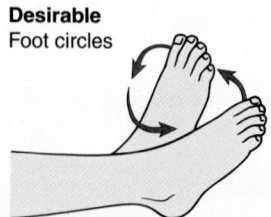

Desirable
Foot circles

Step 1F(2) ■ Foot circles. (From Lewis S and others: *Medical-surgical nursing: assessment and management of clinical problems,* ed 7, St. Louis, 2007, Mosby.)

RECORDING AND REPORTING

- Record which exercises you have demonstrated to patient and if patient performs exercises independently or needs continued assistance.

- Report any problems patient has in practicing exercises to nurse assigned to patient on next shift for follow-up.

UNEXPECTED OUTCOMES AND RELATED INTERVENTIONS

- Patient is unable to perform exercises correctly preoperatively.
  - Assess for the presence of anxiety, pain, and fatigue.
  - Teach patient stress reduction techniques and/or pain management strategies.
  - Repeat teaching using more demonstration or redemonstration at time when family member is present.
- Patient is unwilling to perform exercises postoperatively because of incisional pain of thorax or abdomen (deep breathing, coughing, and turning) or because of surgery in lower abdomen, groin, buttocks, or legs (leg exercises, turning).
  - Instruct patient to ask for pain medication 30 minutes before performing postoperative exercises or to use PCA a few minutes before exercising.
  - Report to surgeon inadequate pain relief and need to change analgesic or increase dose.

- Patient develops pulmonary complications postoperatively.
  - Assess breath sounds in all lobes, and compare bilaterally.
  - Place patient in upright position.
  - Notify surgeon of findings.
  - Be prepared to start oxygen or IV antibiotics as ordered.
- Patient develops circulatory complications, such as venous stasis or thrombophlebitis, postoperatively.
  - Notify health care provider of findings.
  - Place patient on bed rest with affected leg elevated.
  - Continue to have patient do exercises with unaffected leg.

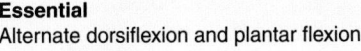
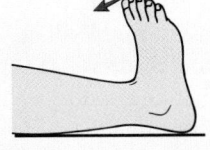
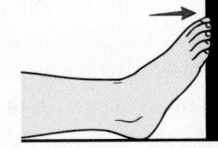
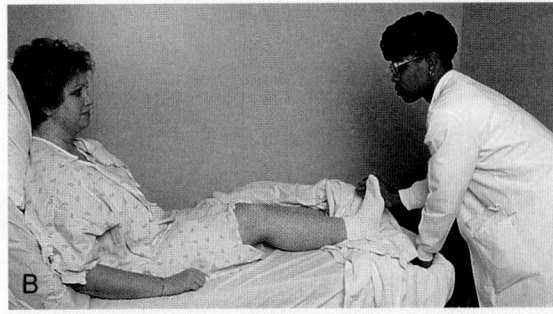

Essential
Alternate dorsiflexion and plantar flexion

Step 1F(3) ■ **A,** Alternate dorsiflexion and plantar flexion. (From Lewis S and others: *Medical-surgical nursing: assessment and management of clinical problems,* ed 7, St. Louis, 2007, Mosby.) **B,** Patient pushes feet to perform plantar flexion.

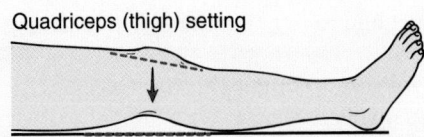

Quadriceps (thigh) setting

Step 1F(4) ■ Quadriceps (thigh) setting. (From Lewis S and others: *Medical-surgical nursing: assessment and management of clinical problems,* ed 7, St. Louis, 2007, Mosby.)

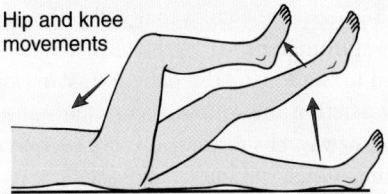

Hip and knee movements

Step 1F(5) ■ Hip and knee movements. (From Lewis S and others: *Medical-surgical nursing: assessment and management of clinical problems,* ed 7, St. Louis, 2007, Mosby.)

KEY POINTS

- Previous illnesses and past surgeries affect the patient's ability to tolerate surgery.
- Older adult patients are at greater surgical risk because of the physiological changes associated with aging.
- All medications taken before surgery are automatically discontinued after surgery unless a health care provider reorders the drugs.
- Family members and significant others are important in assisting patients with physical limitations and in providing emotional support postoperatively.
- Preoperative assessment of vital signs and physical findings provides a baseline with which to compare postoperative assessment data.
- Primary responsibility for informed consent rests with the surgeon.
- Structured preoperative teaching positively influences postoperative recovery.

- In ambulatory surgery, nurses use the limited time available to assess, prepare, and educate patients for surgery.
- Nurses within the operating room focus on protecting the patient from potential harm.
- Postoperative assessment centers on the body systems most likely to be affected by surgery.
- Because a surgical patient's condition may change rapidly during recovery, monitor the patient's status at least every 15 minutes until stable.
- Postoperative nursing interventions focus on prevention of complications.
- The risk for postoperative complications increases when the patient does not become actively involved in recovery.
- From the time of admission the nurse plans for the surgical patient's discharge.

CRITICAL THINKING EXERCISES

As a perioperative nurse, you will care for Mr. Korloff throughout the surgical phases. Recall he is having a laparoscopic gallbladder surgery (cholecystectomy). This procedure will create four small puncture wounds in his right upper quadrant in order for the gallbladder to be removed. You will first care for him in the preoperative holding area.

1. In the preoperative holding area, you conduct an identification of Mr. Korloff. What elements of identification are essential for safety before his surgical procedure?
   a. Two identifiers checked against patient verbal identification, patient armband, and medical record
   b. Two identifiers checked against patient allergy band, surgical consent form, and medical record
   c. Surgical consent form and medical record
   d. Patient name checked against patient armband and allergy band

2. You instruct Mr. Korloff in the use of the incentive spirometer. Considering his history and the type of surgery he is having, describe factors that will influence his ability to use the spirometer postoperatively.

3. On arrival to the PACU, the patient has an oral airway in place. You suction the mucus accumulating in his mouth and in the airway. His respirations are even at a rate of 12 per minute. What nursing diagnosis best relates to the need for an oral airway?
   a. *Ineffective breathing pattern*
   b. *Risk for aspiration*
   c. *Impaired gas exchange*
   d. *Ineffective airway clearance*

Mr. Korloff returns to the surgical unit after an uneventful stay in the PACU.

4. Six hours after he has returned from surgery, you notice that one of Mr. Korloff's dressings has a 3-cm area of serosanguineous drainage on it. What nursing interventions should you take at this time? Select all that apply.
   a. Hold pressure over the incision for 30 minutes.
   b. Notify the surgeon about the bleeding.
   c. Assess Mr. Korloff's vital signs.
   d. Reinforce the dressing with gauze pads.
   e. Remove the dressing, and assess for bleeding.

5. No further bleeding is noted on his dressing. Mr. Korloff is to ambulate and sit in the chair tonight for the first time. What is a priority nursing intervention to perform related to his activity?
   a. Administer oral pain medication 30 minutes before getting him up.
   b. Use a Hoyer lift to transfer him from the bed to the chair.
   c. Have Mr. Korloff pivot on his right foot when moving.
   d. Instruct him to rest 30 minutes before getting up.

evolve *Answers to Critical Thinking Questions can be found on the Evolve website.*

REVIEW QUESTIONS

1. A priority nursing intervention to prevent respiratory complications after surgery in older adults is:
   1. Ambulate the patient every 2 hours
   2. Monitor intake and output every shift
   3. Increase fluid intake during the first 24 hours
   4. Encourage the patient to turn, deep breathe, and cough frequently

2. You must ask each patient preoperatively for the name and dose of all prescription and over-the-counter medications taken before surgery because they:
   1. May cause allergies to develop
   2. May interact with anesthetic agents
   3. Will need to be held for 1 week after surgery
   4. Should be taken the morning of surgery with sips of water

3. A patient with a prothrombin time (PT) or an activated partial thromboplastin time (APTT) greater than normal might develop what clinical sign?
   1. Shortness of breath
   2. Reduced urine output
   3. Reduced oxygen saturation
   4. Bleeding on the operative dressing

4. You review the laboratory results of the patient you are preparing for surgery. Which laboratory value interacts with anesthesia to increase the risk for cardiac dysrhythmias?
   1. Hematocrit 44%
   2. Potassium 3.1 mEq/L
   3. Serum creatinine 0.9 mg/dL
   4. Platelet count 184,000/mm^3

5. You are checking your patient 2 hours after he returns from surgery. Which assessment finding requires immediate attention?
   1. Skin is pale, cool, and dry.
   2. Nasogastric tube drained 50 mL of green drainage.
   3. Foley catheter drained 30 mL of urine for past 2 hours.
   4. Patient is drowsy but responds promptly to nurse's voice.

6. Which factor contributes to the risk for poor wound healing in patients who are obese?
   1. Delay in the resumption of activity.
   2. Decrease in ventilatory capacity.
   3. Delay in intestinal peristalsis.
   4. Fatty tissue has a poor blood supply.

7. Which statement made by the patient having hernia surgery indicates a need for further teaching?
   1. "I'll use a clean disposable razor to shave the hair on my stomach before surgery."
   2. "I will not eat or drink anything after midnight."
   3. "I'll splint my incision with a pillow before I cough to lessen my pain."
   4. "I'll have my wife bring me to the hospital 2 hours before my surgery."

8. In the PACU you note that the patient is having difficulty breathing. You would first:
   1. Suction the pharynx and bronchial tree of secretions to prevent aspiration
   2. Give oxygen through a mask at 10 L/min to prevent decreased tissue perfusion
   3. Ask the patient to use an incentive spirometer to prevent atelectasis
   4. Position the patient so that the tongue falls forward to prevent an airway obstruction

9. Which nursing intervention is **most** effective to prevent the postoperative complication of deep vein thrombosis?
   1. Early ambulation
   2. Use of inspirometer
   3. Turning every 2 hours
   4. Frequent coughing exercises

10. Six hours after abdominal surgery your older adult surgical patient is disoriented to place and time. Considering causative factors for the disorientation, which intervention would you provide?
   1. Further assess patient's pain, and provide pain medication.
   2. Elevate legs, and maintain bed rest.
   3. Provide a sleeping pill at bedtime.
   4. Monitor for bowel sounds and passing of flatus.

Answers to Review Questions can be found on pages 1197-1198.

REFERENCES

Amato-Vealey BJ, Barba MP, Vealey RJ: Hand off communication: a requisite for perioperative patient safety, *AORN J* 88(5):763, 2008.

American Society of Anesthesiologists: Practice guidelines for sedation and analgesia by nonanesthesiologists, *Anesthesiology* 96:1004, 2002.

American Society of Anesthesiologists: *Distinguishing monitored anesthesia care from moderate sedation/analgesia (conscious sedation)*, 2004, http://www.asahq.org/publicationsAndservices/standards/35.htm.

American Society of Anesthesiologists: Practice guidelines for the perioperative management of patients with obstructive sleep apnea: a report by the American Society of Anesthesiologists Task Force on Perioperative Management of Patients With Obstructive Sleep Apnea, *Anesthesiology* 104:1081, 2006.

American Society of Anesthesiologists Task Force on Perioperative Fast: Practice guidelines for preoperative fasting and the use of pharmacologic agents to reduce the risk of pulmonary aspiration: application to healthy patients undergoing elective procedures, *Anesthesiology* 90(3):896, 1999.

Association of periOperative Registered Nurses: *Perioperative Standards and Recommended practices*, Denver, 2009, The Association.

Bernier MR and others: Preoperative teaching received and valued in a day surgery setting, *AORN J* 77(3):563, 2003.

Black JM, Hawks JH: *Medical-surgical nursing: clinical management for positive outcomes*, ed 7, St. Louis, 2005, Saunders.

Blouin MB, Magro S: How to handle the risks of obstructive sleep apnea, *Outpatient Surgery*, December 2005.

Bulechek GM and others, editors: *Nursing interventions classification (NIC)*, ed 5, St. Louis, 2008, Mosby.

Cullum N and others: Pressure sores, *Clin Evid* June (11):2565, 2004.

Fink JB: Forced expiratory technique, directed cough and autogenic drainage, *Respir Care* 52(9):1210, 2007.

Giger JN, Davidhizar RE: *Transcultural nursing: assessment and intervention*, ed 4, St. Louis, 2004, Mosby.

Gupta A: and others. Postoperative analgesia after radical retropubic prostatectomy a double-blind comparison between low thoracic epidural and patient-controlled intravenous analgesia, *Anesthesiology* 105(4):784, 2006.

Heikkinen K and others: Ambulatory orthopaedic surgery patients' knowledge expectations and perceptions of received knowledge, *J Adv Nurs* 60(3):270, 2007.

Jarvis C: *Physical examination and health assessment*, ed 5, St. Louis, 2008, Saunders.

Kaw R, Stoller JK: Pulmonary complications after noncardiac surgery: a review of their frequency and prevention strategies, *Clin Pulm Med* 15(1):18, 2008.

Lewis C and others: Patient knowledge, behavior and satisfaction with the use of a preoperative DVD, *Orthop Nurs* 21(6):41, 2002.

Lewis S and others: *Medical-surgical nursing: assessment and management of clinical problems*, ed 7, St. Louis, 2007, Mosby.

Lowdermilk D, Perry SE: *Maternity and women's health care*, ed 9, St. Louis, 2007, Mosby.

Madsen D and others: Listening to bowel sounds: an evidence-based practice project, *Am J Nurs* 105(12):40, 2005.

McKenry LM, Salerno E: *Mosby's pharmacology in nursing*, ed 21, St. Louis, 2003, Mosby.

Moorhead S and others, editors: *Nursing outcomes classification (NOC)*, ed 4, St. Louis, 2008, Mosby.

Mordiffi SZ and others: Information provided to surgical patients versus information needed, *AORN J* 77(3):546, 2003.

O'Conner-Von S: Preparation of adolescents for outpatient surgery: using an Internet program, *AORN J* 87(2):374, 2008.

Pagana KD, Pagana TJ: *Mosby's diagnostic and laboratory test reference*, ed 9, St. Louis, 2009, Mosby.

Patel KL: Impact of tight glucose control on postoperative infection rates and wound healing in cardiac surgery patients, *J Wound Ostomy Continence Nurs* 35(4):397, 2008.

Phillips N: *Berry and Kohn's operating room technique*, ed 10, St. Louis, 2004, Mosby.

Prouty A and others: Multidisciplinary patient education for total joint replacement surgery, *Orthop Nurs* 25(4):257, 2006.

Pruitt B: Help your patient combat postoperative atelectasis, *Nursing* 36(5):64, 2006.

Ramos M and others: Relationship of perioperative hyperglycemia and postoperative infections in patients who undergo general and vascular surgery, *Ann Surg* 248(4):585, 2008.

Rothrock J: *Alexander's care of the patient in surgery*, ed 13, St. Louis, 2007, Mosby.

Scales BA, Master R: Screening high-risk patients for the ambulatory setting, *J Perianesth Nurs* 18(5):307, 2003.

Schoonhoven L and others: Risk indicators for pressure ulcers during surgery, *Appl Nurs Res* 15(3):163, 2002.

Swan BA: Preparing older patients for ambulatory surgery, *OR Nurse* 2(2):40, 2008.

Taqi A and others: Thoracic epidural analgesia facilitates the restoration of bowel function and dietary intake in patients undergoing laparoscopic colon resection using a traditional, nonaccelerated, perioperative care program, *Surg Endosc* 21(2):247, 2007.

The Joint Commission: *National 2009 National patient safety goals*, 2009, http://www.jointcommission.org.

Warner DO: Helping surgical patients quit smoking: why, when, how, *Anesth Analg* 101(2):481, 2005.

Wu CL and others: Efficacy of postoperative patient-controlled and continuous infusion epidural analgesia versus intravenous patient-controlled analgesia with opioids: a meta-analysis, *Anesthesiology* 103(5):109, 2005.

Glossary

abduction Movement of a limb away from the body.

abrasion Scraping or rubbing away of epidermis; may result in localized bleeding and later weeping of serous fluid.

absorption Passage of drug molecules into the blood. Factors influencing drug absorption include route of administration, ability of the drug to dissolve, and conditions at the site of absorption.

acceptance Fifth stage of Kübler-Ross's stages of grief and dying. An individual comes to terms with a loss rather than submitting to resignation and hopelessness.

accessory muscles Muscles in the thoracic cage that assist with respiration.

accommodation Process of responding to the environment through new activity and thinking and changing the existing schema or developing a new schema to deal with the new information. For example, a toddler whose parent consistently corrected him when he called a horse a "doggie" accommodates and forms a new schema for horses.

accountability State of being answerable for one's actions—a nurse answers to himself or herself, the patient, the profession, the employing institution such as a hospital, and society for the effectiveness of nursing care performed.

accreditation Process whereby a professional association or nongovernmental agency grants recognition to a school or institution for demonstrated ability to meet predetermined criteria.

acculturation The process of adapting to and adopting a new culture.

acne Inflammatory, papulopustular skin eruption, usually occurring on the face, neck, shoulders, and upper back.

acromegaly Chronic metabolic condition caused by overproduction of growth hormone and characterized by gradual, marked enlargement and elongation of bones of the face, jaw, and extremities.

active listening Listening attentively with the whole person—mind, body, and spirit. It includes listening for main and supportive ideas, acknowledging and responding, giving appropriate feedback, and paying attention to the other person's total communication, including the content, the intent, and the feelings expressed.

active range-of-motion (ROM) exercise Completion of exercise to the joint by the patient while doing activities of daily living or during joint assessment.

active strategies of health promotion Activities that depend on the patient's being motivated to adopt a specific health program.

active transport Movement of materials across the cell membrane by means of chemical activity that allows the cell to admit larger molecules than would otherwise be possible.

activities of daily living (ADLs) Activities usually performed in the course of a normal day in the patient's life, such as eating, dressing, bathing, brushing the teeth, or grooming.

activity tolerance Kind or amount of exercise or work a person is able to perform.

actual loss Loss of an object, person, body part or function, or emotion that is overt and easily identifiable.

actual nursing diagnosis A judgment that is clinically validated by the presence of major defining characteristics.

acuity recording Mechanism by which entries describing patient care activities are made over a 24-hour period. The activities are then translated into a rating score, or acuity score, that allows for a comparison of patients who vary by severity of illness.

acute care Pattern of health care in which a patient is treated for an acute episode of illness, for the sequelae of an accident or other trauma, or during recovery from surgery.

acute illness Illness characterized by symptoms that are of relatively short duration, are usually severe, and affect the functioning of the patient in all dimensions.

adduction Movement of a limb toward the body.

adolescence The period in development between the onset of puberty and adulthood. It usually begins between 11 and 13 years of age.

adult day care centers Facility for the supervised care of older adults, providing activities such as meals and socialization during specified day hours.

advanced sleep phase syndrome Common in older adults, a disturbance in sleep manifested as early waking in the morning with an inability to get back to sleep. It is thought that this syndrome is caused by advancing of the body's circadian rhythm.

adventitious sounds Abnormal lung sounds heard with auscultation.

adverse effect Harmful or unintended effect of a medication, diagnostic test, or therapeutic intervention.

adverse reaction Any harmful, unintended effect of a medication, diagnostic test, or therapeutic intervention.

advocacy Process whereby a nurse objectively provides patients with the information they need to make decisions and supports the patients in whatever decisions they make.

afebrile Without fever.

affective learning Acquisition of behaviors involved in expressing feelings in attitudes, appreciation, and values.

afterload Resistance to left ventricular ejection; the work the heart must overcome to fully eject blood from the left ventricle.

age-related macular degeneration Progressive disorder in which the macula (the specialized portion of the retina responsible for central vision) degenerates as a result of aging and loses its ability to function efficiently. First signs include blurring of reading matter, distortion or loss of central vision, sensitivity to glare, and distortion of objects.

agnostic Individual who believes that any ultimate reality is unknown or unknowable.

airborne precautions Safeguards designed to reduce the risk of transmission of infectious agents through the air a person breathes.

alarm reaction Mobilization of the defense mechanisms of the body and mind to cope with a stressor. The initial stage of the general adaptation syndrome.

aldosterone Mineralocorticoid steroid hormone produced by the adrenal cortex with action in the renal tubule to regulate sodium and potassium balance in the blood.

allergic reactions Unfavorable physiological response to an allergen to which a person has previously been exposed and to which the person has developed antibodies.

alopecia Partial or complete loss of hair; baldness.

Alzheimer's disease Disease of the brain parenchyma that causes a gradual and progressive decline in cognitive functioning.

AMBULARM Device used for the patient who climbs out of bed unassisted and is in danger of falling. This device is worn on the leg and signals when the leg is in a dependent position such as over the side rail or on the floor.

amino acid Organic compound of one or more basic groups and one or more carboxyl groups. Amino acids are the building blocks that construct proteins and the end products of protein digestion.

anabolism Constructive metabolism characterized by conversion of simple substances into more complex compounds of living matter.

analgesic Relieving pain; drug that relieves pain.

analogies Resemblances made between things otherwise unlike.

anaphylactic reactions (Chapter 14) Hypersensitive condition induced by contact with certain antigens.

aneurysm (Chapter 13) Localized dilations of the wall of a blood vessel, usually caused by atherosclerosis, hypertension, or a congenital weakness in a vessel wall.

anger Second stage of Kübler-Ross's stages of grief and dying. During this stage an individual resists loss by expressing extreme displeasure, indignation, or hostility.

angiotensin Polypeptide occurring in the blood, causing vasoconstriction, increased blood pressure, and the release of aldosterone from the adrenal cortex.

anion gap Difference between the concentrations of serum cations and anions, determined by measuring the concentrations of sodium cations and chloride and bicarbonate anions.

anions Negatively charged electrolytes.

anthropometric measurements Body measures of height, weight, and skinfolds to evaluate muscle atrophy.

anthropometry Measurement of various body parts to determine nutritional and caloric status, muscular development, brain growth, and other parameters.

antibodies Immunoglobulins, essential to the immune system, that are produced by lymphoid tissue in response to bacteria, viruses, or other antigens.

anticipatory grief Grief response in which the person begins the grieving process before an actual loss.

antidiuretic hormone (ADH) Hormone that decreases the production of urine by increasing the reabsorption of water by the renal tubules. ADH is secreted by cells of the hypothalamus and stored in the posterior lobe of the pituitary gland.

antiembolic stockings Elasticized stockings that prevent formation of emboli and thrombi, especially after surgery or during bed rest.

antigen Substance, usually a protein, that causes the formation of an antibody and reacts specifically with that antibody.

antipyretic Substance or procedure that reduces fever.

anxiolytics Drugs used primarily to treat episodes of anxiety.

aphasia Abnormal neurological condition in which language function is defective or absent; related to injury to speech center in cerebral cortex, causing receptive or expressive aphasia.

apical pulse Heartbeat as listened to with the bell or diaphragm of a stethoscope placed on the apex of the heart.

apnea Cessation of airflow through the nose and mouth.

apothecary system System of measurement. The basic unit of weight is a grain. Weights derived from the grain are the gram, ounce, and pound. The basic measure for fluid is the minim. The fluidram, fluid ounce, pint, quart, and gallon are measures derived from the minim.

approximate To come close together, as in the edges of a wound.

arcus senilis Opaque ring, gray to white in color, that surrounds the periphery of the cornea. The condition is caused by deposits of fat granules in the cornea. Occurs primarily in older adults.

asepsis Absence of germs or microorganisms.

aseptic technique Any health care procedure in which added precautions are used to prevent contamination of a person, object, or area by microorganisms.

assault Unlawful threat to bring about harmful or offensive contact with another.

assertive communication Type of communication based on a philosophy of protecting individual rights and responsibilities. It includes the ability to be self-directive in acting to accomplish goals and advocate for others.

assessment First step of the nursing process; activities required in the first step are data collection, data validation, data sorting, and data documentation. The purpose is to gather information for health problem identification.

assimilation To become absorbed into another culture and to adopt its characteristics.

assisted living Residential living facilities in which each resident has his or her own room and shares dining and social activity areas.

associative play Form of play in which a group of children participates in similar or identical activities without formal organization, direction, interaction, or goals.

atelectasis Collapse of alveoli, preventing the normal respiratory exchange of oxygen and carbon dioxide.

atheist Individual who does not believe in the existence of God.

atherosclerosis Common arterial disorder characterized by yellowish plaques of cholesterol, lipids, and cellular debris in the inner layers of the walls of the large- and medium-size arteries.

atrioventricular (AV) node A portion of the cardiac conduction system located on the floor of the right atrium; it receives electrical impulses from the atrium and transmits them to the bundle of His.

atrophied Wasted or reduced size or physiological activity of a part of the body caused by disease or other influences.

attachment Initial psychosocial relationship that develops between parents and the neonate.

attentional set Internal state of the learner that allows focusing and comprehension.

auditory Related to, or experienced through, hearing.

auscultation Method of physical examination; listening to the sounds produced by the body, usually with a stethoscope.

auscultatory gap (Chapter 12) Disappearance of sound when obtaining a blood pressure; typically occurs between the first and second Korotkoff sounds.

authority The right to act in areas in which an individual has been given and accepts responsibility.

autologous transfusion Procedure in which blood is removed from a donor and stored for a variable period before it is returned to the donor's own circulation.

autonomy Ability or tendency to function independently.

back-channeling Active listening technique that prompts a respondent to continue telling a story or describing a situation. Involves use of phrases such as "Go on," "Uh huh," and "Tell me more."

bacteriuria Presence of bacteria in the urine.

balance Position when the person's center of gravity is correctly positioned so that falling does not occur.

bandages Available in rolls of various widths and materials including gauze, elasticized knit, elastic webbing, flannel, and muslin. Gauze bandages are lightweight and inexpensive, mold easily around contours of the body, and permit air circulation to underlying skin to prevent maceration. Elastic bandages conform well to body parts but can also be used to exert pressure over a body part.

bargaining Third stage of Kübler-Ross's stages of grief and dying. A person postpones the reality of a loss by attempting to make deals in a subtle or overt manner with others or with a higher being.

baridi A condition among the Bena people of Tanzania, this illness is attributed to disrespectful behavior within the family or transgression of cultural taboos. The person experiences physical and psychological symptoms and is usually treated by a traditional healer, who has the person make a public admission or an apology or who treats the person with herbal remedies.

basal cell carcinoma Malignant epithelial cell tumor that begins as a papule and enlarges peripherally, developing a central crater that erodes, crusts, and bleeds. Metastasis is rare.

basal metabolic rate (BMR) Amount of energy used in a unit of time by a fasting, resting subject to maintain vital functions.

battery Legal term for touching of another's body without consent.

bed boards Boards placed under the mattress of a bed that provide extra support to the mattress surface.

bed rest Placement of the patient in bed for therapeutic reasons for a prescribed period.

benchmarking Identifying best practices and comparing them to the organization's current practices for the purpose of improving performance. This process helps to support the institution's claims of quality care delivery.

beneficence Doing good or active promotion of doing good. One of the four principles of the ethical theory of deontology.

benign breast disease (fibrocystic) A benign condition characterized by lumpy, painful breasts and sometimes nipple discharge. Symptoms are more apparent before the menstrual period. Known to be a risk factor for breast cancer.

bereavement Response to loss through death; a subjective experience that a person suffers after losing a person with whom there has been a significant relationship.

biases and prejudices Beliefs and attitudes associating negative permanent characteristics to people who are perceived as different from oneself.

bilineally Kinship that extends to both the mother's and father's sides of the family.

binders Bandages made of large pieces of material to fit specific body parts.

bioethics Branch of ethics within the field of health care.

biological clock Cyclical nature of body functions; functions controlled from within the body are synchronized with environmental factors; same meaning as biorhythm.

biotransformation The chemical changes that a substance undergoes in the body, such as by the action of enzymes.

blanchable hyperemia Redness of the skin due to dilation of the superficial capillaries. When pressure is applied to the skin, the area blanches, or turns a lighter color.

body image Persons' subjective concept of their physical appearance.

body mechanics Coordinated efforts of the musculoskeletal and nervous systems to maintain proper balance, posture, and body alignment.

bone resorption Destruction of bone cells and release of calcium into the blood.

borborygmi Audible abdominal sounds produced by hyperactive intestinal peristalsis.

botanica Place that sells religious and herbal remedies.

bradycardia Slower-than-normal heart rate; heart contracts fewer than 60 times per minute.

bradypnea Abnormally slow rate of breathing.

bronchospasm An excessive and prolonged contraction of the smooth muscle of the bronchi and bronchioles resulting in an acute narrowing and obstruction of the respiratory airway.

bruit Abnormal sound or murmur heard while auscultating an organ, gland, or artery.

buccal Of or pertaining to the inside of the cheek or the gum next to the cheek.

buccal cavity Consists of the lips surrounding the opening of the mouth, the cheeks running along the side walls of the cavity, the tongue and its muscles, and the hard and soft palate.

buffer (Chapter 15) Substance or group of substances that can absorb or release hydrogen ions to correct an acid-base imbalance.

bundle of His A portion of the cardiac conduction system that arises from the distal portion of the atrioventricular (AV) node and extends across the AV groove to the top of the intraventricular septum, where it divides into right and left bundle branches.

cachexia Malnutrition marked by weakness and emaciation, usually associated with severe illness.

capitation Payment mechanism in which a provider (e.g., health care network) receives a fixed amount of payment per enrollee.

carbohydrates Dietary classification of foods comprising sugars, starches, cellulose, and gum.

carbon monoxide Colorless, odorless, poisonous gas produced by the combustion of carbon or organic fuels.

cardiac index The adequacy of the cardiac output for an individual. It takes into account the body surface area (BSA) of the patient.

cardiac output (CO) Volume of blood expelled by the ventricles of the heart, equal to the amount of blood ejected at each beat, multiplied by the number of beats in the period

of time used for computation (usually 1 minute).

cardiopulmonary rehabilitation Actively assisting the patient with achieving and maintaining an optimal level of health through controlled physical exercise, nutrition counseling, relaxation and stress management techniques, prescribed medications and oxygen, and compliance.

cardiopulmonary resuscitation (CPR) Basic emergency procedures for life support consisting of artificial respiration and manual external cardiac massage.

care To feel concern or interest in one who has sorrow or difficulties.

caring Universal phenomenon that influences the way we think, feel, and behave in relation to one another.

carriers Persons or animals who harbor and spread an organism that causes disease in others but do not become ill.

case management Organized system for delivering health care to an individual patient or group of patients across an episode of illness and/or a continuum of care; includes assessment and development of a plan of care, coordination of all services, referral, and followup; usually assigned to one professional.

case management plan A multidisciplinary model for documenting patient care that usually includes plans for problems, key interventions, and expected outcomes for patients with a specific disease or condition.

catabolism Breakdown of body tissue into simpler substances.

cataplexy Condition characterized by sudden muscular weakness and loss of muscle tone.

cataracts An abnormal progressive condition of the lens of the eye characterized by loss of transparency.

cathartics Drugs that act to promote bowel evacuation.

catheterization Introduction of a catheter into a body cavity or organ to inject or remove fluid.

cations Positively charged electrolytes.

center of gravity Midpoint or center of the weight of a body or object.

centigrade Denotes temperature scale in which 0° is the freezing point of water and 100° is the boiling point of water at sea level; also called Celsius.

cerumen Yellowish or brownish waxy secretion produced by sweat glands in the external ear.

chancres Skin lesions or venereal sores (usually primary syphilis) that begin at the site of infection as papules and develop into red, bloodless, painless ulcers with a scooped-out appearance.

change-of-shift report Report that occurs between two scheduled nursing work shifts. Nurses communicate information about their assigned patients to nurses working on the next shift of duty.

channel Method used in the teaching-learning process to present content: visual, auditory, taste, smell. In the communication process, a

method used to transmit a message: visual, auditory, touch.

charting by exception (CBE) Charting methodology in which data are entered only when there is an exception from what is normal or expected. Reduces time spent documenting in charting. It is a shorthand method for documenting normal findings and routine care.

chest percussion Striking of the chest wall with a cupped hand to promote mobilization and drainage of pulmonary secretions.

chest physiotherapy (CPT) Group of therapies used to mobilize pulmonary secretions for expectoration.

chest tube A catheter inserted through the thorax into the chest cavity for removing air or fluid, used after chest or heart surgery or pneumothorax.

chronic illness Illness that persists over a long time and affects physical, emotional, intellectual, social, and spiritual functioning.

circadian rhythm Repetition of certain physiological phenomena within a 24-hour cycle.

circulating nurse Assistant to the scrub nurse and surgeon whose role is to provide necessary supplies, dispose of soiled instruments and supplies, and keep an accurate count of instruments, needles, and sponges used.

civil law Statutes concerned with protecting a person's rights.

climacteric Physiological, developmental change that occurs in the male reproductive system between the ages of 45 and 60.

clinical criteria Objective or subjective signs and symptoms, clusters of signs and symptoms, or risk factors.

clinical decision making A problem-solving approach that nurses use to define patient problems and select appropriate treatment.

closed-ended question A form of question that limits a respondent's answer to one or two words.

clubbing Bulging of the tissues at the nail base that is caused by insufficient oxygenation at the periphery, resulting from conditions such as chronic emphysema and congenital heart disease.

code of ethics Formal statement that delineates a profession's guidelines for ethical behavior; a code of ethics sets standards or expectations for the professional to achieve.

cognitive learning Acquisition of intellectual skills that encompass behaviors such as thinking, understanding, and evaluating.

collaborative interventions Therapies that require the knowledge, skill, and expertise of multiple health care professionals.

collaborative problem Physiological complication that require the nurse to use nursing-prescribed and physician-prescribed interventions to maximize patient outcomes.

colloid osmotic pressure Abnormal condition of the kidney caused by the pressure of concentrations of large particles, such as protein molecules, that will pass through a membrane.

colon Portion of the large intestine from the cecum to the rectum.

colonization The presence and multiplication of microorganisms without tissue invasion or damage.

comforting Acts toward another individual that display both an emotional and physical calm. The use of touch, establishing presence, the therapeutic use of silence, and the skillful and gentle performance of a procedure are examples of comforting nursing measures.

common law One source for law that is created by judicial decisions as opposed to those created by legislative bodies (statutory law).

communicable disease Any disease that can be transmitted from one person or animal to another by direct or indirect contact or by vectors.

communication Ongoing, dynamic series of events that involves the transmission of meaning from sender to receiver.

community health nursing A nursing approach that combines knowledge from the public health sciences with professional nursing theories to safeguard and improve the health of populations in the community.

community-based nursing The acute and chronic care of individuals and families to strengthen their capacity for self-care and promote independence in decision making.

competence Specific range of skills necessary to perform a task.

complete bed bath Bath in which the entire body of a patient is washed in bed.

compress Soft pad of gauze or cloth used to apply heat, cold, or medications to the surface of a body part.

computer-based patient record (CBCR) Comprehensive computerized system used by all health care practitioners to permanently store information pertaining to a patient's health status, clinical problems, and functional abilities.

concentration Relative content of a component within a substance or solution.

concentration gradient Gradient that exists across a membrane separating a high concentration of a particular ion from a low concentration of the same ion.

concept map A care-planning tool that assists in critical thinking and forming associations between a patient's nursing diagnoses and interventions.

confianza Trust.

confidentiality The act of keeping information private or secret; in health care, the nurse only shares information about a patient with other nurses or health care providers who need to know private information about a patient in order to provide care for the patient; information can only be shared with the patient's consent.

conjunctivitis Highly contagious eye infection. The crusty drainage that collects on eyelid margins can easily spread from one eye to the other.

connectedness Having close spiritual relationships with oneself, others, and God or another spiritual being.

connotative meaning The shade or interpretation of a word's meaning influenced by the thoughts, feelings, or ideas people have about the word.

conscious sedation Administration of central nervous system depressant drugs and/or analgesics to provide analgesia, relieve anxiety, and/or provide amnesia during surgical, diagnostic, or interventional procedures.

constipation Condition characterized by difficulty in passing stool or an infrequent passage of hard stool.

consultation Process in which the help of a specialist is sought to identify ways to handle problems in patient management or in the planning and implementing of programs.

contact precautions Safeguards designed to reduce the risk of transmission of epidemiologically important microorganisms by direct or indirect contact.

continent urinary diversion (CUR) Surgical diversion of the drainage of urine from a diseased or dysfunctional bladder. Patient uses a catheter to drain the pouch.

convalescence Period of recovery after an illness, injury, or surgery.

coping Making an effort to manage psychological stress.

core temperature Temperature of deep structures of the body.

cough Sudden, audible expulsion of air from the lungs. The person breathes in, the glottis is partially closed, and the accessory muscles of expiration contract to expel the air forcibly.

counseling A problem-solving method used to help patients recognize and manage stress and to enhance interpersonal relationships; it helps patients examine alternatives and decide which choices are most helpful and appropriate.

crackles Fine bubbling sounds heard on auscultation of the lung; produced by air entering distal airways and alveoli, which contain serous secretions.

crime Act that violates a law and that may include criminal intent.

criminal law Concerned with acts that threaten society but may involve only an individual.

crisis Transition for better or worse in the course of a disease, usually indicated by a marked change in the intensity of signs and symptoms.

crisis intervention Use of therapeutic techniques directed toward helping a patient resolve a particular and immediate problem.

critical pathways Tools used in managed care that incorporate the treatment interventions of caregivers from all disciplines who normally care for a patient. Designed for a specific care type, a pathway is used to manage the care of a patient throughout a projected length of stay.

critical period of development A specific phase or period when the presence of a function or reasoning has its greatest effect on a specific aspect of development.

critical thinking The active, purposeful, organized, cognitive process used to carefully examine one's thinking and the thinking of other individuals.

crutch gait A gait achieved by a person using crutches.

cue Information that a nurse acquires through hearing, visual observations, touch, and smell.

cultural and linguistic competence A set of congruent behaviors, attitudes, and policies that come together in a system, agency, or among professionals that enables effective work in cross-cultural situations.

cultural assessment A systematic and comprehensive examination of the cultural care values, beliefs, and practices of individuals, families, and communities.

cultural awareness Gaining in-depth awareness of one's own background, stereotypes, biases, prejudices, and assumptions about other people.

cultural care accommodation or negotiation Adapting or negotiating with the patient/families to achieve beneficial or satisfying health outcomes.

cultural care preservation or maintenance Retaining and/or preserving relevant care values so that patients are able to maintain their well-being, recover from illness, or face handicaps and/or death.

cultural care repatterning or restructuring Reordering, changing, or greatly modifying a patient's/family's customs for new, different, and beneficial health care pattern.

cultural competence Process in which the health care professional continually strives to achieve the ability and availability to work effectively with individuals, families, and communities.

cultural encounters Engaging in cross-cultural interactions; refining intercultural communication skills; gaining in-depth understanding of others and avoiding stereotypes; and cultural conflict management.

cultural imposition Using one's own values and customs as an absolute guide in interpreting behaviors.

cultural knowledge Obtaining knowledge of other cultures; gaining sensitivity to, respect for, and appreciation of differences.

cultural pain The feeling a patient has after a health care worker disregards the patient's valued way of life.

cultural skills Communication, cultural assessment, and culturally competent care.

culturally congruent care Care that fits the people's valued life patterns and sets of meanings generated from the people themselves. Sometimes this differs from the professionals' perspective on care.

culturally ignorant or blind Uneducated about other cultures.

culture Integrated patterns of human behavior that include the language, thoughts, communications, actions, customs, beliefs, values, and institutions of racial, ethnic, religious, or social groups.

culture-bound syndromes Illnesses restricted to a particular culture or group because of its psychosocial characteristics.

culture care theory Leininger's theory that emphasizes culturally congruent care.

culturological nursing assessment A systematic and comprehensive examination of the cultural care values, beliefs, and practices of individuals, families, and communities.

cutaneous stimulation Stimulation of a person's skin to prevent or reduce pain perception. A massage, warm bath, hot and cold therapies, and transcutaneous electrical nerve stimulation are some ways to reduce pain perception.

cyanosis Bluish discoloration of the skin and mucous membranes caused by an excess of deoxygenated hemoglobin in the blood or a structural defect in the hemoglobin molecule.

DAR (data, action, patient response) The format used in focus charting for recording patient information.

data analysis Logical examination of and professional judgment about patient assessment data; used in the diagnostic process to derive a nursing diagnosis.

data cluster A set of signs or symptoms that are grouped together in logical order.

database Store or bank of information, especially in a form that can be processed by computer.

debridement Removal of dead tissue from a wound.

decentralized management An organizational philosophy that brings decisions down to the level of the staff. Individuals best informed about a problem or issue participate in the decision-making process.

decision making Process involving critical appraisal of information that results from recognition of a problem and ends with the generation, testing, and evaluation of a conclusion. Comes at the end of critical thinking.

defecation Passage of feces from the digestive tract through the rectum.

defendant Individual or organization against whom legal charges are brought in a court of law.

defining characteristics Related signs and symptoms or clusters of data that support the nursing diagnosis.

dehiscence Separation of a wound's edges, revealing underlying tissues.

dehydration Excessive loss of water from the body tissues, accompanied by a disturbance of body electrolytes.

delegation Process of assigning another member of the health care team to be responsible for aspects of patient care; for example, assigning nurse assistants to bathe a patient.

delirium An acute confusional state, which is potentially reversible and is often due to a physical cause.

dementia A generalized impairment of intellectual functioning that interferes with social and occupational functioning.

denial Unconscious refusal to admit an unacceptable idea.

denotative meaning Meaning of a word shared by individuals who use a common language. The word "baseball" has the same meaning for all individuals who speak English, but the word "code" denotes cardiac arrest primarily to health care providers.

dental caries Abnormal destructive condition in a tooth caused by a complex interaction of food, especially starches and sugars, with bacteria that form dental plaque.

deontology Traditional theory of ethics that proposes to define actions as right or wrong based on the characteristics of fidelity to promises, truthfulness, and justice. The conventional use of ethical terms such as *justice, autonomy, beneficence,* and *nonmaleficence* constitutes the practice of deontology.

depression (1) A reduction in happiness and well-being that contributes to physical and social limitations and complicates the treatment of concomitant medical conditions. It is usually reversible with treatment. (2) Fourth stage of Kübler-Ross's stages of grief and dying. In this stage the person realizes the full impact and significance of the loss.

dermis Sensitive vascular layer of the skin directly below the epidermis composed of collagenous and elastic fibrous connective tissues that give the dermis strength and elasticity.

determinants of health The many variables that influence the health status of individuals or communities.

detoxify To remove the toxic quality of a substance; the liver acts to detoxify chemicals in drug compounds.

development Qualitative or observable aspects of the progressive changes one makes in adapting to the environment.

developmental crises Crises associated with normal and expected phases of growth and development, for example, the response to menopause; same as maturational crises.

diabetic retinopathy A disorder of retinal blood vessels. Pathological changes secondary to increased pressure in the blood vessels of the retina result in decreased vision or vision loss due to hemorrhage and macular edema.

diagnosis-related group (DRG) Group of patients classified to establish a mechanism for health care reimbursement based on length of stay; classification is based on the following variables: primary and secondary diagnosis, comorbidities, primary and secondary procedures, and age.

diagnostic process Mental steps (data clustering and analysis, problem identification) that follow assessment and lead directly to the formulation of a diagnosis.

diagnostic reasoning Process that enables an observer to assign meaning and to classify phenomena in clinical situations by integrating observations and critical thinking.

diaphoresis Secretion of sweat, especially profuse secretion associated with an elevated body temperature, physical exertion, or emotional stress.

diaphragmatic breathing Respiration in which the abdomen moves out while the diaphragm descends on inspiration.

diarrhea Increase in the number of stools and the passage of liquid, unformed feces.

diastolic Pertaining to diastole, or the blood pressure at the instant of maximum cardiac relaxation.

dietary reference intake (DRI) Information on each vitamin or mineral to reflect a range of minimum to maximum amounts that avert deficiency or toxicity.

diffusion Movement of molecules from an area of high concentration to an area of lower concentration.

digestion Breakdown of nutrients by chewing, churning, mixing with fluid, and chemical reactions.

direct care interventions Treatments performed through interaction with the patient. For example, a patient may require medication administration, insertion of an intravenous infusion, or counseling during a time of grief.

discharge planning Activities directed toward identifying future proposed therapy and the need for additional resources before and after returning home.

discrimination Prejudicial outlook, action, or treatment.

disease Malfunctioning or maladaptation of biological or psychological processes.

disinfection Process of destroying all pathogenic organisms, except spores.

disorganization and despair One of Bowlby's four phases of mourning in which an individual endlessly examines how and why the loss occurred.

distress Damaging stress; one of the two types of stress identified by Selye.

disuse osteoporosis Reductions in skeletal mass routinely accompanying immobility or paralysis.

diuresis Increased rate of formation and excretion of urine.

documentation Written entry into the patient's medical record of all pertinent information about the patient. These entries validate the patient's problems and care and exist as a legal record.

dominant culture The customs, values, beliefs, traditions, and social and religious views held by a group of people that prevail over another secondary culture.

dorsiflexion Flexion toward the back.

drainage evacuators Convenient portable units that connect to tubular drains lying within a wound bed and exert a safe, constant, low-pressure vacuum to remove and collect drainage.

droplet precautions Safeguards designed to reduce the risk of droplet transmission of infectious agents.

dysmenorrhea Painful menstruation.

dysphagia Difficulty in swallowing, commonly associated with obstructive or motor disorders of the esophagus.

dyspnea Sensation of shortness of breath.

dysrhythmia Deviation from the normal pattern of the heartbeat.

dysuria Painful urination resulting from bacterial infection of the bladder and obstructive conditions of the urethra.

ecchymosis Discoloration of the skin or bruise caused by leakage of blood into subcutaneous tissues as a result of trauma to underlying tissues.

ectropion Eversion of the eyelid, exposing the conjunctival membrane and part of the eyeball.

edema Abnormal accumulation of fluid in interstitial spaces of tissues.

egocentric Developmental characteristic wherein a toddler is only able to assume the view of his or her own activities and needs.

electrocardiogram (ECG) Graphic record of the electrical activity of the myocardium.

electrolyte Element or compound that, when melted or dissolved in water or other solvent, dissociates into ions and can carry an electrical current.

electronic infusion device A piece of medical equipment that delivers intravenous fluids at a prescribed rate through an intravenous catheter.

embolism Abnormal condition in which a blood clot (embolus) travels through the bloodstream and becomes lodged in a blood vessel.

emic worldview An insider or native perspective.

empathy Understanding and acceptance of a person's feelings and the ability to sense the person's private world.

endogenous infections Infections produced within a cell or organism.

endorphins Hormones that act on the mind like morphine and opiates, producing a sense of well-being and reducing pain.

enema Procedure involving introduction of a solution into the rectum for cleansing or therapeutic purposes.

enteral nutrition (EN) Provision of nutrients through the gastrointestinal tract when the patient cannot ingest, chew, or swallow food but can digest and absorb nutrients.

entropion Condition in which the eyelid turns inward toward the eye.

environment All of the many factors, such as physical and psychological, that influence or affect the life and survival of a person.

epidermis Outer layer of the skin that has several thin layers of skin in different stages of maturation; shields and protects the underlying tissues from water loss, mechanical or chemical injury, and penetration by disease-causing microorganisms.

epidural infusion Type of nerve block anesthesia in which an anesthetic is intermittently or continuously injected into the lumbosacral region of the spinal cord.

erythema Redness or inflammation of the skin or mucous membranes that is a result of dilation and congestion of superficial capillaries; sunburn is an example.

eschar A thick layer of dead, dry tissue that covers a pressure ulcer or thermal burn; it may be allowed to be sloughed off naturally or it may need to be surgically removed.

ethical dilemma Dilemma existing when the right thing to do is not clear. Resolution requires the negotiation of differing values among those involved in the dilemma.

ethical principles Set of guidelines for a profession's expectations and standards of behavior for its members.

ethics Principles or standards that govern proper conduct.

ethics of care Delivery of health care based on ethical principles and standards of care.

ethnicity A shared identity related to social and cultural heritage such as values, language, geographical space, and racial characteristics.

ethnocentrism A tendency to hold one's own way of life as superior to others.

ethnohistory Significant historical experiences of a particular group.

etic worldview An outsider's perspective.

etiology Study of all factors that may be involved in the development of a disease.

eupnea Normal respirations that are quiet, effortless, and rhythmical.

eustress Stress that protects health; one of the two types of stress identified by Selye.

evaluation Determination of the extent to which established patient goals have been achieved.

evidence-based knowledge Knowledge that is derived from the integration of best research, clinical expertise, and patient values.

evidence-based practice The use of current best evidence from nursing research, clinical expertise, practice trends, and patient preferences to guide nursing decisions about care provided to patients.

evisceration Protrusion of visceral organs through a surgical wound.

exacerbations Increases in the seriousness of a disease or disorder as marked by greater intensity in signs or symptoms.

excessive daytime sleepiness Extreme fatigue felt during the day. Signs of this include falling asleep at inappropriate times, such as while eating, talking, or driving. May indicate a sleep disorder.

excoriation Injury to the skin's surface caused by abrasion.

exhaustion stage Phase that occurs when the body can no longer resist the stress; when the energy necessary to maintain adaptation is depleted.

exogenous infection Infection originating outside an organ or part.

exostosis An abnormal benign growth on the surface of a bone.

expected outcomes Expected conditions of a patient at the end of therapy or of a disease process, including the degree of wellness and the need for continuing care, medications, support, counseling, or education.

extended care facility An institution devoted to providing medical, nursing, or custodial care for an individual over a prolonged period, such as during the course of a chronic disease or during the rehabilitation phase after an acute illness.

extension Movement by certain joints that increases the angle between two adjoining bones.

extracellular fluid (ECF) Portion of body fluids composed of the interstitial fluid and blood plasma.

exudate Fluid, cells, or other substances that have been slowly discharged from cells or blood vessels through small pores or breaks in cell membranes.

face-saving A way of speaking or acting that preserves dignity.

Fahrenheit Denotes temperature scale in which 32° is the freezing point of water and 212° is the boiling point of water at sea level.

faith Set of beliefs and a way of relating to self, others, and a supreme being.

fajita Cotton binder used on a newborn's abdomen among Hispanics and Filipinos to prevent gas and umbilical hernia.

family Group of interacting individuals composing a basic unit of society.

family as context Nursing perspective in which the family is viewed as a unit of interacting members having attributes, functions, and goals separate from those of the individual family members.

family diversity The unique needs and characteristics of each member in a family.

family durability A system of support for a family that includes immediate and extended family members.

family forms Patterns of people considered by family members to be included in the family.

family functioning Processes families use to achieve their goals.

family hardiness Internal strengths and durability of the family unit; characterized by a sense of control over the outcome of life events and hardships, a view of change as beneficial and growth-producing, and an active rather than passive orientation in responding to stressful life events.

family health Determined by the effectiveness of the family's structure, the processes that the family uses to meet its goals, and internal and external forces.

family as patient A nursing approach that takes into consideration the effect of one intervention on all members of a family.

family resiliency A family's ability to cope with expected and unexpected stressors.

family structure Based on organization (i.e., ongoing membership) of the family and the pattern of relationships.

farmacia Place to obtain prescribed medications.

febrile Pertaining to or characterized by an elevated body temperature.

fecal impaction Accumulation of hardened fecal material in the rectum or sigmoid colon.

fecal incontinence Inability to control passage of feces and gas from the anus.

fecal occult blood test (FOBT) Measures microscopic amounts of blood in the feces.

feces Waste or excrement from the gastrointestinal tract.

feedback Process in which the output of a given system is returned to the system.

felony Crime of a serious nature that carries a penalty of imprisonment or death.

feminist ethics Ethical approach that focuses on relationships of those involved in an ethical dilemma rather than traditional abstract principles of deontology.

fever Elevation in the hypothalamic set point, so that body temperature is regulated at a higher level.

fictive Nonblood kin; considered family in some collective cultures.

fidelity The agreement to keep a promise.

fight-or-flight response The total physiological response to stress that occurs during the alarm reaction stage of the general adaptation syndrome. Massive changes in all body systems prepare a human being to choose to flee or to remain and fight the stressor.

filtration The straining of fluid through a membrane.

fistula Abnormal passage from an internal organ to the body surface or between two internal organs.

flashback A recollection so strong that the individual thinks he or she is actually experiencing the trauma again or seeing it unfold before his or her eyes.

flatus Intestinal gas.

flora Microorganisms that live on or within a body to compete with disease-producing microorganisms and provide a natural immunity against certain infections.

flow sheets Documents on which frequent observations or specific measurements are recorded.

fluid volume deficit (FVD) A fluid and electrolyte disorder caused by failure of the body's homeostatic mechanisms to regulate the retention and excretion of body fluids. The condition is characterized by decreased output of urine, high specific gravity of urine, output of urine that is greater than the intake of fluid in the body, hemoconcentration, and increased serum levels of sodium.

fluid volume excess (FVE) A fluid and electrolyte disorder characterized by an increase in fluid retention and edema, resulting from failure of the body's homeostatic mechanisms to regulate the retention and excretion of body fluids.

focus charting A charting methodology for structuring progress notes according to the focus of the note, for example, symptoms and nursing diagnosis. Each note includes data, actions, and patient response.

focused cultural assessment Method of evaluating a patient's ethnohistory, biocultural history, social organization, and religious and spiritual beliefs to find issues that are most relevant to the problem at hand.

food poisoning Toxic processes resulting from the ingestion of a food contaminated by toxic substances or by bacteria-containing toxins.

foot boots Soft, foot-shaped devices designed to reduce the risk of footdrop by maintaining the foot in dorsiflexion.

footdrop An abnormal neuromuscular condition of the lower leg and foot, characterized by an inability to dorsiflex, or evert, the foot.

friction Effects of rubbing or the resistance that a moving body meets from the surface on which it moves; a force that occurs in a direction to oppose movement.

functional health illiteracy The inability of an individual to obtain, interpret, and understand basic information about health.

functional health patterns Method for organizing assessment data based on the level of patient function in specific areas, for example, mobility.

functional nursing Method of patient care delivery in which each staff member is assigned a task that is completed for all patients on the unit.

future orientation Time dimension emphasized by dominant American culture. It is characterized by direct communication and is focused on task achievement, whereas past orientation communication is circular and indirect and is focused on group harmony.

gait Manner or style of walking, including rhythm, cadence, and speed.

gastrostomy feeding tube The insertion of a feeding tube, through a stoma, into the stomach for the purpose of providing enteral nutrition.

general adaptation syndrome (GAS) Generalized defense response of the body to stress, consisting of three stages: alarm, resistance, and exhaustion.

general anesthesia Intravenous or inhaled medications that cause the patient to lose all sensation and consciousness.

geriatrics Branch of health care dealing with the physiology and psychology of aging and with the diagnosis and treatment of diseases affecting older adults.

gerontology The study of all aspects of the aging process and its consequences.

gingivae Gums of the mouth; a mucous membrane with supporting fibrous tissue that overlies the crowns of unerupted teeth and encircles the necks of those teeth that have erupted.

glaucoma An abnormal condition of elevated pressure within an eye caused by obstruction of the outflow of aqueous humor. Often results in peripheral visual loss, decreased visual acuity with difficulty adapting to darkness, and a halo effect around lights, if untreated.

globalization Worldwide scope or application.

glomerulus Cluster or collection of capillary vessels within the kidney involved in the initial formation of urine.

gluconeogenesis Formation of glucose or glycogen from substances that are not carbohydrates, such as protein or lipid.

glucose The primary fuel for the body, needed to carry out major physiological functions.

glycogen Polysaccharide that is the major carbohydrate stored in animal cells.

glycogenesis The process for storage of glucose in the form of glycogen in the liver.

goals Desired results of nursing actions, set realistically by the nurse and patient as part of the planning stage of the nursing process.

Good Samaritan laws Legislation enacted in some states to protect health care professionals from liability in rendering emergency aid, unless there is proven willful wrong or gross negligence.

graduated measuring container Receptacle for volume measurement.

granny midwives Amateur health practitioners that assist in labor and delivery.

granulation tissue Soft, pink, fleshy projections of tissue that form during the healing process in a wound not healing by primary intention.

graphic record Charting mechanism that allows for the recording of vital signs and weight in such a manner that caregivers can quickly note changes in the patient's status.

grief Form of sorrow involving the person's thoughts, feelings, and behaviors, occurring as a response to an actual or perceived loss.

grieving process Sequence of affective, cognitive, and physiological states through which the person responds to and finally accepts an irretrievable loss.

grounded Connection between the electric circuit and the ground, which becomes part of the circuit.

growth Measurable or quantitative aspect of an individual's increase in physical dimensions as a result of an increase in number of cells. Indicators of growth include changes in height, weight, and sexual characteristics.

guided imagery Method of pain control in which the patient creates a mental image, concentrates on that image, and gradually becomes less aware of pain.

gustatory Pertaining to the sense of taste.

halal Foods permissible for Muslims to eat.

hand rolls Rolls of cloth that keep the thumb slightly adducted and in opposition to the fingers.

hand-wrist splints Splints individually molded for the patient to maintain proper alignment of the thumb, slight adduction of the wrist, and slight dorsiflexion.

haram Foods prohibited by Muslim religious standards.

health Dynamic state in which individuals adapt to their internal and external environments so that there is a state of physical, emotional, intellectual, social, and spiritual well-being.

health belief model Conceptual framework that describes a person's health behavior as an expression of the person's health beliefs.

health beliefs Patient's personal beliefs about levels of wellness, which can motivate or impede participation in changing risk factors, participating in care, and selecting care options.

health care–acquired infection An infection that was not present or incubating at the time of admission to a health care setting.

health care problems Any conditions or dysfunctions that the patient experiences as a result of illness or treatment of an illness.

health promotion Activities such as routine exercise and good nutrition that help patients maintain or enhance their present levels of health and reduce their risk of developing certain diseases.

health promotion model Defines health as a positive, dynamic state, not merely the absence of disease. The health promotion model emphasizes well-being, personal fulfillment, and self-actualization rather than reacting to the threat of illness.

health status Description of health of an individual or community.

heat exhaustion Abnormal condition caused by depletion of body fluid and electrolytes resulting from exposure to intense heat or the inability to acclimatize to heat.

heat stroke Continued exposure to extreme heat raising the core body temperature to 40.5° C (105° F) or higher.

hematemesis Vomiting of blood, indicating upper gastrointestinal bleeding.

hematoma Collection of blood trapped in the tissues of the skin or an organ.

hematuria Abnormal presence of blood in the urine.

hemolysis Breakdown of red blood cells and release of hemoglobin that may occur after administration of hypotonic intravenous solutions, causing swelling and rupture of erythrocytes.

hemoptysis Coughing up blood from the respiratory tract.

hemorrhoids Permanent dilation and engorgement of veins within the lining of the rectum.

hemostasis Termination of bleeding by mechanical or chemical means or by the coagulation process of the body.

hemothorax Accumulation of blood and fluid in the pleural cavity between the parietal and visceral pleurae.

hernia Protrusion of an organ through an abnormal opening in the muscle wall of the cavity that surrounds it.

hilots Amateur health practitioners that assist in labor and delivery among Filipinos.

holistic Of or pertaining to the whole; considering all factors.

holistic health Comprehensive view of the person as a biopsychosocial and spiritual being.

home care Health service provided in the patient's place of residence for the purpose of promoting, maintaining, or restoring health or minimizing the effects of illness and disability.

homeostasis State of relative constancy in the internal environment of the body, maintained naturally by physiological adaptive mechanisms.

hope Confident, yet uncertain, expectation of achieving a future goal.

hospice System of family-centered care designed to help terminally ill persons be comfortable and maintain a satisfactory lifestyle throughout the terminal phase of their illness.

Hoyer lift A mechanical device that uses a canvas sling to easily lift dependent patients for transfer.

humidification Process of adding water to gas.

humor Coping strategy based on an individual's cognitive appraisal of a stimulus that results in behavior such as smiling, laughing, or feelings of amusement that lessen emotional distress.

hydrocephalus Abnormal accumulation of cerebrospinal fluid in the ventricles of the brain.

hydrostatic pressure Pressure caused by a liquid.

hypercalcemia Greater-than-normal amount of calcium in the blood.

hypercapnia Greater-than-normal amounts of carbon dioxide in the blood; also called hypercarbia.

hyperextension Position of maximal extension of a joint.

hyperglycemia Elevated serum glucose levels.

hypertension Disorder characterized by an elevated blood pressure persistently exceeding 120/80 mm Hg.

hyperthermia Situation in which body temperature exceeds the set point.

hypertonic Situation in which one solution has a greater concentration of solute than another solution; therefore the first solution exerts greater osmotic pressure.

hypertonicity Excessive tension of the arterial walls or muscles.

hyperventilation Respiratory rate in excess of that required to maintain normal carbon dioxide levels in the body tissues.

hypnotics Class of drug that causes insensibility to pain and induces sleep.

hypostatic pneumonia Pneumonia that results from fluid accumulation as a result of inactivity.

hypotension Abnormal lowering of blood pressure that is inadequate for normal perfusion and oxygenation of tissues.

hypothermia Abnormal lowering of body temperature below 35° C, or 95° F, usually caused by prolonged exposure to cold.

hypotonic Situation in which one solution has a smaller concentration of solute than another solution; therefore the first solution exerts less osmotic pressure.

hypotonicity Reduced tension of the arterial walls or muscles.

hypoventilation Respiratory rate insufficient to prevent carbon dioxide retention.

hypovolemia Abnormally low circulating blood volume.

hypoxemia Arterial blood oxygen level less than 60 mm Hg; low oxygen level in the blood.

hypoxia Inadequate cellular oxygenation that may result from a deficiency in the delivery or use of oxygen at the cellular level.

identity Component of self-concept characterized by one's persisting consciousness of being oneself, separate and distinct from others.

idiosyncratic reaction Individual sensitivity to effects of a drug caused by inherited or other bodily constitution factors.

illness (1) Abnormal process in which any aspect of a person's functioning is diminished or impaired compared with that person's previous condition. (2) The personal, interpersonal, and cultural reaction to disease.

illness behavior Ways in which people monitor their bodies, define and interpret their symptoms, take remedial actions, and use the health care system.

illness prevention Health education programs or activities directed toward protecting patients from threats or potential threats to health and toward minimizing risk factors.

imam Muslim priest.

immobility Inability to move about freely, caused by any condition in which movement is impaired or therapeutically restricted.

immunity The quality of being insusceptible to or unaffected by a particular disease or condition.

immunization A process by which resistance to an infectious disease is induced or augmented.

implementation Initiation and completion of the nursing actions necessary to help the patient achieve health care goals.

impression management The ability to interpret the others' behavior within their own context of meanings and behave in a culturally congruent way to achieve desired outcomes of communication.

incentive spirometry Method of encouraging voluntary deep breathing by providing visual feedback to patients of the inspiratory volume they have achieved.

incident rates The rate of new cases of a disease in a specified population over a defined period of time.

incident report Confidential document that describes any patient accident while the person is on the premises of a health care agency. (See occurrence report.)

independent practice association (IPA) Managed care organization that contracts with physicians or health care providers who usually are members of groups and whose practices include fee-for-service and capitated patients.

indirect care interventions Treatments performed away from the patient but on behalf of the patient or group of patients.

induration Hardening of a tissue, particularly the skin, because of edema or inflammation.

infection The invasion of the body by pathogenic microorganisms that reproduce and multiply.

inference (1) A judgment or interpretation of informational cues. (2) Taking one proposition as a given and guessing that another proposition follows.

infiltration Dislodging an intravenous catheter or needle from a vein into the subcutaneous space.

inflammation Protective response of body tissues to irritation or injury.

informed consent Process of obtaining permission from a patient to perform a specific test or procedure, after describing all risks, side effects, and benefits.

infusion pump Device that delivers a measured amount of fluid over a period of time.

infusions Introduction of fluid into the vein, giving intravenous fluid over time.

inhalation Method of medication delivery through the patient's respiratory tract. The respiratory tract provides a large surface area for drug absorption. Inhalation can be through the nasal or oral route.

injections Parenteral administration of medication; four major sites of injection: subcutaneous, intramuscular, intravenous, and intradermal.

insensible water loss Water loss that is continuous and is not perceived by the person.

insomnia Condition characterized by chronic inability to sleep or remain asleep through the night.

inspection Method of physical examination by which the patient is visually systematically examined for appearance, structure, function, and behavior.

instillation To cause to enter drop by drop, or very slowly.

institutional ethics committee An interdisciplinary committee that discusses and processes ethical dilemmas that arise within a health care institution.

instrumental activities of daily living (IADLs) Activities that are necessary to be independent in society beyond eating, grooming, transferring, and toileting and include such skills as shopping, preparing meals, banking, and taking medications.

integrated delivery network (IDN) Set of providers and services organized to deliver a coordinated continuum of care to the population of patients served at a capitated cost.

interpersonal communication Exchange of information between two persons or among persons in a small group.

interstitial fluid Fluid that fills the spaces between most of the cells of the body and provides a substantial portion of the liquid environment of the body.

interview Organized, systematic conversation with the patient designed to obtain pertinent health-related subjective information.

intracellular fluid Liquid within the cell membrane.

intradermal (ID) Injection given between layers of the skin, into the dermis. Injections are given at a 5- to 15-degree angle.

intramuscular (IM) Injections given into muscle tissue. The intramuscular route provides a fast rate of absorption that is related to the muscle's greater vascularity. Injections are given at a 90-degree angle.

intraocular Method of medication delivery that involves inserting a medication disk, similar to a contact lens, into the patient's eye.

intrapersonal communication Communication that occurs within an individual; that is, persons "talk with themselves" silently or form an idea in their own mind.

intravascular fluid Fluid circulating within blood vessels of the body.

intravenous Injection directly into the bloodstream. Action of the drug begins immediately when given intravenously.

intubation Insertion of a breathing tube through the mouth or nose into the trachea to ensure a patent airway.

intuition The inner sensing that something is so.

irrigation Process of washing out a body cavity or wounded area with a stream of fluid.

ischemia Decreased blood supply to a body part, such as skin tissue, or to an organ, such as the heart.

isolation Separation of a seriously ill patient from others to prevent the spread of an infection or to protect the patient from irritating environmental factors.

isometric exercises Activities that involve muscle tension without muscle shortening, do not have any beneficial effect on preventing orthostatic hypotension, but may improve activity tolerance.

isotonic Situation in which two solutions have the same concentration of solute; therefore both solutions exert the same osmotic pressure.

jaundice Yellow discoloration of the skin, mucous membranes, and sclera caused by greater-than-normal amounts of bilirubin in the blood.

jejunostomy tube Hollow tube inserted into the jejunum through the abdominal wall for administration of liquefied foods to patients who have a high risk of aspiration.

joint contracture Abnormality that may result in permanent condition of a joint, is characterized by flexion and fixation, and is caused by disuse, atrophy, and shortening of muscle fibers and surrounding joint tissues.

joints Connections between bones; classified according to structure and degree of mobility.

judgment Ability to form an opinion or draw sound conclusions.

justice The ethical standard of fairness.

Kardex Trade name for card-filing system that allows quick reference to the particular need of the patient for certain aspects of nursing care.

karma Asian Indian belief that attributes mental illness to past deeds in one's previous life.

Korotkoff sound Sound heard during the taking of blood pressure using a sphygmomanometer and stethoscope.

kyphosis Exaggeration of the posterior curvature of the thoracic spine.

la cuarentena Period of rest and restricted physical activity after childbirth that usually lasts 40 days.

la dieta Diet.

laceration Torn, jagged wound.

language Code that conveys specific meaning as words are combined.

laryngospasm Sudden uncontrolled contraction of the laryngeal muscles, which in turn decreases airway size.

law Rule, standard, or principle that states a fact or a relationship between factors.

laxatives Drugs that act to promote bowel evacuation.

learning Acquisition of new knowledge and skills as a result of reinforcement, practice, and experience.

learning objective Written statement that describes the behavior a teacher expects from an individual after a learning activity.

left-sided heart failure Abnormal condition characterized by impaired functioning of the left ventricle due to elevated pressures and pulmonary congestion.

leukoplakia Thick, white patches observed on oral mucous membranes.

licensed practical nurse (LPN) Also known as the licensed vocational nurse (LVN), or in Canada, registered nurse's assistant (RNA); trained in basic nursing skills and the provision of direct patient care.

licensed vocational nurse (LVN) The LVN is the same as a licensed practical nurse (LPN), an individual trained in the United States in basic nursing techniques and direct patient care who practices under the supervision of a registered nurse. The LVN is licensed by a board after completing what is usually a 12-month educational program and passing a licensure examination. In Canada an LVN is called a certified nursing assistant.

lipids Compounds that are insoluble in water but soluble in organic solvents.

lipogenesis Process during which fatty acids are synthesized.

living wills Instruments by which a dying person makes wishes known.

local anesthesia Loss of sensation at the desired site of action.

logroll Maneuver used to turn a reclining patient from one side to the other or completely over without moving the spinal column out of alignment.

lordosis Increased lumbar curvature.

maceration Softening and breaking down of skin from prolonged exposure to moisture.

mal de ojo Evil eye.

malignant hyperthermia Autosomal dominant trait characterized by often fatal hyperthermia in affected people exposed to certain anesthetic agents.

malpractice Injurious or unprofessional actions that harm another.

malpractice insurance Type of insurance to protect the health care professional. In case of a malpractice claim, the insurance pays the award to the plaintiff.

managed care Health care system in which there is administrative control over primary health care services. Redundant facilities and services are eliminated, and costs are reduced. Preventive care and health education are emphasized.

Maslow's hierarchy of needs A model, developed by Abram Maslow, used to explain human motivation.

matrilineal Kinship that is limited to only the mother's side.

maturation The genetically determined biological plan for growth and development. Physical growth and motor development are a function of maturation.

maturational loss Loss, usually of an aspect of self, resulting from the normal changes of growth and development.

Medicaid State medical assistance to people with low incomes, based on Title XIX of the Social Security Act. States receive matching federal funds to provide medical care and services to people meeting categorical and income requirements.

medical asepsis Procedures used to reduce the number of microorganisms and prevent their spread.

medical diagnosis Formal statement of the disease entity or illness made by the physician or health care provider.

medical record Patient's chart; a legal document.

Medicare Federally funded national health insurance program in the United States for people over 65 years of age. The program is administered in two parts. Part A provides basic protection against costs of medical, surgical, and psychiatric hospital care. Part B is a voluntary medical insurance program financed in part from federal funds and in part from premiums contributed by people enrolled in the program.

medication abuse Maladaptive pattern of recurrent medication use.

medication allergy Adverse reaction to a medication such as rash, chills, or gastrointestinal disturbances. Once a drug allergy occurs, the patient can no longer receive that particular medication.

medication dependence Maladaptive pattern of medication use in the following patterns: using excessive amounts of the medication, increased activities directed toward obtaining the medication, withdrawal from professional or recreational activities, and so on.

medication error Any event that could cause or lead to a patient's receiving inappropriate drug therapy or failing to receive appropriate drug therapy.

medication interaction The response when one drug modifies the action of another drug. The interaction can potentiate or diminish the actions of another drug, or it may alter the way a drug is metabolized, absorbed, or excreted.

melanoma Group of malignant neoplasms, primarily of the skin, that are composed of melanocytes. Common in fair-skinned people having light-colored eyes and in persons who have had a sunburn.

melena Abnormal black, sticky stool containing digested blood, indicative of gastrointestinal bleeding.

menarche Onset of a girl's first menstruation.

Meniere's disease A chronic disease of the inner ear characterized by recurrent episodes of vertigo, progressive sensorineural hearing loss, which may be bilateral, and tinnitus.

menopause Physiological cessation of ovulation and menstruation that typically occurs during middle adulthood in women.

message Information sent or expressed by sender in the communication process.

metabolic acidosis Abnormal condition of high hydrogen ion concentration in the extracellular fluid caused by either a primary increase in hydrogen ions or a decrease in bicarbonate.

metabolic alkalosis Abnormal condition characterized by the significant loss of acid from the body or by increased levels of bicarbonate.

metabolism Aggregate of all chemical processes that take place in living organisms, resulting in growth, generation of energy, elimination of wastes, and other functions concerned with the distribution of nutrients in the blood after digestion.

metacommunication Dependent not only on what is said but also on the relationship to the other person involved in the interaction. It is a message that conveys the sender's attitude toward the self and the message and the attitudes, feelings, and intentions toward the listener.

metastasize Spread of tumor cells to distant parts of the body from a primary site, for example, lung, breast, or bowel.

metered-dose inhaler (MDI) Device designed to deliver a measured dose of an inhalation drug.

metric system Logically organized decimal system of measurement; metric units can easily be converted and computed through simple multiplication and division. Each basic unit of measurement is organized into units of 10.

microorganisms Microscopic entities, such as bacteria, viruses, and fungi, capable of carrying on living processes.

micturition Urination; act of passing or expelling urine voluntarily through the urethra.

milliequivalent per liter (mEq/L) Number of grams of a specific electrolyte dissolved in 1 L of plasma.

mind mapping A graphic approach to represent the connections between concepts and ideas (e.g., nursing diagnoses) that are related to a central subject (e.g. the patient's health problems).

minerals Inorganic elements essential to the body because of their role as catalysts in biochemical reactions.

minimum data set (MDS) Required by the Omnibus Budget Reconciliation Act of 1987, the MDS is a uniform data set established by the Department of Health and Human Services. The MDS serves as the framework for any state-specified assessment instruments used to develop a written and comprehensive plan of care for newly admitted residents of nursing facilities.

misdemeanor Lesser crime than a felony; the penalty is usually a fine or imprisonment for less than 1 year.

mobility Person's ability to move about freely.

moderate sedation/analgesia/conscious sedation Administration of central nervous system depressant drugs and/or analgesics to provide analgesia, relieve anxiety, and/or provide amnesia during surgical, diagnostic, or interventional procedures. Routinely used for diagnostic or therapeutic procedures that do not require complete anesthesia but simply a decreased level of consciousness.

monosaturated fatty acid A fatty acid in which some of the carbon atoms in the hydrocarbon chain are joined by double or triple bonds. Monounsaturated fatty acids have only one double or triple bond per molecule and are found as components of fats in such foods as fowls, almonds, pecans, cashew nuts, peanuts, and olive oil.

morals Personal conviction that something is absolutely right or wrong in all situations.

motivation Internal impulse that causes a person to take action.

mourning The process of grieving.

murmurs Blowing or whooshing sounds created by changes in blood flow through the heart or by abnormalities in valve closure.

muscle tone Normal state of balanced muscle tension.

myocardial contractility Measure of stretch of the cardiac muscle fiber. It can also affect stroke volume and cardiac output. Poor contraction decreases the amount of blood ejected by the ventricles during each contraction.

myocardial infarction Necrosis of a portion of cardiac muscle caused by obstruction in a coronary artery.

myocardial ischemia Condition that results when the supply of blood to the myocardium from the coronary arteries is insufficient to meet the oxygen demands of the organ.

NANDA International North American Nursing Diagnosis Association, organized in 1973, which formally identifies, develops, and classifies nursing diagnoses.

narcolepsy Syndrome involving sudden sleep attacks that a person cannot inhibit; uncontrollable desire to sleep may occur several times during a day.

nasogastric (NG) tube Tube passed into the stomach through the nose for the purpose of emptying the stomach of its contents or for delivering medication and/or nourishment.

nebulization Process of adding moisture to inspired air by the addition of water droplets.

necessary losses Losses that every person experiences.

necrotic Of or pertaining to the death of tissue in response to disease or injury.

negative health behaviors Practices actually or potentially harmful to health, such as smoking, drug or alcohol abuse, poor diet, and refusal to take necessary medications.

negative nitrogen balance Condition occurring when the body excretes more nitrogen than it takes in.

negligence Careless act of omission or commission that results in injury to another.

neonate Stage of life from birth to 1 month of age.

nephrons Structural and functional units of the kidney containing renal glomeruli and tubules.

neurotransmitter Chemical that transfers the electrical impulse from the nerve fiber to the muscle fiber.

nociceptors Somatic and visceral free nerve endings of thinly myelinated and unmyelinated fibers. They usually react to tissue injury but may also be excited by endogenous chemical substances.

nocturia Urination at night; can be a symptom of renal disease or may occur in persons who drink excessive amounts of fluids before bedtime.

nonblanchable hyperemia Redness of the skin due to dilation of the superficial capillaries. The redness persists when pressure is applied to the area, indicating tissue damage.

nonmaleficence The fundamental ethical agreement to do no harm. Closely related to the ethical standard of beneficence.

nonrapid eye movement (NREM) sleep Sleep that occurs during the first four stages of normal sleep.

nonshivering thermogenesis Occurs primarily in neonates. Because neonates cannot shiver, a limited amount of vascular brown adipose tissue present at birth can be metabolized for heat production.

nonverbal communication Communication using expressions, gestures, body posture, and positioning rather than words.

normal sinus rhythm (NSR) The wave pattern on an electrocardiogram that indicates normal conduction of an electrical impulse through the myocardium.

numbing One of Bowlby's four phases of mourning. It is characterized by the lack of feeling or feeling stunned by the loss. May last a few days or many weeks.

Nurse Practice Acts Statutes enacted by the legislature of any of the states or by the appropriate officers of the districts or possessions that describe and define the scope of nursing practice.

nurse-initiated interventions The response of the nurse to the patient's health care needs and nursing diagnoses. This type of intervention is an autonomous action based on scientific rationale that is executed to benefit the patient in a predicted way related to the nursing diagnosis and patient-centered goals.

nursing diagnosis Formal statement of an actual or potential health problem that nurses can legally and independently treat. The second step of the nursing process, during which the patient's actual and potential unhealthy responses to an illness or condition are identified.

nursing health history Data collected about a patient's present level of wellness, changes in life patterns, sociocultural role, and mental and emotional reactions to illness.

nursing intervention Any treatment, based upon clinical judgment and knowledge, that a nurse performs to enhance patient outcomes.

nursing process Systematic problem-solving method by which nurses individualize care for each patient. The five steps of the nursing process are assessment, diagnosis, planning, implementation, and evaluation.

nursing-sensitive outcomes Outcomes that are within the scope of nursing practice; consequences or effects of nursing interventions that result in changes in the patient's symptoms, functional status, safety, psychological distress, or costs.

nurturant Behavior that involves caring for or fostering the well-being of another individual.

nutrients Foods that contain elements necessary for body function, including water, carbohydrates, proteins, fats, vitamins, and minerals.

obesity Abnormal increase in the proportion of fat cells, mainly in the viscera and subcutaneous tissues of the body.

objective data Information that can be observed by others; free of feelings, perceptions, prejudices.

occurrence report Confidential document that describes any patient accident while the person is on the premises of a health care agency. (See incident report.)

olfactory Pertaining to the sense of smell.

oncotic pressure The total influence of the protein on the osmotic activity of plasma fluid.

open-ended question A form of question that prompts a respondent to answer in more than one or two words.

operating bed Table for surgery.

operating room (1) Room in a health care facility in which surgical procedures requiring anesthesia are performed. (2) Informal: a suite of rooms or an area in a health care facility in which patients are prepared for surgery, undergo surgical procedures, and recover from the anesthetic procedures required for the surgery.

ophthalmic Drugs given into the eye, in the form of either eye drops or ointments.

ophthalmoscope Instrument used to illuminate the structures of the eye in order to examine the fundus, which includes the retina, choroid, optic nerve disc, macula, fovea centralis, and retinal vessels.

opioid Drug substance, derived from opium or produced synthetically, that alters perception of pain and that with repeated use may result in physical and psychological dependence (narcotic).

oral hygiene Condition or practice of maintaining the tissues and structures of the mouth.

orthopnea Abnormal condition in which a person must sit or stand up to breathe comfortably.

orthostatic hypotension Abnormally low blood pressure occurring when a person stands up.

osmolality Concentration or osmotic pressure of a solution expressed in osmoles or milliosmoles per kilogram of water.

osmolarity Osmotic pressure of a solution expressed in osmoles or milliosmoles per kilogram of the solution.

osmoreceptors Neurons in the hypothalamus that are sensitive to the fluid concentration in the blood plasma and regulate the secretion of antidiuretic hormone.

osmosis Movement of a pure solvent through a semipermeable membrane from a solution with a lower solute concentration to one with a higher solute concentration.

osmotic pressure Drawing power for water, which depends on the number of molecules in the solution.

osteoporosis Disorder characterized by abnormal rarefaction of bone, occurring most frequently in postmenopausal women, in sedentary or immobilized individuals, and in patients on long-term steroid therapy.

ostomy Surgical procedure in which an opening is made into the abdominal wall to allow the passage of intestinal contents from the bowel (colostomy) or urine from the bladder (urostomy).

otoscope Instrument, with a special ear speculum, used to examine the deeper structures of the external and middle ear.

ototoxic Having a harmful effect on the eighth cranial (auditory) nerve or the organs of hearing and balance.

outcome Condition of a patient at the end of treatment, including the degree of wellness and the need for continuing care, medication, support, counseling, or education.

outliers Patients with extended lengths of stay beyond allowable inpatient days or costs.

outpatient Patient who has not been admitted to a hospital but receives treatments in a clinic or facility associated with the hospital.

oxygen saturation The amount of hemoglobin fully saturated with oxygen, given as a percent value.

oxygen therapy Procedure in which oxygen is administered to a patient to relieve or prevent hypoxia.

pain Subjective, unpleasant sensation caused by noxious stimulation of sensory nerve endings.

palliative care A level of care that is designed to relieve or reduce intensity of uncomfortable symptoms but not to produce a cure. Palliative care relies on comfort measures and use of alternative therapies to help individuals become more at peace during end of life.

pallor Unnatural paleness or absence of color in the skin.

palpation Method of physical examination whereby the fingers or hands of the examiner are applied to the patient's body for the purpose of feeling body parts underlying the skin.

palpitations Bounding or racing of the heart associated with normal emotions or a heart disorder.

Papanicolaou (Pap) smear Painless screening test for cervical cancer. Specimens are taken of squamous and columnar cells of the cervix.

parallel play Form of play among a group of children, primarily toddlers, in which each one engages in an independent activity that is similar but not influenced by or shared with the others.

paralytic ileus Usually temporary paralysis of intestinal wall that may occur after abdominal surgery or peritoneal injury and that causes cessation of peristalsis. Leads to abdominal distention and symptoms of obstruction.

parenteral administration Giving medication by a route other than the gastrointestinal tract.

parenteral nutrition (PN) The administration of a nutritional solution into the vascular system.

parteras Lay midwives.

partial bed bath Bath in which body parts that might cause the patient discomfort if left unbathed (i.e., face, hands, axillary areas, back, and perineum) are washed in bed.

passive range-of-motion (PROM) exercises Range of movement through which a joint is moved with assistance.

passive strategies of health promotion Activities that involve the patient as the recipient of actions by health care professionals.

pathogenicity Ability of a pathogenic agent to produce a disease.

pathogens Microorganisms capable of producing disease.

pathological fractures Fractures resulting from weakened bone tissue; frequently caused by osteoporosis or neoplasms.

patient-centered care Concept to improve work efficiency by changing the way patient care is delivered.

patient-controlled analgesia (PCA) Drug delivery system that allows patients to self-administer analgesic medications when they want.

patrilineal, patrilineally Kinship that is limited to only the father's side.

perceived loss Loss that is less obvious to the individual experiencing it. Although easily overlooked or misunderstood, a perceived loss results in the same grief process as an actual loss.

perception Persons' mental image or concept of elements in their environment, including information gained through the senses.

percussion Method of physical examination whereby the location, size, and density of a body part is determined by the tone obtained from the striking of short, sharp taps of the fingers.

perfusion (1) Passage of a fluid through a specific organ or an area of the body. (2) Therapeutic measure whereby a drug intended for an isolated part of the body is introduced via the bloodstream.

perineal care Procedure prescribed for cleaning the genital and anal areas as part of the daily bath or after various obstetrical and gynecological procedures.

perioperative nursing Refers to the role of the operating room nurse during the preoperative, intraoperative, and postoperative phases of surgery.

peripherally inserted central catheter (PICC) Alternative intravenous access when the patient requires intermediate-length venous access greater than 7 days to 3 months. Intravenous access is achieved by inserting a catheter into a central vein by way of a peripheral vein.

peristalsis Rhythmical contractions of the intestine that propel gastric contents through the length of the gastrointestinal tract.

peritonitis Inflammation of the peritoneum produced by bacteria or irritating substances introduced into the abdominal cavity by a penetrating wound or perforation of an organ in the gastrointestinal tract or the reproductive tract.

PERRLA Acronym for "pupils equal, round, reactive to light, accommodation"; the acronym is recorded in the physical examination if eye and pupil assessments are normal.

personalismo Personalistic.

petechiae Tiny purple or red spots that appear on skin as minute hemorrhages within dermal layers.

pharmacokinetics Study of how drugs enter the body, reach their site of action, are metabolized, and exit from the body.

phlebitis Inflammation of a vein.

physician-initiated interventions Based on the physician's response to a medical diagnosis, the nurse responds to the physician's written orders.

PIE note Problem-oriented medical record; the four interdisciplinary sections are the database, problem list, care plan, and progress notes.

placebos Dosage form that contains no pharmacologically active ingredients but may relieve pain through psychological effects.

plaintiff Individual who files formal charges against an individual or organization for a legal offense.

planning Process of designing interventions to achieve the goals and outcomes of health care delivery.

plantar flexion Toe-down motion of the foot at the ankle.

pleural friction rub Adventitious lung sound caused by inflamed parietal and visceral pleura rubbing together on inspiration.

pneumothorax Collection of air or gas in the pleural space.

point of maximal impulse (PMI) Point where the heartbeat can most easily be palpated through the chest wall. This is usually the fourth intercostal space at the midclavicular line.

point of view A way of looking at issues that reflects an individual's culture and societal influences.

poison Any substance that impairs health or destroys life when ingested, inhaled, or absorbed by the body in relatively small amounts.

poison control center One of a network of facilities that provides information regarding all aspects of poisoning or intoxication, maintains records of their occurrence, and refers patients to treatment centers.

polypharmacy Use of a number of different drugs by a patient who may have one or several health problems.

polyunsaturated fatty acid Fatty acid that has two or more carbon double bonds.

population A collection of individuals who have in common one or more personal or environmental characteristics.

positive health behaviors Activities related to maintaining, attaining, or regaining good health and preventing illness. Common positive health behaviors include immunizations, proper sleep patterns, adequate exercise, and nutrition.

postanesthesia care unit (PACU) Area adjoining the operating room to which surgical patients are taken while still under anesthesia.

postmortem care Care of a patient's body after death.

postural drainage Use of positioning along with percussion and vibration to drain secretions from specific segments of the lungs and bronchi into the trachea.

postural hypotension Abnormally low blood pressure occurring when an individual assumes the standing posture; also called orthostatic hypotension.

posture Position of the body in relation to the surrounding space.

power of attorney for health care A person designated by the patient to make health care decisions for the patient if the patient becomes unable to make his or her own decisions.

preadolescence Transitional developmental stage that occurs between childhood and adolescence.

preanesthesia care unit Area outside the operating room where preoperative preparations are completed.

preload Volume of blood in the ventricles at the end of diastole, immediately before ventricular contraction.

preoperative teaching Instruction regarding a patient's anticipated surgery and recovery given before surgery. Instruction includes, but is not limited to, dietary and activity restrictions, anticipated assessment activities, postoperative procedures and pain relief measures.

presbycusis Hearing loss associated with aging. It usually involves both a loss of hearing sensitivity and a reduction in the clarity of speech.

presbyopia Gradual decline in ability of the lens to accommodate or to focus on close objects. Reduces ability to see near objects clearly. This condition commonly develops with advancing age.

prescriptions Written directions for a therapeutic agent (e.g., medication, drugs).

presence The deep physical, psychological, and spiritual connection or engagement between a nurse and patient.

present time orientation Time dimension that focuses on what is happening here and now. Communication patterns are circular, and this time orientation is in conflict with the dominant organizational norm in health care that emphasizes punctuality and adherence to appointments.

pressure ulcer Inflammation, sore, or ulcer in the skin over a bony prominence.

presurgical care unit (PSCU) Area outside the operating room where preoperative preparations are completed.

preventive nursing actions Nursing actions directed toward preventing illness and promoting health to avoid the need for primary, secondary, or tertiary health care.

primary appraisal Evaluating an event for its personal meaning related to stress.

primary care First contact in a given episode of illness that leads to a decision regarding a course of action to resolve the health problem.

primary intention Primary union of the edges of a wound, progressing to complete scar formation without granulation.

primary nursing Method of nursing practice in which the patient's care is managed, for the duration, by one nurse, who directs and coordinates other nurses and health care personnel. When on duty, the primary nurse cares for the patient directly.

primary prevention First contact in a given episode of illness that leads to a decision regarding a course of action to prevent worsening of the health problem.

problem identification One of the steps of the diagnostic process in which the patient's health care problem is recognized as a result of data analysis based on professional knowledge and experience.

problem solving Methodical, systematic approach to explore conditions and develop solutions, including analysis of data, determination of causative factors, and selection of appropriate actions to reverse or eliminate the problem.

problem-oriented medical record (POMR) Method of recording data about the health status of a patient that fosters a collaborative problem-solving approach by all members of the health care team.

productive cough Sudden expulsion of air from the lungs that effectively removes sputum from the respiratory tract and helps clear the airways.

professional standards review organization (PSRO) Focuses on evaluation of nursing care provided in a health care setting. The quality, effectiveness, and appropriateness of nursing care for the patient is the focus of evaluation.

prone Position of the patient lying face down.

proprioception The body's ability to sense its position and movement in space.

prospective payment system (PPS) Payment mechanism for reimbursing hospitals for inpatient health care services in which predetermined rate is set for treatment of specific illnesses.

prostaglandins Potent hormonelike substances that act in exceedingly low doses on target organs. They can be used to treat asthma and gastric hyperacidity.

proteins Any of a large group of naturally occurring, complex, organic nitrogenous compounds. Each is composed of large combinations of amino acids containing the elements carbon, hydrogen, nitrogen, oxygen, usually sulfur, and occasionally phosphorus, iron, iodine, or other essential constituents of living cells. Protein is the major source of building material for muscles, blood, skin, hair, nails, and the internal organs.

proteinuria Presence in the urine of abnormally large quantities of protein, usually albumin. Persistent proteinuria is usually a sign of renal disease or renal complications of another disease, or hypertension or heart failure.

protocol Written and approved plan specifying the procedures to be followed during an assessment or in providing treatment.

pruritus Symptom of itching; an uncomfortable sensation leading to the urge to scratch.

psychomotor learning Acquisition of ability to perform motor skills.

ptosis Abnormal condition of one or both upper eyelids in which the eyelid droops, caused by weakness of the levator muscle or paralysis of the third cranial nerve.

puberty Developmental period of emotional and physical changes, including the development of secondary sex characteristics and the onset of menstruation and ejaculation.

public health nursing A nursing specialty that requires the nurse to care for the needs of populations or groups.

public communication Interaction of one individual with large groups of people.

pulmonary hygiene More frequent turning, deep breathing, coughing, use of incentive spirometry, and chest physical therapy (PT) if ordered.

pulse deficit Condition that exists when the radial pulse is less than the ventricular rate as auscultated at the apex or seen on an electrocardiogram. The condition indicates a lack of peripheral perfusion for some of the heart contractions.

pulse pressure Difference between the systolic and diastolic pressures, normally 30 to 40 mm Hg.

Purkinje network Complex network of muscle fibers that spread through the right and left ventricles of the heart and carry the impulses that contract those chambers almost simultaneously.

pursed-lip breathing Deep inspiration followed by prolonged expiration through pursed lips.

pyrexia Abnormal elevation of the temperature of the body above 37° C (98.6° F) because of disease; same as fever.

pyrogens Substances that cause a rise in body temperature, as in the case of bacterial toxins.

quality improvement Monitoring and evaluation of processes and outcomes in health care or any other business to identify opportunities for improvement.

quality indicator Quantitative measure of an important aspect of care that determines whether quality of service conforms to requirements or standards of care.

race The common biological characteristics shared by a group of people.

Ramadan A religious observance held during the ninth month of the Islamic calendar year. It involves fasting from sunrise to sunset.

range of motion (ROM) Range of movement of a joint, from maximum extension to maximum flexion, as measured in degrees of a circle.

rapid eye movement (REM) sleep Stage of sleep in which dreaming and rapid eye movements are prominent; important for mental restoration.

reaction Component of the pain experience that may include both physiological responses, such as in the general adaptation syndrome, and behavioral responses.

reality orientation Therapeutic modality for restoring an individual's sense of the present.

receiver Person to whom message is sent during the communication process.

reception Neurophysiological components of the pain experience, in which nervous system receptors receive painful stimuli and transmit them through peripheral nerves to the spinal cord and brain.

record Written form of communication that permanently documents information relevant to health care management.

recovery A period of time immediately postoperative when the patient is closely observed for effects of anesthesia, changes in vital signs, and bleeding. The area is usually in the postanesthesia care unit.

referent Factor that motivates a person to communicate with another individual.

reflection Process of thinking back or recalling an event to discover the meaning and purpose of that event. Useful in critical thinking.

refractive error Defect in the ability of the lens of the eye to focus light, such as occurs in nearsightedness and farsightedness.

regional anesthesia Loss of sensation in an area of the body supplied by sensory nerve pathways.

registered nurse (RN) In the United States a nurse who has completed a course of study at a state-approved, accredited school of nursing and has passed the National Council Licensure Examination (NCLEX-RN).

regression Return to an earlier developmental stage or behavior.

regulatory agencies Local, state, provincial, or national agencies that inspect and certify health care agencies as meeting specified standards. These agencies can also determine the amount of reimbursement for health care delivered.

rehabilitation Restoration of an individual to normal or near-normal function after a physical or mental illness, injury, or chemical addiction.

reinforcement Provision of a contingent response to a learner's behavior that increases the probability of the behavior's recurring.

related factor Any condition or event that accompanies or is linked with the patient's health care problem.

relaxation Act of being relaxed or less tense.

reminiscence Recalling the past for the purpose of assigning new meaning to past experiences.

remissions Partial or complete disappearances of the clinical and subjective characteristics of chronic or malignant disease; remission may be spontaneous or the result of therapy.

renal calculi Calcium stones in the renal pelvis.

renin Proteolytic enzyme, produced by and stored in the juxtaglomerular apparatus that surrounds each arteriole as it enters a glomerulus. The enzyme affects the blood pressure by catalyzing the change of angiotensinogen to angiotensin, a strong repressor.

reorganization The last phase Bowlby's phases of mourning. During this phase, which sometimes requires a year or more, the person begins to accept unaccustomed roles, acquire new skills, and build new relationships.

reports Transfer of information from the nurses on one shift to the nurses on the following shift. Report may also be given by one of the members of the nursing team to another health care provider, for example, a physician or therapist.

reservoir A place where microorganisms survive, multiply, and await transfer to a susceptible host.

residual urine Volume of urine remaining in the bladder after a normal voiding; the bladder normally is almost completely empty after micturition.

resistance stage Third stage of the stress response, when the person attempts to adapt to the stressor. The body stabilizes, hormone levels stabilize, and heart rate, blood pressure, and cardiac output return to normal.

resource utilization group (RUG) Method of classification for health care reimbursement for long-term care facilities.

respeto Respectful.

respiratory acidosis Abnormal condition characterized by increased arterial carbon dioxide concentration, excess carbonic acid, and increased hydrogen ion concentration.

respiratory alkalosis Abnormal condition characterized by decreased arterial carbon dioxide concentration and decreased hydrogen ion concentration.

respite care Short-term health services to dependent older adults either in their home or in an institutional setting.

responsibility Carrying out duties associated with a particular role.

restorative care Health care settings and services where patients who are recovering from illness or disability receive rehabilitation and supportive care.

restraint Device to aid in the immobilization of a patient or patient's extremity.

return demonstration Demonstration after the patient has first observed the teacher and then practiced the skill in mock or real situations.

rhonchi Abnormal lung sound auscultated when the patient's airways are obstructed with thick secretions.

right-sided heart failure Abnormal condition that results from impaired functioning of the right ventricle characterized by venous congestion in the systemic circulation.

risk factor Any internal or external variable that makes a person or group more vulnerable to illness or an unhealthy event.

risk management A function of administration of a hospital or other health facility directed toward identification, evaluation, and correction of potential risks that could lead to injury of patients, staff members, or visitors and result in property loss or damage.

risk nursing diagnosis Describes human responses to health conditions/life processes that may develop in a vulnerable individual, family, or community.

role performance The way in which a person views his or her ability to carry out significant roles.

root cause analysis A process of data collection and analysis that aids in finding the real cause of the problem and working on dealing with it rather than just dealing with the effects of the problem.

Sabbath From sundown on Friday to sundown on Saturday, this religious observance is a day of rest and worship for Jews and some Christian sects.

sandbags Sand-filled plastic tubes that can be shaped to body contours. They can immobilize an extremity or maintain body alignment.

saturated fatty acid Fatty acid in which each carbon in the chain has an attached hydrogen atom.

scientific method Codified sequence of steps used in the formulation, testing, evaluation, and reporting of scientific ideas.

scientific rationale Reason, based on supporting literature, why a specific nursing action was chosen.

scoliosis Lateral spinal curvature.

scrub nurse Registered nurse or operating room technician who assists surgeons during operations.

secondary appraisal Evaluating one's possible coping strategies when confronted with a stressor.

secondary intention Wound closure in which the edges are separated, granulation tissue develops to fill the gap, and, finally, epithelium grows in over the granulation, producing a larger scar than results with primary intention.

secondary prevention Level of preventive medicine that focuses on early diagnosis, use of referral services, and rapid initiation of treatment to stop the progress of disease processes.

sedatives Medications that produce a calming effect by decreasing functional activity, diminishing irritability, and allaying excitement.

segmentation Alternating contraction and relaxation of gastrointestinal mucosa.

self-concept Complex, dynamic integration of conscious and unconscious feelings, attitudes, and perceptions about one's identity, physical being, worth, and roles; how a person perceives and defines self.

self-esteem Feeling of self-worth characterized by feelings of achievement, adequacy, self-confidence, and usefulness.

self-transcendence An awareness of that which cannot be seen or known in ordinary, physical ways.

sender Person who initiates interpersonal communication by conveying a message.

sensible water loss Loss of fluid from the body through the secretory activity of the sweat glands and the exhalation of humidified air from the lungs.

sensory deficits Defects in the function of one or more of the senses, resulting in visual, auditory, or olfactory impairments.

sensory deprivation State in which stimulation to one or more of the senses is lacking, resulting in impaired sensory perception.

sensory overload State in which stimulation to one or more of the senses is so excessive that the brain disregards or does not meaningfully respond to stimuli.

sequential compression stockings Plastic stockings attached to an air pump that inflates and deflates the stockings, applying intermittent pressure sequentially from the ankle to the knee.

serum half-life Time needed for excretion processes to lower the serum drug concentration by half.

sexual dysfunction Inability or difficulty in sexual functioning caused by physiological or psychological factors or both.

sexual orientation Clear, persistent erotic preference for a person of one sex or the other.

sexuality "A function of the total personality . . . concerned with the biological, psychological, sociological, spiritual and culture variables of life . . ." (Sex Information and Education Council of the United States, 1980).

sexually transmitted infection Infectious process spread through sexual contact, including oral, genital, or anal sexual activity.

shear Force exerted against the skin while the skin remains stationary and the bony structures move.

side effect Any reaction or consequence that results from medication or therapy.

side rails Bars positioned along the sides of the length of the bed or stretcher to reduce the patient's risk of falling.

simpatia Friendly.

sinoatrial (SA) node Called the "pacemaker of the heart" because the origin of the normal heartbeat begins at the SA node. The SA node is in the right atrium next to the entrance of the superior vena cava.

situational crisis Unexpected crisis that arises suddenly in response to an external event or a conflict concerning a specific circumstance.

situational loss Loss of a person, thing, or quality resulting from a change in a life situation, including changes related to illness, body image, environment, and death.

sitz bath Bath in which only the hips or buttocks are immersed in fluid.

skilled nursing facility Institution or part of an institution that meets criteria for accreditation established by the sections of the Social Security Act that determine the basis for Medicaid and Medicare reimbursement for skilled nursing care, including rehabilitation and various medical and nursing procedures.

sleep State marked by reduced consciousness, diminished activity of the skeletal muscles, and depressed metabolism.

sleep apnea Cessation of breathing for a time during sleep.

sleep deprivation Condition resulting from a decrease in the amount, quality, and consistency of sleep.

SOAP note Progress note that focuses on a single patient problem and includes subjective and objective data, analysis, and planning; most often used in the POMR.

socializing Interacting with friends or other people; communicating with others to form relationships and help people feel relaxed.

solute Substance dissolved in a solution.

solution Mixture of one or more substances dissolved in another substance. The molecules of each of the substances disperse homogeneously and do not change chemically. A solution may be a liquid, gas, or solid.

solvent Any liquid in which another substance can be dissolved.

source record Organization of a patient's chart so that each discipline (e.g., nursing, medicine, social work, or respiratory therapy) has a separate section in which to record data. Unlike POMR, the information is not organized by patient problems. The advantage of a source record is that caregivers can easily locate the proper section of the record in which to make entries.

sphygmomanometer Device for measuring the arterial blood pressure that consists of an arm or leg cuff with an air bladder connected to a tube and a bulb for pumping air into the bladder and a gauge for indicating the amount of air pressure being exerted against the artery.

spiritual distress State of being out of harmony with a system of beliefs, a supreme being, or God.

spiritual well-being Individual's spirituality that enables a person to love, have faith and hope, seek meaning in life, and nurture relationships with others.

spirituality Spiritual dimension of a person, including the relationship with humanity, nature, and a supreme being.

standard of care Minimum level of care accepted to ensure high-quality care to patients. Standards of care define the types of therapies typically administered to patients with defined problems or needs.

standard precautions Guidelines recommended by the Centers for Disease Control and Prevention (CDC) to reduce risk of transmission of blood-borne and other pathogens in hospitals.

standardized care plans Written care plans used for groups of patients that have similar health care problems.

standing order Written and approved documents containing rules, policies, procedures, regulations, and orders for the conduct of patient care in various stipulated clinical settings.

statutory law Of or related to laws enacted by a legislative branch of the government.

stenosis Abnormal condition characterized by the constriction or narrowing of an opening or passageway in a body structure.

stereotypes Generalizations that are made about individuals without further assessment.

sterilization (1) Rendering a person unable to produce children; accomplished by surgical, chemical, or other means. (2) A technique for destroying microorganisms using heat, water, chemicals, or gases.

stoma Artificially created opening between a body cavity and the body's surface; for example, a colostomy, formed from a portion of the colon pulled through the abdominal wall.

stress Physiological or psychological tension that threatens homeostasis or a person's psychological equilibrium.

stressor Any event, situation, or other stimulus encountered in a person's external or internal environment that necessitates change or adaptation by the person.

striae Streaks or linear scars that result from rapid development of tension in the skin.

stroke volume (SV) Amount of blood ejected by the ventricles with each contraction. It can be affected by the amount of blood in the left ventricle at the end of diastole (preload), the resistance to left ventricular ejection (afterload), and myocardial contractility.

subacute care Level of medical specialty care provided to patients who need a greater intensity of care than that provided in a skilled nursing facility but who do not require acute care.

subcultures Various ethnic, religious, and other groups with distinct characteristics from the dominant culture.

subcutaneous (Sub-Q) Injection given into the connective tissue, under the dermis. The subcutaneous tissue absorbs drugs more slowly than those injected into muscle. Injections are usually given at an angle of 45 degrees.

subjective data Information gathered from patient statements; the patient's feelings and perceptions. Not verifiable by another except by inference.

sublingual Route of medication administration in which the medication is placed underneath the patient's tongue.

Sunrise Model A model developed by Leininger that aids the health care practitioner in designing care decisions and actions in a culturally congruent fashion.

supine Position of the patient in which the patient is resting on his or her back.

suprainfection Secondary infection usually caused by an opportunistic pathogen.

suprapubic catheter Catheter surgically inserted through abdomen into bladder.

surfactant Chemical produced in the lung by alveolar type 2 cells that maintains the surface tension of the alveoli and keeps them from collapsing.

surgical asepsis Procedures used to eliminate any microorganisms from an area. Also called sterile technique.

sympathy Concern, sorrow, or pity felt by the nurse for the patient in which the nurse personally identifies with the patient's needs. Sympathy is a subjective look at another person's world that prevents a clear perspective of all sides of the issues confronting that person.

synapse Region surrounding the point of contact between two neurons or between a neuron and an effector organ.

syncope A brief lapse in consciousness caused by transient cerebral hypoxia.

synergistic effect Effect resulting from two drugs acting synergistically; the effect of the two drugs combined is greater than the effect that would be expected if the individual effects of the two drugs acting alone were added together.

systolic Pertaining to or resulting from ventricular contraction.

tachycardia Rapid regular heart rate ranging between 100 and 150 beats per minute.

tachypnea Abnormally rapid rate of breathing.

tactile Relating to the sense of touch.

tactile fremitus Tremulous vibration of the chest wall during breathing that is palpable on physical examination.

teaching Implementation method used to present correct principles, procedures, and techniques of health care; to inform patients about their health status; and to refer patients and family to appropriate health or social resources in the community.

team nursing Decentralized system in which the care of a patient is distributed among the members of a team. The charge nurse delegates authority to a team leader, who must be a professional nurse.

teratogens Chemical or physiological agents that may produce adverse effects in the embryo or fetus.

tertiary prevention Activities directed toward rehabilitation rather than diagnosis and treatment.

therapeutic communication Process in which the nurse consciously influences a patient or helps the patient to a better understanding through verbal and/or nonverbal communication.

therapeutic effect Desired benefit of a medication, treatment, or procedure.

thermoregulation Internal control of body temperature.

threshold Point at which a person first perceives a painful stimulus as being painful.

thrill Continuous palpable sensation like the purring of a cat.

thrombus Accumulation of platelets, fibrin, clotting factors, and the cellular elements of the blood attached to the interior wall of a vein or artery, sometimes occluding the lumen of the vessel.

tinnitus Ringing heard in one or both ears.

tissue ischemia Point at which tissues receive insufficient oxygen and perfusion.

tolerance Point at which a person is not willing to accept pain of greater severity or duration.

tort Act that causes injury for which the injured party can bring civil action.

total patient care A nursing delivery of care model originally developed during Florence Nightingale's time. In the model a registered nurse (RN) is responsible for all aspects of care for one or more patients. The nurse works directly with the patient, family, physician or health care provider, and health care team members. The model typically has a shift-based focus.

touch To come in contact with another person, often conveying caring, emotional support, encouragement, or tenderness.

toxic effect Effect of a medication that results in an adverse response.

transcultural Concept of care extending across cultures that distinguishes nursing from other health disciplines.

transcultural nursing A distinct discipline developed by Leininger that focuses on the comparative study of cultures to understand similarities and differences among groups of people.

transcutaneous electrical nerve stimulation (TENS) Technique in which a battery-powered device blocks pain impulses from reaching the spinal cord by delivering weak electrical impulses directly to the skin's surface.

transdermal disk Medication delivery device in which the medication is saturated on a wafer-like disk, which is affixed to the patient's skin. This method ensures that the patient receives a continuous level of medication.

transfer report Verbal exchange of information between caregivers when a patient is moved from one nursing unit or health care setting to another. The report includes information necessary to maintain a consistent level of care from one setting to another.

transfusion reaction Systemic response by the body to the administration of blood incompatible with that of the recipient.

trapeze bar Metal triangular-shaped bar that can be suspended over a patient's bed from an overhanging frame; permits patients to move up and down in bed while in traction or some other encumbrance.

trimester Referring to one of the three phases of pregnancy.

trochanter roll Rolled towel support placed against the hips and upper leg to prevent external rotation of the legs.

turgor Normal resiliency of the skin caused by the outward pressure of the cells and interstitial fluid.

unsaturated fatty acid Fatty acid in which an unequal number of hydrogen atoms are attached and the carbon atoms attach to each other with a double bond.

ureterostomy Diversion of urine away from a diseased or defective bladder through an artificial opening in the skin.

urinal Receptacle for collecting urine.

urinary diversion Surgical diversion of the drainage of urine, such as a ureterostomy.

urinary incontinence Inability to control urination.

urinary reflux Abnormal, backward flow of urine.

urinary retention Retention of urine in the bladder; condition frequently caused by a temporary loss of muscle function.

urine hat Receptacle for collecting urine that fits toilet.

urometer Device for measuring frequent and small amounts of urine from an indwelling urinary catheter system.

urosepsis Organisms in the bloodstream.

utilitarianism Ethic that proposes that the value of something is determined by its usefulness. The greatest good for the greatest number of people constitutes the guiding principle for action in a utilitarian model of ethics.

utilization review (UR) committees Physician-supervised committees to review admissions, diagnostic testing, and treatments provided by physicians or health care providers to patients.

validation Act of confirming, verifying, or corroborating the accuracy of assessment data or the appropriateness of the care plan.

Valsalva maneuver Any forced expiratory effort against a closed airway, such as when an individual holds the breath and tightens the muscles in a concerted, strenuous effort to move a heavy object or to change positions in bed.

value Personal belief about the worth of a given idea or behavior.

valvular heart disease Acquired or congenital disorder of a cardiac valve characterized by stenosis and obstructed blood flow or valvular degeneration and regurgitation of blood.

variances The unexpected event that occurs during patient care and that is different from what is predicted on a CareMap. Variances or exceptions are interventions or outcomes that are not achieved as anticipated. Variance may be positive or negative.

variant Differing from a set standard.

vascular access devices Catheters, cannulas, or infusion ports designed for long-term, repeated access to the vascular system.

vasoconstriction Narrowing of the lumen of any blood vessel, especially the arterioles and the veins in the blood reservoirs of the skin and abdominal viscera.

vasodilation Increase in the diameter of a blood vessel caused by inhibition of its vasoconstrictor nerves or stimulation of dilator nerves.

venipuncture Technique in which a vein is punctured transcutaneously by a sharp rigid stylet (e.g., a butterfly needle), a cannula (e.g., an angiocatheter that contains a flexible plastic catheter), or a needle attached to a syringe.

ventilation Respiratory process by which gases are moved into and out of the lungs.

verbal communication The sending of messages from one individual to another or to a group of individuals through the spoken word.

vertigo Sensation of dizziness or spinning.

vibration Fine, shaking pressure applied by hands to the chest wall only during exhalation.

virulence The ability of an organism to rapidly produce disease.

visual Related to, or experienced through, vision.

vital signs Temperature, pulse, respirations, and blood pressure.

vitamins Organic compounds essential in small quantities for normal physiological and metabolic functioning of the body. With few exceptions, vitamins cannot be synthesized by the body and must be obtained from the diet or dietary supplements.

voiding The process of urinating.

vulnerable populations A collection of individuals who are more likely to develop health problems as a result of excess risks, limits in access to health care services, or being dependent on others for care.

wellness Dynamic state of health in which an individual progresses toward a higher level of functioning, achieving an optimum balance between internal and external environments.

wellness education Activities that teach people how to care for themselves in a healthy manner.

wellness nursing diagnosis Clinical judgment about an individual, group, or community in transition from a specific level of wellness to a higher level of wellness.

wheezes, wheezing Adventitious lung sound caused by a severely narrowed bronchus.

work redesign Formal process used to analyze the work of a certain work group and to change the actual structure of the jobs performed.

worldview A cognitive stance or perspective about phenomena characteristic of a particular cultural group.

wound culture Specimen collected from a wound to determine the specific organism that is causing an infectious process.

yearning and searching The second phase of Bowlby's phases of mourning. It is characterized by emotional outbursts of tearful sobbing and acute distress.

Z-track injection Technique for injecting irritating preparations into muscle without tracking residual medication through sensitive tissues.

Common Abbreviations

Note: Abbreviations in common use can vary widely from place to place. Each institution's list of acceptable abbreviations is the best authority for its records.

°C	degrees centigrade	Cl	chlorine	FHR	fetal heart rate	JRA	juvenile rheumatoid arthritis
°F	degrees Fahrenheit	cm	centimeter	FRC	functional residual capacity		
μm	micrometer	cm³	cubic centimeter			K	potassium
℥	dram	CNS	central nervous system	FSH	follicle-stimulating hormone	kg	kilogram
aa	of each	c/o	complains of			KUB	kidney, ureters, and bladder (radiograph)
ABG	arterial blood gas	CO	carbon monoxide	FUO	fever of unknown origin		
ac	before meals	CO₂	carbon dioxide			KVO	keep vein open
ad lib	freely as desired	COPD	chronic obstructive pulmonary disease	Fx, fx	fracture, fractional urine test	L	liter
ADLs	activities of daily living			g, gm, Gm	gram	L&A	light and accommodation
Ag	silver, antigen	CPK	creatine phosphokinase	Gc, GC	gonococcus		
AIDS	acquired immuno deficiency syndrome	CPR	cardiopulmonary resuscitation	GI	gastrointestinal	LBBB	left bundle branch block
ALS	amyotrophic lateral sclerosis	CSF	cerebrospinal fluid	gr	grain	LE	lupus erythematosus
		CT	computed tomography	grav I, II, III, etc.	pregnancy one, two, three, etc.	LGV	lymphogranuloma venereum
am	morning	CVA	cerebrovascular acci- dent; costovertebral angle	gt, gtt	drop, drops	LLL	left lower lobe
ama	against medical advice			GTT	glucose tolerance test	LLQ	left lower quadrant
AMI	acute myocardial infarction			GU	genitourinary	LMP	last menstrual period
		CVP	central venous pressure	GYN, Gyn	gynecological	LNMP	last normal menstrual period
amp	ampule	D&C	dilation and curettage	h, hr	hour		
ARC	AIDS-related complex	D₅W	5% dextrose in water	H⁺	hydrogen ion	LP	lumbar puncture
ARDS	adult respiratory dis- tress syndrome	db, dB	decibel	H&P	history and physical examination	LUL	left upper lobe
		dc	discontinue			LUQ	left upper quadrant
AS	aortic stenosis	DIC	disseminated intravas- cular coagulation	HAV	hepatitis A virus	LVH	left ventricular hypertrophy
ASD	atrial septal defect			Hb	hemoglobin		
Ba	barium	diff	differential blood count	HBAg	hepatitis B antigen	m	meter
BE	barium enema	dil	dilute	HBV	hepatitis B virus	m, min	minum
bid	two times a day	DJD	degenerative joint disease	Hct, HCT	hematocrit	MAP	mean arterial pressure
BM, bm	bowel movement			HDL	high-density lipoprotein	mcg	microgram
BMR	basal metabolic rate	Dl	deciliter			MCH	mean corpuscular hemoglobin
BP	blood pressure	DNR	do not resuscitate	Hg	mercury		
BPH	benign prostatic hypertrophy	DOE	dyspnea on exertion	Hgb	hemoglobin	MCHC	mean corpuscular hemoglobin concentration
		dx, Dx	diagnosis	HIV	human immunodefi- ciency (AIDS) virus		
BRP	bathroom privileges	EBV	Epstein-Barr virus			MCV	mean cell volume; mean corpuscular volume
BSA	body surface area	ECF	extracellular fluid	HLA	human lymphocyte antigen		
BUN	blood urea nitrogen	ECG	electrocardiogram				
c̄	with	ECHO	echocardiography	h/o	history of	mg	milligram
Ca	calcium, cancer, carcinoma	ECT	electroconvulsive therapy	H₂O	water	Mg	magnesium
				HSV2	herpes simplex virus, type 2	MG	myasthenia gravis
CAD	coronary artery disease	EDC	estimated date of confinement			MI	myocardial infarction
cap	capsule			I&O	intake and output	MICU	medical intensive care unit
CAT	computed axial tomography	EDD	estimated date of delivery	IC	inspiratory capacity		
				ICP	intracranial pressure		
cath	catheter, catheterize	EEG	electroencephalogram	ICU	intensive care unit	ml	milliliter
CBC	complete blood count	EKG	electrocardiogram	IDDM	insulin-dependent diabetes mellitus	mm	millimeter
CBR	complete bed rest	elix	elixir			mm³	cubic millimeter
CC	chief complaint	EMG	electromyogram	IEP	immunoelectrophoresis	mm Hg	millimeters of mercury
CCU	coronary care unit, critical care unit	ENG	electronystagmography	Ig	immunoglobulin	MRI	magnetic resonance imaging
		ER	emergency room	IgA, etc.	immunoglobulin A, etc.		
CDC	Centers for Disease Control and Prevention	ERG	electroretinogram	IM	intramuscular	MW	molecular weight
		ESRD	end-stage renal disease	IOP	intraocular pressure	N	nitrogen
		EST	electroshock therapy	IPPB	intermittent positive pressure breathing	Na	sodium
CEA	carcinoembryonic antigen	℥	fluid ounce			NICU	neonatal intensive care unit
		FANA	fluorescent antinuclear antibody test	IV	intravenous		
CFT	complement-fixation test			IVP	intravenous push; intravenous pyelogram	NIH	National Institutes of Health
		FBS	fasting blood sugar				
cg	centigram	Fe	iron			nm	nanometer
CHF	congestive heart failure	FEV	forced expiratory volume	IVU	intravenous urogram		
CHO	carbohydrate						

NMR — nuclear magnetic resonance

NPO — nothing by mouth

NS — normal saline

O_2 — oxygen

OD — right eye; optical density; overdose

OL — left eye

OOB — out of bed

ORIF — open reduction and internal fixation

OS — left eye

OT — occupational therapy

OTC — over-the-counter

Ou — both eyes

oz, ℥ — ounce

P&A — percussion and auscultation

$PaCO_2$ — partial pressure of carbon dioxide (arterial blood)

PaO_2 — partial pressure of oxygen (arterial blood)

para I, II, etc. — unipara, bipara, etc.

PAT — paroxysmal atrial tachycardia

pc — after meals

PCG — phonocardiogram

PCO_2 — partial pressure of carbon dioxide

PCP — pulmonary capillary pressure, phencyclidine

PCV — packed cell volume

PCWP — pulmonary capillary wedge pressure

PD — interpupillary distance; postural drainage

PE — pulmonary embolism, physical examination

PEEP — positive end-expiratory pressure

PEG — pneumoencephalography

per — through, by way of

PERRLA — pupils equal, round, and reactive to light and accommodation

PET — positron emission tomography

PG — prostaglandin

pH — hydrogen ion concentration (acidity and alkalinity)

PID — pelvic inflammatory disease

PKU — phenylketonuria

PM — postmortem

PM — evening

PMS — premenstrual syndrome

PND — paroxysmal nocturnal dyspnea, postnasal drip

PO, po — orally

PO_2 — partial pressure of oxygen

PPD — purified protein derivative

ppm — parts per million

prn — when required, as often as necessary

PT — physical therapy; prothrombin time

PTT — partial thromboplastin time

PUO — pyrexia of unknown origin

PVC — premature ventricular contraction

q — every

q2h — every 2 hours

q3h — every 3 hours

q4h — every 4 hours

qh — every hour

qid — four times a day

qn — every night

qns — quantity not sufficient

RBBB — right bundle branch block

RBC — red blood cell

RDS — respiratory distress syndrome

Rh+ — positive Rh factor

Rh− — negative Rh factor

RHD — rheumatic heart disease

RLL — right lower lobe

RLQ — right lower quadrant

RML — right middle lobe

R/O — rule out

ROM — range of motion

ROS — review of systems

RS — Reiter's syndrome

RSV — Rous sarcoma virus

RUL — right upper lobe

RUQ — right upper quadrant

Rx — take; treatment

s̄ — without

SB — sternal border

sib — sibling

SICU — surgical intensive care unit

SIDS — sudden infant death syndrome

Sig — write on label

SLE — systemic lupus erythematosus

sol — solution, dissolved

sos — if necessary

sp gr, SG, sg — specific gravity

SR — sedimentation rate

ss — half

SSS — sick sinus syndrome; specific soluble substance; short-stay surgery

stat — immediately

STD — sexually transmitted disease

STS — serologic test for syphilis

Sub-Q — subcutaneous

susp — suspension

SV — stroke volume

T_3 — triiodothyronine

T_4 — tetraiodothyronine

T&A — tonsillectomy and adenoidectomy

TAB — typhoid and paratyphoid A and B

TAH — total abdominal hysterectomy

TAT — tetanus antitoxin; thematic apperception test

TB, TBC — tuberculosis

TBG — thyroxin-binding globulin

TG — triglyceride

TIA — transient ischemic attack

TIBC — total iron-binding capacity

tid — three times a day

TKO — to keep open

TLC — total lung capacity; thin-layer chromatography

TPN — total parenteral nutrition

TPR — temperature, pulse, and respirations

tr, tinct — tincture

TSH — thyroid-stimulating hormone

TST — triple sugar iron test

UA — urinalysis

UGI series — upper gastrointestinal series

UIBC — unsaturated iron-binding capacity

URI — upper respiratory infection

US — ultrasound

UTI — urinary tract infection

V&T — volume and tension

VC — vital capacity

VD — venereal disease

VDA — visual discriminatory acuity

VDH — valvular disease of the heart

VDRL — Venereal Disease Research Laboratories

VLDL — very-low-density lipoprotein

VS — vital signs

VSD — ventricular septal defect

V_T — tidal volume

W/V — weight/volume

WBC — white blood cell, white blood count

WNL — within normal limits

WR — Wassermann reaction

Overview of CDC Hand Hygiene Guidelines

The Centers for Disease Control and Prevention released recommendations for hand hygiene in health care settings in 2002. Hand hygiene is a general term that applies to hand washing, antiseptic hand wash, antiseptic hand rub, or surgical hand antisepsis. Hand washing refers to washing hands thoroughly with plain soap and water. An antiseptic hand wash is defined as washing hands with water and soap containing an antiseptic agent. Antimicrobials effectively reduce bacterial counts on the hands and often have residual antimicrobial effects for several hours. An antiseptic hand rub means to apply an antiseptic alcohol-based waterless product to all surfaces of the hands to reduce the number of microorganisms present. Surgical hand antisepsis is an antiseptic hand wash or antiseptic hand rub performed preoperatively by surgical personnel.

Evidence suggests that hand antisepsis, the cleansing of hands with an antiseptic hand rub, is more effective in reducing nosocomial infections than plain hand washing.

Follow These Guidelines in the Care of *All Patients*

Wash hands when hands are visibly dirty or contaminated with proteinaceous material or are visibly soiled with blood or other body fluids; wash hands preferably with an antimicrobial soap and water or a nonantimicrobial soap and water. The recommended duration for lathering hands is *at least 15 seconds* and preferably 30 seconds.

- Wash hands with soap and water before eating.
- Wash hands with soap and water and after using the restroom.
- Wash hands if exposed to spore-forming organisms such as *Clostridium difficile* or *Bacillus anthracis.* The physical action of washing and rinsing hands is recommended because alcohols, chlorhexidine, iodophors, and other antiseptic agents have poor activity against spores.

If hands are not visibly soiled, use an alcohol-based hand rub for routinely decontaminating the hands in all of the following clinical situations:

- Before having direct contact with patients
- Before donning sterile gloves
- Before inserting indwelling urinary catheters, peripheral vascular catheters, or other invasive devices that do not require a surgical procedure

- After contact with a patient's intact skin (e.g., after taking a pulse or blood pressure, lifting a patient)
- After contact with body fluids or excretions, mucous membranes, nonintact skin, and wound dressings *if hands are not visibly soiled*
- When moving from a contaminated body site to a clean body site during patient care
- After contact with inanimate objects (e.g., medical equipment) in the immediate vicinity of the patient
- After removing gloves

Note that an antiseptic hand wash may be performed in all situations when an alcohol-based hand rub is indicated. Antimicrobial-impregnated wipes (i.e., towelettes) are not a substitute for usizng an alcohol-based hand rub or antimicrobial soap.

Method for Decontaminating Hands

When using an alcohol-based hand rub, apply product to palm of one hand and rub hands together, covering all surfaces of hands and fingers, until hands are dry. Follow the manufacturer's recommendations regarding the volume of product to use.

Follow These Guidelines for Surgical Hand Antisepsis

Surgical hand antisepsis reduces the resident microbial count on the hands to a minimum. See Box 13-9, p. 241, for the surgical hand scrub procedure.

The CDC recommends using an antimicrobial soap and scrubbing hands and forearms for the length of time recommended by the manufacturer, usually 2 to 6 minutes. Refer to agency policy for time required.

When using an alcohol-based surgical hand-scrub product with persistent activity, follow the manufacturer's instructions. Before applying the alcohol solution, prewash hands and forearms with a nonantimicrobial soap and dry hands and forearms completely. After application of the alcohol-based product as recommended, allow hands and forearms to dry thoroughly before donning sterile gloves.

General Recommendations for Hand Hygiene

Use hand lotions or creams to minimize the occurrence of irritant contact dermatitis associated with hand antisepsis or hand washing.

Do not wear artificial fingernails or extenders when having direct contact with patients at high risk (e.g., those in intensive care units or operating rooms).

Keep natural nail tips less than $\frac{1}{4}$ inch long.

Wear gloves when contact with blood or other potentially infectious materials, mucous membranes, and nonintact skin could occur.

Remove gloves after caring for a patient. Do not wear the same pair of gloves for the care of more than one patient.

Change gloves during patient care if moving from a contaminated body site to a clean body site. This includes when working under isolation precautions.

Data from Centers for Disease Control and Prevention, Hospital Infection Control Practice Advisory Committee, HICPAC/SHEA/APIC/IDSA Hand Hygiene Task Force: Guideline for hand hygiene in health-care settings, *MMWR Recommend Rep* 51(RR-16):1, 2002. Available at www.cdc.gov/handhygiene.

Rationales are provided for all answers on the *Basic Nursing* Evolve Site.

CHAPTER 1
1. 2.
2. 1.
3. 3.
4. 1.
5. 1.
6. 1.
7. 4.
8. 2.
9. 3.
10. 2.

CHAPTER 2
1. 4.
2. 2.
3. 3.
4. 2, 3.
5. 2.
6. 2.
7. 1, 2, 3, 5.
8. 4.
9. 4.
10. 3.

CHAPTER 3
1. 4.
2. 2, 3.
3. 1, 2, 3, 4.
4. 2.
5. 4.
6. 1.
7. 4.
8. 4.
9. 1.
10. 3, 4.

CHAPTER 4
1. 3.
2. 3.
3. 2.
4. 4.
5. 4.
6. 4.
7. 2.
8. All answers are correct.
9. 4.
10. 4.

CHAPTER 5
1. 4.
2. 4.
3. 2.
4. 3.
5. 1.
6. 1.
7. 3.
8. 3.

CHAPTER 6
1. 2.
2. 3, 1, 5, 2, 4, 6.
3. 4.
4. 1.
5. 4.
6. 2.
7. 3.
8. 4.

CHAPTER 7
1. 4.
2. 2.
3. 4.
4. 3.
5. 3.
6. 3.
7. 1.
8. 4.

CHAPTER 8
1. 3.
2. 2.
3. 4.
4. 3.
5. 1.
6. 1.
7. 4.

CHAPTER 9
1. 3.
2. 2.
3. 1.
4. 3.
5. 2.
6. 4.
7. 4.
8. 1.
9. 3.
10. 1.

CHAPTER 10
1. 4.
2. 3.
3. 2.
4. 3.
5. 2.
6. 4.
7. 2.
8. 2.
9. 3.
10. 2.

CHAPTER 11
1. 1.
2. 2, 3, 4.
3. 3.
4. 1.
5. 3.
6. 4.
7. 3.
8. 2.
9. 1.
10. 2.

CHAPTER 12
1. 3.
2. 2.
3. 4.
4. 3.
5. 3.
6. 1.
7. 3.
8. 1.
9. 2.
10. 4.

CHAPTER 13
1. 1.
2. 3.
3. 3.
4. 2.
5. 4.
6. 2, 3, 4.
7. 4.
8. 1.
9. 3.
10. 3.

CHAPTER 14
1. 2 and 3.
2. 2.
3. 4.
4. 2.
5. 3.
6. 3.
7. 1.
8. 2.
9. 1.
10. 4.

CHAPTER 15
1. 1, 4.
2. 3.
3. 4.
4. 2.
5. 3.
6. 4.
7. 3.
8. 1.
9. 3.
10. 1.

CHAPTER 16
1. 1.
2. 4.
3. 3.
4. 4.
5. 3.
6. 2.
7. 4.
8. 2.
9. 4.
10. 3.

CHAPTER 17
1. 2.
2. 1.
3. 3.
4. 3, 6, 5, 1, 7, 4, 2, 8.
5. 3.
6. 2.
7. 2.
8. 3.

CHAPTER 18
1. 3.
2. 4.
3. 3.
4. 1.
5. 3.
6. 4.
7. 3.
8. 2.
9. 3.
10. 3.

CHAPTER 19
1. 2.
2. 1.
3. 1.
4. 1.
5. 4.
6. 1.
7. 2.
8. 1.
9. 4.
10. 3.

CHAPTER 20
1. 1.
2. 3.
3. 4.
4. 3.
5. 1, 2, 4.
6. 2.
7. 4.
8. 3.
9. 2.
10. 2.

CHAPTER 21
1. 3.
2. 4.
3. 2.
4. 2.
5. 2.
6. 4.
7. 2.
8. 2.
9. 1, 2, and 4.
10. 2.

CHAPTER 22
1. 2.
2. 4.
3. 3.
4. 1.
5. 1.
6. 1, 2, 3, and 4.
7. 2.
8. 4.
9. 2.
10. 4.

CHAPTER 23
1. 2.
2. 4.
3. 1.
4. 1.
5. 3.
6. 3.
7. 4.
8. 1, 4.
9. 4.
10. 3.

CHAPTER 24
1. 4.
2. 2.
3. 4.
4. 3.
5. 1, 4.
6. 3.
7. 4.
8. 1, 2, 3, and 4.

9. 4.
10. 1.

CHAPTER 25
1. 1.
2. 2.
3. 3, 4, 2, 1, 5.
4. 4.
5. 2, 5, 7.
6. 3.
7. 1.
8. 4.
9. 2.
10. 3.

CHAPTER 26
1. 2.
2. 2.
3. 1.
4. 2.
5. 1.
6. 2.
7. 1.
8. 1.
9. 3.
10. 1.

CHAPTER 27
1. 2.
2. 1.
3. 1.
4. 4.
5. 3, 5, 6.
6. 1.
7. 2.
8. 3.
9. 1.
10. 4.

CHAPTER 28
1. 2.
2. 1, 3.
3. 2.
4. 1, 4.
5. 1.
6. 2, 3, 4, 5.
7. 2, 3, 5.
8. 3.
9. 3.
10. 2.

CHAPTER 29
1. 3.
2. 4.
3. 2.
4. 1, 2, 3.
5. 3.
6. 2.
7. 4.
8. 1.
9. 2, 3, 4.
10. 3.

CHAPTER 30
1. 4.
2. 1.
3. 1.
4. 4.
5. 2.

6. **4.**
7. **1, 2, 6.**
8. **2.**
9. **4.**
10. **2.**

CHAPTER 31

1. **4.**
2. **1.**
3. **2.**
4. **3.**
5. **3.**
6. **2.**
7. **3.**
8. **1.**
9. **1, 3, 4.**
10. **1, 2, 3.**

CHAPTER 32

1. **3, 6, 5, 2, 7, 4, 1.**
2. **1, 3, 5.**
3. **4.**
4. **4.**

5. **3.**
6. **3.**
7. **1.**
8. **2.**
9. **1.**
10. **3.**

CHAPTER 33

1. **4.**
2. **1.**
3. **4.**
4. **1.**
5. **2.**
6. **4.**
7. **1.**
8. **4.**
9. **1.**

CHAPTER 34

1. **2.**
2. **3.**
3. **3.**
4. **1, 2, 3.**

5. **4.**
6. **1.**
7. **2.**
8. **2.**
9. **1, 2, 3.**
10. **1.**

CHAPTER 35

1. **2.**
2. **3.**
3. **1, 3.**
4. **1, 2, 4.**
5. **3.**
6. **1.**
7. **3.**
8. **4.**
9. **4.**
10. **1, 3, 4, 5.**

CHAPTER 36

1. **4.**
2. **3.**
3. **1.**

4. **4.**
5. **3.**
6. **3.**
7. **3, 4.**
8. **4.**
9. **3.**
10. **3.**

CHAPTER 37

1. **1.**
2. **1, 2, 3.**
3. **2, 3.**
4. **4.**
5. **4.**
6. **1, 2, 4.**
7. **1, 3, 5.**
8. **1.**
9. **2.**
10. **4.**

CHAPTER 38

1. **4.**
2. **2.**

3. **4.**
4. **2.**
5. **3.**
6. **4.**
7. **1.**
8. **4.**
9. **1.**
10. **1.**

Page numbers followed by f indicate figures; t, tables; b, boxes.

1199